W9-CDY-798

Quick Table of Contents

Essentials of
PATHOPHYSIOLOGY
Concepts of Altered Health States

Senior Acquisitions Editor: Margaret Zuccarini
Senior Managing Editor: Helen Kogut
Editorial Assistant: Thaddeus Raczkowski
Senior Project Editor: Debra Schiff
Director of Nursing Production: Helen Ewan
Senior Managing Editor/Production: Erika Kors
Art Director: Brett MacNaughton
Design Coordinator: Joan Wendt
Senior Manufacturing Manager: William Alberti
Indexer: Angela Holt
Compositor: Circle Graphics
Printer: RRD-China

2nd Edition

11 10 9 8 7

Library of Congress Cataloging-in-Publication Data

Porth, Carol.
    Essentials of pathophysiology : concepts of altered health states / Carol Mattson
Porth ; consultants, Kathryn J. Gaspard, Glenn Matfin.—2nd ed.
        p. ; cm.
    Abridgement of: Pathophysiology / Carol Mattson Porth. 7th ed. c2005.
    Includes bibliographical references and index.
    ISBN 13: 978-0-7817-7087-3
    ISBN 0-7817-7087-4
    1. Physiology, Pathological. 2. Nursing. I. Porth, Carol. Pathophysiology. II.
Title: Pathophysiology. III. Title.
    [DNLM: 1. Disease—Nurses' Instruction. 2. Pathology—Nurses' Instruction. 3.
Physiology—Nurses' Instruction. QZ 4 P851e 2007]
RB113.P668 2007
616.07—dc22
                                                      2005038066

LWW.com

Essentials of
PATHOPHYSIOLOGY
Concepts of Altered Health States

Second Edition

Carol Mattson Porth, RN, MSN, PhD (Physiology)

Professor Emeritus, College of Nursing
University of Wisconsin-Milwaukee
Milwaukee, Wisconsin

Consultants
Kathryn J. Gaspard, PhD
Clinical Associate Professor
College of Nursing
University of Wisconsin-Milwaukee
Milwaukee, Wisconsin

Glenn Matfin, BSc (Hons), MB ChB, DGM,
MFPM, MRCP (UK), FACE, FACP
Senior Medical Director
Novo Nordisk, Princeton, NJ

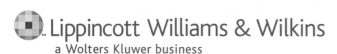
. Lippincott Williams & Wilkins
a Wolters Kluwer business
Philadelphia • Baltimore • New York • London
Buenos Aires • Hong Kong • Sydney • Tokyo

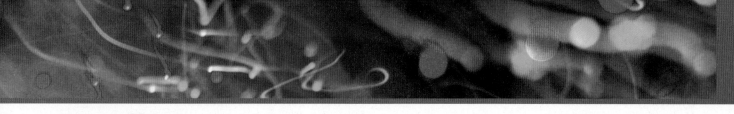

Contributors

Diane Book, MD
Assistant Professor, Neurology
Medical College of Wisconsin
Milwaukee, Wisconsin
(Chapter 36)

Edward W. Carroll, MS, PhD
Clinical Assistant Professor
Department of Biomedical Sciences, College of Health Sciences
Marquette University
Milwaukee, Wisconsin
(Chapters 1, 3, 33, 37)

Robin Curtis, PhD
Professor, Retired
Department of Cellular Biology, Neurobiology, and Anatomy
Medical College of Wisconsin
Milwaukee, Wisconsin
(Chapter 33)

Wm. Michael Dunne Jr., PhD
Professor of Pathology and Immunology and Molecular
  Microbiology
Washington University School of Medicine
Medical Director of Microbiology
Barnes-Jewish Hospital
St. Louis, Missouri
(Chapter 12)

Elizabeth C. Devine, RN, PhD, FAAN
Professor, College of Nursing
University of Wisconsin-Milwaukee
Milwaukee, Wisconsin
(Chapter 34)

Susan A. Fontana, RN, PhD, CS-FNPNET
Certified Family Nurse Practitioner
Associate Professor, College of Nursing
University of Wisconsin-Milwaukee
Milwaukee, Wisconsin
(Chapter 37)

Kathryn J. Gaspard, PhD
Clinical Associate Professor, College of Nursing
University of Wisconsin-Milwaukee
Milwaukee, Wisconsin
(Chapters 9, 10, 11)

Kathleen E. Gunta, RN, MSN, ONC
Clinical Nurse Specialist, Orthopaedics
St. Luke's Medical Center
Milwaukee, Wisconsin
(Chapters 42, 43)

Safak Guven, MD, FACE, FACP
Assistant Professor
Clinical Director
Obesity/Metabolic Syndrome Clinic
Medical College of Wisconsin
Milwaukee, Wisconsin
(Chapters 30, 31, 32)

Julie A. Kuenzi, APRN (BC-ADM), MSN, CDE
Supervisor
Froedtert Hospital and Medical College of Wisconsin
Diabetes and Endocrine Center
Milwaukee, Wisconsin
(Chapters 30, 31, 32)

Mary Pat Kunert, RN, PhD
Associate Professor
College of Nursing
University of Wisconsin-Milwaukee
Milwaukee, Wisconsin
(Chapter 7)

Glenn Matfin, BSc (Hons), MB ChB, DGM, MFPM, MRCP (UK), FACE, FACP
Senior Medical Director
Novo Nordisk
Princeton, New Jersey
(Chapters 6, 16, 17, 18, 19, 30, 31, 32, 38)

Patricia McCowen Mehring, RNC, MSN, OGNP
Nurse Practitioner
Gynecology and Obstetrics
Medical College of Wisconsin
Milwaukee, Wisconsin
(Chapters 39, 40)

Joan Pleuss, MS, RD, CDE
Bionutrition Research Manager
General Clinical Research Center
Medical College of Wisconsin
Milwaukee, Wisconsin
(Chapter 8)

Debra Bancroft Rizzo, RN, MSN, FNP-C
Rheumatology Nurse Practitioner
Rheumatic Disease Center
Milwaukee, Wisconsin
(Chapter 43)

Gladys Simandl, RN, PhD
Professor
Columbia College of Nursing
Milwaukee, Wisconsin
(Chapter 44, 45)

Cynthia V. Sommer, PhD, MT (ASCP)
Associate Professor Emerita, Department of Biological Sciences
University of Wisconsin-Milwaukee
Milwaukee, Wisconsin
(Chapters 13, 14)

Kathleen A. Sweeney, RN, MS, CNS
Advanced Practice Nurse
Froedtert Hospital Cancer Center
Milwaukee, Wisconsin
(Chapter 15)

Kerry Twite, RN, MSN, AOCN
Clinical Nurse Specialist—Oncology
St. Luke's Medical Center
Milwaukee, Wisconsin
(Chapters 5, 9)

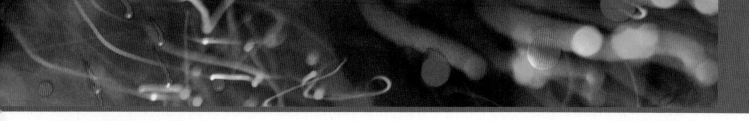

Reviewers

Colleen Anderson, RN, BN, MN
Nursing Faculty
Western Regional School of Nursing
Corner Brook, Newfoundland, Canada

Deborah Armstrong, RN, MSN
Visiting Lecturer, Adult and Child Nursing
University of Massachusetts at Dartmouth
Dartmouth, Massachusetts

Anna Barkman, RN, BN, MN
Nursing Faculty, Undergraduate Nursing Studies
Mount Royal College
Calgary, Alberta, Canada

Donald R. Beadle, CRNP, MSN
Adjunct Instructor
Temple University
College of Allied Health Professions,
    Department of Nursing
Philadelphia, Pennsylvania

Susan Blakey, RN, BSN, MSN
Assistant Professor
Georgia Baptist College of Nursing of Mercer University
Atlanta, Georgia

Sonya H. Blevins, RN, MS
Nursing Instructor, Medical-Surgical Nursing
Central Carolina Technical College
Sumter, South Carolina

Marcia G. Bower, MSN, CRNP, CANP, CMSN
Assistant Professor
Holy Family University
School of Nursing and Allied Health Professions
Philadelphia, Pennsylvania

Patricia S. Bowne, PhD
Professor of Biology
Alverno College
Milwaukee, Wisconsin

Kevin Branch, BHSc, PHC, ACP
Coordinator, Paramedic Program
Cambrian College
Sudbury, Ontario, Canada

Patricia L. Brown, RN, PhD
Director of Nursing Education
Kansas Wesleyan University
Salina, Kansas

Barbara A. Brunow, RN, MSN, CNS
Instructor
Firelands Regional Medical Center
School of Nursing
Huron, Ohio

Theresa Capriotti, RN, MSN, CRNP, DO
Clinical Associate Professor
Villanova University College of Nursing
Villanova, Pennsylvania

Barbara Coles, BS, MS, PhD
Bioscience Instructor
Wake Technical Community College
Raleigh, North Carolina

Zoe Dams, RN, BSN, MSN
Bachelor of Sciences and Nursing Program
Malasina University–College
Nanaimo, British Columbia, Canada

Lynn DiBenedetto, BS, Med, PhD
Assistant Professor
Worcester State College
Worcester, Massachusetts

Shirley Dinkel, ARNP, BC, PhD
Assistant Professor
Washburn University
Topeka, Kansas

Richard L. Doolittle, MS, PhD
Professor and Head, Department of Medical Sciences
Rochester Institute of Technology
Rochester, New York

Karen S. Dunn, RN, PhD
Assistant Professor
Oakland University
Rochester, Michigan

Julie Eggert, PhD, GNP-C, AOCN
Assistant Professor, RN-BS Coordinator
Clemson University
Clemson, South Carolina

Bill Melvin Farnsworth, RN, MSN, FNP-C
Clinical Assistant Professor
University of Texas at El Paso School of Nursing
El Paso, Texas

Kim Garrett, RN, MS, APN-CNP, CCRN, ACNP
Assistant Professor
Rush Medical Center/Rush College of Nursing
Chicago, Illinois

Carol J. Green, RN, MN, PhD
Professor
Johnson County Community College
Overland Park, Kansas

Sheila Grossman, PhD, APRN-BC
Professor and Director, Family Nurse Practitioner Program
Fairfield University School of Nursing
Fairfield, Connecticut

Pamela G. Harrison, RN, MS, EdD, APRN-BC
Associate Professor
Indiana Wesleyan University
Marion, Indiana

Lori Hendricks, RN, EdD, CCRN
Associate Professor
South Dakota State University College of Nursing
Brookings, South Dakota

Karen Hill, RN, BS, MSN, PhD
Associate Professor, School of Nursing
Southeastern Louisiana University
Hammond, Louisiana

Lisa Hopp, RN, MS, PhD
Associate Professor
Purdue University Calumet
Hammond, Indiana

Connie Houser, RN-C, MSN
ADN Instructor
Central Carolina Technical College
FE Debose Career Center
Manning, South Carolina

Jo Ann Jenkins, BSN, MSN
Assistant Professor of Nursing
Central Missouri State University
Warrensburg, Missouri

Judith Jezierski, RN, MSN
Associate Professor and Chair, Department of Nursing
Saint Joseph's College
Rensselaer, Indiana

Karen Johnson, RN, PhD, CCRN
Assistant Professor
University of Maryland School of Nursing
Baltimore, Maryland

Karen C. Johnson-Brennan, RN, EdD
Professor and Associate Director, School of Nursing
San Francisco State University
San Francisco, California

Chris L. Kapicka, PhD
Biology Professor
Northwest Nazerene University
Nampa, Idaho

Karen L. Kearcher, MS, ARNP
Nursing Instructor
Lower Columbia College
Associate's Degree Nursing Program
Longview, Washington

Joyce King, RN, FNP, CNM, PhD
Assistant Professor
Emory University School of Nursing
Atlanta, Georgia

Linda Killian, RN, MSN, CNP
Professor of Nursing
Jackson Community College
Jackson, Michigan

Brenda Lane, RN, BScN, Dip. Ad. Ed., MN
Professor of Nursing
Malaspina University-College
Nanaimo, British Columbia, Canada

Kim Litwack, RN, PhD, FAAN
Associate Professor of Nursing
University of Wisconsin-Milwaukee
Milwaukee, Wisconsin

Elizabeth M. Long, RN, MSN, CGNP, CNS
Instructor
Lamar University
Beaumont, Texas

Joseph P. Maloney, RN, PhD
Professor, School of Nursing
Spalding University
Prospect, Kentucky

Margaret Maag, RN, EdD
Assistant Professor, Adult Health/School of Nursing
University of San Francisco
San Francisco, California

Kim McCarron, RN, MS
Clinical Assistant Professor
Towson University
Towson, Maryland

Leigh Ann McInnis, BSN, MSN
Assistant Professor
Belmont University
Nashville, Tennessee

Julie Nauser, RN, MSN
Assistant Professor
Research College of Nursing
Kansas City, Missouri

Kim A. Noble, RN, MSN, CPAN
Assistant Professor, College of Health Professions
Temple University, Department of Nursing
Philadelphia, Pennsylvania

Betty Norris, DSN, NP
Hospital Education Coordinator
UAB Health System
Birmingham, Alabama

Tommie L. Norris, RN, DNS
Assistant Professor
The University of Memphis
Loewenberg School of Nursing
Memphis, Tennessee

Marilyn Pase, MSN, NMSU
Associate Professor
New Mexico State University
Las Cruces, New Mexico

Sandra Pennington, RN, PhD
Associate Professor of Nursing
Berea College
Berea, Kentucky

Anita K. Reed, RN, MSN
Instructor of Nursing
St. Elizabeth School of Nursing
Lafayette, Indiana

Linda S. Rodebaugh, RN, MSN, EdD
Associate Professor, School of Nursing
University of Indianapolis
Indianapolis, Indiana

Deborah S. Rushing, RN, MSN, CWOCN, SANE
Nursing Instructor, School of Nursing
Troy State University
Troy, Alabama

Julie Sanford, RN, DNS
Assistant Professor of Nursing
Spring Hill College
Mobile, Alabama

Kristen Sethares, RN, PhD
Assistant Professor, College of Nursing
University of Massachusetts at Dartmouth
Dartmouth, Massachusetts

Donald G. Smith, RN, PhD
Assistant Professor of Nursing
Hunter College, CUNY
Hunter-Bellevue School of Nursing
New York, New York

Susan Smith, RN, BSN, MSN-FNP
Department of Nursing
University of British Columbia
Surrey, British Columbia, Canada

Ann Sossong, RN, MSN, MEd, CAS, DNSc
Assistant Professor
University of Maine
Orono, Maine

Nancy Stark, RN, MSN
Instructor
Medical College of Georgia School of Nursing
Augusta, Georgia

Barbara Steuble, RN, MS
Assistant Professor
Samuel Merritt College
Sacramento, California

Joyce Tanaka, RN-C, MSN
Assistant Professor, Nursing
Ohlone College
Fremont, California

Peggy Thweatt, RN, MSN, DrPHc
Nursing Instructor
Medical Careers Institute
Newport News, Virginia

Creina Twomey, RN, MN
Assistant Professor of Nursing
Memorial University of Newfoundland and Labrador
St. John's, Newfoundland, Canada

Joyce Vazzano, RN, MS
Instructor, School of Nursing
Johns Hopkins University
Owings Mills, Maryland

Christine Wade, RN, EDd, PT
Associate Professor of Physical Therapy
Thomas Jefferson University
Philadelphia, Pennsylvania

Sandra Waguespack, RN, BSN, MSN
RN Instructor and Course Director
Health Sciences Center School of Nursing
New Orleans, Louisiana

Elaine Waters, BSN, MSN
Assistant Professor, Department of Baccalaureate Nursing
Eastern Kentucky University
Richmond, Kentucky

Patricia Whelan, RN, BACN
Instructor of Nursing
Grant MacEwan College
University of Alberta
Edmonton, Alberta, Canada

Patricia A. Wessels, RN, MSN
Associate Professor
Viterbo University
La Crosse, Wisconsin

Bernadette White, RN, MSN, APRN, CHTP
Assistant Professor of Nursing
Creighton University
Omaha, Nebraska

Patti Rager Zuzelo, EdD, APRN, BC, CS
Associate Professor of Nursing
La Salle University
Philadelphia, Pennsylvania

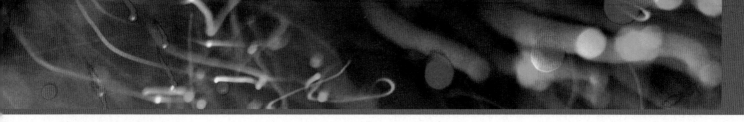

Preface

The enthusiastic reception and acceptance of the first edition of *Essentials of Pathophysiology* fostered the preparation of this second edition. The text, which is based on the seventh edition of *Pathophysiology: Concepts of Altered Health*, has been prepared specifically for those students who do not need the extensive breadth or detail of content provided in the larger book. To accomplish this task, content deemed to be less essential has been omitted, while essential content has been reorganized, revised, and condensed.

Once again, the text was developed with the intent of making the subject of pathophysiology an exciting exploration that relates normal body functioning to the physiologic changes that participate in disease production and occur as a result of disease, as well as the body's remarkable ability to compensate for these changes. While continuing to place a heavy emphasis on the mechanisms of disease and the physiologic basis of signs and symptoms of disease, this edition has been expanded to include additional content on diagnostic strategies and treatment modalities. The presentation again includes integrating the content on children, pregnant women, and elderly adults throughout the text rather than isolating the content in separate chapters. This method allows the reader to contrast and compare information while eliminating the redundancy and contradiction that often occurs when content geared to specific populations is segregated into separate chapters. To aid in the location of this content, an index of specific child, pregnancy, and elderly content is included in the front of this book.

New to the Second Edition

- An Introduction to Pathophysiology that presents a brief description of pathophysiology content areas such as the etiology and pathogenesis of disease, the meaning of mortality and morbidity, and the sources of epidemiologic data presented in the text.
- A new chapter, *Mechanisms of Infectious Diseases*, provides an overview of the various agents of infectious disease, mechanisms of the spread of infection, methods used in the diagnosis of infectious diseases, and concerns related to the global spread of diseases and to bioterrorism.
- Continued seamless integration of text and design in a manner that is designed to aid the reader's exploration and peak learning interest.
- A vibrant new art program complements the text and assists visual learners. The illustrations have been carefully chosen to offer visual appeal and enhance conceptual learning, linking text content to the illustrations. Over 200 new illustrations have been meticulously rendered to better illustrate the complexity of key physiologic processes and disease states. Reader interest is maintained and supported by the variety of styles, including line drawings of anatomic structures and pathophysiologic processes, flow charts, and photographic illustrations of disease states. The flow charts have been completely redone and the content reorganized to reflect two types of learning objectives: *mechanism flow charts* designed to assist the reader in mapping and understanding the molecular and anatomic aspects of normal and abnormal health states; and *category flow charts* designed to assist the reader in organizing and remembering information based on related patterns.
- A new feature called "Understanding" focuses on key physiologic processes and phenomena that form the basis for understanding disorders presented in the text. The feature, introduced as "Understanding . . . ," breaks a process or phenomenon down into its component parts and presents them in a sequential manner, providing an insight into the many opportunities for disease processes to disrupt the sequence.
- Review exercises at the end of each chapter are intended to assist the reader in using the conceptual approach to solving problems related to chapter content.

In addition, supportive features found in the first edition that have been retained include key concept boxes, summary statements, a list of suffixes and prefixes, a table of normal laboratory values, and glossary.

During the entire process of this extensive revision, every attempt has been made to present accurate, up-to-date content in a manner that is logical, understandable, and inspires reader interest. The content has been carefully evaluated to ensure that concepts build on one another. Words are defined as content is presented. Concepts from physiology, biochemistry, physics, and other sciences are reviewed as deemed appropriate. An expansive conceptual model integrates the "what is" with the developmental and preventive aspects of health, yielding a text that has a longevity beyond the classroom. Although material has been added and content has been revised, the text length has been carefully monitored to limit the book size so that it can be effectively used as a textbook and as a reference book that students take with them and use in their practice once the course is finished.

This revision was accomplished through an extensive review of the literature and through the use of in-depth critiques provided by students, faculty, and content specialists to help ensure that the text content is focused correctly to fully meet student learning needs. Readers are encouraged to contact us with any questions relating to this revision. Such feedback is essential to the continual development of the book.

CMP

Student and Instructor Resources

A variety of ancillary materials are available to support students and instructors alike.

Resources for Students

- **Student Resource CD-ROM.** This free CD-ROM is found in the front of the book, and contains
  - **Animations** of selected pathophysiologic processes. (Even more animations are available online at thePoint.LWW.com!)
  - **Student Review Questions** for every chapter
- *Study Guide to Accompany Porth's Essentials of Pathophysiology: Concepts of Altered Health States,* by Kathleen Schmidt Prezbindowski. This study guide reinforces and complements the text using a variety of question styles, including multiple choice, fill-in-the-blank, matching, short answer, and figure-labeling exercises.

Resources for Instructors

- **Instructor's Resource CD-ROM.** This comprehensive resource includes the following:
  - A **Test Generator,** containing more than 400 multiple-choice questions.
  - **Lecture Outlines** with integrated teaching suggestions and learning activities, providing a comprehensive overview to help structure a course.
  - **PowerPoint** presentations with incorporated images.
  - **Worksheets** that can be distributed or posted online as student assignments.
  - An **Image Bank,** containing approximately 300 images from the text in formats suitable for printing, projecting, and incorporating into web sites.
  - **WebCT- and Blackboard-ready materials,** for use with your institution's Learning Management System.
  - and more!

Resources for Students and Instructors

Visit the Porth: *Essentials of Pathophysiology: Concepts of Altered Health States* web site (**http://thePoint.LWW.com/ PorthEssentials**) for additional animations and even more resources.

To The Reader

This book was written with the intent of making the subject of pathophysiology an exciting exploration that relates normal body functioning to the physiologic changes that occur as a result of disease, as well as the body's remarkable ability to compensate for these changes. Indeed, it is these changes that represent the signs and symptoms of disease.

Using a book such as this can be simplified by taking the time to find what is in the book and how to locate information when it is needed. The *table of contents* at the beginning of the book provides an overall view of the organization and content of the book. It also provides clues as to the relationships among areas of content. For example, the location of the chapter on neoplasia within the unit on cell function and growth indicates that neoplasms are products of altered cell growth. The *index,* which appears at the end of the book, can be viewed as a road map for locating content. It can be used to quickly locate related content in different chapters of the book or to answer questions that come up in other courses.

The *introduction* provides an overview of the science and foundations upon which the content of pathophysiology is based. It discusses the meaning of terms such as *morphology* and *histology,* introduces the concept of normality as it relates to diagnostic methods, discusses the methods used in obtaining epidemiologic data, and provides an overview of the evidence-based approach to treatment of disease.

Organization

The book is organized into units and chapters. The *units* identify broad areas of content, such as alterations in the circulatory system. Many of the units start with a chapter that contains essential information about the body systems being discussed in the unit. These chapters provide the foundation for understanding the pathophysiology content presented in the subsequent chapters. The *chapters* focus on specific areas of content, such as heart failure and circulatory shock. The *chapter outline* that appears at the beginning of each chapter provides an overall view of the chapter content and organization. *Icons* identify specific content related to infants and children , pregnant women , and older adults .

Reading and Learning Aids

In an ever-expanding world of information you will not be able to read, let alone remember, everything that is in this book. With this in mind, we have developed a number of special features that will help you focus on and master the essential content for your current as well as future needs. They include

- *Terms in italics* are a signal that a word and the ideas associated with it are important to learn. Because it is essential for any professional to use and understand the vocabulary of his or her profession, two aids are provided to help you expand your vocabulary and improve your comprehension of what you are reading: the glossary and the list of prefixes and suffixes.
- The *glossary* contains concise definitions of frequently encountered terms. If you are unsure of the meaning of a term you encounter in your reading, check the glossary in the back of the book before proceeding.
- The *list of prefixes and suffixes* is a tool to help you derive the meaning of words you may be unfamiliar with and increase your vocabulary. Many disciplines establish a vocabulary by affixing one or more letters to the beginning or end of a word or base to form a derivative word. Prefixes are added to the beginning of a word or base, and suffixes are added to the end. If you know the meanings of common prefixes and suffixes, you can usually derive the meaning of a word, even if you have never encountered it before. A list of prefixes and suffixes can be found on the last page of text and inside back cover.

Boxes

Boxes are used throughout the text to summarize and highlight key information. You will encounter two types of boxes: *Key Concept Boxes* and *Summary Boxes.*

One of the ways to approach learning is to focus on the major ideas or concepts rather than trying to memorize a list of related and unrelated bits of information. As you have probably already discovered, it is impossible to memorize everything that is in a particular section or chapter of the book. Not only does your brain have a difficult time trying to figure out where to store all the different bits of information, but your brain doesn't know how to retrieve the information when you need it. Most important of all, memorized lists of content can seldom, if ever, be applied directly to an actual clinical situation. The *Key Concept Boxes* guide you in identifying the major ideas or concepts that form the foundation for truly understanding the major areas of content. When you understand the concepts in the Key Concept boxes, you will have a framework for remembering and using all of the facts given in the text.

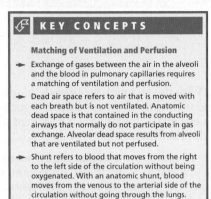

KEY CONCEPTS

Matching of Ventilation and Perfusion

➤ Exchange of gases between the air in the alveoli and the blood in pulmonary capillaries requires a matching of ventilation and perfusion.

➤ Dead air space refers to air that is moved with each breath but is not ventilated. Anatomic dead space is that contained in the conducting airways that normally do not participate in gas exchange. Alveolar dead space results from alveoli that are ventilated but not perfused.

➤ Shunt refers to blood that moves from the right to the left side of the circulation without being oxygenated. With an anatomic shunt, blood moves from the venous to the arterial side of the circulation without going through the lungs. Physiologic shunting results from blood moving through unventilated parts of the lung.

The *Summary Boxes* at the end of each section provide a review and a reinforcement of the main content that has been covered. Use the summaries to assure that you have covered and understand what you have read.

In summary, the arterial system distributes blood to all the tissues of the body, and lesions of the arterial system exert their effects through ischemia or impaired blood flow. Hyperlipidemia, with elevated cholesterol levels, plays a major role in the development of atherosclerotic disorders of the arterial system. Because cholesterol and triglycerides are insoluble in plasma, they are transported as lipoproteins. Elevated blood levels of LDLs, which carry large amounts of cholesterol, are a major risk factor for atherosclerosis. The HDLs, which are protective, remove cholesterol from the tissues and carry it back to the liver for disposal. LDL receptors play a major role in removing cholesterol from the blood; persons with reduced numbers of LDL receptors are at particularly high risk for the development of atherosclerosis.

Tables and Charts

Tables and charts are designed to present complex information in a format that makes it more meaningful and easier to remember. Tables have two or more columns and are often used for the purpose of comparing or contrasting information. Charts have one column and are used to summarize information.

TABLE 6-1	Concentrations of Extracellular and Intracellular Electrolytes in Adults	
Electrolyte	**Extracellular Concentration***	**Intracellular Concentration***
Sodium	135–145 mEq/L	10–14 mEq/L
Potassium	3.5–5.0 mEq/L	140–150 mEq/L
Chloride	98–106 mEq/L	3–4 mEq/L
Bicarbonate	24–31 mEq/L	7–10 mEq/L
Calcium	8.5–10.5 mg/dL	≮1 mEq/L
Phosphate/ phosphorus	2.5–4.5 mg/dL	4 mEq/kg†
Magnesium	1.8–3.0 mg/dL	40 mEq/kg†

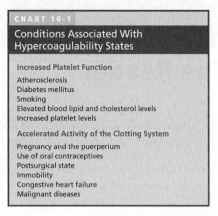

CHART 10-1

Conditions Associated With Hypercoagulability States

Increased Platelet Function

Atherosclerosis
Diabetes mellitus
Smoking
Elevated blood lipid and cholesterol levels
Increased platelet levels

Accelerated Activity of the Clotting System

Pregnancy and the puerperium
Use of oral contraceptives
Postsurgical state
Immobility
Congestive heart failure
Malignant diseases

Illustrations

The full-color illustrations will help you to build your own mental image of the content that is being presented. Each drawing has been developed to fully support and build upon the ideas in the text. Some illustrations are used to help you picture the complex interactions of the multiple phenomena that are involved in the development of a particular disease; others can help you to visualize normal function or understand the mechanisms whereby the disease processes exert their effects. In addition, photographs of pathologic processes and lesions provide a realistic view of selected pathologic processes and lesions.

There are two types of flow charts designed to help you in understanding the relationship among various aspects of normal and abnormal body function:

Mechanism flow charts will assist you in mapping and understanding the molecular and physiologic aspects of normal and abnormal health states.

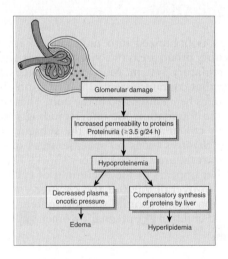

Category flow charts will assist you in understanding and remembering information based on related categories.

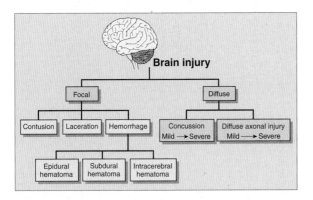

Understanding Physiologic Process

New to this edition is a feature called "Understanding" that focuses on the physiologic processes and phenomena that form the basis for understanding disorders presented in the text. This feature breaks a process or phenomenon down into its component parts and presents them in a sequential manner, providing an insight into the many opportunities for disease processes to disrupt the sequence.

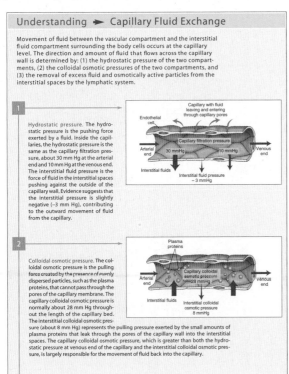

Animations of selected pathophysiologic processes are provided on the Student Resource CD-ROM and will help you to visualize some of these important processes. These animations and more are also available on the *Essentials of Pathophysiology: Concepts of Altered Health States* web site (visit http://thePoint.LWW.com/PorthEssentials).

> **Visit the Porth: Essentials of Pathophysiology: Concepts of Altered Health States web site** (http://thePoint.LWW.com/PorthEssentials) for links to chapter-related resources on the Internet, all-new exclusive animations, chapter review questions, and more!

Materials for Review

Several features have been built into the text to help you verify your understanding of the material presented. After you have finished reading and studying the chapter, work on answering the *review exercises* at the end of the chapter. They are designed to help you integrate and synthesize material. If you are unable to answer a question, reread the relevant section in the chapter.

> A 36-year-old woman enters the clinic complaining of headache and not feeling well. Her blood pressure is 175/90 mm Hg. Her renal test results are abnormal, and follow-up tests confirm that she has a stricture of the left renal artery.
>
> **A.** Would her hypertension be classified as primary or secondary?
> **B.** Explain the physiologic mechanisms underlying her blood pressure elevation.

In addition, you will find *multiple-choice questions* on the Student Resource CD-ROM in the front of your book, as well as on the *Essentials of Pathophysiology: Concepts of Altered Health States* web site (http://thePoint.LWW.com/PorthEssentials). Use these quizzes to review key information and test your knowledge.

Appendix A

Appendix A, *Laboratory Values,* provides rapid access to normal values for many laboratory tests, as well as a description of the prefixes, symbols, and factors (*e.g.,* micro, μ, 10^{-6}) used for describing these values. Knowledge of normal values can help you to put abnormal values in context.

We hope that this guide has given you a clear picture of how to use this book. Good luck and enjoy the journey!

Acknowledgments

As in past editions, many persons participated in the creation of this work. The contributing authors deserve a special mention, for they worked long hours preparing the content for the seventh edition of *Pathophysiology: Concepts of Altered Health States,* which served as the foundation for the preparation of this essentials version of the text. This year the revision has been especially meaningful as it marks a quarter of a century since the first edition of this book was published and many of these authors have been with the book during this time and played an essential role in the genesis of this edition.

I would also like to acknowledge Dr. Kathryn Gaspard and Dr. Glenn Matfin for their consultation and help in making this edition become a reality. Several other persons deserve special recognition. Georgianne Heymann assisted in editing the manuscript. As with previous editions, she provided not only excellent editorial assistance, but also encouragement and support when the tasks associated with manuscript preparation became most frustrating.

Brett MacNaughton deserves recognition for his work in coordinating the development and revision of illustrations in the book. Vicki Heim, CMI, and Anne Rains, CMI, are acknowledged for their talent and expertise in creating the new illustrations for the book. I would also like to recognize the efforts of the editorial and production staff at Lippincott Williams & Wilkins that were directed by Margaret Zuccarini, Senior Acquisitions Editor; Helen Kogut, who served as Senior Managing Editor; and Debra Schiff, for her dedication as Senior Production Editor.

The students in the classes I have taught also deserve a special salute, for they are the inspiration upon which this book is founded. They have provided the questions, suggestions, and contact with the "real world" of patient care that have directed the organization and selection of content for the book.

And last, but not least, I would like to acknowledge my family, my friends, and my colleagues for their patience, their understanding, and their encouragement throughout the entire process.

Index of Specific Content
Child 🧒, Pregnancy 🤰, Elderly 👴

Contents

UNIT *XIII*

Integumentary Function

Introduction to Pathophysiology

The term *pathophysiology*, which is the focus of this book, may be defined as the physiology of altered health. The term combines the words *pathology* and *physiology*. Pathology (from the Greek *pathos*, meaning "disease") deals with the study of the structural and functional changes in cells, tissues, and organs of the body that cause or are caused by disease. Physiology deals with the functions of the human body. Thus, pathophysiology deals not only with the cellular and organ changes that occur with disease, but with the effects that these changes have on total body function. Pathophysiology also focuses on the mechanisms of the underlying disease and provides the background for preventive as well as therapeutic health care measures and practices.

Disease

A *disease* has been defined as an interruption, cessation, or disorder in the function of a body organ or system that is characterized usually by a recognized etiologic agent/s, an identifiable group of signs and symptoms, or consistent anatomic alterations.[1] The aspects of the disease process include the etiology, pathogenesis, morphologic changes, clinical manifestations, diagnosis, and clinical course.

ETIOLOGY

The causes of disease are known as *etiologic factors*. Among the recognized etiologic agents are biologic agents (*e.g.*, bacteria, viruses), physical forces (*e.g.*, trauma, burns, radiation), chemical agents (*e.g.*, poisons, alcohol), and nutritional excesses or deficits. At the molecular level, it is important to distinguish between sick molecules and molecules that cause disease.[2] This is true of diseases such as cystic fibrosis, sickle cell anemia, and familial hypercholesterolemia, in which genetic abnormality of a single amino acid, transporter molecule, or receptor protein produces widespread effects on health.

Most disease-causing agents are nonspecific, and many different agents can cause disease of a single organ. On the other hand, a single agent or traumatic event can lead to disease of a number of organs or systems. Although a disease agent can affect more than a single organ and a number of disease agents can affect the same organ, most disease states do not have a single cause. Instead, the majority of diseases are multifactorial in origin. This is particularly true of diseases such as cancer, heart disease, and diabetes. The multiple factors that predispose to a particular disease often are referred to as *risk factors*.

One way to view the factors that cause disease is to group them into categories according to whether they were present at birth or acquired later in life. *Congenital conditions* are defects that are present at birth, although they may not be evident until later in life. Congenital malformation may be caused by genetic influences, environmental factors (*e.g.*, viral infections in the mother, maternal drug use, irradiation, or intrauterine crowding), or a combination of genetic and environmental factors. *Acquired defects* are those that are caused by events that occur after birth. These include injury, exposure to infectious agents, inadequate nutrition, lack of oxygen, inappropriate immune responses, and neoplasia. Many diseases are thought to be the result of a genetic predisposition and an environmental event or events that serve as a trigger to initiate disease development.

PATHOGENESIS

Pathogenesis is the sequence of cellular and tissue events that take place from the time of initial contact with an etiologic agent until the ultimate expression of a disease. *Etiology* describes what sets the disease process in motion, and pathogenesis, how the disease process evolves. Although the two terms often are used interchangeably, their meanings are quite different. For example, atherosclerosis often is cited as the cause or etiology of coronary heart disease. In reality, the progression from fatty streak to the occlusive vessel lesion seen in persons with coronary heart disease represents the pathogenesis of the disorder. The true etiology of atherosclerosis remains largely uncertain.

MORPHOLOGY

Morphology refers to the fundamental structure or form of cells or tissues. *Morphologic changes* are concerned with both the gross anatomic and microscopic changes that are characteristic of a disease. *Histology* deals with the study of the cells and extracellular matrix of body tissues. The most common method used in the study of tissues is the preparation of histologic sections—thin, translucent sections of human tissues and organs—that can be studied with the aid of a microscope. Histologic sections play an important role in the diagnosis of many types of cancer. A *lesion* represents a pathologic or traumatic discontinuity of a body organ or tissue. Descriptions of lesion size and characteristics often can be obtained through the use of radiographs, ultrasonography, and other imaging methods.

Lesions also may be sampled by biopsy and the tissue samples subjected to histologic study.

CLINICAL MANIFESTATIONS

Disease can be manifest in a number of ways. Sometimes the condition produces manifestations, such as fever, that make it evident that the person is sick. Other diseases are silent at the onset and are detected during examination for other purposes or after the disease is far advanced.

Signs and *symptoms* are terms used to describe the structural and functional changes that accompany a disease. A *symptom* is a subjective complaint that is noted by the person with a disorder, whereas a *sign* is a manifestation that is noted by an observer. Pain, difficulty in breathing, and dizziness are symptoms of a disease. An elevated temperature, a swollen extremity, and changes in pupil size are objective signs that can be observed by someone other than the person with the disease. Signs and symptoms may be related to the primary disorder or they may represent the body's attempt to compensate for the altered function caused by the pathologic condition. Many pathologic states are not observed directly—one cannot see a sick heart or a failing kidney. Instead, what can be observed is the body's attempt to compensate for changes in function brought about by the disease, such as the tachycardia that accompanies blood loss or the increased respiratory rate that occurs with pneumonia.

A *syndrome* is a compilation of signs and symptoms (*e.g.*, chronic fatigue syndrome) that are characteristic of a specific disease state. *Complications* are possible adverse extensions of a disease or outcomes from treatment. *Sequelae* are lesions or impairments that follow or are caused by a disease.

DIAGNOSIS

A *diagnosis* is the designation as to the nature or cause of a health problem (*e.g.*, bacterial pneumonia or hemorrhagic stroke). The diagnostic process usually requires a careful history and physical examination. The history is used to obtain a person's account of his or her symptoms, their progression, and the factors that contribute to a diagnosis. The physical examination is done to observe for signs of altered body structure or function.

The development of a diagnosis involves weighing competing possibilities and selecting the most likely one from among the conditions that might be responsible for the person's clinical presentation. The clinical probability of a given disease in a person of a given age, sex, race, lifestyle, and locality often is influential in arrival at a presumptive diagnosis. Laboratory tests, radiologic studies, computed tomography (CT) scans, and other tests often are used to confirm a diagnosis.

An important factor when interpreting diagnostic test results is the determination of whether they are normal or abnormal. Is a blood count above normal, within the normal range, or below normal? What is termed a *normal* value for a laboratory test is established statistically from test results obtained from a selected sample of people. The normal values refer to the 95% distribution (mean plus or minus two standard deviations [mean ± 2 SD]) of test results for the reference population.[3] Thus, the normal levels for serum sodium (135 to 145 mEq/L) represent the mean serum level for the reference population ± 2 SD. The normal values for some laboratory tests are adjusted for sex or age. For example, the normal hemoglobin range for women is 12.0 to 16.0 g/dL and for men, 14.0 to 17.4 g/dL.[4] Serum creatinine level often is adjusted for age in the elderly, and normal values for serum phosphate differ between adults and children.

The quality of data on which a diagnosis is based may be judged for its reliability, validity, sensitivity, specificity, and predictive value.[5,6] *Reliability* refers to the extent to which an observation, if repeated, gives the same result. A poorly calibrated blood pressure machine may give inconsistent measurements of blood pressure, particularly of pressures in either the high or low range. Reliability also depends on the persons making the measurements. For example, blood pressure measurements may vary from one observer to another because of the technique that is used (*e.g.*, different observers may deflate the cuff at a different rate, thus obtaining different values), the way the numbers on the manometer are read, or differences in hearing acuity. *Validity* refers to the extent to which a measurement tool measures what it is intended to measure. This often is assessed by comparing a measurement method with the best possible method of measure that is available. For example, the validity of blood pressure measurements obtained by a sphygmomanometer might be compared with those obtained by intra-arterial measurements.

Measures of sensitivity and specificity are concerned with determining how well the test or observation identifies people with the disease and people without the disease. *Sensitivity* refers to the proportion of people with a disease who are positive for that disease on a given test or observation (called a *true-positive* result). *Specificity* refers to the proportion of people without the disease who are negative on a given test or observation (called a *true-negative* result). A test that is 95% specific correctly identifies 95 of 100 normal people. The other 5% are *false-positive* results. A false-positive test result can be unduly stressful for the person being tested, whereas a *false-negative* test result can delay diagnosis and jeopardize the outcome of treatment.

Predictive value is the extent to which an observation or test result is able to predict the presence of a given disease or condition. A *positive predictive value* refers to the proportion of true-positive results that occurs in a given population. In a group of women found to have "suspect breast nodules" in a cancer-screening program, the proportion later determined to have breast cancer would constitute the positive predictive value. A *negative predictive value* refers to the true-negative observations in a population. In a screening test for breast cancer, the negative predictive value represents the proportion of women without suspect nodules who do not have breast cancer. Although predictive values rely in part on sensitivity and specificity, they depend more heavily on the prevalence of the condition in the population. Despite unchanging sensitivity and specificity, the positive predictive value of an observation rises with prevalence, whereas the negative predictive value falls.

CLINICAL COURSE

The clinical course describes the evolution of a disease. A disease can have an acute, subacute, or chronic course. An *acute disorder* is one that is relatively severe but self-limiting. *Chronic disease* implies a continuous, long-term process. A chronic disease can run a continuous course or it can present with exacerbations (aggravation of symptoms and severity of the disease) and remissions (a period during which there is a lessening of severity and a decrease in symptoms). *Subacute disease* is intermediate, or between acute and chronic: it is not as severe as an acute disease and not as prolonged as a chronic disease.

The spectrum of disease severity for infectious diseases such as hepatitis B can range from preclinical to persistent chronic infection. During the *preclinical stage,* a disease is not clinically evident but is destined to progress to clinical disease. As with hepatitis B, it is possible to transmit the virus during the preclinical stage. *Subclinical disease* is not clinically apparent and is not destined to become clinically apparent. It is diagnosed with antibody or culture tests. Most cases of tuberculosis are not clinically apparent, and evidence of their presence is established by skin tests. *Clinical disease* is manifested by signs and symptoms. A persistent chronic infectious disease persists for years, sometimes for life. *Carrier status* refers to an individual who harbors an organism but may have few or no laboratory or clinical manifestations. This person still can infect others. Carrier status may be of limited duration or it may be chronic, lasting for months or years.

Perspectives on Health and Disease in Populations

The health of individuals is closely linked to the health of the community and to the population it encompasses. The ability to traverse continents in a matter of hours has opened the world to issues of populations at a global level. Diseases that once were confined to local areas of the world now pose a threat to populations throughout the world.

As we move through the 21st century, we are continually reminded that the health care system and the services it delivers are targeted to particular populations. Managed care systems are focused on a population-based approach to planning, delivering, providing, and evaluating health care. The focus of health care also has begun to emerge as a partnership in which individuals are asked to assume greater responsibility for their own health.

EPIDEMIOLOGY AND PATTERNS OF DISEASE

Epidemiology is the study of disease in populations. It was initially developed to explain the spread of infectious diseases during epidemics and has emerged as a science to study risk factors for multifactorial diseases, such as heart disease and cancer. Epidemiology looks for patterns, such as age, race, dietary habits, lifestyle, or geographic location of persons affected with a particular disorder. In contrast to biomedical researchers, who seek to elucidate the mechanisms of disease production, epidemiologists are more concerned with whether something happens than how it happens.[7] For example, the epidemiologist is more concerned with whether smoking itself is related to cardiovascular disease and whether the risk of heart disease decreases when smoking ceases. On the other hand, the biomedical researcher is more concerned about the causative agent in cigarette smoke and the pathway by which it contributes to heart disease.

Much of our knowledge about disease comes from epidemiologic studies. Epidemiologic methods are used to determine how a disease is spread, how to control it, how to prevent it, and how to eliminate it. Epidemiologic methods also are used to study the natural history of disease, to evaluate new preventative and treatment strategies, to explore the impact of different patterns of health care delivery, and to predict future health care needs. As such, epidemiologic studies serve as a basis for clinical decision making, allocation of health care dollars, and development of policies related to public health issues.

Measures of disease frequency are an important aspect of epidemiology. They establish a means for predicting what diseases are present in a population and provide an indication of the rate at which they are increasing or decreasing. A *disease case* can be either an existing case or the number of new episodes of a particular illness that is diagnosed within a given period. *Incidence* is the number of new cases arising in a population during a specified time. It is determined by dividing the number of new cases of a disease by the population at risk for development of the disease during the same period. *Prevalence* is the number of people in a population who have a particular disease at a given point in time or period. It is determined by dividing the existing number of cases by the population at risk for development of the disorder during the same period. Incidence and prevalence rates always are reported as proportions (*e.g.,* cases per 100 or cases per 100,000).

Morbidity and mortality statistics provide information about the functional effects (morbidity) and death-producing (mortality) characteristics of a disease. These statistics are useful in terms of anticipating health care needs, planning of public education programs, directing health research efforts, and allocating health care dollars.

Mortality, or death, statistics provide information about the trends in the health of a population. In most countries, people are legally required to record certain facts such as age, sex, and cause of death on a death certificate. Internationally agreed classification procedures (the International Classification of Diseases by the World Health Organization [WHO]) are used for coding the cause of death and the data are expressed as death rates.[8] Crude mortality rates (*i.e.,* number of deaths in a given period) do not account for age, sex, race, socioeconomic status, and other factors. For this reason, mortality often is expressed as death rates for a specific population, such as the infant mortality rate. Mortality also can be described in terms of the leading causes of death according to age, sex, race, and ethnicity. Among all persons 65 years of age and older, the five leading causes of death in the United States are heart disease, cancer, stroke, chronic obstructive lung disease, and pneumonia and influenza.[9] In 1997, for example, diabetes was the third leading cause of death among American Indians 65 years of age and older, the fourth leading cause of death among older Hispanic and black persons, and the sixth leading cause of death among older white persons and Asian Americans.[10]

Morbidity describes the effects an illness has on a person's life. Many diseases, such as arthritis, have low death rates but have a significant impact on a person's life. Morbidity is concerned not only with the occurrence or incidence of a disease but also with persistence and the long-term consequences of the disease.

DETERMINATION OF RISK FACTORS

Conditions suspected of contributing to the development of a disease are called *risk factors*. They may be inherent to the person (high blood pressure or overweight) or external (smoking or drinking alcohol). There are different types of studies used to determine risk factors, including cross-sectional studies, case-control studies, and cohort studies. *Cross-sectional studies* use the simultaneous collection of information necessary for classification of exposure and outcome status. They can be used to compare the prevalence of a disease in those with the factor (or exposure) with the prevalence of a disease in those who are unexposed to the factor, such as the prevalence of coronary heart disease in smokers and nonsmokers. *Case-control studies* are designed to compare persons known to have the outcome of interest (*cases*) and those known not to have the outcome of interest (*control*). Information on exposures or characteristics of interest is then collected from persons in both groups. For example, the characteristics of maternal alcohol consumption in infants born with fetal alcohol syndrome (cases) can be compared with those in infants born without the syndrome (control).

A *cohort* is a group of persons who were born at approximately the same time or share some characteristics of interest. Persons enrolled in a cohort study (also called a *longitudinal study*) are followed over a period to observe some health outcome. A cohort may consist of a single group of persons chosen because they have or have not been exposed to suspected risk factors, two groups specifically selected because one has been exposed and the other has not, or a single exposed group in which the results are compared with the general population.

One of the best-known examples of a cohort study is the Framingham Study, which was carried out in Framingham, Massachusetts.[11] Framingham was selected because of the size of the population, the relative ease with which the people could be contacted, and the stability of the population in terms of moving into and out of the area. This longitudinal study, which began in 1950, was set up by the U.S. Public Health Service to study the characteristics of people who would later develop coronary heart disease. The study consisted of 5000 persons, aged 30 to 59 years, selected at random and followed for an initial period of 20 years, during which time it was predicted that 1500 of them would develop coronary heart disease. The advantage of such a study is that it can study a number of risk factors at the same time and determine the relative importance of each. Another advantage is that the risk factors can be related later to other diseases such as stroke.

A second well-known cohort study is the Nurses' Health Study, which was developed by Harvard University and Brigham and Women's Hospital. The study began in 1976 with a cohort of 121,700 female nurses, 30 to 55 years of age, living in the United States.[12] Initially designed to explore the relationship between oral contraceptives and breast cancer, nurses in the study have provided answers to detailed questions about their menstrual cycle, smoking habits, diet, weight and waist measurements, activity patterns, health problems, and medication use. They have collected urine and blood samples, and even provided researchers with their toenail clippings. In selecting the cohort, it was reasoned that nurses would be well organized, accurate, and observant in their responses, and that physiologically they would be no different from other groups of women. It also was anticipated that their childbearing, eating, and smoking patterns would be similar to those of other working women.

NATURAL HISTORY

The *natural history* of disease refers to the progression and projected outcome of a disease without medical intervention. By studying the patterns of a disease over time in populations, epidemiologists can better understand its natural history. A knowledge of the natural history can be used to determine disease outcome, establish priorities for health care services, determine the effects of screening and early detection programs on disease outcome, and compare the results of new treatments with the expected outcome without treatment.

There are some diseases for which there are no effective treatment methods available, or the current treatment measures are effective only in certain people. In this case, the natural history of the disease can be used as a predictor of outcome. For example, the natural history of hepatitis C indicates that 80% of people who become infected with the virus fail to clear the virus and progress to chronic infection.[13] Information about the natural history of a disease and the availability of effective treatment methods provides directions for preventive measures. In the case of hepatitis C, careful screening of blood donations and education of intravenous drug abusers can be used to prevent transfer of the virus. At the same time, scientists are striving to develop a vaccine that will prevent infection in persons exposed to the virus. The development of vaccines to prevent the spread of infectious diseases such as polio and hepatitis B undoubtedly has been motivated by knowledge about the natural history of these diseases and the lack of effective intervention measures. With other diseases, such as breast cancer, early detection through use of breast self-examination and mammography increases the chances for a cure.

Prognosis refers to the probable outcome and prospect of recovery from a disease. It can be designated as chances for full recovery, possibility of complications, or anticipated survival time. Prognosis often is presented in relation to treatment options—that is, the expected outcomes or chances for survival with or without a certain type of treatment. The prognosis associated with a given type of treatment usually is presented along with the risk associated with the treatment.

LEVELS OF PREVENTION

Basically, leading a healthy life contributes to the prevention of disease. There are three fundamental types of prevention: primary prevention, secondary prevention, and tertiary prevention[14] *Primary prevention* is directed at keeping disease from occurring by removing all risk factors. Immunizations are examples of primary prevention. *Secondary prevention* detects disease early when it is still asymptomatic and treatment measures can affect a cure. The use of a Papanicolaou (Pap) smear for early detection of cervical cancer is an example of secondary prevention. *Tertiary prevention* is directed at clinical interventions that prevent further deterioration or reduce the complications of a disease once it has been diagnosed. An example is the use of beta-adrenergic drugs to reduce the risk of death in persons who have had a heart attack. Tertiary prevention measures also include measures to limit physical impairment and social consequences of an illness.

Evidence-Based Practice and Practice Guidelines

Evidence-based practice and evidence-based practice guidelines have recently gained popularity with clinicians, public health practitioners, health care organizations, and the public as a means of improving the quality and efficiency of health care.[15] Their development has been prompted, at least in part, by the enormous amounts of published information about diagnostic and treatment measures for various disease conditions, as well as demands for better and more cost effective health care.

Evidence-based practice has been defined as "the conscientious, explicit, and judicious use of current best evidence in making decisions about the care of individual patients."[15] It is based on the integration of the individual expertise of the practitioner with the best external clinical evidence from systematic research.[15] The term *clinical expertise* implies the proficiency and judgment that individual clinicians gain through clinical experience and clinical practice. The best external clinical evidence relies on the identification of clinically relevant research, often from the basic sciences, but especially from patient-centered clinical studies that focus on the accuracy and precision of diagnostic tests and methods, the power of prognostic indicators, and the effectiveness and safety of therapeutic, rehabilitative, and preventive regimens.

Clinical practice guidelines are systematically developed statements intended to inform practitioners and clients in making decisions about health care for specific clinical circumstances.[16,17] They should not only review various outcomes but also must weigh various outcomes, both positive and negative, and make recommendations. Guidelines are different from systematic reviews. They can take the form of algorithms, which are step-by-step methods for solving a problem; written directives for care; or a combination thereof.

The development of evidence-based practice guidelines often uses methods such as meta-analysis to combine evidence from different studies to produce a more precise estimate of the accuracy of a diagnostic method or the effects of an intervention method.[18] It also requires review: by practitioners with expertise in clinical content, who can verify the completeness of the literature review and ensure clinical sensibility; from experts in guideline development, who can examine the method by which the guideline was developed; and by potential users of the guideline.[16]

Once developed, practice guidelines must be continually reviewed and changed to keep pace with new research findings and with new diagnostic and treatment methods. For example, the Guidelines for the Prevention, Evaluation, and Treatment of High Blood Pressure (Chapter 17), first developed in 1972 by the Joint National Committee, have been revised seven times, and the Guidelines for the Diagnosis and Management of Asthma (Chapter 22), first developed in 1991 by the Expert Panel, have undergone three revisions.

Evidence-based practice guidelines, which are intended to direct client care, are also important in directing research into the best methods of diagnosing and treating specific health problems. This is because health care providers use the same criteria for diagnosing the extent and severity of a particular condition such as hypertension and because they use the same protocols for treatment.

References

1. *Stedman's medical dictionary* (27th ed., p. 509). (2000). Philadelphia: Lippincott Williams & Wilkins.
2. Waldenstrom J. (1989). Sick molecules and our concepts of illness. *Journal of Internal Medicine* 225, 221–227.
3. Brigden M. L., Heathcote J. C. (2000). Problems with interpreting laboratory tests. *Postgraduate Medicine* 107(7), 145–162.
4. Fischbach F. (2004). *A manual of laboratory and diagnostic tests* (7th ed., pp. 964, 974). Philadelphia: Lippincott Williams & Wilkins.

5. Bickley L. (2003). *Bates' A guide to physical assessment and history taking* (6th ed., pp. 641–642). Philadelphia: J. B. Lippincott.

6. Dawson-Saunders B., Trapp R. G. (1990). Evaluating diagnostic procedures. In Dawson-Saunders B., Trapp R. G. (Eds.), *Basic and clinical biostatistics* (pp. 229–244). Norwalk, CT: Appleton & Lange.

7. Vetter N., Mathews I. (1999). *Epidemiology and public health maintenance.* Edinburgh: Churchill Livingstone.

8. World Health Organization. (2001). *About WHO: Definition of health; disease eradication/elimination goals.* [On-line.] Available: http://www.who.int/about/definition/en/. Accessed Feb 19, 2004.

9. Centers for Disease Control. (2003). Death, percent of deaths, and death rates for 15 leading causes of death in selected age groups by race and sex: United States 1999. [On-line.] Available: http://www.cdc.gov/. Accessed October 9, 2005.

10. U.S. Department Health and Human Services. (2000). *Healthy people 2010.* National Health Information Center. [On-line.] Available: http://web.health.gov/healthypeople/. Accessed October 9, 2005.

11. Framingham Heart Study. (2001). *Framingham Heart Study: Design, rationale, objectives, and research milestones.* [On-line.] Available: http://www.nhlbi.nih.gov/about/framingham/design.htm. Accessed October 10, 2005.

12. Channing Laboratory. (2004). Nurses' Health Study. [On-line]. Available: http://www.channing.harvard.edu/nhs/hist.html. Accessed October 10,2005.

13. Liang J., Reherman B., Seeff L. B., Hoofnagle J. H. (2000). Pathogenesis, natural history, treatment, and prevention of hepatitis C. *Annals of Internal Medicine* 132, 296–305.

14. Stanhope M., Lancaster J. (2000). *Community and public health nursing* (5th ed., p. 43). St. Louis: Mosby.

15. Sackett D. L. (1996). Evidence based medicine: What it is and what it isn't. *British Medical Journal* 312, 71–72.

16. Shekelle P. G., Woolff S. H., Eccles M., et al. (1999). Developing guidelines. *British Medical Journal* 318, 593–596.

17. Natsch S., van der Meer J. W. M. (2003). The role of clinical guidelines, policies, and stewardship. *Journal of Hospital Infection* 53, 172–176.

18. Acton G. J. (2001). Meta-analysis: A tool for evidence-based practice. *AACN Clinical Issues* 12, 539–545.

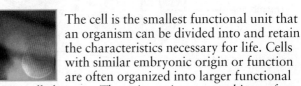

U N I T 1

Cell and Tissue Function

C h a p t e r 1

Cell Structure and Function

The cell is the smallest functional unit that an organism can be divided into and retain the characteristics necessary for life. Cells with similar embryonic origin or function are often organized into larger functional units called *tissues*. These tissues in turn combine to form the various body structures and organs. Although the cells of different tissues and organs vary in structure and function, certain characteristics are common to all cells. Cells are remarkably similar in their ability to exchange materials with their immediate environment, obtaining energy from organic nutrients, synthesizing complex molecules, and replicating themselves. Because most disease processes are initiated at the cellular level, an understanding of cell function is crucial to understanding the disease process. Some diseases affect the cells of a single organ, others affect the cells of a particular tissue type, and still others affect the cells of the entire organism.

Functional Components of the Cell

Although diverse in their organization, all eukaryotic cells (cells with a true nucleus) have in common structures that perform unique functions. Seen under a light microscope, three major components of the eukaryotic cell become evident: the nucleus, the cytoplasm, and the cell membrane (Fig. 1-1).

The internal matrix of the cell is called *protoplasm*. Protoplasm is composed of water, proteins, lipids, carbohydrates, and electrolytes. Water makes up 70% to 85% of the cell's protoplasm. The second most abundant constituents (10% to 20%) of protoplasm are the cell

1

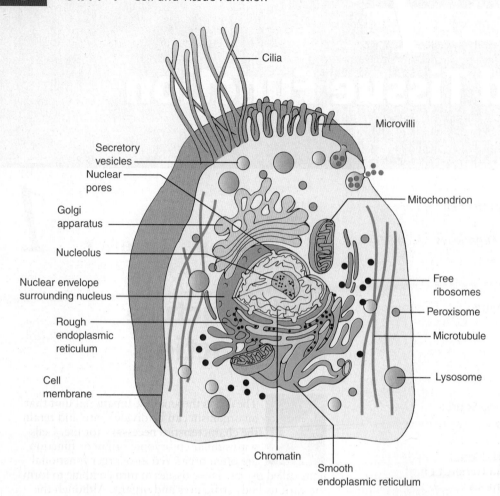

FIGURE 1-1 Composite cell designed to show in one cell all of the various components of the nucleus and cytoplasm.

proteins, which form cell structures and the enzymes necessary for cellular reactions. Proteins can also be found complexed to other compounds such as nucleoproteins, glycoproteins, and lipoproteins. Lipids comprise 2% to 3% of most cells. The most important lipids are the phospholipids and cholesterol, which are mainly insoluble in water; they combine with proteins to form the cell membrane and the membranous barriers that separate different cell compartments. Some cells also contain large quantities of triglycerides. In the fat cells, triglycerides can constitute up to 95% of the total cell mass. The fat stored in these cells represents stored energy, which can be mobilized and used wherever it is needed in the body. Few carbohydrates are found in the cell, and these are used primarily for fuel. Potassium, magnesium, phosphate, sulfate, and bicarbonate ions are the major intracellular electrolytes. Small quantities of sodium, chloride, and calcium ions are also present in the cell. These electrolytes facilitate the generation and transmission of electrochemical impulses in nerve and muscle cells. Intracellular electrolytes participate in reactions that are necessary for cellular metabolism.

THE NUCLEUS

The nucleus of the cell appears as a rounded or elongated structure situated near the center of the cell (see Fig. 1-1).

KEY CONCEPTS

The Functional Organization of the Cell

➤ Cells are the smallest functional unit of the body. They contain structures that are strikingly similar to those needed to maintain total body function.

➤ The nucleus is the control center for the cell. It also contains most of the hereditary material.

➤ The organelles, which are analogous to the organs of the body, are contained in the cytoplasm. They include the mitochondria, which supply the energy needs of the cell; the ribosomes, which synthesize proteins and other materials needed for cell function; and the lysosomes, which function as the cell's digestive system.

➤ The cell membrane encloses the cell and provides for intracellular and intercellular communication, transport of materials into and out of the cell, and maintenance of the electrical activities that power cell function.

It is enclosed in a nuclear membrane and contains chromatin and a distinct region called the *nucleolus*. All eukaryotic cells have at least one nucleus (prokaryotic cells, such as bacteria, lack a nucleus and nuclear membrane). The nucleus can be regarded as the control center for the cell. It contains the deoxyribonucleic acid (DNA) that is essential to the cell because its genes contain the information necessary for the synthesis of proteins that the cell must produce to stay alive. These proteins include structural proteins and enzymes used to synthesize other substances, including carbohydrates and lipids. The genes also represent the individual units of inheritance that transmit information from one generation to another. The nucleus is also the site of ribonucleic acid (RNA) synthesis. There are three types of RNA: messenger RNA (mRNA), which copies and carries the DNA instructions for protein synthesis to the cytoplasm; ribosomal RNA (rRNA), which moves to the cytoplasm and becomes the site of protein synthesis; and transfer RNA (tRNA), which also moves into the cytoplasm, where it transports amino acids to the elongating protein as it is being synthesized (see Chapter 3).

The complex structure of DNA and DNA-associated proteins dispersed in the nuclear matrix is called *chromatin*. Each DNA molecule is made up of two extremely long, double-stranded helical chains containing variable sequences of four nitrogenous bases. These bases form the genetic code. In cells that are about to divide, the DNA must be replicated before *mitosis*, or cell division, occurs. During replication, complementary pairs of DNA are generated such that each daughter cell receives an identical set of genes.

The nucleus also contains the darkly stained round body called the *nucleolus*. Nucleoli are structures composed of regions from five different chromosomes, each with a part of the genetic code needed for the synthesis of rRNA, which is transcribed exclusively in the nucleolus. Cells that are actively synthesizing proteins can be recognized because their nucleoli are large and prominent and the nucleus as a whole is euchromatic or slightly stained.

Surrounding the nucleus is a doubled-layered membrane called the *nuclear envelope* or *nuclear membrane*. The nuclear membrane contains many structurally complex, circular pores where the two membranes fuse to form a gap. Many classes of molecules, including fluids, electrolytes, RNA, some proteins, and perhaps some hormones, can move in both directions through the nuclear pores.

THE CYTOPLASM AND ITS ORGANELLES

The cytoplasm surrounds the nucleus, and it is in the cytoplasm that the work of the cell takes place. Cytoplasm is essentially a colloidal solution that contains water, electrolytes, suspended proteins, neutral fats, and glycogen molecules. Although they do not contribute to the cell's function, pigments may also accumulate in the cytoplasm. Some pigments, such as melanin, which gives skin its color, are normal constituents of the cell.

Embedded in the cytoplasm are various *organelles*, which function as the organs of the cell. These organelles

include the ribosomes, endoplasmic reticulum, Golgi complex, lysosomes and peroxisomes, and mitochondria.

Ribosomes

The ribosomes serve as sites of protein synthesis in the cell. They are small particles of nucleoproteins (rRNA and proteins) that can be found attached to the wall of the endoplasmic reticulum or as free ribosomes. Free ribosomes are scattered singly in the cytoplasm or joined by strands of mRNA to form functional units called *polyribosomes*.

Endoplasmic Reticulum

The endoplasmic reticulum (ER) is an extensive system of paired membranes and flat vesicles that connects various parts of the inner cell (Fig. 1-2). The fluid-filled space between the paired ER membrane layers is connected with the space between the two membranes of the double-layered nuclear membrane, the cell membrane, and various cytoplasmic organelles. It functions as a tubular communication system through which substances can be transported from one part of the cell to another. A large surface area and multiple enzyme systems attached to the ER membranes also provide the machinery for a major share of the metabolic functions of the cell.

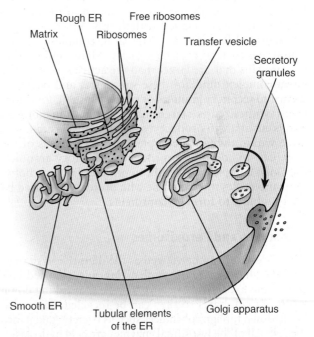

FIGURE 1-2 Three-dimensional view of the rough and smooth endoplasmic reticulum (ER) and the Golgi apparatus. The ER functions as a tubular communication system through which substances can be transported from one part of the cell to another and as the site of protein (rough ER), carbohydrate, and lipid (smooth ER) synthesis. Most of the proteins synthesized by the rough ER are sealed into transfer vesicles and transported to the Golgi apparatus, where they are modified and packaged into secretory granules.

Two forms of ER exist in cells: rough and smooth. Rough ER is studded with ribosomes attached to specific binding sites on the membrane. The ribosomes, with the accompanying strand of mRNA, synthesize proteins. Proteins produced by the rough ER are usually destined for incorporation into cell membranes and lysosomal enzymes or for exportation from the cell. The rough ER segregates these proteins from other components of the cytoplasm and modifies their structure for a specific function. For example, the production of plasma proteins by liver cells takes place in the rough ER. All cells require a rough ER for the synthesis of lysosomal enzymes.

The smooth ER is free of ribosomes and is continuous with the rough ER. It does not participate in protein synthesis; instead, its enzymes are involved in the synthesis of lipid molecules, including lipoproteins and steroid hormones, regulation of intracellular calcium, and metabolism and detoxification of certain hormones and drugs. The sarcoplasmic reticulum of skeletal and cardiac muscle cells is a form of smooth ER. Calcium ions needed for muscle contraction are stored and released from cisternae of the sarcoplasmic reticulum. The smooth ER of liver cells is involved in glycogen storage and metabolism of lipid-soluble drugs.

Golgi Complex

The Golgi apparatus, sometimes called the *Golgi complex,* consists of stacks of thin, flattened vesicles or sacs (see Fig. 1-2). These Golgi bodies are found near the nucleus and function in association with the ER. Substances produced in the ER are carried to the Golgi complex in small, membrane-covered transfer vesicles. Many cells synthesize proteins that are larger than the active product. The Golgi complex modifies these substances and packages them into secretory granules or vesicles. Insulin, for example, is synthesized as a large, inactive proinsulin molecule that is cut apart to produce a smaller, active insulin molecule within the Golgi complex of the beta cells of the pancreas. In addition to producing secretory granules, the Golgi complex is thought to produce large carbohydrate molecules that combine with proteins produced by the rough ER to form glycoproteins.

Lysosomes and Peroxisomes

The lysosomes can be viewed as the digestive system of the cell. They consist of small, membrane-enclosed sacs containing hydrolytic enzymes capable of breaking down worn-out cell parts so they can be recycled. They also break down foreign substances such as bacteria taken into the cell. All of the lysosomal enzymes are acid hydrolases, which means that they require an acid environment. The lysosomes provide this environment by maintaining a pH of approximately 5 in their interior. The pH of the cytoplasm is approximately 7.2, which protects other cellular structures from this activity.

Lysosomal enzymes are synthesized in the rough ER and then transported to the Golgi apparatus, where they are biochemically modified and packaged as lysosomes.

Unlike the sizes and functions of other organelles, those of the lysosomes vary considerably from one cell to another. The type of enzyme packaged in the lysosome by the Golgi complex determines this diversity. Although the lysosomal enzymes can break down most proteins, carbohydrates, and lipids to their basic constituents, some materials remain undigested. These undigested materials may remain in the cytoplasm as *residual bodies* or be extruded from the cell. In some long-lived cells, such as neurons and heart muscle cells, large quantities of residual bodies accumulate as lipofuscin granules or age pigment. Other indigestible pigments, such as inhaled carbon particles and tattoo pigments, also accumulate and may persist in residual bodies for decades.

Lysosomes play an important role in the normal metabolism of certain substances in the body. In some inherited diseases known as *lysosomal storage diseases,* a specific lysosomal enzyme is absent or inactive, in which case the digestion of certain cellular substances does not occur. As a result, these substances accumulate in the cell. In Tay-Sachs disease, an autosomal recessive disorder, the lysosomal enzyme needed for degrading the GM_2 ganglioside found in nerve cell membranes is deficient (see Chapter 4). Although GM_2 ganglioside accumulates in many tissues, such as the heart, liver, and spleen, its accumulation in the nervous system and retina of the eye causes the most damage.

Smaller than lysosomes, spherical membrane-bound organelles called *peroxisomes* contain a special enzyme that degrades peroxides (*e.g.,* hydrogen peroxide). Peroxisomes function in the control of free radicals (see Chapter 2). Unless degraded, these highly unstable chemical compounds would damage other cytoplasmic molecules. For example, catalase degrades toxic hydrogen peroxide molecules to water. Peroxisomes also contain the enzymes needed for breaking down very–long-chain fatty acids, which are ineffectively degraded by mitochondrial enzymes. In liver cells, peroxisomal enzymes are involved in the formation of the bile acids.

Mitochondria

The mitochondria are literally the "power plants" of the cell because they transform organic compounds into energy that is easily accessible to the cell. Energy is not made here but is extracted from organic compounds. Mitochondria contain the enzymes needed for capturing most of the energy in foodstuffs and converting it into cellular energy. This multistep process requires oxygen and is often referred to as *aerobic metabolism.* Much of this energy is stored in the high-energy phosphate bonds of compounds such as adenosine triphosphate (ATP) that power the various cellular activities.

Mitochondria are found close to the site of energy consumption in the cell (*e.g.,* near the myofibrils in muscle cells). The number of mitochondria in a given cell type is largely determined by the type of activity the cell performs and how much energy is needed to undertake this activity. For example, large increases in mitochondria have been observed in skeletal muscle that has been repeatedly stimulated to contract.

The mitochondria are composed of two membranes: an outer membrane that encloses the periphery of the mitochondrion and an inner membrane that forms shelflike projections, called *cristae* (Fig. 1-3). The outer and inner membranes form two spaces: an outer intramembranous space and an inner matrix that is filled with a gel-like material. The outer membrane is involved in lipid synthesis and fatty acid metabolism. The inner membrane contains the respiratory chain enzymes and transport proteins needed for the synthesis of ATP.

Mitochondria contain their own DNA and ribosomes and are self-replicating. The DNA is found in the mitochondrial matrix and is distinct from the chromosomal DNA found in the nucleus. Mitochondrial DNA, known as the "other human genome," is a double-stranded, circular molecule that encodes the rRNA and tRNA required for intramitochondrial synthesis of the proteins needed for the energy-generating function of the mitochondria. Although mitochondrial DNA directs the synthesis of 13 of the proteins required for mitochondrial function, the DNA of the nucleus encodes the structural proteins of the mitochondria and other proteins needed to carry out cellular respiration.

Mitochondrial DNA is inherited matrilineally (*i.e.,* from the mother) and provides a basis for familial lineage studies. Mutations have been found in each of the mitochondrial genes, and an understanding of the role of mitochondrial DNA in certain diseases is beginning to emerge. Most tissues in the body depend to some extent on oxidative metabolism and can therefore be affected by mitochondrial DNA mutations.

THE CYTOSKELETON

In addition to its organelles, the cytoplasm contains a network of microtubules, microfilaments, intermediate filaments, and thick filaments (Fig. 1-4). Because they control cell shape and movement, these structures are a major component of the structural elements called the *cytoskeleton.*

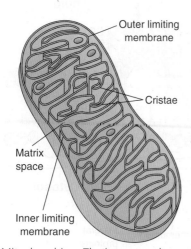

FIGURE 1-3 Mitochondrion. The inner membrane forms transverse folds called cristae, where the enzymes needed for the final step in adenosine triphosphate (ATP) production (*i.e.,* oxidative phosphorylation) are located.

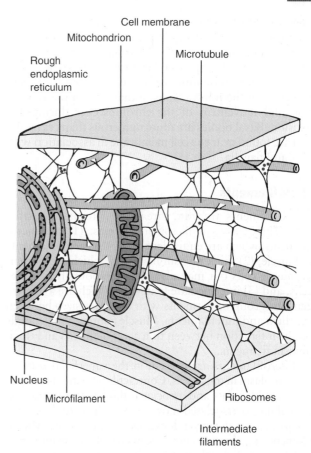

FIGURE 1-4 Microtubules and microfilaments of the cell. The microfilaments are associated with the inner surface of the cell membrane and aid in cell motility. The microtubules form the cytoskeleton and maintain the position of the organelles.

Microtubules

The microtubules are slender tubular structures composed of globular proteins called *tubulin.* Microtubules function in many ways, including the development and maintenance of cell form; participation in intracellular transport mechanisms, including axoplasmic transport in neurons; and formation of the basic structure for several complex cytoplasmic organelles, including the cilia, flagella, centrioles, and basal bodies. Abnormalities of the cytoskeleton may contribute to alterations in cell mobility and function. For example, proper functioning of the microtubules is essential for various stages of leukocyte migration.

Cilia and Flagella. Cilia and flagella are hairlike processes extending from the cell membrane that are capable of sweeping and flailing movements, which can move surrounding fluids or move the cell through fluid media. Cilia are found on the apical or luminal surface of epithelial linings of various body cavities or passages, such as the upper respiratory system. Removal of mucus from the respiratory passages is highly dependent on the proper functioning of the cilia. Flagella form the tail-like structures that provide motility for sperm.

Centrioles and Basal Bodies. Centrioles and basal bodies are structurally identical organelles composed of an array of highly organized microtubules. The centrioles are small, barrel-shaped bodies oriented at right angles to each other. In dividing cells, the two cylindrical centrioles form the mitotic spindle that aids in the separation and movement of the chromosomes during cell division. Basal bodies are more numerous than centrioles and are found near the cell membrane in association with cilia and flagella.

Microfilaments

Microfilaments are thin, threadlike cytoplasmic structures. Three classes of microfilaments exist: (1) thin microfilaments, which are equivalent to the thin actin filaments in muscle; (2) thick myosin filaments, which are present in muscle cells but may also exist temporarily in other cells; and (3) intermediate filaments, which are a heterogeneous group of filaments with diameter sizes between the thick and thin filaments. Muscle contraction depends on the interaction between thin actin filaments and thick myosin filaments.

Microfilaments are present in the superficial zone of the cytoplasm in most cells. Contractile activities involving the microfilaments and associated thick myosin filaments contribute to associated movement of the cytoplasm and cell membrane during endocytosis and exocytosis. Microfilaments are also present in the microvilli of the intestine. The intermediate filaments function in supporting and maintaining the asymmetric shape of cells. Examples of intermediate filaments are the keratin filaments that are found anchored to the cell membrane of epidermal keratinocytes of the skin and the glial filaments that are found in astrocytes and other glial cells of the nervous system. The *neurofibrillary tangle* found in the brain in Alzheimer disease contains microtubule-associated proteins and neurofilaments, evidence of a disrupted neuronal cytoskeleton.

THE CELL MEMBRANE

The cell is enclosed in a thin membrane that separates the intracellular contents from the extracellular environment. To differentiate it from the other cell membranes, such as the mitochondrial or nuclear membranes, the cell membrane is often called the *plasma membrane.* In many respects, the plasma membrane is one of the most important parts of the cell. It acts as a semipermeable structure that separates the intracellular and extracellular environments. It provides receptors for hormones and other biologically active substances, participates in the electrical events that occur in nerve and muscle cells, and aids in the regulation of cell growth and proliferation.

The cell membrane consists of an organized arrangement of lipids (phospholipids, glycolipids, and cholesterol), carbohydrates, and proteins (Fig. 1-5). The lipids form a bilayer structure that is essentially impermeable to all but lipid-soluble substances. About 75% of the lipids are phospholipids, each with a hydrophilic (water-soluble) head and hydrophobic (water-insoluble) tail. The phospholipid molecules along with the glycolipids are aligned

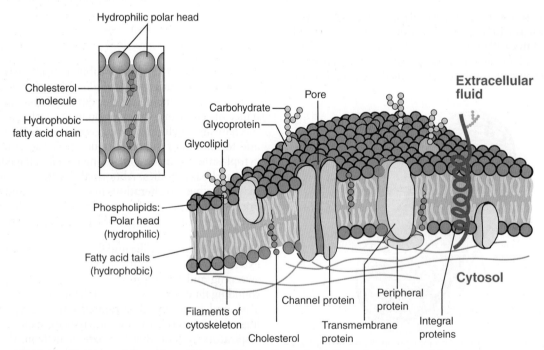

FIGURE 1-5 Structure of the cell membrane, showing the hydrophilic (polar) heads and the hydrophobic (fatty acid) tails (*inset*) and the position of the integral and peripheral proteins in relation to the interior and exterior of the cell.

such that their hydrophilic heads face outward on each side of the membrane and their hydrophobic tails project toward the center of the membrane. The hydrophilic heads retain water and help cells adhere to each other. At normal body temperature, the viscosity of the lipid component of the membrane is equivalent to that of olive oil. The presence of cholesterol stiffens the membrane.

Although the basic structure of the cell membrane is provided by the lipid bilayer, most of the specific functions are carried out by proteins. Some proteins, called *transmembrane proteins*, pass directly through the membrane and communicate with the intracellular and extracellular environments. Many of the transmembrane proteins are tightly bound to lipids in the bilayer and are essentially part of the membrane. These transmembrane proteins are called *integral proteins*. The *peripheral proteins*, a second type of protein, are bound to one or the other side of the membrane and do not pass into the lipid bilayer. Thus, the peripheral proteins are associated with functions involving the inner and outer side of the membrane where they are located. In contrast, the transmembrane proteins can function on both sides of the membrane or transport molecules across it. Many of the integral transmembrane proteins form the ion channels found on the cell surface. These channel proteins have complex structures and are selective with respect to the ions that pass through their channels.

The membrane carbohydrates are incorporated in a fuzzy-looking layer, called the *cell coat* or *glycocalyx*, that surrounds the cell surface. The glycocalyx, which is part of the cell membrane, consists of long, complex carbohydrate chains that are attached to proteins and lipids in the form of glycoproteins and glycolipids. The cell coat participates in cell-to-cell recognition and adhesion. It contains tissue transplant antigens that label cells as self or nonself. ABO blood group antigens are contained in the cell coat of red blood cells.

In summary, the cell is a remarkably autonomous structure that functions in a manner strikingly similar to that of the total organism. The nucleus controls cell function and is the mastermind of the cell. It contains DNA, which provides the information necessary for the synthesis of the various proteins that the cell must produce to stay alive and to transmit information from one generation to another.

The cytoplasm contains the cell's organelles. Ribosomes serve as sites for protein synthesis in the cell. The ER functions as a tubular communication system through which substances can be transported from one part of the cell to another and as the site of protein (rough ER), carbohydrate, and lipid (smooth ER) synthesis. The Golgi apparatus modifies materials synthesized in the ER and packages them into secretory granules for transport within the cell or export from the cell. Lysosomes, which can be viewed as the digestive system of the cell, contain hydrolytic enzymes that digest worn-out cell parts and foreign materials. The mitochondria serve as power plants for the cell because they transform food energy into ATP, which is used to power cell activities. Mitochondria contain their own extrachromosomal DNA, which is used in the synthesis of mitochondrial RNAs and proteins used in oxidative metabolism. Microtubules are slender, stiff tubular structures that influence cell shape, provide a means of moving organelles through the cytoplasm, and effect movement of the cilia and of chromosomes during cell division. Several types of threadlike filaments, including actin and myosin filaments, participate in muscle contraction.

The plasma membrane is a lipid bilayer that surrounds the cell and separates it from its surrounding external environment. It contains receptors for hormones and other biologically active substances, participates in the electrical events that occur in nerve and muscle cells, and aids in the regulation of cell growth and proliferation. The cell surface is surrounded by a fuzzy-looking layer called the cell coat or glycocalyx. The cell coat participates in cell-to-cell recognition and adhesion, and it contains tissue transplant antigens.

Cell Metabolism and Energy Sources

Energy metabolism refers to the processes by which fats, proteins, and carbohydrates from the foods we eat are converted into energy or complex energy sources in the cell. Catabolism and anabolism are the two phases of metabolism. *Catabolism* consists of breaking down stored nutrients and body tissues to produce energy. *Anabolism* is a constructive process in which more complex molecules are formed from simpler ones.

The special carrier for cellular energy is ATP. ATP molecules consist of adenosine, a nitrogenous base; ribose, a five-carbon sugar; and three phosphate groups (Fig. 1-6). The last two phosphate groups are attached to the remainder of the molecule by two high-energy bonds. Each bond releases a large amount of energy when hydrolyzed. ATP is hydrolyzed to form adenosine diphosphate (ADP) with the loss of one high-energy bond and to adenosine monophosphate (AMP) with the loss of two such bonds. The energy liberated from the hydrolysis of ATP is used to drive reactions that require free energy, such as muscle contraction and active transport mechanisms. Energy from foodstuffs is used to convert ADP back to ATP. ATP is often called the *energy currency* of the cell; energy can be "saved" or "spent" using ATP as an exchange currency.

Two types of energy production are present in the cell: the anaerobic (*i.e.*, without oxygen) glycolytic pathway, occurring in the cytoplasm, and the aerobic (*i.e.*, with oxygen) pathways occurring in the mitochondria. The glycolytic pathway serves as the prelude to the aerobic pathways.

Understanding ➤ Cell Metabolism

Cell metabolism is the process that converts carbohydrates, proteins, and fats into adenosine triphosphate (ATP), which is the major source of energy for all body cells. ATP is formed through three main pathways: (1) the glycolytic pathway, (2) the citric acid cycle, and (3) the electron transport chain. The glycolytic pathway is anaerobic and the citric acid cycle and electron transport chain are aerobic or require oxygen. Two coenzymes, nicotinamide-adenine-dinucleotide (NAD) and flavin adenine dinucleotide (FAD), serve as hydrogen carriers and have unique roles in the generation of ATP from the oxidation of fuels.

1

Glycolytic pathway. Glycolysis, which occurs in the cytoplasm of the cell, involves the splitting of a 6-carbon molecule of glucose into two 3-carbon molecules of pyruvic acid. Each glucose molecule is first split into two 3-carbon molecules, each of which is then converted to pyruvic acid. Because the reactions that split glucose require two molecules of ATP, there is a net gain of only two molecules of ATP (one from each of the 3-carbon molecules) for each molecule of glucose that is metabolized. The process is anaerobic and does not use oxygen or generate carbon dioxide. When oxygen is present, pyruvic acid moves into the mitochondria, where it enters the aerobic citric acid cycle. Under anaerobic conditions, pyruvate is converted to lactic acid. This allows glycolysis to continue as a means of supplying cells with ATP when oxygen is lacking.

2

Citric acid cycle. Under aerobic conditions, each of the two pyruvate molecules formed by glycolysis enters the mitochondria and combines with acetyl coenzyme to form acetyl-coenzyme A (acetyl-CoA). The formation of acetyl-CoA begins the reactions that occur in the citric acid cycle. Some reactions release carbon dioxide (CO_2) and some release hydrogen, which is transferred to NAD or FADH. Each of the two molecules of pyruvate from the glycolytic pathway yields one molecule of ATP and two molecules of CO_2. In addition to pyruvate from the glycolysis of glucose, products from amino acid and fatty acid breakdown can also enter the citric acid cycle and transfer their energy to ATP.

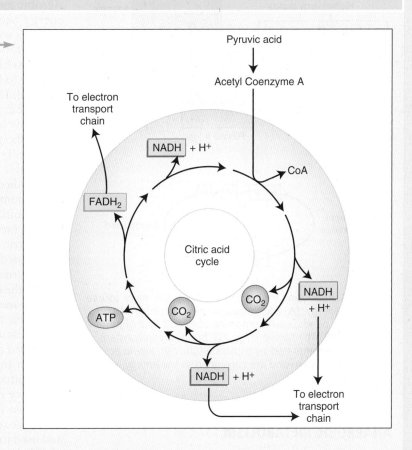

3

Electron transport chain. At the completion of the citric acid cycle, each glucose molecule has yielded only four new molecules of ATP (two from the glycolytic pathway and two from the citric acid cycle). In fact, the principal function of these earlier stages is to make the hydrogen from glucose or other food substrates available for oxidation. Oxidation of the hydrogen carried by NADH or FADH$_2$ is accomplished through a series of enzymatically catalyzed reactions in the mitochondrial electron transport chain. These reactions split each hydrogen atom into a hydrogen ion (H^+) and an electron (e^-) and facilitate the combination of the hydrogen ions with oxygen (O_2) to form water (2 H [$2H^+ + 2e^-$] + 1/2 O_2 = H_2O. During this sequence of oxidative reactions, large amounts of energy are released and used to convert adenosine diphosphate (ADP) to ATP (total of 36 ATP molecules from one molecule of glucose [2 from glycolysis, 2 from the citric acid cycle, and 32 from the electron transport chain]).

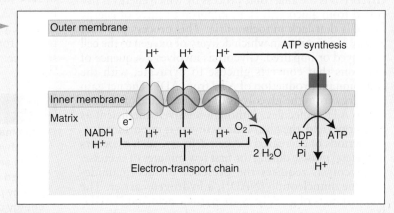

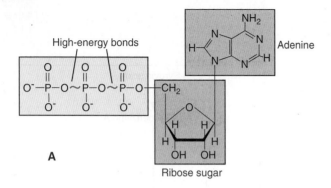

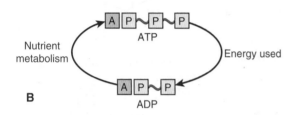

FIGURE 1-6 Adenosine triphosphate (ATP) is the major source of cellular energy. (**A**) Each molecule of ATP contains two high-energy bonds, each containing about 12 kcal of potential energy. (**B**) The high-energy ATP bonds are in constant flux. They are generated by substrate (glucose, amino acid, and fat) metabolism and are consumed as the energy is expended.

ANAEROBIC METABOLISM

Glycolysis is the anaerobic process by which energy is liberated from glucose. It is an important source of energy for cells that lack mitochondria. This process provides energy in situations in which delivery of oxygen to the cell is delayed or impaired. Glycolysis involves a sequence of reactions that converts glucose to pyruvate, with the concomitant production of ATP from ADP. The net gain of energy from the glycolysis of one molecule of glucose is two ATP molecules. Although relatively inefficient as to energy yield, the glycolytic pathway is important during periods of decreased oxygen delivery, such as occurs in skeletal muscle during the first few minutes of exercise.

Glycolysis requires the presence of nicotinamide-adenine dinucleotide (NAD⁺), a hydrogen carrier. The end products of glycolysis are pyruvic acid and NADH. When oxygen is present, pyruvic acid moves into the aerobic mitochondrial pathway, and NADH subsequently enters into oxidative chemical reactions that remove the hydrogen atoms. The transfer of hydrogen from NADH during the oxidative reactions allows the glycolytic process to continue by facilitating the regeneration of NAD⁺. Under anaerobic conditions, such as cardiac arrest or circulatory shock, the hydrogen from NADH is transferred to pyruvic acid, converting it to lactic acid. Conversion of pyruvic acid to lactic acid is reversible, and after the oxygen supply has been restored, lactic acid is converted back to pyruvic acid and used directly for energy or to synthesize glucose.

AEROBIC METABOLISM

Aerobic metabolism, which supplies 90% of the body's energy needs, occurs in the cell's mitochondria and requires oxygen. It is here that hydrogen and carbon molecules from dietary fats, proteins, and carbohydrates are broken down and combined with molecular oxygen to form carbon dioxide and water as energy is released. Unlike lactic acid, which is an end product of anaerobic metabolism, carbon dioxide and water are relatively harmless and easily eliminated from the body. In a 24-hour period, oxidative metabolism produces 150 to 300 mL of water.

Aerobic metabolism uses the *citric acid cycle*, sometimes called the *tricarboxylic acid* or *Krebs cycle*, as the final common pathway for the metabolism of nutrients. In the initial stage of the citric acid cycle, acetyl coenzyme A (acetyl-CoA) combines with oxaloacetic acid to form citric acid. The coenzyme A portion of acetyl-CoA can be used again and again to generate more acetyl-CoA from pyruvic acid, whereas the acetyl portion becomes part of the citric acid cycle and moves through a series of enzyme-mediated steps that produce carbon dioxide and hydrogen atoms.

Oxidation of electrons from the hydrogen atoms generated during glycolysis and the citric acid cycle takes place in the electron transport system located on the inner mitochondrial membrane. The electrons are used to reduce elemental oxygen, which combines with the hydrogen ions to form water. During this sequence of oxidative reactions, large amounts of energy are released and used to convert ADP to ATP. Because the formation of ATP involves the addition of a high-energy phosphate bond to ADP, the process is called *oxidative phosphorylation*. Cyanide poisoning kills by binding to the enzymes needed for a final step in the oxidative phosphorylation sequence.

In summary, metabolism is the process whereby the carbohydrates, fats, and proteins we eat are broken down and subsequently converted into the energy needed for cell function. Energy is stored in the high-energy phosphate bonds of ATP, which serves as the energy currency for the cell. Two sites of energy conversion are present in cells: the glycolytic or anaerobic pathway in the cell's cytoplasmic matrix and the aerobic or citric acid cycle in the mitochondria. The most efficient of these pathways is the citric acid pathway. This pathway, which requires oxygen, produces carbon dioxide and water as end products and results in the release of large amounts of energy that is used to convert ADP to ATP. The glycolytic pathway, which is located in the cytoplasm, involves the breakdown of glucose to form ATP. This pathway can function without oxygen by producing lactic acid.

Cell Membrane Transport, Signal Transduction, and Generation of Membrane Potentials

MOVEMENT ACROSS THE CELL MEMBRANE

The unique properties of the cell's membrane are responsible for differences in the composition of the intracellular and extracellular fluids. However, a constant movement of molecules and ions across the cell membrane is required to maintain the functions of the cell. Movement through the cell membrane occurs in essentially two ways: passively, without an expenditure of energy, or actively, using energy-consuming processes. The cell membrane can also engulf substances, forming a membrane-coated vesicle; this membrane-coated vesicle is moved into the cell by *endocytosis* or out of the cell by *exocytosis*.

Passive Movement

The passive movement of particles or ions across the cell membrane is directly influenced by chemical or electrical gradients and does not require an expenditure of energy. A difference in the number of particles on either side of the membrane creates a chemical gradient, and a difference in charged particles or ions creates an electrical gradient. Chemical and electrical gradients are often linked and are called *electrochemical gradients*.

Diffusion. *Diffusion* refers to the process by which molecules and other particles in a solution become widely dispersed and reach a uniform concentration because of energy created by their spontaneous kinetic movements (Fig. 1-7). In the process of reaching a uniform concentration, these molecules and particles move from an area of higher to an area of lower concentration. With ions, diffusion is affected by energy supplied by their electrical charge. Lipid-soluble molecules, such as oxygen, carbon dioxide, alcohol, and fatty acids, become dissolved in the lipid matrix of the cell membrane and diffuse through the membrane in the same manner that diffusion occurs in water. Other substances diffuse through minute pores of the cell membrane. The rate of movement depends on how many particles are available for diffusion and the velocity of the kinetic movement of the particles.

Facilitated Diffusion. Like simple diffusion, facilitated diffusion occurs down a concentration gradient; thus, it does not require input of metabolic energy (see Fig. 1-7). Unlike simple diffusion, however, facilitated diffusion requires a transport protein. Some substances, such as glucose, cannot pass unassisted through the cell membrane because they are not lipid soluble or they are too large to pass through the membrane's pores. These substances combine with special transport proteins at the membrane's outer surface, are carried across the membrane attached to the transporter, and then are released. In facilitated diffusion, a substance can move only from an area of higher concentration to one of lower concentration. The rate at

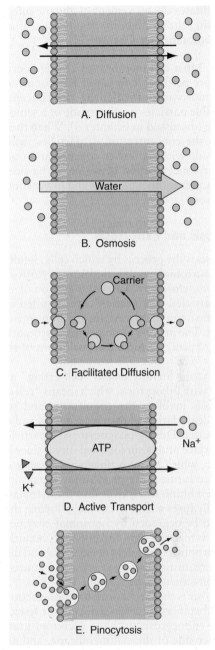

FIGURE 1-7 Mechanisms of membrane transport. (**A**) Diffusion, in which particles move to become equally distributed across the membrane. (**B**) The osmotically active particles regulate the flow of water. (**C**) Facilitated diffusion uses a carrier system. (**D**) In active transport, selected molecules are transported across the membrane using the energy-driven (ATPase) pump. (**E**) In pinocytosis, the membrane forms a vesicle that engulfs the particle and transports it across the membrane, where it is released.

which a substance moves across the membrane because of facilitated diffusion depends on the difference in concentration between the two sides of the membrane. Also important are the availability of transport proteins and the rapidity with which they can bind and release the substance being transported. It is thought that insulin, which facilitates the movement of glucose into cells, acts by increasing the availability of glucose transporters in the cell membrane (see Chapter 32).

Osmosis. Most cell membranes are semipermeable in that they are permeable to water but not all solute particles. Osmosis is controlled by the concentration of nondiffusible particles on either side of a semipermeable membrane (discussed in Chapter 6). When there is a difference in the concentration of particles, water moves from the side with the lower concentration of particles and higher concentration of water to the side with the higher concentration of particles and lower concentration of water (see Fig. 1-7).

Endocytosis and Exocytosis

Endocytosis is the process by which cells engulf materials from their surroundings. It includes pinocytosis and phagocytosis. *Pinocytosis* involves the ingestion of small solid or fluid particles. The particles are engulfed into small, membrane-surrounded vesicles for movement into the cytoplasm. The process of pinocytosis is important in the transport of proteins and strong solutions of electrolytes (see Fig. 1-7).

Phagocytosis literally means "cell eating" and can be compared with pinocytosis, which means "cell drinking." Phagocytosis involves the engulfment and subsequent killing or degradation of microorganisms and other particulate matter. During phagocytosis, a particle contacts the cell surface and is surrounded on all sides by the cell membrane, which forms a phagocytic vesicle or phagosome. Once formed, the phagosome breaks away from the cell membrane and moves into the cytoplasm, where it eventually fuses with a lysosome, allowing the ingested material to be degraded by lysosomal enzymes. Certain cells, such as macrophages and polymorphonuclear leukocytes (neutrophils), are adept at engulfing and disposing of invading organisms, damaged cells, and unneeded extracellular constituents (see Chapter 14).

Exocytosis is the mechanism for the secretion of intracellular substances into the extracellular spaces. It is the reverse of endocytosis in that a secretory granule fuses to the inner side of the cell membrane, and an opening occurs in the cell membrane. This opening allows the contents of the granule to be released into the extracellular fluid. Exocytosis is important in removing cellular debris and releasing substances, such as hormones, synthesized in the cell.

During endocytosis, portions of the cell membrane become an endocytotic vesicle. During exocytosis, the vesicular membrane is incorporated into the plasma membrane. In this way, cell membranes can be conserved and reused.

Active Transport and Cotransport

The process of diffusion describes particle movement from an area of higher concentration to one of lower concentration, resulting in an equal distribution across the cell membrane. However, sometimes different concentrations of a substance are needed in the intracellular and extracellular fluids. For example, the intracellular functioning of the cell requires a much higher concentration of potassium than is present in the extracellular fluid while maintaining a much lower concentration of sodium than in the extracellular fluid. In these situations, energy is required to pump the ions "uphill" or against their concentration gradient. When cells use energy to move ions against an electrical or chemical gradient, the process is called *active transport.*

The active transport system studied in the greatest detail is the sodium–potassium membrane pump, or Na^+/K^+ ATPase membrane pump (see Fig. 1-7). The Na^+/K^+ ATPase membrane pump moves sodium from inside the cell to the extracellular region, where its concentration is approximately 14 times greater than inside; the pump also returns potassium to the inside, where its concentration is approximately 35 times greater than it is outside the cell. If it were not for the activity of the Na^+/K^+ ATPase membrane pump, the osmotically active sodium particles would accumulate in the cell, causing cellular swelling because of an accompanying influx of water.

There are two types of active transport: primary active transport and secondary active transport. In *primary active transport,* the source of energy (*e.g.,* ATP) is used directly in the transport of a substance. *Secondary active transport* mechanisms harness the energy derived from the primary active transport of one substance, usually sodium ions, for the cotransport of a second substance. For example, when sodium ions are actively transported out of a cell by primary active transport, a large concentration gradient develops (*i.e.,* high concentration on the outside and low on the inside). This concentration gradient represents a large storehouse of energy because sodium ions are always attempting to diffuse into the cell. Similar to facilitated diffusion, secondary transport mechanisms use membrane transport proteins. These proteins have two binding sites: one for sodium ions and the other for the substance undergoing secondary transport. Secondary transport systems are classified into two groups: *cotransport,* in which the sodium ion and solute are transported in the same direction, and *countertransport,* in which sodium ions and the solute are transported in opposite directions (Fig. 1-8). An example of cotransport occurs in the intestine, where the absorption of glucose and amino acids is coupled with sodium transport.

Ion Channels

The electrical charge on small ions such as Na^+ and K^+ makes it difficult for these ions to move across the lipid layer of the cell membrane. However, rapid movement of these ions is required for many types of cell functions, such as nerve activity. This is accomplished by facilitated diffusion through selective ion channels. Ion channels are made up of integral proteins that span the width of the cell membrane and are normally composed of several polypeptides or protein subunits that form a gating system. Specific stimuli cause the protein subunits to undergo

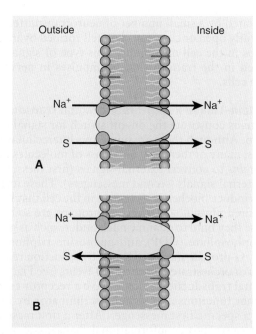

FIGURE 1-8 (**A**) Secondary active transport systems carry the transported solute (*S*) in the same direction as the Na$^+$ ion. (**B**) Countertransport carries the solute and Na$^+$ in opposite directions.

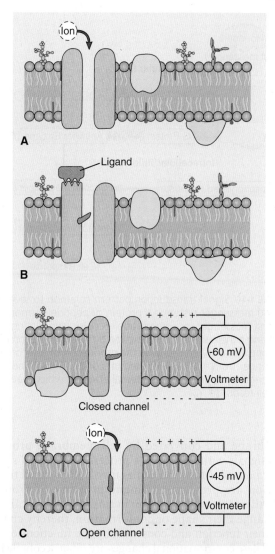

FIGURE 1-9 Ion channels. (**A**) Nongated ion channel remains open, permitting free movement of ions across the membrane. (**B**) Ligand-gated channel is controlled by ligand binding to the receptor. (**C**) Voltage-gated channel is controlled by a change in membrane potential. (From Rhoades R. A., Tanner G. A. [1996]. *Medical physiology.* Boston: Little, Brown.)

conformational changes to form an open channel or gate through which the ions can move. In this way, ions do not need to cross the lipid-soluble portion of the membrane but can remain in the aqueous solution that fills the ion channel. Ion channels are highly selective; some channels allow only for passage of sodium ions, and others are selective for potassium, calcium, or chloride ions.

The plasma membrane contains two basic groups of ion channels: nongated and gated channels (Fig. 1-9). Nongated or leakage channels are open even in the unstimulated state, whereas gated channels open and close in response to specific stimuli. There are two types of gated channels: voltage-gated and ligand-gated channels. Voltage-gated channels have electrically operated gates that open when the membrane potential changes beyond a certain point. Ligand-gated channels have chemically operated gates that respond to specific receptor-bound ligands, such as the neurotransmitter acetylcholine.

SIGNAL TRANSDUCTION AND CELL COMMUNICATION

Cells in multicellular organisms need to communicate with one another to coordinate their function and control their growth. Cells communicate with each other by means of chemical messenger systems. In some tissues, messengers move from cell to cell through gap junctions without entering the extracellular fluid. In other tissues, cells communicate by chemical messengers secreted into the extracellular fluid. Many types of chemical messengers that cannot cross the cell membrane bind to receptors on or near the cell surface. These chemical messengers are

sometimes called *first messengers* because, by one means or another, their external signals are converted into internal signals carried by second chemicals called *second messengers* (Fig. 1-10). It is the second messenger that triggers the intracellular changes that produce the desired physiologic effect. Some lipid-soluble chemical messengers move through the membrane and bind to cytoplasmic or nuclear receptors to exert their physiologic effects.

Cell Membrane Receptors

Neurotransmitters, protein and peptide hormones, and other chemical messengers do not exert their effects by entering cells. Instead, they attach to receptors on the cell surface, and their messages are conveyed across the

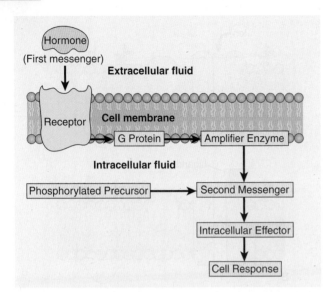

FIGURE 1-10 Signal transduction pattern common to several second messenger systems. A protein or peptide hormone is the first messenger to a membrane receptor, stimulating or inhibiting a membrane-bound enzyme by means of a G protein. The amplifier enzyme catalyzes the production of a second messenger from a phosphorylated precursor. The second messenger then activates an internal effector, which leads to the cell response.

membrane and converted by cell membrane proteins into signals within the cell, a process often called *signal transduction*. Many molecules involved in signal transduction are proteins. A unique property of proteins that allows them to function in this way is their ability to change their shape or conformation, thereby changing their function and consequently the functions of the cell. These conformational changes are often accomplished through enzymes called *protein kinases* that catalyze the phosphorylation of amino acids in the protein structure.

Each cell type in the body contains a distinctive set of receptor proteins that enables it to respond to a complementary set of signaling molecules in a specific, pre-programmed way. These receptors, which span the cell membrane, relay information to a series of intracellular intermediates that eventually pass the signal to its final destination. Many receptors for chemical messengers have been isolated and characterized. These proteins are not static components of the cell membrane; they increase or decrease in number, according to the needs of the cell. When excess chemical messengers are present, the number of active receptors decreases in a process called *down-regulation;* when there is a deficiency of the messenger, the number of active receptors increases through *up-regulation*. There are three known classes of cell surface receptor proteins: ion channel linked, G protein linked, and enzyme linked.

Ion-Channel–Linked Receptors. Ion-channel–linked receptors are involved in the rapid synaptic signaling between electrically excitable cells. This type of signaling is mediated by a small number of neurotransmitters that transiently open or close ion channels formed by integral proteins in the cell membrane. This type of signaling is involved in the transmission of impulses in nerve and muscle cells.

G-Protein–Linked Receptors and Signal Transduction. G proteins constitute the on–off switch for signal transduction. Although there are numerous intercellular messengers, many of them rely on a class of molecules called *G proteins* to convert external signals (first messengers) into internal signals (second messengers). These internal signals induce biochemical changes in the cell that lead to the desired physiologic effects. G proteins are so named because they bind to guanine nucleotides, such as guanosine diphosphate (GDP) and guanosine triphosphate (GTP). G-protein–mediated signal transduction relies on a series of orchestrated biochemical events (see Fig. 1-10). All signal transduction systems have a receptor component that functions as a signal discriminator by recognizing a specific first messenger. After a first messenger binds to a receptor, conformational changes occur in the receptor, which activates the G protein. The activated G protein, in turn, acts on other membrane-bound intermediates called *effectors*. Often, the effector is an enzyme that converts an inactive precursor molecule into a second messenger, which diffuses into the cytoplasm and carries the signal beyond the cell membrane.

Although there are differences among the G proteins, all share a number of features. All are found on the cytoplasmic side of the cell membrane, and all incorporate the GTPase cycle, which functions as the on–off switch for G-protein activity. Certain bacterial toxins can bind to the G protein, causing inhibition or stimulation of its signal function. One such toxin, the toxin of *Vibrio cholerae*, binds and activates the stimulatory G protein linked to the cyclic AMP (cAMP) system that controls the secretion of fluid into the intestine. In response to the cholera toxin, these cells overproduce fluid, leading to severe diarrhea and life-threatening depletion of extracellular fluid volume. There is also interest in the role that G-protein signaling may play in the pathogenesis of cancer.

Enzyme-Linked Receptors. The receptors for certain protein hormones, such as insulin, and peptide growth factors activate an intracellular enzyme such as protein-tyrosine kinase. The enzyme catalyzes the phosphorylation of tyrosine residues on specific intracellular proteins, thereby transferring an external message to the cell interior. Enzyme-linked receptors mediate cellular responses such as calcium influx, increased sodium–potassium exchange, and stimulation of the uptake of sugars and amino acids.

Messenger-Mediated Control of Nuclear Function

Some messengers, such as thyroid hormone and steroid hormones, do not bind to membrane receptors but move directly across the lipid layer of the cell membrane and are carried to the cell nucleus, where they influence DNA activity. Many of these hormones bind to a cytoplasmic receptor, and together they are carried to the nucleus. In the nucleus, the receptor–hormone complex binds to DNA, thereby increasing transcription of mRNA. The mRNAs are translated in the ribosomes, with the production of increased amounts of proteins that alter cell function.

GENERATION OF MEMBRANE POTENTIALS

The human body runs on a system of self-generated electricity. Electrical potentials exist across the membranes of most cells in the body. Because these potentials occur at the level of the cell membrane, they are called *membrane potentials*. In excitable tissues, such as nerve or muscle cells, changes in the membrane potential are necessary for generation and conduction of nerve impulses and muscle contraction. In other types of cells, such as glandular cells, changes in the membrane potential contribute to hormone secretion and other functions.

Electrical Potential

Electrical potential, measured in volts (V), describes the ability of separated electrical charges of opposite polarity (+ and −) to do work. In regard to cells, the opposite charged particles are ions, and the barrier that separates them is the cell membrane. Because the total amount of charge that can be separated by the cell membrane is small, the potential differences are small and are measured in *millivolts* (1/1000 of a volt).

In their resting state, all body cells exhibit a resting membrane potential that typically ranges from −20 to −100 mV, depending on cell type. Hence, all cells are said to be polarized (negative on the inside and positive on the outside). Usually, a small excess of positive charges on the outside of the membrane is balanced by an equal number of negative charges on the inside. Because of the extreme thinness of the cell membrane, the accumulation of these ions at the surfaces of the membrane contributes to the establishment of a membrane potential.

There are two main factors that alter membrane excitability: the difference in the concentration of ions on the inside and outside of the membrane and the permeability of the membrane to the ions. Extracellular and intracellular fluids are electrolyte solutions containing approximately 150 to 160 mmol/L of positively charged ions and an equal number of negatively charged ions. It is the diffusion of these current-carrying ions that is responsible for generating and conducting membrane potentials. Because the resting cell membrane is more permeable to potassium than sodium, the resting cell membrane reflects the diffusion of potassium. The Na^+/K^+ ATPase membrane pump, which removes three Na^+ from inside the cell membrane while returning two K^+ to the inside, assists in maintaining the resting membrane potential. During an action potential, the cell membrane becomes more permeable to sodium, causing its polarity to change so that it becomes positive on the inside and negative on the outside (discussed in Chapter 33).

In summary, the movement of materials across the cell's membrane is essential for survival of the cell. Diffusion is a process by which substances such as ions move from areas of greater concentration to areas of lesser concentration in an attempt to reach a uniform distribution. Osmosis refers to the diffusion of water molecules through a semipermeable membrane along a concentration gradient. Facilitated diffusion is a passive process, in which molecules that cannot normally pass through the cell's membranes do so with the assistance of a carrier molecule. Another type of transport, called active transport, requires the cell to expend energy in moving ions against a concentration gradient. The Na^+/K^+ ATPase membrane pump is the best-known type of active transport. Endocytosis is a process by which cells engulf materials from the surrounding medium. Small particles are ingested by a process called pinocytosis; larger particles are engulfed by a process called phagocytosis. Exocytosis involves the removal of large particles from the cell and is essentially the reverse of endocytosis. Ion channels are integral transmembrane proteins that span the width of the cell membrane to form a gating system that controls the movement of ions across the cell membrane.

Cells communicate with each other by means of chemical messenger systems. In some tissues, chemical messengers move from cell to cell through gap junctions without entering the extracellular fluid. Other types of chemical messengers bind to receptors on or near the cell surface. There are three known classes of cell surface receptor proteins: ion channel linked, G protein linked, and enzyme linked. Ion-channel–linked signaling is mediated by neurotransmitters that transiently open or close ion channels formed by integral proteins in the cell membrane. G-protein–linked receptors rely on a class of molecules called G proteins that function as on–off switches to convert external signals (first messengers) into internal signals (second messengers). Enzyme-linked receptors interact with certain peptide hormones (*e.g.*, insulin and growth factors) to initiate directly the activity of an intracellular enzyme, which in turn triggers multiple cellular responses, such as stimulation of glucose and amino acid uptake or transcription of certain genes that control cell proliferation.

Electrical potentials (negative on the inside and positive on the outside) exist across the membranes of most cells in the body. There are two main factors that contribute to the generation of a membrane potential: a difference in the concentration of ions on the inside and outside of the membrane and the permeability of the membrane to the ions. At rest, the cell membrane is more permeable to potassium than to sodium; thus, the resting membrane potential reflects the diffusion of potassium. During an action potential, the cell membrane becomes more permeable to sodium, which causes it to depolarize, becoming negative on the outside and positive on the inside.

Understanding ➤ Membrane Potentials

Electrochemical potentials are present in virtually all cells of the body. Some cells, such as nerve and muscle cells, are capable of generating rapidly changing impulses at their membrane, and these impulses are used to transmit signals along nerve and muscle membranes. In other cells, such as glandular cells, membrane potentials are used to signal the release of hormones or activate other functions of the cell. Membrane potentials, (1) which are measured in millivolts, rely on the (2) diffusion of electrically changed ions and the establishment of an (3) equilibrium or (4) resting membrane potential.

1

Membrane potentials. A membrane potential represents the potential difference in charge across a cell membrane, with the inside being negative (having less charge) in relation to the outside. This potential difference is measured in millivolts (mV) or thousandths of a volt. The greater the potential difference, the greater the voltage.

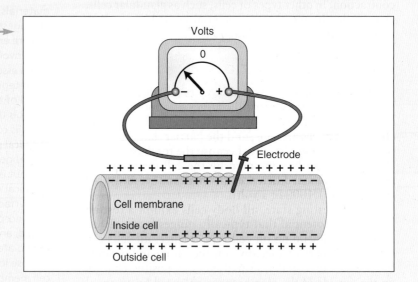

2

Diffusion potentials. A diffusion potential is a membrane potential that is generated when a charged particle (ion), such as a sodium (Na^+) or a potassium (K^+) ion, diffuses across a membrane based on a concentration gradient. Two conditions are necessary for this to occur: (1) the membrane must be selectively permeable to a particular current-carrying ion, and (2) the concentration of the diffusible ion must be greater on one side

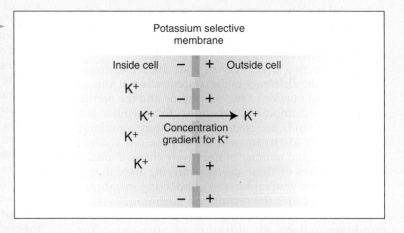

of the membrane than on the other. The sign (+ or −) or polarity of the potential depends on the diffusing ion. It is negative on the inside when a positively charged ion such as K^+ diffuses from the inside to the outside of the membrane carrying its charge with it, and it is positive when a positively charged ion such as Na^+ diffuses from the outside to the inside of the membrane.

3

Equilibrium potentials. An equilibrium potential is the membrane potential that exactly balances and opposes the net diffusion of an ion down its concentration gradient. As a cation diffuses down its concentration gradient, it carries its positive charge across the membrane generating an electrical force, which will eventually retard and stop its diffusion. The same will occur with diffusion of an anion. An *electrochemical* equilibrium is one in which the driving chemical diffusion and electrical forces are exactly balanced so that no further diffusion occurs. The equilibrium potential (EMF, electromotive force) can be calculated by inserting the inside and outside concentrations of the ion into the *Nernst equation* on the right.

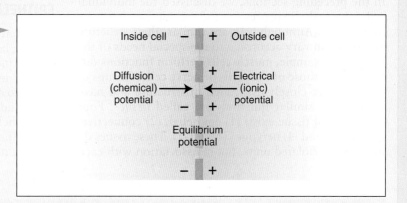

Nernst equation

$$EMF\ (mV) = -61 \times \log_{10}\ (\text{ion concentration inside/ion concentration outside})$$

4

Resting membrane potentials. The resting membrane potential occurs when an excitable tissue, such as a nerve cell, is not transmitting impulses. Because the resting cell membrane is much more permeable to K^+ than Na^+, the resting membrane potential is essentially a K^+ equilibrium potential. This can be explained in terms of the large K^+ concentration gradient (*e.g.*, 140 mEq/L inside and 4 mEq/L outside), which causes the positively charged K^+ to diffuse outward leaving the nondiffusible negatively charged anions (A^-) behind. This creates a state of electronegativity on the inside and electropositivity on the outside. The Na^+/K^+ membrane pump, which removes three Na^+ from inside the membrane while returning only two K^+ to the inside, contributes to the maintenance of the resting membrane potential.

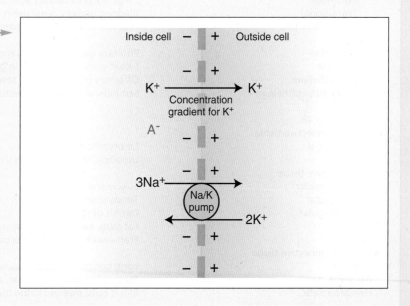

Body Tissues

In the preceding sections, we discussed the individual cell, its metabolic processes, and mechanisms of communication. Although cells are similar, their structure and function vary according to the special needs of the body. For example, muscle cells perform functions different from those of skin cells or nerve cells. Groups of cells that are closely associated in structure and have common or similar functions are called *tissues*. Four categories of tissue exist: (1) epithelial, (2) connective, (3) muscle, and (4) nervous (Table 1-1). These tissues do not exist in isolated units, but in association with each other and in variable proportions, forming different structures and organs.

EPITHELIAL TISSUE

Epithelial tissue forms sheets that cover the body's outer surface, line the internal surfaces, and form the glandular tissue. Underneath all types of epithelial tissue is an extracellular matrix, called the *basement membrane*, which serves to attach the epithelial cells to adjacent connective tissue and provides them with flexible support.

Epithelial cells have strong intracellular protein filaments (*i.e.*, cytoskeleton) that are important in transmitting mechanical stresses from one cell to another.

TABLE 1-1	Classification of Tissue Types
Tissue Type	**Location**
Epithelial Tissue	
Covering and lining of body surfaces	
Simple epithelium	
Squamous	Lining of blood vessels, body cavities, alveoli of lungs
Cuboidal	Collecting tubules of kidney; covering of ovaries
Columnar	Lining of intestine and gallbladder
Stratified epithelium	
Squamous keratinized	Skin
Squamous nonkeratinized	Mucous membranes of mouth, esophagus, and vagina
Cuboidal	Ducts of sweat glands
Columnar	Large ducts of salivary and mammary glands; also found in conjunctiva
Transitional	Bladder, ureters, renal pelvis
Pseudostratified	Tracheal and respiratory passages
Glandular	
Endocrine	Pituitary gland, thyroid gland, adrenal, and other glands
Exocrine	Sweat glands and glands in gastrointestinal tract
Neuroepithelium	Olfactory mucosa, retina, tongue
Reproductive epithelium	Seminiferous tubules of testis; cortical portion of ovary
Connective Tissue	
Embryonic connective tissue	
Mesenchymal	Embryonic mesoderm
Mucous	Umbilical cord (Wharton's jelly)
Adult connective tissue	
Loose or areolar	Subcutaneous areas
Dense regular	Tendons and ligaments
Dense irregular	Dermis of skin
Adipose	Fat pads, subcutaneous layers
Reticular	Framework of lymphoid organs, bone marrow, liver
Specialized connective tissue	
Bone	Long bones, flat bones
Cartilage	Tracheal rings, external ear, articular surfaces
Hematopoietic	Blood cells, myeloid tissue (bone marrow)
Muscle Tissue	
Skeletal	Skeletal muscles
Cardiac	Heart muscles
Smooth	Gastrointestinal tract, blood vessels, bronchi, bladder, and others
Nervous Tissue	
Neurons	Central and peripheral neurons and nerve fibers
Supporting cells	Glial and ependymal cells in central nervous system; Schwann and satellite cells in peripheral nervous system

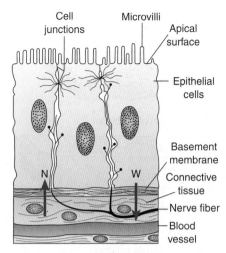

FIGURE 1-11 Typical arrangement of epithelial cells in relation to underlying tissues and blood supply. Epithelial tissue has no blood supply of its own but relies on the blood vessels in the underlying connective tissue for nutrition (*N*) and elimination of wastes (*W*).

The cells of epithelial tissue are tightly bound together by specialized junctions. These specialized junctions enable these cells to form barriers to the movement of water, solutes, and cells from one body compartment to the next. Epithelial tissue is avascular (*i.e.,* without blood vessels) and must therefore receive oxygen and nutrients from the capillaries of the connective tissue on which the epithelial tissue rests (Fig. 1-11). To survive, the epithelial cells must be kept moist. Even the seemingly dry skin epithelium is kept moist by a nonvitalized waterproof layer of superficial skin cells called *keratin,* which prevents evaporation of moisture from the deeper living cells. Epithelium is able to regenerate quickly when injured.

Epithelial tissues are classified according to the shape of the cells and the number of layers that are present: simple, stratified, and pseudostratified. Glandular epithelial tissue is formed by cells specialized to produce a fluid secretion. The terms *squamous* (thin and flat), *cuboidal* (cube shaped), and *columnar* (resembling a column) refer to the cells' shape (Fig. 1-12).

Simple Epithelium

Simple epithelium contains a single layer of cells, which rests on the basement membrane. Simple squamous epithelium is adapted for filtration; it is found lining the blood vessels, lymph nodes, and alveoli of the lungs. The single layer of squamous epithelium lining the heart and blood vessels is known as the *endothelium.* A similar type of layer, called the *mesothelium,* forms the serous membranes that line the pleural, pericardial, and peritoneal cavities and covers the organs of these cavities. A *simple cuboidal epithelium* is found on the surface of the ovary and in the thyroid. *Simple columnar epithelium* lines the intestine. One form of a simple columnar epithelium has hairlike projections called *cilia,* often with specialized mucus-secreting cells called *goblet cells.* This form of simple columnar epithelium lines the airways of the respiratory tract.

Stratified and Pseudostratified Epithelium

Stratified epithelium contains more than one layer of cells, with only the deepest layer resting on the basement membrane. It is designed to protect the body surface. *Stratified squamous keratinized* epithelium makes up the epidermis of the skin. Keratin is a tough, fibrous protein existing as filaments in the outer cells of skin. A stratified squamous keratinized epithelium is made up of many layers. The layers closest to the underlying tissues are cuboidal or columnar. The cells become more irregular and thinner as they move closer to the surface. Surface cells become totally filled with keratin and die, are sloughed off, and then replaced by the deeper cells. A stratified squamous non-keratinized epithelium is found on moist surfaces, such as the mouth and tongue. Stratified cuboidal and columnar epithelia are found in the ducts of salivary glands and the

Simple squamous

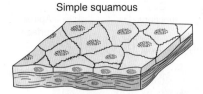

Simple cuboidal

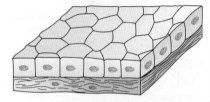

Simple columnar

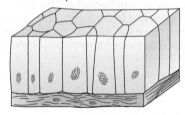

Pseudostratified columnar
ciliated

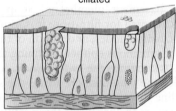

Transitional

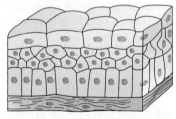

Stratified squamous

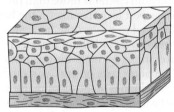

FIGURE 1-12 Representation of the various epithelial tissue types.

larger ducts of the mammary glands. In smokers, the normal columnar ciliated epithelial cells of the trachea and bronchi are often replaced with stratified squamous epithelium cells that are better able to withstand the irritating effects of cigarette smoke.

Pseudostratified epithelium is a type of epithelium in which all of the cells are in contact with the underlying intercellular matrix, but some do not extend to the surface. A pseudostratified ciliated columnar epithelium with goblet cells forms the lining of most of the upper respiratory tract. All of the tall cells reaching the surface of this type of epithelium are either ciliated cells or mucus-producing goblet cells. The basal cells that do not reach the surface serve as stem cells for ciliated and goblet cells. *Transitional epithelium* is a stratified epithelium characterized by cells that can change shape and become thinner when the tissue is stretched. Such tissue can be stretched without pulling the superficial cells apart. Transitional epithelium is well adapted for the lining of organs that are constantly changing their volume, such as the urinary bladder.

Glandular Epithelium

Glandular epithelial tissue is formed by cells specialized to produce a fluid secretion. This process is usually accompanied by the intracellular synthesis of macromolecules. The chemical nature of these macromolecules is variable. The macromolecules typically are stored in the cells in small, membrane-bound vesicles called *secretory granules*. For example, glandular epithelia can synthesize, store, and secrete proteins (*e.g.*, insulin), lipids (*e.g.*, adrenocortical hormones, secretions of the sebaceous glands), and complexes of carbohydrates and proteins (*e.g.*, saliva). Less common are secretions such as those produced by the sweat glands, which require minimal synthetic activity.

All glandular cells arise from surface epithelia by means of cell proliferation and invasion of the underlying connective tissue. Epithelial glands can be divided into two groups: exocrine and endocrine glands. *Exocrine glands*, such as the sweat glands and lactating mammary glands, retain their connection with the surface epithelium from which they originated. This connection takes the form of epithelium-lined tubular ducts through which the secretions pass to reach the surface. *Endocrine glands* are epithelial structures that have had their connection with the surface obliterated during development. These glands are ductless and produce secretions (*i.e.*, hormones) that move directly into the bloodstream.

Epithelial Cell Junctions

Cell junctions occur at many points in cell-to-cell contact, but they are particularly plentiful and important in epithelial tissue. Three basic types of intercellular junctions are observed: continuous tight junctions, adhering junctions, and gap junctions (Fig. 1-13). Often, the cells in epithelial tissue are joined by all three types of junctions.

Continuous tight or *occluding junctions* (*i.e.*, zonula occludens), which are found only in epithelial tissue, seal the surface membranes of adjacent cells together. This

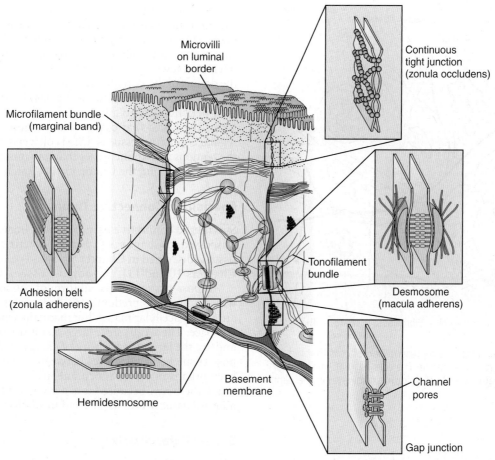

FIGURE 1-13 Three types of intercellular junctions found in epithelial tissue: the continuous tight junction (zonula occludens); the adhering junction, which includes the adhesion belt (zonula adherens), desmosomes (macula adherens), and hemidesmosomes; and the gap junction.

type of intercellular junction prevents materials such as macromolecules present in the intestinal contents from entering the intercellular space.

Adhering junctions represent a site of strong adhesion between cells. The primary role of adhering junctions may be that of preventing cell separation. Adhering junctions are not restricted to epithelial tissue; they provide adherence between adjacent cardiac muscle cells as well. Adhering junctions are found as continuous, beltlike adhesive junctions (*i.e.*, zonula adherens), or scattered, spotlike adhesive junctions called *desmosomes* (*i.e.*, macula adherens). A special feature of the adhesion belt junction is that it provides a site for anchorage of microfilaments to the cell membrane. In epithelial desmosomes, bundles of keratin-containing intermediate filaments (*i.e.*, tonofilaments) are anchored to the junction on the cytoplasmic area of the cell membrane. Hemidesmosomes are another type of junction. They are found at the base of epithelial cells and help attach the epithelial cell to the underlying connective tissue. They resemble half a desmosome, thus their name.

Gap or *nexus junctions* involve the close adherence of adjoining cell membranes with the formation of channels that link the cytoplasm of the two cells. Gap junctions are not unique to epithelial tissue; they play an essential role in many types of cell-to-cell communication. Because they are low-resistance channels, gap junctions are important in cell-to-cell conduction of electrical signals (*e.g.*, between cells in sheets of smooth muscle or between adjacent cardiac muscle cells, where they function as electrical synapses). These multiple communication channels also enable ions and small molecules to pass directly from one cell to another.

CONNECTIVE OR SUPPORTIVE TISSUE

Connective tissue is the most abundant tissue in the body. As its name suggests, it connects and binds or supports the various tissues. In general, connective tissue consists of cells and an extracellular matrix that includes fibers, ground substance, and tissue fluid. The functions of the various connective tissues are reflected by the types of cells and fibers present in the tissue and the character of the extracellular matrix (Fig. 1-14). One type of cell, the fibroblast, is responsible for synthesis of collagen, elas-

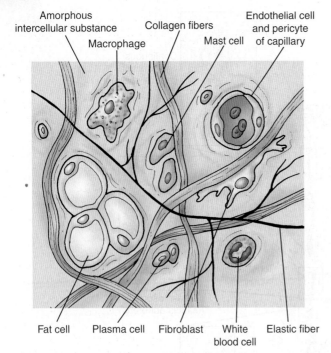

Amorphous intercellular substance   Collagen fibers   Endothelial cell and pericyte of capillary

Macrophage   Mast cell

Fat cell   Plasma cell   Fibroblast   White blood cell   Elastic fiber

FIGURE 1-14 Diagrammatic representation of cells that may be seen in loose connective tissue. The cells lie in an intercellular matrix that is bathed in tissue fluid that originates in the capillaries.

tic, reticular fibers, and ground substance of the extracellular matrix. Other cells, such as lymphocytes, plasma cells, macrophages, and eosinophils, are associated with body defense systems.

Connective tissue is generally divided into two main types: connective tissue proper and specialized connective tissue. Another type of connective tissue, embryonic connective tissue, is present in the embryo and umbilical cord.

Connective Tissue Proper

There are three types of connective tissue proper: loose, reticular, and dense connective tissue. Loose connective tissue is soft and pliable and its cells secrete substances that form the extracellular matrix. Fibroblasts are the most abundant of these cells. They are responsible for the synthesis of the fibrous gel-like substance that fills the intercellular spaces of the body and for the production of collagen, elastic, and reticular fibers. Although loose connective tissue is more cellular than dense connective tissue, it contains large amounts of intercellular substance. It fills spaces between muscle sheaths and forms a layer that encases blood and lymphatic vessels. Reticular tissue is characterized by a network of reticular fibers associated with reticular cells. Reticular fibers provide the framework for capillaries, nerves, and muscle cells. They also constitute the main supporting elements for the blood-forming tissues and the liver.

Dense connective tissue exists in two forms: dense irregular and dense regular. Dense irregular connective tissue consists of the same components found in loose connective tissue, but there is a predominance of collagen fibers and fewer cells. This type of tissue can be found in the dermis of the skin (*i.e.,* reticular layer), the fibrous capsules of many organs, and the fibrous sheaths of cartilage (*i.e., perichondrium*) and bone (*i.e., periosteum*). It also forms the fascia that covers muscles and organs. Dense regular connective tissue is rich in collagen fibers and forms the tendons and aponeuroses that join muscles to bone or other muscles and the ligaments that join bone to bone.

Specialized Connective Tissue

Specialized connective tissue includes bone and cartilage (discussed in Chapter 41), hematopoietic and lymphatic tissues (discussed in Chapter 9), blood cells (discussed in Chapters 10 and 11), and adipose tissue.

Adipose tissue is a special form of connective tissue in which adipocytes predominate. Adipocytes do not generate an extracellular matrix but maintain a large intracellular space. These cells store large quantities of triglycerides and are the largest repository of energy in the body. Adipose tissue helps fill spaces between tissues and helps to keep organs in place. Subcutaneous layers of fat help to shape the body. Because fat is a poor conductor of heat, adipose tissue serves as thermal insulation for the body.

Extracellular Matrix

The extracellular matrix is composed of a variety of proteins and polysaccharides (*i.e.,* a molecule made up of many sugars). These proteins and polysaccharides are secreted locally and are organized into a supportive meshwork in close association with the cells that produced them. Two main groups of extracellular macromolecules make up the extracellular matrix. The first group consists of fibrous proteins (*i.e.,* collagen and elastin) and fibrous adhesive proteins (*i.e.,* fibronectin and laminin), which are found in the basement membrane. The second is composed of polysaccharide chains of proteins called *glycosamino-glycans* (GAGs), which are usually found linked to protein as proteoglycans.

Three types of fibers are found in the extracellular space: collagen, elastin, and reticular fibers. *Collagen* is the most common protein in the body. It is a tough, nonliving white fiber that serves as the structural framework for skin, ligaments, tendons, and many other structures. *Elastin* acts like a rubber band; it can be stretched and then returns to its original form. Elastin fibers are abundant in structures subjected to frequent stretching, such as the aorta and some ligaments. *Reticular fibers* are extremely thin fibers that create a flexible network in organs subjected to changes in form or volume, such as the spleen, liver, uterus, or intestinal muscle layer.

The proteoglycan and GAG molecules in connective tissue form a highly hydrated, gel-like substance, or tissue gel, in which the fibrous proteins are embedded. The polysaccharide gel resists compressive forces, the collagen fibers strengthen and help organize the matrix, the rubber-like elastin adds resilience, and the adhesive proteins help cells attach to the appropriate part of the matrix. Polysaccharides in the tissue gel are highly hydrophilic, and they form gels even at low concentrations. They also accumulate a negative charge that attracts cations such as sodium, which are osmotically active, causing large amounts of water to be sucked into the matrix. This creates a swelling pressure, or turgor, that enables the matrix to withstand extensive compressive forces. This is in contrast to collagen, which resists stretching forces. For example, the cartilage matrix that lines the knee joint can support pressures of hundreds of atmospheres by this mechanism.

MUSCLE TISSUE

Three types of muscle tissues exist: *skeletal, cardiac,* and *smooth*. Skeletal and cardiac muscles are striated muscles. The actin and myosin filaments, which are contractile elements, are arranged in large parallel arrays in bundles, giving the muscle fibers a striped or striated appearance when they are viewed through a microscope. Most skeletal muscles are attached to bones, and their contractions are responsible for movements of the skeleton. Cardiac muscle, which is found in the heart, is designed to pump blood continuously. Smooth muscle lacks striations and is found in the walls of hollow organs such as the gastrointestinal tract and urinary bladder, as well as the blood vessels, the ureters, the bronchioles, and the iris of the eye.

Although the three types of muscle tissues differ significantly in structure, contractile properties, and control mechanisms, they have many similarities. In the following section, the structural properties of skeletal muscle are presented using striated muscle tissue as the prototype. Smooth muscle and the ways in which it differs from skeletal muscle are also discussed. Cardiac muscle is described in Chapter 16.

Skeletal Muscle

Skeletal muscle is the most abundant tissue in the body, accounting for 40% to 45% of the total body weight. Skeletal muscle tissue is packaged into skeletal muscles that attach to and cover the body skeleton. Each skeletal muscle is a discrete organ made up of hundreds of thousands of muscle fibers. Even though muscle fibers predominate, substantial amounts of connective tissue, blood vessels, and nerve fibers are present. In an intact muscle, several different layers of connective tissue hold the individual muscle fibers together. A dense connective tissue covering called the *epimysium* forms the outermost layer surrounding the whole muscle (Fig. 1-15). Each muscle is subdivided into smaller bundles called *fascicles*, which are surrounded by a connective tissue covering called the *perimysium*. The number of fascicles and their size vary among muscles. Fascicles consist of many elongated structures called *muscle fibers*, each of which is surrounded by connective tissue called the *endomysium*.

Skeletal muscles are syncytial or multinucleated structures, meaning there are no true cell boundaries within a skeletal muscle fiber. The cytoplasm or sarcoplasm of the muscle fiber is contained within the sarcolemma, which represents the cell membrane. Embedded throughout the sarcoplasm are the contractile elements actin and myosin, which are arranged in parallel bundles (*i.e., myofibrils*). The thin, lighter-staining myofilaments are composed of actin, and the thicker, darker-staining myofilaments are composed of myosin. Each myofibril consists of regularly repeating units along the length of the myofibril; each of these units is called a *sarcomere* (see Fig. 1-15). Sarcomeres are the structural and functional units of cardiac and skeletal muscle.

A sarcomere extends from one Z line to another Z line. Within the sarcomere are alternating light and dark bands. The central dark band (A band) contains mainly myosin filaments, with some overlap with actin filaments. The lighter I band contains only actin filaments and straddles the Z band; therefore, it takes two sarcomeres to complete an I band. An H zone is found in the middle of the A band and represents the region where only myosin filaments are found. In the center of the H zone is a thin dark band, the M band or line that is produced by linkages between the myosin filaments. Z bands consist of short elements that interconnect and provide the thin actin filaments from two adjoining sarcomeres with an anchoring point.

The *sarcoplasmic reticulum*, which is comparable to the smooth ER, is composed of longitudinal tubules that run parallel to the muscle fiber and surround each myofibril. This network ends in enlarged, saclike regions called the *lateral sacs* or *terminal cisternae*. These sacs store calcium to be released during muscle contraction. A second system of tubules consists of the *transverse* or *T tubules,* which are extensions of the plasma membrane and run perpendicular to the muscle fiber. The hollow portion or lumen of the transverse tubule is continuous with the extracellular fluid compartment. Action potentials, which are rapidly conducted over the surface of the muscle fiber, are in turn propagated by the T tubules and into the sarcoplasmic reticulum. As the action potential moves through the lateral sacs, the sacs release calcium, initiating muscle contraction. The membrane of the sarcoplasmic reticulum also has an active transport mechanism for pumping calcium ions back into the reticulum. This prevents interactions between calcium ions and the actin and myosin myofilaments after cessation of a muscle contraction.

Skeletal Muscle Contraction. Muscle contraction involves the sliding of the thick myosin and thin actin filaments over each other to produce shortening of the muscle fiber, while the actual length of the individual thick and thin filaments remains unchanged. The thick myosin filaments consist of a thin tail, which provides the structural backbone for the filament, and a globular head that forms cross-bridges with the thin actin filaments (Fig. 1-16). Myosin molecules are bundled together side by side in the thick filaments such that one half have their heads toward one end of the filament and their tails toward the other

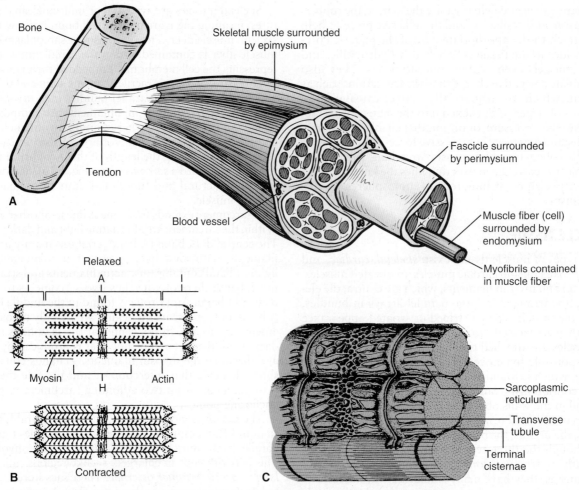

FIGURE 1-15 (**A**) Connective tissue components of a skeletal muscle. (**B**) Structure of the myofibril and the relationship between actin and myosin myofilaments during muscle relaxation and contraction. (**C**) Sarcoplasmic reticulum and system of transverse tubules in the myofibril.

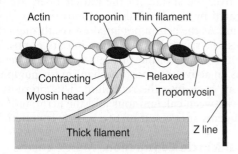

FIGURE 1-16 Molecular structure of the thin actin filament and the thicker myosin filament of striated muscle. The thin filament is a double-stranded helix of actin molecules with tropomyosin and troponin molecules lying along the grooves of the actin strands. During muscle contraction, the ATP-activated heads of the thick myosin filament swivel into position, much like the oars on a boat, form a cross-bridge with a reactive site on tropomyosin, and then pull the actin filament forward. During muscle relaxation, the troponin molecules cover the reactive sites on tropomyosin.

end; the other half are arranged in the opposite manner. Each globular myosin head contains a binding site able to bind to a complementary site on the actin molecule. In addition to the binding site for actin, each myosin head has a separate active site that catalyzes the breakdown of ATP to provide the energy needed to activate the myosin head so it can form a cross-bridge with actin. After contraction, myosin also binds ATP, thus breaking the linkage between actin and myosin.

The thin filaments are composed mainly of actin, a globular protein lined up in two rows that coil around each other to form a long helical strand. Associated with each actin filament are two regulatory proteins, tropomyosin and troponin. *Tropomyosin*, which lies in grooves of the actin strand, provides the site for attachment of the globular heads of the myosin filament. In the noncontracted state, *troponin* covers the tropomyosin binding sites and prevents formation of cross-bridges between the actin and myosin. During an action potential, calcium ions released from the sarcoplasmic reticulum diffuse to the adjacent myofibrils, where they bind to troponin. The binding of calcium to troponin uncovers the tropomyosin binding sites such that the myosin heads can attach and form cross-bridges.

Muscle contraction begins with activation of the cross-bridges from the myosin filaments and uncovering of the tropomyosin binding sites on the actin filament. When activated by ATP, the heads of the myosin filaments swivel in a fixed arc, much like the oars of a boat, as they become attached to the actin filament. During contraction, each myosin head undergoes its own cycle of movement, forming a bridge attachment and releasing it, and moving to another site where the same sequence of movement occurs. This pulls the thin and thick filaments past each other. Energy from ATP is used to break the actin and myosin cross-bridges, stopping the muscle contraction. With the breaking of the linkage between actin and myosin, the concentration of calcium around the myofibrils decreases as calcium is actively transported into the sarcoplasmic reticulum by a membrane pump that uses energy derived from ATP.

Smooth Muscle

Smooth muscle is often called *involuntary muscle* because its activity arises spontaneously or through the activity of the autonomic nervous system. Smooth muscle is usually arranged in sheets or bundles and its contractions are slower and more sustained than skeletal or cardiac muscle contractions.

Smooth muscle cells are spindle shaped and smaller than skeletal muscle fibers. Each smooth muscle cell has one centrally positioned nucleus. Z bands or M lines are not present in smooth muscle fibers, and the cross-striations are absent because the bundles of filaments are not parallel but crisscross obliquely through the cell. Instead, the actin filaments are attached to structures called *dense bodies*. Some of the dense bodies are attached to the cell membrane, and others are dispersed in the cell and linked together by structural proteins (Fig. 1-17).

The lack of Z lines and regular overlapping of the contractile elements provides a greater range of tension development. This is important in hollow organs that undergo changes in volume, with consequent changes in the length of the smooth muscle fibers in their walls. Even with the distention of a hollow organ, the smooth muscle fiber retains some ability to develop tension, whereas such distention would stretch skeletal muscle beyond the area where the thick and thin filaments overlap.

Smooth Muscle Contraction. As with cardiac and skeletal muscle, smooth muscle contraction is initiated by an increase in intracellular calcium. However, smooth muscle differs from skeletal muscle in the way its cross-bridges are formed. The sarcoplasmic reticulum of smooth muscle is less developed than in skeletal muscle, and no transverse tubules are present. Thus, smooth muscle relies heavily on the entrance of extracellular calcium for muscle contraction. This dependence on movement of extracellular calcium across the cell membrane during muscle

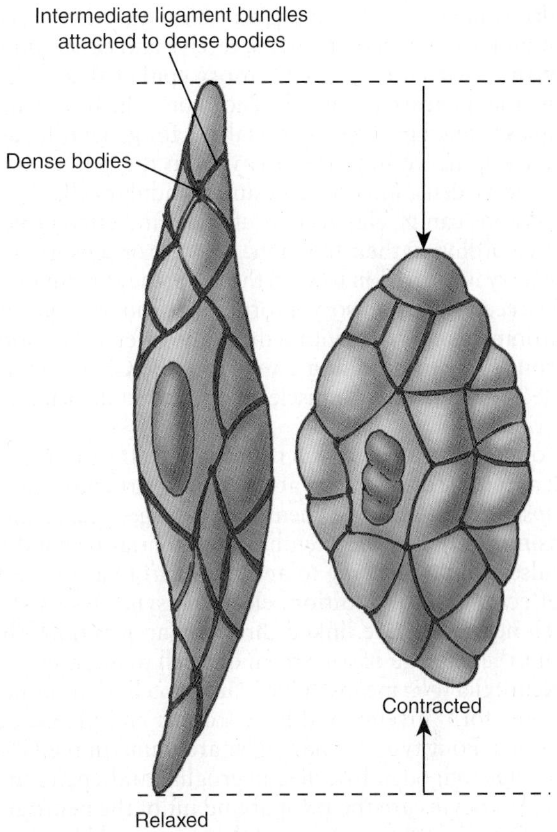

FIGURE 1-17 Structure of smooth muscle showing the dense bodies. In smooth muscle, the force of contraction is transmitted to the cell membrane by bundles of intermediate fibers.

contraction is the basis for the action of calcium-blocking drugs used in the treatment of cardiovascular disease.

Smooth muscle also lacks the calcium-binding regulatory protein troponin, which is found in skeletal and cardiac muscle. Instead, it relies on another cytoplasmic protein called *calmodulin*. The calcium–calmodulin complex binds to and activates the myosin-containing thick filaments, which interact with actin.

NERVOUS TISSUE

Nervous tissue is distributed throughout the body as an integrated communication system. Anatomically, the nervous system is divided into the central nervous system (CNS), which consists of the brain and spinal cord, and the peripheral nervous system (PNS), composed of nerve fibers and ganglia that exist outside the CNS. Nerve cells develop from the embryonic ectoderm. Nerve cells are highly differentiated and therefore incapable of regeneration in postnatal life. Embryonic development of the nervous system and the structure and functions of the nervous system are discussed more fully in Chapter 33.

Structurally, nervous tissue consists of two cell types: nerve cells or neurons and supporting cells or neuroglia. Most nerve cells consist of three parts: soma or cell body, dendrites, and axon. The cytoplasm-filled dendrites, which are multiple elongated processes, receive and carry stimuli from the environment, from sensory epithelial cells, and from other neurons to the cell. The axon, which is a single cytoplasm-filled process, is specialized for generating and conducting nerve impulses away from the cell body to other nerve cells, muscle cells, and glandular cells.

Neurons can be classified as afferent and efferent neurons according to their function. Afferent or sensory neurons carry information toward the CNS; they are involved in the reception of sensory information from the external environment and from within the body. Efferent or motor neurons carry information away from the CNS; they are needed for control of muscle fibers and endocrine and exocrine glands.

Communication between neurons and effector organs, such as muscle cells, occurs at specialized structures called *synapses*. At the synapse, chemical messengers (*i.e.*, neurotransmitters) alter the membrane potential to conduct impulses from one nerve to another or from a neuron to an effector cell. In addition, electrical synapses exist in which nerve cells are linked through gap junctions that permit the passage of ions from one cell to another.

Neuroglia (*glia* means "glue") are the cells that support neurons, form myelin, and have trophic and phagocytic functions. Four types of neuroglia are found in the CNS: astrocytes, oligodendrocytes, microglia, and ependymal cells. Astrocytes are the most abundant of the neuroglia. They have many long processes that surround blood vessels in the CNS. They provide structural support for the neurons, and their extensions form a sealed barrier that protects the CNS. The oligodendrocytes provide myelination of neuronal processes in the CNS. The microglia are phagocytic cells that represent the mononuclear phagocytic system in the nervous system. Ependymal cells line the cavities of the brain and spinal cord and are in contact with the cerebrospinal fluid. In the PNS, supporting cells consist of the Schwann and satellite cells. The Schwann cells provide myelination of the axons and dendrites, and the satellite cells enclose and protect the dorsal root ganglia and autonomic ganglion cells.

In summary, body cells are organized into four basic tissue types: epithelial, connective, muscle, and nervous. The epithelium covers and lines the body surfaces and forms the functional components of glandular structures. Epithelial tissue is classified into three types according to the shape of the cells and the number of layers that are present: simple, stratified, and pseudostratified. The cells in epithelial tissue are held together by three types of intercellular junctions: tight, adhering, and gap. They are attached to the underlying tissue by hemidesmosomes.

Connective tissue supports and connects body structures; it forms the bones and skeletal system, the joint structures, the blood cells, and the cells that produce the extracellular matrix. Fibroblasts are the most abundant of these cells. They are responsible for the synthesis of collagen, elastic, and reticular fibers and the gel-like substance that fills the intercellular spaces of the body. Specialized connective tissue includes bone and cartilage, hematopoietic and lymphatic tissue, blood cells, and adipose tissue.

Muscle tissue is a specialized tissue designed for contractility. Three types of muscle tissue exist: skeletal, cardiac, and smooth. Actin and myosin filaments interact to produce muscle shortening, a process activated by the presence of calcium. In skeletal muscle, calcium is released from the sarcoplasmic reticulum in response to an action potential. Smooth muscle is often called *involuntary muscle* because it contracts spontaneously or through the activity of the autonomic nervous system. It differs from skeletal muscle in that its sarcoplasmic reticulum is less defined and it depends on the entry of extracellular calcium ions for muscle contraction.

Nervous tissue is designed for communication purposes and includes the neurons, the supporting neural structures, and the ependymal cells that line the ventricles of the brain and the spinal canal.

Review Exercises

Tattoos consist of pigments that have been injected into the skin.

A. Explain what happens to the dye once it has been injected and why it does not eventually wash away.

Insulin is synthesized in the beta cells of the pancreas as a prohormone and then secreted as an active hormone.

A. Using your knowledge of the function of DNA, the RNAs, the endoplasmic reticulum, and the Golgi complex, propose a pathway for the synthesis of insulin.

Persons who drink sufficient amounts of alcohol display rapid changes in central nervous system function, including both motor and behavioral changes, and the odor of alcohol can be detected on their breath.

A. Use the concepts related to the lipid bilayer structure of the cell membrane to explain these observations.

The absorption of glucose from the intestine involves a cotransport mechanism in which the active primary transport of sodium is used to provide for the secondary transport of glucose.

A. Hypothesize how this information might be used to design an oral rehydration solution for someone who is suffering from diarrhea.

Visit the Porth: Essentials of Pathophysiology: Concepts of Altered Health States web site (http://thePoint.LWW.com/PorthEssentials) for links to chapter-related resources on the Internet, all-new exclusive animations, chapter review questions, and more!

BIBLIOGRAPHY

Alberts B., Johnson A., Lewis J., et al. (2002). *Molecular biology of the cell* (4th ed.). New York and London: Garland Publishing.

Ashcroft F. M. (2000). *Ion channels and disease.* San Diego: Academic Press.

Cormack D. H. (2001). *Essential histology.* (2nd ed.). Philadelphia: Lippincott Williams & Wilkins.

Costanzo L. S. (2002). *Physiology* (2nd ed.). Philadelphia: W. B. Saunders.

Gartner L. P., Hiatt J. L. (2001). *Color textbook of histology* (2nd ed.). Philadelphia: W. B. Saunders.

Guyton A. C., Hall J. E. (2006). *Textbook of medical physiology* (11th ed.). Philadelphia: Elsevier Saunders.

Joachim F. (1998). How the ribosome works. *American Scientist* 86, 428–439.

Kerr J. B. (1999). *Atlas of functional histology.* London: Mosby.

Kumar V., Abbas A. K., Fausto N. (Eds.). (2005). *Robbins and Cotran pathologic basis of disease* (7th ed). Philadelphia: Elsevier Saunders.

Mathews C. K., van Holde K. E., Ahern K. G. (2000). *Biochemistry.* San Francisco: Benjamin/Cummings.

Nelson D. L., Cox M. M. (2000). *Lehninger's principles of biochemistry* (3rd ed.). New York: Worth.

Rhoades R. A., Tanner G. A. (2003). *Medical physiology* (2nd ed.). Philadelphia: Lippincott Williams & Wilkins.

Ross M. H., Kaye G. I., Pawlina W. (2003). *Histology: A text and atlas* (4th ed.). Philadelphia: Lippincott Williams & Wilkins.

Rubin E., Gorstein F., Rubin R., et al. (Eds.). (2005). *Rubin's pathology: Clinicopathologic foundations of medicine* (4th ed.). Philadelphia: Lippincott Williams & Wilkins.

Tortora G. J., Grabowski S. R. (2000). *Principles of anatomy and physiology.* New York: John Wiley & Sons.

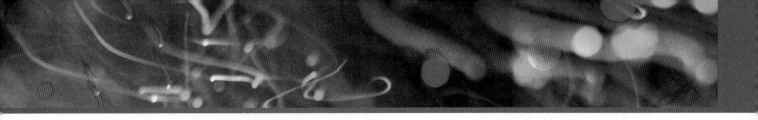

Chapter 2

Cellular Responses to Stress, Injury, and Aging

 In their simplest form, all diseases exert their effects on the smallest living unit of the body, namely, the cell. When confronted with stresses that endanger its normal structure and function, the cell undergoes adaptive changes that permit survival and maintenance of function. It is only when the stress is overwhelming or adaptation is ineffective that injury, maladaptive changes, and cell death occur. Biologic aging produces its own changes in cell structure and function.

Cellular Responses to Stress

Cells adapt to changes in the internal environment, just as the total organism adapts to changes in the external environment. Cells may adapt by undergoing changes in size, number, and type. These changes, occurring singly or in combination, may lead to atrophy, hypertrophy, hyperplasia, metaplasia, and dysplasia (Fig. 2-1). Cellular stresses also include intracellular accumulations and storage of products in abnormal amounts.[1,2]

ADAPTATIONS OF GROWTH AND DIFFERENTIATION

There are numerous molecular mechanisms mediating cellular adaptation, including factors produced by other cells or by the cells themselves. These mechanisms depend largely on signals transmitted by chemical messengers that exert their effects by altering gene function. In general, the genes expressed in all cells fall into two categories: "housekeeping" genes that are necessary for the normal function of a cell, and genes that determine the differentiating characteristics of a particular cell type. In many adaptive cellular responses, the expression of the differentiation genes is altered, whereas that of the housekeeping genes remains unaffected.[1] Thus, a cell is able to change size or form without compromising its housekeeping function. Once

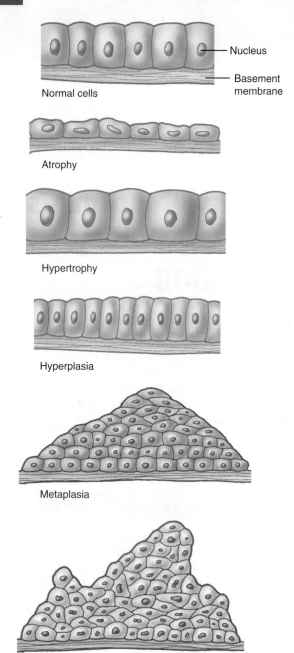

FIGURE 2-1 Adaptive tissue cell responses involving a change in cell size (atrophy and hypertrophy), number (hyperplasia), cell type (metaplasia), or size, shape, and organization (dysplasia). (From Anatomical Chart Company. [2002]. *Atlas of pathophysiology* [p. 4]. Springhouse, PA: Springhouse.)

the stimulus for adaptation is removed, the effect on expression of the differentiating genes is removed and the cell resumes its previous state of specialized function. Whether adaptive cellular changes are normal or abnormal depends on whether the response was mediated by an appropriate stimulus. Normal adaptive responses occur in response to need and an appropriate stimulus. After the need has been removed, the adaptive response ceases.

Atrophy

Atrophy is a decrease in the size of a tissue organ resulting from a decrease in cell size of the individual cells or in the number of cells. It is important to note that atrophy, which occurs in normally formed organs, is distinct from aplasia or hypoplasia, which are abnormalities of organ development. It is also important to distinguish cellular atrophy from organ atrophy that is due to irreversible loss of cells. For example, atrophy of the brain in Alzheimer disease is secondary to extensive cell death, and the size of the organ cannot be restored. The general causes of cell atrophy include disuse and reduced functional demand, loss of trophic stimuli, insufficient nutrients, decreased blood flow, persistent cell injury, and aging.

Disuse atrophy, particularly in muscle tissue, is related to workload. When confronted with a decrease in work demands or adverse environmental conditions, most cells are able to revert to a smaller size and a lower and more efficient level of functioning that is compatible with survival. As the workload of a cell diminishes, oxygen consumption and protein synthesis decrease. Cells that are atrophied reduce their oxygen consumption and other cellular functions by decreasing the number and size of their organelles and other structures. There are fewer mitochondria, myofilaments, and endoplasmic reticulum structures. An extreme example of disuse atrophy is seen in the muscles of extremities that have been encased in plaster casts. Because atrophy is adaptive and reversible, muscle size is restored after the cast is removed and muscle use is resumed.

The functions of many cells depend on trophic signals such as those transmitted by the nervous and endocrine systems. Denervation atrophy is a form of atrophy in paralyzed limbs that results from loss of nervous system stimulation. Lack of endocrine stimulation produces a form of disuse atrophy. In women, the loss of estrogen stimulation during menopause results in atrophic changes in the reproductive organs.

With malnutrition and decreased blood flow, cells decrease their size and energy requirements as a means of survival. Persistent cell injury is most commonly caused by chronic inflammation associated with prolonged viral or bacterial infections. Chronic inflammation may also occur in other conditions, such as immunologic and granulomatous disorders. Villous atrophy of the small intestinal mucosa follows the chronic inflammation characteristic of celiac disease (see Chapter 28).

One of the hallmarks of aging, particularly in non-replicating cells such as the brain and heart, is cell atrophy. There is a decrease in the size of most body organs. The size of the brain is invariably decreased, and in the very old, the size of the heart may be greatly diminished.

Hypertrophy

Hypertrophy represents an increase in cell size as well as an increase in the amount of functioning tissue mass. It results from an increased workload imposed on an organ or body part and is commonly seen in cardiac and skeletal muscle tissue, which cannot adapt to an increase in workload through mitotic division and formation of more cells. Hypertrophy involves an increase in the functional components of the cell that allows it to achieve equilibrium between demand and functional capacity. For example, as muscle cells hypertrophy, additional actin and myosin filaments, cell enzymes, and adenosine triphosphate (ATP) are synthesized.

Hypertrophy may occur as the result of normal physiologic or abnormal pathologic conditions. The increase in muscle mass associated with exercise is an example of physiologic hypertrophy. Pathologic hypertrophy occurs as the result of disease conditions and may be adaptive or compensatory. Examples of adaptive hypertrophy are the thickening of the urinary bladder from long-continued obstruction of urinary outflow and the myocardial hypertrophy that results from valvular heart disease or hypertension. Compensatory hypertrophy is the enlargement of a remaining organ or tissue after a portion has been surgically removed or rendered inactive. For instance, if one kidney is removed, the remaining kidney enlarges to compensate for the loss.

The precise signal for hypertrophy is unknown. It may be related to ATP depletion, mechanical forces such as stretching of the muscle fibers, activation of cell degradation products, or hormonal factors.[1] Whatever the mechanism, a limit is eventually reached beyond which further enlargement of the tissue mass is no longer able to compensate for the increased work demands. The limiting factors for continued hypertrophy might be related to limitations in blood flow. For example, in hypertension the increased workload required to pump blood against an elevated arterial pressure results in a progressive increase in left ventricular muscle mass (Fig. 2-2).

There has been recent interest in the signaling pathways that control the arrangement of contractile elements in myocardial hypertrophy. Research suggests that certain signal molecules can alter gene expression controlling the size and assembly of the contractile proteins in hypertrophied myocardial cells. For example, the hypertrophied myocardial cells of well-trained athletes have proportional increases in width and length. This is in contrast to the hypertrophy that develops in dilated cardiomyopathy, in which the hypertrophied cells have a relatively greater increase in length than width (see Chapter 19). In pressure

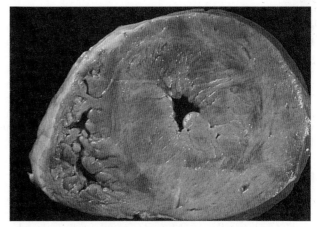

FIGURE 2-2 Myocardial hypertrophy. Cross-section of the heart in a patient with long-standing hypertension. (From Rubin E., Gorstein E., Rubin R., et al. [2005]. *Rubin's pathology: Clinico-pathologic foundations of medicine* [4th ed., p. 7]. Philadelphia: Lippincott Williams & Wilkins.)

overload, as occurs with hypertension, the hypertrophied cells have greater width than length.[3] It is anticipated that further elucidation of the signal pathways that determine the adaptive and nonadaptive features of cardiac hypertrophy will lead to new targets for treatment.

Hyperplasia

Hyperplasia refers to an increase in the number of cells in an organ or tissue. It occurs in tissues with cells that are capable of mitotic division, such as the epidermis, intestinal epithelium, and glandular tissue. Nerve cells and skeletal and cardiac muscle cells do not divide and therefore have no capacity for hyperplastic growth. There is evidence that hyperplasia involves activation of genes controlling cell proliferation. As with other normal adaptive cellular responses, hyperplasia is a controlled process that occurs in response to an appropriate stimulus and ceases after the stimulus has been removed.

The stimuli that induce hyperplasia may be physiologic or nonphysiologic. Physiologic hyperplasia can occur as the result of hormonal stimulation or increased functional demands, or as a compensatory mechanism. Breast and uterine enlargement during pregnancy are examples of a physiologic hyperplasia that results from estrogen stimulation. An increased demand for parathyroid hormone, as occurs in chronic renal failure, results in hyperplasia of the parathyroid gland. The regeneration of the liver that occurs after partial hepatectomy (*i.e.*, partial removal of the liver) is an example of compensatory hyperplasia. Hyperplasia is also an important response of connective tissue in wound healing, during which proliferating fibroblasts and blood vessels contribute to wound repair. Although hypertrophy and hyperplasia are two distinct processes, they may occur together and are often triggered by the same mechanism.[1] For example, the pregnant uterus undergoes both hypertrophy and hyperplasia as the result of estrogen stimulation.

Most forms of nonphysiologic hyperplasia are due to excessive hormonal stimulation or the effects of growth factors on target tissues.[2] Excessive estrogen production can cause endometrial hyperplasia and abnormal menstrual bleeding (see Chapter 39). Benign prostatic hyperplasia, which is a common disorder of men older than 50 years of age, is thought to be related to the synergistic action of estrogen and androgens (see Chapter 38). Skin warts are an example of hyperplasia caused by growth factors produced by the human papillomaviruses.

Metaplasia

Metaplasia represents a reversible change in which one adult cell type (epithelial or mesenchymal) is replaced by another adult cell type. Metaplasia is thought to involve the reprogramming of undifferentiated stem cells that are present in the tissue undergoing the metaplastic changes.

Metaplasia usually occurs in response to chronic irritation and inflammation and allows for substitution of cells that are better able to survive under circumstances in which a more fragile cell type might succumb. However, the conversion of cell types never oversteps the boundaries of the primary groups of tissue (*e.g.,* one type of epithelial cell may be converted to another type of epithelial cell, but not to a connective tissue cell). An example of metaplasia is the adaptive substitution of stratified squamous epithelial cells for the ciliated columnar epithelial cells in the trachea and large airways of a habitual cigarette smoker. Although the squamous epithelium is better able to survive in these situations, the protective function that the ciliated epithelium provides for the respiratory tract is lost. In addition, continued exposure to the influences that cause metaplasia may predispose to cancerous transformation of the metaplastic epithelium.

Dysplasia

Dysplasia is characterized by deranged cell growth of a specific tissue that results in cells that vary in size, shape, and appearance. Minor degrees of dysplasia are associated with chronic irritation or inflammation. The pattern is most frequently encountered in metaplastic squamous epithelium of the respiratory tract and uterine cervix. Dysplasia is strongly implicated as a precursor of cancer.

Similar to the development of cancer, dysplasia involves sequential mutations in proliferating cell populations. Through the use of the Papanicolaou (Pap) smear, it has been documented that cancer of the uterine cervix develops in a series of incremental epithelial changes ranging from severe dysplasia to invasive cancer. Because of these and other observations, dysplasia is now included in the morphologic classification of the stages of intraepithelial cancer of the cervix, prostate, and bladder.[1] Accordingly, severe dysplasia is considered an indication for aggressive preventative therapy to remove the underlying cause or to surgically remove the affected tissue. However, it is important to point out that dysplasia is an adaptive process and as such does not necessarily lead to cancer. In many cases, the dysplastic cells revert to their former structure and function.

INTRACELLULAR ACCUMULATIONS

Intracellular accumulations represent the buildup of substances that cells cannot immediately use or dispose of. The substances may accumulate in the cytoplasm (frequently in the lysosomes) or in the nucleus. In some cases the accumulation may be an abnormal substance that the cell has produced, and in other cases the cell may be storing exogenous materials or products of pathologic processes occurring elsewhere in the body. These substances can be grouped into three categories: (1) normal body substances, such as lipids, proteins, carbohydrates, melanin, and bilirubin, that are present in abnormally large amounts; (2) abnormal products from inside the body, such as those resulting from inborn errors of metabolism; and (3) products from outside the body, such as environmental agents and pigments, that cannot be broken down by the cell.[2] These substances may accumulate transiently or permanently, and they may be harmless or, in some cases, toxic.

Lipids

The accumulation of normal cellular constituents occurs when a substance is produced at a rate that exceeds its metabolism or removal. An example of this type of process is fatty changes in the liver caused by intracellular accumulation of triglycerides. Liver cells normally contain some fat, which is either oxidized and used for energy or converted to triglycerides. This fat is derived from free fatty acids released from adipose tissue. Abnormal accumulation occurs when the delivery of free fatty acids to the liver is increased, as in starvation and diabetes mellitus, or when the intrahepatic metabolism of lipids is disturbed, as in alcoholism.

Glycogen

Intracellular accumulation can result from genetic disorders that disrupt the metabolism of selected substances. A normal enzyme may be replaced with an abnormal one, resulting in the formation of a substance that cannot be used or eliminated from the cell, or an enzyme may be missing, so that an intermediate product accumulates in the cell. For example, there are at least 10 genetic disorders that affect glycogen metabolism, most of which lead to the accumulation of intracellular glycogen stores. In the most common form of this disorder, von Gierke disease, large amounts of glycogen accumulate in the liver and kidneys because of a deficiency of the enzyme glucose-6-phosphatase. Without this enzyme, glycogen cannot be broken down to form glucose. The disorder leads not only to an accumulation of glycogen but to a reduction in blood glucose levels.

Abnormal Proteins

A number of acquired or inherited diseases are characterized by intracellular accumulation of abnormal proteins. The deviant protein structure may result from an inherited mutation that alters a normal amino acid sequence or may reflect an acquired defect in protein folding. After newly assembled polypeptides emerge from ribosomes, they fold to assume the structure of mature proteins. Misfolded proteins can lead to loss of cell function, extracellular deposition of aggregated proteins, retention of secretory proteins, or formation of toxic proteins that accumulate in the cell. Aggregations of abnormally folded proteins caused by genetic mutations, aging, or unknown environmental insults are now recognized as a feature of some neurodegenerative disorders, including Alzheimer disease and Parkinson disease.

Pigments

Pigments are colored substances that may accumulate in cells. They can be endogenous (*i.e.*, arising from within the body) or exogenous (*i.e.*, arising from outside the body). Icterus, also called *jaundice,* is a yellow discoloration of tissue caused by the retention of bilirubin, an endogenous bile pigment. This condition may result from increased bilirubin production from red blood cell destruction, obstruction of bile passage into the intestine, or toxic diseases that affect the liver's ability to remove bilirubin from the blood. Lipofuscin is a yellow-brown pigment that results from the accumulation of the indigestible residues produced during normal turnover of cell structures. The accumulation of lipofuscin increases with age and is sometimes referred to as the *wear-and-tear pigment*. It is more common in heart, nerve, and liver cells than other tissues and is seen most often in conditions associated with atrophy of an organ.

One of the most common exogenous pigments is carbon in the form of coal dust. In coal miners or persons exposed to heavily polluted environments, the accumulation of carbon dust blackens the lung tissue and may cause serious lung disease. The formation of a blue lead line along the margins of the gum is one of the diagnostic features of lead poisoning. Tattoos are the result of insoluble pigments introduced into the skin, where they are engulfed by macrophages and persist for a lifetime.

The significance of intracellular accumulations depends on the cause and severity of the condition. Many accumulations, such as lipofuscin and mild fatty change, have no effect on cell function. Some conditions, such as the hyperbilirubinemia that causes jaundice, are reversible. Other disorders, such as glycogen storage diseases, produce accumulations that result in organ dysfunction and other alterations in physiologic function.

PATHOLOGIC CALCIFICATIONS

Pathologic calcification involves the abnormal tissue deposition of calcium salts, together with smaller amounts of iron, magnesium, and other minerals. It is known as *dystrophic calcification* when it occurs in dead or dying tissue and as *metastatic calcification* when it occurs in normal tissue.[1,2]

Dystrophic Calcification

Dystrophic calcification represents the macroscopic deposition of calcium salts in injured tissue. The pathogenesis of dystrophic calcification involves the intracellular or

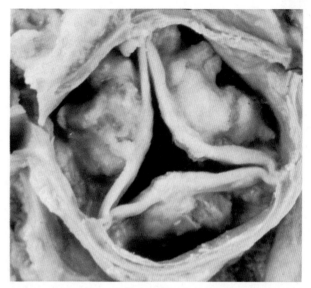

FIGURE 2-3 Calcific aortic stenosis. Large deposits of calcium salts are evident in the cusps and free margins of the thickened aortic valve as viewed from above. (From Rubin E., Gorstein E., Rubin R., et al. [2005]. *Rubin's pathology: Clinicopathologic foundations of medicine* [4th ed., p. 14]. Philadelphia: Lippincott Williams & Wilkins.)

extracellular formation of crystalline calcium phosphate. The components of the calcium deposits are derived from the bodies of dead or dying cells as well as from the circulation and interstitial fluid. Dystrophic calcification is commonly seen in atheromatous lesions of advanced atherosclerosis, areas of injury in the aorta and large blood vessels, and damaged heart valves. Although the presence of calcification may only indicate the presence of previous cell injury, as in healed tuberculosis lesions, it is also a frequent cause of organ dysfunction. For example, calcification of the aortic valve is a frequent cause of aortic stenosis in the elderly (Fig. 2-3).

Metastatic Calcification

In contrast to dystrophic calcification, which occurs in injured tissues, metastatic calcification occurs in normal tissues as the result of increased serum calcium levels (hypercalcemia). Almost any condition that increases the serum calcium level can lead to calcification in inappropriate sites such as the lung, renal tubules, and blood vessels. The major causes of hypercalcemia are hyperparathyroidism, either primary or secondary to phosphate retention in renal failure; increased mobilization of calcium from bone as in Paget disease, cancer with metastatic bone lesions, or immobilization; and vitamin D intoxication.

In summary, cells adapt to changes in their environment and in their work demands by changing their size, number, and type. These adaptive changes are consistent with the needs of the cell and occur in response to an appropriate stimulus. The changes are usually reversed after the stimulus has been withdrawn.

When confronted with a decrease in work demands or adverse environmental conditions, cells atrophy or reduce their size and revert to a lower and more efficient level of functioning. Hypertrophy results from an increase in work demands and is characterized by an increase in tissue size brought about by an increase in cell size and functional cell components. An increase in the number of cells in an organ or tissue that is still capable of mitotic division is called hyperplasia. Metaplasia occurs in response to chronic irritation and represents the substitution of cells of a type that are better able to survive under circumstances in which a more fragile cell type might succumb. Dysplasia is characterized by deranged cell growth of a specific tissue that results in cells that vary in size, shape, and appearance. It is a precursor of cancer.

Under some circumstances, cells may accumulate abnormal amounts of various substances such as lipids, glycogen, proteins, and pigments. If the accumulation reflects a correctable systemic disorder, such as the hyperbilirubinemia that causes jaundice, the accumulation is reversible. If the disorder cannot be corrected, as often occurs in many inborn errors of metabolism, the cells become overloaded, causing cell injury and death.

Pathologic calcification involves the abnormal tissue deposition of calcium salts. Dystrophic calcification occurs in dead or dying tissue. Although the presence of dystrophic calcification may only indicate the presence of previous cell injury, it is also a frequent cause of organ dysfunction (*e.g.*, when it affects the heart valves). Metastatic calcification occurs in normal tissues as the result of elevated serum calcium levels.

KEY CONCEPTS

Cell Injury

➤ Cells can be damaged in a number of ways, including physical trauma, extremes of temperature, electrical injury, exposure to damaging chemicals, radiation damage, injury from biologic agents, and nutritional factors.

➤ Most injurious agents exert their damaging effects through uncontrolled free radical production, impaired oxygen delivery or utilization, or the destructive effects of uncontrolled intracellular calcium release.

➤ Cell injury can be reversible, allowing the cell to recover, or it can be irreversible, causing cell death and necrosis.

➤ In contrast to necrosis, which results from tissue injury, apoptosis is a normal physiologic process designed to remove injured or worn-out cells.

Cell Injury and Death

Cells can be injured in many ways. The extent to which any injurious agent can cause cell injury and death depends in large measure on the intensity and duration of the injury and the type of cell that is involved. Cell injury is usually reversible to a certain point, after which irreversible cell injury and death occur. Whether a specific stress causes irreversible or reversible cell injury depends on the severity of the insult and on variables such as blood supply, nutritional status, and regenerative capacity. Cell injury and death are ongoing processes, and in the healthy state, they are balanced by cell renewal.

REVERSIBLE AND IRREVERSIBLE CELL INJURY

The mechanisms of cell injury can produce sublethal and reversible cellular damage or lead to irreversible injury with cell destruction or death. Reversible cell injury, although impairing cell function, does not result in cell death. Two patterns of reversible cell injury can be observed under the microscope: cellular swelling and fatty change.

Cellular swelling occurs with impairment of cellular volume regulation, a process that mediates the electrolyte concentrations in the cytoplasm. Impairment of this mechanism, particularly regarding sodium concentrations, involves disruption of cell membrane permeability, thus allowing passive entry of sodium into the cell; impaired functioning of the energy-dependent sodium/potassium (Na^+/K^+) ATPase membrane pump, which is necessary for the removal of sodium from inside the cell; and impaired synthesis of adenosine triphosphate (ATP), which provides the energy for the Na^+/K^+ ATPase pump.[1] There is increased intracellular volume, dilation of the endoplasmic reticulum, swelling of the mitochondria, aggregation of cytoskeletal elements, and formation of blebs on the plasma membrane (Fig. 2-4). In the nucleus, reversible injury is reflected principally in nucleolar changes. These changes in the cell organelles are reflected mainly in decreased protein synthesis and energy production. After withdrawal of the event that led to the reversible cell injury, the cell returns to its normal state.

Fatty changes are linked to intracellular accumulation of fat. When fatty changes occur, small vacuoles of fat disperse throughout the cytoplasm. The process is usually more ominous than cellular swelling, and although it is reversible, it usually indicates more severe injury. These fatty changes may occur because normal cells are presented with an increased fat load or because injured cells are unable to metabolize the fat properly. In obese persons, fatty infiltrates often occur within and between the cells of the liver and heart because of an increased fat load. Pathways for fat metabolism may be impaired during cell injury, and fat may accumulate in the cell as production exceeds use and export. The liver, where most fats are

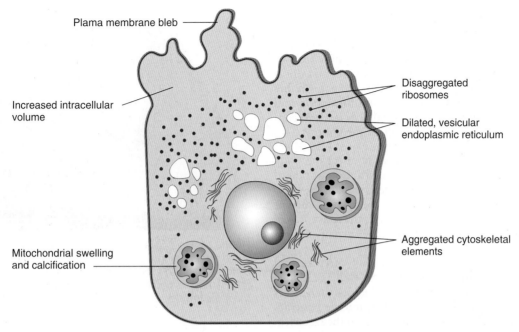

FIGURE 2-4 Ultrastructural features of reversible cell injury. (From Rubin E., Gorstein E., Rubin R., et al. [2005]. *Rubin's pathology: Clinicopathologic foundations of medicine* [4th ed., p. 17]. Philadelphia: Lippincott Williams & Wilkins.)

synthesized and metabolized, is particularly susceptible to fatty change, but fatty changes may also occur in the kidney, the heart, and other organs.

CAUSES OF CELL INJURY

The causes of cell injury can range from the gross physical effects of an automobile accident to the subtle changes that result from the lack of an essential nutrient. In general, the causes of cell injury can be grouped into the following broad categories: hypoxia, physical agents, chemical agents and drugs, biologic agents, ionizing radiation, and nutritional imbalances. Ultraviolet radiation injury is discussed in Chapter 45.

Hypoxia

Hypoxia deprives the cell of oxygen and interrupts oxidative metabolism and the generation of ATP. Hypoxia can result from an inadequate amount of oxygen in the air, respiratory disease, ischemia (*i.e.,* decreased blood flow caused by circulatory disorders), anemia, edema, or inability of the cells to use oxygen. Ischemia is characterized by impaired oxygen delivery and impaired removal of metabolic end-products, such as lactic acid. In contrast to pure hypoxia, which affects the oxygen content of the blood and affects all of the cells in the body, ischemia commonly affects blood flow through small numbers of blood vessels and produces local tissue injury.

Hypoxia literally causes a power failure in the cell, with widespread effects on the cell's functional and structural components. As oxygen tension in the cell falls, oxidative metabolism ceases, and the cell reverts to anaerobic metabolism, using its limited glycogen stores in an attempt to maintain vital cell functions. Cellular pH falls as lactic acid accumulates in the cell. This reduction in pH can have profound effects on intracellular structures. The nuclear chromatin clumps and myelin figures, which derive from destructive changes in cell membranes and intracellular structures, are seen in the cytoplasm and extracellular spaces.

Physical Agents

Physical agents responsible for cell and tissue injury include mechanical forces, extremes of temperature, and electrical forces. They are common causes of injuries due to environmental exposure, occupational and transportation accidents, and physical violence and assault.

Mechanical Forces. Injury or trauma caused by mechanical forces occurs as the result of body impact with another object. The body or the object can be in motion or, as sometimes occurs, both can be in motion at the time of impact. These types of injuries split and tear tissue, fracture bones, injure blood vessels, and disrupt blood flow.

Extremes of Temperature. Extremes of heat and cold cause damage to the cell, its organelles, and its enzyme systems. Exposure to low-intensity heat (43°C to 46°C), such as occurs with partial-thickness burns and severe heat stroke, causes cell injury by inducing vascular injury, accelerating cell metabolism, inactivating temperature-sensitive enzymes, and disrupting the cell membrane. With more intense heat, coagulation of blood vessels and tissue proteins occurs.

Exposure to cold increases blood viscosity and induces vasoconstriction by direct action on blood vessels and through reflex activity of the sympathetic nervous system. The resultant decrease in blood flow may lead to hypoxic tissue injury, depending on the degree and duration of cold exposure. Injury from freezing probably results from a combination of ice crystal formation and vasoconstriction. The decreased blood flow leads to capillary stasis and arteriolar and capillary thrombosis.

Electrical Injuries. Electrical forces can affect the body through extensive tissue injury and disruption of neural and cardiac impulses. The effect of electricity on the body is mainly determined by its voltage, the type of current (*i.e.,* direct or alternating), its amperage, the resistance of the intervening tissue, the pathway of the current, and the duration of exposure.[4–6]

Lightning and high-voltage wires that carry several thousand volts produce the most severe damage. Alternating current (AC) is usually more dangerous than direct current (DC) because it causes violent muscle contractions, preventing the person from releasing the electrical source and sometimes resulting in fractures and dislocations. In electrical injuries, the body acts as a conductor of the electrical current. The current enters the body from an electrical source, such as an exposed wire, and passes through the body and exits to another conductor, such as the moisture on the ground or a piece of metal the person is holding. The pathway that a current takes is critical because the electrical energy disrupts impulses in excitable tissues. Current flow through the brain may interrupt impulses from respiratory centers in the brain stem, and current flow through the chest may cause fatal cardiac arrhythmias.

The resistance to the flow of current in electrical circuits transforms electrical energy into heat. Much of the tissue damage produced by electrical injuries is caused by heat production in tissues that have the highest electrical resistance.[4–6] Resistance to electrical current varies from the greatest to the least in bone, fat, tendons, skin, muscles, blood, and nerves. The most severe tissue injury usually occurs at the skin sites where the current enters and leaves the body (Fig. 2-5). After electricity has penetrated the skin, it passes rapidly through the body along the lines of least resistance—through body fluids and nerves. Degeneration of vessel walls may occur, and thrombi may form as current flows along the blood vessels. This can cause extensive muscle and deep tissue injury. Thick, dry skin is more resistant to the flow of electricity than thin, wet skin. It is generally believed that the greater the skin resistance, the greater is the amount of local skin burn, and the less the resistance, the greater are the deep and systemic effects.

Chemical Agents and Drugs

Chemicals capable of damaging cells are everywhere around us. Air and water pollution contain chemicals capable of tissue injury, as do tobacco smoke and some processed or preserved foods. Chemical agents can injure

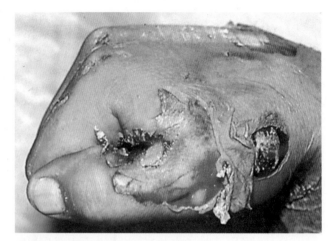

FIGURE 2-5 Electrical burn of the skin. The victim was electrocuted after attempting to stop a fall from a ladder by grasping a high-voltage line. (From Rubin E., Gorstein E., Rubin R., et al. [2005]. *Rubin's pathology: Clinicopathologic foundations of medicine* [4th ed., p. 337]. Philadelphia: Lippincott Williams & Wilkins.)

the cell membrane and other cell structures, block enzymatic pathways, coagulate cell proteins, and disrupt the osmotic and ionic balance of the cell. Corrosive substances such as strong acids and bases destroy cells as the substances come into contact with the body. Other chemicals may injure cells in the process of metabolism or elimination. For example, carbon tetrachloride (CCl_4) causes little damage until it is metabolized by liver enzymes to a highly reactive free radical ($CCl_3\cdot$). Carbon tetrachloride is extremely toxic to liver cells.

Some of the most damaging chemicals exist in our environment, including gases such as carbon monoxide, insecticides, and trace metals such as lead. Lead is a particularly toxic metal. Small amounts accumulate to reach toxic levels.[4,5,7] There are innumerable sources of lead in the environment, including flaking paint, lead-contaminated dust and soil, lead-contaminated root vegetables, lead water pipes or soldered joints, pottery glazes, and newsprint. Children are exposed to lead through ingestion of peeling lead paint, by breathing dust from lead paint (*e.g.,* during remodeling), or from playing in contaminated soil.[7] Lead crosses the placenta, exposing the fetus to lead levels comparable with those of the mother. The toxicity of lead is related to its multiple biochemical effects. It has the ability to inactivate enzymes, compete with calcium for incorporation into bone, and interfere with nerve transmission and brain development. The major targets are the red blood cells, the gastrointestinal tract, the kidneys, and the nervous system.[4,5,7] Some of the manifestations of lead toxicity include anemia, acute abdominal pain, signs of kidney damage, and cognitive deficits and neuropathies resulting from demyelination of cerebral and cerebellar white matter and death of cortical nerve cells.

Many drugs—alcohol, prescription drugs, over-the-counter drugs, and street drugs—also are capable of directly or indirectly damaging tissues. Ethyl alcohol can harm the gastric mucosa, liver (see Chapter 29), developing fetus (see Chapter 4), and other organs. Antineoplastic (anticancer) and immunosuppressant drugs can directly injure cells. Other drugs produce metabolic end-products that are toxic to cells. Acetaminophen, a commonly used analgesic drug, is detoxified in the liver, where small amounts of the drug are converted to a highly toxic metabolite.[4,5] This metabolite is detoxified by a metabolic pathway that uses a substance (i.e., glutathione) normally present in the liver. When large amounts of the drug are ingested, this pathway becomes overwhelmed and toxic metabolites accumulate, causing massive liver necrosis.

Biologic Agents

Biologic agents differ from other injurious agents in that they are able to replicate and can continue to produce their injurious effects. These agents range from submicroscopic viruses to the larger parasites. Biologic agents injure cells by diverse mechanisms. Viruses enter the cell and become incorporated into its deoxyribonucleic acid (DNA) synthetic machinery. Certain bacteria elaborate exotoxins that interfere with cellular production of ATP. Other bacteria, such as the gram-negative bacilli, release endotoxins that cause cell injury and increased capillary permeability.

Ionizing Radiation

Ionizing radiation affects cells by causing ionization of molecules and atoms in the cell, by directly hitting the target molecules in the cell, or by producing free radicals that interact with critical cell components.[4,5] It can immediately kill cells, interrupt cell replication, or cause a variety of genetic mutations, which may or may not be lethal. Most radiation injury is caused by localized irradiation that is used in the treatment of cancer (see Chapter 5).

The injurious effects of ionizing radiation vary with the dose, the dose rate (a single dose can cause greater injury than divided or fractionated doses), and the differential sensitivity of the exposed tissue to radiation injury. Because of the effect on DNA synthesis and interference with mitosis, rapidly dividing cells of the bone marrow and intestine are much more vulnerable to radiation injury than are tissues such as bone and skeletal muscle. Over time, occupational and accidental exposure to ionizing radiation can result in increased risk for the development of various types of cancers, including skin cancers, leukemia, osteogenic sarcomas, and lung cancer.

Many of the manifestations of radiation therapy result from acute cell injury, dose-dependent changes in the blood vessels that supply the irradiated tissues, and fibrotic tissue replacement. The cell's initial response to radiation injury involves swelling, disruption of the mitochondria and other organelles, alterations in the cell membrane, and marked changes in the nucleus. The endothelial cells in blood vessels are particularly sensitive to irradiation as evidenced by the vessel dilation (e.g., the initial erythema of the skin after radiation therapy) that occurs during the immediate postirradiation period. Later or with higher levels of radiation, destructive changes occur in small blood vessels such as the capillaries and venules. Acute reversible necrosis is represented by such disorders as radiation cystitis, dermatitis, and diarrhea from enteritis. More persistent damage can be attributed to acute necrosis of tissue cells that are not capable of regeneration and chronic ischemia. Chronic effects of radiation damage are characterized by fibrosis and scarring of tissues and organs in the irradiated area (e.g., interstitial fibrosis of the heart and lungs after irradiation of the chest). Because the radiation delivered in radiation therapy inevitably travels through the skin, radiation dermatitis is common. There may be necrosis of the skin, impaired wound healing, and chronic radiation dermatitis.

Nutritional Imbalances

Nutritional excesses and nutritional deficiencies predispose cells to injury. Obesity and diets high in saturated fats are thought to predispose persons to atherosclerosis. The body requires more than 60 organic and inorganic substances in amounts ranging from micrograms to grams. These nutrients include minerals, vitamins, certain fatty acids, and specific amino acids. Dietary deficiencies can occur in the form of starvation, in which there is a deficiency of all nutrients and vitamins, or because of a selective deficiency of a single nutrient or vitamin. Iron-deficiency anemia, scurvy, beriberi, and pellagra are examples of injury caused by the lack of specific vitamins or minerals. The protein and calorie deficiencies that occur with starvation cause widespread tissue damage.

MECHANISMS OF CELL INJURY

The mechanisms by which injurious agents cause cell injury and death are complex. Some agents, such as heat, produce direct cell injury; other factors, such as genetic derangement, produce their effects indirectly through metabolic disturbances and altered immune responses. There seem to be at least three major mechanisms whereby most injurious agents exert their effects: depletion of ATP, free radical formation, and disruption of intracellular calcium homeostasis.

Depletion of ATP

ATP depletion and decreased ATP synthesis are associated with hypoxia and chemical (toxic) cell injury. High-energy phosphate in the form of ATP is required for many synthetic and degradative processes in the cells. One of the earliest effects of reduced ATP is acute cellular swelling caused by failure of the energy-dependent Na^+/K^+ ATPase membrane pump, which extrudes sodium from and returns potassium to the cell.[1,2] With impaired function of this pump, intracellular potassium levels decrease, and sodium and water accumulate in the cell. The movement of fluid and ions into the cell is associated with dilation of the endoplasmic reticulum, increased membrane permeability, and decreased mitochondrial function. To this point, the cellular changes caused by ischemia are reversible if oxygenation is restored. However, if the oxygen supply is not restored, there is a continued loss of essential enzymes, proteins, and ribonucleic acid through the hyperpermeable membrane of the cell. Injury to the lysosomal membranes results in leakage of destructive lysosomal enzymes into the cytoplasm and enzymatic digestion of cell components. Many of the intracellular enzymes that leak into the extracellular fluids can be measured by laboratory tests. Because cells from different tissues have their own particular type of enzymes, the type and level of serum enzymes provide valuable diagnostic information regarding the site and extent of tissue injury.

Free Radical Injury

Many injurious agents exert their damaging effects through a reactive chemical species called a *free radical*.[1,2,8–13] In most atoms, the outer electron orbits are filled with paired electrons moving in opposite directions to balance their spins. A free radical is a highly reactive chemical species arising from an atom that has a single unpaired electron in an outer orbit. In this state, the radical is highly unstable and can enter into reactions with cellular constituents, particularly key molecules in cell membranes and nucleic acids. Moreover, free radicals can establish chain reactions, sometimes thousands of events long, as the molecules they react with in turn form free radicals. Chain reactions may branch, causing even greater damage. Uncontrolled free radical production causes damage to cell membranes, cross-linking of cell proteins, inactivation of enzyme systems, or damage to the nucleic acids that make up DNA.

Free radical formation is a byproduct of many normal cellular reactions in the body, including energy generation, breakdown of lipids and proteins, and inflammatory processes (Fig. 2-6). For example, free radical generation is the main mechanism for killing microbes by phagocytic white blood cells. Molecular oxygen (O_2) with its two unpaired outer electrons is the main source of free radicals. During the course of normal respiration, molecular oxygen is sequentially reduced in the mitochondria by the addition of four electrons to produce water. During the process, small amounts of partially reduced intermediate species are converted to free radicals by oxidative enzymes in the cytoplasm, endoplasmic reticulum, mitochondria, plasma membrane, lysosomes, and peroxisomes. These reactive species include the superoxide anion (O_2^-), hydrogen peroxide (H_2O_2), and hydroxyl radical ($\cdot OH$). Transition metals such as copper and iron, which can accept or donate free electrons during intracellular reactions, are also a source of free radicals.

Although the effects of these reactive species are wide-ranging, three types of effects are particularly important in cell injury: lipid peroxidation, oxidative modification of proteins, and DNA effects (Fig. 2-7). Destruction of the phospholipids in cell membranes, including the outer plasma membrane and those of the intracellular organelles, results in loss of membrane integrity. Free radical attack on cell proteins, particularly those of critical enzymes, can interrupt vital processes throughout the cell. DNA is an important target of the hydroxyl free radical. Damage can involve single-stranded breaks in DNA, modification of base pairs, and cross-links between strands. In most cases, various DNA repair pathways can repair the damage. However, if the damage is extensive, the cell dies. The effects of free radical–mediated DNA changes have also been implicated in aging and malignant transformation of cells.

Under normal conditions, most cells have chemical mechanisms that protect them from the injurious effects of free radicals. These mechanisms commonly break down when the cell is deprived of oxygen or exposed to certain chemical agents, radiation, or other injurious agents. Free radical formation is a particular threat to tissues in which the blood flow has been interrupted and then restored.[10] During the period of interrupted flow, the

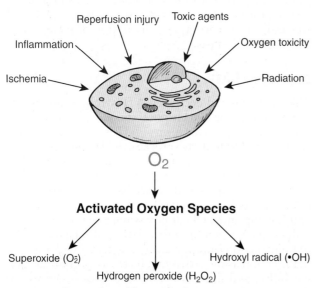

FIGURE 2-6 Generation of free radicals.

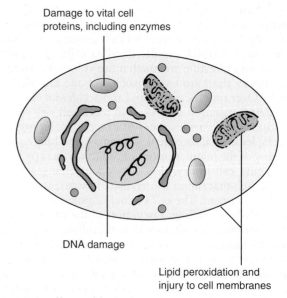

FIGURE 2-7 Effects of free radical cell damage.

intracellular mechanisms that control free radicals are inactivated or damaged. When blood flow is restored, the cell is suddenly confronted with an excess of free radicals that it cannot control.

Scientists continue to investigate the use of free radical scavengers to protect against cell injury during periods when protective cellular mechanisms are impaired. Defenses against free radicals include vitamins E and A as well as ascorbic acid.[1,2] Vitamin E is the major lipid-soluble antioxidant present in all cellular membranes. Retinoids, the precursors of vitamin A, are lipid soluble, and act as chain-breaking antioxidants. Vitamin C is an important water-soluble, cytosolic, chain-breaking antioxidant; it acts directly with superoxide and singlet oxygen radicals.

Impaired Calcium Homeostasis

Calcium functions as a messenger for the release of many intracellular enzymes. Normally, intracellular calcium levels are kept extremely low compared with extracellular levels. These low intracellular levels are maintained by energy-dependent, membrane-associated calcium/magnesium (Ca^{2+}/Mg^{2+}) ATPase exchange systems.[1,2] Ischemia and certain toxins lead to an increase in cytosolic calcium because of increased influx across the cell membrane and the release of calcium stored in the mitochondria and endoplasmic reticulum. The increased calcium level activates a number of enzymes with potentially damaging effects. The enzymes include the phospholipases, which are responsible for damaging the phospholipids in the cell membrane; the proteases, which damage the cytoskeleton and membrane proteins; ATPase, which breaks down ATP and hastens its depletion; and the endonucleases, which fragment chromatin.

CELL DEATH

In each cell line, the control of cell number is regulated by a balance of cell proliferation and cell death. Cell death can involve apoptosis or necrosis. Apoptotic cell death involves controlled cell destruction and is involved in normal cell deletion and renewal. For example, blood cells that undergo constant renewal from progenitor cells in the bone marrow are removed by apoptotic cell death. By contrast, necrotic cell death is a pathologic form of cell death that is unregulated and invariably injurious to the organism. It may result from a number of insults to cell integrity, including ischemia, extremes of temperature, and toxins. It is characterized by cell swelling, rupture of the cell membrane, and inflammation.

Apoptosis

Apoptosis, from Greek *apo* for "apart" and *ptosis* for "fallen," means "fallen apart." Apoptotic cell death, which is equated with cell suicide, eliminates cells that are worn out, have been produced in excess, have developed improperly, or have genetic damage. In normal cell turnover, this process provides the space needed for cell replacement. The process, which was first described in

1972, has become one of the most vigorously investigated processes in biology.[1,2,14–17]

Apoptotic cell death is induced by a tightly regulated intracellular program in which cells destined to die activate enzymes that degrade the cells' own nuclear DNA and cytoplasmic proteins. The cell's plasma membrane remains intact, but its structure is altered in such a way that the apoptotic cell becomes an avid target for phagocytosis (Fig. 2-8). The dead cell is rapidly cleared before its contents have leaked out; therefore, cell death by this pathway does not elicit an inflammatory response.

Apoptosis is induced by a cascade of molecular events that may be induced by a number of different stimuli and propagated by a family of proteases called *caspases.* The process of apoptosis may be divided into an *initiation phase,* during which the caspases become activated, and an *execution phase,* during which they act to cause cell death. Initiation of apoptosis occurs principally by signals from two pathways: the extrinsic, or receptor-initiated, pathway and the intrinsic, or mitochondrial, pathway. Both pathways converge to activate caspases. The extrinsic pathway is initiated by the engagement of cell surface receptors on a variety of cells. These transmembrane receptor proteins have amino acid sequences, termed *death domains,* on the cytoplasmic side of the cell membrane that participate in the signaling process leading to apoptosis. The intrinsic pathway involves the mitochondrial membrane and proapoptotic or antiapoptotic signaling proteins. Activation of the tumor-suppressor p53 gene by DNA damage or other means also initiates apoptosis through the mitochondria. The p53 gene plays a pivotal role in the life–death cycle of a cell. It preserves the viability of an injured cell when DNA damage can be repaired and it propels the cell toward apoptosis when irreparable harm has occurred.

Apoptosis is thought to be responsible for several normal physiologic processes, including programmed destruction of cells during embryonic development; hormone-dependent involution of tissues; removal of proliferating cell populations, such as those of the intestinal epithelia,

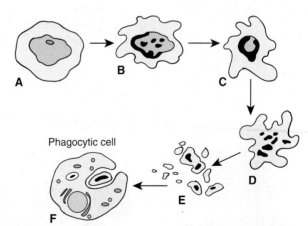

FIGURE 2-8 Apoptotic cell removal: (**A**) shrinking of the cell structures, (**B** and **C**) condensation and fragmentation of the nuclear chromatin, (**D** and **E**) separation of nuclear fragments and cytoplasmic organelles into apoptotic bodies, and (**F**) engulfment of apoptotic fragments by phagocytic cell.

to maintain a constant number; death of host cells that have served their useful purpose, such as the neutrophils in an acute inflammatory process; and elimination of potentially harmful self-reactive lymphocytes. During embryogenesis, in the development of a number of organs such as the heart, which begins as a single pulsating tube and is gradually modified to become a four-chambered pump, apoptotic cell death allows the next stage of organ development. It also separates the webbed fingers and toes of the developing embryo (Fig. 2-9). The control of immune cell numbers and destruction of autoreactive T cells in the thymus have been credited to apoptosis. Cytotoxic T cells and natural killer cells are thought to destroy target cells by inducing apoptotic cell death. Apoptotic cell death occurs in the hormone-dependent involution of endometrial cells during the menstrual cycle and in the regression of breast tissue after weaning from breast-feeding.

Apoptosis has also been linked to a number of pathologic processes. For example, suppression of apoptosis may be a determinant in the growth of cancers (see Chapter 5). Apoptosis is also thought to be involved in the cell death associated with certain viral infections, such as hepatitis B and C, and in cell death caused by a variety of injurious agents, such as mild thermal injury and radiation injury. Apoptosis may also be involved in neurodegenerative disorders manifested by an excessive loss of specific sets of neurons, such as in spinal muscular atrophy.[1] The loss of cells in these disorders does not induce inflammation; although the initiating event is unknown, apoptosis appears to be the mechanism of cell death.[16] As in the case of programmed cell death, the signals that induce apoptosis may be the lack of a growth factor or hormone, specific engagement of death receptors, or exposure to an injurious agent. In hepatitis B and C, the virus seems to sensitize the hepatocytes to apoptosis.[17]

Necrosis

Necrosis refers to cell death in an organ or tissue that is still part of a living person.[2] Necrosis differs from apoptosis in that it involves unregulated enzymatic digestion of cell components, loss of cell membrane integrity with uncontrolled release of the products of cell death into the intracellular space, and initiation of the inflammatory response.[18] In contrast to apoptosis, which functions to remove cells so they can be replaced by new cells, necrosis often interferes with cell replacement and tissue regeneration.

With necrotic cell death, there are marked changes in the appearance of the cytoplasmic contents and the nucleus. These changes often are not visible, even under the microscope, for hours after cell death. The dissolution of the necrotic cell or tissue can follow several paths. The cell can undergo liquefaction (*i.e.,* liquefaction necrosis); it can be transformed to a gray, firm mass (*i.e.,* coagulation necrosis); or it can be converted to a cheesy material by infiltration of fatlike substances (*i.e.,* caseous necrosis). *Liquefaction necrosis* occurs when some of the cells die but their catalytic enzymes are not destroyed. An example of liquefaction necrosis is the softening of the center of an abscess with discharge of its contents. During *coagulation necrosis,* acidosis develops and denatures the enzymatic and structural proteins of the cell. This type of necrosis is characteristic of hypoxic injury and is seen in infarcted areas. *Infarction (i.e.,* tissue death) occurs when

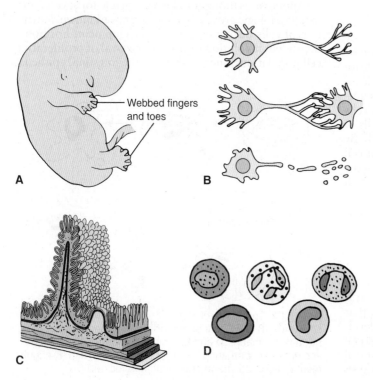

FIGURE 2-9 Examples of apoptosis: (**A**) separation of webbed fingers and toes in embryo, (**B**) development of neural connections, (**C**) removal of cells from intestinal villa, and (**D**) removal of senescent blood cells.

an artery supplying an organ or part of the body becomes occluded and no other source of blood supply exists. As a rule, the infarct's shape is conical and corresponds to the distribution of the artery and its branches. An artery may be occluded by an embolus, a thrombus, disease of the arterial wall, or pressure from outside the vessel. *Caseous necrosis* (*i.e.*, soft, cheeselike center) is a distinctive form of coagulation necrosis. It is most commonly associated with tubercular lesions and is thought to result from immune mechanisms.

Gangrene. The term *gangrene* is applied when a considerable mass of tissue undergoes necrosis. Gangrene may be classified as dry or moist. In dry gangrene, the part becomes dry and shrinks, the skin wrinkles, and its color changes to dark brown or black. The spread of dry gangrene is slow, and its symptoms are not as marked as those of wet gangrene. The irritation caused by the dead tissue produces a line of inflammatory reaction (*i.e.*, line of demarcation) between the dead tissue of the gangrenous area and the healthy tissue (Fig. 2-10). Dry gangrene usually results from interference with arterial blood supply to a part without interference with venous return and is a form of coagulation necrosis.

In moist or wet gangrene, the area is cold, swollen, and pulseless. The skin is moist, black, and under tension. Blebs form on the surface, liquefaction occurs, and a foul odor is caused by bacterial action. There is no line of demarcation between the normal and diseased tissues, and the spread of tissue damage is rapid. Systemic symptoms are usually severe, and death may occur unless the condition can be arrested. Moist or wet gangrene primarily results from interference with venous return from the part. Bacterial invasion plays an important role in the development of wet gangrene and is responsible for many of its prominent symptoms. Dry gangrene is confined almost exclusively to the extremities, but moist gangrene may affect the internal organs or the extremities. If bacteria invade the necrotic tissue, dry gangrene may be converted to wet gangrene.

Gas gangrene is a special type of gangrene that results from infection of devitalized tissues by one of several species of *Clostridium* bacteria. These anaerobic and spore-forming organisms are widespread in nature, particularly in soil; gas gangrene is prone to occur in trauma and compound fractures in which dirt and debris are embedded. Some species have been isolated in the stomach, gallbladder, intestine, vagina, and skin of healthy persons. The bacteria produce toxins that dissolve the cell membranes, causing death of muscle cells, massive spreading edema, hemolysis of red blood cells, hemolytic anemia, hemoglobinuria, and renal toxicity.[19] Characteristic of this disorder are the bubbles of hydrogen sulfide gas that form in the muscle. Gas gangrene is a serious and potentially fatal disease. Because the organism is anaerobic, oxygen is sometimes administered in a hyperbaric chamber.

In summary, cell injury can be caused by a number of agents. Among the physical agents that generate cell injury are mechanical forces that produce tissue trauma, extremes of temperature, electricity, radiation, and nutritional disorders. Chemical agents can cause cell injury through several mechanisms: they can block enzymatic pathways, cause coagulation of tissues, or disrupt the osmotic or ionic balance of the cell. Ionizing radiation affects cells by causing ionization of molecules and atoms in the cell, by directly hitting the target molecules in the cell, or by producing free radicals that interact with critical cell components. Biologic agents differ from other injurious agents in that they are able to replicate and continue to produce injury. Among the nutritional factors that contribute to cell injury are excesses and deficiencies of nutrients, vitamins, and minerals.

Injurious agents exert their effects largely through the production of cell hypoxia, generation of free radicals, and unregulated intracellular calcium levels. Lack of oxygen underlies the pathogenesis of cell injury in hypoxia and ischemia. Hypoxia can result from inadequate oxygen in the air, cardiorespiratory disease, anemia, or the inability of the cells to use oxygen. Partially reduced oxygen species called *free radicals* are important mediators of cell injury in many pathologic conditions. They are an important cause of cell injury in hypoxia and after exposure to radiation and certain chemical agents. Increased intracellular calcium activates a number of enzymes with potentially damaging effects.

Injurious agents may produce sublethal and reversible cellular damage or may lead to irreversible cell injury and death. Cell death can involve two mechanisms: apoptosis or necrosis. Apoptosis involves controlled cell destruction and is the means by which the body removes and replaces cells that have been produced in excess, developed improperly, have genetic damage, or are worn out. Necrosis refers to cell death that is characterized by cell swelling, rupture of the cell membrane, and inflammation.

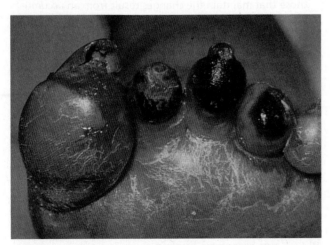

FIGURE 2-10 Gangrenous toes. (Biomedical Communications Group, Southern Illinois University School of Medicine, Springfield, IL.)

Cellular Aging

Although the causes of aging are obscure, there is general consensus that its elucidation should be sought at the cellular level. A number of cell functions decline with age. Oxidative phosphorylation by the mitochondria is reduced, as is synthesis of nucleic acids and structural and enzymatic proteins, cell receptors, and transcription factors. At the functional level, there is a decline in muscular strength, cardiac reserve, nerve conduction time, vital capacity, glomerular filtration rate, and vascular elasticity.[1]

Theories formulated to explain the aging processes have been grouped into several categories, some of the most widely used being the programmed change and stochastic, or error, theories.[20-23] The programmed change theories propose that aging changes are genetically programmed, whereas stochastic or error theories maintain that the changes result from an accumulation of random events or damage from environmental agents or influences. It is accepted now that the process of aging and longevity is multifaceted, with both genetic and environmental factors playing a role.

PROGRAMMED CHANGE THEORIES

The programmed change theories focus on genetic influences that determine physical condition, occurrence of disease, age of death, cause of death, and other factors contributing to longevity. A straightforward theory of programmed cell senescence envisions the activation of a particular gene (or genes) after a number of cell divisions. Hayflick and Moorhead observed more than 35 years ago that cultured human fibroblasts have a limited ability to replicate (approximately 50 population doublings) before dying.[20] As they approach this maximum, the cells slow their rate of division and manifest identifiable and predictable morphologic changes characteristic of senescent cells.

Werner syndrome is an autosomally inherited disease, evidenced by premature development of atherosclerosis, glucose intolerance, osteoporosis, early graying, loss of hair, skin atrophy, and menopause. Most persons with Werner syndrome die in the fifth decade of either cancer or cardiovascular disease.[1] The gene responsible for the disorder has been localized to chromosome 8 and appears to code for an enzyme involved in unwinding DNA, a process that is necessary for DNA repair and replication.[1,22]

ERROR THEORIES

The stochastic, or error, theories propose that aging is caused by random damage to vital cell molecules.[5] The damage eventually accumulates to a level sufficient to result in the physiologic decline associated with aging. The most prominent example of the stochastic theory is the somatic mutation theory of aging, which states that the longevity and function of cells in various tissues of the body are determined by the double-stranded DNA molecule and its specific repair enzymes. DNA undergoes continuous change in response both to exogenous agents and intrinsic processes. It has been suggested that aging results from conditions that produce mutations in DNA or deficits in DNA repair mechanisms.

The oxidative free radical explanation of aging is a stochastic theory in which aging is thought to result partially from oxidative metabolism and the effects of free radical damage. The major byproducts of oxidative metabolism include superoxides that react with DNA, ribonucleic acid, proteins, and lipids, leading to cellular damage and aging. Another damage theory, the wear and tear theory, proposes that accumulated damage to vital parts of the cell leads to aging and death. Cellular DNA is cited as an example. If repair to damaged DNA is incomplete or defective, as is thought to occur with aging, declines in cellular function might occur.

Another explanation of cellular aging resides with an enzyme called *telomerase* that is believed to govern chromosomal aging through its action on telomeres, the outermost extremities of the chromosome arms. The telomeres are not replicated with the rest of the genome but are enzymatically added to the ends of the chromosome by the telomerase enzyme. Unless a cell has a constant supply of telomerase, a small segment of telomeric DNA is lost with each cell division. In the absence of telomerase, the telomeres shorten, resulting in senescence-associated decline in gene expression and inhibition of cell replication. Currently, there is interest in developing telomerase therapy that could be used to initiate cell death in selected targets, such as cancer cells, and to prevent cell senescence in other cell types, such as chondrocytes in joints, retinal epithelial cells in the eye, and lymphocytes in the immune system.

In summary, a number of cell functions decline with age. Oxidative phosphorylation by the mitochondria is reduced, as is synthesis of nucleic acids and structural and enzymatic proteins, cell receptors, and transcription factors. The theories of cellular aging include those that propose the changes are genetically programmed and those that maintain the changes result from an accumulation of random events or damage from environmental influences.

Review Exercises

A 30-year-old man sustained a fracture of his leg 2 months ago. The leg has been encased in a cast and he has just had the cast removed. He is amazed at the degree to which the muscles in his leg have shrunk.

A. Would you consider this to be a normal adaptive response? Explain.
B. Will these changes have an immediate/long-term effect on the function of the leg?

C. What type of measures can be taken to restore full function to the leg?

A 45-year-old woman has been receiving radiation therapy for breast cancer.

A. Explain the effects of ionizing radiation in eradicating the tumor cells.
B. Why is the radiation treatment given in small divided, or fractionated, doses rather than as a single large dose?
C. Part way through the treatment schedule, the woman notices that her skin over the irradiated area has become reddened and irritated. What is the reason for this?

People who have had a heart attack may experience additional damage once blood flow has been restored, a phenomenon referred to as *reperfusion injury*.

A. What is the proposed mechanism underlying reperfusion injury?
B. What factors might influence this mechanism?

Every day blood cells in our body become senescent and die without producing signs of inflammation; yet, massive injury or destruction of tissue, such as occurs with a heart attack, produces significant signs of inflammation.

A. Explain.

Visit the Porth: Essentials of Pathophysiology: Concepts of Altered Health States web site (http://thePoint.LWW.com/PorthEssentials) for links to chapter-related resources on the Internet, all-new exclusive animations, chapter review questions, and more!

REFERENCES

1. Rubin E., Strayer D. S. (2005). Cell injury. In Rubin E., Gorstein F., Rubin R., et al. (Eds.), *Rubin's pathology: Clinicopathologic foundations of medicine* (4th ed., pp. 3–39). Philadelphia: Lippincott Williams & Wilkins.
2. Kumar V., Abbas A. K., Fausto N. (2005). *Robbins and Cotran pathologic basis of disease* (7th ed., pp. 3–46). Philadelphia: Elsevier Saunders.
3. Hunter J. J., Chien K. R. (1999). Signaling pathways in cardiac hypertrophy and failure. *New England Journal of Medicine* 341, 1276–1283.
4. Rubin E., Strayer D. S. (2005). Environmental and nutritional pathology. In Rubin E., Gorstein F., Rubin R., et al. (Eds.), *Rubin's pathology: Clinicopathologic foundations of medicine* (4th ed., pp. 313–335). Philadelphia: Lippincott Williams & Wilkins.
5. Kane A. B., Kumar V. (2005). Environmental and nutritional pathology. In Kumar V., Abbas A. K., Fausto N. (Eds.), *Robbins and Cotran pathologic basis of disease* (7th ed., pp. 3–46). Philadelphia: Elsevier Saunders.
6. Koumbourlis A. G. (2002). Electrical injury. *Critical Care Medicine* 30(Suppl.), S424–S430.
7. Markowitz M. (2004). Lead poisoning. In Behrman R. E., Kliegman R. M., Jenson H. B. (Eds.), *Nelson textbook of pediatrics* (17th ed., pp. 2359–2362). Philadelphia: W. B. Saunders.
8. McCord J. M. (2000). The evolution of free radicals and oxidative stress. *American Journal of Medicine* 108, 652–659.
9. Kerr M. E., Bender C. M., Monti E. J. (1996). An introduction to oxygen free radicals. *Heart and Lung* 25, 200–209.
10. Li C., Jackson R. M. (2002). Reactive species mechanisms of cellular hypoxia-reoxygenation injury. *American Journal of Physiology, Cell Physiology* 282, C227–C241.
11. Martindale J. L., Holbrook N. J. (2002). Cellular response to oxidative stress: Signaling for suicide and survival. *Journal of Cell Physiology* 192, 1–15.
12. Betteridge D. J. (2000). What is oxidative stress? *Metabolism* 49(2), 3–8.
13. Dröge W. (2002). Free radicals in the physiological control of cell function. *Physiological Reviews* 82, 47–95.
14. Lawen A. (2003). Apoptosis: An introduction. *Bioessays* 25, 888–896.
15. Skikumar P., Dong Z., Mikhailov V., et. al. (1999). Apoptosis: Definitions, mechanisms, and relevance to disease. *American Journal of Medicine* 107, 490–505.
16. Thompson C. B. (1995). Apoptosis in the pathogenesis and treatment of disease. *Science* 267, 1456–1462.
17. Rust C., Gores G. J. (2000). Apoptosis and liver disease. *American Journal of Medicine* 108, 568–575.
18. Proskuryakov S. Y., Konoplyannikov A. G., Gabai V. L. (2003). Necrosis: A specific form of programmed death. *Experimental Cell Research* 283, 1–16.
19. Corry M., Montoya L. (1990). Gas gangrene: Certain diagnosis or certain death. *Critical Care Nursing* 9(10), 30–38.
20. Weinert B., Timiras P. S. (2003). Invited review: Theories of aging. *Journal of Applied Physiology* 95, 1706–1716.
21. Dice J. F. (1993). Cellular and molecular mechanisms of aging. *Physiological Reviews* 73, 149–159.
22. Troen B. R. (2003). The biology of aging. *Mount Sinai Journal of Medicine* 70, 3–22.
23. Ben-Porath I., Weinberg R. A. (2004). When cells get stressed: An integrative view of cellular senescence. *Journal of Clinical Investigation* 113, 8–13.

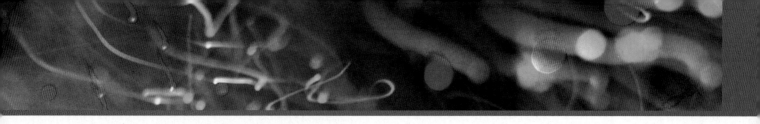

C h a p t e r *3*

Genetic Control of Cell Function and Inheritance

 Our genetic information is found in the nucleus of each cell stored in the structure of *deoxyribonucleic acid* (DNA). The term *gene* is used to describe a part of the DNA molecule that contains the information needed to code for the types of proteins and enzymes needed for the day-to-day function of the cells in the body. For example, genes control the type and quantity of hormones a cell produces, the antigens and receptors present on the cell membrane, and the synthesis of enzymes necessary for metabolism. In addition, a gene is the unit of heredity passed from generation to generation. This chapter includes discussions of genetic regulation of cell function, chromosomal structure, patterns of inheritance, and gene technology.

Genetic Control of Cell Function

The genetic information needed for protein synthesis is encoded in the DNA contained in the cell nucleus. A second type of nucleic acid, *ribonucleic acid* (RNA), is involved in the actual synthesis of cellular enzymes and proteins. Cells contain several types of RNA: messenger RNA, transfer RNA, and ribosomal RNA. *Messenger RNA* (mRNA) contains the transcribed instructions for protein synthesis obtained from the DNA molecule and carries them into the cytoplasm. Transcription is followed by translation, the synthesis of proteins according to the instructions carried by mRNA. *Ribosomal RNA* (rRNA) provides the machinery needed for protein synthesis. *Transfer RNA* (tRNA) reads the instructions and delivers the appropriate amino acids to the ribosome, where they are incorporated into the protein being synthesized.

The nuclei of all the cells in an organism contain the same accumulation of genes derived from the gametes (ovum and sperm) of the two parents. This means that liver cells contain the same genetic information as skin and

Understanding ➤ DNA-Directed Protein Synthesis

Deoxyribonucleic acid (DNA) directs the synthesis of the many thousands of proteins that are contained in the different cells of the body. While some of the proteins are structural proteins, the majority are enzymes that catalyze the different chemical reactions in the cell. Because DNA is located in the cell's nucleus and protein synthesis takes place in the cytoplasm, a second type of nucleic acid—ribonucleic acid (RNA)—participates in the actual assembly of the proteins. There are three types of RNA: messenger RNA (mRNA), ribosomal RNA (rRNA), and transfer RNA (tRNA) that participate in (1) the transcription of the DNA instructions for protein synthesis and (2) the translation of those instructions into the assembly of the polypeptides that make up the various proteins.

1

Transcription. Transcription involves copying of the genetic code containing the instructions for protein synthesis from DNA to a complementary strand of mRNA. The genetic code is a successive sequence of four bases (adenine [A], thymine [T], guanine [G], and cytosine [C], with thymine in DNA being replaced by uracil [U] in RNA) that control the sequence of amino acids in a protein molecule that is being synthesized in a cell. Once mRNA has transcribed the genetic code for the amino acids used in the synthesis of a protein, it detaches from DNA and diffuses through the nuclear pores into the cytoplasm, where it controls the assembly of the protein.

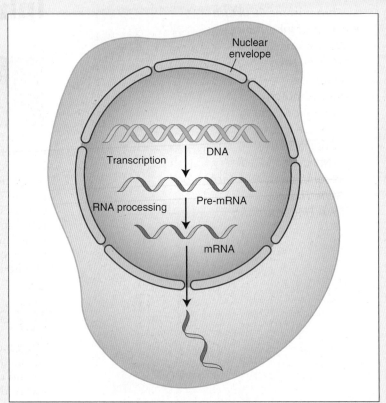

muscle cells. For this to be true, the molecular code must be duplicated before each succeeding cell division, or mitosis. Each particular cell type in a tissue uses only part of the information stored in the genetic code. Although information required for the development and differentiation of the other cell types is still present, it is repressed.

Besides DNA located in the nucleus, part of the DNA of a cell resides outside of the nucleus in the mitochondria (see Chapter 4). Mitochondrial DNA is inherited from the mother by her offspring (*i.e.*, matrilineal inheritance). Several genetic disorders are attributed to defects in mitochondrial DNA. Leber hereditary optic neuropathy was the first human disease attributed to mutation in mitochondrial DNA.

GENE STRUCTURE

The structure that stores the genetic information in the nucleus is a long, double-stranded, helical molecule of DNA. DNA is composed of *nucleotides*, which consist of phosphoric acid, a five-carbon sugar called *deoxyribose*, and one of four nitrogenous bases. These nitrogenous bases carry the genetic information and are divided into two groups: the *purine bases*, adenine and guanine, which

2

Translation. The process of translation involves taking the instructions transcribed from DNA to mRNA and transferring them to the rRNA of ribosomes located in the cytoplasm. When the mRNA carrying the instructions for a particular protein comes in contact with a ribosome, it binds to a small subunit of the rRNA. It then travels through the ribosome where the transcribed instructions are communicated to tRNA, which delivers and transfers the correct amino acid to its proper position on the growing peptide chain. There are 20 types of tRNA, one for each of the 20 different types of amino acid. Each type of tRNA carries an anticodon complementary to the mRNA codon calling for the amino acid carried by the tRNA, and it is the recognition of the mRNA codon by the tRNA anticodon that ensures the proper sequence of amino acids in a synthesized protein.

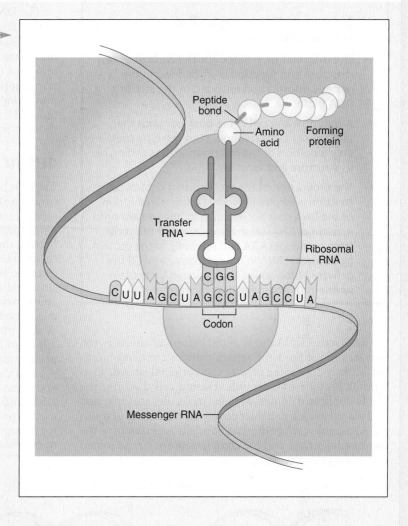

have two nitrogen ring structures, and the *pyrimidine bases,* thymine and cytosine, which have one ring. The backbone of DNA consists of alternating groups of sugar and phosphoric acid; the paired bases project inward from the sides of the sugar molecule. DNA resembles a spiral staircase, with the paired bases representing the steps (Fig. 3-1A). A precise complementary pairing of purine and pyrimidine bases, called a *base pair,* occurs in the double-stranded DNA molecule. Adenine is paired with thymine, and guanine is paired with cytosine. Each nucleotide in a pair is on one strand of the DNA molecule, bound together with the bases on the opposite DNA

strand by hydrogen bonds that are extremely stable under normal conditions. Enzymes called *DNA helicases* separate the two strands so that the genetic information can be duplicated or transcribed.

Several hundred to almost one million base pairs can represent a gene; the size is proportional to the protein product it encodes. Of the two DNA strands, only one is used in transcribing the information for the cell's polypeptide-building machinery. The genetic information of one strand is meaningful and is used as a template for transcription; the complementary code of the other strand does not make sense and is ignored. Both strands, however,

together as a double helix. In 1958, Meselson and Stahl characterized this replication of DNA as *semiconservative* as opposed to conservative (Fig. 3-2).

The DNA molecule is combined with several types of protein and small amounts of RNA into a complex known as *chromatin*. Chromatin is the readily stainable portion of the cell nucleus. Some DNA proteins form binding sites for repressor molecules and hormones that regulate genetic transcription; others may block genetic transcription by preventing access of nucleotides to the surface of the DNA molecule. A specific group of proteins called *histones* are thought to control the folding of the DNA strands.

GENETIC CODE

The four bases—guanine, adenine, cytosine, and thymine (uracil is substituted for thymine in RNA)—make up the alphabet of the genetic code. A sequence of three of these bases forms the fundamental triplet code used in transmitting the genetic information needed for protein synthesis. This triplet code is called a *codon* (Table 3-1). An example is the nucleotide sequence GCU (guanine, cytosine, and uracil), which is the triplet RNA code for the amino acid alanine. The genetic code is a universal language used by most living cells (*i.e.*, the code for the amino acid tryptophan is the same in a bacterium, a plant, and a human being). *Stop codes*, which signal the end of a protein molecule, are also present. Mathematically, the 4 bases can be arranged in 64 different combinations. Sixty-one of the triplets correspond to particular amino acids, and three are stop signals. Only 20 amino acids are used in protein synthesis in humans. Several triplets code for the same amino acid; therefore, the genetic code is said to be *redundant* or *degenerate*. For example, AUG is a

are involved in DNA duplication. Before cell division, the two strands of the helix separate and a complementary molecule is duplicated next to each original strand. Two strands become four strands. During cell division, the newly duplicated double-stranded molecules are separated and placed in each daughter cell by the mechanics of mitosis. As a result, each of the daughter cells again contains the meaningful strand and the complementary strand joined

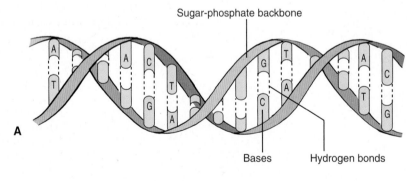

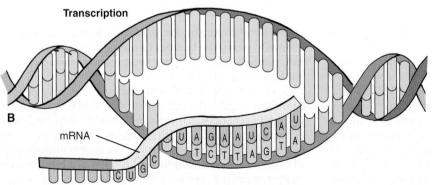

FIGURE 3-1 The DNA double helix and transcription of messenger RNA (mRNA). The top panel (**A**) shows the sequence of four bases (adenine [A], cytosine [C], guanine [G], and thymine [T]) that determines the specificity of genetic information. The bases face inward from the sugar–phosphate backbone and form pairs (*dashed lines*), with complementary bases on the opposing strand. In the bottom panel (**B**), transcription creates a complementary mRNA copy from one of the DNA strands in the double helix.

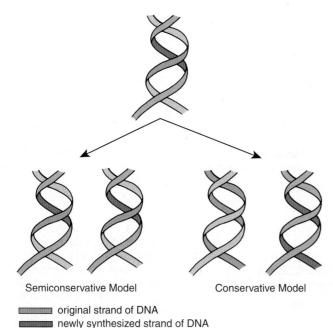

Semiconservative Model   Conservative Model

▨ original strand of DNA
▨ newly synthesized strand of DNA

FIGURE 3-2 Semiconservative vs. conservative models of DNA replication as proposed by Meselson and Stahl in 1958. In semiconservative DNA replication, the two original strands of DNA unwind and a complementary strand is formed along each original strand.

part of the initiation, or start, signal and the codon for the amino acid methionine. Codons that specify the same amino acid are called *synonyms*. Synonyms usually have the same first two bases but differ in the third base.

TABLE 3-1	Triplet Codes for Amino Acids				
Amino Acid	**RNA Codons**				
Alanine	GCU	GCC	GCA	GCG	
Arginine	CGU	CGC	CGA	CGG	AGA	AGG
Asparagine	AAU	AAC			
Aspartic acid	GAU	GAC			
Cysteine	UGU	UGC			
Glutamic acid	GAA	GAG			
Glutamine	CAA	CAG			
Glycine	GGU	GGC	GGA	GGG	
Histidine	CAU	CAC			
Isoleucine	AUU	AUC	AUA		
Leucine	CUU	CUC	CUA	CUG	UUA	UUG
Lysine	AAA	AAG			
Methionine	AUG				
Phenylalanine	UUU	UUC			
Proline	CCU	CCC	CCA	CCG	
Serine	UCU	UCC	UCA	UCG	AGC	AGU
Threonine	ACU	ACC	ACA	ACG	
Tryptophan	UGG				
Tyrosine	UAU	UAC			
Valine	GUU	GUC	GUA	GUG	
Start (CI)	AUG				
Stop (CT)	UAA	UAG	UGA		

PROTEIN SYNTHESIS

Although DNA determines the type of biochemical product that the cell synthesizes, the transmission and decoding of information needed for protein synthesis are carried out by RNA, the formation of which is directed by DNA (Fig. 3-3). The general structure of RNA differs from DNA in three respects: RNA is a single-stranded rather than a double-stranded molecule; the sugar in each nucleotide of RNA is ribose instead of deoxyribose; and the pyrimidine base thymine in DNA is replaced by uracil in RNA. All three types of RNA (mRNA, tRNA, and rRNA) are synthesized in the nucleus by RNA polymerase enzymes that take directions from DNA. Because the ribose sugars found in RNA are more susceptible to degradation than the sugars in DNA, the types of RNA molecules in the cytoplasm can be altered rapidly in response to extracellular signals.

Messenger RNA

Messenger RNA is the template for protein synthesis. It is a long molecule containing several hundred to several thousand nucleotides. Each group of three nucleotides forms a codon that is exactly complementary to the triplet of nucleotides of the DNA molecule. Messenger RNA is formed by a process called *transcription*. In this process, the weak hydrogen bonds of the DNA are broken so that free RNA nucleotides can pair with their exposed DNA counterparts on the meaningful strand of the DNA molecule (see Fig. 3-1B). As with the base pairing of the DNA strands, complementary RNA bases pair with the DNA bases. In RNA, uracil replaces thymine and pairs with adenine.

During transcription, a specialized nuclear enzyme, called *RNA polymerase*, recognizes the beginning, or start, sequence of a gene (see Fig. 3-3). The RNA polymerase attaches to the double-stranded DNA and proceeds to copy the meaningful strand into a single strand of RNA as it travels along the length of the gene. On reaching the stop signal, the enzyme leaves the gene and releases the RNA strand. The RNA strand then is processed. Processing involves the addition of certain nucleic acids at the ends of the RNA strand and cutting and splicing of certain internal sequences. Splicing often involves the removal of stretches of RNA (Fig. 3-4). Because of the splicing process, the final mRNA sequence is different from the original DNA template. RNA sequences that are retained are called *exons,* and those excised are called *introns.* The functions of the introns are unknown. They are thought to be involved in the activation or deactivation of genes during various stages of development.

Splicing permits a cell to produce a variety of mRNA molecules from a single gene. By varying the splicing segments of the initial mRNA, different mRNA molecules are formed. For example, in a muscle cell, the original tropomyosin mRNA is spliced in as many as 10 different ways, yielding distinctly different protein products. This permits different proteins to be expressed from a single gene and reduces how much DNA must be contained in the genome.

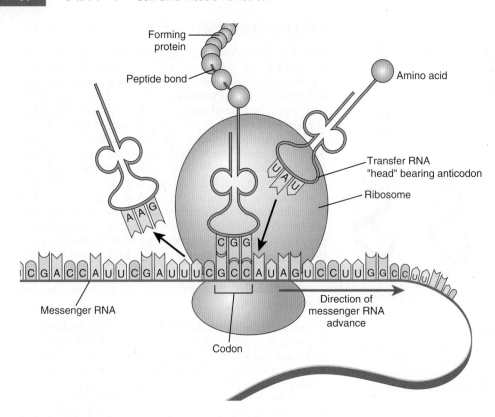

Forming protein

Peptide bond

Amino acid

Transfer RNA "head" bearing anticodon

Ribosome

Messenger RNA

Direction of messenger RNA advance

Codon

FIGURE 3-3 Protein synthesis. A messenger RNA (mRNA) strand is shown moving along a small ribosomal subunit in the cytoplasm. As the mRNA codon passes along the ribosome, a new amino acid is added to the growing peptide chain by the transfer RNA (tRNA) bearing the anticodon for the mRNA-designated amino acid. As each amino acid is bound to the next by a peptide bond, its tRNA is released.

Transfer RNA

The clover-shaped tRNA molecule contains only 80 nucleotides, making it the smallest RNA molecule. Its function is to deliver the activated form of amino acids to protein molecules in the ribosomes (see Fig. 3-3). At least 20 different types of tRNA are known, each of which recognizes and binds to only one type of amino acid. Each tRNA molecule has two recognition sites: the first is complementary (anticodon) for the mRNA codon, the second for the amino acid itself. Each type of tRNA carries its own specific amino acid to the ribosomes, where protein synthesis is taking place; there it recognizes the appropriate codon on the mRNA and delivers the amino acid to the newly forming protein molecule.

Ribosomal RNA

The ribosome is the physical structure in the cytoplasm where protein synthesis takes place. Ribosomal RNA forms 60% of the ribosome, with the remainder of the ribosome composed of the structural proteins and enzymes needed for protein synthesis. As with the other types of RNA, rRNA is synthesized in the nucleus. Unlike mRNA and tRNA, ribosomal RNA is produced in a specialized nuclear structure called the *nucleolus*. The formed rRNA combines with ribosomal proteins in the nucleus to produce the ribosome, which is then transported into the cytoplasm. On reaching the cytoplasm, most ribosomes become attached to the endoplasmic reticulum and begin the task of protein synthesis.

Proteins are made from a standard set of amino acids, which are joined end-to-end to form the long polypeptide chains of protein molecules. Each polypeptide chain may have as many as 100 to more than 300 amino acids in it. The process of protein synthesis is called *translation* because the genetic code is translated into the production language needed for polypeptide assembly. Besides rRNA, translation requires the coordinated actions of mRNA and tRNA (see Fig. 3-3). Each of the 20 different tRNA molecules transports its specific amino acid to the ribosome

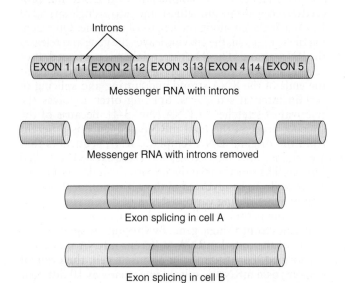

Introns

EXON 1 | 11 | EXON 2 | 12 | EXON 3 | 13 | EXON 4 | 14 | EXON 5

Messenger RNA with introns

Messenger RNA with introns removed

Exon splicing in cell A

Exon splicing in cell B

FIGURE 3-4 In different cells, an RNA strand may eventually produce different proteins depending on the sequencing of exons during gene splicing. This variation allows a gene to code for more than one protein. (Courtesy of Edward W. Carroll.)

for incorporation into the developing protein molecule. Messenger RNA provides the information needed for placing the amino acids in their proper order for each specific type of protein. During protein synthesis, mRNA passes through the ribosome, which "reads" the directions for protein synthesis in much the same way that a tape is read as it passes through a tape player. As mRNA passes through the ribosome, tRNA delivers the appropriate amino acids for attachment to the growing polypeptide chain. The long mRNA molecule usually travels through and directs protein synthesis in more than one ribosome at a time. After the first part of the mRNA is read by the first ribosome, it moves onto a second and a third. As a result, ribosomes that are actively involved in protein synthesis are often found in clusters called *polyribosomes*.

REGULATION OF GENE EXPRESSION

Although all cells contain the same genes, not all genes are active all of the time, nor are the same genes active in all cell types. On the contrary, only a small, select group of genes is active in directing protein synthesis in the cell, and this group varies from one cell type to another. For the differentiation process of cells to occur in the various organs and tissues of the body, protein synthesis in some cells must be different from that in others. To adapt to an ever-changing environment, certain cells may need to produce varying amounts and types of proteins. The degree to which a gene or particular group of genes is active is called *gene expression*. A phenomenon termed *induction* is an important process by which gene expression is increased. Except in early embryonic development, induction is promoted by some external influence. *Gene repression*, or inhibition, is a process by which a regulatory gene acts to reduce or prevent gene expression. Some genes are normally dormant but can be activated by inducer substances; other genes are naturally active and can be inhibited by repressor substances.

GENE MUTATIONS

Rarely, accidental errors in duplication of DNA occur. These errors are called *mutations*. Mutations result from the substitution of one base pair for another, the loss or addition of one or more base pairs, or rearrangements of base pairs. Many of these mutations occur spontaneously; others occur because of environmental agents, chemicals, and radiation. Mutations may arise in somatic cells or in germ cells. Only those DNA changes that occur in germ cells can be inherited. A somatic mutation affects a cell line that differentiates into one or more of the many tissues of the body and is not transmissible to the next generation. Somatic mutations that do not have an impact on the health or functioning of a person are called *polymorphisms*. Occasionally, a person is born with one brown eye and one blue eye because of a somatic mutation. The change or loss of gene information is just as likely to affect the fundamental processes of cell function or organ differentiation. Such somatic mutations in the early embryonic period can result in embryonic death or congenital malformations.

Somatic mutations are important causes of cancer and other tumors in which cell differentiation and growth get out of control. Each year, hundreds of thousands of random changes occur in the DNA molecule because of environmental events or metabolic accidents. Fortunately, less than 1 in 1000 base pair changes results in serious mutations. Most of these defects are corrected by DNA repair mechanisms (see Chapter 5). Several mechanisms exist, and each depends on specific enzymes such as DNA repair nucleases. Fishermen, farmers, and others who are excessively exposed to the ultraviolet radiation of sunlight have an increased risk for development of skin cancer because of potential radiation damage to the genetic structure of the skin-forming cells.

In summary, genes are the fundamental unit of information storage in the cell. They determine the types of proteins and enzymes made by the cell and therefore control inheritance and day-to-day cell function. Genes store information in a stable macromolecule called *DNA*. Genes transmit information contained in the DNA molecule as a triplet code. The genetic code is determined by the arrangement of the nitrogenous bases of the four nucleotides (*i.e.*, adenine, guanine, thymine [or uracil in RNA], and cytosine). The transfer of stored information into production of cell products is accomplished through a second type of macromolecule called *RNA*. Messenger RNA transcribes the instructions for product synthesis from the DNA molecule and carries them into the cell's cytoplasm, where ribosomal RNA uses the information to direct product synthesis. Transfer RNA acts as a carrier system for delivering the appropriate amino acids to the ribosomes, where the synthesis of cell products occurs. Although all cells contain the same genes, only a small, select group of genes is active in a given cell type. In all cells, some genetic information is repressed, whereas other information is expressed. Gene mutations represent accidental errors in duplication, rearrangement, or deletion of parts of the genetic code. Fortunately, most mutations are corrected by DNA repair mechanisms in the cell.

Chromosomes

Most genetic information of a cell is organized, stored, and retrieved in small intracellular structures called *chromosomes*. Although the chromosomes are visible only in dividing cells, they retain their integrity between cell divisions. The chromosomes are arranged in pairs: one member of the pair is inherited from the father, the other from the mother. The maternal and paternal chromosomes of a pair are called homologous chromosomes (homologs). Each species has a characteristic number of chromosomes. In the human, 46 single or 23 pairs of chromosomes are present. Of the 23 pairs of human chromosomes, 22 are called *autosomes* and are alike in both males and females.

Each of the 22 pairs of autosomes has the same appearance in all individuals, and each has been given a numeric designation for classification purposes (Fig. 3-5). The sex chromosomes make up the 23rd pair of chromosomes. Two sex chromosomes determine the sex of a person. All males have an X and Y chromosome (*i.e.*, an X chromosome from the mother and a Y chromosome from the father); all females have two X chromosomes (*i.e.*, one from each parent). The much smaller Y chromosome contains the *male-specific region* (MSY) that determines sex. This region comprises more than 90% of the length of the Y chromosome.

Only one X chromosome in the female is active in controlling the expression of genetic traits; however, both X chromosomes are activated during gametogenesis. In the female, the active X chromosome is invisible, but the inactive X chromosome can be demonstrated with appropriate nuclear staining. This inactive chromatin mass is seen as the *Barr body* in epithelial cells or as the drumstick body in the chromatin of neutrophils. The genetic sex of a child can be determined by microscopic study of cell or tissue samples. The total number of X chromosomes is equal to the number of Barr bodies plus one (*i.e.*, an inactive plus an active X chromosome). For example, the cells of a normal female have one Barr body and therefore a total of two X chromosomes. A normal male has no Barr bodies. Males with Klinefelter syndrome (one Y, an inactive X, and an active X chromosome) exhibit one Barr body. In the female, whether the X chromosome derived from the mother or that derived from the father is active

is randomly determined within a few days after conception. This random selection is called the *Lyon principle*, after Mary Lyon, the British geneticist who described it.

CELL DIVISION

Cells reproduce by duplicating their chromosomes and dividing in two. There are two types of cell division: mitosis and meiosis. *Mitosis* is the cell cycle process in which nongerm cells are replicated (see Chapter 5). It provides a way for the body to replace cells that have a limited life span, such as skin and blood cells; increase tissue mass during periods of growth; and repair tissue, such as in wound healing.

Meiosis is limited to replicating germ cells and takes place only once in a cell line. It results in the formation of gametes or reproductive cells (*i.e.*, ovum and sperm), each of which has only a single set of 23 chromosomes. Meiosis is typically divided into two distinct phases: meiotic divisions I and II (Fig. 3-6). During meiotic division I, homologous chromosomes pair up, forming a synapsis or tetrad (two chromatids per chromosome). They are sometimes called *bivalents*. The X and Y chromosomes are not homologs and do not form bivalents. While in meiosis I, an interchange of chromatid segments can occur. This process is called *crossing over* (Fig. 3-7). Crossing over allows for new combinations of genes, increasing genetic variability. After cell division I, each of the two daughter cells contains one member of each homologous pair of chromosomes and a sex chromosome (23 double-stranded

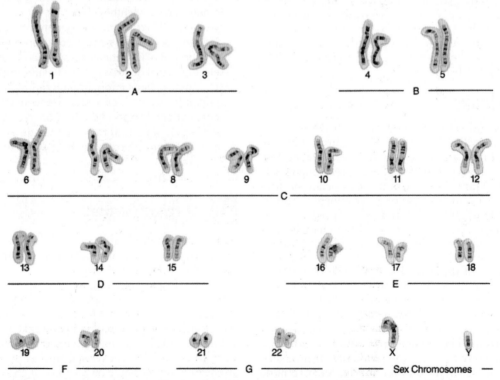

FIGURE 3-5 Karyotype of normal human boy. (Courtesy of the Prenatal Diagnostic and Imaging Center, Sacramento, CA. Frederick W. Hansen, MD, Medical Director.)

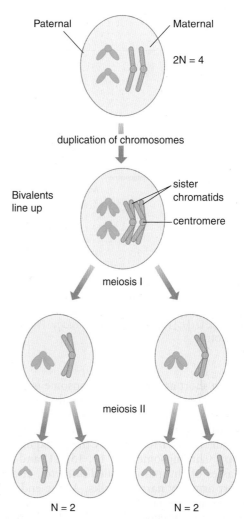

<table>
</table>

KEY CONCEPTS

Chromosome Structure

➤ The DNA that stores genetic material is organized into 23 pairs of chromosomes. There are 22 pairs of autosomes, which are alike for males and females, and one pair of sex chromosomes, with XX pairing in females and XY pairing in males.

➤ Mitosis refers to the duplication of chromosomes in somatic cell lines, in which each daughter cell receives a pair of 23 chromosomes.

➤ Meiosis is limited to replicating germ cells and results in the formation of a single set of 23 chromosomes.

FIGURE 3-6 Separation of chromosomes at the time of meiosis in germ cells. Meiosis, or reduction division, occurs in two steps: meiosis I, during which the number of chromosomes is reduced to half, but the chromatid pairs remain together, and meiosis II, during which the chromatids split apart.

chromosomes). No DNA synthesis occurs before meiotic division II. During cell division II, the 23 double-stranded chromosomes (two chromatids) of each of the two daughter cells from meiosis I divide at their centromeres. Each subsequent daughter cell receives 23 single-stranded chromatids. Thus, a total of four daughter cells are formed by a meiotic division of one cell.

CHROMOSOME STRUCTURE

Cytogenetics is the study of the structure and numeric characteristics of the cell's chromosomes. Chromosome studies can be done on any tissue or cell that grows and divides in culture. Lymphocytes from venous blood are frequently used for this purpose. After the cells have been cultured, a drug called *colchicine* is used to arrest mitosis before the chromosomes separate. A chromosome spread is prepared by fixing and spreading the chromosomes on a slide. Subsequently, appropriate staining techniques show the chromosomal banding patterns so they can be identified. The chromosomes are photographed, and the photomicrograph of each chromosome is cut out and arranged in pairs according to a standard classification system (see Fig. 3-5). The completed picture is called a *karyotype*, and the procedure for preparing the picture is called *karyotyping*. A uniform system of chromosome classification was originally formulated at the 1971 Paris Chromosome Conference and was later revised to describe the chromosomes as seen in preparations of more elongated mitotic stages.

While the chromosomes are aligned on the equatorial plate of the cell, each chromosome takes the form of chromatids to form an "X" or "wishbone" pattern. Human chromosomes are divided into three types according to the position of the centromere (Fig. 3-8). If the centromere is in the center and the arms are of approximately the same length, the chromosome is said to be *metacentric*; if it is not centered and the arms are of clearly different lengths, it is *submetacentric*; and if it is near one end, it is *acro-*

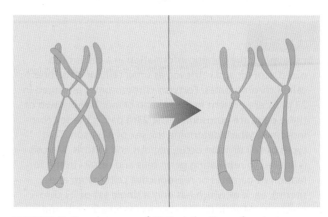

FIGURE 3-7 Crossing over of DNA at the time of meiosis.

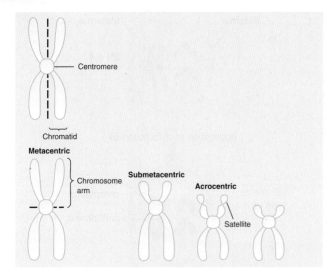

FIGURE 3-8 Three basic shapes and the component parts of human metaphase chromosomes. The relative size of the satellite on the acrocentric is exaggerated for visibility. (Adapted from Cormack D. H. [1993]. *Essential histology*. Philadelphia: J. B. Lippincott.)

centric. The short arm of the chromosome is designated as "p" for "petite," and the long arm is designated as "q" for no other reason than it is the next letter of the alphabet. The arms of the chromosome are indicated by the chromosome number followed by the p or q designation (*e.g.,* 15p). Chromosomes 13, 14, 15, 21, and 22 have small masses of chromatin, called *satellites,* attached to their short arms by narrow stalks. At the ends of each chromosome are special DNA sequences called *telomeres.* Telomeres allow the end of the DNA molecule to be replicated completely.

The banding patterns of a chromosome are used in describing the position of a gene on the chromosome. Each arm of a chromosome is divided into regions, which are numbered from the centromere outward (*e.g.,* 1, 2). The regions are further divided into bands, which are also numbered (Fig. 3-9). These numbers are then used to designate the position of a gene on a chromosome. For example, Xp22, refers to band 2, region 2 of the short arm (p) of the X chromosome.

In summary, the genetic information in a cell is organized, stored, and retrieved as small cellular structures called *chromosomes.* Forty-six chromosomes arranged in 23 pairs are present in the human being. Twenty-two of these pairs are autosomes. The 23rd pair is the sex chromosomes, which determine the sex of a person. Two types of cell division occur, meiosis and mitosis. Meiosis is limited to replicating germ cells and results in the formation of gametes or reproductive cells (ovum and sperm), each of which has only a single set of 23 chromosomes. Mitotic division occurs in somatic cells and

results in the formation of 23 pairs of chromosomes. A karyotype is a photograph of a person's chromosomes. It is prepared by special laboratory techniques in which body cells are cultured, fixed, and then stained to display identifiable banding patterns. A photomicrograph is then made. Often the individual chromosomes are cut out and regrouped according to chromosome number.

Patterns of Inheritance

The characteristics inherited from a person's parents are inscribed in gene pairs found along the length of the chromosomes. Alternate forms of the same gene are possible (*i.e.,* one inherited from the mother and the other from the father), and each may produce a different aspect of a trait.

DEFINITIONS

Genetics has its own set of definitions. The *genotype* of a person is the genetic information stored in the base sequence triplet code. The *phenotype* refers to the recognizable traits, physical or biochemical, associated with a specific genotype. Often, the genotype is not evident by available detection methods. More than one genotype may have the same phenotype. Some brown-eyed persons are carriers of the code for blue eyes, and other brown-eyed persons are not. Phenotypically, these two types of brown-eyed persons are the same, but genotypically they are different.

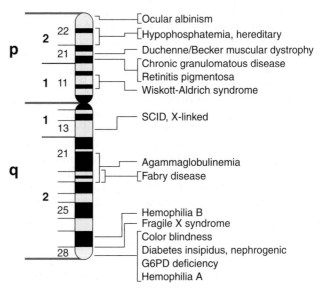

FIGURE 3-9 The localization of inherited diseases as represented on the banded karyotype of the X chromosome. Notice the nomenclature of arms (p, q), regions (1, 2), and bands (*e.g.,* 22 [region 2, band 2]). (Adapted from Rubin E., Farber J. L. [1999]. *Pathology* [3rd ed., p. 260]. Philadelphia: Lippincott Williams & Wilkins.)

KEY CONCEPTS

Transmission of Genetic Information

➤ The transmission of information from one generation to the next is vested in genetic material transferred from each parent at the time of conception.

➤ Alleles are the alternate forms of a gene (one from each parent), and the locus is the position that they occupy on the chromosome.

➤ The genotype of a person represents the sum total of the genetic information in the cells and the phenotype the physical manifestations of that information.

➤ Penetrance is the percentage in a population with a particular genotype in which that genotype is phenotypically manifested, whereas expressivity is the manner in which the gene is expressed.

When it comes to a genetic disorder, not all persons with a mutant gene are affected to the same extent. *Expressivity* refers to the manner in which the gene is expressed in the phenotype, which can range from mild to severe. *Penetrance* represents the ability of a gene to express its function. Seventy-five percent penetrance means 75% of persons of a particular genotype present with a recognizable phenotype. Syndactyly (webbed fingers or toes) and blue sclera are genetic mutations that often do not exhibit 100% penetrance.

The position of a gene on a chromosome is called its *locus*, and alternate forms of a gene at the same locus are called *alleles*. When only one pair of genes is involved in the transmission of information, the term *single-gene trait* is used. Single-gene traits follow the mendelian laws of inheritance (to be discussed).

Polygenic inheritance involves multiple genes at different loci, with each gene exerting a small additive effect in determining a trait. Most human traits are determined by multiple pairs of genes, many with alternate codes, accounting for some dissimilar forms that occur with certain genetic disorders. Polygenic traits are predictable, but with less reliability than single-gene traits. *Multifactorial* inheritance is similar to polygenic inheritance in that multiple alleles at different loci affect the outcome; the difference is that multifactorial inheritance includes environmental effects on the genes.

Many other gene–gene interactions are known. These include *epistasis*, in which one gene masks the phenotypic effects of another nonallelic gene; *multiple alleles*, in which more than one allele affects the same trait (*e.g.*, ABO blood types); *complementary genes*, in which each gene is mutually dependent on the other; and *collaborative genes*, in which two different genes influencing the same trait interact to produce a phenotype neither gene alone could produce.

MENDEL LAWS

A main feature of inheritance is predictability: given certain conditions, the likelihood of the occurrence or recurrence of a specific trait is remarkably predictable. The units of inheritance are the genes, and the pattern of single-gene expression can often be predicted using the Mendel laws of genetic transmission. Techniques and discoveries since Gregor Mendel's original work was published in 1865 have led to some modification of his original laws.

Mendel discovered the basic pattern of inheritance by conducting carefully planned experiments with simple garden peas. Experimenting with several phenotypic traits in peas, Mendel proposed that inherited traits are transmitted from parents to offspring by means of independently inherited factors—now known as genes—and that these factors are transmitted as recessive and dominant traits. Mendel labeled dominant factors (his round peas) "A" and recessive factors (his wrinkled peas) "a." Geneticists continue to use capital letters to designate dominant traits and lowercase letters to identify recessive traits. The possible combinations that can occur with transmission of single-gene dominant and recessive traits can be described by constructing a figure called a *Punnett square* using capital and lowercase letters (Fig. 3-10).

The observable traits of single-gene inheritance are inherited by the offspring from the parents. During maturation, the primordial germ cells (*i.e.*, sperm and ovum) of both parents undergo reduction division, in which the number of chromosomes is divided in half (from 46 to 23). At this time, the two alleles from a gene locus separate so that each germ cell receives only one allele from each pair (*i.e.*, Mendel first law). According to Mendel second

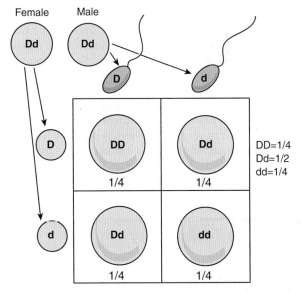

FIGURE 3-10 The Punnett square showing all possible combinations for transmission of a single gene trait (dimpled cheeks). The example shown is when both parents are heterozygous (dD) for the trait. The alleles carried by the mother are on the left and those carried by the father are on the top. The D allele is dominant and the d allele is recessive. The DD and Dd offspring have dimples, and the dd offspring does not.

law, the alleles from the different gene loci segregate independently and recombine randomly in the zygote. Persons in whom the two alleles of a given pair are the same (AA or aa) are called *homozygotes*. *Heterozygotes* have different alleles (Aa) at a gene locus. A *recessive trait* is one expressed only in a homozygous pairing; a *dominant trait* is one expressed in either a homozygous or a heterozygous pairing. All persons with a dominant allele (depending on the penetrance of the genes) manifest that trait. A *carrier* is a person who is heterozygous for a recessive trait and does not manifest the trait. For example, the genes for blond hair are recessive and those for brown hair are dominant. Therefore, only persons with a genotype having two alleles for blond hair would be blond; persons with either one or two brown alleles would have dark hair.

PEDIGREE

A *pedigree* is a graphic method for portraying a family history of an inherited trait. It is constructed from a carefully obtained family history and is useful for tracing the pattern of inheritance for a particular trait.

In summary, inheritance represents the likelihood of the occurrence or recurrence of a specific genetic trait. The genotype refers to information stored in the genetic code of a person, whereas the phenotype represents the recognizable traits, physical and biochemical, associated with the genotype. Expressivity refers to the expression of a gene in the phenotype, and penetrance is the ability of a gene to express its function. The point on the DNA molecule that controls the inheritance of a particular trait is called a *gene locus*. Alternate forms of a gene at a gene locus are called *alleles.* The alleles at a gene locus may carry recessive or dominant traits. A recessive trait is one expressed only when two copies (homozygous pairing) of the recessive allele are present. Dominant traits are expressed with either homozygous or heterozygous pairing of the alleles. A pedigree is a graphic method for portraying a family history of an inherited trait.

 Gene Technology

GENOMIC MAPPING

The genome is the gene complement of an organism. Genomic mapping is the assignment of genes to specific chromosomes or parts of the chromosome. The Human Genome Project, which started in 1990 and was completed in 2003, was an international project to identify and localize the over 30,000 genes in the human genome. This was a phenomenal undertaking because approxi-

mately three million base pairs are present in the human genome. The results of the project are expected to reveal the chemical basis for as many as 4000 genetic diseases, provide information needed for developing screening and diagnosing disorders, and generate new treatment methods for these disorders.

Two types of genomic maps exist: genetic maps and physical maps. Genetic maps are like highway maps. They use linkage studies (*e.g.,* dosage, hybridization) to estimate the distances between chromosomal landmarks (*i.e.,* gene markers). Physical maps are similar to a surveyor's map. They measure the actual physical distance between chromosomal elements in biochemical units, the smallest being the nucleotide base.

Genetic maps and physical maps have been refined over the decades. The earliest mapping efforts localized genes on the X chromosome. The initial assignment of a gene to a particular chromosome was made in 1911 for the color blindness gene inherited from the mother (*i.e.,* following the X-linked pattern of inheritance). In 1968, the specific location of the Duffy blood group on the long arm of chromosome 1 was determined. The locations of more than 12,000 expressed human genes have been mapped to a specific chromosome, and most of them to a specific region on the chromosome. However, genetic mapping is continuing at such a rapid pace that these numbers are constantly being updated. Documentation of gene assignments to specific human chromosomes is updated almost daily in *Online Mendelian Inheritance in Man* (www.ncbi.nlm.nih.gov/Omim), an encyclopedia of expressed gene loci. Many methods have been used for developing genetic maps. The most important ones are family linkage studies, gene dosage methods, and hybridization studies. Often, the specific assignment of a gene is made using information from several mapping techniques.

Most of the genome mapping has been accomplished by a method called *transcript mapping.* The two-part process begins with isolating mRNAs immediately after they are transcribed. Next, the complementary DNA molecule is prepared. Although transcript mapping may provide knowledge of the gene sequence, it does not automatically mean that the function of the genetic material has been determined.

Linkage Studies

Mendel laws were often insufficient to explain the transmission of several well-known traits such as color blindness and hemophilia A. In some families it was noted that these two conditions were transmitted together. In 1937, Bell and Haldane concluded that somehow the two mutations were coupled or "linked." Detailed analyses of other familial conditions have concluded that several exceptions to Mendel laws exist.

Linkage studies assume that genes occur in a linear array along the chromosomes. During meiosis, the paired chromosomes of the diploid germ cell exchange genetic material because of the crossing-over phenomenon (see Fig. 3-7). This exchange usually involves more than one gene; large blocks of genes (representing large portions of the chromosome) are usually exchanged. Although the point at which the block separates from another occurs randomly, the closer together two genes are on the same chromosome, the greater the chance is that they will be passed on together to the offspring. When two inherited traits occur together at a rate greater than would occur by chance alone, they are said to be *linked*.

Several methods take advantage of the crossing over and recombination of genes to map a particular gene. In one method, any gene that is already assigned to a chromosome can be used as a marker to assign other linked genes. For example, it was found that an extra long chromosome 1 and the Duffy blood group were inherited as a dominant trait, placing the position of the blood group gene close to the extra material on chromosome 1. Color blindness has been linked to classic hemophilia A (*i.e.*, lack of factor VIII) in some pedigrees; hemophilia A has been linked to glucose-6-phosphate dehydrogenase deficiency in others; and color blindness has been linked to glucose-6-phosphate dehydrogenase deficiency in still others. Because the gene for color blindness is found on the X chromosome, all three genes must be found in a small section of the X chromosome. Linkage analysis can be used clinically to identify affected persons in a family with a known genetic defect. Males, because they have one X and one Y chromosome, are said to be *hemizygous* for sex-linked traits. Females can be homozygous (normal or mutant) or heterozygous for sex-linked traits. Heterozygous females are known as *carriers* for X-linked defects.

Dosage Studies

Dosage studies involve measuring enzyme activity. Autosomal genes are normally arranged in pairs, and normally both are expressed. If both alleles are present and both are expressed, the activity of the enzyme should be 100%. If one member of the gene pair is missing, only 50% of the enzyme activity is present, reflecting the activity of the remaining normal allele.

Hybridization Studies

A recent biologic discovery revealed that two somatic cells from different species, when grown together in the same culture, occasionally fuse to form a new hybrid cell. Two types of hybridization methods are used in genomic studies: somatic cell hybridization and in situ hybridization.

Somatic cell hybridization involves the fusion of human somatic cells with those of a different species (typically, the mouse) to yield a cell containing the chromosomes of both species. Because these hybrid cells are unstable, they begin to lose chromosomes of both species during subsequent cell divisions. This makes it possible to obtain cells with different partial combinations of human chromosomes. By studying the enzymes that these cells produce, it is possible to determine that a specific enzyme is produced only when a certain chromosome is present; the coding for that enzyme must be located on that chromosome.

In situ hybridization involves the use of specific sequences of DNA or RNA to locate genes that do not express themselves in cell culture. DNA and RNA can be chemically tagged with radioactive or fluorescent markers. These chemically tagged DNA or RNA sequences are used as probes to detect gene location. The probe is added to a chromosome spread after the DNA strands have been separated. If the probe matches the complementary DNA of a chromosome segment, it hybridizes and remains at the precise location (therefore the term *in situ*) on a chromosome. Radioactive or fluorescent markers are used to find the location of the probe.

RECOMBINANT DNA TECHNOLOGY

During the past several decades, genetic engineering has provided the methods for manipulating nucleic acids and recombining genes (recombinant DNA) into hybrid molecules that can be inserted into unicellular organisms and reproduced many times over. Each hybrid molecule produces a genetically identical population or *clone* that reflects its common ancestor.

Gene isolation and cloning techniques rely on the fact that the genes of all organisms, from bacteria through mammals, are based on similar molecular organization. Gene cloning requires cutting a DNA molecule apart, modifying and reassembling its fragments, and producing copies of the modified DNA, its mRNA, and its gene product. The DNA molecule is cut apart by a bacterial enzyme, called a *restriction enzyme,* which binds to DNA wherever a particular short sequence of base pairs is found and cleaves the molecule at a specific nucleotide site. In this way, a long DNA molecule can be broken down into smaller, discrete fragments with the intent that one fragment contains the gene of interest. More than 100 restriction enzymes are commercially available that cut DNA at different recognition sites.

The selected gene fragment is replicated through insertion into a unicellular organism, such as a bacterium. To do this, a cloning vector such as a bacterial virus or a *plasmid*, a small DNA circle found in most bacteria, is used. Viral and plasmid vectors replicate autonomously in the host bacterial cell. During gene cloning, a bacterial vector and the DNA fragment are mixed and joined by a special enzyme called a *DNA ligase*. The recombinant vectors formed are then introduced into a suitable culture of bacteria, and the bacteria are allowed to replicate and express the recombinant vector gene. Sometimes mRNA taken from a tissue that expresses a high level of the gene is used to produce a complementary DNA molecule, which is then used in the cloning process. Because the fragments of the entire DNA molecule are used in the cloning process, additional steps are taken to identify and separate the clone that contains the gene of interest.

As for biologic research and technology, cloning makes it possible to identify the DNA sequence in a gene and produce the protein product encoded by a gene. The specific nucleotide sequence of a cloned DNA fragment can often be identified by analyzing the amino acid sequence and mRNA codons of its protein product. Short sequences of base pairs can be synthesized, radioactively labeled, and subsequently used to identify their complementary sequence. In this way, identifying normal and abnormal gene structures is possible. Proteins that formerly were available only in small amounts can now be made in large quantities once their respective genes have been isolated. For example, genes encoding for an insulin and growth hormone have been cloned to produce these hormones for pharmacologic use.

GENE THERAPY

Although quite different from inserting genetic material into a unicellular organism such as bacteria, techniques are available for inserting genes into the genome of intact multicellular plants and animals. Promising delivery vehicles for these genes are the adenoviruses. These viruses are ideal vehicles because their DNA does not become integrated into the host genome; however, repeated inoculations are often needed because the body's immune system usually targets cells expressing adenovirus proteins. Sterically stable liposomes also show promise as DNA delivery mechanisms. This type of therapy is one of the more promising methods for the treatment of genetic disorders, certain cancers, cystic fibrosis, and many infectious diseases. Two main approaches are used in gene therapy: transferred genes can replace defective genes or they can selectively inhibit deleterious genes. Cloned DNA sequences or ribosomes are usually the compounds used in gene therapy. However, the introduction of the cloned gene into the multicellular organism can influence only the few cells that get the gene. An answer to this problem would be the insertion of the gene into a sperm or ovum; after fertilization, the gene would be replicated in all of the differentiating cell types. Even so, techniques for cell insertion are limited. Not only are moral and ethical issues involved, but these techniques cannot direct the inserted DNA to attach to a particular chromosome or supplant an existing gene by knocking it out of its place.

DNA FINGERPRINTING

The technique of DNA fingerprinting is based in part on those techniques used in recombinant DNA technology and those originally used in medical genetics to detect slight variations in the genomes of different individuals. Using restrictive endonucleases, DNA is cleaved at specific regions. The DNA fragments are separated according to size by electrophoresis (i.e., Southern blot) and transferred to a nylon membrane. The fragments are then broken apart and subsequently annealed with a series of radioactive probes specific for regions in each fragment. An autoradiograph reveals the DNA fragments on the membrane. When used in forensic pathology, this procedure is undertaken on specimens from the suspect and the forensic specimen. Banding patterns are then analyzed to see if they match. With conventional methods of analysis of blood and serum enzymes, a 1 in 100 to 1000 chance exists that the two specimens match because of chance. With DNA fingerprinting, these odds are 1 in 100,000 to 1 million.

In summary, the genome is the gene complement of an organism. Genomic mapping is a method used to assign genes to particular chromosomes or parts of a chromosome. The most important ones used are family linkage studies, gene dosage methods, and hybridization studies. Often the specific assignment of a gene is determined by using information from several mapping techniques. Linkage studies assign a chromosome location to genes based on their close association with other genes of known location. Recombinant DNA studies involve the extraction of specific types of mRNA used in synthesis of complementary DNA strands. The complementary DNA strands, labeled with a radioisotope, bind with the genes for which they are complementary and are used as gene probes. An international project established to identify and localize all 30,000 estimated genes in the human genome, the Human Genome Project, was started in 1990 and completed in 2003. Genetic engineering has provided the methods for manipulating nucleic acids and recombining genes (recombinant DNA) into hybrid molecules that can be inserted into unicellular organisms and reproduced many times over. As a result, proteins that formerly were available only in small amounts can now be made in large quantities once their respective genes have been isolated. DNA fingerprinting, which relies on recombinant DNA technologies and those of genetic mapping, is often used in forensic investigations.

Review Exercises

Cystic fibrosis is a disorder of a cell membrane chloride channel that causes the exocrine glands of the body to produce abnormally thick mucus with the resultant development of chronic obstructive lung disease, pancreatitis, and infertility in men.

A. Explain how a single mutant gene can produce such devastating effects.
B. The disease is transmitted as a single-gene recessive trait. Describe the inheritance of the disorder using Figure 3-10.

Adult polycystic kidney disease is transmitted as an autosomal dominant trait.

A. Explain the parent-to-child transmission of this disorder.
B. Although the disease is transmitted as an autosomal dominant trait, some people who inherit the gene may develop symptoms early in life, others may develop them later in life, and still others may never develop significant symptoms of the disease during their lifetime. Explain.

Human insulin, prepared by recombinant DNA technology, is now available for treatment of diabetes mellitus.

A. Explain the techniques for producing a human hormone using this technology.

Visit the Porth: Essentials of Pathophysiology: Concepts of Altered Health States web site (http://thePoint.LWW.com/PorthEssentials) for links to chapter-related resources on the Internet, all-new exclusive animations, chapter review questions, and more!

BIBLIOGRAPHY

Alberts B., Johnson A., Lewis J., et al. (2002). *Molecular biology of the cell* (4th ed., pp. 191–468, 386–387). New York: Garland Science.

Aparicio S. A. J. R. (2000). How to count human genes. *Nature Genetics* 25, 129–130. [On-line]. Available: www.nature.com. Accessed July 13, 2000.

Ewing B., Green P. (2000). Analysis of expressed sequence tags indicates 35,000 human genes. *Nature Genetics* 25, 232–234.

Guyton A. C., Hall J. E. (2006). *Textbook of medical physiology* (11th ed., pp. 27–42). Philadelphia: Elsevier Saunders.

Hattori M., Fujyama A., Taylor H., et al. (2000). The DNA sequence of human chromosome 21. *Nature* 405, 311–319.

International RH Mapping Consortium. (2000). *A new gene map of the human genome*. [On-line]. Available: www.ncbi.nlm.nih.gov/genemap99. Accessed September 9, 2005.

Jegalian K., Lahn B. T. (2001). Why the Y is so weird. *Scientific American* 284(2), 56–61.

Kierszenbaum A. L. (2003). *Histology and cell biology: An introduction to pathology* (pp. 87–88). St. Louis: Mosby.

Liang F., Holt I., Pertea G., et al. (2000). Gene index analysis of the human genome estimates approximately 120,000 genes. *Nature Genetics* 25, 239–240.

Naussbaum R. L., McInnes R. R., Willard H. F. (2001). *Thompson & Thompson genetics in medicine* (6th ed.). Philadelphia: W. B. Saunders.

Sadler R. W. (2003). *Langman's medical embryology* (9th ed., pp. 3–30). Philadelphia: Lippincott Williams & Wilkins.

Skaletsky H., Kuroda-Kawaguchi T., Minx P., et. al. (2003). The male-specific region of the Y chromosome is a mosaic of discrete sequence classes. *Nature* 423, 825–837.

Snustad D. P., Simmons J. M. (Eds.). (2000). *Principles of genetics* (2nd ed., pp. 3–21, 52–71, 91–115, 665–669). New York: John Wiley & Sons.

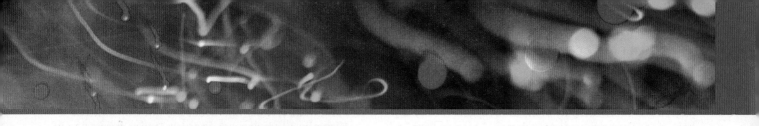

C h a p t e r *4*

Genetic and Congenital Disorders

 Genetic and congenital defects are important at all levels of health care because they affect all age groups and can involve almost any of the body tissues and organs. Congenital disorders, sometime called *birth defects,* are defects that are present at birth, whether the result of genetic or nongenetic factors (*i.e.,* maternal disease, infections, or drugs taken during pregnancy). Birth defects, which affect more than 150,000 infants each year, are the leading cause of infant death.[1] Genetic disorders, which involve a permanent change (or mutation) in the genome, may be apparent at birth or, as in Huntington disease, may not become apparent until later in life.

Genetic and Chromosomal Disorders

A genetic disorder can be described as a discrete event that affects gene expression in a group of cells related to each other by gene linkage. It can involve a single-gene trait or multifactorial inheritance. Most genetic disorders are caused by an alteration in deoxyribonucleic acid (DNA) sequences that alter the synthesis of a single gene product. However, some genetic disorders are caused by chromosome rearrangements that result in deletion or duplication of a group of closely linked genes or by mistakes during meiosis that result in an abnormal number of chromosomes.[2]

The genes on each chromosome are arranged in pairs and in strict order, with each gene occupying a specific location or *locus.* The alternate members of a gene pair, one inherited from the mother and the other from the father, are called *alleles.* If the members of a gene pair are identical (*i.e.,* code the exact same gene product), the person is *homozygous,* and if the two members are different, the person is *heterozygous.* The genetic composition of a person is called a *genotype,* whereas the *phenotype* is the observable expression of a genotype in terms of morphologic, biochemical, or molecular traits.

If the trait is expressed in the heterozygote (one member of the gene pair codes for the trait), it is said to be *dominant*; if it is expressed only in the homozygote (both members of the gene pair code for the trait), it is *recessive*.

SINGLE-GENE DISORDERS

Single-gene disorders are caused by a single defective or mutant gene. The defective gene may be present on an autosome or the X chromosome and it may affect only one member of an autosomal gene pair (matched with a normal gene) or both members of the pair. Single-gene defects follow the mendelian patterns of inheritance (see Chapter 3) and are often called *mendelian disorders*. At last count, there were more than 8000 single-gene disorders, many of which have been mapped to a specific chromosome.[3]

A single mutant gene may be expressed in many different parts of the body. Marfan syndrome is a defect in connective tissue that has widespread effects involving skeletal, eye, and cardiovascular structures. In other single-gene disorders, the same defect can be caused by mutations at several different loci. Childhood deafness can result from 16 different types of autosomal recessive mutations.

Single-gene disorders are characterized by their patterns of transmission, which usually are obtained through a family genetic history. The patterns of inheritance depend on whether the phenotype is dominant or recessive, and whether the gene is located on an autosomal or sex chromosome. Disorders of autosomal inheritance include autosomal dominant and autosomal recessive traits. Among the approximate 8000 single-gene disorders, more than half are autosomal dominant. Autosomal recessive phenotypes are less common, accounting for approximately one third of single-gene disorders.[4] Currently, all sex-linked genetic disorders are thought to be X-linked and most are recessive. The only mutations affecting the Y-linked genes are involved in spermatogenesis and male fertility and hence are not transmitted.

Virtually all single-gene disorders lead to formation of an abnormal protein or decreased production of a gene product. The defect can result in defective or decreased amounts of an enzyme, defects in receptor proteins and their function, alterations in nonenzyme proteins, or mutations resulting in unusual reactions to drugs.

Autosomal Dominant Disorders

Autosomal dominant disorders involve a single mutant allele that is transmitted from an affected parent to an offspring regardless of sex. The affected parent has a 50% chance of transmitting the disorder to each offspring (Fig. 4-1). The unaffected relatives of the parent or unaffected siblings of the offspring do not transmit the disorder. In many conditions, the age of onset is delayed, and the signs and symptoms of the disorder do not appear until later in life, as in Huntington disease (see Chapter 36).

Autosomal dominant disorders also may manifest as a new mutation. Whether the mutation is passed on to the next generation depends on the affected person's reproductive capacity. Many new autosomal dominant mutations are accompanied by reduced reproductive capacity; therefore, the defect is not perpetuated in future generations. If an autosomal defect is accompanied by a total inability to reproduce, essentially all new cases of the disorder will be due to new mutations. If the defect does not affect reproductive capacity, it is more likely to be inherited.

Although there is a 50% chance of inheriting a dominant genetic disorder from an affected parent, there can be wide variation in gene penetration and expression. When a person inherits a dominant mutant gene but fails to express it, the trait is described as having *reduced penetrance*. Penetrance is expressed in mathematical terms; a 50% penetrance indicates that a person who inherits the defective gene has a 50% chance of expressing the disorder. The person who has a mutant gene but does not express it is an important exception to the rule that unaffected persons do not transmit an autosomal dominant

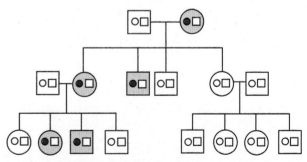

FIGURE 4-1 Simple pedigree for inheritance of an autosomal dominant trait. The *small colored circle* represents the mutant gene. An affected parent with an autosomal dominant trait has a 50% chance of passing the mutant gene on to each child, regardless of sex.

trait. These persons can transmit the gene to their descendants and so produce a skipped generation. Autosomal dominant disorders also can display *variable expressivity,* meaning that they can be expressed differently among individuals. For example, polydactyly or the presence of more than the usual number of digits may be expressed in the fingers or the toes.

The gene products of autosomal dominant disorders usually are regulatory proteins involved in rate-limiting components of complex metabolic pathways or key components of structural proteins such as collagen.[5,6] Two disorders of autosomal inheritance, Marfan syndrome and neurofibromatosis (NF), are described in this chapter.

Marfan Syndrome. Marfan syndrome is a connective tissue disorder that is manifested by changes in the skeleton, eyes, and cardiovascular system. The cause of Marfan syndrome has been mapped to a gene that codes for a connective tissue protein, fibrillin-1 (FBN1), on the long arm of chromosome 15.[5]

There is a wide range of variation in gene expression in persons with Marfan syndrome. Persons may have abnormalities of one or all three systems. The skeletal deformities, which are the most obvious features of the disorder, include a long, thin body with exceptionally long extremities and long, tapering fingers, sometimes called *arachnodactyly* or *spider fingers* (Fig. 4-2), hyperextensible joints, and a variety of spinal deformities including kyphoscoliosis. Chest deformity, pectus excavatum (*i.e.,* deeply depressed sternum), or pigeon chest deformity, often is present. The most common eye disorder is bilateral dislocation of the lens caused by weakness of the suspensory ligaments. Myopia and predisposition to retinal detachment also are common, the result of increased optic globe length due to altered connective tissue support of ocular structures. However, the most life-threatening aspects of the disorder are the cardiovascular defects, which include mitral valve prolapse, progressive dilation of the aortic valve ring, and weakness of the aorta and other arteries. Dissection and rupture of the aorta often lead to premature death. The average age of death in persons with Marfan syndrome is 30 to 40 years.[5]

Neurofibromatosis. Neurofibromatosis is a condition involving neurogenic tumors that arise from Schwann cells and other elements of the peripheral nervous system.[5,6] There are at least two genetically and clinically distinct forms of the disorder: type 1 NF (NF-1), also known as *von Recklinghausen disease,* and type 2 bilateral acoustic NF (NF-2). Both of these disorders result from a genetic defect in a tumor suppressor protein that regulates cell growth.[5] The gene for NF-1 has been mapped to chromosome 17, and the gene for NF-2 has been mapped to chromosome 22.

NF-1 is characterized by the presence of disfiguring neurofibromas, areas of dark pigmentation of the skin, and pigmented lesions of the iris of the eye. NF-1 is a relatively common disorder with a frequency of 1 in 3000.[6] Approximately 50% of cases have a family history of autosomal dominant transmission, and the remaining 50% appear to represent a new mutation.

The cutaneous neurofibromas, which vary in number from a few to many hundreds, manifest as soft, pedunculated lesions that project from the skin. They are the most common type of lesion, often are not apparent until puberty, and are present in greatest density over the trunk (Fig. 4-3). The subcutaneous lesions grow just below the skin; they are firm and round, and may be painful. Plexiform neurofibromas involve the larger peripheral nerves. They tend to form large tumors that cause severe disfigurement of the face or an extremity. The pigmented skin lesions, known as *café-au-lait spots,* consist of large (usually ≥15 mm in diameter), flat cutaneous pigmentations. The lesions tend to be ovoid, with the longer axis oriented

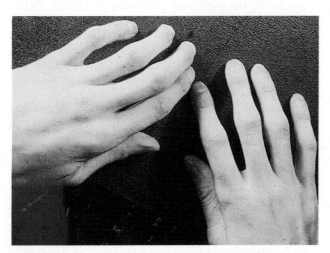

FIGURE 4-2 Long, slender fingers (arachnodactyly) in a patient with Marfan syndrome. (From Rubin E., Gorstein F., Rubin R., et al. [2005]. *Rubin's pathology: Clinicopathologic foundations of medicine* [4th ed., p. 244]. Philadelphia: Lippincott Williams & Wilkins.)

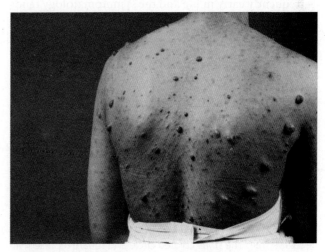

FIGURE 4-3 Neurofibromatosis, type I. Multiple cutaneous neurofibromas are noted on the trunk. (From Rubin E., Gorstein F., Rubin R., et al. [2005]. *Rubin's pathology: Clinicopathologic foundations of medicine* [4th ed., p. 246]. Philadelphia: Lippincott Williams & Wilkins.)

in the direction of the cutaneous nerve. Pigmented nodules of the iris (Lisch nodules), which are specific for NF-1, usually are present after 6 years of age. They do not present any clinical problem but are useful in establishing a diagnosis. Persons with NF-1 may also have a variety of other associated lesions, the most common being skeletal lesions such as scoliosis and erosive bone defects.

One of the major complications of NF-1, occurring in 3% to 5% of persons with the disease, is the appearance of a neurosarcoma in a neurofibroma.[5] NF-1 is also associated with an increased risk for development of other nervous system tumors such as meningiomas, optic gliomas, and pheochromocytomas (discussed in Chapter 17).

NF-2 is characterized by tumors of the acoustic nerve. It is much less common than NF-1, occurring in about 1 in 50,000 persons. Most often, the disorder is asymptomatic through the first 15 years of life. The most frequently reported symptoms are headaches, hearing loss, and tinnitus (*i.e.*, ringing in the ears). There may be associated intracranial and spinal meningiomas. The condition is made worse by pregnancy, and oral contraceptives may increase the growth and symptoms of tumors. Persons with the disorder should be warned that severe disorientation may occur during diving or swimming underwater, and drowning may result. Surgery may be indicated for debulking or removal of the tumors.

Autosomal Recessive Disorders

Autosomal recessive disorders are manifested only when both members of the gene pair are affected. In this case, both parents may be unaffected but are carriers of the defective gene. Autosomal recessive disorders affect both sexes. The occurrence risk in each pregnancy is one in four for an affected child, two in four for a carrier child, and one in four for a normal (noncarrier, unaffected) homozygous child (Fig. 4-4).

With autosomal recessive disorders, the age of onset is frequently early in life and the symptomatology tends to be more uniform than with autosomal dominant dis-

orders. The disorders are characteristically caused by deficiencies in enzymes rather than abnormalities in structural proteins. In the case of a heterozygous carrier, the presence of a mutant gene usually does not produce symptoms because equal amounts of normal and defective enzymes are synthesized. By contrast, the inactivation of both alleles in a homozygote results in complete loss of enzyme activity. Autosomal recessive disorders include almost all inborn errors of metabolism. Enzyme disorders that impair catabolic pathways result in an accumulation of dietary substances (*e.g.*, phenylketonuria [PKU]) or cellular constituents (*e.g.*, lysosomal storage diseases). Other disorders result from a defect in the enzyme-mediated synthesis of an essential protein (*e.g.*, the cystic fibrosis transmembrane conductance regulator in cystic fibrosis). Two examples of autosomal recessive disorders that are not covered elsewhere in this book are PKU and Tay-Sachs disease.

Phenylketonuria. Phenylketonuria is a relatively rare metabolic disorder caused by a deficiency of the liver enzyme that converts the amino acid phenylalanine to tyrosine. As a result of this deficiency, toxic levels of the amino acid phenylalanine accumulate in the blood and other tissues. The disorder, which affects approximately 1 in every 15,000 infants in the United States, is usually inherited as a recessive trait and is manifested only in the homozygote.[7] If untreated, the disorder results in mental retardation, microcephaly, delayed speech, and other signs of impaired neurologic development.

Because the symptoms of untreated PKU develop gradually and would often go undetected until irreversible mental retardation had occurred, newborn infants are routinely screened for abnormal levels of serum phenylalanine. It also is possible to identify carriers of the trait by subjecting them to a phenylalanine test, in which a large dose of phenylalanine is administered orally and the rate at which it disappears from the bloodstream is measured.

In 2000, the National Institutes of Health (NIH) released a consensus statement on the screening and management of PKU.[7] This statement emphasized the need for a nationwide approach to newborn screening that includes appropriate specimen collection; specimen tracking; laboratory analysis; data collection and analysis; locating and notifying families with abnormal results; diagnosis; treatment; and long-term management consisting of psychological, nursing, and social services, as well as nutritional therapy and genetic and family counseling.

Infants with the disorder are treated with a special diet that restricts phenylalanine intake. The results of dietary therapy of children with PKU have been impressive. The diet can prevent mental retardation as well as other neurodegenerative effects of untreated PKU. However, dietary treatment must be started early in neonatal life to prevent brain damage. Infants with elevated phenylalanine levels (>10 mg/dL) should begin treatment by 7 to 10 days of age. Evidence suggests that high levels of phenylalanine even during the first 2 weeks of life can affect the structural development of the visual system, although visual deficits are usually mild.[7] Women with PKU who wish to have

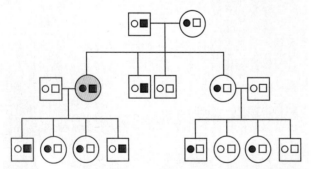

FIGURE 4-4 Simple pedigree for inheritance of an autosomal recessive trait. The *small colored circle* and *square* represent a mutant gene. When both parents are carriers of a mutant gene, there is a 25% chance of having an affected child, a 50% chance of a carrier child, and a 25% chance of a nonaffected or noncarrier child, regardless of sex. All children (100%) of an affected parent are carriers.

children require careful attention to their diet, both before conception and during pregnancy, as a means of controlling their phenylalanine levels.[7]

Tay-Sachs Disease. Tay-Sachs disease is a variant of a class of lysosomal storage diseases, known as *gangliosidoses*, in which substances (gangliosides) found in membranes of nervous tissue are deposited in neurons of the central nervous system (CNS) and retina because of a failure of lysosomal degradation.[5,6] The disease is particularly prevalent among eastern European (Ashkenazi) Jews. Infants with Tay-Sachs disease appear normal at birth but begin to manifest progressive weakness, muscle flaccidity, and decreased attentiveness at approximately 6 to 10 months of age. This is followed by rapid deterioration of motor and mental function, often with the development of generalized seizures. Retinal involvement leads to visual impairment and eventual blindness. Death usually occurs before 4 years of age. Although there is no cure for the disease, analysis of the blood serum for a deficiency of the lysosomal enzyme, hexosaminidase A, which is deficient in Tay-Sachs disease, allows for accurate identification of the genetic carriers for the disease.

X-Linked Disorders

Sex-linked disorders are almost always associated with the X, or female, chromosome, and the inheritance pattern is predominantly recessive. Because of a normal paired gene, female heterozygotes rarely experience the effects of a defective gene. The common pattern of inheritance is one in which an unaffected mother carries one normal and one mutant allele on the X chromosome. This means that she has a 50% chance of transmitting the defective gene to her sons, and her daughters have a 50% chance of being carriers of the mutant gene (Fig. 4-5). When the affected son procreates, he transmits the defective gene to all of his daughters, who become carriers of the mutant gene. Because the genes of the Y chromosome are unaffected, the affected male does not transmit the defect to any of his sons, and they will not be carriers or transmit the disorder to their children. X-linked recessive disorders include glucose-6-phosphate dehydrogenase deficiency (see Chapter 11), hemophilia A (see Chapter 10), and X-linked agammaglobulinemia (see Chapter 15).

Fragile X Syndrome. Fragile X syndrome is an X-linked disorder associated with a fragile site on the X chromosome. As with other X-linked disorders, fragile X syndrome affects males more often than females. The disorder, which affects approximately 1 in 1250 males and 1 in 2500 females, is the second most common cause of mental retardation, after Down syndrome.[5]

In 1991, the fragile X syndrome was mapped to a small area on the X chromosome (Xq27), now designated the site of the fragile X mental retardation-1 (FMR1) gene.[8] Researchers believe that the FMR1 gene codes for a protein that may regulate the amount of communication between brain cells. The mechanism by which the normal FMR1 gene is converted to an altered, or mutant, gene capable of producing disease symptoms involves an increase in the length of the gene. A small region of the gene that contains a CCG triplet code undergoes repeated duplication, resulting in a longer gene (Fig. 4-6). The longer gene is susceptible to methylation, a chemical process that results in inactivation of the FMR1 gene. When the number of repeats is small (<200), the person often has few or no manifestations of the disorder, compared with those evidenced in persons with a larger number of repeats.

Affected males, although appearing normal at birth, are mentally retarded and share a common physical phenotype that includes a long face with large mandible; large, everted ears; and large testicles (macroorchidism). Hyperextensible joints, a high-arched palate, and mitral

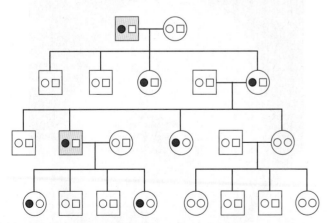

FIGURE 4-5 Simple pedigree for inheritance of an X-linked recessive trait. X-linked recessive traits are expressed phenotypically in the male offspring. A *small colored circle* represents the X chromosome with the defective gene, and the *larger colored square* the affected male. The affected male passes the mutant gene to all of his daughters, who become carriers of the trait and have a 50% chance of passing the gene to their sons and their daughters, who in turn have a 50% chance of being carriers of the gene.

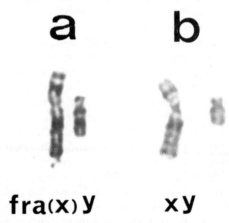

FIGURE 4-6 Fragile X [fra(x)y] chromosome. Note the increased length of the fragile X chromosome (**A**) compared with normal X chromosome (**B**). (From Rubin E., Gorstein F., Rubin R., et al. [2005]. *Rubin's pathology: Clinicopathologic foundations of medicine* [4th ed., p. 265]. Philadelphia: Lippincott Williams & Wilkins.)

valve prolapse, which are observed in some cases, mimic a connective tissue disorder. Some physical abnormalities may be subtle or absent.[5,8]

In fragile X families, the probability of being affected with the disorder is related to the position in the pedigree: later generations are more likely to be affected than earlier ones. This phenomenon reflects the progressive nature of the repeated expansion of the genes on the fragile site of the X chromosome. Approximately 20% of males who have been shown to carry the fragile X mutation are clinically and cytogenetically normal. Because male carriers transmit the trait through all their daughters (who are phenotypically normal) to affected grandchildren, they are called *transmitting males.* Approximately one third of female carriers are affected (mentally retarded), a proportion that is higher than with other X-linked disorders.[5] It is thought that the variability in disease expression in females may relate to the pattern of X inactivation (see discussion of the Lyon principle in Chapter 3).

Multifactorial Inheritance Disorders

Multifactorial inheritance disorders are caused by multiple genes and, in many cases, environmental factors. The exact number of genes contributing to multifactorial traits is not known, and these traits do not follow a clear-cut pattern of inheritance, as do single-gene disorders. Disorders of multifactorial inheritance can be expressed during fetal life and be present at birth, or they may be expressed later in life. Congenital disorders that are thought to arise through multifactorial inheritance include cleft lip or palate, clubfoot, congenital dislocation of the hip, congenital heart disease, pyloric stenosis, and urinary tract malformation. Environmental factors are thought to play a significant role in disorders of multifactorial inheritance that develop in adult life, such as coronary artery disease, diabetes mellitus, hypertension, cancer, and common psychiatric disorders such as manicdepressive psychoses and schizophrenia.

Although multifactorial traits cannot be predicted with the same degree of accuracy as disorders caused by single-gene mutations, characteristic patterns exist. First, multifactorial congenital malformations tend to involve a single organ or tissue derived from the same embryonic developmental field. Second, the risk of recurrence in future pregnancies is for the same or a similar defect. This means that parents of a child with a cleft palate defect have an increased risk of having another child with a cleft palate, but not with spina bifida. Third, the increased risk (compared with the general population) among first-degree relatives of the affected person is 2% to 7%, and among second-degree relatives it is approximately one half that amount.[5] The risk increases with increasing incidence of the defect among relatives. This means that the risk is greatly increased when a second child with the defect is born to a couple. The risk also increases with severity of the disorder and when the defect occurs in the sex not usually affected by the disorder.

Cleft Lip and Cleft Palate. Cleft lip with or without cleft palate is one of the most common birth defects. It is one of the more conspicuous birth defects, resulting in abnormal facial appearance and defective speech. The incidence varies among ethnic groups, ranging from 3.6 per 1000 live births among Native Americans to 2.0 per 1000 among Asians, 1.0 per 1000 among people of European ancestry, to 0.3 per 1000 among Africans.[9] Cleft lip with or without cleft palate is more frequent among boys, whereas isolated cleft palate is twice as common among girls.

Developmentally, the defect has its origin at about the 35th day of gestation when the frontal prominences of the craniofacial structures fuse with the maxillary process to form the upper lip.[5] This process is under the control of many genes, and the disturbances in gene expression (hereditary or environmental) at this time may result in cleft lip with or without cleft palate (Fig. 4-7). The defect may also be caused by teratogens (*e.g.,* rubella, anticonvulsant drugs) and is often encountered in children with chromosomal abnormalities.

Cleft lip and palate defects may vary from a small notch in the vermilion border of the lip to complete separation involving the palate and extending into the floor of the nose. The clefts may be unilateral or bilateral and may involve the alveolar ridge. The condition may be accompanied by deformed, supernumerary, or absent teeth. Isolated cleft palate occurs in the midline and may involve only the uvula or may extend into or through the soft and hard palates.

A child with cleft lip or palate may require years of special treatment by medical and dental specialists, including

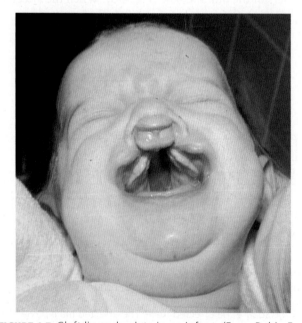

FIGURE 4-7 Cleft lip and palate in an infant. (From Rubin E., Gorstein F., Rubin R., et al. [2005]. *Rubin's pathology: Clinicopathologic foundations of medicine* [4th ed., p. 268]. Philadelphia: Lippincott Williams & Wilkins.)

a plastic surgeon, pediatric dentist, orthodontist, speech therapist, and nurse specialist. The immediate problem in an infant with cleft lip or palate is feeding. This is often accomplished through construction of a plastic obturator or use of specially constructed nipples with large openings and a squeezable bottle.[10]

Major advances in the care of children born with cleft lip and palate were made in the last quarter of the 20th century.[11] During the past decade, the older staged operations have been superseded by synchronous repair of bilateral cleft lip, gums, and nasal deformity. Earlier and more effective surgical procedures have also reduced the prevalence of the "cleft-palate speech" that can present as a problem in children with the disorder.

Mitochondrial Gene Disorders

The mitochondria contain their own DNA, which is distinct from the DNA contained in the cell nucleus (see Chapter 1). Mitochondrial DNA, which is packaged in a double-stranded circular chromosome located inside the mitochondria, is often referred to as the "other human genome."[12,13] Mitochondrial DNA is subject to mutations at a higher rate than nuclear DNA and it has no repair mechanisms. It is inherited maternally and does not recombine; thus, mothers transmit mitochondrial genes to all their offspring—male and female. However, although daughters transmit the DNA further to their offspring, sons do not.

Mitochondrial DNA contains 37 genes, which encode 2 types of ribosomal RNA, 22 types of transfer RNA, and 13 polypeptides that participate in oxidative phosphorylation.[5] Another 74 polypeptides that participate in oxidative phosphorylation are encoded by the nuclear genes. Consequently, disorders of mitochondrial function can result from mutations in either mitochondrial DNA or nuclear DNA. Oxidative phosphorylation is central to three major functions of the mitochondria: (1) production of cell energy, (2) generation of reactive oxygen species, and (3) generation of apoptosis signals.[5] Diseases associated with mitochondrial inheritance are rare and many affect the neuromuscular system.

Our understanding of the role of mitochondrial DNA has evolved since 1988, when the first mutation of mitochondrial DNA was discovered.[12] Since that time, more than 100 different disease-related rearrangements and point mutations have been identified.[5] Table 4-1 describes representative examples of disorders due to mutations in mitochondrial DNA.

CHROMOSOMAL DISORDERS

Chromosomal disorders form a major category of genetic disease, accounting for a large proportion of reproductive wastage (early gestational abortions), congenital malformations, and mental retardation. Specific chromosomal abnormalities can be linked to more than 60 identifiable syndromes that are present in 0.7% of all live births, 2% of all pregnancies in women older than 35 years of age, and 50% of all first-term abortions.[3]

During mitotic cell division in nongerm cells, the chromosomes replicate so that each cell receives a full diploid number. In germ cells, a different form of reduction division (i.e., meiosis) takes place (see Chapter 3, Fig. 3-6). During meiosis, the double sets of 22 autosomes and the 2 sex chromosomes (normal diploid number) are reduced to single sets (haploid number) in each gamete. At the time of conception, the haploid number in the ovum and that in the sperm join and restore the diploid number of chromosomes. Chromosomal defects usually develop during meiosis because of failure of chromosome separation (nondisjunction), rearrangement of genetic constituents, or breakage of a chromosome with loss or translocation of genetic material.

Chromosome abnormalities are commonly described according to the shorthand description of the karyotype. In this system, the total number of chromosomes is given first, followed by the sex chromosome complement, and then the description of any abnormality. For example, a male with trisomy 21 is designated 47, XY, +21.

TABLE 4-1	**Some Disorders of Organ Systems Associated With Mitochondrial DNA Mutations**
Disorder	**Manifestations**
Leigh disease	Proximal muscle weakness, sensory neuropathy, developmental delay, ataxia, seizures, dementia, and visual impairment due to retinal pigment degeneration
Myoclonic epilepsy with ragged red fibers	Myoclonic seizures, cerebellar ataxia, mitochondrial myopathy (muscle weakness, fatigue)
Leber hereditary optic neuropathy	Painless, subacute, bilateral visual loss, with central blind spots (scotomas) and abnormal color vision
MELAS	*Mitochondrial Encephalomyopathy* (cerebral structural changes), *Lactic Acidosis*, and *Strokelike* syndrome, seizures, and other clinical and laboratory abnormalities. May manifest only as diabetes mellitus
MERRF	*Myoclonic Epilepsy, Ragged Red Fibers* in muscle, ataxia, sensorineural deafness
Deafness	Progressive sensorineural deafness, often associated with aminoglycoside antibiotics
Chronic progressive external ophthalmoplegia	Progressive weakness of the extraocular muscles
Kearns-Sayre syndrome	Progressive weakness of the extraocular muscles of early onset with heart block, retinal pigmentation

Alterations in Chromosome Structure

Aberrations in chromosome structure occur when there is a break in one or more of the chromosomes followed by rearrangement or deletion of the chromosome parts. Among the factors believed to cause chromosome breakage are exposure to radiation sources, such as x-rays; influence of certain chemicals; extreme changes in the cellular environment; and viral infections. Several patterns of chromosome breakage and rearrangement can occur[5] (Fig. 4-8). There can be a *deletion* of the broken portion of the chromosome. When one chromosome is involved, the broken parts may be *inverted. Isochromosome formation* occurs when the centromere, or central portion, of the chromosome separates horizontally instead of vertically. *Ring formation* results when deletion is followed by uniting of the chromatids to form a ring. *Translocation* occurs when there are simultaneous breaks in two chromosomes from different pairs, with exchange of chromosome parts. With a balanced reciprocal translocation, no genetic information is lost; therefore, persons with translocations usually are normal. However, these persons are translocation carriers and may have normal and abnormal children.

A special form of translocation called a *centric fusion* or *robertsonian translocation* involves two acrocentric chromosomes in which the centromere is near the end. Typically, the break occurs near the centromere, affecting the short arm in one chromosome and the long arm in the other. Transfer of the chromosome fragments leads to one long and one extremely short chromosome. The short fragments commonly are lost. In this case, the person has only 45 chromosomes, but the amount of genetic material that is lost is so small that it often goes unnoticed. However, difficulty arises during meiosis; the result is gametes with an unbalanced number of chromosomes. A rare form of Down syndrome can occur in the offspring of persons in whom there has been a translocation involving the long arm of chromosome 21q and the long arm of one of the acrocentric chromosomes (most often 14 or 22). The translocation adds to the normal long arm of chromosome 21; therefore, the person with this type of Down syndrome has 46 chromosomes, but essentially a trisomy of 21q.[6]

The manifestations of aberrations in chromosome structure depend to a great extent on the amount of genetic material that is lost. Many cells sustaining unrestored breaks are eliminated within the next few mitoses because of deficiencies that may in themselves be fatal. This is beneficial because it prevents the damaged cells from becoming a permanent part of the organism or, if it occurs in the gametes, from giving rise to grossly defective, nonviable zygotes. Some altered chromosomes, such as those that occur with translocations, are passed on to the next generation.

Alterations in Chromosome Duplication

Mosaicism is the presence in one individual of two or more cell lines characterized by distinctive karyotypes. This defect results from an accident during chromosomal duplication. Sometimes, mosaicism consists of an abnor-

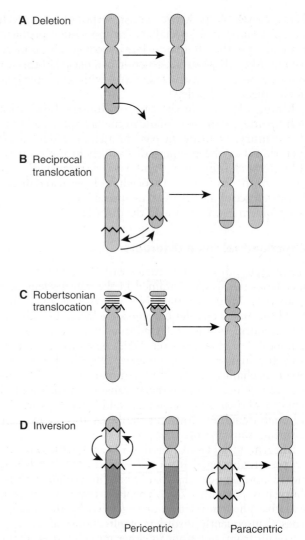

FIGURE 4-8 Examples of structural abnormalities of human chromosomes: (**A**) deletion of part of a chromosome leads to loss of genetic material and shortening of the chromosome; (**B**) a reciprocal translocation involves breaks in two nonhomologous chromosomes, with exchange of the acentric segment; (**C**) robertsonian translocation in which two nonhomologous chromosomes break near their centromeres, after which the long arms fuse to form one large metacentric chromosome; (**D**) inversion requires two breaks in a single chromosome with inversion to the opposite side of the centromere (pericentric), or paracentric if the breaks are on the same arm. (Adapted from Rubin E., Gorstein F., Rubin R., et al. [2005]. *Rubin's pathology: Clinicopathologic foundations of medicine* [4th ed., p. 228]. Philadelphia: Lippincott Williams & Wilkins.)

mal karyotype and a normal one, in which case the physical deformities caused by the abnormal cell line usually are less severe.

Alterations in Chromosome Number

A change in chromosome number is called *aneuploidy*. Among the causes of aneuploidy is failure of the chromosomes to separate during oogenesis or spermatogenesis.

This can occur in the autosomes or the sex chromosomes and is called *nondisjunction*. Nondisjunction can occur during the first or second meiotic division and gives rise to germ cells that have an even number of chromosomes (22 or 24) instead of 23. The products of conception formed from this even number of chromosomes have an uneven number of chromosomes, 45 or 47. *Monosomy* refers to the presence of only one member of a chromosome pair. The defects associated with monosomy of the autosomes are severe and usually cause abortion. Monosomy of the X chromosome (45, X/0), or Turner syndrome, causes less severe defects. *Polysomy*, or the presence of more than two chromosomes to a set, occurs when a germ cell containing more than 23 chromosomes is involved in conception. This defect has been described for the autosomes and the sex chromosomes. Trisomies of chromosomes 18 and 21 are the most common forms of polysomy of the autosomes. There are several forms of polysomy of the sex chromosomes in which extra X or Y chromosomes are present.

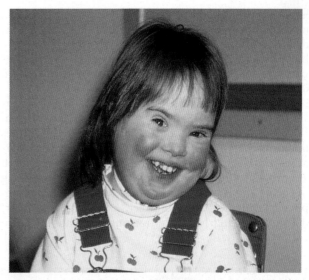

FIGURE 4-9 A child with Down syndrome. (Courtesy of March of Dimes Birth Defects Foundation, White Plains, NY.)

Down Syndrome (Trisomy 21). First described in 1866 by John Langdon Down, trisomy 21, or Down syndrome, causes a combination of birth defects, including characteristic facial features, some degree of mental retardation, and other health problems. According to the National Down Syndrome Association, it is the most common chromosomal disorder, occurring approximately once in every 800 to 1000 births. Currently, there are approximately 350,000 people in the United States with Down syndrome.[14]

Approximately 95% of cases of Down syndrome are caused by nondisjunction during the first meiotic division, resulting in a trisomy of chromosome 21.[5] Most of the remaining cases are due to a translocation in which part of chromosome 21 breaks off and attaches to another chromosome (usually chromosome 14). Although there still are only 46 chromosomes in the cell, the presence of the extra part of chromosome 21 causes the features of Down syndrome.

The risk of having a child with Down syndrome increases with maternal age: it is 1/1300 at 25 years of age, 1/365 at 35 years, and 1/30 at 45 years of age.[15] The reason for the correlation between maternal age and nondisjunction is unknown, but is thought to reflect some aspect of aging of the oocyte. Although males continue to produce sperm throughout their reproductive life, females are born with all the oocytes they ever will have. These oocytes may change as a result of the aging process. With increasing age, there is also a greater chance of a woman having been exposed to damaging environmental agents such as drugs, chemicals, and radiation.

The physical features of a child with Down syndrome are distinctive, and therefore the condition usually is apparent at birth.[15] These features include a small and rather square head. There is upward slanting of the eyes; small, low-set, and malformed ears; a fat pad at the back of the neck; an open mouth; and a large, protruding tongue (Fig. 4-9). The child's hands usually are short and stubby, with fingers that curl inward, and there usually is only a single palmar (*i.e.*, simian) crease. Hypotonia and joint laxity also are present in infants and young children. There often are accompanying congenital heart defects and an increased risk of gastrointestinal malformations. About one third of children with Down syndrome suffer from a congenital heart disorder. Of particular concern is the much greater risk of development of acute leukemia among children with Down syndrome.[5] With increased life expectancy due to improved health care, it has been found that there is an increased risk of Alzheimer disease among older persons with Down syndrome.

There are several prenatal screening tests that can be done to determine the risk of having a child with Down syndrome. The most commonly used test is the triple screen—α-fetoprotein (AFP), human chorionic gonadotropin (HCG), and unconjugated estriol.[16] Although neural tube defects have been associated with elevated levels of AFP, decreased levels have been associated with Down syndrome. The single maternal serum marker that yields the highest detection rate in Down syndrome is an elevated level of HCG. The combined use of these three maternal tests at between 15 to 20 weeks' gestation, together with the woman's age, has been shown to detect as many as 60% of Down syndrome pregnancies. Another test, nuchal translucency (sonolucent space at the back of the fetal neck), uses ultrasonography and can be performed between 10 and 13 weeks gestation.[18] The fetus with Down syndrome tends to have a larger area of translucency compared with the chromosomally normal infant. The nuchal transparency test is usually used in combination with other screening tests. The only way accurately to determine the presence of Down syndrome in the fetus is through chromosome analysis using chorionic villus sampling, amniocentesis, or percutaneous umbilical blood sampling.

Turner Syndrome (Monosomy X). Turner syndrome describes an absence of all (45, X/0) or part of the X chromosome.[17–20] Some women with Turner syndrome may have part of the X chromosome and some may display a mosaicism with one or more additional cells lines.[17] This disorder affects approximately 1 of every 2500 live births, and it has been estimated that almost all fetuses with the 45, X/0 karyotype are spontaneously aborted during the first trimester.[5]

Characteristically, the girl with Turner syndrome is short in stature, but her body proportions are normal (Fig. 4-10). Because of the absence of ovaries, she does not menstruate and shows no signs of secondary sex characteristics. There are variations in the syndrome, with abnormalities ranging from essentially none to webbing of the neck with redundant skin folds, nonpitting lymphedema of the hands and feet, and congenital heart defects, particularly coarctation of the aorta. There also

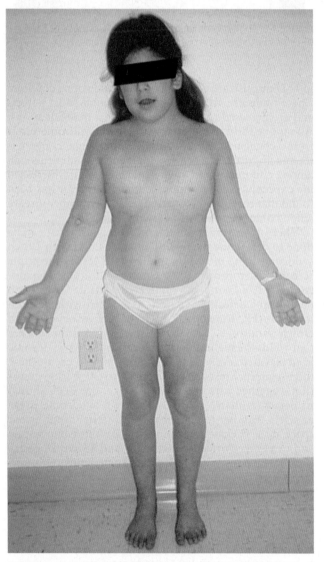

FIGURE 4-10 Turner syndrome. Short stature, stocky build, crest chest, lack of breast development, and cubitus valgus are evident in this 13-year-old girl. (From Shulman D., Beru B. [2000]. *Atlas of clinical endocrinology: Neuroendocrinology and pituitary disease.* Philadelphia: Current Medicine.)

may be abnormalities in kidney development (*i.e.,* abnormal location, abnormal vascular supply, or double collecting system). There may be other abnormalities, such as changes in nail growth, high-arched palate, short fourth metacarpal, and strabismus. Although intelligence is normal, individuals with the disorder may have problems with spatial perception, visual-motor coordination, mathematics, and other learning abilities.

The diagnosis of Turner syndrome often is delayed until late childhood or early adolescence in girls who do not present with the classic features of the syndrome.[20] Only about one fifth to one third of affected girls receive a diagnosis as a newborn because of puffy hands and feet or redundant nuchal skin; another one third receive a diagnosis in mid-childhood because of short stature; and the rest are mainly diagnosed in adolescence when they fail to enter puberty. Early diagnosis is an important aspect of treatment for Turner syndrome. It allows for counseling about the phenotypic characteristics of the disorder; screening for cardiac, renal, thyroid, and other abnormalities; and provision of emotional support for the girl and her family. Because of the potential for delay in diagnosis, it has been recommended that girls with unexplained short stature (height below the fifth percentile), webbed neck, peripheral lymphedema, coarctation of the aorta, or delayed puberty have chromosome studies done. In addition, chromosome analysis should be considered for girls who remain above the fifth percentile but have two or more features of Turner syndrome, including high palate, nail deformities, short fourth metacarpal, and strabismus.

The medical care of children with Turner syndrome requires ongoing assessment and treatment. Growth hormone is standard treatment for a child with Turner syndrome. Administration of female sex hormones (*i.e.,* estrogens) is used to promote development of secondary sexual characteristics and produce additional skeletal growth in women with Turner syndrome.

Klinefelter Syndrome (Polysomy X). Klinefelter syndrome is a condition of testicular dysgenesis accompanied by the presence of one or more extra X chromosomes in excess of the normal male XY complement.[21,22] Most males with Klinefelter syndrome have one extra X chromosome (XXY). In rare cases, there may be more than one extra X chromosome (XXXY). Regardless of the number of X chromosomes present, the male phenotype is retained.

Based on studies conducted in the 1970s, including one sponsored by the National Institute of Health and Human Development that checked the chromosomes of more than 40,000 infants, it has been estimated that the XXY syndrome is one of the most common genetic abnormalities known, occurring as frequently as 1 in 500 to 1 in 1000 male births.[21] Although the presence of the extra chromosome is fairly common, the syndrome with its accompanying signs and symptoms that may result from the extra chromosome is uncommon. Many men live their lives without being aware that they have an additional chromosome. For this reason, it has been suggested that the term *Klinefelter syndrome* be replaced with *XXY male.*[21]

Klinefelter syndrome is characterized by enlarged breasts, sparse facial and body hair, small testes, and the inability to produce sperm.[21,22] The condition often goes undetected at birth. The infant usually has normal male genitalia, with a small penis and small, firm testicles. At puberty, the intrinsically abnormal testes do not respond to stimulation from the gonadotropins and undergo degeneration. This leads to a tall stature with abnormal body proportions in which the lower part of the body is longer than the upper part. Later in life, the body build may become heavy, with a female distribution of subcutaneous fat and variable degrees of breast enlargement. There may be deficient secondary male sex characteristics, such as a voice that remains feminine in pitch and sparse beard and pubic hair. There may be sexual dysfunction along with the complete infertility that occurs owing to the inability to produce sperm. Regular administration of testosterone, beginning at puberty, can promote more normal growth and development of secondary sexual characteristics. Although the intellect usually is normal, most XXY males have some degree of language impairment. They often learn to talk later than other children and often have difficulty learning to read and write.

In summary, genetic disorders involve a permanent change or mutation in the genome. They can involve a single gene (mendelian inheritance) or multifactorial inheritance. Single-gene disorders may be present on an autosome or on the X chromosome and they may be expressed as a dominant or recessive trait. In autosomal dominant disorders, a single mutant allele from an affected parent is transmitted to an offspring regardless of sex. The affected parent has a 50% chance of transmitting the disorder to each offspring. Autosomal recessive disorders are manifested only when both members of the gene pair are affected. Usually, both parents are unaffected but are carriers of the defective gene. Their chances of having an affected child are one in four; of having a carrier child, two in four; and of having a noncarrier unaffected child, one in four. Sex-linked disorders, which are associated with the X chromosome, are those in which an unaffected mother carries one normal and one mutant allele on the X chromosome. She has a 50% chance of transmitting the defective gene to her sons, and her daughters have a 50% chance of being carriers of the mutant gene. Because of a normal paired gene, female heterozygotes rarely experience the effects of a defective gene. Multifactorial inheritance disorders are caused by multiple genes and, in many cases, environmental factors.

Chromosomal disorders result from a change in chromosome structure or number that occurs during meiosis. Alterations in chromosome structure involve deletion or addition of genetic material, which may involve a translocation of genetic material from one chromosome

pair to another. *Monosomy* involves the presence of only one member of a chromosome pair; it is seen in Turner syndrome, in which there is monosomy of the X chromosome. *Polysomy* refers to the presence of more than two chromosomes in a set. Trisomy 21 (*i.e.,* Down syndrome) is the most common form of chromosome disorder. Klinefelter syndrome involves polysomy of the X chromosome.

Disorders Due to Environmental Influences

The developing embryo is subject to many nongenetic influences. After conception, development is influenced by the environmental factors the embryo shares with the mother. The physiologic status of the mother—her hormone balance, her general state of health, her nutritional status, and the drugs she takes—undoubtedly influences the development of the unborn child. For example, diabetes mellitus is associated with increased risk of congenital anomalies. Smoking is associated with lower than normal neonatal weight. Alcohol, in the context of chronic alcoholism, is known to cause fetal abnormalities. Some agents cause early abortion. Measles and other infectious agents cause congenital malformations. Other agents, such as radiation, can cause chromosomal and genetic defects and produce developmental disorders.

PERIOD OF VULNERABILITY

The embryo's development is most easily disturbed during the period when differentiation and development of the organs are taking place. This time interval, which is often referred to as the period of *organogenesis*, extends from day 15 to day 60 after conception.[5] Environmental influences during the first 2 weeks after fertilization may interfere with implantation and result in abortion or early resorption of the products of conception. Each organ has a critical period during which it is highly susceptible to environmental derangements (Fig. 4-11). Often, the effect is expressed at the biochemical level just before the organ begins to develop. The same agent may affect different organ systems that are developing at the same time.

TERATOGENIC AGENTS

A teratogenic agent is an environmental agent that produces abnormalities during embryonic or fetal development. It is important to remember that, in this case, the environment is that of the embryo and fetus. For discussion purposes, teratogenic agents have been divided into three groups: radiation, drugs and chemical substances, and infectious agents. Chart 4-1 lists commonly identified agents in each of these groups. Theoretically, environmental agents can cause birth defects in three ways: by direct exposure of the pregnant woman and the embryo

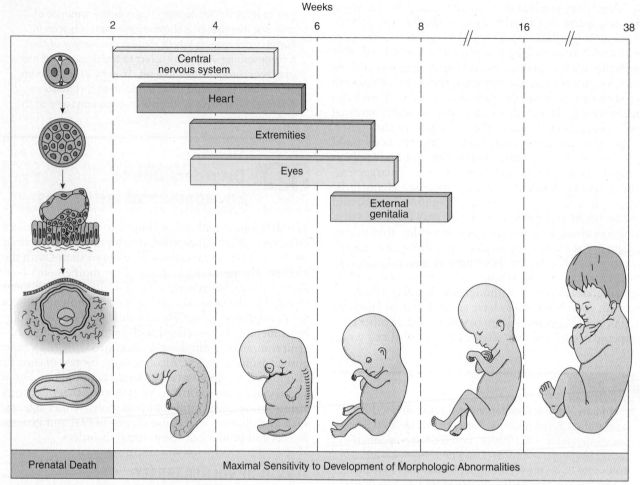

Weeks

FIGURE 4-11 Sensitivity of specific organs to teratogenic agents at critical periods in embryogenesis. Exposure to adverse influences in the preimplantation and early postimplantation stages of development (*far left*) leads to prenatal death. Periods of maximal sensitivity to teratogens (*horizontal bars*) vary for different organ systems, but overall are limited to the first 8 weeks of pregnancy. (From Rubin E., Gorstein F., Rubin R., et al. [2005]. *Rubin's pathology: Clinicopathologic foundations of medicine* [4th ed., p. 218]. Philadelphia: Lippincott Williams & Wilkins.)

or fetus to the agent; through exposure of the soon-to-be-pregnant woman to an agent that has a slow clearance rate such that a teratogenic dose is retained during early pregnancy; or as a result of mutagenic effects of an environmental agent that occur before pregnancy, causing permanent damage to a woman's (or a man's) reproductive cells.

Radiation

Heavy doses of ionizing radiation have been shown to cause microcephaly, skeletal malformations, and mental retardation. There is no evidence that diagnostic levels of radiation cause congenital abnormalities. However, because the question of safety remains, many agencies require that the day of a woman's last menstrual period be noted on all radiologic requisitions. Other institutions may require a pregnancy test before any extensive diagnostic x-ray studies are performed. Radiation is teratogenic

and mutagenic, and there is the possibility of effecting inheritable changes in genetic materials. Administration of therapeutic doses of radioactive iodine (^{131}I) during the 13th week of gestation, the time when the fetal thyroid is beginning to concentrate iodine, has been shown to interfere with thyroid development.

Chemicals and Drugs

Environmental chemicals and drugs can cross the placenta and cause damage to the developing embryo and fetus. Some of the best-documented environmental teratogens are the organic mercurials, which cause neurologic deficits and blindness. Sources of exposure to mercury include contaminated food (fish) and water.[23] The precise mechanism by which chemicals and drugs exert their teratogenic effects is largely unknown. They may have cytotoxic (cell-killing), antimetabolic, or growth-inhibiting properties. Often their effects depend on the time of exposure (in

CHART 4-1

Teratogenic Agents*

Radiation

Drugs and Chemical Substances

Alcohol
Anticoagulants
  Warfarin
Anticonvulsants
Cancer drugs
  Aminopterin
  Methotrexate
  6-Mercaptopurine
Isotretinoin (Accutane)
Propylthiouracil
Tetracycline
Thalidomide

Infectious Agents

Viruses
  Cytomegalovirus
  Herpes simplex virus
  Measles (rubella)
  Mumps
  Varicella-zoster virus (chickenpox)
Nonviral factors
  Syphilis
  Toxoplasmosis

*Not inclusive.

---

terms of embryonic and fetal development) and extent of exposure (dosage).

Drugs, including alcohol and illicit drugs, top the list of chemical teratogens. Most drugs can cross the placenta and expose the fetus to both the pharmacologic and teratogenic effects. Factors that affect placental drug transfer and drug effects on the fetus include the rate at which the drug crosses the placenta, the duration of exposure, and the stage of placental and fetal development at the time of exposure.[24] Lipid-soluble drugs tend to cross the placenta more readily and enter the fetal circulation. The molecular weight of a drug also influences the rate of transfer and the amount of drug transferred across the placenta. Drugs with a molecular weight less than 500 can cross the placenta easily, depending on lipid solubility and degree of ionization; those with a molecular weight of 500 to 1000 cross the placenta with more difficulty; and those with molecular weights greater than 1000 cross very poorly.

A number of drugs are suspected of being teratogens, but only a few have been identified with certainty.[25] Perhaps the best known of these drugs is thalidomide, which was shown to give rise to a full range of malformations, including phocomelia (*i.e.*, short, flipper-like appendages) of all four extremities. Other drugs known to cause fetal abnormalities are the antimetabolites that are used in the treatment of cancer, the anticoagulant drug warfarin, several of the anticonvulsant drugs, ethyl alcohol, and cocaine. Some drugs affect a single developing structure; for example, propylthiouracil can impair thyroid development and tetracycline can interfere with the mineralization phase of tooth development. More recently, vitamin A and its derivatives (the retinoids) have been targeted for concern because of their teratogenic potential. Concern over the teratogenic effects of vitamin A derivatives became evident with the introduction of the acne drug isotretinoin (Accutane). Fetal abnormalities such as cleft palate, heart defects, retinal and optic nerve abnormalities, and CNS malformations were observed in women ingesting therapeutic doses of the drug during the first trimester of pregnancy.[26] There also is concern about the teratogenic effects when a woman consumes high doses of vitamin A, such as those contained in some dietary supplements or vitamin pills. It is currently recommended that doses greater than 10,000 IU should be avoided.[27]

In 1983, the U.S. Food and Drug Administration established a system for classifying drugs according to probable risks to the fetus. According to this system, drugs are put into five categories: A, B, C, D, and X.[28] Drugs in category A are the least dangerous, and categories B, C, and D are increasingly more dangerous. Those in category X are contraindicated during pregnancy because of proven teratogenicity. The law does not require classification of drugs that were in use before 1983.

Because many drugs are suspected of causing fetal abnormalities, and even those that were once thought to be safe are now being viewed critically, it is recommended that women in their childbearing years avoid unnecessary use of drugs. This pertains to nonpregnant women as well as pregnant women because many developmental defects occur early in pregnancy. As happened with thalidomide, the damage to the embryo may occur before pregnancy is suspected or confirmed.

Fetal Alcohol Syndrome. The term *fetal alcohol syndrome* (FAS) refers to a constellation of physical, behavioral, and cognitive abnormalities resulting from maternal

---

 KEY CONCEPTS

Teratogenic Agents

➤ Teratogenic agents such as radiation, chemicals and drugs, and infectious organisms are agents that produce abnormalities in the developing embryo.

➤ The stage of development of the embryo determines the susceptibility to teratogens. The period during which the embryo is most susceptible to teratogenic agents is when rapid differentiation and development of body organs and tissues are taking place, usually from days 15 to 60 postconception.

alcohol consumption. It has been reported that 1–2 in 1000 infants born in the United States manifests some characteristics of the syndrome.[29–31] Alcohol, which is lipid soluble and has a molecular weight between 600 and 1000, passes freely across the placental barrier; concentrations of alcohol in the fetus are at least as high as in the mother. Unlike other teratogens, the harmful effects of alcohol are not restricted to the sensitive period of early gestation but extend throughout pregnancy.

Alcohol has widely variable effects on fetal development, ranging from minor abnormalities to FAS. There may be prenatal or postnatal growth retardation; CNS involvement, including neurologic abnormalities, developmental delays, behavioral dysfunction, intellectual impairment, and skull and brain malformation; and a characteristic face with short palpebral fissures (i.e., eye openings), a thin upper lip, and an elongated, flattened midface and philtrum (i.e., the groove in the middle of the upper lip; Fig. 4-12). The facial features of FAS may not be as apparent in the newborn but become more prominent as the infant develops. As the children grow into adulthood, the facial features become more subtle, making diagnosis of FAS in older individuals more difficult. Each of these defects can vary in severity, probably reflecting the timing of alcohol consumption in terms of the period of fetal development, amount of alcohol consumed, and hereditary and environmental influences.

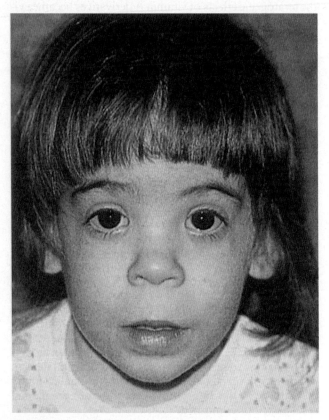

FIGURE 4-12 Fetal alcohol syndrome. (From Clarren S. K., Smith D. W. [1978]. The fetal alcohol syndrome. *New England Journal of Medicine* 298, 1065. © 1978 Massachusetts Medical Society.)

In 2004, the National Task Force on Fetal Alcohol Syndrome and Fetal Alcohol Effect published guidelines for the referral and diagnosis of FAS.[30] The diagnosis of FAS requires the documented presence of the following findings: (1) three facial abnormalities (smooth philtrum, thin vermillion, and small palpebral fissures); (2) growth deficits (prenatal or postnatal height or weight, or both, below the 10th percentile); and (3) CNS abnormalities (e.g., head circumference below 10th percentile, global cognitive or intellectual deficits, motor functioning delays, problems with attention or hyperactivity).

The amount of alcohol that can be safely consumed during pregnancy is unknown. Animal studies suggest that the fetotoxic effects of alcohol are dose dependent, rather than threshold dependent. Studies suggest that even three drinks per day may be associated with a lower IQ at 4 years of age.[32] However, it may be that the time during which alcohol is consumed is equally important. Even small amounts of alcohol consumed during critical periods of fetal development may be teratogenic. For example, if alcohol is consumed during the period of organogenesis, a variety of skeletal and organ defects may result. When alcohol is consumed later in gestation, when the brain is undergoing rapid development, there may be behavioral and cognitive disorders in the absence of physical abnormalities. Chronic alcohol consumption throughout pregnancy may result in a variety of effects, ranging from physical abnormalities to growth retardation and compromised CNS functioning. Evidence suggests that short-lived high concentrations of alcohol such as those that occur with binge drinking may be particularly significant, with abnormalities being unique to the period of exposure. Because of the possible effect on the fetus, it is recommended that women abstain from alcohol during pregnancy.

Folic Acid Deficiency. Although most birth defects are related to exposure to a teratogenic agent, deficiencies of nutrients and vitamins also may be a factor. Folic acid deficiency has been implicated in the development of neural tube defects (e.g., anencephaly, spina bifida, encephalocele). Studies have shown a reduction in neural tube defects when folic acid was taken before conception and continued during the first trimester of pregnancy.[33,34] The Public Health Service recommends that all women of childbearing age should take 400 micrograms (µg) of folic acid daily. It has been suggested that this recommendation may help to prevent as much as 50% of neural tube defects.[33] These recommendations are particularly important for women who have previously had an affected pregnancy, for couples with a close relative with the disorder, and for women with diabetes mellitus and those taking anticonvulsant drugs who are at increased risk for having infants with birth defects.

Since 1998, all enriched cereal grain products in the United States have been fortified with folic acid. To achieve an adequate intake of folic acid, pregnant women should couple a diet that contains folate-rich foods (e.g., orange juice, dark, leafy green vegetables, and legumes) with sources of synthetic folic acid, such as fortified food products.[35]

Infectious Agents

Many microorganisms cross the placenta and enter the fetal circulation, often producing multiple malformations. The acronym TORCH stands for *t*oxoplasmosis, *o*ther, *r*ubella (*i.e.*, German measles), *c*ytomegalovirus, and *h*erpes, which are the agents most frequently implicated in fetal anomalies.[5] Other infections include varicella-zoster virus infection, listeriosis, leptospirosis, Epstein-Barr virus infection, tuberculosis, and syphilis. The TORCH screening test examines the infant's serum for the presence of antibodies to these agents. These infections tend to cause similar clinical manifestations, including microcephaly, hydrocephalus, defects of the eye, and hearing problems.

Toxoplasmosis is a protozoal infection that can be contracted by eating raw or poorly cooked meat.[35] The domestic cat also seems to carry the organism, excreting the protozoa in its stools. It has been suggested that pregnant women should avoid contact with excrement from the family cat. The introduction of the rubella vaccine in the United States has virtually eliminated congenital rubella. The epidemiology of cytomegalovirus infection is largely unknown. Some infants are severely affected at birth, and others, although having evidence of the infection, have no symptoms. In some symptom-free infants, brain damage becomes evident over a span of several years. There also is evidence that some infants contract the infection during the first year of life, and in some of them the infection leads to retardation a year or two later. Herpes simplex type 2 infection is considered to be a genital infection and usually is transmitted through sexual contact. The infant acquires this infection in utero or in passage through the birth canal.

> **In summary,** a teratogenic agent is one that produces abnormalities during embryonic or fetal life. It is during the early part of pregnancy (15 to 60 days after conception) that environmental agents are most apt to produce their deleterious effects on the developing embryo. A number of environmental agents can be damaging to the unborn child, including radiation, drugs and chemicals, and infectious agents. Because many drugs have the potential for causing fetal abnormalities, often at an early stage of pregnancy, it is recommended that women of childbearing age avoid unnecessary use of drugs. FAS is a risk for infants of women who regularly consume alcohol during pregnancy. It also has been shown that folic acid deficiency can contribute to neural tube defects. The acronym TORCH stands for *toxoplasmosis, other, rubella, cytomegalovirus,* and *herpes,* which are the infectious agents most frequently implicated in fetal anomalies.

Prenatal Diagnosis

Prenatal diagnosis should begin with measures to identify pregnancies in which there is a recognizable risk of diagnosable fetal disorder.[4,16] Among the methods used for fetal diagnosis are ultrasonography, maternal blood screening, amniocentesis, chorionic villus sampling, and percutaneous umbilical fetal blood sampling.

ULTRASONOGRAPHY

Ultrasonography has become the primary method used to determine gestational age, number of fetuses, fetal position, amount of amniotic fluid, and placental location. It also is possible to assess fetal movement, breathing movements, and heart pattern. In some countries, including the United States, it is common practice to perform ultrasonographic examination at some time during the second trimester. Improved resolution and real-time units have enhanced the ability of ultrasound scanners to detect congenital anomalies. With this more sophisticated equipment, it is possible to obtain information such as measurements of hourly urine output in a high-risk fetus. Ultrasonography makes possible the in utero diagnosis of hydrocephalus, spina bifida, facial defects, congenital heart defects, congenital diaphragmatic hernias, disorders of the gastrointestinal tract, and skeletal anomalies. A four-chamber view of the fetal heart improves the detection of cardiac malformations. Intrauterine diagnosis of congenital abnormalities permits planning of surgical correction shortly after birth, preterm delivery for early correction, selection of cesarean section to reduce fetal injury, and, in some cases, intrauterine therapy. When a congenital abnormality is suspected, a diagnosis made using ultrasonography usually can be obtained by weeks 16 to 18 of gestation.

Fetal echocardiography is used in the diagnosis of fetal heart defects and rhythm disturbances. It can be performed after 20 weeks' gestation and is used along with ultrasonography.

MATERNAL SERUM MARKERS

Maternal serum can provide useful indicators such as α-fetoprotein (AFP), human chorionic gonadotropin (HCG), and unconjugated estriol. AFP is a major fetal plasma protein and has a structure similar to the albumin that is found in postnatal life. AFP is made initially by the yolk sac and later by the liver. It peaks at approximately 12 to 14 weeks in the fetus and falls thereafter. The normal maternal serum AFP level rises from 13 weeks and peaks at 32 weeks of gestation. In pregnancies where the fetus has a neural tube defect (*i.e.*, anencephaly and open spina bifida) or certain other malformations such as an anterior abdominal wall defect, maternal and amniotic levels of AFP are elevated because open neural tube and ventral wall defects are associated with exposed fetal membrane and blood vessel surfaces that increase the AFP in the amniotic fluid and maternal blood. Screening of maternal blood samples usually is done between weeks 16 and 18 of gestation.

INVASIVE TESTING

Amniocentesis

Amniocentesis involves the withdrawal of a sample of amniotic fluid from the pregnant uterus by means of a needle inserted through the abdominal wall. The procedure is useful in women older than 35 years of age, who have an increased risk of giving birth to an infant with Down syndrome; in parents who have another child with chromosomal abnormalities; and in situations in which a parent is known to be a carrier of an inherited disease. Ultrasonography is used to gain additional information and to guide the placement of the amniocentesis needle. The amniotic fluid and cells that have been shed by the fetus are studied. Usually, a determination of fetal status can be made by the 15th to 18th week of pregnancy.[16] The amniotic fluid also can be tested using various biochemical tests.

Chorionic Villus Sampling

Sampling of the chorionic villi usually is performed at 10 to 12 weeks' gestation. Doing the test earlier is not recommended because of the danger of limb reduction defects in the fetus. The chorionic villi are the site of exchange of nutrients between the maternal blood and the embryo—the chorionic sac encloses the early amniotic sac and fetus, and the villi are the primitive blood vessels that develop into the placenta. The sampling procedure usually is performed using a transabdominal approach. The tissue that is obtained can be used for fetal chromosome studies, DNA analysis, and biochemical studies.

Percutaneous Umbilical Blood Sampling

Percutaneous umbilical blood sampling involves the transcutaneous insertion of a needle through the uterine wall and into the umbilical artery. It is performed under ultrasonographic guidance and is usually performed at 19 to 21 weeks of gestation.[4] It is used for prenatal diagnosis of hemoglobinopathies, coagulation disorders, metabolic and cytogenic disorders, and immunodeficiencies. Fetal infections such as rubella and toxoplasmosis can be detected through measurement of immunoglobulin M antibodies or direct blood cultures. Because the procedure carries a greater risk of pregnancy loss than amniocentesis, it usually is reserved for situations in which rapid cytogenic analysis is needed or in which diagnostic information cannot be obtained by other methods.

CYTOGENIC AND BIOCHEMICAL ANALYSES

Amniocentesis and chorionic villus sampling yield cells that can be used for cytogenetic and DNA analyses. Bio-

chemical analyses can be used to detect abnormal levels of AFP and abnormal biochemical products in the maternal blood and in specimens of amniotic fluid and fetal blood.

Cytogenetic studies are used for fetal karyotyping to determine the chromosomal makeup of the fetus. They are done to detect abnormalities of chromosome number and structure. Karyotyping also reveals the sex of the fetus. This may be useful when an inherited defect is known to affect only one sex.

Analysis of DNA is done on cells extracted from the amniotic fluid, chorionic villus sampling, or fetal blood from percutaneous umbilical sampling to detect genetic defects such as inborn errors of metabolism. The defect may be established through direct demonstration of the molecular defect or through methods that break the DNA into fragments, which are studied to determine the presence of an abnormal gene. Direct demonstration of the molecular defect is done by growing the amniotic fluid cells in culture and measuring the enzymes that the cultured cells produce. Many of the enzymes are expressed in the chorionic villi; this permits earlier prenatal diagnosis because the cells do not need to be subjected to prior culture. DNA studies are used to detect genetic defects that cause inborn errors of metabolism, such as Tay-Sachs disease, glycogen storage diseases, and familial hypercholesterolemia.

In summary, prenatal diagnosis includes the use of ultrasonography, maternal blood screening, amniocentesis, chorionic villus sampling, and percutaneous umbilical fetal blood sampling. Ultrasonography is used for determination of fetal size and position and for the presence of structural anomalies. Maternal blood screening, which measures AFP, unconjugated estriol, and HCG, is used to assess for neural tube defects (AFP) and Down syndrome (AFP, unconjugated estriol, and HCG). Amniocentesis, chorionic villus sampling, and percutaneous umbilical blood sampling are used to obtain specimens for cytogenetic and biochemical studies.

Review Exercises

A 23-year-old woman with sickle cell anemia and her husband want to have a child, but worry that their child will be born with the disease.

A. What is the mother's genotype in terms of the sickle cell gene? Is she heterozygous or homozygous?
B. If the father is found not to have the sickle cell gene, what is the probability of their child

having the disease or being a carrier of the disease?

C. If both the mother and father were heterozygous (carriers) of the sickle cell gene, what are the chances that their child would have sickle cell disease or be a carrier of the trait?

A couple has a child who was born with a congenital heart defect.

A. Would you consider the defect to be the result of a single gene or a polygenetic trait?

B. Would these parents be at greater risk of having another child with a heart defect or would they be at equal risk for having a child with a defect in another organ system, such as a cleft palate?

A 26-year-old woman is planning to become pregnant.

A. What information would you give her regarding the effects of medications and drugs on the fetus? What stage of fetal development is associated with greatest risk?

B. What is the rationale for ensuring that she has an adequate intake of folic acid before conception and during pregnancy?

C. She and her husband have an indoor cat. What precautions should she use in caring for the cat?

Visit the Porth: Essentials of Pathophysiology: Concepts of Altered Health States web site (http://thePoint.LWW.com/PorthEssentials) for links to chapter-related resources on the Internet, all-new exclusive animations, chapter review questions, and more!

REFERENCES

1. March of Dimes Birth Defects Foundation. (2003). Birth defects information. [On-line]. Available: www.modimes.org.
2. Barsch G. (2002). Genetic diseases. In McPhee S. J., Linappa V. R., Ganong W. F., et al. (Eds.), *Pathology of disease* (4th ed., pp. 2–27). New York: McGraw-Hill.
3. *Online Mendelian Inheritance in Man* (OMIN). (2003). Baltimore, MD: McKusick-Nathans Institute of Genetic Medicine, John Hopkins University; and Bethesda, MD: National Center for Biotechnology Information, National Library of Medicine. [On-line]. Available: www.ncbi.nlm.nih.gov/omim.
4. Nussbaum R. L., McInnes R. R., Willard H. F. (2001). *Thompson and Thompson genetics in medicine* (6th ed., pp. 51–78, 135, 159, 173–176, 244–249, 359–388). Philadelphia: W. B. Saunders.
5. Rubin E., Killeen N. (2005). Developmental and genetic disease. In Rubin E., Gorstein F., Rubin R., et al. (Eds.), *Rubin's pathology: Clinicopathologic foundations of medicine* (4th ed., pp. 215–279). Philadelphia: Lippincott Williams & Wilkins.
6. Kumar V., Abbas A. K., Fausto N. (2005). *Robbins and Cotran pathologic basis of disease* (7th ed., pp. 145–192). Philadelphia: Elsevier Saunders.
7. National Institutes of Health Consensus Development Panel. (2001). National Institutes of Health Consensus Development Conference Statement. Phenylketonuria: Screening and management, October 16–18, 2000. *Pediatrics* 108, 972–982.
8. National Institutes of Health. (2003). *Families and fragile X syndrome*. NIH Publication no. 96-3402. Bethesda, MD: U.S. Department of Health and Human Services, Public Health Services, National Institutes of Health.
9. Schutte B. C., Murray J. C. (1999). The many faces and factors of orofacial clefts. *Human Molecular Genetics* 10, 1853–1859.
10. Tinanoff N. (2004). Cleft lip and palate. In Behrman R. E., Kliegman R. M., Jensen H. B. (Eds.), *Nelson textbook of pediatrics* (17th ed., pp. 1207–1208). Philadelphia: Elsevier Saunders.
11. Mulliken J. B. (2004). The changing faces of children with cleft lip and palate. *New England Journal of Medicine* 351, 745–747.
12. Johns D. R. (1995). Mitochondrial DNA and disease. *New England Journal of Medicine* 333, 638–644.
13. DiMauro S., Schon E. A. (2003). Mitochondrial respiratory chain disease. *New England Journal of Medicine* 348, 2656–2668.
14. March of Dimes. (2003). Down syndrome. [On-line]. Available: www.modimes.com.
15. Roizen N. J., Patterson D. (2003). Down's syndrome. *Lancet* 361, 1281–1289.
16. Cunniff C., and the American Academy Committee of Pediatrics Committee on Genetics. (2004). Prenatal screening and diagnosis for pediatricians. *Pediatrics* 114, 889–894.
17. Sybert V. P., McCauley E. (2004). Turner's syndrome. *New England Journal of Medicine* 351, 1227–1238.
18. American Academy of Pediatrics. (2005). Clinical report: Health supervision of children with Turner syndrome. *Pediatrics* 111, 691–702.
19. Rosenfeld R. G. (2000). Turner's syndrome: A growing concern. *Pediatrics* 137, 443–444.
20. Savendahl L., Davenport M. (2000). Delayed diagnoses of Turner's syndrome: Proposed guidelines for change. *Journal of Pediatrics* 137, 455–459.
21. National Institute of Child Health and Human Development. (2000). A guide for XXY males and their family. [On-line]. Available: www.nichd.nih.gov/publications/pubs/klinefelter.htm.
22. Lanfranco F., Kamischke A., Zitzmann M., Nieschlag E. (2004). Klinefelter syndrome. *Lancet* 364, 273–283.
23. Steurerwald U., Weibe P., Jorgensen P. J., et al. (2000). Maternal seafood diet, methylmercury exposure, and neonatal neurologic function. *Journal of Pediatrics* 136, 599–605.
24. Koda-Kimble M. A., Young L., Kradian W. A. (Eds.). (2005). *Applied therapeutics: The clinical use of drugs* (8th ed., pp. 47-1–47-15). Philadelphia: Lippincott Williams & Wilkins.
25. Koren G., Pstuszak A., Ito S. (1998). Drugs in pregnancy. *New England Journal of Medicine* 338, 1128–1137.
26. Ross S. A., McCaffery P. J., Drager U. C., et al. (2000). Retinoids in embryonal development. *Physiological Reviews* 80, 1021–1055.
27. Oakley G. P., Erickson J. D. (1995). Vitamin A and birth defects. *New England Journal of Medicine* 333, 1414–1415.

28. U.S. Food and Drug Administration. (2000). Pregnancy categories. [On-line]. Available: www.fda.gov.

29. Stoll B. V., Kliegman R. M. (2004). Metabolic disturbances. In Behrman R. E., Kliegman R. M., Jensen H. L. (Eds.), *Nelson textbook of Pediatrics* (17th ed., p. 612). Philadelphia: Elsevier Saunders.

30. National Task Force on Fetal Alcohol and Fetal Alcohol Effects. (2004). *Fetal alcohol guidelines for referral and diagnosis.* [On-line]. Available: http:www.cdc.gov/ncbddd/fas/documents/FAS_guidelines_accessible.pdf. Accessed September 3, 2005.

31. American Academy of Pediatrics. (2000). Fetal alcohol syndrome and alcohol-related neurodevelopmental disorders. *Pediatrics* 106, 358–361.

32. Ernhart C. B., Bowden D. M., Astley S. J. (1987). Alcohol teratogenicity in the human: A detailed assessment of specificity, critical period, and threshold. *American Journal of Obstetrics and Gynecology* 156, 33–39.

33. Centers for Disease Control and Prevention. (1992). Recommendations for use of folic acid to reduce the number of cases of spina bifida and other neural tube defects. *Morbidity and Mortality Weekly Report* 41, 1–8.

34. Scholl T. O., Johnson W. G. (2000). Folic acid: Influence on outcome of pregnancy. *American Journal of Clinical Nutrition* 71 (Suppl.), 1295S–1303S.

35. Jones J., Lopez A., Wilson M. (2003). Congenital toxoplasmosis. *American Family Physician* 67, 2131–2138.

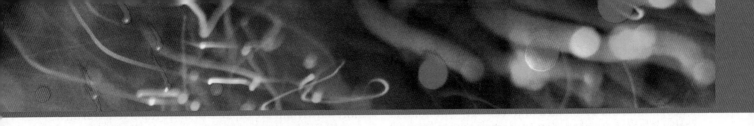

Chapter 5

Neoplasia: A Disorder of Cell Proliferation and Differentiation

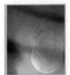 Cancer is the second leading cause of death in the United States after cardiovascular disease. The disease affects all age groups, causing more death in children 3 to 15 years of age than any other disease. According to the American Cancer Society, an estimated 1.3 million Americans were newly diagnosed with cancer in 2005 and approximately 570,300 persons died of the disease during the same year.[1] As age-adjusted cancer mortality rates increase and heart disease mortality decreases, it is predicted that cancer will become the leading cause of death in a few decades. The good news, however, is that the survival rates have improved to the extent that almost 64% of people who develop cancer each year will be alive 5 years later.[1]

Cancer is not a single disease. Cancer can originate in almost any organ, with the prostate being the most common site in men and the breast in women. The ability of cancer to be cured varies considerably and depends on the type of cancer and the extent of the disease at diagnosis. Some cancers, such as acute lymphocytic leukemia, Hodgkin disease, and testicular cancer, are highly curable, whereas others, such as cancer of the pancreas and lung, have a high mortality rate.

This chapter is divided into six sections: concepts of cell growth, benign and malignant neoplasms, etiology of cancer, clinical manifestations, diagnosis and treatment, and childhood cancers. Hematologic malignancies (lymphomas, leukemia, and myeloma) are presented in Chapter 9.

Concepts of Cell Growth

Cancer is a disorder of altered cell differentiation and growth. The resulting process is called *neoplasia,* and the tissue, a *neoplasm,* which comes from a Greek word meaning "new formation." Unlike the tissue growth that occurs with hypertrophy and hyperplasia, the growth of a neoplasm is uncoordinated and relatively autonomous in that it lacks normal regulatory controls over cell growth and division. Neoplasms tend to increase in size and continue to grow after the stimulus has ceased or the needs of the organism have been met.

Tissue renewal and repair, as well as the pathogenesis of cancer, involves cell proliferation and differentiation. *Proliferation*, or the process of cell division, is an inherent adaptive mechanism for replacing body cells when old cells die or additional cells are needed. *Differentiation* is the process of specialization whereby new cells acquire the structure and function of the cells they replace. In adult tissues, the size of a population of cells is determined by the rates of cell proliferation, differentiation, and death by apoptosis.[2] *Apoptosis*, which is discussed in Chapter 2, is a form of programmed cell death designed to eliminate senescent or unwanted cells. In some instances, the accumulation of cancer cells reflects an aberration in apoptosis.

CELL PROLIFERATION

Cell proliferation is an orderly process that provides the body with the means for replacing cells, such as skin and blood cells, that have a limited life span, increasing tissue mass during periods of growth, and providing for tissue repair and wound healing. In normal tissue, cell proliferation is regulated so that the number of cells actively dividing is equivalent to the number dying or being shed.

In terms of cell proliferation, the 200 or more cell types of the body can be divided into 3 large groups: the *permanent cells*, such as neurons and cardiac muscle cells that are unable to divide and reproduce; the *labile cells*, such as the cells forming the epithelial lining of the gastrointestinal tract and the cells of the hematopoietic system,

---

> ### ⚑ KEY CONCEPTS
>
> **Cell Proliferation and Growth**
>
> ➤ Tissue growth and repair involve cell proliferation and differentiation.
>
> ➤ Cell proliferation is the process whereby tissues acquire new or replacement cells through cell division.
>
> ➤ Cell differentiation is the orderly process in which proliferating cells are transformed into different and more specialized types. It determines the microscopic characteristics of the cell, how the cell functions, and how long it will live.
>
> ➤ Cells that are fully differentiated are no longer capable of cell division.

---

that are in a constant state of renewal; and the *stable cells*, such as those in the liver, that are normally renewed more slowly but are capable of more rapid renewal after tissue loss. In most tissues, the rate of cell reproduction is greatly increased when tissue is injured or lost. For example, bleeding stimulates the rapid reproduction of the blood-forming cells of the bone marrow.

CELL DIFFERENTIATION

Cell differentiation is the process whereby proliferating cells are transformed into different and more specialized cell types. This process leads to a fully differentiated adult cell type that has achieved its specific set of structural, functional, and life expectancy characteristics. For example, a red blood cell is programmed to develop into a concave disk that functions as a vehicle for oxygen transport and lives approximately 120 days.

The process of differentiation occurs in orderly steps; with each progressive step, increased specialization is exchanged for a loss of ability to develop different cell characteristics and different cell lines. The more highly specialized a cell becomes, the more likely it is to lose its ability to undergo mitosis. Neurons, which are the most highly specialized cells in the body, lose their ability to divide and reproduce once development of the nervous system is complete. Although there are no reserve or parent cells to direct their replacement, adequate numbers of these cell types are generated in the embryo and in early postnatal life so that the loss of a certain percentage of cells does not affect the total cell population.

Even in the continuously renewing cell populations, the more specialized cells are unable to divide. An alternative mechanism provides for their replacement. There are *progenitor* or *parent cells* of the same lineage that have not yet differentiated to the extent that they have lost their ability to divide. These cells are sufficiently differentiated that their daughter cells are limited to the same cell line, but they are insufficiently differentiated to preclude the potential for active proliferation. As a result, these progenitor cells are able to provide large numbers of replacement cells.

Another type of cell, called a *stem cell*, remains incompletely differentiated throughout life. Stem cells are reserve cells that remain quiescent until there is a need for cell replenishment, in which case they divide, thereby producing other stem cells and cells that can carry out the functions of the differentiated cell (Fig. 5-1). There are several types of stem cells. Embryos contain pluripotent stem cells, which give rise to all the tissues of the human body. In postnatal life, many fully developed tissues continue to contain reservoirs of stem cells called *adult stem cells*. Compared with embryonic stem cells, adult stem cells have more restricted differentiation capacity and are usually lineage specific. However, recent research has shown that stem cells with broad differentiation potential exist in adult bone marrow and perhaps in other tissues as well.[2] It is now recognized that bone marrow contains hematopoietic stem cells as well as stromal cells capable of differenti-

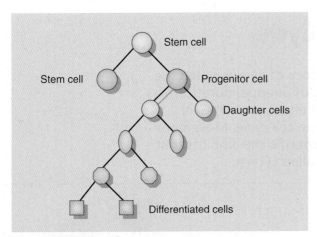

FIGURE 5-1 Mechanism of stem cell–mediated cell replacement. Division of a stem cell with an unlimited potential for proliferation results in one daughter cell, which retains the characteristics of a stem cell, and a second daughter cell, which differentiates into a progenitor or parent cell, with a limited potential for differentiation and proliferation. As the daughter cells of the progenitor cell proliferate, they become more differentiated, until reaching the stage where they are fully differentiated and no longer able to divide.

ating into various lineages. The hematopoietic stem cells generate all of the blood cells and are the primary component of bone marrow transplantation. Although work is still in the experimental stages, stromal bone marrow cells have been shown to generate osteoblasts, adipocytes, myoblasts, and endothelial cell precursors.[2]

THE CELL CYCLE

The cell cycle, which is the interval between each cell division, regulates the duplication of genetic information and appropriately aligns the duplicated chromosomes to be received by the daughter cells.[2–4] Many of the molecular events that occur in the pathogenesis of cancer involve aberrations in the cell cycle.

The cell cycle is divided into four distinct phases referred to as G_1, S, G_2, and M. G_1 (*gap 1*) is the postmitotic phase during which deoxyribonucleic acid (DNA) synthesis ceases while ribonucleic acid (RNA) and protein synthesis and cell growth take place. During the *S phase*, DNA synthesis occurs, giving rise to two separate sets of chromosomes, one for each daughter cell. G_2 (*gap 2*) is the premitotic phase and is similar to G_1 in that DNA synthesis ceases while RNA and protein synthesis continues. The *M phase* is the phase of cellular division or mitosis. Cells that are not actively dividing are quiescent and reside in G_0 (*gap 0*) or the resting phase of the cell cycle. These quiescent cells reenter the cell cycle in response to extracellular nutrients, growth factors, hormones, and other signals such as blood loss or tissue injury that signal for cell renewal.

Movement through the cell cycle is controlled by a family of proteins called *cyclins, cyclin-dependent kinases*

(*CDKs*), and their inhibitors. CDKs are enzymes that phosphorylate specific target proteins. Different combinations of cyclins and CDKs are associated with each of the stages of the cell cycle. One of the cyclin-kinase complexes (D-CDK4 complex), which is activated during G_1, plays a critical role in phosphorylating the retinoblastoma susceptibility protein (RB). Phosphorylation of RB is the molecular on-off switch for the cell cycle and alterations in its function are thought to play a role in the etiology of certain types of cancers (to be discussed). The activity of the cyclin-CDK complexes is tightly regulated by inhibitors, called *CDK inhibitors*. These inhibitors, which bind to the complexes formed between cyclins and CDKs to inactivate them, function as tumor suppressors and are frequently altered in tumors. The function of one of these suppressors is under the control of the p53 gene, which is mutated in a large number of human cancers (to be discussed).

In addition, pauses or checkpoints in the cell cycle determine the fidelity or accuracy with which DNA is duplicated. There are two main checkpoints, one at the transition from G_1 to S and another at G_2 to M. These checkpoints allow for any DNA defects to be edited and repaired, thereby ensuring that the daughter cells receive the full complement of genetic information, identical to that of the parent cell.[3] Defects in cell cycle checkpoint components are thought to play a major role in the genetic instability of cancer cells.

In summary, cancers result from disorders of cell proliferation, differentiation, and apoptosis. Cell proliferation is the process whereby cells divide and bear offspring; it normally is regulated so that the number of cells that are actively dividing is equal to the number dying or being shed. There are three types of cells based on their proliferative capacity: permanent cells that are unable to divide and reproduce; labile cells that are in a constant state of renewal; and stable cells that are normally renewed more slowly but are capable of more rapid renewal after tissue loss. Differentiation is the process whereby proliferating cells are transformed into different and more specialized cell types as they proliferate. This process leads to a fully differentiated, adult cell type that has achieved its specific set of structural, functional, and life expectancy characteristics. Apoptosis is a form of programmed cell death designed to eliminate senescent cells or unwanted cells.

The process of cell growth and division is called the cell cycle. The entry into and the progression through the various stages of the cell cycle are controlled by cyclins, CDKs, and CDK inhibitors. In addition, pauses or checkpoints in the cell cycle determine the accuracy with which DNA is duplicated. Defects in the cyclin-CDK regulation of movement through the cell cycle or in the accuracy of DNA replication at cell cycle checkpoints can contribute to the development of cancer.

Understanding ➤ The Cell Cycle

A cell reproduces by performing an orderly sequence of events called the *cell cycle.* The cell cycle is divided into five phases of unequal duration: (1) the synthesis and mitosis phases, (2) gaps (G) 1 and 2, and (3) G₀ or dormant phase during which the cell may leave the cell cycle. Movement through each of these phases is mediated (4) by specific checkpoints that are controlled by specific enzymes and proteins called *cyclins.*

1

Synthesis and mitosis. Synthesis (S) and mitosis (M) represent the two major phases of the cell cycle. The S phase, which takes about 10 to 12 hours, is the period of DNA synthesis and replication of the chromosomes. The M phase, which usually takes less than an hour, involves formation of the mitotic spindle and cell division with formation of two daughter cells.

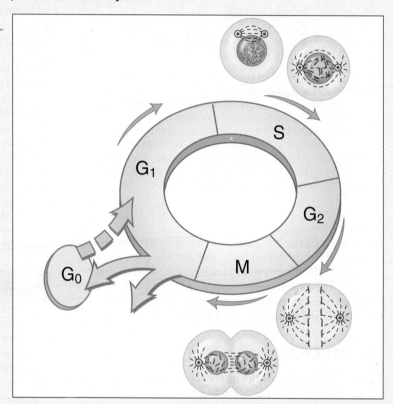

2

Gaps 1 and 2. Because most cells require time to grow and double their mass of proteins and organelles, extra gaps (G) are inserted into the cell cycle. G₁ is the stage during which the cell is starting to prepare for DNA replication and mitosis through protein synthesis and an increase in organelle and cytoskeletal elements. G₂ is the premitotic phase. During this phase, enzymes and other proteins needed for cell division are synthesized and moved to their proper sites.

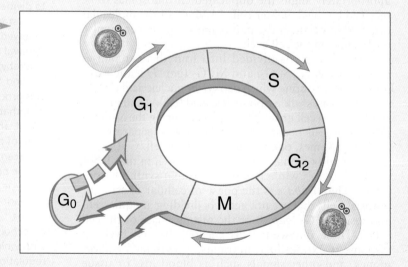

3

Gap 0. G_0 is the stage after mitosis during which a cell may leave the cell cycle and either remain in a state of inactivity or reenter the cell cycle at another time. Labile cells, such as blood cells and those that line the gastrointestinal tract, do not enter G_0 but continue cycling. Stable cells, such as hepatocytes, enter G_0 after mitosis but can reenter the cell cycle when stimulated by the loss of other cells. Permanent cells, such as neurons that become terminally differentiated after mitosis, leave the cell cycle and are no longer capable of cell renewal.

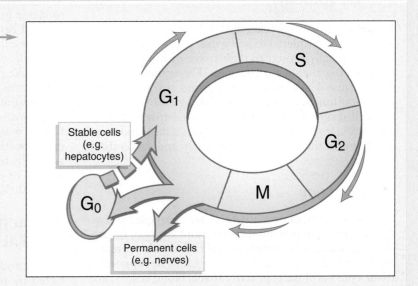

4

Checkpoints and cyclins. In most cells there are several checkpoints in the cell cycle, at which time the cycle can be arrested if previous events have not been completed. For example, the G_1/S checkpoint monitors whether the DNA in the chromosomes is damaged by radiation or chemicals, and the G_2/M checkpoint prevents entry into mitosis if DNA replication is not complete.

The cyclins are a family of proteins that control entry and progression of cells through the cell cycle. They act by activating proteins called *cyclin-dependent kinases* (CDKs). Different combinations of cyclins and CDKs are associated with each stage of the cell cycle. In addition to the synthesis and degradation of the cyclins, the cyclin-CDK complexes are regulated by the binding of CDK inhibitors. The CDK inhibitors are particularly important in regulating cell cycle checkpoints during which mistakes in DNA replication are repaired.

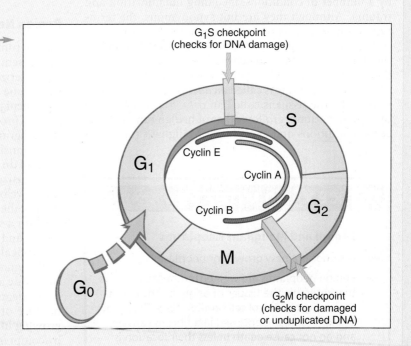

Benign and Malignant Neoplasms

Neoplasms usually are classified as benign or malignant. Tumors are considered to be *benign* when their cells are microscopically similar to their tissue of origin and are clustered together in a single mass. These tumors usually do not cause death unless their location or size interferes with vital functions. In contrast, *malignant neoplasms,* also called *cancers,* tend to invade and destroy surrounding tissues, spread to distant sites (metastasize), and cause death unless they are discovered early and successfully treated.

TERMINOLOGY

All tumors, benign or malignant, are composed of two types of tissue: parenchymal tissue and stromal, or supporting, tissue. The *parenchymal* tissue cells represent the functional components of an organ. The *supporting* tissue consists of the connective tissue, blood vessels, and lymph structure. The parenchymal cells of a tumor determine its behavior and are the component for which a tumor is named.

By definition, a *tumor* is a swelling that can be caused by a number of conditions, including inflammation and trauma. Although they are not synonymous, the terms *tumor* and *neoplasm* often are used interchangeably.

In general, benign tumors usually are named by adding the suffix *-oma* to the parenchymal tissue type from which the growth originated.[2,5] Thus, a benign tumor of glandular epithelial tissue is called an *adenoma,* and a benign tumor of bone tissue is called an *osteoma.* The naming of malignant tumors follows that of benign tumors, with certain additions and exceptions. Malignant tumors of

epithelial cell origin are called *carcinoma.* In the case of a malignant adenoma, the term *adenocarcinoma* is used. Malignant tumors of mesenchymal origin are called *sarcomas* (*e.g.,* osteosarcoma). Table 5-1 lists the names of selected benign and malignant tumors according to tissue types.

Papillomas are benign microscopic or macroscopic finger-like projections that grow on any surface. A *polyp* is a growth that projects from a mucosal surface, such as the intestine. Although the term usually implies a benign neoplasm, some malignant tumors also appear as polyps.[3] *Cancer in situ* is a localized preinvasive lesion. Depending on its location, this type of lesion usually can be removed surgically or treated so that the chances of recurrence are small. For example, cancer in situ of the cervix is essentially 100% curable.

CHARACTERISTICS OF BENIGN AND MALIGNANT NEOPLASMS

Benign and malignant neoplasms usually are differentiated by their (1) level of differentiation, (2) rate of growth, (3) local invasion, (4) capacity for metastasizing and spreading to other parts of the body, and (5) potential for causing death. The characteristics of benign and malignant neoplasms are summarized in Table 5-2.

Benign Neoplasms

Benign tumors are composed of well-differentiated cells that resemble the cells of the tissues of origin and are characterized by a slow, progressive rate of growth that may come to a standstill or regress. For unknown reasons, benign tumors have lost the ability to suppress the genetic program for cell proliferation but have retained the program for normal cell differentiation. They grow by expansion and remain localized to their site of origin and do not have the capacity to infiltrate, invade, or metastasize to distant sites. Because they expand slowly, they develop a surrounding rim of compressed connective tissue called a *fibrous capsule.*[2,5] The capsule is responsible for a sharp line of demarcation between the benign tumor and the adjacent tissues, a factor that facilitates its surgical removal.

Benign tumors do not undergo degenerative changes as readily as malignant tumors, and they usually do not cause death unless they interfere with vital functions because of their location. For instance, a benign tumor growing in the cranial cavity can eventually cause death by compressing brain structures. Benign tumors also can cause disturbances in the function of adjacent or distant structures by producing pressure on tissues, blood vessels, or nerves. Some benign tumors are also known for their ability to cause alterations in body function through abnormal elaboration of hormones.

Malignant Neoplasms

Malignant neoplasms are noted for their lack of differentiation, rapid rate of growth, ability to invade surrounding

KEY CONCEPTS

Benign and Malignant Neoplasms

➤ A tumor is a new growth or neoplasm.

➤ Benign neoplasms are well-differentiated tumors that resemble the tissues of origin but have lost the ability to control cell proliferation. They grow by expansion, are enclosed in a fibrous capsule, and do not cause death unless their location is such that it interrupts vital body functions.

➤ Malignant neoplasms are less well-differentiated tumors that have lost the ability to control both cell proliferation and differentiation. They grow in a crablike manner to invade surrounding tissues, have cells that break loose and travel to distant sites to form metastases, and inevitably cause suffering and death unless their growth can be controlled through treatment.

TABLE 5-1   Names of Selected Benign and Malignant Tumors According to Tissue Types

Tissue Type	Benign Tumors	Malignant Tumors
Epithelial		
Surface	Papilloma	Squamous cell carcinoma
Glandular	Adenoma	Adenocarcinoma
Connective		
Fibrous	Fibroma	Fibrosarcoma
Adipose	Lipoma	Liposarcoma
Cartilage	Chondroma	Chondrosarcoma
Bone	Osteoma	Osteosarcoma
Blood vessels	Hemangioma	Hemangiosarcoma
Lymph vessels	Lymphangioma	Lymphangiosarcoma
Lymph tissue		Lymphosarcoma
Muscle		
Smooth	Leiomyoma	Leiomyosarcoma
Striated	Rhabdomyoma	Rhabdomyosarcoma
Neural		
Nerve cell	Neuroma	Neuroblastoma
Glial tissue	Glioma (benign)	Glioblastoma, astrocytoma, medulloblastoma, oligodendroglioma
Nerve sheaths	Neurilemmoma	Neurilemmal sarcoma
Meninges	Meningioma	Meningeal sarcoma
Hematologic		
Granulocytic		Myelocytic leukemia
Erythrocytic		Erythrocytic leukemia
Plasma cells		Multiple myeloma
Lymphocytic		Lymphocytic leukemia or lymphoma
Monocytic		Monocytic leukemia
Endothelial		
Blood vessels	Hemangioma	Hemangiosarcoma
Lymph vessels	Lymphangioma	Lymphangiosarcoma

tissues, and metastasis to distant sites.[2,5] Because of their rapid rate of growth, malignant tumors tend to compress blood vessels and outgrow their blood supply, causing ischemia and tissue necrosis; rob normal tissues of essential nutrients; and liberate enzymes and toxins that destroy tumor tissue and normal tissue.

There are two categories of malignant neoplasms—solid tumors and hematologic cancers. Solid tumors initially are confined to a specific tissue or organ. As the growth of a solid tumor progresses, cells are shed from the original tumor mass and travel through the blood and lymph system to produce metastasis in distant sites. Hematologic cancers involve the blood-forming cells that naturally migrate to the blood and lymph systems, thereby making them disseminated diseases from the beginning.

Cancer Cell Characteristics. Cancer cells, unlike normal cells, fail to undergo normal cell proliferation and differentiation. It is thought that cancer cells develop from mutations that occur during the differentiation process.

TABLE 5-2   Characteristics of Benign and Malignant Neoplasms

Characteristics	Benign	Malignant
Cell characteristics	Well-differentiated cells that resemble cells in the tissue of origin	Cells are undifferentiated, with anaplasia and atypical structure that often bears little resemblance to cells in the tissue of origin
Rate of growth	Usually progressive and slow; may come to a standstill or regress	Variable and depends on level of differentiation; the more anaplastic the cells, the more rapid the rate of growth
Mode of growth	Grows by expansion without invading the surrounding tissues; usually encapsulated	Grows by invasion, sending out processes that infiltrate the surrounding tissues
Metastasis	Does not spread by metastasis	Gains access to blood and lymph channels to metastasize to other areas of the body

When the mutation occurs early in the process, the resulting tumor is poorly differentiated and highly malignant; when it occurs later in the process, the tumor is more fully differentiated and less malignant (Fig. 5-2).

The term *anaplasia* is used to describe the lack of cell differentiation in cancerous tissue. Undifferentiated cancer cells display marked variations in size and shape. Their nuclei are variable in size and bizarre in shape, the chromatin is coarse and clumped, and the nucleoli are often exceedingly large. In descending the scale of differentiation, enzymes and specialized pathways of metabolism are lost and cells undergo functional simplification.[2] Highly anaplastic cancer cells, whatever their tissue of origin, begin to resemble each other more than they do their tissue of origin. For example, when examined under the microscope, anaplastic cancerous tissue that originates in the liver does not have the appearance of normal liver tissue. Some cancers display only slight anaplasia, and others display marked anaplasia. The cytologic-histologic grading of tumors is based on the degree of differentiation and the number of proliferating cells. The closer the tumor cells resemble comparable normal cells, both morphologically and functionally, the lower the grade. Accordingly, grade I neoplasms are well differentiated and grade IV are poorly differentiated and display marked anaplasia.

Because cancer cells lack differentiation, they do not function properly, nor do they die according to the time frame of normal cells. In some types of leukemia, for example, the lymphocytes do not follow the normal developmental process. They do not differentiate fully, acquire the ability to destroy bacteria, or die on schedule. Instead, these long-lived, defective cells continue to grow, crowding the normal developing blood cells and thereby affecting the development of other cell lineages such as the erythrocytes, platelets, and other white blood cells. This results in reduced numbers of mature, effectively functioning cells, producing immature white blood cells that cannot effectively fight infection, a decreased pool of erythrocytes that cannot effectively transport oxygen to tissues, and a diminished number of platelets that cannot participate in the clotting system.

Alterations in cell differentiation also are accompanied by changes in cell characteristics and cell function that distinguish cancer cells from their fully differentiated normal counterparts. These changes include alterations in contact inhibition, loss of cohesiveness and adhesion, impaired cell-to-cell communication, expression of altered tissue antigens, and elaboration of degradative enzymes that enable invasion and metastatic spread.

Contact inhibition is the cessation of growth after a cell comes in contact with another cell. Contact inhibition usually switches off cell growth by blocking the synthesis of DNA, RNA, and protein. In wound healing, contact inhibition causes fibrous tissue growth to cease at the point where the edges of the wound come together. Cancer cells, however, tend to grow rampantly without regard for adjacent tissue. The reduced tendency of cancer cells to stick together (*i.e., cohesiveness* and *adhesiveness*) permits shedding of the tumor's surface cells; these cells appear in the surrounding body fluids or secretions and often can be detected by cytologic examination. Impaired cell-to-cell communication may interfere with formation of intercellular connections and responsiveness to membrane-derived signals.

Cancer cells also express a number of cell surface molecules or antigens that are immunologically identified as foreign. These *tissue antigens* are coded by the genes of a cell. Many transformed cancer cells revert to earlier stages of gene expression and produce antigens that are immunologically distinct from the antigens that are expressed by cells of the well-differentiated tissue from which the cancer originated. Some cancers express fetal antigens that are not produced by comparable cells in the adult. Tumor antigens may be clinically useful as markers to indicate the presence, recurrence, or progressive growth of a cancer. Response to treatment can be evaluated based on an increase or decrease in tumor antigens.

Cancers may also engage in the abnormal production of substances that affect body function. For example, nonendocrine tumors may assume hormone synthesis, or cancer cells may produce procoagulant materials that affect the clotting mechanisms. These conditions are often referred to as *paraneoplastic syndromes* (to be discussed).

Invasiveness and Metastasis. Unlike benign tumors, which grow by expansion and usually are surrounded by a capsule, malignant tumors grow by extensive infiltration and invasion of the surrounding tissues. The word *cancer* is derived from the Latin word meaning "crablike" because cancerous growth spreads by sending crablike projections into the surrounding tissues. Most cancers synthesize and secrete enzymes that break down proteins

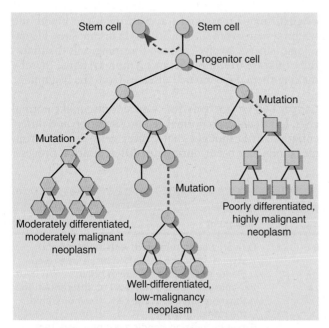

FIGURE 5-2 Mutation of a cell line. In general, mutations that occur early in the differentiation process result in poorly differentiated neoplasms and those that appear late in the differentiation process result in relatively well-differentiated neoplasms.

Labels in figure:
Stem cell
Stem cell
Progenitor cell
Mutation
Mutation
Mutation
Moderately differentiated, moderately malignant neoplasm
Poorly differentiated, highly malignant neoplasm
Well-differentiated, low-malignancy neoplasm

and contribute to the infiltration, invasion, and penetration of the surrounding tissues. The lack of a sharp line of demarcation separating them from the surrounding tissue makes the complete surgical removal of malignant tumors more difficult than removal of benign tumors.

The seeding of cancer cells into body cavities occurs when a tumor erodes into these spaces. Most often, the peritoneal cavity is involved, but other spaces such as the pleural cavity, pericardial cavity, and joint spaces may be involved. Seeding into the peritoneal cavity is particularly common with ovarian cancers.

The term *metastasis* is used to describe the development of a secondary tumor in a location distant from the primary tumor. Metastatic tumors retain many of the characteristics of the primary tumor from which they were derived. Because of this, it usually is possible to determine the site of the primary tumor from the cellular characteristics of the metastatic tumor. Some tumors tend to metastasize early in their developmental course, but others do not metastasize until later. Occasionally, the metastatic tumor is far advanced before the primary tumor becomes clinically detectable.

Metastasis occurs by way of the lymph channels (*i.e.,* lymphatic spread) and the blood vessels (*i.e.,* hematogenic spread).[2,5,6] Lymphatic spread is more typical of carcinomas and hematogenic spread of sarcomas. In many types of cancer, the first evidence of disseminated disease is the presence of tumor cells in the lymph nodes that drain the tumor area. When metastasis occurs by way of the lymphatic channels, the tumor cells lodge first in the regional lymph nodes that receive drainage from the tumor site. Once in the lymph node, the cells may die because of the lack of a proper environment, grow into a discernible mass, or remain dormant for unknown reasons. Because the lymphatic channels empty into the venous system, cancer cells that survive may eventually break loose and gain access to the circulatory system. In patients with breast cancer, lymphatic spread and, therefore, extent of disease may be determined by performing a sentinel lymph node biopsy, which is done by injecting a radioactive tracer and blue dye into the tumor to determine the first lymph node in the route of lymph drainage from the cancer. Once the sentinel lymph node is identified, it is examined to determine the presence or absence of cancer cells.

Hematogenous spread is typical of sarcomas but is also seen with carcinomas. With this type of spread, the blood-borne cancer cells typically follow the venous flow that drains the site of the neoplasm. Before entering the general circulation, venous blood from the gastrointestinal tract, pancreas, and spleen is routed through the portal vein to the liver. Thus, the liver is a common site for metastatic spread of cancers that originate in these organs. Although the site of hematologic spread is usually related to vascular drainage of the primary tumor, some tumors metastasize to distant and unrelated sites. One explanation is that cells of different tumors tend to metastasize to specific target organs that provide substances such as hormones or growth factors that are needed for their survival.[2]

The selective nature of hematologic spread indicates that metastasis is a finely orchestrated, multistep process, and only a small, select clone of cancer cells has the right combination of gene products to perform all of the steps needed for establishment of a secondary tumor (Fig. 5-3). To metastasize, a cancer cell must be able to break loose from the primary tumor, invade the surrounding extracellular matrix, gain access to a blood vessel, survive its passage in the bloodstream, emerge from the bloodstream at a favorable location, invade the surrounding tissue, and begin to grow.

Considerable evidence suggests that cancer cells capable of metastasis secrete enzymes that break down the surrounding extracellular matrix, allowing them to move through the degraded matrix and gain access to a blood vessel. Once in the circulation, the tumor cells are vulnerable to destruction by host immune cells. Some tumor cells gain protection from the antitumor host cells by aggregating and adhering to circulating blood components, particularly platelets, to form tumor emboli. Tumor cells that survive their travel in the circulation must be able to halt their passage by adhering to the vessel wall. Tumor cells express various cell surface attachment factors, such as laminin receptors that facilitate their anchoring to laminin in the basement membrane. After attachment, the tumor cells secrete proteolytic enzymes that degrade the basement membrane and facilitate their migration through the capillary wall into the surrounding tissue, where they subsequently establish growth of a secondary tumor.

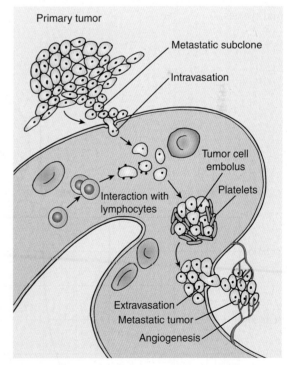

FIGURE 5-3 The pathogenesis of metastasis. (Adapted from Kumar V., Abbas A. K., Fausto N. [Eds.]. [2005]. *Robbins and Cotran pathologic basis of disease* [7th ed., p. 311]. Philadelphia: Elsevier Saunders.)

Once in the target tissue, metastasis depends on local factors that promote proliferation of the tumor cells. However, a new vascular supply is necessary for the tumor to grow. Hence, many tumors secrete growth factors, which trigger and regulate the development of new blood vessels, a process termed *angiogenesis*.[6] The presence of stimulatory or inhibitory growth factors correlates with the site-specific pattern of metastasis. One example is transferrin, a growth-promoting substance isolated from lung tissue. It has been found to stimulate the growth of extremely malignant cells that typically metastasize to the lungs. Other organs that are preferential sites for metastasis contain their own specific types of growth-promoting substances.

Tumor Growth. The rate of tissue growth in normal and cancerous tissue depends on three factors: (1) the number of cells that are actively dividing and moving through the cell cycle, (2) the duration of the cell cycle, and (3) the number of cells that are lost compared with the number of new cells that are produced. Although it was once believed that cancer resulted from totally unregulated growth and that neoplastic cells proliferated more rapidly than normal cells, it is now known that one of the reasons that cancerous tumors often seem to grow so rapidly relates to the size of the cell pool that is actively engaged in cycling. It has been shown that the cell cycle time of cancerous tissue cells is not necessarily shorter than that of normal cells; rather, cancer cells do not die on schedule. Also, the growth factors that allow cells to enter the resting, or G_0, phase when they are not needed for cell replacement are often lacking. Thus, a greater percentage of cells is actively engaged in moving through the cell cycle than occurs in normal tissues.

The ratio of dividing cells to resting cells in a tissue mass is called the *growth fraction*. The *doubling time* is the length of time it takes for the total mass of cells in a tumor to double. As the growth fraction increases, the doubling time decreases. When normal tissues reach their adult size, equilibrium between cell birth and cell death is reached. However, cancer cells continue to divide until limitations in blood supply and nutrients inhibit their growth. When this occurs, the doubling time for cancer cells decreases. If tumor growth is plotted against time on a semilogarithmic scale, the initial growth rate is exponential and then tends to decrease or flatten out over time. This characterization of tumor growth is called the *Gompertzian model*.[7]

A tumor usually is undetectable until it has doubled 30 times and contains more than 1 billion (10^9) cells. At this point, it is approximately 1 cm in size (Fig. 5-4). After 35 doublings, the mass contains more than 1 trillion (10^{12}) cells, which is a sufficient number to kill the host.

In summary, the term *neoplasm* refers to a tumor or abnormal mass of tissue in which the growth exceeds and is uncoordinated with that of normal tissue. Neoplasms may be benign or malignant. Tumors usually are named by adding the suffix *-oma* to the parenchymal tissue type from which the growth originated. A benign tumor of glandular epithelial tissue is called an *adenoma,* and one of bone tissue, an *osteoma.* Malignant tumors of epithelial tissue origin are called *carcinomas* (*e.g.,* adenocarcinoma) and those of mesenchymal origin are called *sarcomas* (*e.g.,* osteosarcoma).

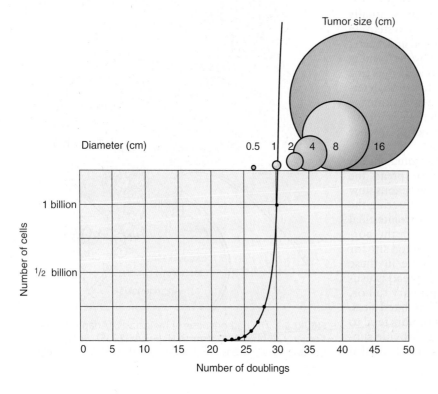

FIGURE 5-4 Growth curve of a hypothetical tumor on arithmetic coordinates. Notice the number of doubling times before the tumor reaches an appreciable size. (Adapted from Collins V. P., Loeffler R. K., Tivey H. [1956]. Observations of growth rates of human tumors. *American Journal of Roentgenology, Radium Therapy and Nuclear Medicine* 76, 988.)

Benign and malignant neoplasms usually are differentiated by their cell characteristics (differentiation or anaplasia), rate of growth, ability to invade surrounding tissues, capacity to metastasize and spread to other parts of the body, and potential for causing death. Benign tumors are composed of well-differentiated cells that bear a close resemblance to the cells of the tissue of origin, their growth is restricted to the site of origin, and the tumor usually does not cause death unless it interferes with vital functions.

Cancers or malignant neoplasms have cells that often are poorly differentiated, grow wildly and without organization, and metastasize and spread to distant parts of the body. There are two types of cancers: solid tumors and hematologic cancers. Solid tumors initially are confined to a specific organ or tissue, whereas hematologic cancers are disseminated from the onset. The spread of solid tumors occurs through three pathways: direct invasion and extension, seeding of cancer cells in body cavities, and metastatic spread through vascular or lymphatic pathways. To invade the surrounding tissues and form metastases, a cancer cell must be able to break loose from the primary tumor, invade the surrounding extracellular matrix, gain access to a blood vessel, survive its passage in the bloodstream, emerge from the bloodstream at a favorable location, invade the surrounding tissue, and begin to grow. The rapid rate of growth in malignant neoplasms is related to factors such as the number of cells that are dividing and moving through the cell cycle, the duration of the cell cycle, and the rate of apoptotic cell death.

Etiology of Cancer

The cause of cancer can be viewed from two perspectives: a molecular origin within cells and an external origin in which factors such as age, heredity, and environmental agents influence its inception and growth. Together, both mechanisms contribute to a multidimensional web of causation by which cancers develop and progress over time.

THE MOLECULAR BASIS OF CANCER

The term *oncogenesis* refers to the genetic mechanism whereby normal cells are transformed into cancer cells. Three kinds of genes control cell growth and replication: *proto-oncogenes*, *tumor suppressor genes*, and genes that control programmed cell death, or *apoptosis*.[2,5,8] In addition to these three classes of genes, a fourth category of genes, those that regulate repair of damaged DNA, is also implicated in the process of oncogenesis (Fig. 5-5). The DNA repair genes affect cell proliferation and survival indirectly through their ability to repair nonlethal damage in other genes, including proto-oncogenes, tumor suppressor genes, and the genes that control apoptosis.[2] These genes have been implicated as the principal targets of genetic damage occurring during the development of

 KEY CONCEPTS

Oncogenesis

➤ Normal cell growth is controlled by growth-promoting proto-oncogenes and growth-suppressing antioncogenes (tumor-suppressor genes). Normally, cell growth is genetically controlled so that potentially malignant cells are targeted for elimination by tumor-suppressing genes.

➤ Oncogenesis is a genetic process whereby normal cells are transformed into cancer cells. It involves mutations in the normal growth-regulating genes.

➤ The transformation of normal cells into cancer cells is multifactorial, involving the inheritance of cancer susceptibility genes and environmental factors such as chemicals, radiation, and viruses.

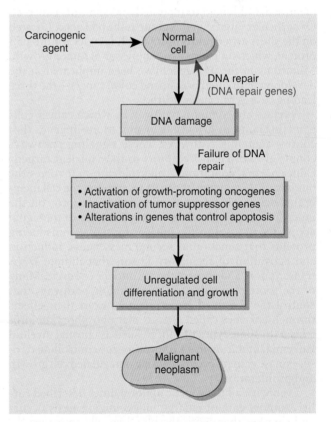

FIGURE 5-5 Flowchart depicting the stages in the development of a malignant neoplasm resulting from exposure to an oncogenic agent that produces DNA damage. When DNA repair genes are present (*red arrow*), the DNA is repaired and gene mutation does not occur.

cancer cells.[8] Such genetic damage may be caused by the action of chemicals, radiation, or viruses, or it may be inherited in the germ line. Significantly, it appears that the acquisition of a single-gene mutation is not sufficient to transform normal cells into cancer cells. Instead, cancerous transformation appears to require the activation of many independently mutated genes.

Genes that promote autonomous cell growth in cancer cells are called *oncogenes*. They are derived from mutations in proto-oncogenes and are characterized by the ability to promote cell growth in the absence of normal growth-promoting signals. A key feature of oncogene activity is that a single altered copy of a gene regulating any of the steps in this process leads to unregulated cell growth. Selected oncogenes have been associated with numerous cancer types. For example, the human epidermal growth factor receptor-2 (*HER-2/neu*) gene is amplified in up to 30% of breast cancers and indicates a tumor that is aggressive with a poor prognosis.[9] One of the newer cancer drugs is trastuzumab (Herceptin), a monoclonal antibody that selectively binds to HER-2, inhibiting the proliferation of tumor cells that overexpress HER-2.

Tumor suppressor genes, or antioncogenes, inhibit the proliferation of cells in a tumor. When this type of gene is inactivated, a genetic signal that normally inhibits proliferation is removed, thereby causing unregulated growth to begin. Numerous tumor suppressor genes have been identified and linked to inherited and sporadic cancers.[2] Of particular interest in this group is the p53 gene. Located on the short arm of chromosome 17, it codes for the p53 protein, which functions as a suppressor of tumor growth. Mutations in the p53 gene have been implicated in the development of lung, breast, and colon cancer—the three leading causes of cancer death.[2]

A relatively common pathway by which cancer cells gain autonomous growth is by mutations in genes that control signaling pathways. These signaling pathways couple growth factor receptors to their nuclear targets. Under normal conditions, cell proliferation involves the binding of a growth factor to its receptor on the cell membrane, activation of the growth factor receptor on the inner surface of the cell membrane, transfer of the signal across the cytosol to the nucleus by signal-transducing proteins that function as second messengers, induction and activation of regulatory factors that initiate DNA transcription, and entry of the cell into the cell cycle. Many of the proteins involved in the signaling pathways that control the action of growth factors exert their effects through enzymes called *kinases* that phosphorylate proteins.[2,5] In some types of cancer, such as chronic myeloid leukemia, mutation in a proto-oncogene controlling tyrosine kinase activity occurs, causing unregulated cell growth and proliferation.

Even with all the genetic abnormalities described earlier, tumors cannot enlarge unless angiogenesis occurs and supplies them with the blood vessels necessary for survival. Angiogenesis is required not only for continued tumor growth but for metastasis. The molecular basis for the angiogenic switch is unknown, but it appears to involve increased production of angiogenic factors or loss of angiogenic inhibitors. Because of the crucial role of angiogenic factors in tumor growth, much interest is focused on the development of antiangiogenesis therapy.

Tumor Cell Transformation

The transformation of normal cells to cancer cells by carcinogenic agents is a multistep process that can be divided into three stages: initiation, promotion, and progression[2] (Fig. 5-6). *Initiation* involves the exposure of cells to appropriate doses of a carcinogenic agent that makes them susceptible to malignant transformation. The carcinogenic agents can be chemical, physical, or biologic, and they produce irreversible changes in the genome of a previously normal cell. Because the effects of initiating agents are irreversible, multiple divided doses may achieve the same effects as single exposures of the same comparable dose or small amounts of highly carcinogenic substances. The most susceptible cells for mutagenic alterations in the genome are the cells that are actively synthesizing DNA.[10]

Promotion involves the induction of unregulated accelerated growth in already initiated cells by various chemicals and growth factors. Promotion is reversible if the promoter substance is removed. Cells that have been irreversibly initiated may be promoted even after long latency

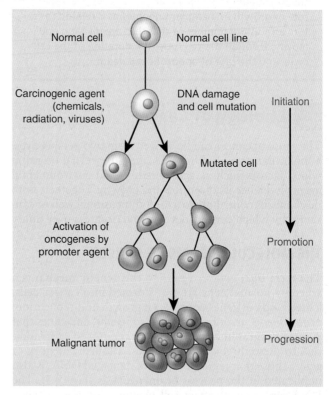

FIGURE 5-6 The process of initiation, promotion, and progression in the clonal evolution of malignant tumors. Initiation involves the exposure of cells to appropriate doses of a carcinogenic agent; promotion, the unregulated and accelerated growth of the mutated cells; and progression, the acquisition of malignant characteristics by the tumor cells.

periods. The latency period varies with the type of agent, the dosage, and the characteristics of the target cells. *Progression* is the process whereby tumor cells acquire malignant phenotypic changes that promote invasiveness, metastatic competence, autonomous growth tendencies, and increased karyotypic instability.[11]

HOST AND ENVIRONMENTAL FACTORS

Because cancer is not a single disease, it is reasonable to assume that it does not have a single cause. More likely, cancer occurs because of interactions among multiple risk factors or repeated exposure to a single carcinogenic (cancer-producing) agent. Among the host factors that have been linked to cancer are heredity, hormonal factors, and immunologic mechanisms.

Heredity

A hereditary predisposition to approximately 50 types of cancer has been observed in families. Breast cancer, for example, occurs more frequently in women whose grandmothers, mothers, aunts, and sisters also have experienced a breast malignancy. The genetic predisposition to development of cancer has been documented for a number of

cancerous and precancerous lesions that follow mendelian inheritance patterns. Cancer is found in approximately 10% of persons having one affected first-degree relative, in approximately 15% of persons having two affected family members, and in 30% of persons having three affected family members. The risk increases to approximately 50% in women 65 years of age who have multiple family members with breast cancer. Two genes, called *BRCA-1* (breast carcinoma-1) and *BRCA-2* (breast carcinoma-2), have been implicated in a genetic susceptibility to breast cancer and several other cancers, including epithelial ovarian cancers.[2,5] Approximately 10% to 20% of breast cancers are familial; mutations in *BRCA-1* and *BRCA-2* account for 80% of the familial cases in families with multiple affected members, but less than 3% in all breast cancers.[2]

Several cancers exhibit an autosomal dominant inheritance pattern that greatly increases the risk of developing a tumor. The inherited mutation is usually a point mutation occurring in a single allele of a tumor suppressor gene. Persons who inherit the mutant gene are born with one normal and one mutant copy of the gene (Fig. 5-7). For cancer to develop, the normal gene must be inactivated, usually through a somatic mutation. Retinoblastoma, a rare childhood tumor of the retina, is an example of a cancer that follows an autosomal dominant inheri-

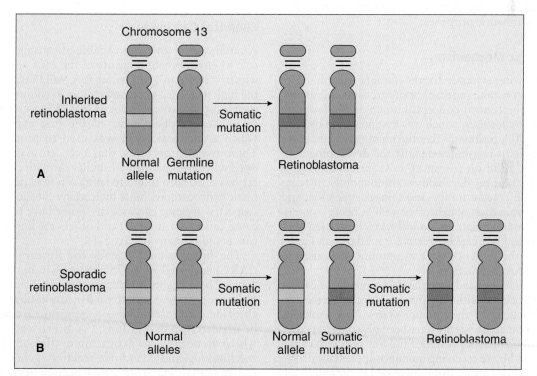

FIGURE 5-7 The "two-hit" origin of retinoblastoma. (**A**) A child with an inherited form of retinoblastoma is born with a germline mutation in one allele of the retinoblastoma (*Rb*) gene located on the long arm of chromosome 13. A second somatic mutation in the retina leads to inactivation of the normally functioning *Rb* allele and subsequent development of retinoblastoma. (**B**) In sporadic (noninherited) cases of retinoblastoma, the child is born with two normal *Rb* alleles. It requires two independent somatic mutations to inactivate *Rb* gene function and allow for appearance of a neoplastic clone. (From Rubin E., Rubin R., Aaronson S. [2005]. Neoplasia. In Rubin E., Gorstein F., Rubin R., et al. [Eds.], *Rubin's pathology: Clinicopathologic foundations of medicine* [4th ed., p. 171]. Philadelphia: Lippincott Williams & Wilkins.)

tance pattern. Approximately 40% of retinoblastomas are inherited, and carriers of the mutant retinoblastoma (RB) suppressor gene have a 10,000-fold increased risk for development of retinoblastoma; usually the affected person has bilateral disease.[2] They are also at risk for development of a second cancer, particularly osteosarcoma. In sporadic (noninherited) retinoblastoma, which accounts for 60% of cases, children are born with two normal copies of the RB gene, but both copies are inactivated through somatic mutations. Familial adenomatous polyposis of the colon also follows an autosomal dominant inheritance pattern. In people who inherit this gene, hundreds of adenomatous polyps may develop, some of which inevitably become malignant.[2]

Hormones

Hormones have received considerable research attention with respect to cancer of the breast, ovary, and endometrium in women and of the prostate and testis in men. Although the link between hormones and the development of cancer is unclear, it has been suggested that it may reside with the ability of hormones to drive the cell division of a malignant phenotype. Because of the evidence that endogenous hormones affect the risk of these cancers, concern exists regarding the effects on cancer risk if the same or closely related hormones are administered for therapeutic purposes.

Immunologic Mechanisms

There is growing evidence for the immune system's participation in resistance against the progression and spread of cancer. The central concept, known as the *immune surveillance hypothesis,* which was first proposed by Paul Ehrlich in 1909, postulates that the immune system plays a central role in resistance against the development of tumors.[12] In addition to cancer–host interactions as a mechanism of cancer development, immunologic mechanisms provide a means for the detection, classification, and prognostic evaluation of cancers as well as being a potential method of treatment. *Immunotherapy* (discussed later in this chapter) is a cancer treatment modality designed to heighten the patient's general immune responses to increase tumor destruction.

It has been suggested that the development of cancer might be associated with impairment or decline in the surveillance capacity of the immune system. For example, increases in cancer incidence have been observed in people with immunodeficiency diseases and in those with organ transplants who are receiving immunosuppressant drugs. The incidence of cancer also is increased in the elderly, in whom there is a known decrease in immune activity. The association of Kaposi sarcoma with acquired immunodeficiency syndrome (AIDS) further emphasizes the role of the immune system in preventing malignant cell proliferation (see Chapter 15).

It has been shown that most tumor cells express antigens that can be specifically recognized by immune T cells or by antibodies and hence are termed *tumor antigens.*

The most relevant tumor antigens fall into two categories: unique tumor-specific antigens found only on tumor cells, and tumor-associated antigens found on tumor cells and on normal cells. Quantitative and qualitative differences permit the use of these tumor-associated antigens to distinguish cancer cells from normal cells.[13]

Virtually all components of the immune system have the potential for eradicating cancer cells, including T lymphocytes, B lymphocytes, and natural killer (NK) cells (see Chapter 13). Neoplastic transformation results in genetic alterations, some of which may result in the expression of cell surface antigens that are seen as foreign by the immune system. The CD8+ lymphocytes, which have been shown to play a protective role against virus-induced neoplasms (*e.g.,* Epstein-Barr virus–induced Burkitt lymphoma), have been demonstrated in the blood and tumor infiltrates of some patients with cancer.[2] The finding of tumor-reactive antibodies in the serum of people with cancer supports the role of the B cell as a member of the immune surveillance team. Antibodies can destroy cancer cells through complement-mediated mechanisms or through antibody-dependent cellular cytotoxicity, in which the antibody binds the cancer cell to another effector cell, such as the NK cell, that does the actual killing of the cancer cell. NK cells do not require antigen recognition and can lyse a wide variety of target cells.[13]

Chemical Carcinogens

A carcinogen is an agent capable of causing cancer. The role of environmental agents in the causation of cancer was first noted in 1775 by Sir Percivall Pott, who related the high incidence of scrotal cancer in chimney sweeps to their exposure to coal soot.[2,5] In 1915, a group of Japanese investigators conducted the first experiments in which a chemical agent was used to produce cancer. These investigators found that a cancerous growth developed when they painted a rabbit's ear with coal tar. Coal tar has since been found to contain potent polycyclic aromatic hydrocarbons. Since then, many chemicals have been suspected of being carcinogens. Some have been found to cause cancers in animals, and others are known to cause cancers in humans (Chart 5-1).

The International Agency for Research in Cancer (IARC) has listed about 75 chemicals as human carcinogens.[5] These agents include carcinogens such as natural plant products (*e.g.,* aflatoxin B_1), aromatic amines, vinyl chloride, and insecticides.[2] Chemical carcinogens can be divided into two groups: (1) direct-reacting agents, which do not require activation in the body to become carcinogenic; and (2) indirect-reacting agents, called *procarcinogens* or *initiators,* which become active only after metabolic conversion. Direct- and indirect-acting initiators form highly reactive species (*i.e.,* electrophiles and free radicals) that bind with the nucleophilic residues on DNA, RNA, or cellular proteins. The action of these reactive species tends to cause cell mutation or alteration in the synthesis of cell enzymes and structural proteins in a manner that alters cell replication and interferes with cell regulatory controls. The carcinogenicity of some chemi-

CHART 5-1

Chemical and Environmental Agents Known to be Carcinogenic in Humans

Polycyclic Hydrocarbons

Soots, tars, and oils
Cigarette smoke

Industrial Agents

Aniline and azo dyes
Arsenic compounds
Asbestos
β-Naphthylamine
Benzene
Benzo[a]pyrene
Carbon tetrachloride
Insecticides, fungicides
Nickel and chromium compounds
Polychlorinated biphenyls
Vinyl chloride

Food and Drugs

Smoked foods
Nitrosamines
Aflatoxin B$_1$
Diethylstilbestrol
Anticancer drugs (e.g., alkylating agents, cyclophosphamide, chlorambucil, nitrosourea)

cals is augmented by agents called *promoters* that, by themselves, have little or no cancer-causing ability. It is believed that promoters exert their effect by changing the expression of genetic material in a cell, increasing DNA synthesis, enhancing gene amplification (*i.e.*, number of gene copies that are made), and altering intercellular communication.

The exposure to many chemical carcinogens is associated with lifestyle risk factors, such as smoking, dietary factors, and alcohol consumption. Cigarette smoke contains both procarcinogens and promoters. It is directly associated with lung and laryngeal cancer and has been linked with cancers of the oropharynx, esophagus, stomach, pancreas, bladder, and kidney, as well as myeloid leukemias.[1] Chewing tobacco or tobacco products increases the risk of cancers of the oral cavity and esophagus. Not only is the smoker at risk, but others passively exposed to cigarette smoke are also at risk.

There is strong evidence that certain elements in the diet contain chemicals that contribute to cancer risk. Most known dietary carcinogens occur naturally in plants (*e.g.*, aflatoxins) or are produced during food preparation.[14] For example, benzo[a]pyrene and other polycyclic hydrocarbons are converted to carcinogens when foods are fried in fat that has been reused multiple times. Among the most potent of the procarcinogens are the polycyclic aromatic hydrocarbons, which are of particular interest

because they are produced from animal fat in the process of charcoal-broiling meats and are present in smoked meats and fish. They also are produced in the combustion of tobacco and are present in cigarette smoke. Nitrosamines, which are powerful carcinogens, are formed in foods that are smoked, salted, cured, or pickled using nitrites or nitrates as preservatives.[14]

Alcohol modifies the metabolism of some carcinogens in the liver and esophagus.[7] It is believed to influence the transport of carcinogens, increasing the contact between an externally induced carcinogen and the stem cells that line the upper oral cavity, larynx, and esophagus. The carcinogenic effect of cigarette smoke can be enhanced by concomitant consumption of alcohol; persons who smoke and drink considerable amounts of alcohol are at increased risk for development of cancer of the oral cavity, larynx, and esophagus.

The effects of carcinogenic agents usually are dose dependent—the larger the dose or the longer the duration of exposure, the greater the risk that cancer will develop. Some chemical carcinogens may act in concert with other carcinogenic influences, such as viruses or radiation, to induce neoplasia. There usually is a time delay ranging from 5 to 30 years from the time of chemical carcinogen exposure to the development of overt cancer. This is unfortunate because many people may have been exposed to the agent and its carcinogenic effects before the association was recognized. This occurred, for example, with the use of diethylstilbestrol, which was widely used in the United States from the mid-1940s to 1970 to prevent miscarriages. But it was not until the late 1960s that many cases of vaginal adenosis and adenocarcinoma in young women were found to be the result of their exposure in utero to diethylstilbestrol.[15]

Radiation

The effects of *ionizing radiation* in carcinogenesis have been well documented in atomic bomb survivors, in patients diagnostically exposed, and in industrial workers, scientists, and physicians who were exposed during employment. Malignant epitheliomas of the skin and leukemia were significantly elevated in these populations. Between 1950 and 1970, the death rate from leukemia alone in the most heavily exposed population groups of the atomic bomb survivors in Hiroshima and Nagasaki was 147 per 100,000 persons, 30 times the expected rate.[16]

The type of cancer that developed depended on the dose of radiation, the sex of the person, and the age at which exposure occurred. For instance, approximately 25 to 30 years after total-body or trunk irradiation, there were increased incidences of leukemia and cancers of the breast, lung, stomach, thyroid, salivary gland, gastrointestinal system, and lymphoid tissues. The length of time between exposure and the onset of cancer is related to the age of the individual. For example, children exposed to ionizing radiation in utero have an increased risk for developing leukemias and childhood tumors, particularly 2 to 3 years after birth. This latency period for leukemia extends to 5 to 10 years if the child was exposed after birth and to 20 years for certain solid tumors.[17] As another example, the latency period for the development of thyroid cancer in infants and small children who received radiation to the head and neck to decrease the size of the tonsils or thymus was as long as 35 years after exposure.

The association between sunlight and the development of skin cancer has been reported for more than 100 years. *Ultraviolet radiation* emits relatively low-energy rays that do not deeply penetrate the skin (see Chapter 45). As with other carcinogens, the effects of ultraviolet radiation usually are additive, and there usually is a long delay between the time of exposure and the time that cancer can be detected.

Oncogenic Viruses

An oncogenic virus is one that can induce cancer. Viruses, which are small particles containing genetic (DNA or RNA) material, enter a host cell and become incorporated into its chromosomal DNA or take control of the cell's machinery for the purpose of producing viral proteins. A large number of DNA and RNA viruses (*i.e.*, retroviruses) have been shown to be oncogenic in animals. However, only a few viruses have been directly linked to cancer in humans.[2] Among the recognized oncogenic viruses in humans are the human papilloma virus (HPV), Epstein-Barr virus (EBV), hepatitis B virus (HBV), and human T-cell leukemia virus-1 (HTLV-1). There is also an association between infection with the bacterium *Helicobacter pylori* and gastric tumors[2,5] (discussed in Chapter 28).

Four DNA viruses have been implicated in human cancers: HPV, EBV, HBV, and the Kaposi sarcoma herpesvirus (discussed in Chapter 15). Although not a DNA virus, hepatitis C is associated with cancer. The transforming DNA viruses form stable associations with the human genome, using genes that allow them to complete their replication cycle and be expressed in transformed cells. There is strong evidence to suggest that the DNA viruses act in concert with other factors to cause cancer.

There are more than 60 genetically different types of HPV. Some types (*i.e.*, types 1, 2, 3, 4, and 10) have been shown to cause benign squamous papillomas (*i.e.*, warts). HPVs also have been implicated in squamous cell carcinoma of the cervix and anogenital region. HPV types 16 and 18 and, less commonly, types 31, 33, 35, and 51 have been found in approximately 85% of squamous cell carcinomas of the cervix and presumed precursors (*i.e.*, severe cervical dysplasia and carcinoma in situ).[2] Because only some women who are infected with HPV develop cervical cancer, other factors, such as cigarette smoking, coexisting microbial infections, dietary deficiencies, and hormonal changes, may be necessary for malignant transformation.[2]

EBV is a member of the herpesvirus family. It has been implicated in the pathogenesis of four human cancers: Burkitt lymphoma, nasopharyngeal cancer, B-cell lymphomas in immunosuppressed individuals such as those with AIDS, and in some cases of Hodgkin lymphoma. Burkitt lymphoma, a tumor of B lymphocytes, is endemic in parts of East Africa and occurs sporadically in other areas worldwide. In persons with normal immune function, the EBV-driven B-cell proliferation is readily controlled, and the person becomes asymptomatic or experiences a self-limited episode of infectious mononucleosis (see Chapter 9). In regions of the world where Burkitt lymphoma is endemic, concurrent malaria or other infections cause impaired immune function, allowing sustained B-lymphocyte proliferation. The incidence of nasopharyngeal cancer is high in some areas of China, particularly southern China, and in the Cantonese population in Singapore.

HBV is the etiologic agent in the development of hepatitis B, cirrhosis, and hepatocellular carcinoma. There is a significant correlation between elevated rates of hepatocellular carcinoma worldwide and the prevalence of HBV carriers. The precise mechanism whereby HBV induces hepatocellular cancer has not been determined. It has been suggested that the effect is indirect and multifactorial. By causing chronic liver injury and accompanying regenerative hyperplasia, HBV expands the pool of cycling cells at risk for subsequent genetic changes. In the mitotically active liver cells, mutations may arise spontaneously or be brought about by other environmental agents, such as aflatoxin. HBV also encodes a regulatory protein that disrupts several normal growth-regulating genes, such as the p53 tumor-suppressor gene.

HTLV-1, a retrovirus, is associated with a form of T-cell leukemia that is endemic in certain parts of Japan and some areas of the Caribbean and Africa, and is found sporadically elsewhere, including the United States and Europe.[2] Similar to the human immunodeficiency virus (HIV) that causes AIDS, HTLV-1 is attracted to CD4+ T cells, and this subset of T cells is therefore the major target for cancerous transformation. The virus requires transmission of infected T cells through sexual intercourse, infected blood, or breast milk.

In summary, the cause of cancer can be viewed from two perspectives: a molecular origin within cells and an external origin in which factors such as age, heredity, and environmental agents influence its inception and growth. The molecular pathogenesis of cancer is thought to have its origin in genetic damage or mutation (oncogenesis) and changes in cell physiology that transform a normally functioning cell into a cancer cell. There are four kinds of genes that control cell growth and replication: growth-promoting regulatory genes (proto-oncogenes), growth-inhibiting tumor suppressor genes (antioncogenes), genes that control programmed cell death (apoptosis genes), and genes that regulate the repair of damaged DNA.

Because cancer is not a single disease, it is likely that multiple factors interact at the genetic level to transform normal cells into cancer cells. Such genetic damage may result from interactions between multiple risk factors or repeated exposure to a single carcinogenic (cancer-producing) agent. Among the risk factors that have been linked to cancer are host factors such as heredity, hormonal factors, and immunologic mechanisms, and environmental agents such as chemicals, radiation, and cancer-causing viruses.

Clinical Manifestations

There probably is no single body function left unaffected by the presence of cancer. Because tumor cells replace normally functioning parenchymal tissue, the initial manifestations of cancer usually reflect the primary site of involvement. For example, cancer of the lung initially produces impairment of respiratory function; as the tumor grows and metastasizes, other body structures become affected. Cancer also produces generalized manifestations such as fatigue, anorexia and involuntary weight loss, anemia, and other symptoms unrelated to the tumor site. Many of these manifestations are compounded by the side effects of methods used to treat the disease.

TISSUE INTEGRITY

Cancer disrupts tissue integrity. As cancers grow, they compress and erode blood vessels, causing ulceration and necrosis along with frank bleeding and sometimes hemorrhage. One of the early warning signals of colorectal cancer is blood in the stool. Cancer cells also may produce enzymes and metabolic toxins that are destructive to the surrounding tissues. Usually, tissue damaged by cancerous growth does not heal normally. Instead, the damaged area persists and often continues to grow; a sore that does not heal is another warning signal of cancer. Cancer has no regard for normal anatomic boundaries; as it grows, it invades and compresses adjacent structures. Abdominal cancer, for example, may compress the viscera and cause bowel obstruction. Cancer may also obstruct lymph flow and penetrate serous cavities, causing pleural effusion or ascites.

In its late stages, cancer often causes pain (see Chapter 34). Pain is probably one of the most dreaded aspects of cancer, and pain management is one of the major treatment concerns for persons with incurable cancers.

CANCER CACHEXIA

Many cancers are associated with weight loss and wasting of body fat and muscle tissue, accompanied by profound weakness, anorexia, and anemia. This wasting syndrome is often referred to as the cancer anorexia-cachexia syndrome.[18,19] It is a common manifestation of most solid tumors with the exception of breast cancer. It has been estimated that 80% of persons with upper gastrointestinal cancer and 60% of persons with lung cancer have already experienced substantial weight loss at the time of diagnosis.[18] It is more common in children and elderly persons and becomes more pronounced as the disease progresses. The condition contributes to disease outcome and survival time. Persons with cancer cachexia also respond less well to chemotherapy and experience increased toxicity.

The cause of the cancer anorexia-cachexia syndrome is probably multifactorial, resulting from tumor- or host-derived factors that cause anorexia directly by acting on satiety centers in the hypothalamus or indirectly by injuring tissues that subsequently release anorexigenic substances. Although anorexia, reduced food intake, and abnormalities of taste are common in people with cancer and often are accentuated by treatment methods, the extent of weight loss and protein wasting cannot be explained in terms of diminished food intake alone. There also is a disparity between the size of the tumor and the severity of cachexia, which supports the existence of other mediators in the development of cachexia. It has been demonstrated that tumor necrosis factor (TNF)-α and other cytokines (interferons, interleukin-6) can produce the wasting syndrome in experimental animals.[5]

PARANEOPLASTIC SYNDROMES

In addition to signs and symptoms at the sites of primary and metastatic disease, cancer can produce manifestations in sites that are not directly affected by the disease. Such manifestations are collectively referred to as *paraneoplastic syndromes*.[2,20,21] Some of these manifestations are caused by the elaboration of hormones by cancer cells, and others result from the production of circulating factors that produce hematopoietic, neurologic, and dermatologic syndromes (Table 5-3). These syndromes are most commonly associated with lung, breast, and hematologic malignancies.[2]

A variety of peptide hormones are produced by both benign and malignant tumors. The biochemical pathways for the synthesis and release of peptide hormones (*e.g.*, antidiuretic [ADH], adrenocorticotropic [ACTH], and parathyroid [PTH] hormones) are present, although repressed, in most cells. Thus, the three most common endocrine syndromes associated with cancer are the syndrome of inappropriate ADH secretion (see Chapter 6), Cushing syndrome due to ectopic ACTH production (see Chapter 31), and hypercalcemia[2,20,21] (see Chapter 6). Hypercalcemia of malignancy does not appear to be related to PTH but to a PTH-related protein, which shares several biologic actions with PTH. Hypercalcemia also can be caused by osteolytic (bone breakdown) processes induced by cancers such as multiple myeloma or bony metastases from other cancers.

Some paraneoplastic syndromes are associated with the production of circulating mediators that produce hematologic complications. For example, a variety of cancers may produce procoagulation factors that contribute to an increased risk of venous thrombosis and nonbacterial thrombotic endocarditis. Sometimes unexplained thrombotic events are the first indication of undiagnosed malignancy. The precise relationship between coagulation disorders and cancer is largely unknown. Several malignancies, such as mucin-producing adenocarcinomas, release thromboplastic materials that may activate the clotting system.

The symptomatic paraneoplastic neurologic disorders are relatively rare with the exception of the Lambert-Eaton myasthenic syndrome, which is a disease of the myoneural junction that is distinct from myasthenia gravis. The disorder, which occurs primarily as a paraneoplastic process in persons with small cell lung cancer, produces proximal muscle weakness with autonomic dysfunction.[22]

TABLE 5-3	Common Paraneoplastic Syndromes	
Type of Syndrome	**Associated Tumor Type**	**Proposed Mechanism**
Endocrinologic		
Syndrome of inappropriate ADH	Small cell lung cancer, others	Production and release of ADH by tumor
Cushing syndrome	Small cell lung cancer, bronchial carcinoid cancers	Production and release of ACTH by tumor
Hypercalcemia	Squamous cell cancers of lung, head, neck, ovary	Production and release of polypeptide factor with close relationship to PTH
Hematologic		
Venous thrombosis	Pancreatic, lung, other cancers	Production of procoagulation factors
Nonbacterial thrombolytic endocarditis	Advanced cancers	Hypercoagulability
Neurologic		
Eaton-Lambert syndrome	Small cell lung cancer	Autoimmune production of antibodies to motor end-plate structures
Myasthenia gravis	Thymoma	

ADH, antidiuretic hormone; ACTH, adrenocorticotropic hormone; PTH, parathyroid hormone.

Unlike myasthenia gravis, no clinical improvement occurs with administration of anticholinergic drugs.

The paraneoplastic syndromes may be the earliest indication that a person has cancer, and should be regarded as such. They may also represent significant clinical problems, may be potentially lethal in persons with cancer, and may mimic metastatic disease and confound treatment.[2] Diagnostic methods focus both on identifying the cause of the presenting symptoms as well as locating the malignancy responsible for the disorder. The treatment of paraneoplastic syndromes involves concurrent treatment of the underlying cancer and suppression of the mediator causing the syndrome.

In summary, although the clinical manifestations vary with the type of cancer and the organ that is involved, there are some general manifestations related to the effects of tumor growth. Cancer compresses blood vessels, obstructs lymph flow, disrupts tissue integrity, invades serous cavities, and compresses visceral organs. It produces chemical mediators, such as TNF-α, that produce pain, sap energy reserves, and cause weight loss and tissue wasting. Paraneoplastic syndromes arise from the ability of cancers to elaborate hormones and other chemical messengers that produce nonmetastatic endocrine, hematopoietic, neurologic, and dermatologic syndromes.

Diagnosis and Treatment

DIAGNOSTIC METHODS

The methods used in the diagnosis and staging of cancer are determined largely by the location and type of cancer suspected. A number of diagnostic procedures are used in the diagnosis of cancer, including x-ray studies, endoscopic examinations, urine and stool tests, blood tests for tumor markers, bone marrow aspirations, ultrasound imaging, magnetic resonance imaging (MRI), computed tomography (CT) scan, and positron emission tomography (PET) scan.

The Papanicolaou Test

The Papanicolaou (Pap) test is a cytologic method that is used for detecting cancer cells. It consists of a microscopic examination of a properly prepared slide by a cytotechnologist or pathologist for the purpose of detecting the presence of abnormal cells. The usefulness of the Pap test relies on the fact that the cancer cells lack the cohesive properties and intercellular junctions that are characteristic of normal tissue; without these characteristics, cancer cells tend to exfoliate and become mixed with secretions surrounding the tumor growth. Although the Pap test is widely used as a screening test for cervical cancer (see Chapter 39), it can be performed on other body secretions, including nipple drainage, pleural or peritoneal fluid, and gastric washings.

Biopsy

Tissue biopsy is the removal of a tissue specimen for microscopic study. Biopsies are obtained in a number of ways, including needle aspiration (*i.e.*, fine, percutaneous, or core needle); endoscopic methods, such as bronchoscopy or cystoscopy, which involve the passage of an endoscope through an orifice and into the involved structure; or laparoscopic methods. In some instances, a surgical incision is made from which biopsy specimens are obtained. Excisional biopsies are those in which the entire tumor is removed. The tumors usually are small, solid, palpable masses. If the tumor is too large to be completely removed, a wedge of tissue from the mass can be excised for examination. Tissue diagnosis is of critical importance in designing the treatment plan should cancer cells be found.

Tumor Markers

Tumor markers are antigens that are expressed on the surface of tumor cells or substances released from normal cells in response to the presence of tumor.[2,23] Some substances, such as hormones and enzymes, are produced normally by the tissue involved but become overexpressed as a result of cancer. Other tumor markers, such as oncofetal protein, are produced during fetal development and are induced to reappear later in life as a result of benign and malignant neoplasms. Tumor markers are used for screening, diagnosis, establishing prognosis, monitoring treatment, and detecting recurrent disease.

The markers that have been most useful in clinical practice have been human chorionic gonadotropin (hCG), CA-125, prostate-specific antigen (PSA), α-fetoprotein (AFP), and carcinoembryonic antigen (CEA). A hormone normally produced by the placenta, hCG is used as a marker for diagnosing, prescribing treatment, and following the disease course in persons with high-risk gestational trophoblastic tumors. PSA is used as a marker in prostate cancer, and CA-125 is used as a marker in ovarian cancer. Table 5-4 identifies some of the more commonly used tumor markers and summarizes their source and the cancers associated with them.

Nearly all tumor markers can be elevated in benign conditions, and most are not elevated in the early stages of malignancy. Hence, tumor markers have limited value as screening tests. Extremely elevated levels of a tumor marker can indicate a poor prognosis or the need for more aggressive treatment. Perhaps the greatest value of tumor markers is in monitoring therapy in people with widespread cancer. Nearly all markers show an association with the clinical course of the disease. The levels of most markers are decreased with successful treatment and increased with recurrence or spread of the tumor.

Staging and Grading of Tumors

The two basic methods for classifying cancers are *grading* according to the histologic or cellular characteristics of the tumor and *staging* according to the clinical spread of the disease. Both methods are used to determine the course of the disease and aid in selecting an appropriate treatment or management plan. Grading of tumors involves the microscopic examination of cancer cells to determine their level of differentiation and the number of mitoses. Cancers are classified as grades I, II, III, and IV with increasing anaplasia or lack of differentiation. Staging of cancers uses methods to determine the extent and spread of the disease. Surgery may be used to determine tumor size and lymph node involvement.

The clinical staging of cancer is intended to group patients according to the extent of their disease. It is useful in determining the choice of treatment for individual patients, estimating prognosis, and comparing the results of different treatment regimens. The TNM system of the American Joint Committee on Cancer (AJCC) is used by most cancer facilities.[24] This system, which is briefly described in Chart 5-2, classifies the disease into stages using three tumor components: *T* stands for the size and local spread of the primary tumor, *N* refers to the involvement of the regional lymph nodes, and *M* describes the extent of metastatic involvement. The time of staging is indicated as clinical-diagnostic staging (cTNM); postsurgical resection-pathologic staging (pTNM); surgical-evaluative staging (sTNM); retreatment staging (rTNM); and autopsy staging (aTNM).[24]

TABLE 5-4	Tumor Markers	
Marker	**Source**	**Associated Cancers**
Oncofetal Antigens		
α-Fetoprotein (AFP)	Fetal yolk sac and gastrointestinal structures early in fetal life	Primary liver cancers; germ cell cancer of the testis
Carcinoembryonic antigen (CEA)	Embryonic tissues in gut, pancreas, and liver	Colorectal cancer and cancers of the pancreas, lung, and stomach
Hormones		
Human chorionic gonadotropin (hCG)	Hormone normally produced by placenta	Gestational trophoblastic tumors; germ cell cancer of testis
Calcitonin	Hormone produced by thyroid parafollicular cells	Thyroid cancer
Catecholamines (epinephrine, norepinephrine) and metabolites	Hormones produced by chromaffin cells of the adrenal gland	Pheochromocytoma and related tumors
Specific Proteins		
Monoclonal immunoglobulin	Abnormal immunoglobulin produced by neoplastic cells	Multiple myeloma
Prostate-specific antigen (PSA)	Produced by the epithelial cells lining the acini and ducts of prostate.	Prostate cancer
Mucins and Other Glycoproteins		
CA-125	Produced by müllerian cells of ovary	Ovarian cancer
CA-19-9	Produced by alimentary tract epithelium	Cancer of the pancreas, colon

---

CHART 5-2

TNM Classification System

T (tumor)

Tx	Tumor cannot be adequately assessed
T0	No evidence of primary tumor
Tis	Carcinoma in situ
T1–4	Progressive increase in tumor size or involvement

N (nodes)

Nx	Regional lymph nodes cannot be assessed
N0	No evidence of regional node metastasis
N 1–3	Increasing involvement of regional lymph nodes

M (metastasis)

Mx	Not assessed
M0	No distant metastasis
M1	Distant metastasis present, specify sites

CANCER TREATMENT

The goals of cancer treatment methods fall into three categories: curative, control, and palliative. The most common modalities are surgery, radiation, chemotherapy, hormonal therapy, and biotherapy. Gene therapy, although investigational, may provide a foundation for the development of more effective treatments in the future. Bone marrow transplantation and peripheral blood stem cell transplantation are two treatment approaches for leukemias, certain solid tumors, and other cancers previously thought to be incurable.

Surgery

Surgery is used for diagnosis and staging of cancer; tumor removal or as a component of adjuvant therapy when used in combination with chemotherapy or radiation therapy; control of oncologic emergencies, such as gastrointestinal hemorrhages; and palliation (*i.e.*, relief of symptoms) when a cure cannot be achieved. The type of surgery to be used is determined by the extent of the disease, the location and structures involved, the tumor growth rate and invasiveness, the surgical risk to the patient, and the quality of life the patient will experience after the surgery. If the tumor is small and has well-defined margins, the entire tumor often can be removed. If, however, the tumor is large or involves vital tissues, surgical removal may be difficult or impossible.

Radiation Therapy

Radiation can be used as the primary method of treatment, as preoperative or postoperative treatment, with chemotherapy, or with chemotherapy and surgery. It can also be used as a palliative treatment to reduce symptoms in persons with advanced cancers. It is effective in reducing the pain associated with bone metastasis and, in some cases, improves mobility. Radiation also is used to treat several oncologic emergencies, such as superior vena cava syndrome, spinal cord compression, bronchial obstruction, and hemorrhage.[25]

Radiation therapy exerts its effects through ionizing radiation, which affects cells by direct ionization of molecules or, more commonly, by indirect ionization. Indirect ionization produced by x-rays or gamma rays causes cellular damage when these rays are absorbed into tissue and give up their energy by producing fast-moving electrons. These electrons interact with free or loosely bonded electrons of the absorber cells and subsequently produce free radicals that interact with critical cell components (see Chapter 2). It can immediately kill cells, delay or halt cell cycle progression, or, at dose levels commonly used in radiation therapy, cause damage to the cell nucleus resulting in cell death after replication. Cell damage can be sublethal, in which case a single break in the strand can repair itself before the next radiation insult. Double-stranded breaks in DNA are generally believed to be the primary damage that leads to cell death. Cells with unrepaired DNA damage may continue to function until they undergo cell mitosis, at which time the genetic damage causes cell death.

The therapeutic effects of radiation therapy derive from the fact that the rapidly proliferating and poorly differentiated cells of a cancerous tumor are more likely to be injured by radiation therapy than are the more slowly proliferating cells of normal tissue. To some extent, however, radiation is injurious to all rapidly proliferating cells, including those of the bone marrow and the mucosal lining of the gastrointestinal tract. This results in many of the common adverse effects of radiation therapy, including infection, bleeding, and anemia due to loss of blood cells and nausea and vomiting due to loss of gastrointestinal cells. In addition to its lethal effects, radiation also produces sublethal injury. Recovery from sublethal doses of radiation occurs in the interval between the first dose of radiation and subsequent doses. This is why large total doses of radiation can be tolerated when they are divided into multiple smaller, fractionated doses. Normal tissue is usually able to recover from radiation damage more readily than is cancerous tissue.

Chemotherapy

Cancer chemotherapy has evolved as one of the major systemic treatment modalities. Unlike surgery and radiation, cancer chemotherapy is a systemic treatment that enables drugs to reach the site of the tumor as well as distant sites. More than 50 different chemotherapeutic drugs are used alone or in various combinations.[26] Chemotherapeutic drugs may be the primary form of treatment, or they may be used as part of a multimodal treatment plan. Chemotherapy is the primary treatment for most hematologic and some solid tumors, including choriocarcinoma, testicular cancer, acute and chronic leukemia, Burkitt lymphoma, Hodgkin disease, and multiple myeloma.

Most cancer drugs are more toxic to rapidly proliferating cells than to those incapable of replication or in phase G_0 of the cell cycle. Because of their mechanism of action, they are more effective against tumors with a high growth fraction.[26,27] By the time many cancers reach a size that is clinically detectable, the growth fraction has decreased considerably. In this case, reduction in tumor size through the use of surgical debulking procedures or radiation therapy often causes tumor cells residing in G_0 to reenter the cell cycle. Thus, surgery or radiation therapy may be used to increase the effectiveness of chemotherapy or chemotherapy may be given to patients with no overt evidence of residual disease after local treatment (*e.g.*, surgical resection of a primary breast cancer).

For most chemotherapy drugs, the relationship between tumor cell survival and drug dose is exponential, with the number of cells surviving being proportional to drug dose, and the number of cells at risk for exposure being proportional to the destructive action of the drug. Exponential killing implies that a proportion or percentage of tumor cells is killed, rather than an absolute number (Fig. 5-8).

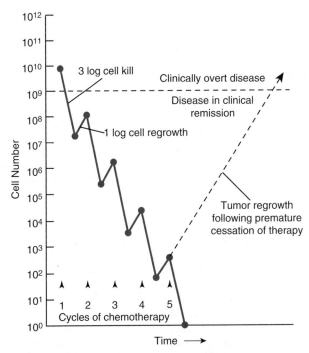

FIGURE 5-8 Relationship between tumor cell survival and administration of chemotherapy. The exponential relationship between drug dose and tumor cell survival dictates that a constant proportion, not number, of tumor cells is killed with each treatment cycle. In this example, each cycle of drug administration results in 99.9% (3 log) of cells killed, and 1 log of cell growth occurs between cycles. The *broken line* indicates what would occur if the last cycle of therapy were omitted: despite complete clinical remission of disease, the tumor ultimately would recur. (From Cooper M. R., Cooper M. R. [2001]. Basis for current major therapies for cancer: Systemic therapy. In Lenhard R. E., Osteen R. T., Gansler T. [Eds.], *The American Cancer Society's clinical oncology* [p. 181]. Atlanta: American Cancer Society.)

This proportion is a constant percentage of the total number of cells. For this reason, multiple courses of treatment are needed if the tumor is to be eradicated.[27]

Cancer chemotherapy drugs may be classified as either cell cycle specific or cell cycle nonspecific. Drugs are cell cycle specific if they exert their action during a specific phase of the cell cycle. For example, methotrexate, an antimetabolite, acts by interfering with DNA synthesis and thereby interrupts the S phase of the cell cycle. Cell cycle–nonspecific drugs exert their effects throughout all phases of the cell cycle. The alkylating agents, which are cell cycle nonspecific, act by disrupting DNA when cells are in the resting state as well as when they are dividing. The site of action of chemotherapeutic drugs varies. Chemotherapy drugs that have similar structures and effects on cell function usually are grouped together, and these drugs usually have similar side effect profiles. Because chemotherapy drugs differ in their mechanisms of action, cell cycle–specific and cell cycle–nonspecific agents are often combined to treat cancer.

Combination chemotherapy has been found to be more effective than treatment with a single drug. With this method, several drugs with different mechanisms of action, metabolic pathways, times of onset of action and recovery, side effects, and onset of side effects are used. Drugs used in combinations are individually effective against the tumor and synergistic with each other. The regimens for combination therapy often are referred to by acronyms. Two well-known combinations are CHOP (cyclophosphamide, doxorubicin, Oncovin [vincristine], and prednisone), used in the treatment of Hodgkin disease, and CMF (cyclophosphamide, methotrexate, and 5-fluorouracil), used in the treatment of breast cancer. The maximum possible drug doses usually are used to ensure the maximum cell killing. Routes of administration and dosage schedules are carefully designed to ensure optimal delivery of the active forms of the drugs to the tumor during the sensitive phase of the cell cycle.

Unfortunately, chemotherapeutic drugs affect both cancer cells and the rapidly proliferating cells of normal tissue, producing undesirable side effects. Some side effects appear immediately or after a few days (acute), some within a few weeks (intermediate), and others months to years after chemotherapy administration (long-term). Most chemotherapeutic drugs suppress bone marrow function and formation of blood cells, leading to anemia, neutropenia, and thrombocytopenia. With neutropenia, there is risk for developing serious infections, whereas thrombocytopenia increases the risk of bleeding. Anorexia, nausea, and vomiting are common problems associated with cancer chemotherapy. These symptoms can occur within minutes or hours of drug administration and are thought to be due to activation of the chemoreceptor trigger zone in the medulla that stimulates vomiting.[28] Some drugs also cause stomatitis and damage to the rapidly proliferating cells of the gastrointestinal tract's mucosal lining. Fatigue, the cause of which is multifactorial, is one of the most prevalent problems experienced by patients with cancer and is estimated to occur in 96% of individuals receiving chemotherapy. Hair loss results from impaired proliferation of the hair follicles and is a side effect of a number of cancer drugs; it usually is temporary, and the hair tends to regrow when treatment is stopped. The rapidly proliferating structures of the reproductive system are also sensitive to the action of cancer drugs. Women may experience changes in menstrual flow or have amenorrhea. Men may have a decreased sperm count (*i.e.*, oligospermia) or absence of sperm (*i.e.*, azoospermia). Many chemotherapeutic agents also may have teratogenic or mutagenic effects leading to fetal abnormalities.[29]

Chemotherapy drugs are toxic to all cells. Because they are potentially mutagenic, carcinogenic, and teratogenic, special care is required when handling or administering the drugs. Drugs, drug containers, and administration equipment require special disposal as hazardous waste.[29–31] There is also risk of second malignancies, such as acute leukemia, as a result of chemotherapy administered for hematologic malignancies and solid tumors.[32] Although the cause of these second malignancies is unclear, the mutagenicity of these drugs seems to be a contributing factor. Most persons who have developed second malignancies related to chemotherapy have been treated with alkylating agents, which damage the cross-linking DNA during the resting phase of the cell cycle.[32]

Hormone and Antihormone Therapy

Hormonal therapy consists of administration of drugs designed to alter the hormonal environment of cancer cells negatively. It is used for cancers that are responsive to or dependent on hormones for growth. The actions of hormones and antihormones depend on the presence of specific receptors in the tumor. Among the tumors that are known to be responsive to hormonal manipulation are those of the breast, prostate, and endometrium. Other cancers, such as Kaposi sarcoma and renal, liver, ovarian, and pancreatic cancer, are also responsive to hormonal manipulation, but to a lesser degree.[33]

The therapeutic options for altering the hormonal environment in the woman with breast cancer or the man with prostate cancer include surgical and pharmacologic measures.[33] Surgery involves the removal of the organ (*e.g.*, oophorectomy in women or orchiectomy in men) responsible for producing the hormone that is stimulating the target tissue. Pharmacologic methods focus largely on reducing circulating hormone levels or changing the hormone receptors so they no longer respond to the hormone. Pharmacologic suppression of circulating hormone levels can be effected through pituitary desensitization, as with the administration of androgens, or through the administration of gonadotropin-releasing hormone (GnRH) analogs that act at the level of the hypothalamus to inhibit gonadotropin production and release. Another class of drugs, the aromatase inhibitors, is used to treat breast cancer; these drugs act by interrupting the biochemical processes that convert androstenedione, an adrenally generated androgen, to estradiol in the peripheral tissues. Hormone receptor function can be altered by the administration of pharmacologic doses of exogenous hormones that act by producing a decrease in hormone receptors or by antihormone drugs that complex with hormone receptors (antiestrogens [*e.g.*, tamoxifen] and antiandrogens [*e.g.*, flutamide]), making them inaccessible to hormone stimulation.

Biotherapy

Biotherapy involves the use of immunotherapy and biologic response modifiers as a means of changing the person's own immune response to cancer.[34,35] The major mechanisms by which biotherapy exerts its effects are modification of host responses, direct destruction of cancer cells by suppressing tumor growth or killing the tumor cell, and modification of tumor cell biology.[35]

Immunotherapy. Immunotherapy techniques include active and passive, or adoptive, immunotherapy. Active immunotherapy involves nonspecific techniques such as bacillus Calmette-Guérin (BCG). BCG is an attenuated strain of the bacterium that causes bovine tuberculosis. It acts as a nonspecific stimulant of the immune system and is instilled into the bladder as a means of treating superficial bladder cancer. Passive or adoptive immunotherapy involves the transfer of cultured immune cells into a tumor-bearing host. Early research efforts with adoptive immunotherapy involved the transfer of sensitized NK cells or T lymphocytes combined with cytokines to the tumor-bearing host in an attempt to augment the host's immune response. However, randomized clinical trials demonstrated no benefit from the addition of the cellular component beyond the benefit from the cytokine alone. Further research has focused on using antigen-presenting dendritic cells as delivery vehicles for tumor antigens. Dendritic cells are efficient at activating not only CD4+ helper cells and CD8+ killer T cells but B cells and innate effectors such as NK cells.[35]

Biologic Response Modifiers. Biologic response modifiers can be grouped into three types: cytokines, which include the interferons and interleukins; monoclonal antibodies; and hematopoietic growth factors. The *interferons* (IFNs) are endogenous polypeptides that are synthesized by a number of cells in response to a variety of cellular or viral stimuli. The three major types of interferons are alpha (IFN-α), beta (IFN-β), and gamma (IFN-γ), with each group differing in terms of their cell surface receptors.[36] The IFNs appear to inhibit viral replication and also may be involved in inhibiting tumor protein synthesis and in prolonging the cell cycle and increasing the percentage of cells in the G_0 phase. Interferons also stimulate NK cells and cytotoxic T cells.[36] The *interleukins* (ILs) are cytokines that enable communication between cells by binding to receptor sites on the cell surface membranes of the target cells. Of the 18 known interleukins (see Chapter 13), IL-2 has been the most widely studied. A recombinant human IL-2 (rIL-2 aldesleukin) has been approved by the U.S. Food and Drug Administration (FDA) and is being used for the treatment of metastatic renal cell carcinoma and metastatic melanoma.[37]

Monoclonal antibodies (MoAbs) are highly specific antibodies derived from cloned cells or hybridomas. Scientists have been able to produce large quantities of these MoAbs that are specific for tumor cells.[38,39] For a MoAb to be therapeutic as a cancer treatment modality, a specific target antigen should be present on cancer cells only. Therapeutic MoAbs can be combined with a toxin, chemotherapy drug, or radioisotope to increase their effectiveness.[38]

Hematopoietic growth factors are growth and maturation factors that include the colony-stimulating factors (CSFs). The CSFs are factors that control the production of granulocytes (granulocyte CSF), granulocytes and macrophages (granulocyte-macrophage CSF), erythrocytes (erythropoietin), and platelets (thrombopoietin).

Targeted Therapy

Researchers have been working diligently to produce drugs that target the processes of cancer cells specifically, leaving normal cells unharmed. The characteristics and capabilities of cancer cells have been used to establish a framework for the development of such targeted agents, including those that disrupt molecular signaling pathways, inhibit angiogenesis, and harness the body's immune system. The first targeted therapies were the MoAbs. Researchers now are working to design new drugs that can disrupt molecular signaling pathways such as those that use protein tyrosine kinase. Imatinib mesylate is a protein tyrosine kinase inhibitor indicated in the treatment of chronic myeloid leukemia.[40] Thalidomide is an antiangiogenic agent that is used to interfere with tumor neovascularization.[41] Its use as an antiangiogenic agent was suggested when researchers considered that the characteristic phocomelia ("seal limbs") produced by its use during pregnancy may have resulted from toxicity to blood vessels in the fetal limb buds.[41] Cancer vaccines attempt to boost the immune system's recognition of tumor antigens. A number of vaccines for melanoma and prostate cancer are in research development.[40]

In summary, the methods used in the diagnosis of cancer vary with the type of cancer and its location. Because many cancers are curable if diagnosed early, health care practices designed to promote early detection are important. Pap smears, tissue biopsies, and tumor markers are used to detect the presence of cancer cells and in diagnosis. There are two basic methods of classifying tumors: grading according to histologic or tissue characteristics and clinical staging according to spread of the disease. Histologic studies are done in the laboratory using cells or tissue specimens. The TNM system for clinical staging of cancer uses tumor size, lymph node involvement, and presence of metastasis.

Treatment plans that use more than one type of therapy, often in combination, are providing cures for a number of cancers that a few decades ago had a poor prognosis, and are increasing the life expectancy in other types of cancer. Surgical procedures are more precise and less invasive, preserving organ function and resulting in better quality-of-life outcomes. Newer radiation equipment and techniques permit greater and more controlled destruction of cancer cells while sparing normal tissues. Chemotherapy involves the use of drugs that exert their effects at the cellular level to prevent cell replication. Successes with biotherapy techniques offer hope that the body's own defenses can be used in fighting cancer. Hybridoma technology has forged the frontier of the "magic bullet," where therapy is targeted to specific tumor antigens.

 ## Childhood Cancers

In the United States, cancer is the second leading cause of death by disease in children 1 to 14 years of age.[42] An estimated 9500 children were diagnosed with childhood cancer in 2005, and approximately 1500 died of the disease during the same year. Mortality rates from childhood cancer have declined by about 49% since 1979. The spectrum of cancers that affect children differs markedly from those that affect adults. Although most adult cancers are of epithelial cell origin (*e.g.,* lung cancer, breast cancer, colorectal cancers), childhood cancers usually involve the hematopoietic system, nervous system, or connective tissue. Chart 5-3 lists the most common forms of solid childhood cancers.

As with adult cancers, there probably is no one cause of childhood cancer. However, many forms of childhood cancer repeat in families and may result from polygenic or single-gene inheritance, chromosomal aberrations (*e.g.,* translocations, deletions, insertions, inversions, duplications), exposure to mutagenic environmental agents, or a combination of these factors. If cancer develops in one child, the risk of cancer in siblings is approximately twice that of the general population, and if the disease develops in two children, the risk is even greater.

Heritable forms of cancer tend to have an earlier age of onset, a higher frequency of multifocal lesions in a

---

CHART 5-3

Common Solid Tumors of Childhood

Brain and nervous system tumors
   Medulloblastoma
   Glioma
Neuroblastoma
Wilms tumor
Rhabdomyosarcoma and embryonal sarcoma
Retinoblastoma
Osteosarcoma
Ewing sarcoma

single organ, and bilateral involvement of paired organs or multiple primary tumors. The two-hit hypothesis has been used as one explanation of heritable cancers such as retinoblastoma.[2] The first "hit" or mutation occurs prezygotically (*i.e.*, in germ cells before conception) and is present in the genetic material of all somatic cells (see Fig. 5-6). Cancer subsequently develops in one or several somatic cell lines that undergo a second mutation.

Children with heritable disorders are at increased risk for developing certain forms of cancer. For example, Down syndrome is associated with increased risk of leukemia; primary immunodeficiency disorders (see Chapter 15) are associated with lymphoma, leukemia, and brain cancer; and xeroderma pigmentosum is associated with basal and squamous cell carcinoma and melanoma.

DIAGNOSIS AND TREATMENT

The early diagnosis of childhood cancers often is overlooked because the signs and symptoms often are similar to those of common childhood diseases and because cancer occurs less frequently in children than in adults.[42] Symptoms of prolonged fever, unexplained weight loss, and growing masses (especially in association with weight loss) should be viewed as warning signs of cancer in children. Diagnosis of childhood cancers involves many of the same methods that are used in adults. Accurate disease staging is especially beneficial in childhood cancers, in which the potential benefits of treatment must be carefully weighed against potential long-term effects.

ADULT SURVIVORS OF CHILDHOOD CANCER

With improvement in treatment methods, the number of children who survive childhood cancer is continuing to increase.[43] Unfortunately, therapy may produce late sequelae, such as impaired growth, neurologic dysfunction, hormonal dysfunction, cardiomyopathy, pulmonary fibrosis, and risk for second malignancies. Although cures for large numbers of children have been possible only since the 1970s, much already is known about the potential for delayed effects.

Children reaching adulthood after cancer therapy may have reduced physical stature because of the therapy they received, particularly radiation, which retards the growth of normal tissues along with cancer tissue. The younger the age and the higher the radiation dose, the greater the deviation from normal growth. There also is concern that central nervous system radiation as a prophylactic measure in childhood leukemia has an effect on cognition and learning. Children younger than 6 years of age at the time of radiation and those receiving the highest radiation doses are most likely to have subsequent cognitive difficulties.

Delayed sexual maturation in both boys and girls can result from irradiation of the gonads. Delayed sexual maturation also is related to the treatment of children with alkylating agents. Cranial irradiation may result in premature menarche in girls, with subsequent early closure of the epiphysis and a reduction in final growth achieved. Data related to fertility and health of the offspring of childhood cancer survivors is just becoming available.

Vital organs such as the heart and lungs may be affected by cancer treatment. Children who received anthracyclines (*i.e.*, doxorubicin or daunorubicin) may be at risk for developing cardiomyopathy and congestive heart failure. Pulmonary irradiation may cause lung dysfunction and restrictive lung disease. Drugs such as bleomycin, methotrexate, and busulfan also can cause lung disease.

For survivors of childhood cancers, the risk of second cancers is reported to range from 3% to 12%. There is a special risk of second cancers in children with the retinoblastoma gene. Because of this risk, children who have been treated for cancer should be followed up routinely.

In summary, although most adult cancers are of epithelial cell origin, most childhood cancers usually involve the hematopoietic system, nervous system, or connective tissue. Heritable forms of cancer tend to have an earlier age of onset, a higher frequency of multifocal lesions in a single organ, and bilateral involvement of paired organs or multiple primary tumors. The early diagnosis of childhood cancers often is overlooked because the signs and symptoms often are similar to those of other childhood diseases. With improvement in treatment methods, the number of children who survive childhood cancer is continuing to increase. As these children approach adulthood, there is continued concern that the life-saving therapy they received during childhood may produce late sequelae, such as impaired growth, neurologic dysfunction, hormonal dysfunction, cardiomyopathy, pulmonary fibrosis, and risk of second malignancies.

Review Exercises

A 30-year-old woman has experienced heavy menstrual bleeding and is told she has a uterine tumor called a *leiomyoma*. She is worried she has cancer.

A. What is the difference between a leiomyoma and leiomyosarcoma?

B. How would you go about explaining the difference to her?

The American Cancer Society recommends that all women have a yearly Pap test to screen for cervical cancer.

A. Use the characteristics of cancer cells to explain how this relatively simple test can be used as a screening method for cervical cancer.

A 48-year-old man presents at his health care clinic with complaints of leg weakness. He is a heavy smoker and has had a productive cough for years. Subsequent diagnostic tests reveal he has a small cell lung cancer with brain metastasis. His proposed plan of treatment includes chemotherapy and radiation therapy.

A. What is the probable cause of the leg weakness, and is it related to the lung cancer?
B. Relate this man's smoking history to the development of lung cancer.
C. Explain the mechanism of cancer metastasis.
D. Explain the mechanisms whereby chemotherapy and irradiation are able to destroy cancer cells while having a lesser or no effect on normal cells.

Visit the Porth: Essentials of Pathophysiology: Concepts of Altered Health States web site (http://thePoint.LWW.com/PorthEssentials) for links to chapter-related resources on the Internet, all-new exclusive animations, chapter review questions, and more!

REFERENCES

1. American Cancer Society. (2005). *Cancer facts 2005*. Atlanta: Author.
2. Kumar V., Abbas A. K., Fausto N. (Eds.). (2005). *Robbins and Cotran pathologic basis of disease* (7th ed., pp. 87–101, 269–342). Philadelphia: Elsevier Saunders.
3. Kasten M. B., Skopek S. X. (2001). Molecular basis of cancer: The cell cycle. In DeVita V. T., Jr., Hellman S., Rosenberg S. A. (Eds.), *Cancer: Principles and practice of oncology* (6th ed., pp. 91–108). Philadelphia: Lippincott Williams & Wilkins.
4. Sephel G. C., Woodward C. (2005). Repair, regeneration, and fibrosis. In Rubin E., Gorstein F., Rubin R., et al. (Eds.), *Rubin's pathology: Clinicopathologic foundations of medicine* (4th ed., pp. 85–109). Philadelphia: Lippincott Williams & Wilkins.
5. Rubin E., Rubin R., Aaronson S. (2005). Neoplasia. In Rubin E., Gorstein F., Rubin R., et al. (Eds.), *Rubin's pathology: Clinicopathologic foundations of medicine* (4th ed., pp. 165–213). Philadelphia: Lippincott Williams & Wilkins.
6. Stetler W. G., Kliener D. E. (2001). Molecular biology of cancer: Invasion and metastasis. In DeVita V. T., Jr., Hellman S., Rosenberg S. A. (Eds.), *Cancer: Principles and practice of oncology* (6th ed., pp. 121–136). Philadelphia: Lippincott Williams & Wilkins.
7. Yaeger T. E., Brady L. W. (2001). Basis for current major therapies in cancer. In Lenhard R. E., Osteen R. T., Gansler T. (Eds.), *The American Cancer Society's clinical oncology* (pp. 159–229). Atlanta: American Cancer Society.
8. Heath C. W., Fontham E. T. (2001). Cancer etiology. In Lenhard R. E., Osteen R. T., Gansler T. (Eds.), *The American Cancer Society's clinical oncology* (pp. 38–54). Atlanta: American Cancer Society.
9. Zhou B. P., Hung M. C. (2003). Dysregulation of cellular signaling by HER2/neu in breast cancer. *Seminars in Oncology* 30(5 Suppl. 16), 38–48.
10. Levine A. J. (1996). Tumor suppressor genes. In Pusztai L., Lewis C. E., Yap E. (Eds.), *Cell proliferation in cancer: Regulatory mechanisms of neoplastic cell growth* (pp. 86–104), Oxford: Oxford University Press.
11. Pusztai L., Cooper K. (1996). Introduction: Cell proliferation and carcinogenesis. In Pusztai L., Lewis C. E., Yap E. (Eds.), *Cell proliferation in cancer: Regulatory mechanisms of neoplastic cell growth* (pp. 3–24), Oxford: Oxford University Press.
12. Burnett F. M. (1967). Immunologic aspects of malignant disease. *Lancet* 1, 1171.
13. Abbas A. K., Lichtman A. (2003). *Cellular and molecular immunology* (5th ed., pp. 391–410). Philadelphia: W. B. Saunders.
14. Willett W. C. (2001). Cancer prevention: Diet and chemopreventive agents. In DeVita V. T., Jr., Hellman S., Rosenberg S. A. (Eds.), *Cancer: Principles and practice of oncology* (6th ed., pp. 561–614). Philadelphia: Lippincott Williams & Wilkins.
15. Poskanzer D. C., Herbst A. (1977). Epidemiology of vaginal adenosis and adenocarcinoma associated with exposure to stilbestrol in utero. *Cancer* 39, 1892–1895.
16. Jablon S., Kato H. (1972). Studies of the mortality of A-bomb survivors: 5. Radiation dose and mortality, 1950–1970. *Radiation Research* 50, 649–698.
17. Ruddon R. W. (Ed.). (1995). *Cancer biology* (pp. 3–60, 141–276). New York and Oxford: Oxford University Press.
18. Imui A. (2002). Cancer anorexia-cachexia syndrome: Current issues in research and management. *CA A Cancer Journal for Clinicians* 52(2), 72–91.
19. Rubin H. (2003). Cancer cachexia: Its correlations and causes. *Proceedings of the National Academy of Science* 100, 5384–5389.
20. Zumsteg M. M., Casperson D. S. (1998). Paraneoplastic syndromes in metastatic disease. *Seminars in Oncology Nursing* 14(3), 220–229.
21. Rosenthal P. E. (2001). Paraneoplastic and endocrine syndromes. In Lenhard R. E., Osteen R. T., Gansler T. (Eds.), *The American Cancer Society's clinical oncology* (pp. 721–732). Atlanta: American Cancer Society.
22. Darnell R. B., Posner J. B. (2003). Paraneoplastic syndromes involving the nervous system. *New England Journal of Medicine* 349, 1543–1554.
23. Pfiefer J. D., Wick M. R. (2001). Pathologic evaluation of neoplastic diseases. In Lenhard R. E., Osteen R. T., Gansler T. (Eds.), *The American Cancer Society's clinical oncology* (pp. 123–147). Atlanta: American Cancer Society.
24. Green F. L., Page D. L., Fleming I. D. (2002). *AJCC cancer staging manual* (6th ed.). New York: Springer-Verlag.
25. Dunne-Daley C. F. (1999). Principles of radiotherapy and radiobiology. *Seminars in Oncology Nursing* 15(4), 250–259.
26. Miaskowski C., Viele C. (1999). Cancer chemotherapy. In Miaskowski C., Buchsel P. (Eds.), *Oncology nursing: Assessment and clinical care* (pp. 83–106). St. Louis: Mosby.
27. Cooper M. R., Cooper M. R. (2001). Basis for current major therapies for cancer: Systemic therapy. In Lenhard R. E., Osteen R. T., Gansler T. (Eds.), *The American Cancer Society's clinical oncology* (pp. 175–215). Atlanta: American Cancer Society.
28. Schnell F. M. (2003). Chemotherapy-induced nausea and vomiting: The importance of acute antiemetic control. *Oncologist* 8, 187–198.
29. Oncology Nursing Society. (2002). *Cancer chemotherapy and biotherapy guidelines: Recommendations for practice.* Pittsburgh: Author.
30. U.S. Department of Labor, Office of Occupational Medicine, Occupational Safety and Health Administration (OSHA). (1986). *Work practice guidelines for personnel dealing with*

cytotoxic (antineoplastic) drugs. Publication no. 8-1.1. Washington, DC: Author.

31. Polovich M. (2003). *Safe handling of hazardous drugs.* Pittsburgh: Oncology Nursing Society.

32. Rosenthal P. E. (2001). Complications of cancer and cancer treatment. In Lenhard R. E., Osteen R. T., Gansler T. (Eds.), *The American Cancer Society's clinical oncology* (p. 246). Atlanta: American Cancer Society.

33. Hawkins R. (2002). Hormone therapy in cancer. *Oncology Nursing Updates* 9(3), 1–16.

34. DeMeyer E., Stein B. A. (1999). Biotherapy. In Miakowski C., Buchsel P. (Eds.), *Oncology nursing: Assessment and clinical care* (pp. 119–141). St. Louis: Mosby.

35. Reiger P. T. (2001). Biotherapy: An overview. In Reiger P. T. (Ed.), *Biotherapy: A comprehensive overview* (2nd ed., pp. 3–37). Sudbury, MA: Jones and Bartlett.

36. Kirkwood J. M. (2001). Interferons. In DeVita V. T., Jr., Hellman S., Rosenberg S. A. (Eds.), *Cancer: Principles and practice of oncology* (7th ed., pp. 461–471). Philadelphia: Lippincott Williams & Wilkins.

37. Mier J. W., Atkins M. B. (2001). Interleukin-2. In DeVita V. T., Jr., Hellman S., Rosenberg S. A. (Eds.), *Cancer: Principles and practice of oncology* (7th ed., pp. 471–478). Philadelphia: Lippincott Williams & Wilkins.

38. Schmidt K. V., Wood B. A. (2003). Trends in cancer therapy: Role of monoclonal antibodies. *Seminars in Oncology Nursing* 19(3), 169–179.

39. Von Mehren M., Adams G. P., Weiner L. M. (2003). Monoclonal antibody therapy for cancer. *Annual Review of Medicine* 54, 343–369.

40. Davey M. P. (2002). Imatinib mesylate. *Clinical Journal of Oncology Nursing* 6(2), 118–120.

41. Waldman A. R. (2000). Thalidomide. *Clinical Journal of Oncology Nursing* 4(2), 99–100.

42. Behrman R. E., Kliegman R. M., Jenson H. B. (Eds.). (2004). *Nelson textbook of pediatrics* (17th ed., pp. 1679–1693). Philadelphia: Elsevier Saunders.

43. Rowland J. H., Asis N., Tesauro G., et al. (2001). The changing face of cancer survivorship. *Seminars in Oncology Nursing* 17(4), 236–240.

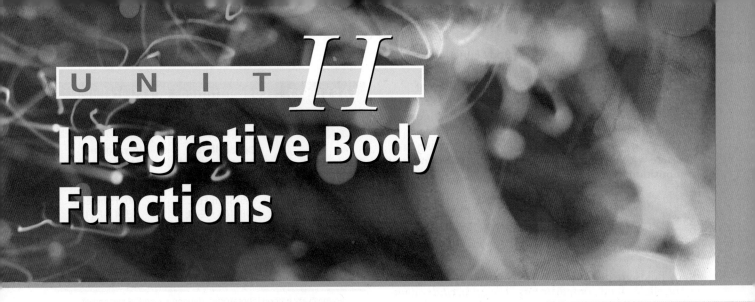

Chapter 6

Disorders of Fluid, Electrolyte, and Acid-Base Balance

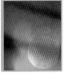

Fluids and electrolytes are present in body cells, in the tissue spaces between the cells, and in the blood that fills the vascular compartment. Body fluids serve to transport gases, nutrients, and wastes; help to generate the electrical activity needed to power body functions; take part in the transformation of food into energy; and otherwise maintain the overall function of the body. Although the volume and composition of body fluids remain relatively constant in the presence of a wide range of changes in intake and output, conditions such as environmental stresses and disease can increase fluid loss, impair its intake, and otherwise interfere with mechanisms that regulate fluid volume, composition, and distribution.

Composition and Compartmental Distribution of Body Fluids

Body fluids are distributed between the intracellular and extracellular fluid compartments. The *intracellular compartment* (ICF) consists of fluid contained within all of the billions of cells in the body. The ICF contains approximately two thirds of the body water in healthy adults, and is the larger of the two compartments. The remaining one third of body water is in the *extracellular compartment* (ECF), which contains all the fluids outside the cells, including that in the interstitial or tissue spaces and blood vessels (Fig. 6-1). The ECF, including the plasma and interstitial fluids, contains large amounts of sodium and chloride, moderate amounts of bicarbonate, but only small quantities of potassium, magnesium, calcium, and phosphate. In contrast to the ECF, the ICF contains almost no calcium; small amounts of sodium, chloride, bicarbonate, and phosphate; moderate amounts of magnesium; and large amounts of potassium (Table 6-1). It is the ECF levels of electrolytes in the blood or blood plasma that are measured clinically (this text uses the term *serum* rather than *plasma* in reference to laboratory values of electrolytes). Although blood levels usually are representative of the total body levels of an electrolyte, this is not always the case, particularly with potassium, which is more concentrated inside the cell than outside.

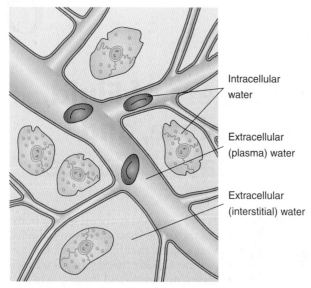

FIGURE 6-1 Distribution of body water. The extracellular space includes the vascular compartment (plasma water) and the interstitial spaces.

Intracellular water

Extracellular (plasma) water

Extracellular (interstitial) water

TABLE 6-1	Concentrations of Extracellular and Intracellular Electrolytes in Adults	
Electrolyte	**Extracellular Concentration***	**Intracellular Concentration***
Sodium	135–145 mEq/L	10–14 mEq/L
Potassium	3.5–5.0 mEq/L	140–150 mEq/L
Chloride	98–106 mEq/L	3–4 mEq/L
Bicarbonate	24–31 mEq/L	7–10 mEq/L
Calcium	8.5–10.5 mg/dL	<1 mEq/L
Phosphate/ phosphorus	2.5–4.5 mg/dL	4 mEq/kg†
Magnesium	1.8–3.0 mg/dL	40 mEq/kg†

*Values may vary among laboratories, depending on the method of analysis used.

†Values vary among various tissues and with nutritional status.

INTRODUCTORY CONCEPTS

Dissociation of Electrolytes

Body fluids contain water and electrolytes. Electrolytes are substances that dissociate in solution to form charged particles, or *ions*. For example, a sodium chloride (NaCl) molecule dissociates to form a positively charged Na^+ and a negatively charged Cl^- ion. Particles that do not dissociate into ions such as glucose and urea are called *nonelectrolytes*. Positively charged ions are called *cations* because they are attracted to the cathode of a wet electric cell, and negatively charged ions are called *anions* because they are attracted to the anode. The ions found in body fluids carry one charge (*i.e.*, monovalent ion) or two charges (*i.e.*, divalent ion). Because of their attraction forces, positively charged cations are always accompanied by negatively charged anions. The distribution of electrolytes between body compartments is influenced by their electrical charge. However, one cation may be exchanged for another, provided it carries the same charge. For example, a positively charged H^+ ion may be exchanged for a positively charged K^+ ion and a negatively charged bicarbonate (HCO_3^-) ion may be exchanged for another negatively charged Cl^- anion.

Diffusion and Osmosis

Diffusion is the movement of charged or uncharged particles along a concentration gradient. All molecules and ions, including water and dissolved molecules, are in constant random motion. It is the motion of these particles, each colliding with one another, that supplies the energy for diffusion. Because there are more molecules in constant motion in a concentrated solution, particles move from an area of higher concentration to one of lower concentration. The concentrations of electrolytes and solutes can be expressed in several ways, for example, milligrams per deciliter (mg/dL), milliequivalents per liter (mEq/L), or millimoles per liter (mmol/L).

Osmosis is the movement of water across a semipermeable membrane (*i.e.,* one that is permeable to water but impermeable to most solutes). As with solute particles, water diffuses down its concentration gradient, moving from the side of the membrane with the lesser number of particles and greater concentration of water to the side with the greater number of particles and lesser concentration of water (Fig. 6-2). As water moves across the semipermeable membrane, it generates a pressure, called the *osmotic pressure.* The osmotic pressure represents the pressure (measured in millimeters of mercury [mm Hg]) needed to oppose the movement of water across the membrane.

The osmotic activity that nondiffusible particles exert in pulling water from one side of the semipermeable membrane to the other is measured by a unit called an *osmole.* The osmole is derived from the gram molecular weight of a substance (*i.e.,* 1 gram molecular weight of a nondiffusible and nonionizable substance is equal to 1 osmole). In the clinical setting, osmotic activity usually is expressed in milliosmoles (mOsm) or one thousandth of an osmole. Each nondiffusible particle, large or small, is equally effective in its ability to pull water through a semipermeable membrane. Thus, it is the number, rather than the size, of the nondiffusible particles that determines the osmotic activity of a solution.

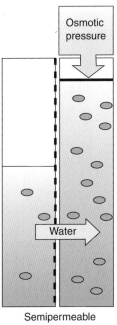

FIGURE 6-2 Movement of water across a semipermeable membrane. Water moves from the side that has fewer nondiffusible particles to the side that has more. The osmotic pressure is equal to the hydrostatic pressure needed to oppose water movement across the membrane.

Measurement Units

Laboratory measurements of electrolytes in body fluids are expressed as a concentration or amount of solute in a given volume of fluid, such as milligrams per deciliter (mg/dL), milliequivalents per liter (mEq/L), or millimoles per liter (mmol/L).

The use of *milligrams (mg) per deciliter* expresses the weight of the solute in one tenth of a liter (dL). The concentration of electrolytes, such as calcium, phosphate, and magnesium, is often expressed in mg/dL.

The *milliequivalent* is used to express the charge equivalency for a given weight of an electrolyte: 1 mEq of sodium has the same number of charges as 1 mEq of chloride, regardless of molecular weight. The number of milliequivalents of an electrolyte in a liter of solution can be derived from the following equation:

$$mEq = \frac{mg/100\ mL \times 10 \times valence}{atomic\ weight}$$

The Système Internationale (SI) units express electrolyte concentration in *millimoles per liter* (mmol/L). A millimole is one thousandth of a mole, or the molecular weight of a substance expressed in milligrams. The number of millimoles of an electrolyte in a liter of solution can be calculated using the following equation:

$$mmol/L = \frac{mEq/L}{valence}$$

The osmotic activity of a solution may be expressed in terms of either its osmolarity or osmolality. *Osmolarity* refers to the osmolar concentration in 1 L of solution (mOsm/L) and *osmolality* to the osmolar concentration in 1 kg of water (mOsm/kg of H_2O). Osmolarity is usually used when referring to fluids outside the body and osmolality for describing fluids inside the body. Because 1 L of water weighs 1 kg, the terms *osmolarity* and *osmolality* are often used interchangeably.

Serum osmolality, which is largely determined by sodium and its attendant anions (Cl^- and HCO_3^-), normally ranges from 280 to 295 mOsm/kg. Blood urea nitrogen (BUN) and glucose, which also are osmotically active, account for less than 5% of the total osmotic pressure in the ECF compartment. However, this can change, such as when blood glucose levels are elevated in persons with diabetes mellitus or when BUN levels rise rapidly in persons with renal failure.

The term *tonicity* refers to the tension or effect that the effective osmotic pressure of a solution with impermeable solutes exerts on cell size because of water movement across the cell membrane. Solutions to which body cells are exposed can be classified as isotonic, hypotonic, or hypertonic, depending on whether they cause cells to swell or shrink (Fig. 6-3). Cells placed in an isotonic solution (*e.g.,* 0.9% sodium chloride or 5% dextrose in water), which has the same effective osmolality as the ICF (*i.e.,* 280 mOsm/L), neither shrink nor swell. These solutions are important in the clinical setting because they can be infused into the blood without danger of upsetting the

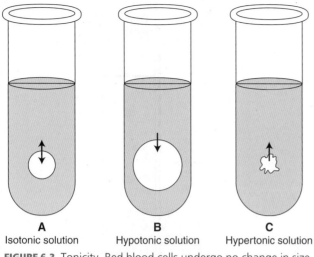

FIGURE 6-3 Tonicity. Red blood cells undergo no change in size in isotonic solutions (**A**). They increase in size in hypotonic solutions (**B**) and decrease in size in hypertonic solutions (**C**).

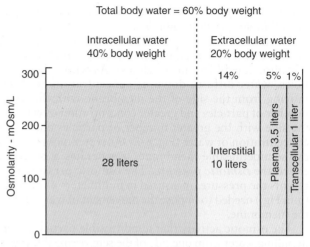

FIGURE 6-4 Approximate size of body compartments in a 70-kg adult.

osmotic equilibrium between the ICF and ECF. When cells are placed in a hypotonic solution (*e.g.*, distilled water), which has a lower effective osmolality than the ICF, they swell as water moves into the cell; when they are placed in a hypertonic solution (*e.g.*, 3% normal saline or 10% glucose), which has a greater effective osmolality than ICF, they shrink as water is pulled out of the cell.

COMPARTMENTAL DISTRIBUTION OF BODY FLUIDS

Body water is distributed between the ICF and ECF compartments. In the adult, the fluid in the ICF compartment constitutes approximately 40% of body weight.[1] The fluid in the ECF compartment is further divided into two major subdivisions: the plasma compartment, which constitutes approximately 5% of body weight, and the interstitial fluid compartment, which constitutes approximately 14% of body weight (Fig. 6-4).

The fluid in the interstitial compartment acts as a transport vehicle for gases, nutrients, wastes, and other materials that move between the vascular compartment and body cells. The interstitial fluid compartment also provides a reservoir from which vascular volume can be maintained during periods of hemorrhage or loss of vascular volume. A tissue gel, which is a spongelike material composed of large quantities of mucopolysaccharides, fills the tissue spaces and aids in even distribution of interstitial fluid. Normally, most of the fluid in the interstitium is in gel form. The tissue gel is supported by collagen fibers that hold the gel in place. The tissue gel, which has a firmer consistency than water, opposes the outflow of water from the capillaries and prevents the accumulation of free water in the interstitial spaces.

A third, usually minor, subdivision of the ECF compartment is the transcellular compartment. It includes the cerebrospinal fluid and fluid contained in the various body spaces, such as the peritoneal, pleural, and pericar-

dial cavities, and joint spaces. Normally, only about 1% of ECF is in the transcellular space. This amount can increase considerably in conditions such as ascites, in which large amounts of fluid are sequestered in the peritoneal cavity. When the transcellular fluid compartment becomes considerably enlarged, it is referred to as a *third space*, because this fluid is not readily available for exchange with the rest of the ECF.

CAPILLARY/INTERSTITIAL FLUID EXCHANGE

The transfer of water between the vascular and interstitial compartments occurs at the capillary level. Four forces control the movement of water between the capillary and interstitial spaces: (1) the capillary filtration pressure, which pushes water out of the capillary into the interstitial spaces; (2) the capillary colloidal osmotic pressure, which pulls water back into the capillary; (3) the interstitial hydrostatic pressure, which opposes the movement of water out of the capillary; and (4) the tissue colloidal osmotic pressure, which pulls water out of the capillary into the interstitial spaces. Normally, the combination of these four forces is such that only a small excess of fluid remains in the interstitial compartment. This excess fluid is removed from the interstitium by the lymphatic system and returned to the systemic circulation.

Capillary filtration refers to the movement of water through capillary pores because of a mechanical, rather than an osmotic, force. The capillary filtration pressure (about 30 to 40 mm Hg at the arterial end, 10 to 15 mm Hg at the venous end, and 25 mm Hg in the middle), sometimes called the *capillary hydrostatic pressure*, is the pressure pushing water out of the capillary into the interstitial spaces. It reflects the arterial and venous pressures, the precapillary (arterioles) and postcapillary (venules) resistances, and the force of gravity.[2] A rise in arterial or venous pressure increases capillary pressure. The force of gravity increases capillary pressure in the dependent parts of the body. In a person who is standing absolutely still, the weight of blood in the vascular column causes an increase of 1 mm Hg in pressure for every 13.6 mm of distance from the heart.[2] This pressure results from the weight of water and is therefore called *hydrostatic pressure*. In the adult who is standing absolutely still, the pressure in the veins of feet can reach 90 mm Hg. This pressure is then transmitted to the capillaries.

The *capillary colloidal osmotic pressure* (about 28 mm Hg) is the osmotic pressure generated by the plasma proteins that are too large to pass through the pores of the capillary wall.[2] The term *colloidal osmotic pressure* differentiates this type of osmotic pressure from the osmotic pressure that develops at the cell membrane from the presence of electrolytes and non-electrolytes. Because plasma proteins do not normally penetrate the capillary pores and because their concentration is greater in the plasma than in the interstitial fluids, it is capillary colloidal osmotic pressure that pulls fluids back into the capillary.

The interstitial fluid pressure (about −3 mm Hg) and the tissue colloidal osmotic pressure (about 8 mm Hg) contribute to movement of water into and out of the interstitial spaces.[2] The interstitial fluid pressure, which is normally negative, contributes to the outward movement of water into the interstitial spaces. The tissue colloidal osmotic pressure, which reflects the small amount of plasma proteins that normally escape into the interstitial spaces from the capillary, also pulls water out of the capillary into the tissue spaces.

The lymphatic system represents an accessory route whereby fluid from the interstitial spaces can return to the circulation. More importantly, the lymphatics afford a means for removing plasma proteins and osmotically active particulate matter from the tissue spaces, neither of which can be reabsorbed into the capillaries.

Edema

Edema can be defined as palpable swelling produced by expansion of the interstitial fluid volume. Edema does not become evident until the interstitial fluid volume has been increased by 2.5 to 3 L.[3] The physiologic mechanisms that contribute to edema formation include factors that (1) increase the capillary filtration pressure, (2) decrease the capillary colloidal osmotic pressure, (3) increase capillary permeability, or (4) produce obstruction to lymph flow. The causes of edema are summarized in Chart 6-1.

Increased Capillary Filtration Pressure. As the capillary filtration pressure rises, the movement of vascular fluid into the interstitial spaces increases. Among the factors that increase capillary pressure are (1) a decrease in the resistance to flow through the precapillary sphincters, (2) an increase in venous pressure or resistance to outflow at the postcapillary sphincters, and (3) capillary distention caused by increased vascular volume.

Edema can be either localized or generalized. The localized edema that occurs with urticaria (*i.e.*, hives) or other allergic or inflammatory conditions results from the release of histamine and other inflammatory mediators that cause dilation of the precapillary sphincters and arterioles that supply the swollen lesions. Thrombophlebitis obstructs venous flow, producing an elevation of venous pressure and edema of the affected part, usually one of the lower extremities.

Generalized edema is usually the result of increased vascular volume. The swelling of hands and feet that occurs in healthy persons during hot weather is an example of edema that is caused by the vasodilation of superficial blood vessels along with sodium and water retention. Generalized edema is common in conditions such as congestive heart failure that produce fluid retention and venous congestion. In right-sided heart failure, blood dams up throughout the entire venous system, causing organ congestion and edema of the dependent extremities (discussed in Chapter 19).

Because of the effects of gravity, edema resulting from increased capillary pressure commonly causes fluid to accumulate in the dependent parts of the body, a condition referred to as *dependent edema*. For example, edema of the ankles and feet becomes more pronounced during prolonged periods of standing.

Decreased Capillary Colloidal Osmotic Pressure. Plasma proteins exert the osmotic force needed to pull fluid back into the capillary from the tissue spaces. The plasma proteins constitute a mixture of proteins, including albumin, globulins, and fibrinogen. Albumin, the smallest of the plasma proteins, has a molecular weight of 69,000; globulins have molecular weights of approximately 140,000; and fibrinogen has a molecular weight of 400,000.[2] Because of its lower molecular weight, 1 g of albumin has approximately twice as many osmotically active molecules as 1 g of globulin and almost six times as many osmotically active molecules as 1 g of fibrinogen. In addition, the concentration of albumin (approximately 4.5 g/dL) is greater than that of the globulins (2.5 g/dL) and fibrinogen (0.3 mg/dL).

Edema caused by decreased capillary colloidal osmotic pressure usually is the result of inadequate production or abnormal loss of plasma proteins, mainly albumin. The plasma proteins are synthesized in the liver. In persons with severe liver failure, the impaired synthesis of albumin results in a decrease in colloidal osmotic pressure. In starvation and malnutrition, edema develops because there is a lack of the amino acids needed in plasma protein synthesis. The most common site of plasma protein loss is the kidney. In kidney diseases such as nephrosis, the glomerular capillaries become permeable to the plasma proteins, particularly albumin, which is the smallest of the proteins. When this happens, large amounts of albumin are filtered out of the blood and lost in the urine. An excessive loss of plasma proteins also occurs when large areas of skin are injured or destroyed. Edema is a common problem during the early stages of a burn, resulting from capillary injury and loss of plasma proteins.

Because the plasma proteins are evenly distributed throughout the body and are not affected by the force of

Understanding ➤ Capillary Fluid Exchange

Movement of fluid between the vascular compartment and the interstitial fluid compartment surrounding the body cells occurs at the capillary level. The direction and amount of fluid that flows across the capillary wall is determined by: (1) the hydrostatic pressure of the two compartments, (2) the colloidal osmotic pressures of the two compartments, and (3) the removal of excess fluid and osmotically active particles from the interstitial spaces by the lymphatic system.

1

Hydrostatic pressure. The hydrostatic pressure is the pushing force exerted by a fluid. Inside the capillaries, the hydrostatic pressure is the same as the capillary filtration pressure, about 30 mm Hg at the arterial end and 10 mm Hg at the venous end. The interstitial fluid pressure is the force of fluid in the interstitial spaces pushing against the outside of the capillary wall. Evidence suggests that the interstitial pressure is slightly negative (−3 mm Hg), contributing to the outward movement of fluid from the capillary.

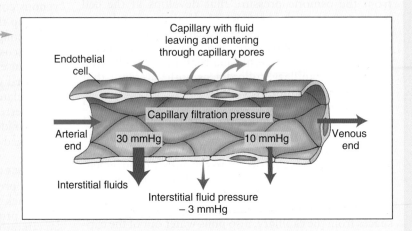

2

Colloidal osmotic pressure. The colloidal osmotic pressure is the pulling force created by the presence of evenly dispersed particles, such as the plasma proteins, that cannot pass through the pores of the capillary membrane. The capillary colloidal osmotic pressure is normally about 28 mm Hg throughout the length of the capillary bed. The interstitial colloidal osmotic pressure (about 8 mm Hg) represents the pulling pressure exerted by the small amounts of plasma proteins that leak through the pores of the capillary wall into the interstitial spaces. The capillary colloidal osmotic pressure, which is greater than both the hydrostatic pressure at venous end of the capillary and the interstitial colloidal osmotic pressure, is largely responsible for the movement of fluid back into the capillary.

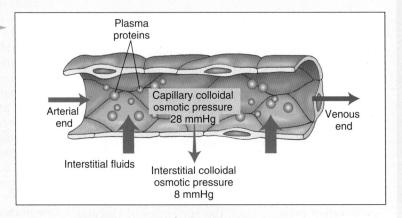

3

Lymph drainage. The lymphatic system represents an accessory system by which fluid can be returned to the circulatory system. Normally the forces moving fluid out of the capillary into the interstitium are greater than those returning fluid to the capillary. Any excess fluids and osmotically active plasma proteins that may have leaked into the interstitium are picked up by vessels of the lymphatic system and returned to the circulation. Without the function of the lymphatic system, excessive amounts of fluid would accumulate in the interstitial spaces.

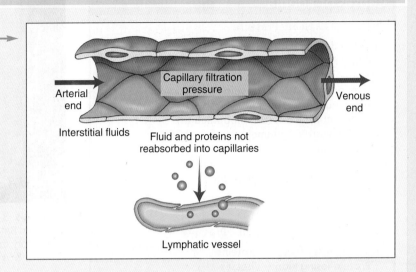

gravity, edema caused by decreased capillary colloidal osmotic pressure tends to affect tissues in nondependent as well as dependent parts of the body. There is swelling of the face as well as the legs and feet.

Increased Capillary Permeability. When the capillary pores become enlarged or the integrity of the capillary wall is damaged, capillary permeability is increased. When this happens, plasma proteins and other osmotically active particles leak into the interstitial spaces, increasing the tissue colloidal osmotic pressure and thereby contributing to the accumulation of interstitial fluid. Among the conditions that increase capillary permeability are trauma, burn injury, inflammation, and immune responses.

Obstruction of Lymph Flow. Osmotically active plasma proteins and other large particles that cannot be reabsorbed through the pores in the capillary membrane rely on the lymphatic system for movement back into the circulatory system. Edema caused by impaired lymph

flow is commonly referred to as *lymphedema*. Malignant involvement of lymph structures and removal of lymph nodes at the time of cancer surgery are common causes of lymphedema. Another cause of lymphedema is infection involving the lymphatic channels and lymph nodes.

Manifestations. The effects of edema are determined largely by its location. Edema of the brain, larynx, or lungs is an acute, life-threatening condition. Although not life threatening, edema may interfere with movement by limiting joint motion. Swelling of the ankles and feet often is insidious in onset and may or may not be associated with disease. At the tissue level, edema increases the distance for diffusion of oxygen, nutrients, and wastes. Edematous tissues usually are more susceptible to injury and the development of ischemic tissue damage, including pressure ulcers. Edema can also compress blood vessels. For example, the skin of a severely swollen finger can act as a tourniquet, shutting off the blood flow to the finger. Edema can also be disfiguring, causing psychological effects and disturbances in self-concept.

CHART 6-1

Causes of Edema

Increased Capillary Pressure

Decreased arteriolar resistance
  Calcium channel–blocking drug responses
Venous obstruction
  Liver disease with portal vein obstruction
  Acute pulmonary edema
  Venous thrombosis (thrombophlebitis)
Increased vascular volume
  Heart failure
  Kidney disease
  Premenstrual sodium retention
  Pregnancy
  Environmental heat stress

Decreased Colloidal Osmotic Pressure

Increased loss of plasma proteins
  Protein-losing kidney diseases
  Extensive burns
Decreased production of plasma proteins
  Liver disease
  Starvation, malnutrition

Increased Capillary Permeability

Inflammation
Allergic reactions (*e.g.*, hives, angioneurotic edema)
Malignancy (*e.g.*, ascites, pleural effusion)
Tissue injury and burns

Obstruction of Lymphatic Flow

Malignant obstruction of lymphatic structures
Surgical removal of lymph nodes

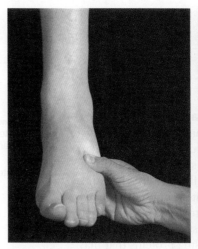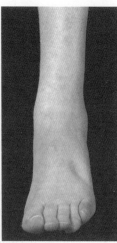

FIGURE 6-5 3+ pitting edema of the left foot. (Used with permission from Bates B. [1999]. *Bates' guide to physical examination and history taking* [7th ed., p. 472]. Philadelphia: Lippincott Williams & Wilkins.)

Assessment and Treatment. Methods for assessing edema include daily weight, visual assessment, measurement of the affected part, and application of finger pressure to assess for pitting edema. Daily weight performed at the same time each day with the same amount of clothing provides a useful index of water gain (1 L of water weighs 2.2 lb) attributable to edema. Visual inspection and measurement of the circumference of an extremity can also be used to assess the degree of swelling. This is particularly useful when swelling is caused by thrombophlebitis. Pitting edema occurs when the accumulation of interstitial fluid exceeds the absorptive capacity of the tissue gel. In this form of edema, the tissue water becomes mobile and can be translocated with pressure exerted by a finger. Finger pressure can be used to assess the degree of pitting edema. If an indentation remains after the finger has been removed, pitting edema is identified. It is evaluated on a scale of +1 (minimal) to +4 (severe; Fig. 6-5).

Treatment of edema usually is directed toward maintaining life when the swelling involves vital structures, correcting or controlling the cause, and preventing tissue injury. Diuretic therapy commonly is used to treat edema.

Edema of the lower extremities may respond to simple measures such as elevating the feet.

Elastic support stockings and sleeves increase interstitial fluid pressure and resistance to outward movement of fluid from the capillary into the tissue spaces. These support devices typically are prescribed for patients with conditions such as lymphatic or venous obstruction and are most efficient if applied before the tissue spaces have filled with fluid, such as in the morning, before the effects of gravity have caused fluid to move into the ankles.

Third-Space Accumulation

Third spacing represents the loss or trapping of ECF in the transcellular space. The serous cavities are part of the transcellular compartment (*i.e.*, third space) located in strategic body areas where there is continual movement of body structures—the pericardial sac, the peritoneal cavity, and the pleural cavity. The exchange of ECF among the capillaries, the interstitial spaces, and the transcellular space of the serous cavity uses the same mechanisms as capillaries elsewhere in the body. The serous cavities are closely linked with lymphatic drainage systems. The milking action of the moving structures, such as the lungs, continually forces fluid and plasma proteins back into the circulation, keeping these cavities empty. Any obstruction to lymph flow causes fluid accumulation in the serous cavities. As with edema fluid, third-space fluids represent an accumulation or trapping of body fluids that contribute to body weight but not to fluid reserve or function.

The prefix *hydro-* may be used to indicate the presence of excessive fluid, as in *hydrothorax*, which means excessive fluid in the pleural cavity. The accumulation of fluid in the peritoneal cavity is called *ascites*. The transudation of fluid into the serous cavities is also referred to as *effusion*. Effusion can contain blood, plasma proteins, inflammatory cells (*i.e.*, pus), and ECF.

In summary, body fluids are distributed between the ICF and ECF compartments of the body. Two thirds of body fluids are contained in the body cells of the ICF compartment, and one third is contained in the vascular compartment, interstitial spaces, and third-space areas of the ECF compartment. *Diffusion* is the movement of charged or uncharged particles along a concentration gradient. *Osmosis* refers the movement of water across a semipermeable membrane, with water moving from the side with the lesser number to side with the greater number of particles. The osmotic tension or effect that a solution exerts on cell volume in terms of causing the cell to swell or shrink is called *tonicity.*

Edema represents an increase in interstitial fluid volume. The physiologic mechanisms that predispose to edema formation are increased capillary filtration pressure, decreased capillary colloidal osmotic pressure, increased capillary permeability, and obstruction of lymphatic flow. The effect that edema exerts on body function is determined largely by its location. Edema of the brain, larynx, or lungs is an acute, life-threatening condition, whereas swelling of the ankles and feet can be a normal discomfort that accompanies hot weather. Fluid can also accumulate in the transcellular compartment—the joint spaces, pericardial sac, the peritoneal cavity, and the pleural cavity. Because this fluid is not easily exchanged with the rest of the ECF, it is often referred to as third-space fluid.

Sodium and Water Balance

REGULATION OF SODIUM AND WATER BALANCE

The movement of body fluids between the ICF and ECF compartments occurs at level of the cell membrane and depends on regulation of ECF water and sodium. Water provides approximately 90% to 93% of the volume of body fluids and sodium salts approximately 90% to 95% of the ECF solutes. Normally, equivalent changes in sodium and water are such that the volume and osmolality of the ECF is maintained within a normal range. Because it is the concentration of sodium (in milligrams per liter) that controls ECF osmolality, changes in sodium are normally accompanied by proportionate changes in water volume.

Regulation of Body Water Balance

Total body water (TBW) varies with sex and weight. These differences can be explained by differences in body fat, which is essentially water free. In men, body water approximates 60% of body weight during young adulthood and decreases to approximately 50% in old age. In young women, it is approximately 50%, and in elderly women,

approximately 40%.[3] Obesity produces further decreases in body water, sometimes reducing these levels to values as low as 30% to 40% of body weight in adults (Fig. 6-6).

Infants have a high TBW content. TBW constitutes approximately 75% to 80% of body weight in full-term infants and is even greater in premature infants. In addition to having proportionately more body water than adults, infants have relatively more water in their ECF compartment. Infants have more than half of their TBW in the ECF compartment, whereas adults have only approximately a third.[4] The greater extracellular water content of an infant can be explained in terms of its higher metabolic rate, larger surface area in relation to its body mass, and its inability to concentrate its urine because of immature kidney structures. Because ECF is more easily lost from the body, infants are more vulnerable to fluid deficit than are older children and adults. As an infant grows older, TBW decreases, and by the second year of life, the percentages and distribution of body water approach those of an adult.[5]

Gains and Losses. Regardless of age, all healthy persons require approximately 100 mL of water per 100 calories metabolized for dissolving and eliminating metabolic wastes. This means that a person who expends 1800 calories for energy requires approximately 1800 mL of water for metabolic purposes. The metabolic rate increases with fever; it rises approximately 12% for every 1°C (7% for every 1°F) increase in body temperature.[2] Fever also increases the respiratory rate, resulting in additional loss of water vapor through the lungs.

The main source of water gain is through oral intake and metabolism of nutrients. Water, including that obtained from liquids and solid foods, is absorbed from

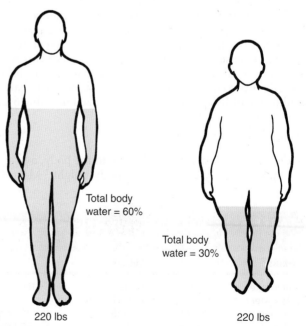

FIGURE 6-6 Body composition of a lean and an obese individual. (Adapted with permission from Statland H. [1963]. *Fluids and electrolytes in practice.* [3rd ed.]. Philadelphia: J. B. Lippincott.)

the gastrointestinal tract. Metabolic processes also generate a small amount of water. The amount of water gained from these processes varies from 150 to 300 mL/day, depending on metabolic rate.

The loss of body water occurs through the kidneys, gastrointestinal tract, skin, and respiratory tract. The kidneys are the main source of water loss. The kidneys normally regulate the volume and solute concentration of the extracellular fluid, promoting diuresis in conditions of water excess and conserving water when extracellular fluid volume is decreased. Even when oral or parenteral fluids are withheld, the kidneys continue to produce urine as a means of ridding the body of metabolic wastes. The urine output that is required to eliminate these wastes is called the *obligatory urine output.* The obligatory urine loss is approximately 300 to 500 mL/day.

There is a continuous exchange of fluid between the extracellular compartment and the gastrointestinal tract. In a single day, 8 to 10 L of ECF is secreted into the gastrointestinal tract. Most of it is reabsorbed in the ileum and proximal colon, and only about 150 to 200 mL per day is eliminated in the feces. Vomiting and diarrhea interrupt the reabsorption process, causing increased loss of fluid from the gastrointestinal tract. In many forms of diarrhea, the rate of fluid secretion into the intestine is further increased because of the osmotic or irritating effects of the causative agent. Gastrointestinal suction, fistulas, and drainage tubes can also disrupt the absorptive process by removing large amounts of fluid from the gastrointestinal tract.

Water also leaves the body through the skin and respiratory tract. Evaporative water losses from the respiratory tract and skin are referred to as *insensible water losses* because they occur without a person's awareness. The insensible water loss that occurs through the skin, sometimes referred to as *perspiration,* occurs by diffusion through the skin surface and is independent of water loss that occurs through the sweat glands.[2] The loss of skin integrity, such as occurs with extensive burns, increases evaporative water losses. For this reason, burn victims must be given large amounts of fluid, usually intravenously, to balance fluid loss. The gains and losses of body water are summarized in Table 6-2.

Regulation of Sodium Balance

Sodium is the most abundant cation in the body, averaging approximately 60 mEq/kg of body weight.[2] Most of

the body's sodium (135 to 145 mEq/L) is in the ECF compartment, with only a small amount (10 to 14 mEq/L) located in the ICF compartment.

Sodium functions mainly in regulating extracellular fluid volume, including that in the vascular compartment. As the major cation in the ECF compartment, Na^+ and its attendant anions (Cl^- and HCO_3^-) account for most of the osmotic activity in the ECF. Because sodium is part of the sodium bicarbonate molecule, it also is important in regulating acid-base balance, and as a current-carrying ion, it contributes to the function of the nervous system and other excitable tissues.

Gains and Losses. Sodium normally enters the body through the gastrointestinal tract and is eliminated by the kidneys or lost through the gastrointestinal tract or skin. Sodium intake normally is derived from dietary sources. Body needs for sodium usually can be met by as little as 500 mg/day. In the United States, the average salt intake is approximately 6 to 15 g/day, or 12 to 30 times the daily requirement. Dietary intake, which frequently exceeds the amount needed by the body, is often influenced by culture and food preferences rather than need. As package labels indicate, many commercially prepared foods and soft drinks contain considerable amounts of sodium. Other sources of sodium are intravenous saline infusions and medications that contain sodium.

Most sodium losses occur through the kidney. The kidney is extremely efficient in regulating sodium output, and when sodium intake is limited or conservation of sodium is needed, it is able to reabsorb almost all the sodium that has been filtered by the glomerulus. This results in production of essentially sodium-free urine. The rate at which the kidney excretes or conserves sodium is coordinated by the sympathetic nervous system and the renin-angiotensin-aldosterone system. The sympathetic nervous system responds to changes in arterial pressure and blood volume by adjusting the glomerular filtration rate and the rate at which sodium is filtered from the blood. Sympathetic activity also regulates tubular reabsorption of sodium and renin release. The renin-angiotensin-aldosterone system exerts its action through angiotensin II and aldosterone (see Chapter 17). Angiotensin II acts directly on the renal tubules to increase sodium reabsorption. It also acts to constrict renal blood vessels, thereby decreasing the glomerular filtration rate and slowing renal blood flow so that less sodium is filtered and more is reabsorbed. Angiotensin II is also a powerful regulator of aldosterone, a hormone secreted by the adrenal cortex. Aldosterone acts at the level of the cortical collecting tubules of the kidneys to increase sodium reabsorption while increasing potassium elimination.

Usually less than 10% of sodium intake is lost through the gastrointestinal tract and skin. Although the sodium concentration of fluids in the upper part of the gastrointestinal tract approaches that of the extracellular fluid, sodium is reabsorbed as the fluids move through the lower part of the bowel, so that the concentration of sodium in the stool is only approximately 40 mEq/L. Sodium losses

TABLE 6-2	Sources of Body Water Gains and Losses in the Adult		
Gains		**Losses**	
Oral intake		Urine	1500 mL
As water	1000 mL	Insensible losses	
In food	1300 mL	Lungs	300 mL
Water of	200 mL	Skin	500 mL
oxidation		Feces	200 mL
Total	2500 mL	Total	2500 mL

increase with conditions such as vomiting, diarrhea, fistula drainage, and gastrointestinal suction that remove sodium from the stomach or small intestine.

Sodium leaves the skin by way of the sweat glands. Sweat is a hypotonic solution containing both sodium and chloride. Although sodium losses due to sweating are usually negligible, they can increase greatly during exercise and periods of exposure to a hot environment. A person who sweats profusely can lose up to 15 to 30 g of salt each day for first few days of exposure to a hot environment. This amount usually drops to less than 3 to 5 g a day after 4 to 6 weeks of acclimatization.[2]

DISORDERS OF THIRST AND ANTIDIURETIC HORMONE

There are two main physiologic mechanisms that assist in regulating body water: thirst and antidiuretic hormone (ADH). Thirst is primarily a regulator of water intake and ADH a regulator of water output (Fig. 6-7). Both mechanisms respond to changes in extracellular osmolality and volume and both contribute indirectly to the regulation of the sodium concentration of the ECF.

Disorders of Thirst

Like appetite and eating, thirst and drinking behavior are two separate entities. Thirst is a conscious sensation of the need to obtain and drink fluids high in water content. Drinking of water or other fluids often occurs as the result of habit or for reasons other than those related to thirst. Most people drink without being thirsty, and water is consumed before it is needed. As a result, thirst is basically an emergency response. It usually occurs only when the need for water has not been anticipated.

Thirst is controlled by the thirst center in the hypothalamus. There are two stimuli for true thirst based on water need: (1) cellular dehydration caused by an increase in extracellular osmolality; and (2) a decrease in blood volume, which may or may not be associated with a decrease in serum osmolality.[6] Sensory neurons, called *osmoreceptors,* which are located in or near the thirst center in the hypothalamus, respond to changes in extracellular osmolality by stimulating the sensation of thirst (see Fig. 6-7). Stretch receptors in the vascular system that are sensitive to changes in arterial blood pressure (baroreceptors) and central blood volume (cardiopulmonary receptors) also aid in the regulation of thirst. A third important stimulus for thirst is angiotensin II, which becomes increased in response to low blood volume and low blood pressure. Dryness of the mouth produces a sensation of thirst that is not necessarily associated with the body's hydration status. Thirst sensation also occurs in those who breathe through their mouths, such as smokers and persons with chronic respiratory disease or hyperventilation syndrome.

Hypodipsia. Hypodipsia represents a decrease in the ability to sense thirst. It is commonly associated with cere-

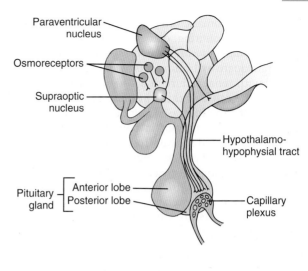

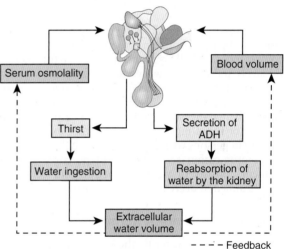

FIGURE 6-7 (Top) sagittal section through the pituitary and anterior hypothalamus. Antidiuretic hormone (ADH) is formed primarily in the supraoptic nucleus and to a lesser extent in the paraventricular nucleus of the hypothalamus. It is then transported down the hypothalamohypophysial tract and stored in secretory granules in the posterior pituitary, where it can be released into the blood. **(Bottom)** pathways for regulation of extracellular water volume by thirst and ADH.

bral lesions in the area of the hypothalamus (*e.g.,* head trauma, meningioma, occult hydrocephalus, subarachnoid hemorrhage).[6] There is also evidence that thirst is decreased and water intake reduced in elderly persons, despite higher serum sodium and osmolality levels.[7,8] The inability to perceive and respond to thirst is compounded in elderly persons who have had a stroke and may be further influenced by confusion and sensory disturbances.

Polydipsia. Polydipsia, or excessive thirst, can be classified into three categories: (1) symptomatic or true thirst, (2) inappropriate or false thirst that occurs despite normal levels of body water and serum osmolality, and (3) compulsive water drinking. *Symptomatic thirst* develops when there is a loss of body water and resolves after the loss has been replaced. Among the most common causes of symptomatic thirst are water losses associated with diarrhea, vomiting, diabetes mellitus, and diabetes insipidus. *Inappropriate* or *excessive thirst* may persist despite adequate hydration. It is a common complaint in persons with renal failure and congestive heart failure. Although the cause of thirst in these persons is unclear, it may result from increased angiotensin levels. Thirst is also a common complaint in persons with dry mouth caused by decreased salivary function or treatment with drugs with an anticholinergic action (*e.g.*, antihistamines, atropine) that lead to decreased salivary flow.

Psychogenic polydipsia involves compulsive water drinking and is usually seen in persons with psychiatric disorders, most commonly schizophrenia. Persons with the disorder drink large amounts of water and excrete large amounts of urine. The cause of excessive water drinking in these persons is uncertain. It has been suggested that the compulsive water drinking may share the same pathologic basis as the psychosis because persons with the disorder often increase their water drinking during periods of exacerbation of their psychotic symptoms.[9] The condition may be compounded by antipsychotic medications that increase ADH levels and interfere with water excretion by the kidneys. Cigarette smoking, which is common among persons with psychiatric disorders, also stimulates ADH secretion. Excessive water ingestion coupled with impaired water excretion (or rapid ingestion at a rate that exceeds renal excretion) in persons with psychogenic polydipsia can lead to water intoxication (see section on Hyponatremia, later). Treatment consists of water restriction and behavioral measures aimed at decreasing water consumption.[10]

Disorders of Antidiuretic Hormone

The reabsorption of water by the kidneys is regulated by ADH, also known as *vasopressin*. ADH is synthesized by cells in the supraoptic and paraventricular nuclei of the hypothalamus; transported along a neural pathway (*i.e.*, hypothalamo-hypophysial tract) to the neurohypophysis (*i.e.*, posterior pituitary); and then released into the circulation[11,12] (see Fig. 6-7).

As with thirst, ADH levels are controlled by extracellular volume and osmolality. Osmoreceptors in the hypothalamus sense changes in extracellular osmolality and stimulate the production and release of ADH. A blood volume decrease of as little as 5% to 10% produces maximal changes in ADH levels.[13] Likewise, stretch receptors sensitive to changes in blood pressure and central blood volume aid in the regulation of ADH release. As with many other homeostatic mechanisms, acute conditions produce greater changes in ADH levels than do chronic conditions; long-term changes in blood volume or blood pressure may exist without affecting ADH levels.

An abnormal increase in ADH synthesis and release occurs in a number of stress situations. Severe pain, nausea, trauma, surgery, certain anesthetic agents, and some narcotics (*e.g.*, morphine and meperidine) increase ADH levels. Among the drugs that affect ADH are nicotine, which stimulates its release, and alcohol, which inhibits it. Two important conditions alter ADH levels: diabetes insipidus and inappropriate secretion of ADH.

Diabetes Insipidus. Diabetes insipidus (DI) is caused by a deficiency of or a decreased response to ADH.[14] Persons with DI are unable to concentrate their urine during periods of water restriction; they excrete large volumes of urine, usually 3 to 20 L/day, depending on the degree of ADH deficiency or renal insensitivity to ADH. This large urine output is accompanied by excessive thirst. As long as the thirst mechanism is normal and fluid is readily available, there is little or no alteration in the fluid levels of persons with DI. The danger arises when the condition develops in someone who is unable to communicate the need for water or is unable to secure the needed water. In such cases, inadequate fluid intake rapidly leads to hypertonic dehydration and increased serum osmolality.

There are two types of DI: neurogenic or central DI and nephrogenic DI. Neurogenic DI occurs because of a defect in the synthesis or release of ADH and nephrogenic DI occurs because the kidneys do not respond to ADH. In neurogenic DI, loss of 75% to 80% of ADH-secretory neurons in the hypothalamus is necessary before polyuria becomes evident. Most persons with neurogenic DI have an incomplete form of the disorder and retain some ability to concentrate their urine. Temporary neurogenic DI may follow head injury or surgery near the hypophysial tract. Nephrogenic DI is characterized by impairment of the urine-concentrating ability of the kidney and free-water conservation. It may occur as a genetic trait that affects the ADH receptors in the kidney, as a side effect of drugs such as lithium,[15] or as the result of electrolyte disorders such as potassium depletion or chronic hypercalcemia.

The manifestations of DI are complaints of polyuria and intense thirst, with the volume of ingested fluids ranging from 2 to 20 L. DI may present with hypernatremia and dehydration, especially after hypothalamic damage due to shock and anoxia.

The management of central DI depends on the cause and severity of the disorder. Many persons with incomplete neurogenic DI maintain near-normal water balance when permitted to ingest water in response to thirst. Pharmacologic preparations of ADH are available for persons who cannot be managed by conservative measures. The oral antidiabetic agent chlorpropamide may be used to stimulate ADH release in partial neurogenic DI. Both neurogenic and nephrogenic forms of the disorder respond partially to the thiazide diuretics (*e.g.*, hydrochlorothiazide). These diuretics are thought to act by increasing sodium excretion by the kidneys, thus producing a decrease in the glomerular filtration rate and an increase in water reabsorption in the proximal tubule.

Syndrome of Inappropriate Secretion of ADH. The syndrome of inappropriate secretion of ADH (SIADH) results from a failure of the negative feedback system that regulates the release and inhibition of ADH.[16,17] In persons with this syndrome, ADH secretion continues even when serum osmolality is decreased, causing marked water retention and dilutional hyponatremia.

SIADH may occur as a transient condition, such as in a stress situation, or as a chronic condition, resulting from disorders such as a lung tumor. Stimuli, such as surgery, pain, stress, and temperature changes, are capable of stimulating ADH release through the central nervous system (CNS). Drugs induce SIADH in different ways; some drugs are thought to increase hypothalamic production and release of ADH, and others are believed to act directly on the renal tubules to enhance the action of ADH. More chronic forms of SIADH may be the result of lung tumors, chest lesions, and CNS disorders. Tumors, particularly bronchogenic carcinoma and cancers of the lymphoid tissues, prostate, and pancreas, are known to produce and release ADH independent of normal hypothalamic control mechanisms. Other intrathoracic conditions, such as advanced tuberculosis, severe pneumonia, and positive-pressure breathing, can also cause SIADH. The suggested mechanism for SIADH in positive-pressure ventilation is activation of stretch receptors (*e.g.*, aortic baroreceptors, cardiopulmonary receptors) that respond to marked changes in intrathoracic pressure. Human immunodeficiency virus (HIV) infection is emerging as a new cause of SIADH. It has been reported that as many as 35% of persons with acquired immunodeficiency syndrome (AIDS) who are admitted to the acute care setting have SIADH related to *Pneumocystis carinii* pneumonia, CNS infections, or malignancies.[18]

The manifestations of SIADH are those of dilutional hyponatremia (to be discussed). Urine output decreases despite adequate or increased fluid intake. Urine osmolality is high, and serum osmolality is low. Hematocrit and the serum sodium and BUN levels are all decreased because of the expansion of the ECF volume. The severity of symptoms usually is proportional to the extent of sodium depletion and water intoxication.

The treatment of SIADH depends on its severity. In mild cases, treatment consists of fluid restriction. If fluid restriction is not sufficient, diuretics such as furosemide (Lasix) may be given to promote diuresis and free-water clearance. Lithium and the antibiotic demeclocycline inhibit the action of ADH on the renal collecting ducts and sometimes are used in treating the disorder. In cases of severe water intoxication, a hypertonic (*e.g.*, 3%) sodium chloride solution may be administered intravenously. New antagonists to the antidiuretic action of ADH (aquaretics) offer a novel therapeutic approach.[17]

DISORDERS OF SODIUM AND WATER BALANCE

Disorders of sodium and water balance can be divided into two main categories: (1) isotonic contraction or expansion of ECF volume, and (2) hypotonic dilution (hyponatremia) or hypertonic concentration (hypernatremia) of sodium brought about by changes in extracellular water (Fig. 6-8). Isotonic disorders usually are confined to the ECF compartment, producing a contraction (fluid volume deficit) or expansion (fluid volume excess) of the interstitial and vascular fluids. Disorders of sodium concentration produce a change in the osmolality of the ECF with movement of water from the ECF compartment into the ICF compartment (hyponatremia) or from the ICF compartment into the ECF compartment (hypernatremia).

Isotonic Fluid Volume Deficit

Fluid volume deficit is characterized by a decrease in the ECF, including the circulating blood volume. The term *isotonic fluid volume deficit* is used to differentiate this type of fluid deficit in which there are proportionate losses in sodium and water from water deficit and the hyperosmolar state associated with hypernatremia. Unless other fluid and electrolyte imbalances are present, the concentration of serum electrolytes remains essentially unchanged. When

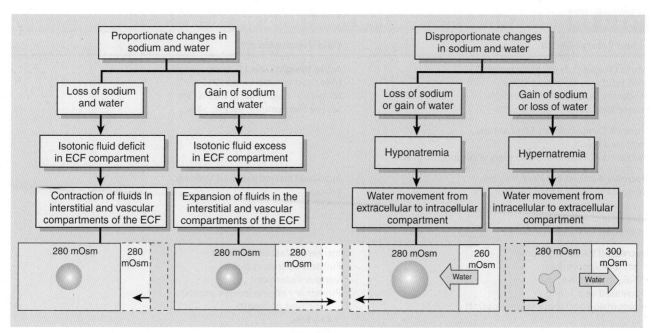

FIGURE 6-8 Effect of isotonic fluid volume deficit and excess and of hyponatremia and hypernatremia on extracellular (ECF) and intracellular fluid volume.

KEY CONCEPTS

Sodium and Water Balance

➤ It is the amount of water and its effect on sodium concentration in the ECF that serves to regulate the distribution of fluid between the ICF and the ECF compartments.

➤ Isotonic changes in body fluids that result from proportionate gains or losses of sodium and water are largely confined to the ECF compartment. Many of the manifestations of isotonic fluid deficit or excess reflect changes in vascular and interstitial fluid volume.

➤ Hyponatremia or hypernatremia that is brought about by disproportionate losses or gains in sodium or water exert their effects on the ICF compartment, causing water to move in or out of body cells. Many of the manifestations of changes in sodium concentration reflect changes in the intracellular volume of cells, particularly those in the nervous system.

and exercise. Third-space losses can cause sequestering of ECF in the serous cavities, extracellular spaces in injured tissues, or lumen of the gut.

Excess urinary losses can result from kidney disease, osmotic diuresis, or injudicious use of diuretics. Certain forms of kidney disease are characterized by salt wasting caused by impaired sodium reabsorption. Glucose in the urine filtrate prevents reabsorption of water by the renal tubules, causing osmotic diuresis with loss of sodium and water. In Addison disease, a condition of chronic adrenocortical insufficiency, there is unregulated loss of sodium in the urine with a resultant loss of ECF volume (see Chapter 31).

Manifestations. The manifestations of fluid volume deficit, which reflect a decrease in ECF volume, include thirst, signs of water conservation by the kidney, loss of body weight, impaired temperature regulation, and signs of reduced interstitial and vascular volume (Table 6-3).

A loss in fluid volume is characterized by a decrease in body weight. One liter of water weighs 1 kg (2.2 lb). A mild ECF deficit exists when weight loss equals 2% of body weight.[5] In a person who weighs 68 kg (150 lb), this percentage of weight loss equals 1.4 L of water. A moderate deficit equates to a 5% loss in weight and a severe deficit to an 8% or greater loss in weight.[5] To be accurate, weight must be measured at the same time each day with the person wearing the same amount of clothing. Because the fluid is trapped in the body in persons with third-space losses, their body weight may not decrease.

Thirst is a common symptom of fluid deficit, although it is not always present during early stages of isotonic fluid deficit. It develops as the effective circulating volume decreases to a point sufficient to stimulate the thirst mechanism. Urine output decreases and urine osmolality

the effective circulating blood volume is compromised, the condition is often referred to as *hypovolemia*.

Isotonic fluid volume deficit results when water and electrolytes are lost in isotonic proportions. It is almost always caused by a loss of body fluids and is often accompanied by a decrease in fluid intake. It can occur because of a loss of gastrointestinal fluids as with vomiting or diarrhea, polyuria, or excessive sweating caused by fever

TABLE 6-3 Manifestations of Isotonic Fluid Volume Deficit and Excess	
Fluid Volume Deficit	**Fluid Volume Excess**
Acute Weight Loss (% body weight) Mild fluid volume deficit: 2% Moderate fluid volume deficit: 5% Severe fluid volume deficit: >8%	**Acute Weight Gain (% body weight)** Mild fluid volume excess: 2% Moderate fluid volume excess: 5% Severe fluid volume excess: >8%
Signs of Compensatory Mechanisms Increased thirst Increased ADH: oliguria and high urine-specific gravity	
Decreased Interstitial Fluid Volume Decreased skin and tissue turgor Dry mucous membranes Sunken and soft eyeballs Depressed fontanel in infants	**Increased Interstitial Fluid Volume** Edema

Decreased Vascular Volume
Postural hypotension
Weak, rapid pulse
Decreased vein filling
Hypotension and shock (severe deficit)
	Increased Vascular Volume
	Full and bounding pulse
	Venous distention
	Pulmonary edema (severe excess)
	    Shortness of breath
	    Crackles
	    Dyspnea
	    Cough

and specific gravity increase as ADH levels rise because of a decrease in vascular volume. Although there is an isotonic loss of sodium and water from the vascular compartment, other substances such as hematocrit and BUN become more concentrated.

The fluid content of body tissues decreases as fluid is removed from the interstitial spaces. The eyes assume a sunken appearance and feel softer than normal as the fluid content in the anterior chamber of the eye is decreased. Fluids add resiliency to the skin and underlying tissues that is referred to as *skin* or *tissue turgor*.[5] Pinching a fold of skin between the thumb and forefinger provides a means for assessing tissue turgor. The skin should immediately return to its original configuration when the fingers are released. A loss of 3% to 5% of body water in children causes the resiliency of the skin to be lost. Decreased tissue turgor is less predictive of fluid deficit in older persons (>65 years) because of the loss of tissue elasticity. In infants fluid deficit may be evidenced by depression of the anterior fontanel because of a decrease in cerebrospinal fluid. Body temperature may be subnormal because of decreased metabolism.[5]

Arterial and venous volumes decline during periods of fluid deficit, as does filling of the capillary circulation. As the volume in the arterial system declines, the blood pressure decreases, the heart rate increases, and the pulse become weak and thready. Postural hypotension (a drop in blood pressure on standing) is an early sign of fluid deficit. On the venous side of the circulation, the veins become less prominent. When volume depletion becomes severe, signs of hypovolemic shock and vascular collapse appear (discussed in Chapter 19).

Diagnosis and Treatment. Diagnosis of fluid volume deficit is based on a history of conditions that predispose to sodium and water losses, weight loss, intake and output measurements, and observations of altered physiologic function indicative of decreased fluid volume. Measurement of heart rate and blood pressure provides useful information about vascular volume. A simple test to determine venous refill time consists of compressing the distal end of a vein on the dorsal aspect of the hand when it is not in the dependent position. The vein is then emptied by "milking" the blood toward the heart. The vein should refill almost immediately when the occluding finger is removed. When there is a decrease in venous volume, as occurs in fluid deficit, venous refill time increases. Capillary refill time is also increased. Capillary refill can be assessed by applying pressure to a fingernail for 5 seconds and then releasing the pressure and observing the time (normally 1 to 2 seconds) it takes for the color to return to normal.[5]

Treatment of fluid volume deficit consists of fluid replacement and measures to correct the underlying cause. Usually, isotonic electrolyte solutions are used for fluid replacement. Acute hypovolemia and hypovolemic shock can cause renal damage; therefore, prompt assessment of the degree of fluid deficit and adequate measures to resolve the deficit and treat the underlying cause are essential.

Isotonic Fluid Volume Excess

Fluid volume excess represents an isotonic expansion of the ECF compartment with increases in both interstitial and vascular volumes. Although increased fluid volume is usually the result of a disease condition, this is not always true. For example, a compensatory isotonic expansion of body fluids can occur in healthy persons during hot weather as a mechanism for increasing body heat loss.

Isotonic fluid volume excess almost always results from an increase in total body sodium that is accompanied by a proportionate increase in body water. Although it can occur as the result of excessive sodium intake, it is most commonly caused by a decrease in sodium and water elimination by the kidney. Among the causes of decreased sodium and water elimination are disorders of renal function, heart failure, liver failure, and corticosteroid hormone excess.

Heart failure (see Chapter 19) produces a decrease in renal blood flow and a compensatory increase in sodium and water retention. Persons with severe congestive heart failure maintain a precarious balance between sodium and water intake and output. Even small increases in sodium intake can precipitate a state of fluid volume excess and a worsening of heart failure. Liver failure impairs aldosterone metabolism and alters renal perfusion, leading to increased salt and water retention. The corticosteroid hormones increase sodium reabsorption by the kidneys. Persons taking corticosteroid medications and those with Cushing disease (see Chapter 31) often have problems with sodium retention.

Manifestations. Isotonic fluid volume excess is characterized by an increase in interstitial and vascular fluids. It is manifested by weight gain over a short period of time. A mild fluid volume excess represents a 2% weight gain; moderate fluid volume excess, a 5% weight gain; and severe fluid volume excess, a weight gain of 8% or more[5] (see Table 6-3). The presence of edema is characteristic of isotonic fluid volume excess. When the excess fluid accumulates gradually, as often happens in debilitating diseases and starvation, edema fluid may mask the loss of tissue mass. As the vascular volume increases, the jugular veins become distended, the pulse becomes full and bounding, and the central venous pressure becomes elevated. The BUN and hematocrit may be decreased as a result of the expanded plasma volume. When excess fluid accumulates in the lungs (*i.e.*, pulmonary edema), there is shortness of breath, complaints of difficult breathing, respiratory crackles, and a productive cough. Ascites and pleural effusion may occur with severe fluid volume excess.

Diagnosis and Treatment. Diagnosis of fluid volume excess is usually based on a history of factors that predispose to sodium and water retention, weight gain, and manifestations such as edema and cardiovascular symptoms indicative of an expanded extracellular fluid volume.

The treatment of fluid volume excess focuses on providing a more favorable balance between sodium intake and output. A sodium-restricted diet is often prescribed. Diuretic therapy may be used to increase sodium elimination.

Hyponatremia

The normal serum sodium ranges from 135 to 145 mEq/L (135 to 145 mmol/L). Serum sodium values, expressed in milliequivalents per liter (mEq/L), reflect the concentration or dilution of sodium by water, rather than its absolute value. Because sodium and its attendant anions account for 90% to 95% of the osmolality of the ECF (normal, 275 to 295 mOsm/kg), changes in serum sodium usually are accompanied by changes in serum osmolality.

Hyponatremia represents a serum sodium concentration below 135 mEq/L (135 mmol/L). It is one of the most common electrolyte disorders seen in hospitalized patients and is also common in the outpatient population, particularly in the elderly population. A number of age-related events make the elderly population more vulnerable to hyponatremia, including a decrease in renal function accompanied by limitations in sodium conservation. Although older people maintain body fluid homeostasis under most circumstances, the ability to withstand environmental, drug-related, and disease-associated stresses becomes progressively limited.

Because of the effects of osmotically active particles such as glucose, hyponatremia can present as a hypertonic or hypotonic state.[19–21] *Hypertonic (translocational) hyponatremia* results from an osmotic shift of water from ICF to the ECF, such as occurs with hyperglycemia. In this case, the sodium in the ECF becomes diluted as water moves out of cells in response to the osmotic effects of the elevated blood glucose level. *Hypotonic (dilutional) hyponatremia,* by far the most common type of hyponatremia, is caused by water retention. It can be classified as hypovolemic, euvolemic, or hypervolemic based on accompanying ECF fluid volumes.[20] Because of its effect on both sodium and water elimination, diuretic therapy can cause either hypovolemic or euvolemic hyponatremia.

Hypovolemic hypotonic hyponatremia occurs when water is lost along with sodium but to a lesser extent. Among the causes of hypovolemic hyponatremia are excessive sweating in hot weather, particularly during heavy exercise, which leads to loss of salt and water. Hyponatremia develops when water, rather than electrolyte-containing liquids, is used to replace fluids lost in sweating. Another potential cause of hypovolemic hyponatremia is the loss of sodium from the gastrointestinal tract caused by frequent gastrointestinal irrigations with distilled water. Iso-osmotic fluid loss, such as occurs in vomiting or diarrhea, does not usually lower serum sodium levels unless these losses are replaced with disproportionate amounts of orally ingested or parenterally administered water. Gastrointestinal fluid loss and ingestion of excessively diluted formula are common causes of acute hyponatremia in infants and children. Hypovolemic hyponatremia is also a common complication of adrenal insufficiency and is attributable to a decrease in aldosterone levels. A lack of aldosterone increases renal losses of sodium, and a cortisol deficiency leads to increased release of ADH with water retention.

Euvolemic or *normovolemic hypotonic hyponatremia* represents retention of water with dilution of sodium while maintaining the ECF volume within a normal range. It is usually the result of SIADH. The risk of normovolemic hyponatremia is increased during the postoperative period. During this time ADH levels are often high, producing an increase in water reabsorption by the kidney (see section on SIADH, earlier). Although these elevated levels usually resolve in about 72 hours, they can persist for as long as 5 days. The hyponatremia becomes exaggerated when electrolyte-free fluids (*e.g.,* 5% glucose in water) are used for fluid replacement.

Hypervolemic hypotonic hyponatremia is seen when hyponatremia is accompanied by edema-associated disorders such as heart failure, cirrhosis, nephrotic syndrome, and advanced renal disease. Although the total body sodium is increased in heart failure, the effective circulating blood volume is often sensed as inadequate by the baroreceptors, resulting in increased ADH levels.

Manifestations. The manifestations of hyponatremia vary depending on the serum osmolality, ECF fluid volume status, rapidity of onset, and severity of sodium dilution[19–22] (Table 6-4). The signs and symptoms may be acute, as in severe water intoxication, or more insidious in onset and less severe, as in chronic hyponatremia. Because of water movement, hypotonic hyponatremia produces an increase in intracellular water, which is responsible for many of the clinical manifestations of the disorder.

Muscle cramps, weakness, and fatigue reflect the effects of hyponatremia on skeletal muscle function and are often early signs of hyponatremia. These effects commonly are observed in persons with hyponatremia that occurs during heavy exercise in hot weather. Gastrointestinal manifestations such as nausea and vomiting, abdominal cramps, and diarrhea may develop.

The brain and nervous system are the most seriously affected by pronounced increases in intracellular water. Symptoms include lethargy and headache, which can progress to disorientation, confusion, gross motor weakness, and depression of deep tendon reflexes. Seizures and coma occur when serum sodium levels reach extremely low levels. These severe effects, which are caused by brain swelling, may be irreversible. If the condition develops slowly, signs and symptoms do not usually develop until serum sodium levels approach 120 mEq/L.[19] The term *water intoxication* is often used to describe the neurologic effects of acute hypotonic hyponatremia.

Diagnosis and Treatment. Diagnosis of hyponatremia is based on laboratory reports of serum sodium concentration and osmolality, the presence of conditions that predispose to sodium loss or water retention, and signs and symptoms indicative of the disorder.

The treatment of hyponatremia with water excess focuses on the underlying cause and the rapidity with which it developed. When hyponatremia is caused by water retention, limiting water intake or discontinuing medications that contribute to water retention may be sufficient. The management of hypervolemic hyponatremia requires both water and salt restrictions. In many cases a loop diuretic (*e.g.,* furosemide [Lasix]) may be needed to increase sodium excretion by the kidney.

The administration of saline solution orally or intravenously may be needed in severe hyponatremia caused by sodium deficiency. There is concern about the rapidity

TABLE 6-4	Manifestations of Hyponatremia and Hypernatremia
Hyponatremia (Hypotonic)	**Hypernatremia**
Laboratory Values Serum sodium <135 mEq/L Decreased serum osmolality Dilutional decrease in blood components, including 　hematocrit, blood urea nitrogen (BUN)	**Laboratory Values** Serum sodium >145 mEq/L Increased serum osmolality Increased concentrations of blood components, including hematocrit, BUN **Compensatory Mechanisms** Increased thirst Increased ADH with oliguria and high urine-specific gravity **Decreased Intracellular Fluid** Dry skin and mucous membranes Decreased tissue turgor Decreased salivation and lacrimation
Hypo-osmolality and Movement of Water Into Muscle, Neural, and Gastrointestinal Tract Tissue *Muscle* 　Muscle cramps and weakness 　Depressed deep tendon reflexes *Central Nervous System* 　Headache 　Disorientation 　Lethargy 　Seizures and coma (severe) *Gastrointestinal Tract* 　Anorexia, nausea, vomiting 　Abdominal cramps, diarrhea	**Hyperosmolality and Movement of Water Out of Neural Tissue** Headache Disorientation and agitation Decreased reflexes Seizures and coma (severe) **Decreased Vascular Volume** Weak, rapid pulse Possible impaired temperature regulation with fever Decreased blood pressure Vascular collapse (severe)

with which plasma sodium levels are corrected, particularly in persons with chronic symptomatic hyponatremia. Cells, particularly those in the brain, tend to defend against changes in cell volume caused by a decrease in ECF osmolality by decreasing the number of intracellular osmoles.[20] It takes several days for brain cells to restore the osmoles lost during hyponatremia. Thus, treatment measures that produce rapid changes in serum osmolality when brain cells have already undergone volume regulation may cause a dramatic change in cell volume. One of the reported effects of rapid treatment of hyponatremia is an osmotic demyelinating condition called *central pontine myelosis*, which produces serious neurologic sequelae and sometimes causes death.[20,21]

Hypernatremia

Hypernatremia implies a serum sodium level above 145 mEq/L and a serum osmolality greater than 295 mOsm/kg. Because sodium is functionally an impermeable solute, it contributes to the tonicity and movement of water across cell membranes. Hypernatremia is characterized by hypertonicity of the ECF and almost always causes cellular dehydration.[22]

Causes. Hypernatremia represents a deficit of water in relation to the body's sodium levels. It can be caused by net gain of sodium or net loss of water. Rapid ingestion or infusion of sodium with insufficient time or opportunity for water ingestion can produce a disproportionate gain in sodium. A defect in thirst or inability to obtain or drink water can interfere with water replacement.

Hypernatremia occurs when there is an excess loss of body fluids that have a lower than normal concentration of sodium so that water is lost in excess of sodium. This can result from increased losses from the respiratory tract during fever or strenuous exercise, from watery diarrhea, or when osmotically active tube feedings are given with inadequate amounts of water.

Normally, water deficit stimulates thirst and increases water intake. Therefore, hypernatremia is more likely to occur in infants and in persons who cannot express their thirst or obtain water to drink. With hypodipsia, or impaired thirst, the need for fluid intake does not activate the thirst response. Hypodipsia is particularly prevalent among the elderly. In persons with diabetes insipidus, hypernatremia can develop when thirst is impaired or access to water is impeded.

The therapeutic administration of sodium-containing solutions may also cause hypernatremia. For example, the administration of sodium bicarbonate during cardiopulmonary resuscitation increases body sodium levels because each 50-ml ampule of 7.5% sodium bicarbonate contains 892 mEq of sodium.[5] Rarely, salt intake occurs rapidly, as in taking excess salt tablets or during near-drowning in salt water.

Manifestations. The clinical manifestations of hypernatremia caused by water loss are largely those of ECF fluid loss and cellular dehydration (see Table 6-4). The severity of signs and symptoms is greatest when the increase in serum sodium is large and occurs rapidly. Body weight is decreased in proportion to the amount of water that has been lost. Because blood plasma is roughly 90% to 93%

water, the concentrations of blood cells, hematocrit, BUN, and other solutes increase as ECF water decreases.

Thirst is an early symptom of water deficit, occurring when water losses are equal to 0.5% of body water. Urine output is decreased and urine osmolality increased because of renal water-conserving mechanisms. Body temperature frequently is elevated, and the skin becomes warm and flushed. As the vascular volume decreases, the pulse becomes rapid and thready, and the blood pressure drops. Hypernatremia produces an increase in serum osmolality and results in water being pulled out of body cells. As a result, the skin and mucous membranes become dry, and salivation and tearing of the eyes are decreased. The mouth becomes dry and sticky, and the tongue becomes rough and fissured. Swallowing is difficult. The subcutaneous tissues assume a firm, rubbery texture. Most significantly, water is pulled out of the cells in the CNS, causing decreased reflexes, agitation, headache, and restlessness. Coma and seizures may develop as hypernatremia progresses.

Diagnosis and Treatment. The diagnosis of hypernatremia is based on history, physical examination findings indicative of dehydration, and results of laboratory tests. Treatment includes measures to treat the underlying cause of the disorder and fluid replacement therapy to treat the accompanying dehydration. Replacement fluids can be given orally or intravenously. The oral route is preferable. Oral glucose–electrolyte replacement solutions are available for the treatment of infants with diarrhea. Until recently, these solutions were used only early in diarrheal illness or as a first step in reestablishing oral intake after parenteral replacement therapy. These solutions are now widely available in grocery stores and pharmacies for use in the treatment of diarrhea and other dehydrating disorders in infants and young children.

In summary, body fluids are distributed between the ICF and ECF compartments. Regulation of fluid volume, solute concentration, and distribution between the two compartments depends on water and sodium balance. Water provides approximately 90% to 93% of fluid volume, and sodium salts, approximately 90% to 95% of extracellular solutes. Sodium is ingested in the diet and eliminated by the kidneys under the influence of the sympathetic nervous system and the renin-angiotensin-aldosterone system. Body water is regulated by thirst, which controls water intake, and ADH, which controls urine concentration and renal output.

Isotonic fluid disorders result from contraction or expansion of ECF volume brought about by proportionate losses of sodium and water. *Isotonic fluid volume deficit* is characterized by a decrease in ECF volume. It causes thirst, decreased vascular volume and circulatory function, decreased urine output, and increased urine specific gravity. *Isotonic fluid volume excess* is characterized by an increase in ECF volume. It is manifested by signs of increased vascular volume and edema.

Alterations in extracellular sodium concentration are brought about by a disproportionate gain (hyponatremia) or loss (hypernatremia) of water. As the major cation in the ECF compartment, sodium controls the ECF osmolality and its effect on cell volume. *Hyponatremia* can present as a hypertonic (translocational) hyponatremia in which water moves out of the cell in response to elevated blood glucose levels, or as a hypotonic (dilutional) hyponatremia, which is caused by retention of water by the body in excess of sodium. Hypovolemic hypotonic hyponatremia is characterized by water being pulled into the cell from the extracellular compartment, causing cells to swell. It is manifested by muscle cramps and weakness; nausea, vomiting, abdominal cramps, and diarrhea; and CNS signs such as headache, lethargy, depression of deep tendon reflexes, and, in severe cases, seizure and coma. *Hypernatremia* represents a disproportionate loss of body water in relation to sodium. It is characterized by intracellular water being pulled into the extracellular compartment, causing cells to shrink. It is manifested by thirst and decreased urine output; dry mouth and decreased tissue turgor; signs of decreased vascular volume (tachycardia, weak and thready pulse); and CNS signs, such as decreased reflexes, agitation, headache, and, in severe cases, seizures and coma.

Potassium Balance

REGULATION OF POTASSIUM BALANCE

Potassium is the second most abundant cation in the body and the major cation in the ICF compartment. Approximately 98% of body potassium is contained within body cells, with an intracellular concentration of about 140 to 150 mEq/L.[23] The potassium content of ECF (3.5 to 5.0 mEq/L) is considerably lower. Because potassium is an intracellular ion, total body stores of potassium are related to body size and muscle mass. In adults, total body potassium ranges from 50 to 55 mmol/kg body weight.[24] Approximately 65% to 75% of potassium is in muscle.[25] Thus, total body potassium declines with age, mainly as a result of a decrease in muscle mass.

Gains and Losses

Potassium intake is normally derived from dietary sources. In healthy persons, potassium balance usually can be maintained by a daily dietary intake of 50 to 100 mEq. Additional amounts of potassium are needed during periods of trauma and stress. The kidneys are the main source of potassium loss. Approximately 80% to 90% of potassium losses occur in the urine, with the remainder being lost in stools or sweat.

Mechanisms of Regulation

Normally, the ECF concentration of potassium is precisely regulated at levels of about 3.5 to 4.5 mEq/mL.

The precise control is necessary because many cell functions are sensitive to even small changes in ECF potassium levels.

Serum potassium levels are largely regulated through two mechanisms: (1) renal mechanisms that conserve or eliminate potassium, and (2) a transcellular shift of potassium between the ICF and ECF compartments.

Renal Regulation. The kidney provides the major route for potassium elimination.[26] Potassium is filtered in the glomerulus, reabsorbed along with sodium and water in the proximal tubule and with sodium and chloride in the thick ascending loop of Henle, and then secreted into the late distal and cortical collecting tubules for elimination in the urine. The latter mechanism serves to "fine-tune" the concentration of potassium in the ECF.

Aldosterone plays an essential role in regulating potassium elimination by the kidney (see Chapter 23). In the presence of aldosterone, sodium is transported back into the blood and potassium is secreted into the tubular filtrate for elimination in the urine. There is also a potassium–hydrogen exchange system in the collecting tubules of the kidney. When serum potassium levels are increased, potassium is secreted into the urine and hydrogen is reabsorbed into the blood, producing a decrease in pH and metabolic acidosis. Conversely, when potassium levels are low, potassium is reabsorbed and hydrogen is secreted into the urine, leading to metabolic alkalosis.

Extracellular–Intracellular Shifts. Normally, it takes 6 to 8 hours to eliminate 50% of potassium intake.[3] To avoid an increase in extracellular potassium levels during this time, excess potassium is temporarily shifted into red blood cells and other cells such as those of muscle, liver, and bone. This movement is controlled by the func-

tion of the Na^+/K^+ adenosine triphosphatase (ATPase) membrane pump and the permeability of the ion channels in the cell membrane.

Among the factors that alter the intracellular/extracellular distribution of potassium are acid-base disorders, serum osmolality, insulin, and β-adrenergic stimulation (Fig. 6-9). The hydrogen and potassium ions, which are positively charged, can be exchanged between the ICF and ECF in a cation shift. In metabolic acidosis, for example, hydrogen ions move into body cells for buffering, causing potassium to leave the cells and move into the ECF. Acute increases in serum osmolality cause water to leave the cell. The loss of cell water produces an increase in intracellular potassium, causing it to move out of the cell into the ECF.

Both insulin and the catecholamines (*e.g.*, epinephrine) increase cellular uptake of potassium by increasing the activity of the Na^+/K^+ ATPase membrane pump.[26,27] Insulin produces an increase in cellular uptake of potassium after a meal. The catecholamines, particularly epinephrine, facilitate the movement of potassium into muscle tissue during periods of physiologic stress. β-Adrenergic agonist drugs, such as pseudoephedrine and albuterol, have a similar effect on potassium distribution.[24]

Exercise can also produce compartmental shifts in potassium. Repeated muscle contraction causes potassium to be released into the ECF. Although the increase usually is small with modest exercise, it can be considerable during exhaustive exercise. Even the repeated clenching and unclenching of the fist during a blood draw can cause potassium to move out of cells and artificially elevate serum potassium levels.

DISORDERS OF POTASSIUM BALANCE

As the major intracellular cation, potassium is critical to many body functions. It is involved in a wide range of body functions, including the maintenance of the osmotic integrity of cells, acid-base balance, and the kidney's

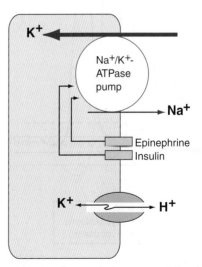

FIGURE 6-9 Mechanism for regulating transcellular shifts in potassium.

ability to concentrate urine. Potassium is necessary for growth, and it contributes to the intricate chemical reactions that transform carbohydrates into energy, change glucose into glycogen, and convert amino acids to proteins. Potassium also plays a critical role in conducting nerve impulses and the excitability of skeletal, cardiac, and smooth muscle (see Chapter 1). It does this by regulating (1) the resting membrane potential, (2) the opening of the sodium channels that control the flow of current during the action potential, and (3) the rate of repolarization.[12] Changes in nerve and muscle excitability are particularly important in the heart, where alterations in serum potassium can produce serious arrhythmias and conduction defects.

The *resting membrane potential* is determined by the ratio of intracellular to extracellular potassium. A decrease in serum potassium causes the resting membrane potential to become more negative (hyperpolarization), moving further from the threshold for excitation (Fig. 6-10). Thus, it takes a greater stimulus to reach threshold and open the sodium channels that are responsible for the action potential. An increase in serum potassium has the opposite effect; it causes the resting membrane potential to become more positive (hypopolarized), moving closer to threshold. This change initially increases membrane excitability, such that a lesser stimulus is needed to generate an action potential. However, the later effects are different because persistent depolarization inactivates the sodium channels in the membrane, producing a decrease in excitability. The *rate of repolarization* also varies with serum potassium levels.[12] It is more rapid in hyperkalemia and delayed in hypokalemia. Both the inactivation of the sodium channels and the rate of repolarization are important clinically because they predispose to conduction defects and arrhythmias in the heart.

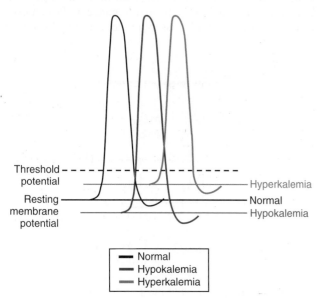

Threshold potential
Resting membrane potential
Hyperkalemia
Normal
Hypokalemia

—— Normal
—— Hypokalemia
—— Hyperkalemia

FIGURE 6-10 Effect of changes in serum hypokalemia (red) and hyperkalemia (blue) on the resting membrane potential.

Hypokalemia

Hypokalemia refers to a serum potassium level below 3.5 mEq/L (3.5 mmol/L). Because of transcellular shifts, temporary changes in serum potassium may occur as the result of movement between the ICF and ECF compartments.

Causes. The causes of potassium deficit can be grouped into three categories: (1) inadequate intake; (2) excessive losses through the kidney, skin, and gastrointestinal tract; and (3) redistribution between the ICF and ECF compartments.

Inadequate intake is a frequent cause of hypokalemia. A potassium intake of at least 10 to 30 mEq/day is needed to compensate for obligatory urine losses.[27] A person on a potassium-free diet continues to lose approximately 5 to 15 mEq of potassium daily. Insufficient dietary intake may result from the inability to obtain or ingest food or from a diet that is low in potassium-containing foods.

Excessive renal losses can occur with diuretic use, metabolic alkalosis, magnesium depletion, trauma and stress, and increased levels of aldosterone. Diuretic therapy, with the exception of potassium-sparing diuretics, is the most common cause of hypokalemia. Both thiazide and loop diuretics increase the loss of potassium in the urine.[23] Magnesium depletion, which often coexists with potassium depletion due to diuretic therapy, produces additional renal potassium losses. Renal losses of potassium are also accentuated by aldosterone and cortisol. Trauma and surgery produce a stress-related increase in these hormones. Primary aldosteronism, caused by an aldosterone-secreting tumor of the adrenal cortex, can produce severe urinary losses of potassium.

Although potassium losses from the gastrointestinal tract and the skin usually are minimal, these losses can become excessive under certain conditions. Vomiting and gastrointestinal suction lead to hypokalemia, partly because of actual potassium losses and partly because of renal losses associated with metabolic alkalosis (see section on Metabolic Alkalosis, under Acid-Base Balance, later). Excessive skin losses occur with loss of the protective skin surface and sweating. Burns and other types of skin injury increase the loss of potassium through wound drainage.

Because of the high ratio of intracellular to extracellular potassium, a redistribution of potassium from the ECF to the ICF compartment can produce marked decreases in the serum potassium levels. A wide variety of β_2-adrenergic agonist drugs (*e.g.*, decongestants and bronchodilators) shift potassium into cells and cause transient hypokalemia. Insulin also increases the movement of potassium into the cell. Because insulin increases the movement of glucose and potassium into cells, potassium deficit often develops during treatment of diabetic ketoacidosis.

Manifestations. The manifestations of hypokalemia include the effect of altered membrane potentials and excitability on cardiovascular, neuromuscular, and gastrointestinal function (Table 6-5). The signs and symptoms

TABLE 6-5	Manifestations of Hypokalemia and Hyperkalemia
Hypokalemia	**Hyperkalemia**
Laboratory Values Serum potassium <3.5 mEq/L	**Laboratory Values** Serum potassium >5.0 mEq/L
Thirst and Urine Increased thirst Inability to concentrate urine with polyuria and 　urine with low specific gravity	
Effects of Changes in Membrane Potentials on Neural and Muscle Function *Gastrointestinal* 　Anorexia, nausea, vomiting 　Abdominal distention 　Paralytic ileus (severe hypokalemia) *Neuromuscular* 　Muscle weakness, flabbiness, fatigue 　Muscle cramps and tenderness 　Paresthesias 　Paralysis (severe hypokalemia) *Central Nervous System* 　Confusion, depression *Cardiovascular* 　Postural hypotension 　Predisposition to digitalis toxicity 　Electrocardiogram changes 　Cardiac arrhythmias	**Effects of Changes in Membrane Potentials on Neural and Muscle Function** *Gastrointestinal* 　Nausea, vomiting 　Intestinal cramps 　Diarrhea *Neuromuscular* 　Weakness, dizziness 　Muscle cramps 　Paresthesias 　Paralysis (severe hyperkalemia) *Cardiovascular* 　Electrocardiogram changes 　Risk of cardiac arrest with severe hyperkalemia
Acid-Base Balance Metabolic alkalosis	

of potassium deficit seldom develop until the serum potassium level has fallen to less than 3.0 mEq/L. They are typically gradual in onset; therefore, the disorder may go undetected for some time.

The renal processes that conserve potassium during hypokalemia interfere with the kidney's ability to concentrate urine. As a result, urine output and serum osmolality are increased, urine specific gravity is decreased, and polyuria, nocturia, and thirst are common. Metabolic alkalosis and renal chloride wasting are signs of severe hypokalemia.

There are numerous signs and symptoms associated with altered gastrointestinal function, including anorexia, nausea, and vomiting. Atony of the gastrointestinal smooth muscle can cause constipation, abdominal distention, and, in severe hypokalemia, paralytic ileus. When gastrointestinal symptoms occur gradually and are not severe, they often impair potassium intake and exaggerate the condition.

The most serious effects of hypokalemia are those affecting cardiovascular function. Postural hypotension is common. Most persons with a serum potassium level less than 3.0 mEq/L demonstrate electrocardiographic (ECG) changes typical of hypokalemia. These changes include prolongation of the PR interval, depression of the ST segment, flattening of the T wave, and appearance of a prominent U wave (Fig. 6-11). Although these ECG

changes usually are not serious, they may predispose to sinus bradycardia and ectopic ventricular arrhythmias. Digitalis toxicity can be provoked in persons treated with this drug, and there is an increased risk of ventricular arrhythmias, particularly in persons with underlying heart disease. The dangers associated with digitalis toxicity are compounded in persons who are receiving diuretics that increase urinary losses of potassium.

Complaints of weakness, fatigue, and muscle cramps, particularly during exercise, are common in moderate hypokalemia (serum potassium 3.0 to 2.5 mEq/L). Muscle paralysis with life-threatening respiratory insufficiency can occur with severe hypokalemia (serum potassium <2.5 mEq/L). Leg muscles, particularly the quadriceps, are most prominently affected. Some persons complain of muscle tenderness and paresthesias rather than weakness. In chronic potassium deficiency, muscle atrophy may contribute to muscle weakness.

In a rare condition called *hypokalemic familial periodic paralysis,* episodes of hypokalemia cause attacks of flaccid paralysis that last 6 to 48 hours if untreated.[3] The paralysis may be precipitated by situations that cause severe hypokalemia by producing an intracellular shift in potassium, such as ingestion of a high-carbohydrate meal or administration of insulin, epinephrine, or glucocorticoid drugs. The paralysis often can be reversed by potassium replacement therapy. A similar condition can

Normal

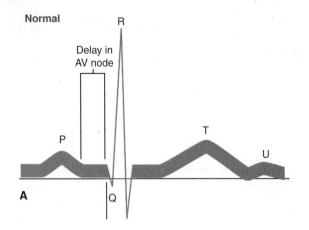

Hypokalemia

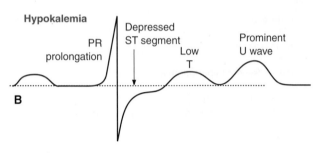

Hyperkalemia

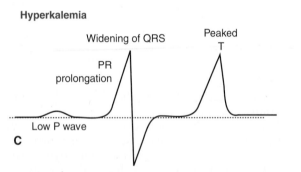

FIGURE 6-11 Effect of serum potassium levels on the cardiac conduction system as evidenced by changes in the electrocardiogram: (**A**) normal, (**B**) hypokalemia, and (**C**) hyperkalemia. AV, atrioventricular.

occur with poorly controlled hyperthyroidism (thyrotoxic hypokalemic periodic paralysis), especially in persons of Asian descent. Treatment is with potassium replacement and appropriate therapy for the underlying thyroid disorder.[28]

Diagnosis and Treatment. Diagnosis of hypokalemia is based on clinical manifestations and serum potassium levels. When possible, hypokalemia caused by potassium deficit is treated by increasing the intake of foods high in potassium content. Oral potassium supplements are prescribed for persons whose intake of potassium is insufficient in relation to losses. This is particularly true of persons who are receiving diuretic therapy and those who are taking digitalis.

Potassium may be given intravenously when the oral route is not tolerated or when rapid replacement is needed.

Magnesium deficiency may impair potassium correction; in such cases, magnesium replacement is indicated.[29] The excessively rapid infusion of a concentrated potassium solution can cause death from cardiac arrest. Health care personnel who assume responsibility for administering potassium-containing intravenous solutions should be fully aware of all the precautions pertaining to potassium dilution and infusion rate.

Hyperkalemia

Hyperkalemia refers to an increase in serum levels of potassium above 5.0 mEq/L (5.0 mmol/L). It seldom occurs in healthy persons because the body is extremely effective in preventing excess potassium accumulation in the ECF.

Causes. The three major causes of potassium excess are (1) decreased renal elimination, (2) excessively rapid administration, and (3) movement of potassium from the ICF to ECF compartment.

The most common cause of hyperkalemia is decreased renal function. Chronic hyperkalemia is almost always associated with renal failure. Usually, the glomerular filtration rate must decline to less than 10 mL/minute before hyperkalemia develops. Some renal disorders, such as sickle cell nephropathy, lead nephropathy, and systemic lupus nephritis, can selectively impair tubular secretion of potassium without causing renal failure. As discussed previously, acidosis diminishes potassium elimination by the kidney. Persons with acute renal failure accompanied by lactic acidosis or ketoacidosis are at increased risk for the development of hyperkalemia. Correcting the acidosis usually helps to correct the hyperkalemia.[30]

Aldosterone acts at the level of the distal tubular sodium/potassium exchange system to increase potassium excretion while facilitating sodium reabsorption. A decrease in aldosterone-mediated potassium elimination can result from adrenal insufficiency (*i.e.*, Addison disease), depression of aldosterone release caused by a decrease in renin or angiotensin II, or impaired ability of the kidneys to respond to aldosterone. Potassium-sparing diuretics (*e.g.*, spironolactone, amiloride, triamterene) can produce hyperkalemia by means of the latter mechanism. Because of their ability to decrease aldosterone levels, angiotensin-converting enzyme inhibitors also can produce an increase in serum potassium levels.

Potassium excess can result from excessive oral ingestion or intravenous administration of potassium. It is difficult to increase potassium intake to the point of causing hyperkalemia when renal function is adequate and the aldosterone sodium–potassium exchange system is functioning. An exception to this rule is the intravenous route of administration. In some cases, severe and fatal incidents of hyperkalemia have occurred when intravenous potassium solutions were infused too rapidly. Because the kidneys control potassium elimination, the administration of potassium-containing intravenous solutions should not be initiated until urine output has been assessed and renal function has been deemed adequate.

The movement of potassium out of body cells into the ECF also can lead to elevated serum potassium levels. Tissue injury, such as that caused by burns and crushing injuries, causes release of intracellular potassium into the ECF compartment. The same injuries often diminish renal function, which contributes to the development of hyperkalemia. Transient hyperkalemia may be induced during extreme exercise or seizures, when muscle cells are permeable to potassium.

Manifestations. The signs and symptoms of potassium excess are closely related to the alterations in neuromuscular excitability (see Table 6-5). The neuromuscular manifestations of potassium excess usually are absent until the serum concentration exceeds 6 mEq/L. The first symptom associated with hyperkalemia typically is paresthesia. There may be complaints of generalized muscle weakness or dyspnea secondary to respiratory muscle weakness.

The most serious effect of hyperkalemia is on the heart. As potassium levels increase, disturbances in cardiac conduction occur. The earliest changes are peaked, narrow T waves and widening of the QRS complex. If serum levels continue to rise, the PR interval becomes prolonged and is followed by the disappearance of P waves (see Fig. 6-11). The heart rate may be slow. Ventricular fibrillation and cardiac arrest are terminal events. Detrimental effects of hyperkalemia on the heart are most pronounced when the serum potassium level rises rapidly.

Diagnosis and Treatment. The diagnosis of hyperkalemia is based on clinical manifestations and serum potassium levels. The treatment of potassium excess varies with the severity of the disturbance and focuses on decreasing or curtailing intake or absorption, increasing renal excretion, and increasing cellular uptake. Decreased intake can be achieved by restricting dietary sources of potassium. The major ingredient in most salt substitutes is potassium chloride, and such substitutes should not be given to patients with renal problems. Increasing potassium output often is more difficult. People with renal failure may require hemodialysis or peritoneal dialysis to reduce serum potassium levels. Most emergency methods focus on measures that cause serum potassium to move from the ECF into the ICF compartment. An intravenous infusion of insulin and glucose is often used for this purpose.

In summary, potassium, which is the major intracellular cation, contributes to the maintenance of intracellular osmolality, is necessary for normal neuromuscular function, and influences acid-base balance. Potassium levels are influenced by dietary intake and elimination by the kidney. A transcellular shift can produce a redistribution of potassium between the ECF and ICF compartments, causing blood levels to increase or decrease.

Hypokalemia is characterized by serum potassium levels less than 3.5 mEq/L. It can result from inadequate intake, excessive losses, or redistribution between the ICF and ECF compartments. The manifestations of potassium deficit include alterations in renal, skeletal muscle, gastrointestinal, and cardiovascular function, reflecting the crucial role that potassium plays in cell metabolism and neuromuscular function. *Hyperkalemia* is manifested by serum potassium levels greater than 5.0 mEq/L. It seldom occurs in healthy persons because the body is extremely effective in preventing excess potassium accumulation in the ECF. The major causes of potassium excess are decreased renal elimination of potassium, excessively rapid intravenous administration of potassium, and a transcellular shift of potassium out of the cell to the ECF compartment. The most serious effect of hyperkalemia is cardiac arrest.

Calcium and Magnesium Balance

DISORDERS OF CALCIUM BALANCE

Calcium is one of the major divalent cations in the body. Approximately 99% of body calcium is found in bone, where it provides the strength and stability for the skeletal system and serves as an exchangeable source to maintain extracellular calcium levels. Most of the remaining calcium (approximately 0.7%) is located inside cells, and only 0.1% to 0.3% is present in the ECF.

Extracellular calcium exists in three forms: (1) protein bound, (2) complexed, and (3) ionized (Fig. 6-12). Approximately 40% of serum calcium is bound to plasma

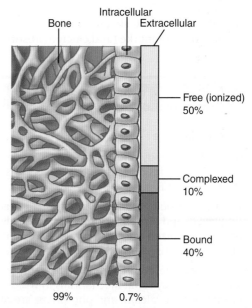

FIGURE 6-12 Distribution of body calcium between the bone and the intracellular (ICF) and extracellular (ECF) fluids. The percentages of free (ionized), complexed, and protein-bound calcium in extracellular fluids are indicated.

proteins, mostly albumin. Another 10% is complexed (*i.e.,* chelated) with substances such as citrate, phosphate, and sulfate. This form is not ionized.[5] The remaining 50% of serum calcium is present in the ionized form. It is the ionized form of calcium that is free to leave the vascular compartment and participate in cellular functions. The total plasma calcium level fluctuates with changes in plasma albumin and pH. As a rule, the total plasma calcium level is decreased 0.75 to 1.0 mg/dL for every 1-g/dL decrease from normal in the plasma albumin level, and by 0.16 mg/dL for each 0.1-unit rise in pH.[5]

Ionized calcium serves a number of functions. It participates in many enzyme reactions; exerts an important effect on membrane potentials and neuronal excitability; is necessary for contraction in skeletal, cardiac, and smooth muscle; participates in the release of hormones, neurotransmitters, and other chemical messengers; influences cardiac contractility and automaticity by way of slow calcium channels; and is essential for blood clotting. Calcium is required for all but the first two steps of the intrinsic pathway for blood coagulation. Because of its ability to bind calcium, citrate often is used to prevent clotting in blood that is to be used for transfusions.

Regulation of Calcium

Calcium enters the body through the gastrointestinal tract, is absorbed from the intestine under the influence of vitamin D, is stored in bone, and is excreted by the kidney. The major sources of calcium are milk and milk products. Only 30% to 50% of dietary calcium is absorbed from the duodenum and upper jejunum; the remainder is eliminated in the stool. There is a calcium influx of approximately 150 mg/day into the intestine from the blood. Net absorption of calcium is equal to the amount that is absorbed from the intestine less the amount that moves into the intestine. Calcium balance can become negative when dietary intake (and calcium absorption)

is less than intestinal secretion. A dietary intake of less than 400 mg/day can be associated with negative calcium balance.[5]

Calcium is filtered in the glomerulus of the kidney and then selectively reabsorbed back into the blood. Approximately 60% to 65% of filtered calcium is passively reabsorbed in the proximal tubule, driven by the reabsorption of sodium chloride; 15% to 20% is reabsorbed in the thick ascending loop of Henle, driven by the $Na^+/K^+/2Cl^-$ cotransport system; and 5% to 10% is reabsorbed in the distal convoluted tubule (see Chapter 23). The distal convoluted tubule is an important regulatory site for controlling the amount of calcium that enters the urine. Thiazide diuretics, which exert their effects in the distal convoluted tubule, enhance calcium reabsorption.

Serum calcium, which is responsible for the physiologic functions of calcium, is directly or indirectly regulated by parathyroid hormone (PTH) and vitamin D.[31] The main function of PTH is to maintain the calcium concentration of the ECF (to be discussed). It performs this function by promoting the release of calcium from bone, increasing the activation of vitamin D as a means of enhancing intestinal absorption of calcium, and stimulating calcium conservation by the kidney while increasing phosphate excretion. The major action of the activated form of vitamin D is to increase the absorption of calcium from the intestine (discussed in Chapter 41). Calcitonin, a hormone produced by C cells in the thyroid, is thought to act on the kidney and bone to remove calcium from the circulation.

A calcium-sensing receptor that functions in the regulation of extracellular calcium levels has been identified in the parathyroid gland, the renal tubular cells, and the calcitonin-producing C cells in the thyroid.[32] Some diseases associated with disturbed calcium metabolism (*e.g.,* familial hypocalcemia) are due to defects in this receptor.

The regulation of serum calcium is strongly influenced by serum phosphate levels. The extracellular concentrations of calcium and phosphate are reciprocally regulated such that calcium levels fall when phosphate levels are high, and vice versa. Normal serum levels of calcium (8.5 to 10.5 mg/dL in adults) and phosphate (2.5 to 4.5 mg/dL in adults) are regulated so that the product of the two concentrations ($[Ca^{2+}] \times [PO_4^{2-}]$) is normally maintained at less than 70.[33] Maintenance of the calcium-phosphate product within this range is important in preventing the deposition of $CaPO_4$ salts in soft tissue, damaging the kidneys, blood vessels, and lungs.

Hypocalcemia

Hypocalcemia represents a serum calcium level of less than 8.5 mg/dL. Hypocalcemia occurs in many forms of critical illness and affects as much as 70% to 90% of patients in intensive care units.[34,35]

Causes. The causes of hypocalcemia can be divided into three categories: (1) abnormal losses of calcium from the kidney, (2) impaired ability to mobilize calcium bone stores, and (3) increased protein binding such that greater

---

KEY CONCEPTS

Calcium Balance

➤ About 99% of body calcium is stored in bone; 0.7% is located inside cells; and 0.2 to 0.3% is found in the ECF.

➤ ECF calcium levels are made up of free (ionized), complexed, and protein-bound fractions. Only the free or ionized calcium ions play an essential role in neuromuscular and cardiac excitability.

➤ Serum calcium levels are regulated by parathyroid hormone and by renal mechanisms in which serum levels of calcium and phosphate are reciprocally regulated to prevent the damaging deposition of calcium phosphate crystals in the soft tissues of the body.

proportions of calcium are in the nonionized form. A pseudohypocalcemia is caused by hypoalbuminemia. It results in a decrease in protein-bound, rather than ionized, calcium and usually is asymptomatic. Calcium deficit caused by dietary deficiency exerts its effects on bone stores, rather than extracellular calcium levels.

An important cause of hypocalcemia is renal failure, in which decreased production of activated vitamin D and hyperphosphatemia both play a role (see Chapter 25). Because of the inverse relation between calcium and phosphate, serum calcium levels fall as phosphate levels rise in renal failure. Hypocalcemia and hyperphosphatemia occur when the glomerular filtration rate falls to less than 25 to 30 mL/minute (normal is 100 to 120 mL/minute).

The ability to mobilize calcium from bone depends on adequate levels of PTH. Decreased levels of PTH may result from primary or secondary forms of hypoparathyroidism (to be discussed). Suppression of PTH release may also occur when vitamin D levels are elevated. Magnesium deficiency inhibits PTH release and impairs the action of PTH on bone resorption. This form of hypocalcemia is difficult to treat with calcium supplementation alone and requires correction of the magnesium deficiency.

Disorders of acid-base balance can change the proportion of calcium that is in the bound and ionized forms. A decrease in pH as occurs in acidosis increases protein binding, resulting in an increase in ionized calcium, while the total serum calcium remains unchanged. An increase in pH as occurs in alkalosis has the opposite effect. As an example, hyperventilation sufficient to cause respiratory alkalosis can produce a decrease in ionized calcium sufficient to cause tetany. Free fatty acids also increase protein binding, causing a reduction in ionized calcium. Elevations in free fatty acids sufficient to alter calcium binding may occur during stressful situations that cause elevations of epinephrine, glucagon, growth hormone, and adrenocorticotropin levels.

Hypocalcemia is also a common finding in a patient with acute pancreatitis. Inflammation of the pancreas causes release of proteolytic and lipolytic enzymes. It is thought that the calcium ion combines with free fatty acids released by lipolysis in the pancreas, forming soaps and removing calcium from the circulation.

Manifestations. Hypocalcemia can manifest as an acute or chronic condition. The severity of the manifestations depends on the underlying cause, rapidity of onset, accompanying electrolyte disorders, and extracellular pH.

Hypocalcemia increases excitation of nerve and muscle cells, primarily affecting the neuromuscular and cardiovascular systems (Table 6-6). Increased neuromuscular excitability can manifest as paresthesias (*i.e.*, tingling around the mouth and in the hands and feet) and tetany (*i.e.*, muscle spasms of the muscles of the face, hands, and feet). Severe hypocalcemia can lead to laryngeal spasm, seizures, and even death. The cardiovascular effects of

---

TABLE 6-6	Manifestations of Hypocalcemia and Hypercalcemia
Hypocalcemia	**Hypercalcemia**
Laboratory Serum calcium <8.5 mg/dL	**Laboratory** Serum calcium >10.5 mg/dL
	Inability to Concentrate Urine and Exposure of Kidney to Increased Concentration of Calcium Polyuria Increased thirst Flank pain Signs of acute renal insufficiency Signs of kidney stones
Neural and Muscle Effects (Increased Excitability) Paresthesias, especially numbness and tingling Skeletal muscle cramps Abdominal muscle spasms and cramps Hyperactive reflexes Carpopedal spasm Tetany Laryngeal spasm	**Neural and Muscle Effects (Decreased Excitability)** Muscle weakness Ataxia, loss of muscle tone Lethargy Personality and behavioral changes Stupor and coma
Cardiovascular Effects Hypotension Signs of cardiac insufficiency Decreased response to drugs that act by calcium-mediated mechanisms Prolongation of the QT interval predisposes to ventricular arrhythmias	**Cardiovascular Effects** Hypertension Shortening of the QT interval Atrioventricular block
Skeletal Effects (Chronic Deficiency) Osteomalacia Bone pain	**Gastrointestinal Effects** Anorexia Nausea, vomiting Constipation

acute hypocalcemia include hypotension, cardiac arrhythmias (particularly heart block and ventricular fibrillation), and failure to have a response to drugs such as digitalis, norepinephrine, and dopamine that act through calcium-mediated mechanisms.[35]

Chronic hypocalcemia is often accompanied by skeletal manifestations and skin changes. There may be bone pain, fragility, deformities, and fractures. The skin may be dry and scaling, the nails brittle, and hair dry. The development of cataracts is common. A person with chronic hypocalcemia may also present with mild diffuse brain disease mimicking depression, dementia, or psychoses.

Diagnosis and Treatment.

The diagnosis of hypocalcemia is initially based on serum calcium levels and signs of increased neuromuscular excitability. Chvostek's and Trousseau's tests can be used to assess for an increase in neuromuscular excitability and tetany.[5] *Chvostek's sign* is elicited by tapping the face just below the temple at the point where the facial nerve emerges. Tapping the face over the facial nerve causes spasm of the lip, nose, or face when the test result is positive. An inflated blood pressure cuff is used to test for *Trousseau's sign*. The cuff is inflated above systolic blood pressure for 3 minutes. Contraction of the fingers and hands (*i.e.,* carpopedal spasm) indicates the presence of tetany (Fig. 6-13).

Acute hypocalcemia is an emergency situation, requiring prompt treatment. An intravenous infusion containing calcium is used when tetany or acute symptoms are present or anticipated because of a decrease in the serum calcium level.

Chronic hypocalcemia is treated with oral intake of calcium. One glass of milk contains approximately 300 mg of calcium. Oral calcium supplements may be used. In some cases, long-term treatment may require the use of vitamin D preparations. The active form of vitamin D is administered when the liver or kidney mechanisms needed for hormone activation are impaired.

Hypercalcemia

Hypercalcemia represents a total serum calcium concentration greater than 10.5 mg/dL.[36,37] Falsely elevated

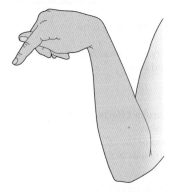

FIGURE 6-13 Trousseau's sign. Ischemia-induced carpal spasm can occur with hypocalcemia or hypomagnesemia. (From Smeltzer S. C., Bare B. G. [2003]. *Medical-surgical nursing* [10th ed., p. 271]. Philadelphia: Lippincott Williams & Wilkins.)

levels of calcium can result from prolonged drawing of blood with an excessively tight tourniquet. Increased plasma proteins (*e.g.,* hyperalbuminemia, hyperglobulinemia) may elevate the total serum calcium but not affect the ionized calcium concentration.

Causes.

A serum calcium excess (*i.e.,* hypercalcemia) results when calcium movement into the circulation overwhelms the calcium regulatory hormones or the ability of the kidney to remove excess calcium ions. The most common causes of hypercalcemia are increased bone resorption caused by neoplasms or hyperparathyroidism.[36,37] Hypercalcemia is a common complication of cancer, occurring in approximately 10% to 20% of persons with advanced disease.[36] A number of malignant tumors, including carcinoma of the lungs, have been associated with hypercalcemia. Some tumors destroy the bone, but others produce humoral agents that stimulate osteoclastic activity, increase bone resorption, or inhibit bone formation.

Less common causes of hypercalcemia are prolonged immobilization, increased intestinal absorption of calcium, and excessive doses of vitamin D.[37] Prolonged immobilization and lack of weight bearing cause demineralization of bone and release of calcium into the bloodstream. Intestinal absorption of calcium can be increased by excessive doses of vitamin D or as a result of a condition called the *milk-alkali syndrome*.[37] The milk-alkali syndrome is caused by excessive ingestion of calcium (often in the form of milk) and absorbable antacids. Because of the advent of nonabsorbable antacids, the condition is seen less frequently than in the past, but it may occur in women who are overzealous in taking calcium preparations for osteoporosis prevention.

A variety of drugs elevate calcium levels. The use of lithium to treat bipolar disorders has caused hypercalcemia and hyperparathyroidism. The thiazide diuretics increase calcium reabsorption in the distal convoluted tubule of the kidney. Although the thiazide diuretics seldom cause hypercalcemia, they can unmask hypercalcemia from other causes such as underlying bone disorders and conditions that increase bone resorption.

Manifestations.

The signs and symptoms associated with calcium excess originate from three sources: (1) changes in neural excitability, (2) alterations in smooth and cardiac muscle function, and (3) exposure of the kidneys to high concentrations of calcium[36,37] (see Table 6-6).

Neural excitability is decreased in patients with hypercalcemia. There may be a dulling of consciousness, stupor, weakness, and muscle flaccidity. Behavioral changes may range from subtle alterations in personality to acute psychoses.

The heart responds to elevated levels of calcium with increased contractility and ventricular arrhythmias. Digitalis accentuates these responses. Gastrointestinal symptoms reflect a decrease in smooth muscle activity and include constipation, anorexia, nausea, and vomiting. Pancreatitis is another potential complication of hypercalcemia and is probably related to stones in the pancreatic ducts.[38]

High calcium concentrations in the urine impair the ability of the kidneys to concentrate urine by interfering with the action of ADH. This causes salt and water diuresis and an increased sensation of thirst. Hypercalciuria also predisposes to the development of renal calculi.

Hypercalcemic crisis describes an acute increase in the serum calcium level.[36] Malignant disease and hyperparathyroidism are major causes of hypercalcemic crisis. In hypercalcemic crisis, polyuria, excessive thirst, volume depletion, fever, altered levels of consciousness, azotemia (*i.e.*, nitrogenous wastes in the blood), and a disturbed mental state accompany other signs of calcium excess. Symptomatic hypercalcemia is associated with a high mortality rate; death often is caused by cardiac arrest.

Treatment. The diagnosis of hypercalcemia is based on history, clinical manifestations, and serum calcium levels. The treatment of calcium excess usually is directed toward rehydration and measures to increase urinary excretion of calcium and inhibit release of calcium from bone. Fluid replacement is needed in situations of volume depletion. The excretion of sodium is accompanied by calcium excretion. Diuretics and sodium chloride can be administered to increase urinary elimination of calcium after the ECF volume has been restored. Loop diuretics commonly are used, rather than thiazide diuretics, which increase calcium reabsorption.

The initial lowering of calcium levels is followed by measures to inhibit bone reabsorption. Drugs that are used to inhibit calcium mobilization include bisphosphonates, calcitonin, and the glucocorticosteroids. The bisphosphonates are a relatively new group of drugs that act mainly by inhibiting osteoclastic activity. Calcitonin also inhibits osteoclastic activity, thereby decreasing resorption. The glucocorticosteroids inhibit the conversion of vitamin D to its active form and are used to treat hypercalcemia due to vitamin D toxicity and hematologic malignancies.[37]

Disorders of Parathyroid Function

Parathyroid hormone (PTH), a major regulator of plasma calcium and phosphate, is secreted by the parathyroid glands (Fig. 6-14). There are four parathyroid glands located on the dorsal surface of the thyroid gland. The dominant regulator of PTH is the plasma calcium concentration, which is sensed by calcium-sensing receptors located on the cell membrane of the parathyroid gland cells.[32] When the plasma calcium level is high, PTH secretion is inhibited and the calcium is deposited in the bones. When the level is low, PTH secretion is increased and calcium is mobilized from the bones. The response to a decrease in plasma calcium is prompt, occurring within seconds. The synthesis and release of PTH from the parathyroid gland is influenced by magnesium.[39] Because of its function in regulating PTH release, severe and prolonged hypomagnesemia can markedly inhibit PTH levels.

The main function of PTH is to maintain the calcium concentration of the ECF. It performs this function by

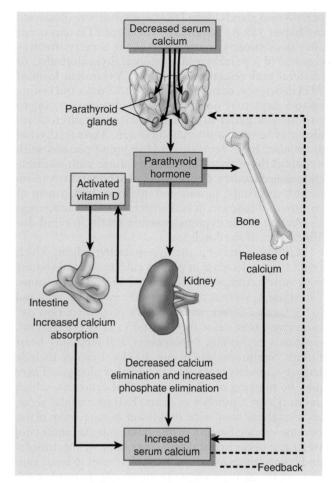

FIGURE 6-14 Regulation of serum calcium concentration by parathyroid hormone.

promoting the release of calcium from bone, increasing the activation of vitamin D as a means of enhancing intestinal absorption of calcium, and stimulating calcium conservation by the kidney while increasing phosphate excretion (see Fig. 6-14). The skeletal response to PTH is a two-step process. There is an immediate response in which calcium that is present in bone fluid is released into the ECF, and a second, more slowly developing response in which completely mineralized bone is resorbed, resulting in the release of both calcium and phosphate. The activation of vitamin D by the kidney is enhanced by the presence of PTH, and it is through the activation of vitamin D that PTH increases intestinal absorption of calcium and phosphate. PTH acts directly on the kidney to increase tubular reabsorption of calcium and magnesium while increasing phosphate elimination. The accompanying increase in phosphate elimination ensures that calcium released from bone does not produce hyperphosphatemia and increase the risk of soft tissue deposition of calcium phosphate crystals.

Hypoparathyroidism. Hypoparathyroidism reflects deficient PTH secretion, resulting in hypocalcemia. PTH deficiency may be caused by a congenital absence of all of the parathyroid glands, as in DiGeorge syndrome (discussed in Chapter 15). An acquired deficiency of PTH may occur after neck surgery, particularly if the surgery involves removal of a parathyroid adenoma, thyroidectomy, or bilateral neck resection for cancer. A transient form of PTH deficiency, occurring within 1 to 2 days and lasting up to 5 days, may occur after thyroid surgery owing to parathyroid gland suppression.[5] Hypoparathyroidism also may have an autoimmune origin. Antiparathyroid antibodies have been detected in some persons with hypoparathyroidism, particularly those with multiple endocrine disorders. Other causes of hypoparathyroidism include metastatic tumors and infection. Impairment of parathyroid function occurs with magnesium deficiency. Correction of the hypomagnesemia results in rapid disappearance of the condition.

Manifestations of acute hypoparathyroidism, which result from a decrease in plasma calcium, include tetany with muscle cramps, carpopedal spasm, and convulsions. Paresthesias, such as tingling of the circumoral area and in the hands and feet, are almost always present. Low calcium levels may cause prolongation of the QT interval, resistance to digitalis, hypotension, and refractory heart failure. Symptoms of chronic PTH deficiency include lethargy, anxiety state, and personality changes. There may be blurring of vision because of cataracts, which develop over a number of years. Extrapyramidal signs, such as those seen with Parkinson disease, may occur because of calcification of the basal ganglia. Successful treatment of the hypocalcemia may improve the disorder and is sometimes associated with decreases in basal ganglia calcification on x-ray. Teeth may be defective if the disorder occurs during childhood.

Diagnosis of hypoparathyroidism is based on low plasma calcium levels, high plasma phosphate levels, and low plasma PTH levels. Plasma magnesium levels usually are measured to rule out hypomagnesemia as a cause of the disorder. Treatment of acute hypoparathyroidism includes administration of intravenous calcium gluconate followed by oral administration of calcium salts and vitamin D. Magnesium supplementation is used when the disorder is caused by magnesium deficiency. Persons with chronic hypoparathyroidism are treated with oral calcium and vitamin D. Plasma calcium levels are monitored at regular intervals (at least every 3 months) as a means of maintaining plasma calcium within a slightly low but asymptomatic range.

Pseudohypoparathyroidism is a rare familial disorder characterized by target tissue resistance to PTH. It is characterized by hypocalcemia, increased parathyroid function, and a variety of congenital defects in the growth and development of the skeleton, including short stature and short metacarpal and metatarsal bones. There are variants in the disorder, with some persons having the pseudohypoparathyroidism with the congenital defects and others having the congenital defects with normal calcium and phosphate levels. The manifestations of the disorder are due primarily to chronic hypocalcemia. Treatment is similar to that for hypoparathyroidism.

Hyperparathyroidism. Hyperparathyroidism, which involves the hypersecretion of PTH, can present as a primary or secondary disorder. Secondary hyperparathyroidism involves hyperplasia of the parathyroid glands and occurs primarily in persons with renal failure (see Chapter 25). Primary hyperparathyroidism is relatively common disorder, with an incidence of 1 in 500 to 1000. It is seen more commonly after 50 years of age and is more common in women than men.[40] It can be caused by hyperplasia of the parathyroid glands (15%), an adenoma of a single parathyroid gland (85%), or rarely parathyroid carcinoma.[40]

Primary hyperparathyroidism causes hypercalcemia and increased calcium in the urine filtrate, resulting in hypercalciuria and the potential for development of kidney stones. Chronic bone resorption may produce diffuse demineralization, pathologic fractures, and cystic bone lesions. Manifestations of the disorder are related to skeletal abnormalities, exposure of the kidney to high calcium levels, and elevated plasma calcium levels (see section on Hypercalcemia). Most persons with primary hyperparathyroidism are asymptomatic, and the disorder is discovered in the course of routine biochemical blood tests.

Diagnostic procedures include serum calcium and PTH levels and imaging studies of the parathyroid area. Parathyroid surgery is usually the treatment of choice. Calcimimetics, which increase the sensitivity of the parathyroid calcium-sensing receptor to extracellular calcium, are being developed to control primary and secondary hyperparathyroidism.[32]

DISORDERS OF MAGNESIUM BALANCE

Magnesium is the second most abundant intracellular cation. The average adult has approximately 24 g of magnesium distributed throughout the body. Of the total magnesium content, approximately 50% to 60% is stored in bone, 39% to 49% is contained in the body cells, and the remaining 2% is dispersed in the ECF.[41] Approximately 20% to 30% of the extracellular magnesium is protein bound, and only a small fraction of intracellular magnesium (15% to 30%) is exchangeable with the ECF. The normal serum concentration of magnesium is 1.8 to 2.7 mg/dL.

Only recently has the importance of magnesium to the overall function of the body been recognized.[42] Magnesium acts as a cofactor in many intracellular enzyme reactions, including those related to transfer of phosphate groups. It is essential to all reactions that require ATP, for every step related to replication and transcription of DNA, and for the translation of messenger RNA. It is required for cellular energy metabolism; nerve conduction; and cell membrane function, including activity of the sodium-potassium membrane pump, ion transport, and calcium channel activity. Magnesium binds to calcium receptors, and it has been suggested that alterations in magnesium levels may exert their effects through calcium-mediated mechanisms. Magnesium may bind competitively to calcium binding sites, producing the appropriate response; it may compete with calcium for a binding site but not exert an effect; or it may alter the distribution of calcium by interfering with its movement across the cell membrane.

Regulation of Magnesium

Magnesium is ingested in the diet, absorbed from the intestine, and excreted by the kidneys. Intestinal absorption is not closely regulated, and approximately 30% to 40% of the normal dietary intake of magnesium is absorbed.[41] Magnesium is contained in all green vegetables, grains, nuts, meats, and seafood. Magnesium is also present in much of the groundwater in North America.

The kidney is the principal organ of magnesium regulation. Magnesium is a unique electrolyte in that only approximately 30% to 40% of the filtered amount is reabsorbed in the proximal tubule. The greatest quantity, approximately 50% to 70%, is reabsorbed in the thick ascending loop of Henle. The distal tubule, which reabsorbs a small amount of magnesium, is the major site of magnesium regulation. Magnesium reabsorption is decreased in the presence of increased serum levels, stimulated by PTH, and inhibited by increased calcium levels. The major driving force for magnesium absorption is the $Na^+/K^+/2Cl^-$ cotransport system in the thick ascending loop of Henle[41] (see Chapter 23). This is also the site where the loop diuretics (*e.g.*, furosemide [Lasix]) exert their actions. Thus, inhibition of this transport system by loop diuretics lowers magnesium reabsorption.

Hypomagnesemia

Hypomagnesemia represents a serum magnesium concentration of less than 1.8 mg/dL[43] (Table 6-7). It is seen in conditions that limit intake or increase intestinal or renal losses, and is a common finding in emergency department and critical care patients.

Causes. Magnesium deficiency can result from insufficient intake, excessive losses, or movement between the ECF and ICF compartments. It can result from conditions that directly limit intake, such as malnutrition, starvation,

or prolonged maintenance of magnesium-free parenteral nutrition. Other conditions, such as diarrhea, malabsorption syndromes, prolonged nasogastric suction, or laxative abuse can serve to decrease intestinal absorption. Excessive calcium intake impairs intestinal absorption of magnesium by competing for the same transport site. Another common cause of magnesium deficiency is chronic alcoholism. There are many factors that contribute to hypomagnesemia in alcoholism, including low intake and gastrointestinal losses from diarrhea.

Although the kidneys are able to defend against hypermagnesemia, they are less able to conserve magnesium and prevent hypomagnesemia. Urine losses are increased in diabetic ketoacidosis, hyperparathyroidism, and hyperaldosteronism. Some drugs increase renal losses of magnesium, including diuretics (particularly loop diuretics) and nephrotoxic drugs such as aminoglycoside antibiotics, cyclosporine, cisplatin, and amphotericin B.

A relative hypomagnesemia may also develop in conditions that promote movement of magnesium between the ECF and ICF compartments, including rapid administration of glucose, insulin-containing parenteral solutions, and alkalosis. Although transient, these conditions can cause serious alterations in body function.

Manifestations. Signs of magnesium deficiency are not usually apparent until the serum magnesium is less than 1.2 mEq/dL. Hypomagnesemia is characterized by an increase in neuromuscular excitability as evidenced by muscle weakness and tremors. Other manifestations may include hyperactive deep tendon reflexes, paresthesias (*e.g.*, numbness, pricking, tingling sensation), muscle fasciculations, and tetanic muscle contractions. A positive Chvostek's or Trousseau's sign may be present, particularly if hypocalcemia is present. Because decreased serum magnesium increases irritability in nervous tissue, seizures may occur. Other manifestations may include ataxia, vertigo, disorientation, depression, and psychotic symptoms.

Cardiovascular manifestations include tachycardia, hypertension, and ventricular arrhythmias. There may be ECG changes such as widening of the QRS complex, appearance of peak T waves, prolongation of the PR

TABLE 6-7   Manifestations of Hypomagnesemia and Hypermagnesemia

Hypomagnesemia	Hypermagnesemia
Laboratory Values	**Laboratory Values**
Serum magnesium <1.8 mg/dL	Serum magnesium >2.7 mg/dL
Neural and Muscle Effects	**Neural and Muscle Effects**
Personality changes	Lethargy
Athetoid or choreiform movements	Hyporeflexia
Nystagmus	Confusion
Tetany	Coma
Cardiovascular Effects	**Cardiovascular Effects**
Tachycardia	Hypotension
Hypertension	Cardiac arrhythmias
Cardiac arrhythmias	Cardiac arrest

interval, T-wave inversion, and appearance of U waves. Ventricular arrhythmias, particularly in the presence of digitalis, may be difficult to treat unless magnesium levels are normalized.

Magnesium deficiency often occurs in conjunction with hypocalcemia and hypokalemia, producing a number of related neurologic and cardiovascular manifestations. Hypocalcemia is typical of severe hypomagnesemia. Most persons with hypomagnesemia-related hypocalcemia have decreased PTH levels, probably as a result of impaired magnesium-dependent mechanisms that control PTH release and synthesis. Hypokalemia also is a typical feature of hypomagnesemia. It leads to a reduction in intracellular potassium and impairs the ability of the kidney to conserve potassium. When hypomagnesemia is present, hypokalemia is unresponsive to potassium replacement therapy.

Diagnosis and Treatment. The diagnosis of hypomagnesemia is based on clinical manifestations and laboratory findings. Treatment consists of magnesium replacement. The route of administration depends on the severity of the condition. Symptomatic, moderate to severe magnesium deficiency is treated by parenteral administration. Treatment must be continued for several days to replace stored and plasma levels. In conditions of chronic intestinal or renal loss, maintenance support with oral magnesium may be required. Patients with any degree of renal failure must be carefully monitored to prevent magnesium excess.

Hypermagnesemia

Hypermagnesemia represents a serum magnesium concentration in excess of 2.7 mg/dL (see Table 6-7). Because of the ability of the normal kidney to excrete magnesium, hypermagnesemia is rare. When hypermagnesemia does occur, it usually is related to renal insufficiency or the injudicious use of magnesium-containing medications such as antacids, mineral supplements, or laxatives. The elderly are particularly at risk because they have age-related reductions in renal function and tend to consume more magnesium-containing medications. Magnesium may be used therapeutically to treat cardiac arrhythmia, myocardial infarct, angina, and pregnancy complicated by preeclampsia or eclampsia—in which case, caution to prevent hypermagnesemia is essential.

Hypermagnesemia affects neuromuscular and cardiovascular function. The signs and symptoms occur only when serum magnesium levels exceed 4.9 mg/dL (2 mmol/L).[43] Hypermagnesemia diminishes neuromuscular transmission, causing hyporeflexia, muscle weakness, and confusion. Magnesium decreases acetylcholine release at the myoneural junction and may cause neuromuscular blockade and respiratory paralysis. Cardiovascular effects are related to the calcium channel–blocking effects of magnesium. Blood pressure is decreased, and the ECG shows an increase in the PR interval, a shortening of the QT interval, T-wave abnormalities, and prolongation of the QRS and PR intervals. Hypotension caused by vasodilation and cardiac arrhythmias can occur with moderate hypermagnesemia (≥5 to 10 mg/dL), and confusion and coma can occur with severe hypermagnesemia (≥10 mg/dL). Very severe hypermagnesemia (≥15 mg/dL) may cause cardiac arrest.

Diagnosis and Treatment. The diagnosis of hypermagnesemia is based on clinical manifestations and laboratory findings. Treatment is directed toward alleviating renal insufficiency and avoidance of magnesium-containing medications. Calcium is a direct antagonist of magnesium, and intravenous administration of calcium may be used. Peritoneal dialysis or hemodialysis may be required.

In summary, calcium is one of the major divalent ions in the body. Approximately 99% of body calcium is found in bone; about 1% is in the ICF and 0.1% to 0.2% is in the ECF. The calcium in bone is in dynamic equilibrium with extracellular calcium. Of the three forms of ECF calcium (*i.e.,* protein bound, complexed, and ionized), only the ionized form can cross the cell membrane and contribute to cellular function. Ionized calcium has a number of functions. It stabilizes neuromuscular excitability, thereby making nerve cells less sensitive to stimuli; it plays a vital role in the blood clotting process; and it participates in a number of enzyme reactions. Acute alterations in ionized calcium levels are evidenced mainly by changes in neural excitability, being increased in hypocalcemia and decreased in hypercalcemia.

Parathyroid hormone, a major regulator of serum calcium and phosphate, is secreted by the parathyroid glands. The main function of PTH is to maintain the calcium concentration of the ECF. It performs this function by promoting the release of calcium from bone, increasing the activation of vitamin D as a means of enhancing intestinal absorption of calcium, and stimulating calcium conservation by the kidney while increasing phosphate elimination. Hypoparathyroidism, which is characterized by hypocalcemia, reflects deficient PTH secretion, resulting in hypocalcemia. Hyperparathyroidism, which is caused by hypersecretion of PTH, is manifest by signs and symptoms related to skeletal abnormalities, exposure of the kidney to high calcium levels, and elevated plasma calcium levels.

Magnesium is the second most abundant intracellular cation. It acts as a cofactor in many enzyme reactions and affects neuromuscular function in the same manner as the calcium ion. Magnesium deficiency can result from insufficient intake, excessive losses, or movement between the ECF and ICF compartments. The manifestations of hypomagnesemia are characterized by a decrease in neuromuscular excitability as evidenced by paresthesias and hyperactive reflexes. Cardiovascular effects include tachycardia, hypertension, and ventricular arrhythmias. Hypermagnesemia usually is related to renal insufficiency and the injudicious use of magnesium-containing medications such as antacids, mineral supplements, or laxatives. It diminishes neuromuscular transmission, leading to hyporeflexia, muscle weakness, and confusion.

Acid-Base Balance

Metabolic activities of the body require the precise regulation of acid-base balance, which is reflected by the pH of ECF.[44-47] Membrane excitability, enzyme systems, and chemical reactions depend on pH being regulated within a narrow physiologic range. Many conditions, pathologic or otherwise, can alter body pH.

INTRODUCTORY CONCEPTS

Normally, the concentration of body acids and bases is regulated so that the pH of ECF is maintained within the very narrow range of 7.35 to 7.45. This balance is maintained through mechanisms that generate, buffer, and eliminate acids and bases.

Acid-Base Chemistry

An *acid* is a molecule that can release a hydrogen ion (H^+), and a *base* is a molecule that can accept or combine with an H^+. Most of the body's acids and bases are weak acids and bases; the most important are *carbonic acid* (H_2CO_3), which is a weak acid derived from carbon dioxide (CO_2), and *bicarbonate* (HCO_3^-), which is a weak base.

The concentration of H^+ in body fluids is low compared with other ions. For example, the sodium ion (Na^+) is present at a concentration approximately 1 million times that of the H^+. Because of its low concentration in body fluids, the H^+ concentration is commonly expressed in terms of pH. Specifically, *pH* represents the negative logarithm (p) of the H^+ concentration in mEq/L. A pH value of 7.0 implies an H^+ concentration of 10^{-7} (0.0000001 mEq/L). Because the pH is inversely related to the H^+ concentration, a low pH indicates a high concentration of H^+, and a high pH, a low concentration.[2]

Metabolic Acid and Bicarbonate Production

Acids are continuously generated as byproducts of metabolic processes. Physiologically, these acids fall into two groups: the volatile carbonic acid (H_2CO_3) and all other nonvolatile or fixed acids (Fig. 6-15). The difference between the two types of acids arises because H_2CO_3 is in equilibrium with the volatile CO_2, which leaves the body by way of the lungs. Therefore, the H_2CO_3 concentration is determined by the lungs and their respiratory capacity. The *noncarbonic acids* (*e.g.*, sulfuric, hydrochloric, phosphoric) are *nonvolatile* and are not eliminated by the lungs. Instead, they are buffered by body proteins or extracellular buffers, such as HCO_3^-, and then excreted by the kidney.

Carbon Dioxide and Bicarbonate Production. Body metabolism results in the production of approximately 15,000 mmol of CO_2 each day.[12] Carbon dioxide is transported in the circulation in three forms: (1) attached to hemoglobin, (2) as dissolved CO_2 (*i.e.*, PCO_2), and as (3) HCO_3^-. Collectively, PCO_2 and HCO_3^- constitute approximately 77% of the CO_2 that is transported in the ECF; the remaining CO_2 travels attached to hemoglobin.

Although CO_2 is not an acid, a small percentage of the gas combines with water in the bloodstream to form H_2CO_3 ($CO_2 + H_2O \leftrightarrow H_2CO_3$). The reaction between CO_2 and water (H_2O) is catalyzed by an enzyme, called *carbonic anhydrase*, which is present in large quantities in red blood cells, renal tubular cells, and other tissues in the body.

Because it is almost impossible to measure H_2CO_3, dissolved PCO_2 measurements are commonly substituted when calculating pH. The H_2CO_3 content of the blood can be calculated by multiplying the partial pressure of the CO_2 (PCO_2) in the blood by its solubility coefficient, which is 0.03. This means that the concentration of H_2CO_3 in venous blood, which normally has a PCO_2 of approximately 45 mm Hg, is 1.35 mEq/L ($45 \times 0.03 = 1.35$).

Production of Metabolic Acids. The metabolism of dietary proteins is the major source of strong *inorganic acids*—sulfuric acid, hydrochloric acid, and phosphoric acid.[12,47] Oxidation of the sulfur-containing amino acids (*e.g.*, methionine, cysteine, cystine) results in the production of sulfuric acid. Oxidation of arginine and lysine produces hydrochloric acid, and oxidation of phosphorus-containing nucleic acids yields phosphoric acid. Incomplete oxidation of glucose results in the formation of lactic acid, and incomplete oxidation of fats results in the production of ketoacids. The major source of base is the metabolism of amino acids such as aspartate and glutamate and the metabolism of certain organic anions (*e.g.*, citrate, lactate, acetate). Acid production normally exceeds base production, with the net effect being the addition of approximately 1 mmol/kg body weight of nonvolatile acid to the body each day.[12] A vegetarian diet, which contains large amounts of organic anions, results in the net production of base.

Calculation of pH

The pH can be calculated with the *Henderson-Hasselbalch equation* using the dissociation constant for the bicarbonate buffer system (6.1) and the HCO_3^- to PCO_2 (used as a measure of H_2CO_3) ratio. When the ratio is 20:1, the pH is within the normal range at 7.4 (Fig. 6-16). Because the ratio is used, a change in HCO_3^- will have little or no effect on pH, as long as there is an accompanying change in PCO_2. Likewise, a change in PCO_2 will have little effect on pH, as long as there is an accompanying change in HCO_3^-.

Regulation of pH

The pH of body fluids is regulated by three major mechanisms: (1) intracellular and extracellular buffering systems; (2) the lungs, which control the elimination of CO_2; and (3) the kidneys, which reabsorb HCO_3^- and eliminate H^+.

Intracellular and Extracellular Buffer Systems. The moment-by-moment regulation of pH depends on the intracellular and extracellular buffer systems. A *buffer system* consists of a weak acid and the base salt of that

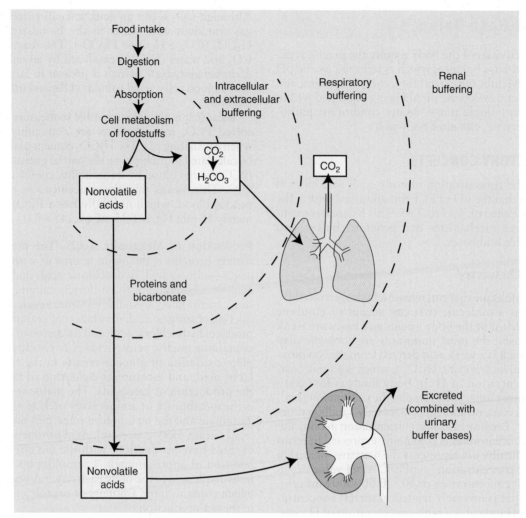

FIGURE 6-15 Role of intracellular and extracellular buffer, respiratory, and renal mechanisms in maintaining normal blood pH. (From Rhoades R. A., Tanner G. A. [1996]. *Medical physiology* [p. 468]. Boston: Little, Brown.)

KEY CONCEPTS

Mechanisms of Acid-Base Balance

➤ The pH is determined by the ratio of the HCO_3^- base to CO_2 (H_2CO_3). At a pH of 7.4, the ratio is normally 20 to 1.

➤ The HCO_3^- part of the pH equation reflects the generation of nonvolatile metabolic acids that are buffered in intracellular and extracellular buffers and eliminated by the kidney.

➤ The H_2CO_3 or volatile acid part of the equation represents the level of dissolved CO_2 ($H_2O + CO_2 \leftrightarrow H_2CO_3$) in the blood. It is regulated by the elimination of CO_2 by the lungs.

acid or of a weak base and its acid salt. In the process of preventing large changes in pH, the system trades a strong acid for a weak acid or a strong base for a weak base.

The three major buffer systems that protect the pH of body fluids are (1) body proteins, (2) the bicarbonate buffer system, and (3) the transcellular hydrogen–potassium exchange system.[2] These buffer systems are immediately available to combine with excess acids or bases and prevent large changes in pH from occurring during the time it takes for the respiratory and renal mechanisms to become effective. Bone also represents an important site for the buffering of acids and bases.[12] The role of bone buffers is even greater in chronic acid-base disorders. One consequence of bone buffering is the release of calcium from bone and increased renal excretion of calcium. In addition to causing demineralization of bone, it also predisposes to kidney stones.

Proteins are the largest buffer system in the body. Proteins are *amphoteric*, meaning that they can function as

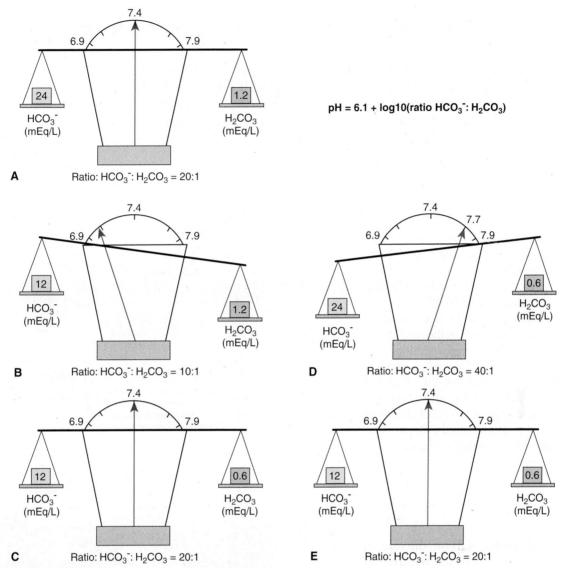

$$pH = 6.1 + log10(ratio\ HCO_3^-:H_2CO_3)$$

FIGURE 6-16 Normal and compensated states of pH and acid-base balance represented as a balance scale. (**A**) When the ratio of bicarbonate (HCO_3^-) to carbonic acid (H_2CO_3, arterial $CO_2 \times 0.03$) = 20:1, the pH = 7.4. (**B**) Metabolic acidosis with an HCO_3^- : H_2CO_3 ratio of 10:1 and a pH of 7.1. (**C**) Respiratory compensation lowers the H_2CO_3 to 0.6 mEq/L and returns the HCO_3^- : H_2CO_3 ratio to 20:1 and the pH to 7.4. (**D**) Respiratory alkalosis with an HCO_3^- : H_2CO_3 ratio of 40:1 and a pH of 7.7. (**E**) Renal compensation eliminates HCO_3^-, reducing serum levels to 12 mEq/L and returning the HCO_3^- : H_2CO_3 ratio to 20:1 and the pH to 7.4. Normally, these compensatory mechanisms are capable of buffering large changes in pH, but do not return the pH completely to normal as illustrated here.

either acids or bases. They contain many ionizable groups that can release or bind H^+. The protein buffers are largely located within cells, and H^+ ions and CO_2 diffuse across cell membranes for buffering by intracellular proteins. Albumin and plasma globulins are the major protein buffers in the vascular compartment.

The *bicarbonate buffer system* uses H_2CO_3 as its weak acid and HCO_3^- as its weak base. It substitutes the weak carbonic acid for a strong acid such as hydrochloric acid or the weak bicarbonate base for a strong base such as sodium hydroxide. The bicarbonate/carbonic acid buffer system is a particularly efficient system because the buffer components can be readily added or removed from the body.[47] Metabolism provides an ample supply of CO_2, which can replace any H_2CO_3 that is lost when excess base is added, and CO_2 can be readily eliminated by the lungs when excess acid is added. Likewise, the kidney can form new HCO_3^- when excess acid is added, and it can excrete HCO_3^- when excess base is added.

Understanding ➤ Carbon Dioxide Transport

Body metabolism results in a continuous production of carbon dioxide (CO_2). As CO_2 is formed during the metabolic process, it diffuses out of body cells into the tissue spaces and then into the circulation. It is transported in the circulation in three forms: (1) dissolved in the plasma, (2) as bicarbonate, and (3) attached to hemoglobin.

1

Plasma. A small portion (about 10%) of the CO_2 that is produced by body cells is transported in the dissolved state to the lungs and then exhaled. The amount of dissolved CO_2 that can be carried in plasma is determined by the partial pressure of the gas (PCO_2) and its solubility coefficient (0.03 mL/ 100 mL plasma for each 1 mm Hg PCO_2). Thus, each 100 mL of arterial blood with a PCO_2 of 40 mm Hg would contain 1.2 mL of dissolved CO_2. It is the dissolved CO_2 that contributes to the pH of the blood.

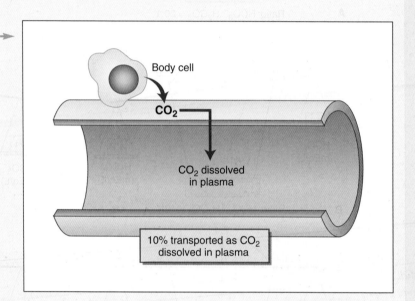

2

Bicarbonate. Carbon dioxide in excess of that which can be carried in the plasma moves into the red blood cells, where the enzyme carbonic anhydrase (CA) catalyzes its conversion to carbonic acid (H_2CO_3). The H_2CO_3, in turn, dissociates into hydrogen (H^+) and bicarbonate (HCO_3^-) ions. The H^+ combines with hemoglobin and the HCO_3^- diffuses into plasma, where it participates in acid-base balance. The movement of HCO_3^- into the plasma is made possible by a special transport system on the red blood cell membrane in which HCO_3^- ions are exchanged for chloride ions (Cl^-).

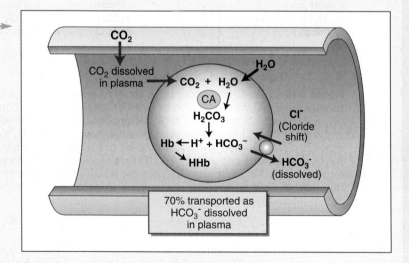

3

Hemoglobin. The remaining CO_2 in the red blood cells combines with hemoglobin to form carbaminohemoglobin ($HbCO_2$). The combination of CO_2 with hemoglobin is a reversible reaction characterized by a loose bond, so that CO_2 can be easily released in the alveolar capillaries and exhaled from the lung.

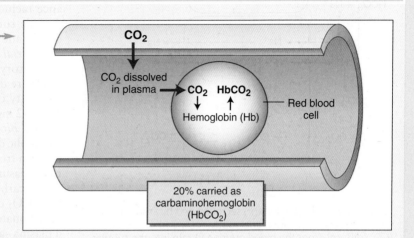

The transcompartmental hydrogen–potassium exchange system is important in the regulation of acid-base balance. Both ions are positively charged, and both ions move freely between the intracellular and extracellular compartments (see Fig. 6-9). When excess H^+ is present in the ECF, it moves into the body cells in exchange for potassium (K^+). Likewise, when excess K^+ is present in the ECF, it moves into the cell in exchange for H^+. On the average, serum potassium levels increase by approximately 0.6 mEq/L for every 0.1-unit fall in pH.[12] Thus, alterations in potassium levels can affect acid-base balance, and changes in acid-base balance can influence potassium levels.

Respiratory Control Mechanisms. The respiratory system provides for the elimination of CO_2 into the air and plays a major role in acid-base regulation. The respiratory control of pH is rapid, occurring within minutes, and is maximal within 12 to 24 hours and then gradually declines over the next 1 to 2 days.[12] Because the lungs cannot eliminate H^+, they cannot return the pH to a completely normal range.

Renal Control Mechanisms. The kidneys play two major roles in acid-base regulation. The first role is accomplished through the reabsorption of bicarbonate so this important buffer is not lost in the urine. The second is through the excretion of H^+ from fixed acids that result from protein and lipid metabolism. The renal mechanisms for regulating acid-base balance cannot adjust the pH within minutes, as respiratory mechanisms can, but they continue to function for days until the pH has returned to normal or near-normal range.

Bicarbonate Reabsorption. The kidneys regulate bicarbonate by reclaiming the HCO_3^- that has been filtered in the glomerulus. Mechanistically, each HCO_3^- that is reclaimed requires the secretion of one H^+, a process that is tightly coupled with sodium reabsorption[45] (Fig. 6-17). Bicarbonate reabsorption also requires the presence of carbonic anhydrase to catalyze the combining of CO_2 with H_2O to form H_2CO_3. Carbonic anhydrase is present both intracellularly as well as on the tubular surface, allowing the secreted H^+ to combine with the tubular fluid HCO_3^- to form H_2CO_3. The H_2CO_3 rapidly dissociates to form CO_2 and H_2O that can readily cross the tubular cell membrane. Inside the cell, carbonic anhydrase again catalyzes the formation of H_2CO_3, which subsequently dissociates into HCO_3^- and H^+. The HCO_3^- then leaves the tubular cell and enters the ECF, and the H^+ is secreted into the tubular fluid to begin another cycle of HCO_3^- reclamation.

Phosphate and Ammonia Buffers. Because extremely acidic urine would be damaging to structures in the urinary tract, the elimination of H^+ requires a buffering system. There are two important intratubular buffer systems: the phosphate buffer system and the ammonia buffer system. The phosphate buffer system uses HPO_4^{2-} and $H_2PO_4^-$ that are present in the tubular filtrate to buffer H^+. The combination of H^+ with HPO_4^{2-} to form $H_2PO_4^-$ allows the kidneys to increase their secretion of H^+ ions. Because the phosphates are poorly absorbed, they become more concentrated as they move through the tubules. The other important but more complex buffer system is the *ammonia buffer system*. Renal tubular cells are able to use the amino acid glutamine to synthesize ammonia (NH_3) and secrete it into the tubular fluid. The H^+ ions then combine with the NH_3 to form an ammonium ion (NH_4^+). The NH_4^+ ions combine with Cl^- ions (Cl^-), which are present in the tubular fluid, to form ammonium chloride (NH_4Cl), which is then excreted in the urine.

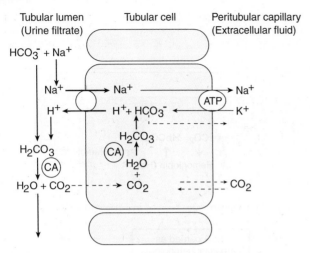

Tubular lumen (Urine filtrate)   Tubular cell   Peritubular capillary (Extracellular fluid)

FIGURE 6-17 Hydrogen ion (H⁺) secretion and bicarbonate ion (HCO₃⁻) reabsorption in a renal tubular cell. Carbon dioxide (CO₂) diffuses from the blood or urine filtrate into the tubular cell, where it combines with water in a carbonic anhydrase–catalyzed reaction that yields carbonic acid (H₂CO₃). The H₂CO₃ dissociates to form H⁺ and HCO₃⁻. The H⁺ is secreted into the tubular fluid in exchange for Na⁺. The Na⁺ and HCO₃⁻ enter the extracellular fluid. ATP, adenosine triphosphate.

Potassium–Hydrogen Exchange. Serum potassium (K⁺) levels influence renal elimination of H⁺ ions. When there is a fall in potassium levels, K⁺ moves from body cells into the ECF and there is a reciprocal movement of H⁺ ions from the ECF into body cells. In the kidney, these movements lower the intracellular pH of tubular cells, producing an increase in H⁺ ion secretion. Potassium depletion also stimulates ammonia synthesis by the kidney as a means of buffering the excess H⁺ ions. The net result is an increased reabsorption of the filtered HCO₃⁻ ions and the development of metabolic alkalosis. An elevation in plasma K⁺ levels has the opposite effect. Plasma K⁺ levels are similarly altered by acid-base balance (*e.g.*, acidosis tends to increase potassium levels and alkalosis to decrease potassium levels).

Aldosterone also influences H⁺ ion elimination by the kidney. It acts in the collecting duct indirectly to stimulate H⁺ ion secretion, while increasing Na⁺ ion reabsorption and K⁺ ion secretion. Hyperaldosteronism tends to lead to a decrease in plasma K⁺ levels and increased pH and alkalosis because of increased H⁺ ion secretion. Hypoaldosteronism has the opposite effect, leading to increased K⁺ levels, decreased H⁺ ion secretion, and acidosis.

Bicarbonate–Chloride Exchange. Another mechanism that the kidney uses in regulating HCO₃⁻ is the bicarbonate–chloride anion exchange that occurs in association with Na⁺ reabsorption. Chloride is absorbed along with Na⁺ throughout the kidney nephron. In situations of volume depletion due to vomiting and Cl⁻ depletion, the kidney increases its absorption of HCO₃⁻. *Hypochloremic alkalosis* refers to an increase in pH induced by excess HCO₃⁻ reabsorption due to a decrease in Cl⁻ levels, and *hyperchloremic acidosis* to a decrease in pH due to decreased HCO₃⁻ reabsorption because of an increase in Cl⁻ levels.

Laboratory Tests

Laboratory tests that are used in assessing acid-base balance include arterial blood gas measurements, carbon dioxide content and bicarbonate levels, base excess or deficit, and the anion gap.

Arterial blood gases provide a means of assessing the respiratory component of acid-base balance. H₂CO₃ levels are determined from arterial PCO₂ levels and the solubility coefficient for CO₂ (normal arterial PCO₂ is 38 to 42 mm Hg). Arterial blood gases are used because *venous blood gases* are highly variable, depending on metabolic demands of the various tissues that empty into the vein from where the sample is being drawn. Laboratory measurements of electrolytes include the CO₂ content and bicarbonate levels. The *CO₂ content* refers to the total CO₂ content of blood, including that contained in bicarbonate. It is determined by adding a strong acid to a plasma sample and measuring the amount of CO₂ generated. More than 70% of the CO₂ in the blood is in the form of bicarbonate.[2] The serum *bicarbonate* is then determined from the total CO₂ content of the blood.

Base excess or *deficit* is a measurement of HCO₃⁻ excess or deficit. It describes the amount of a fixed acid or base that must be added to a blood sample to achieve a pH of 7.4 (normal, ±3.0 mEq/L).[12] A base excess is indicative of metabolic alkalosis, and a base deficit, metabolic acidosis.

The *anion gap* describes the difference between the plasma concentration of the major measured cation (Na⁺) and the sum of the measured anions (Cl⁻ and HCO₃⁻). This difference represents the concentration of unmeasured anions, such as phosphates, sulfates, organic acids, and proteins (Fig. 6-18). Normally, the anion gap ranges between 8 and 12 mEq/L (a value of 16 mEq is normal if Na⁺ and K⁺ concentrations are used in the calculation). The anion gap is increased in conditions such as lactic aci-

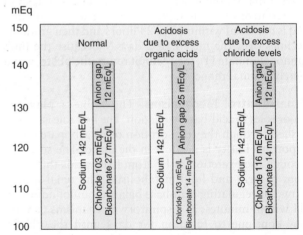

FIGURE 6-18 The anion gap in acidosis due to excess metabolic acids and excess serum chloride levels. Unmeasured anions such as phosphates, sulfates, and organic acids increase the anion gap because they replace bicarbonate. This assumes there is no change in sodium content.

dosis and ketoacidosis that result in a decrease of HCO_3^-, and it is normal in hyperchloremic acidosis, where Cl^- replaces the HCO_3^- anion.

ALTERATIONS IN ACID-BASE BALANCE

The terms *acidosis* and *alkalosis* describe the clinical conditions that arise as a result of changes in PCO_2 and HCO_3^- concentrations. An alkali represents a combination of one or more alkali metals such as sodium or potassium with a highly basic ion such as a hydroxyl ion (OH^-). Sodium bicarbonate ($NaHCO_3$) is the main alkali in the ECF. Although the definitions differ somewhat, the terms *alkali* and *base* are often used interchangeably. Thus, the term *alkalosis* has come to mean the opposite of *acidosis*.

Metabolic Versus Respiratory Acid-Base Disorders

There are two types of acid-base disorders: metabolic and respiratory. Metabolic disorders produce an alteration in HCO_3^- concentration and result from the addition or loss of nonvolatile acid or alkali to or from the ECF. A decrease in pH caused by a decrease in HCO_3^- is called *metabolic acidosis*, and an elevated pH caused by increased HCO_3^- is called *metabolic alkalosis*. Respiratory disorders involve changes in the PCO_2, reflecting an increase or decrease in alveolar ventilation. *Respiratory acidosis* is characterized by a decrease in pH, reflecting a decrease in ventilation and an increase in PCO_2. *Respiratory alkalosis* involves an increase in pH, resulting from an increase in alveolar ventilation and a decrease in PCO_2.

Primary Versus Compensatory Mechanisms

Acidosis and alkalosis typically involve a *primary* or *initiating event* and a *compensatory state* that results from

KEY CONCEPTS

Acid-Base Disorders

➤ The manifestations of acid-base disorders can be divided into three groups: (1) those due to the primary cause of the imbalance, (2) those due to the changed pH, and (3) those due to the elicited compensatory mechanisms.

➤ Metabolic acidosis represents a decrease in HCO_3^- that is caused by an excess of nonvolatile acids or loss of bicarbonate, and metabolic alkalosis represents an increase in HCO_3^- caused by a decrease in nonvolatile acids or increase in HCO_3^- intake or generation.

➤ Respiratory acidosis represents an increase in H_2CO_3 that is caused by respiratory conditions that interfere with the elimination of CO_2, and respiratory alkalosis represents a decrease in H_2CO_3 that is caused by excess elimination of CO_2.

homeostatic mechanisms that attempt to correct or prevent large changes in pH. For example, a person may have a primary metabolic acidosis as a result of overproduction of ketoacids and respiratory alkalosis because of a compensatory increase in ventilation (Table 6-8).

Compensatory mechanisms adjust the pH toward a more normal level without correcting the underlying cause of the disorder. Often, compensatory mechanisms are interim measures that permit survival while the body attempts to correct the primary disorder. Compensation requires the use of mechanisms that are different from those that caused the primary disorder. In other words, the lungs cannot compensate for respiratory acidosis that is caused by lung disease, nor can the kidneys compensate for metabolic acidosis that occurs because of renal failure. Because compensatory mechanisms often become more effective with time, there are often differences between the level of pH change that occurs with acute and chronic acid-base disorders.

Metabolic Acidosis

Metabolic acidosis involves a primary deficit in base bicarbonate along with a decrease in serum pH. In metabolic acidosis, the body compensates for the decrease in pH by increasing the respiratory rate in an effort to decrease PCO_2 and H_2CO_3 levels. The PCO_2 can be expected to fall by 1 to 1.5 mm Hg for each 1 mEq/L fall in HCO_3^-.[44,45]

Causes. Metabolic acidosis can be caused by one of four mechanisms: increased production of nonvolatile metabolic acids, decreased acid secretion by the kidney, excessive loss of bicarbonate, or an increase in Cl^-.[46,48] The anion gap is often useful in determining the cause of the metabolic acidosis (Chart 6-2). The presence of excess metabolic acids produces an increase in the anion gap as sodium bicarbonate is replaced by the sodium salt of the offending acid (*e.g.*, sodium lactate). When acidosis results from increased Cl^- levels (*e.g.*, hyperchloremic acidosis), the anion gap remains within normal levels.

Increased Production of Metabolic Acids. Metabolic acids increase when there is an accumulation of lactic acid or overproduction of ketoacids.

Acute lactic acidosis is one of the most common types of metabolic acidosis.[43] Lactic acidosis develops when there is excess production of lactic acid or diminished lactic acid removal from the blood. Lactic acid is produced by the anaerobic metabolism of glucose and is removed by the liver and, to a lesser extent, by the kidneys. Virtually all tissues can produce lactic acid under appropriate circumstances. Tissues such as red blood cells, intestine, and skeletal muscle do so under normal conditions. For example, excess lactate is produced with vigorous exercise, during which there is a local disproportion between oxygen supply and demand in the contracting muscles.

Most cases of lactic acidosis are caused by inadequate oxygen delivery, as in shock or cardiac arrest.[43] Such conditions increase lactic acid production, and they

TABLE 6-8	Summary of Acid-Base Imbalances		
Acid-Base Imbalance	Primary Disturbance	Respiratory Compensation	Renal Compensation
Metabolic acidosis	Decrease in bicarbonate	Hyperventilation to decrease PCO_2	If no renal disease, increased H^+ excretion and increased HCO_3^- reabsorption
Metabolic alkalosis	Increase in bicarbonate	Hypoventilation to increase PCO_2	If no renal disease, decreased H^+ excretion and decreased HCO_3^- reabsorption
Respiratory acidosis	Increase in PCO_2	None	Increased H^+ excretion and increased HCO_3^- reabsorption
Respiratory alkalosis	Decrease in PCO_2	None	Decreased H^+ excretion and decreased HCO_3^- reabsorption

impair lactic acid clearance because of poor liver perfusion. Mortality rates are high for persons with lactic acidosis because of shock and tissue hypoxia.[43] Lactic acidosis is also associated with disorders in which tissue hypoxia does not appear to be present. It has been reported in patients with leukemia, lymphomas, and other cancers; those with poorly controlled diabetes; and pa-

tients with severe liver failure. Mechanisms causing lactic acidosis in these conditions are poorly understood. Some conditions such as neoplasms may produce local increases in tissue metabolism and lactate production or interfere with blood flow to noncancerous cells. Ethanol produces a slight elevation in lactic acid, but clinically significant lactic acidosis does not occur in alcohol intoxication unless other problems such as liver failure are present.

Ketoacids (*i.e.*, acetoacetic and β-hydroxybutyric acid), produced in the liver from fatty acids, are the source of fuel for many body tissues. An overproduction of ketoacids occurs when carbohydrate stores are inadequate or when the body cannot use available carbohydrates as a fuel. Under these conditions, fatty acids are mobilized from adipose tissue and delivered to the liver, where they are converted to ketones. Ketoacidosis develops when ketone production exceeds tissue use. The most common cause of ketoacidosis is uncontrolled diabetes mellitus, in which an insulin deficiency leads to the release of fatty acids from adipose cells with subsequent production of excess ketoacids (see Chapter 32). Ketoacidosis may also develop as the result of fasting or food deprivation, during which the lack of carbohydrates produces a self-limited state of ketoacidosis (self-limited because the resultant decrease in insulin release suppresses the release of fatty acids for fat cells).

CHART 6-2

The Anion Gap in Differential Diagnosis of Metabolic Acidosis

Decreased Anion Gap (<8 mEq/L)

Hypoalbuminemia (decrease in unmeasured anions)
Multiple myeloma (increase in unmeasured cationic IgG paraproteins)
Increased unmeasured cations (hyperkalemia, hypercalcemia, hypermagnesemia, lithium intoxication)

Increased Anion Gap (>12 mEq/L)

Presence of unmeasured metabolic anion
  Diabetic ketoacidosis
  Alcoholic ketoacidosis
  Lactic acidosis
  Starvation
  Renal insufficiency
Presence of drug or chemical anion
  Salicylate poisoning
  Methanol poisoning
  Ethylene glycol poisoning

Normal Anion Gap (8–12 mEq/L)

Loss of bicarbonate
  Diarrhea
  Pancreatic fluid loss
  Ileostomy (unadapted)
Chloride retention
  Renal tubular acidosis
  Ileal loop bladder
  Parenteral nutrition (arginine and lysine)

Decreased Renal Function. Kidney failure is the most common cause of chronic metabolic acidosis. The kidneys normally conserve HCO_3^- and secrete H^+ ions into the urine as a means of regulating acid-base balance. In renal failure, there is loss of glomerular and tubular function, with retention of nitrogenous wastes and metabolic acids. In a condition called *renal tubular acidosis*, glomerular function is normal, but the tubular secretion of H^+ or reabsorption of HCO_3^- is abnormal.

Increased Bicarbonate Losses. Increased HCO_3^- losses occur with the loss of bicarbonate-rich body fluids or with impaired conservation of HCO_3^- by the kidney. Intestinal secretions have a high HCO_3^- concentration. Consequently, excessive losses of HCO_3^- ions occur with severe diarrhea; small bowel, biliary, or ileostomy drainage; and intestinal suction. In diarrhea of microbial origin, HCO_3^- is secreted into the bowel to neutralize the metabolic acids produced by the microorganisms causing the diarrhea.

Hyperchloremic Acidosis. Hyperchloremic acidosis occurs when serum Cl^- ion levels are increased. Because Cl^- and HCO_3^- are anions, the serum HCO_3^- ion concentration decreases when there is an increase in Cl^- ions. Hyperchloremic acidosis can occur as the result of abnormal absorption of Cl^- by the kidneys or as a result of treatment with chloride-containing medications (*i.e.*, sodium chloride, amino acid–chloride hyperalimentation solutions, and ammonium chloride). The administration of intravenous sodium chloride or parenteral hyperalimentation solutions that contain an amino acid–chloride combination can cause acidosis in a similar manner.[49] With hyperchloremic acidosis, the anion gap is within the normal range, but the Cl^- levels are increased and HCO_3^- levels are decreased.

Manifestations. Metabolic acidosis is characterized by a decrease in pH (<7.35) and a decrease in serum HCO_3^- levels (<24 mEq/L). Acidosis typically produces a compensatory increase in respiratory rate with a decrease in PCO_2 (Table 6-9).

The manifestations of metabolic acidosis fall into three categories: signs and symptoms of the disorder causing the acidosis, changes in body function related to recruitment of compensatory mechanisms, and alterations in cardiovascular, neurologic, and musculoskeletal function resulting from the decreased pH. The signs and symptoms of metabolic acidosis usually begin to appear when the plasma HCO_3^- concentration falls to 20 mEq/L or less. A fall in pH to less than 7.0 to 7.10 can reduce cardiac contractility and predispose to potentially fatal cardiac dysrhythmias.[12]

Metabolic acidosis is seldom a primary disorder; it usually develops during the course of another disease. The manifestations of metabolic acidosis frequently are superimposed on the symptoms of the contributing health problem. With diabetic ketoacidosis, which is a common cause of metabolic acidosis, there is an increase in blood and urine glucose and a characteristic smell of ketones to the breath. In metabolic acidosis that accompanies renal failure, blood urea nitrogen levels are elevated and other tests of renal function yield abnormal results.

Manifestations related to respiratory and renal compensatory mechanisms usually occur early in the course of metabolic acidosis. In situations of acute metabolic acidosis, the respiratory system compensates for a decrease

TABLE 6-9	Manifestations of Metabolic Acidosis and Alkalosis
Metabolic Acidosis	**Metabolic Alkalosis**
Laboratory Tests pH decreased Bicarbonate (primary) decreased PCO_2 (compensatory) decreased	**Laboratory Tests** pH increased Bicarbonate (primary) increased PCO_2 (compensatory) increased
Signs of Compensation Increased respirations (rate and depth) Hyperkalemia Acid urine Increased ammonia in urine	**Signs of Compensation** Decreased respirations (rate and depth) with various degrees of hypoxia and respiratory acidosis
Gastrointestinal Effects Anorexia Nausea and vomiting Abdominal pain	
Nervous System Effects Weakness Lethargy Confusion Stupor Coma Depression of vital functions	**Nervous System Effects** Hyperactive reflexes Tetany Confusion Seizures
Cardiovascular Effects Peripheral vasodilation Decreased heart rate Cardiac arrhythmias	**Cardiovascular Effects** Hypotension Cardiac arrhythmias
Skin Warm and flushed	
Skeletal System Effects Bone disease (chronic acidosis)	

in pH by increasing ventilation to reduce PCO_2; this is accomplished through deep and rapid respirations. In diabetic ketoacidosis, this breathing pattern is referred to as *Kussmaul breathing*. For descriptive purposes, it can be said that Kussmaul breathing resembles the hyperpnea of exercise—the person breathes as though he or she had been running. There may be complaints of difficult breathing or dyspnea with exertion; with severe acidosis, dyspnea may be present even at rest. Respiratory compensation for acute acidosis tends to be somewhat greater than for chronic acidosis. When kidney function is normal, H^+ ion excretion increases promptly in response to acidosis, and the urine becomes more acid.

Changes in pH have a direct effect on body function that can produce signs and symptoms common to most types of metabolic acidosis, regardless of cause. A person with metabolic acidosis often complains of weakness, fatigue, general malaise, and a dull headache. The person also may have anorexia, nausea, vomiting, and abdominal pain. Tissue turgor is impaired, and the skin is dry when fluid deficit accompanies acidosis. In persons with undiagnosed diabetes mellitus, the nausea, vomiting, and abdominal symptoms may be misinterpreted as being caused by gastrointestinal flu or other abdominal disease, such as appendicitis. Acidosis depresses neuronal excitability and it decreases binding of calcium to plasma proteins so that more free calcium is available to decrease neural activity. As acidosis progresses, the level of consciousness declines, and stupor and coma develop. The skin is often warm and flushed because skin vessels become less responsive to sympathetic stimulation and lose tone.

When the pH falls to 7.0 to 7.1, cardiac contractility and cardiac output decrease, the heart becomes less responsive to catecholamines (*i.e.*, epinephrine and norepinephrine), and arrhythmias, including fatal ventricular arrhythmias, can develop. A decrease in ventricular function may be particularly important in perpetuating shock-induced lactic acidosis, and partial correction of the acidemia may be necessary before tissue perfusion can be restored.[12]

Chronic acidemia, as in renal failure, can lead to a variety of musculoskeletal problems, some of which result from the release of calcium and phosphate during bone buffering of excess H^+ ions.[50] Of particular importance is impaired growth in children. In infants and children, acidemia may be associated with a variety of nonspecific symptoms such as anorexia, weight loss, muscle weakness, and listlessness.[12] Muscle weakness and listlessness may result from alterations in muscle metabolism.

Treatment. Treatment of metabolic acidosis focuses on correcting the condition that caused the disorder and restoring the fluids and electrolytes that have been lost from the body. The treatment of diabetic ketoacidosis is discussed in Chapter 32.

The use of supplemental sodium bicarbonate ($NaHCO_3$) may be indicated in the treatment of some forms of normal anion gap acidosis. However, its use in treatment of metabolic acidosis with an increased anion gap is controversial, particularly in cases of impaired tissue perfusion. In most patients with cardiac arrest, shock, or sepsis, impaired oxygen delivery is the primary cause of lactic acidosis. In these situations, the administration of large amounts of $NaHCO_3$ does not improve oxygen delivery and may produce hypernatremia, hyperosmolality, and decreased oxygen release by hemoglobin because of a shift in the oxygen dissociation curve (see Chapter 20).[51]

Metabolic Alkalosis

Metabolic alkalosis is a systemic disorder caused by an increase in pH due to a primary excess of plasma HCO_3^- ions.[52,53] It is reported to be the second most common acid-base disorder in hospitalized adults, accounting for about 32% of all acid-base disorders.[54]

Causes. Most of the body's plasma HCO_3^- is obtained from three sources: from CO_2 that is produced during metabolic processes, from reabsorption of filtered HCO_3^-, or from generation of new HCO_3^- by the kidney. Usually, HCO_3^- production and renal reabsorption are balanced in a manner that prevents alkalosis from occurring. The proximal tubule reabsorbs 99.9% of the filtered HCO_3^-. When the plasma levels of HCO_3^- rise above the threshold for tubular reabsorption, the excess is excreted in the urine. Many of the conditions that increase plasma HCO_3^- also raise the level for HCO_3^- reabsorption, and thus an increase in HCO_3^- contributes not only to the generation of metabolic alkalosis but to its maintenance.

Metabolic alkalosis is caused by factors that generate a loss of H^+ or gain of HCO_3^- ions and those that maintain it by interfering with excretion of the excess HCO_3^-. They include excess alkali intake, HCO_3^- excess associated with H^+, Cl^-, and K^+ loss; and maintenance of increased HCO_3^- by volume contraction, hypokalemia, and hypochloremia.

Excess Alkali Intake. Excess alkali intake, as in the use of bicarbonate-containing antacids (*e.g.*, Alka-Seltzer) or $NaHCO_3$ administration during cardiopulmonary resuscitation, can cause metabolic alkalosis. Other sources of alkali intake are acetate in hyperalimentation solutions, lactate in intravenous solutions such as Ringer lactate, and citrate used in blood transfusions. A condition called the *milk-alkali syndrome* may develop in persons who consume excess amounts of milk along with an antacid such as calcium carbonate (discussed previously in the section on Hypercalcemia).

Bicarbonate Retention. Vomiting, removal of gastric secretions through use of nasogastric suction, and low potassium levels resulting from diuretic therapy are the most common causes of metabolic alkalosis in hospitalized patients.

Hypokalemia is a potent stimulus for H^+ secretion and HCO_3^- reabsorption by the kidney. The mechanisms by which hypokalemia increases HCO_3^- reabsorption are likely the effects of tubular K^+/H^+ ion exchange. In hypokalemia, K^+ moves out of the tubular cell into the blood and is replaced by the H^+ ion. This results in intracellular acidosis and increased HCO_3^- reabsorption.

The binge-purge syndrome, or self-induced vomiting, also is associated with metabolic alkalosis.[52] Gastric secretions contain high concentrations of HCl and lesser concentrations of potassium chloride (KCl). As Cl^- is taken from the blood and secreted into the stomach with the H^+ ion, it is replaced by HCO_3^-. Under normal conditions, each 1 mEq of H^+ ion that is secreted into the stomach generates 1 mEq of plasma HCO_3^-.[52] Because the entry of acid into the duodenum stimulates an equal amount of pancreatic HCO_3^- secretion, the increase in plasma HCO_3^- concentration is usually transient and pH returns to normal within hours. However, loss of H^+ and Cl^- ions from the stomach due to vomiting or gastric suction stimulates continued production of gastric acid and thus the addition of more bicarbonate into the blood.

Metabolic alkalosis can also result from excessive adrenocorticosteroid hormones (*e.g.*, hyperaldosteronism, Cushing syndrome). The hormone aldosterone increases tubular secretion of H^+ into the urine filtrate as it increases Na^+ and HCO_3^- ion reabsorption. In hyperaldosteronism, the concurrent loss of K^+ in the urine serves to perpetuate the alkalosis.

Maintenance of Metabolic Alkalosis. Extracellular volume depletion is one of the most important factors resulting in continued absorption of HCO_3^- by the kidney. A decrease in extracellular fluid volume activates the renin-angiotensin-aldosterone system, which increases Na^+ reabsorption as a means of maintaining extracellular fluid volume. The reabsorption of Na^+ requires concomitant anion reabsorption; because there is a Cl^- deficit, HCO_3^- is reabsorbed along with Na^+.

Vomiting, which results in loss of water, hydrochloric acid, sodium, and potassium, is an important cause of metabolic alkalosis (Fig. 6-19). The volume depletion, hypokalemia, and hypochloremia that occur with vomiting serve to maintain the generated metabolic alkalosis by increasing the renal reabsorption of HCO_3^- ion.

The use of diuretics is often associated with metabolic alkalosis. Loop diuretics (*e.g.*, furosemide [Lasix]) decrease Na^+, K^+, and Cl^- reabsorption, leading to volume contraction and hypokalemia. The thiazide diuretics (*e.g.*, hydrochlorothiazide) increase renal K^+ loss, leading to increased HCO_3^- reabsorption.

Chronic respiratory acidosis produces a compensatory loss of H^+ and Cl^- ions in the urine along with HCO_3^- retention. When respiratory acidosis is corrected abruptly, as with mechanical ventilation, a "posthypercapneic" metabolic alkalosis may develop because of a rapid drop in PCO_2, while the concentration of HCO_3^- ions, which are eliminated renally, remains elevated.

Manifestations. Metabolic alkalosis is characterized by a serum pH above 7.45, plasma HCO_3^- level above 29 mEq/L (29 mmol/L), and base excess above 3.0 mEq/L (3 mmol/L; see Table 6-9). Persons with metabolic alkalosis often are asymptomatic or have signs related to volume depletion or hypokalemia. Neurologic signs and symptoms (*e.g.*, hyperexcitability) occur less frequently with metabolic alkalosis than with other acid-base disorders because the HCO_3^- ion enters the CSF more slowly

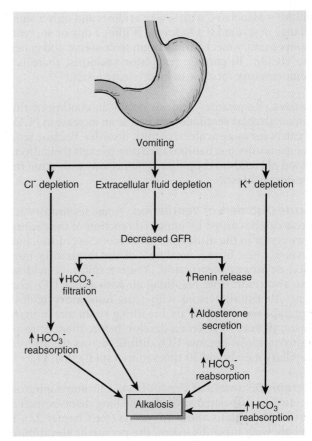

FIGURE 6-19 Renal mechanisms for bicarbonate (HCO_3^-) reabsorption and maintenance of metabolic alkalosis after depletion of extracellular fluid volume, chloride (Cl^-), and potassium (K^+) due to vomiting.

than CO_2. When neurologic manifestations do occur, as in acute and severe metabolic alkalosis, they include mental confusion, hyperactive reflexes, tetany, and carpopedal spasm. Metabolic alkalosis also leads to a compensatory hypoventilation with development of various degrees of hypoxemia and respiratory acidosis. Significant morbidity occurs with severe metabolic alkalosis (pH >7.55), including respiratory failure, arrhythmias, seizures, and coma.

Treatment. The treatment of metabolic alkalosis usually is directed toward correcting the cause of the condition. A chloride deficit requires correction. Potassium chloride usually is the treatment of choice for metabolic alkalosis when there is an accompanying potassium deficit. When potassium chloride is used as a therapy, Cl^- replaces HCO_3^- and the administration of K^+ corrects the potassium deficit, allowing the kidneys to conserve H^+ while eliminating the K^+. Fluid replacement with normal saline or one-half normal saline often is used in the treatment of patients with volume contraction alkalosis.

Respiratory Acidosis

Respiratory acidosis involves an increase in PCO_2 and H_2CO_3 along with a decrease in pH. Acute respiratory failure is associated with severe acidosis and only a small change in serum HCO_3^- levels. Within a day or so, renal compensatory mechanisms begin to conserve and generate HCO_3^-. In chronic respiratory acidosis, there is a compensatory increase in bicarbonate levels.[55,56]

Causes. Respiratory acidosis occurs in conditions that impair alveolar ventilation and cause an increase in PCO_2. It can occur as an acute or chronic disorder. Because renal compensatory mechanisms take time to exert their effects, blood pH tends to drop sharply in persons with acute respiratory acidosis.

Acute Disorders of Ventilation. Acute respiratory acidosis can be caused by impaired function of the respiratory center in the medulla (as in narcotic overdose), lung disease, chest injury, weakness of the respiratory muscles, or airway obstruction. Acute respiratory acidosis can also result from breathing air with a high CO_2 content. Almost all persons with acute respiratory acidosis are hypoxemic if they are breathing room air. In many cases, signs of hypoxemia develop before those of respiratory acidosis because CO_2 diffuses across the alveolar capillary membrane 20 times more rapidly than O_2.[2,12]

Chronic Disorders of Ventilation. Chronic respiratory acidosis is associated with chronic lung diseases such as chronic bronchitis and emphysema (see Chapter 22). In people with these disorders, the persistent elevation of PCO_2 stimulates renal H^+ ion secretion and HCO_3^- reabsorption. The effectiveness of these compensatory mechanisms can often return the pH to near-normal values as long as O_2 levels are maintained within a range that does not unduly suppress the chemoreceptor-mediated control of ventilation.

An acute episode of respiratory acidosis can develop in persons with chronic lung disease who receive oxygen therapy at a flow rate sufficient to raise the PO_2 to a level that produces a decrease in ventilation (discussed in Chapter 22). In these persons, the respiratory center has become adapted to the elevated levels of PCO_2 and no longer responds to increases in PCO_2. Instead, the PO_2 content of their blood becomes the major stimulus for respiration. If oxygen is administered at a flow rate that is sufficient to suppress this stimulus, the rate and depth of respiration decrease, and the PCO_2 increases.

Increased Carbon Dioxide Production. Carbon dioxide is a product of the body's metabolic processes, generating a substantial amount of acid that must be excreted by the lungs or kidney to prevent acidosis. An increase in CO_2 production can result from numerous processes, including exercise, fever, sepsis, and burns. For example, CO_2 production increases by approximately 13% for each 1°C rise in temperature above normal.[57] Nutrition also affects the production of CO_2. A carbohydrate-rich diet produces larger amounts of CO_2 than one containing reasonable amounts of protein and fat. Although excess CO_2 production can lead to an increase in PCO_2, it seldom does. In healthy persons, an increase in CO_2 is usually matched by an increase in CO_2 elimination by the lungs. In contrast, persons with respiratory diseases may be unable to eliminate the excess CO_2.

Manifestations. Respiratory acidosis is associated with a serum pH less than 7.35 and an arterial PCO_2 greater than 50 mm Hg (Table 6-10). The signs and symptoms

TABLE 6-10	Manifestations of Respiratory Acidosis and Alkalosis	
Respiratory Acidosis		**Respiratory Alkalosis**
Laboratory Tests		**Laboratory Tests**
pH decreased		pH increased
PCO_2 (primary) increased		PCO_2 (primary) decreased
Bicarbonate (compensatory) increased		Bicarbonate (compensatory) decreased
Signs of Compensation		**Signs of Compensation**
Acid urine		Alkaline urine
Nervous System Effects		**Nervous System Effects**
Dilation of cerebral vessels and decreased neuronal activity		Constriction of cerebral vessels and increased neuronal activity
Headache		Dizziness, panic, light-headedness
Behavioral changes		Tetany
Confusion		Numbness and tingling of fingers and toes
Depression		Seizures (severe)
Paranoia		
Hallucinations		
Weakness		
Tremors		
Paralysis		
Stupor and coma		
Skin		**Cardiovascular Effects**
Warm and flushed		Cardiac arrhythmias

of respiratory acidosis depend on the rapidity of onset and whether the condition is acute or chronic. Because respiratory acidosis often is accompanied by hypoxemia, the manifestations of respiratory acidosis often are intermixed with those of oxygen deficit.

Sudden elevations in arterial PCO_2 can cause headache, blurred vision, an increase in heart rate and blood pressure, warm and flushed skin, irritability, muscle twitching, and psychological disturbances. Carbon dioxide readily crosses the blood-brain barrier, exerting its effects by changing the pH of brain fluids. Elevated levels of PCO_2 produce vasodilation of cerebral blood vessels. If the condition is severe and prolonged, it can cause an increase in cerebrospinal fluid pressure and papilledema. Impaired consciousness, ranging from lethargy to coma, develops as the PCO_2 rises. Paralysis of extremities may occur, and there may be respiratory depression.

Treatment. The treatment of acute and chronic respiratory acidosis is directed toward improving ventilation (see Chapter 22). In severe cases, mechanical ventilation may be necessary.

Respiratory Alkalosis

Respiratory alkalosis involves a decrease in PCO_2 and a primary deficit in H_2CO_3 along with an increase in pH.[57,58] Because respiratory alkalosis can occur suddenly, a compensatory decrease in HCO_3^- may not occur before respiratory correction has been accomplished. The increase in pH is less in chronic compensated respiratory alkalosis, and the fall in HCO_3^- is greater.

Causes. Respiratory alkalosis is caused by hyperventilation or a respiratory rate in excess of that needed to maintain normal plasma PCO_2 levels. It may occur as the result of central stimulation of the medullary respiratory center or stimulation of peripheral (*e.g.*, carotid chemoreceptor) pathways to the medullary respiratory center.[55]

Mechanical ventilation may produce respiratory alkalosis if the rate and tidal volume are set so that CO_2 elimination exceeds CO_2 production. Carbon dioxide crosses the alveolar capillary membrane 20 times more rapidly than oxygen. Therefore, the increased minute ventilation may be necessary to maintain adequate oxygen levels while producing a concomitant decrease in CO_2 levels. In some cases, respiratory alkalosis may be induced medically as a means of controlling disorders such as severe intracranial hypertension.[57]

Central stimulation of the medullary respiratory center occurs with anxiety, pain, pregnancy, febrile states, sepsis, encephalitis, and salicylate toxicity. Respiratory alkalosis has long been recognized as a common acid-base disorder in critically ill patients, and is a consistent finding in both septic shock and the systemic inflammatory response syndrome[57] (see Chapter 19). Progesterone increases ventilation in women; during the progesterone phase of the menstrual cycle, normal women increase their PCO_2 values by 2 to 4 mm Hg and their pH by 0.01 to .02.[3] Women also develop substantial hypocapnia dur-

ing pregnancy, most notably during the last trimester, with PCO_2 values of 29 to 32 mm Hg.[3,57]

One of the most common causes of respiratory alkalosis is the hyperventilation syndrome, which is characterized by recurring episodes of overbreathing often associated with anxiety. Persons experiencing panic attacks frequently present in the emergency department with manifestations of acute respiratory alkalosis.

Hypoxemia exerts its effect on pH through the peripheral chemoreceptors in the carotid bodies. Stimulation of peripheral chemoreceptors occurs in conditions that cause hypoxemia with relatively unimpaired CO_2 transport such as exposure to high altitudes, asthma, and respiratory disorders that decrease lung compliance.

Manifestations. Respiratory alkalosis manifests with a decrease in PCO_2 and a deficit in H_2CO_3 (see Table 6-10). In respiratory alkalosis, the pH is above 7.45, arterial PCO_2 is below 35 mm Hg, and serum HCO_3^- levels usually are below 24 mEq/L (24 mmol/L).

The signs and symptoms of respiratory alkalosis are those associated with hyperexcitability of the nervous system and a decrease in cerebral blood flow. Alkalosis increases protein binding of extracellular calcium. This reduces ionized calcium levels, causing an increase in neuromuscular excitability. A decrease in the CO_2 content of the blood causes constriction of cerebral blood vessels. Because CO_2 crosses the blood-brain barrier rather quickly, the manifestations of acute respiratory alkalosis are usually of sudden onset. The person often experiences light-headedness, dizziness, tingling, and numbness of the fingers and toes. These manifestations may be accompanied by sweating, palpitations, panic, air hunger, and dyspnea. Chvostek's and Trousseau's signs may be positive, and tetany and convulsions may occur. Because CO_2 provides the stimulus for short-term regulation of respiration, short periods of apnea may occur in persons with acute episodes of hyperventilation.

Treatment. The treatment of respiratory alkalosis focuses on measures to increase the PCO_2. Attention is directed toward correcting the disorder that caused the overbreathing. Rebreathing of small amounts of expired air (breathing into a paper bag) may prove useful in restoring PCO_2 levels in persons with anxiety-produced respiratory alkalosis.

In summary, normal body function depends on the precise regulation of acid-base balance to maintain a pH within the narrow physiologic range of 7.35 to 7.45. Metabolic processes produce volatile and nonvolatile metabolic acids that must be buffered and eliminated from the body. The volatile acid H_2CO_3 is in equilibrium with dissolved PCO_2, which is eliminated through the lungs. The nonvolatile acids, which are derived mainly from protein metabolism and incomplete carbohydrate and fat metabolism, are excreted by the kidneys. It is the ratio of the HCO_3^- concentration to H_2CO_3 (PCO_2)

that determines body pH. When this ratio is 20:1, the pH is 7.4. The ability of the body to maintain pH within the normal physiologic range depends on respiratory and renal mechanisms and on intracellular and extracellular buffers, the most important being the bicarbonate buffer system. The respiratory regulation of pH is rapid but does not return the pH completely to normal. The kidney aids in regulation of pH by eliminating H^+ ions or conserving HCO_3^- ions. In the process of eliminating H^+, it uses the phosphate and ammonia buffer systems. Body pH is also affected by the distribution of exchangeable cations (K^+ and H^+) and anions (Cl^- and HCO_3^-).

Metabolic acidosis is defined as a decrease in HCO_3^- and metabolic alkalosis as an increase in HCO_3^-. Metabolic acidosis is caused by an excessive production and accumulation of metabolic acids or excessive loss of HCO_3^-. Metabolic alkalosis is caused by an increase in HCO_3^- or from a decrease in H^+ or Cl^-, with a resultant increase in renal reabsorption of HCO_3^-. Respiratory acidosis reflects a decrease in pH that is caused by conditions that produce hypoventilation, with a resultant increase in PCO_2 levels. Respiratory alkalosis reflects an increase in pH that is caused by conditions that produce hyperventilation, with a resultant decrease in PCO_2 levels.

The signs and symptoms of acidosis and alkalosis reflect alterations in body function associated with the disorder causing the acid-base disturbance, the effect of the change of pH on body function, and the body's attempt to correct and maintain the pH within a normal physiologic range. In general, neuromuscular excitability is decreased in acidosis and increased in alkalosis.

Review Exercises

A 40-year-old man with advanced acquired immunodeficiency syndrome (AIDS) presents with an acute lung infection. Investigators confirm a diagnosis of *P. carinii* pneumonia. Although he is being treated appropriately, his serum sodium level is 118 mEq/L. Results of tests of adrenal function are normal.

A. What is the likely cause of this man's electrolyte disorder?
B. What are the five cardinal features of this condition?

A 70-year-old woman who is taking furosemide (a loop diuretic) for congestive heart failure complains of weakness, fatigue, and cramping in the muscles of her legs. Her serum potassium is 2.0 mEq/L, and her serum sodium is 140 mEq/L. She also complains that she experiences a "strange heartbeat" at times.

A. What is the likely cause of this woman's symptoms?
B. An ECG shows depressed ST segment and low T-wave changes. Explain the physiologic mechanisms underlying these changes.
C. What would be the appropriate treatment for this woman?

A 50-year-old woman presents with symptoms of hypercalcemia. She has a recent history of breast cancer treatment.

A. How would you evaluate this woman for increased calcium levels?
B. What is the significance of the recent history of malignancy?
C. What further tests may be indicated?

A 34-year-old woman with diabetes is admitted to the emergency department in a stuporous state. Her skin is flushed and warm, her breath has a sweet odor, her pulse is rapid and weak, and her respirations are rapid and deep. Her initial laboratory tests indicate a blood sugar of 320 mg/dL, serum bicarbonate of 12 mEq/L (normal, 24 to 27 mEq/L), and a pH of 7.1 (normal, 7.35 to 7.45).

A. What is the most likely cause of her lowered pH and bicarbonate levels?
B. How would you account for her rapid and deep respirations?
C. Using the Henderson-Hasselbalch equation and the solubility coefficient for carbon dioxide given in this chapter, what would you expect her PCO_2 to be?
D. How would you explain her warm, flushed skin and stuporous mental state?

A 65-year-old man with chronic obstructive lung disease has been using low-flow oxygen therapy because of difficulty in maintaining adequate oxygenation of his blood. He has recently had a severe respiratory tract infection and has had difficulty breathing. He is admitted to the emergency department because he became increasingly lethargic and his wife has had trouble arousing him. His respirations are 12 breaths/minute. She relates that he had "turned his oxygen way up" because of difficulty breathing.

A. What is the most likely cause of this man's problem?
B. How would you explain the lethargy and difficulty in arousal?

C. Arterial blood gases, drawn on admission to the emergency department, indicated a PO_2 of 85 mm Hg (normal, 90 to 95 mm Hg) and a PCO_2 of 90 mm Hg (normal, 40 mm Hg). His serum bicarbonate levels were 34 mEq/L (normal, 24 to 48 mEq/L). What is his pH?

D. What would be the main goal of treatment for this man in terms of acid-base balance?

Visit the Porth: Essentials of Pathophysiology: Concepts of Altered Health States web site
(http://thePoint.LWW.com/PorthEssentials) for links to chapter-related resources on the Internet, all-new exclusive animations, chapter review questions, and more!

REFERENCES

1. Schrier R. W., Gurevich A. K., Abraham W. T. (2003). Renal sodium excretion, edematous disorders, and diuretic use. In Schrier R. W. (Ed.), *Renal and electrolyte disorders* (6th ed., pp. 64–114). Philadelphia: Lippincott Williams & Wilkins.
2. Guyton A., Hall J. E. (2006). *Textbook of medical physiology* (11th ed., pp. 177–178, 183–190, 291–306, 358–363, 383–401, 893–894). Philadelphia: Elsevier Saunders.
3. Cogan M. G. (1991). *Fluid and electrolytes* (pp. 1, 43, 80–84, 100–111, 112–123, 125–130, 242–245). Norwalk, CT: Appleton & Lange.
4. Stearns R. H., Spital A., Clark E. C. (1996). Disorders of water balance. In Kokko J., Tannen R. L. (Eds.), *Fluids and electrolytes* (3rd ed., pp. 65, 69, 95). Philadelphia: W. B. Saunders.
5. Metheney N. M. (2000). *Fluid and electrolyte balance* (4th ed., pp. 3, 16, 18, 43, 47, 56, 162, 256). Philadelphia: Lippincott Williams & Wilkins.
6. Beri T., Schrier R. W. (2003). Disorders of water balance. In Schrier R. W. (Ed.), *Renal and electrolyte disorders* (6th ed., pp. 1-63). Philadelphia: Lippincott Williams & Wilkins.
7. Kugler J. P., Hustead T. (2000). Hyponatremia and hypernatremia in the elderly. *American Family Physician* 61, 3623–3630.
8. Luckey A. E., Parsa C. J. (2003). Fluids and electrolytes in the aged. *Archives of Surgery* 138, 1005–1060.
9. Illowsky B. P., Kirch D. G. (1988). Polydipsia and hyponatremia in psychiatric patients. *American Journal of Psychiatry* 145, 675–683.
10. Vieweg W. V. R. (1994). Treatment strategies for polydipsia-hyponatremia syndrome. *Journal of Clinical Psychiatry* 55(4), 154–159.
11. Antunes-Rodrigues J., DeCastro M., Elias L. L., et al. (2004). Neuroendocrine control of body fluid metabolism. *Physiological Reviews* S4, 169–208.
12. Rose B. D., Post T. W. (2001). *Clinical physiology of acid-base and electrolyte disorders* (5th ed., pp. 168–178, 822, 835, 858, 909). New York: McGraw-Hill.
13. Berne R. M., Levy M. (2000). *Principles of physiology* (3rd ed., p. 438). St. Louis: Mosby.
14. Robertson G. L. (1995). Diabetes insipidus. *Endocrinology and Metabolic Clinics of North America* 24, 549–571.
15. Bendz H., Aurell M. (1999). Drug-induced diabetes insipidus. *Drug Safety* 21, 449–456.
16. Baylis P. (2003). The syndrome of inappropriate antidiuretic hormone secretion. *International Journal of Biochemistry and Cellular Biology* 35, 1495–1499.
17. Costello-Boerrigter L. C., Boerrigter G., Burnett J. C. (2003). Revisiting salt and water retention, aquaretics, and natriuretics. *Medical Clinics of North America* 87, 475–491.
18. Kumar S., Beri T. (1998). Sodium. *Lancet* 352, 220–228.
19. Gohl K. P. (2004). Management of hyponatremia. *American Family Physician* 69, 2387–2394.
20. Palmer B. F., Gates J. R., Lader M. (2003). Causes and management of hyponatremia. *Annals of Pharmacotherapy* 37, 1694–1702.
21. Adrogué H. J. (2000). Hyponatremia. *New England Journal of Medicine* 343, 1581–1589.
22. Adrogué H. J. (2000). Hypernatremia. *New England Journal of Medicine* 342, 1493–1499.
23. Gennari F. J. (2002). Disorders of potassium homeostasis: Hypokalemia and hyperkalemia. *Critical Care Clinics of North America* 18, 273–288.
24. Mandell A. K. (1997). Hypokalemia and hyperkalemia. *Medical Clinics of North America* 81, 611–639.
25. Gennari F. J. (1998). Hypokalemia. *New England Journal of Medicine* 339, 451–458.
26. Peterson L. N., Levi M. (2003). Disorders of potassium metabolism. In Schrier R. W. (Ed.), *Renal and electrolyte disorders* (6th ed., pp. 171–215). Philadelphia: Lippincott Williams & Wilkins.
27. Tannen R. L (1996). Potassium disorders. In Kokko J., Tannen R. L. (Eds.), *Fluids and electrolytes* (3rd ed., pp. 116–118). Philadelphia: W. B. Saunders.
28. Matfin G., Durand D., D'Agostino A., et al. (1998). Thyrotoxic hypokalemic periodic paralysis. *Hospital Practice* 1, 23–26.
29. Whang G., Whang G. G., Ryan M. P. (1992). Refractory potassium repletion: A consequence of magnesium deficiency. *Archives of Internal Medicine* 152, 40–45.
30. Clark B. A., Brown R. S. (1995). Potassium homeostasis and hyperkalemic syndromes. *Endocrinology and Metabolic Clinics of North America* 24, 573–590.
31. Popovtzer M. M. (2003). Disorders of calcium, phosphorus, vitamin D, and parathyroid hormone activity. In Schrier R. W. (Ed.), *Renal and electrolyte disorders* (6th ed., pp. 216–277). Philadelphia: Lippincott Williams & Wilkins.
32. Quarles L. D. (2003) Extracellular calcium-sensing receptors in the parathyroid gland, kidney, and other tissues. *Current Opinions in Nephrology and Hypertension* 12, 349–355.
33. Llach F. (1999). Hyperphosphatemia in end-stage renal disease patients: Pathological consequences. *Kidney International* 56(Suppl. 73), S31–S37.
34. Zaloga G. F. (1992). Hypocalcemia in critically ill patients. *Critical Care Medicine* 20, 251–262.
35. Reber R. M., Heath H. (1995). Hypocalcemic emergencies. *Medical Clinics of North America* 79, 93–165.
36. Barnett M. L. (1999). Hypercalcemia. *Seminars in Oncology Nursing* 15, 190–201.
37. Carroll M. F., Schade D. S. (2003). A practical approach to hypercalcemia. *American Family Physician* 67, 1959–1966.
38. Inzucchi S. E. (2004). Understanding hypercalcemia. *Postgraduate Medicine* 115(4), 27–36.
39. Korbin S. M., Goldfarb S. (1990). Magnesium deficiency. *Seminars in Nephrology* 10, 525–535.
40. Tangiera E. D. (2004). Hyperparathyroidism. *American Family Physician* 69, 333–340.
41. Alfrey A. C. (2003). Normal and abnormal magnesium metabolism. In Schrier R. W. (Ed.), *Renal and electrolyte disorders* (6th ed., pp. 278–302). Philadelphia: Lippincott Williams & Wilkins.
42. Swain R., Kaplan-Machlis B. (1999). Magnesium for the next millennium. *Southern Medical Journal* 92, 1040–1046.
43. Topf J. M., Murray P. T. (2003) Hypomagnesemia and hypermagnesemia. *Reviews in Endocrine and Metabolic Disorders* 4, 195–206.

44. Adrogué H. E., Adrogué H. J. (2001). Acid-base physiology. *Respiratory Care* 46, 328–341.

45. Shapiro J. I., Kaehny W. D. (2003). Pathogenesis and management of metabolic acidosis and alkalosis. In Schrier R. W. (Ed.), *Renal and electrolyte disorders* (6th ed., pp. 115–153). Philadelphia: Lippincott Williams & Wilkins.

46. Kraut J. A., Madias N. E. (2001). Approach to patients with acid-base disorders. *Respiratory Care* 46, 392–402.

47. Abelow B. (1998). *Understanding acid-base* (pp. 43–49, 83–93, 139–169, 171–188, 189–198, 224–230). Baltimore: Williams & Wilkins.

48. Gauthier P. M., Szerlip H. M. (2002). Metabolic acidosis in the intensive care unit. *Critical Care Medicine* 18, 289–308.

49. Powers F. (1999). The role of chloride in acid-base balance. *Journal of Intravenous Nursing* 22, 286–291.

50. Alpern R. J., Sakhaee K. (1997). The clinical spectrum of chronic metabolic acidosis: Homeostatic mechanisms produce significant morbidity. *American Journal of Kidney Diseases* 29, 291–302.

51. Forsythe S. M., Schmidt G. A. (2000). Sodium bicarbonate for the treatment of lactic acidosis. *Chest* 117, 260–267.

52. Khanna A., Kurtzman N. A. (2001). Metabolic alkalosis. *Respiratory Care* 46, 354–365.

53. Galla J. H. (2000). Metabolic alkalosis. *Journal of the American Society of Nephrology* 11, 369–375.

54. Adrogué H. J., Madias N. E. (1998). Management of life-threatening acid-base disorders. *New England Journal of Medicine* 338, 107–111.

55. Kaehny W. D. (2003). Pathogenesis and management of respiratory and mixed acid-base disorders. In Schrier R. W. (Ed), *Renal and electrolyte disorders* (6th ed., pp. 154–170). Philadelphia: Lippincott Williams & Wilkins.

56. Epstein S. K., Singh N. (2001). Respiratory acidosis. *Respiratory Care* 46, 366–383.

57. Laffey J. H., Kavenaugh B. P. (2002). Hypocapnia. *New England Journal of Medicine* 347, 43–53.

58. Foste G. T., Vaziri N. D., Sassoon C. S. H. (2001). Respiratory alkalosis. *Respiratory Care* 46, 384–391.

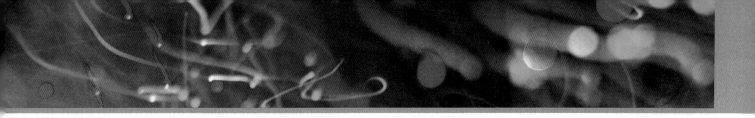

Stress and Adaptation

 Stress has become an increasingly discussed topic in today's world. The concept is discussed extensively in the health care fields, and it is found as well in economics, political science, business, and education. At the level of the popular press, the term is exploited with messages about how stress can be prevented, managed, and even eliminated.

Whether stress is more prevalent today than it was in centuries past is uncertain. Certainly, the pressures that existed were equally challenging, although of a different type. Social psychologists Richard Lazarus and Susan Folkman related that as early as the 14th century the term was used to indicate hardship, straits, adversity, or affliction.[1] In the 17th century, *stress* and related terms appeared in the context of physical sciences: *load* was defined as an external force, *stress* as the ratio of internal force created by the load to the area over which the force acted, and *strain* was the deformation or distortion of the object.[1] These concepts are still used in engineering today.

The concepts of stress and strain survived, and throughout the 19th and early 20th centuries, stress and strain were thought to be the cause of "ill health" and "mental disease."[2] By the 20th century, stress had drawn considerable attention both as a health concern and as a research focus. In 1910, when Sir William Osler delivered his Lumleian Lectures on "angina pectoris," he described the relationship of stress and strain to angina pectoris.[3] Approximately 15 years later, Walter Cannon, well known for his work in physiology, began to use the word *stress* in relation to his laboratory experiments on the "fight-or-flight" response. It seems possible that the term emerged from his work with the homeostatic features of living organisms and their tendency to "bound back" and "resist disruption" when acted on by an "external force."[4] At about the same time, Hans Selye, who became known for his research and publications on stress, began using the term *stress* in a very special way to mean an orchestrated set of bodily responses to any form of noxious stimulus.[5]

151

The content in this chapter has been organized into two sections: the first focuses on stress and adaptation and the second on disorders of the stress response.

 ## Stress and Adaptation

A variety of definitions have been given to the phenomenon of stress. The concept of stress has been studied extensively by physiologists, psychologists, sociologists, and members of the health care professions. The nature of these of these disciplines and the individual work of its members has to some extent influenced the approaches used, leading to rather disparate bodies of knowledge about stress.[6] Despite this disparity, the definition of stress seems to encompass three basic concepts: homeostasis, stress and the stress response, and adaptation and coping.

HOMEOSTASIS

The concepts of stress and adaptation have their origin in the complexity of the human body and the interactions between the body's cells and its many organ systems. The body requires that a level of homeostasis or constancy be maintained during the many changes that occur in the internal and external environments. Stress and adaptation involve feedback control systems that regulate cellular function and integrate the function of the different body system. Homeostasis can also be expanded to include the neuroendocrine control systems that influence behavior.

Constancy of the Internal Environment

Claude Bernard, a 19th century physiologist, was the first to describe clearly the central importance of a stable internal environment, which he termed the *milieu intérieur*. Bernard recognized that body fluids surrounding the cells and the various organ systems provide the means for exchange between the external and the internal environments. He also emphasized that a multicellular organism is able to survive only as long as the composition of the internal environment is compatible with the survival needs of the individual cells.

The concept of a stable internal environment was supported by Walter B. Cannon. He proposed that this kind of stability, which he called *homeostasis,* was achieved through a system of carefully coordinated physiologic processes that oppose change.[4,7] Cannon pointed out that these processes were largely automatic and emphasized that homeostasis involves resistance to both internal and external disturbances.

In his book *The Wisdom of the Body,* published in 1939, Cannon presented four tentative propositions to describe the general features of homeostasis.[7] With this set of propositions, Cannon emphasized that when a factor is known to shift homeostasis in one direction, it is reasonable to expect the existence of mechanisms that have the opposite effect. In the homeostatic regulation of blood sugar, for example, mechanisms that both raise and lower blood sugar would be expected to play a part. As long as the responding mechanism to the initiating disturbance can recover homeostasis, the integrity of the body and the status of normality are retained.

Control Systems

The ability of the body to function and maintain homeostasis under conditions of change in the internal and external environment depends on the thousands of physiologic *control systems* that function to keep a physical or chemical parameter of the body relatively constant. These control systems are composed of sensors that detect changes in a physiologic function, an integrator or comparator that sums and compares the sensed changes with a set point, and an effector system that returns the sensed function to within the range of the set point. The body's control systems regulate cellular function, control life processes, and integrate functions of the different organ systems.

Of recent interest have been the neuroendocrine control systems that influence behavior. Biochemical messengers that exist in our brain control nerve activity, information flow, and, ultimately, behavior.[8] These control systems function in producing the emotional reactions to stressors. In persons with mental health disorders, they can interact in the production of symptoms associated with the disorder. The field of neuropharmacology has focused on the modulation of the endogenous messengers and signaling systems that control behavior in the treatment of mental disorders such as anxiety disorders, depression, and schizophrenia.

Constancy of the Internal Environment

1. Constancy in an open system, such as our bodies represent, requires mechanisms that act to maintain this constancy. Cannon based this proposition on insights into the ways by which steady states such as glucose concentrations, body temperature, and acid-base balance were regulated.
2. Steady-state conditions require that any tendency toward change automatically meet with factors that resist change. An increase in blood sugar results in thirst as the body attempts to dilute the concentration of sugar in the extracellular fluid.
3. The regulating system that determines the homeostatic state consists of a number of cooperating mechanisms acting simultaneously or successively. Blood sugar is regulated by insulin, glucagon, and other hormones that control its release from the liver or its uptake by the tissues.
4. Homeostasis does not occur by chance, but is the result of organized self-government.

(Cannon W. B. [1932]. *The wisdom of the body* (pp. 299–300). New York: W.W. Norton.)

Allostasis

A different view of factors affecting constancy involves the concept of *allostasis*. In contrast to homeostasis, in which stability is achieved through processes that oppose change, allostasis describes the ability to achieve stability through change.[9] Also in contrast to homeostasis, which is based in the physiologic responses, allostasis involves both the person's perception of the situation and the ability to mount an appropriate response. In allostasis, previous experience and learning serve as the control system for a person's perception of the situation. Formally, instability occurs whenever there is a discrepancy between what the person perceives the situation should be and what it is. This has been termed the *cognitive activation theory of stress*.[10]

THE STRESS RESPONSE

In the early 1930s, the world-renowned endocrinologist Hans Selye was the first to describe a group of specific anatomic changes that occurred in rats that were exposed to a variety of different experimental stimuli. He came to an understanding that these changes were manifestations of the body's attempt to adapt to stimuli. Selye described *stress* as "a state manifested by a specific syndrome of the body developed in response to any stimuli that made an intense systemic demand on it."[5]

In his early career as an experimental scientist, Selye noted that a triad of adrenal enlargement, thymic atrophy, and gastric ulcer appeared in rats he was using for his studies. These same three changes developed in response to many different or nonspecific experimental challenges. He assumed that the hypothalamic-pituitary-adrenal (HPA) axis played a pivotal role in the development of this response. To Selye, the response to stressors was a process that enabled the rats to resist the experimental challenge by using the function of the system best able to respond to it. He labeled the response the *general adaptation syndrome* (GAS): *general* because the effect was a general systemic reaction, *adaptive* because the response was in reaction to a stressor, and *syndrome* because the physical manifestations were coordinated and dependent on each other.[5]

According to Selye, the GAS involves three stages: the alarm stage, the stage of resistance, and the stage of exhaustion. The *alarm stage* is characterized by a generalized stimulation of the sympathetic nervous system and the HPA axis, resulting in the release of catecholamines, which are the neuromediators of the sympathetic nervous system, and the hormone cortisol, which is released from adrenal cortex. During the *resistance stage,* the body selects the most effective and economic channels of defense. During this stage, the increased cortisol levels present during the first stage drop because they are no longer needed. If the stressor is prolonged or overwhelms the ability of the body to defend itself, the *stage of exhaustion* ensues, during which resources are depleted and signs of "wear and tear" or systemic damage appear.[11] Selye contended that many ailments, such as various emotional disturbances, mildly annoying headaches, insomnia, upset stomach, gastric and duodenal ulcers, certain types of rheumatic disorders, and cardiovascular and kidney diseases appear to be initiated or encouraged by the "body itself because of its faulty adaptive reactions to potentially injurious agents."[12]

The events or environmental agents responsible for initiating the stress response were called *stressors*. According to Selye, stressors could be endogenous, arising from within the body, or exogenous, arising from outside the body.[12] Stressors tend to produce different responses in different persons or in the same person at different times, indicating the influence of the adaptive capacity of the person, or what Selye called *conditioning factors*. These conditioning factors may be internal (*e.g.*, genetic predisposition, age, sex) or external (*e.g.*, exposure to environmental agents, life experiences, dietary factors, level of social support).[12]

Selye emphasized the role of an integrated response of multiple systems rather than isolated reflexes. Although virtually all organs are affected by exposure to stress, the neuroendocrine and immune systems are the first to experience functional changes. These responses are further exemplified by the neuroendocrine responses that interact with the immune system and affect the cardiovascular, gastrointestinal, reproductive, and other body systems.

Neuroendocrine Responses

The manifestations of the stress response are strongly influenced by both the nervous and endocrine systems.[13] The neuroendocrine systems integrate signals received along neurosensory pathways and from circulating mediators that are carried in the bloodstream. In addition, the immune system both affects and is affected by the stress response. Table 7-1 summarizes the action of hormones involved in the neuroendocrine response to stress.

The stress response is meant to protect the person against acute threats to homeostasis and is normally time limited. Therefore, under normal circumstances, the neural responses and the hormones that are released during the response are not present long enough to cause damage to vital tissues. However, in situations in which the stress response is hyperactive or becomes habituated, the physiologic and behavioral changes (*e.g.*, immunosuppression, sympathetic system activation) induced by the response can themselves become a threat to homeostasis. If the stress response is hypoactive, the person may be more susceptible to diseases associated with overactivity of the immune response.[14]

The integration of the stress responses, which occurs at the level of the central nervous system (CNS), is complex and not completely understood. It relies on communication along neuronal pathways of the cerebral cortex, the limbic system, the thalamus, the hypothalamus, the pituitary gland, and the reticular activating

TABLE 7-1	Hormones Involved in the Neuroendocrine Response to Stress	
Hormones Associated With the Stress Response	Source of the Hormone	Physiologic Effects
Catecholamines (norepinephrine, epinephrine)	Locus ceruleus, adrenal medulla	Produces a decrease in insulin release and an increase in glucagon release resulting in increased glycogenolysis, gluconeogenesis, lipolysis, proteolysis, and decreased glucose uptake by the peripheral tissues; an increase in heart rate, cardiac contractility, and vascular smooth muscle contraction; and relaxation of bronchial smooth muscle
Corticotropin-releasing factor (CRF)	Hypothalamus	Stimulates ACTH release from anterior pituitary and increased activity of neurons in locus ceruleus
Adrenocorticotropic hormone (ACTH)	Anterior pituitary	Stimulates the synthesis and release of cortisol
Glucocorticoid hormones (e.g., cortisol)	Adrenal cortex	Potentiates the actions of epinephrine and glucagon; inhibits the release and/or actions of the reproductive hormones and thyroid-stimulating hormone; and produces a decrease in immune cells and inflammatory mediators
Mineralocorticoid hormones (e.g., aldosterone)	Adrenal cortex	Increases sodium absorption by the kidney
Antidiuretic hormone (ADH, vasopressin)	Hypothalamus, posterior pituitary	Increases water absorption by the kidney, produces vasoconstriction of blood vessels; and stimulates the release of ACTH

system (RAS) (Fig. 7-1). The cerebral cortex is involved with vigilance, cognition, and focused attention, and the limbic system with emotional components (e.g., fear, excitement, rage, anger) of the stress response. The thalamus functions as the relay center and is important in receiving, sorting out, and distributing sensory input. The hypothalamus coordinates the responses of the endocrine and autonomic nervous systems (ANS). The RAS modulates mental alertness, ANS activity, and skeletal muscle tone, using input from other neural structures. The musculoskeletal tension that occurs during the stress response reflects the increased activity of the RAS and its influence on the reflex circuits that control muscle tone.

Locus Ceruleus. Central to the neural component of the neuroendocrine response to the stress is an area in the brain stem called the locus ceruleus (LC).[15] The locus ceruleus is densely populated with neurons that produce norepinephrine (NE) and is thought to be the central integrating site for the ANS response to stressful stimuli (Fig. 7-2). The LC-NE system has afferent pathways to the hypothalamus, the limbic system, the hippocampus, and the cerebral cortex.

The LC-NE system confers an adaptive advantage during a stressful situation. The sympathetic nervous system manifestation of the stress reaction has been called the *fight-or-flight response.* This is the most rapid of the stress responses and represents the basic survival response of our primitive ancestors when confronted with the perils of the wilderness and its inhabitants. The increase in sympathetic activity in the brain increases attention and arousal and thus probably intensifies memory. The heart and respiratory rates increase, the hands and feet become moist, the pupils dilate, the mouth becomes dry, and the activity of the gastrointestinal tract decreases.

Corticotropin-Releasing Factor. Corticotropin-releasing factor (CRF) is central to the endocrine component of the neuroendocrine response to stress (see Fig. 7-2). CRF is a small peptide hormone found in both the hypothalamus and in extrahypothalamic structures, such as the limbic system and the brain stem. It is both an important endocrine regulator of pituitary and adrenal activity and a neurotransmitter involved in autonomic nervous system activity, metabolism, and behavior.[16–19] Receptors for CRF are distributed throughout the brain as well as many peripheral sites. CRF (also called corticotropin-releasing hormone) from the hypothalamus induces the secretion of the adrenocorticotropic hormone (ACTH) from the anterior pituitary gland. ACTH, in turn, stimulates the adrenal gland to synthesize and secrete the glucocorticoid hormones, about 95% of which is cortisol.

The glucocorticoid hormones have a number of direct or indirect effects that help mediate the ongoing or pending stress response, enhance the action of other stress hormones, or suppress other components of the stress response. In this regard, cortisol acts both as a mediator of the stress response and an inhibitor of the stress response such that overactivation does not occur.[18] Cortisol maintains blood glucose levels by antagonizing the effects of insulin and enhances the effect of catecholamines on the cardiovascular system. It also suppresses osteoblast activity, hematopoiesis, protein and collagen synthesis, and immune responses. All of these functions are meant to protect the organism against the effects of a stressor and to focus energy on regaining balance in the face of an acute challenge to homeostasis. Cortisol also plays an

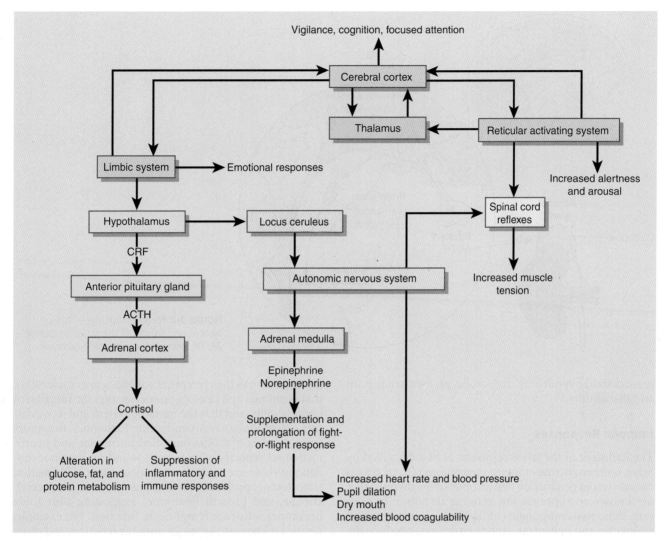

FIGURE 7-1 Neuroendocrine pathways and physiologic responses to stress. CRF, corticotropin-releasing factor; ACTH, adrenocorticotropic hormone.

important regulatory role in the neuroendocrine control of the HPA axis on termination of the stress response by exerting negative feedback at all levels of the hypothalamus and pituitary.

Other Hormones. A wide variety of other hormones, including growth hormones, thyroid hormone, and the reproductive hormones, also are responsive to stressful situations. Systems responsible for reproduction, growth, and immunity are directly linked to the stress system, and the hormonal effects of the stress response profoundly influence these systems.

Although growth hormone is initially elevated at the onset of stress, the prolonged presence of cortisol leads to suppression of growth hormone, insulinlike growth factor-I (IGF-I), and other growth factors, exerting a chronically inhibitory effect on growth. In addition, CRF directly increases somatostatin, which in turn inhibits growth hormone secretion. Although the connection is speculative, the effects of stress on growth hormone may

provide one of the vital links to understanding failure to thrive in some children.

Stress-induced cortisol secretion also is associated with decreased levels of thyroid-stimulating hormone and inhibition of conversion of thyroxine to the more biologically active triiodothyronine in peripheral tissues. Both changes may serve as a means to conserve energy at times of stress.

Antidiuretic hormone (ADH) also is involved in the stress response, particularly in hypotensive stress or stress caused by fluid volume loss. ADH, also known as vasopressin, increases water retention by the kidneys, produces vasoconstriction of blood vessels, and appears to synergize CRF's capacity to increase the release of ACTH.

The reproductive hormones are inhibited by CRF at the hypophysial level and by cortisol at the pituitary, gonadal, and target tissue levels.[19] Sepsis and severe trauma can induce anovulation and irregular menstrual cycles in women and decreased spermatogenesis and decreased levels of testosterone in men. In addition, emotional and life stresses can influence the severity of

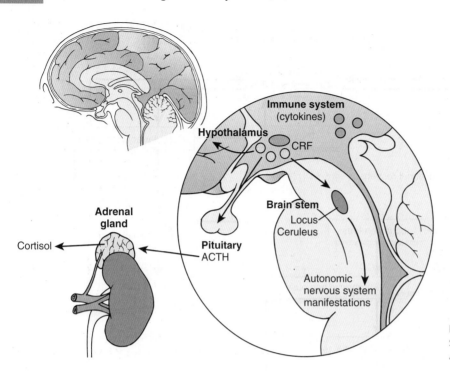

FIGURE 7-2 Neuroendocrine–immune system regulation of the stress response. ACTH, adrenocorticotropic hormone.

premenstrual syndrome and cyclic premenstrual pain and discomfort.[19]

Immune Responses

The hallmark of the stress response, as first described by Selye, is the endocrine–immune interactions (*i.e.*, increased corticosteroid production and atrophy of the thymus) that are known to suppress the immune response. In concert, these two components of the stress system, through endocrine and neurotransmitter pathways, produce the physical and behavioral changes designed to adapt to acute stress. Much of the literature regarding stress and the immune response focuses on the causal role of stress in immune-related diseases. It has also been suggested that the reverse may occur; emotional and psychological manifestations of the stress response may be a reflection of alterations in the CNS resulting from the immune response (see Fig. 7-2). Immune cells such as monocytes and lymphocytes can penetrate the blood-brain barrier and take up residence in the brain, where they secrete cytokines and other inflammatory mediators that influence the stress response. In the case of cancer, this could mean that the subjective feelings of helplessness and hopelessness that have been repeatedly related to the onset and progression of cancers may arise secondary to the CNS effects of products released by immune cells during the early stage of the disease.[20]

The exact mechanism by which stress produces its effect on the immune response is unknown and probably varies from person to person, depending on genetic endowment and environmental factors. The three most significant arguments for interactions between the neuroendocrine and immune systems derive from evidence that the immune and neuroendocrine systems share common signal pathways (*i.e.*, receptors and messenger molecules), that hormones and neuropeptides can alter the function of immune cells, and that the immune system and its mediators can modulate neuroendocrine function.[21] Receptors for a number of CNS-controlled hormones and neuromediators reportedly have been found on lymphocytes. Among these are receptors for glucocorticoids, insulin, testosterone, prolactin, catecholamines, estrogens, acetylcholine, and growth hormone, suggesting that these hormones influence lymphocyte function. For example, cortisol is known to suppress immune function, and pharmacologic doses of cortisol are used clinically to suppress the immune response. There also is evidence that the immune system, in turn, influences neuroendocrine function.[22] It has been observed that the HPA axis is activated by cytokines such as interleukin-1, interleukin-6, and tumor necrosis factor that are released from immune cells (see Chapter 13).

A second possible route for neuroendocrine regulation of immune function is through the sympathetic nervous system and the release of catecholamines. The lymph nodes, thymus, and spleen are supplied with ANS nerve fibers. Thus, centrally acting CRF can act synergistically with cortisol to inhibit the immune system by activating the ANS.

Not only is the quantity of immune response changed because of stress, but the type of response may be changed. The messenger molecules associated with stress response may differentially affect the proliferation of different subtypes of T-helper lymphocytes. Because these T-helper cell subtypes secrete different cytokines, they stimulate different aspects of the immune response. One subtype tends to stimulate the cell-mediated immune responses, whereas a second type tends to activate B lymphocytes and humoral-mediated immune responses.

ADAPTATION TO STRESS

The ability to adapt to a wide range of environments and stressors is not peculiar to humans. According to René Dubos (a microbiologist noted for his study of human responses to the total environment), "adaptability is found throughout life and is perhaps the one attribute that distinguishes most clearly the world of life from the world of inanimate matter."[23] Living organisms, no matter how primitive, do not submit passively to the impact of environmental forces. They attempt to respond adaptively, each in its own unique and most suitable manner. The higher the organism is on the evolutionary scale, the larger its repertoire of adaptive mechanisms and its ability to select and limit aspects of the environment to which it responds. The most fully evolved mechanisms are the social responses through which individuals or groups modify their environments, their habits, or both to achieve a way of life that is best suited to their needs.

Human beings, because of their highly developed nervous system and intellect, usually have alternative mechanisms for adapting and have the ability to control many aspects of their environment. Air conditioning and central heating limit the need to adapt to extreme changes in environmental temperature. The availability of antiseptic agents, immunizations, and antibiotics eliminates the need to respond to common infectious agents. At the same time, modern technology creates new challenges for adaptation and provides new sources of stress, such as increased noise, air pollution, exposure to harmful chemicals, and changes in biologic rhythms imposed by shift work and transcontinental air travel.

Of particular interest are the differences in the body's response to events that threaten the integrity of the body's physiologic environment and those that threaten the integrity of the person's psychosocial environment. Many of the body's responses to physiologic disturbances are controlled on a moment-by-moment basis by feedback mechanisms that limit their application and duration of action. For example, the baroreflex-mediated rise in heart rate that occurs when a person moves from the recumbent to the standing position is almost instantaneous and subsides within seconds. Furthermore, the response to physiologic disturbances that threaten the integrity of the internal environment is specific to the threat; the body usually does not raise the body temperature when an increase in heart rate is needed. In contrast, the response to psychological disturbances is not regulated with the same degree of specificity and feedback control; instead, the effect may be inappropriate and sustained.

Factors Affecting the Ability to Adapt

Adaptation implies that an individual has successfully created a new balance between the stressor and the ability to deal with it. The means used to attain this balance are called *coping strategies* or *coping mechanisms*. Coping mechanisms are the emotional and behavioral responses used to manage threats to our physiologic and psychological homeostasis. According to Lazarus, how we cope with stressful events depends on how we perceive and interpret the event.[24] Is the event perceived as a threat of harm or loss? And, is the event perceived as a challenge rather than a threat? Physiologic reserve, time, genetic endowment and age, health status, nutrition, sleep–wake cycles, hardiness, and psychosocial factors all influence a person's appraisal of a stressor and the coping mechanisms used to adapt to the new situation (Fig. 7-3).

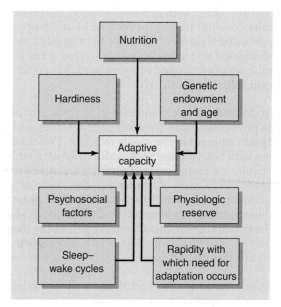

FIGURE 7-3 Factors affecting adaptation.

KEY CONCEPTS

Stress and Adaptation

➤ Stress is a state manifested by symptoms that arise from the coordinated activation of the neuroendocrine and immune systems, which Selye called the *general adaptation syndrome.*

➤ The hormones and neurotransmitters (catecholamines and cortisol) that are released during the stress response function to alert the individual to a threat or challenge to homeostasis, to enhance cardiovascular and metabolic activity in order to manage the stressor, and to focus the energy of the body by suppressing the activity of other systems that are not immediately needed.

➤ Adaptation is the ability to respond to challenges of physical or psychological homeostasis and to return to a balanced state.

➤ The ability to adapt is influenced by previous learning, physiologic reserve, time, genetic endowment, age, health status and nutrition, sleep–wake cycles, and psychosocial factors.

Physiologic and Anatomic Reserve. The safety margin for adaptation of most body systems is considerably greater than that needed for normal activities. The trained athlete is able to increase cardiac output sixfold to sevenfold during exercise. The red blood cells carry more oxygen than the tissues can use, the liver and fat cells store excess nutrients, and bone tissue stores calcium in excess of that needed for normal neuromuscular function. The ability of body systems to increase their function given the need to adapt is known as the *physiologic reserve.* Many of the body organs, such as the lungs, kidneys, and adrenals, are paired to provide anatomic reserve as well. Both organs are not needed to ensure the continued existence and maintenance of the internal environment. Many persons function normally with only one lung or one kidney.

Time. Adaptation is most efficient when changes occur gradually, rather than suddenly. For instance, it is possible to lose a liter or more of blood through chronic gastrointestinal bleeding during the period of a week or more without manifesting signs of shock. However, a sudden hemorrhage that causes rapid loss of an equal amount of blood is likely to cause hypotension and shock.

Genetic Endowment. Adaptation is further affected by the availability of adaptive responses and flexibility in selecting the most appropriate and economical response. The greater the number of available responses, the more effective is the capacity to adapt.

Genetic endowment can ensure that the systems that are essential to adaptation function adequately. Even a gene that has deleterious effects may prove adaptive in some environments. In Africa, the gene for sickle cell anemia persists in some populations because it provides some resistance to infection with the parasite that causes malaria.

Age. The capacity to adapt is decreased at the extremes of age. The ability to adapt is impaired by the immaturity of an infant, much as it is by the decline in functional reserve that occurs with age. For example, the infant has difficulty concentrating urine because of immature renal structures and therefore is less able than an adult to cope with decreased water intake or exaggerated water losses. A similar situation, caused by age-related changes in renal function, exists in the elderly.

Health Status. Physical and mental health status determines physiologic and psychological reserves and is a strong determinant of the ability to adapt. For example, persons with heart disease are less able to adjust to stresses that require the recruitment of cardiovascular responses. Severe emotional stress often produces disruption of physiologic function and limits the ability to make appropriate choices related to long-term adaptive needs. Those who have worked with acutely ill persons know that the will to live often has a profound influence on survival during life-threatening illnesses.

Nutrition. There are 50 to 60 essential nutrients, including minerals, lipids, certain fatty acids, vitamins, and specific amino acids. Deficiencies or excesses of any of these nutrients can alter a person's health status and impair the ability to adapt. The importance of nutrition to enzyme function, immune response, and wound healing is well known. On a worldwide basis, malnutrition may be one of the most common causes of immunodeficiency.

Among the problems associated with dietary excess are obesity and alcohol abuse. Obesity is becoming an increasingly common problem in industrialized societies. It predisposes to a number of health problems, including atherosclerosis and hypertension. Alcohol is commonly used in excess. It acutely affects brain function and, with long-term use, can seriously impair the function of the liver, brain, and other vital structures.

Sleep–Wake Cycles. Sleep is considered to be a restorative function in which energy is restored and tissues are regenerated.[25] Sleep occurs in a cyclic manner, alternating with periods of wakefulness and increased energy use. Biologic rhythms play an important role in adaptation to stress, development of illness, and response to medical treatment. Many rhythms, such as rest and activity, work and leisure, and eating and drinking, oscillate with a frequency similar to that of the 24-hour light–dark solar day. The term *circadian,* from the Latin *circa* ("about") and *dies* ("day"), is used to describe these 24-hour diurnal rhythms.

Sleep disorders and alterations in the sleep–wake cycle have been shown to alter immune function, the normal circadian pattern of hormone secretion, and physical and psychological functioning.[26] The two most common manifestations of an alteration in the sleep–wake cycle are insomnia and sleep deprivation or increased somnolence. In some persons, stress may produce sleep disorders, and in others, sleep disorders may lead to stress. Acute stress and environmental disturbances, loss of a loved one, recovery from surgery, and pain are common causes of transient and short-term insomnia. Air travel and jet lag constitute additional causes of altered sleep–wake cycles, as does shift work. In persons with chronic insomnia, the bed often acquires many unpleasant secondary associations and becomes a place of stress and worry, rather than a place of rest.[27]

Hardiness. Studies by social psychologists have focused on individuals' emotional reactions to stressful situations and their coping mechanisms to determine those characteristics that help some people remain healthy despite being challenged by high levels of stressors. For example, the concept of *hardiness* describes a personality characteristic that includes a sense of having control over the environment, a sense of having a purpose in life, and an ability to conceptualize stressors as a challenge, rather than a threat.[28] Many studies by nurses and social psychologists suggest that hardiness is correlated with positive health outcomes.[28]

Psychosocial Factors. Several studies have related social factors and life events to illness. Scientific interest in the social environment as a cause of stress has gradually broadened to include the social environment as a resource that modulates the relation between stress and health. Presumably, persons who can mobilize strong supportive resources from within their social relationships are better able to withstand the negative effects of stress on their health. Studies suggest that social support has direct and indirect positive effects on health status and serves as a buffer or modifier of the physical and psychosocial effects of stress.[29]

Social networks contribute in a number of ways to a person's psychosocial and physical integrity. The configuration of significant others that constitutes this network functions to mobilize the resources of the person; these friends, colleagues, and family members share the person's tasks and provide monetary support, materials and tools, and guidance in improving problem-solving capabilities.[30] Persons with ample social networks are not as likely to experience many types of stress, such as being homeless or being lonely. There is also evidence that persons who have social supports or social assets may live longer and have a lower incidence of somatic illness.[30]

Social support has been viewed in terms of the number of relationships a person has and the person's perception of these relationships.[31] Close relationships with others can involve positive effects as well as the potential for conflict and may, in some situations, leave the person less able to cope with life stressors.

In summary, physiologic and psychological adaptation involves the ability to maintain the constancy of the internal environment (homeostasis) and behavior in the face of a wide range of changes in the internal and external environments. It involves control systems that regulate cellular function, control life's processes, regulate behavior, and integrate the function of the different body systems. In contrast to homeostasis, allostasis describes the ability to achieve stability through processes that oppose change; instability occurs whenever there is a discrepancy between what the person perceives the situation should be and what it is.

The stress response, as described by the late Hans Selye, is a state manifested by the body's response to any stimulus that makes an intense systemic demand on it. Selye called this response the *general adaptation syndrome.* The stress response is divided into three stages: the *alarm stage,* with activation of the sympathetic nervous system and the HPA axis; the *resistance stage,* during which the body selects the most effective defenses; and the *stage of exhaustion,* during which physiologic resources are depleted and signs of systemic damage appear. The activation and control of the stress response are mediated by the combined efforts of the nervous and endocrine systems. The neuroendocrine systems integrate signals received along neurosensory pathways and from circulating mediators that are carried in the bloodstream. In addition, the immune system both affects and is affected by the stress response.

Adaptation to stress and the stress response is affected by a number of factors, including experience and previous learning, the rapidity with which the need to adapt occurs, genetic endowment and age, health status, nutrition, sleep–wake cycles, hardiness, and psychosocial factors.

 # Disorders of the Stress Response

For the most part, the stress response is meant to be acute and time limited. The time-limited nature of the process renders the accompanying catabolic and immunosuppressive effects advantageous. It is the chronicity of the response that is thought to be disruptive to physical and mental health.

Stressors can assume a number of patterns in relation to time. They may be classified as acute time-limited, chronic intermittent, or chronic sustained. An acute time-limited stressor is one that occurs over a short time and does not recur; a chronic intermittent stressor is one to which a person is chronically exposed. The frequency or chronicity of circumstances to which the body is asked to respond often determines the availability and efficiency of the stress responses. For example, the response of the immune system is more rapid and efficient on second exposure to an infectious agent than it is on first exposure.

EFFECTS OF ACUTE STRESS

The reactions to acute stress are those associated with the autonomic nervous system, the fight-or-flight response. The manifestations of the stress response—a pounding headache, cold, moist skin, a stiff neck—are all part of the acute stress response. Centrally, there is facilitation of neural pathways mediating arousal, alertness, vigilance, cognition, and focused attention, as well as appropriate aggression. The acute stress response can result from either psychologically or physiologically threatening events. In situations of life-threatening trauma, these acute responses may be lifesaving in that they divert blood from less essential to more essential body functions. Increased alertness and cognitive functioning enables rapid processing of information and arrival at the most appropriate solution to the threatening situation.

However, for persons with limited coping abilities, either because of physical or mental health, the acute stress response may be detrimental. This is true of persons with preexisting heart disease in whom the overwhelming sympathetic behaviors associated with the stress response can lead to dysrhythmias. For people with other chronic health problems, such as headache disorder, acute stress may precipitate a recurrence. In healthy individuals, the acute stress response can redirect attention from behaviors that promote health, such as attention to proper meals and getting adequate sleep. For those with health problems, it can interrupt compliance with medication regimens and exercise programs. In some situations, the acute arousal state actually can be life threatening, physically immobilizing the person when movement would avert catastrophe (*e.g.*, moving out of the way of a speeding car).

EFFECTS OF CHRONIC STRESS

The stress response is designed to be an acute self-limited response in which activation of the ANS and the HPA axis is controlled in a negative feedback manner. As with all negative feedback systems, including the stress response system, pathophysiologic changes can occur. Function can be altered in several ways, including when a component of the system fails; when the neural and hormonal connections among the components of the system are dysfunctional; and when the original stimulus for the activation of the system is prolonged or of such magnitude that it overwhelms the ability of the system to respond appropriately. In these cases, the system may become overactive or underactive.

Chronicity and excessive activation of the stress response can result from chronic illnesses as well as contribute to the development of long-term health problems. Chronic activation of the stress response is an important public health issue from both a health and a cost perspective. The National Institute for Occupational Safety and Health declared stress a hazard of the workplace.[32] It is linked to a myriad of health disorders, such as diseases of the cardiovascular, gastrointestinal, immune, and neurologic systems, as well as depression, chronic alcoholism and drug abuse, eating disorders, accidents, and suicide.

Occurrence of the oral disease acute necrotizing gingivitis, in which the normal bacterial flora of the mouth become invasive, is known by dentists to be associated with acute stress, such as final examinations.[33] Similarly, herpes simplex type 1 infection (*i.e.*, cold sores) often develops during periods of inadequate rest, fever, ultraviolet radiation, and emotional upset. The resident herpes-virus is kept in check by body defenses, probably T lymphocytes, until a stressful event occurs that causes suppression of the immune system. Psychological stress is associated in a dose–response manner with an increased risk for development of the common cold, and this risk is attributable to increased rates of infection, rather than frequency of symptoms after infection.[34]

In a study in which participants were infected with the influenza virus, persons who reported the greatest amount of premorbid stress also reported the most intense influenza symptoms and had a statistically greater production of interleukin-6, a cytokine that acts as a chemotactic agent for immune cells.[35] Elderly caregivers of a spouse with dementia had a significantly higher score for emotional distress and higher salivary cortisol than did matched control subjects. The higher stress was correlated with a decreased immune response to the influenza vaccine.[36] The experience of stress also has been associated with delays in wound healing.[37]

POST-TRAUMATIC STRESS DISORDER

The post-traumatic stress disorder (PTSD) is an example of chronic activation of the stress response as a result of experiencing a potentially life-threatening event. It was formerly called *battle fatigue* or *shell shock* because it was first characterized in men and women returning from combat. Although war is still a significant cause of PTSD, other major catastrophic events, including major weather-related disasters such as hurricanes and tsunamis, airplane crashes, terrorist bombings, and rape or child abuse, also may result in the development of the disorder. The terrorist attack on the World Trade Center and Pentagon on September 11, 2001, represented an amalgam of interpersonal violence, loss, and threat to tens of thousands of people.[38] These events have influenced and will continue to influence the development of PTSD in a substantial number of people. Past exposure to war increases the risk of PTSD. Witnessing atrocities, seeing the death of children, seeing friends killed and wounded, and feeling responsibility for the death of a friend are especially disturbing elements of combat and war environments for both military and civilian persons.[39]

PTSD is characterized by a constellation of three types of symptoms that are experienced as states of intrusion, avoidance, and hyperarousal. *Intrusion* refers to the reexperiencing of an event through the occurrence of "flashbacks" during waking hours or nightmares in which the past traumatic event is relived, often in vivid and frightening detail. *Avoidance* refers to the emotional numbing that accompanies this disorder and disrupts important personal relationships. Because a person with PTSD has not been able to resolve the painful feelings associated with the trauma, depression is commonly a part of the clinical picture. Survivor guilt also may be a product of traumatic situations in which the person survived the disaster but loved ones did not. *Hyperarousal* refers to the presence of increased irritability, concentration difficulties, exaggerated startle reflex, and increased vigilance and concern over safety. In addition, memory problems, sleep disturbances, and excessive anxiety are commonly experienced by persons with PTSD.

To be given a diagnosis of PTSD, a person has to have been exposed to an extreme stress or a traumatic event and have symptoms that focus on reexperiencing the event, avoidance of stimuli associated with the trauma, and persistent symptoms of increased arousal. The three types of symptoms must be present together for at least 1 month and the disorder must have caused clinically significant distress or impairment in social, occupational, and other areas of functioning.[40]

Although the pathophysiology of PTSD is not completely understood, the revelation of physiologic changes related to the disorder has shed light on why some people recover from the disorder, whereas others do not. It has been hypothesized that the intrusive symptoms of PTSD may arise from exaggerated sympathetic nervous system activation in response to the traumatic event. Persons with chronic PTSD have been shown to have increased levels of norepinephrine and increased activity of α_2-adrenergic receptors.[41] The increase in catecholamines, in tandem with increased thyroid hormone levels in persons with PTSD, is thought to explain some of the intrusive and somatic symptoms of the disorder.[41,42]

Recent neuroanatomic studies have identified alterations in two brain structures (the amygdala and hippocampus) in persons with PTSD. Positron emission tomography (PET) and functional magnetic resonance imaging (fMRI) have shown increased reactivity of the amygdala and hippocampus and decreased reactivity of the anterior cingulate and orbitofrontal areas. These areas of the brain are involved in fear responses. The hippocampus also functions in memory processes. Differences in hippocampal function and memory processes suggest a neuroanatomic basis for the intrusive recollections and other cognitive problems that characterize PTSD.[38]

Importantly, the observed neuroanatomic changes in persons with PTSD do not uniformly resemble those seen with other types of stress.[42] For example, persons with PTSD demonstrate decreased cortisol levels, increased sensitivity of cortisol receptors, and an enhanced negative feedback inhibition of cortisol release with the dexamethasone suppression test. Dexamethasone is a synthetic glucocorticoid that mimics the effects of cortisol and directly inhibits the action of CRF and ACTH. This is in contrast to persons with major depression, who have a decreased sensitivity of glucocorticoid receptors, a high plasma level of cortisol, and a decreased dexamethasone suppression of cortisol release.[42] The hypersuppression of cortisol observed with the dexamethasone test suggests that persons with PTSD do not exhibit a classic stress response as described by Selye. Because this hypersuppression has not been described in other psychiatric disorders, it may serve as a relatively specific marker for PTSD.

Little is known about the risk factors that predispose people to the development of PTSD. Less than half of all people who are exposed to a traumatic event develop PTSD; for example, only 15% to 30% of soldiers exposed to combat develop the disorder.[43] It also has been found that children exposed to violent events but who have strong family relationships rarely develop PTSD.[44] Statistics indicate there is a need for studies to determine risk factors for PTSD as a means of targeting individuals who may need intensive therapeutic measures after a life-threatening event. Research also is needed to determine the mechanisms by which the disorder develops so that it can be prevented, or if that is not possible, so that treatment methods can be created to decrease the devastating effects that this disorder has on affected individuals and their families.[41]

It is suggested that health care professionals need to be aware that clients who present with symptoms of depression, anxiety, and alcohol or drug abuse may in fact be suffering from PTSD. The client history should include questions concerning recent or remote trauma exposure, although the method used may vary depending on the recency of the traumatic event.[39] The first interventions in the aftermath of acute trauma consist of emergency medical and supportive psychological support. Crisis teams are often among the first people to attend to the emotional needs of those caught in catastrophic events. In these situations, diagnostic evaluation may be continued after the initial period has passed and a physically and psychologically safe environment has been provided. It is important for this diagnostic assessment to include a complete evaluation for PTSD.

The general goals for treatment of PTSD include measures to reduce the severity of the disorder, prevent or treat trauma-related disorders that may be present or emerge, improve adaptive functioning and restore a psychological sense of safety and trust, limit generalization of the danger experienced as a result of the traumatic situation, and protect against relapse.[39] Debriefing, or talking about the traumatic event at the time it happens, often is an effective therapeutic tool. Some people may need continued individual or group therapy. Often concurrent pharmacotherapy with antidepressant and antianxiety agents is useful and helps the individual participate more fully in therapy.

TREATMENT OF STRESS DISORDERS

The treatment of stress should be directed toward helping people avoid coping behaviors that impose a risk to their health and providing them with alternative stress-reducing strategies. Purposeful priority setting and problem solving can be used by persons who are overwhelmed by the number of life stresses to which they have been exposed. Other nonpharmacologic methods used for stress reduction are relaxation techniques, guided imagery, music therapy, massage, and biofeedback.

The Relaxation Response

Practices for evoking the relaxation response are numerous.[45] They are found in virtually every culture and are credited with producing a generalized decrease in sympathetic system activity and musculoskeletal tension. According to Herbert Benson, a physician who worked in developing the technique, four elements are integral to the various relaxation techniques: a repetitive mental device, a passive attitude, decreased muscle tension, and a quiet environment.[46] Benson developed a noncultural method that is commonly used for achieving relaxation (see accompanying box).

Progressive muscle relaxation, originally developed by Edmund Jacobson, who did extensive research on the muscle correlates of anxiety and tension, is another method of relieving tension. He observed that tension can be defined physiologically as the inappropriate contraction of muscle fibers. His procedure, which has been modified by a number of therapists, consists of systematic contraction and relaxation of major muscle groups.[47] As the person learns to relax, the various muscle groups are combined. Eventually, the person learns to relax individual muscle groups without first contracting them.

Imagery

Guided imagery is another technique that can be used to achieve relaxation. One method is scene visualization, in which the person is asked to sit back, close the eyes, and

The Relaxation Response

- Sit quietly in a comfortable position.
- Deeply relax all your muscles, beginning at your feet and progressing up to your face.
- Breathe through your nose. Become aware of your breathing. As you breathe out, say the word "one" silently to yourself. Continue for 20 minutes. When you have finished, sit quietly for several minutes, first with your eyes closed and then with them open.
- Do not worry about whether you are successful in achieving a deep level of relaxation. Maintain a positive attitude and permit the relaxation to occur at its own rate. Expect distracting thoughts, ignore them, and continue repeating "one" as you breathe out.

(Modified from Benson H. [1977]. Systemic hypertension and the relaxation response. *New England Journal of Medicine* 296, 1152.)

concentrate on a scene narrated by the therapist. Whenever possible, all five senses are involved: the person attempts to see, feel, hear, touch, and taste aspects of the visual experience. Other types of imagery involve imagining the appearance of each of the major muscle groups and how they feel during tension and relaxation.

Music Therapy

Music therapy is used for both its physiologic and psychological effects. It involves listening to selected pieces of music as a means of ameliorating anxiety or stress, reducing pain, decreasing feelings of loneliness and isolation, buffering noise, and facilitating expression of emotion. Music is defined as having three components: rhythm, melody, and harmony.[48,49] Rhythm is the order in the movement of the music. Rhythm is the most dynamic aspect of music, and particular pieces of music often are selected because they harmonize with body rhythms such as heart rhythm, respiratory rhythm, or gait. The melody is created by the musical pitch and distance (or interval) between the musical tones. The melody contributes to the listener's emotional response to the music. The harmony results from the way pitches are blended together, with the combination of sounds described as consonant or dissonant by the listener.

Music selection usually is based on a person's musical preference and past experiences with music. Depending on the setting, headphones may be used to screen out other distracting noises. Radio and television music is inappropriate for music therapy because of the inability to control the selection of pieces that are played, the interruptions that occur (*e.g.*, commercials and announcements), and the quality of the reception.

Massage Therapy

Massage is the manipulation of the soft tissues of the body to promote relaxation and relief of muscle tension. The technique that is used may involve a gentle stroking along the length of a muscle, application of pressure across the width of a muscle, deep massage movements applied by a circular motion of the thumbs or fingertips, squeezing across the width of a muscle, or use of light slaps or chopping actions.[50] Massage may be administered by practitioners who have received special training in its use or by less prepared persons such as parents of small children[51,52] or caregivers of confused elders.[53] It often is used as a means of physiologic relaxation and stress relief in critically ill patients.[54]

Biofeedback

Biofeedback is a technique in which an individual learns to control physiologic functioning. It involves electronic monitoring of one or more physiologic responses to stress with immediate feedback of the specific response to the person undergoing treatment. Several types of responses are used: electromyographic (EMG), electrothermal, and electrodermal (EDR).[55] The EMG response involves the measurement of electrical potentials from muscles, usually the forearm extensor or frontalis. This is used to gain control over the contraction of skeletal muscles that occurs with anxiety and tension. The electrodermal sensors monitor skin temperature in the fingers or toes. The sympathetic nervous system exerts significant control over blood flow in the distal parts of the body such as the digits of the hands and feet. Consequently, anxiety often is manifested by a decrease in skin temperature in the fingers and toes. EDR sensors measure conductivity of skin (usually the hands) in response to anxiety. Fearful and anxious people often have cold and clammy hands, which lead to a decrease in conductivity.

In summary, stress in itself is neither negative nor deleterious to health. The stress response is designed to be time limited and protective, but in situations of prolonged activation of the response because of overwhelming or chronic stressors, it could be damaging to health. PTSD is an example of chronic activation of the stress response as a result of experiencing a severe trauma. It is characterized by a constellation of symptoms that focus on reexperiencing the event, avoidance of stimuli associated with the trauma, and persistent symptoms of increased arousal that cause clinically significant distress or impairment of social, occupational, or other important areas of function.

Treatment of stress should be aimed at helping people avoid coping behaviors that can adversely affect their health and providing them with other ways to reduce stress. Nonpharmacologic methods used in the treatment of stress include relaxation techniques, guided imagery, music therapy, massage techniques, and biofeedback.

Review Exercises

A 21-year-old college student notices that she frequently develops "cold sores" during stresses involved in final examination week.

A. What is the association between stress and the immune system?

B. One of her classmates suggests that she listen to music or try relaxation exercises as a means of relieving stress. Explain how these interventions might work in relieving stress.

A 75-year-old woman with congestive heart failure complains that her condition gets worse when she worries and is under a lot of stress.

A. Relate the effects of stress on the neuroendocrine control of cardiovascular function and its possible relationship to a worsening of the woman's congestive heart failure.

B. She tells you that she dealt with much worse stresses when she was younger and never had any problems. How would you explain this?

A 30-year-old woman who was rescued from a collapsed building has been having nightmares recalling the event, excessive anxiety, and loss of appetite, and is afraid to leave her home for fear something will happen.

A. Given her history and symptoms, what is the likely diagnosis?

B. How might she be treated?

Visit the Porth: Essentials of Pathophysiology: Concepts of Altered Health States web site

(http://thePoint.LWW.com/PorthEssentials) for links to chapter-related resources on the Internet, all-new exclusive animations, chapter review questions, and more!

REFERENCES

1. Lazarus R. S., Folkman S. (1984). *Stress, appraisal, and coping*. New York: Springer.
2. Hinkle L. E. (1977). The concept of "stress" in the biological and social sciences. In Lipowskin Z. J., Lipsitt D. R., Whybrow P. C. (Eds.), *Psychosomatic medicine* (pp. 27–49). New York: Oxford University Press.
3. Osler W. (1910). The Lumleian lectures in angina pectoris. *Lancet* 1, 696–700, 839–844, 974–977.
4. Cannon W. B. (1935). Stresses and strains of homeostasis. *American Journal of Medical Science* 189, 1–5.
5. Selye H. (1976). *The stress of life* (rev. ed.). New York: McGraw-Hill.
6. Page G. G., Lindsey A. M. (2003). Stress response. In Carrieri-Kohlman V., Lindsey A. M., West C. M. (Eds.), *Pathophysiological phenomena in nursing: Human responses to illness* (3rd ed., pp. 275–296). St. Louis: Mosby.
7. Cannon W. B. (1939). *The wisdom of the body* (pp. 299–300). New York: W. W. Norton.
8. Wilcox R. E., Gonzales R. A. (1995). Introduction to neurotransmitters, receptors, signal transduction, and second messengers. In Schatzberg A. F., Nemeroff C. B. (Eds.), *Textbook of psychopharmacology* (pp. 3–29). Washington, DC: American Psychiatric Press.
9. McEwen B. S. (1998). Protective and damaging effects of stress mediators. *New England Journal of Medicine* 338, 171–179.
10. Ursin H., Erickson H. R. (2004). The cognitive activation theory of stress. *Psychoneuroendocrinology* 29, 567–592.
11. Selye H. (1974). *Stress without distress* (p. 6). New York: New American Library.
12. Selye H. (1973). The evolution of the stress concept. *American Scientist* 61, 692–699.
13. Carrasco G. A., Van de Kar L. D. (2003). Neuroendocrine pharmacology of stress. *European Journal of Pharmacology* 463, 235–272.
14. Chrousos G. P. (1998). Stressors, stress, and neuroendocrine integration of the adaptive response. *Annals of the New York Academy of Sciences* 851, 311–335.
15. Lopez J. F., Akil H., Watson S. J. (1999). Neural circuits mediating stress. *Biological Psychiatry* 46, 1461–1471.
16. Koob G. F. (1999). Corticotropin-releasing factor, norepinephrine, and stress. *Biological Psychiatry* 46, 1167–1180.
17. Lehnert H., Schulz C., Dieterich K. (1998). Physiological and neurochemical aspects of corticotrophin-releasing factor actions in the brain: The role of the locus ceruleus. *Neurochemical Research* 23, 1039–1052.
18. Sapolsky R. M., Romero L. M., Munck A. U. (2000). How do glucocorticoids influence stress responses? Integrating permissive, suppressive, stimulatory, and preparative actions. *Endocrine Reviews* 21, 55–89.
19. Hertig V. (2004). Stress, stress response, and health. *Nursing Clinics of North America* 39, 1–17.
20. Dantzer R., Kelley K. W. (1989). Stress and immunity: An integrated view of relationships between the brain and immune system. *Life Sciences* 44, 1995–2008.
21. Falaschi P., Martocchia A., Proietti A., et al. (1994). Immune system and the hypothalamus-pituitary-adrenal axis. *Annals of the New York Academy of Sciences* 741, 223–231.
22. Woiciechowsky C., Schoning F., Lanksch W. R., et al. (1999). Mechanisms of brain mediated systemic anti-inflammatory syndrome causing immunodepression. *Journal of Molecular Medicine* 77, 769–780.
23. Dubos R. (1965). *Man adapting* (pp. 256, 258, 261, 264). New Haven, CT: Yale University Press.
24. Lazarus R. (2000). Evolution of a model of stress, coping, and discrete emotions. In Rice V. H. (Ed.), *Handbook of stress, coping, and health* (pp. 195–222). Thousand Oaks, CA: Sage.
25. Adams K., Oswold I. (1983). Protein synthesis, bodily renewal and sleep-wake cycle. *Clinical Science* 65, 561–567.
26. Gillin J. C., Byerley W. F. (1990). The diagnosis and management of insomnia. *New England Journal of Medicine* 322, 239–248.
27. Moldofsky H., Lue F. A., Davidson J. R., et al. (1989). Effects of sleep deprivation on human immune functions. *FASEB Journal* 3, 1972–1977.
28. Ford-Gilboe M., Cohen J. A. (2000). Hardiness: A model of commitment, challenge, and control. In Rice V. H. (Ed.),

Handbook of stress, coping, and health (pp. 425–436). Thousand Oaks, CA: Sage.

29. Broadhead W. E., Kaplan B. H., James S. A., et al. (1983). The epidemiologic evidence for a relationship between social support and health. *American Journal of Epidemiology* 117, 521–537.

30. Greenblatt M., Becerra R. M., Serafetinides E. A. (1982). Social networks and mental health: An overview. *American Journal of Psychiatry* 139, 977–984.

31. Tilden V. P., Weinert C. (1987). Social support and the chronically ill individual. *Nursing Clinics of North America* 33, 613–620.

32. National Institute for Occupational Safety and Health. (1999). *Stress at work* (pp. 1–26). Publication no. 99-101, HE 20.7102:ST 8/4. Bethesda, MD: U.S. Department of Health and Human Services.

33. Dworkin S. F. (1969). Psychosomatic concepts and dentistry: Some perspectives. *Journal of Periodontology* 40, 647.

34. Cohen S., Tyrrell D. A. J., Smith A. P. (1991). Psychological stress and susceptibility to the common cold. *New England Journal of Medicine* 325, 606–612.

35. Cohen S., Doyle W. J., Skoner D. P. (1999). Psychological stress, cytokine production, and severity of upper respiratory illness. *Psychosomatic Medicine* 61, 175–180.

36. Vedhara K., Wilcock G. K., Lightman S. L., et al. (1999). Chronic stress in elderly carers of dementia patients and antibody response to influenza vaccination. *Lancet* 353, 627–631.

37. Rozlog L. A., Kiecolt-Glaser J. K., Marucha P. T., et al. (1999). Stress and immunity: Implication for viral disease and wound healing. *Journal of Periodontology* 70, 786–792.

38. Yehuda R. (2002). Post-traumatic stress disorder. *New England Journal of Medicine* 346, 108–114.

39. Ursano R. J., Bell C., Eth S., et al., Steering Committee on Practice Guidelines. (2004). Practice guidelines for the treatment of patients with acute stress disorder and posttraumatic stress disorder. *American Journal of Psychiatry Supplement* 11, 3–31.

40. American Psychiatric Association. (2000). *Diagnostic and statistical manual of mental disorders* (DSM-IV) (4th ed., text rev.). Washington, DC: American Psychiatric Press.

41. Yehuda R. (2000). Biology of posttraumatic stress disorder. *Journal of Clinical Psychiatry* 61(Suppl. 7), 14–21.

42. Yehuda, R. (1998). Psychoneuroendocrinology of posttraumatic stress disorder. *Psychiatric Clinics of North America* 21, 359–379.

43. Sapolsky R. (1999). Stress and your shrinking brain (posttraumatic stress disorder's effect on the brain). *Discover* 20(3), 116.

44. McCloskey L. A. (2000). Posttraumatic stress in children exposed to family violence and single event trauma. *Journal of the American Academy of Child and Adolescent Psychiatry* 39, 108–115.

45. Esch T., Fricchione G. L., Stefano G. B. (2003). The therapeutic use of the relaxation response in stress-related diseases. *Medical Science Monitor* 9(2), RA23–RA34.

46. Benson H. (1977). Systemic hypertension and the relaxation response. *New England Journal of Medicine* 296, 1152–1154.

47. Jacobson E. (1958). *Progressive relaxation.* Chicago: University of Chicago Press.

48. Chlan L., Tracy M. F. (1999). Music therapy in critical care: Indications and guidelines for intervention. *Critical Care Nurse* 19(3), 35–41.

49. White J. M. (1999). Effects of relaxing music on cardiac autonomic balance and anxiety after acute myocardial infarction. *American Journal of Critical Care* 8, 220–230.

50. Vickers A., Zollman C. (1999). ABC of complementary therapies: Massage therapies. *British Medical Journal* 319, 1254–1257.

51. Rusy L. M., Weisman S. J. (2000). Complementary therapies for acute pediatric pain management. *Pediatric Clinics of North America* 47, 589–599.

52. Huhtala V., Lehtonen L., Heinonen R., et al. (2000). Infant massage compared with crib vibrator in treatment of colicky infants. *Pediatrics* 105(6), E84.

53. Rowe M., Alfred D. (1999). The effectiveness of slow-stroke massage in diffusing agitated behaviors in individuals with Alzheimer's disease. *Journal of Gerontological Nursing* 25(6), 22–34.

54. Richards K. C. (1998). Effect of back massage and relaxation intervention on sleep in critically ill patients. *American Journal of Critical Care* 7, 288–299.

55. Fischer-Williams M., Nigl A. J., Sovine D. L. (1986). *A textbook of biological feedback.* New York: Human Sciences Press.

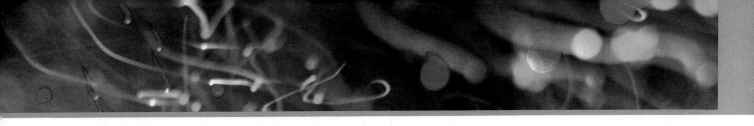

C h a p t e r 8

Alterations in Body Nutrition

 Nutritional status describes the condition of the body related to the availability and use of nutrients. Intake of nutrients provides energy for performing various body functions or storage for future use. The stability and composition of body weight over time requires that a person's energy intake be balanced with energy expenditure. Also, because different foods contain different amounts of proteins, fats, carbohydrates, vitamins, and minerals, appropriate amounts of these dietary elements must be maintained to ensure proper body functioning.

Regulation of Food Intake and Energy Metabolism

Energy is measured in heat units called *calories*. A calorie, spelled with a small "c" and also called a *gram calorie,* is the amount of heat or energy required to raise the temperature of 1 g of water by 1°C. A *kilocalorie* (kcal), or *large calorie* (spelled with a capital C), is the amount of energy needed to raise the temperature of 1 kg of water by 1°C. Because a calorie is so small, kilocalories often are used in nutritional and physiologic studies.

Metabolism is the organized process through which nutrients such as carbohydrates, fats, and proteins are broken down, transformed, or otherwise converted into cellular energy. The oxidation of proteins provides 4 kcal/g; fats, 9 kcal/g; carbohydrates, 4 kcal/g; and alcohol, 7 kcal/g.

The process of metabolism is unique in that it enables the continual release of energy, and it couples this energy with physiologic functioning. For example, the energy used for muscle contraction is derived largely from energy sources that are stored in muscle cells and then released as the muscle contracts. Because most of our energy sources come from the nutrients in the food that is eaten, the ability to store energy and control its release is important. Normally, energy utilization is balanced with energy expenditure. When a person is overfed and intake of food

KEY CONCEPTS

Energy Metabolism

➤ Energy is required for all the body's activities. Food is the source of the body's energy, which is measured in kilocalories (kcal).

➤ Fats, which are a concentrated water-free energy source, contain 9 kcal/g. They are stored in fat cells as triglycerides, which are the main storage sites for energy.

➤ Carbohydrates are hydrated fuels, which supply 4 kcal/g. They are stored in limited quantities as glycogen and can be converted to fatty acids and stored in fat cells as triglycerides.

➤ Amino acids, which supply 4 kcal/g, are used in building body proteins. Amino acids in excess of those needed for protein synthesis are converted to fatty acids, ketones, or glucose and are stored or used as metabolic fuel.

consistently exceeds energy expenditure, the excess energy is stored as fat, and the person becomes overweight. Conversely, when food intake is less than energy expenditure, fat stores and other body tissues are broken down, and the person loses weight.

ENERGY STORAGE

Adipose Tissue

More than 90% of body energy is stored in the adipose tissues of the body. *Adipocytes*, or fat cells, occur singly or in small groups in loose connective tissue. In many parts of the body, they cushion body organs such as the kidneys. In addition to isolated groups of fat cells, entire regions of fat tissue are committed to fat storage. Collectively, fat cells constitute a large body organ that is metabolically active in the uptake, synthesis, storage, and mobilization of lipids, which are the main source of fuel storage for the body. Some tissues, such as liver cells, are able to store small amounts of lipids, but when these lipids accumulate, they begin to interfere with cell function. Adipose tissue not only serves as a storage site for body fuels, it provides insulation for the body, fills body crevices, and protects body organs. Adipose tissue is now also recognized as an endocrine and paracrine organ that secretes a number of important factors. These include leptin, certain cytokines (*e.g.*, tumor necrosis factor-α), growth factors, and adiponectin (important in insulin resistance).

Studies of adipocytes in the laboratory have shown that fully differentiated cells do not divide. However, such cells have a long life span, and anyone born with large numbers of adipocytes runs the risk of becoming obese. Some immature adipocytes (termed *pre-adipocytes*) capable of division are present in postnatal life; these cells are the potential source of additional fat cells during postnatal

life.[1] Fat deposition results from proliferation of these existing immature adipocytes and can occur as a consequence of excessive caloric intake when a woman is breast-feeding or during estrogen stimulation around the time of puberty. An increase in fat cells also may occur during late adolescence and in middle-aged persons who already are overweight. Some medications can also have an important effect on fat cell numbers. The thiazolidinedione (TZD) class of antidiabetic drugs can also stimulate the formation of new fat cells from pre-adipocytes, allowing increased uptake of glucose into these cells (and storage as fat) and resulting in reduced serum glucose levels. In contrast, some drugs can cause loss of fat cells, resulting in lipodystrophy. This occurs in human immunodeficiency virus (HIV)–associated lipodystrophy in persons treated with highly active antiretroviral therapy (HAART). Although the mechanism of fat loss is not known, it may be due to increased programmed cell death of the adipocytes (*i.e.*, increased apoptosis).

There are two types of adipose tissue: white fat and brown fat. White fat, which despite its name is cream colored or yellow, is the prevalent form of adipose tissue in postnatal life. It constitutes 10% to 20% of body weight in adult men and 15% to 25% in adult women. At body temperature, the lipid content of fat cells exists as an oil. It consists of triglycerides, which are three molecules of fatty acids esterified to a glycerol molecule. Triglycerides, which contain no water, have the highest caloric content of all nutrients and are an efficient form of energy storage. Fat cells synthesize triglycerides, the major fat storage form, from dietary fats and carbohydrates. Insulin is required for transport of glucose into fat cells. When calorie intake is restricted for any reason, fat cell triglycerides are broken down, and the resultant fatty acids and glycerol are released as energy sources.

Brown fat differs from white fat in terms of its thermogenic capacity, or ability to produce heat. Brown fat, the site of diet-induced thermogenesis and nonshivering thermogenesis, is found primarily in early neonatal life in humans and in animals that hibernate. In humans, brown fat decreases with age but is still detectable in the sixth decade. This small amount of brown fat has a minimal effect on energy expenditure.

NUTRITIONAL NEEDS

Recommended Dietary Allowances and Dietary Reference Intakes

The *Recommended Dietary Allowances* (RDAs) define the average daily intakes that meet the nutrient needs of almost all healthy persons in a specific age and sex group.[2] The RDAs, which are periodically updated, have been published since 1941 by the National Academy of Sciences. The RDA is used in advising persons about the level of nutrient intake they need to decrease the risk of chronic disease.

The *Dietary Reference Intake* (DRI) includes a set of at least four nutrient-based reference values: the RDA, the Adequate Intake, the Estimated Average Requirement, and the Tolerable Upper Intake Level, each of which has specific uses.[3] The *United States RDA* (USRDA) was established for the purpose of labeling foods. It takes the highest recommended daily intake of each nutrient for children older than 4 years of age and for adults (excluding those pregnant or lactating); therefore, the USRDA sometimes provides a margin of nutritional safety higher than the RDA.

The *Adequate Intake* (AI) is the amount of intake necessary to prevent a deficiency state. An *Estimated Average Requirement* is the intake that meets the estimated nutrient need of half of the persons in a specific group. This figure is used as the basis for developing the RDA and is expected to be used by nutrition policy makers in the evaluation of the adequacy of a nutrient for a specific group and for planning how much of the nutrient the group should consume. The *Tolerable Upper Intake Level* is the maximum intake that is judged unlikely to pose a health risk in almost all healthy persons in a specified group. It refers to the total intakes from food, fortified food, and nutrient supplements. This value is not intended to be a recommended level of intake, and there is no established benefit for persons who consume nutrients above the RDA or AI levels. The DRIs are regularly reviewed and updated by the Food and Nutrition Board of the Institute of Medicine and the National Academy of Science.

Food and supplement labels use *Daily Values* (DVs), which are set by the U.S. Food and Drug Administration (FDA). However, the DVs are based on data that are older than the data used to determine the DRIs. Percent Daily Value (% DV) tells the consumer what percentage of the DV one serving of a food or supplement supplies.

Proteins, fats, carbohydrates, vitamins, and minerals each have their own function in providing the body with what it needs to maintain life and health. Recommended allowances have not been established for every nutrient; some are given as a safe and adequate intake, but others, such as carbohydrates and fats, are expressed as a percentage of the calorie intake.

Calories

Energy requirements are greater during growth periods. Children require approximately 115 kcal/kg at birth, 105 kcal/kg at 1 year, and 80 kcal/kg of body weight between 1 to 10 years of age. During adolescence, boys require 45 kcal/kg of body weight and girls require 38 kcal/kg of body weight. During pregnancy, a woman needs an extra 300 kcal/day above her usual requirement, and during the first 3 months of breast-feeding, she requires an additional 500 kcal.[2] Table 8-1 can be used to predict the caloric requirements of healthy adults.

Proteins, Fats, and Carbohydrates

Proteins are required for growth and maintenance of body tissues, formation of enzymes and antibodies, fluid and electrolyte balance, and nutrient transport. Proteins are composed of amino acids, nine of which are essential

TABLE 8-1	Caloric Requirements Based on Body Weight and Activity Level		
	Sedentary	**Moderate**	**Active**
Overweight	20–25 kcal/kg	30 kcal/kg	35 kcal/kg
Normal	30 kcal/kg	35 kcal/kg	40 kcal/kg
Underweight	30 kcal/kg	40 kcal/kg	45–50 kcal/kg

(Adapted from Goodhart R.S., Shils M.E. [1980]. *Modern nutrition in health and disease* [6th ed.]. Philadelphia: Lea and Febiger.)

to the body. These are leucine, isoleucine, methionine, phenylalanine, threonine, tryptophan, valine, lysine, and histidine. The foods that provide these essential amino acids in adequate amounts are milk, eggs, meat, fish, and poultry. Dried peas and beans, nuts, seeds, and grains contain all the essential amino acids but in less than adequate proportions. The proteins in these foods need to be combined with each other or with complete proteins to meet the amino acid requirements for protein synthesis.

Unlike carbohydrates and fats, which are composed of hydrogen, carbon, and oxygen, proteins contain 16% nitrogen; therefore, nitrogen excretion is an indicator of protein intake. If the amount of nitrogen taken in by way of protein is equivalent to the nitrogen excreted, the person is said to be in *nitrogen balance*. A person is in positive nitrogen balance when the nitrogen consumed by way of protein is greater than the amount excreted. This occurs during growth, pregnancy, or healing after surgery or injury. A negative nitrogen balance often occurs with fever, illness, infection, trauma, or burns, when more nitrogen is excreted than is consumed. It represents a state of tissue breakdown.

Dietary fats are composed primarily of triglycerides (*i.e.,* a mixture of fatty acids and glycerol). The fatty acids are saturated (*i.e.,* no double bonds), monounsaturated (*i.e.,* one double bond), or polyunsaturated (*i.e.,* two or more double bonds). The saturated fatty acids elevate blood cholesterol, whereas the monounsaturated and polyunsaturated fats lower blood cholesterol. Saturated fats usually are from animal sources and remain solid at room temperature. With the exception of coconut and palm oils (which are saturated), unsaturated fats are found in plant oils and usually are liquid at room temperature.

Dietary fats provide energy, serve as carriers for the fat-soluble vitamins, are precursors of prostaglandins, and are a source of fatty acids. The polyunsaturated fatty acid linoleic acid is the only fatty acid that is required. A deficiency of linoleic acid results in dermatitis. The daily requirement is 5 g or 1% to 2% of the total daily calories. Because vegetable oils are rich sources of linoleic acid, this level can be met by including two teaspoons of oil in the daily diet.

Other than the requirement for linoleic acid, there is no specific requirement for dietary fat, provided there is adequate nutrition available for energy. Fat is the most concentrated source of energy. It is recommended that 30% or less of the calories in the diet should come from fats (with <10% of calories being saturated fat).

Cholesterol is the major constituent of cell membranes and is synthesized by the body. Cholesterol metabolism and transport are discussed in Chapter 17. The daily dietary recommendation for cholesterol is less than 300 mg.

Dietary carbohydrates are composed of simple sugars, complex carbohydrates, and undigested carbohydrates (*i.e.*, fiber). Within the body, carbohydrate is transformed into glucose, a six-carbon molecule. Excess glucose is stored as glycogen or converted to triglycerides for storage in fat cells. Because of their vitamin, mineral, and fiber content, it is recommended that the bulk of the carbohydrate content in the diet be in the complex form, rather than as simple sugars that contain few nutrients. Sucrose (*i.e.*, table sugar) is implicated in the development of dental caries.

There is no specific dietary requirement for carbohydrates. All of the energy requirements can be met by dietary fats and proteins. Although some tissues, such as the nervous system, require glucose as an energy source, this need can be met through the conversion of amino acids and the glycerol part of the triglyceride molecule to glucose. A carbohydrate-deficient diet usually results in the loss of tissue proteins and the development of ketosis. Because protein and fat metabolism increases the production of osmotically active metabolic wastes that must be eliminated through the kidneys, there is a danger of dehydration and electrolyte imbalances. The amount of carbohydrate needed to prevent tissue wasting and ketosis is 50 to 100 g/day. In practice, most of the daily energy requirement should be from carbohydrate. This is because protein is an expensive source of calories and because it is recommended that no more than 30% of the calories in the diet be derived from fat. The current recommendation is that the diet should provide 50% to 60% of the calories as carbohydrates.

Vitamins and Minerals

Vitamins are a group of organic compounds that act as catalysts in various chemical reactions. A compound cannot be classified as a vitamin unless it is shown that a deficiency of it causes disease. Contrary to popular belief, vitamins do not provide energy directly. As catalysts, they are part of the enzyme systems required for the release of energy from protein, fat, and carbohydrates. Vitamins also are necessary for the formation of red blood cells, hormones, genetic materials, and the nervous system. They are essential for normal growth and development.

There are two types of vitamins: fat soluble and water soluble. The four fat-soluble vitamins are vitamins A, D, E, and K. The nine required water-soluble vitamins are thiamine, riboflavin, niacin, pyridoxine (vitamin B_6), pantothenic acid, vitamin B_{12}, folic acid, biotin, and vitamin C. Because the water-soluble vitamins are excreted in the urine, it is less likely that they may become toxic to the body, but the fat-soluble vitamins are stored in the body, and they may reach toxic levels.

Minerals serve many functions. They are involved in acid-base balance and in the maintenance of osmotic pressure in body compartments. Minerals are components of vitamins, hormones, and enzymes. They maintain normal hemoglobin levels, play a role in nervous system function, and are involved in muscle contraction and skeletal development and maintenance. Minerals that are present in relatively large amounts in the body are called *macrominerals*. These include calcium, phosphorus, sodium, chloride, potassium, magnesium, and sulfur. The remainder are classified as *trace minerals;* they include iron, manganese, copper, iodine, zinc, cobalt, fluorine, and selenium.

REGULATION OF FOOD INTAKE AND ENERGY STORAGE

Stability of body weight and composition over time requires that energy intake matches energy utilization. Environmental, cultural, genetic, and psychological factors all influence food intake and energy expenditure. In addition, powerful physiologic control systems contribute to the regulation of hunger and food intake.[1]

Hunger, Appetite, and Food Intake

The sensation of *hunger* is associated with several sensory perceptions, such as the rhythmic contractions of the stomach and that "empty feeling" in the stomach that stimulates a person to seek food. A person's *appetite* is the desire for a particular type of food. It is useful in helping the person determine the type of food that is eaten. Satiety is the feeling of fullness or decreased desire for food.

The hypothalamus contains the feeding center for hunger and satiety (Fig. 8-1). It receives neural input from the gastrointestinal tract that provides information about stomach filling, chemical signals from the blood about the nutrients in food, and input from the cerebral cortex regarding the smell, sight, and taste of the food. Centers in the hypothalamus also control the secretion

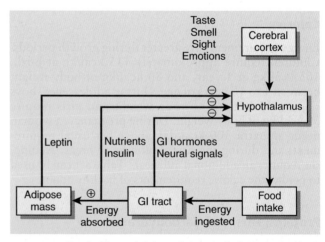

FIGURE 8-1 Feedback mechanisms for control of energy intake. GI, gastrointestinal. (Adapted from Guyton A., Hall J. E. [2000]. *Textbook of medical physiology* [10th ed., p. 805]. Philadelphia: W. B. Saunders, with permission from Elsevier Science.)

of several hormones (*e.g.*, thyroid and adrenocortical hormones) that regulate energy balance and metabolism.

The control of food intake can be divided into short-term regulation, which is concerned with the amount of food that is consumed at a meal or snack, and intermediate and long-term regulation, which is concerned with the maintenance of energy stores over time.[1]

The short-term regulation of food intake provides a person with the feeling of satiety and turns off the desire for eating when adequate food has been consumed. It requires rapid feedback mechanisms that signal the adequacy of food intake before digestion has taken place and nutrients have been absorbed into the blood. These mechanisms include receptors that monitor filling of the gastrointestinal tract, gastrointestinal tract hormones, and oral receptors that monitor food intake. Stretch receptors in the gastrointestinal tract monitor gastrointestinal filling and send inhibitory impulses by way of the vagus nerve to the feeding center to suppress the desire for food. The gastrointestinal hormones cholecystokinin (which is released in response to fat in the duodenum), and glucagon-like peptide-1 (which is released from the lower small bowel in response to nutrients, especially carbohydrates) have a strong suppressant effect on the feeding center. The presence of food in the stomach increases the release of insulin and glucagon, both of which suppress the neurogenic feeding signals from the brain.[1] The act of tasting, chewing, and swallowing also appears to suppress the feeling of hunger.

The intermediate and long-term regulation of food intake is determined by the amount of nutrients that are in the blood and in storage sites. It has long been known that a decrease in blood glucose causes hunger. In contrast, an increase in breakdown products of lipids such as ketoacids produces a decrease in appetite. The ketogenic weight-loss diet relies partly on the appetite-suppressant effects of ketones in the blood. Recent evidence suggests that the hypothalamus also senses the amount of energy that is stored in fat cells through a hormone called *leptin*. Increased amounts of leptin are released from the adipocytes when fat stores are increased. The stimulation of leptin receptors in the hypothalamus produces a decrease in appetite and food intake as well as an increase in metabolic rate and energy consumption. It also produces a decrease in insulin release from the beta cells, which decreases energy storage in fat cells.

ASSESSMENT OF ENERGY STORES AND NUTRITIONAL STATUS

Anthropometric measurements provide a means for assessing body composition, particularly fat stores and skeletal muscle mass. This is done by measuring height, weight, body circumferences, and thickness of various skinfold areas. These measurements commonly are used to determine growth patterns in children and appropriateness of current weight in adults.

Body weight is the most frequently used method of assessing nutritional status; it should be used in combination with measurements of body height to establish whether a person is underweight or overweight.

Relative weight is the actual weight divided by the desirable weight and multiplied by 100. A relative weight greater than 120% is indicative of obesity. Recent changes in weight are probably a better indication of undernutrition than a low relative weight. An unintentional loss of 10% of body weight or more within the past 6 months usually is considered predictive of a poor clinical outcome, especially if weight loss is continuing.[4] The body mass index (BMI) uses height and weight to determine healthy weight (Table 8-2). It is calculated by dividing the weight in kilograms by the height in meters squared (BMI = weight [kg]/height [m^2]). A BMI between 18.5 and 25 has the lowest statistical health risk.[5] A BMI of 25 to 29.9 is considered overweight; a BMI of 30 or greater as obese; and a BMI greater than 40 as very or morbidly obese.[6]

TABLE 8-2	Classification of Overweight and Obesity by BMI, Waist Circumference, and Associated Disease Risk*			
			Disease Risk* Relative to Normal Weight and Waist Circumference	
	BMI (kg/m²)	Obesity Class	*Men ≤102 cm (≤40 in)* *Women ≤88 cm (≤35 in)*	*Men >102 cm (>40 in)* *Women >88 cm (>35 in)*
Underweight	<18.5		—	—
Normal†	18.5–24.9		—	—
Overweight	25.0–29.9		Increased	High
Obesity	30.0–34.9	I	High	Very high
	35.0–39.9	II	Very high	Very high
Extreme obesity	≥40	III	Extremely high	Extremely high

BMI, body mass index.
*Disease risk for type 2 diabetes, hypertension, and cardiovascular disease.
†Increased waist circumference also can be a marker for increased risk, even in persons of normal weight.
(Expert Panel. [1998]. Clinical guidelines on the identification, evaluation, and treatment of overweight and obesity in adults. National Institutes of Health. [On-line.] Available: http://nhlbi.nih.gov/guidelines/ob_gdlns.htm.)

Body weight reflects both lean body mass and adipose tissue and cannot be used as a method for describing body composition or the percentage of fat tissue present. Statistically, the best percentage of body fat for men is between 12% and 20%, and for women, between 20% and 30%.[7] During physical training, body fat usually decreases and lean body mass increases.

Among the methods used to estimate body fat are skinfold thickness, body circumferences, bioelectrical impedance, computed tomography (CT), and magnetic resonance imaging (MRI). The measurement of *body circumferences,* most commonly waist and hip, provides an objective measurement of body fat and supplies the information needed to calculate the ratio of waist circumference to hip circumference (to be discussed).

Bioelectrical impedance involves the use of electrodes attached to the wrist and ankles to send a harmless current through the body. The flow of the current is affected by the amount of water in the body. Because fat-free tissue contains virtually all the water and current-conducting electrolytes, measurements of the resistance (*i.e.,* impedance) can be used to estimate the percentage of body fat present.[8]

Computed tomography and *MRI* can be used to provide quantitative pictures from which the thickness of fat can be determined. CT scans also can be used to provide quantitative estimates of regional fat and give a ratio of intra-abdominal to extra-abdominal fat. Because these methods are costly, they usually are reserved for research studies.

Various laboratory tests can aid in evaluating nutritional status. Some of the most commonly performed tests are serum albumin to assess the protein status, total lymphocyte count and delayed hypersensitivity reaction to assess cellular immunity, and creatinine–height index to assess skeletal muscle protein.

In summary, nutritional status describes the condition of the body related to the availability and use of nutrients. Metabolism is the organized process whereby nutrients such as carbohydrates, fats, and proteins are broken down, transformed, or otherwise converted to cellular energy. Glucose, fats, and amino acids from proteins serve as fuel sources for cellular metabolism. These fuel sources are ingested during meals and stored for future use. Glucose is stored as glycogen or converted to triglycerides in fat cells for storage. Fats are stored in adipose tissue as triglycerides. Amino acids are the building blocks of proteins, and most of the stored amino acids are contained in body proteins and as fuel sources for cellular metabolism. Energy is measured in heat units called *kilocalories.* The RDA is the recommended *dietary* allowance needed to meet the known nutritional needs of healthy persons.

Nutritional status reflects the continued daily intake of nutrients over time and the deposition and use of these nutrients in the body. When a person is consis-

tently overfed, the excess energy is stored as fat, and the person gains weight. When energy expenditure exceeds food intake, body fat and other tissues are broken down, and the person loses weight. The nutritional status of a person can be assessed by evaluation of dietary intake, anthropometric measurements, health assessment, and laboratory tests. Anthropometric measurements are used for assessing body composition; they include height and weight measurements and measurements to determine the composition of the body in relation to lean body mass and fat tissue (*e.g.,* skinfold thickness, body circumferences, bioelectrical impedance, and CT scans).

Overnutrition and Obesity

Obesity is defined as a condition characterized by excess body fat. Clinically, obesity and overweight have been defined in terms of the BMI. Historically, various world organizations have used different BMI cutoff points to define obesity. In 1997, the World Health Organization defined the various classifications of overweight (BMI ≥ 25) and obesity (BMI ≥ 30). This classification system was subsequently adopted by the National Institutes of Health.[6] The use of a BMI cutoff of 25 as a measure of overweight raised some concern that the BMI in some men might be attributable to muscle mass, rather than adipose tissue. However, it has been shown that a BMI cutoff of 25 can sensitively detect most overweight people and does not erroneously detect overlean people.[9]

Overweight and obesity have become national health problems, increasing the risk of hypertension, hyperlipidemia, type 2 diabetes, coronary heart disease, and other health problems. Sixty-five percent of the U.S. popula-

---

KEY CONCEPTS

Obesity

➤ Obesity results from an imbalance between energy intake and energy consumption. Because fat is the main storage form of energy, obesity represents an excess of body fat.

➤ Overweight and obesity are determined by measurements of body mass index (BMI; weight [kg]/height [m²]) and waist circumference. A BMI of 25 to 29.9 is considered overweight; a BMI of 30 or greater, obese; and a BMI greater than 40, very or morbidly obese.

➤ Waist circumference is used to determine the distribution of body fat. Central, or abdominal, obesity is an independent predictor of morbidity and mortality associated with obesity.

tion is estimated to be overweight (BMI ≥ 25). Obesity is particularly prevalent among some minority groups, lower-income groups, and people with less education. The prevalence of obesity (BMI ≥ 30) in the United States is estimated at 30.5% of adults (over 61 million people), whereas morbid obesity (BMI > 40) was found in 4.7%.[10]

CAUSES OF OBESITY

The excess body fat of obesity often significantly impairs health. This excess body fat is generated when the calories consumed exceed those expended through exercise and activity.[11] The physiologic mechanisms that lead to this imbalance are poorly understood. They probably exist in different combinations among obese persons.

Although factors that lead to the development of obesity are not understood, they are thought to involve the interaction of the person's genotype with environmental influences such as social, behavioral, and cultural factors.[12] Obesity is known to run in families, suggesting a hereditary component. The question that surrounds this observation is whether the disorder arises because of genetic endowment or environmental influences. Studies of twin and adopted children have provided evidence that heredity contributes to the disorder.[13]

Although genetic factors may explain some of the individual variations in terms of excess weight, environmental influences also must be taken into account. These influences include family dietary patterns, decreased level of activity because of labor-saving devices and time spent using the computer, reliance on the automobile for transportation, easy access to food, energy density of food, and large food portions. The obese may be greatly influenced by the availability of food, the flavor of food, time of day, and other cues. The composition of the diet also may be a causal factor, and the percentage of dietary fat or carbohydrate independent of total calorie intake may play a part in the development of obesity. Psychological factors include using food as a reward, comfort, or means of getting attention. Eating may be a way to cope with tension, anxiety, and mental fatigue. Some persons may overeat and use obesity as a means of avoiding emotionally threatening situations. A growing number of medications have been implicated in causing weight gain in some or most patients for whom they are prescribed. These include antidiabetic agents (*e.g.*, insulin, sulfonylureas, and TZDs), steroid hormones, and some antipsychotic, antidepressant, and antiepileptic agents.

TYPES OF OBESITY

Two types of obesity based on distribution of fat have been described: upper body and lower body obesity (Fig. 8-2). *Upper body obesity* is also referred to as *central, abdominal,* or *male* obesity. Lower body obesity is known as *peripheral, gluteal-femoral,* or *female* obesity. The obesity type is determined by dividing the waist by the hip circumference. A waist–hip ratio greater than 1.0 in men and 0.8 in women indicates upper body obesity.[14] Research

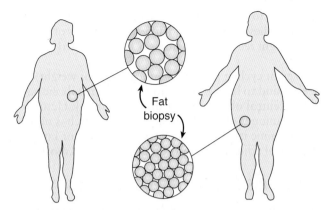

FIGURE 8-2 Distribution of body fat and size of fat cells in persons with upper and lower body obesity. (Courtesy of Ahmed Kissebah, M. D., Ph.D., Medical College of Wisconsin, Milwaukee, WI.)

suggests that fat distribution may be a more important factor for morbidity and mortality than overweight or obesity.

The presence of excess fat in the abdomen out of proportion to total body fat is an independent predictor of risk factors and mortality. Waist circumference is positively correlated with abdominal fat content. Waist circumference 35 inches or greater in women and 40 inches or greater in men has been associated with increased health risk[6] (see Table 8-2). Central obesity can be further differentiated into intra-abdominal, or visceral, fat and subcutaneous fat by the use of CT or MRI scans. However, intra-abdominal fat usually is synonymous with central fat distribution. One of the characteristics of intra-abdominal fat is that free fatty acids released from the viscera go directly to the liver before entering the systemic circulation, having a potentially greater impact on hepatic function. Higher levels of circulating free fatty acids in obese persons, particularly those with upper body obesity, are thought to be associated with many of the adverse effects of obesity.[11]

In general, men have more intra-abdominal fat and women more subcutaneous fat. As men age, the proportion of intra-abdominal fat to subcutaneous fat increases. After menopause, women tend to acquire more central fat distribution. Increasing weight gain, alcohol, and low levels of activity are associated with upper body obesity. These changes place persons with upper body obesity at greater risk for ischemic heart disease, stroke, and death independent of total body fat. They also tend to exhibit hypertension, elevated levels of triglycerides and decreased levels of high-density lipoproteins, hyperinsulinemia, and diabetes mellitus (this combination of cardiovascular risk factors is also known as the *metabolic syndrome;* see Chapter 32).

Weight reduction causes a loss of intra-abdominal fat and has resulted in improvements in metabolic and hormonal abnormalities.[15] In terms of weight reduction, some studies have shown that persons with upper body obesity are easier to treat than those with lower body obesity. Other studies have shown no difference in terms of success with weight reduction programs between the two types of obesity.

Weight cycling (the losing and gaining of weight) has been found to have little or no effect on metabolic variables, central obesity, or cardiovascular risk factors or future amount of weight loss.[16] More research is needed to determine its effect on dietary preference for fat, psychological adjustment, disordered eating, and mortality.

HEALTH RISKS ASSOCIATED WITH OBESITY

Obese persons are more likely to have high blood pressure, hyperlipidemia, cardiovascular disease, insulin resistance, and type 2 diabetes. They are also more prone to develop gallbladder disease, menstrual irregularities and infertility, cancer of the endometrium, prostate, colon, and, in postmenopausal women, cancer of the breast.[6] The increased weight associated with obesity stresses the bones and joints, increasing the likelihood of arthritis. Other conditions associated with obesity include sleep apnea and pulmonary dysfunction, nonalcoholic steatohepatitis (also known as "fatty liver"), carpal tunnel syndrome, venous insufficiency and deep vein thrombosis, and poor wound healing.[6] Because some drugs are lipophilic and exhibit increased distribution in fat tissue, the administration of these drugs, including some anesthetic agents, can be more dangerous in obese persons. If surgery is required, the obese person tends to heal more slowly than a nonobese person of the same age.

Massive obesity, because of its close association with so many health problems, can be regarded as a disease in its own right.[17] It is the second leading cause of preventable death. In men who have never smoked, the risk of death increases from 1.06 at a BMI of 24.5 to 1.67 at a BMI higher than 26.[18]

PREVENTION AND TREATMENT

It has been theorized that obesity is preventable because the effect of hereditary factors is no more than moderate. A more active lifestyle together with a low-fat diet (<30% of calories) is seen as the strategy for prevention. The target audience should be young children, adolescents, and young adults.[19] Tools needed to achieve this goal include promotion of regular low-fat meals, avoidance of snacking, substitution of water for calorie-containing beverages, reduction of time spent in sedentary activities, such as television viewing, and an increase in activity. Other high-risk periods are from 25 to 35 years of age, at menopause,[19] and the year after successful weight loss.

The goals for weight loss are, at a minimum, prevention of further weight gain, reduction of current weight, and maintenance of a lowered body weight indefinitely. An algorithm has been designed for use in treating overweight and obesity. The initial goal in treatment is to lower body weight by 10% from baseline during a 6-month period. This degree of weight loss requires a calorie reduction of 300 to 500 kcal/day in individuals with a BMI of 27 to 35. For those persons with a BMI greater than 35, the calorie intake needs to be reduced by 500 to 1000 kcal/day. After 6 months, the person should be given strategies for maintaining the new weight. The person who is unable to achieve significant weight loss should be enrolled in a weight management program to prevent further weight gain.

There are many ways to treat obesity. It is currently recommended that treatment should focus on lifestyle modification through a combination of a low-calorie diet, increased physical activity, and behavior therapy.[6]

Dietary therapy should be individually prescribed based on the person's overweight status and risk profile. The diet should be a personalized plan that is 300 to 1000 kcal/day less than the current dietary intake. If the patient's risk status warrants it, the diet also should be decreased in saturated fat and contain 30% or less of total calories from fat. Reduction of dietary fat without a calorie deficit will not result in weight loss.

Physical activity is important in the prevention of weight gain. In addition, it reduces cardiovascular and diabetes risk beyond that achieved by weight loss alone. Although physical activity is an important part of weight loss therapy, it does not lead to a significant weight loss. Exercise should be started slowly, with the duration and intensity increased independent of each other. The goal should be 30 minutes or more of moderate-intensity activity on most days of the week. The activity can be performed at one time or intermittently over the day.

Techniques for changing behavior include self-monitoring of eating habits and physical activity (including the use of pedometers, which counts the number of steps taken in a day), stress management, stimulus control, problem solving, contingency management, cognitive restructuring, and social support.

Pharmacotherapy and surgery are available as an adjunct to lifestyle changes in individuals who meet specific criteria.[20] Pharmacotherapy is usually considered only after combined diet, exercise, and behavioral therapy has been in effect for a minimum of 6 months. Weight loss surgery is limited to persons with a BMI greater than 40; those with a BMI greater than 35 who have comorbid conditions and in whom efforts at medical therapy have failed; and those who have complications of extreme obesity.

 ## CHILDHOOD OBESITY

Obesity is the most prevalent nutritional disorder affecting the pediatric population in the United States. The findings from the National Health and Nutrition Examination Survey (NHANES) III, conducted between 1999 and 2000, indicated that 15% of children from ages 6 to 19 years were overweight.[21] This was a 4% increase from the previous NHANES study. Ten percent of children 2 to 5 years of age were overweight. The increase in prevalence was greater for those of African-American and Hispanic ethnicity. The definition for overweight for the NHANES III study was a BMI at or above the sex- and age-specific 95th percentile. Those who were between the 85th and 95th percentiles were defined as at risk for overweight.

The major concern of childhood obesity is that obese children will grow up to become obese adults. Pediatricians are now beginning to see hypertension, dyslipidemia, and type 2 diabetes in obese children and adolescents. In North America, type 2 diabetes now accounts for half of all new diagnoses of diabetes (types 1 and 2) in some populations of adolescents.[22] In addition, there is a growing concern that childhood and adolescent obesity may be associated with negative psychosocial consequences, such as low self-esteem and discrimination by adults and peers.[23]

Childhood obesity is determined by a combination of hereditary and environmental factors. It is associated with obese parents, higher socioeconomic status, increased parental education, small family size, and sedentary lifestyle.[24] Children with overweight parents are at highest risk; the risk for those with two overweight parents is much higher than for children in families in which neither parent is obese. One of the trends leading to childhood obesity is the increase in inactivity. Increasing perceptions that neighborhoods are unsafe has resulted in less time spent outside playing and walking and more time spent indoors engaging in sedentary activities such as television viewing and computer usage. Television viewing is associated with consumption of calorie-dense snacks and decreased indoor activity. Studies have shown a 10% decrease in obesity risk for each hour per day of moderate to vigorous physical activity, whereas the risk increased by 12% for each hour per day of television viewing.[25] Obese children also may have a deficit in recognizing hunger sensations, stemming perhaps from parents who use food as gratification. Fast food, increased portion size and energy density, sugar-sweetened soft drinks, and high–glycemic-index foods all are likely contributing to the increased weights in children and adolescents.

Because adolescent obesity is predictive of adult obesity, prevention and treatment of childhood obesity are desirable. The goals of therapy in uncomplicated obesity are directed toward healthy eating and activity, not achievement of ideal body weight.[26] Maintenance of baseline weight should be the initial step in weight control for all overweight children 2 years of age or older.[26] The weight loss interventions should include all family members and caregivers; begin early at the point when the family is ready for change; assist the family in learning to monitor eating and activity patterns and make small and acceptable changes in these patterns; and they should encourage and emphasize, not criticize. Approaches can include a reduction of inactivity by limitation of television, computer, and video games and by building activity into daily routine, encouraging 30 minutes of unstructured outdoor play on most days. Specific strategies can include reduction of certain high-calorie foods or an appropriate balance of low-, medium-, and high-calorie foods. Commercial diets are not recommended.

In summary, obesity is defined as excess body fat resulting from the consumption of calories in excess of those expended for exercise and activities. Heredity, socioeconomic, cultural, and environmental factors, psychological influences, and activity levels have been implicated as causative factors in the development of obesity. The health risks associated with obesity include hypertension and cardiovascular disease, hyperlipidemia, insulin resistance, and type 2 diabetes mellitus. Other risks include menstrual irregularities and infertility, cancer of the endometrium, breast, prostate, and colon, and gallbladder disease. There are two types of obesity—upper body and lower body obesity. Upper body obesity is associated with a higher incidence of complications. The treatment of obesity focuses on nutritionally adequate weight-loss diets, behavior modification, exercise, social support, and, in situations of marked obesity, surgical methods. Obesity is the most prevalent nutritional disorder affecting the pediatric population in the United States.

Undernutrition

Undernutrition ranges from the selective deficiency of a single nutrient to starvation, in which there is deprivation of all ingested nutrients. Undernutrition can result from willful eating behaviors, as in anorexia nervosa and the binge-eating/purging syndrome; lack of food availability; or health problems that impair food intake and decrease its absorption and use. Weight loss and malnutrition are common during illness, recovery from trauma, and hospitalization.

The prevalence of malnutrition in children is substantial. Globally, nearly 195 million children younger than 5 years of age are undernourished.[27] Malnutrition is most obvious in developing countries of the world, where the condition takes severe forms. Even in developed nations, malnutrition remains a problem. In 1992, it was estimated that 12 million American children consumed diets that were significantly below the recommended allowances of the National Academy of Sciences.[27]

MALNUTRITION AND STARVATION

Malnutrition and starvation are conditions in which a person does not receive or is unable to use an adequate amount of calories and nutrients for body function. Among the many causes of starvation, some are willful, such as occurs in persons with anorexia nervosa who do not consume enough food to maintain weight and health, and some are due to disease conditions, such as occurs in persons with Crohn disease who are unable to absorb nutrients from the food they eat. Most cases of food deprivation result in semistarvation with protein and calorie (protein-calorie) malnutrition.

In malnutrition and starvation, the amount of food consumed and absorbed is drastically reduced. It may be primary, due to inadequate food intake, or secondary to disease conditions that produce tissue wasting. Most of the literature on malnutrition and starvation has dealt with infants and children in underdeveloped countries. Malnutrition in this population commonly is divided into two distinct conditions: marasmus and kwashiorkor.

Marasmus represents a progressive loss of muscle mass and fat stores due to inadequate food intake that is equally deficient in calories and protein. The person appears emaciated, with sparse, dry, and dull hair and depressed heart rate, blood pressure, and body temperature. The child with marasmus has a wasted appearance, with stunted growth and loss of subcutaneous fat, but with relatively normal skin, hair, liver function, and affect. *Kwashiorkor* is caused by protein deficiency. The term *kwashiorkor* comes from the African word meaning "the disease suffered by the displaced child," because the condition develops soon after a child is displaced from the breast after the arrival of a new infant and placed on a starchy gruel feeding. The child with kwashiorkor is characterized by edema, desquamating skin, discolored hair, enlarged abdomen, anorexia, and extreme apathy. There is less weight loss and wasting of skeletal muscles than in marasmus. Other manifestations include skin lesions, easily pluckable hair, enlarged liver and distended abdomen, cold extremities, and decreased cardiac output and tachycardia. *Marasmus-kwashiorkor* is an advanced protein-calorie deficit together with increased protein requirement or loss. This results in a rapid decrease in anthropometric measurements with obvious edema and wasting and loss of organ mass.

Protein-Calorie Malnutrition

Protein-calorie malnutrition represents a depletion of the body's lean tissues caused by starvation or a combination of starvation and catabolic stress. The lean tissues are the fat-free, metabolically active tissues of the body; namely, the skeletal muscles, viscera, and cells of the blood and immune system. They account for 35% to 50% of the total weight in the healthy young adult, with fat (20% to 30%), extracellular fluid (20%), and skeletal and connective tissues (10% to 15%).[28] Because the lean tissues are the largest body compartment, their rate of loss is the main determinant of total body weight in most cases of protein-calorie malnutrition.

Protein-calorie malnutrition is common in persons with trauma, sepsis, and serious illnesses such as cancer and acquired immunodeficiency syndrome. Approximately half of all persons with cancer experience tissue wasting in which the tumor induces metabolic changes leading to a loss of adipose tissue and muscle mass.[29] In healthy adults, body protein homeostasis is maintained by a cycle in which the net loss of protein in the postabsorptive state is matched by a net postprandial gain of protein.[30,31] In persons with severe injury or illness, net protein breakdown is accelerated and protein rebuilding disrupted. Consequently, these persons may lose up to 20% of body protein, much of which originates in skeletal muscle. Protein mass is lost from the liver, gastrointestinal tract, kidneys, and heart. As protein is lost from the liver, hepatic synthesis of serum proteins decreases and decreased levels of serum proteins are observed. There is a decrease in immune cells. Wound healing is poor, and the body is unable to fight off infection because of multiple immunologic malfunctions throughout the body. The gastrointestinal tract undergoes mucosal atrophy with loss of villi in the small intestine, resulting in malabsorption. The loss of protein from cardiac muscle leads to a decrease in myocardial contractility and cardiac output. The muscles used for breathing become weakened, and respiratory function becomes compromised as muscle proteins are used as a fuel source. A reduction in respiratory function has many implications, especially for persons with burns, trauma, infection, or chronic respiratory disease and for persons who are being mechanically ventilated because of respiratory failure.

In hospitalized patients, malnutrition increases morbidity and mortality rates, the incidence of complications, and length of stay. Malnutrition may present at the time of admission or develop during hospitalization. The hospitalized patient often finds eating a healthful diet difficult and commonly has restrictions on food and water intake in preparation for tests and surgery. Pain, medications, special diets, and stress can decrease appetite. Even when the patient is well enough to eat, being alone in a room where unpleasant treatments may be given is not conducive to eating. Although hospitalized patients may appear to need fewer calories because they are on bed rest, their actual need for caloric intake may be higher because of other energy expenditures. For example, more calories are expended during fever, when the metabolic rate is increased. There also may be an increased need for protein to support tissue repair after trauma or surgery.

Diagnosis

No single diagnostic measure is sufficiently accurate to serve as a reliable test for malnutrition. Techniques of nutritional assessment include evaluation of dietary intake, anthropometric measurements, clinical examination, and laboratory tests. Evaluation of weight is particularly important. Body weight can be assessed in relation to height using the BMI. Evaluation of body composition can be performed by inspection or using anthropometric measurements such as skinfold thickness. Serum albumin and prealbumin are used in the diagnosis of protein-calorie malnutrition. Albumin, which historically has been used as a determinant of nutrition status, has a relatively large body pool and a half-life of 20 days and is less sensitive to changes in nutrition than prealbumin, which has a shorter half-life and a relatively small body pool.[32]

Treatment

The treatment of severe protein-calorie malnutrition involves the use of measures to correct fluid and electrolyte abnormalities and replenish proteins, calories, and micronutrients. Treatment is started with modest quantities of proteins and calories based on the person's actual weight. Concurrent administration of vitamins and minerals is needed. Either the enteral or parenteral route can be used. The treatment should be undertaken slowly to avoid complications. The administration of water and sodium with carbohydrates can overload a heart that has been weakened by malnutrition and result in congestive failure. Enteral feedings can result in malabsorptive symptoms because of abnormalities in the gastrointestinal tract. Refeeding edema is benign dependent edema that results from renal sodium reabsorption and poor skin and blood vessel integrity. It is treated by elevation of the dependent area and modest sodium restrictions. Diuretics are ineffective and may aggravate electrolyte deficiencies.

EATING DISORDERS

Eating disorders affect an estimated 5 million Americans each year.[33] These illnesses, which include anorexia nervosa, bulimia nervosa, and binge-eating disorder and their variants, incorporate serious disturbances in eating, such as restriction of intake and binging, with an excessive concern over body shape or body weight. Eating disorders typically occur in adolescent girls and young women, although 5% to 15% of cases of anorexia nervosa and 40% of cases of binge-eating disorder occur in boys and men.[33] The mortality rate from anorexia nervosa, 0.56% per year, is more than 12 times the mortality rate among young women in the general population.[33]

KEY CONCEPTS

Eating Disorders

➤ Eating disorders are serious disturbances in eating, such as willful restriction of intake and binge eating, as well as excessive concern over body weight and shape.

➤ Anorexia nervosa is characterized by a refusal to maintain a minimally normal body weight (e.g., at least 85% of minimal expected weight); an excessive concern over gaining weight and how the body is perceived in terms of size and shape; and amenorrhea (in girls and women after menarche).

➤ Bulimia nervosa is characterized by recurrent binge eating; inappropriate compensatory behaviors, such as self-induced vomiting, fasting, or excessive exercise that follow the binge-eating episode; and extreme concern over body shape and weight.

➤ Binge eating consists of consuming unusually large quantities of food during a discrete period (e.g., within any 2-hour period) along with a lack of control over the binge-eating episode.

Eating disorders are more prevalent in industrialized societies and occur in all socioeconomic and major ethnic groups. A combination of genetic, neurochemical, developmental, and sociocultural factors is thought to contribute to the development of the disorders.[34,35] The American Psychiatric Society's *Diagnostic and Statistical Manual of Mental Disorders, 4th Edition, Text Revision* (DSM-IV-TR) has established criteria for the diagnosis of anorexia nervosa and bulimia nervosa.[36] Although these criteria allow clinicians to make a diagnosis in persons with a specific eating disorder, the symptoms often occur along a continuum between those of anorexia nervosa and bulimia nervosa. Preoccupation with weight and excessive self-evaluation of weight and shape are common to both disorders, and persons with eating disorders may demonstrate a mixture of both disorders.[36] The female athlete triad, which includes disordered eating, amenorrhea, and osteoporosis, does not meet the strict DSM-IV-TR criteria for anorexia nervosa or bulimia nervosa, but shares many of the characteristics and therapeutic concerns of the two disorders (see Chapter 43). Persons with eating disorders may require concomitant evaluation for psychiatric illness because eating disorders often are accompanied by mood, anxiety, and personality disorders. Suicidal behavior may accompany anorexia nervosa and bulimia nervosa and should be ruled out.[33]

Anorexia Nervosa

Anorexia nervosa was first described in the scientific literature over 100 years ago by Sir William Gull.[37] The DSM-IV-TR diagnostic criteria for anorexia nervosa are (1) a refusal to maintain a minimally normal body weight for age and height (e.g., at least 85% of minimal expected weight or BMI ≥ 17.5); (2) an intense fear of gaining weight or becoming fat; (3) a disturbance in the way one's body size, weight, or shape is perceived; and (4) amenorrhea (in girls and women after menarche).[36] Anorexia nervosa is more prevalent among young women than men. The disorder typically begins in teenaged girls who are obese or perceive themselves as being obese. An interest in weight reduction becomes an obsession, with severely restricted caloric intake and frequently with excessive physical exercise. The term *anorexia,* meaning "loss of appetite," is a misnomer because hunger is felt, but in this case is denied.

Many organ systems are affected by the malnutrition that occurs in persons with anorexia nervosa. The severity of the abnormalities tends to be related to the degree of malnutrition and is reversed by refeeding. The most frequent complication of anorexia is amenorrhea and loss of secondary sex characteristics with decreased levels of estrogen, which can eventually lead to osteoporosis. Bone loss can occur in young women after as short a period of illness as 6 months.[33] Symptomatic compression fractures and kyphosis have been reported. Constipation, cold intolerance and failure to shiver in cold, bradycardia, hypotension, decreased heart size, electrocardiographic changes, blood and electrolyte abnormalities, and skin with lanugo (i.e., increased amounts of fine hair) are common. Unexpected sudden deaths have been reported; the risk appears to increase as weight drops to less than 35% to 40% of ideal weight. It is believed that these deaths are caused by myocardial degeneration and heart failure rather than dysrhythmias.

The most exasperating aspect of the treatment of anorexia is the inability of the person with anorexia to recognize there is a problem. Because anorexia is a form of starvation, it can lead to death if left untreated. A multidisciplinary approach appears to be the most effective method of treating persons with the disorder.[38,39] The goals of treatment are eating and weight gain, resolution of issues with the family, healing of pain from the past, and efforts to work on psychological, relationship, and emotional issues.

Bulimia Nervosa and Binge Eating

Bulimia nervosa and binge eating are eating disorders that encompass an array of distinctive behaviors, feelings, and thoughts. Binge eating is characterized by the consumption of an unusually large quantity of food during a discrete time (*e.g.*, within any 2-hour period) along with lack of control over the binge-eating episode. A binge-eating/purging subtype of anorexia nervosa also exists.[36] Low body weight is the major factor that differentiates this subtype of anorexia nervosa from bulimia nervosa.

Bulimia Nervosa. Bulimia nervosa is 10 times more common in women than men; it usually begins between 13 and 20 years of age, and affects up to 3% of young women.[40] The DSM-IV-TR criteria for bulimia nervosa are (1) recurrent binge eating (at least two times per week for 3 months); (2) inappropriate compensatory behaviors such as self-induced vomiting, abuse of laxatives or diuretics, fasting, or excessive exercise that follow the binge-eating episode; (3) self-evaluation that is unduly influenced by body shape and weight; and (4) a determination that the eating disorder does not occur exclusively during episodes of anorexia nervosa.[36] The diagnostic criteria for bulimia nervosa now include subtypes to distinguish patients who compensate by purging (*e.g.*, vomiting or abuse of laxatives or diuretics) and those who use nonpurging behaviors (*e.g.*, fasting or excessive exercise). The disorder may be associated with other psychiatric disorders, such as substance abuse.[33,40,41]

The complications of bulimia nervosa include those resulting from overeating, self-induced vomiting, and cathartic and diuretic abuse.[33,40–42] Among the complications of self-induced vomiting are dental disorders, parotitis, and fluid and electrolyte disorders. Dental abnormalities, such as sensitive teeth, increased dental caries, and periodontal disease, occur with frequent vomiting because the high acid content of the vomitus causes tooth enamel to dissolve. Esophagitis, dysphagia, and esophageal stricture are common. With frequent vomiting, there often is reflux of gastric contents into the lower esophagus because of relaxation of the lower esophageal sphincter. Vomiting may lead to aspiration pneumonia,

especially in intoxicated or debilitated persons. Potassium, chloride, and hydrogen are lost in the vomitus, and frequent vomiting predisposes to metabolic acidosis with hypokalemia (see Chapter 6). An unexplained physical response to vomiting is the development of benign, painless parotid gland enlargement.

The weights of persons with bulimia nervosa may fluctuate, although not to the dangerously low levels seen in anorexia nervosa. Their thoughts and feelings range from fear of not being able to stop eating to a concern about gaining too much weight. They also experience feelings of sadness, anger, guilt, shame, and low self-esteem.

Treatment strategies include psychological and pharmacologic treatments. Unlike persons with anorexia nervosa, persons with bulimia nervosa or binge eating are upset by the behaviors practiced and the thoughts and feelings experienced, and they are more willing to accept help. Pharmacotherapeutic agents include the tricyclic antidepressants (*e.g.*, desipramine, imipramine), the selective serotonin reuptake inhibitors (*e.g.*, fluoxetine), and other antidepressant medications.[42]

Binge Eating. Binge eating is characterized by recurrent episodes of binge eating at least 2 days per week for 6 months and at least three of the following: (1) eating rapidly; (2) eating until becoming uncomfortably full; (3) eating large amounts when not hungry; (4) eating alone because of embarrassment; and (5) disgust, depression, or guilt because of eating episodes.[36,38,41] The great majority of persons with binge-eating disorder are overweight and, in turn, obese persons have a higher prevalence of binge-eating disorder than the nonobese populations.[42]

The primary goal of therapy for binge-eating disorders is to establish a regular, healthful eating pattern. Persons with binge-eating disorders who have been successfully treated for their eating disorder have reported that making meal plans, eating a balanced diet at three regular meals a day, avoiding high-sugar foods and other binge foods, recording food intake and binge-eating episodes, exercising regularly, finding alternative activities, and avoiding alcohol and drugs are helpful in maintaining their more healthful eating behaviors after treatment.

In summary, Undernutrition can range from a selective deficiency of a single nutrient to starvation, in which there is deprivation of all ingested nutrients. Malnutrition and starvation are among the most widespread causes of morbidity and mortality in the world. The body adapts to starvation through the use of fat stores and glucose synthesis to supply the energy needs of the central nervous system. Malnutrition is common during illness, recovery from trauma, and hospitalization. The effects of malnutrition and starvation on body function are widespread. They include loss of muscle mass, impaired wound healing, impaired immunologic function, decreased appetite, loss of calcium and phosphate from bone, anovulation and amenorrhea in women, and decreased testicular function in men.

Anorexia nervosa, bulimia nervosa, and binge eating are eating disorders that result in malnutrition. In persons with anorexia nervosa, a distorted attitude about eating leads to serious weight loss and malnutrition. Bulimia nervosa is characterized by secretive episodes or binges of eating large quantities of easily consumed, high-calorie foods, followed by compensatory behaviors such as fasting, self-induced vomiting, or abuse of laxatives or diuretics. Binge-eating disorder is characterized by eating large quantities of food but is not accompanied by purging and other inappropriate compensatory behaviors seen in persons with bulimia nervosa.

Review Exercises

A 25-year-old woman is 65 inches tall and weighs 300 pounds. She works as a receptionist in an office, brings her lunch to work with her, spends her evenings watching television, and gets very little exercise. She reports that she has been fat ever since she was a little girl, she has tried "every diet under the sun," and when she diets she loses some weight, but gains it all back again.

A. Calculate her BMI.
B. How would you classify her obesity?
C. What are her risk factors for obesity?
D. What would be one of the first steps in helping her develop a plan to lose weight?

A 16-year-old high school student is brought into the physician's office by her mother, who is worried because her daughter insists on dieting because she thinks she is too fat. The daughter is 67 inches tall and weighs 96 pounds. Her history reveals that she is a straight-A student, plays in the orchestra, and is on the track team. Although she had been having regular menstrual periods, she has not had a period in 4 months. She is given a tentative diagnosis of anorexia nervosa.

A. What are the criteria for a diagnosis of anorexia nervosa?
B. What is the physiologic reason for her amenorrhea?
C. What are some of the physiologic manifestations associated with malnutrition and severe weight loss?

Visit the Porth: Essentials of Pathophysiology: Concepts of Altered Health States web site (http://thePoint.LWW.com/PorthEssentials) for links to chapter-related resources on the Internet, all-new exclusive animations, chapter review questions, and more!

REFERENCES

1. Guyton A. C., Hall J. E. (2006). *Textbook of medical physiology* (11th ed., pp. 865–875). Philadelphia: Elsevier Saunders.
2. Subcommittee on the Tenth Edition of the RDAs. (1989). *Recommended dietary allowances* (10th ed.). Commission on Life Sciences–National Council. Washington, DC: National Academy Press.
3. National Academy Press. (2000). Introduction to dietary references intakes. In *Dietary reference intakes for vitamin C, vitamin E, selenium, and carotenoids*. Washington, DC: National Academy Press. [On-line.] Available: www.nap.edu/books/0309069351/html.
4. Detsky A. S., Smalley P. S., Chang J. (1994). Is this patient malnourished? *Journal of the American Medical Association* 271, 54–58.
5. World Health Organization. (1989). *Measuring obesity: Classification and description of anthropometric data.* Copenhagen: World Health Organization.
6. North American Association for Study of Obesity. (1998). Clinical guidelines on the identification, evaluation, and treatment of overweight and obesity in adults. NIH publication no. 98-4083. *Obesity Research* 6(Suppl. 2), 51S–209S. [On-line.] Available: www.nhlbi.nih.gov/guidelines/ob_gdlns.htm.
7. Abernathy R. P., Black D. R. (1996). Healthy body weight: An alternative perspective. *American Journal of Clinical Nutrition* 63(Suppl.), 448S–451S.
8. Willett W. C., Dietz W. H., Colditz G. A. (1999). Guidelines to healthy weight. *New England Journal of Medicine* 341, 427–434.
9. Mokdad A. H., Serdula M. K., Dietz W. H., et al. (1999). The spread of the obesity epidemic in the United States, 1991–1998. *Journal of the American Medical Association* 282, 1519–1522.
10. Flegal K. M., Carroll M. D., Kuczmarski R. J., et al. (2002). Prevalence and trends in obesity among US adults, 1999–2000. *Journal of the American Medical Association* 288, 2793–2796.
11. Goran M. I. (2000). Energy metabolism and obesity. *Medical Clinics of North America* 84, 347–362.
12. Hill J. O., Wyatt H. R., Melanson E. L. (2000). Genetic and environmental contributions to obesity. *Medical Clinics of North America* 84, 333–346.
13. Soreneson T. J., Holst C., Stunkard A. J., et al. (1992). Correlations of body mass index of adult adoptees and their biological and adoptive relatives. *International Journal of Obesity and Related Metabolic Disorders* 16, 227–236.
14. Kissebah A. H., Krakower G. R. (1994). Regional adiposity and morbidity. *Physiological Reviews* 74, 761–811.
15. Pleuss J. A., Hoffman R. G., Sonnentag G. E., et al. (1993). Effects of abdominal fat on insulin and androgen levels. *Obesity Research* 1(Suppl. 1), 25F.
16. Jeffery R. W. (1996). Does weight cycling present a health risk? *American Journal of Clinical Nutrition* 63(Suppl. 3), 452S–455S.
17. Dwyer J. (1996). Policy and healthy weight. *American Journal of Nutrition* 63(Suppl. 3), 415S–418S.
18. Lee I., Manson J. E., Hennekens C. H., et al. (1993). Body weight and mortality: A 27-year follow-up of middle-aged men. *Journal of the American Medical Association* 270, 2823–2828.

19. Task Force on Prevention and Treatment of Obesity. (1994). Towards prevention of obesity: Research directives. *Obesity Research* 2, 571.

20. Berke E. M., Morden N. E. (2000). Medical management of obesity. *American Family Physician* 62, 419–426.

21. Ogden C. L., Flegal K. M., Carroll M. D., et al. (2002). Prevalence and trends in overweight among US children and adolescents, 1999–2000. *Journal of the American Medical Association* 288, 1728–1732.

22. Fagot-Campagna A., Pettitt D. J., Engelgau N. M., et al. (2000). Type 2 diabetes among North American children and adolescents: An epidemiologic review and a public health perspective. *Journal of Pediatrics* 136, 664–672.

23. Hill J. O., Trowbridge F. L. (1998). Childhood obesity: Future directions and research priorities. *Pediatrics* 101(Suppl. 3), 570–574.

24. Birch L. L., Fisher J. O. (1998). Development of eating behaviors among children and adolescents. *Pediatrics* 101(Suppl. 3), 539–554.

25. Ebbeling C. B., Pawlak D. B., Ludwig D. S. (2002). Childhood obesity: Public-health crisis, common sense cure. *Lancet* 360, 473–482.

26. Schonfeld-Warden N., Warden C. H. (1997). Childhood obesity. *Pediatric Clinics of North America* 44, 339–361.

27. Brown J. L., Pollitt E. (1996). Malnutrition, poverty, intellectual development. *Scientific American* 274(2), 38–43.

28. Hoffer I. J. (2001). Clinical nutrition: 1. Protein-energy malnutrition in the inpatient. *Canadian Medical Association Journal* 165, 1345–1349.

29. Tisdale M. J. (1999). Wasting in cancer. *Journal of Nutrition* 129(IS Suppl.), 43S–46S.

30. Chiolero R., Revelly J., Tappy L. (1999). Energy metabolism in sepsis and injury. *Journal of Nutrition* 129(IS Suppl.), 45S–51S.

31. Biolo G., Gabriele T., Ciccchi B., et al. (1999). Metabolic response to injury and sepsis: Changes in protein metabolism. *Journal of Nutrition* 129(IS Suppl.), 53S–57S.

32. Beck F. E., Rosenthal T. C. (2002). Prealbumin: A marker for nutritional evaluation. *American Family Physician* 65, 1575–1578.

33. Becker A., Grinspoon S. K., Klibanski A., et al. (1999). Eating disorders. *New England Journal of Medicine* 340, 1092–1098.

34. Pritt S. D. (2003). Diagnosis of eating disorders in primary care. *American Family Physician* 67, 304–312.

35. Fairburn C. G., Harrison P. J. (2003). Eating disorders. *Lancet* 361, 407–416.

36. American Psychiatric Society. (2000). Practice guideline for treatment of patients with eating disorders (revision). *American Journal of Psychiatry* 157, 1–38.

37. Gull W. W. (1868). Anorexia nervosa. *Transactions of the Clinical Society of London* 7, 22–27.

38. Kreipe R. E., Birndorf S. A. (2000). Eating disorders in adolescents and young adults. *Medical Clinics of North America* 84, 1027–1049.

39. Gordon A. (2001). Eating disorders: Anorexia nervosa. *Hospital Practice* 36(2), 36–38.

40. McGilley B. M., Pryor T. L. (1998). Assessment and treatment of bulimia nervosa. *American Family Physician* 57, 2743–2750.

41. Mehler P. S. (2003). Bulimia nervosa. *New England Journal of Medicine* 349, 875–881.

42. Schneider M. (2003). Bulimia nervosa and binge-eating disorders in adolescents. *Adolescent Medicine* 14, 119–131.

C h a p t e r 9

Disorders of White Blood Cells and Lymphoid Tissues

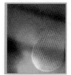

The hematopoietic system and lymphoid tissues are responsible for the generation and regulation of the blood cells that function in the transport of oxygen, defense against microorganisms, and preservation of the integrity of the vascular system. The discussion in this chapter is divided into two parts: the first provides an introduction to the hematopoietic system, lymphoid tissues, and the white blood cells, and the second focuses on disorders of the white blood cells, including those of non-neoplastic (neutropenia and infectious mononucleosis) and neoplastic (lymphomas, leukemias, and multiple myeloma) origin. The megakaryocytes and platelets are discussed in Chapter 10, the red cells in Chapter 11, and the immune cells (lymphocytes and monocytes) in Chapter 13.

Hematopoietic and Lymphoid Tissue

Blood consists of blood cells (*i.e.,* leukocytes or white blood cells, thrombocytes or platelets, and erythrocytes or red blood cells) and the plasma in which the cells are suspended. The generation of blood cells takes place in the *hematopoietic* (from the Greek *haima* for "blood" and *poiesis* for "making") system. These cells all derive from a single pool of pluripotent stem cells in the bone marrow, which give rise to two types of multipotential stem cells: the hematopoietic stem cells, which remain in the bone marrow, and the lymphopoietic stem cells, which migrate to the lymphoid tissues in the thymus, lymph nodes, and spleen.

THE BONE MARROW AND HEMATOPOIESIS

The bone marrow consists of hematopoietic or blood-forming cells and stromal tissue that provides support for the blood-forming cells. The blood-forming population of bone marrow is made up of three types of cells: pluripotent stem cells, multipotent stem cells, and committed progenitor cells that develop into the various types of blood cells (Fig. 9-1). The pluripotent stem cells give rise to two types of multipotential stem cells, the common lymphoid and the common myeloid stem cells. The common lymphoid stem cells, in turn, differentiate into lineage-specific precursor cells that develop into T lymphocytes (T cells), B lymphocytes (B cells), and natural killer cells. From the common myeloid stem cells arise precursor cells capable of differentiating along the erythrocyte/megakaryocytic, eosinophilic, and granulocyte-monocyte pathways.

A committed stem cell that forms a specific type of blood cell is called a *colony-forming unit* (CFU). Under normal conditions, the numbers and total mass for each type of circulating blood cell remain relatively constant. The blood cells are produced in different numbers according to needs and regulatory factors. This regulation of blood cells is controlled by a group of short-acting soluble mediators, called *cytokines*, that stimulate the proliferation, differentiation, and functional activation of the various blood cell precursors in bone marrow.[2] The cytokines that stimulate hematopoiesis are called *colony-stimulating factors* (CSFs), based on their ability to stimulate the growth of the hematopoietic cell colonies from bone marrow precursors. Lineage-specific CSFs that act on committed progenitor cells include erythropoietin (EPO), granulocyte-monocyte colony-stimulating factor (GM-CSF), and thrombopoietin (TPO). The major sources of the CSFs are the lymphocytes and stromal cells of the bone marrow. Other cytokines, such as the interleukins, support the development of lymphocytes and act synergistically to aid the functions of the CSFs (see Chapter 13).

LYMPHOID TISSUES

The lymphoid tissues represent the structures where lymphocytes proliferate, mature, and interact with antigens. Lymphoid tissues can be classified into two groups: the central or generative organs and peripheral lymphoid organs. The central lymphoid structures consist of the bone marrow, where all lymphocytes arise, and the thy-

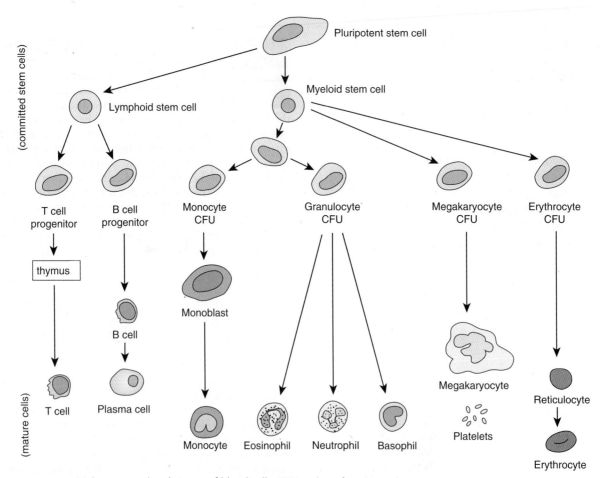

FIGURE 9-1 Major maturational stages of blood cells. CFU, colony-forming units.

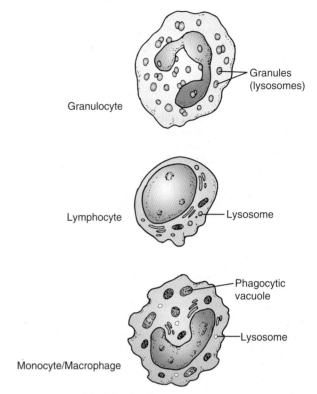

FIGURE 9-2 White blood cells.

mus, where T cells mature and self-reactive T cells are eliminated. The peripheral lymphoid organs are the sites where mature lymphocytes respond to foreign antigens. They include the lymph nodes, the spleen, the mucosa-associated lymphoid tissues, and the cutaneous immune system. In addition, poorly defined aggregates of lymphocytes are found in connective tissues and virtually all organs of the body.

LEUKOCYTES (WHITE BLOOD CELLS)

The white blood cells, or leukocytes, which constitute only 1% of the total blood volume, originate in the bone marrow and circulate throughout the lymphoid tissues of the body. There they function in the inflammatory and immune processes. They include the granulocytes, the lymphocytes, and the monocytes (Fig. 9-2).

Granulocytes

The granulocytes are all phagocytic cells and are identifiable because of their cytoplasmic granules. These white blood cells are spherical and have distinctive multilobar nuclei. The granulocytes are divided into three types (neutrophils, eosinophils, and basophils) according to the staining properties of the granules.

Neutrophils. The neutrophils, which constitute 55% to 65% of the total number of white blood cells, have granules that are neutral and thus do not stain with an acidic or a basic dye. Because their nuclei are divided into three to five lobes, they are often called polymorphonuclear leukocytes (PMNs).

The neutrophils are primarily responsible for maintaining normal host defenses against pathogens that have breached the physical barriers of skin and mucous membranes. The cytoplasm of mature neutrophils contains fine granules. These granules contain degrading enzymes that are used in destroying foreign substances and correspond to lysosomes found in other cells. The degradative functions of the neutrophil are important in maintaining normal host defenses and in mediating the inflammatory response (see Chapter 14).

The neutrophil has a short life span. After release from the marrow, the neutrophils spend only about 4 to 8 hours in the circulation before moving into the tissues.[1] Their survival in the tissues lasts about 4 to 5 days. They die in the tissues while discharging their phagocytic function or die of senescence. The pool of circulating neutrophils (*i.e.,* those that appear in the blood count) is in rapid equilibrium with a similar-sized pool of cells marginating along the walls of small blood vessels. These are the neutrophils that respond to chemotactic factors and migrate into the tissues toward the offending agent during an inflammatory response.

Eosinophils. The cytoplasmic granules of the eosinophils stain red with the acidic dye eosin. These leukocytes constitute 1% to 3% of the total number of white blood cells and increase in number during allergic reactions. They are thought to release enzymes or chemical mediators that detoxify agents associated with allergic reactions. Eosinophils are also involved in parasitic infections. Although most parasites are too large to be phagocytized by eosinophils, the eosinophils attach themselves to the parasite by special surface molecules and release hydrolytic enzymes and other substances from their granules that kill the parasite.

Basophils. The granules of the basophils stain blue with a basic dye. These cells constitute only about 0.3% to 0.5% of the white blood cells. The basophils in the circulating blood are similar to the large mast cells located immediately outside the capillaries in body tissues. Both the basophils and mast cells release heparin, an anticoagulant, into the blood. The mast cells and basophils also release histamine, a vasodilator, and other inflammatory mediators. The mast cells and basophils play an exceedingly important role in allergic reactions (see Chapter 15).

Lymphocytes

The lymphocytes have their origin in the lymphoid stem cells that are found in the bone marrow. The lymphocytes constitute 20% to 30% of the white blood cell count. They have no identifiable granules in the cytoplasm and are sometimes referred to as *agranulocytes*. They move between blood and lymphoid tissues, where they may be stored for hours or years. Their function in the lymph nodes or spleen is to defend against foreign microbes in the immune response.

Lymphocytes consist of three distinct subsets that are morphologically indistinguishable, but different in terms of function and protein products. One subset, the B lymphocytes, differentiates into antibody-producing plasma cells that are involved in humoral-mediated immunity. A second subset, the T lymphocytes, is responsible for orchestrating the immune response and effecting cell-mediated immunity. Natural killer (NK) cells are a third subset of lymphocytes whose receptors are different from those of B and T cells and whose major function is in innate immunity. These different types of lymphocytes are distinguished by their cell surface molecules or markers, which can be identified through use of monoclonal antibodies.[2] These molecules, which are called *clusters of differentiation* (CD), can be grouped into categories that are specific for cells of different lineages, maturational pathways, or activation states. For example, helper T cells express the CD4+ surface marker and the effector T cells express the CD8+ marker. The classification of lymphocytes by CD markers is now widely used to identify the different cells and define their function, and to help diagnose different diseases such as lymphoma and leukemia.

Monocytes and Macrophages

Monocytes are the largest of the white blood cells and constitute about 3% to 8% of the total leukocyte count. They have abundant cytoplasm and a darkly stained nucleus, which has a distinctive "U" or kidney shape. The circulating life span of the monocyte is about 1 to 3 days, three to four times longer than that of the granulocytes. These cells survive for months to years in the tissues. The monocytes, which are phagocytic cells, are often referred to as *macrophages* when they enter the tissues. The mono-

cytes engulf larger and greater quantities of foreign material than do the neutrophils. These leukocytes play an important role in chronic inflammation and are also involved in the immune response by activating lymphocytes and by presenting antigen to T cells. When the monocyte leaves the vascular system and enters the tissues, it functions as a macrophage with specific activity. The macrophages are known as *histiocytes* in loose connective tissue, *microglial cells* in the brain, and *Kupffer cells* in the liver.

In summary, the hematopoietic system consists of the different types of blood cells generated from the pluripotent stem cells in the bone marrow. These cells differentiate into committed cell lines that develop into red blood cells, platelets, and a variety of white blood cells. The development of the different types of blood cells is supported by chemical messengers called colony-stimulating factors. The lymphoid tissues represent the structures where lymphocytes proliferate, mature, and interact with antigens. They include the bone marrow and thymus, where the lymphocytes originate and differentiate, and peripheral lymphoid organs (lymph nodes, spleen, mucosa-associated lymphoid tissues), where the mature lymphocytes respond to foreign antigens.

The white blood cells or leukocytes originate in the bone marrow and circulate throughout the lymphoid tissues of the body. They include the granulocytes, lymphocytes, and monocytes. The neutrophils, the predominant type of granulocyte, are phagocytic cells responsible for maintaining normal host defenses against pathogens that have gotten past the physical barriers of skin and mucous membranes. The lymphocytes are responsible for acquired immunity (T and B cells) and innate immunity (NK cells). The circulating monocytes and tissue macrophages are phagocytic cells that play an important role in chronic inflammation and are also involved in the immune response by activating lymphocytes and presenting antigen to T cells.

Non-neoplastic Disorders of White Blood Cells

The number of leukocytes, or white blood cells, in the peripheral circulation normally ranges from 5000 to 10,000/µL of blood. The non-neoplastic disorders of white blood cells include a deficiency of leukocytes (leukopenia) and proliferative disorders in which there are increased numbers of leukocytes.

NEUTROPENIA (AGRANULOCYTOSIS)

The term *leukopenia* describes an absolute decrease in white blood cell numbers. The disorder may affect any of the specific types of white blood cells, but most often it affects the neutrophils, which are the predominant type of granulocyte. *Neutropenia* refers specifically to a decrease in neutrophils. It commonly is defined as a circulating neutrophil count of less than 1500 cells/μL. Agranulocytosis, which denotes a severe neutropenia, is characterized by a circulating neutrophil count of less than 200 cells/μL.[3] In *aplastic anemia,* all of the myeloid stem cells are affected, resulting in anemia, thrombocytopenia, and agranulocytosis.

Pathogenesis

The reduction in the number of granulocytes in the blood (neutropenia) can be seen in a wide variety of circumstances (Table 9-1). A number of conditions, including aplastic anemia and treatment with cancer chemotherapeutic drugs and irradiation, may cause suppression of bone marrow stem cells, with decreased production of all blood cell types. Overgrowth of neoplastic cells in cases of nonmyelogenous leukemia and lymphoma also may suppress the function of neutrophil precursors. Autoimmune disorders or idiosyncratic drug reactions may cause increased and premature destruction of neutrophils. In splenomegaly, neutrophils may be trapped in the spleen along with other blood cells. In Felty syndrome, a variant of rheumatoid arthritis, there is increased destruction of neutrophils in the spleen. Infections by viruses or bacteria may drain neutrophils from the blood faster than they can be replaced, thereby depleting the neutrophil storage pool in the bone marrow.[3] Neutropenia is also a feature of a group of rare inherited disorders such as Kostmann syndrome.

Most cases of neutropenia are drug related. Chemotherapeutic drugs used in the treatment of cancer (*e.g.,* alkylating agents, antimetabolites) cause predictable dose-dependent suppression of bone marrow function. The term *idiosyncratic* is used to describe drug reactions that are different from the effects obtained in most persons and that cannot be explained in terms of allergy. A number of drugs, such as chloramphenicol (an antibiotic), phenothiazines (antipsychotic agents), propylthiouracil (used in the treatment of hyperthyroidism), and phenylbutazone (used in the treatment of arthritis), may cause idiosyncratic depression of bone marrow function. Many idiosyncratic cases of drug-induced neutropenia are thought to be caused by immunologic mechanisms, with the drug or its metabolites acting as antigens (*i.e.,* haptens) to incite the production of antibodies reactive against the neutrophils. Neutrophils possess human leukocyte antigens (HLA) and other antigens specific to a given leukocyte line. Antibodies to these specific antigens have been identified in some cases of drug-induced neutropenia.[3]

Clinical Course

The clinical features of neutropenia usually depend on the severity of neutropenia and the cause of the disorder. Neutropenia from any cause places persons at risk for infection by gram-positive and gram-negative bacteria and by fungi. The risk of infection is related to the severity of the neutropenia. Persons with chronic benign neutropenia are often free of infection despite low neutrophil counts.

Neutrophils provide the first line of defense against organisms that inhabit the skin and gastrointestinal tract. Thus, skin infections and ulcerative necrotizing lesions of the mouth are common types of infection in neutropenia.[3] The most frequent site of serious infection is the respiratory tract, a result of bacteria or fungi that frequently colonize the airways. Untreated infections can be rapidly fatal, particularly if the neutrophil count is less than 250/μL. In the presence of severe neutropenia, the usual signs of inflammatory response to infection may be absent.

Antibiotics are used to treat infections in those situations in which neutrophil destruction can be controlled or the neutropoietic function of the bone marrow can be recovered. Hematopoietic growth factors such as recombinant human granulocyte colony-stimulating factor (rhG-CSF) may be used to stimulate the maturation and differentiation of the polymorphonuclear cell lineage.[3]

TABLE 9-1	Causes of Neutropenia	
Cause	**Mechanism**
Accelerated removal (*e.g.,* inflammation and infection)	Removal of neutrophils from the circulation exceeds production
Drug-induced granulocytopenia	
Cytotoxic drugs used in cancer therapy	Depressed bone marrow function with decreased production of all blood cells.
Phenothiazines, propylthiouracil, and others	Toxic effect on bone marrow precursors
Aminopyrine, certain sulfonamides, phenylbutazone, and others	Immune-mediated destruction
Periodic or cyclic neutropenia (occurs during infancy and later)	Unknown
Neoplasms involving bone marrow (*e.g.,* leukemias and lymphomas)	Overgrowth of neoplastic cells, which crowd out granulopoietic precursors
Idiopathic neutropenia that occurs in the absence of other disease or provoking influence	Autoimmune reaction
Felty syndrome	Intrasplenic destruction of neutrophils

Congenital Neutropenia

A decreased production of granulocytes is a feature of a group of hereditary hematologic disorders, including cyclic neutropenia and Kostmann syndrome. *Periodic* or *cyclic neutropenia* is an autosomal dominant disorder with variable expression that begins in infancy and persists for decades. It is characterized by periodic neutropenia that develops every 18 to 24 days and lasts approximately 3 to 6 days. Although the cause is undetermined, it is thought to result from impaired feedback regulation of granulocyte production and release. *Kostmann syndrome*, which occurs sporadically or as an autosomal recessive disorder, causes severe neutropenia while preserving the erythroid and megakaryocyte cell lineages that result in red blood cell and platelet production. The total white blood cell count may be within normal limits, but the neutrophil count is less than 200/µL. Monocyte and eosinophil levels may be elevated. Treatment includes the administration of rhG-CSF.[4]

A transient neutropenia may occur in neonates whose mothers have hypertension. It usually lasts from 1 to 60 hours but can persist for 3 to 30 days. This type of neutropenia, which is associated with increased risk of nosocomial infection, is thought to result from transiently reduced neutrophil production.

INFECTIOUS MONONUCLEOSIS

Infectious mononucleosis is a self-limiting lymphoproliferative disorder caused by the Epstein-Barr virus (EBV), a member of the herpesvirus family.[5-7] (*EBV-associated infectious mononucleosis* is often used to designate infectious mononucleosis caused by EBV as opposed to the non–EBV-associated clinical syndrome of infectious mononucleosis caused by other agents.) EBV is one of the most successful viruses in evading the immune system, infecting 90% of humans and persisting for the lifetime of the person.[5] Infectious mononucleosis may occur at any age, but occurs principally in adolescents and young adults among upper socioeconomic classes in developed nations. In other populations, the primary infection occurs in childhood and usually is asymptomatic.

Pathogenesis

Infectious mononucleosis is largely transmitted through oral contact with EBV-contaminated saliva. The virus initially penetrates the nasopharyngeal, oropharyngeal, and salivary epithelial cells. It then spreads to the underlying oropharyngeal lymphoid tissue and, more specifically, to B lymphocytes, all of which have receptors for EBV. Infection of the B cells may take one of two forms—it may kill the infected B cell or it may become incorporated into its genome. The B cells that harbor the EBV genome proliferate in the circulation and produce the well-known *heterophil* antibodies that are used for the diagnosis of infectious mononucleosis.[5,6] A heterophil antibody is an immunoglobulin that reacts with antigens from another species—in this case, sheep red blood cells.

The normal immune response is important in controlling the proliferation of the EBV-infected B cells and free virus. Most important in controlling the proliferation of EBV-infected B cells are the cytotoxic CD8+ T cells and natural killer (NK) cells. The virus-specific T cells appear as large, atypical lymphocytes that are characteristic of the infection. In otherwise healthy persons, the humoral and cellular immune responses serve to control viral shedding by limiting the number of infected B cells rather than eliminating them.

Although infectious B cells and free virions disappear from the blood after recovery from the disease, the virus remains in a few transformed B cells in the oropharyngeal region and is shed in the saliva. Once infected with the virus, persons remain asymptomatically infected for life, and a few intermittently shed EBV. Immunosuppressed persons shed the virus more frequently. Asymptomatic shedding of EBV by healthy persons is thought to account for most of the spread of infectious mononucleosis, despite the fact that it is not a highly contagious disease.

Clinical Course

The onset of infectious mononucleosis usually is insidious. The incubation period lasts 4 to 8 weeks.[7,8] A prodromal period, which lasts for several days, follows and is characterized by malaise, anorexia, and chills. The prodromal period precedes the onset of fever, pharyngitis, and lymphadenopathy. Occasionally, the disorder comes on abruptly with a high fever. Most persons seek medical attention for severe pharyngitis, which usually is most severe on days 5 to 7 and persists for 7 to 14 days. The lymph nodes are typically enlarged throughout the body, particularly in the cervical, axillary, and groin areas. Hepatitis and splenomegaly are common manifestations of the disease and are thought to be immune mediated. Hepatitis is characterized by hepatomegaly, nausea, anorexia, and jaundice. Although uncomfortable, it usually is a benign condition that resolves without causing permanent liver damage. The spleen may be enlarged two to three times its normal size, and rupture of the spleen is an infrequent complication. In less than 1% of cases, mostly in the adult age group, complications of the central nervous system (CNS) develop. These complications include cranial nerve palsies, encephalitis, meningitis, transverse myelitis, and Guillain-Barré syndrome.

The peripheral blood usually shows an increase in the number of leukocytes, with a white blood cell count between 12,000 and 18,000/µL, 60% of which are lymphocytes.[6] The rise in white blood cells begins during the first week, continues during the second week of the infection, and then returns to normal around the fourth week. Although leukocytosis is common, leukopenia may be seen in some persons during the first 3 days of the illness. Atypical lymphocytes are common, constituting more than 20% of the total lymphocyte count. Heterophil antibodies usually appear during the second or third week and decline after the acute illness has subsided. They may, however, be detectable for up to 9 months after onset of the disease.

Most persons with infectious mononucleosis recover without incident. The acute phase of the illness usually lasts for 2 to 3 weeks, after which recovery occurs rapidly. Some degree of debility and lethargy may persist for 2 to 3 months. Treatment is primarily symptomatic and supportive. It includes bed rest and analgesics such as aspirin to relieve the fever, headache, and sore throat.[7]

In persons with immunodeficiency disorders that lead to defects in cellular immunity (*e.g.*, human immunodeficiency virus [HIV] infection, immunosuppressant-treated recipients of organ or bone marrow transplants), EBV infection may contribute to the development of lymphoproliferative disorders (*e.g.*, non-Hodgkin lymphoma).[5,6] These persons have impaired T-cell immunity and are unable to control the proliferation of EBV-infected T cells.

In summary, neutropenia, a marked reduction in the number of circulating neutrophils, is one of the major disorders of the white blood cells. It can result from a number of mechanisms, including conditions in which there is reduced or ineffective production of neutrophils, immunologically mediated injury to the neutrophils, splenic sequestration, increased peripheral utilization, or rare inherited disorders such as Kostmann syndrome. Because the neutrophil is essential to host defenses against bacterial and fungal infections, severe and often life-threatening infections are common in persons with neutropenia.

Infectious mononucleosis is a self-limited lymphoproliferative disorder caused by the B-lymphocytotropic EBV, a member of the herpesvirus family. The highest incidence of infectious mononucleosis is found in adolescents and young adults, and it is seen more frequently in the upper socioeconomic classes of developed countries. The virus is usually transmitted in the saliva. The disease is characterized by fever, generalized lymphadenopathy, sore throat, and the appearance in the blood of atypical lymphocytes and several antibodies, including the well-known heterophil antibodies that are used in the diagnosis of infectious mononucleosis. Most persons with infectious mononucleosis recover without incident. Treatment is largely symptomatic and supportive.

Neoplastic Disorders of Hematopoietic and Lymphoid Origin

The neoplastic disorders of hematopoietic and lymphoid origin represent the most important of the white cell disorders. They include somewhat overlapping categories: the lymphomas (Hodgkin lymphoma and the non-Hodgkin lymphomas), the acute and chronic leukemias, and the plasma cell dyscrasias (multiple myeloma). The clinical features of these neoplasms are largely determined by their site of origin, the progenitor cell from which they originated, and the molecular events involved in their transformation into a malignant neoplasm. The lymphomas originate in peripheral lymphoid structures such as the lymph nodes, where B and T lymphocytes undergo further differentiation and proliferation as they interact with antigens. The leukemias, which arise from hematopoietic precursors in the bone marrow, can involve lymphocytes, granulocytes, and other blood cells. The plasma cell dyscrasias originate in the bone marrow where B cells differentiate into plasma cells. Because blood cells circulate throughout the body, these neoplasms are disseminated from the onset.

MALIGNANT LYMPHOMAS

The lymphomas, Hodgkin lymphoma and the non-Hodgkin lymphomas, represent solid tumors derived from neoplastic lymphoid tissue cells (*i.e.*, lymphocytes or histiocytes) and their precursors or derivatives. The sixth most common cancer in the United States, the lymphomas are among the most studied human tumors and among the most curable.

Hodgkin Lymphoma

Hodgkin lymphoma (HL), previously known as Hodgkin disease, is a specialized form of lymphoma that features the presence of an abnormal cell called a *Reed-Sternberg cell*.[9] It was estimated that approximately 7300 new cases of HL would be diagnosed in 2005, with 1400 deaths.[10] Distribution of the disease is bimodal; the incidence rises

KEY CONCEPTS

Malignant Lymphomas

➥ The lymphomas represent malignancies of cells derived from lymphoid cells and tissues.

➥ Hodgkin lymphoma is a type of cancer characterized by Reed-Sternberg cells that begins as a malignancy in a single lymph node and then spreads to contiguous lymph nodes.

➥ Non-Hodgkin lymphomas represent a group of heterogeneous lymphocytic cancers that are multicentric in origin and spread to various tissues throughout the body, including the bone marrow.

➥ Both types of lymphomas are characterized by manifestations related to uncontrolled lymph node and lymphoid tissue growth, bone marrow involvement, and constitutional symptoms (fever, fatigue, weight loss) related to the rapid growth of abnormal lymphoid cells and tissues.

sharply after 10 years of age, peaks in the early 20s, and then declines until 50 years of age. After 50 years of age, the incidence again increases steadily with age. The younger adult group consists equally of men and women, but after age 50 years, the incidence is higher among men.[11]

The cause of HL is unknown. Although exposure to carcinogens and viruses as well as genetic and immune mechanisms have been proposed as causes, none has been proven to be involved in the pathogenesis of HL. There is an increased frequency in persons with acquired immunodeficiency syndrome (AIDS) and after bone marrow transplantation.[9,12]

Hodgkin lymphoma is characterized by painless and progressive enlargement of a single node or group of nodes. It is believed to originate in one area of the lymphatic system, and if unchecked, it spreads throughout the lymphatic network. The initial lymph node involvement typically is above the level of the diaphragm. An exception is in elderly persons, in whom the subdiaphragmatic lymph nodes may be the first to be involved. Involvement of the retroperitoneal lymph nodes, liver, spleen, and bone marrow occurs after the disease becomes generalized.

A distinctive tumor cell, the Reed-Sternberg cell, is considered to be the true neoplastic element in HL[9,12,13] (Fig. 9-3). These malignant proliferating cells, which have been shown to be of B-cell origin, may invade almost any area of the body and may produce a wide variety of signs and symptoms. The spleen is involved in one third of the cases at the time of diagnosis.

Manifestations. Persons with HL commonly present with painless lymph node enlargement, involving a single lymph node or groups of lymph nodes. The cervical and mediastinal nodes are involved most frequently. Less commonly, the axillary, inguinal, and retroperitoneal nodes are initially involved. Accompanying constitutional symptoms may include fevers, night sweats, chills, and weight loss. An unusual symptom of HL is pain in an involved lymph node following ingestion of alcohol. Persons with HL are designated as stage A if they lack constitutional symptoms and stage B if constitutional symptoms

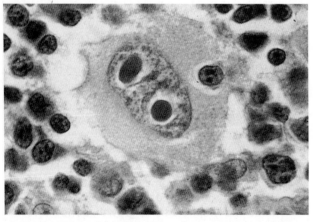

FIGURE 9-3 Classic Reed-Sternberg cell. Mirror-image nuclei contain large eosinophilic nucleoli. (From Rubin E., Gorstein F., Rubin R., et al. [Eds.]. [2005]. *Rubin's pathology: Clinicopathologic foundations of medicine* [4th ed., p. 1112]. Philadelphia: Lippincott Williams & Wilkins.)

are present. Approximately 40% of persons with HL exhibit the B symptoms.[12]

In the advanced stages of HL, the liver, lungs, digestive tract, and, occasionally, the CNS may be involved. As the disease progresses, the rapid proliferation of abnormal lymphocytes leads to an immunologic defect, particularly in cell-mediated responses, rendering the person more susceptible to viral, fungal, and protozoal infections. Anergy, or the failure to develop a positive response to skin tests, such as the tuberculin test, is common early in the course of the disease. An increased neutrophil count and mild anemia are often noted.

Diagnosis and Treatment. A definitive diagnosis of HL requires that the Reed-Sternberg cell be present in a biopsy specimen of lymph node tissue. Computed tomography (CT) scans of the chest and abdomen commonly are used to assess for involvement of mediastinal, abdominal, and pelvic lymph nodes.[14] A bipedal lymphangiogram may detect structural changes in the lymph nodes too small to visualize on CT scan. If with initial screenings the extent of lymph node involvement cannot be determined, a positron emission tomography (PET) scan may be helpful. A bilateral bone marrow biopsy is usually performed on patients who are suspected of having disseminated disease.

Persons with HL are staged according to the number of lymph nodes that are involved, whether the lymph nodes are on one or both sides of the diaphragm, and whether there is disseminated disease involving the bone marrow, liver, lung, or skin. The staging of HL is of great clinical importance because the choice of treatment and the prognosis ultimately are related to the distribution of the disease.

Irradiation and chemotherapy are used in treating the disease. Most people with localized disease are treated with radiation therapy. A combined approach using radiation and chemotherapy is used when the patient has adverse prognostic factors such as B symptoms, bulky masses, or disease involving nodes in the lower abdomen. As the accuracy of staging techniques, delivery of radiation, and curative efficacy of combination chemotherapy regimens have improved, the survival of people with HL also has improved. With modern treatment methods, a 5-year cure rate of 85% can be achieved.[10]

Non-Hodgkin Lymphomas

The non-Hodgkin lymphomas (NHLs) are a heterogeneous group of solid tumors composed of neoplastic lymphoid cells. The heterogeneity reflects the potential for malignant transformation at any stage of B- and T-lymphocyte differentiation. Non-Hodgkin lymphoma occurs three times more frequently than HL. In 2005, an estimated 56,400 new cases of NHL were diagnosed in the United States, with approximately 19,000 deaths resulting from these disorders.[10] Since the early 1970s, incidence rates for NHL have nearly doubled. More recently, incidence rates have stabilized, primarily because of the decline in HIV-related NHL.

The etiology of most of the NHLs is unknown. However, impairment of the immune system and infectious agents may play a role. There is evidence of EBV infection

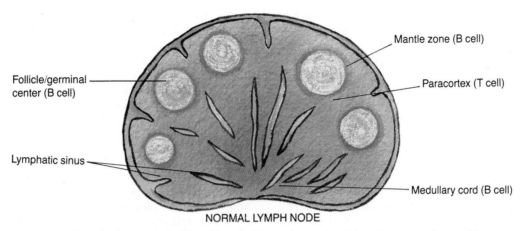

FIGURE 9-4 Sites of origin of B- and T-cell lymphoid neoplasms. B-cell lymphomas tend to proliferate in the B-cell areas of the lymph nodes (germinal center and mantle zone of secondary follicles), and T-cell lymphomas grow in the paracortical T-cell areas.

in essentially all people with Burkitt lymphoma, which is endemic to some parts of Africa.[9,12] A second virus, the human T-cell lymphotropic virus (HTLV-1), which is endemic in the southwestern islands of Japan, has been associated with adult T-cell leukemia/lymphoma. The NHLs are also seen with increased frequency in persons infected with HIV, in those who have received chronic immunosuppressive therapy after organ transplantation, and in individuals with acquired or congenital immunodeficiencies.[13,15] There is also a reported association between chronic *Helicobacter pylori* infection and low-grade, mucosa-associated lymphoid tissue (MALT) lymphoma of the stomach.[15]

Non-Hodgkin lymphomas can originate from malignant transformation of either the T or B cells during their differentiation in the peripheral lymphoid tissues.[9,12,13] Although the NHLs can originate in any of the lymphoid tissues, they most commonly originate in the lymph nodes. Most (80% to 85%) are of B-cell origin, with the remainder being largely of T-cell origin. Like normal lymphocytes, transformed B and T cells tend to home to particular lymph node sites, leading to characteristic patterns of involvement. For example, B-cell lymphomas tend to proliferate in the B-cell areas of the lymph node, whereas T-cell lymphomas typically grow in the paracortical T-cell areas (Fig. 9-4). All have the potential to spread to various lymphoid tissues throughout the body, especially the liver, spleen, and bone marrow. The classification of NHLs remains a controversial area and is still evolving. A commonly used classification is the Revised European-American Lymphoma/World Health Organization (REAL/WHO) classification, which sorts the types of lymphomas by the appearance of the lymphoma cells, the presence of surface markers (*e.g.*, antigens, CD markers), and genetic features.[16] In addition, the many specific types are sometimes grouped together into low-grade, aggressive, and very aggressive categories.

Manifestations. The manifestations of NHL depend on lymphoma type and the stage of the disease. For example, the small lymphocyte tumors are low-grade tumors that tend to progress slowly and are often asymptomatic for long periods. With or without treatment, the natural course of the disease may fluctuate over 5 to 10 or more years. Low-grade lymphomas eventually transform into more aggressive forms of lymphoma/leukemia and cause the death of the patient. The diffuse large B-cell lymphomas, which account for about 50% of all NHLs, are particularly aggressive tumors.[9] They are diagnosed with significant symptoms, grow, metastasize rapidly, and are fatal if not treated. Because of their high growth fraction, these lymphomas tend to be radiosensitive and chemosensitive. Hence, with intensive combination chemotherapy, complete remission can be achieved in 60% to 80% of cases.[17]

The most frequently occurring clinical manifestation of NHL is painless, superficial lymphadenopathy. There may be noncontiguous nodal spread of the disease with involvement of the gastrointestinal tract, lung, liver, testes, and bone marrow. Frequently, there is increased susceptibility to bacterial, viral, and fungal infections associated with hypogammaglobulinemia and a poor humoral antibody response, rather than the impaired cellular immunity seen with HL. Leukemic transformation with high peripheral lymphocytic counts occurs in a small percentage of persons with NHL.[9]

Diagnosis and Treatment. A lymph node biopsy is used to confirm the diagnosis of NHL and immunophenotyping is used to determine the lineage and clonality of the lymphoma cell. Lymphomas can be grouped according to surface markers or phenotypic markers (*e.g.*, CD20).[14] Staging of the disease is important in selecting a treatment for persons with NHL. Bone marrow biopsy, blood studies, chest and abdominal CT scans, magnetic resonance imaging (MRI), PET, gallium scans, and bone scans may be used to determine the stage of the disease.[16]

Treatment of NHL depends on the histologic type and stage of the disease. For early-stage disease, localized radiation may be used as a single treatment modality. However, because most people present with late-stage disease, combination chemotherapy, combined adjuvant radiation therapy, or both are recommended. Persons with lymphomas that carry a risk of CNS involvement usually receive CNS prophylaxis with high doses of chemotherapeutic agents or cranial irradiation. About 30% to 60% of patients do not achieve a complete response or relapse after standard-dose chemotherapy.[17]

Several monoclonal antibodies (MOAs) have recently become available for use in the treatment of NHL. Rituximab (Rituxan), which was the first to be approved by the U.S. Food and Drug Administration (FDA), recognizes and attaches to the CD20 antigen found on most B-cell lymphomas.[18,19] For aggressive lymphomas, the combination of chemotherapy and rituximab has shown dramatic response rates, indicating a synergistic effect. Because lymphoma cells tend to be very sensitive to radiation, newer forms of MOAs have been developed that are similar to rituximab, but with radioactive isotope such as ^{131}I and ^{90}Y attached to them. Bone marrow and peripheral stem cell transplantation are potentially curative treatments for people with highly resistant forms of the disease.

LEUKEMIAS

The leukemias are malignant neoplasms of cells originally derived from hematopoietic stem cells. They are characterized by diffuse replacement of bone marrow with unregulated, proliferating, immature neoplastic cells. In most cases, the leukemic cells spill out into the blood, where they are seen in large numbers. The term *leukemia* (*i.e.,* "white blood") was first used by Virchow to describe a reversal of the usual ratio of red blood cells to white blood cells. The leukemic cells may also infiltrate the liver, spleen, lymph nodes, and other tissues throughout the body, causing enlargement of these organs.

An estimated 35,000 new cases of leukemia were diagnosed in 2005 and approximately 22,500 persons died of the disease.[10] More children are stricken with leukemia than with any other form of cancer, and it is the leading cause of death in children between the ages of 1 and 14 years. Although commonly thought of as a childhood disease, leukemia is diagnosed 10 times more frequently in adults than children. Since the early 1990s, there has been a decrease in the incidence of leukemia in both men and women, with a slower decrease in deaths from leukemia.[10]

Classification

The leukemias commonly are classified according to their predominant cell type (*i.e.,* lymphocytic or myelocytic) and whether the condition is acute or chronic. Biphenotypic leukemias demonstrate characteristics of both lymphoid and myeloid lineages. A rudimentary classification system divides leukemia into four types: acute lymphocytic (lymphoblastic) leukemia (ALL), chronic lymphocytic leukemia (CLL), acute myelogenous (myeloblastic) leukemia (AML), and chronic myelogenous leukemia (CML). The *lymphocytic leukemias* involve immature lymphocytes and their progenitors that originate in the bone marrow but infiltrate the spleen, lymph nodes, CNS, and other tissues. The *myelogenous leukemias*, which involve the pluripotent myeloid stem cells in bone marrow, interfere with the maturation of all blood cells, including the granulocytes, erythrocytes, and thrombocytes.

Etiology and Molecular Biology

The causes of leukemia are largely unknown. The incidence of leukemia among persons who have been exposed to high levels of radiation is unusually high. An increased incidence of leukemia also is associated with exposure to benzene and the use of antitumor drugs (*i.e.,* mechlorethamine, procarbazine, cyclophosphamide, chloramphenicol, and the epipodophyllotoxins).[20] Leukemia may occur as a second cancer after aggressive chemotherapy for other cancers, such as HL.[21] The existence of a genetic predisposition to develop acute leukemia is suggested by the increased leukemia incidence among a number of congenital disorders, including Down syndrome, von Recklinghausen disease, and Fanconi anemia. In individuals with Down syndrome, the incidence of acute leukemia is 10 times that of the general population.[22] Also, there are numerous reports of multiple cases of acute leukemia occurring within the same family.

The molecular biology of leukemia suggests that the event or events causing the disorders exert their effects through disruption or dysregulation of genes that normally regulate blood cell development, blood cell homeostasis, or both.[23] Cytogenetic studies have shown that recurrent chromosomal changes occur in over one half of all cases of leukemia.[24] Most commonly these are structural changes, classified as translocations, inversions, or deletions (see Chapter 4). It is the disruption or dysregulation of specific genes and gene products occurring at the site of these chromosomal aberrations that contributes to the development of leukemia.[23] In many instances, these genes have also been found to be directly or indirectly

---

KEY CONCEPTS

Leukemias

➤ Leukemias are malignant neoplasms arising from the transformation of a single blood cell line derived from hematopoietic stem cells.

➤ The leukemias are classified as acute and chronic lymphocytic (lymphocytes) or myelogenous (granulocytes, monocytes) leukemias, according to their cell lineage.

➤ Because leukemic cells are immature and poorly differentiated, they proliferate rapidly and have a long life span; they do not function normally; they interfere with the maturation of normal blood cells; and they circulate in the bloodstream, cross the blood-brain barrier, and infiltrate many body organs.

involved in the normal development or maintenance of the hematopoietic system. Thus, it would appear that leukemia results, at least in part, from disruption in the activity of genes that normally regulate blood cell development. Currently, more than 500 recurring translocations have been described in hematologic malignancies.[24] One of the more studied is the reciprocal translocation from the long arm of chromosome 22 to the long arm of chromosome 9 that occurs in the Philadelphia (Ph) chromosome (to be discussed). Advances in the understanding of the molecular biology of leukemia are beginning to provide a more complete understanding of the molecular complexity of leukemia for the purposes of diagnosis, classification, treatment, and monitoring of clinical outcomes.

Acute Leukemias

Acute leukemia is a cancer of the hematopoietic stem cells.[25,26] It usually has a sudden and stormy onset with signs and symptoms related to depressed bone marrow function (Table 9-2). Acute lymphocytic leukemia (ALL) is the most common leukemia in childhood, comprising 80% to 85% of leukemia cases.[25] The peak incidence occurs between 2 and 4 years of age. Acute myelogenous leukemia (AML) is chiefly an adult disease; however, it is also seen in children and young adults. The incidence steadily increases after middle age, with a median age of 60 to 65 years for adult AML.[25]

Acute lymphoblastic leukemia encompasses a group of neoplasms composed of immature precursor B or T lymphocytes. Most cases (about 85%) of ALL are of pre–B-cell origin.[9] The AMLs are an extremely heterogeneous group of disorders. Some arise from the pluripotent stem cells in which myeloblasts predominate, and others arise from the monocyte-granulocyte precursor,

which is the cell of origin for myelomonocytic leukemia. Of all the leukemias, AML is most strongly linked with toxins and underlying congenital and hematologic disorders. It is the type of leukemia associated with Down syndrome.

Manifestations. Although ALL and AML are distinct disorders, they typically present with similar clinical features. The warning signs and symptoms of acute leukemia are fatigue, pallor, weight loss, repeated infections, easy bruising, and epistaxis (nosebleeds) and other types of hemorrhage. These features often appear suddenly in children.

Persons with acute leukemia usually present for medical evaluation within 3 months of the onset of symptoms. Both ALL and AML are characterized by fatigue resulting from anemia; low-grade fever, night sweats, and weight loss due to the rapid proliferation and hypermetabolism of the leukemic cells; bleeding because of a decreased platelet count; and bone pain and tenderness due to bone marrow expansion.[25] Infection results from neutropenia, with the risk of infection becoming high as the neutrophil count falls below 500 cells/μL. Generalized lymphadenopathy, splenomegaly, and hepatomegaly caused by infiltration of leukemic cells occur in all acute leukemias but are more common in ALL. In addition to the common manifestations of acute leukemia (i.e., fatigue, weight loss, fever, easy bruising), infiltration of malignant cells in the skin, gums, and other soft tissue is particularly common in the monocytic form of AML. The leukemic cells may also cross the blood-brain barrier and establish sanctuary in the CNS. CNS involvement is more common in ALL than AML, and is more common in children than adults. Signs and symptoms of CNS involvement include cranial nerve palsies, headache, nausea, vomiting, papilledema, and occasionally seizures and coma.

TABLE 9-2 **Clinical Manifestations of Acute Leukemia and Their Pathologic Basis***

Clinical Manifestations	Pathologic Basis
Bone marrow depression	
Malaise, easy fatigability	Anemia
Fever	Infection or increased metabolism by neoplastic cells
Bleeding	Decreased thrombocytes
Petechiae	
Ecchymosis	
Gingival bleeding	
Epistaxis	
Bone pain and tenderness upon palpation	Subperiosteal bone infiltration, bone marrow expansion, and bone resorption
Headache, nausea, vomiting, papilledema, cranial nerve palsies, seizures, coma	Leukemic infiltration of central nervous system
Abdominal discomfort	Generalized lymphadenopathy, hepatomegaly, splenomegaly due to leukemic cell infiltration
Increased vulnerability to infections	Immaturity of the white cells and ineffective immune function
Hematologic abnormalities	Physical and metabolic encroachment of leukemia cells on red blood cell and thrombocyte precursors
Anemia	
Thrombocytopenia	
Hyperuricemia and other metabolic disorders	Abnormal proliferation and metabolism of leukemic cells

*Manifestations vary with the type of leukemia.

Leukostasis is a condition in which the circulating blast count is markedly elevated (usually 100,000 cells/μL). The high number of circulating leukemic blasts increases blood viscosity and predisposes to the development of leuko-blastic emboli with obstruction of small vessels in the pulmonary and cerebral circulations. Occlusion of the pulmonary vessels leads to vessel rupture and infiltration of lung tissue, resulting in sudden shortness of breath and progressive dyspnea. Cerebral leukostasis leads to diffuse headache and lethargy, which can progress to confusion and coma. Once identified, leukostasis requires immediate and effective treatment to lower the blast count rapidly. Initial treatment uses apheresis to remove excess blast cells, followed by chemotherapy to stop leukemic cell production in the marrow.[25]

Hyperuricemia occurs as the result of increased pro-liferation or increased breakdown of purine nucleotides (*i.e.*, one of the compounds of nucleic acid) secondary to leukemic cell death that results from chemotherapy. It may increase before and during treatment. Prophylactic therapy with allopurinol, a drug that inhibits uric acid syn-thesis, is routinely administered to prevent renal compli-cations secondary to uric acid crystallization in the urine.

Diagnosis and Staging. A definitive diagnosis of acute leukemia is based on blood and bone marrow studies; it requires the demonstration of leukemic cells in the periph-eral blood, bone marrow, or extramedullary tissue. Lab-oratory findings reveal the presence of immature (blasts) white blood cells in the circulation and bone marrow, where they may constitute 60% to 100% of the cells. As these cells proliferate and begin to crowd the bone mar-row, the development of other blood cell lines in the mar-row is suppressed. Consequently, there is a loss of mature myeloid cells, such as erythrocytes, granulocytes, and platelets. Anemia is almost always present, and the platelet count is decreased. Bone marrow specimens are used to determine the molecular characteristics of the leukemia, the degree of bone marrow involvement, and the mor-phology and histology of the disease. Immunopheno-typing is performed to determine the lineage subtype of the leukemia.[25] In ALL, the staging includes a lumbar punc-ture to assess CNS involvement. Imaging studies that include CT scans of the chest, abdomen, and pelvis may also be obtained to identify additional sites of disease.

Treatment. Treatment of ALL and AML consists of several phases and includes induction therapy, which is designed to elicit a remission; intensification therapy, which is used to produce a further reduction in leukemic cells after a remission is achieved; and maintenance ther-apy, which serves to maintain the remission. The goal of induction therapy is the production of a severe bone mar-row response with destruction of leukemic progenitor cells followed by normal bone marrow recovery. The likelihood of achieving a remission depends on a number of factors, including age, type of leukemia, and stage of the disease at time of presentation. Of these factors, age is probably the most significant prognostic variable.

Treatment of ALL usually consists of four phases: induction therapy designed to elicit a remission; CNS prophylaxis; consolidation or intensification therapy; and maintenance therapy. Induction therapy incorporates a number of chemotherapeutic agents designed to achieve remission. CNS prophylaxis may be accomplished through the administration of intrathecal chemotherapy by lumbar puncture or by cranial irradiation concurrent with systemic chemotherapy.[25] Because of its side effects, CNS irradia-tion is being used less frequently than in the past. The use of high-dose chemotherapy that crosses the blood-brain barrier may make separate CNS treatment unnecessary in the future. Although CNS involvement is a major problem in children, the incidence in adults at the time of diagnosis is less than 10%. Consolidation therapy consists of high doses of chemotherapy given to patients who have achieved remission with their induction therapy. Mainte-nance therapy usually is accomplished with lower doses of chemotherapy given over a long period (*e.g.*, 2 years) to patients after consolidation therapy. Although almost 80% of children with ALL are cured, only about 30% to 40% of adults achieve long-term disease-free survival.[26,27]

Massive necrosis of malignant cells can occur during the initial phase of treatment. This phenomenon, known as *tumor lysis syndrome*, can lead to life-threatening metabolic disorders, including hyperkalemia, hyperphos-phatemia, hyperuricemia, hypomagnesemia, hypocal-cemia, and acidosis, with the potential for causing acute renal failure. Aggressive prophylactic hydration with alka-line solutions and administration of allopurinol to reduce uric acid levels are used to counteract these effects.

As with ALL, treatment of AML consists of a number of phases. Treatment usually consists of induction ther-apy followed by intensive consolidation therapy. Induc-tion therapy consists of intensive chemotherapy to effect aplasia of the bone marrow. During this period, support-ive transfusion and antibiotic therapy often are needed. A monoclonal antibody conjugated with a chemotherapeutic agent (gemtuzumab ozogamicin) that targets the CD33 antigen found on 90% of AML blast cells is another treatment option for patients older than 60 years of age who are not candidates for intensive chemotherapy.[27]

Bone marrow or stem cell transplantation may be con-sidered for persons with ALL and AML who have failed to respond to other forms of therapy.[25] Because of the risk of complications, bone marrow transplantation is not usually recommended for patients older than 50 to 55 years of age.[20]

Chronic Leukemias

In contrast to acute leukemias, chronic leukemias are malignancies involving the proliferation of well-differentiated myeloid and lymphoid cells. The two major types of chronic leukemia are chronic lymphocytic leukemia (CLL) and chronic myelogenous leukemia (CML). CLL is mainly a disorder of older persons; fewer than 10% of those who develop the disease are younger than 50 years of age. Men are affected twice as frequently as women. CML accounts for 15% to 20% of all leukemias in adults.[22] It is predominantly a disorder of adults between the ages of 30 and 50 years, but it can affect children as well. The incidence is slightly higher in men than women.

Chronic lymphocytic leukemia is a lymphoproliferative disorder characterized by lymphocytosis, lymphadenopathy, and splenomegaly. The majority (95%) of cases result from the malignant transformation of relatively mature B lymphocytes that are immunologically incompetent. The leukemic B cells fail to respond to antigenic stimulation; hence, persons with CLL have hypogammaglobulinemia. Infections remain a major cause of morbidity and mortality. Immunologic abnormalities, including autoimmune hemolytic anemia and immune-mediated thrombocytopenia, are also common, reflecting the abnormal immunoregulation inherent in the lymphocytic origin of the disorder.

Chronic myelogenous leukemia is a myeloproliferative disorder that results from the malignant transformation of a pluripotent hematopoietic stem cell. CML is associated with the presence of the Philadelphia (Ph) chromosome, arising from a reciprocal translocation between the long arm of chromosome 22 and the long arm of chromosome 9.[9,12] During the translocation, a large portion of 22q is translocated to 9q and a smaller piece of 9q is moved to 22q (Fig. 9-5). The portion of 9q that is translocated contains ABL, a proto-oncogene that is the cellular homolog of the Abelson murine leukemic virus. The ABL gene is received at a specific site on 22q called the *breakpoint cluster* (BCR). The BCR-ABL fusion gene codes for a novel protein that differs from that of the normal ABL gene in that it possesses tyrosine kinase activity (a characteristic activity of transforming genes).[9,12,28] It is generally believed that CML develops when a single, pluripotential hematopoietic stem cell acquires a Ph chromosome carrying the BCR-ABL fusion gene. The presence of the tyrosine kinase generated by the fusion gene in turn allows the affected cells to bypass the regulated signals that control normal cell growth and differentiation and instead undergo malignant transformation to become leukemic cells. Although CML originates in the pluripotent stem cells, granulocyte precursors remain the dominant leukemic cell type.

Manifestations. Both CLL and CML have a more insidious onset than acute leukemias and may be discovered during a routine medical examination by a blood count. The two types of chronic leukemias differ, however, in their manifestations and clinical course.

CLL typically follows a slow and indolent course. The clinical signs and symptoms are largely related to the progressive infiltration of neoplastic lymphocytes in the bone marrow and extramedullary tissue and to secondary

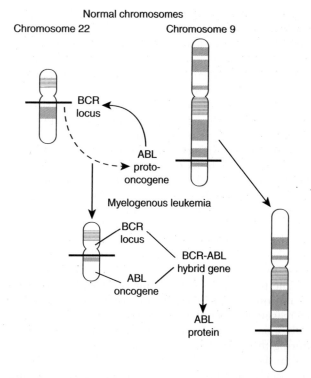

FIGURE 9-5 The Philadelphia (Ph) chromosome, which is formed by breaks at the end of the long arms of chromosome 9 and 22, allowing the ABL proto-oncogene on chromosome 9 to be translocated to the breakpoint cluster region (BCR) on chromosome 22. The result is a new fusion gene coding for the BCR-ABL protein, which is presumably involved in the pathogenesis of chronic myelogenous leukemia.

immunologic defects. Often affected persons are asymptomatic at the time of diagnosis, and lymphocytosis is noted on a complete blood count obtained for another, unrelated disorder. Fatigue, reduced exercise tolerance, enlargement of superficial lymph nodes, or splenomegaly usually reflects a more advanced stage. As the disease progresses, lymph nodes gradually increase in size and new nodes are involved, sometimes in unusual areas such as the scalp, orbit, pharynx, pleura, gastrointestinal tract, liver, prostate, and gonads. Severe fatigue, recurrent or persistent infections, pallor, edema, thrombophlebitis, and pain are also experienced. As the malignant cell population increases, the proportion of normal marrow precursors is reduced until only lymphocytes remain in the marrow.

Typically CML follows a triphasic course: (1) a chronic phase of variable length, (2) a short accelerated phase, and (3) a terminal blast crisis phase. The onset of the chronic phase is usually slow with nonspecific symptoms such as weakness and weight loss. The most characteristic laboratory finding at the time of presentation is leukocytosis with immature granulocyte cell types in the peripheral blood. Anemia and, eventually, thrombocytopenia develop. Anemia causes weakness, easy fatigability, and exertional dyspnea. Splenomegaly is often present at the time of diagnosis; hepatomegaly is less common; and lymphadenopathy is relatively uncommon. Although persons in the early chronic phase of CML usually are asymptomatic, without effective treatment most enter the accelerated phase within 4 years.[29]

The accelerated phase of CML is characterized by enlargement of the spleen and progressive symptoms. Splenomegaly often causes a feeling of abdominal fullness and discomfort. An increase in basophil count and more immature cells in the blood or bone marrow confirm transformation to the accelerated phase. During this phase, constitutional symptoms such as low-grade fever, night sweats, bone pain, and weight loss develop because of rapid proliferation and hypermetabolism of the leukemic cells. Bleeding and easy bruising may arise from dysfunctional platelets. The accelerated phase usually is short (6 to 12 months).[28]

The terminal blast crisis phase of CML represents evolution to acute leukemia and is characterized by an increasing number of myeloid precursors, especially blast cells. Constitutional symptoms become more pronounced during this period, and splenomegaly may increase significantly. Isolated infiltrates of leukemic cells can involve the skin, lymph nodes, bones, and CNS. With very high blast counts (100,000/µL), symptoms of leukostasis may occur. The prognosis for patients who are in the blast crisis phase is poor, with a median survival of 3 months.[29]

Diagnosis and Treatment. The diagnosis of chronic leukemia is based on blood and bone marrow studies. The treatment varies with the type of leukemic cell, the stage of the disease, other health problems, and the person's age.

Most early cases of CLL require no specific treatment. Reassurance that persons with the disorder can live a normal life for many years is important. Indications for chemotherapy or monoclonal antibodies include progressive fatigue, troublesome lymphadenopathy, anemia, and thrombocytopenia, and a lymphocyte count over 150,000/µL. Initially, chemotherapy is used. The monoclonal antibody (alemtuzumab), directed against the CD52 cell surface antigen present on lymphocytes of almost all persons with B- and T-cell CLL, may be used to treat those who have not responded to chemotherapy.[29] Complications such as autoimmune hemolytic anemia or thrombocytopenia may require treatment with corticosteroids or splenectomy. In younger patients with aggressive disease, an allogeneic ablative (destruction of bone marrow cells with irradiation or chemotherapy) or nonmyeloablative stem cell transplant is a treatment option. In a nonmyeloablative transplant, the goal is marrow suppression; destruction of leukemia cells by the donor's lymphocytes, known as "graft-versus-leukemia" effect; and marrow recovery with donor cells.

The goals of treatment for CML include a hematological response characterized by normalized blood counts; a cytogenetic response demonstrated by the reduction or elimination of the Ph chromosome from the bone marrow; and a molecular response confirmed by the elimination of the BCR-ABL fusion protein.[29] In the past, standard treatment included the use of single-agent chemotherapy (hydroxyurea) as well as alpha interferon. In patients in the chronic phase, both agents normalized blood counts and reduced symptoms, but cytogenetic and molecular responses were rare. With its FDA approval in 2001, imatinib mesylate, a specifically designed inhibitor of the tyrosine kinase activity of the BCR-ABL oncogene, has largely replaced hydroxyurea and interferon as standard therapy for CML.[30,31] Its side effect profile and ease of administration (oral route) have dramatically changed the treatment of CML.

The only available cure for CML is allogeneic bone marrow or stem cell transplantation. In most transplantation centers, full myoablative transplants are available to children and adults younger than 60 years of age who have a HLA-matched sibling donor or molecular-matched unrelated donor. Nonmyeloablative or "mini" transplants are available to patients younger than 70 years of age who have an HLA-matched sibling or molecular-matched donor.

PLASMA CELL DYSCRASIAS

Plasma cell dyscrasias are characterized by expansion of a single clone of immunoglobulin-producing plasma cells and a resultant increase in serum levels of a single monoclonal immunoglobulin or its fragments. The plasma cell dyscrasias include multiple myeloma, localized plasmacytoma (solitary myeloma), lymphoplasmacytic lymphoma, primary or immunocyte amyloidosis due to excessive production of light chains, and monoclonal gammopathy of undetermined significance. *Monoclonal gammopathy of undetermined significance* (MGUS) is characterized by the presence of M proteins (discussed later) in the serum without other findings of multiple myeloma. M proteins can be detected in the serum of 1% to 3% of healthy persons older than 50 years of age. MGUS is considered a premalignant condition.[32,33] Approximately 20% of persons with MGUS go on to develop a plasma cell dyscrasia (multiple myeloma, lymphoplasmacytic lymphoma, or amyloidosis) over a period of 10 to 15 years.

Multiple Myeloma

Multiple myeloma is by far the most frequent of the malignant plasma cell dyscrasias, accounting for 1% of all cancers and 10% of all hematologic malignancies in whites and 20% in African Americans.[34] It occurs most frequently in persons older than 60 years of age; the median age of patients with multiple myeloma is 71 years. The disease tends to occur more frequently in men than in women.

The cause of multiple myeloma is unknown. Risk factors are thought to include chronic immune stimulation, autoimmune disorders, exposure to ionizing radiation, and occupational exposure to pesticides or herbicides (*e.g.*, dioxin).[32] Myeloma has been associated with exposure to Agent Orange during the Vietnam War. A number of viruses have been associated with the pathogenesis of myeloma. There is a 4.5-fold increased likelihood of developing myeloma for persons with HIV infection.[32] Hereditary and genetic factors may predispose to myeloma development. From family studies, researchers have identified 20 families in France where the risk of developing myeloma is as high as 5%.

Pathogenesis. Multiple myeloma is characterized by proliferation of malignant plasma cells in the bone marrow and osteolytic bone lesions throughout the skeletal system. As with other hematopoietic malignancies, it is now recognized that multiple myeloma is associated with chromosomal translocations, specifically those involving the immunoglobulin G (IgG) locus on chromosome 14. One fusion partner is a fibroblast growth factor receptor gene on chromosome 4, which is truncated to produce a constitutively active receptor. There is also a reported overexpression by myeloma cells of a gene, called the *dickkopf 1* (DKK1) gene, that codes for a protein product that inhibits differentiation of osteoblast precursor cells, thereby contributing to the osteolytic lesions that occur with the disease.[35]

One of the characteristics of multiple myelomas is the unregulated production of a monoclonal antibody referred to as the *M protein* because it is detected as an M spike on protein electrophoresis. In most cases the M protein is either IgG (60%) or IgA (20% to 25%).[36] In the remaining 15% to 20% of cases, the plasma cells produce only *Bence Jones proteins*, abnormal proteins that consist of light chains of the immunoglobulin molecule. Because of their low molecular weight, the Bence Jones proteins are readily excreted in the urine. Persons with this form of the disease (light-chain disease) have Bence Jones proteins in their serum, but lack the M component. However, up to 80% of myeloma cells produce both complete immunoglobulins as well as excess light chains; therefore, both M proteins and Bence Jones proteins are present. Many of the light-chain proteins are directly toxic to renal tubular structures, which may lead to tubular destruction and, eventually, to renal failure.

Cytokines are important in the pathogenesis of the disorder. The multiple myeloma cell has a surface-membrane receptor for interleukin-6, which is known to be a growth factor for the disorder. Another important growth factor for the myeloma cell is interleukin-1, which has important osteoclastic activity.[33] Other growth factors that are implicated in multiple myeloma include granulocyte colony-stimulating factor, interferon-α, and interleukin-10. Replacement of the bone marrow (and perhaps humoral suppression of myelopoiesis) leads initially to anemia and later to general bone marrow failure. The proliferation of neoplastic myeloma cells is supported by the cytokine interleukin-6 produced by fibroblasts and macrophages in the bone marrow stroma.

Manifestations. The main sites involved in multiple myeloma are the bones and bone marrow. In addition to the abnormal proliferation of marrow plasma cells, there is proliferation and activation of osteoclasts that leads to bone resorption and destruction (Fig. 9-6). The increased bone resorption predisposes the individual to pathologic fractures and hypercalcemia. Paraproteins secreted by the plasma cells may cause a hyperviscosity of body fluids and may break down into amyloid, a proteinaceous substance deposited between cells, causing heart failure and neuropathy. Although multiple myeloma is characterized by excessive production of monoclonal immunoglobulin, levels of normal immunoglobulins are usually depressed. This contributes to a general susceptibility to recurrent bacterial infections.

The malignant plasma cells also can form plasmacytomas in bone and soft tissue sites. The most common site of soft tissue plasmacytomas is the gastrointestinal tract. The development of plasmacytomas in bone tissue is associated with bone destruction and localized pain. Osteolytic lesions and compression fractures may be seen in the axial skeleton and proximal long bones. Occasionally, the lesions may affect the spinal column, causing vertebral collapse and spinal cord compression.[32]

Bone pain is one of the first symptoms occurring in approximately three fourths of all individuals diagnosed with multiple myeloma. Bone destruction also impairs the production of erythrocytes and leukocytes and predisposes the patient to anemia and recurrent infections. Many patients experience weight loss and weakness. Renal

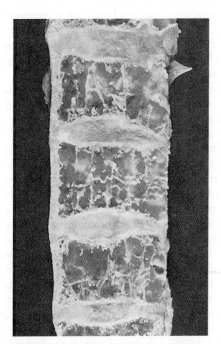

FIGURE 9-6 Multiple myeloma. Multiple lytic lesions of the vertebrae are present. (From Rubin E., Gorstein F., Rubin R., et al. [Eds.]. [2005]. *Rubin's pathology: Clinicopathologic foundations of medicine* [4th ed., p. 1100]. Philadelphia: Lippincott Williams & Wilkins.)

insufficiency occurs in 50% of patients. Neurologic manifestations caused by neuropathy or spinal cord compression also may be present.

Diagnosis and Treatment.

Diagnosis of multiple myeloma is based on clinical manifestations, blood tests, and bone marrow examination. The classic triad of bone marrow plasmacytosis (>10% plasma cells), lytic bone lesions, and either the serum M-protein spike or the presence of Bence Jones proteins in the urine is definitive for a diagnosis of multiple myeloma. Bone radiographs, skeletal survey, and MRI are important in establishing the presence of bone lesions. The Durie and Salmon staging system correlates clinical parameters with the burden of myeloma disease by examining the levels of M and Bence Jones proteins, assessing the presence and location of bone lesions, and evaluating the patient for hypercalcemia and anemia.[33]

For several decades, the combination of melphalan and prednisone has remained the cornerstone for treatment of multiple myeloma. The overall response rate for this regimen was about 50%. The addition of anthracyclines, alternative alkylating agents, and interferon has yielded minimal improvement in treatment outcomes. Although multiple myeloma is a radiosensitive disease, radiation therapy provides only supportive therapy or pain relief from lytic bone lesions and compression fractures.

High-dose chemotherapy with autologous stem cell transplantation is now considered appropriate front-line therapy for patients with newly diagnosed multiple myeloma who are younger than 70 years of age. Allogeneic transplantation offers prolonged disease-free outcomes and potential cure, but at a high cost of treatment-related mortality. Because of this, "mini-transplants" using non–marrow-ablative chemotherapy may be used to provide sufficient immune suppression to allow donor engraftment and subsequent graft-versus-tumor effect.

Almost all persons with multiple myeloma have a risk of eventual relapse. Recently, thalidomide, an agent with antiangiogenic properties, emerged as an active agent for relapsed and refractory multiple myeloma.[33,37] Thalidomide combined with dexamethasone pulsing has shown promising results in previously treated and in newly diagnosed patients, and the combination of dexamethasone and thalidomide was added to the list of options for the primary treatment of advanced disease.[33,37] Because of its teratogenicity, the use of thalidomide in pregnant women is absolutely contraindicated. Another agent, bortesomib, a reversible 26S proteasome inhibitor, was recently approved for treatment of progressive myeloma after previous treatment failures. Proteasomes are intracellular enzymes that degrade many proteins regulating the cell cycle, ribonucleic acid (RNA) transcription, apoptosis, cell adhesion, angiogenesis, and antigen presentation.[33,37] Proteolysis by the 26S proteasome is fundamental to multiple signaling pathways in the cell, and disruption of this homeostatic pathway by bortesomib can lead to cell death and a delay in tumor growth.

In summary, the lymphomas (HL and NHL) represent malignant neoplasms of cells native to lymphoid tissue (*i.e.,* lymphocytes and histiocytes) that have their origin in the secondary lymphoid structures such as the lymph nodes and mucosa-associated lymphoid tissues. HL is characterized by painless and progressive enlargement of a single node or group of nodes. It is believed to originate in one area of the lymphatic system and, if unchecked, spreads throughout the lymphatic network. The NHLs are a group of neoplastic disorders that originate in the lymphoid tissues, usually the lymph nodes. The NHLs are multicentric in origin and spread early to various lymphoid tissues throughout the body, especially the liver, spleen, and bone marrow.

The leukemias are malignant neoplasms of the hematopoietic stem cells that originate in the bone marrow. They are classified according to cell type (*i.e.,* lymphocytic or myelogenous) and whether the disease is acute or chronic. The lymphocytic leukemias involve immature lymphocytes and their progenitors that originate in the bone marrow but infiltrate the spleen, lymph nodes, CNS, and other tissues. The myelogenous leukemias involve the pluripotent myeloid stem cells in bone marrow and interfere with the maturation of all blood cells, including the granulocytes, erythrocytes, and thrombocytes.

The acute leukemias (*i.e.,* ALL, which primarily affects children, and AML, which primarily affects adults) have a sudden and stormy onset with symptoms of depressed bone marrow function (anemia, fatigue, bleeding, and infections); bone pain; and generalized lymphadenopathy, splenomegaly, and hepatomegaly. The chronic leukemias, which largely affect adults, have a more insidious onset. CLL often has the most favorable clinical course, with many persons living long enough to die of other, unrelated causes. The course of CML is slow and progressive, with transformation to a course resembling that of AML.

Multiple myeloma is a plasma cell dyscrasia characterized by expansion of a single clone of immunoglobulin-producing plasma cells and a resultant increase in serum levels of a single monoclonal immunoglobulin or its fragments. The main sites involved in multiple myeloma are the bones and bone marrow. In addition to the abnormal proliferation of marrow plasma cells, there is proliferation and activation of osteoclasts that leads to bone resorption and destruction, and predisposes to increased risk for pathologic fractures and development of hypercalcemia. Paraproteins secreted by the plasma cells may cause a hyperviscosity of body fluids and may break down into amyloid, a proteinaceous substance deposited between cells, causing heart failure and neuropathy. Bone marrow involvement leads to increased risk of infection due to suppressed humoral and cell-mediated immunity and anemia due to impaired red cell production.

Review Exercises

Many of the primary immunodeficiency disorders, in which there is a defect in the development of the T- or B-lymphocyte immune cells, can be cured by an allogeneic stem cell transplant from an unaffected donor.

A. Explain why stem cells are used rather than mature lymphocytes. You might want to refer to Figure 9-1.
B. Explain how the stem cells would go about the process of repopulating the bone marrow.

A mother brings her 4-year-old son into the pediatric clinic because of irritability, loss of appetite, low-grade fever, pallor, and complaints that his legs hurt. Blood tests reveal anemia, thrombocytopenia, and an elevated leukocyte count with atypical lymphocytes. A diagnosis of acute lymphocytic leukemia (ALL) is confirmed with bone marrow studies.

A. What is the origin of the anemia, thrombocytopenia, elevated leukocyte count, and atypical lymphocytes seen in this child?
B. Explain the cause of the child's fever, pallor, increased bleeding, and bone pain.
C. The parents are informed the preferred treatment for ALL consists of aggressive chemotherapy with the purpose of achieving a remission. Explain the rationale for using chemotherapy to treat leukemia.
D. The parents are also told that the child will need intrathecal chemotherapy administered by a lumbar puncture. Why is this treatment necessary?

A 36-year-old man presents to his health care clinic with fever, night sweats, weight loss, and feeling of fullness in his abdomen. Subsequent lymph node biopsy reveals a diagnosis of non-Hodgkin lymphoma (NHL).

A. Although lymphomas can originate in any of the lymphoid tissues of the body, most originate in the lymph nodes, and most (80% to 85%) are of B-cell origin. Hypothesize as to why B cells are more commonly affected than T cells.
B. A newly developed monoclonal antibody, rituximab, is being used in the treatment of NHL. Explain how this agent exerts its effect and why it is specific for B-cell lymphomas.

Visit the Porth: Essentials of Pathophysiology: Concepts of Altered Health States web site (http://thePoint.LWW.com/PorthEssentials) for links to chapter-related resources on the Internet, all-new exclusive animations, chapter review questions, and more!

REFERENCES

1. Guyton A. C., Hall J. E. (2006). *Textbook of medical physiology* (11th ed. pp. 429–456). Philadelphia: Elsevier Saunders.
2. Abbas A. K., Lichtman A. H. (2003). *Cellular and molecular immunology* (5th ed., pp. 3–39, 273). Philadelphia: Elsevier Saunders.
3. Curnutte J. T., Coates T. D. (2000). Disorders of phagocyte function and number. In Hoffman R., Benz E. K., Shattil S. J., et al. (Eds.), *Hematology: Basic principles and practice* (3rd ed., pp. 720–762). New York: Churchill Livingstone.
4. Boxer L. A. (2004). Leukopenia. In Behrman R. E., Kliegman R. M., Jenson H. B. (Eds.), *Nelson textbook of pediatrics* (17th ed., pp. 717–723). Philadelphia: Elsevier Saunders.
5. Cohen J. I. (2000). Epstein-Barr virus infection. *New England Journal of Medicine* 343, 481–492.
6. McAdam A. J., Sharpe A. H. (2005). Infectious diseases. In Kumar V., Abbas A. K., Fausto N. (Eds.), *Robbins and Cotran pathologic basis of disease* (7th ed., pp. 369–371). Philadelphia: Elsevier Saunders.
7. Godshall S. E., Kirscher J. T. (2000). Infectious mononucleosis: Complexities of a common syndrome. *Postgraduate Medicine* 107(7), 175–186.
8. Ebell M. H. (2004). Epstein-Barr virus infectious mononucleosis. *American Family Physician* 7, 1279–1287, 1289–1290.
9. Aster J. (2005). Diseases of the white blood cells, lymph nodes, spleen, and thymus. In Kumar V., Abbas A. K., Fausto N. (Eds.), *Robbins and Cotran pathologic basis of disease* (7th ed., pp. 661–695). Philadelphia: Elsevier Saunders.
10. American Cancer Society. (2005). *Cancer facts and figures 2005*. Atlanta: American Cancer Society.
11. Diehl, V., Mauch P. M., Harris N. L. (2001). Hodgkin's disease. In DeVita V. T., Hellman S., Rosenberg S. A. (Eds.), *Cancer: Principles and practice of oncology* (6th ed., pp. 2339–2387). Philadelphia: Lippincott Williams & Wilkins.
12. Schwarting R., Kocher W. D., McKenzie S., et al. (2005). Hematopathology. In Rubin E., Gorstein F., Rubin R., et al. (Eds.), *Rubin's pathology: Clinicopathologic foundations of medicine* (4th ed., pp. 1063–1117). Philadelphia: Lippincott Williams & Wilkins.
13. Cheson B. D. (2001). Hodgkin's and non-Hodgkin's lymphomas. In Lenbard R. E., Jr., Osteen R. T., Gansler T. (Eds.), *The American Cancer Society's clinical oncology* (pp. 497–516). Atlanta: American Cancer Society.
14. National Comprehensive Cancer Network. (2003). *NCCN clinical practice guidelines in oncology: Hodgkin's disease*. Jenkintown, PA: National Comprehensive Cancer Network.
15. Vose J. M., Chiu B. C.-H., Cheson B. D., et al. (2002). Update on epidemiology and therapeutics in non-Hodgkin's lymphoma. *Hematology* 241–268.
16. American Cancer Society and National Comprehensive Cancer Network. (2003). *Non-Hodgkin's lymphomas: Treatment guidelines for patients*. Atlanta: American Cancer Society.
17. Reiser M., Diehl V. (2002). Current treatment of follicular non-Hodgkin's lymphoma. *European Journal of Cancer* 38, 1167–1172.

18. Bilodeau, B. A., Fessele, K. L. (1998). Non-Hodgkin's lymphoma. *Seminars in Oncology Nursing* 14, 273–283.
19. Vose, J. M. (2002). Immunotherapy for non-Hodgkin's lymphoma. *Clinical Oncology Updates* 5(4), 1–15.
20. Scheinberg D. A., Maslak P., Weiss M. (2001). Acute leukemias. In DeVita V. T., Hellman S., Rosenberg S. A. (Eds.), *Cancer: Principles and practice of oncology* (6th ed., pp. 2404–2433). Philadelphia: Lippincott Williams & Wilkins.
21. Kaldor J. M., Day N. E., Clarke E. A., et al. (1990). Leukemia following Hodgkin's. *New England Journal of Medicine* 322, 1–6.
22. Miller K. B., Grodman H. M. (2001). Leukemia. In Lenbard R. E., Jr., Osteen R. T., Gansler T. (Eds.), *The American Cancer Society's clinical oncology* (pp. 527–551). Atlanta: American Cancer Society.
23. Bloomfield C. D., Caligiuri M. A. (2001). Biology of leukemias. In DeVita V. T., Hellman S., Rosenberg S. A. (Eds.), *Cancer: Principles and practice of oncology* (6th ed., pp. 2390–2402). Philadelphia: Lippincott Williams & Wilkins.
24. Wujcik D. (2003). Molecular biology of leukemia. *Seminars in Oncology Nursing* 19, 83–89.
25. Viele, C. S. (2003). Diagnosis, treatment, and nursing care of acute leukemia. *Seminars in Oncology Nursing* 19, 98–108.
26. Faderi S., Jeha S., Kantajian H. M. (2003). The biology and therapy of adult acute lymphoblastic leukemia. *Cancer* 98, 1337–1354.
27. Stull, D. M. (2003). Targeted therapies for the treatment of leukemia. *Seminars in Oncology Nursing* 19, 90–97.
28. Thijsen S. F. T., Schuurhuis G. J., van Oostveen J. W., et al. (1999). Chronic myeloid leukemia: From basics to bedside. *Leukemia* 13, 1646–1674.
29. Breed, C. D. (2003). Diagnosis, treatment, and nursing care of patients with chronic leukemia. *Seminars in Oncology Nursing* 19, 109–117.
30. Vlahorvic G., Crawford J. (2003). Activation of tyrosine kinases in cancer. *Oncologist* 8, 531–538.
31. Goldman J. M., Melo J. V. (2003). Chronic myeloid leukemia: Advances in biology and new approaches to treatment. *New England Journal of Medicine* 349, 1451–1464.
32. Zaidi, A. A., Vesole, D. H. (2001). Multiple myeloma: An old disease with new hope for the future. *CA: A Cancer Journal for Clinicians* 51, 273–285.
33. Kyle R. A., Rajkumar S. V. (2004). Multiple myeloma. *New England Journal of Medicine* 351, 1860–1873.
34. Rosenthal D. S., Schnipper L. E., McCaffrey R. P., et al. (2001). Multiple myeloma. In Lenbard R. E., Jr., Osteen R. T., Gansler T. (Eds.), *The American Cancer Society's clinical oncology* (pp. 516–525). Atlanta: American Cancer Society.
35. Triko G. (2000). Multiple myeloma and other plasma cell disorders. In Hoffman R., Benz E. K., Shattil S. J., et al. (Eds.), *Hematology: Basic principles and practice* (3rd ed., pp. 1398–1416). New York: Churchill Livingstone.
36. Glass D. A., Patel M. S., Karsenty G. (2003). A new insight into the formation of osteolytic lesions in multiple myeloma. *New England Journal of Medicine* 349, 2479–2481.
37. Rajkumar S. V., Gertz M. A., Kyle R. A., et al. (2002). Current therapy for multiple myeloma. *Mayo Clinic Proceedings* 77, 813–822.

Chapter *10*

Alterations in Hemostasis

 The term *hemostasis* refers to the stoppage of blood flow. The normal process of hemostasis is regulated by a complex array of activators and inhibitors that maintain blood fluidity and prevent blood from leaving the vascular compartment. Hemostasis is normal when it seals a blood vessel to prevent blood loss and hemorrhage. It is abnormal when it causes inappropriate blood clotting or when clotting is insufficient to stop the flow of blood from the vascular compartment. Disorders of hemostasis fall into two main categories: the inappropriate formation of clots within the vascular system (*i.e.*, thrombosis) and the failure of blood to clot in response to an appropriate stimulus (*i.e.*, bleeding).

Mechanisms of Hemostasis

Hemostasis is a multistep process that transforms blood into a semisolid clot with erythrocytes trapped in its fibrin meshwork (Fig. 10-1). It involves platelets, plasma clotting factors, naturally occurring anticoagulants, and the inherent properties of the blood vessels themselves.

Platelets, also called *thrombocytes,* are large fragments from the cytoplasm of bone marrow cells called *megakaryocytes.*[1] Platelets have a cell membrane but no nucleus and cannot reproduce. There are normally 150,000 to 400,000 platelets in each microliter (μL) of blood. The life span of a platelet is only 8 to 9 days. Platelets do not leave the blood as white blood cells do, but at any time about one third of them are in storage in blood-filled spaces in the spleen. These stored platelets can be released from the spleen into the circulation as needed. Platelet production is controlled by a protein called *thrombopoietin* that causes proliferation and maturation of megakaryocytes.[2] The sources of thrombopoietin include the liver, kidney, smooth muscle, and bone marrow. Its production and release are regulated by the number of platelets in the circulation.

Although platelets lack a nucleus, they have many of the structural and functional characteristics of a whole cell.[1,3,4]

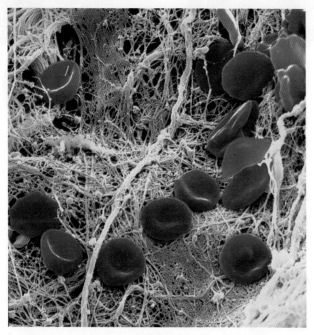

FIGURE 10-1 Scanning electron micrograph of a blood clot (×3600). The fibrous bridges that form a meshwork between red blood cells are fibrin fibers. (© Oliver Meckes, Science Source/Photo Researchers.)

They contain an outer cell membrane, microtubular structures, and inner organelles (see Chapter 1). The platelet cell membrane is covered with a surface coat of glycocalyx, consisting of glycoproteins, glycosaminoglycans, and several coagulation factors adsorbed from the plasma.[3] The glycoproteins function as receptors in platelet function. For example, glycoprotein IIb/IIIa binds fibrinogen and forms bridges between adjacent platelets when activated. The cell membrane is supported by a network of microtubules, actin filaments, myosin, and actin-binding proteins. They are arranged circumferentially and are responsible for maintaining the platelet's disk shape.

KEY CONCEPTS

Hemostasis

➤ Hemostasis is the orderly, stepwise process for stopping bleeding that involves vasospasm, formation of a platelet plug, and the development of a fibrin clot.

➤ The blood clotting process requires the presence of platelets produced in the bone marrow, von Willebrand factor generated by the vessel endothelium, and clotting factors synthesized in the liver, using vitamin K.

➤ The final step of the process involves fibrinolysis or clot dissolution, which prevents excess clot formation.

The central part of the platelet contains mitochondria, enzymes needed for synthesis of adenosine diphosphate (ADP) and the prostaglandin thromboxane A_2 (TXA_2), glycogen, and two specific types of granules (α- and δ-granules) that release mediators for hemostasis.[3] The α-granules contain fibrinogen, coagulation factors, plasminogen, plasminogen activator inhibitor, and platelet-derived growth factors. The contents of these granules play an important role in the initial phase of vessel repair, blood coagulation, and platelet aggregation. The release of growth factors causes vascular endothelial cells, smooth muscle cells, and fibroblasts to proliferate and grow. The δ-granules, or dense granules, mainly contain ADP, adenosine triphosphate (ATP), serotonin, and histamine, which facilitate platelet adhesion and vasoconstriction in the area of the injured vessel.

The coagulation factors are plasma proteins that are present as inactive procoagulation factors. Each of the procoagulation or coagulation factors, identified by Roman numerals, performs a specific step in the coagulation process. The activation of one procoagulation factor or proenzyme is designed to activate the next factor in the sequence (*i.e.*, cascade effect). Because most of the inactive procoagulation factors are present in the blood at all times, the multistep process ensures that a massive episode of intravascular clotting does not occur by chance. Most of the coagulation factors are proteins synthesized in the liver. Vitamin K is necessary for the synthesis of factors VII, IX, and X, prothrombin, and protein C.

Calcium (factor IV) is required in all but the first two steps of the clotting process. The body usually has sufficient amounts of calcium for these reactions. Inactivation of the calcium ion prevents blood from clotting when it is removed from the body. The addition of citrate to blood stored for transfusion purposes prevents clotting by chelating ionic calcium. EDTA, another chelator, is often added to blood samples used for analysis in the clinical laboratory.

A clot is not meant to be a permanent solution to vessel injury; thus, blood clotting is accompanied by processes designed to control the coagulation process and dissolve the clot once bleeding has been controlled. Blood coagulation is regulated by several natural anticoagulants, including antithrombin III and proteins C and S, which act as anticoagulants by inactivating some of the clotting factors (to be discussed).[4] The plasma also contains a plasma protein called *plasminogen*, that when activated is converted to plasmin, an enzyme capable of digesting the fibrin strands of the clot. In addition to removing clots that are no longer needed, plasmin functions continually to prevent clots from forming inappropriately.

The blood vessels themselves also play an important role in preventing and controlling the formation of blood clots. Probably the most important factor in preventing blood clotting is the normal smoothness of the endothelial surface that lines the blood vessels and prevents adherence of platelets and clotting factors. Vascular neural reflexes and humoral factors also cause the smooth muscle in the vessel wall to contract when a vessel is injured.

HEMOSTASIS AND FORMATION OF THE BLOOD CLOT

Hemostasis is divided into five stages: (1) vessel spasm, (2) formation of the platelet plug, (3) blood coagulation or development of an insoluble fibrin clot, (4) clot retraction, and (5) clot dissolution.[1,4]

Vessel Spasm

Vessel spasm is initiated by endothelial injury and caused by local and humoral mechanisms. It is a transient event, usually lasting less than 1 minute, that results from neural reflexes and humoral factors released from the traumatized tissue and blood platelets. For smaller vessels, release of the vasoconstrictor TXA_2 is responsible for much of the vessel spasm.

Formation of the Platelet Plug

The platelet plug, the second line of defense, is initiated as platelets come in contact with the vessel wall. Tiny breaks in the vessel wall are often sealed with the platelet plug rather than a blood clot. Platelet plug formation involves adhesion and aggregation of platelets. Platelets are attracted to a damaged vessel wall, become activated, and change from smooth disks to spiny spheres, exposing receptors on their surfaces. *Platelet adhesion* requires a protein molecule called *von Willebrand factor* (vWF). This factor is produced by the endothelial cells of blood vessels and circulates in the blood as a carrier protein for coagulation factor VIII. Adhesion to the vessel subendothelial layer occurs when the platelet receptor binds to vWF at the injury site, linking the platelet to exposed collagen fibers.

Platelet aggregation occurs soon after adhesion. It is mediated by the release of ADP from the platelet granules. ADP release also facilitates the release of ADP from other platelets, leading to amplification of the aggregation process. Besides ADP, platelets also release TXA_2, which is an important stimulus for platelet aggregation. The combined actions of ADP and TXA_2 lead to the buildup of the enlarging platelet aggregate, which becomes the primary hemostatic plug. Stabilization of the platelet plug occurs as the coagulation pathway is activated on the platelet surface and fibrinogen is converted to fibrin, thereby creating a fibrin meshwork that cements the platelets and other blood components together. The primary aggregation and formation of the platelet plug is reversible up to the point where the coagulation cascade has been activated and the platelets have been irreversibly fused together by the fibrin meshwork.

The platelet membrane plays an important role in platelet adhesion and the coagulation process. Platelets normally avoid adherence to the endothelium but interact with injured areas of the vessel wall and the deeper exposed collagen.[1] Glycoprotein (GpIIb/IIIa) receptors on the platelet membrane bind fibrinogen and link platelets together. Drugs that act as glycoprotein receptor ago-

nists have been developed for use in the treatment of acute myocardial infarction[4] (see Chapter 18).

Mechanisms of Blood Coagulation

The coagulation cascade is the third component of the hemostatic process. It is a stepwise process resulting in the conversion of the soluble plasma protein, fibrinogen, into fibrin. The insoluble fibrin strands create a meshwork that cements platelets and other blood components together to form the clot.

The coagulation process results from the activation of what have traditionally been designated the *intrinsic* or the *extrinsic* pathways (Fig. 10-2). The intrinsic pathway, which is a relatively slow process, begins in the circulation and is initiated by the activation of circulating factor XII. The extrinsic pathway, which is a much faster process, is activated by a cellular lipoprotein, called *tissue factor,* that becomes exposed when tissues are injured. The terminal steps in both pathways are the same: the activation of factor X and the conversion of prothrombin to thrombin. Thrombin then acts as an enzyme to convert fibrinogen to fibrin, the material that stabilizes a clot. Both pathways are needed for normal hemostasis, and many interrelations exist between them. Bleeding that occurs because of defects in the extrinsic system usually is not as severe as that which results from defects in the intrinsic pathway.

The coagulation process is regulated by both procoagulation factors that promote clotting and naturally occurring anticoagulants that inhibit it. Under most circumstances, the endothelial cells of blood vessels maintain an environment that is conducive to blood flow by mechanisms that interfere with the blood coagulation process. These effects are mediated by heparin molecules on endothelial cells, a specific thrombin receptor called *thrombomodulin,* an α-globulin called *antithrombin III,* and plasma proteins C and S.[4] The heparin molecules act indirectly by serving as cofactors that interact with antithrombin III to inactivate thrombin, factor Xa, and several other coagulation factors. Thrombomodulin also acts indirectly by binding to thrombin, converting it to an anticoagulant capable of activating protein C. Protein C acts as an anticoagulant by inactivating factors V and VIII. Protein S, in turn, accelerates the action of protein C.

The anticoagulant drugs warfarin and heparin are used to prevent thromboembolic disorders such as deep vein thrombosis and pulmonary embolism. Warfarin acts by decreasing prothrombin and other procoagulation factors. It alters vitamin K such that it reduces its availability to participate in synthesis of the vitamin K–dependent coagulation factors in the liver. Heparin, which is available as a pharmacologic preparation, acts in the same manner as natural heparin on the endothelial cells. Heparin is unable to cross the membranes of the gastrointestinal tract and must be given by injection, usually by intravenous infusion. Because heparin levels can be highly variable, achieving this goal is often difficult, and requires careful control of dosage based on frequent tests of coagulation (*e.g.,* activated partial thromboplastin time [APTT]). Low–molecular-weight (LMW) heparins that are composed of molecules that are

Understanding ➤ Hemostasis

Hemostasis, which refers to the stoppage of blood flow, is divided into five stages: (1) vessel spasm, (2) formation of the platelet plug, (3) development of a blood clot as a result of blood coagulation, (4) clot retraction, and (5) clot dissolution.

1

Vessel spasm. Injury to a blood vessel causes vascular smooth muscle in the vessel wall to contract. This instantaneously reduces the flow of blood from the vessel rupture. Both local nervous reflexes and local humoral factors such as thromboxane A_2 (TXA$_2$), which is released from platelets, contribute to the vasoconstriction.

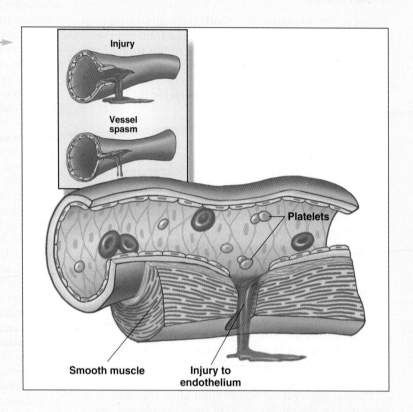

2

Formation of the platelet plug. Seconds after vessel injury, von Willebrand factor, released from the endothelium, binds to platelet receptors, causing adhesion of the platelets to the exposed collagen fibers *(inset)*. As the platelets adhere to the collagen fibers on the damaged vessel wall, they become activated and release adenosine diphosphate (ADP) and TXA$_2$. The ADP and TXA$_2$ attract additional platelets, leading to platelet aggregation.

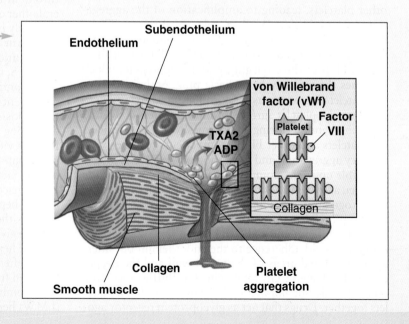

3

Blood coagulation. Blood coagulation is a complex process involving the sequential activation of various factors in the blood. There are two coagulation pathways: (1) the intrinsic pathway begins in the circulation and is initiated by activation of circulating factor XII, and (2) the extrinsic pathway, which is activated by a cellular lipoprotein, called *tissue factor,* that becomes exposed when tissues are injured. Both pathways lead to the activation of factor X, the conversion of prothrombin to thrombin, and conversion of fibrinogen to the insoluble fibrin threads that hold the clot together.

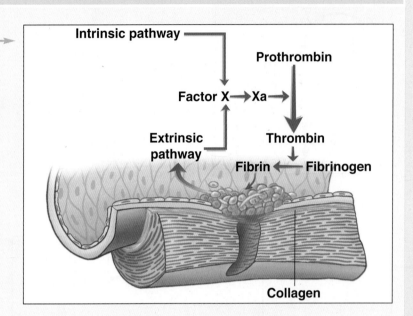

4

Clot retraction. Within a few minutes after a clot is formed, the actin and myosin in the platelets that are trapped in the clot begin to contract in a manner similar to that in muscles. As a result, the fibrin strands of the clot are pulled toward the platelets, thereby squeezing serum (plasma without fibrinogen) from the clot and causing it to shrink.

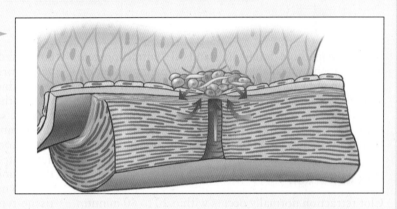

5

Clot dissolution or lysis. Clot dissolution begins shortly after a clot is formed. It begins with activation of plasminogen, an inactive precursor of the proteolytic enzyme, plasmin. When a clot is formed, large amounts of plasminogen are trapped in the clot. The slow release of a very powerful activator called tissue plasminogen activator (t-PA) from injured tissues and vascular endothelium converts plasminogen to plasmin, which digests the fibrin strands, causing the clot to dissolve.

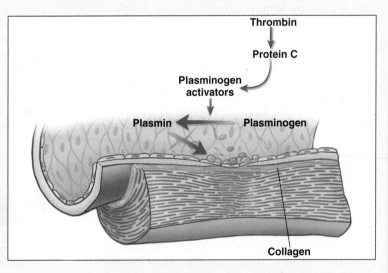

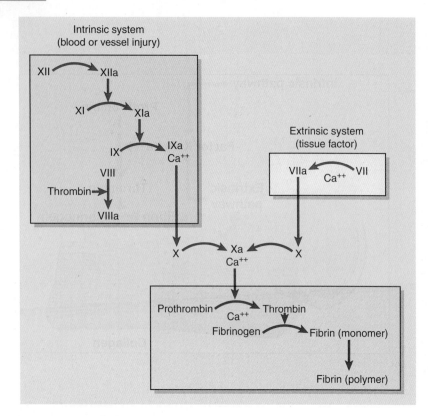

Intrinsic system
(blood or vessel injury)

XII → XIIa

XI → XIa

IX → IXa
Ca++

VIII

Thrombin →

VIIIa

Extrinsic system
(tissue factor)

VIIa ← VII
Ca++

X → Xa ← X
Ca++

Prothrombin → Thrombin
Ca++
Fibrinogen → Fibrin (monomer)

Fibrin (polymer)

FIGURE 10-2 The intrinsic and extrinsic coagulation pathways. The terminal steps in both pathways are the same. Calcium, factors X and V, and platelet phospholipids combine to form prothrombin activator, which then converts prothrombin to thrombin. This interaction causes conversion of fibrinogen into the fibrin strands that create the insoluble blood clot.

shorter than those found in standard (unfractionated) heparin are now available. The LMW heparins inhibit the activation of factor Xa, but have little effect on thrombin and other coagulation factors. They are given by subcutaneous injection and require less frequent administration than the standard form of heparin. They also do not require the frequent monitoring of coagulation blood tests.

Clot Retraction

Clot retraction normally occurs within 20 to 60 minutes after a clot has formed, contributing to hemostasis by squeezing serum from the clot and joining the edges of the broken vessel. Platelets contribute directly to clot contraction through the action of their actin and myosin filaments, which cause contraction of the fibrin strands attached to their cell membrane. As the clot retracts, the edges of the broken blood vessel are pulled together, thus contributing to the hemostasis process. Adequate numbers of platelets are necessary for clot retraction to occur.

CLOT DISSOLUTION AND PREVENTION OF BLOOD CLOTTING

The dissolution of a blood clot begins shortly after its formation; this allows blood flow to be reestablished and permanent tissue repair to take place. The process by which a blood clot dissolves is called *fibrinolysis*. The process involves a plasma protein called *plasminogen*, the proenzyme for the fibrinolytic process, which is normally present in the blood in its inactive form. It is

converted to its active form, plasmin, by plasminogen activators formed in the vascular endothelium, liver, and kidneys. The plasmin formed from plasminogen digests the fibrin strands of the clot and certain clotting factors, such as fibrinogen, factor V, factor VIII, prothrombin, and factor XII. Circulating plasmin is rapidly inactivated by α_2-plasmin inhibitor, which confines its action to the local clot and prevents it from moving throughout the entire circulation.

Two naturally occurring plasminogen activators are tissue-type plasminogen activator and urokinase-type plasminogen activator. The liver, plasma, and vascular endothelium are the major sources of physiologic activators. These activators are released in response to a number of stimuli, including vasoactive drugs, venous occlusion, elevated body temperature, and exercise. The activators are unstable and rapidly inactivated by inhibitors synthesized by the endothelium and the liver. For this reason, chronic liver disease may cause altered fibrinolytic activity. A major inhibitor, plasminogen activator inhibitor-1, in high concentrations has been associated with deep vein thrombosis, coronary artery disease, and myocardial infarction.[5]

In summary, hemostasis is designed to maintain the integrity of the vascular compartment. The process is divided into five phases: vessel spasm, which constricts the size of the vessel and reduces blood flow; platelet adherence and formation of the platelet plug; formation of the fibrin clot, which cements the platelet plug together; clot retraction, which pulls the edges of the injured vessel together; and clot dissolution, which involves the action of plasmin to dissolve the clot and allow blood flow to be reestablished and tissue healing to take place. Blood coagulation requires the stepwise activation of coagulation factors, carefully controlled by activators and inhibitors.

Hypercoagulability States

Hypercoagulability represents hemostasis in an exaggerated form and predisposes to thrombosis. Arterial thrombi caused by turbulence are composed of platelet aggregates, and venous thrombi caused by stasis of flow are largely composed of platelet aggregates and fibrin complexes that result from excess coagulation. There are two general forms of hypercoagulability states: conditions that trigger increased platelet function and conditions that accelerate the activity of the coagulation system. Chart 10-1 summarizes conditions commonly associated with hypercoagulability states.

INCREASED PLATELET FUNCTION

Increased platelet function predisposes to platelet adhesion, formation of platelet clots, and the disruption of blood flow. The causes of increased platelet function include an increase in platelet numbers and disturbances in blood flow, damage to the vascular endothelium, and increased sensitivity of platelets to factors that cause adhesiveness and aggregation.

CHART 10-1

Conditions Associated With Hypercoagulability States

Increased Platelet Function

Atherosclerosis
Diabetes mellitus
Smoking
Elevated blood lipid and cholesterol levels
Increased platelet levels

Accelerated Activity of the Clotting System

Pregnancy and the puerperium
Use of oral contraceptives
Postsurgical state
Immobility
Congestive heart failure
Malignant diseases

KEY CONCEPTS

Hypercoagulability States

➤ Hypercoagulability states increase the risk of clot or thrombus formation in either the arterial or venous circulations.

➤ Arterial thrombi are associated with conditions that produce turbulent blood flow and platelet adherence.

➤ Venous thrombi are associated with conditions that cause stasis of blood flow with increased concentrations of coagulation factors.

The term *thrombocytosis* is used to describe elevations in the platelet count above 1,000,000/μL.[1] This occurs in some malignancies and chronic inflammatory states, and after splenectomy. Myeloproliferative disorders such as polycythemia vera produce excess platelets that may predispose to thrombosis or, paradoxically, bleeding when the rapidly produced platelets are defective.

Atherosclerotic plaques disturb flow, cause endothelial damage, and promote platelet adherence. Platelets that adhere to the vessel wall release growth factors that cause proliferation of smooth muscle and thereby contribute to the development of atherosclerosis (discussed in Chapter 17). Smoking, elevated levels of blood lipids and cholesterol, hemodynamic stress, diabetes mellitus, and immune mechanisms may also contribute to vessel damage, platelet adherence, and, eventually, thrombosis.

INCREASED CLOTTING ACTIVITY

Thrombus formation due to activation of the coagulation system can result from primary (genetic) or secondary (acquired) disorders affecting the coagulation components of the blood (*i.e.*, an increase in procoagulation factors or a decrease in anticoagulation factors).

Hereditary Disorders

Of the inherited causes of hyperactivity, mutations in the factor V gene and prothrombin gene are the most common.[4] In persons with inherited defects in factor V, the mutant factor Va cannot be inactivated by protein C; as a result, an important antithrombotic counter-regulatory mechanism is lost. Approximately 2% to 10% of the white population carries a specific factor V mutation (referred to as the Leiden mutation, after the Dutch city where it was first discovered).[4] The defect predisposes to recurrent deep vein thrombosis. Thromboses often occur during early adulthood rather than in childhood and are often precipitated by factors such as trauma and pregnancy. Less common primary hypercoagulable states include inherited deficiencies of anticoagulants such as antithrombin III, protein C, and protein S.[4] Another hereditary defect resulting in high circulating levels of homocysteine also predisposes to venous and arterial thrombosis by activating platelets and altering antithrombotic mechanisms.[4]

Acquired Disorders

Among the acquired or secondary factors that lead to increased coagulation and thrombosis are stasis due to prolonged bed rest or immobilization, myocardial infarction, cancer, hyperestrogenic states, and oral contraceptives. Smoking and obesity also promote hypercoagulability for unknown reasons.

Stasis causes the accumulation of platelets and activated clotting factors. Slow and disturbed flow is a common cause of venous thrombosis in the immobilized or postsurgical patient. Heart failure also contributes to venous congestion and thrombosis. Hyperviscosity syndromes (polycythemia) and deformed red cells in sickle cell anemia increase the resistance to flow and cause small vessel stasis.

Elevated levels of estrogen increase hepatic synthesis of many coagulation factors and decrease the synthesis of antithrombin III.[6] The incidence of stroke, thromboemboli, and myocardial infarction is greater in women who use oral contraceptives, particularly in women who are older than 35 years of age and smoke.[6] Clotting factors are also increased during normal pregnancy. These changes, along with limited activity during the puerperium (immediate postpartum period), predispose to venous thrombosis.

Hypercoagulability is common in cancer and sepsis. Many tumor cells are thought to release tissue factor molecules that, along with the increased immobility and sepsis seen in patients with malignant disease, contribute to thrombosis in these patients.

Antiphospholipid Syndrome. Another cause of increased venous and arterial clotting is the *antiphospholipid syndrome,* a condition associated with antibodies directed against phospholipid-binding proteins that function as anticoagulants.[7,8] The disorder can be manifest as a primary condition occurring in isolation with signs of hypercoagulability or as a secondary condition usually associated with systemic lupus erythematosus.

Persons with the disorder present with a variety of clinical manifestations; these are typically characterized by recurrent venous and arterial thrombi, but also include cardiac valvular vegetations associated with thrombi adherence, and thrombocytopenia due to excessive platelet consumption. In most persons with antiphospholipid syndrome, the thrombotic events occur as a single episode at one anatomic site. Occasionally, someone may present with multiple vascular occlusions involving many organ systems. This rapid-onset condition is termed *catastrophic antiphospholipid syndrome* and is associated with a high mortality rate. Women with the disorder commonly have a history of recurrent pregnancy losses after the 10th week of gestation because of ischemia and thrombosis of the placental vessels. These women also have an increased risk of giving birth to a premature infant because of pregnancy-associated hypertension and uteroplacental insufficiency.

Treatment focuses on removal or reduction in factors that predispose to thrombosis, including advice to stop smoking and counseling against use of estrogen-containing oral contraceptives by women. The acute thrombotic event is treated with anticoagulants (heparin and warfarin) and immune suppression in refractory cases. Aspirin and anticoagulant drugs may be used to prevent future thrombosis.

In summary, hypercoagulability causes excessive clotting and contributes to thrombus formation. It results from conditions leading to increased platelet function or accelerated activity of the coagulation system. Increased platelet function usually results from disorders such as atherosclerosis that damage the vessel endothelium and disturb blood flow or from conditions such as smoking that produce increased sensitivity of platelets to factors that promote adhesiveness and aggregation. Factors that cause accelerated activity of the coagulation system include blood flow stasis, resulting in an accumulation of coagulation factors, and alterations in the components of the coagulation system (*i.e.,* an increase in procoagulation factors or a decrease in anticoagulation factors). The antiphospholipid syndrome is another cause of venous and arterial clotting and is manifest as a primary disorder or a secondary disorder associated with systemic lupus erythematosus. It is associated with antiphospholipid antibodies that promote thrombosis and can affect many organs.

 ## Bleeding Disorders

Bleeding disorders or impairment of blood coagulation can result from defects in any of the factors that contribute to hemostasis. Defects are associated with platelets, coagulation factors, and vascular integrity.

PLATELET DISORDERS

Bleeding can occur as a result of a decrease in the number of circulating platelets or impaired platelet function. Because platelets form temporary hemostatic plugs that quickly stop bleeding and promote key reactions in the coagulation cascade, spontaneous bleeding associated with platelet disorders most often involves small blood vessels. The most common sites are the skin and mucous membranes of the gastrointestinal and genitourinary tracts.[4] Petechiae (*i.e.,* pinpoint purplish-red spots) and purpura (*i.e.,* purple areas of bruising) are common manifestations resulting from bleeding into the skin (Fig. 10-3). Bleeding of the intracranial vessels is a rare danger with severe platelet depletion.

Thrombocytopenia

Thrombocytopenia is a decrease in the number of circulating platelets to a level less than 100,000/µL.[9] How-

KEY CONCEPTS

Bleeding Disorders

→ Bleeding disorders are caused by defects associated with platelets, coagulation factors, and vessel integrity.

→ Disorders of platelet plug formation include a decrease in platelet numbers due to inadequate platelet production (bone marrow dysfunction), excess platelet destruction (thrombocytopenia), abnormal platelet function (thrombocytopathia), or defects in von Willebrand factor.

→ Impairment of the coagulation stage of hemostasis is caused by a deficiency in one or more of the clotting factors.

→ Disorders of blood vessel integrity result from structurally weak vessels or vessel damage due to inflammation and immune mechanisms.

ever, spontaneous bleeding usually does not occur until the platelet count falls below 20,000/μL.[9] It can result from decreased platelet production by the bone marrow, decreased platelet survival time, sequestration of platelets in the spleen, or dilutional thrombocytopenia.

Decreased platelet production is usually caused by diseases of the bone marrow such as aplastic anemia (see Chapter 11) or replacement of bone marrow by malignant cells, such as occurs in leukemia. Infection with human immunodeficiency virus (HIV) suppresses the production of megakaryocytes, the platelet precursors. Radiation therapy and drugs such as those used in the treatment of cancer may depress bone marrow function and reduce platelet production.

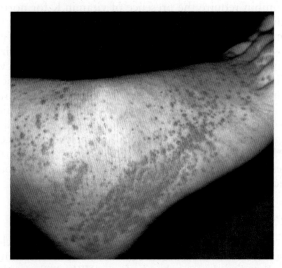

FIGURE 10-3 Foot with acute purpura and petechiae. (From Hall J. C. [2000]. *Sauer's manual of skin diseases* [8th ed., p. 112]. Philadelphia: Lippincott Williams & Wilkins.)

Reduced platelet survival occurs by a variety of immune and nonimmune mechanisms. Platelet destruction may be caused by antiplatelet antibodies. The antibodies may be directed against the platelet self-antigens or against antigens on the platelets due to blood transfusions or pregnancy. The antibodies target the platelet membrane glycoproteins. Nonimmune destruction of platelets results from mechanical injury due to prosthetic heart valves or malignant hypertension, which results in small vessel narrowing. In acute disseminated intravascular coagulation (DIC) or thrombotic thrombocytopenic purpura (TTP), excessive platelet consumption leads to a deficiency.

There may be normal production of platelets but excessive pooling of platelets in the spleen. Although the spleen normally sequesters 30% to 40% of the platelets before release into the circulation, this can be increased to as much as 90% when the spleen is enlarged in splenomegaly.[1] When necessary, hypersplenic thrombocytopenia may be treated with splenectomy. Massive blood or plasma transfusions may cause a dilutional thrombocytopenia because blood stored for more than 24 hours and red cell mass reconstituted for transfusion have no viable platelets.

Idiopathic Thrombocytopenic Purpura. Idiopathic thrombocytopenic purpura (ITP), an autoimmune disorder, results in platelet antibody formation and excess destruction of platelets. The immunoglobulin G (IgG) antibody commonly binds to two identified membrane glycoproteins (IIb/IIIa and Ib/IX) while in the circulation. The platelets, which are made more susceptible to phagocytosis because of the antibody, are destroyed in the spleen and the liver.

Half of the cases of ITP occur as an acute disorder in young children (5 years of age) and usually follow a viral infection.[10] It is characterized by sudden onset of petechiae and purpura and is a self-limited disorder with no treatment. Most children recover in a few weeks. In contrast, ITP in adults is a chronic disorder with insidious onset and seldom follows an infection. It is a disease of young people, with a peak incidence between the ages of 18 and 40 years, and is seen twice as often in women as in men.

Secondary forms of ITP may be associated with acquired immunodeficiency syndrome (AIDS), systemic lupus erythematosus, antiphospholipid syndrome, lymphoproliferative disorders, hepatitis C, and drugs such as heparin and quinidine. The condition may be discovered incidentally or as a result of signs of bleeding, often into the skin (*i.e.,* purpura and petechiae) or oral mucosa. There is commonly a history of bruising, bleeding from gums, epistaxis (*i.e.,* nosebleeds), and abnormal menstrual bleeding in those with moderately reduced platelet counts. Because the spleen is the site of platelet destruction, splenic enlargement may occur.

Diagnosis usually is based on severe thrombocytopenia (platelet counts <20,000/μL), and exclusion of other causes. Tests for the platelet-bound antibodies are available but lack specificity (*e.g.,* they react with platelet antibodies from other sources). Treatment includes the initial use of corticosteroid drugs, intravenous immune globulin, and splenectomy for those who relapse or do not respond to drugs.[10]

Drug-Induced Thrombocytopenia. Some drugs, such as quinine, quinidine, and certain sulfa-containing antibiotics, may induce thrombocytopenia. These drugs act as haptens and induce antigen–antibody responses and formation of immune complexes that cause platelet destruction by complement-mediated lysis (see Chapter 13). In persons with drug-associated thrombocytopenia, there is a rapid fall in platelet count within 2 to 3 days of resuming a drug or 7 or more days (*i.e.*, the time needed to mount an immune response) after starting a drug for the first time. The platelet count rises rapidly after the drug is discontinued.

The anticoagulant drug heparin has been increasingly implicated in thrombocytopenia and, paradoxically, in thrombosis. The complications typically occur 5 days after the start of therapy and result from heparin-dependent antiplatelet antibodies that cause aggregation of platelets and their removal from the circulation. The antibodies often bind to vessel walls, causing thrombosis and complications such as stroke and myocardial infarction. The newer LMW heparin has been shown to be effective in reducing the incidence of heparin-induced complications compared with the older high–molecular-weight form of the drug.[11]

Thrombotic Thrombocytopenic Purpura. Thrombotic thrombocytopenic purpura (TTP) is a microvascular disorder characterized by widespread platelet thrombi in arterioles and capillaries of the heart, brain, and kidneys; thrombocytopenia; and fragmentation of erythrocytes as they circulate through the partly occluded vessels, causing hemolytic anemia and jaundice. The pathogenesis of TTP is unclear, but appears to involve the introduction of one or more platelet-aggregating substances into the circulation.[1] It is a rare disorder occurring predominantly in adults between 20 and 50 years of age, with a slight predominance in women. The syndrome is occasionally precipitated by estrogen use, pregnancy, drugs, or infections and may occur in association with HIV infection. Toxins produced by some strains of *Escherichia coli* (*e.g., E. coli* 0157:H7) cause endothelial injury and are responsible for a similar condition, *hemolytic uremic syndrome* (discussed in Chapter 28).

Clinical manifestations include purpura, petechiae, and vaginal bleeding and neurologic symptoms ranging from headache to seizures and altered consciousness. The onset is usually abrupt and the outcome may be fatal. The disorder is similar to DIC but does not involve the clotting system.

Treatment for TTP includes *plasmapheresis,* a procedure that involves removal of plasma from withdrawn blood and replacement with fresh-frozen plasma. The treatment is continued until remission occurs. With plasmapheresis treatment, there is a complete recovery in about 80% of cases.[1]

Impaired Platelet Function

Impaired platelet function (also called *thrombocytopathia*) may result from inherited disorders of adhesion (*e.g.,* von Willebrand disease) or acquired defects caused by drugs, disease, or extracorporeal circulation. Defective platelet function is common in end-stage renal disease, presumably because of the retention of uremic waste products. Cardiopulmonary bypass also causes platelet defects and destruction.

The use of aspirin and other nonsteroidal anti-inflammatory drugs (NSAIDs) is the most common cause of impaired platelet function. Aspirin produces irreversible acetylation of platelet cyclooxygenase activity and consequently the synthesis of the prostaglandin TXA_2, which is required for platelet aggregation. The effect of aspirin on platelet aggregation lasts for the life of the platelet—usually approximately 8 to 9 days. In contrast to the effects of aspirin, the inhibition of cyclooxygenase by other NSAIDs is reversible and lasts only for the duration of drug action.[12] Aspirin (81 mg/day) commonly is used to prevent formation of arterial thrombi and reduce the risk for heart attack and stroke.

COAGULATION DEFECTS

Blood coagulation defects can result from deficiencies or impairment of one or more of the clotting factors. Deficiencies can arise because of defective synthesis, inherited disease, or increased consumption of the clotting factors. Bleeding resulting from a clotting factor deficiency typically occurs after injury or trauma, with large bruises, hematomas, or prolonged bleeding into the gastrointestinal tract, urinary tract, or joints being the most common manifestations.

Impaired Synthesis of Coagulation Factors

Coagulation factors V, VII, IX, X, XI, and XII, prothrombin, and fibrinogen are synthesized in the liver. In liver disease, synthesis of these clotting factors is reduced, and bleeding may result. Of the coagulation factors synthesized in the liver, factors VII, IX, and X and prothrombin require the presence of vitamin K for normal activity. In vitamin K deficiency, the liver produces the clotting factor, but in an inactive form. Vitamin K is a fat-soluble vitamin that is continuously being synthesized by intestinal bacteria. This means that a deficiency in vitamin K is not likely to occur unless intestinal synthesis is interrupted or absorption of the vitamin is impaired. Because vitamin K is a fat-soluble vitamin that requires bile salts for absorption, a deficiency can be caused by liver or gallbladder disease. Vitamin K deficiency can occur in the newborn infant before the establishment of the intestinal flora or as the result of treatment with broad-spectrum antibiotics that destroy intestinal flora.

Hereditary Disorders

Hereditary defects have been reported for each of the clotting factors, but most are rare diseases. The most common bleeding disorders involve the factor VIII–vWF complex; Hemophilia A affects 1 in 5000 male live births, and von Willebrand disease may affect more than 1 in 1000.[13] Factor IX deficiency (*i.e.*, hemophilia B) occurs in approximately 1 in 30,000 persons and is genetically and clinically similar to hemophilia A.

Circulating factor VIII is part of a complex molecule, bound to vWF. Factor VIII coagulant protein is the functional portion produced by the liver and endothelial cells. The vWF, synthesized by the endothelium and megakaryocytes, binds and stabilizes factor VIII in the circulation by preventing proteolysis. It is also required for platelet adhesion to the subendothelial layer.

Hemophilia A. Hemophilia A is an X-linked recessive disorder that primarily affects males. Although it is a hereditary disorder, there is no family history of the disorder in approximately 30% of newly diagnosed cases, suggesting that it has arisen as a new mutation in the factor VIII gene.[13] The percentage of normal factor VIII activity in the circulation depends on the genetic defect and determines the severity of hemophilia (*i.e.*, 6% to 30% in mild hemophilia, 2% to 5% in moderate hemophilia, and 1% or less in severe forms of hemophilia). In mild or moderate forms of the disease, bleeding usually does not occur unless there is a local lesion or trauma such as surgery or dental procedures. The mild disorder may not be detected in childhood. In severe hemophilia, bleeding usually occurs in childhood (*e.g.*, it may be noticed at the time of circumcision) and is spontaneous and severe, often occurring several times a month.

Characteristically, bleeding occurs in soft tissues, the gastrointestinal tract, and the hip, knee, elbow, and ankle joints. Joint bleeding usually begins when a child begins to walk. Often, a target joint is prone to repeated bleeding. The bleeding causes inflammation of the synovium, with acute pain and swelling. Without proper treatment, chronic bleeding and inflammation cause joint fibrosis and contractures, resulting in major disability. Muscle hematomas may be present in 30% of episodes, and intracranial hemorrhage is an important cause of death.[14]

Factor VIII replacement therapy is initiated when bleeding occurs or as prophylaxis with repeated bleeding episodes. Highly purified factor VIII concentrates prepared from human plasma are the usual replacement products for persons with severe hemophilia. Before blood was tested for infectious diseases, these products were prepared from multiple donor samples and carried a high risk of exposure to hepatitis viruses and HIV. Donor screening and the development of effective virus-inactivation procedures have effectively reduced the transmission of hepatitis viruses and HIV through clotting concentrates. Recombinant factor VIII, although expensive, is now available and should reduce the risk of transmitting HIV or other viruses. Desmopressin acetate (DDAVP, 1-desamino-8-D-arginine vasopressin) may be used to prevent bleeding in persons with mild hemophilia.[15] It stimulates the release of vWF (the carrier for factor VIII) from the endothelium, thus increasing factor VIII levels two- to threefold for several hours.

The cloning of the factor VIII gene and progress in gene delivery systems have led to the hope that hemophilia A may be cured by gene therapy. Carrier detection and prenatal diagnosis can now be done by analysis of direct gene mutation or DNA linkage studies.

Von Willebrand Disease. Von Willebrand disease, which typically is diagnosed in adulthood, is the most common hereditary bleeding disorder. Transmitted as an autosomal trait, it is caused by a deficiency of or defect in vWF. This deficiency results in reduced platelet adhesion. There are many variants of the disease, and manifestations range from mild to severe. Because vWF carries factor VIII, its deficiency may also be accompanied by reduced levels of factor VIII, contributing to defective clot formation. Symptoms include bruising, excessive menstrual flow, and bleeding from the nose, mouth, and gastrointestinal tract. Many persons with the disorder are diagnosed when surgery or dental extraction results in prolonged bleeding. Most cases are mild and untreated. In severe cases, life-threatening gastrointestinal bleeding and joint hemorrhage may resemble hemophilia.

Treatment for all forms of the disease includes factor VIII products that contain vWF. The disorder also responds to desmopressin acetate (DDAVP), a synthetic analog of the hormone vasopressin, which stimulates the endothelial cells to release vWF and plasminogen activator. DDAVP can also be used to treat mild hemophilia A and platelet dysfunction caused by uremia, heart bypass, and the effects of aspirin.[15,16]

DISSEMINATED INTRAVASCULAR COAGULATION

Disseminated intravascular coagulation is a paradox in the hemostatic sequence and is characterized by widespread coagulation and bleeding in the vascular compartment.[17] It is not a primary disease but occurs as a complication of a wide variety of conditions. DIC begins with massive activation of the coagulation sequence as a result of unregulated generation of thrombin, resulting in systemic formation of fibrin. In addition, levels of all the major anticoagulants are reduced (Fig. 10-4). The microthrombi that result cause vessel occlusion and tissue ischemia. Multiple organ failure may ensue. Clot formation consumes all available coagulation proteins and platelets, and severe hemorrhage results.

The disorder can be initiated by activation of the intrinsic or extrinsic pathways. Activation through the extrinsic pathway occurs with liberation of tissue factors, as in obstetric complications, trauma, bacterial sepsis, and cancers. The intrinsic pathway may be activated through extensive endothelial damage caused by viruses, infections, immune mechanisms, stasis of blood, or temperature extremes. Common clinical conditions that may cause DIC include obstetric disorders, accounting for 50% of cases, massive trauma, shock, infections, and malignant disease. Chart 10-2 summarizes the conditions associated with DIC.

The factors involved in the conditions that cause DIC are often interrelated. In obstetric complications, tissue factors released from necrotic placental or fetal tissue or amniotic fluid may enter the circulation, inciting the DIC. Hypoxia, shock, and acidosis, which may coexist, also

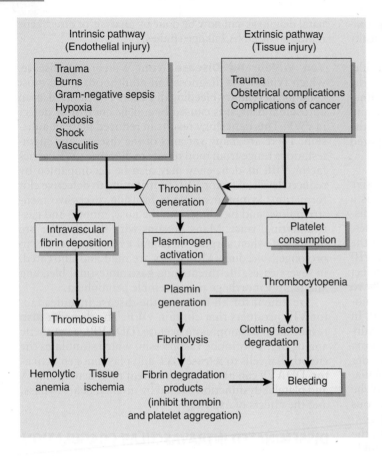

FIGURE 10-4 Pathophysiology of disseminated intravascular coagulation.

contribute by causing endothelial injury. Gram-negative bacterial infections result in the release of endotoxins, which activate both the extrinsic pathway by release of tissue factors and the intrinsic pathway through endothelial damage. Endotoxins also inhibit the activity of protein C, an anticoagulant. Antigen–antibody complexes associated with infection can activate platelets through complement fragments.[9]

There is increasing evidence that the underlying cause of DIC is infection or inflammation and that the cytokines liberated in the process are the pivotal mediators.[18] Cytokines and endotoxins activate the fibrinolytic system early in DIC. They later activate the coagulation system and inhibit fibrinolysis, causing a procoagulant state.[18]

Although coagulation and formation of microemboli characterize DIC, its acute manifestations usually are more directly related to the bleeding problems that occur. The bleeding may be present as petechiae, purpura, oozing from puncture sites, or severe hemorrhage. Uncontrolled postpartum bleeding may indicate DIC. Microemboli may obstruct blood vessels and cause tissue hypoxia and necrotic damage to organ structures, such as the kidneys, heart, lungs, and brain. As a result, common clinical signs may be due to renal, circulatory, or respiratory failure or convulsions and coma. A form of hemolytic anemia may develop as red cells are damaged as they pass through vessels partially blocked by thrombus.

The treatment of DIC is directed toward managing the primary disease, replacing clotting components, and preventing further activation of clotting mecha-

nisms. Transfusions of fresh-frozen plasma, platelets, or fibrinogen-containing cryoprecipitate may correct the clotting factor deficiency. Heparin may be given to decrease blood coagulation, thereby interrupting the clotting process. Tissue factor pathway inhibitors, antithrombin, and protein C concentrates are being evaluated as potential therapies.[17]

VASCULAR DISORDERS

Bleeding from small blood vessels may result from vascular disorders. These disorders may occur because of structurally weak vessel walls or because of damage to vessels by inflammation or immune responses. Among the vascular disorders that cause bleeding are hemorrhagic telangiectasia, an uncommon autosomal dominant disorder characterized by thin-walled, dilated capillaries and arterioles; vitamin C deficiency (*i.e.*, scurvy), resulting in poor collagen synthesis and failure of the endothelial cells to be cemented together properly, which causes a fragile wall; Cushing disease, causing protein wasting and loss of vessel tissue support because of excess cortisol; and senile purpura (*i.e.*, bruising in elderly persons) caused by the aging process. Vascular defects also occur in the course of DIC as a result of the presence of microthrombi and corticosteroid therapy.

Vascular disorders are characterized by easy bruising and the spontaneous appearance of petechiae and purpura of the skin and mucous membranes. In persons with bleeding disorders caused by vascular defects, the platelet

CHART 10-2

Conditions That Have Been Associated With DIC

Obstetric Conditions

Abruptio placentae
Dead fetus syndrome
Preeclampsia and eclampsia
Amniotic fluid embolism

Cancers

Metastatic cancer
Leukemia

Infections

Acute bacterial infections (*e.g.*, meningococcal meningitis)
Acute viral infections
Rickettsial infections (*e.g.*, Rocky Mountain spotted fever)
Parasitic infection (*e.g.*, malaria)

Shock

Septic shock
Severe hypovolemic shock

Trauma or Surgery

Burns
Massive trauma
Surgery involving extracorporeal circulation
Snake bite
Heatstroke

Hematologic Conditions

Blood transfusion reactions

count and results of other tests for coagulation factors are normal.

In summary, bleeding disorders or impairment of blood coagulation can result from defects in any of the factors that contribute to hemostasis: platelets, coagulation factors, or vascular integrity. The number of circulating platelets can be decreased (*i.e.*, thrombocytopenia) or platelet function can be impaired (*i.e.*, thrombocytopathia). Impairment of blood coagulation can result from deficiencies of one or more of the known clotting factors. Deficiencies can arise because of defective synthesis (*i.e.*, liver disease or vitamin K deficiency), inherited diseases (*i.e.*, hemophilia A or von Willebrand disease), or increased consumption of the clotting factors (*i.e.*, DIC). Bleeding may also occur from structurally weak vessels that result from impaired synthesis of vessel wall components (*i.e.*, vitamin C deficiency,

excessive cortisol levels as in Cushing disease, or the aging process) or from damage by genetic mechanisms (*i.e.*, hemorrhagic telangiectasia) or the presence of microthrombi.

Review Exercises

A 55-year-old man has begun taking one 81-mg aspirin tablet daily on the recommendation of his physician. The physician had told him that this would help to prevent heart attack and stroke.

A. What is the action of aspirin in terms of heart attack and stroke prevention?
B. The drug clopidogrel ([Plavix] an inhibitor of ADP-induced platelet aggregation) is often prescribed along with aspirin to prevent thrombosis in persons with severe atherosclerotic disease who are at risk for myocardial infarction or stroke. Explain the rationale for using the two drugs.

The drug desmopressin acetate (DDAVP), which is a synthetic analog of arginine vasopressin, increases the half-life of factor VIII and is sometimes used to treat bleeding in patients with mild hemophilia.

A. Explain.

A 29-year-old new mother, who delivered her baby 3 days ago, is admitted to the hospital with chest pain and is diagnosed as having venous thrombosis with pulmonary emboli.

A. What factors would contribute to this woman's risk for development of thromboemboli?

She is admitted to the intensive care unit and started on low–molecular-weight heparin and warfarin. She is told that she will be discharged in a day or two and will remain on the heparin for 5 days and the warfarin for at least 3 months.

A. Use Figure 10-2 to explain the action of heparin and warfarin. Why is heparin administered for 5 days during the initiation of warfarin treatment?
B. Anticoagulation with heparin and warfarin is not a definitive treatment for clot removal in pulmonary emboli, but a form of secondary prevention. Explain.

REFERENCES

1. Schwarting R., Kocher W. D., McKenzie S., et al. (2005). Hematopathology. In Rubin E., Gorstein F., Rubin R., et al. (Eds.), *Rubin's pathology: Clinicopathologic foundations of medicine* (4th ed., pp. 1048–1062). Philadelphia: Lippincott Williams & Wilkins.

2. Kaushansky K. (1998). Thrombopoietin. *New England Journal of Medicine* 339, 746–754.

3. Ross M. H. (2003). *Histology: A text and atlas* (4th ed., pp. 229–231). Philadelphia: Lippincott Williams & Wilkins.

4. Mitchell R. N. (2005). Hemodynamic disorders, thrombosis, and shock. In Kumar V., Abbas A. K., Fausto N. (Eds.), *Robbins and Cotran pathologic basis of disease* (7th ed., pp. 124–135). Philadelphia: Elsevier Saunders.

5. Kohler H. P., Grant P. J. (2000). Plasminogen-activator inhibitor type 1 and coronary artery disease. *New England Journal of Medicine* 342, 1792–1801.

6. Chrousos G. P., Zoumakis E. N., Gravania A. (2001). The gonadal hormones and inhibitors. In Katzung B. G. (Ed.), *Basic and clinical pharmacology* (8th ed., pp. 683–684). Norwalk, CT: Appleton & Lange.

7. Levine J. S., Branch D. W., Rausch J. (2002). The antiphospholipid syndrome. *New England Journal of Medicine* 346, 752–763.

8. Hanly J. C. (2003). Antiphospholipid syndrome: An overview. *Canadian Medical Association Journal* 168, 1675–1682.

9. Aster J. C. (2005). Red cells and bleeding disorders. In Kumar V., Abbas A. K., Fausto N. (Eds.), *Robbins and Cotran pathologic basis of disease* (7th ed., pp. 649–659). Philadelphia: Elsevier Saunders.

10. Cines D. B., Blanchette V. S. (2002). Immune thrombocytopenic purpura. *New England Journal of Medicine* 346, 995–1008.

11. Warkentin T. E., Chong B. H., Greinacher A. (1998). Heparin-induced thrombocytopenia: Towards consensus. *Thrombosis and Haemostasis* 79, 1–7.

12. George J. N., Shattil S. J. (2000). Acquired disorders of platelet function. In Hoffman R., Benz E. J., Shattil S. J., et al. (Eds.), *Hematology* (3rd ed., p. 2176). New York: Churchill Livingstone.

13. Mannucci P. M., Tuddenham E. G. D. (2001). The hemophilias: From royal genes to gene therapy. *New England Journal of Medicine* 344, 1773–1779.

14. Klinge J., Ananyeva N. M., Hauser C., et al. (2002). Hemophilia A: From basic science to clinical practice. *Seminars in Thrombosis and Hemostasis* 28, 309–322.

15. Mannucci P. M. (1997). Desmopressin (DDAVP) in the treatment of bleeding disorders: The first 20 years. *Blood* 90, 2515–2521.

16. Mannucci P. M. (2004). Treatment of von Willebrand's disease. *New England Journal of Medicine* 351, 683–694.

17. Levi M., Jonge E., van der Poll T., et al. (2001). Advances in the understanding of the pathogenetic pathways of disseminated intravascular coagulation result in more insight in the clinical picture and better management strategies. *Seminars in Thrombosis and Hemostasis* 27, 569–575.

18. Van der Poll T., Jonge E., Levi M. (2001). Regulatory role of cytokines in disseminated intravascular coagulation. *Seminars in Thrombosis and Hemostasis* 27, 639–651.

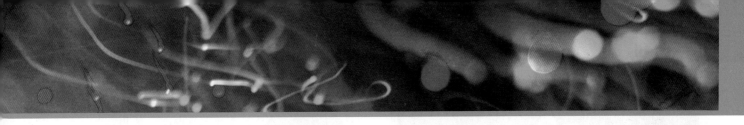

Chapter *11*

The Red Blood Cell and Alterations in Oxygen Transport

 Although the lungs provide the means for gas exchange between the external and internal environment, it is the hemoglobin in the red blood cells that transports oxygen to the tissues. The red blood cells also function as carriers of carbon dioxide and participate in acid-base balance. The function of the red blood cells, in terms of oxygen transport, is discussed in Chapter 20, and acid-base balance is covered in Chapter 6. This chapter focuses on the red blood cell, anemia, and polycythemia.

The Red Blood Cell

The erythrocytes or mature red blood cells are the most common type of blood cell, being 500 to 1000 times more numerous than other blood cells. The erythrocyte is a non-nucleated, thin, biconcave disk (Fig. 11-1). This unique shape contributes in two ways to the oxygen (O_2) transport function of the erythrocyte. The biconcave shape provides a larger surface area for O_2 diffusion than would a spherical cell of the same volume, and the thinness of the cell membrane enables O_2 to diffuse rapidly between the exterior and innermost regions of the cell. Another structural feature that facilitates the transport function of the red blood cell is the flexibility of its membrane. The biconcave shape and flexibility of the red cell membrane are maintained by a network of fibrous proteins, especially one called *spectrin*, attached to the cytoplasmic side of the cell membrane. This complex arrangement allows for the inherent deformability of red cells as they squeeze through capillaries one-third their diameter without rupturing.

The most important anatomic feature that enables the red blood cell to transport O_2 is the hemoglobin it contains. Because O_2 is poorly soluble in plasma, about 95% to 98% is carried bound to hemoglobin. The hemoglobin molecule is composed of two pairs of structurally different alpha (α)

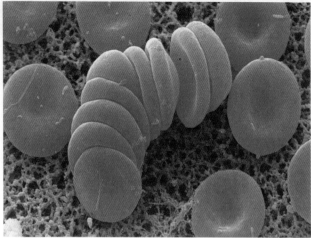

FIGURE 11-1 Scanning electron micrograph of normal red blood cells showing their normal concave appearance (×3000). (© Andrew Syred, Science Photo Lab, Science Source/Photo Researchers.)

Plasma membrane

Hemoglobin

β₂   β₁

Heme

α₂   α₁

A Red blood cell   **B**   Hemoglobin

FIGURE 11-2 (**A**) Biconcave structure of the red blood cell as shown in cross-sectional side view and in lateral surface view. (**B**) Hemoglobin molecule, showing the four iron-containing heme subunits.

and beta (β) polypeptide chains (Fig. 11-2). Each of the four polypeptide chains consists of a globin (protein) portion and heme unit, which surrounds an atom of iron that binds oxygen.[1] Thus, each molecule of hemoglobin can carry four molecules of oxygen. Hemoglobin is a natural pigment; because of its iron content, it appears reddish when oxygen is attached and has a bluish cast when deoxygenated.

There are two major types of normal hemoglobin—adult hemoglobin (HbA) and fetal hemoglobin (HbF). HbA consists of a pair of α chains and a pair of β chains. HbF is the predominant hemoglobin in the fetus from the third through the ninth month of gestation. It has a pair of gamma (γ) chains substituted for the α chains. Because of this chain substitution, HbF has a high affinity for oxygen. This affinity facilitates the transfer of oxygen across the placenta from the HbA in the mother's blood to the HbF in the fetus's blood. HbF is replaced within 6 months of birth by HbA.

HEMOGLOBIN SYNTHESIS

The rate at which hemoglobin is synthesized depends on the availability of iron for heme synthesis. A lack of iron results in relatively small amounts of hemoglobin in the red blood cells. The amount of iron in the body is approximately 2 g in women and up to 6 g in men.[2] Body iron is found in several compartments. About 80% is complexed to heme in hemoglobin, and most of the remaining iron (about 20%) is stored in the bone marrow, liver, spleen, and other organs. Iron in the hemoglobin compartment is recycled. When red blood cells age and are destroyed in the spleen, the iron from their hemoglobin is released into the circulation and returned to the bone marrow for incorporation into new red blood cells, or to the liver and other tissues for storage.

Dietary iron helps to maintain body stores. Iron, principally derived from meat, is absorbed in the small intestine, especially the duodenum (Fig. 11-3). When body stores of iron are diminished or erythropoiesis is stimulated, absorption is increased. Normally, some iron is sequestered in the intestinal epithelial cells and is lost in the feces as these cells slough off. The iron that is absorbed enters the circulation, where it attaches a transport protein called *transferrin*. From the circulation, iron can be deposited in tissues such as the liver, where it is stored as *ferritin*, a protein–iron complex, which can easily return to the circulation. Serum ferritin levels, which can be

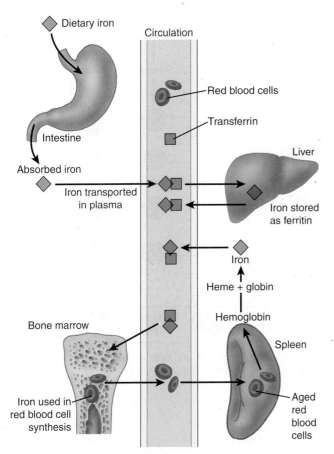

FIGURE 11-3 Diagrammatic representation of the iron cycle, including its absorption from the gastrointestinal tract, transport in the circulation, storage in the liver, recycling from aged red cells destroyed in the spleen, and use in the bone marrow synthesis of red blood cells.

measured in the laboratory, provide an index of body iron stores.

RED CELL PRODUCTION

Erythropoiesis is the production of red blood cells. After birth, red cells are produced in the red bone marrow. Until age 5 years, almost all bones produce red cells to meet growth needs. After this period, bone marrow activity gradually declines. After 20 years of age, red cell production takes place mainly in the membranous bones of the vertebrae, sternum, ribs, and pelvis. With this reduction in activity, the red bone marrow is replaced with fatty yellow bone marrow.

The red blood cells are derived from precursor cells called *erythroblasts*, which are continuously being formed from the pluripotent stem cells in the bone marrow (Fig. 11-4). The red cell precursors move through a series of divisions, each producing a smaller cell as they continue to develop into mature red blood cells. Hemoglobin synthesis begins at the early erythroblast stage and continues until the cell becomes a mature erythrocyte. During

its transformation from normoblast to reticulocyte, the red blood cell accumulates hemoglobin as the nucleus condenses and is finally lost. The period from stem cell to emergence of the reticulocyte in the circulation normally takes approximately 1 week. Maturation of reticulocyte to erythrocyte takes approximately 24 to 48 hours.[1] During this process, the red cell loses its mitochondria and ribosomes, along with its ability to produce hemoglobin and engage in oxidative metabolism. Most maturing red cells enter the blood as reticulocytes. Approximately 1% of the body's total complement of red blood cells is generated from bone marrow each day, and the reticulocyte count therefore serves as an index of the erythropoietic activity of the bone marrow.

Erythropoiesis is governed for the most part by tissue oxygen needs. Any condition that causes a decrease in the amount of oxygen that is transported in the blood produces an increase in red cell production. The oxygen content of the blood does not act directly on the bone marrow, but is sensed by the kidneys, which produce and release a hormone called *erythropoietin* into the blood, and this hormone in turn stimulates erythropoiesis in the bone marrow. In the absence of erythropoietin, as in kidney failure, hypoxia has little or no effect on red blood cell production. Human erythropoietin can be produced by recombinant deoxyribonucleic acid (DNA) technology. It is used for the management of anemia in conditions such as chronic renal failure and chemotherapy-induced anemia in persons with cancer.

RED CELL DESTRUCTION

Mature red blood cells have a life span of approximately 4 months, or 120 days. Without DNA and ribonucleic acid (RNA), red blood cells cannot synthesize the proteins needed for cellular repair, growth, or renewal of enzymes. As the red blood cell ages, its metabolic activity decreases, its enzyme activity declines, and its nonreparable membrane becomes fragile and prone to rupture as it travels through narrow spaces in the circulation and small trabecular spaces in the spleen. The rate of red cell destruction (1% per day) normally is equal to red cell production, but in conditions such as hemolytic anemia, the cell's life span may be shorter.

The destruction of red blood cells is accomplished by a group of large phagocytic cells found in the spleen, liver, bone marrow, and lymph nodes. During red blood cell destruction, amino acids from the globin chains and iron from the heme units are salvaged and reused, whereas the bulk of the heme unit is converted to bilirubin, the pigment of bile (Fig. 11-5). Bilirubin, which is insoluble in plasma, attaches to plasma proteins for transport to the liver, where it removed from the blood and conjugated with glucuronide to render it water soluble so that it can be excreted in the bile. The plasma-insoluble form of bilirubin is referred to as *unconjugated bilirubin;* the water-soluble form is referred to as *conjugated bilirubin.* Serum levels of conjugated and unconjugated bilirubin can be measured in the laboratory and are reported as direct and

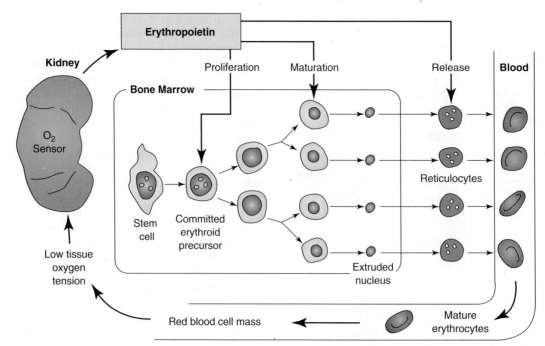

FIGURE 11-4 Red blood cell development. Committed bone marrow cells proliferate and differentiate through the erythroblast and normoblast stages to reticulocytes, which are released into the bloodstream and finally become erythrocytes.

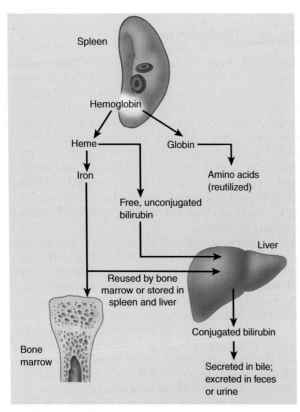

FIGURE 11-5 Destruction of red blood cells and fate of hemoglobin.

indirect, respectively. If red cell destruction and consequent bilirubin production are excessive, unconjugated bilirubin accumulates in the blood. This results in a yellow discoloration of the skin, called *jaundice.*

When red blood cell destruction takes place in the circulation, as in hemolytic anemia, the hemoglobin remains in the plasma. The plasma contains a hemoglobin-binding protein called *haptoglobin.* Other plasma proteins, such as albumin, can also bind hemoglobin. With extensive intravascular destruction of red blood cells, hemoglobin levels may exceed the hemoglobin-binding capacity of haptoglobin and other plasma proteins. When this happens, free hemoglobin appears in the blood (*i.e.,* hemoglobinemia) and is excreted in the urine (*i.e.,* hemoglobinuria). Because excessive red blood cell destruction can occur in hemolytic transfusion reactions, urine samples are tested for free hemoglobin after a transfusion reaction.

RED CELL METABOLISM

The red blood cell, which lacks mitochondria, relies on glucose and the glycolytic pathway for its metabolic needs (see Chapter 1). The enzyme-mediated anaerobic metabolism of glucose generates the adenosine triphosphate (ATP) needed for normal membrane function and ion transport. The depletion of glucose or the functional deficiency of one of the glycolytic enzymes leads to the premature death of the red blood cell. A hereditary deficiency of glucose-6-phosphate dehydrogenase (G6PD; to be discussed) predisposes to oxidative denaturation of hemoglobin, with resultant red cell injury and lysis.

LABORATORY TESTS

Red blood cells can be studied by means of a sample of blood (Table 11-1). In the laboratory, automated blood cell counters rapidly provide accurate measurements of red cell content and cell indices. The *red blood cell count* (RBC) measures the total number of red blood cells in 1 mm³ of blood. The *percentage of reticulocytes* (normally approximately 1%) provides an index of the rate of red cell production. The *hemoglobin* (grams per dL of blood) measures the hemoglobin content of the blood. The major components of blood are the red cell mass and plasma volume. The *hematocrit* measures the percentage of red cell mass in 100 mL of blood (Fig. 11-6). To determine the hematocrit, a sample of blood is placed in a glass tube, which is then centrifuged to separate the cells and the plasma. The hematocrit may be deceptive because it varies with the quantity of extracellular fluid, rising with dehydration and falling with overexpansion of extracellular fluid volume.

Red cell indices are used to differentiate types of anemias by size or color of red cells. The *mean corpuscular volume* (MCV) reflects the volume or size of the red cells. The MCV falls in microcytic (small cell) anemia and rises in macrocytic (large cell) anemia. Some anemias are normocytic (*i.e.*, cells are of normal size or MCV). The *mean corpuscular hemoglobin concentration* (MCHC) is the concentration of hemoglobin in each cell. Hemoglobin accounts for the color of red blood cells. Anemias are described as *normochromic* (normal color or MCHC) or *hypochromic* (decreased color or MCHC). *Mean cell hemoglobin* (MCH) refers to the mass of the red cell and is less useful in classifying anemias.

A stained blood smear provides information about the size, color, and shape of red cells and the presence of immature or abnormal cells. If blood smear results are abnormal, examination of the bone marrow may be important. Marrow commonly is aspirated with a special needle from the posterior iliac crest or the sternum. The aspirate is stained and observed for number and maturity of cells and abnormal types.

In summary, red blood cells with their hemoglobin provide the means for transporting oxygen from the lungs to the tissues. The biconcave shape of the red blood cell increases its surface area for diffusion, the thinness of the cell membrane allows oxygen to move readily to the interior of the cell, and the membrane structure of the red cell allows it to be deformed while moving through the smallest of capillaries. The hemoglobin molecule is composed of two pairs of α and β chains, each of which consists of a globin (protein) portion and heme unit, which surrounds an atom of iron that binds oxygen. Red cells develop from stem cells in the bone marrow and are released as reticulocytes into the blood, where they become mature erythrocytes. Red blood cell production is regulated by the hormone erythropoietin, which is produced by the kidney in response to a decrease in oxygen levels.

The life span of a red blood cell is approximately 120 days. Red cell destruction normally occurs in the spleen, liver, bone marrow, and lymph nodes. In the process of destruction, the heme portion of the hemoglobin molecule is converted to bilirubin and its iron is salvaged and reused. Bilirubin, which is insoluble in plasma, attaches to plasma proteins for transport in the blood. It is removed from the blood by the liver and conjugated to a water-soluble form so that it can be excreted in the bile.

In the laboratory, automated blood cell counters rapidly provide accurate measurements of red cell content and cell indices. A stained blood smear provides information about the size, color, and shape of red cells, and the presence of immature or abnormal cells. If blood smear results are abnormal, examination of the bone marrow may be important.

TABLE 11-1	Standard Laboratory Values for Red Blood Cells	
Test	**Normal Values**	**Significance**
Red blood cell count (RBC)		
Men	$4.2–5.4 \times 10^6/\mu L$	Number of red cells in the blood
Women	$3.6–5.0 \times 10^6/\mu L$	
Reticulocytes	1.0%–1.5% of total RBC	Rate of red cell production
Hemoglobin		
Men	14–16.5 g/dL	Hemoglobin content of the blood
Women	12–15 g/dL	
Hematocrit		
Men	40%–50%	Volume of cells in 100 mL of blood
Women	37%–47%	
Mean corpuscular volume	85–100 fL/red cell	Size of the red cell
Mean corpuscular hemoglobin concentration	31–35 g/dL	Concentration of hemoglobin in the red cell
Mean cell hemoglobin	27–34 pg/cell	Red cell mass

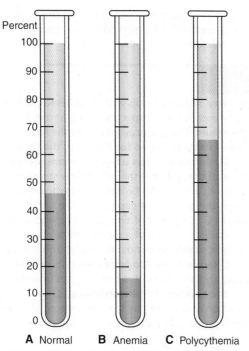

FIGURE 11-6 Hematocrit. The hematocrit measures the percentage of cells in 100 mL of blood: (**A**) normal, (**B**) decreased in anemia, and (**C**) increased in polycythemia.

Anemia

Anemia is defined as an abnormally low hemoglobin level, number of circulating red blood cells, or both, resulting in diminished oxygen-carrying capacity of the blood. Anemia usually results from excessive loss (*i.e.*, bleeding) or destruction (*i.e.*, hemolysis) of red blood cells or from deficient red blood cell production because of a lack of nutritional elements or bone marrow failure.

Anemia is not a disease, but an indication of some disease process or alteration in body function. The manifestations of anemia can be grouped into three categories: (1) those resulting from tissue hypoxia due to decreased oxygen delivery, (2) those due to compensatory mechanisms, and (3) the signs and symptoms associated with the pathologic process causing the anemia. The manifestations of anemia depend on its severity, the rapidity of its development, and the affected person's age and health status.[1]

In anemia, the oxygen-carrying capacity of hemoglobin is reduced, causing tissue hypoxia. Tissue hypoxia can give rise to fatigue, weakness, dyspnea, and sometimes angina. Brain hypoxia results in headache and faintness. The redistribution of the blood from cutaneous tissues or a lack of hemoglobin causes pallor of the skin, mucous membranes, conjunctiva, and nail beds. Tachycardia and palpitations may occur as the body tries to compensate with an increase in cardiac output. A flow-type systolic heart murmur may result from the turbulence caused by a decrease in blood viscosity. Ventricular hypertrophy and high-output heart failure may develop in persons

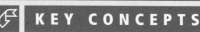

KEY CONCEPTS

Anemia

➤ Anemia, which is a deficiency of red cells or hemoglobin, results from excessive loss (blood loss anemia), increased destruction (hemolytic anemia), or impaired production of red blood cells (iron-deficiency, megaloblastic, and aplastic anemias).

➤ Blood loss anemia is characterized by loss of iron-containing red blood cells from the body; hemolytic anemia involves destruction of red blood cells in the body with iron being retained in the body.

➤ Manifestations of anemia are caused by the decreased presence of hemoglobin in the blood (pallor), tissue hypoxia due to deficient oxygen transport (weakness and fatigue), and recruitment of compensatory mechanisms (tachycardia and palpitations) designed to increase oxygen delivery to the tissues.

with severe anemia, particularly those with preexisting heart disease. Erythropoiesis is accelerated and may be recognized by diffuse bone pain and sternal tenderness. In addition to the common manifestations of anemia, hemolytic anemias are often accompanied by jaundice caused by increased blood levels of bilirubin. In aplastic anemia, petechiae and purpura (*i.e.*, red spots caused by small-vessel bleeding) are the result of reduced platelet function.

Laboratory tests are useful in determining the severity and cause of the anemia. The red cell count and hemoglobin levels provide information about the severity of the anemia, whereas red cell characteristics such as size (normocytic, microcytic, macrocytic), color (normochromic, hypochromic), and shape often provide information about the cause of anemia (Fig. 11-7).

BLOOD LOSS ANEMIA

The clinical and red cell manifestations associated with blood loss anemia depend on the rate of hemorrhage and whether the bleeding loss is internal or external. With rapid blood loss, circulatory shock and circulatory collapse may occur. With more slowly developing anemia, the amount of red cell mass lost may reach 50% without the occurrence of signs and symptoms.[1] The effects of acute blood loss are mainly due to loss of intravascular volume, which can lead to cardiovascular collapse and shock (see Chapter 19). A fall in the red blood cell count, hematocrit, and hemoglobin is caused by hemodilution resulting from movement of fluid into the vascular compartment. Initially, the red cells are normal in size and color (normocytic, normochromic). The hypoxia that results

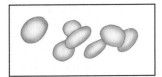
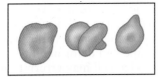

A Iron-deficiency anemia   **B** Megaloblastic anemia

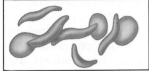
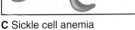
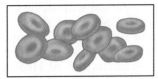

C Sickle cell anemia   **D** Normal

FIGURE 11-7 Red cell characteristics seen in different types of anemia: (**A**) microcytic and hypochromic red cells, characteristic of iron-deficiency anemia; (**B**) macrocytic and misshaped red blood cells, characteristic of megaloblastic anemia; (**C**) abnormally shaped red blood cells seen in sickle cell disease; and (**D**) normocytic and normochromic red blood cells, as a comparison.

from blood loss stimulates proliferation of committed erythroid stem cells in the bone marrow. It takes about 5 days for the progeny of stem cells to fully differentiate, an event that is marked by increased reticulocytes in the blood.[3] If the bleeding is controlled and sufficient iron stores are available, the red cell concentration returns to normal within 3 to 4 weeks. External bleeding leads to iron loss and possible iron deficiency, which can hamper restoration of red cell counts.

Chronic blood loss does not affect blood volume but instead leads to iron-deficiency anemia when iron stores are depleted. Because of compensatory mechanisms, patients are commonly asymptomatic until the hemoglobin level is less than 8 g/dL. The red cells that are produced have too little hemoglobin, giving rise to microcytic hypochromic anemia.

HEMOLYTIC ANEMIAS

Hemolytic anemia is characterized by the premature destruction of red cells, retention in the body of iron and other products of hemoglobin destruction, and an increase in erythropoiesis to compensate for the loss of red cells. Because of the red blood cell's shortened life span, the bone marrow usually is hyperactive, resulting in an increase in the number of reticulocytes in the circulating blood. As with other types of anemias, the person experiences easy fatigability, dyspnea, and other signs and symptoms of impaired oxygen transport.

As with physiologic destruction of senescent red cells, in the great majority of hemolytic anemias, the premature destruction of red cells occurs in the spleen (extravascular hemolysis). Much less commonly, red cell lysis occurs in the vascular compartment (intravascular hemolysis) and is related to acquired conditions such as mechanical injury, complement fixation, or exogenous toxic factors. Intravascular hemolysis is characterized by presence of hemoglobin in the blood (hemoglobinemia), hemoglobin in the urine (hemoglobinuria), the intracellular storage form of iron in the urine (hemosiderinuria), and jaundice. In extravascular hemolysis, premature destruction of red cells takes place in the thin-walled splenic sinusoids, a spongelike labyrinth of macrophages with long dendritic processes. It occurs whenever red cells are rendered "foreign" or become less deformable. Because extreme alterations in shape are required to navigate these sinusoids, cells with reduced deformability become sequestered and are phagocytosed by macrophages. With extravascular hemolysis, hemoglobinemia and hemoglobinuria are not observed, and the principal features are anemia and jaundice.

Hemolytic anemia can be further classified as to whether the underlying cause of the disorder is inherited or acquired. Inherited disorders include the inherited disorders of the red cell membrane, hemoglobinopathies (*e.g.*, sickle cell anemia and thalassemias), and inherited enzyme disorders. Acquired forms of hemolytic anemia are caused by agents extrinsic to the red blood cell, such as drugs, bacterial and other toxins, antibodies, and physical trauma.

Inherited Disorders of the Red Cell Membrane

Hereditary spherocytosis, transmitted as an autosomal dominant trait, is the most common inherited disorder of the red cell membrane. The disorder is a deficiency of membrane proteins (*e.g.*, spectrin) that leads to the gradual loss of the membrane surface during the life span of the red blood cell, resulting in a tight sphere instead of a concave disk. Although the spherical cell retains its ability to transport oxygen, it is poorly deformable and susceptible to destruction as it passes through the venous sinuses of the splenic circulation. Clinical signs are variable but typically include mild anemia, jaundice, splenomegaly, and bilirubin gallstones. A life-threatening aplastic crisis may occur when a sudden disruption of red cell production (in most cases from a viral infection) causes a rapid drop in hematocrit and the hemoglobin level. The disorder usually is treated with splenectomy to reduce red cell destruction.

Hemoglobinopathies

The hemoglobinopathies represent disorders of the hemoglobin molecule, most being caused by point mutations in a globin chain gene. The production of each type of globin chain is controlled by individual structural genes with five different gene loci. Mutations can occur anywhere in these five loci.

Sickle Cell Disease. Sickle cell disease is a chronic disorder resulting in anemia, and pain and organ failure due to vessel occlusion. Affected persons experience severe hemolytic anemia, chronic hyperbilirubinemia, and vaso-occlusive crises. Hemolysis produces an anemia with hematocrit values ranging from 18% to 30%.[4] The hyperbilirubinemia that results from the breakdown products of hemoglobin often leads to jaundice and the production of pigment stones in the gallbladder.

Sickle cell disease is an inherited disease that is caused by the presence of an abnormal hemoglobin S (HbS), which upon deoxygenation transforms the erythrocyte into a sickle shape (see Fig. 11-7). HbS is transmitted by recessive inheritance and can manifest as sickle cell trait (*i.e.*, heterozygote with one HbS gene) or sickle cell disease (*i.e.*, homozygote with two HbS genes). Sickle cell disease affects approximately 50,000 (0.1% to 0.2%) African Americans, and about 10% of African Americans carry the trait.[4] In parts of Africa, where malaria is endemic, the gene frequency approaches 30%, attributed to the slight protective effect it confers against *Plasmodium falciparum* malaria.[5]

The abnormal structure in HbS results from a point mutation in the β chain of the hemoglobin molecule, with an abnormal substitution of a single amino acid, valine, for glutamic acid (Fig. 11-8). In the heterozygote, only approximately 40% of the hemoglobin is HbS, but in the homozygote, 80% to 95% of the hemoglobin is HbS. Variations in proportions exist, and the concentration of HbS correlates with the risk of sickling.[5] Under conditions of deoxygenation, HbS in the homozygote with sickle cell disease aggregates and polymerizes in the cytoplasm, creating a semisolid gel that changes the shape and deformability of the cell (see Fig. 11-7). The sickled cell may return to normal shape with oxygenation in the lungs. However, after repeated episodes of deoxygenation, the cells remain permanently sickled. The person with sickle cell trait who has less HbS has little tendency to sickle except during severe hypoxia and is virtually asymptomatic. Fetal hemoglobin (HbF), with its high affinity for oxygen, inhibits the polymerization of HbS; therefore, most infants with sickle cell disease do not begin to experience the effects of the sickling until sometime after 4 to 6 months of age, when the HbF has been replaced by HbS.

There are two major consequences of red blood cell sickling: hemolysis of the sickled cells and vessel occlusion (see Fig. 11-8). The increased rigidity of the sickled cells results in obstruction of the microcirculation and ischemic injury to many tissues. The inflexibility of the sickled cells also makes them more susceptible to destruction (hemolysis) during circulation through the spleen. The sickled cells also demonstrate membrane changes, leading to increased adhesiveness and adherence, producing further complications of capillary blood flow.[2]

Blood vessel occlusion causes most of the severe complications of sickle cell disease. An acute pain episode results from vessel occlusion and can occur suddenly in almost any part of the body.[6] Common sites obstructed by sickled cells include the abdomen, chest, bones, and joints. Many areas may be affected simultaneously. Infarctions caused by sluggish blood flow may cause chronic damage to the liver, spleen, heart, kidneys, retina, and other organs. *Acute chest syndrome* is an atypical pneumonia resulting from pulmonary infarction. It is the second leading cause of hospitalization in persons with sickle cell disease and is characterized by pulmonary infiltrates, shortness of breath, fever, chest pain, and cough.[6,7] The syndrome can cause chronic respiratory insufficiency and is a leading cause of death in sickle cell disease. Children may experience growth retardation and susceptibility to osteomyelitis. Painful bone crises may be caused by marrow infarcts of the bones of the hands and feet, resulting in swelling of those extremities. Twenty-five percent of persons with sickle cell disease have neurological complications related to vessel occlusion.[7] Stroke occurs in children 1 to 15 years of age and may recur in two thirds of those afflicted. Transient ischemic attack or cerebral hemorrhage may precede the stroke.

The spleen is especially susceptible to damage by HbS. Because of the spleen's sluggish blood flow and low oxygen tension, hemoglobin is deoxygenated and causes ischemia. Splenic injury begins as early as 3 to 6 months of age with intense congestion and is usually asymptomatic.[8] The congestion causes functional asplenia and predisposes the person to life-threatening infections by encapsulated organisms such as *Streptococcus pneumoniae*, *Haemophilus influenzae* type b, and *Klebsiella* species. Neonates and small children have not had time to create antibodies to these organisms and rely on the

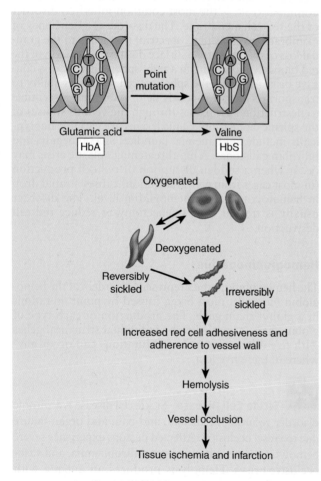

FIGURE 11-8 Mechanism of sickling and its consequences in sickle cell disease.

spleen for their removal. In the absence of specific antibodies to the polysaccharide capsular antigens of these organisms, splenic activity is essential for removing these organisms when they enter the blood.

The factors associated with sickling and vessel occlusion include cold, stress, physical exertion, infection, and illnesses that cause hypoxia, dehydration, or acidosis. The rate of HbS polymerization is affected by the concentration of hemoglobin in the cell. Dehydration increases the hemoglobin concentration and contributes to the polymerization and resulting sickling. Acidosis reduces the affinity of hemoglobin for oxygen, resulting in more deoxygenated hemoglobin and increased sickling. Even such trivial incidents as reduced oxygen tension induced by sleep may contribute to the sickling process.

The signs and symptoms of sickle cell disease make their appearance during infancy. Neonatal diagnosis of sickle cell disease is made on the basis of clinical findings and hemoglobin solubility results, which are confirmed by hemoglobin electrophoresis. Prenatal diagnosis is done by the analysis of fetal DNA obtained by amniocentesis.[4]

In the United States, screening programs have been implemented to detect newborns with sickle cell disease and other hemoglobinopathies. Cord blood or heel stick samples are subjected to electrophoresis to separate the HbF from the small amounts of HbA and HbS. Other hemoglobins may be detected and quantified by further laboratory evaluation. Many states mandate neonatal screening of all newborns, regardless of ethnic origin. Ideally, the effective screening program also includes expert genetic counseling and education about pregnancy options.

There is no known cure for sickle cell anemia, so treatment to reduce symptoms includes pain control, hydration, and management of complications. The person is advised to avoid situations that precipitate sickling episodes, such as infections, cold exposure, severe physical exertion, acidosis, and dehydration. Infections are aggressively treated, and blood transfusions may be warranted in a crisis or given chronically in severe disease. Most children with sickle cell disease are at risk for fulminant septicemia and death during the first 3 years of life, when bacteremia from encapsulated organisms occurs commonly even in normal children. Prophylactic penicillin should be begun as early as 2 months of age and continued until at least 5 years of age.[9] Maintaining full immunization, including *H. influenzae* vaccine and hepatitis B vaccine, is recommended. The National Institutes of Health Committee on Management of Sickle Cell Disease also recommends administration of the 7-valent pneumococcal vaccine beginning at 2 to 6 months of age.[9] The 7-valent vaccine should be followed by immunization with the 23-valent pneumococcal vaccine at 24 months of age or later.

Hydroxyurea is a cytotoxic drug used to prevent complications of sickle cell disease. The drug allows synthesis of more HbF and less HbS, thereby decreasing sickling. Long-term effects on organ damage, growth and development, and risk of malignancies are unknown.[6] Bone marrow or stem cell transplantation has the potential for cure in symptomatic children but carries the risk of graft-versus-host disease.

Thalassemias. The thalassemias are a group of inherited disorders of hemoglobin synthesis due to absent or defective synthesis of the α or β chains of adult hemoglobin. The defect is inherited as a mendelian trait, and a person may be heterozygous for the trait and have a mild form of the disease or be homozygous and have the severe form of the disease. Like sickle cell disease, the thalassemias occur with a high degree of frequency in certain populations. The β-thalassemias, sometimes called *Cooley anemia* or *Mediterranean anemia,* are most common in the Mediterranean populations of southern Italy and Greece, and the α-thalassemias are most common among Asians. Both α- and β-thalassemias are common in Africans and African Americans.

Two factors contribute to the anemia that occurs in thalassemia: (1) the direct effect of gene mutation on production of α or β chains of the hemoglobin molecule, and (2) the indirect effect resulting from the continued production of the unaffected chain. Defective production of α or β chains leads to deficient hemoglobin production and the development of a hypochromic microcytic anemia. Although there is impaired production of the affected chain, the unaffected type of chain continues to be synthesized and accumulates in the red cell, interfering with normal maturation, and generating oxygen free radicals that contribute to red cell hemolysis and anemia.

The β-*thalassemias* result from one of nearly 200 point mutations in the β-globin gene, causing a defect in β-chain synthesis.[10] In β-thalassemia, the excess α chains are denatured to form precipitates (*i.e.,* Heinz bodies) in the bone marrow red cell precursors. These Heinz bodies impair DNA synthesis and cause damage to the red cell membrane. Severely affected red cell precursors are destroyed in the bone marrow, and those that escape intramedullary death are at increased risk of destruction in the spleen. In addition to the anemia, persons with moderate to severe forms of the disease suffer from coagulation abnormalities. Thrombotic events (stroke and pulmonary embolism) appear to be related to altered platelet function, endothelial activation, and an imbalance of procoagulants and anticoagulants.[10]

The clinical manifestations of β-thalassemias are based on the severity of the anemia. The presence of one normal gene in heterozygous persons (thalassemia minor) usually results in sufficient normal hemoglobin synthesis to prevent severe anemia. Persons who are homozygous for the trait (thalassemia major) have severe, transfusion-dependent anemia that is evident at 6 to 9 months of age. If transfusion therapy is not started early in life, severe growth retardation occurs in children with the disorder. Increased hematopoiesis, in response to erythropoietin, causes bone marrow expansion, impairs bone growth, and causes bone abnormalities. Bone marrow expansion leads to thinning of the cortical bone, with new bone formation evident on the maxilla and frontal bones of the face (*i.e.,* chipmunk facies). The long bones, ribs, and vertebrae may become vulnerable to fracture. Splenomegaly and hepatomegaly result from increased red cell destruction. Iron overload is a major complication of β-thalassemia. Excess iron stores, which accumulate from increased dietary absorption and repeated transfusions, are deposited in the myocardium, liver, and endocrine organs and induce organ damage. Cardiac and hepatic disease are common causes of death from iron overload. Disorders of the pituitary, thyroid, and adrenal glands and the pancreas result in significant morbidity.[11]

Frequent transfusions (every 3 to 4 weeks) prevent most of the complications, and iron chelation therapy can reduce the iron overload and extend life expectancy.[11] Bone marrow transplantation is a potential cure for some patients, particularly in younger persons with no complications of the disease or its treatment.[11] In the future, stem cell gene replacement may provide a cure for many with the disease.

The α-*thalassemias* are caused by a gene deletion that results in defective α-chain synthesis. Synthesis of the α-globin chains of hemoglobin is controlled by two pairs of genes; hence, α-thalassemia shows great variations in severity. Silent carriers who have a deletion of a single α-globin gene are asymptomatic, and those with deletion of two genes have mild hemolytic anemia. Deletion of three of the four α-chain genes lead to unstable aggregates of α chains called *hemoglobin H* (HbH). This disorder is the most important clinical form and is common in Asians. The β chains are more soluble than the α chains, and their accumulation is less toxic to the red cells, so that senescent rather than precursor red cells are affected. Most persons with HbH have chronic moderate hemolytic anemia and may require transfusions during febrile illnesses or with certain medications.[11] The most severe form of α-thalassemia occurs in infants in whom all four α-globin genes are deleted. Such a defect results in a hemoglobin molecule (Hb Bart's) that is formed exclusively from the chains of HbF. Hb Bart's, which has an extremely high oxygen affinity, cannot release oxygen in the tissues. This disorder usually results in death in utero or shortly after birth.[10]

Inherited Enzyme Defects

The most common inherited enzyme defect that results in hemolytic anemia is a deficiency of G6PD. The gene that determines this enzyme is located on the X chromosome, and the defect is expressed only in males and homozygous females. There are more than 350 genetic variants of this disorder found in all populations. The African variant has been found in 10% of African Americans.[2] The disorder makes red cells more vulnerable to oxidants and causes direct oxidation of hemoglobin to methemoglobin and the denaturing of the hemoglobin molecule to form Heinz bodies, which are precipitated in the red blood cell. Hemolysis usually occurs as the damaged red blood cells move through the narrow vessels of the spleen, causing hemoglobinemia, hemoglobinuria, and jaundice. The hemolysis is short-lived, occurring 2 to 3 days after the trigger event. In persons of African descent, the defect is mildly expressed and is not associated with chronic hemolytic anemia unless triggered by oxidant drugs, acidosis, or infection.

The antimalarial drug primaquine, the sulfonamides, nitrofurantoin, aspirin, phenacetin, some chemotherapeutic agents, and other drugs cause hemolysis. Free radicals generated by phagocytes during infections also are possible triggers. A more severe deficiency of G6PD is found in people of Mediterranean descent (*e.g.*, Sardinians, Sephardic Jews, Arabs). In some of these persons, chronic hemolysis occurs in the absence of exposure to oxidants. The disorder can be diagnosed through the use of a G6PD assay or screening test.

Acquired Hemolytic Anemias

Several acquired factors exogenous to the red blood cell produce hemolysis by direct membrane destruction or by antibody-mediated lysis. Various drugs, chemicals, toxins, venoms, and infections such as malaria destroy red cell membranes. Hemolysis can also be caused by mechanical factors such as prosthetic heart valves, vasculitis, and severe burns. Obstructions in the microcirculation, as in disseminated intravascular coagulation, thrombotic thrombocytopenic purpura, and renal disease, may traumatize the red cells by producing turbulence and changing pressure gradients.

Many hemolytic anemias are immune mediated, caused by antibodies that damage or destroy the red cell membrane. Antibodies may be produced by a person in response to drugs and disease (autoantibodies) or may come from an exogenous source (alloantibodies), such as those that are responsible for transfusion reactions and hemolytic disease of the newborn.

The autoantibodies that cause red cell destruction are of two types: warm-reacting antibodies of the immunoglobulin G (IgG) and sometimes IgA types, which are maximally active at 37°C, and cold-reacting antibodies of the IgM type, which are optimally active at or near 4°C.[2]

The warm-reacting antibodies react with antigens on the red cell membrane, causing destructive changes that lead to spherocytosis, with subsequent phagocytic destruction in the spleen or liver. They lack specificity for the ABO antigens but may react with the Rh antigens. The reactions are typically of rapid onset that may be life threatening in severity. Patients complain of fatigue and may present with angina or heart failure. On physical examination, jaundice and splenomegaly are usually present. There are varied causes. In approximately half the cases, the cause is idiopathic or unknown, and the other half are related to cancers of the lymphoproliferative system (*e.g.*, chronic lymphocytic leukemia, lymphoma), collagen diseases (*e.g.*, systemic lupus erythematosus), viral infections, and inflammatory disorders (*e.g.*, ulcerative colitis).[2] The antihypertensive drug α-methyldopa and the antiarrhythmic drug quinidine account for a small number of cases.[2] The drug-induced hemolysis is commonly benign.

The cold-reacting antibodies activate complement. Chronic hemolytic anemia caused by cold-reacting antibodies occurs with lymphoproliferative disorders and as an idiopathic disorder of unknown cause. The hemolytic process occurs in distal body parts, where the temperature may fall below 30°C. Vascular obstruction by red cells results in pallor, cyanosis of the body parts exposed to cold temperatures, and Raynaud phenomenon (see Chapter 17). Hemolytic anemia caused by cold-reacting antibodies develops in only a few persons and is rarely severe.

Coombs' test, or the antiglobulin test, is used to diagnose immune hemolytic anemias. It detects the presence of antibody or complement on the surface of the red cell. The direct antiglobulin test detects the antibody on red blood cells and is positive in cases of autoimmune hemolytic anemia, erythroblastosis fetalis (*i.e.*, Rh disease of the newborn), transfusion reactions, and drug-induced hemolysis. The indirect antiglobulin test detects antibody in the serum, and the result is positive for specific antibodies. It is used for antibody detection and cross-matching before transfusion.

ANEMIAS OF DEFICIENT RED CELL PRODUCTION

Anemia may result from the decreased production of erythrocytes by the bone marrow. A deficiency of nutrients for hemoglobin synthesis (iron) or DNA synthesis (cobalamin or folic acid) may reduce red cell production by the bone marrow. A deficiency of red cells also results when the marrow itself fails or is replaced by nonfunctional tissue.

Iron-Deficiency Anemia

Iron deficiency is a common worldwide cause of anemia affecting persons of all ages. The anemia results from dietary deficiency, loss of iron through bleeding, or increased demand. Because iron is a component of heme, a deficiency leads to decreased hemoglobin synthesis and consequent impairment of oxygen delivery.

Body iron is used repeatedly. When red cells become senescent and are broken down, their iron is released and reused in the production of new red cells. Despite this efficiency, small amounts of iron are lost in the feces and need to be replaced by dietary uptake. Iron balance is maintained by the absorption of 0.5 to 1.5 mg daily to replace the 1 mg lost in the feces. The average Western diet supplies this amount. The absorbed iron is more than sufficient to supply the needs of most individuals, but may be barely adequate in toddlers, adolescents, and women of childbearing age.

The usual reason for iron deficiency in adults is chronic blood loss because iron cannot be recycled to the pool. In men and postmenopausal women, blood loss may occur from gastrointestinal bleeding because of peptic ulcer, intestinal polyps, hemorrhoids, or cancer. Excessive aspirin intake may cause undetected gastrointestinal bleeding. In women, menstruation may account for an average of 1.5 mg of iron lost per day, causing a deficiency.[12] Although cessation of menstruation removes a major source of iron loss in the pregnant woman, iron requirements increase at this time, and deficiency is common. The expansion of the mother's blood volume requires

approximately 500 mg of additional iron, and the growing fetus requires approximately 360 mg during pregnancy. In the postnatal period, lactation requires approximately 1 mg of iron daily.[12]

A child's growth places extra demands on the body. Blood volume increases, with a greater need for iron. Iron requirements are proportionally higher in infancy (3 to 24 months) than at any other age, although they are also increased in childhood and adolescence. In infancy, the two main causes of iron-deficiency anemia are low iron levels at birth because of maternal deficiency and a diet consisting mainly of cow's milk, which is low in absorbable iron. Adolescents are also susceptible to iron deficiency because of high requirements due to growth spurts, dietary deficiencies, and menstrual loss.[13]

Iron-deficiency anemia is characterized by low hemoglobin and hematocrit levels, decreased iron stores, and low serum iron and ferritin levels. The red cells are decreased in number and are microcytic and hypochromic. Poikilocytosis (irregular shape) and anisocytosis (irregular size) are also present (see Fig. 11-7). The laboratory values indicate reduced MCHC and MCV. Membrane changes may predispose to hemolysis, causing further loss of red cells.

The manifestations of iron-deficiency anemia are related to impaired oxygen transport and lack of hemoglobin. Depending on the severity of the anemia, fatigability, palpitations, dyspnea, angina, and tachycardia may occur. Epithelial atrophy is common and results in waxy pallor, brittle hair and nails, smooth tongue, sores in the corners of the mouth, and sometimes in dysphagia and decreased acid secretion. A poorly understood symptom that sometimes is seen is pica, the bizarre compulsive eating of ice, dirt, or other abnormal substances. Iron deficiency in children may also result in neurologic manifestations such as developmental delay, stroke, and cranial nerve palsies.[14]

Prevention of iron deficiency is a primary concern in infants and children. Iron supplementation is recommended at 4 to 6 months of age in breast-fed infants, and use of iron-fortified formulas (rather than cow's milk) and cereals is recommended for infants younger than 1 year of age.[15] In the second year, a diet rich in iron-containing foods and use of iron-fortified vitamins will help prevent iron deficiency. The treatment of iron-deficiency anemia is directed toward controlling chronic blood loss, increasing dietary intake of iron, and administering supplemental iron. Ferrous sulfate, which is the usual oral replacement therapy, replenishes iron stores in several months. Parenteral iron (iron dextran) therapy may be used when oral forms are not tolerated or are ineffective. Caution is required because of the possibility of severe hypersensitivity reactions.

Megaloblastic Anemias

Megaloblastic anemias are caused by abnormal nucleic acid synthesis that results in enlarged red cells (MCV >100 fL) and deficient nuclear maturation. Cobalamin (vitamin B_{12}) and folic acid deficiencies are the most common megaloblastic anemias. Because megaloblastic anemias develop slowly, there are often few symptoms until the anemia is far advanced.

Cobalamin (Vitamin B₁₂)–Deficiency Anemia.

Vitamin B₁₂ serves as a cofactor for two important reactions in humans. It is essential for the synthesis of DNA. When it is deficient, nuclear maturation and cell division, especially of the rapidly proliferating red cells, fail to occur. It is also involved in a reaction that prevents abnormal fatty acids from being incorporated into neuronal lipids. This abnormality may predispose to myelin breakdown and produce some of the neurologic complications of vitamin B₁₂ deficiency.

Vitamin B₁₂ is found in all foods of animal origin. Dietary deficiency is rare and usually found only in strict vegetarians who avoid all dairy products as well as meat and fish. It is absorbed by a unique process. After release from the animal protein, vitamin B₁₂ is bound to intrinsic factor, a protein secreted by the gastric parietal cells (Fig. 11-9). The vitamin B₁₂–intrinsic factor complex travels to the ileum, where membrane receptors allow the binding of the complex to the epithelial cells. Vitamin B₁₂ is then separated from intrinsic factor and transported across the membrane into the circulation. There it is bound to its carrier protein, transcobalamin II, which transports vitamin B₁₂ to its storage and tissue sites. Any defects in this pathway may cause a vitamin B₁₂ deficiency. An important cause of vitamin B₁₂ deficiency is pernicious anemia, resulting from a hereditary atrophic gastritis. As discussed in Chapter 28, immune-mediated chronic atrophic gastritis is a disorder that destroys the gastric mucosa, with loss of parietal cells and production of antibodies that interfere with the binding of vitamin B₁₂ to the intrinsic factor. Other causes of vitamin B₁₂ deficiency anemia include gastrectomy, ileal resection, inflammation or neoplasms in the terminal ileum, and malabsorption syndromes in which vitamin B₁₂ and other B-vitamin compounds are poorly absorbed.

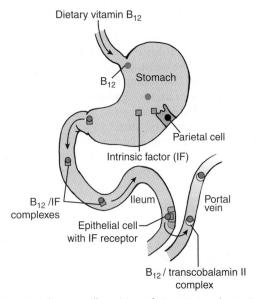

Dietary vitamin B₁₂

B₁₂

Stomach

Parietal cell

Intrinsic factor (IF)

B₁₂ /IF complexes

Ileum

Portal vein

Epithelial cell with IF receptor

B₁₂ / transcobalamin II complex

FIGURE 11-9 Schematic illustration of vitamin B₁₂ absorption.

The hallmark of vitamin B₁₂ deficiency is megaloblastic anemia. When vitamin B₁₂ is deficient, the red cells that are produced are abnormally large because of excess RNA production of hemoglobin and structural protein (see Fig. 11-7). The cells have immature nuclei and show evidence of cellular destruction. They have flimsy membranes and are oval rather than biconcave. These oddly shaped cells have a short life span that can be measured in weeks rather than months. The MCV is elevated, and the MCHC is normal.

Neurologic changes that accompany the disorder are caused by deranged methylation of myelin protein. Demyelination of the dorsal and lateral columns of the spinal cord causes symmetric paresthesias of the feet and fingers, loss of vibratory and position sense, and eventual spastic ataxia. In more advanced cases, cerebral function may be altered. In some cases, dementia and other neuropsychiatric changes may precede hematologic changes.

Vitamin B₁₂ deficiency is diagnosed by finding an abnormally low vitamin B₁₂ serum level. The Schilling test, which measures the 24-hour urinary excretion of radiolabeled vitamin B₁₂ administered orally, has been commonly used in the past to document decreased absorption of vitamin B₁₂. Currently, the diagnosis of pernicious anemia is usually made by the detection of parietal cell and intrinsic factor antibodies.[16] Lifelong treatment consisting of intramuscular injections of vitamin B₁₂ reverses the anemia and improves the neurologic changes.

Folic Acid–Deficiency Anemia.

Folic acid (folate) is also required for DNA synthesis and red cell maturation, and its deficiency produces the same type of megaloblastic red cell changes that occur in vitamin B₁₂–deficiency anemia (i.e., increased MCV and normal MCHC). Symptoms are also similar, but the neurologic manifestations are not present.

Folic acid is readily absorbed from the intestine. It is found in vegetables (particularly the green leafy types), fruits, cereals, and meats. Much of the vitamin, however, is lost in cooking. The most common causes of folic acid deficiency are malnutrition or dietary lack, especially in the elderly or in association with alcoholism. Total body stores of folic acid amount to 2000 to 5000 micrograms (μg), and 50 μg is required in the daily diet.[3] A dietary deficiency may result in anemia in a few months. Malabsorption of folic acid may be due to syndromes such as sprue or other intestinal disorders. Some drugs used to treat seizure disorders (e.g., primidone, phenytoin, phenobarbital) and triamterene, a diuretic, predispose to a deficiency by interfering with folic acid absorption. In neoplastic disease, tumor cells compete for folate, and deficiency is common. Methotrexate, a folic acid analog used in the treatment of cancer, impairs the action of folic acid by blocking its conversion to the active form.

Because pregnancy increases the need for folic acid 5- to 10-fold, a deficiency commonly occurs. Poor dietary habits, anorexia, and nausea are other reasons for folic acid deficiency during pregnancy. Studies also show an association between folate deficiency and neural tube defects.[17] The U.S. Public Health Service recommends that all women of childbearing age should take 400 µg of folic acid daily. It is estimated that 50% of neural tube defects could thus be prevented.[18] To ensure adequate folate consumption, the U.S. Food and Drug Administration mandated the addition of folate to cereal grain products effective January 1, 1998.

Aplastic Anemia

Aplastic anemia (*i.e.*, bone marrow depression) describes a primary condition of bone marrow stem cells that results in a reduction of all three hematopoietic cell lines—red blood cells, white blood cells, and platelets—with fatty replacement of bone marrow. Pure red cell aplasia, in which only the red cells are affected, rarely occurs.

Anemia results from the failure of the marrow to replace senescent red cells that are destroyed and leave the circulation, although the cells that remain are of normal size and color. At the same time, because the leukocytes, particularly the neutrophils, and the thrombocytes have a short life span, a deficiency of these cells usually is apparent before the anemia becomes severe.

The onset of aplastic anemia may be insidious, or it may strike with suddenness and great severity. It can occur at any age. The initial presenting symptoms include weakness, fatigability, and pallor caused by anemia. Petechiae (*i.e.*, small, punctate skin hemorrhages) and ecchymoses (*i.e.*, bruises) often occur on the skin, and bleeding from the nose, gums, vagina, or gastrointestinal tract may occur because of decreased platelet levels. The decrease in the number of neutrophils increases susceptibility to infection.

The causes of aplastic anemia include exposure to high doses of radiation, chemicals, and toxins that suppress hematopoiesis directly or through immune mechanisms. Chemotherapy and irradiation commonly result in bone marrow depression, which causes anemia, thrombocytopenia, and neutropenia. Identified toxic agents include benzene, the antibiotic chloramphenicol, and the alkylating agents and antimetabolites used in the treatment of cancer (see Chapter 5). Aplastic anemia caused by exposure to chemical agents may be an idiosyncratic reaction because it affects only certain susceptible persons. It typically occurs weeks after a drug is initiated. Such reactions often are severe and sometimes irreversible and fatal. Aplastic anemia can also develop in the course of many infections and has been reported most often as a complication of viral hepatitis, mononucleosis, and other viral illnesses, including acquired immunodeficiency syndrome (AIDS). In two thirds of cases, the cause is unknown, and these are called *idiopathic aplastic anemia*.

For young and severely affected individuals, the treatment of aplastic anemia can include the use of stem cell replacement by bone marrow or peripheral blood transplantation. Histocompatible donors supply the stem cells to replace the patient's destroyed marrow cells. Graft-versus-host disease, rejection, and infections are major risks of the procedure, yet 70% or more survive.[19] For those who are not transplantation candidates, immunosuppressive therapy with lymphocyte immune globulin (*i.e.*, antithymocyte globulin) prevents suppression of proliferating stem cells, producing remission in up to 50% of patients.[19] Patients with aplastic anemia should avoid the offending agents and be treated with antibiotics for infection. Red cell transfusions to correct the anemia and platelets and corticosteroid therapy to minimize bleeding may also be required.

Chronic Disease Anemias

Anemia often occurs as a complication of chronic infections, inflammation, and cancer. Chronic diseases commonly associated with anemia include tuberculosis, AIDS, osteomyelitis, rheumatoid arthritis, systemic lupus erythematosus, and Hodgkin disease. It is thought that the short life span, deficient red cell production in response to erythropoietin, and low serum iron are caused by actions of macrophages and lymphocytes in response to cell injury. Macrophages sequester iron in the spleen and contribute to red cell destruction. The lymphocytes release cytokines (*e.g.*, interleukin-1 and interferon) that suppress the erythropoietin response, inhibit erythroid precursors, and reduce iron transport.[20] The moderate to severe anemia is similar to iron-deficiency anemia with microcytic, hypochromic red cells. The anemia may be reversed when the underlying disease is treated, or with erythropoietin therapy.[20]

Chronic renal failure almost always results in a normocytic, normochromic anemia, primarily because of a deficiency of erythropoietin. Unidentified uremic toxins and retained nitrogen also interfere with the actions of erythropoietin, and red cell production and survival. Hemolysis and blood loss associated with hemodialysis and bleeding tendencies also contribute to the anemia of renal failure. In persons whose hematocrits are 30% to 35%, recombinant erythropoietin injected several times a week eliminates the need for transfusions.[20] Oral iron is sometimes required for a good response.

In summary, anemia is a condition of an abnormally low number of circulating red blood cells or low hemoglobin level, or both. It is not a disease, but manifestation of a disease process or alteration in body function. Anemia can result from excessive blood loss, red cell destruction due to hemolysis, or deficient hemoglobin or red cell production. Blood loss anemia can be acute or chronic. With bleeding, iron and other components of the erythrocyte are lost from the body. Hemolytic anemia is characterized by the premature destruction of red cells, with retention in the body of iron and the other products of red cell destruction. Hemolytic anemia can be caused by defects in the red cell membrane, hemoglobinopathies (sickle cell anemia or thalassemia), or inherited enzyme defects (G6PD deficiency). Acquired forms of hemolytic anemia are caused by agents extrinsic to the red blood cell, such as drugs, bacterial and other toxins, antibodies, and physical trauma. Iron-deficiency anemia, which is characterized by decreased hemoglobin synthesis, can result from dietary deficiency, loss of iron through bleeding, or increased demands for red cell production. Vitamin B_{12} and folic acid deficiencies impair red cell production by interfering with DNA synthesis. Aplastic anemia is caused by bone marrow suppression and usually results in a reduction of white blood cells and platelets, as well as red blood cells.

The manifestations of anemia are those associated with impaired oxygen transport; alterations in red blood cell number, hemoglobin content, and cell structure; and the signs and symptoms of the underlying process causing the anemia.

Polycythemia

Polycythemia is an abnormally high total red blood cell mass with a hematocrit greater than 50%. It is categorized as relative or absolute. In relative polycythemia, the hematocrit rises because of a loss of plasma volume without a corresponding decrease in red cells. This may occur with water deprivation, excess use of diuretics, or gastrointestinal losses. Relative polycythemia is corrected by increasing the vascular fluid volume.

Absolute polycythemia is a rise in hematocrit due to an increase in total red cell mass and is classified as primary or secondary. Primary polycythemia, or polycythemia vera, is a proliferative disease of the pluripotent cells of the bone marrow characterized by an absolute increase in total red blood cell mass accompanied by elevated white cell and platelet counts. It most commonly is seen in men between the ages of 40 and 60 years. In polycythemia vera, the manifestations are related to an increase in the red cell count, hemoglobin level, and hematocrit with increased blood volume and viscosity. Viscosity rises exponentially with the hematocrit and interferes with cardiac output and blood flow. Hypertension is common and there may be complaints of headache, inability to concentrate, and some difficulty with hearing and vision because of decreased cerebral blood flow. Venous stasis gives rise to a plethoric appearance or dusky redness—even cyanosis—particularly of the lips, fingernails, and mucous membranes. Because of the increased concentration of blood cells, the person may experience itching and pain in the fingers or toes, and the hypermetabolism may induce night sweats and weight loss. Thromboembolism occurs in 15% to 60% of persons with polycythemia vera and contributes to death in 10% to 40% of the cases.[21] Hemorrhage, due to platelet abnormalities, occurs in 15% to 35% of cases and is also an important cause of death. The goal of treatment in primary polycythemia is to reduce blood viscosity. This can be done by withdrawing blood by means of periodic phlebotomy to reduce red cell volume. Control of platelet and white cell counts is accomplished by suppressing bone marrow function with chemotherapy.

Secondary polycythemia results from a physiologic increase in the level of erythropoietin, commonly as a compensatory response to hypoxia. Conditions causing hypoxia include living at high altitudes, chronic heart and lung disease, and smoking. The resultant release of erythropoietin by the kidney causes the increased formation of red blood cells in the bone marrow. Neoplasms that secrete erythropoietin may also cause a secondary polycythemia. Treatment of secondary polycythemia focuses on relieving hypoxia. For example, continuous low-flow oxygen therapy can be used to correct the severe hypoxia that occurs in some persons with chronic obstructive lung disease.

In summary, polycythemia describes a condition in which the red blood cell mass is increased. It can present as a relative, primary, or secondary disorder. Relative polycythemia results from a loss of vascular fluid and is corrected by replacing the fluid. Primary polycythemia, or polycythemia vera, is a proliferative disease of the bone marrow with an absolute increase in total red blood cell mass accompanied by elevated white cell and platelet counts. Secondary polycythemia results from increased erythropoietin levels caused by hypoxic conditions such as chronic heart and lung disease. Many of the manifestations of polycythemia are related to increased blood volume and viscosity that lead to hypertension and stagnation of blood flow.

Age-Related Changes in Red Blood Cells

RED CELL CHANGES IN THE NEONATE

At birth, changes in the red blood cell indices reflect the transition to extrauterine life and the need to transport oxygen from the lungs (Table 11-2). Hemoglobin concentrations at birth are high, reflecting the high synthetic activity in utero to provide adequate oxygen delivery. Toward the end of the first postnatal week, hemoglobin concentration begins to decline, gradually falling to a minimum value at approximately 2 months of age.[22] The red cell count, hematocrit, and MCV likewise fall. The factors responsible for the decline include reduced red cell production and plasma dilution caused by increased blood volume with growth. Neonatal red cells also have a shorter life span of 50 to 70 days and are thought to be more fragile than those of older persons. During the early neonatal period, there is also a switch from HbF to HbA. The amount of HbF in term infants averages about 70% of the total hemoglobin and declines to trace amounts by 6 to 12 months of age.[22] The switch to HbA provides greater unloading of oxygen to the tissues because HbA has a lower affinity for oxygen compared with HbF. Infants who are small for gestational age, born to diabetic or smoking mothers, or who experienced hypoxia in utero

TABLE 11-2	Red Cell Values for Term Infants			
Age	RBC × 10⁶/μL Mean ± SD	Hb (g/dL) Mean ± SD	Hct (%) Mean ± SD	MCV (fL) Mean ± SD
Days				
1	5.14 ± 0.7	19.3 ± 2.2	61 ± 7.4	119 ± 9.4
4	5.00 ± 0.6	18.6 ± 2.1	57 ± 8.1	114 ± 7.5
7	4.86 ± 0.6	17.9 ± 2.5	56 ± 9.4	118 ± 11.2
Weeks				
1–2	4.80 ± 0.8	17.3 ± 2.3	54 ± 8.3	112 ± 19.0
3–4	4.00 ± 0.6	14.2 ± 2.1	43 ± 5.7	105 ± 7.5
8–9	3.40 ± 0.5	10.7 ± 0.9	31 ± 2.5	93 ± 12.0
11–12	3.70 ± 0.3	11.3 ± 0.9	33 ± 3.3	88 ± 7.9

Hb, hemoglobin; Hct, hematocrit; MCV, mean corpuscular volume.
(Adapted from Matoth Y., Zaizor R., Varsano I. [1971]. Postnatal changes in some red cell parameters. *Acta Paediatrica Scandinavica 60*, 317.)

have higher total hemoglobin levels, higher HbF levels, and a delayed switch to HbA.

A physiologic anemia of the newborn develops at approximately 2 months of age. It seldom produces symptoms and cannot be altered by nutritional supplements. Anemia of prematurity, an exaggerated physiologic response in low–birth-weight infants, is thought to result from a poor erythropoietin response. A contributing factor is the frequent blood sampling that is often necessary to stabilize these infants.[22] The hemoglobin level rapidly declines after birth to a low of 7 to 10 g/dL at approximately 6 weeks of age. Signs and symptoms include apnea, poor weight gain, pallor, decreased activity, and tachycardia. In infants born before 33 weeks' gestation or those with hematocrits below 33%, the clinical features are more evident.

Anemia at birth, characterized by pallor, congestive heart failure, or shock, usually is caused by hemolytic disease of the newborn. Bleeding from the umbilical cord, internal hemorrhage, congenital hemolytic disease, or frequent blood sampling are other possible causes of anemia. The severity of symptoms and presence of coexisting disease may warrant red cell transfusion.

Hyperbilirubinemia in the Neonate

Hyperbilirubinemia, an increased level of serum bilirubin, is a common cause of jaundice in the neonate. A benign, self-limited condition, it most often is related to the developmental state of the neonate. Rarely, cases of hyperbilirubinemia are pathologic and may lead to kernicterus and serious brain damage.

In the first week of life, approximately 60% of term and 80% of preterm neonates are jaundiced.[23] This physiologic jaundice appears in term infants on the second or third day of life. Ordinarily, the indirect bilirubin in umbilical cord blood is 1 to 3 mg/dL and rises at a rate of less than 5 mg/dL in 24 hours, peaking at 5 to 6 mg/dL between the second and fourth days and decreasing to less than 2 mg/dL between the fifth and seventh days of life.[23] The increase in bilirubin is related to the increased

red cell breakdown and the inability of the immature liver to conjugate bilirubin. Premature infants exhibit a slower rise and longer duration in serum bilirubin levels, perhaps because of poor hepatic uptake and reduced albumin binding of bilirubin. Most neonatal jaundice resolves within 1 week and is untreated.

Many factors can contribute to elevated bilirubin levels in the neonate, including breast-feeding, hemolytic disease of the newborn, hypoxia, infections, and acidosis. Bowel or biliary obstruction and liver disease are less common causes. Associated risk factors include prematurity, Asian ancestry, and maternal diabetes. Breast milk jaundice occurs in approximately 2% of breast-fed infants.[23] These neonates accumulate significant levels of unconjugated bilirubin 7 days after birth and reach maximum levels of 10 to 30 mg/dL in the third week of life. It is thought that the breast milk contains fatty acids that inhibit bilirubin conjugation in the neonatal liver. A factor in breast milk is also thought to increase the absorption of bilirubin in the duodenum. This type of jaundice disappears if breast-feeding is discontinued. Nursing can be resumed in 3 to 4 days without any hyperbilirubinemia ensuing.

Hyperbilirubinemia places the neonate at risk for the development of a neurologic syndrome called *kernicterus*. This condition is caused by the accumulation of unconjugated bilirubin in brain cells. Unconjugated bilirubin is lipid soluble, crosses the permeable blood-brain barrier of the neonate, and is deposited in cells of the basal ganglia, causing brain damage. Asphyxia and hyperosmolality may also contribute by damaging the blood-brain barrier and allowing bilirubin to cross and enter the cells. The level of unconjugated bilirubin and the duration of exposure that will be toxic to the infant are unknown. The less mature infant, however, is at greater risk for kernicterus.[23] The manifestations of kernicterus may appear 2 to 5 days after birth in term infants or by day 7 in premature infants. Lethargy, poor feeding, and short-term behavioral changes may be evident in mildly affected infants. Severe manifestations include rigidity, tremors, ataxia, and hearing loss. Extreme cases cause seizures and death. Most survivors are seriously damaged and by

3 years of age exhibit involuntary muscle spasm, seizures, mental retardation, and deafness.

The diagnosis of neonatal jaundice is made on the basis of history and clinical and laboratory findings. Treatment usually consists of phototherapy. Exposure to fluorescent light in the blue range of the visible spectrum (420- to 470-nm wavelength) reduces bilirubin levels.[23] Bilirubin in the skin absorbs the light energy and is converted to a structural isomer that is more water soluble and can be excreted in the stool and urine. Effective treatment depends on the area of skin exposed and the infant's ability to metabolize and excrete bilirubin. Frequent monitoring of bilirubin levels, body temperature, and hydration is critical to the infant's care. Exchange transfusion is considered when signs of kernicterus are evident or hyperbilirubinemia is sustained or rising and unresponsive to phototherapy.

Hemolytic Disease of the Newborn

Erythroblastosis fetalis, or hemolytic disease of the newborn, occurs in Rh-positive infants of Rh-negative mothers who have been sensitized. The mother can produce anti-Rh antibodies from pregnancies in which the infants are Rh positive or by blood transfusions of Rh-positive blood. The Rh-negative mother usually becomes sensitized during the first few days after delivery, when fetal Rh-positive red cells from the placental site are released into the maternal circulation. Because the antibodies take several weeks to develop, the first Rh-positive infant of an Rh-negative mother usually is not affected. Infants with Rh-negative blood have no antigens on their red cells to react with the maternal antibodies and are not affected.

After an Rh-negative mother has been sensitized, the Rh antibodies from her blood are transferred to subsequent infants through the placental circulation. These antibodies react with the red cell antigens of the Rh-positive infant, causing agglutination and hemolysis. This leads to severe anemia with compensatory hyperplasia and enlargement of the blood-forming organs, including the spleen and liver, in the fetus. Liver function may be impaired, with decreased production of albumin causing massive edema, called *hydrops fetalis*. If blood levels of unconjugated bilirubin are abnormally high because of red cell hemolysis, there is a danger of kernicterus developing in the infant, resulting in severe brain damage or death.

Several advances have served significantly to decrease the threat to infants born to Rh-negative mothers: prevention of sensitization, antenatal identification of the at-risk fetus, and intrauterine transfusion to the affected fetus. The injection of Rh immune globulin (*i.e.*, gammaglobulin–containing Rh antibody) prevents sensitization in Rh-negative mothers who have given birth to Rh-positive infants if administered at 28 weeks' gestation and within 72 hours of delivery, abortion, genetic amniocentesis, or fetal-maternal bleeding. After sensitization has developed, the immune globulin is of no value. Since 1968, the year Rh immune globulin was introduced, the incidence of sensitization of Rh-negative women has dropped dramatically. Early prenatal care and screening of maternal blood continue to be important in reducing immunization. Efforts to improve therapy are aimed at production of monoclonal anti-D, the Rh antibody.

In the past, approximately 20% of erythroblastotic fetuses died in utero. Fetal Rh phenotyping can now be performed to identify at-risk fetuses in the first trimester using fetal blood or amniotic cells.[24] Hemolysis in these fetuses can be treated by intrauterine transfusions of red cells through the umbilical cord. Exchange transfusions are administered after birth by removing and replacing the infant's blood volume with type O Rh-negative blood. The exchange transfusion removes most of the hemolyzed red cells and some of the total bilirubin, treating the anemia and hyperbilirubinemia.

RED CELL CHANGES WITH AGING

Anemia is an increasingly common health problem in the elderly, affecting approximately 12% of persons aged 60 years and older.[25] Its prevalence is known to increase with age, the highest prevalence occurring in men aged 85 years and older. Undiagnosed and untreated anemia can have severe consequences and is associated with increased risk of mortality, lower functional ability, self-care deficits, and depression. It can also cause neurologic and cognitive disorders and cardiovascular complications.

Hemoglobin levels decline after middle age. In studies of men older than 60 years of age, mean hemoglobin levels ranged from 15.3 to 12.4 g/dL, with the lowest levels found in the oldest persons. The decline is less in women, with mean levels ranging from 13.8 to 11.7 g/dL.[26] In most asymptomatic elderly persons, lower hemoglobin levels result from iron deficiency and anemia of chronic disease. Anemia of chronic disease is associated with a number of conditions such as acute infections, chronic infections (tuberculosis), chronic inflammatory disorders (rheumatoid arthritis), malignancy, and protein-calorie malnutrition.[25]

As with other body systems, the capacity for red cell production changes with aging. The location of bone cells involved in red cell production shifts toward the axial skeleton and the number of progenitor cells declines from approximately 50% at age 65 to approximately 30% at age 75 years.[26] Despite these changes, the elderly are able to maintain hemoglobin and hematocrit levels within a range that is similar to that in younger adults.[27] However, during a stress situation such as bleeding, the red blood cells of the elderly are not replaced as promptly as those of their younger counterparts. This inability to replace red blood cells closely correlates with the increased prevalence of anemia in the elderly.

Although the age-associated decline in the hematopoietic reserve in the elderly is not completely understood, several factors seem to play a role, including a reduction in hematopoietic progenitors, reduced production of hematopoietic growth factors, and reduced sensitivity of hematopoietic progenitors (*e.g.*, erythropoietin).[25,28] Inflammatory cytokines, which have been found to increase with age, may mediate this reduced sensitivity to erythropoietin.

The diagnosis of anemia in the elderly requires a complete physical examination, a complete blood count, and studies to rule out comorbid conditions such as malignancy, gastrointestinal conditions that cause bleeding, and pernicious anemia. The complete blood count should include a peripheral blood smear and a reticulocyte count and index. If the reticulocyte index is appropriately increased for the level of anemia, then blood loss or red cell destruction should be suspected. If the reticulocyte index is inappropriately low, then decreased red cell production is indicated.[28]

The treatment of anemia in the elderly should focus on the underlying cause and correction of the red cell deficit. An important aspect of anemia of chronic disease is the inability to use and mobilize iron effectively.[25] Orally administered iron is poorly used in older adults, despite normal iron absorption.[26] Although erythropoietin remains the treatment of choice for anemias associated with cancer and renal disease, its potential use in treating anemias associated with aging remains to be established.

In summary, hemoglobin concentrations at birth are high, reflecting the in utero need for oxygen delivery; toward the end of the first postnatal week, these levels begin to decline, gradually falling to a minimum value at approximately 2 months of age. During the early neonatal period, there is a shift from fetal to adult hemoglobin. Many infants have physiologic jaundice because of hyperbilirubinemia during the first week of life, probably related to increased red cell breakdown and the inability of the infant's liver to conjugate bilirubin. The term *kernicterus* describes elevated levels of lipid-soluble, unconjugated bilirubin, which can be toxic to brain cells. Depending on severity, it is treated with phototherapy or exchange transfusions (or both). Hemolytic disease of the newborn occurs in Rh-positive infants of Rh-negative mothers who have been sensitized. It involves hemolysis of infant red cells in response to maternal Rh antibodies that have crossed the placenta. Administration of Rh immune globulin to the mother within 72 hours of delivery of an Rh-positive infant, abortion, or amniocentesis prevents sensitization.

Anemia is an increasingly common health problem in the elderly, affecting approximately 12% of persons aged 60 years and older. As with cells in other tissues, the capacity for red cell replacement decreases with aging. Although most elderly persons are able to maintain their hemoglobin and hematocrit levels within a normal range, they are unable to replace their red cells as promptly as their younger counterparts during a stress situation such as bleeding. This inability to replace red blood cells closely correlates with the increased prevalence of anemia in the elderly, which is usually the result of bleeding, infection, malignancy, or chronic disease.

Review Exercises

A 29-year-old woman complains of generalized fatigue. Her physical examination reveals a heart rate of 115 beats/minute, BP 115/75, and respiratory rate of 28 breaths/minute. Her skin and nail beds are pale. Her laboratory results include RBC $3.0 \times 10^6/\mu L$, hematocrit 30%, hemoglobin 9 g/dL, and decreased serum ferritin levels.

A. What disorder do you suspect this woman has?
B. What additional data would be helpful in determining the etiology of her condition?
C. Which of her signs reflect the body's attempt to compensate for the disorder?
D. What is the significance of the low ferritin level, and how could it be used to make decisions related to her treatment?

A 65-year-old woman is being seen in the clinic because of numbness in her lower legs and feet and difficulty in walking. She has no other complaints. She takes a blood pressure pill, two calcium pills, and a multivitamin pill daily. Her laboratory results include RBC $3.0 \times 10^6/\mu L$, hematocrit 20%, hemoglobin 9 g/dL, and a markedly elevated MVC.

A. What type of anemia does she have?
B. What is the reason for her neurologic symptoms?
C. What type of treatment would be appropriate?

A 12-year-old boy with sickle cell disease presents in the emergency department with severe chest pain. His mother reports that he was doing well until he came down with a respiratory tract infection. She also says he insisted on playing basketball with the other boys in the neighborhood even though he wasn't feeling well.

A. What is the most likely cause of pain in this boy?
B. Infections and aerobic-type exercise that increase the levels of deoxygenated hemoglobin produce sickling in persons who are homozygous for the sickle cell gene and have sickle cell disease, but not in persons who are heterozygous and have sickle cell trait. Explain.
C. People with sickle cell disease experience anemia but not iron deficiency. Explain.

REFERENCES

1. Guyton A. C., Hall J. E. (2006). *Textbook of medical physiology* (11th ed., pp. 419–438). Philadelphia: W. B. Saunders.
2. Aster J. C. (2005). Red blood cell and bleeding disorders. In Kumar V., Abbas A. K., Fausto N. (Eds.), *Robbins and Cotran pathologic basis of disease* (7th ed., pp. 619–649). Philadelphia: Elsevier Saunders.
3. Beck W. S. (1991). Erythropoiesis and introduction to the anemias. In Beck W. S. (Ed.), *Hematology* (5th ed., pp. 27, 29). Cambridge, MA: MIT Press.
4. Schwarting R., Kocher W. D., McKenzie S., et al. (2005). Hematopathology. In Rubin E., Gorstein F., Rubin R., et al. (Eds.), *Rubin's pathology: Clinicopathologic foundations of medicine* (4th ed., pp. 1026–1051). Philadelphia: Lippincott Williams & Wilkins.
5. Steinberg M. H., Rodgers G. P. (2001). Pathophysiology of sickle cell disease: Role of cellular and genetic modifiers. *Seminars in Hematology* 38, 299–306.
6. Stuart M. J., Nagel R. L. (2004). Sickle-cell disease. *Lancet* 364, 1343–1360.
7. Ballas S. K. (2001). Sickle cell disease. *Seminars in Hematology* 38, 307–314.
8. Lane P. (1996). Sickle cell disease. *Pediatric Clinics of North America* 43, 639–666.
9. National Institutes of Health. (2002). *The management of sickle cell disease.* NIH publication no. 02-2117. [On-line.] Available at www.nhlbi.nih.gov/health/prof/blood/sickle/index.htm.
10. Rund D., Rachmilewitz E. (2001). Pathophysiology of α- and β-thalassemia: Therapeutic implications. *Seminars in Hematology* 38, 343–349.
11. Lo L., Singer S. T. (2002). Thalassemia: Current approach to an old disease. *Pediatric Clinics of North America* 49, 1165–1191.
12. Brittenham G. M. (2000). Disorders of iron metabolism: Iron deficiency and overload. In Hoffman R., Benz E. J., Shattil S. J., et al. (Eds.), *Hematology: Basic principles and practice* (3rd ed., pp. 405, 413). New York: Churchill Livingstone.
13. Glader B. (2004). Anemia of inadequate production. In Behrman R. E., Kliegman R. M., Jenson H. B. (Eds.), *Nelson textbook of pediatrics* (17th ed., pp. 1606–1607). Philadelphia: W. B. Saunders.
14. Yager J. Y., Hartfield D. S. (2002). Neurologic manifestations of iron deficiency in childhood. *Pediatric Neurology* 27, 85–92.
15. Kazal L. A. (2002). Prevention of iron deficiency in infants and toddlers. *American Family Physician* 66, 1217–1224.
16. Oh R., Brown D. L. (2003). Vitamin B$_{12}$ deficiency. *American Family Physician* 67, 979–986.
17. Hoffbrand A. V., Herbert V. (1999). Nutritional anemias. *Seminars in Hematology* 36(Suppl. 7), 13–23.
18. Johnston M. V., Kinsman S. (2004). Congenital anomalies of the central nervous system. In Behrman R. E., Kliegman R. M., Jenson H. B. (Eds.), *Nelson textbook of pediatrics* (17th ed., pp. 1983–1984). Philadelphia: W. B. Saunders
19. Young N. S., Maciejewski J. P. (2000). Aplastic anemias. In Hoffman R., Benz E. J., Shattil S. J., et al. (Eds.), *Hematology: Basic principles and practice* (3rd ed., pp. 316, 318). New York: Churchill Livingstone.
20. Hillman R. S., Ault K. A. (2002). *Hematology in clinical practice* (3rd ed., pp. 12, 46). New York: McGraw-Hill.
21. Hocking W. G. (2002). Primary and secondary erythrocytosis. In Mazza J. J. (Ed.), *Manual of clinical hematology* (3rd ed., p. 80). Philadelphia: Lippincott Williams & Wilkins.
22. Ohls R. K., Christensen R. D. (2004). Development of the hematopoietic system. In Behrman R. E., Kliegman R. M., Jenson H. B. (Eds.), *Nelson textbook of pediatrics* (17th ed., pp. 1599–1604). Philadelphia: W. B. Saunders.
23. Stoll B. J., Kliegman R. M. (2004). Jaundice and hyperbilirubinemia in the newborn. In Behrman R. E., Kliegman R. M., Jenson H. B. (Eds.), *Nelson textbook of pediatrics* (17th ed., pp. 592–599). Philadelphia: W. B. Saunders.
24. Kramer K., Cohen H. J. (2000). Antenatal diagnosis of hematologic disorders. In Hoffman R., Benz E. J., Shattil S. J., et al. (Eds.), *Hematology: Basic principles and practice* (3rd ed., p. 2495). New York: Churchill Livingstone.
25. Williams W. J. (1995). Hematology in the aged. In Beutler E., Lichtman A., Coller B. S., et al. (Eds.), *Williams' hematology* (5th ed., p. 73). New York: McGraw-Hill.
26. Balducci L. (2003). Epidemiology of anemia in the elderly: Information on diagnostic evaluation. *Journal of the American Geriatrics Society* 51(Suppl. 3), S2–S9.
27. Rothstein G. (2003). Disordered hematopoiesis and myelodysplasia in the elderly. *Journal of the American Geriatrics Society* 51(Suppl. 3), S22–S26.
28. Lipschitz D. (2003). Medical and functional consequences of anemia in the elderly. *Journal of the American Geriatrics Society* 51(Suppl. 3), S10–S13.

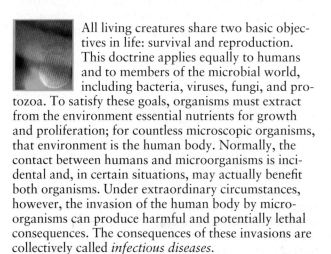

UNIT *IV*

Infection, Inflammation, and Immunity

Chapter *12*

Mechanisms of Infectious Disease

All living creatures share two basic objectives in life: survival and reproduction. This doctrine applies equally to humans and to members of the microbial world, including bacteria, viruses, fungi, and protozoa. To satisfy these goals, organisms must extract from the environment essential nutrients for growth and proliferation; for countless microscopic organisms, that environment is the human body. Normally, the contact between humans and microorganisms is incidental and, in certain situations, may actually benefit both organisms. Under extraordinary circumstances, however, the invasion of the human body by microorganisms can produce harmful and potentially lethal consequences. The consequences of these invasions are collectively called *infectious diseases.*

Infectious Diseases

TERMINOLOGY

All scientific disciplines evolve with a distinct vocabulary, and the study of infectious diseases is no exception. The most appropriate way to approach this subject is with a brief discussion of the terminology used to characterize interactions between humans and microbes.

Any organism capable of supporting the nutritional and physical growth requirements of another is called a *host.* Throughout this chapter, the term *host* most often

229

refs to humans supporting the growth of microorganisms. The term *infection* describes the presence and multiplication of a living organism on or within the host. Occasionally, *infection* and *colonization* are used interchangeably.

One common misconception should be dispelled right away: not all interactions between microorganisms and humans are detrimental. The internal and external exposed surfaces of the human body are normally and harmlessly inhabited by a multitude of bacteria, collectively referred to as the normal *microflora*, many of which serve important functions for their hosts, such as aiding in the digestion of food, producing vitamins (*e.g.*, vitamin K), and protecting the host from colonization by pathogenic microbes. Although many of these organisms can cause disease, they normally reside in locations such as the skin, gastrointestinal tract, and upper respiratory tract that are technically outside the body.

The severity of an infectious disease can range from mild to life threatening, depending on many variables, including the health of the host at the time of infection and the *virulence* (disease-producing potential) of the microorganism. A select group of microorganisms called *pathogens* are so virulent that they are rarely found in the absence of disease. Fortunately, there are few human pathogens in the microbial world. Most microorganisms are harmless, free-living organisms (*i.e.*, *saprophytes*) obtaining their growth from dead or decaying organic material from the environment. All microorganisms, even saprophytes and members of the normal flora, can be *opportunistic pathogens*, capable of producing an infectious disease when the health and immunity of the host have been severely weakened by illness, famine, or medical therapy.

AGENTS OF INFECTIOUS DISEASE

The agents of infectious disease can be arranged in order of increasing complexity, beginning with prions and proceeding through viruses, bacteria, rickettsiae and chlamydiae, fungi, and parasites. Infectious agents can be further classified in terms of their ability to multiply inside or outside body cells. *Obligate intracellular organisms* can grow and multiply only in host cells and require the metabolic apparatus of the host cell for growth. *Extracellular organisms* can grow and multiply outside cells. Most extracellular organisms can be cultured on artificial media.

Prions

Can a protein alone cause a transmissible infectious disease? Until recently, microbiologists assumed that all infectious agents must possess a genetic master plan (a genome of either ribonucleic acid [RNA] or deoxyribonucleic acid [DNA]) that codes for the production of the essential proteins and enzymes necessary for survival and reproduction. Prions, which are composed of a small modified infectious host protein (PrP) and lack any kind of demonstrable genome, appear to be an exception to this rule. Prions are derived from a protein normally found in

> ## ⚗ KEY CONCEPTS
>
> ### Agents of Infectious Disease
>
> ➤ The agents of infectious disease represent a diversity of microorganisms that are not visible to the human eye.
>
> ➤ Microorganisms can be separated into eukaryotes (fungi and parasites), organisms containing a membrane-bound nucleus, and prokaryotes (bacteria), organisms in which the nucleus is not separated.
>
> ➤ Eukaryotes and prokaryotes are organisms because they contain all the enzymes required for their replication and possess all the biologic equipment necessary for exploiting metabolic energy.
>
> ➤ Viruses, which are the smallest pathogens, have no organized cellular structure, but consist of a protein coat surrounding a nucleic acid core of DNA or RNA. Unlike eukaryotes and prokaryotes, viruses are incapable of replication outside of a living cell.
>
> ➤ Parasites (protozoa, helminths, and arthropods) are members of the animal kingdom that infect and cause disease in other animals, which then transmit them to humans.

neurons. Disease occurs when the normal protein undergoes changes that render it resistant to the action of proteases (enzymes that break polypeptide chains), causing it to accumulate and produce neuronal damage. The protease-resistant PrP promotes conversion of the normal protease-sensitive protein to the abnormal form, explaining the infectious nature of the disease.

A number of prion-associated diseases have been identified, the most famous of which include Creutzfeldt-Jacob disease (see Chapter 36) and kuru (associated with human cannibalism) in humans, and scrapie and bovine spongiform encephalopathy (BSE or mad cow disease) in animals. The various prion-associated diseases produce very similar symptomatology and pathology in the host and are collectively called *transmissible neurodegenerative diseases*. All are characterized by a slowly progressive, noninflammatory neuronal degeneration, leading to loss of coordination (ataxia), dementia, and death over a period ranging from months to years.

Prions are transmitted predominantly by injection, transplantation of contaminated tissue (corneal transplants), contact with contaminated medical devices (*e.g.*, brain electrodes), and possibly food (contaminated beef). Because prions lack reproductive and metabolic functions, the currently available antibacterial and antiviral agents are useless. Prions also fail to elicit an immune response and are extremely resistant to inactivation by heat, disinfectants, and radiation.

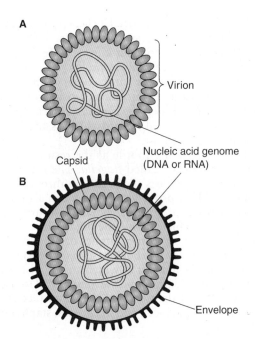

FIGURE 12-1 (**A**) The basic structure of a virus includes a protein coat surrounding an inner core of nucleic acid (DNA or RNA). (**B**) Some viruses may also be enclosed in a lipoprotein outer envelope.

Viruses

Viruses are the smallest obligate intracellular pathogens. They have no organized cellular structures but instead consist of a protein coat, or capsid, surrounding a nucleic acid core, or genome, of RNA or DNA—never both (Fig. 12-1). Some viruses are enclosed within a lipoprotein envelope derived from the cell membrane of the parasitized host cell. Enveloped viruses include members of the herpesvirus group, paramyxoviruses such as influenza, and poxviruses. Certain enveloped viruses are continuously shed from the infected cell surface enveloped in

buds pinched from the cell membrane. The viruses of humans and animals have been categorized somewhat arbitrarily according to various characteristics. These include the type of viral genome (single-stranded or double-stranded DNA or RNA), the mechanism of replication (*e.g.*, retroviruses), the mode of transmission (*e.g.*, arthropod-borne viruses, enteroviruses), and the type of disease produced (*e.g.*, hepatitis A, B, C, D, and E viruses), to name just a few.

Viruses are incapable of replication outside of a living cell. They must penetrate a susceptible living cell and use the biosynthetic machinery of the cell to produce viral progeny. The process of viral replication is shown in Figure 12-2. Not every viral agent causes lysis and death of the host cell during the course of replication. Some viruses enter the host cell and insert their genome into the host cell chromosome, where it remains in a latent, nonreplicating state for long periods without causing disease. Under the appropriate stimulation, the virus undergoes active replication and produces symptoms of disease months to years later. For example, the varicella-zoster virus, the cause of chickenpox, can enter dorsal root ganglia and establish latency there, with later periodic activation causing herpes zoster (shingles), a painful skin disease (see Chapter 45).

Since the early 1980s, members of the retrovirus group have received considerable attention after identification of the human immunodeficiency virus (HIV) as the causative agent of acquired immunodeficiency syndrome (AIDS). The retroviruses have a unique mechanism of replication. After entry into the host cell, the viral RNA genome is first translated into DNA by a viral enzyme called *reverse transcriptase*. The viral DNA copy is integrated into the host chromosome and exists in a latent state, similar to the herpesviruses. Reactivation and replication require reversal of the entire process. Some retroviruses lyse the host cell during the process of replication. In the case of HIV, the infected cells regulate the immunologic defense system of the host and their lysis leads to a permanent suppression of the immune response.

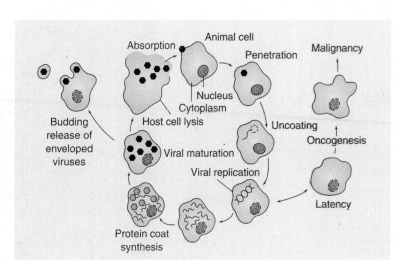

FIGURE 12-2 Schematic representation of the many possible consequences of viral infection of host cells, including cell lysis (poliovirus), continuous release of budding viral particles, or latency (herpesviruses) and oncogenesis (papovaviruses).

Bacteria

Bacteria are autonomously replicating unicellular organisms known as *prokaryotes* because they lack an organized nucleus. Compared with nucleated eukaryotic cells (see Chapter 1), the bacterial cell is small and structurally relatively primitive (Fig. 12-3). Similar to eukaryotic cells, but unlike viruses, bacteria contain DNA and RNA. They usually contain no organized intracellular organelles, and the genome consists of only a single chromosome of DNA. Many bacteria transiently harbor smaller extrachromosomal pieces of circular DNA called *plasmids*. Occasionally, plasmids contain genetic information that increases the virulence of the organism.

The prokaryotic cell is organized into an internal compartment called the *cytoplasm*, which contains the reproductive and metabolic machinery of the cell (Fig. 12-4). The cytoplasm is surrounded by a flexible lipid membrane, called the *cytoplasmic membrane*. This in turn is enclosed in a rigid cell wall. The structure and synthesis of the cell wall determine the microscopic shape of the bacterium (*e.g.*, spherical [cocci], helical [spirilla], or elongate [bacilli]). Most bacteria produce a cell wall composed of a distinctive polymer known as *peptidoglycan*. This polymer is produced only by prokaryotes and is therefore an attractive target for antibacterial therapy. Several bacteria synthesize an extracellular capsule composed of protein or carbohydrate. The capsule protects the organism from environmental hazards such as the immunologic defenses of the host.

Certain bacteria are motile as the result of external whiplike appendages called *flagella*. The rotary action of the flagella transports the organism through a liquid environment like a propeller. Bacteria can also produce hairlike structures projecting from the cell surface called *pili* or *fimbriae*, which enable the organism to adhere to surfaces such as mucous membranes or other bacteria.

Most prokaryotes reproduce asexually by simple cellular division. The manner in which an organism divides can influence the microscopic morphology. For instance, when the cocci divide in chains, they are called streptococci; in pairs, diplococci; and in clusters, staphylococci.

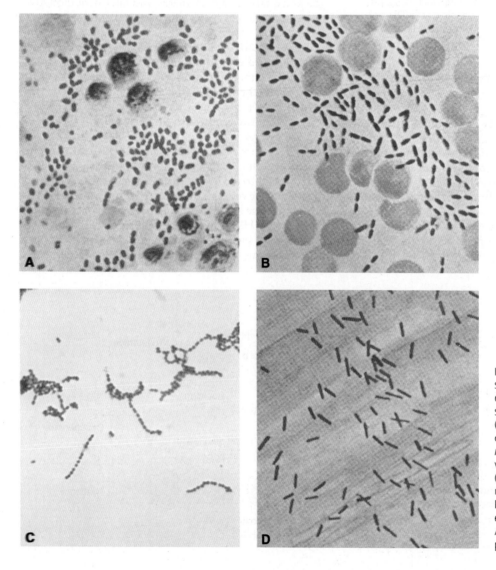

FIGURE 12-3 A sampling of microscopic morphology of bacteria demonstrating the variability of size and shape: (**A**) *Yersinia pestis;* (**B**) gram-positive diplococci typical of *Streptococcus pneumoniae;* (**C**) *Streptococcus species* visualized using Gram stain; (**D**) *Escherichia coli* visualized using Gram stain. (From Public Images Library, Centers for Disease Control and Prevention. Available: http://phil.cdc.gov/phil/detail.?id=2170.)

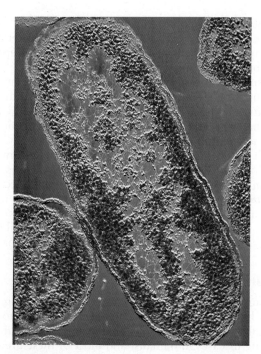

FIGURE 12-4 False-color transmission electron micrograph of the rod-shaped, gram-negative bacterium *Escherichia coli,* showing the simple prokaryotic cell structure, including the cytoplasm, the cytoplasmic membrane, and the rigid cell wall. (© Science Source/Photo Researchers.)

The growth rate of bacteria varies significantly among different species and depends greatly on physical growth conditions and the availability of nutrients. In the laboratory, a single bacterium placed in a suitable growth environment, such as an agar plate, reproduces to the extent that it forms a visible colony composed of millions of bacteria within a few hours.

In nature, however, bacteria rarely exist as single cells floating in an aqueous environment. Rather, bacteria prefer to stick to and colonize environmental surfaces, producing structured communities called *biofilms.* The organization and structure of biofilms permit access to available nutrients and elimination of metabolic waste. Within the biofilm, individual organisms use chemical signaling as a form of primitive intercellular communication to represent the state of the environment. These signals inform members of the community when sufficient nutrients are available for proliferation or when environmental conditions warrant dormancy or evacuation. Examples of biofilms abound in nature and are found on surfaces of aquatic environments and on humans. One has only to disassemble a clogged sink drain to see a perfect example of a bacterial biofilm.

The physical appearance of a colony of bacteria grown on an agar plate can be quite distinctive for different species. Some produce pigments that give colonies a unique color. Some bacteria produce highly resistant spores when faced with an unfavorable environment. The spores can exist in a quiescent state almost indefinitely until suitable growth conditions are encountered,

at which time the spores germinate and the organism resumes normal metabolism and replication.

Bacteria are extremely adaptable life forms. They inhabit almost every environmental extreme on earth, including humans. However, each individual bacterial species has a well-defined set of growth parameters, including nutrition, temperature, light, humidity, and atmosphere. For example, *Neisseria gonorrhoeae,* the bacterium that causes gonorrhea, cannot live for extended periods outside the human body. Some bacteria require oxygen for growth and metabolism and are called *aerobes;* others cannot survive in an oxygen-containing environment and are called *anaerobes.* An organism capable of adapting its metabolism to aerobic or anaerobic conditions is called *facultatively anaerobic.*

In the laboratory, bacteria are generally classified according to the microscopic appearance and staining properties of the cell. Gram stain, originally developed in 1884 by the Danish bacteriologist Christian Gram, is still the most widely used staining procedure. Bacteria are designated as *gram-positive* organisms if they are stained purple by a primary basic dye (usually crystal violet); those that are not stained by the crystal violet but are counterstained red by a second dye (safranin) are called *gram-negative* organisms. Staining characteristics and microscopic morphology are used in combination to describe bacteria. For example, *Streptococcus pyogenes,* the agent of scarlet fever and rheumatic fever, is a gram-positive streptococcal organism that is spherical, grows in chains, and stains purple by Gram stain. *Legionella pneumophila,* the bacterium responsible for Legionnaires disease, is a gram-negative rod.

Another means of classifying bacteria according to microscopic staining properties is afforded by the *acid-fast stain.* Because of their unique cell membrane fatty acid content and composition, certain bacteria are resistant to the decolorization of a primary stain (either carbol fuchsin or a combination of auramine and rhodamine) when treated with a solution of acid alcohol. These organisms are termed *acid-fast* and include a number of significant human pathogens, most notably *Mycobacterium tuberculosis* (the cause of tuberculosis) and other mycobacteria.

For purposes of taxonomy (*e.g.,* identification and classification), each member of the bacterial kingdom is categorized into a small group of biochemically and genetically related organisms called the *genus,* and further subdivided into distinct individuals within the genus called *species.* The genus and species assignment of the organism is reflected in its name (*e.g., Staphylococcus* [genus] *aureus* [species]).

Spirochetes. The spirochetes are an eccentric category of bacteria that are mentioned separately because of their unusual cellular morphology and distinctive mechanism of motility. Technically, the spirochetes are gram-negative rods but are unique in that the cell's shape is helical and the length of the organism is many times its width. A series of filaments are wound about the cell wall and extend the entire length of the cell. These filaments propel the organism through an aqueous environment in a corkscrew motion.

Spirochetes are anaerobic organisms and contain three genera: *Leptospira*, *Borrelia*, and *Treponema*. Each genus has saprophytic and pathogenic strains. The pathogenic leptospires infect a wide variety of wild and domestic animals. Infected animals shed the organisms into the environment through the urinary tract. Transmission to humans occurs by contact with infected animals or urine-contaminated surroundings. In contrast, the borreliae are transmitted from infected animals to humans through the bite of an arthropod vector such as lice or ticks. Included among the genus *Borrelia* is *Borrelia burgdorferi*, the agent of Lyme disease. Pathogenic *Treponema* species require no intermediates and are spread from person to person by direct contact. The most important member of the genus is *Treponema pallidum*, the cause of syphilis (see Chapter 40).

Mycoplasmas. The mycoplasmas are unicellular prokaryotes capable of independent replication. These organisms are less than one-third the size of bacteria and contain a small DNA genome approximately one-half the size of the bacterial chromosome. The cell is composed of cytoplasm surrounded by a membrane but, unlike bacteria, the mycoplasmas do not produce a rigid peptidoglycan cell wall. As a consequence, the microscopic appearance of the cell is highly variable, ranging from coccoid forms to filaments, and the mycoplasmas are resistant to cell-wall–inhibiting antibiotics such as penicillins and cephalosporins.

The mycoplasmas of humans are divided into three genera: *Mycoplasma*, *Ureaplasma*, and *Acholeplasma*. The first two require cholesterol from the environment to produce the cell membrane; the acholeplasmas do not. In the human host, mycoplasmas are commensals. However, a number of species are capable of producing serious diseases, including pneumonia (*Mycoplasma pneumoniae*), genital infections (*Mycoplasma hominis* and *Ureaplasma urealyticum*), and maternally transmitted respiratory infections to low–birth-weight infants (*U. urealyticum*).

Rickettsiae and Chlamydiae

This interesting group of organisms combines the characteristics of viral and bacterial agents to produce disease in humans. All are obligate intracellular pathogens, like the viruses, but produce a rigid peptidoglycan cell wall, reproduce asexually by cellular division, and contain RNA and DNA, similar to the bacteria.

The rickettsiae depend on the host cell for essential vitamins and nutrients, but the chlamydiae appear to scavenge intermediates of energy metabolism such as adenosine triphosphate (ATP). The rickettsiae infect but do not produce disease in the cells of certain arthropods such as fleas, ticks, and lice. The organisms are incidentally transmitted to humans through the bite of the arthropod (*i.e.*, vector) and produce a number of potentially lethal diseases, including Rocky Mountain spotted fever and epidemic typhus.

The chlamydiae are slightly smaller than the rickettsiae but are structurally similar. Unlike the rickettsiae, chlamydiae are transmitted directly between susceptible vertebrates without an intermediate arthropod host. Transmission and replication of chlamydiae occur through a defined life cycle. The infectious form, called an *elementary body*, attaches to and enters the host cell, where it transforms into a larger *reticulate body*. This undergoes active replication into multiple elementary bodies, which are then shed into the extracellular environment to initiate another infectious cycle. Chlamydial diseases of humans include sexually transmitted genital infections (*Chlamydia trachomatis*; see Chapter 40); ocular infections and pneumonia of newborns (*C. trachomatis*); and upper and lower respiratory tract infections in children, adolescents, and young adults (*Chlamydia pneumoniae*).

Fungi

The fungi are free-living, eukaryotic saprophytes found in every habitat on earth. Some are members of the normal human microflora. Fortunately, few fungi are capable of causing diseases in humans, and most of these are incidental, self-limited infections of skin and subcutaneous tissue. Serious fungal infections are rare and usually initiated through puncture wounds or inhalation. Despite their normally harmless nature, fungi can cause serious, life-threatening opportunistic diseases when host defense capabilities have been disabled.

The fungi can be separated into two groups, yeasts and molds, based on rudimentary differences in their morphology (Fig. 12-5). The yeasts are single-celled organisms, approximately the size of red blood cells, that reproduce by a budding process. The buds separate from the parent cell and mature into identical daughter cells. Molds produce long, hollow, branching filaments called *hyphae*. Some molds produce cross-walls, which segregate the hyphae into compartments, and others do not. A limited number of fungi are capable of growing as yeasts at one temperature and as molds at another. These organisms are called *dimorphic fungi* and include a number of human pathogens such as the agents of blastomycosis, histoplasmosis, and coccidioidomycosis (San Joaquin fever).

The appearance of a fungal colony tends to reflect its cellular composition. Colonies of yeast are usually smooth with a waxy or creamy texture. Molds tend to produce cottony or powdery colonies composed of mats of hyphae collectively called a *mycelium*. The mycelium can penetrate the growth surface or project above the colony like the roots and branches of a tree. Yeasts and molds produce a rigid cell wall layer that is chemically unrelated to the peptidoglycan of bacteria and is therefore not susceptible to the effects of penicillin-like antibiotics.

Most fungi are capable of sexual or asexual reproduction. The former process involves the fusion of zygotes with the production of a recombinant zygospore. Asexual reproduction involves the formation of highly resistant spores called *conidia* or *sporangiospores*, which are borne by specialized structures that arise from the hyphae. Molds are identified in the laboratory by the characteristic

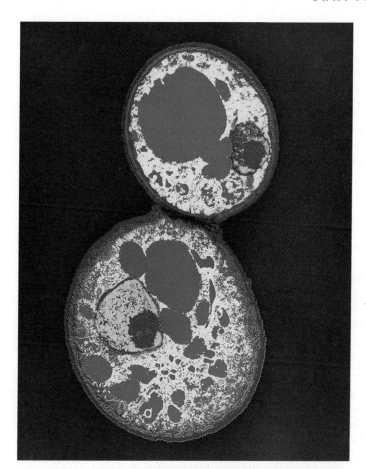

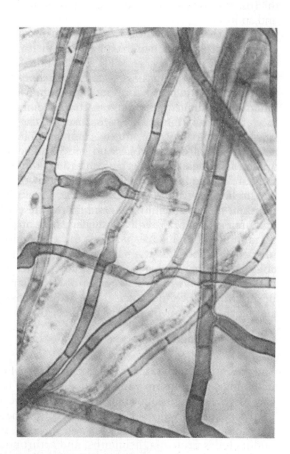

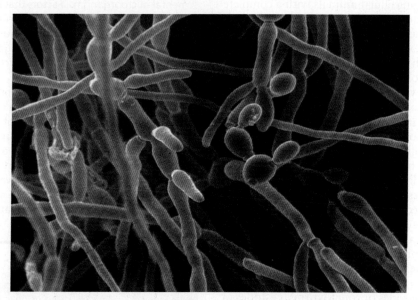

FIGURE 12-5 The microscopic morphology of fungal pathogens in humans. The yeasts are single-celled organisms that reproduce by the budding process (**top left**). The molds (**top right**) produce long branched or unbranched filaments called *hyphae. Candida albicans* (**bottom left**) is a budding yeast that produces pseudohyphae both in culture and in tissues and exudates. (Top left and bottom left © Science Source/Photo Researchers.)

microscopic appearance of the asexual fruiting structures and spores.

Like the bacterial pathogens of humans, fungi can produce disease in the human host only if they can grow at the temperature of the infected body site. For example, a number of fungal pathogens called the *dermatophytes* are incapable of growing at core body temperature (37°C), and the infection is limited to the cooler cutaneous surfaces (see Chapter 45). Diseases caused by these organisms, including ringworm, athlete's foot, and jock itch, are collectively called *superficial mycoses*. Systemic mycoses are serious fungal infections of deep tissues and, by definition, are caused by organisms capable of growth at 37°C. Yeasts such as *Candida albicans* are commensal flora of the skin, mucous membranes, and gastrointestinal tract and are capable of growth at a wider range of temperatures. Intact immune mechanisms and competition for nutrients provided by the bacterial flora normally keep colonizing fungi in check. Alterations in either of these components by disease states or antibiotic therapy can upset the balance, permitting fungal overgrowth and setting the stage for opportunistic infections.

Parasites

In a strict sense, any organism that derives benefits from its biologic relationship with another organism is a parasite. In the study of clinical microbiology, however, the term *parasite* has come to designate members of the animal kingdom that infect and cause disease in other animals and includes protozoa, helminths, and arthropods.

The protozoa are unicellular animals with a complete complement of eukaryotic cellular machinery, including a well-defined nucleus and organelles. Reproduction may be sexual or asexual, and life cycles may be simple or complicated, with several maturation stages requiring more than one host for completion. Most are saprophytes, but a few have adapted to the accommodations of the human environment and produce a variety of diseases, including malaria, amebic dysentery, and giardiasis. Protozoan infections can be passed directly from host to host such as through sexual contact, indirectly through contaminated water or food, or by way of an arthropod vector. Direct or indirect transmission results from the ingestion of highly resistant cysts or spores that are shed in the feces of an infected host. When the cysts reach the intestine, they mature into vegetative forms called *trophozoites*, which are capable of asexual reproduction or cyst formation. Most trophozoites are motile by means of flagella, cilia, or ameboid motion.

The helminths are a collection of wormlike parasites that include the nematodes or roundworms, cestodes or tapeworms, and trematodes or flukes. The helminths reproduce sexually in the definitive host, and some require an intermediate host for the development and maturation of offspring. Humans can serve as the definitive or intermediate host and, in certain diseases such as trichinosis, as both. Transmission of helminth diseases occurs primarily through the ingestion of fertilized eggs (ova) or the penetration of infectious larval stages through the skin—

directly or with the aid of an arthropod vector. Helminth infections can involve many organ systems and sites, including the liver and lung, urinary and intestinal tracts, circulatory and central nervous systems, and muscle. Although most helminth diseases have been eradicated from the United States, they are still a major health concern of developing nations.

The parasitic arthropods of humans and animals include the vectors of infectious diseases (*e.g.*, ticks, mosquitoes, biting flies) and the ectoparasites. The ectoparasites infest external body surfaces and cause localized tissue damage or inflammation secondary to the bite or burrowing action of the arthropod. The most prominent human ectoparasites are mites (scabies), chiggers, lice (head, body, and pubic), and fleas. Transmission of ectoparasites occurs directly by contact with immature or mature forms of the arthropod or its eggs found on the infested host or the host's clothing, bedding, or grooming articles such as combs and brushes. Many of the ectoparasites are vectors of other infectious diseases, including endemic typhus and bubonic plague (fleas) and epidemic typhus (lice).

In summary, throughout life, humans are continuously and harmlessly exposed to and colonized by a multitude of microscopic organisms. This relationship is kept in check by the intact defense mechanisms of the host (*e.g.*, mucosal and cutaneous barriers, normal immune function) and the innocuous nature of most environmental microorganisms. Factors that weaken the resistance of the host or increase the virulence of colonizing microorganisms can disturb the equilibrium of the relationship and cause disease. The degree to which the balance is shifted in favor of the microorganism determines the severity of illness.

There is an extreme diversity of prokaryotic and eukaryotic microorganisms capable of causing infectious diseases in humans. With the advent of immunosuppressive medical therapy and immunosuppressive diseases such as AIDS, the number and type of potential microbial pathogens, the so-called opportunistic pathogens, have increased dramatically. However, most infectious illnesses in humans continue to be caused by only a small fraction of the organisms that comprise the microscopic world.

 Mechanisms of Infection

EPIDEMIOLOGY OF INFECTIOUS DISEASES

Epidemiology, in the context of this chapter, is the study of factors, events, and circumstances that influence the transmission of infectious diseases among humans (see chapter introduction). The ultimate goal of the epidemiologist is to devise strategies that interrupt or eliminate the spread of an infectious agent. To accomplish this, infectious diseases must be classified according to incidence, portal of entry, source, symptoms, disease course, site of infection, and virulence factors so that potential outbreaks may be predicted and averted or appropriately treated.

PORTAL OF ENTRY

The portal of entry refers to the process by which a pathogen enters the body, gains access to susceptible tissues, and causes disease. Among the potential modes of transmission are penetration, direct contact, ingestion, and inhalation. The portal of entry does not necessarily dictate the site of infection. Ingested pathogens may penetrate the intestinal mucosa, disseminate through the circulatory system, and cause diseases in other organs such as the lung or liver. Whatever the mechanisms of entry, the transmission of infectious agents is directly related to the number of infectious agents absorbed by the host.

Penetration

Any disruption in the integrity of the body's surface barrier—the skin or mucous membranes—is a potential site for invasion of microorganisms. The break may be the result of an injury causing abrasions, burns, or penetrating wounds, medical procedures such as surgery or catheterization, a primary infectious process that produces surface lesions such as chickenpox or impetigo, or direct inoculation from intravenous drug use or from animal or arthropod bites. The latter mode of transmission can be extremely dangerous because large numbers of organisms can gain access directly to vital sites, thus bypassing the host's primary immune defense systems.

Direct Contact

Some pathogens are transmitted directly from infected tissue or secretions to exposed, intact mucous membranes without a prerequisite for damaged mucosal barriers. This is especially true of certain sexually transmitted diseases (STDs) such as gonorrhea, syphilis, chlamydia, and herpes, for which exposure of uninfected membranes to pathogens occurs during intimate contact.

The transmission of STDs is not limited to sexual contact. *Vertical transmission* of these agents, from mother to child, can occur across the placenta or during birth when the mucous membranes of the child come in contact with infected vaginal secretions of the mother. When an infectious disease is transmitted from mother to child during gestation or birth, it is classified as a *congenital infection*. The most frequently observed congenital infections include the parasite *Toxoplasma gondii*, other infections (most commonly syphilis), rubella, cytomegalovirus, and herpes simplex virus (the so-called *TORCH* infections); varicella-zoster (chickenpox); parvovirus B19; group B streptococci (*Streptococcus agalactiae*); and HIV. Of these, cytomegalovirus is by far the most com-

mon cause of congenital infection in the United States, affecting nearly 1% of all newborns. However, more than 6000 HIV-infected women give birth each year in the United States, and the numbers are likely far greater in developing nations. With a 13% to 30% chance of vertical transmission, HIV disease is rapidly gaining in stature as a congenitally transmitted infection (see Chapter 15).

Ingestion

The entry of pathogenic microorganisms or their toxic products through the oral cavity and gastrointestinal tract represents one of the more efficient means of disease transmission in humans. Many bacterial, viral, and parasitic infections, including cholera, typhoid fever, dysentery (amebic and bacillary), food poisoning, traveler's diarrhea, cryptosporidiosis, and hepatitis A, are initiated through the ingestion of contaminated food and water. This mechanism of transmission necessitates that an infectious agent survive the low pH and enzyme activity of gastric secretions and the peristaltic action of the intestines in numbers sufficient to establish infection, deemed an *infectious dose*. Ingested pathogens also must compete successfully with the normal bacterial flora of the bowel for nutritional needs. Persons with reduced gastric acidity (called *achlorhydria*) because of disease or medication are more susceptible to infection by this route because the number of ingested microorganisms surviving the gastric environment is greater. Ingestion has also been postulated as a means of transmission of HIV infection from mother to child through breast-feeding.

Inhalation

The respiratory tract of healthy persons is equipped with a multitiered defense system to prevent potential pathogens from entering the lungs. The surface of the respiratory tree is lined with a layer of mucus that is continuously swept up and away from the lungs and toward the mouth by the beating motion of ciliated epithelial cells. Humidification of inspired air increases the size of aerosolized particles, which are effectively filtered by the mucous membranes of the upper respiratory tract. Coughing also aids in the removal of particulate matter from the lower respiratory tract. Respiratory secretions contain antibodies and enzymes capable of inactivating infectious agents. Particulate matter and microorganisms that ultimately reach the lung are cleared by phagocytic cells.

Despite this impressive array of protective mechanisms, a number of pathogens can invade the human body through the respiratory tract, including agents of bacterial pneumonia (*S. pneumoniae, L. pneumophila*), meningitis and sepsis (*N. meningitidis* and *Haemophilus influenzae*), and tuberculosis, as well as the viruses responsible for measles, mumps, chickenpox, influenza, and the common cold. Defective pulmonary function or mucociliary clearance caused by noninfectious processes such as cystic fibrosis, emphysema, or smoking can increase the risk of inhalation-acquired diseases.

SOURCE

The source of an infectious disease refers to the location, host, object, or substance from which the infectious agent was acquired: essentially the who, what, where, and when of disease transmission. The source may be endogenous (acquired from the host's own microbial flora, as would be the case in an opportunistic infection) or exogenous (acquired from sources in the external environment, such as the water, food, soil, or air). The infectious agent can originate from another human being, as from mother to child during gestation (congenital infections) or birth (perinatal infections). *Zoonoses* are a category of infectious diseases passed from other animal species to humans. Examples of zoonoses include cat-scratch disease, rabies, and visceral or cutaneous larval migrans. The spread of infectious diseases such as Lyme disease through biting arthropod vectors has already been mentioned.

Source can denote a place. For instance, infections that develop in patients while they are hospitalized are called *nosocomial*, and those that are acquired outside of health care facilities are called *community acquired*. The source may also pertain to the body substance that is the most likely vehicle for transmission, such as feces, blood, body fluids, respiratory secretions, and urine. Infections can be transmitted from person to person through shared inanimate objects (fomites) contaminated with infected body fluids. An example of this mechanism of transmission would include the spread of HIV and hepatitis B virus through the use of shared syringes by intravenous drug users. Infection can also be spread through a complex combination of source, portal of entry, and vector. The well-publicized 1993 outbreak of hantavirus pulmonary syndrome in the southwestern United States is a prime example. This viral illness was transmitted to humans by inhalation of dust contaminated with saliva, feces, and urine of infected rodents.

SYMPTOMATOLOGY

Symptomatology refers to the collection of signs and symptoms expressed by the host during the disease course. This is also known as the *clinical picture* or *disease presentation*, and can be characteristic of any given infectious agent. In terms of pathophysiology, symptoms are the outward expression of the struggle between invading organisms and the retaliatory inflammatory and immune responses of the host. The symptoms of an infectious disease may be specific and reflect the site of infection (*e.g.*, diarrhea, rash, convulsions, hemorrhage, pneumonia). Conversely, symptoms such as fever, myalgia, headache, and lethargy are relatively nonspecific and can be shared by a number of diverse infectious diseases. The symptoms of a diseased host can be obvious, as in the cases of chickenpox or measles. Other covert symptoms, such as increased white blood cell count, may require laboratory testing to detect. Accurate recognition and documentation of symptomatology can aid in the diagnosis of an infectious disease.

DISEASE COURSE

The course of any infectious disease can be divided into several distinct stages after the point in which the potential pathogen enters the host. These stages are the incubation period, the prodromal stage, the acute stage, the convalescent stage, and the resolution stage (Fig. 12-6). The stages are based on the progression and intensity of the host's symptoms over time. The duration of each phase and the pattern of the overall illness can be specific for different pathogens, thereby aiding in the diagnosis of an infectious disease.

The *incubation period* is the phase during which the pathogen begins active replication without producing recognizable symptoms in the host. The incubation period may be short, as in the case of salmonellosis (6 to 24 hours), or prolonged, such as that of hepatitis B (50 to 180 days) or HIV (months to years). The duration of the incubation period can be influenced by additional factors, including the general health of the host, the portal of entry, and the infectious dose of the pathogen.

The hallmark of the *prodromal stage* is the initial appearance of symptoms in the host, although the clinical presentation during this time may consist only of a vague sense of malaise. The host may experience mild fever, myalgia, headache, and fatigue. These are constitutional changes common to a great number of disease processes. The duration of the prodromal stage can vary considerably from host to host.

The *acute stage* is the period during which the host experiences the maximum impact of the infectious process, corresponding to rapid proliferation and dissemination of the pathogen. During this phase, toxic byproducts of microbial metabolism, cell lysis, and the immune

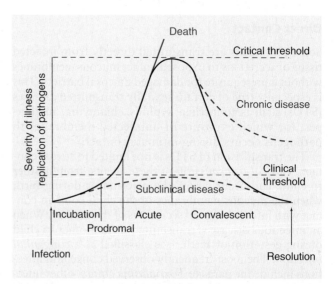

FIGURE 12-6 The stages of a primary infectious disease as they appear in relation to the severity of symptoms and the numbers of infectious agents. The clinical threshold corresponds with the initial expression of recognizable symptoms, whereas the critical threshold represents the peak of disease intensity.

response mounted by the host combine to produce tissue damage and inflammation. The symptoms of the host are pronounced and more specific than in the prodromal stage, usually typifying the pathogen and sites of involvement.

The *convalescent period* is characterized by the containment of infection, progressive elimination of the pathogen, repair of damaged tissue, and resolution of associated symptoms. Similar to the incubation period, the time required for complete convalescence may be days, weeks, or months, depending on the type of pathogen and the efficacy of the host's immune response. The *resolution* is the total elimination of a pathogen from the body without residual signs or symptoms of disease.

Several notable exceptions to the classic presentation of an infectious process have been recognized. Chronic infectious diseases have a markedly protracted and sometimes irregular course. The host may experience symptoms of the infectious process continuously or sporadically for months or years without a convalescent phase. In contrast, *subclinical* or *subacute illness* progresses from infection to resolution without clinically apparent symptoms. A disease is called *insidious* if the prodromal phase is protracted; a *fulminant* illness is characterized by abrupt onset of symptoms with little or no prodrome. Fatal infections are variants of the typical disease course.

SITE OF INFECTION

Inflammation of an anatomic location is usually designated by adding the suffix *-itis* to the name of the involved tissue (*e.g.,* bronchitis, infection of the bronchi and bronchioles; encephalitis, brain infection; carditis, infection of the heart). These are general terms, however, and they apply equally to inflammation from infectious and noninfectious causes. The suffix *-emia* is used to designate the presence of a substance in the blood (*e.g., bacteremia, viremia,* and *fungemia* describe the presence of these infectious agents in the bloodstream). The term *sepsis,* or *septicemia,* refers to the presence of microbial toxins in the blood.

The site of an infectious disease is determined ultimately by the type of pathogen, the portal of entry, and the competence of the host's immunologic defense system. Many pathogenic microorganisms are restricted in their capacity to invade the human body. *M. pneumoniae,* influenza viruses, and *L. pneumophila* rarely cause disease outside the respiratory tract; infections caused by *N. gonorrhoeae* are usually confined to the genitourinary tract; and shigellosis and giardiasis seldom extend beyond the gastrointestinal tract. These are considered localized infectious diseases. The bacterium *Helicobacter pylori* is an extreme example of a site-specific pathogen (see Chapter 28). *H. pylori* is a significant cause of gastric ulcers and has not been implicated in disease processes elsewhere in the human body. Bacteria such as *N. meningitidis,* a prominent pathogen of children and young adults; *Salmonella typhi,* the cause of typhoid fever; and *B. burgdorferi,* the agent of Lyme disease, tend to disseminate from the primary site of infection to involve other locations and organ systems. These are examples of systemic pathogens disseminated throughout the body by the circulatory system.

An *abscess* is a localized pocket of infection composed of devitalized tissue, microorganisms, and the host's phagocytic white blood cells: in essence, a stalemate in the infectious process. In this case, the dissemination of the pathogen has been contained by the host, but white cell function within the toxic environment of the abscess is hampered, and the elimination of microorganisms is retarded. Abscesses usually must be surgically drained to effect a complete cure. Similarly, infections of biomedical implants such as catheters, artificial heart valves, and prosthetic bone implants are seldom cured by the host's immune response and antimicrobial therapy. The infecting organism colonizes the surface of the implant, producing a dense matrix of cells, host proteins, and capsular material—a *biofilm*—necessitating the removal of the device.

VIRULENCE FACTORS

Virulence factors are substances or products generated by infectious agents that enhance their ability to cause disease. Although many different types of microbial products fit this description, they can generally be grouped into four categories: toxins, adhesion factors, evasive factors, and invasive factors.

Toxins

Toxins are substances that alter or destroy the normal function of the host or host's cells. Toxin production is a trait chiefly monopolized by bacterial pathogens, although certain fungal and protozoan pathogens also elaborate substances toxic to humans. Bacterial toxins have a diverse spectrum of activity and exert their effects on a wide variety of host target cells. For classification purposes, however, the bacterial toxins can be divided into two main types: exotoxins and endotoxins.

Exotoxins. Exotoxins are proteins released from the bacterial cell during growth. Bacterial exotoxins enzymatically inactivate or modify key cellular constituents, leading to cell death or dysfunction. Diphtheria toxin, for example, inhibits cellular protein synthesis; botulism toxin decreases the release of neurotransmitter from cholinergic neurons, causing flaccid paralysis; tetanus toxin decreases the release of neurotransmitter from inhibitory neurons, producing spastic paralysis; and cholera toxin induces fluid secretion into the lumen of the intestine, causing diarrhea. Other examples of exotoxin-induced diseases include pertussis (whooping cough), anthrax, traveler's diarrhea, toxic shock syndrome, and a host of foodborne illnesses (*i.e.,* food poisoning).

Bacterial exotoxins that produce vomiting and diarrhea are sometimes referred to as *enterotoxins*. There has been a resurgent interest in streptococcal pyrogenic exotoxin A

(SPEA), an exotoxin produced by certain strains of group A, beta-hemolytic streptococci (*S. pyogenes*) that causes a life-threatening toxic shock–like syndrome similar to the disease associated with tampon use produced by *S. aureus*. Other exotoxins that have gained notoriety include the Shiga toxins produced by *Escherichia coli* 0157:H7 and other select strains. The ingestion of undercooked hamburger meat or unpasteurized fruit juices contaminated with this organism produces hemorrhagic colitis and a sometimes fatal illness called *hemolytic-uremic syndrome* (HUS), characterized by vascular endothelial damage, acute renal failure, and thrombocytopenia. HUS occurs primarily in infants and young children who have not developed antibodies to the Shiga toxins.

Endotoxins. Endotoxins do not contain protein, are not actively released from the bacterium during growth, and have no enzymatic activity. Rather, endotoxins are complex molecules composed of lipid and polysaccharides found in the cell wall of gram-negative bacteria. Studies of different endotoxins have indicated that the lipid portion of the endotoxin confers the toxic properties to the molecule. Endotoxins are potent activators of a number of regulatory systems in humans. A small amount of endotoxin in the circulatory system (endotoxemia) can induce clotting, bleeding, inflammation, hypotension, and fever. The sum of the physiologic reactions to endotoxins is sometimes called *endotoxic shock*.

Adhesion Factors

No interaction between microorganisms and humans can progress to infection or disease if the pathogen is unable to attach to and colonize the host. The process of microbial attachment may be site specific (*e.g.*, mucous membranes, skin surfaces), cell specific (*e.g.*, T lymphocytes, respiratory epithelium), or nonspecific (*e.g.*, moist areas, charged surfaces). In any of these cases, adhesion requires a positive interaction between the surfaces of host cells and the infectious agent.

The site to which microorganisms adhere is called a *receptor*, and the reciprocal molecule or substance that binds to the receptor is called a *ligand* or *adhesin*. Receptors may be proteins, carbohydrates, lipids, or complex molecules composed of all three. Similarly, ligands may be simple or complex molecules and, in some cases, highly specific structures. Ligands that bind to specific carbohydrates are called *lectins*. Certain bacteria produce pili or fimbriae, which anchor the organism to receptors on host cell membranes to establish an infection. Many viral agents, including influenza, mumps, and measles viruses and adenoviruses, produce filamentous appendages or spikes called *hemagglutinins*, which recognize carbohydrate receptors on the surfaces of specific cells in the upper respiratory tract of the host.

After initial attachment, a number of bacterial agents become embedded in a gelatinous matrix of polysaccharides called a *slime* or *mucous layer*. The slime layer serves two purposes: it anchors the agent firmly to host tissue surfaces and it protects the agent from the immunologic defenses of the host.

Evasive Factors

A number of factors produced by microorganisms enhance virulence by evading various components of the host's immune system. Extracellular polysaccharides, including capsules and slime or mucous layers, discourage engulfment and killing of pathogens by the host's phagocytic white blood cells (*i.e.*, neutrophils and macrophages). Encapsulated organisms such as *S. agalactiae, S. pneumoniae, N. meningitidis,* and *H. influenzae* type b (before the vaccine) are a cause of significant morbidity and mortality in neonates and children who lack protective anticapsular antibodies. Certain bacterial, fungal, and parasitic pathogens avoid phagocytosis by excreting leukocidin C toxins, which cause specific and lethal damage to the cell membrane of host neutrophils and macrophages. Other pathogens, such as the bacterial agents of listeriosis and Legionnaires disease, are adapted to survive and reproduce within phagocytic white blood cells after ingestion, avoiding or neutralizing the usually lethal products contained in the lysosomes of the cell.

Other unique strategies used by pathogenic microbes to evade immunologic surveillance have evolved solely to avoid recognition by host antibodies. Strains of *S. aureus* produce a surface protein (protein A) that immobilizes immunoglobulin G, holding the antigen-binding region harmlessly away from the organisms. This pathogen also secretes a unique enzyme called *coagulase*. Coagulase converts soluble human coagulation factors into a solid clot, which envelops and protects the organism from phagocytic host cells and antibodies. *H. influenzae* and *N. gonorrhoeae* secrete enzymes that cleave and inactivate secretory immunoglobulin A, neutralizing the primary defense of the respiratory and genital tracts at the site of infection. *H. pylori*, the infectious cause of gastritis and gastric ulcers, produces a urease enzyme on its outer cell wall. The urease converts gastric urea into ammonia, thus neutralizing the acidic environment of the stomach and allowing the organism to survive in this hostile environment. *Borrelia* species, including the agents of Lyme disease and relapsing fever, alter their surface antigens during the disease course to avoid immunologic detection.

Invasive Factors

Invasive factors are products produced by infectious agents that facilitate the penetration of anatomic barriers and host tissue. Most invasive factors are enzymes capable of destroying cellular membranes (*e.g.*, phospholipases), connective tissue (*e.g.*, elastases, collagenases), intercellular matrices (*e.g.*, hyaluronidase), and structural protein complexes (*e.g.*, proteases). It is the combined effects of invasive factors, toxins, and antimicrobial and inflammatory substances released by host cells to counter infection that mediate the tissue damage and pathophysiology of infectious diseases.

In summary, epidemiology is the study of factors, events, and circumstances that influence the transmission of disease. *Incidence* refers to the number of new cases of an infectious disease that occur in a defined population and *prevalence* to the number of active cases that are present at any given time. Infectious diseases are considered endemic in a geographic area if the incidence and prevalence are expected and relatively stable. An epidemic refers to an abrupt and unexpected increase in the incidence of a disease over endemic rates, and a pandemic to the spread of disease beyond continental boundaries.

The ultimate goal of epidemiology and epidemiologic studies is to devise strategies to interrupt or eliminate the spread of infectious disease. To accomplish this, infectious diseases are classified according to incidence, portal of entry, source, symptoms, disease course, site of infection, and virulence factors.

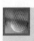

Diagnosis and Treatment of Infectious Diseases

DIAGNOSTIC METHODS

The diagnosis of an infectious disease requires two criteria: the recovery of a probable pathogen or evidence of its presence from the infected sites of a diseased host, and accurate documentation of clinical signs and symptoms (symptomatology) compatible with an infectious process. In the laboratory, the diagnosis of an infectious agent is accomplished using three basic techniques: culture, serology, or the detection of characteristic antigens, genomic sequences, or metabolites produced by the pathogen.

Culture

Culture refers to the propagation of a microorganism outside of the body, usually on or in artificial growth media such as agar plates or broth (Fig. 12-7). The specimen from the diseased host is inoculated into broth or onto the surface of an agar plate, and the culture is placed in a controlled environment such as an incubator until the growth of microorganisms becomes detectable. In the case of a bacterial pathogen, identification is based on microscopic appearance and Gram's stain reaction; shape, texture, and color (*i.e.*, morphology) of the colonies; and by a panel of reactions that fingerprint salient biochemical characteristics of the organism. Certain bacteria such as *Mycobacterium leprae*, the agent of leprosy, and *T. pallidum*, the syphilis spirochete, do not grow on artificial media and require additional methods of identification. Fungi and mycoplasmas are cultured in much the same way as bac-

teria but with more reliance on microscopic and colonial morphology for identification.

Chlamydiae, rickettsiae, and all human viruses are obligate intracellular pathogens. As a result, the propagation of these agents in the laboratory requires the inoculation of eukaryotic cells grown in culture (cell cultures). A cell culture consists of a flask containing a single layer, or monolayer, of eukaryotic cells covering the bottom and overlaid with broth containing essential nutrients and growth factors. When a virus infects and replicates in cultured eukaryotic cells, it produces pathologic changes in the appearance of the cell called the *cytopathic effect* (CPE). The CPE can be detected microscopically, and the pattern and extent of cellular destruction is often characteristic of a particular virus.

Although culture media have been developed for the growth of certain human protozoa and helminths in the laboratory, the diagnosis of parasitic infectious diseases has traditionally relied on microscopic, or in the case of worms, visible identification of organisms, cysts, or ova directly from infected patient specimens.

Serology

Serology—literally, "the study of serum"—is an indirect means of identifying infectious agents by measuring serum antibodies in the diseased host. A tentative diagnosis can be made if the antibody level, also called *antibody titer,* against a specific pathogen rises during the acute phase of the disease and falls during convalescence. Serologic identification of an infectious agent is not as accurate as culture, but it may be a useful adjunct, especially for the diagnosis of diseases caused by pathogens such as the hepatitis B virus that cannot be cultured. The measurement of antibody titers has another advantage in that specific antibody types such as immunoglobulin M (IgM) and IgG are produced by the host during different phases of an infectious process. IgM-specific antibodies usually rise and fall during the acute phase of the disease, whereas the synthesis of the IgG class of antibodies increases during the acute phase and remains elevated until or beyond resolution. Measurements of class-specific antibodies are also useful in the diagnosis of congenital infections. IgM antibodies do not cross the placenta, but certain IgG antibodies are transferred passively from mother to child during the final trimester of gestation. Consequently, an elevated level of pathogen-specific IgM antibodies in the serum of a neonate must have originated from the child and therefore indicates congenital infection. A similarly increased IgG titer in the neonate does not differentiate congenital from maternal infection.

The technology of *direct antigen detection* has evolved rapidly over the past decade and in the process has revolutionized the diagnosis of certain infectious diseases. Antigen detection incorporates features of culture and serology but reduces to a fraction the time required for diagnosis. In principle, this method relies on purified antibodies to detect antigens of infectious agents in specimens

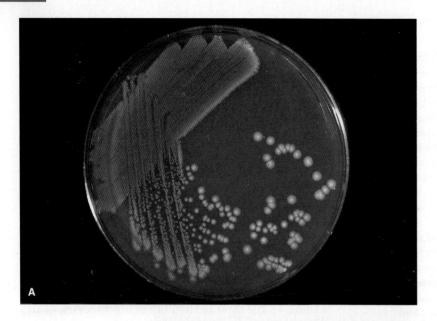

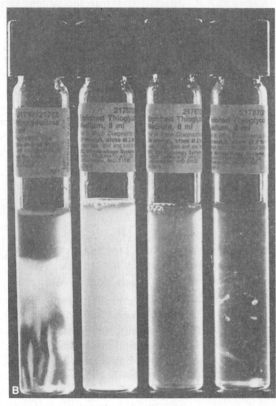

FIGURE 12-7 Variability of the macroscopic appearance of bacteria cultured on solid, agar-containing medium (**A**) and liquid broth medium (**B**). On solid surfaces, bacteria form distinct colonies, as demonstrated by the beta-hemolytic streptococcus, *Streptococcus pyogenes,* on sheep blood agar (**A**). Bacteria cultured in broth form a variety of growth patterns, ranging from particulate to homogeneous, turbid suspensions (**B**). Anaerobic bacteria cultured in liquid medium tend to grow best at the bottom of the tube, where the concentration of molecular oxygen is lowest. (**A** © Science Source/Photo Researchers.)

obtained from the diseased host. The source of antibodies used for antigen detection can be animals immunized against a particular pathogen or *hybridomas*. Hybridomas are created by fusing normal antibody-producing spleen cells from an immunized animal with malignant myeloma cells, which synthesize large quantities of antibody. The result is a cell that produces an antibody called a *monoclonal antibody,* which is highly specific for a single antigen and a single pathogen. Regardless of the source, the antibodies are labeled with a substance that allows micro-

scopic or overt detection when bound to the pathogen or its products. In general, the three types of labels used for this purpose are fluorescent dyes, enzymes, and particles such as latex beads. Fluorescent antibodies allow visualization of an infectious agent with the aid of fluorescence microscopy. Depending on the type of fluorescent dye used, the organism may appear as bright green or orange against a black background, making detection extremely easy. Enzyme-labeled antibodies function in a similar manner. The enzyme is capable of converting a colorless compound into a colored substance, thereby permitting detection of antibody bound to an infectious agent without the use of fluorescence microscopy. Particles coated with antibodies clump together, or agglutinate, when the appropriate antigen is present in a specimen. Particle agglutination is especially useful when examining infected body fluids such as urine, serum, or spinal fluid.

DNA and RNA Sequencing

Methods for identifying infectious agents through the detection of DNA or RNA sequences unique to a single agent have undergone rapid development since the mid-1990s, and are increasingly used. Several techniques have been devised to accomplish this goal, each having different degrees of sensitivity regarding the number of organisms that need to be present in a specimen for detection. The first of these methods is called *DNA probe hybridization*. Small fragments of DNA are cut from the genome of a specific pathogen and labeled with compounds (photo-emitting chemicals or antigens) that allow detection. The labeled DNA probes are added to specimens from an infected host. If the pathogen is present, the probe attaches to the complementary strand of DNA on the genome of the infectious agent, permitting rapid diagnosis. The use of labeled probes has allowed visualization of particular agents within and around individual cells in histologic sections of tissue.

A second and more sensitive method of DNA detection, the *polymerase chain reaction* (PCR), can detect single copies of viral DNA by amplifying the DNA many millionfold (Fig. 12-8). It also allows for the diagnosis of infections caused by microorganisms that are impossible or difficult to grow in culture. PCR uses two unique reagents: a specific pair of oligonucleotides called *primers*, which are complementary to the ends of the known genetic sequence in the virus, and a heat-stable DNA polymerase. To perform the assay, the primers are added to the specimen containing the suspect pathogen, and the sample is heated to melt the DNA in the specimen, and then allowed to cool. The primers locate and bind only to the complementary target DNA of the pathogen in question. The heat-stable polymerase begins to replicate the DNA from the point at which the primers attached, similar to two trains approaching one another on separate but converging tracks. After the initial cycle, DNA polymerization ceases at the point where the primers were located, producing a strand of DNA with a distinct size, depending on the distance separating the two primers. The specimen is heated again, and the process starts anew. After many cycles of heating, cooling, and polymerization, a large number of uniformly sized DNA fragments are produced only if the specific pathogen (or its DNA) is present in the specimen. The polymerized DNA fragments are separated by electrophoresis and visualized with a dye or identified by hybridization with a specific probe.

Several variations of molecular gene detection techniques in addition to PCR have been developed and incorporated into diagnostic kits for use in the clinical laboratory. Many of the newer gene detection technologies have been adapted for quantitation of the target DNA

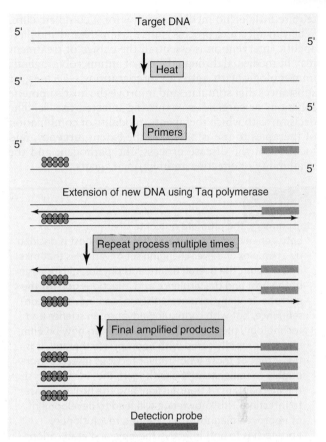

FIGURE 12-8 The polymerase chain reaction. The target DNA is first melted using heat (generally around 94°C) to separate the strands of DNA. Primers that recognize specific sequences within the target DNA are allowed to bind as the reaction cools. Using a unique, thermostable DNA polymerase called Taq and an abundance of deoxynucleoside triphosphates, new DNA strands are amplified from the point of the primer attachment. The process is repeated many times (called cycles) until millions of copies of DNA are produced, all of which have the same length defined by the distance (in base pairs) between the primer binding sites. These copies are then detected by electrophoresis and staining or through the use of labeled DNA probes that, similar to the primers, recognize a specific sequence located within the amplified section of DNA.

or RNA in serum specimens of patients infected with viruses such as HIV and hepatitis C. If therapy is effective, viral replication is suppressed and the viral load (level of viral genome) in the peripheral blood is low. Conversely, if mutations in the viral genome lead to resistant strains or if the antiviral therapy is ineffective, viral replication and the patient's viral load rise, indicating a need to change the therapeutic approach.

TREATMENT

The goal of treatment for an infectious disease is complete removal of the pathogen from the host and the restoration of normal physiologic function to damaged tissues. Most infectious diseases of humans are self-limiting in that they require little or no medical therapy for a complete cure. When an infectious process gains the upper hand and therapeutic intervention is essential, the choice of treatment may be medicinal through the use of antimicrobial agents; immunologic with antibody preparations, vaccines, or substances that stimulate and improve the host's immune function; or surgical by removing infected tissues. The decision as to which therapeutic modality or combination of therapies to use is based on the extent, urgency, and location of the disease process, the pathogen, and the availability of effective antimicrobial agents.

In summary, the ultimate outcome of any interaction between microorganisms and the human host is decided by a complex and ever-changing set of variables that take into account the overall health and physiologic function of the host and the virulence and infectious dose of the microbe. In many instances, disease is an inevitable consequence, but with continuing advances in science and technology, the vast majority of cases can now be eliminated or rapidly cured with appropriate therapy. It is the intent of those who study infectious diseases thoroughly to understand the pathogen, the disease course, the mechanisms of transmission, and the host response to infection. This knowledge will lead to development of improved diagnostic techniques, revolutionary approaches to anti-infective therapy, and eradication or control of microscopic agents that cause frightening devastation and loss of life throughout the world.

Bioterrorism and Emerging Global Infectious Diseases

BIOTERRORISM

In October of 2001, less than 1 month after the tragedy of September 11th, the world became instantly acquainted with the term *bioterrorism.* By the end of November of that year, 22 cases of human anthrax (11 cutaneous and 11 inhalation) had been identified, resulting in 5 deaths, and all cases were associated with exposure to 4 intentionally contaminated envelopes delivered through the U.S. Postal Service. Although the possibility of such an attack had been discussed in a workshop hosted by the Centers for Disease Control and Prevention (CDC) 3 years earlier, the reality of the 2001 outbreak brought a new awareness concerning the use of microorganisms as weapons.

Anthrax is an ancient disease caused by the cutaneous inoculation, inhalation, or ingestion of the spores of *Bacillus anthracis,* a gram-positive bacillus. Anthrax is more commonly known as a disease of herbivores that can be transmitted to humans through contact with infected secretions, soil, or animal products. It is a rare disease in the United States, and so the sudden increase

in cases over a short period of time was a chilling indication that the spread of the organism had been intentional. Fortunately, the number of deaths was limited thanks to prompt recognition of cases by private physicians and public health personnel and rapid institution of antimicrobial prophylaxis to exposed individuals.

To prepare for the possibility of secondary bioterrorist attacks, the CDC (www.cdc.gov), along with other federal, state, and local agencies, has created the laboratory response network (LRN). The LRN is a tiered structure consisting of laboratories with ever-increasing expertise, responsibility, and biocontainment facilities that allows for the rapid and coordinated detection and identification of bioterrorism events under safe working conditions.

Potential agents of bioterrorism have been categorized into three levels (A, B, C) based on risk of use, transmissibility, invasiveness, and mortality rate. The agents considered to be in the highest biothreat level include *B. anthracis, Yersinia pestis* (the cause of bubonic plague), *Francisella tularensis* (the cause of tularemia), variola major virus (smallpox), and several hemorrhagic fever viruses (Ebola, Marburg, Lassa, and Junin). The toxin of the anaerobic gram-positive organism *Clostridium botulinum,* which causes the neuromuscular paralysis termed *botulism,* is also listed as a category A agent. Interestingly, purified *C. botulinum* toxins A and B are finding increasing use under the trade names of Botox, Myobloc, and Neurobloc for various medicinal and cosmetic purposes. The category B agents include agents of foodborne and waterborne disease (*Salmonella, Shigella, Vibrio cholerae, E. coli* O157:H7), agents of zoonotic infections (*Brucella* species, *Coxiella burnetii, Burkholderia mallei*), viral encephalitides (Venezuelan, Western, and Eastern equine encephalitis viruses), as well as toxins from *S. aureus, Clostridium perfringens,* and *Ricinus communis* (the castor bean). Category C agents are defined as emerging pathogens and potential risks for the future even though many of these organisms are causes of ancient diseases. Category C agents include *M. tuberculosis,* Nipah virus, Hantavirus, tickborne and Yellow fever viruses, and the only protozoan of the group, *Cryptosporidium parvum.*

The potential for bioterrorism using smallpox virus pilfered from frozen stocks maintained in unsecured laboratory facilities has reinvigorated a national vaccination program in the United States that ended with the last reported human case of smallpox in 1978. Because the availability of smallpox vaccine is limited, a tiered approach to vaccination has been undertaken to protect individuals most likely to encounter sentinel cases of the disease should an outbreak occur (*e.g.,* emergency department personnel, infectious diseases physicians, laboratory personnel, and public health workers). Efforts are also underway to engineer and rapidly manufacture a safer form of the vaccine to avoid the side effects associated with the older vaccinia virus vaccine.

GLOBAL INFECTIOUS DISEASES

Aided by a global market and the ease of international travel, the past decade has witnessed the importation or emergence of a host of novel infectious diseases. During the late summer and early fall of 1999, West Nile virus (WNV; an arthropod-borne flavivirus) was identified as the cause of an epidemic involving 56 patients in the New York City area. This outbreak, which led to seven deaths (primarily in the elderly) marked the first time that WNV had been recognized in the Western hemisphere since its discovery in Uganda nearly 60 years earlier. Because WNV is a mosquito-borne disease and is transmitted to a number of susceptible avian (*e.g.*, blue jays, crows, and hawks) and equine hosts, the potential for rapid and sustained spread of the disease across the United States was appreciated early. By the fall of 2002, a national surveillance network had detected WNV activity in 2289 counties from 44 states, including Los Angeles County, California, and had identified more than 3000 human cases. The disease ranges in intensity from nonspecific febrile illness to fulminant meningoencephalitis. In 2002 alone, 3389 cases of WNV-associated illness were identified in the United States with 201 deaths, making this the largest arboviral meningoencephalitis outbreak ever described in the Western hemisphere. Efforts to prevent further spread of the disease are currently centered on surveillance of WNV-associated illness in birds, humans, and other mammals, as well as mosquito control.

In the winter of 2003, the Ministry of Health of China reported 305 cases of a mysterious and virulent respiratory tract illness that had appeared in Guangdong province in southern China over the previous 4 months. The illness was highly transmissible as evidenced by the spread of the disease to household contacts of sick individuals and medical personnel caring for patients with the disease. In a very short time, patients with compatible symptoms were recognized in Hong Kong and Vietnam. The illness was called *severe acute respiratory syndrome* (SARS), and the World Health Organization (WHO) promptly issued a global alert and started international surveillance for patients with typical symptomatology with a history of travel to the endemic region. As of June 2003, more than 8000 cases of SARS from 29 countries and 809 deaths were reported to WHO. In a remarkable feat of molecular technology, the etiology of SARS was quickly determined to be a novel coronavirus possibly of mammalian or avian origin, and its entire genome was sequenced by the end of May 2003. Because of the intense effort by WHO in conjunction with international health agencies, the SARS epidemic was held in check (temporary or permanent) through the use of intense infection control strategies, and by the summer of 2003, most travel restrictions to countries with high levels of endemic disease were lifted.

In May of 2003, a child was seen in central Wisconsin for fever, lymphadenopathy, and a papular rash. Electron microscopic examination of tissue from one of the patient's skin lesions revealed a virus that morphologically resembled poxvirus, generating immediate concern because of the awareness of the potential for bioterrorism using smallpox virus. However, the same virus was identified from a lymph node biopsy of the patient's ill pet prairie dog. Additional testing of the patient and the prairie dog

specimens indicated that the virus was a monkeypox virus, a member of the orthopoxvirus family of viruses. By the beginning of June, 53 possible cases of monkeypox infection were being followed in Wisconsin, Illinois, and Indiana. Epidemiologic investigations conducted by state and federal health care agencies identified the potential source of the virus as nine different species of small mammals, including Gambian giant rats that had been imported from Ghana in April and were housed in common facilities with prairie dogs. A number of these animals were then shipped to a pet distributor in Illinois and subsequently sold to the public.

These three scenarios highlight the rapidity with which novel or exotic diseases can be introduced into nonindigenous regions of the world and to a susceptible population. Although great strides in molecular microbiology have allowed for the rapid identification of new or rare microorganisms, the potential devastation in terms of human and economic loss is great, underscoring the need to maintain resources for public health surveillance and intervention.

In summary, the challenges associated with maintaining health throughout a global community are becoming increasingly apparent. Aided by a global market and the ease of international travel, the past decade has witnessed the importation and emergence of a host of novel infectious diseases. There is also the potential threat for the deliberate use of microorganisms as weapons of bioterrorism.

Review Exercises

Microorganisms are capable of causing infection only if they can grow at the temperature of the infected body site.

A. Using this concept, explain the different sites of fungal infections due to the dermatophyte fungal species that causes tinea pedis (athlete's foot) and *Candida albicans*, which causes infections of the mouth (thrush) and female genitalia (vulvovaginitis).

The threat of global infections, such as severe acute respiratory syndrome (SARS), continues to grow.

A. What would you propose to be one of the most important functions of health care professionals in terms of controlling the spread of such infections?

BIBLIOGRAPHY

Butler J. C., Peters C. J. (1994). Hantaviruses and hantavirus pulmonary syndrome. *Clinical Infectious Diseases* 19, 387–395.

Centers for Disease Control and Prevention. (2003). Multistate outbreak of monkeypox—Illinois, Indiana, and Wisconsin, 2003. *MMWR Morbidity and Mortality Weekly Report* 52, 537–540.

Centers for Disease Control and Prevention. (1999). Outbreak of West Nile–like viral encephalitis—New York. *MMWR Morbidity and Mortality Weekly Report* 48, 845–849.

Centers for Disease Control and Prevention. (2002). Provisional surveillance summary of the West Nile virus epidemic—United States, January–November 2002. *MMWR Morbidity and Mortality Weekly Report* 51, 1129–1133.

Centers for Disease Control and Prevention. (2003). Update: Severe acute respiratory syndrome—worldwide and United States, 2003. *MMWR Morbidity and Mortality Weekly Report* 52, 664–665.

Dunne W. M., Jr. (2002). Bacterial adhesion: Seen any good biofilms lately? *Clinical Microbiology Review* 15, 155–166.

Jernigan D. M., Raghunathan P. L., Bell B. P., et al. (2002). Investigation of bioterrorism-related anthrax, United States, 2001: Epidemiologic findings. *Emerging Infectious Diseases* 8, 1019–1028.

McAdam A. J., Sharpe A. H. (2005). Infectious diseases. In Kumar V., Abbas A. K., Fausto N. (Eds.), *Robbins and Cotran pathologic basis of disease* (7th ed., pp. 343–414). Philadelphia: Elsevier Saunders.

Murray P. R., Rosenthal K. S., Kohayashi G. S., et al. (2001). *Medical microbiology* (4th ed.). St. Louis: Mosby.

O'Brien K. K., Higdon M. L., Halverson J. J. (2003). Recognition and management of bioterrorism infections. *American Family Physician* 67, 1927–1934.

Ryan E. T., Wilson M. E., Kain K. C. (2002). Illness after international travel. *New England Journal of Medicine* 347, 505–516.

Tyler K. L. (2000). Prions and prion diseases of the central nervous system (neurodegenerative diseases). In Mandell G. L., Bennett J. E., Dolin R. (Eds.), *Mandell, Douglas, and Bennett's principles and practice of infectious diseases* (5th ed., pp. 1971–1985). Philadelphia: Churchill Livingstone.

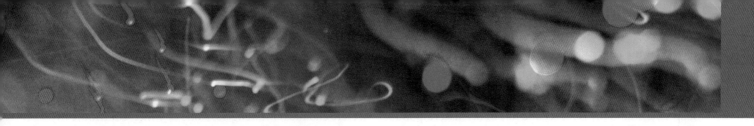

Chapter *13*

The Immune Response

The immune system is clearly essential for survival. It constantly defends the body against bacteria, viruses, and other foreign substances it encounters. It also defends against abnormal cells and molecules that periodically develop in the body, such as cancer cells. An essential aspect of the immune response is the ability to distinguish self from nonself; to discriminate potentially harmful agents from nonharmful agents; to recall previous encounters with the same agent; and to mount an effective response.

The major focus of this chapter is to present an overview of the immune system, its cells, and the tissues in which they develop, and to describe the mechanisms used to protect the body against foreign substances.

The Immune System

The term *immunity* has come to mean the protection from disease and, more specifically, infectious disease. The collective, coordinated response of the cells and molecules of the immune system is called the *immune response*. Although the relationship between microbes and infectious diseases dates far back in history, it has only been within the last 50 to 60 years that an understanding of the cellular and biochemical mechanisms involved in the immune response has begun to emerge. Advances in cell culture techniques, immunochemistry, recombinant deoxyribonucleic acid (DNA) technology, and the creation of genetically altered animals, such as "transgenic" and "knockout" mice, have transformed immunology from a largely descriptive science to one of immune phenomena that can be explained in structural and biochemical terms.

INNATE AND ADAPTIVE IMMUNE DEFENSES

There are two types of immune defenses; the early reactions of innate immunity and the later responses of adaptive immunity. As a first line of defense, the innate immune system is able to distinguish self from nonself but is unable to distinguish between pathogens. Adaptive, or specific, immunity is the second line of defense, responding less rapidly than innate immunity but more effectively. Adaptive immunity responds through focused recognition and an amplified response to each unique type of foreign agent.

Innate and adaptive immune responses form a dynamic network in which numerous cells and molecules function cooperatively. Innate immunity produces an immediate response and serves to control or contain an infection while the adaptive immune responses are being produced. The many microorganisms not controlled by innate immunity require the more specific functions of adaptive immunity. There are two powerful links between innate and adaptive immunities. First, the innate immune response stimulates and influences the nature of adaptive immune responses. Second, adaptive immune responses use many of the effector mechanisms of innate immunity to eliminate microbes, and they often function by enhancing the antimicrobial defenses of innate immunity.

Innate Immunity

Innate immunity (also called *natural* or *native immunity*) consists of cellular and biochemical defenses that are in place before infection and respond rapidly to it. These mechanisms normally respond only to microbes, and they respond in essentially the same way to different types of infections. The major components of the innate immune system are the epithelial barriers that block entry of infectious agents; phagocytic cells (mainly neutrophils and macrophages); natural killer (NK) cells; several types of plasma proteins, including members of the complement system and other mediators of inflammation; and cell messengers, called *cytokines,* that regulate and coordinate many of the activities of the cells of innate immunity.

The epithelial surfaces of the body keep pathogens out and protect against colonization by preventing pathogen adherence and by secreting antimicrobial enzymes and peptides. Microorganisms that overcome this barrier are faced immediately with destruction by phagocytic tissue macrophages that can engulf and destroy many different types of pathogens. This, in turn, leads to an inflammatory response, which causes accumulation of plasma proteins, including the complement components (to be discussed), and phagocytic neutrophils at the site of infection. Activated NK cells can also serve to contain certain pathogens.

The various innate immune responses are set in motion by generic molecules associated with threatening pathogens, such as the carbohydrates typically found in bacterial cell walls but not in mammalian cells. These molecules are recognized by a recently discovered family of membrane proteins, called *Toll-like receptors,* that are present on phagocytic cells of the innate immune system. The Toll-like receptors, which have been described as the eyes of the innate immune system, recognize and bind with telltale pathogen markers, allowing the effector cells of the innate immune system to "see" the pathogens as distinct from self-cells. Recognition of a pathogen by the receptor triggers the phagocyte to engulf and destroy the infectious agent. It also triggers the phagocytic cell to secrete chemical messengers, some of which contribute to inflammation—an important innate response to microbial invasion. Still other chemicals secreted by the phagocytes are important in recruiting cells of the adaptive immune system.

Adaptive Immunity

Adaptive immunity (also known as *acquired,* or *specific, immunity*) is able to recognize and react to a large number of microbes and nonmicrobial substances. In addition, it is able to distinguish among the different, even closely related, microbes and molecules. The components of the adaptive immune system are white blood cells, called *lymphocytes,* and their products. Foreign substances that elicit specific responses are called *antigens.* There are two types of adaptive immune responses: humoral and cell-mediated. *Humoral immunity* is mediated by molecules in the blood and is the principal defense against extracellular microbes and toxins. *Cell-mediated immunity,* or *cellular immunity,* is mediated by specific T lymphocytes and defends against intracellular microbes such as viruses. In contrast to innate immunity, adaptive immunity exhibits exact or specific recognition of the microbe, can amplify and sustain its responses, and has the unique ability to "remember" the pathogen and quickly produce a heightened immune response on subsequent encounters with the same agent. By convention, the terms *immune responses* and *immune system* usually refer to adaptive immunity.

ANTIGENS

Before discussing the cells and responses inherent to immunity, it is important to understand the substances that elicit a response from the host. *Antigens,* or *immunogens,* are substances foreign to the host that can stimulate an immune response. These foreign molecules are recognized by receptors on immune cells and by proteins, called *antibodies* or *immunoglobulins,* which are secreted in response to the antigen. Antigens include components of the microbial world, including those found on bacteria, fungi, viruses, protozoa, and parasites. Nonmicrobial agents, such as plant pollens, poison ivy resin, insect venom, and transplanted organs, can also act as antigens. Most antigens are macromolecules, although lipids and nucleic acids occasionally can serve as antigens.

Antigens, which are large and chemically complex molecules, are biologically degraded into smaller chemical units or peptides. These discrete, immunologically active sites on antigens are called *antigenic determinants* or *epitopes* (Fig. 13-1). It is the unique molecular shape of an epitope that is recognized by a specific immunoglobulin receptor found on the surface of the lymphocyte or by an antigen-binding site of a secreted antibody. A single antigen may contain multiple antigenic determinants, each stimulating a distinct clone of lymphocytes to produce a unique type of antibody. For example, different proteins that comprise a virus may function as unique antigens, each of which contains several antigenic determinants. Hundreds of antigenic determinants are found on structures such as the bacterial cell wall.

Smaller substances (molecular masses <10,000 daltons) usually are unable to stimulate an adequate immune response by themselves. When these low–molecular-weight compounds, known as *haptens*, combine with larger protein molecules, they function as antigens. The proteins act as carrier molecules for the haptens to form antigenic hapten–carrier complexes. An allergic response to the antibiotic penicillin is an example of a medically important reaction due to hapten–carrier complexes. Penicillin (molecular mass of approximately 350 daltons) is normally a nonantigenic molecule. However, in some individuals, it can chemically combine with body proteins to form larger complexes that can then generate a potentially harmful immune allergic response.

IMMUNE CELLS

The principal cells of the immune system are the lymphocytes, antigen-presenting cells, and effector cells. Lymphocytes are the cells that specifically recognize and respond to foreign antigens. Accessory cells, such as macrophages and dendritic cells, function as antigen-presenting cells (APCs) by the processing of a complex antigen into epitopes required for the activation of lymphocytes. Functionally, there are two types of immune cells: regulatory cells and effector cells. The *regulatory cells* assist in orchestrating and controlling the immune response. For example, helper T lymphocytes activate other lymphocytes and phagocytes. The final stages of the immune response are accomplished with the elimination of the antigen by *effector cells*. Activated T lymphocytes, mononuclear phago-

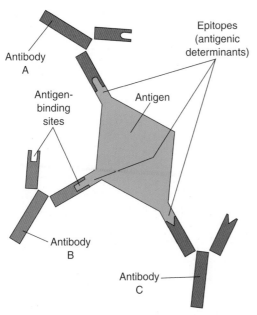

FIGURE 13-1 Multiple epitopes on a complex antigen being recognized by their respective (A, B, C) antibodies.

Labels in figure:
Antibody A
Antigen-binding sites
Antibody B
Antibody C
Epitopes (antigenic determinants)
Antigen

cytes, and other leukocytes (*e.g.*, neutrophils) function as effector cells in different immune responses.

Lymphocytes represent 25% to 35% of blood leukocytes, and 99% of the lymphocytes reside in the lymph. Like other blood cells, lymphocytes are generated from stem cells in the bone marrow (Fig. 13-2). One class of lymphocyte, the *B lymphocytes* (B cells), matures in the bone marrow and is essential for *humoral, or antibody-mediated, immunity*. The other class of lymphocyte, the *T lymphocytes* (T cells), completes its maturation in the thymus and functions in the peripheral tissues to produce *cell-mediated immunity*, as well as aiding antibody production. Approximately 60% to 70% of blood lymphocytes are T cells and 10% to 20% are B cells. The various types of lymphocytes are distinguished by their function and response to antigen, their cell membrane molecules and receptors, their types of secreted proteins, and their tissue location.

The key trigger for the activation of B and T cells is the recognition of the antigen by unique surface receptors. The B-cell antigen receptor consists of membrane-bound immunoglobulin molecules that can bind to a specific epitope on the antigen surface. The T-cell receptor recognizes a processed antigen peptide in association with a self-recognition protein, called a *major histocompatibility complex* (MHC) molecule (to be discussed).

Activation of the lymphocytes depends on the appropriate processing and presentation of antigen to the T lymphocytes by APCs such as macrophages (Fig. 13-3). On recognition of antigen and after additional stimulation

Understanding ➡ Innate and Adaptive Immunity

The body's defense against microbes is mediated by two types of immunity: (1) innate immunity and (2) adaptive immunity. Both types of immunity are members of an integrated system in which numerous cells and molecules function cooperatively to protect the body against foreign invaders. The innate immune system stimulates adaptive immunity and influences the nature of the adaptive immune responses to make them more effective. While they use different mechanisms of pathogen recognition, both types of immunity use many of the same effector mechanisms, including destruction of the pathogen by phagocytosis and the complement system.

1

Innate immunity. Innate immunity (also called natural or inborn immunity) consists of the cellular and biochemical defenses that are in place before an encounter with an infectious agent and that provide rapid protection against infection. The major effector components of innate immunity include epithelial cells, which block the entry of infectious agents; phagocytic neutrophils and macrophages, which engulf and digest microbes; natural killer (NK) cells, which kill foreign cells; complement proteins, which produce an inflammatory response; and cytokines, which influence adaptive immune responses. The innate immune system uses pattern recognition receptors to recognize structures that are shared by microbes and are often essential to their survival, but are not present on human cells. Thus, the innate immune system is able to distinguish between self and nonself, but lacks the ability to differentiate between agents.

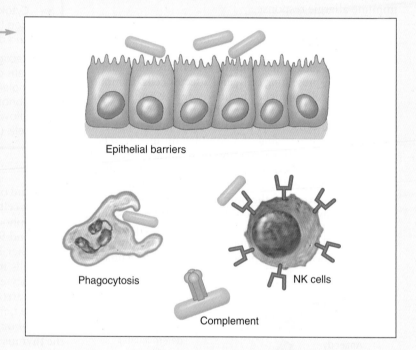

Epithelial barriers

Phagocytosis

NK cells

Complement

2

Adaptive immunity. Adaptive immunity (also called acquired immunity) refers to immunity that is acquired through previous exposure to infectious and other foreign agents. A defining characteristic of adaptive immunity is the ability not only to distinguish self from nonself, but to recognize and destroy specific foreign agents based on their distinct antigenic properties. The components of the adaptive immune system are the T and B lymphocytes and their products. There are two types of adaptive immune responses, humoral and cell-mediated immunity, that function to eliminate different types of microbes.

Humoral immunity is mediated by the B lymphocytes (B cells) and is the principal defense against extracellular microbes and their toxins. The B cells differentiate into antibody-secreting plasma cells. The circulating antibodies then interact with and destroy the microbes that are present in the blood or mucosal surfaces.

Cell-mediated, or cellular, immunity is mediated by the cytotoxic T lymphocytes (T cells) and functions in the elimination of intracellular pathogens (e.g., viruses). T cells develop receptors that recognize the viral peptides displayed on the surface of infected cells and then signal destruction of the infected cells.

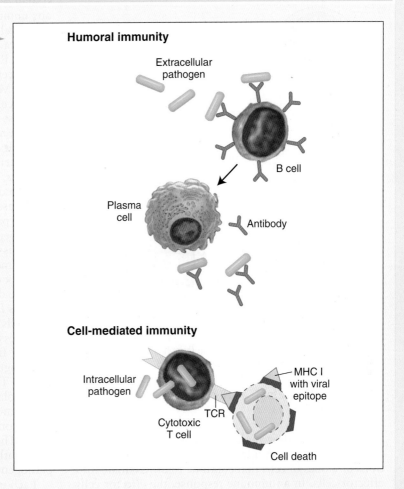

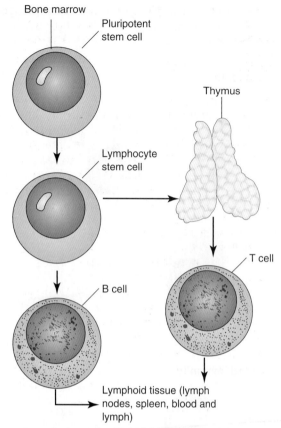

FIGURE 13-2 Pathway for T- and B-cell differentiation.

by secreted signaling molecules called *cytokines*, the T and B lymphocytes divide several times to form populations or clones of cells that continue to differentiate into effector cells. In an immune response, the effector cells destroy the antigen and the memory cells retain the information needed for future encounters with the antigen.

Clusters of Differentiation

T and B cells display additional membrane molecules called *clusters of differentiation* (CD). These molecules aid the function of immune cells and also serve to define functionally distinct subsets of cells, such as CD4+ helper T cells and CD8+ cytotoxic T cells. The many cell surface CD molecules detected on immune cells have allowed scientists to identify distinct subsets of lymphocytes and study both the normal and abnormal developmental processes displayed by these cells.

Major Histocompatibility Complex Molecules

An essential feature of adaptive immunity is the ability to discriminate between the body's own molecules and foreign antigens. Key recognition molecules essential for distinguishing self from nonself are the cell surface MHC molecules. These proteins, which in humans are coded by closely linked genes on chromosome 6, were first identified because of their role in organ and tissue transplanta-

tion. When cells are transplanted between individuals who are not identical for their MHC molecules, the immune system recognizes them as foreign and produces a vigorous immune response, leading to rejection of the transferred cells or organs. MHC molecules did not evolve to reject transplanted tissues, a situation not encountered in nature. Rather, these molecules are essential for correct cell-to-cell interactions among immune and body cells.

The MHC molecules involved in self-recognition and cell-to-cell communication fall into two classes, class I and class II (Fig. 13-4). The class I molecules are involved in the recognition of intracellular antigens and the class II molecules in the recognition of extracellular antigens that have been endocytosed by immune cells.

Class I MHC molecules are found on virtually all nucleated cells in the body. Antigen peptides associate with class I molecules in cells that are infected by intracellular pathogens, such as a virus. As the virus multiplies, small peptides from degraded viral proteins associate with class I MHC molecules and are then transported to the cell membrane of the infected cell. This MHC–antigen complex communicates to cytotoxic T cells that the cell must be destroyed for the overall survival of the host.

Class II MHC molecules are found primarily on phagocytic cells such as macrophages, dendritic cells, and B lymphocytes that engulf extracellular antigens. Class II MHC binds a fragment of antigen from pathogens that have been engulfed and digested during the process of phagocytosis. The engulfed pathogen is degraded into peptides in cytoplasmic vesicles and then complexed with class II MHC molecules. Helper T cells recognize these complexes on the surface of APCs and then become activated. These triggered helper T cells multiply quickly and direct other immune cells to respond to the invading pathogen through the secretion of cytokines.

Each individual has a unique collection of MHC proteins, and a variety of MHC molecules can exist in a population. Because of the number of MHC genes and the possibility of several alleles for each gene, it is almost impossible for any two individuals to be identical, except if they are identical twins.

Human MHC proteins are called *human leukocyte antigens* (HLA) because they were first detected on white blood cells. Because these molecules play a role in transplant rejection and are detected by immunologic tests, they are commonly called *antigens*. The human class I MHC molecules are divided into types called HLA-A, HLA-B, and HLA-C, and the class II MHC molecules are identified as HLA-DR, HLA-DP, and HLA-DQ (Table 13-1). Each of the gene loci that describe HLA molecules can be occupied by multiple alleles or alternate genes. For example, there are more than 120 possible genes for the A locus and 250 genes for the B locus. The genes and their expressed molecule are designated by a letter and numbers (*i.e.*, HLA-B27).

Because the class I and class II MHC genes are closely linked on one chromosome, the combination of HLA genes usually is inherited as a unit, called a *haplotype*. Each person inherits a chromosome from each parent and therefore has two HLA haplotypes. The identifica-

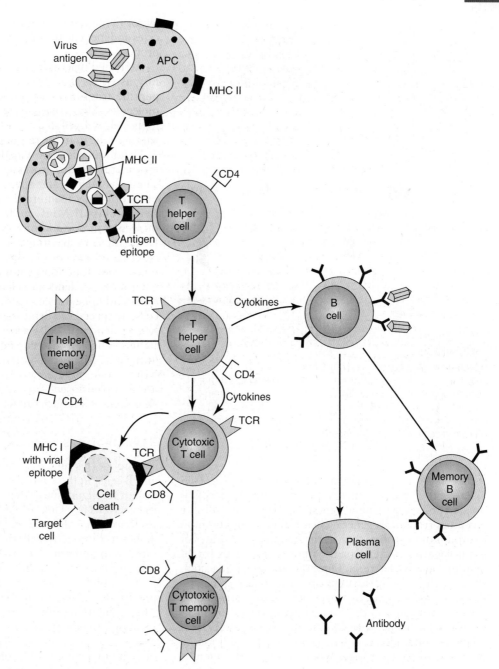

FIGURE 13-3 Pathway for immune cell participation in an immune response.

tion or typing of HLA molecules is important in tissue or organ transplantation, forensics, and paternity evaluations. In organ or tissue transplantation, the closer the matching of HLA types, the greater is the probability of identical antigens and the lower the chance of rejection.

Monocytes, Macrophages, and Dendritic Cells

Monocytes, tissue macrophages, and most dendritic cells arise from a common precursor in the bone marrow. Monocytes and macrophages are key members of the mononuclear phagocytic system that engulf and digest microbes and other foreign substances. The monocytes migrate from the blood to various tissues where they mature into the major tissue phagocytes, the macrophages. As the general scavenger cells of the body, macrophages can be fixed in a tissue or free to migrate from an organ to lymphoid tissues. The tissue macrophages are scattered in connective tissue or clustered in organs such as the lung (*i.e.*, alveolar macrophages), liver (*i.e.*, Kupffer cells), spleen, lymph nodes, peritoneum, central nervous system (*i.e.*, microglial cells), and other areas.

Macrophages are activated to engulf and digest antigens that come in contact with their cell membrane. The initial attachment of the microbe to the phagocyte can be aided by antibody or complement-coated microbes or by

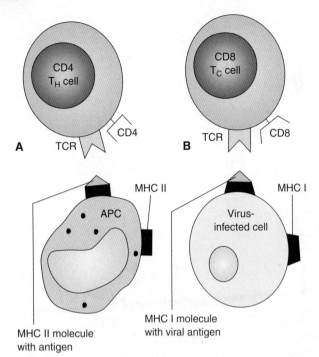

FIGURE 13-4 (**A**) Recognition by a T-cell receptor (TCR) on a CD4 helper T (T$_H$) cell of an epitope associated with a class II major histocompatibility complex (MHC) molecule on an antigen-presenting cell (APC). (**B**) Recognition by a TCR on a CD8 cytotoxic T cell (T$_C$) of a viral antigen associated with a class I MHC molecule on a virus-infected cell.

pathogen-associated molecular pattern receptors (*i.e.*, Toll-like receptors) that are integral to innate immune recognition. On phagocyte membranes, the family of Toll-like receptors recognizes general chemical patterns common to groups of microbes, such as the lipopolysaccharides of gram-negative bacteria or the lipoteichoic acids found in gram-positive bacteria. Once the microbe is ingested, the cell generates digestive enzymes and toxic oxygen and nitrogen products (*i.e.*, hydrogen peroxide or nitric oxide) through metabolic pathways). The phagocytic killing of microorganisms helps to contain infectious agents until adaptive immunity can be marshaled. In addition to phagocytosis, macrophages function early in the immune response to amplify the inflammatory response and initiate adaptive immunity. Macrophages direct these processes through the secretion of cytokines (*e.g.*, tumor necrosis

factor [TNF], interleukin-1 [IL-1]) that activate lymphocytes and mediate the different aspects of the inflammatory process.

Activated macrophages also influence adaptive immunity as APCs that break down complex antigens into peptide fragments for association with class II MHC molecules. Macrophages can then present these complexes to the helper T cell so that self–nonself recognition and activation of the immune response can occur (Fig. 13-3).

Dendritic cells share with the macrophage the important task of presenting processed antigen to T lymphocytes. These distinctive, star-shaped cells with long extensions of cytoplasmic membrane provide an extensive surface rich in class II MHC molecules and other membrane molecules important for initiation of adaptive immunity. Dendritic cells are found in most tissues where antigen enters the body and in the peripheral lymphoid tissues where they function as potent APCs. In these different environments, dendritic cells can acquire specialized functions and appearances, as do macrophages. Langerhans cells are specialized dendritic cells in the skin, whereas follicular dendritic cells are found in the lymph nodes. Langerhans cells are constantly surveying the skin for antigen and can transport foreign material to a nearby lymph node. Skin dendritic cells and macrophages also are involved in cell-mediated immune reactions of the skin such as allergic contact dermatitis.

T Lymphocytes

T lymphocytes function in the activation of other T cells and B cells, in the control of viral infections, in the rejection of foreign tissue grafts, and in delayed hypersensitivity reactions (see Chapter 15). Collectively, these immune responses are called *cell-mediated immunity*. Besides the ability to respond to cell-associated antigens, the T cell is integral to immunity because it regulates self-recognition and amplifies the response of B and T lymphocytes.

T lymphocytes arise from bone marrow stem cells as pre-T cells and migrate to the thymus for their maturation. There, the immature T lymphocytes undergo rearrangement of the genes needed for expression of a unique T-cell antigen receptor. The T-cell receptor (TCR) is composed of two polypeptides that fold to form a groove that recognizes processed antigen peptide–MHC complexes. The TCR–antigen–MHC complex is further stabilized by the CD4+ molecule on helper T cells or the CD8+ molecule on

TABLE 13-1	**Properties of MHC Class I and MHC Class II Molecules**	
Properties	**MHC Class I**	**MHC Class II**
HLA antigens	HLA-A, HLA-B, HLA-C	HLA-DR, HLA-DP, HLA-DQ
Distribution	Virtually all nucleated cells	Restricted to immune cells, antigen-presenting cells, B cells, and macrophages
Functions	Present processed antigen to cytotoxic CD8+ T cells; restrict cytolysis to virus-infected cells, tumor cells, transplanted cells	Present processed antigenic fragments to CD4+ T cells; necessary for effective interaction among immune cells

HLA, human leukocyte antigen; MHC, major histocompatibility complex.

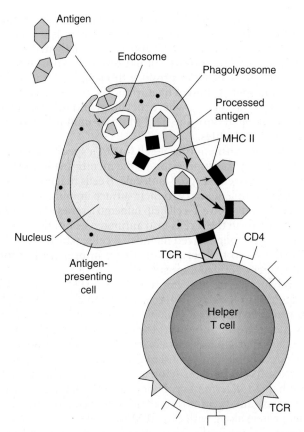

FIGURE 13-5 Processing and presentation of antigen associated with a class II major histocompatibility complex (MHC) molecule to a helper T cell by an antigen-presenting cell.

cytotoxic T cells. Maturation of subpopulations of T cells (*i.e.*, CD4+ and CD8+) also occurs in the thymus. Mature T cells migrate to the peripheral lymphoid tissues and, on encountering antigen, multiply and differentiate into memory T cells and various effector T cells.

There are two types of T cells: the CD4+ helper T cell and the CD8+ cytotoxic T cell. The CD4+ helper T cell (T_H) serves as a master regulator for the immune system. Activation of helper T cells depends on the recognition of antigen in association with class II MHC molecules on APCs. Once activated, the cytokines they secrete influence the function of nearly all other cells of the immune system. These cytokines activate and regulate B cells, cytotoxic T cells, natural killer (NK) cells, macrophages, and other immune cells. The activated helper T cell can differentiate into two distinct subpopulations of helper T cells (*i.e.*, T_H1 or T_H2). The T_H1 differentiation pathway is the response to microbes that infect or activate macrophages and those that induce activation of NK cells (Table 13-2). The T_H2 pathway is activated in response to allergens and helminths (intestinal parasites), which cause chronic T-lymphocyte stimulation, often without significant innate immune response or macrophage activation. The T_H1 and T_H2 subsets develop from the same precursor CD4+ T lymphocytes, with the pattern of differentiation determined by the type of stimuli present early in the immune response. In most immune responses, a balanced response of T_H1 and T_H2 cells occurs, but extensive immunization or other factors can skew the response to one or the other subset. For example, the extensive exposure to an allergen in atopic individuals has been shown to shift the naive helper T-cell differentiation toward a T_H2 response with the production of the cytokines that influence immunoglobulin E (IgE) production and mast cell priming (see Chapter 15).

Activated CD8+ T cells become cytotoxic T lymphocytes (CTLs) after recognition of class I MHC–antigen complexes on target cell surfaces, such as body cells, infected by viruses or transformed by cancer (Fig. 13-6). The recognition of class I MHC–antigen complexes on infected target cells ensures that uninfected host cells are not indiscriminately destroyed. The CD8+ cytotoxic T lymphocytes destroy target cells by releasing cytolytic enzymes, toxic cytokines, and pore-forming molecules (*i.e.*, perforins), or through apoptotic cell death. The perforin proteins produce pores in the target cell membrane, allowing entry of toxic molecules and loss of cell constituents. The CD8+ cytotoxic T cells are especially important in controlling replicating viruses and intracellular bacteria because antibody cannot readily penetrate the membrane of living cells.

B Lymphocytes

B lymphocytes can be identified by the presence of membrane immunoglobulin that functions as the antigen receptor, class II MHC proteins, complement receptors,

TABLE 13-2	**Comparison of Properties of Helper T-Cell Subtypes 1 (T_H1) and 2 (T_H2)**	
	T_H1	**T_H2**
Stimulus for differentiation to T_H subtype	Microbes	Allergens and parasitic worms
Cells and cytokines influencing T_H subtype maturation	Macrophages, NK cells, IL-12	Mast cells, IL-4
Cytokines secreted by T_H subtype	IFN-γ	IL-4, IL-5
Effector functions	Phagocyte-mediated defense against infections, especially intracellular microbes. Stimulates production of IgG	IgE- and eosinophil/mast cell-mediated immune reactions. Stimulates production of IgE

NK, natural killer; IL, interleukin; IFN, interferon; Ig, immunoglobulin.

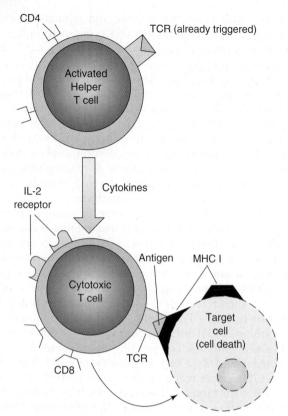

FIGURE 13-6 Destruction of target cell by cytotoxic T cell. Cytokines released from the activated helper T cell enhance the potential of the cytotoxic T cell in destruction of the target cell.

bone marrow, enters the circulation, and migrates to the various peripheral lymphoid tissues, where it is stimulated to respond to a specific antigen. The activated B cell divides and undergoes terminal differentiation into a plasma cell, which can produce thousands of antibody molecules per second. The antibodies are released into the blood and lymph, where they bind and remove their unique antigen with the help of other immune effector cells and molecules.

The commitment of a B-cell line to a specific antigen is evident by the expression of the membrane immunoglobulin antigen receptor molecule. B cells that encounter antigen complementary to their surface immunoglobulin receptor and receive T-cell help undergo a series of changes that transform the B cells into antibody-secreting plasma cells or into longer-lived memory B cells, which are then distributed to the peripheral tissues in preparation for subsequent antigen exposure (Fig. 13-7).

B lymphocytes also can function as APCs in humoral responses to haptens. Haptens are small chemicals, such as penicillin and plant pollens, that are not immunogenic by themselves. If, however, the haptens are coupled with proteins that serve as carriers, the B lymphocytes are able to induce antibody responses against the haptens. Hapten-specific B cells bind the hapten–protein complex through the hapten determinant, endocytose the hapten–carrier complex, and present the peptides derived from the carrier protein along with class II MHC molecules to carrier-specific helper T cells. Thus, the two cooperating types of lymphocytes are responsible for mounting an antibody response to haptens—the hapten-specific B cell is responsible for recognizing the hapten and the carrier-specific helper T cell for stimulating the differentiation of B cells into immunoglobulin-producing plasma cells.

and specific CD molecules. During the maturation of B cells in the bone marrow, stem cells change into immature precursor (pre-B) cells. A rearrangement of immunoglobulin genes produces in each cell a unique membrane receptor and secreted effector antibody (*e.g.*, IgM or IgD). This stage of maturation is programmed into the B cells and does not require antigen. The mature B cell leaves the

Immunoglobulins. Antibodies comprise a class of proteins called *immunoglobulins*. The immunoglobulins have been divided into five classes: IgG, IgA, IgM, IgD, and IgE, each with a different role in the immune defense strategy (Table 13-3). Each immunoglobulin is composed

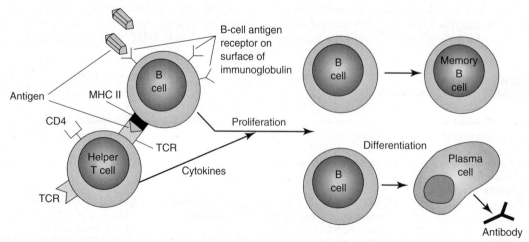

FIGURE 13-7 Pathway for B-cell differentiation.

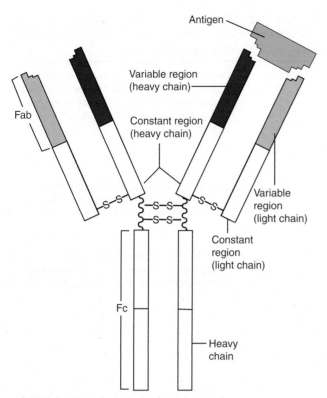

Antigen

Variable region
(heavy chain)

Constant region
(heavy chain)

Fab

Variable
region
(light chain)

Constant
region
(light chain)

Fc

Heavy
chain

FIGURE 13-8 Schematic model of an immunoglobulin G molecule showing the constant and variable regions of the light and dark chains.

of two identical light (L) chains and two identical heavy (H) chains to form a Y-shaped molecule (Fig. 13-8). The two forked ends of the immunoglobulin molecule bind antigen and are called *Fab* (*i.e.,* antigen-binding) fragments, and the tail of the molecule, which is called the *Fc* fragment, determines the biologic properties that are characteristic of a particular class of immunoglobulins. The amino acid sequence of the heavy and light chains shows constant (C) regions and variable (V) regions. The *constant regions* have sequences of amino acids that vary little among the antibodies of a particular class of immunoglobulin. The constant regions allow separation of immunoglobulins into classes (*e.g.,* IgM, IgG) and allow each class of antibody to interact with certain effectors cells and molecules. For example, the constant region on IgG can tag an antigen for recognition and destruction by phagocytes. The *variable regions* contain the antigen-binding sites of the molecule. The wide variation in the amino acid sequence of the variable regions seen from antibody to antibody allows this region to recognize its complementary epitope. A unique amino acid sequence in this region determines a distinctive three-dimensional pocket that is complementary to the antigen, allowing recognition and binding. Each B-cell clone produces antibody with one specific antigen-binding variable region or domain. During the course of the immune response, class switching (*e.g.,* from IgM to IgG) can occur, causing the B-cell clone to produce one of the different antibody types.

IgG (gamma globulin) is the most abundant of the circulating immunoglobulins. It is present in body fluids and readily enters the tissues. IgG is the only immunoglobulin that crosses the placenta and can transfer immunity from the mother to the fetus. This class of immunoglobulin protects against bacteria, toxins, and viruses in body fluids and activates the complement system. There are four subclasses of IgG (*i.e.,* IgG_1, IgG_2, IgG_3, and IgG_4) that have some restrictions in their response to certain types of antigens. For example, IgG_2 appears to be responsive to bacteria that are encapsulated with a polysaccharide layer, such as *Streptococcus pneumoniae*, *Haemophilus influenzae*, and *Neisseria meningitidis*.

IgM is a macromolecule that forms a polymer of five basic immunoglobulin units. It cannot cross the placenta and does not transfer maternal immunity. It is the first circulating immunoglobulin to appear in response to an antigen and is the first antibody type made by a newborn. This is diagnostically useful because the presence of IgM suggests a current infection in the infant by a specific pathogen. The identification of newborn IgM rather than maternally transferred IgG to the specific pathogen is indicative of an in utero or newborn infection.

IgA, a secretory immunoglobulin, is found in saliva, tears, colostrum (*i.e.,* first milk of a nursing mother), and in bronchial, gastrointestinal, prostatic, and vaginal secretions. This dimeric secretory immunoglobulin is considered a primary defense against local infections in mucosal tissues. IgA prevents the attachment of viruses and bacteria to epithelial cells.

IgD is found primarily on the cell membranes of B lymphocytes. It serves as an antigen receptor for initiating the differentiation of B cells.

IgE is involved in inflammation, allergic responses, and combating parasitic infections. It binds to mast cells and basophils. The binding of antigen to mast cell– or basophil-bound IgE triggers these cells to release histamine and other mediators important in inflammation and allergies.

Natural Killer Cells

Natural killer cells are lymphocytes that are functionally and phenotypically distinct from T cells, B cells, and monocyte-macrophages. The NK cell is an effector cell important in innate immunity that can kill tumor cells, virus-infected cells, or intracellular microbes. They are called *natural killer cells* because, unlike cytotoxic T cells, they do not need to recognize a specific antigen before being activated. Both NK cells and cytotoxic T cells kill after contact with a target cell. The NK cell is programmed to automatically kill foreign cells, in contrast to the CD8+ T cell, which needs to be activated to become cytotoxic. However, programmed killing is inhibited in the NK cell if its cell membrane receptors contact MHC self-molecules on normal host cells.

The mechanism of NK cell cytotoxicity is similar to T-cell cytotoxicity in that it depends on the production of pore-forming proteins (*i.e.,* NK perforins), enzymes,

TABLE 13-3	Classes and Characteristics of Immunoglobulins		
Figure	Class	Percentage of Total	Characteristics
	IgG	75.0	Displays antiviral, antitoxin, and antibacterial properties; only Ig that crosses the placenta; responsible for protection of newborn; activates complement and binds to macrophages
	IgA	15.0	Predominant Ig in body secretions, such as saliva, nasal and respiratory secretions, and breast milk; protects mucous membranes
	IgM	10.0	Forms the natural antibodies such as those for ABO blood antigens; prominent in early immune responses; activates complement
	IgD	0.2	Found on B lymphocytes; needed for maturation of B cells
	IgE	0.004	Binds to mast cells and basophils; involved in parasitic infections, allergic and hypersensitivity reactions

and toxic cytokines. NK cell activity can be enhanced in vitro on exposure to IL-2, a phenomenon called *lymphokine-activated killer activity*. NK cells also participate in *antibody-dependent cellular cytotoxicity*, a mechanism by which a cytotoxic effector cell can kill an antibody-coated target cell. The role of NK cells is believed to be one of immune surveillance for cancerous or virus-infected cells.

LYMPHOID ORGANS

The cells of the immune system are present in large numbers in the central and peripheral lymphoid organs. These organs and tissues are widely distributed in the body and provide different, but often overlapping, functions (Fig. 13-9). The central lymphoid organs, the bone marrow and the thymus, provide the environment for immune cell production and maturation. The peripheral lymphoid organs function to trap and process antigen and promote its interaction with mature immune cells. Lymph nodes, spleen, tonsils, appendix, Peyer patches in the intestine, and mucosa-associated lymphoid tissues in the respiratory, gastrointestinal, and reproductive systems comprise the peripheral lymphoid organs. The lymphoid organs are connected by networks of lymph channels, blood vessels, and capillaries. The immune cells continuously circulate through the various tissues and organs to seek out and destroy foreign material. The structure and organization of the cellular components of the peripheral lymphoid tissues ensure that the rare antigen-specific B and T cells will see each other and antigen– and peptide-MHC–coated antigen-presenting cells (*e.g.*, dendritic cells).

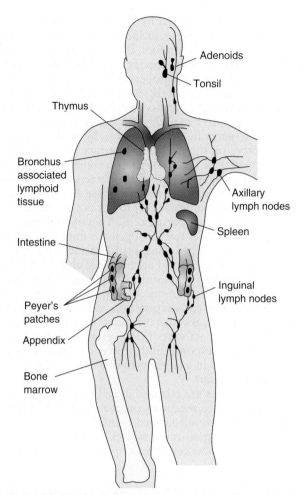

FIGURE 13-9 Central and peripheral lymphoid organs and tissues.

Thymus

The thymus is an elongated, bilobed structure that is located in the neck region above the heart. The function of the thymus is central to the development of the immune system because it generates mature immunocompetent T lymphocytes. The thymus is a fully developed organ at birth, weighing approximately 15 to 20 g. At puberty, when the immune cells are well established in peripheral lymphoid tissues, the thymus begins regressing and is replaced by adipose tissue. Nevertheless, some thymus tissue persists into old age. Precursor T (pre-T) cells enter the thymus as functionally and phenotypically immature T cells. They progressively differentiate into mature T cells under the influence of the thymic hormones and cytokines. As the T cells multiply and mature, they acquire T-cell receptors, surface markers that distinguish among the different types of T cells, and antigens that distinguish self from nonself. More than 95% of the thymocytes die in the thymus because they do not produce the appropriate type of self-antigens. Only those T cells able to recognize foreign antigen and not react to self-antigens are allowed to mature. This process is called *thymic selection*. Mature immunocompetent T cells leave the thymus

in 2 to 3 days and enter the peripheral lymphoid tissues through the bloodstream.

Lymph Nodes

Lymph nodes are small aggregates of lymphoid tissue located along lymphatic vessels throughout the body. Each lymph node processes lymph from a discrete, adjacent anatomic site. Many lymph nodes are in the axillae, groin, and along the great vessels of the neck, thorax, and abdomen. These tissues are located along the lymph ducts, which lead from the tissues to the thoracic duct. Lymph nodes have two functions: removing foreign material from lymph before it enters the bloodstream and serving as centers for proliferation of immune cells.

A lymph node is a bean-shaped tissue surrounded by a connective tissue capsule. Lymph enters the node through afferent channels that penetrate the capsule, and the lymph leaves through the efferent lymph vessels located in the deep indentation of the hilus (Fig. 13-10). Lymphocytes and macrophages flow slowly through the node, which allows trapping and interaction of antigen and immune cells. The reticular meshwork serves as a surface on which macrophages can more easily phagocytize antigens. Dendritic cells, which also permeate the lymph node, aid antigen presentation.

Spleen

The spleen is a large, ovoid secondary lymphoid organ located high in the left abdominal cavity. The spleen filters antigens from the blood and is important in the response to systemic infections. The spleen is composed of red and white pulp. The red pulp is well supplied with arteries and is the area where senescent and injured red blood cells are removed. The white pulp contains concentrated areas of B and T lymphocytes permeated by macrophages and dendritic cells. A sequence of activation events similar to that seen in the lymph nodes occurs in the spleen.

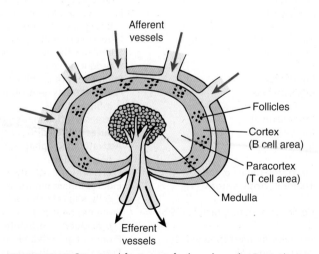

FIGURE 13-10 Structural features of a lymph node. Bacteria that gain entry to the body are filtered out of the lymph as it flows through the node.

Other Secondary Lymphoid Tissues

Other secondary lymphoid tissues include the *mucosa-associated lymphoid tissues*. These nonencapsulated clusters of lymphoid tissues are located around membranes lining the respiratory, digestive, and urogenital tracts. These gateways into the body must contain the immune cells needed to respond to a large and diverse population of microorganisms. In some tissues, the lymphocytes are organized in loose clusters, but in other tissues such as the tonsils, Peyer patches in the intestine, and the appendix, organized structures are evident (see Fig. 13-9). These tissues contain all the necessary cell components (*i.e.*, T cells, B cells, macrophages, and dendritic cells) for an immune response. Because of the continuous stimulation of the lymphocytes in these tissues by microorganisms constantly entering the body, large numbers of plasma cells are evident. Immunity at the mucosal layers helps to exclude many pathogens and thus protects the vulnerable internal organs.

CYTOKINES AND THE IMMUNE RESPONSE

Cytokines can be described as low–molecular-weight proteins made by cells that affect the behavior of other cells. They are made primarily by and act primarily on immune cells, especially activated helper T cells and macrophages. Cytokines were originally named for the general cell type that produces them (*e.g.*, lymphokines, monokines). With the development of anticytokine antibodies and other methods of identification, it has become clear that the same

protein may be synthesized by lymphocytes, monocytes, and a variety of tissue types, including endothelial cells and some epithelial cells. Therefore, the generic term *cytokine* is preferred. The names of specific types of cytokines were derived from the biologic properties first ascribed to them. For example, *interleukins* (IL) were found to be made by leukocytes and to act on leukocytes, and *interferons* (IFNs) were found to interfere with virus multiplication.

Cytokines generate their responses by binding to specific receptors on the membrane surface of their target cells. Many of these receptors share a common structural shape and a cytoplasmic tail that interacts with a family of intracellular signaling proteins. These signaling molecules are very potent, act at very low concentrations, and usually regulate neighboring cells. They modulate reactions of the host to foreign antigens or injurious agents by regulating the movement, proliferation, and differentiation of leukocytes and other cells (Table 13-4). The actions of cytokines commonly affect more than one cell type and have more than one biologic effect. For example, IFN-γ inhibits virus replication and is a potent activator of macrophages and NK cells. Specific cytokines can have biologic activities that overlap. Maximization of the immune response and protection against detrimental mutations in a single cytokine are possible benefits of this redundancy.

Most cytokines are released at cell-to-cell interfaces, where they bind to receptors on nearby cells. Cytokine secretion is a brief, self-limited event. Cytokines are not usually stored as preformed molecules and their synthesis is initiated by new gene transcription as a result of cel-

TABLE 13-4	Characteristic Biologic Properties of Selected Human Cytokines
Cytokines	**Biologic Activity**
Interleukin-1 (α and β)	Wide variety of biologic effects; activates endothelium and lymphocytes; induces fever and acute-phase response; stimulates neutrophil production
Interleukin-2	Growth factor for activated T cells; induces synthesis of other cytokines; activates cytotoxic T lymphocytes and NK cells
Interleukin-3	Growth factor for progenitor hematopoietic cells
Interleukin-4	Promotes growth and survival of T, B, and mast cells; causes T_H2 cell differentiation; activates B cells and eosinophils and induces IgE-type responses
Interleukin-5	Induces eosinophil growth and differentiation; induces IgA production in B cells
Interleukin-6	Stimulates the liver to produce acute-phase response; induces proliferation of antibody-producing cells
Interleukin-7	Stimulates pre-B cells and thymocyte development and proliferation
Interleukin-8	Chemoattracts neutrophils and T lymphocytes; regulates lymphocyte homing and neutrophil infiltration
Interleukin-10	Decreases inflammation by inhibiting T_H1 cells and release of IL-12 from macrophages
Interleukin-12	Induces T_H1 cell differentiation and IFN-γ synthesis by T and NK cells; enhances NK cytotoxicity
Interferon-γ	Activates macrophages; increases expression of class I and II and MHC antigen processing and presentation
Interferon (type I α and β)	Exerts antiviral activity in body cells; induces class I antigen expression; activates NK cells
Tumor necrosis factor-α	Induces inflammation, fever, and acute-phase response; activates neutrophils and endothelial cells; kills cells through apoptosis
Colony-stimulating factors (CSFs)	Promotes neutrophil, eosinophil, and macrophage maturation and growth; activates mature granulocytes; promotes growth and maturation of monocytes
Granulocyte-macrophage CSF	Promotes growth and maturation of neutrophils
Macrophage CSF	Promotes growth and maturation of monocytes

Ig, Immunoglobulin; IL, interleukin; IFN, interferon; NK, natural killer; MHC, major histocompatibility complex; T_H, helper T.

lular activation. The short half-life of cytokines ensures that excessive immune responses and systemic activation do not occur. The biologic responses associated with cytokines are also regulated by the time of expression of the cytokine receptor. External signals often regulate the expression of cytokine receptors. For example, stimulation of T and B lymphocytes by antigens leads to increased expression of cytokine receptors. For this reason, during an immune response, the antigen-specific lymphocytes are the preferential responders to secreted cytokines.

The production of cytokines often occurs in a cascade in which one cytokine affects the production of subsequent cytokines or cytokine receptors. Some cytokines function as antagonists to inhibit the biologic effects of earlier cytokines. This pattern of expression and feedback ensures appropriate control of cytokine synthesis and subsequently of the immune response. Excessive cytokine production can have serious adverse effects, including those associated with septic shock, food poisoning, and types of cancer.

The biologic properties of cytokines fall into several major functional groups. One group of cytokines (*e.g.*, IL-1, IL-6, TNF) mediates inflammation by producing fever and the acute-phase response and by attracting and activating phagocytes (*e.g.*, IL-8, IFN-γ). Depending on the concentration of these cytokines, the biologic changes can be seen as local inflammation (low concentration), systemic inflammation (moderate concentration), or even septic shock (high concentration). Other cytokines are maturation factors for the hematopoiesis of white or red blood cells (*e.g.*, IL-3, granulocyte-macrophage colony-stimulating factor [GM-CSF]; see Chapter 9). Recombinant CSF molecules are being used to increase the success rates of bone marrow transplantations. Most of the IL cytokines and IFN-γ function in adaptive immunity as intercellular communication molecules among T cells, B cells, macrophages, and other immune cells. The availability of recombinant cytokines offers the possibility of several clinical therapies in which stimulation or inhibition of the immune response or cell production is desirable. IL-2 therapy for several malignancies has led to some clinical success.

In summary, immunity is the resistance to a disease that is provided by the immune system. Immune mechanisms can be divided into two types: innate or nonspecific and adaptive or specific. Innate immunity is the first line of defense against microbial agents. It can distinguish between self and nonself through recognition of conserved patterns on microbes but cannot differentiate among unique antigens. Adaptive, or specific, immunity involves humoral and cellular mechanisms that respond to a unique antigen, can amplify and sustain its responses, distinguish self from nonself, and remember the antigen to produce a heightened response quickly on subsequent encounters with the same agent.

Antigens are substances foreign to the host that can stimulate an immune response. They have antigenic determinant sites or epitopes, which the immune system recognizes with specific receptors that distinguish the antigens as nonself and as unique foreign molecules.

The principal cells of the immune system are the lymphocytes, antigen-presenting cells, and effector cells that eliminate the antigen. There are two classes of lymphocytes: T lymphocytes and B lymphocytes. B lymphocytes differentiate into plasma cells that produce antibodies and provide for the elimination of microbes in the extracellular fluids (humoral immunity). T lymphocytes differentiate into regulatory (helper T cells) and effector (cytotoxic T cells) cells. Natural killer cells are lymphocytes that are functionally and phenotypically distinct from T cells, B cells, and monocyte-macrophages. They are nonspecific in their action and able to recognize antigen without being activated. Antigen-presenting cells consist of monocytes, tissue macrophages, and dendritic cells. They engulf and process antigens and present them to helper T cells.

Central to the identity of the immune cells are the CD molecules that distinguish between the different immune cells and their levels of differentiation. The regulatory CD4+ helper T cells serve as a trigger for the immune response and are essential to the differentiation of B cells into antibody-producing plasma cells and the differentiation of T lymphocytes into effector CD8+ cytotoxic T cells that eliminate intracellular microbes such as viruses. The cell surface MHC molecules are key recognition molecules that the immune system uses in distinguishing self from nonself. Class I MHC molecules, which are present on almost all cells, interact with CD8+ cytotoxic T cells in the destruction of cells that have been affected by intracellular pathogens or cancer. Class II MHC molecules, found on immune cells, aid in receptor communication between different members of the immune system.

Effector Responses of the Immune System

The effector functions of the immune system rely on humoral and cell-mediated immune responses, chemical messengers and signal systems, and the complement system. They involve both active and passive immunities. The humoral immune response involves secreted antibodies produced by activated B lymphocytes. Cell-mediated immunity depends on T-cell responses to cellular antigens. The complement system, which is a primary effector system for both the innate and adaptive immune systems, consists of a group of proteins that are present in the circulation as functionally inactive precursors.

ACTIVE VERSUS PASSIVE IMMUNE RESPONSES

Adaptive, or specific, immune responses are designed to protect the body against potentially harmful foreign substances, infections, and other sources of nonself antigens. It is the specific protection that is induced after exposure to antigens (active immunity) or through transfer of protective antibodies against an antigen (passive immunity).

Active immunity is acquired through immunization or actually having a disease. It is called *active immunity* because it depends on a response to the antigen by the person's immune system. Active immunity, although long lasting once established, requires a few days to weeks after a first exposure before the immune response is sufficiently developed to contribute to the destruction of the pathogen. However, the immune system usually is able to react within hours to subsequent exposure to the same agent because of the presence of memory B and T lymphocytes and circulating antibodies. The process of acquiring the ability to respond to an antigen after administration by vaccines is known as *immunization*. An acquired immune response can improve on repeated exposures to an injected antigen or a natural infection. The immune response describes the interaction between an antigen (*i.e.*, immunogen) and an antibody (*i.e.*, immunoglobulin) or reactive T lymphocyte.

Passive immunity is immunity transferred from another source. An infant receives passive immunity naturally from the transfer of antibodies from its mother in utero and through the mother's breast milk. Maternal IgG crosses the placenta and protects the newborn during the first few months of life. Normally, an infant has few infectious diseases during the first 3 to 6 months owing to the protection provided by the mother's antibodies. Passive immunity also can be artificially provided by the transfer of antibodies produced by other people or

animals. Some protection against infectious disease can be provided by the injection of hyperimmune serum, which contains high concentrations of antibodies for a specific disease, or immune serum or gamma globulin, which contains a pool of antibodies from many individuals providing protection against many infectious agents. Passive immunity produces only short-term protection that lasts weeks to months.

HUMORAL IMMUNITY

The B lymphocytes are responsible for humoral immunity. Humoral immunity depends on maturation of B lymphocytes into plasma cells, which produce and secrete antibodies. The combination of antigen with antibody can result in several effector responses, such as precipitation of antigen–antibody complexes, agglutination or clumping of cells, neutralization of bacterial toxins and viruses, lysis and destruction of pathogens or cells, adherence of antigen to immune cells, facilitation of phagocytosis, and complement activation. For example, antibodies can neutralize a virus by blocking the sites on the virus that it uses to bind to the host cell, thereby negating its ability to infect the cell.

Two types of responses occur in the development of humoral immunity: primary and secondary (Fig. 13-11). A *primary immune response* occurs when the antigen is first introduced into the body. During the primary response, there is a latent period or lag before the antibody can be detected in the serum. During this latent period, B cells are activated to proliferate and differentiate into antibody-secreting plasma cells and memory cells. Recovery from many infectious diseases occurs at the time during the primary response when the antibody concentration is reaching its peak. The *secondary*, or *memory*, *response* occurs on second or subsequent exposures to the antigen. During the secondary response, the rise in antibody occurs sooner and reaches a higher level because of the available memory cells. The booster immunization given for some infectious diseases, such as tetanus, makes use of the memory response. For a person who has been

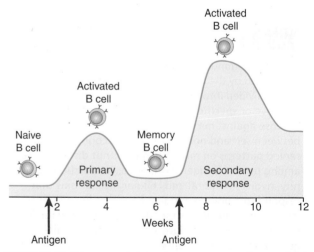

FIGURE 13-11 Primary and secondary or memory phases of the humoral immune response to the same antigen.

previously immunized, administration of a booster shot causes an almost immediate rise in antibody to a level sufficient to prevent development of the disease.

CELL-MEDIATED IMMUNITY

Cell-mediated immunity provides protection against viruses, intracellular bacteria, and cancer cells. In cell-mediated immunity, the actions of T lymphocytes and effector macrophages predominate. The most aggressive phagocyte, the macrophage, becomes activated after exposure to T-cell cytokines, especially IFN-γ. As in humoral immunity, the initial stages of cell-mediated immunity are directed by an APC displaying the antigen peptide–class II MHC complex to the helper T cell. Helper T cells become activated after antigen recognition and by induction with IL-12. The activated helper T cell then synthesizes IL-2 or IL-4. These molecules drive the multiplication of clones of helper T cells, which amplify the response. Further differentiation of the helper T cells leads to production of additional cytokines (*e.g.*, IFN-γ), which enhance the activity of cytotoxic T cells and effector macrophages. A cell-mediated immune response usually occurs through the cytotoxic activity of cytotoxic T cells and the enhanced engulfment and killing by macrophages. This type of defense is important against intracellular pathogens such as *Mycobacterium* species and *Listeria monocytogenes*. A similar sequence of T-cell and macrophage activation, but with sustained inflammation, is elicited in delayed hypersensitivity reactions (see Chapter 15). Contact dermatitis due to poison ivy sensitivity is an example of cell-mediated hypersensitivity caused by hapten–carrier complexes.

THE COMPLEMENT SYSTEM

The complement system is a primary mediator of both innate and adaptive immunity that enables the body to produce an inflammatory response, lyse foreign cells, and increase phagocytosis. The complement system, like the blood coagulation system, consists of a group of proteins (C1 through C9) that normally are present in the circulation as functionally inactive precursors. For a complement reaction to occur, the complement components must be activated in the proper sequence. Modified or split complement proteins (*e.g.*, C3b, C3a, C5a) released during activation function in the next step of the pathway or are released into the tissue fluid to produce biologic effects important in inflammation. Uncontrolled activation of the complement system is prevented by inhibitor proteins and the instability of the activated complement proteins at each step of the process.

There are three parallel but independent mechanisms for recognizing microorganisms that result in the activation of the complement system: the classic, the alternative, and the lectin pathways. All three pathways generate a series of enzymatic reactions that proteolytically cleave successive complement proteins in the pathway. The classic pathway of complement activation is initiated by antibody bound to antigens on the surface of microbes or through soluble immune complexes. The alternative and the lectin pathways do not use antibodies and are part of the innate immune defenses. The alternative pathway of complement activation is initiated by the interaction with certain polysaccharide molecules characteristic of bacterial surfaces. The lectin-mediated pathway is initiated after the binding of a mannose-binding protein to mannose-containing molecules commonly present on the surface of bacteria and yeast.

All three pathways converge with formation of a C3 convertase enzyme, which cleaves C3 to produce the active complement component C3b. The activation of complement can result in formation of products that produce or enhance opsonization, chemotaxis, inflammation, and cell membrane attack. A major biologic function of complement activation is opsonization—the coating of antigen–antibody complexes such that antigens are engulfed and cleared more efficiently by macrophages. Chemotactic complement products (C3a and C5a) can trigger an influx of leukocytes. These white blood cells remain fixed in the area of complement activation through attachment to specific sites on C3b and C4b molecules. Activation of C3a and C5a leads to activation of basophils and mast cells and release of inflammatory mediators that produce smooth muscle contraction and increased vascular permeability. The late phase of the complement cascade triggers the assembly of a membrane attack complex (MAC) that leads to the lytic destruction of many kinds of cells, including red blood cells, platelets, bacteria, and lymphocytes.

Regulation of the Immune Response

Self-regulation is an essential property of the immune system. An inadequate immune response may lead to immunodeficiency, but an inappropriate or excessive response may lead to conditions varying from allergic reactions to autoimmune diseases. This regulation is not well understood and involves all aspects of the immune response—antigen, antibody, cytokines, regulatory T cells, and the neuroendocrine system.

With each exposure to antigen, the immune system must determine which of its branches to activate and the extent and duration of the immune response. After exposure to an antigen, the immune response to that antigen develops after a brief lag, reaches a peak, and then recedes. Normal immune responses are self-limited because the response eliminates the antigen, and the products of the response, such as cytokines and antibodies, have a short or limited life span and are secreted only for brief periods after antigen recognition. Evidence suggests that cytokine feedback from the helper T or regulatory T cells controls several aspects of the immune response.

Another facet of immune self-regulation is inhibition of immune responses by tolerance. The term *tolerance* is used to define the ability of the immune system to be nonreactive to self-antigens while producing immunity to foreign agents (see Chapter 15). Tolerance to self-antigens protects an individual from harmful autoimmune reactions. Exposure of an individual to foreign antigens may lead to tolerance and the inability to respond to potential pathogens that cause infection. Tolerance exists not only to self-tissues but also to maternal-fetal tissues. Spe-

Understanding ➡ The Complement System

The complement system provides one of the major effector mechanisms of both humoral and innate immunity. The system consists of a group of proteins (complement proteins C1 through C9) that are normally present in the plasma in an inactive form. Activation of the complement system is a highly regulated process, involving the sequential breakdown of the complement proteins to generate a cascade of cleavage products capable of proteolytic enzyme activity. This allows for tremendous amplification because each enzyme molecule activated by one step can generate multiple activated enzyme molecules at the next step. Complement activation is inhibited by proteins that are present on normal host cells; thus, its actions are limited to microbes and other antigens that lack these inhibitory proteins.

The reactions of the complement system can be divided into three phases: (1) the initial activation phase, (2) the early-step inflammatory responses, and (3) the late-step membrane attack responses.

1

Initial activation phase. There are three pathways for recognizing microbes and activating the complement system: (1) the alternative pathway, which is activated on microbial cell surfaces in the absence of antibody and is a component of innate immunity; (2) the classic pathway, which is activated by certain types of antibodies bound to antigen and is part of humoral immunity; and (3) the lectin pathway, which is activated by a plasma lectin that binds to mannose on microbes and activates the classic system pathway in the absence of antibody.

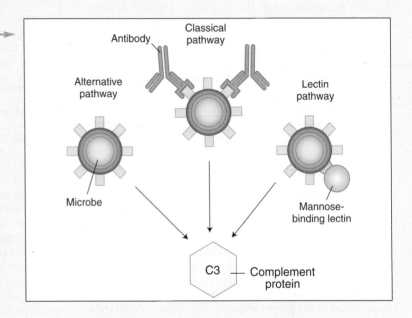

2

Early-step inflammatory responses. The central component of complement for all three pathways is the activation of the complement protein C3 and its enzymatic cleavage into a large C3b fragment and a smaller C3a fragment. The smaller 3a fragment stimulates inflammation by acting as a chemoattractant for neutrophils. The larger 3b fragment becomes attached to the microbe and acts as an opsonin for phagocytosis. It also acts as an enzyme to cleave C5 into two components: a C5a fragment, which produces vasodilation and increases vascular permeability; and a C5b fragment, which leads to the late-step membrane attack responses.

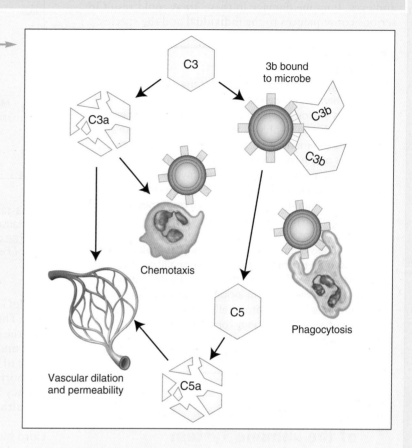

3

Late-step membrane attack. In the late-step responses, C3b binds to other complement proteins to form an enzyme that cleaves C5, generating C5a and C5b fragments. C5a stimulates the influx of neutrophils and the vascular phase of acute inflammation. The C5b fragment, which remains attached to the microbe, initiates the formation of a complex of complement proteins C6, C7, C8, and C9 into a membrane attack protein, or pore, that allows fluids and ions to enter and cause cell lysis.

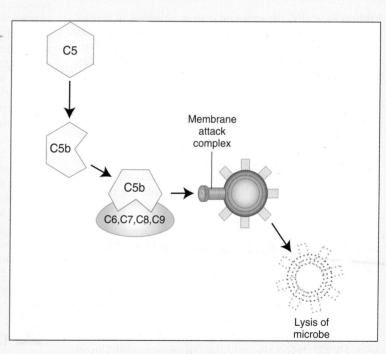

cial regulation of the immune system is evident in defined immune-privileged sites such as the brain, testes, ovaries, and eyes. Immune damage in these areas could result in serious consequences to the individual and the species.

In summary, the effector functions of the immune system rely on chemical messengers and signal systems. Cytokines are low–molecular-weight proteins that are produced during all phases of the immune response and serve as a communication system for coordinating the functions of the various members of the immune system. The humoral immune response involves secreted antibodies produced by activated B lymphocytes. Cell-mediated immunity depends on T-cell responses to cellular antigens. The complement system, which is a primary effector system for both the innate and adaptive immune system, consists of a group of proteins that are present in the circulation as functionally inactive precursors. The effector functions of activated members of the complement system include (1) chemotaxis with recruitment of inflammatory cells, (2) opsonization or coating of antigen–antibody complexes so they can be more efficiently cleared by macrophages, and (3) formation of a membrane attack complex and pathogen lysis.

Developmental Aspects of the Immune System

Embryologically, the immune system develops in several stages, beginning at 5 to 6 weeks as the fetal liver becomes active in hematopoiesis. Development of the primary lymphoid organs (*i.e.*, thymus and bone marrow) begins during the middle of the first trimester and proceeds rapidly. Secondary lymphoid organs (*i.e.*, spleen, lymph nodes, and mucosa-associated lymphoid tissues) develop soon after. These secondary lymphoid organs are rather small but well developed at birth and mature rapidly after exposure to microorganisms during the postnatal period. The thymus at birth is the largest lymphoid tissue relative to body size and normally is approximately two thirds of its mature weight, which it achieves during the first year of life.

TRANSFER OF IMMUNITY FROM MOTHER TO INFANT

Protection of a newborn against antigens occurs through transfer of maternal antibodies. Maternal IgG antibodies cross the placenta during fetal development and remain functional in the newborn for the first months of life (Fig. 13-12). IgG is the only class of immunoglobulins to cross the placenta. Levels of maternal IgG decrease significantly during the first 3 to 6 months of life, while infant synthesis of immunoglobulins increases. Maternally trans-

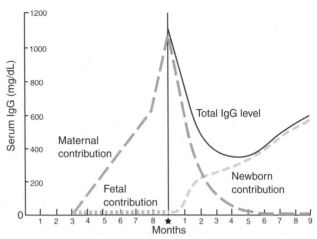

FIGURE 13-12 Maternal/neonatal serum immunoglobulin levels. (From Allansmith M., McClellan B. H., Butterworth M., et al. [1968]. The development of immunoglobulin levels in man. *Journal of Pediatrics* 72, 289.)

mitted IgG is effective against most microorganisms and viruses. The largest amount of IgG crosses the placenta during the last weeks of pregnancy and is stored in fetal tissues, and infants born prematurely may be deficient. Because of transfer of the IgG antibodies to the fetus, an infant born to a mother infected with human immunodeficiency virus (HIV) has a positive HIV antibody test result, although the child may not be infected with the virus.

Cord blood does not normally contain IgM or IgA. If present, these antibodies are of fetal origin and represent exposure to intrauterine infection. The infant begins producing IgM antibodies shortly after birth, in response to the immense antigenic stimulation of his or her new environment. Premature infants appear to be able to produce IgM as well as term infants. At approximately 6 days of age the IgM rises sharply, and this rise continues until approximately 1 year of age, when the adult level is achieved.

Serum IgA normally is first detected at approximately 13 days after birth. The level increases during early childhood until adult levels are reached between the sixth and seventh year. Maternal IgA also is transferred to the infant in colostrum, or milk, by breast-feeding. These antibodies provide local immunity for the intestinal system and have been shown to decrease diarrheal infections in underdeveloped countries. These evolutionary adaptations of the immune system have increased the survival of our species and optimized the development of other important organs in the early months of life.

IMMUNE RESPONSE IN THE ELDERLY

Aging is characterized by a declining ability to adapt to environmental stresses. One of the factors thought to contribute to this problem is a decline in immune responsiveness. This includes changes in cell-mediated and humoral immune responses. Elderly persons tend to be more susceptible to infections, have more evidence of auto-immune and immune complex disorders than younger persons, and have a higher incidence of cancer. Experimental evidence suggests that vaccination is less successful in inducing immunization in older persons than younger adults. However, the effect of altered immune function on the health of elderly persons is clouded by the fact that age-related changes or disease may affect the immune response.

The alterations in immune function that occur with advanced age are not fully understood. There is a decrease in the size of the thymus gland, which is thought to affect T-cell function. The size of the gland begins to decline shortly after sexual maturity, and by 50 years of age, it usually has diminished to 15% or less of its maximum size. There are conflicting reports regarding age-related changes in the peripheral lymphocytes. The suggestion of a biologic clock in T cells that determines the number of times the T cell divides may regulate cell number with age. Some researchers have reported a decrease in the absolute number of lymphocytes, and others have found little, if any, change. The most common finding is a slight decrease in the proportion of T cells to other lymphocytes and a decrease in CD4+ and CD8+ cells.

More evident are altered responses of the immune cells to antigen stimulation; increasing proportions of lymphocytes become unresponsive, whereas the remainder continue to function relatively normally. T and B cells show deficiencies in activation. In the T-cell types, the CD4+ subset is most severely affected. Evidence indicates that aged T cells have a decreased rate of synthesis of the cytokines that drive the proliferation of lymphocytes and a diminished expression of the receptors that interact with those cytokines. For example, it has been shown that IL-2, IL-4, and IL-12 levels decrease with aging. Although B-cell function is compromised with age, the range of antigens that can be recognized is not diminished. If anything, the repertoire, including outgrowths of autoreactive B-cell clones, is increased to the extent that B cells begin to recognize some self-antigens as foreign antigens. This may be the basis for the increased incidence of autoimmune disease in the elderly.

In summary, a newborn is protected against antigens in early life by passive transfer of maternal antibodies through the placenta (IgG) and in colostrum (IgA) through breast-feeding. Some changes are seen with aging, including an increase in autoimmune diseases. The impact of alterations in immune function that occur with aging is not fully understood.

Review Exercises

A nursing student is working in a community clinic as a volunteer. Each time she enters the clinic, she suffers bouts of sneezing and runny eyes. She has a history of mold allergy and her younger brother has asthma. Analysis at the allergy clinic indicates a strong reaction to latex. It is recommended that she avoid exposure to all forms of latex.

A. What class of immunoglobulin and what type of mediator cells are responsible for the symptoms expressed in this individual?

B. What type of T-helper cell and cytokines direct the expression of this humoral immune response?

C. Is this an example of active or passive immunity? Is this likely to be a primary or secondary immune response?

A young child at 5 months of age presents with thrush, a yeast infection of the mouth. He also has had recurrent bouts of otitis media in the last 2 months. His tonsils were very small. Laboratory analysis indicates a low lymphocyte count and no T lymphocytes. Further analysis indicates a genetic mutation in the T-cell receptor molecule complex (TCR–CD3) that affected the maturation of all T cells. The final diagnosis is severe combined immunodeficiency disease. A bone marrow transplant is being pursued with cells from his HLA-matched sibling.

A. Why were infections not present in the first few months of this child's life?

B. What would be the impact of an absence of T cells on both humoral and cell-mediated immunity?

C. Why would it not be advisable to administer a live virus vaccine to this child?

Visit the Porth: Essentials of Pathophysiology: Concepts of Altered Health States web site (http://thePoint.LWW.com/PorthEssentials) for links to chapter-related resources on the Internet, all-new exclusive animations, chapter review questions, and more!

BIBLIOGRAPHY

Abbas A. K., Lichtman A. H. (2003). *Cellular and molecular immunology* (5th ed.). Philadelphia: W. B. Saunders.

Benjamini E., Cioco R., Sunshine G. (2003). *Immunology: A short course* (5th ed.). New York: John Wiley & Sons.

Chaplin D. D. (2003). Overview of the immune response. *Journal of Allergy and Clinical Immunology* 111, S442–S459.

Goldsby R. A., Kindt T. J., Osborne B. A., et al. (2003). *Immunology* (5th ed.). San Francisco: W. H. Freeman.

Janeway C. A., Jr., Travers P., Walport M., et al. (2001). *Immunobiology: The immune system in health and disease* (5th ed.). New York: Garland.

Levinson W., Jawetz E. (2002). *Medical microbiology and immunology* (7th ed.). East Norwalk, CT: McGraw Hill/Appleton & Lange.

Lui, Y. J. (2001). Dendritic cell subsets and lineages and their functions in innate and adaptive immunity. *Cell* 106, 259–262.

Nairn R., Helbert M. (2002). *Immunology for medical students.* New York: Mosby/Elsevier.

Natarajan K., Dimasi N., Wang J., et al. (2002). Structure and function of natural killer cell receptors: Multiple molecular solutions to self, nonself discrimination. *Annual Review of Immunology* 20, 853–885.

Roitt I., Rabson A. (2002). *Really essential immunology.* London: Blackwell Science.

Russell J. H., Ley T. J. (2002). Lymphocyte mediated cytotoxicity. *Annual Review of Immunology* 20, 323–370.

Sunyer J. O., Boshra H., Lorenzo G., et al. (2003). Evolution of complement as an effector system in innate and adaptive immunity. *Immunologic Research* 27, 549–564.

Szabo S. J., Sullivan B. M., Peng S. L., et al. (2003). Molecular mechanisms regulating Th1 immune responses. *Annual Review of Immunology* 21, 713–758.

Takeda K., Kaisho T., Akira S. (2003). Toll-like receptors. *Annual Review of Immunology* 21, 335–376.

Underhill D. M., Ozinski A. (2002). Phagocytosis of microbes: Complexity in action. *Annual Review of Immunology* 20, 825–852.

Walport M. J. (2001). Complement. *New England Journal of Medicine* 344, 1058–1066, 1141–1144.

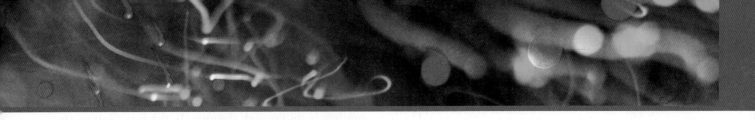

Chapter *14*

Inflammation, Tissue Repair, and Fever

 The ability of the body to sustain injury, resist attack by microbial agents, and repair damaged tissue depends on the inflammatory reaction, immune response, and tissue repair and wound healing. Inflammation is a protective response intended to eliminate the initial cause of cell injury as well as the necrotic cells and tissues resulting from that injury. It accomplishes this by diluting, destroying, or otherwise neutralizing the harmful agents. It then sets the stage for the events that will eventually heal and reconstitute the sites of injury. During repair, the injured tissue is replaced by regeneration of the damaged cells or by filling in the defect with fibrous scar tissue.

This chapter focuses on the manifestations of acute and chronic inflammation, tissue repair and wound healing, and temperature regulation and fever. The immune response is discussed in Chapter 13.

The Inflammatory Response

The inflammatory response, first described over 2000 years ago, has evoked renewed interest during the past several decades. As a result, a number of diseases are now known to have a basis in the inflammatory response. For example, the role of the inflammatory response in producing the incapacitating effects of bronchial asthma and the crippling effects of rheumatoid arthritis has been well established. There is also emerging evidence that the inflammatory response may play a role in the pathogenesis of a number of other diseases, such as atherosclerosis and Alzheimer disease. Thus, what was once narrowly viewed as a local response to injury is today becoming an engaging problem in inflammatory mediators as well as fueling a multi-billion-dollar market for the anti-inflammatory drugs produced by the pharmaceutical industry.

Inflammatory conditions are commonly named by adding the suffix *-itis* to the affected organ or system. For example, *appendicitis* refers to inflammation of the appendix, *pericarditis* to inflammation of the pericardium, and *neuritis* to inflammation of a nerve. More descriptive expressions of the inflammatory process might indicate whether the process was acute or chronic and what type of exudate was formed (*e.g.*, acute fibrinous pericarditis).

Inflammation can be divided into two basic patterns: acute and chronic.[1,2] Acute inflammation is of relatively short duration, lasting from a few minutes to several days, and is characterized by the exudation of fluid and plasma components and emigration of leukocytes, predominantly neutrophils, into the extravascular tissues. Chronic inflammation is of a longer duration, lasting for days to years, and is associated with the presence of lymphocytes and macrophages, proliferation of blood vessels, fibrosis, and tissue necrosis. These basic forms of inflammation often overlap, however, and many factors may influence their course.

ACUTE INFLAMMATION

Acute inflammation is the early (almost immediate) reaction of local tissues and their blood vessels to injury. It typically occurs before the immune response becomes established and is aimed primarily at removing the injurious agent and limiting the extent of tissue damage. Acute inflammation can be triggered by a variety of stimuli, including infections, immune reactions, blunt and penetrating trauma, physical or chemical agents (*e.g.*, burns, frostbite, irradiation, caustic chemicals), and tissue necrosis from any cause.

KEY CONCEPTS

The Inflammatory Response

➤ Inflammation represents the response of body tissue to immune reactions, injury, or ischemic damage.

➤ The classic response to inflammation includes redness, swelling, heat, pain or discomfort, and loss of function.

➤ The manifestations of an acute inflammatory response can be attributed to the immediate vascular changes that occur (vasodilation and increased capillary permeability), the influx of inflammatory cells such as neutrophils, and, in some cases, the widespread effects of inflammatory mediators, which produce fever and other systemic signs and symptoms.

➤ The manifestations of chronic inflammation are due to infiltration with macrophages, lymphocytes, and fibroblasts, leading to persistent inflammation, fibroblast proliferation, and scar formation.

Cardinal Signs

The classic description of acute inflammation has been handed down through the ages. In the first century AD, the Roman physician Celsus described the local reaction to injury in terms now known as the *cardinal signs* of inflammation.[1] These signs are *rubor* (redness), *tumor* (swelling), *calor* (heat), and *dolor* (pain). In the second century AD, the Greek physician Galen added a fifth cardinal sign, *functio laesa* (loss of function). These signs and symptoms, which are apparent when inflammation occurs on the surface of the body, may not be present when internal organs are involved. Inflammation of the lung, for example, usually does not cause pain unless the pleura, where pain receptors are located, is affected. Also, an increase in heat is uncommon in inflammation involving internal organs, where tissues are normally maintained at core temperature.

In addition to the cardinal signs that appear at the site of injury, systemic manifestations (*e.g.*, fever) may occur as chemical mediators produced at the site of inflammation gain entrance to the circulatory system. The constellation of systemic manifestations that may occur during an acute inflammation is known as the *acute-phase response*.

Acute inflammation involves two major components: the vascular and cellular stages.[1–3] Both the vascular and cellular reactions of the inflammatory response are mediated by chemical factors that are derived from plasma proteins or cells and are produced in response to or activated by the inflammatory stimulus.

Vascular Stage

The vascular, or hemodynamic, changes that occur with inflammation begin almost immediately after injury and are initiated by a momentary constriction of small blood vessels in the area. This vasoconstriction is followed rapidly by vasodilatation of the arterioles and venules that supply the area. As a result, the area becomes congested, causing the redness (erythema) and warmth associated with acute inflammation. Accompanying this hyperemic response is an increased permeability of vessels in the microcirculation, with the outpouring of a protein-rich fluid (exudate) into the extravascular spaces. The loss of plasma proteins and accompanying decrease in capillary colloidal osmotic pressure and the increase in interstitial fluid colloidal osmotic pressure coupled with the increase in capillary pressure causes fluid to move into the tissues and produce swelling (*i.e.*, edema), pain, and impaired function. The exudation of fluid into the tissue spaces also serves to dilute the offending agent. As fluid moves out of the blood vessels, stagnation of flow and clotting of blood occurs at the site of injury. This aids in localizing the spread of infectious microorganisms.

Depending on the severity of injury, the vascular changes that occur with inflammation follow one of three patterns of response.[3] The first is an immediate transient response, which occurs with minor injury. The second is an immediate sustained response, which occurs with more serious injury, continues for several days, and damages the vessels in the area. The third is a delayed hemodynamic response, which involves an increase in capillary permeability that occurs 4 to 24 hours after injury. A delayed response often accompanies injuries due to irradiation, such as sunburn.

Cellular Stage

The cellular stage of acute inflammation is marked by movement of white blood cells, or leukocytes, into the area of injury. Two types of leukocytes participate in the acute inflammatory response—granulocytes and monocytes. Although attention has focused on the recruitment of leukocytes from the blood, a rapid response also requires the release of chemical mediators from tissue cells (mast cells and macrophages) that are prepositioned in the tissues.[4]

Granulocytes. Granulocytes are identifiable because of their characteristic cytoplasmic granules. These white blood cells have distinctive multilobed nuclei. The granulocytes are divided into three types (*i.e.,* neutrophils, eosinophils, and basophils) according to the staining properties of their granules (Fig. 14-1). The *neutrophil* is the primary phagocyte that arrives early at the site of inflammation, usually within 90 minutes of injury. Their cytoplasmic granules, which resist staining and remain a neutral color, contain enzymes and other antibacterial substances that are used in destroying and degrading the engulfed particles. They also have oxygen-dependent metabolic pathways that generate toxic oxygen (*e.g.,* hydrogen peroxide) and nitrogen (*e.g.,* nitric oxide) products that aid in the destruction of pathogens.

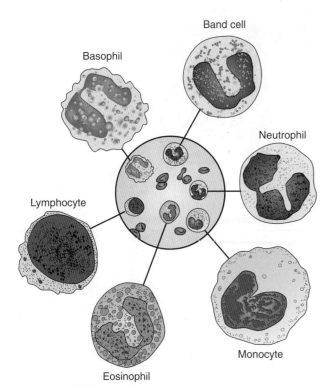

Band cell

Basophil

Neutrophil

Lymphocyte

Monocyte

Eosinophil

FIGURE 14-1 White blood cells.

Because these white blood cells have nuclei that are divided into three to five lobes, they often are called *polymorphonuclear neutrophils* (PMNs) or *segmented neutrophils* (segs). The neutrophil count in the blood often increases greatly during the inflammatory process, especially with bacterial infections. After being released from the bone marrow, circulating neutrophils have a life span of only approximately 10 hours and therefore must be constantly replaced if their numbers are to remain adequate. This requires an increase in circulating white blood cells, a condition called *leukocytosis*. With excessive demand for phagocytes, immature forms of neutrophils are released from the bone marrow. These immature cells often are called *bands* because of their horseshoe-shaped nuclei.

The cytoplasmic granules of the *eosinophils* stain red with the acid dye eosin. These granulocytes increase in the blood during allergic reactions and parasitic infections. The granules of eosinophils contain a protein that is highly toxic to large parasitic worms that cannot be phagocytized. They also play an important role in allergic reactions by controlling the release of specific chemical mediators.

The granules of the *basophils,* which stain blue with a basic dye, contain histamine and other bioactive mediators of inflammation. The *mast cell,* which resides in connective tissues throughout the body, is very similar in many of its properties to the basophil. Mast cells are particularly prevalent along mucosal surfaces of the lung and gastrointestinal tract and the dermis of the skin. This distribution places the mast cell in a sentinel position between environmental antigens and the host for a variety of acute and chronic inflammatory conditions.[2] Both the basophils and mast cells are involved in producing the symptoms associated with allergic reactions (see Chapter 15).

Mononuclear Phagocytes. The monocytes are the largest of the circulating white blood cells and constitute 3% to 8% of the total blood leukocytes. The circulating life span of the monocyte is three to four times longer that of the granulocytes. These longer-lived phagocytes help to destroy the causative agent, aid in the signaling processes of immunity, and serve to resolve the inflammatory process.

The monocytes, which have their origin in the bone marrow, exit the circulation in response to inflammatory stimuli and become macrophages. Within 24 hours, mononuclear cells arrive at the inflammatory site, and by 48 hours, monocytes and macrophages are the predominant cell types. The macrophages engulf larger quantities of foreign material than the neutrophils. They also play an important role in chronic inflammation, where they can surround and wall off foreign material that cannot be digested.

Leukocyte Response. The sequence of events in the leukocyte response to inflammation includes leukocyte (1) margination and adhesion, (2) emigration, (3) chemotaxis, and (4) activation and phagocytosis. During the early stages of the inflammatory response, fluid leaves

Understanding ➤ Acute Inflammation

Acute inflammation is the immediate and early response to an injurious agent. The response, which serves to control and eliminate the source of injury, occurs in two phases: (1) the vascular phase, which leads to an increase in blood flow and changes in the small blood vessels of the microcirculation; and the (2) cellular phase, which leads to the emigration of leukocytes from the microcirculation and their activation to eliminate the injurious agent.

1

Vascular phase. The vascular phase of acute inflammation is characterized by changes in the small blood vessels at the site of injury. It begins with momentary vasoconstriction followed rapidly by vasodilation. Vasodilation involves the arterioles and venules with a resultant increase in capillary blood flow, causing heat and redness, which are two of the cardinal signs of inflammation. This is accompanied by an increase in vascular permeability with outpouring of protein-rich fluid (exudate) into the extravascular spaces. The loss of proteins reduces the capillary osmotic pressure and increases the interstitial osmotic pressure. This, coupled with an increase in capillary pressure, causes a marked outflow of fluid and its accumulation in the tissue spaces, producing the swelling, pain, and impaired function that represent the other cardinal signs of acute inflammation. As fluid moves out of the vessels, stagnation of flow and clotting of blood occurs. This aids in localizing the spread of infectious microorganisms.

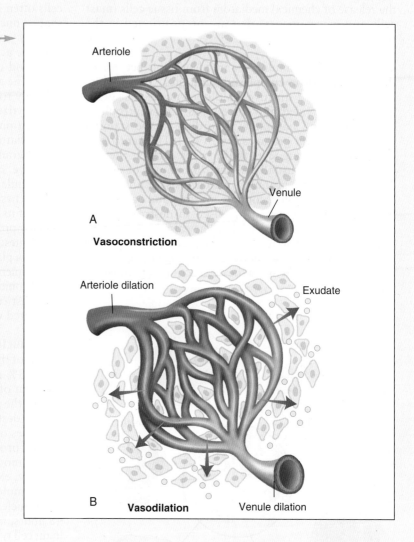

A
Vasoconstriction

B   **Vasodilation**

2

Cellular phase. The cellular phase of acute inflammation involves the delivery of leukocytes, mainly neutrophils, to the site of injury so they can perform their normal functions in host defense. The delivery and activation of leukocytes can be divided into the following steps: margination and adhesion, emigration, chemotaxis, leukocyte activation, and phagocytosis. The recruitment of leukocytes to the postcapillary venules, where they make their exit, is facilitated by the slowing of blood flow. Margination and adhesion to the vessel endothelium facilitate leukocyte movement or emigration from the vascular space into the extravascular tissue. After extravasation, leukocytes emigrate in the tissues toward the site of injury by chemotaxis, or locomotion oriented along a chemical gradient. Once at the site of injury, the products generated by tissue injury induce a number of leukocyte responses, including phagocytosis. Phagocytosis and the release of enzymes by neutrophils and macrophages are responsible for eliminating the injurious agents.

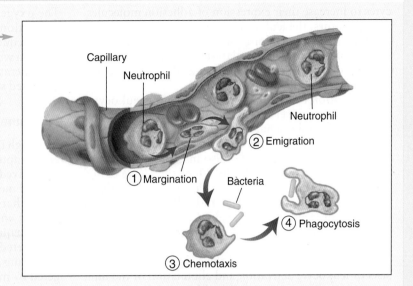

the capillaries, causing an increase in blood viscosity. The release of chemical mediators and cytokines affects the endothelial cells of the capillaries and causes the leukocytes to increase their expression of adhesion molecules. As this occurs, the leukocytes slow their movement and begin to accumulate along the endothelial surface. This process of leukocyte accumulation is called *margination*. As the leukocytes accumulate, they also begin to adhere to the vessel endothelium.

Emigration is a mechanism by which the leukocytes change shape, insert pseudopods into the junctions between the endothelial cells, and squeeze through the interendothelial junctions into the extravascular space. The emigration of leukocytes also may be accompanied by an escape of red blood cells. Once they have exited the capillary, the leukocytes wander through the tissue guided by cytokines, bacterial and cellular debris, and complement fragments (*e.g.*, C3a, C5a). The process by which leukocytes migrate in response to a chemical signal is called *chemotaxis*.

The next and final stage of the cellular response consists of leukocyte activation and elimination of the injurious agent. This is accomplished largely phagocytosis, a process in which activated leukocytes engulf and degrade the bacteria and cellular debris. Phagocytosis involves three distinct steps: (1) adherence plus opsonization, (2) engulfment, and (3) intracellular killing (Fig. 14-2). Contact of the bacteria or antigen with the phagocyte cell membrane is essential for trapping the agent and triggering the final steps of phagocytosis. If the antigen is coated with antibody or complement, its adherence is increased because of binding to complement. The enhanced binding of an antigen due to antibody or complement is called *opsonization*. Engulfment follows the recognition of the agent as foreign. During the process of engulfment, extensions of cytoplasm move around and eventually enclose the particle in a membrane-surrounded phagosome. The phagosome then fuses with a membrane of a lysosome (see Chapter 1), resulting in the formation of a phagolysosome.

Intracellular killing of pathogens by phagocytic cells is accomplished through several mechanisms, including lysosomal enzymes and oxygen-dependent mechanisms. The oxygen-dependent mechanisms, which involve the generation of reactive oxygen intermediates (free radicals), require a number of metabolic enzymes. Individuals born with genetic defects affecting the enzymes needed for generation of the reactive oxygen intermediates have increased susceptibility to recurrent bacterial infection.

Inflammatory Mediators

Although inflammation is precipitated by injury, its signs and symptoms are produced by chemical mediators that are derived either from the plasma or from cells. Plasma-derived mediators are present in the plasma in precursor forms that must be activated, usually by a series of proteolytic enzymes. The cell-derived mediators are normally sequestered in intracellular granules that need to be secreted, or they are newly synthesized in response to a stimulus. The production of active mediators is triggered by microbial products or by host proteins, such as proteins of the coagulation or complement systems.

Plasma-Derived Mediators of Inflammation. The plasma is the source of three major mediators of inflammation, including the kinins, the products of the coagulation/fibrinolysis system, and the proteins of the complement system. One kinin, bradykinin, causes increased capillary permeability and pain. The clotting system (see Chapter 10) contributes to the vascular phase of inflammation, mainly through fibrin products formed during the final steps of the clotting process. The complement system consists of a cascade of plasma proteins that plays an important role in both immunity and inflammation. Complement proteins contribute to the inflammatory response by (1) causing vasodilation and increasing vascular permeability; (2) promoting leukocyte activation, adhesion, and chemotaxis; and (3) augmenting phagocytosis (see Chapter 13).

Cell-Derived Mediators of Inflammation. The cell-derived mediators include histamine and serotonin, which are preformed and stored in intracellular granules, and arachidonic acid metabolites, platelet-activating factors, cytokines, and nitric oxide, all of which are rapidly synthesized in response to an appropriate stimulus.

Histamine and Serotonin. *Histamine* is widely distributed throughout the body. Preformed histamine is found in high concentrations in the mast cells of connective tissues adjacent to blood vessels. It is also found in blood basophils and platelets. Histamine is released in response to a variety of stimuli, including trauma and immune reactions involving binding of immunoglobulin E (IgE) antibodies to mast cells. It is one of the first mediators of an inflammatory response. Histamine causes dilatation of arterioles and increases the permeability of venules. *Serotonin* is a preformed mediator, found in platelets, that has actions similar to those of histamine.

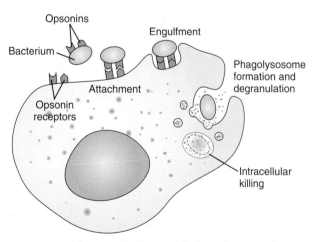

FIGURE 14-2 Phagocytosis of a particle (*e.g.*, bacterium): opsonization, attachment, engulfment, and intracellular killing.

Arachidonic Acid Metabolites. Arachidonic acid is a 20-carbon unsaturated fatty acid found in phospholipids of cell membranes. The release of arachidonic acid from membrane phospholipids in mast cells and basophils is accomplished through the enzymatic action of phospholipases. The synthesis of arachidonic acid mediators follows one of two pathways: the cyclooxygenase pathway, which culminates in the synthesis of the prostaglandins, and the lipoxygenase pathway, which culminates in the synthesis of the leukotrienes (Fig. 14-3). The corticosteroid drugs block the inflammatory effects of both pathways by inhibiting phospholipase activity and thus preventing the release of arachidonic acid.

Several prostaglandins are synthesized from arachidonic acid through the cyclooxygenase pathway. The stable prostaglandins (PGE_1 and PGE_2) induce inflammation and potentiate the effects of histamine and other inflammatory mediators. The prostaglandin thromboxane A_2 promotes platelet aggregation and vasoconstriction. Aspirin and the nonsteroidal anti-inflammatory drugs (NSAIDs) reduce inflammation by inactivating the first enzyme in the cyclooxygenase pathway for prostaglandin synthesis (see Fig. 14-3).

Like the prostaglandins, the leukotrienes are formed from arachidonic acid, but through the lipoxygenase pathway. Histamine and leukotrienes are complementary in action in that they have similar functions. Histamine is produced rapidly and transiently while the more potent leukotrienes are being synthesized. The leukotrienes also have been reported to affect the permeability of the postcapillary venules, the adhesion properties of endothelial cells, and the chemotaxis and extravasation of neutrophils, eosinophils, and monocytes. The leukotrienes LTC_4, LTD_4, and LTE_4, collectively known as the *slow-reacting substance of anaphylaxis* (SRS-A), cause slow and sustained constriction of the bronchioles and are important inflammatory mediators in bronchial asthma and anaphylaxis.

Platelet-Activating Factor. Platelet-activating factor (PAF), a potent inflammatory mediator, is generated from a complex lipid stored in cell membranes. It is synthesized by virtually all inflammatory cells, endothelial cells, and injured tissue cells. It causes platelet aggregation, primes and enhances the functions of neutrophils and monocytes, and is a potent eosinophil chemoattractant. It is also an extremely potent vasodilator, augmenting the permeability of small blood vessels at the site of injury.

Cytokines. Cytokines are polypeptide products synthesized by many cell types, but primarily by lymphocytes and macrophages, that modulate the function of other cell types. They include the colony-stimulating factors that direct the growth of immature marrow precursor cells and the interleukins (IL), interferons (IFN), and tumor necrosis factor (TNF) that are important in the inflammatory response. The actions of the various cytokines are summarized in Chapter 13, Table 13-4.

Nitric Oxide. Nitric oxide, which is produced by a variety of cells, plays multiple roles in inflammation. It relaxes vascular smooth muscle, reduces platelet aggregation

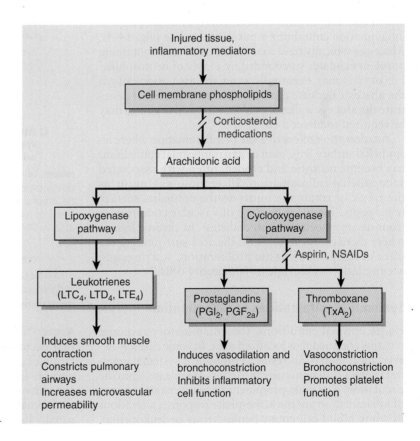

FIGURE 14-3 The pathways for production of the arachidonic acid-derived mediators where the corticosteroids and nonsteroidal anti-inflammatory drugs (NSAIDs) exert their action.

and adhesion, serves as a regulator of leukocyte recruitment, and aids in the killing of microbial agents by phagocytic cells.

MANIFESTATIONS OF INFLAMMATION

Local Manifestations of Inflammation

The local manifestations of inflammation depend on its cause and the particular tissue involved. These manifestations can range from swelling and the formation of exudates to abscess formation or ulceration.

Characteristically, the acute inflammatory response involves production of exudates that vary in terms of fluid, plasma proteins, and cellular debris. Acute inflammation can produce serous, hemorrhagic, fibrinous, membranous, or purulent exudates. Inflammatory exudates often are composed of a combination of these types. *Serous exudates* are watery fluids low in protein content that result from plasma entering the inflammatory site. *Hemorrhagic exudates* occur when there is severe tissue injury that causes damage to blood vessels or when there is significant leakage of red cells from the capillaries. *Fibrinous exudates* contain large amounts of fibrinogen and form a thick and sticky meshwork, much like the fibers of a blood clot. *Membranous* or *pseudomembranous exudates* develop on mucous membrane surfaces and are composed of necrotic cells enmeshed in a fibropurulent exudate.

A *purulent* or *suppurative exudate* contains pus, which is composed of degraded white blood cells, proteins, and tissue debris. Certain microorganisms, such as staphylococci, are more likely to induce localized suppurative inflammation than others. An abscess is a localized area of inflammation containing a purulent exudate (Fig. 14-4). Abscesses typically have a central necrotic core containing purulent exudates surrounded by a layer of neutrophils.[2] Fibroblasts may eventually enter the area and wall off the abscess. Because antimicrobial agents cannot penetrate the abscess wall, surgical incision and drainage may be required to effect a cure.

An *ulceration* refers to a site of inflammation where an epithelial surface (*e.g.*, skin or gastrointestinal epithelium) has become necrotic and eroded, often with associated subepithelial inflammation. Ulceration may occur as the result of traumatic injury to the epithelial surface (*e.g.*, peptic ulcer) or because of vascular compromise (foot ulcers associated with diabetes). In chronic lesions where there is repeated insult, the area surrounding the ulcer develops fibroblastic proliferation, scarring, and accumulation of chronic inflammatory cells.[2]

Systemic Manifestations of Inflammation

Under optimal conditions, the inflammatory response remains confined to a localized area. In some cases, however, local injury can result in prominent systemic manifestations as inflammatory mediators are released into the circulation. The most prominent systemic manifestations of inflammation are the acute-phase response, alterations in white blood cell count (leukocytosis or leukopenia),

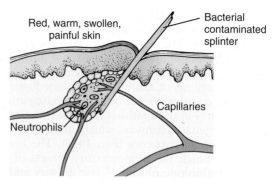

A Inflammation
Capillary dilation, fluid exudation, neutrophil migration

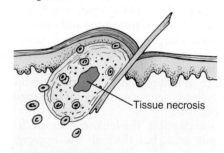

B Suppuration
Development of suppurative or purulent exudate containing degraded neutrophils and tissue debris

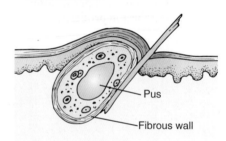

C Abscess formation
Walling off of the area of purulent (pus) exudate to form an abscess

FIGURE 14-4 Abscess formation. (**A**) Bacterial invasion and development of inflammation. (**B**) Continued bacterial growth, neutrophil migration, liquefaction tissue necrosis, and development of a purulent exudate. (**C**) Walling off of the inflamed area with its purulent exudate to form an abscess.

and fever. Sepsis and septic shock, also called the *systemic inflammatory response*, represent the severe systemic manifestations of inflammation (see Chapter 19).

Acute-Phase Response.   Along with the cellular responses that occur during the inflammatory response, a constellation of systemic effects called the *acute-phase response* occurs. In general, the acute-phase response serves to coordinate the various changes in body activity to enable an optimal host response. The acute-phase response, which usually begins within hours or days of the onset of inflammation or infection, includes changes in the concentrations of plasma proteins, increased erythrocyte sedimentation rate (ESR), fever, increased leukocyte count, skeletal muscle catabolism, and negative nitrogen balance. These responses are generated by the release of cytokines, particularly IL-1, IL-6, and TNF-α. These cytokines affect the thermoregulatory center in the hypothalamus to produce fever, the most obvious sign of the acute-phase response. IL-1 and other cytokines induce an increase in the number and immaturity of circulating neutrophils by stimulating their production in the bone marrow. Lethargy, a common feature of the acute-phase response, results from the effects of IL-1 and TNF-α on the central nervous system. The metabolic changes, including skeletal muscle catabolism, provide amino acids that can be used in the immune response and for tissue repair.

During the acute-phase response, the liver dramatically increases the synthesis of acute-phase proteins, such as fibrinogen and C-reactive protein (CRP), that serve several different nonspecific defense functions. Increased plasma levels of some acute-phase proteins are reflected in an accelerated ESR.

C-reactive protein, first described in 1930, is the classic acute-phase reactant. It was originally named *C precipitant* or *C-reactive substance* because it precipitated with the C fraction (C-polypeptide) of pneumococci. Ultimately, it was determined to be a protein; hence, its permanent designation became *C-reactive protein*.[5] The complete amino acid sequence of CRP has been described, and it can be accurately measured in the laboratory. Everyone maintains a low level of CRP; this level rises when there is an acute inflammatory response, sometimes to a factor of 500 or more. The function of CRP is thought to be protective, in that it binds to the surface of invading microorganisms and targets them for destruction by complement and phagocytosis. It is also thought to have an anti-inflammatory function, neutralizing inflammatory mediators, proteases, and oxidants released into the blood from inflamed tissues. Recent interest has focused on the use of CRP as a predictor of risk for cardiovascular events in persons with atherosclerotic heart disease.[6,7]

The ESR, which measures the rate at which erythrocytes settle out of anticoagulated blood, is used as a qualitative index to monitor the activity of many inflammatory diseases. The presence of increased levels of acute-phase proteins is associated with an increase in the ESR. The increased levels of acute-phase proteins are thought to dampen the repulsive effects of like charges on red blood cells, causing them to clump or aggregate, forming stacks (rouleau formation).

White Blood Cell Response (Leukocytosis and Leukopenia). Leukocytosis, or the increase in white blood cells, is a common feature of the inflammatory response, especially when it is caused by bacterial infection. The white blood cell count commonly increases to 15,000 to 20,000 cells/μL (normal, 4000 to 10,000 cells/μL) in acute inflammatory conditions. After being released from the bone marrow, circulating neutrophils have a life span of only about 10 hours and therefore must be constantly replaced if their numbers are to be adequate. With excessive demand for phagocytes, immature forms of neutrophils (bands) are released from the bone marrow. The phase, which is referred to as a *shift to the left* in a white blood cell differential count, refers to the increase in immature neutrophils seen in severe infections.

Bacterial infections produce a relatively selective increase in neutrophils (neutrophilia), whereas parasitic and allergic responses induce eosinophilia. Viral infections tend to produce a decrease in neutrophils (neutropenia) and an increase in lymphocytes (lymphocytosis).[3] Leukopenia is also encountered in infections that overwhelm persons with other debilitating diseases, such as cancer.

Lymphadenitis. Localized acute and chronic inflammation may lead to a reaction in the lymph nodes that drain the affected area. This reaction represents a nonspecific response to mediators released from the injured tissue or an immunologic response to a specific antigen. Painful, palpable nodes are more commonly associated with inflammatory processes, whereas nonpainful lymph nodes are more characteristic of neoplasms.[1]

CHRONIC INFLAMMATION

In contrast to acute inflammation, which is usually self-limited and brief, chronic inflammation is self-perpetuating and may last for weeks, months, or even years. It may develop as the result of a recurrent or progressive acute inflammatory process or from low-grade, smoldering responses that fail to evoke an acute response.

Characteristic of chronic inflammation is an infiltration by mononuclear cells (macrophages) and lymphocytes instead of the neutrophils commonly seen in acute inflammation. Chronic inflammation also involves the proliferation of fibroblasts instead of exudates. As a result, the risk of scarring and deformity usually is considered greater than in acute inflammation. Agents that evoke chronic inflammation typically are low-grade, persistent irritants that are unable to penetrate deeply or spread rapidly. Among the causes of chronic inflammation are foreign bodies such as talc, silica, asbestos, and surgical suture materials. Many viruses provoke chronic inflammatory responses, as do certain bacteria, fungi, and larger parasites of moderate to low virulence. Examples are the tubercle bacillus and the treponeme of syphilis. The presence of injured tissue such as that surrounding a healing fracture also may incite chronic inflammation. Immunologic mechanisms are thought to play an important role in chronic inflammation. The two patterns of chronic inflammation are a nonspecific chronic inflammation and granulomatous inflammation.

Nonspecific Chronic Inflammation

Nonspecific chronic inflammation involves a diffuse accumulation of macrophages and lymphocytes at the site of injury. Ongoing chemotaxis causes macrophages to

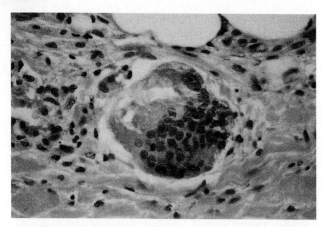

FIGURE 14-5 Foreign body giant cell. The numerous nuclei are randomly arranged in the cytoplasm. (Rubin E., Farber J. L. [1999]. *Pathology* [3rd ed., p. 40]. Philadelphia: Lippincott Williams & Wilkins.)

infiltrate the inflamed site, where they accumulate owing to prolonged survival and immobilization. These mechanisms lead to fibroblast proliferation, with subsequent scar formation that in many cases replaces the normal connective tissue or the functional parenchymal tissues of the involved structures. For example, scar tissue resulting from chronic inflammation of the bowel causes narrowing of the bowel lumen.

Granulomatous Inflammation

A granulomatous lesion is a distinctive form of chronic inflammation. A *granuloma* typically is a small, 1- to 2-mm lesion in which there is a massing of macrophages surrounded by lymphocytes. These modified macrophages resemble epithelial cells and sometimes are called *epithelioid cells*. Like other macrophages, these epithelioid cells are derived originally from blood monocytes. Granulomatous inflammation is associated with foreign bodies such as splinters, sutures, silica, and asbestos and with microorganisms that cause tuberculosis, syphilis, sarcoidosis, deep fungal infections, and brucellosis. These types of agents have one thing in common: they are poorly digested and usually are not easily controlled by other inflammatory mechanisms. The epithelioid cells in granulomatous inflammation may clump in a mass or coalesce, forming a multinucleated giant cell that attempts to surround the foreign agent (Fig. 14-5). A dense membrane of connective tissue eventually encapsulates the lesion and isolates it. These cells are often referred to as *foreign body giant cells*.

In summary, inflammation describes a local response to tissue injury and can present as an acute or chronic condition. The classic signs of inflammation are redness, swelling, local heat, pain, and loss of function. It involves a vascular phase during which blood flow and capillary permeability are increased, and a cellular phase during which phagocytic white blood cells move into the area to engulf and degrade the inciting agent. The inflammatory response is orchestrated by chemical mediators such as histamine, prostaglandins, PAF, complement fragments, and reactive molecules that are liberated by leukocytes.

Acute inflammation may involve the production of exudates containing serous fluid (serous exudate), red blood cells (hemorrhagic exudate), fibrinogen (fibrinous exudate), or tissue debris and white blood cell breakdown products (purulent exudate). The manifestations of inflammation include the systemic effects of the acute-phase response, such as fever and lethargy; increased ESR and levels of CRP and other acute-phase proteins; leukocytosis or, in some cases, leukopenia; and enlargement of the lymph nodes that drain the affected area.

In contrast to acute inflammation, which is self-limiting, chronic inflammation is prolonged and usually is caused by persistent irritants, most of which are insoluble and resistant to phagocytosis and other inflammatory mechanisms. Chronic inflammation involves the presence of mononuclear cells (lymphocytes and macrophages) rather than granulocytes.

Tissue Repair and Wound Healing

TISSUE REPAIR

Tissue repair, which overlaps the inflammatory process, is a response to tissue injury and represents an attempt to maintain normal tissue structure and function. It can take the form of regeneration in which the injured cells are replaced with cells of the same type, sometimes leaving no residual trace of previous injury, or it can take the form of replacement by connective tissue, which leaves a permanent scar. Both regeneration and repair by connective tissue replacement involve similar mechanisms, including cell migration, proliferation, and differentiation, as well as the action of chemical mediators and growth factors, and interaction with the extracellular matrix.

Tissue Regeneration

Tissue regeneration involves replacement of the injured tissue with cells of the same type, leaving little or no evidence of the previous injury. The capacity for regeneration varies with the tissue and cell type. Body cells are divided into three types according to their ability to undergo regeneration:[2,8] labile, stable, or permanent cells. *Labile cells* are those that continue to divide and replicate throughout life, replacing cells that are continually being destroyed. They include the surface epithelial cells of the skin, oral cavity, vagina, and cervix; the columnar epithelium of the gastrointestinal tract, uterus, and fallopian tubes; the transitional epithelium of the urinary tract; and bone

KEY CONCEPTS

Tissue Repair and Wound Healing

➤ Injured tissues can be repaired by regeneration of the injured tissue cells with cells of the same tissue or parenchymal type, or by connective repair processes in which scar tissue is used to effect healing.

➤ Regeneration is limited to tissues with cells that are able to undergo mitosis.

➤ Connective tissue repair occurs by primary or secondary intention and involves the inflammatory phase, the proliferative phase, and remodeling phases of the wound healing process.

➤ Wound healing is impaired by conditions that diminish blood flow and oxygen delivery, restrict nutrients and other materials needed for healing, and depress the inflammatory and immune responses; and by infection, wound separation, and the presence of foreign bodies.

marrow cells. *Stable cells* are those that normally stop dividing when growth ceases. However, these cells are capable of undergoing regeneration when confronted with an appropriate stimulus. *Permanent* or *fixed cells* cannot undergo mitotic division. The fixed cells include nerve cells, skeletal muscle cells, and cardiac muscle cells. These cells cannot regenerate; once destroyed, they are replaced with fibrous scar tissue that lacks the functional characteristics of the destroyed tissue.

Fibrous Tissue Repair

Severe or persistent injury with damage to both the parenchymal cells and extracellular matrix (ECM) leads to a situation in which the repair cannot be accomplished with regeneration alone. Under these conditions, repair occurs by replacement with connective tissue, a process that involves generation of granulation tissue and formation of scar tissue.

Granulation tissue is a glistening red, moist connective tissue that contains newly formed capillaries, proliferating fibroblasts, and residual inflammatory cells. The development of granulation tissue involves the growth of new capillaries (angiogenesis) and fibrogenesis, and formation of scar tissue. Angiogenesis involves the generation and sprouting of new blood vessels from preexisting vessels. These sprouting capillaries tend to protrude from the surface of the wound as minute red granules, imparting the name *granulation tissue*. Eventually, portions of the new capillary bed differentiate into arterioles and venules.

Fibrogenesis involves the influx of activated fibroblasts. Activated fibroblasts secrete components of the ECM, including fibronectin, hyaluronic acid, proteoglycans, and collagen (to be discussed). Fibronectin and hyaluronic acid are the first to be deposited in the healing wound, and proteoglycans appear later. Because the proteoglycans are hydrophilic, their accumulation contributes to the edematous appearance of the wound. The initiation of collagen synthesis contributes to the subsequent formation of scar tissue.

Scar formation builds on the granulation tissue framework of new vessels and loose ECM. The process occurs in two phases: (1) emigration and proliferation of fibroblasts into the site of injury, and (2) deposition of extracellular matrix by these cells. As healing progresses, the number of proliferating fibroblasts and new vessels decreases and there is increased synthesis and deposition of collagen. Collagen synthesis is important to the development of strength in the healing wound site. Ultimately, the granulation tissue scaffolding evolves into a scar composed of largely inactive spindle-shaped fibroblasts, dense collagen fibers, fragments of elastic tissue, and other ECM components. As the scar matures, vascular degeneration eventually transforms the highly vascular granulation tissue into a pale, largely avascular scar.

Regulation of the Healing Process

Tissue healing is regulated by the action of chemical mediators and growth factors that mediate the healing process as well as orchestrate the interactions between the extracellular and cell matrix.

Chemical Mediators and Growth Factors. Considerable research has contributed to the understanding of chemical mediators and growth factors that orchestrate the healing process. These chemical mediators and growth factors are released in an orderly manner from many of the cells that participate in tissue regeneration and the healing process. The chemical mediators include the interleukins, interferons, TNF, and arachidonic acid derivatives (prostaglandins and leukotrienes) that participate in the inflammatory response. The growth factors are hormone-like molecules that interact with specific cell surface receptors to control processes involved in tissue repair and wound healing.[2,8,9] They may act on adjacent cells or on the cell producing the growth factor. The growth factors are named for their tissue of origin (*e.g.,* platelet-derived growth factor [PDGF], fibroblast growth factor [FGF]), their biologic activity (*e.g.,* transforming growth factor [TGF]), or the cells on which they act (*e.g.,* epithelial growth factor [EGF]). The growth factors control the proliferation, differentiation, and metabolism of cells during wound healing. They assist in regulating the inflammatory process; serve as chemoattractants for neutrophils, monocytes (macrophages), fibroblasts, and epithelial cells; stimulate angiogenesis; and contribute to the generation of the ECM.

Extracellular Matrix. The understanding of tissue regeneration and repair has expanded over the past several decades to encompass the complex environment of the ECM. The ECM is secreted locally and assembles into a network of spaces surrounding tissue cells. There are three basic components of the ECM: fibrous structural proteins (*e.g.*, collagen and elastin fibers), water-hydrated gels (*e.g.*, proteoglycans and hyaluronan) that permit resilience and lubrication, and adhesive glycoproteins (*e.g.*, fibronectin and laminin) that connect the matrix elements one to another and to cells[2,8] (see Chapter 1). The ECM occurs in two basic forms: (1) the *basement membrane* that surrounds epithelial, endothelial, and smooth muscle cells; and (2) the *interstitial matrix* that is present in the spaces between cells in connective tissue and between the epithelium and supporting cells of blood vessels

The ECM provides turgor to soft tissue and rigidity to bone; it supplies the substratum for cell adhesion; it is involved in the regulation of growth, movement, and differentiation of the cells surrounding it; and it provides for the storage and presentation of regulatory molecules that control the repair process. The ECM also provides the scaffolding for tissue renewal. Although the cells in many tissues are capable of regeneration, injury does not always result in restoration of normal structure unless the ECM is intact. The integrity of the underlying basement membrane, in particular, is critical to the regeneration of tissue. When the basement membrane is disrupted, cells proliferate in a haphazard way, resulting in disorganized and nonfunctional tissues.

Critical to the process of wound healing is the transition from granulation tissue to scar tissue, which involves shifts in the composition of the ECM. In the transitional process, the ECM components are degraded by proteases (enzymes) that are secreted locally by a variety of cells (fibroblasts, macrophages, neutrophils, synovial cells, and epithelial cells). Some of the proteases, such as the collagenases, are highly specific, cleaving particular proteins at a small number of sites.[10] This allows for the structural integrity of the ECM to be retained while cell migration occurs. Because of their potential to produce havoc in tissues, the actions of the proteases are tightly controlled. They are typically elaborated in an inactive form that must be activated by certain chemicals or proteases that are likely to be present at the site of injury, and they are rapidly inactivated by tissue inhibitors. Recent research has focused on the unregulated action of the proteases in disorders such as cartilage matrix breakdown in arthritis and neuroinflammation in multiple sclerosis.[10]

WOUND HEALING

Because of its visibility, the healing of a skin wound is often used to illustrate the general principles of repair that apply in most tissues. Although more difficult to study, healing of visceral structures parallels the repair sequence in skin.

Healing by Primary and Secondary Intention

Depending on the extent of tissue loss, wound closure and healing occur by *primary* or *secondary* intention (Fig. 14-6). A sutured surgical incision is an example of

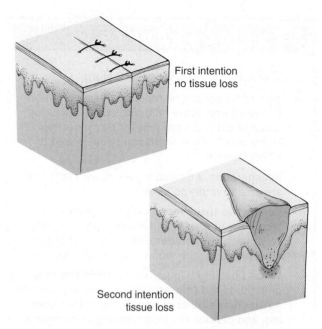

FIGURE 14-6 Healing of a skin wound by first and second intention.

healing by primary intention. Larger wounds (*e.g.*, burns and large surface wounds) that have a greater loss of tissue and wound contamination heal by secondary intention. Healing by secondary intention is slower than healing by primary intention and results in the formation of larger amounts of scar tissue. A wound that might otherwise have healed by primary intention may become infected and heal by secondary intention.

Phases of Wound Healing

Healing of a cutaneous wound is commonly divided into three phases: (1) the inflammatory phase, (2) the proliferative phase, and (3) the maturational or remodeling phase.[2,8,11,12] The duration of these phases is fairly predictable in wounds healing by primary intention. In wounds healing by secondary intention, the process depends on the extent of injury and the healing environment.

Inflammatory Phase. The inflammatory phase of wound healing begins at the time of injury and is a critical period because it prepares the wound environment for healing. It includes hemostasis (see Chapter 10) and the vascular and cellular phases of inflammation. Hemostatic processes are activated immediately at the time of injury. There is constriction of injured blood vessels and initiation of blood clotting through platelet activation and aggregation. After a brief period of constriction, these same vessels dilate and capillaries increase their permeability, allowing plasma and blood components to leak into the injured area. In small surface wounds, the clot loses fluid and becomes a hard, desiccated scab that protects the area.

The cellular phase of inflammation follows and is evidenced by the migration of phagocytic white blood cells that digest and remove invading organisms, fibrin, extracellular debris, and other foreign matter. The neutrophils are the first cells to arrive and are usually gone by day 3 or 4. They ingest bacteria and cellular debris. After approximately 24 hours, macrophages, which are larger and less specific phagocytic cells, enter the wound area and remain for an extended period. These cells, arising from blood monocytes, are essential to the healing process. Their functions include phagocytosis and release of growth factors that stimulate epithelial cell growth and angiogenesis and attract fibroblasts. When a large defect occurs in deeper tissues, neutrophils and macrophages are required to remove the debris and facilitate wound closure. Although a wound may heal in the absence of neutrophils, it cannot heal in the absence of macrophages.

Proliferative Phase. The proliferative phase of healing usually begins within 2 to 3 days of injury and may last as long as 3 weeks in wounds healing by primary intention. The primary processes during this time focus on the building of new tissue to fill the wound space. As early as 24 to 48 hours after injury, fibroblasts and vascular endothelial cells begin proliferating to form the granulation tissue that serves as the foundation for scar tissue development.

The final component of the proliferative phase is epithelialization, which is the migration, proliferation, and differentiation of the epithelial cells at the wound edges to form a new surface layer that is similar to that destroyed by the injury. In wounds that heal by primary intention, these epidermal cells proliferate and seal the wound within 24 to 48 hours.[2] Because epithelial cell migration requires a moist vascular wound surface and is impeded by a dry or necrotic wound surface, epithelialization is delayed in open wounds until a bed of granulation tissue has formed. When a scab has formed on the wound, the epithelial cells migrate between it and the underlying viable tissue; when a significant portion of the wound has been covered with epithelial tissue, the scab lifts off.

At times, excessive granulation tissue, sometimes called *proud flesh*, may form and extend above the edges of wound, preventing reepithelialization from taking place.[2] Surgical removal or cautery of the defect allows healing to proceed.

As the proliferative phase progresses, there is continued accumulation of collagen and proliferation of fibroblasts. Collagen synthesis reaches a peak within 5 to 7 days and continues for several weeks, depending on wound size. By the second week, the white blood cells have largely left the area, the edema has diminished, and the wound begins to blanch as the small blood vessels become thrombosed and degenerate.

Remodeling Phase. The third phase of wound healing, the remodeling process, begins approximately 3 weeks after injury and can continue for 6 months or longer, depending on the extent of the wound. As the term implies, there is continued remodeling of scar tissue by simultaneous synthesis of collagen by fibroblasts and lysis by collagenase enzymes. As a result of these two processes, the architecture of the scar becomes reoriented to increase the tensile strength of the wound.

Most wounds do not regain the full tensile strength of unwounded skin after healing is completed. Carefully sutured surgical wounds have approximately surgical 70% of the strength of unwounded skin, largely because of the placement of the sutures. This allows the person to move about freely after surgery without fear of wound separation. When the sutures are removed, usually at the end of the first week, wound strength is approximately 10%. It increases rapidly over the next 4 weeks and then slows, reaching a plateau of approximately 70% to 80% of the tensile strength of unwounded skin at the end of 3 months.[2] An injury that heals by secondary intention undergoes wound contraction during the proliferative and remodeling phases. As a result, the scar that forms is considerably smaller than the original wound. Cosmetically, this may be desirable because it reduces the size of the visible defect. However, contraction of scar tissue over joints and other body structures tends to limit movement and cause deformities. As a result of loss of elasticity, scar tissue that is stretched fails to return to its original length.

An abnormality in healing by scar tissue repair is *keloid* formation. Keloids are tumor-like masses caused by excess production of scar tissue (Fig. 14-7). The tendency toward development of keloids is more common in African Americans and seems to have a genetic basis.

Factors that Affect Wound Healing

Among the causes of impaired wound healing are malnutrition; impaired blood flow and oxygen delivery; impaired inflammatory and immune responses; infection, wound separation, and foreign bodies; and age effects.

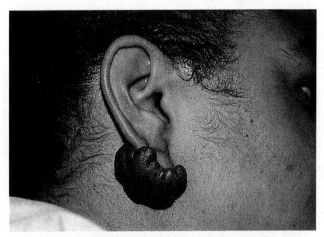

FIGURE 14-7 A keloid developed in this light-skinned black woman after ear piercing. (From Rubin E., Gorstein F., Rubin R., et al. [Eds.]. [2005]. *Rubin's pathology: Clinicopathologic foundations of medicine* [4th ed., p. 115]. Philadelphia: Lippincott Williams & Wilkins.)

Understanding ➤ Wound Healing

Wound healing involves the restoration of the integrity of injured tissue. The healing of skin wounds, which are commonly used to illustrate the general principles of wound healing, is generally divided into three phases: (1) the inflammatory phase, (2) the proliferative phase, and (3) the wound contraction and remodeling phase. Each of these phases is mediated through cytokines and growth factors.

1

Inflammatory phase. The inflammatory phase begins at the time of injury with the formation of a blood clot and the migration of phagocytic white blood cells into the wound site. The first cells to arrive, the neutrophils, ingest and remove bacteria and cellular debris. After 24 hours, the neutrophils are joined by macrophages, which continue to ingest cellular debris and play an essential role in the production of growth factors for the proliferative phase.

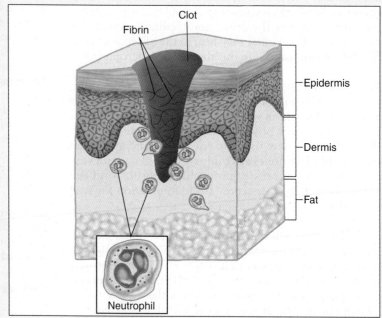

2

Proliferative phase. The primary processes during this phase focus on the building of new tissue to fill the wound space. The key cell during this phase is the *fibroblast*, a connective tissue cell that synthesizes and secretes the collagen, proteoglycans, and glycoproteins needed for wound healing. Fibroblasts also produce a family of growth factors that induce angiogenesis (growth of new blood vessels) and endothelial cell proliferation and migration. The final component of the proliferative phase is epithelialization, during which epithelial cells at the wound edges proliferate to form a new surface layer that is similar to that which was destroyed by the injury.

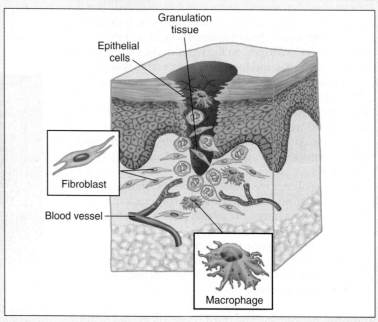

3

Wound contraction and remodeling phase. This phase begins approximately 3 weeks after injury with the development of the fibrous scar, and can continue for 6 months or longer, depending on the extent of the wound. During this phase, there is a decrease in vascularity and continued remodeling of scar tissue by simultaneous synthesis of collagen by fibroblasts and lysis by collagenase enzymes. As a result of these two processes, the architecture of the scar becomes reoriented to increase its tensile strength, and the size of the scar shrinks so it is less visible.

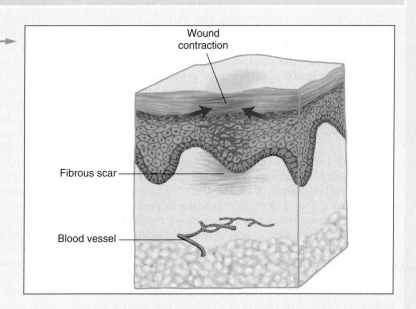

Malnutrition. Successful wound healing depends in part on adequate stores of proteins, carbohydrates, fats, vitamins, and minerals. It is well recognized that malnutrition slows the healing process, causing wounds to heal inadequately or incompletely.[13–15] Protein deficiencies prolong the inflammatory phase of healing and impair fibroblast proliferation, collagen and protein matrix synthesis, angiogenesis, and wound remodeling. Carbohydrates are needed as an energy source for white blood cells. Carbohydrates also have a protein-sparing effect and help to prevent the use of amino acids for fuel when they are needed for the healing process. Fats are essential constituents of cell membranes and are needed for the synthesis of new cells.

Although most vitamins are essential cofactors for the daily functions of the body, vitamins A and C play an essential role in the healing process. Vitamin C is needed for collagen synthesis. In vitamin C deficiency, improper sequencing of amino acids occurs, proper linking of amino acids does not take place, the byproducts of collagen synthesis are not removed from the cell, new wounds do not heal properly, and old wounds may fall apart. Vitamin A functions in stimulating and supporting epithelialization, capillary formation, and collagen synthesis. Vitamin A also has been shown to counteract the anti-inflammatory effects of corticosteroid drugs and can be used to reverse these effects in persons who are on chronic steroid therapy. The B vitamins are important cofactors in enzymatic reactions that contribute to the wound-healing process. All are water soluble, and with the exception of vitamin B_{12}, which is stored in the liver, almost all must be replaced daily. Vitamin K plays an indirect role in wound healing by preventing bleeding disorders that contribute to hematoma formation and subsequent infection.

The role of minerals in wound healing is less clearly defined. The macrominerals, including sodium, potassium, calcium, and phosphorus, as well as the microminerals, such as copper and zinc, must be present for normal cell function. Zinc is a cofactor in a variety of enzyme systems responsible for cell proliferation and reepithelialization.

Blood Flow and Oxygen Delivery. For healing to occur, wounds must have adequate blood flow to supply the necessary nutrients and to remove the resulting waste, local toxins, bacteria, and other debris. Impaired wound healing due to poor blood flow may occur as a result of wound conditions (*e.g.,* swelling) or preexisting health problems. Arterial disease and venous pathology are well-documented causes of impaired wound healing. In situations of severe trauma, a decrease in blood volume may cause a reduction in blood flow to injured tissues.

Molecular oxygen is required for collagen synthesis. It has been shown that even a temporary lack of oxygen can result in the formation of less stable collagen.[16,17] Wounds in ischemic tissue become infected more frequently than wounds in well-vascularized tissue. PMNs and macrophages require oxygen for destruction of microorganisms that have invaded the area. Although these cells can accomplish phagocytosis in a relatively anoxic environment, they cannot digest bacteria.

Hyperbaric oxygen is a treatment in which 100% oxygen is delivered at greater than twice the normal atmospheric pressure at sea level.[18] The goal is to increase oxygen delivery to tissues by increasing the partial pressure of oxygen dissolved in the plasma. An increase in tissue oxygen tension by hyperbaric oxygen enhances wound healing by a number of mechanisms, including the increased killing of bacteria by neutrophils, impaired growth of anaerobic bacteria, and the promotion of angiogenesis and fibroblast activity. Hyperbaric oxygen is currently reserved for the treatment of problem wounds in which hypoxia and infection interfere with healing.

Impaired Inflammatory and Immune Responses. Inflammatory and immune mechanisms function in wound healing. Inflammation is essential to the first phase of wound healing, and immune mechanisms prevent infections that impair wound healing. Among the conditions that impair inflammation and immune function are disorders of phagocytic function, diabetes mellitus, and therapeutic administration of corticosteroid drugs.

Phagocytic disorders may be divided into extrinsic and intrinsic defects. Extrinsic disorders are those that impair attraction of phagocytic cells to the wound site, prevent engulfment of bacteria and foreign agents by the phagocytic cells (*i.e.*, opsonization), or suppress the total number of phagocytic cells (*e.g.*, immunosuppressive agents). Intrinsic phagocytic disorders are the result of enzymatic deficiencies in the metabolic pathway for destroying the ingested bacteria by the phagocytic cell. The intrinsic phagocytic disorders include chronic granulomatous disease, an X-linked inherited disease in which there is a deficiency of enzymes needed for the generation of the superoxide free radical and hydrogen peroxide needed for killing bacteria.

Wound healing is a problem in persons with diabetes mellitus, particularly those who have poorly controlled blood glucose levels.[19,20] Of particular importance is the effect of hyperglycemia on phagocytic function. Neutrophils, for example, have diminished chemotactic and phagocytic function, including engulfment and intracellular killing of bacteria, when exposed to elevated blood glucose levels. Small blood vessel disease is also common among persons with diabetes, impairing the delivery of inflammatory cells, oxygen, and nutrients to the wound site.

The therapeutic administration of corticosteroid drugs decreases the inflammatory process and may delay the healing process. These hormones decrease capillary permeability during the early stages of inflammation, impair the phagocytic property of leukocytes, and inhibit fibroblast proliferation and function.

Wound Separation, Infection, and Foreign Bodies. Wound separation, contamination, and foreign bodies delay wound healing. Approximation of the wound edges (*i.e.*, suturing of an incision type of wound) greatly enhances healing and prevents infection. Large, gaping wounds tend to heal more slowly because it is often impossible to effect wound closure with this type of wound. Mechanical factors such as increased local pressure or torsion can cause wounds to pull apart, or *dehisce*. Foreign bodies tend to invite bacterial contamination and delay healing. Fragments of wood, steel, glass, and other compounds that may have entered the wound at the site of injury can be difficult to locate when the wound is treated. Sutures are also foreign bodies, and although needed for the closure of surgical wounds, they may serve as an impediment to healing. This is why sutures are removed as soon as possible after surgery.

Infection impairs all dimensions of wound healing.[2] It prolongs the inflammatory phase, impairs the formation of granulation tissue, and inhibits proliferation of fibroblasts and deposition of collagen fibers. All wounds are considered to be contaminated at the time of injury. Although body defenses can handle the invasion of microorganisms at the time of wounding, badly contaminated wounds can overwhelm host defenses. Trauma and existing impairment of host defenses also can contribute to the development of wound infections. Wound infections are of special concern in persons with implanted foreign bodies such as orthopedic devices (*e.g.*, pins, stabilization devices), cardiac pacemakers, and shunt catheters. These infections are difficult to treat and may require removal of the device.

In summary, the ability of tissues to repair damage due to injury depends on the body's ability to replace the parenchymal cells and organize them as they were originally. Body cells are divided into types according to their ability to regenerate: labile cells, such as the epithelial cells of the skin and gastrointestinal tract, which continue to regenerate throughout life; stable cells, such as those in the liver, which normally do not divide but are capable of regeneration when confronted with an appropriate stimulus; and permanent or fixed cells, such as nerve cells, which are unable to regenerate. Regeneration describes the process by which tissue is replaced with cells of a similar type and function. Healing by regeneration is limited to tissue with cells that are able to divide and replace the injured cells. Scar tissue repair involves the substitution of fibrous connective tissue for injured tissue that cannot be repaired by regeneration. Both tissue regeneration and healing by fibrous tissue repair depend on the action of chemical mediators and growth factors as well as interactions between the tissue cells and the ECM.

Wound healing occurs by primary and secondary intention and is commonly divided into three phases: the inflammatory phase, the proliferative phase, and the maturational or remodeling phase. In wounds healing by primary intention, the duration of the phases is fairly predictable. In wounds healing by secondary intention, the process depends on the extent of injury and the healing environment. Wound healing can be impaired or complicated by factors such as malnutrition; restricted blood flow and oxygen delivery; diminished inflammatory and immune responses; and infection, wound separation, and the presence of foreign bodies.

Temperature Regulation and Fever

Fever is a clinical hallmark of infection and inflammation. This section of the chapter focuses on regulation of body temperature and fever caused by infectious and noninfectious conditions.

BODY TEMPERATURE REGULATION

The temperature in the deep tissues of the body (core temperature) is normally maintained within a range of 36.0°C to 37.5°C (97.0°F to 99.5°F).[21–23] Within this range, there are individual differences and diurnal variations; internal core temperatures reach their highest point in late afternoon and evening and their lowest point in the early morning hours (Fig. 14-8). Virtually all biochemical processes in the body are affected by changes in temperature. Metabolic processes speed up or slow down, depending on whether body temperature is rising or falling.

Body temperature, which reflects the difference between heat production and heat loss, is regulated by the *thermoregulatory center* in the hypothalamus. Body heat is generated in the tissues of the body, transferred to the skin surface by the blood, and then released into the environment surrounding the body. It is the temperature of the deep body tissues, or "core" of the body, rather than the surface temperature, that is regulated by the thermoregulatory center. The temperature of the body is regulated almost entirely by nervous system feedback mechanisms, with the thermoregulatory center integrating input from cold and warmth receptors located throughout the body. The *thermostatic set point* of the thermoregulatory center is the level at which body temperature is regulated so that core temperature is maintained within the normal range. When body temperature begins to rise above this set point, heat-dissipating behaviors are initiated, and when the temperature falls below the set point, heat production is increased. A core temperature greater than 41°C (105.8°F) or less than 34°C (93.2°F) usually indicates that the body's ability to thermoregulate is impaired (Fig. 14-9). Body responses that produce, conserve, and

dissipate heat are described in Table 14-1. Spinal cord injuries that transect the cord at T6 or above can seriously impair temperature regulation because the hypothalamus no longer can control skin blood flow or sweating.

In addition to physiologic thermoregulatory mechanisms, humans engage in voluntary behaviors to help regulate body temperature. These behaviors include the

---

KEY CONCEPTS

Fever

→ Fever represents an increase in body temperature due to resetting of the hypothalamic thermoregulatory set point as the result of endogenous pyrogens released from host macrophages or endothelial cells.

→ In response to the increase in set point, the hypothalamus initiates physiologic responses to increase core temperature to match the new set point.

→ Fever is an adaptive response to bacterial and viral infections or to tissue injury. The growth rate of microorganisms is inhibited, and immune function is enhanced.

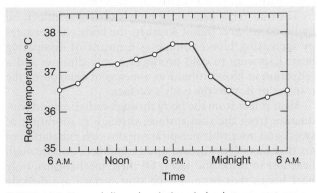

FIGURE 14-8 Normal diurnal variations in body temperature.

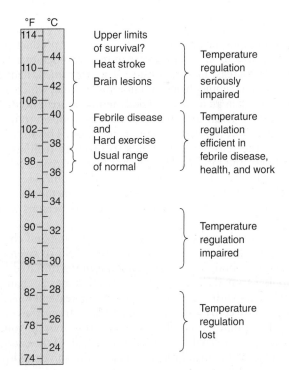

FIGURE 14-9 Body temperatures under different conditions. (From Dubois E. F. [1948]. *Fever and the regulation of body temperature.* Courtesy of Charles C Thomas, Publisher, Ltd., Springfield, IL.)

TABLE 14-1	Heat Gain and Heat Loss Responses Used in Regulation of Body Temperature		
Heat Gain		**Heat Loss**	
Body Response	*Mechanism of Action*	*Body Response*	*Mechanism of Action*
Vasoconstriction of the superficial blood vessels	Confines blood flow to the inner core of the body, with the skin and subcutaneous tissues acting as insulation to prevent loss of core heat	Dilatation of the superficial blood vessels	Delivers blood containing core heat to the periphery where it is dissipated through radiation, conduction, and convection
Contraction of the pilomotor muscles that surround the hairs on the skin	Reduces the heat loss surface of the skin	Sweating	Increases heat loss through evaporation
Assumption of the huddle position with the extremities held close to the body	Reduces the area for heat loss		
Shivering	Increases heat production by the muscles		
Increased production of epinephrine	Increases the heat production associated with metabolism		
Increased production of thyroid hormone	Is a long-term mechanism that increases metabolism and heat production		

selection of proper clothing and regulation of environmental temperature through heating systems and air conditioning. Body positions that hold the extremities close to the body (*e.g.,* huddling) prevent heat loss and are commonly assumed in cold weather.

Mechanisms of Heat Production

Metabolism is the body's main source of heat production. There is a 0.56°C (1°F) increase in body temperature for each 7% increase in metabolism.[21] The sympathetic neurotransmitters, epinephrine and norepinephrine, which are released when an increase in body temperature is needed, act at the cellular level to shift body metabolism to heat production rather than energy generation. This may be one of the reasons fever tends to produce feelings of weakness and fatigue. Thyroid hormone increases cellular metabolism, but this response usually requires several weeks to reach maximal effectiveness. The metabolic rate is typically 45% or more above normal in persons with hyperthyroidism.

Fine involuntary actions such as shivering and chattering of the teeth can produce a threefold to fivefold increase in body temperature. *Shivering* is initiated by impulses from the hypothalamus. The first muscle change that occurs with shivering is a general increase in muscle tone, followed by an oscillating rhythmic tremor involving the spinal-level reflex that controls muscle tone. Because no external work is performed, all of the energy liberated by the metabolic processes from shivering is in the form of heat.

Physical exertion also increases body temperature. With strenuous exercise, more than three fourths of the increased metabolism resulting from muscle activity

appears as heat within the body, and the remainder appears as external work.

Mechanisms of Heat Loss

Most of the body's heat is produced by the deeper core tissues (*i.e.,* muscles and viscera), and then transferred in the blood to the body surface, where it is released into the environment. Contraction of the *pilomotor muscles* of the skin, which raises the skin hair and produces goose bumps, reduces the surface area available for heat loss.

There are numerous *arteriovenous (AV) shunts* under the skin surface that allow blood to move directly from the arterial to the venous system.[21] These AV shunts are much like the radiators in a heating system. When the shunts are open, body heat is freely dissipated to the skin and surrounding environment; when the shunts are closed, heat is retained in the body. The blood flow in the AV shunts is controlled almost exclusively by the sympathetic nervous system in response to changes in core temperature and environmental temperature.

The transfer of heat to the body's surface is influenced by blood volume. In hot weather, the body compensates by increasing blood volume as a means of dissipating heat. Exposure to cold produces a cold diuresis and a reduction in blood volume as a means of controlling the transfer of heat to the body's surface.

Heat is lost from the body through radiation and conduction from the skin surface; through evaporation of sweat and insensible perspiration; through exhalation of air that has been warmed and humidified; and through heat lost in urine and feces. Of these mechanisms, only heat losses that occur at the skin surface are directly under hypothalamic control.

Radiation. Radiation involves the transfer of heat through the air or a vacuum. Heat loss through radiation varies with the temperature of the environment. Environmental temperature must be less than that of the body for heat loss to occur. About 60% to 70% of body heat loss typically occurs through radiation.

Conduction. Conduction involves the direct transfer of heat from one molecule to another. Blood carries, or conducts, heat from the inner core of the body to the skin surface. Normally, only a small amount of body heat is lost through conduction to a cooler surface. Cooling blankets and mattresses that are used for reducing fever rely on conduction of heat from skin to the cooler surface of the mattress or blanket. Heat can also be conducted in the opposite direction—from the external environment to the body surface. For instance, body temperature may rise slightly after a hot bath.

Water has a specific heat several times greater than air, so water absorbs far greater amounts of heat than air does. The loss of body heat can be excessive and life threatening in situations of cold-water immersion or cold exposure in damp or wet clothing.

Convection. Convection refers to heat transfer through the circulation of air currents. Normally, a layer of warm air tends to remain near the body's surface; convection causes continual removal of the warm layer and replacement with air from the surrounding environment. The wind-chill factor that often is included in the weather report combines the effect of convection caused by wind with the still-air temperature.

Evaporation. Evaporation involves the use of body heat to convert water on the skin to water vapor. Water that diffuses through the skin independent of sweating is called *insensible perspiration*. Insensible perspiration losses are greatest in a dry environment. Sweating occurs through the sweat glands and is controlled by the sympathetic nervous system. In contrast to other sympathetically mediated functions, sweating relies on acetylcholine as a neurotransmitter, rather than the catecholamines. This means that anticholinergic drugs, such as atropine, can interfere with heat loss by interrupting sweating.

Evaporative heat losses involve insensible perspiration and sweating, with 0.58 calorie being lost for each gram of water that is evaporated.[21] As long as body temperature is greater than the atmospheric temperature, heat is lost through radiation. However, when the temperature of the surrounding environment becomes greater than skin temperature, evaporation is the only way the body can rid itself of heat. Any condition that prevents evaporative heat losses causes the body temperature to rise.

FEVER

Fever, or *pyrexia*, describes an elevation in body temperature that is caused by a cytokine-induced upward displacement of the set point of the hypothalamic thermoregulatory center. Fever is resolved or "broken" when the factor that caused the increase in the set point is removed. Fevers that are regulated by the hypothalamus usually do not rise above 41°C (105.8°F), suggesting a built-in thermostatic safety mechanism. Temperatures above that level are usually the result of superimposed activity, such as convulsions, hyperthermic states, or direct impairment of the temperature control center.

Fever can be caused by a number of microorganisms and substances that are collectively called *pyrogens* (Fig. 14-10). Many proteins, breakdown products of proteins, and certain other substances, including lipopolysaccharide toxins released from bacterial cell membranes, can

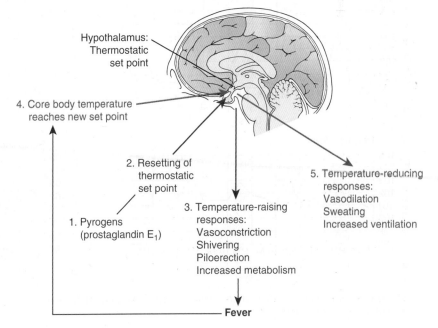

FIGURE 14-10 Mechanisms of fever. (1) Release of endogenous pyrogen from inflammatory cells, (2) resetting of hypothalamic thermostatic set point to a higher level (prodrome), (3) generation of hypothalamus-mediated responses that raise body temperature (chill), (4) development of fever with elevation of body temperature to new thermostatic set point, and (5) production of temperature-lowering responses (flush and defervescence) and return of body temperature to a lower level.

Hypothalamus: Thermostatic set point

4. Core body temperature reaches new set point

2. Resetting of thermostatic set point

1. Pyrogens (prostaglandin E₁)

3. Temperature-raising responses: Vasoconstriction Shivering Piloerection Increased metabolism

5. Temperature-reducing responses: Vasodilation Sweating Increased ventilation

Fever

raise the set point of the hypothalamic thermostat. Some pyrogens can act directly and immediately on the hypothalamic thermoregulatory center to increase its set point. Other pyrogens, sometimes called *exogenous pyrogens,* act indirectly and may require several hours to produce their effect.[21]

Exogenous pyrogens induce host cells, such as blood leukocytes and tissue macrophages, to produce fever-producing mediators called *endogenous pyrogens* (e.g., IL-1). For example, the phagocytosis of bacteria and breakdown products of bacteria that are present in the blood lead to the release of endogenous pyrogens into the circulation. The endogenous pyrogens are thought to increase the set point of the hypothalamic thermoregulatory center through the action of prostaglandin E_2.[21] In response to the sudden increase in set point, the hypothalamus initiates heat production behaviors (shivering and vasoconstriction) that increase the core body temperature to the new set point, and fever is established. In addition to their fever-producing actions, the endogenous pyrogens mediate a number of other responses. For example, IL-1 is an inflammatory mediator that produces other signs of inflammation, such as leukocytosis, anorexia, and malaise.

Many noninfectious disorders, such as myocardial infarction, pulmonary emboli, and neoplasms, produce fever. In these conditions, the injured or abnormal cells incite the production of pyrogen. For example, trauma and surgery can be associated with several days of fever. Some malignant cells, such as those of leukemia and Hodgkin disease, secrete pyrogen.

A fever that has its origin in the central nervous system is sometimes referred to as a *neurogenic fever.*[24] It usually is the result of damage to the hypothalamus caused by central nervous system trauma, intracerebral bleeding, or an increase in intracranial pressure. Neurogenic fevers are characterized by a high temperature that is resistant to antipyretic therapy and is not associated with sweating.

The purpose of fever is not completely understood. However, from a purely practical standpoint, fever is a valuable index to health status. For many, fever signals the presence of an infection and may legitimize the need for medical treatment. In ancient times, fever was thought to "cook" the poisons that caused the illness. With the availability of antipyretic drugs in the late 19th century, the belief that fever was useful began to wane, probably because most antipyretic drugs also had analgesic effects.

There is little research to support the belief that fever is harmful unless the temperature rises to extreme levels. It has been shown that small elevations in temperature, such as those that occur with fever, enhance immune function. There is increased motility and activity of the white blood cells, stimulation of interferon production, and activation of T cells.[25,26] Many of the microbial agents that cause infection grow best at normal body temperatures, and their growth is inhibited by temperatures in the fever range. For example, the rhinoviruses responsible for the common cold are cultured best at 33°C (91.4°F), which is close to the temperature in the nasopharynx. Temperature-sensitive mutants of the virus that cannot grow at temperatures greater than 37.5°C (99.5°F) produce fewer signs and symptoms.[27]

Patterns

The patterns of temperature change in persons with fever vary and may provide information about the nature of the causative agent.[28,29] These patterns can be described as intermittent, remittent, sustained, or relapsing (Fig. 14-11). An *intermittent fever* is one in which temperature

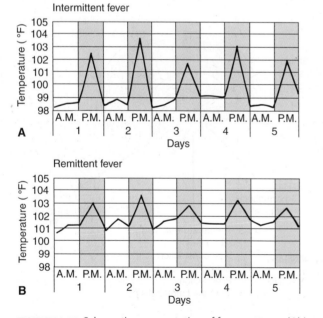

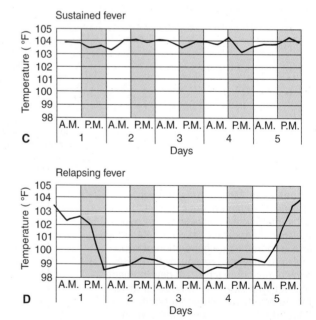

FIGURE 14-11 Schematic representation of fever patterns: (**A**) intermittent, (**B**) remittent, (**C**) sustained, and (**D**) recurrent or relapsing.

returns to normal at least once every 24 hours. Intermittent fevers are commonly associated with conditions such as gram-negative/positive sepsis, abscesses, and acute bacterial endocarditis. In a *remittent fever*, the temperature does not return to normal and varies a few degrees in either direction. It is associated with viral upper respiratory tract, *Legionella*, and mycoplasma infections. In a *sustained* or *continuous* fever, the temperature remains above normal with minimal variations (usually less than 0.55°C or 1°F). Sustained fevers are seen in persons with drug fever. A *recurrent* or *relapsing fever* is one in which there is one or more episodes of fever, each as long as several days, with one or more days of normal temperature between episodes. Relapsing fevers may be caused by a variety of infectious diseases, including tuberculosis, fungal infections, Lyme disease, and malaria.

Critical to the analysis of a fever pattern is the relation of heart rate to the level of temperature elevation. Normally, a 1°C rise in temperature produces a 15-bpm (beats per minute) increase in heart rate (1°F, 10 bpm).[28] Most persons respond to an increase in temperature with an appropriate increase in heart rate. The observation that a rise in temperature is not accompanied by the anticipated change in heart rate can provide useful information about the cause of the fever. For example, a heart rate that is slower than would be anticipated can occur with Legionnaires disease and drug fever, and a heart rate that is more rapid than anticipated can be symptomatic of hyperthyroidism.

Manifestations

The physiologic behaviors that occur during the development of fever can be divided into four successive stages: a prodrome; a chill, during which the temperature rises; a flush; and defervescence. During the *first* or *prodromal* period, there are nonspecific complaints, such as mild headache and fatigue, general malaise, and fleeting aches and pains. During the *second stage* or *chill*, there is the uncomfortable sensation of being chilled and the onset of generalized shaking, although the temperature is rising. Vasoconstriction and piloerection usually precede the onset of shivering. At this point the skin is pale and covered with goose flesh. There is a feeling of being cold and an urge to put on more clothing or covering and to curl up in a position that conserves body heat. When the shivering has caused the body temperature to reach the new set point of the temperature control center, the shivering ceases, and a sensation of warmth develops. At this point, the *third stage* or *flush* begins, during which cutaneous vasodilatation occurs and the skin becomes warm and flushed. The *fourth,* or *defervescence,* stage of the febrile response is marked by the initiation of sweating. Not all persons proceed through the four stages of fever development. Sweating may be absent, and fever may develop gradually, with no indication of a chill or shivering.

Common manifestations of fever are anorexia, myalgia, arthralgia, and fatigue. These discomforts are worse when the temperature rises rapidly or exceeds 39.5°C (103.1°F). Respiration is increased, and the heart rate usually is elevated. Dehydration occurs because of sweating and the increased vapor losses caused by the rapid respiratory rate. The occurrence of chills commonly coincides with the introduction of pyrogen into the circulation. This is one of the reasons that blood cultures to identify the organism causing the fever are usually drawn during the first signs of a chill.

Many of the manifestations of fever are related to the increases in the metabolic rate, increased need for oxygen, and use of body proteins as an energy source. During fever, the body switches from using glucose (an excellent medium for bacterial growth) to metabolism based on protein and fat breakdown. With prolonged fever, there is increased breakdown of endogenous fat stores. If fat breakdown is rapid, metabolic acidosis may result (see Chapter 6).

Headache is a common accompaniment of fever and is thought to result from the vasodilatation of cerebral vessels occurring with fever. Delirium is possible when the temperature exceeds 40°C (104°F). In the elderly, confusion and delirium may follow moderate elevations in temperature. Because of the increasingly poor oxygen uptake by the aging lung, pulmonary function may prove to be a limiting factor in the hypermetabolism that accompanies fever in older persons. Confusion, incoordination, and agitation commonly reflect cerebral hypoxemia. Febrile seizures can occur in some children.[30] They usually occur with rapidly rising temperatures or at a threshold temperature that differs with each child.

Herpetic lesions, or fever blisters, develop in some persons during fever. They are caused by a separate infection by the type 1 herpes simplex virus that established latency in the regional ganglia and is reactivated by a rise in body temperature.

Diagnosis and Treatment

Fever usually is a manifestation of a disease state, and as such, determining the cause of a fever is an important aspect of its treatment. Sometimes it is difficult to establish the cause of a fever. A prolonged fever for which the cause is difficult to ascertain is often referred to as *fever of unknown origin* (FUO). FUO is defined as a temperature elevation of 38.3°C (101°F) or higher that is present for 3 weeks or longer.[31] Among the causes of FUO are malignancies (*i.e.*, lymphomas, metastases to the liver and central nervous system); infections such as human immunodeficiency virus or tuberculosis, or abscessed infections; and drug fever. Malignancies, particularly non-Hodgkin lymphoma, are important causes of FUO in the elderly. Cirrhosis of the liver is another cause of FUO.

The methods of fever treatment focus on modifications of the external environment intended to increase heat transfer from the internal to the external environment, support of the hypermetabolic state that accompanies fever, protection of vulnerable body organs and systems, and treatment of the infection or condition causing the fever. Because fever is a disease symptom, its manifestation suggests the need for treatment of the primary cause.

Modification of the environment ensures that the environmental temperature facilitates heat transfer away from the body. Sponge baths with cool water or an alcohol solution can be used to increase evaporative heat losses. More profound cooling can be accomplished through the use of a cooling blanket or mattress, which facilitates the conduction of heat from the body into the coolant solution that circulates through the mattress. Care must be taken so that cooling methods do not produce vasoconstriction and shivering that decrease heat loss and increase heat production.

Adequate fluids and sufficient amounts of simple carbohydrates are needed to support the hypermetabolic state and prevent the tissue breakdown that is characteristic of fever. Additional fluids are needed for sweating and to balance the insensible water losses from the lungs that accompany an increase in respiratory rate. Fluids also are needed to maintain an adequate vascular volume for heat transport to the skin surface.

Antipyretic drugs, such as aspirin and acetaminophen, often are used to alleviate the discomforts of fever and protect vulnerable organs, such as the brain, from extreme elevations in body temperature. These drugs act by resetting the hypothalamic temperature control center to a lower level, presumably by blocking the activity of cyclooxygenase, an enzyme that is required for the conversion of arachidonic acid to prostaglandin E_2.

Fever in Children

The mechanisms for controlling temperature are not well developed in the infant. In infants younger than 3 months, a mild elevation in temperature (i.e., rectal temperature of 38°C [100.4°F]) can indicate serious infection that requires immediate medical attention.[32–35] Fever without a source occurs frequently in infants and children and is a common reason for visits to the clinic or emergency department.

Both minor and life-threatening infections are common in the infant to 3-year age group.[34,35] The most common causes of fever in children are minor or more serious infections of the respiratory system, urinary system, gastrointestinal tract, or central nervous system. Occult bacteremia and meningitis also occur in this age group and should be excluded as diagnoses. The Agency for Health Care Policy and Research Expert Panel has developed clinical guidelines for use in the treatment of infants and children 0 to 36 months of age with fever without a source.[35] The guidelines define fever in this age group as a rectal temperature of at least 38°C (100.4°F). The guidelines also point out that fever may result from overbundling or a vaccine reaction. When overbundling is suspected, it is suggested that the infant be unbundled and the temperature retaken after 15 to 30 minutes.

Fever in infants and children can be classified as low risk or high risk, depending on the probability of the infection progressing to bacteremia or meningitis. Infants usually are considered at low risk if they were delivered at term and sent home with their mother without complications and have been healthy with no previous hospital-

izations or previous antimicrobial therapy. A white blood cell count and urinalysis are recommended as a means of confirming low-risk status. Signs of toxicity (and high risk) include lethargy, poor feeding, hypoventilation, poor tissue oxygenation, and cyanosis. Blood and urine cultures, chest radiographs, and lumbar puncture usually are done in high-risk infants and children to determine the cause of fever.

Infants with fever who are considered to be at low risk usually are managed on an outpatient basis provided the parents or caregivers are deemed reliable. Older children with fever without source also may be treated on an outpatient basis. Parents or caregivers require full instructions, preferably in writing, regarding assessment of the febrile child. They should be instructed to contact their health care provider should their child show signs suggesting sepsis. Infants younger than 3 months are evaluated carefully. Infants and children with signs of toxicity or petechiae (a sign of meningitis) usually are hospitalized for evaluation and treatment.[34,35] Parenteral antimicrobial therapy usually is initiated after samples for blood, urine, and spinal fluid cultures have been taken.

Fever in the Elderly

In the elderly, even slight elevations in temperature may indicate serious infection or disease. This is because the elderly often have a lower baseline temperature, and although they increase their temperature during an infection, it may fail to reach a level that is equated with significant fever.[36–38]

Normal body temperature and the circadian pattern of temperature variation often are altered in the elderly. Elderly persons are reported to have a lower basal temperature (36.4°C [97.6°F] in one study) than do younger persons.[36] It has been recommended that the definition of fever in the elderly be expanded to include an elevation of temperature of at least 1.1°C (2°F) above baseline values.[37]

It has been suggested that 20% to 30% of elders with serious infections present with an absent or blunted febrile response.[36] When fever is present in the elderly, it usually indicates the presence of serious infection, most often caused by bacteria. The absence of fever may delay diagnosis and initiation of antimicrobial treatment. Unexplained changes in functional capacity, worsening of mental status, weakness and fatigue, and weight loss are signs of infection in the elderly. They should be viewed as possible signs of infection and sepsis when fever is absent. The probable mechanisms for the blunted fever response include a disturbance in sensing of temperature by the thermoregulatory center in the hypothalamus, alterations in release of endogenous pyrogens, and the failure to elicit responses such as vasoconstriction of skin vessels, increased heat production, and shivering that increase body temperature during a febrile response.

Another factor that may delay recognition of fever in the elderly is the method of temperature measurement. Oral temperature remains the most commonly used method for measuring temperature in the elderly.

It has been suggested that rectal and tympanic membrane methods may be more effective in detecting fever in the elderly. This is because conditions such as mouth breathing, tongue tremors, and agitation often make it difficult to obtain accurate oral temperatures in the elderly.

In summary, body temperature is normally maintained within a range of 36.0°C to 37.4°C (97.0°F to 99.5°F). Body heat is produced by metabolic processes that occur within deep core structures of the body and is lost at the body's surface when core heat is transported to the skin by the circulating blood. The transfer of heat from the skin to the environment occurs through radiation, conduction, convection, and evaporation. The thermoregulatory center in the hypothalamus functions to modify heat production and heat losses as a means of regulating body temperature. Fever represents an increase in body temperature outside the normal range. Fever can be caused by a number of factors, including microorganisms, trauma, and drugs or chemicals, all of which incite the release of endogenous pyrogens and subsequent resetting of the hypothalamic thermoregulatory center. The reactions that occur during fever consist of four stages: a prodrome, a chill, a flush, and defervescence. Many of the manifestations of fever are related to the increases in the metabolic rate, increased need for oxygen, and use of body proteins as an energy source.

Fever in infants and children can be classified as low risk or high risk, depending on the probability of the infection progressing to bacteremia or meningitis. Infants younger than 28 days and those at high risk usually are hospitalized for evaluation of their fever and treatment. In the elderly, even slight elevations in temperature may indicate serious infection or disease. The elderly often have a lower baseline temperature, so serious infections may go unrecognized because of the perceived lack of a significant fever.

Review Exercises

A 15-year-old boy presents with abdominal pain, a temperature of 38°C (100.5°F), and an elevated white blood cell count of 13,000/μL, with an increase in neutrophils. A tentative diagnosis of appendicitis is made.

A. Explain the significance of pain as it relates to the inflammatory response.
B. What is the cause of the fever and elevated white blood cell count?
C. What would be the preferred treatment for this boy?

Aspirin and other NSAIDs are used to control the manifestations of chronic inflammatory disorders such as arthritis.

A. Explain their mechanism of action in terms of controlling the inflammatory response.

After a heart attack, the area of heart muscle that has undergone necrosis because of a lack of blood supply undergoes healing by replacement with scar tissue.

A. Compare the functioning of the heart muscle that has been replaced by scar tissue with that of the normal surrounding heart muscle.

A 35-year-old man with a large abscess on his leg is seen in the outpatient department. He tells you he injured his leg while doing repair work on his house and he thinks there might be a wood sliver in the infected area.

A. Explain the events that participate in formation of an abscess.
B. He is told that incision and drainage of the lesion will be needed so healing can take place. Explain.
C. He is reluctant to have the procedure done and asks whether an antibiotic would work as well. Explain why antibiotics alone are usually not effective in eliminating the microorganisms contained in an abscess.

A 3-year-old child is seen in a pediatric clinic with a temperature of 39°C (103°F) temperature. Her skin is warm and flushed, her pulse is 120 bpm, and her respirations are shallow and rapid at 32 breaths per minute. Her mother states that she has complained of a sore throat and has refused to drink or take medications to bring her temperature down.

A. Explain the physiologic mechanisms of fever generation.
B. Are the warm and flushed skin, rapid heart rate, and respirations consistent with this level of fever?
C. After receiving an appropriate dose of acetaminophen, the child begins to sweat, and the temperature drops to 37.2°C. Explain the physiologic mechanisms responsible for the drop in temperature.

REFERENCES

1. Murphy H. S., Ward P. A. (2005). Inflammation. In Rubin E., Gorstein F., Rubin R., et al. (Eds.), *Rubin's pathology: Clinicopathologic foundations of medicine* (4th ed., pp. 41–83). Philadelphia: Lippincott Williams & Wilkins.

2. Kumar V., Abbas A. K., Fausto N. (Eds.). (2005). *Robbins and Cotran pathologic basis of disease* (7th ed., pp. 47–86, 87–118). Philadelphia: Elsevier Saunders.

3. Chandrasoma P., Taylor C. R. (1998). *Concise pathology* (3rd ed., pp. 31–92). Stamford, CT: Appleton & Lange.

4. Nathan C. (2002). Points of control in inflammation. *Nature* 420, 848–852.

5. Gewurz H. (1982). Biology of C-reactive protein and the acute phase response. *Hospital Practice* 17(6), 67–81.

6. Haverkate F., Thompson S. G., Pyke S. D., et al. (1997). Production of C-reactive protein and risk of coronary events in stable and unstable angina. *Lancet* 349, 462–466.

7. Ridker P. M., Hennekens C. H., Buring J. E., et al. (2000). C-reactive protein and other markers of inflammation in prediction of cardiovascular disease in women. *New England Journal of Medicine* 342, 836–843.

8. Sephel G. C., Woodward S. C. (2005). Repair, regeneration, and fibrosis. In Rubin E., Gorstein F., Rubin R., et al. (Eds.), *Rubins' pathology: Clinicopathologic foundations of medicine* (4th ed., pp. 85–116). Philadelphia: Lippincott Williams & Wilkins.

9. Robson M. C. (2003). Cytokine manipulation of the wound. *Clinical Plastic Surgery* 30, 57–65.

10. Parks W. C. (1999). Matrix metalloproteinases in repair. *Wound Repair and Regeneration* 7, 423–432.

11. Singer A. J., Clark R. A. F. (1999). Cutaneous wound healing. *New England Journal of Medicine* 341, 738–746.

12. Monaco J. L., Lawrence W. T. (2003). Acute wound healing: An overview. *Clinical Plastic Surgery* 30, 1–12.

13. Harding K. G., Morris H. L., Patel K. G. (2002). Healing chronic wounds. *British Medical Journal* 324, 160–163.

14. Burns J. L., Mancoll J. S., Phillips L. G. (2003). Impairments of wound healing. *Clinical Plastic Surgery* 30, 47–56.

15. Albina J. E. (1995). Nutrition and wound healing. *Journal of Parenteral and Enteral Nutrition* 18, 367–376.

16. Whitney J. D. (1990). The influence of tissue oxygenation and perfusion on wound healing. *Clinical Issues in Critical Care Nursing* 1, 578–584.

17. Whitney J. D. (1989). Physiologic effects of tissue oxygenation on wound healing. *Heart and Lung* 18, 466–474.

18. Zamboni W. A., Browder L. K., Martinez J. (2003). Hyperbaric oxygen and wound healing. *Clinics in Plastic Surgery* 30, 67–75.

19. King L. (2000). Impaired wound healing in patients with diabetes. *Nursing Standards* 15(38), 39–45.

20. Greenhalgh D. G. (2003). Wound healing and diabetes mellitus. *Clinics in Plastic Surgery* 30, 37–45.

21. Guyton A. C., Hall J. E. (2006). *Textbook of medical physiology* (11th ed., pp. 889–901). Philadelphia: Elsevier Saunders.

22. Wenger C. B. (2003). The regulation of body temperature. In Rhoades R. A., Tanner G. A. (Eds.), *Medical physiology* (2nd ed., pp. 527–550). Philadelphia: Lippincott Williams & Wilkins.

23. Gisolfi C. V., Mora F. (2000). *The hot brain: Survival, temperature, and the human body.* Cambridge, MA: MIT Press.

24. Saper C. B., Breder C. D. (1994). The neurologic basis of fever. *New England Journal of Medicine* 330, 1880–1886.

25. Dinarello C. A., Gatti S., Bartfai T. (1999). Fever: Links with an ancient receptor. *Current Biology,* 9, R147–R150.

26. Blatteis C. M. (1998). Fever. In Blatteis C. M. (Ed.), *Physiology and pathophysiology of temperature regulation* (pp. 178–192). River Edge, NJ: World Scientific Publishing.

27. Rodbard D. (1981). The role of regional temperature in the pathogenesis of disease. *New England Journal of Medicine* 305, 808–814.

28. McGee Z. A., Gorby G. L. (1987). The diagnostic value of fever patterns. *Hospital Practice* 22(10), 103–110.

29. Cunha B. A. (1996). The clinical significance of fever patterns. *Infectious Disease Clinics of North America* 10, 33–43.

30. Champi C., Gaffney-Yocum P. A. (1999). Managing febrile seizures in children. *Nurse Practitioner* 24(10), 28–30, 34–35.

31. Cunha B. A. (1996). Fever without source. *Infectious Disease Clinics of North America* 10, 111–127.

32. Baker M. D. (1999). Evaluation and management of infants with fever. *Pediatric Clinics of North America* 46, 1061–1072.

33. Park J. W. (2000). Fever without source in children. *Postgraduate Medicine* 107, 259–266.

34. Luszczak M. (2001). Evaluation and management of infants and young children with fever. *American Family Physician* 64, 1219–1226.

35. Baraff L. J., Bass J. W., Fleisher G. R., et al. (1993). Practice guidelines for the management of infants and children 0 to 36 months of age with fever without source. Agency for Health Care Policy and Research. (Erratum appears in *Annals of Emergency Medicine* [1993]. 22, 1490.) *Annals of Emergency Medicine* 22, 1198–1210.

36. Yoshikawa T. T., Norman D. C. (1996). Approach to fever and infections in the nursing home. *Journal of the American Geriatrics Society* 44, 74–82.

37. Yoshikawa T. T., Norman D. C. (1998). Fever in the elderly. *Infectious Medicine* 15, 704–706, 708.

38. Castle S. C., Yeh M., Toledo S., et al. (1993). Lowering the temperature criterion improves detection of infections in nursing home residents. *Aging: Immunology and Infectious Disease* 4, 67–76.

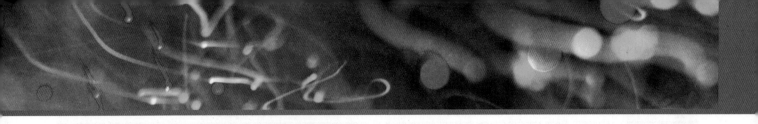

C h a p t e r *15*

Alterations in the Immune Response

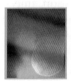 The immune system is a multifaceted defense network that has evolved to protect against invading microorganisms, prevent the proliferation of cancer cells, and mediate the healing of damaged tissue. Under normal conditions, the immune response deters or prevents disease. Occasionally, however, the inadequate, inappropriate, or misdirected activation of the immune system can lead to debilitating or life-threatening illnesses, typified by allergic or hypersensitivity reactions, autoimmune disorders, transplantation rejection, and immunodeficiency states.

 ## Hypersensitivity Disorders

Hypersensitivity disorders refer to excessive or inappropriate activation of the immune system. Although activation of the immune system normally leads to production of antibodies and T-cell responses that protect the body against attack by microorganisms, it is also capable of causing tissue injury and disease. Disorders caused by immune responses are collectively referred to as *hypersensitivity reactions*.

Hypersensitivity disorders are commonly divided into four types: type I, immediate hypersensitivity disorders; type II, antibody-mediated disorders; type III, immune complex–mediated disorders; and type IV, T-cell–mediated disorders[1,2] (Table 15-1). These categories differ in terms of type of immune response and location of the antigen that is the target of the response.

TYPE I IMMEDIATE HYPERSENSITIVITY

Type I reactions are immunoglobulin E (IgE)–mediated hypersensitivity reactions that begin rapidly, often within minutes of antigen challenge. These types of reactions are often referred to as *allergic reactions* and the antigens causing the response as *allergens*. Typical allergens include the protein in pollen, house dust mites, animal dander, foods, and chemicals like the antibiotic penicillin. Exposure to

TABLE 15-1	Classification of Hypersensitivity Responses	
Type	**Mechanism**	**Examples**
I Immediate hypersensitivity	IgE-mediated—mast cell degranulation	Hay fever, asthma, anaphylaxis
II Antibody-mediated hypersensitivity	Formation of antibodies (IgG, IgM) against cell surface antigens. Complement usually is involved.	Autoimmune hemolytic anemia, hemolytic disease of the newborn, Goodpasture disease
III Immune complex-mediated hypersensitivity	Formation of antibodies (IgG, IgM, IgA) that interact with exogenous or endogenous antigens to form antigen–antibody complexes that cause vessel or tissue injury.	Arthus reaction, autoimmune diseases (systemic lupus erythematosus, rheumatoid arthritis), certain forms of acute glomerulosclerosis
IV Cell-mediated hypersensitivity	Sensitized T lymphocytes release cytokines that cause direct cell-mediated cytotoxicity or delayed-type hypersensitivity disorders.	Tuberculosis, contact dermatitis, transplant rejection

the allergen can be through inhalation, ingestion, injection, or skin contact.

Two types of cells are central to a type I hypersensitivity reaction: CD4+ helper T cells of the T_H2 type and mast cells or basophils.[1–3] In contrast to CD4+ helper T cells of the T_H1 type that differentiate in response to microbes and stimulate IgG production, T_H2 cells differentiate in response to allergens and helminths (intestinal parasites). Cytokines (cell messengers) produced by T_H2 cells stimulate the differentiation of B cells into IgE-producing plasma cells, act as growth factors for mast cells, and recruit and activate eosinophils[1] (Fig. 15-1).

Mast cells, which are tissue cells, and basophils, which are blood cells, are derived from hematopoietic (blood)

precursor cells. Mast cells normally are distributed throughout connective tissue, especially areas beneath the skin and mucous membranes of the respiratory, gastrointestinal, and genitourinary tracts, and adjacent to blood and lymph vessels.[4,5] This location places mast cells near surfaces that are exposed to environmental antigens and parasites. Mast cells have preformed granules containing mediators that initiate the early events in type I hypersensitivity reactions.

Type I hypersensitivity reactions begin with mast cell sensitization. During the sensitization or priming stage, allergen-specific IgE antibodies attach to receptors on the surface of mast cells.[6] With subsequent exposure, the sensitizing allergen binds to the cell-associated IgE and triggers a series of events that ultimately lead to degranulation of the sensitized mast cells, causing release of their preformed mediators (see Fig. 15-1). Mast cells are also the source of prostaglandins, leukotrienes (derived from lipids in their cell membrane), and cytokines that participate in the continued response to the allergen.

Many type I hypersensitivity reactions such as bronchial asthma have two well-defined phases: (1) an initial, or early, response characterized by vasodilatation, vascular leakage, and smooth muscle contraction; and (2) a secondary, or late-phase, response characterized by more intense infiltration of tissues with eosinophils and other acute and chronic inflammatory cells, as well as tissue destruction in the form of epithelial cell damage.

The initial, or early, response usually occurs within 5 to 30 minutes of exposure to antigen and subsides within 60 minutes. It is mediated by mast cell degranulation and the release of preformed mediators. These mediators include histamine, acetylcholine, and enzymes such as chymase and trypsin that lead to generation of kinins. Histamine is a potent vasodilator that increases the permeability of capillaries and venules and causes smooth muscle contraction and bronchial constriction. The parasympathetic nervous system neurotransmitter, acetylcholine, produces bronchial smooth muscle contraction and dilatation of small blood vessels. The kinins, which are a group of potent inflammatory peptides, require activation through enzymatic modification. Once acti-

KEY CONCEPTS

Allergic and Hypersensitivity Disorders

➤ Allergic and hypersensitivity disorders result from immune responses to exogenous and endogenous antigens that produce inflammation and cause tissue damage.

➤ Type I hypersensitivity is an IgE-mediated immune response that leads to the release of inflammatory mediators from sensitized mast cells.

➤ Type II disorders involve humoral antibodies that participate directly in injuring cells by predisposing them to phagocytosis or lysis.

➤ Type III disorders result in the generation of immune complexes in which humoral antibodies bind antigen and activate complement. The fractions of complement attract inflammatory cells that release tissue-damaging products.

➤ Type IV disorders involve tissue damage in which cell-mediated immune responses with sensitized T lymphocytes cause cell and tissue injury.

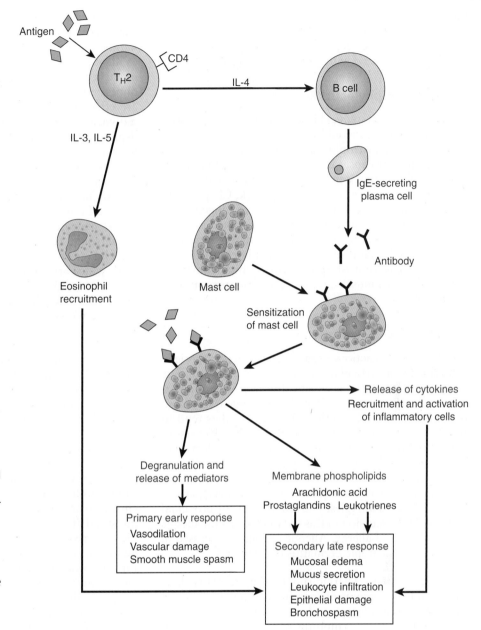

FIGURE 15-1 Type I, IgE-mediated hypersensitivity reaction. The stimulation of B-cell differentiation by an antigen-stimulated type 2 helper (T$_H$2) T cell leads to plasma cell production of IgE and mast cell sensitization. Subsequent binding of the antigen produces degranulation of the sensitized mast cell with release of preformed mediators that leads to a primary, or early-phase, response. T$_H$2 T-cell recruitment of eosinophils along with the release of cytokines and membrane phospholipids from the mast cell leads to a secondary, or late-phase, response.

vated, these peptide mediators produce vasodilatation and smooth muscle contraction.

The secondary, or late-phase, response sets in about 2 to 8 hours later and lasts for several days. It results from the action of lipid mediators and cytokines involved in the inflammatory response. The lipid mediators are derived from mast cell membrane phospholipids, which are broken down to form arachidonic acid. Arachidonic acid, in turn, is the parent compound from which the leukotrienes and prostaglandins are synthesized (see Chapter 14). The leukotrienes and prostaglandins produce responses similar to histamine and acetylcholine, although their effects are delayed and prolonged by comparison. Mast cells also produce cytokines and chemotactic factors that prompt the influx of eosinophils and leukocytes to the site of allergen contact, contributing to the inflammatory response. The late-phase response is an important cause of many serious long-term illnesses, such as bronchial asthma.

The clinical effects of allergic reactions vary according to the site of allergen exposure and the type of mast cell that is activated. A systemic or anaphylactic reaction occurs with activation of mast cells in the vascular system. Local or atopic reactions occur when the action of the antigen is confined to a particular site by virtue of exposure.

Not all IgE-mediated responses produce discomfort and disease, however. Type I hypersensitivity, particularly the late-phase response, plays a protective role in the control of parasitic infections. IgE antibodies directly damage the larvae of these parasites by recruiting inflammatory cells and causing antibody-dependent cell-mediated cytotoxicity. This kind of type I hypersensitivity reaction is particularly important in developing countries, where much of the population is infected with intestinal parasites.

Systemic (Anaphylactic) Reactions

Anaphylaxis is a systemic, life-threatening hypersensitivity reaction characterized by widespread vasodilatation that leads to a catastrophic fall in blood pressure, airway constriction that causes difficulty breathing, and vascular permeability that causes swelling and obstruction of the upper airway (see Anaphylactic Shock, Chapter 19). It results from the intravascular presence of antigen introduced by injection, insect sting, or absorption across the epithelial surface of the skin or gastrointestinal mucosa. This potentially fatal reaction is usually controlled by immediate injection of epinephrine, which constricts vascular smooth muscle and relaxes respiratory smooth muscle.

Local (Atopic) Reactions

Local or atopic reactions usually occur when the antigen is confined to a particular site by virtue of exposure. The term *atopic* refers to a genetically determined hypersensitivity to common environmental allergens mediated by an IgE–mast cell reaction. Atopic disorders tend to run in families and affect approximately 1 in 10 persons in the United States.[2] Persons with atopic disorders commonly are allergic to more than one, and often many, environmental allergens. The most common atopic disorders are urticaria (hives), allergic rhinitis (hay fever), atopic dermatitis, food allergies, and some forms of bronchial asthma. The discussion in this section focuses on allergic rhinitis and food allergy. Allergic asthma is discussed in Chapter 22 and atopic dermatitis in Chapter 45.

Allergic Rhinitis. Allergic rhinitis (hay fever) is characterized by symptoms of sneezing, itching, and watery discharge from the eyes and nose. Allergic rhinitis not only produces nasal symptoms but frequently is associated with other chronic airway disorders, such as sinusitis and bronchial asthma.[7,8] Severe attacks may be accompanied by systemic malaise, fatigue, and muscle soreness from sneezing. Fever is absent. Sinus obstruction may cause headache. Typical allergens include pollens from ragweed, grasses, trees, and weeds; fungal spores; house dust mites; animal dander; and feathers. Allergic rhinitis can be divided into perennial and seasonal allergic rhinitis depending on the chronology of symptoms. Persons with the perennial type of allergic rhinitis experience symptoms throughout the year, but those with seasonal allergic rhinitis (i.e., hay fever) are plagued with intense symptoms in conjunction with periods of high allergen (e.g., pollens, fungal spores) exposure. Symptoms that become worse at night suggest a household allergen, and symptoms that disappear on weekends suggest occupational exposure.

Diagnosis depends on a careful history and physical examination, microscopic identification of an increased number of eosinophils on a nasal smear, and skin testing to identify the offending allergens. Treatment is symptomatic in most cases and includes the use of oral antihistamines and decongestants.[8] Intranasal corticosteroids often are effective when used appropriately. Intranasal cromolyn, a drug that stabilizes mast cells and prevents their degranulation, may be useful, especially when administered before expected contact with an offending allergen. The anticholinergic agent ipratropium, which is available as a nasal spray, also may be used. When possible, avoidance of the offending allergen is recommended. A program of specific immunotherapy or desensitization (allergy shots) may be used when symptoms are particularly bothersome. Desensitization involves frequent (usually weekly) injections of the offending antigens.[7–9] The antigens, which are given in increasing doses, stimulate production of high levels of IgG, which acts as a blocking antibody by combining with the antigen before it can combine with the cell-bound IgE antibodies.

Food Allergies. Virtually any food can produce atopic or nonatopic allergies. The primary target of food allergy may be the skin, the gastrointestinal tract, or the respiratory system. The foods most commonly causing these reactions in children are milk, eggs, peanuts, soy, tree nuts, fish, and shellfish (i.e., crustaceans and mollusks).[10] In adults, they are peanuts,[11] shellfish, and fish.[10] The allergenicity of a food may be changed by heating or cooking. A person may be allergic to drinking milk but may not have symptoms when milk is included in cooked foods. Both acute reactions (hives and anaphylaxis) and chronic reactions (asthma, atopic dermatitis, and gastrointestinal disorders) can occur. The foods most responsible for anaphylaxis are peanuts, tree nuts (e.g., walnuts, almonds, pecans, cashews, hazelnuts), and shellfish. One form of food-associated anaphylaxis occurs when exercise follows ingestion of the incriminated food.[10,12]

Food allergies can occur at any age but, similar to atopic dermatitis and rhinitis, they tend to manifest during childhood. The allergic response is thought to occur after contact between specific food allergens and sensitizing IgE found in the intestinal mucosa causes local and systemic release of histamine and other mediators of the allergic response. In this disorder, allergens usually are food proteins and partially digested food products. Carbohydrates, lipids, or food additives, such as preservatives, colorings, or flavorings, also are potential allergens. Closely related food groups can contain common cross-reacting allergens. For example, some persons are allergic to all legumes (i.e., beans, peas, and peanuts).

Diagnosis of food allergies usually is based on careful food history and provocative diet testing. Provocative testing involves careful elimination of a suspected allergen from the diet for a time to see if the symptoms disappear and reintroducing the food to see if the symptoms reappear. Only one food should be tested at a time. Treatment focuses on avoidance of the food or foods responsible for the allergy. However, avoidance may be difficult for persons who are exquisitely sensitive to a particular food protein because foods may be contaminated with the protein during processing or handling of the food. For example, contamination may occur when chocolate candies without peanuts are processed with the same equipment used for making candies with peanuts.

TYPE II ANTIBODY-MEDIATED HYPERSENSITIVITY

Type II (cytotoxic) hypersensitivity reactions are mediated by IgG or IgM antibodies directed against target antigens on the surface of cells or other tissue components. The reaction can involve either complement-mediated cell destruction or antibody-mediated cytotoxicity that does not require the complement system (Fig. 15-2). The antigens may be endogenous antigens that are present on the membranes of body cells or exogenous antigens that are adsorbed on the membrane surface. Examples of type II reactions include mismatched blood transfusion reactions, hemolytic disease of the newborn due to ABO or Rh incompatibility (see Chapter 11), and certain drug reactions. In the latter, the binding of certain drugs or drug metabolites to the surface of red or white blood cells elicits an antibody response that lyses the drug-coated cell. Lytic drug reactions can produce transient anemia, leukopenia, or thrombocytopenia, which are corrected by the removal of the offending drug.

TYPE III IMMUNE COMPLEX–MEDIATED HYPERSENSITIVITY

Immune complex disorders are mediated by the formation of insoluble antigen–antibody complexes, complement fixation, and localized inflammation (Fig. 15-3). Immune complexes formed in the circulation produce damage when they come in contact with the vessel lining or are deposited in tissues, including the glomeruli of the kidney, skin vessels, and joint synovium. Once deposited, the immune complexes elicit an inflammatory response by activating complement, thereby leading to chemotactic recruitment of neutrophils and other inflammatory cells. The activation of these inflammatory cells by immune complexes and complement, accompanied by the release of potent inflammatory mediators, is directly responsible for the injury.

Type III reactions are responsible for the vasculitis (*i.e.*, inflammation of a blood vessel) seen in certain autoimmune diseases such as systemic lupus erythematosus (SLE) and the kidney damage seen with acute glomerulonephritis. Unlike type II reactions, in which the damage is caused by direct and specific binding of antibody to tissue, the harmful effects of type III reactions are indirect (*i.e.*, secondary to the inflammatory response induced by activated complement). As with type I hypersensitivity reactions, type III immune complex disorders can present

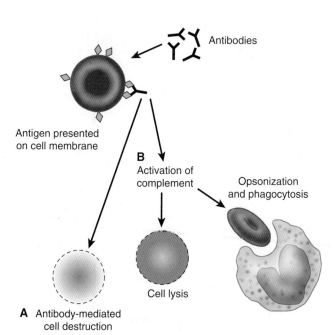

FIGURE 15-2 Type II, cytotoxic hypersensitivity reactions involve formation of immunoglobins (IgG and IgM) against cell surface antigens. The antigen-antibody response leads to (**A**) antibody-mediated toxicity that does not require the complement system or (**B**) complement-mediated cell lysis or opsonization and phagocytosis.

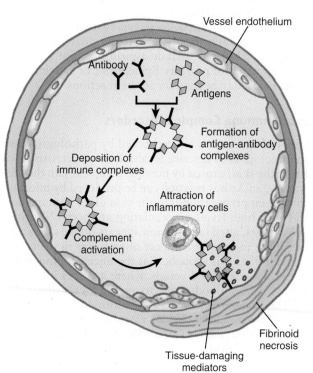

FIGURE 15-3 Type III, immune complex reactions involve complement-activating IgG and IgM immunoglobulins with formation of blood-borne immune complexes that are eventually deposited in tissues. Complement activation at the site of immune complex deposition leads to recruitment of leukocytes, which are eventually responsible for vessel and tissue injury.

with systemic manifestations, as in serum sickness, or as a local reaction, as in the Arthus reaction.

Systemic Immune Complex Disorders

Serum sickness is a systemic immune complex disorder that is triggered by the deposition of insoluble antigen–antibody (IgM and IgG) complexes in blood vessels, joints, and glomeruli of the kidney. The deposited complexes activate complement, increase vascular permeability, and recruit phagocytic cells, all of which can promote focal tissue damage and edema. The term *serum sickness* was originally coined to describe a syndrome consisting of rash, lymphadenopathy, arthralgias, and occasionally neurologic disorders that appeared 7 or more days after injections of tetanus antisera obtained from horses. Although this therapy is not used today, the name remains. Currently, the most common causes of this disorder are antibiotics (especially penicillin), various foods, drugs, and insect venoms.

The signs and symptoms of serum sickness include urticaria, patchy or generalized rash, extensive edema (usually of the face, neck, and joints), and fever. In most cases, the damage is temporary, and symptoms resolve within a few days. However, a prolonged and continuous exposure to the sensitizing antigen can lead to irreversible damage. In previously sensitized persons, severe and even fatal forms of serum sickness may occur immediately or within several days after the sensitizing drug or serum is administered.

Treatment of serum sickness usually is directed toward removal of the sensitizing antigen and providing symptom relief. This may include aspirin for joint pain and antihistamines for pruritus. Epinephrine or systemic corticosteroids may be used for severe reactions.

Local Immune Complex Disorders

The *Arthus reaction* is a term used by pathologists and immunologists to describe localized tissue necrosis (usually in the skin) caused by immune complexes. In the laboratory, an Arthus reaction can be produced by injecting an antigen preparation into the skin of an immune animal with high levels of circulating antibody. Within 4 to 10 hours, a red raised lesion appears on the skin at the site of the injection.[2] An ulcer often forms in the center of the lesion. It is thought that the injected antigen diffuses into local blood vessels, where it comes in contact with specific antibody (IgG) to incite a localized vasculitis. This experimental model of localized vasculitis is the prototype of many forms of vasculitis seen in humans, such as the cutaneous vasculitides that characterize certain drug reactions.

TYPE IV CELL-MEDIATED HYPERSENSITIVITY

Type IV hypersensitivity reactions involve cell-mediated rather than antibody-mediated immune responses.[2,6] Cell-mediated immunity is the principal mechanism of response to a variety of microorganisms, including intracellular pathogens such as *Mycobacterium tuberculosis* and viruses, as well as extracellular agents such as fungi, protozoa, and parasites. It can also lead to cell death and tissue injury in response to chemical antigens (contact dermatitis) or self-antigens (autoimmunity).

Type IV hypersensitivity reactions, which are mediated by specifically sensitized T lymphocytes, can be divided into two basic types: direct cell-mediated cytotoxicity and delayed-type hypersensitivity (Fig. 15-4).

Direct Cell-Mediated Cytotoxicity

In direct cell-mediated cytotoxicity, CD8+ cytotoxic T lymphocytes (CTLs) directly kill the antigen-presenting target cells. In viral infections, CTL responses can lead to tissue injury by killing infected target cells even if the virus itself has no cytotoxic effects.[2,6] Some viruses directly injure infected cells and are said to be cytopathic, whereas other, noncytopathic viruses do not. Because CTLs cannot distinguish between cytopathic and noncytopathic viruses, they kill virtually all infected cells regardless of whether the

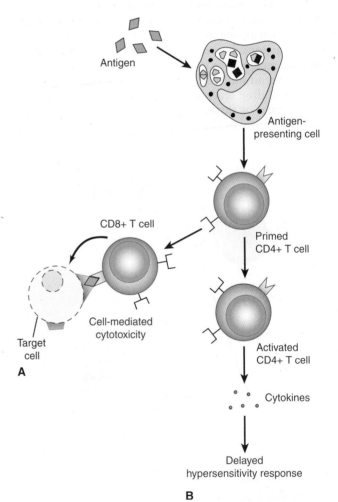

FIGURE 15-4 Type IV, direct cell-mediated cytotoxicity (**A**) or delayed-type hypersensitivity (**B**) reactions involve sensitization of T lymphocytes with the subsequent formation of cytotoxic T cells that lyse target cells, or T cells that release cell-damaging cytokines.

infection is harmful. In certain forms of hepatitis, for example, the destruction of liver cells is due to the host CTL response and not the virus.

Delayed-Type Hypersensitivity Disorders

Delayed-type hypersensitivity (DTH) reactions occur in response to soluble protein antigens and primarily involve antigen-presenting cells such as macrophages and CD4+ helper T cells of the T_H1 type. During the reaction T_H1 cells are activated and secrete an array of cytokines that recruit and activate monocytes, lymphocytes, fibroblasts, and other inflammatory cells.[2,6] These T-cell–mediated responses require the synthesis of effector molecules and take 24 to 72 hours to develop, which is why they are called delayed-type hypersensitivity disorders.

The best-known type of DTH response is the reaction to the tuberculin test, in which inactivated tuberculin or purified protein derivative is injected under the skin. In a person who has been sensitized by previous infection, a local area of redness and induration develops within 8 to 12 hours, reaching a peak in 24 to 72 hours. The tuberculin reaction is characterized by perivascular accumulation of T_H1 cells and, to a lesser extent, macrophages. Local secretion of cytokines by these mononuclear inflammatory cells leads to increased microvascular permeability with local redness and swelling. A positive tuberculin test indicates that a person has had sufficient exposure to the *M. tuberculosis* organism to incite a hypersensitivity reaction; it does not mean that the person has tuberculosis.

The sequence of events in DTH, as demonstrated by the tuberculin reaction, begins with the first exposure to the tuberculin bacilli. The T_H1 cells recognize the peptide antigens of the tuberculin bacilli in association with class II major histocompatibility complex (MHC) antigens on the surface of macrophages and antigen-presenting cells that have processed the mycobacterial antigens. This process leads to sensitized T_H1 memory cells that remain in the circulation for years. Subsequent injection of tuberculin into such an individual results in the secretion of T_H1 cell cytokines that increase blood vessel permeability, allowing plasma and inflammatory cells to enter the site and cause visible swelling.

Allergic Contact Dermatitis. Allergic contact dermatitis denotes an inflammatory response confined to the skin that is initiated by reexposure to an allergen to which a person had previously become sensitized (*e.g.*, cosmetics, hair dyes, topical drugs). The most common form of this condition is the dermatitis that follows exposure to poison ivy or poison oak antigens.

Contact dermatitis is characterized by erythematous, papular, and vesicular lesions associated with intense pruritus and weeping. The affected area often becomes swollen and warm, with exudation, crusting, and development of a secondary infection. The location of the lesions often provides a clue about the nature of the antigen causing the disorder. The severity of the reaction associated with contact dermatitis ranges from mild to intense, depending on the person and the allergen. Because

this condition follows the mechanism of a DTH response, the reaction does not become apparent for at least 12 hours and usually more than 24 hours after exposure. Depending on the antigen and the duration of exposure, the reaction may last from days to weeks.

Diagnosis of contact dermatitis is made by observing the distribution of lesions on the skin surface and associating a particular pattern with exposure to possible allergens. If a particular allergen is suspected, a patch test can be used to confirm the suspicion. Treatment usually is limited to removal of the irritant and application of topical preparations (*e.g.*, corticosteroid creams or ointments) to relieve symptomatic skin lesions and prevent secondary bacterial infections. Severe reactions may require systemic corticosteroid therapy.

Hypersensitivity Pneumonitis. Hypersensitivity pneumonitis, which is associated with exposure to inhaled organic dusts or related occupational antigens, is another example of a DTH reaction. The disorder is thought to involve a susceptible host and activation of pulmonary T cells, followed by the release of cytokine mediators of inflammation.[13] The inflammatory response that ensues (usually several hours after exposure) produces labored breathing, dry cough, chills and fever, headache, and malaise. The symptoms usually subside within hours after the sensitizing antigens are removed. A primary example of hypersensitivity pneumonitis is "farmer's lung," a condition resulting from exposure to moldy hay. Other sensitizing antigens include tree bark, sawdust, animal danders, and *Actinomycetes* bacteria that are occasionally found in humidifiers, hot tubs, and swimming pools. Exposure to small amounts of antigen for a long period may lead to chronic lung disease with minimal reversibility. This can happen to persons exposed to avian or animal antigens or a contaminated home air humidifier.[13]

The most important element in the diagnosis of hypersensitivity pneumonitis is to obtain a good history (occupational and otherwise) of exposure to possible antigens. Treatment consists of identifying and avoiding the offending antigens. Severe forms of the disorder may be treated with systemic corticosteroid therapy.

In summary, hypersensitivity and allergic disorders are responses to environmental, food, or drug antigens that would not affect most of the population. There are four basic categories of hypersensitivity responses: (1) type I responses, which are mediated by the IgE antibodies and include anaphylactic shock, hay fever, and bronchial asthma; (2) type II cytotoxic reactions, which are mediated by IgG antibodies directed against antigens on the surface of cells such as those on the red cells of donor blood that cause hemolytic transfusion reactions; (3) type III reactions, which involve IgG and IgM antibodies and result from the formation of insoluble antigen–antibody complexes that become deposited in blood vessels or in the kidney and cause localized tissue injury; and (4) type

IV, T-cell–mediated hypersensitivity responses in which CD8+ cytotoxic T cells directly kill the antigen-presenting target cells or activated CD4+ T cells secrete cytokines that recruit and activate tissue damaging inflammatory cells.

Type 2 helper T cells and mast cells play a pivotal role in the pathogenesis of type I reactions. Type II and type III hypersensitivity responses involve T_H1 cells and IgG and IgM antibodies. Type IV hypersensitivity reactions involve cell-mediated (macrophages and lymphocytes) rather than antibody-mediated responses.

 ## Autoimmune Disease

Autoimmune diseases represent a group of disorders that are caused by a breakdown in the ability of the immune system to differentiate between self and nonself antigens. Autoimmune diseases can affect almost any cell or tissue in the body. Some autoimmune disorders, such as Hashimoto thyroiditis, are tissue specific; whereas others, such as SLE, affect multiple organs and systems. The mechanisms of tissue damage in autoimmune disease are essentially the same as those involved in protective immunity and hypersensitivity reactions.[14] Chart 15-1 lists some of the probable autoimmune diseases, many of which are discussed elsewhere in this book.

IMMUNOLOGIC TOLERANCE

Immunologic tolerance is a state in which a person is incapable of developing an immune response to a specific antigen. *Self-tolerance* refers to the inability to mount an immune response against a person's own antigens.[14] It is the human leukocyte antigens (HLA) encoded by MHC genes that serve as recognition markers of self for the immune system (see Chapter 13). To elicit an immune response, an antigen must first be processed by an antigen-presenting cell (APC), such as a macrophage, which then presents the antigenic determinants along with an MHC II molecule to a CD4+ helper T cell for binding to its T-cell receptor (TCR). It is the dual recognition of the MHC–antigen complex by the TCR acting as a security check that affects all T cells, including CD4+ helper T cells, which orchestrate the immune responses, and CD8+ cytotoxic T cells, which act directly to destroy target cells. A number of chemical messengers (*e.g.*, interleukins) and costimulatory signals are essential to the activation of immune responses and the preservation of self-tolerance.

Several mechanisms have been postulated to explain the tolerant state, including central tolerance and peripheral tolerance.[2,15] Central tolerance refers to the elimination of self-reactive T cells in the thymus and B cells in the bone marrow. Peripheral tolerance refers to the deletion or inactivation of autoreactive T cells or B cells that escaped elimination in the central lymphoid organs. Autoreactive B cells are deleted in the spleen and lymph nodes. Autoreactive T cells that have escaped deletion in the thymus may undergo long-term inactivation (anergy) to the extent that

---

CHART 15-1

Probable Autoimmune Disease*

Systemic

Mixed connective tissue disease
Polymyositis-dermatomyositis
Rheumatoid arthritis
Scleroderma
Sjögren syndrome
Systemic lupus erythematosus

Blood

Autoimmune hemolytic anemia
Autoimmune neutropenia and lymphopenia
Idiopathic thrombocytopenic purpura

Other Organs

Acute idiopathic polyneuritis
Atrophic gastritis and pernicious anemia
Autoimmune adrenalitis
Goodpasture syndrome
Hashimoto thyroiditis
Insulin-dependent diabetes mellitus
Myasthenia gravis
Premature gonadal (ovarian) failure
Primary biliary cirrhosis
Sympathetic ophthalmia
Temporal arteritis
Thyrotoxicosis (Graves disease)
Ulcerative colitis

*Examples are not inclusive.

---

they cannot recognize self-antigens, or may experience activation-induced cell death; their activity also may be suppressed by other regulatory T cells.[2]

MECHANISMS OF AUTOIMMUNE DISEASE

It is not known what triggers autoimmunity, but both inheritance of susceptibility genes that contribute to the maintenance of self-tolerance and environmental factors, such as infections that promote the activation of self-reactive lymphocytes, are clearly important.[2,16,17] Gender may also play a role in the development of autoimmune disorders. A number of autoimmune disorders such as SLE occur more commonly in women than men, suggesting that estrogens may play a role in the development of autoimmune disease. Evidence suggests that estrogens stimulate and androgens suppress the immune response.[18]

Genetic Susceptibility

Genetic factors can increase the incidence and severity of autoimmune diseases, as shown by the familial clustering of several autoimmune diseases and the observation that certain inherited HLA genotypes occur more frequently in persons with a variety of autoimmune disorders.[2,16,17] For example, 90% of persons with ankylosing spondylitis carry the HLA-B27 antigen. Other HLA-associated diseases are Reiter syndrome and HLA-B27, rheumatoid arthritis and HLA-DR4, and SLE and HLA-DR3 (see Chapter 43). Although these examples provide insights into the mechanisms of autoimmunity, it should be emphasized that most autoimmune disorders have complex, multigenic patterns of inheritance and are not attributable to a single gene mutation.

Environmental Factors

Although environmental factors, such as infectious agents, appear to be involved in the pathogenesis of autoimmune disorders, their precise role in initiating or perpetuating the autoreactive response is largely unknown. Among the proposed mechanisms involved in loss of self-tolerance are breakdown of T-cell anergy, release of sequestered antigens, molecular mimicry, and superantigens.

Breakdown in T-Cell Anergy. *Anergy* is a state of unresponsiveness to antigen. It involves the prolonged or irreversible inactivation of lymphocytes, such as that induced by an encounter with self-antigens. Activation of antigen-specific CD4+ helper T cells requires two signals: (1) recognition of the antigen in association with class II MHC molecules on the surface of an APC, and (2) a set of *costimulatory signals* provided by the APC. If the second costimulatory signal is not delivered, the T cell becomes anergic.[2] Most normal tissues do not express the costimulatory molecules and thus are protected from autoreactive T cells. However, this protection can be broken if the normal cells that do not normally express the costimulatory molecules are induced to do so. Some inductions can occur after an infection or in situations where there is tissue necrosis and local inflammation.

Release of Sequestered Antigens. Normally, the body does not produce antibodies against self-antigens. Thus, any self-antigen that was completely sequestered during development and then reintroduced to the immune system is likely to be regarded as foreign. Among the sequestered tissues that could be regarded as foreign are spermatozoa and ocular antigens such as those found in the uvea. Post-traumatic orchiditis after vasectomy and uveitis may fall into this category.

Changes in antigen structure or release of hidden antigens may also account for the persistence of autoimmune disorders. Once an autoimmune disorder has been induced, it tends to be progressive, sometimes with sporadic relapses and remissions. A possible mechanism for the persistence and evolution of autoimmunity is the phenomenon of epitope reading.[2] Infections, and even the initial autoimmune episode, may release and damage self-antigens and expose epitopes of the antigen that have been hidden from the immune system. The result is continued activation of new lymphocytes that recognize the previously hidden epitopes.

Molecular Mimicry. Some microbes may express antigens that have the same amino acid sequence as self-antigens, a phenomenon sometimes referred to as *molecular mimicry*. In this case, immune responses against the microbial antigens may result in the activation of self-reactive lymphocytes.[2,19,20] For example, in rheumatic fever and acute glomerulonephritis, a protein in the cell wall of group A beta-hemolytic streptococci has considerable similarity with antigens in heart and kidney tissue, respectively. After infection, antibodies directed against the microorganism cause a classic case of mistaken identity, which leads to inflammation of the heart or kidney. Not everyone exposed to group A beta-hemolytic streptococci has an autoimmune reaction, indicating that the MHC (HLA) genotype is important. The HLA type determines exactly which fragments of a pathogen are displayed on the cell surface for presentation to T cells. One individual's HLA may bind self-mimicry molecules for presentation to T cells, and another's HLA type may not.

Superantigens. Superantigens are a family of related substances, including staphylococcal and streptococcal exotoxins, that can short-circuit the normal sequence of events in an immune response and lead to inappropriate activation of CD4+ helper T cells.[19,21] Superantigens do not require processing and presentation of antigen by APCs to induce a T-cell response. Instead, they activate T cells through the variable domain of the TCR. This distinctive mode of activation, together with the ability of superantigens to bind to a wide variety of MHC class II molecules, leads to activation of large numbers of T cells regardless of their MHC/peptide specificity. Superantigens are involved in several diseases, including food poisoning and toxic shock syndrome. Recently, a bacterial superantigen was isolated that may be important in the pathogenesis of Crohn disease[19] (see Chapter 28).

DIAGNOSIS AND TREATMENT

The suggested criteria for determining that a disorder is an autoimmune disorder are evidence of an autoimmune reaction, determination that the immunologic findings are not secondary to another condition, and the lack of other identified causes for the disorder.[2,6] Currently, the diagnosis of autoimmune disease is based primarily on clinical findings and serologic testing. In the future, it is likely that autoimmune disorders will be diagnosed by directly identifying the genes responsible for the condition. The basis for most serologic assays is the demonstration of antibodies directed against tissue antigens or cellular components.

Treatment of autoimmune disease is based on the tissue or organ that is involved, the effector mechanism involved, and the magnitude and chronicity of the effector processes. Ideally, treatment should focus on the mechanism underlying the autoimmune disorder. Corticosteroids and immunosuppressive drugs may be used to arrest or reverse the downhill course of some autoimmune disorders. Plasma exchange therapy (*i.e.,* plasmapheresis) to remove circulating autoreactive cells is also an option in some severe cases of autoimmunity.[16]

Recent research has focused on the cytokines involved in the inflammatory response that accompanies many of the autoimmune disorders. Two new agents, interferon-β for multiple sclerosis and tumor necrosis factor (TNF)-α antibodies (*e.g.,* infliximab) for rheumatoid arthritis and Crohn disease, are the first new treatments for autoimmunity approved by the U.S. Food and Drug Administration (FDA) in the past 30 years.[16] Finally, research into the development of vaccines to target critical pathways in the emergence of autoimmune responses is ongoing.

In summary, autoimmune diseases represent a disruption in self-tolerance that results in damage to body tissues by the immune system. Autoimmune diseases can affect almost any cell or tissue of the body. The ability of the immune system to differentiate self from nonself is called *self-tolerance.* Normally, self-tolerance is maintained through central and peripheral mechanisms that delete autoreactive B or T cells or suppress or inactivate immune responses that would be destructive to host tissues. Defects in any of these mechanisms could impair self-tolerance and predispose to the development of autoimmune disease.

It is not known what triggers autoimmunity, but both environmental and genetic factors, especially MHC genotype, are clearly important. Genetic factors can increase the incidence and severity of autoimmune diseases, as shown by the familial clustering of several autoimmune diseases. Gender may also play a role in the development of autoimmune disorders. Among the proposed environmental mechanisms involved in loss of self-tolerance are breakdown of T-cell anergy, release of sequestered antigens, molecular mimicry, and superantigens.

The suggested criteria for determining that a disorder results from autoimmunity are evidence of an autoimmune reaction, determination that the immunologic findings are not secondary to another condition, and the lack of other identifiable causes for the disorder.

Transplantation Immunopathology

A relatively short time ago, transplantation of solid organs (*e.g.,* liver, kidney, heart) and bone marrow was considered experimental and reserved for persons for whom alternative methods of therapy were exhausted and survival was unlikely. However, with a greater understanding of humoral and cellular immune regulation, the development of immunosuppressive drugs such as cyclosporine, and an appreciation of the role of the MHC antigens, transplantation is becoming a more common treatment option for many diseases that lead to organ failure.

The cell surface antigens that determine whether transplanted tissue is recognized as foreign are the MHC or human leukocyte antigens (HLA; see Chapter 13). Transplanted tissue can be categorized as *allogeneic* if the donor and recipient are related or unrelated but share similar HLA types, *syngeneic* if the donor and recipient are identical twins, and *autologous* if donor and recipient are the same person. Donors of solid organ transplants can be living or dead (cadaver) and related or unrelated (heterologous). When cells bearing foreign MHC antigens are transplanted, the recipient's immune system attempts to eliminate the donor cells, a process referred to as *host-versus-graft disease* (HVGD). Conversely, the cellular immune system of the transplanted tissue can attack unrelated recipient tissue, causing a *graft-versus-host disease* (GVHD; Fig. 15-5). The likelihood of rejection varies indirectly with the degree of MCH or HLA relatedness between donor and recipient.

HOST-VERSUS-GRAFT DISEASE

In HVGD, the immune cells of the transplant recipient attack the donor cells of the transplanted organ. HVGD usually is limited to allogeneic organ transplants, although even HLA-identical siblings may differ in some minor HLA loci, which can evoke slow rejection. Rejection due to HVGD is a complex process that involves cell-mediated and circulating antibodies. Although many cells may participate in the process of acute transplant rejection, only the T lymphocytes seem to be absolutely required.[22,23] The activation of CD4+ helper T cells and CD8+ cytotoxic T cells is triggered in response to the donor's HLA. Activation of CD4+ helper cells leads to proliferation of B-cell–mediated antibody production and T-cell–mediated

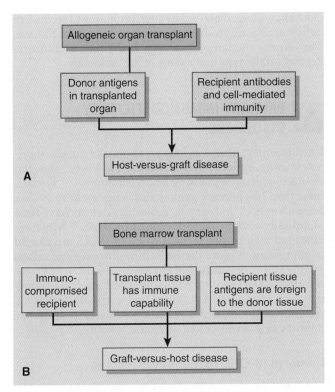

FIGURE 15-5 Mechanism of host-versus-graft disease in allogeneic organ transplant (**A**) and graft-versus-host disease in bone marrow transplant (**B**).

DTH or CTL hypersensitivity reactions. There are three basic patterns of transplant rejection: hyperacute, acute, and chronic.[1,2]

A *hyperacute reaction* occurs almost immediately after transplantation. In kidney transplants, it can often be seen at the time of surgery. As soon as blood flow from the recipient to the donor kidney begins, it takes on a cyanotic, mottled appearance. At other times, the reaction may take hours or days to develop. The hyperacute response is produced by existing recipient antibodies to graft antigens that initiate a type III, Arthus-type hypersensitivity reaction in the blood vessels of the graft. These antibodies usually have developed in response to previous blood transfusions, pregnancies in which the mother makes antibodies to fetal antigens, or infections with bacteria or viruses possessing antigens that mimic MHC antigens of the donor.

Acute rejection usually occurs within the first few months after transplantation and is evidenced by signs of organ failure. It also may occur suddenly months or even years later, after immunosuppression has been used and terminated. T lymphocytes play a central role in acute rejection, responding to antigens in the graft tissue. The activated T cells cause direct lysis of graft cells and recruit and activate inflammatory cells that injure the graft. In vascularized grafts such as kidney grafts, the endothelial cells of blood vessels are the earliest targets of acute rejection.

Chronic host-versus-graft rejection occurs over a prolonged period. It manifests with dense intimal fibro-

sis of blood vessels of the transplanted organ. In renal transplantation, it is characterized by a gradual rise in serum creatinine over a period of 4 to 6 months. The actual mechanism of this type of response is unclear but may include release of cytokines that stimulate fibrosis.

GRAFT-VERSUS-HOST DISEASE

Graft-versus-host disease occurs when immunologically competent cells or precursors are transplanted into recipients who are immunologically compromised. Although GVHD occurs most often in persons who have undergone allogeneic bone marrow transplantation, it may also follow transplantation of organs rich in lymphoid tissue (*e.g.*, the liver) or transfusions with nonirradiated blood.[2,24,25]

Three basic requirements are necessary for GVHD to develop: (1) the transplant must have a functional cellular immune component, (2) the recipient tissue must bear antigens foreign to the donor tissue, and (3) the recipient immunity must be compromised to the point that it cannot destroy the transplanted cells.[1,2,24] The primary agents of GVHD are the donor immunocompetent T cells derived from the donor marrow and the recipient tissue that they recognize as foreign and react against.[2] GVHD results in activation of both CD4+ and CD8+ T cells with ultimate generation of type IV, cell-mediated DTH and CTL hypersensitivity reactions. The greater the difference in tissue antigens between the donor and recipient, the greater is the likelihood of GVHD.

GVHD can occur as an acute or chronic reaction. Acute GVHD, which develops within days to weeks after transplantation, involves the epithelial cells of the skin, liver, and gastrointestinal tract.[2,24] The organ most commonly affected in acute GVHD is the skin. There is development of a pruritic, maculopapular rash, which begins on the palms and soles and frequently extends over the entire body, with subsequent desquamation. Involvement of the gastrointestinal tract usually parallels the development of skin and liver involvement. Gastrointestinal symptoms include nausea, bloody diarrhea, and abdominal pain. GVHD of the liver is heralded by painless jaundice, hyperbilirubinemia, and abnormal liver function test results. Liver involvement can progress to the development of venoocclusive disease, drug toxicity, viral infection, iron overload, extrahepatic biliary obstruction, sepsis, and coma. Venoocclusive disease is characterized by obliteration of the small hepatic veins and venules with centrilobular congestion and death of liver cells. As the disease progresses, fibrous tissue is deposited in the lumen of venules. The incidence of venoocclusive disease approaches 25% of recipients of allogenic marrow transplants, with mortality rates of more than 30%.[26]

GVHD is considered chronic if symptoms persist or begin 100 days or more after transplantation. Chronic GVHD may follow acute GVHD, or it may develop insidiously. Although persons with chronic GVHD are profoundly immunocompromised, they develop skin lesions resembling systemic sclerosis (discussed in Chapter 43) and manifestations mimicking other autoimmune diseases.

A second type of GVHD can follow the transplantation of genetically identical tissue (*i.e.*, syngeneic or autologous). This type of GVHD stems from the use of pretreatment conditioning regimens (*e.g.*, total-body irradiation or treatment with cytotoxic drugs). The conditioning therapy disrupts the normal immune surveillance system and allows "rogue" autoreactive T cells to proliferate and attack native tissue. This type of GVHD usually is self-limited and not severe.

GVHD can be prevented by blocking any of the three steps of pathogenesis. For example, donor T cells can be selectively removed from the transplanted tissue or destroyed using various treatments such as monoclonal antibodies with attached toxins, equivalent to heat-seeking missiles. Alternatively, immunosuppressive or anti-inflammatory drugs such as cyclosporine and tacrolimus or glucocorticoids can be used to block T-cell activation and the action of cytokines.

In summary, organ and bone marrow transplantation has been enhanced by a greater understanding of humoral and cellular immune regulation, the development of immunosuppressive drugs (*e.g.*, cyclosporine or tacrolimus), and an appreciation of the role of the MHC antigens. The likelihood of rejection varies with the degree of HLA (or MHC) relatedness between donor and recipient. A rejection can involve an attempt by the recipient's immune system to eliminate the donor cells, as in HVGD, or an attack by the cellular immunity of the transplanted tissue on the unrelated recipient tissue, as in GVHD.

Immunodeficiency Disorders

Immunodeficiency can be defined as an abnormality in one or more branches of the immune system that renders a person susceptible to diseases normally prevented by an intact immune system. Two major categories of immune mechanisms defend the body against infectious or neoplastic disease: humoral or antibody-mediated immunity (*i.e.*, B lymphocytes) and cell-mediated immunity (*i.e.*, T lymphocytes and lymphokines).

Abnormalities of the immune system can be classified as primary (*i.e.*, congenital or inherited) or secondary if the immunodeficiency is acquired later in life. Secondary immunodeficiencies are more common than primary disorders of genetic origin. Secondary deficiencies in humoral immunity can develop as a consequence of selective loss of immunoglobulins through the gastrointestinal or genitourinary tracts. Secondary deficiencies of T-cell function have been described in conjunction with acute viral infections (*e.g.*, measles virus, cytomegalovirus) and with certain malignancies (*e.g.*, Hodgkin disease and other lymphomas). Human immunodeficiency virus (HIV)/acquired immunodeficiency syndrome (AIDS; to be discussed) is the most devastating example of a secondary immuno-

deficiency. Regardless of the cause, primary and secondary deficiencies can produce the same spectrum of disease. The severity and symptomatology of the various disorders depend on the type and extent of the deficiency.

 PRIMARY IMMUNODEFICIENCY DISORDERS

Until recently, little was known about the causes of primary immunodeficiency diseases. However, this has changed with advances in genetic technology.[27–29] To date, more than 100 primary immunodeficiency syndromes have been identified, and specific molecular defects have been identified in more than one third of these.[28] Most are inherited as recessive traits, several of which are caused by mutations in genes on the X chromosomes and others by mutations on autosomal chromosomes. Many of these disorders have been traced to mutations affecting signaling pathways (*e.g.*, cytokines and cytokine signaling, receptor subunits, and metabolic pathways) that dictate immune cell development and their function.[30]

Humoral (B-Cell) Immunodeficiencies

Humoral immunodeficiencies involve B-cell function and immunoglobulin or antibody production. Defects in humoral immunity increase the risk of recurrent pyogenic

 KEY CONCEPTS

Primary Immunodeficiency Disorders

➤ Primary immunodeficiency disorders are congenital or inherited abnormalities of immune function that render a person susceptible to diseases normally prevented by an intact immune system.

➤ Disorders of B-cell function impair the ability to produce antibodies and defend against microorganisms and toxins that circulate in body fluids (IgM and IgG) or enter the body through the mucosal surface of the respiratory or gastrointestinal tract (IgA). Persons with primary B-cell immunodeficiency are particularly prone to infections due to encapsulated organisms.

➤ Disorders of T-cell function impair the ability to orchestrate the immune response (CD4+ helper T cells) and to protect against fungal, protozoan, viral, and intracellular bacterial infections (CD8+ cytotoxic T cells).

➤ Combined T-cell and B-cell immunodeficiency states affect all aspects of immune function. Severe combined immunodeficiency represents a life-threatening absence of immune function that requires bone marrow transplantation for survival.

infections, including those caused by *Streptococcus pneumoniae*, *Haemophilus influenzae*, *Staphylococcus aureus*, and by gram-negative organisms such as *Pseudomonas* species. Humoral immunity usually is not as important in defending against intracellular bacteria (mycobacteria), fungi, and protozoa. Viruses usually are handled normally, except for the enteroviruses that cause gastrointestinal infections.

Humoral immunodeficiency can range from a transient decrease in immunoglobulin levels during early infancy to inherited disorders that interrupt the production of one or all of the immunoglobulins. During the first few months of life, infants are protected from infection by IgG class antibodies that have been transferred from the maternal circulation during fetal life. IgA, IgM, IgD, and IgE do not normally cross the placenta (see Chapter 13). An infant's level of maternal IgG gradually declines during a period of approximately 6 months. Concomitant with the loss of maternal antibody, the infant's immature humoral immune system begins to function, and between the ages of 1 and 2 years, the child's antibody production reaches that of adult levels.

Any abnormality that blocks or prevents the maturation of B-lymphocyte stem cells can produce a state of immunodeficiency. For example, certain infants may experience a delay in the maturation process of B cells that leads to a prolonged deficiency in IgG levels (IgM and IgA levels are normal) beyond 6 months of age. The total number and antigenic response of circulating B cells are normal, but the chemical communication between B and T cells that leads to clonal proliferation of antibody-producing plasma cells seems to be reduced.[31] This condition is referred to as *transient hypogammaglobulinemia*

of infancy. The result of this condition usually is limited to repeated bouts of upper respiratory and middle ear infections. This condition usually resolves by the time the child is 2 to 4 years of age.

Primary humoral immunodeficiency disorders are genetic disorders of the B lymphocytes. They are the most frequent type of primary immunodeficiencies, accounting for 70% of all primary immunodeficiency disorders.[32] Immunoglobulin production depends on the differentiation of stem cells to mature B lymphocytes and the generation of immunoglobulin-producing plasma cells (Fig. 15-6). This maturation cycle initially involves the production of surface IgM, migration from the marrow to the peripheral lymphoid tissue, and switching to the specialized production of IgG, IgA, IgD, IgE, or IgM antibodies after antigenic stimulation. Primary humoral immunodeficiency disorders can interrupt the production of one or all of the immunoglobulins.

X-Linked Agammaglobulinemia. X-linked or Bruton agammaglobulinemia is a recessive trait that affects only males.[28,29,31] As the name implies, persons with this disorder have essentially undetectable levels of all serum immunoglobulins. Therefore, they are susceptible to meningitis and recurrent otitis media and to sinus and pulmonary infections with encapsulated organisms such as *S. pneumoniae*, *H. influenzae* type b, *S. aureus*, and *Neisseria meningitidis*.[29] Many boys with this disorder have severe tooth decay.

The central defect in this syndrome is a genetic mutation that blocks the differentiation of pre-B cells, creating an absence of mature circulating B cells and plasma cells. T lymphocytes, however, are normal in number

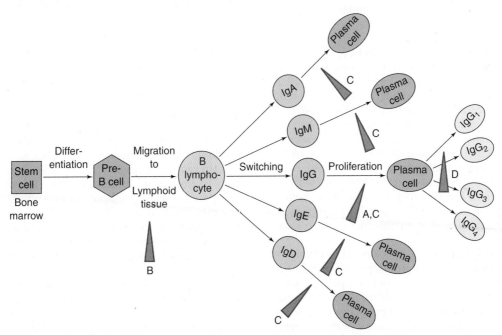

FIGURE 15-6 Stem cells to mature immunoglobulin-secreting plasma cells. *Arrows* indicate the stage of the maturation process that is interrupted in (**A**) transient hypogammaglobulinemia, (**B**) X-linked hypogammaglobulinemia, (**C**) common variable immunodeficiency, and (**D**) IgG subclass deficiency.

and function. Symptoms of the disorder usually coincide with the loss of maternal antibodies. A clue to the presence of the disorder is the failure of an infection to respond completely and promptly to antibiotic therapy.

Diagnosis is based on demonstration of low or absent serum immunoglobulins. Therapy consists of prophylaxis with intravenous immunoglobulin and prompt antimicrobial therapy for suspected infections. The prognosis of this condition depends on the prompt recognition and treatment of infections. Chronic pulmonary disease is an ever-present danger.

Common Variable Immunodeficiency. Another disorder of B-cell maturation that is similar to X-linked agammaglobulinemia is a condition called *common variable immunodeficiency*. In this syndrome, the terminal differentiation of mature B cells to plasma cells is blocked. The result is markedly reduced serum immunoglobulin levels, normal numbers of circulating B lymphocytes, and the complete absence of germinal centers and plasma cells in lymph nodes and the spleen.

The symptomatology of common variable immunodeficiency is similar to that of X-linked agammaglobulinemia (*i.e.*, recurrent otitis media and sinus and pulmonary infections with encapsulated organisms), but the onset of symptoms occurs much later, usually between the ages of 15 and 35 years, and distribution of disease between the sexes is equal. Persons with late-onset hypogammaglobulinemia also have an increased tendency toward development of chronic lung disease, autoimmune disorders, hepatitis, gastric carcinoma, and chronic diarrhea with associated intestinal malabsorption. Approximately one half of persons with the disorder have evidence of abnormal T-cell immunity, suggesting that this syndrome is a complex immunodeficiency. Treatment methods for late-onset hypogammaglobulinemia are similar to those used for X-linked hypogammaglobulinemia.

Selective Immunoglobulin A Deficiency. Selective IgA deficiency is the most common type of immunoglobulin deficiency, affecting 1 in 400 to 1 in 1000 persons.[28] The syndrome is characterized by moderate to marked reduction in levels of serum and secretory IgA. The cause of this deficiency is a block in the pathway that promotes terminal differentiation of mature B cells to IgA-secreting plasma cells. The occurrence of IgA deficiency in both boys and girls and in members of successive generations within families suggests autosomal inheritance with variable expressivity. The disorder has also been noted in persons treated with certain drugs (*e.g.*, phenytoin, sulfasalazine), suggesting that environmental factors may trigger the disorder.[28]

Approximately two thirds of persons with selective IgA deficiency have no overt symptoms, presumably because IgG and IgM levels are normal and compensate for the defect. At least 50% of affected children overcome the deficiency by the age of 14 years. Persons with markedly reduced levels of IgA often experience repeated upper respiratory and gastrointestinal infections and have increased incidence of allergic manifestations, such as asthma, and autoimmune disorders. Persons with IgA deficiency also can develop antibodies against IgA, which can lead to severe anaphylactic reactions when blood components containing IgA are given.[28] Therefore, only specially washed erythrocytes from normal donors or erythrocytes from IgA-deficient donors should be used.

There is no treatment available for selective IgA deficiency unless there is a concomitant reduction in IgG levels. Administration of IgA immunoglobulin is of little benefit because it has a short half-life and is not secreted across the mucosa. There also is the risk of anaphylactic reactions associated with IgA antibodies in the immunoglobulin.

Immunoglobulin G Subclass Deficiency. An IgG subclass deficiency can affect one or more of the IgG subtypes, despite normal levels or elevated serum concentrations of IgG. As discussed in Chapter 13, IgG immunoglobulins can be divided into four subclasses (IgG_1 through IgG_4) based on structure and function. Most circulating IgG belongs to the IgG_1 (70%) and IgG_2 (20%) subclasses. In general, antibodies directed against protein antigens belong to the IgG_1 and IgG_3 subclasses, and antibodies directed against carbohydrate and polysaccharide antigens are primarily IgG_2 subclass. As a result, persons who are deficient in IgG_2 subclass antibodies can be at greater risk for development of sinusitis, otitis media, and pneumonia caused by polysaccharide-encapsulated microorganisms such as *S. pneumoniae*, *H. influenzae* type b, and *N. meningitidis*.

Children with mild forms of the deficiency can be treated with prophylactic antibiotics to prevent repeated infections. Intravenous immune globulin can be given to children with severe manifestations of this deficiency.

Cellular (T-Cell) Immunodeficiencies

There are few primary forms of T-cell immunodeficiency, probably because persons with defects in this branch of the immune response rarely survive beyond infancy or childhood. However, exceptions are being recognized as newer T-cell defects, such as X-linked immunodeficiency with hyper-IgM and CD2, are being identified. Other primary T-cell immunodeficiency disorders result from defective expression of the T-cell receptor complex, defective cytokine production, and defects in T-cell activation.

Unlike the B-cell lineage, in which a well-defined series of differentiation steps ultimately leads to the production of immunoglobulins, mature T lymphocytes are composed of distinct subpopulations whose immunologic assignments are diverse. T cells can be functionally divided into helper and cytotoxic subtypes and a population of T cells that promote delayed hypersensitivity reactions. Collectively, T lymphocytes protect against fungal, protozoan, viral, and intracellular bacterial infections; control malignant cell proliferation; and are responsible for coordinating the overall immune response.

DiGeorge Syndrome. DiGeorge syndrome stems from a developmental defect that occurs while the thymus gland, parathyroid gland, and parts of the head, neck, and heart are developing (*i.e.*, before the 12th week of gestation).

The disorder affects both sexes. Formerly thought to be caused by a variety of factors, including extrinsic teratogens, this defect has been traced to a gene on chromosome 22 (22q11).[27,31–33]

Infants born with this defect have partial or complete failure of development of the thymus and parathyroid glands and have congenital defects of the head, neck, and heart (Fig. 15-7). The extent of immune and parathyroid abnormalities is highly variable, as are the other defects. Occasionally, a child has no heart defect. In some children, the thymus is not absent but is in an abnormal location and is extremely small. These infants also can have partial DiGeorge syndrome, in which hypertrophy of the thymus occurs with development of normal immune function. The facial disorders can include hypertelorism (*i.e.*, increased distance between the eyes); micrognathia (*i.e.*, fish mouth); low-set, posteriorly angulated ears;

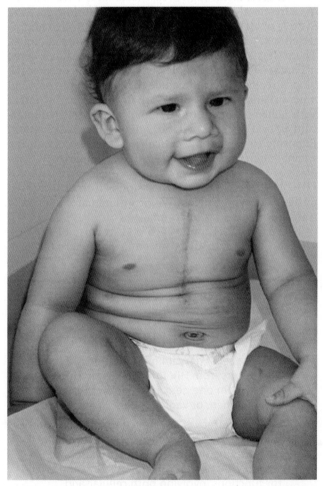

FIGURE 15-7 An infant with DiGeorge syndrome. The surgical scar on the chest indicates repair of heart disease caused by truncus arteriosus or interrupted aortic arch, which is common in this syndrome. The infant also has the facial features of a child with DiGeorge syndrome: hypertelorism, low-set ears, hypoplastic mandible, and bowing upward of the upper lip. (From Roberts R. [1998]. *Atlas of infectious diseases.* Edited by Gerald Mandell (series editor), Catherine M. Wilfert. © 1998 Current Medicine, Inc.)

split uvula; and high-arched palate. Urinary tract abnormalities also are common. The most common presenting sign is hypocalcemia and tetany that develops during the first 24 hours of life. It is caused by the absence of the parathyroid gland and is resistant to standard therapy.

Children who survive the immediate neonatal period may have recurrent or chronic infections because of impaired T-cell immunity. Without helper T-cell function, children also may lack immunoglobulin production. For children who do require treatment, thymus transplantation can be performed to reconstitute T-cell immunity. Bone marrow transplantation also has been successfully used to restore normal T-cell populations. If blood transfusions are needed, as during corrective heart surgery, special processing is required to prevent graft-versus-host disease.

X-Linked Immunodeficiency With Hyper-IgM. The X-linked immunodeficiency of hyper-IgM, also known as the *hyper-IgM syndrome*, is characterized by low IgG and IgA levels with normal or, more frequently, high IgM concentrations. Being X-linked, the disorder is confined to boys. Formerly classified as a B-cell defect, it now has been traced to a T-cell defect. The disorder results from the inability of T cells to signal B cells to undergo isotype switching to IgG and IgA; thus, they produce only IgM.[18]

Like boys with X-linked agammaglobulinemia, affected boys become symptomatic during the first and second years of life. They have recurrent pyogenic infections, including otitis media, sinusitis, tonsillitis, and pneumonia. They are also more susceptible to *Pneumocystis carinii* infection. Thymus-dependent lymphoid tissues and T-cell function usually are normal, as are B-cell counts. Hemolytic anemia and thrombocytopenia may occur, and transient, persistent, or cyclic neutropenia is a common feature. The occurrence of concomitant autoimmune disorders is higher than with other immunoglobulin deficiency disorders.[18]

Combined T-Cell and B-Cell Immunodeficiencies

Disorders that affect both B and T lymphocytes, with resultant defects in both humoral and cell-mediated immunity, fall under the broad classification of combined immunodeficiency syndrome (CIDS). A single mutation in any one of the many genes that influence lymphocyte development or response, including lymphocyte receptors, cytokines, or major histocompatibility antigens, can lead to combined immunodeficiency. Regardless of the affected gene, the net result is a disruption in the normal communication system of B and T lymphocytes and deregulation of the immune response. The spectrum of disease resulting from combined immunodeficiency disorders ranges from mild to severe to ultimately fatal forms.

Severe Combined Immunodeficiency. The most pronounced form of the combined immunodeficiencies often is referred to as *severe combined immunodeficiency syndrome* (SCIDS). SCIDS is caused by diverse genetic mutations that lead to the absence of all immune function and, in some cases, a lack of natural killer (NK) cells.[28,29]

Affected infants have a disease course that resembles AIDS, with failure to thrive, chronic diarrhea, and opportunistic infections that usually lead to death by the age of 2 years. If recognized at birth or within the first 3 months of life, 95% of infants can be successfully treated with bone marrow or stem cell transplantation.[29] A family history of similarly affected relatives occurs in approximately 50% of cases.[33] Both X-linked and autosomal recessive inheritances are involved.

X-linked SCIDS are due to mutations in the gene encoding the common gamma chain (γ_c) shared by receptors for many of the cytokines that direct the differentiation and maturation of both T and B lymphocytes.[27] These mutations are recessive, so that heterozygous girls are usually normal carriers of the gene, whereas boys who inherit the abnormal chromosome manifest the disease. Children with this disorder appear similar to those with other forms of SCIDS except for having uniformly low percentages of T and NK cells and an elevated percentage of B cells. However, the B cells do not produce immunoglobulin in a normal manner because of a lack of T-cell help.

The recent successful correction of T and NK cell defects using gene transfer therapy (insertion of exogenous genetic material into the infant's bone marrow cells) offers hope that this method will eventually become the treatment of choice for this form of SCIDS.[34]

About 50% of persons with SCIDS show an autosomal recessive pattern of inheritance, and about half of these are due to a deficiency in adenosine deaminase (ADA).[1] Absence of this enzyme leads to the accumulation of toxic metabolites that kill dividing and resting T cells. Infants with ADA-deficiency SCIDS, who typically manifest absolute lymphocyte counts of less than 500/mm³, usually have a much more profound lymphopenia than do infants with other forms of SCIDS. The absolute numbers of both T and B cells are very low. Although the number of NK cells is low, their function is normal. Other distinguishing features of the ADA deficiency include the presence of rib cage deformity and numerous skeletal deformities.

Bone marrow transplantation has been successful in treating children with ADA-negative SCIDS.[29,33,34] Enzyme replacement therapy also may be used in the management of persons with this form of SCIDS.[29,34] However, it should not be used if bone marrow transplantation is anticipated because it can predispose to graft rejection.

ACQUIRED IMMUNODEFICIENCY SYNDROME

The acquired immunodeficiency syndrome (AIDS) is a disease caused by infection with the human immunodeficiency virus (HIV) and is characterized by profound immunosuppression with associated opportunistic infections, malignancies, wasting, and central nervous system degeneration. Because the disease affects an exceptionally high proportion of the population throughout the world, it is often referred to as a *pandemic*.[35]

As a national and global epidemic, the degree of morbidity and mortality caused by HIV, as well as its impact on health care resources and the economy, is tremendous—and unrelenting. Most of the new infections worldwide are in people younger than 25 years of age who live in developing countries. Sub-Saharan Africa has been hardest hit by HIV. There are over 29.4 million people living with HIV infection in Africa, with a reported 3.5 million new infections in 2002. Eastern Europe and central Asia have the world's fastest-growing HIV-positive population.[36] In the United States, there had been over 816,000 cases and more than 467,000 deaths from HIV at the end of 2000, with racial and ethnic minorities being disproportionately affected.[37]

Transmission of HIV Infection

HIV is transmitted from one person to another through sexual contact or blood-to-blood contact, and from infected women to their offspring in utero or during labor and delivery, or through breast-feeding. It is transmitted most frequently through sexual contact. Worldwide, 75% to 85% of HIV infections are transmitted through unprotected sex.[38] HIV is present in semen and vaginal fluids. There is risk of transmitting HIV when these fluids come in contact with a part of the body that lets them enter the bloodstream. This can include the vaginal mucosa, anal mucosa, and wounds or a sore on the skin.[38] Contact with semen occurs during vaginal and anal sexual intercourse, oral sex (*i.e.*, fellatio), and donor insemination. Exposure to vaginal or cervical secretions occurs during vaginal intercourse and oral sex (*i.e.*, cunnilingus). Condoms are highly effective in preventing transmission of HIV. The risk of HIV transmission is further increased in the presence of ulcerative or inflammatory sexually transmitted diseases or trauma.

Because HIV is found in blood, the use of needles, syringes, and other drug injection paraphernalia pro-

---

> **KEY CONCEPTS**
>
> **Acquired Immunodeficiency Syndrome**
>
> ➤ AIDS is a secondary immunodeficiency disorder that results from HIV infection, which is transmitted from one person to another through blood, semen, or vaginal fluids.
>
> ➤ The main effect of HIV infection is the destruction of CD4+ T cells, which constitutes an attack on the entire immune system, because this subset of T cells exerts critical regulatory and effector functions involving both cellular and humoral immunity.
>
> ➤ The three phases of HIV are primary HIV, latency, and overt AIDS. The classification of HIV/AIDS is based on laboratory counts of CD4+ T cells and the manifestations of the immunodeficiency state (development of opportunistic infections, neoplasms, and other related problems).

vides a direct route for transmission. HIV-infected injecting drug users can pass the virus to their needle-sharing and sex partners and, in the case of pregnant women, to their offspring. Although alcohol, cocaine, and other non-injected drugs do not directly transmit infection, their use alters perception of risk and reduces inhibitions about engaging in behaviors that pose a high risk of transmitting HIV infection.

Transfusions of whole blood, plasma, platelets, or blood cells before 1985 resulted in the transmission of HIV. Since 1985, all blood donations in the United States have been screened for HIV, so the risk of transmission has virtually been eliminated. The clotting factor used by persons with hemophilia is derived from the pooled plasma of hundreds of donors. Before HIV testing of plasma donors was implemented in 1985, the virus was transmitted to persons with hemophilia through infusions of these clotting factors. Clotting factors are now heat-treated to reduce further the likelihood of HIV transmission.

Occupational HIV infection among health care workers is uncommon.[39] Universal Blood and Body Fluid Precautions should be used in encounters with all patients in the health care setting because HIV status is not always known. The occupational risk of infection for health care workers most often is associated with percutaneous inoculation (i.e., needle stick) of blood from a patient with HIV.

The HIV-infected person can transmit the virus even when no symptoms are present and the antibody test is negative. The point at which an infected person converts from being negative for the presence of HIV antibodies in the blood to being positive is called *seroconversion.* Seroconversion typically occurs within 1 to 3 months after exposure to HIV but can take up to 6 months.[40] The time after infection and before seroconversion is known as the *window period.* During the window period, an HIV-infected person could transmit the virus through the blood. Blood collection centers have implemented more stringent processes to avoid HIV transmission from a donor who has not seroconverted. Potential donors are now screened through interviews designed to identify risk behaviors for HIV infection, and blood is tested for the HIV antibody as well as viral nucleic acid.

Pathophysiology of AIDS

The primary etiologic agent of AIDS is HIV, an enveloped ribonucleic acid (RNA) retrovirus that carries its genetic material in RNA rather than deoxyribonucleic acid (DNA). Two genetically different but antigenically related forms of HIV, HIV-1 and HIV-2, have been isolated in people with AIDS.[2] HIV-1 is the type most commonly associated with AIDS in the United States, Europe, and central Africa, whereas HIV-2 causes a similar disease principally in western Africa. HIV-2 appears to be transmitted in the same manner as HIV-1; it can also cause immunodeficiency as evidenced by a reduction in the number of CD4+ T cells and the development of AIDS. Although the spectrum of disease for HIV-2 is similar to that of HIV-1, it spreads more slowly and causes disease more slowly than HIV-1. Specific tests are now available for HIV-2, and blood collected for transfusion is routinely screened for HIV-2. The remaining discussion focuses on HIV-1, but the information is generally applicable to HIV-2 as well.

HIV infects a limited number of cell types in the body, including CD4+ helper T cells (also known as CD4+ T cells), macrophages, and dendritic cells[2,6] (see Chapter 13). The CD4+ T cells are necessary for normal immune function. Among other functions, the CD4+ T cell recognizes foreign antigens and helps activate antibody-producing B-lymphocytes.[2] The CD4+ T cells also orchestrate cell-mediated immunity, in which cytotoxic CD8+ T cells and NK cells directly destroy virus-infected cells, tubercle bacilli, and foreign antigens. The phagocytic function of monocytes and macrophages is also influenced by CD4+ T cells.

The HIV is spherical in shape and contains an electron-dense core surrounded by a lipid envelope (Fig. 15-8). The virus core contains the major capsid protein p24, two copies of the genomic RNA, and three viral enzymes (protease, reverse transcriptase, and integrase). Because p24 is the most readily detected antigen, it is the target for the antibodies used in screening for HIV infection.[2] The viral core is surrounded by a matrix protein called p17, which lies beneath the viral envelope. The viral envelope is studded with two viral glycoproteins, gp120 and gp41, which are critical for the infection of cells.

Replication of HIV occurs in eight steps[1,2,6] (see Fig. 15-8). Each of these steps provides insights into the development of methods used for preventing or treating the infection. The *first step* involves the binding of the virus to the CD4+ T cell. Once HIV has entered the bloodstream, it attaches to the surface of a CD4+ T cell by binding to a CD4 receptor that has a high affinity for HIV. However, binding to the CD4+ T-cell receptor is not sufficient for infection; the virus must also bind with other surface molecules (chemokine coreceptors) that bind the gp120 and gp41 envelope glycoproteins. This process is known as *attachment.* The chemokine coreceptors are critical components of the HIV infection process. It has recently been found that people with defective coreceptors are more resistant to HIV infection, despite repeated exposure.[2] The *second step* allows for the internalization of the virus. After attachment, the viral envelope peptides fuse to the CD4+ T-cell membrane. Fusion results in an *uncoating* of the virus, allowing the contents of the viral core (the two single strands of viral RNA and the reverse transcriptase, integrase, and protease enzymes) to enter the host cell.

The *third step* consists of DNA synthesis. For the HIV to reproduce, it must change its single-stranded RNA into double-stranded DNA. It does this by using the *reverse transcriptase* enzyme. Reverse transcriptase makes a copy of the viral RNA, and then in reverse makes another, mirror-image copy. The result is double-stranded DNA that carries instructions for viral replication. The *fourth step* is called *integration.* During integration, the new DNA

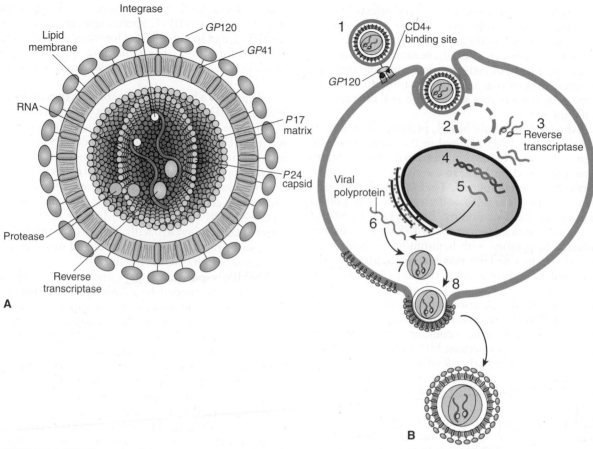

FIGURE 15-8 (**A**) Life cycle of the type 1 human immunodeficiency virus (HIV-1). (**B**) (**1**) Attachment of HIV to CD4+ T-cell receptor; (**2**) internalization and uncoating of the virus with viral RNA and reverse transcriptase; (**3**) reverse transcription, which produces a mirror image of the viral RNA and double-stranded DNA molecule; (**4**) integration of viral DNA into host DNA using the integrase enzyme; (**5**) transcription of the inserted viral DNA to produce viral messenger RNA; (**6**) translation of viral messenger RNA to create viral polyprotein; (**7**) cleavage of viral polyprotein into individual viral proteins that make up the new virus; and (**8**) assembly and release of the new virus from the host cell.

enters the nucleus of the CD4+ T cell and, with the help of the enzyme integrase, is inserted into the cell's DNA.

The *fifth step* involves *transcription* of the double-stranded viral DNA to form a single-stranded messenger RNA (mRNA) with the instructions for building new viruses. Transcription involves activation of the T cell and induction of host cell transcription factors. The *sixth step* includes translation of mRNA. During *translation*, ribosomal RNA (rRNA) uses the instructions in the mRNA to create a chain of proteins and enzymes called a *polyprotein*. These polyproteins contain the components needed for the next stages in the construction of new viruses. The *seventh step* is called *cleavage*. During cleavage, the protease enzyme cuts the polyprotein chain into the individual proteins that will make up the new viruses. Finally, during the *eighth step*, the proteins and viral RNA are assembled into new HIV viruses and released from the CD4+ T cell.

The replication of HIV results in the killing of the CD4+ T cell and the release of copies of the HIV into the bloodstream. These viral particles, or *virions*, invade other CD4+ T cells, allowing the infection to progress. Although it is estimated that millions of infected CD4+ T cells are destroyed daily and billions of viral particles are released into the bloodstream, nearly all the CD4+ T cells are replaced and nearly all the viral particles are destroyed. Over years, however, the CD4+ cell count gradually decreases and the number of viruses detected in the blood of persons infected with HIV increases. Until the CD4+ cell count falls to a very low level, a person infected with HIV can remain asymptomatic although active viral replication is still taking place and serologic tests can identify antibodies to HIV.

Classification and Course of Infection

Classification. In January of 1993, the U.S. Centers for Disease Control and Prevention (CDC) implemented a classification system for HIV infection and expanded surveillance case definition for AIDS in adolescents and adults based on HIV-related clinical conditions and CD4+ T-cell count. The classification system defines three laboratory test categories that correspond to CD4+ cell counts per microliter (µL) of blood: *category 1:* >500 cells/µL, *category 2:* 200 to 499 cells/µL, and *category 3:* <200 cells/µL. The HIV-related clinical conditions include the opportunistic infections, malignancies, dementia, and wasting (documented weight loss) that rarely occur in the absence of severe immunodeficiency.[41] The clinical manifestations are also divided into three categories. *Clinical category A* includes persons who have no symptoms or have persistent generalized lymphadenopathy or symptoms of primary HIV infection (*i.e.,* acute seroconversion illness). *Clinical category B* includes persons with symptoms of immune deficiency not serious enough to be defined as AIDS. *Clinical category C* includes AIDS-defining illnesses that are listed in the AIDS surveillance case definition shown in Chart 15-2. Each HIV-infected person has a CD4+ T-cell category and a clinical category. According to the 1993 case definition, persons in laboratory category 3 or clinical category C are considered to have AIDS.

Dramatic increases in the efficacy of HIV treatment regimens have improved the prognosis of persons with HIV/AIDS. As a result, fewer persons with HIV infection experience opportunistic infections or have low enough CD4+ counts to classify them has having AIDS, which means that the CDC definition has become a less useful measure of the impact of HIV/AIDS in the United States. In an effort to obtain data representing the increasing number of HIV-infected persons who do not meet the AIDS-defining criteria, the CDC issued a revised surveillance case definition that incorporates the criteria for HIV infection (*i.e.,* laboratory evidence of HIV) and AIDS-defining conditions into a single case definition.[42]

Course of Infection. The typical course of HIV infection is defined by three phases: the primary infection phase, the chronic asymptomatic or latency phase, and the overt AIDS phase[43] (Fig. 15-9). These phases usually occur over a period of 8 to 12 years.

When they initially become infected with HIV, many persons have an acute mononucleosis-like syndrome known as the *primary infection phase.* This acute phase may include fever, fatigue, myalgias, sore throat, night sweats, gastrointestinal problems, lymphadenopathy, maculopapular rash, and headache (Chart 15-3). During the primary infection phase, there is an increase in viral replication, which leads to very high viral loads, sometime greater than 1,000,000 copies/mL, and a decrease in the CD4+ cell count. The signs and symptoms of primary HIV infection usually appear 2 to 4 weeks after exposure to HIV, and last for a few days to 2 weeks.[41] After several weeks, the immune system acts to control viral replication and reduces the viral load to a lower level, where it often remains for several years. People who are diagnosed with HIV while they are in the primary infection phase appear to have a unique opportunity for treatment. It seems possible that, if started early, treatment may reduce the number of long-living HIV-infected cells (*e.g.,* CD4+ memory cells).

CHART 15-2

Conditions Included in the 1993 AIDS Surveillance Case Definition

Candidiasis of bronchi, trachea, or lungs
Candidiasis, esophageal
Cervical cancer, invasive*
Coccidioidomycosis, disseminated or extrapulmonary
Cryptococcosis, extrapulmonary
Cryptosporidiosis, chronic intestinal (>1 month's duration)
Cytomegalovirus disease (other than liver, spleen, or nodes)
Cytomegalovirus retinitis (with loss of vision)
Encephalopathy, HIV-related
Herpes simplex: chronic ulcer(s) (>1 month's duration) or bronchitis, pneumonitis, or esophagitis
Histoplasmosis, disseminated or extrapulmonary
Isosporiasis, chronic intestinal (>1 month's duration)
Kaposi sarcoma
Lymphoma, Burkitt (or equivalent term)
Lymphoma, immunoblastic (or equivalent term)
Lymphoma, primary, of brain
Mycobacterium avium-intracellulare complex or *M. kansasii,* disseminated or extrapulmonary
Mycobacterium tuberculosis, any site (pulmonary* or extrapulmonary)
Mycobacterium, other species or unidentified species, disseminated or extrapulmonary
Pneumocystis carinii pneumonia
Pneumonia, recurrent*
Progressive multifocal leukoencephalopathy
Salmonella septicemia, recurrent
Toxoplasmosis of brain
Wasting syndrome due to HIV

*Added to the 1993 expansion of the AIDS surveillance case definition.
(Centers for Disease Control and Prevention. [1992]. 1993 Revised classification system for HIV infection and expanded surveillance case definition for AIDS among adolescents and adults. *MMWR Morbidity and Mortality Weekly Report* 41 [RR-17], 19.)

The primary phase is followed by a *latency phase* during which the person has no signs or symptoms of illness. The median time of the latent period is about 10 years. During this time, the CD4+ cell count falls until it reaches a critical level below which there is substantial risk of opportunistic infection.[2] Lymphadenopathy develops in some persons with HIV infection during this phase. Persistent generalized lymphadenopathy usually is defined as lymph nodes that are chronically swollen for more than 3 months in at least two locations, not including the groin. The lymph nodes may be sore or visible externally.

The *overt AIDS phase* occurs when a person has a CD4+ cell count less than 200 cells/µL or an AIDS-defining illness.[43] Without antiretroviral therapy, this phase can lead to death within 2 to 3 years. The risk of opportunistic

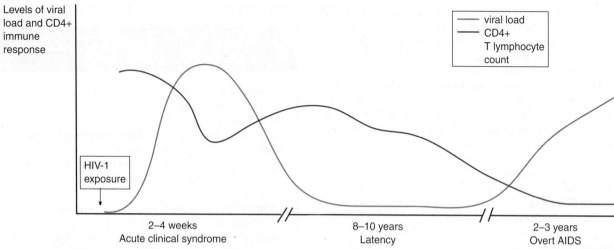

FIGURE 15-9 Viral load and CD4+ T-cell count during the phases of HIV infection.

infections and death is increased significantly when the CD4+ cell count reaches this level. In the United States, the typical adult with overt AIDS presents with fever, diarrhea, weight loss and the wasting syndrome, generalized lymphadenopathy, multiple opportunistic infections, and, in many cases, secondary neoplasms.

The clinical course of HIV varies from person to person. Most (60% to 70%) of those infected with HIV develop overt AIDS 10 to 11 years after infection. These people are the *typical progressors*.[43] Another 10% to 20% of those infected experience more rapid progression. They develop overt AIDS in less than 5 years and are called *rapid progressors*. The final 5% to 15% are *slow progressors*, who do not experience progression to overt AIDS for more than 15 years. There is a subset of slow progressors, called *long-term nonprogressors*, who account for 1% of all HIV infections. These people have been infected for at least 8 years, are antiretroviral naive, have high CD4+ counts, and usually have very low viral loads.

Opportunistic Infections

Opportunistic infections account for the majority of deaths from AIDS.[1] In the United States, the most common opportunistic infections are *Pneumocystis carinii* pneumonia (PCP), oropharyngeal or esophageal candidiasis (thrush), cytomegalovirus (CMV) infection, and infections caused by *Mycobacterium avium-intracellulare* complex (MAC).[44]

Respiratory Tract Infections. The most common causes of respiratory disease in persons with HIV infection are PCP and pulmonary tuberculosis (TB). Other organisms that cause opportunistic pulmonary infections in persons with AIDS include CMV, MAC, *Toxoplasma gondii*, and *Cryptococcus neoformans*. Pneumonia also may occur because of more common bacterial pulmonary pathogens, including *Streptococcus pneumoniae, Haemophilus influenzae*, and *Legionella pneumophila*.

P. carinii pneumonia was the most common presenting manifestation of AIDS during the first decade of the epidemic. Since highly active antiretroviral therapy (HAART) and prophylaxis for PCP was instituted, the incidence has decreased.[2] PCP still is common in people who do not know their HIV status, in those who choose not to treat their HIV infection, and in those with poor access to health care. The best predictor of PCP is a CD4+ cell count below 200 cell/μL,[45] and it is at this point that prophylaxis with trimethoprim-sulfamethoxazole is started. PCP is caused by *P. carinii*, an organism that is common in soil, houses, and many other places in the environment. In persons with healthy immune systems, *P. carinii* does not cause infection or disease. In persons with HIV, *P. carinii* can multiply quickly in the lungs and cause pneumonia. As the disease progresses, the alveoli become filled with a foamy, protein-rich fluid that impairs gas exchange. The symptoms of PCP may be acute or gradually progressive. Patients may present with complaints of a mild cough, fever, shortness of breath, and weight loss. Physical examination may demonstrate only fever and tachypnea, and breath sounds may be normal. Diagnosis of PCP is made on recognition of the organism in pulmonary secretions. This can be done through examination of induced sputum, bronchoalveolar lavage, occasionally bronchoscopy, and, rarely, lung biopsy.[45]

Tuberculosis is the leading cause of death for people with HIV worldwide. There are over 80,000 people coinfected with HIV and TB in North America and another 5 million in the rest of the world.[46] Although the lungs are the most common site of *M. tuberculosis* infection, extrapulmonary infection of the kidney, bone marrow, and other organs also occurs in people with HIV infection. Whether a person has pulmonary or extrapulmonary TB, most patients present with fever, night sweats, cough, and weight loss. Persons infected with *M. tuberculosis* (*i.e.*, those with positive tuberculin skin tests) are more likely to develop reactivated TB if they become infected with HIV. Coinfected individuals are also more likely to have a rapidly progressive form of TB. Equally important, HIV-infected persons with TB coinfection usually have an increase in viral load, which decreases the success of TB therapy. They also have an increased number of other opportunistic infections and an increased mortality rate.

Since the late 1960s, most persons with TB have responded well to therapy. However, in 1991, there were outbreaks of multidrug-resistant TB.[46] Many cases of drug-resistant TB occur in HIV-infected persons.

Gastrointestinal Infections. Diseases of the gastrointestinal tract are some of the most frequent complications of HIV and AIDS. Esophageal candidiasis (thrush), CMV infection, and herpes simplex virus infection are common opportunistic infections that cause esophagitis in people with HIV infection.[47] Persons experiencing these infections usually complain of painful swallowing or retrosternal pain. The clinical presentation can range from asymptomatic to a complete inability to swallow and consequent dehydration. Endoscopy or barium esophagography is required for definitive diagnosis.

Diarrhea or gastroenteritis is a common complaint in persons with HIV. The most common protozoal infection that causes diarrhea is *Cryptosporidium parvum*. The clinical features of cryptosporidiosis can range from mild diarrhea to severe, watery diarrhea with a loss of up to several liters of water per day. The most severe form usually occurs in persons with a CD4+ cell count less than 50 cells/μL. Other organisms that cause gastroenteritis and diarrhea are *Salmonella*, CMV, *Clostridium difficile*, *Escherichia coli*, *Shigella*, *Giardia*, and Microsporida.[47] These organisms are identified by examination of stool cultures or endoscopy.

Nervous System Infections. HIV infection, particularly in its late stages of severe immunocompromise, leaves the nervous system vulnerable to an array of neurologic disorders, including AIDS dementia complex (ADC), toxoplasmosis, and progressive multifocal leukoencephalopathy (PML). These disorders can affect the peripheral or central nervous system (CNS) and contribute to the morbidity and mortality of persons with HIV.

AIDS dementia complex, or HIV-associated dementia, is a syndrome of cognitive and motor dysfunction.[48] ADC is caused by HIV itself, rather than an opportunistic infection, and usually is a late complication of HIV infection. The clinical features of ADC are impairment of attention and concentration, slowing of mental speed and agility, slowing of motor speed, and apathetic behavior. The diagnosis of ADC can be based on these clinical findings. Treatment of ADC consists of HAART to decrease symptoms, but there is no cure.

Toxoplasmosis is a common opportunistic infection in persons with AIDS. The organism responsible, *T. gondii*, is a parasite that most often affects the CNS. Toxoplasmosis usually is a reactivation of a latent *T. gondii* infection that has been dormant in the CNS. The typical presentation includes fever, headaches, and neurologic dysfunction, including confusion and lethargy, visual disturbances, and seizures. Computed tomography (CT) scanning or magnetic resonance imaging (MRI) is usually performed to detect the presence of neurologic lesions.

Progressive multifocal leukoencephalopathy is a demyelinating disease of the white matter of the brain caused by the JC virus, a DNA papovavirus that attacks the oligodendrocytes. PML advances slowly, and it can be weeks to months before the patient seeks medical care. PML is characterized by progressive limb weakness, sensory loss, difficulty controlling the digits, visual disturbances, subtle alterations in mental status,[49] hemiparesis, ataxia, diplopia, and seizures. The mortality rate is high, and the average survival time is 2 to 4 months. Diagnosis is based on clinical findings and an MRI, and confirmed by the presence of the JC virus.

Malignancies

Persons with AIDS have a high incidence of certain malignancies, especially Kaposi sarcoma (KS), non-Hodgkin lymphoma, and noninvasive cervical carcinoma. The increased incidence of malignancies is thought to be a function of impaired cell-mediated immunity.

Kaposi sarcoma is a malignancy of the endothelial cells that line small blood vessels.[50] It was one of the first opportunistic cancers associated with AIDS and still is the most frequent malignancy related to HIV infection. There is evidence linking KS to a herpes virus (herpes virus 8, also called KS-associated herpes virus [KSHV]).[50] Over 95% of KS lesions, regardless of the source or clinical subtype, have reportedly been found to be infected with KSHV. The virus is readily transmitted through homosexual and heterosexual activities. Maternal–infant transmission also occurs. The lesions of KS can be found on the skin and in the oral cavity, gastrointestinal tract, and lungs. The disease usually begins as one or more macules, papules, or violet skin lesions that enlarge and become darker (Fig. 15-10). They may enlarge to form raised plaques or tumors. Tumor nodules frequently are located on the trunk, neck, and head, especially the tip of the nose. They usually are painless in the early stages, but discomfort may ensue as the tumor develops. Invasion of internal organs, including the lungs, gastrointestinal

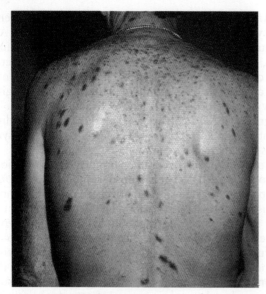

FIGURE 15-10 Disseminated Kaposi sarcoma. Multiple red to brown papules are distributed along the skin tension lines in a man with AIDS. (From Hall J. C. [2000]. *Sauer's manual of skin* [p. 197]. Philadelphia: Lippincott Williams & Wilkins.)

tract, and lymphatic system, commonly occurs. Gastrointestinal tract KS is often asymptomatic, but can cause pain, bleeding, or obstruction.[50] Pulmonary KS usually is a late development of the disease and causes dyspnea, cough, and hemoptysis.

With prolonged survival, the number of persons with AIDS who develop non-Hodgkin lymphoma has increased steadily.[2] The clinical features are fever, night sweats, and weight loss (see Chapter 9). Because the manifestations of non-Hodgkin lymphoma are similar to those of other opportunistic infections, diagnosis often is difficult. Treatment includes aggressive combination chemotherapy with intrathecal chemotherapy to prevent or treat meningeal involvement.

In addition to KS and lymphomas, women with HIV infection also have a higher incidence of cervical dysplasia[51] (see Chapter 39). These lesions, which are thought to result from infection with the human papillomavirus, are usually a slowly developing precursor to cervical carcinoma and progress rapidly in women with HIV infection. For this reason, HIV-infected women should have Papanicolaou smears every 6 months rather than every 12 months. In addition to the rapid progression from mild dysplasia to carcinoma in situ, women with HIV infection may be less responsive to standard treatments and have a poorer prognosis than uninfected women.[51]

Wasting Syndrome and Metabolic Disorders

In 1997, the wasting syndrome became an AIDS-defining illness. The syndrome is characterized by involuntary weight loss of at least 10% of baseline body weight in the presence of diarrhea, more than two stools per day, or chronic weakness and a fever. This diagnosis is made when no other opportunistic infections or neoplasms can

be identified as causing these symptoms. Factors that contribute to wasting are anorexia, metabolic abnormalities, endocrine dysfunction, malabsorption, and cytokine dysregulation. Treatment for wasting includes nutritional interventions such as oral supplements or enteral or parenteral nutrition. There also are numerous pharmacologic agents used to treat wasting, including appetite stimulants, cannabinoids, and megestrol acetate.[52]

A number of metabolic abnormalities have been linked to the protease inhibitors and nucleoside analogs that are used to treat HIV infection. These abnormalities include insulin resistance and impaired glucose tolerance, elevated cholesterol and triglyceride levels, and changes in body composition.[53] The combination of lipid abnormalities and changes in body composition is referred to as *lipodystrophy*. The alterations in body composition include an increase in abdominal girth, buffalo hump development (abnormal distribution of fat in the supraclavicular area), wasting of fat from the face and extremities, and breast enlargement in men and women. Originally attributed to the use of protease inhibitors, the pathogenesis of lipodystrophy is still not understood.[54] It may be due to protease inhibitor therapy or nucleoside reverse transcriptase inhibitor therapy, or may arise simply because people are living longer with HIV infection.

Diagnosis and Treatment

Diagnostic Methods. The most accurate and inexpensive method for identifying HIV infection is the HIV antibody test. The first commercial assays for HIV were introduced in 1985 to screen donated blood. Since then, the use of antibody detection tests has been expanded to include evaluating persons at increased risk for HIV infection. The HIV antibody test procedure consists of screening with an *enzyme immunoassay* (EIA), also known as *enzyme-linked immunosorbent assay* (ELISA), followed by a confirmatory test, the *Western blot* assay, which is performed if the EIA is positive. The EIA is based on the reaction of antibodies to HIV in the blood sample with viral proteins in the test material. The Western blot is a more sensitive assay that looks for the presence of antibodies to specific viral antigens.

Millions of HIV antibody tests are performed in the United States each year. New technology has led to new forms of testing, like the oral test, home testing kits, and the new rapid blood test. Oral fluids contain antibodies to HIV. In the late 1990s, the FDA approved the OraSure test.[55] The OraSure uses a cotton swab that is inserted into the mouth for 2 minutes, placed in a transport container with preservative, and then sent to a laboratory for EIA and Western blot testing. Home HIV testing kits can be bought over the counter. The kits, approved by the FDA, allow persons to collect their own blood sample through a fingerstick process, mail the specimen to a laboratory for EIA and confirmatory Western blot tests, and receive results by telephone in 3 to 7 days. In November 2002, the FDA approved the Ora Quick Rapid HIV-1 Antibody Test.[56] The Ora Quick test uses a whole-blood specimen from a fingerstick and can provide results in about 20 minutes. Reactive, or positive, test results require confirmation using Western blot testing. A person with a reactive result needs to be told that their preliminary test was positive, but they need a confirmatory test.

Polymerase chain reaction (PCR) is a technique for detecting HIV DNA. PCR detects the presence of the virus, rather than the antibody to the virus, which the EIA and Western blot tests detect.[2] PCR is useful in diagnosing HIV infection in infants born to infected mothers because these infants have their mothers' HIV antibody, regardless of whether the children are infected.

Treatment. There is no cure for HIV infection. The medications that are currently available to treat HIV infection decrease the amount of HIV in the body, but they do not get rid of the virus. Because different drugs act on different stages of the replication cycle, optimal treatment includes a combination of at least three drugs, often referred to as HAART.[57] The goal of HAART is a sustained suppression of HIV replication, resulting in an undetectable viral load and an increasing CD4+ cell count. In general, antiviral therapies are prescribed to slow the progression to AIDS and improve the overall quality of life and survival time of persons with HIV infection.

There currently are five different types of HIV antiretroviral medications: nucleoside reverse transcriptase inhibitors; nucleoside analog reverse transcriptase inhibitors; non-nucleoside reverse transcriptase inhibitors; protease inhibitors; and the newest class, fusion inhibitors. Each type of agent attempts to interrupt the life cycle of HIV at a different point (see Fig. 15-7). *Reverse transcriptase inhibitors* inhibit HIV replication by acting on the enzyme reverse transcriptase. *Nucleoside reverse transcriptase inhibitors* act by blocking the elongation of the DNA chain by stopping more nucleosides from being added. *Non-nucleoside reverse transcriptase inhibitors* work by binding to the reverse transcriptase enzyme so it cannot copy the virus's RNA into DNA. *Protease inhibitors* bind to the protease enzyme and inhibit its action. This inhibition prevents the cleavage of the polyprotein chain into individual proteins, which would be used to construct the new virus. Because the information inside the nucleus is not put together properly, the new viruses that are released into the body are immature and noninfectious. The newest class of antiretroviral therapy consists of the *fusion inhibitors*, which prevent HIV from fusing with the CD4+ T cell, thus blocking the virus from inserting its genetic information into the CD4+ cell.

Drugs and vaccines commonly are used for the prevention and treatment of opportunistic infections and conditions, including PCP, toxoplasmosis, MAC, candidiasis, CMV infection, influenza, hepatitis B, and *S. pneumoniae* infections.

 Infection in Pregnancy and in Infants and Children

Early in the epidemic, children who contracted HIV could have become infected through blood products or perinatally. Now, almost all children who become infected with HIV at a young age in the United States get infected perinatally. Infected women may transmit the virus to their offspring in utero, during labor and delivery, or through breast milk.[58] The risk of transmission of HIV from mother to infant is approximately 25%, with estimates ranging from 15% to 45%, depending on the country in which they reside.[59] The risk of transmission is increased if the mother has advanced HIV disease as evidenced by low CD4+ cell counts or high levels of HIV in the blood (high viral load); if there is prolonged time from rupture of membranes to delivery; if the mother breast-feeds the child[12]; or if there is increased exposure of the fetus to maternal blood.[60]

Diagnosis of HIV infection in children born to HIV-infected mothers is complicated by the presence of maternal HIV IgG antibody, which crosses the placenta to the fetus.[58] Consequently, infants born to HIV-infected women can be HIV antibody positive by ELISA up to 18 months of age even though they are not HIV infected. PCR testing for HIV DNA is used most often to diagnose HIV infection in infants younger than 18 months of age. Two positive PCR tests for HIV DNA are needed to diagnose a child with HIV infection. Children born to mothers with HIV infection are considered uninfected if they become HIV antibody negative after 6 months of age, have no other laboratory evidence of HIV infection, and have not met the surveillance case definition criteria for AIDS in children.

The landmark PACTG 076 trial of 1994 found that perinatal transmission could be lowered by two thirds, from 26% to 8%, by administering zidovudine to the mother during pregnancy and labor and delivery and to the infant when it is born.[61] The U.S. Public Health Service therefore recommends that HIV counseling and testing should be offered to all pregnant women.[62] The recommendations also stress that women who test positive for HIV antibodies should be informed of the perinatal prevention benefits of zidovudine therapy and offered HAART, which often includes zidovudine. This is done because it has now been found that women receiving antiretroviral therapy who also have a viral load of less than 1000 copies/mL have very low rates of perinatal transmission. Benefits of voluntary testing for mothers and newborns include reduced morbidity because of intensive treatment and supportive health care, the opportunity for early antiviral therapy for mother and child, and information regarding the risk of transmission from breast milk.

Because pregnant women in less developed countries do not always have access to zidovudine, studies are being conducted in Africa to determine if any other simple and less expensive antiretroviral regimen can be used to decrease transmission from mother to infant. One such study, HIVNET 012, looked at single-dose nevirapine compared with zidovudine. It found that nevirapine lowered the risk of HIV transmission by almost 50%.[63]

Children have a very different pattern of HIV infection than adults. Failure to thrive, CNS abnormalities, and developmental delays are the most prominent primary manifestations of HIV infection in children.[59] Children born infected with HIV usually weigh less and are shorter than noninfected infants. A major cause of early mortality for HIV-infected children is PCP. As opposed to adults, in whom PCP occurs in the late stages, PCP occurs early in children, with the peak age of onset at 3 to 6 months. For this reason, prophylaxis with trimethoprim-sulfamethoxazole is started by 4 to 6 weeks for all infants born to HIV-infected mothers, regardless of their CD4+ cell count or infection status.

In summary, an immunodeficiency is defined as an absolute or partial loss of the normal immune response, which places a person in a state of compromise and increases the risk for development of infections or malignant complications. The defect may be classified as a primary or secondary disorder and may affect any components of the immune response, including antibody or humoral (B-cell) immunity, cellular or T-cell immunity, or a combination of B-cell and T-cell immunity.

Most primary immunodeficiency states are inherited and are either present at birth or become apparent shortly after birth. Primary immunodeficiencies can be categorized into three types: humoral (B-cell) immunodeficiencies, cellular (T-cell) immunodeficiencies, and combined (B-cell and T-cell) immunodeficiencies. B-cell immunodeficiencies can selectively affect a single type of immunoglobulin (*e.g.,* IgA immunodeficiency) or all of the immunoglobulins. Defects in B-cell function increase the risk of recurrent pyogenic infections, including those caused by *S. pneumoniae, H. influenzae,* and *S. aureus,* and by gram-negative organisms such as *Pseudomonas* species. There are few primary forms of T-cell immunodeficiency, probably because persons with defects in this branch of the immune response rarely survive beyond infancy or childhood. Combined immunodeficiency disorders involve both B-cell and T-cell dysfunction and include a spectrum of inherited (autosomal recessive and X-linked) conditions. The spectrum of disease resulting from combined immunodeficiency ranges from mild to severe to ultimately fatal forms.

AIDS, the most common type of secondary immunodeficiency, is caused by HIV infection. The virus is most commonly transmitted from one person to another through sexual contact, blood exchange, or perinatally. HIV is a retrovirus that infects the body's CD4+ T cells and macrophages. The destruction of CD4+ T cells constitutes an attack on the entire immune system because this subset of lymphocytes exerts critical regulatory and effector functions that involve both humoral and cellular immunity. The clinical course of HIV infection can be divided into three phases: a primary phase that occurs shortly after infection and is usually manifested with mononucleosis-like symptoms, a latency phase that may last for many years, and an overt AIDS phase that is characterized by a marked decrease in CD4+ T cells and

the development of opportunistic infections of the respiratory, gastrointestinal, and nervous systems, malignancies such as Kaposi sarcoma and non-Hodgkin lymphoma, wasting syndrome, and metabolic disorders. There is no cure for AIDS. Treatment largely involves the use of drugs that interrupt replication of HIV and prevention or treatment of complications such as opportunistic infections.

Infected women may transmit the virus to their offspring in utero, during labor and delivery, or through breast milk. Diagnosis of HIV infection in children born to HIV-infected mothers is complicated by the presence of maternal HIV antibody, which crosses the placenta to the fetus. This antibody usually disappears within 18 months in uninfected children. The administration of zidovudine to the mother during pregnancy and labor and delivery and to the infant after birth can decrease perinatal transmission.

Review Exercises

A 32-year-old man presents in the allergy clinic with complaints of allergic rhinitis or hay fever. His major complaints are those of nasal pruritus (itching), nasal congestion with profuse watery drainage, sneezing, and eye irritation. The physical examination reveals edematous and inflamed nasal mucosa and redness of the ocular conjunctiva. He relates that this happens every fall during "ragweed season."

A. Explain the immunologic mechanisms that are responsible for this man's symptoms.
B. What type of diagnostic tests might be used?
C. What type of treatment(s) might be used to relieve his symptoms?

Persons with intestinal parasites and those with allergies may both have elevated levels of eosinophils in their blood.

A. Explain.

A 20-year-old woman has been diagnosed with IgA deficiency. She has been plagued with frequent bouts of bronchitis and sinus infections.

A. Why are these types of infections particularly prominent in persons with an IgA deficiency?
B. She has been told she needs to be aware that she could have a severe reaction if given unwashed blood transfusions. Explain.

Persons with impaired cellular immunity may not respond to the tuberculin test, even when infected with *Mycobacterium tuberculosis.*

A. Explain.

A 29-year-old woman presents to the clinic for her initial obstetric visit, about 10 weeks into her pregnancy.

A. This woman is in a monogamous relationship. Should an HIV test be a part of her initial blood work? Why?
B. The woman's HIV test comes back positive. What should be done to decrease the risk of her passing on HIV to her child?
C. The infant is born, and its initial antibody test is positive. Does this mean the infant is infected? How is the diagnosis of HIV infection in a child younger than 18 months made, and why is this different than the diagnosis for adults?

A 40-year-old man presents to the clinic very short of breath, and after X-ray and examination, he is diagnosed with *Pneumocystis carinii* pneumonia (PCP). His provider does an HIV test, which comes up positive. Upon further testing, the man's CD4+ cell count is found to be 100 cells/μL and his viral load is 250,000 copies/mL.

A. Why did the provider do an HIV test after the man was diagnosed with PCP?
B. Is there a way to prevent PCP?
C. What classification does this man fall into based on his CD4+ count and symptomatology, and why?

Visit the Porth: Essentials of Pathophysiology: Concepts of Altered Health States web site (http://thePoint.LWW.com/PorthEssentials) for links to chapter-related resources on the Internet, all-new exclusive animations, chapter review questions, and more!

REFERENCES

1. Abbas A. K., Lichtman A. H. (2003). *Cellular and molecular immunology* (5th ed., pp. 369–389, 453–464). Philadelphia: W. B. Saunders.
2. Abbas A. K. (2005). Diseases of immunity. In Kumar V., Abbas A. K., Fausto N. (Eds.), *Robbins and Cotran pathologic basis of disease* (7th ed., pp. 193–268). Philadelphia: Elsevier Saunders.
3. Kay A. B. (2001). Allergy and allergic disease (first of two parts). *New England Journal of Medicine* 344, 30–37.
4. Galli S. J. (1993). New concepts about the mast cell. *New England Journal of Medicine* 328, 257–265.
5. Benoist C., Mathias D. (2003). Mast cells in autoimmune disease. *Nature* 420, 875–878.
6. Warren J. S. (2005). Immunopathology. In Rubin E., Gorstein F., Rubin R., et al. (Eds.), *Rubin's pathology: Clinicopathologic foundations of medicine* (4th ed., pp. 118–163). Philadelphia: Lippincott Williams & Wilkins.
7. Kay A. B. (2001). Allergy and allergic disease (second of two parts). *New England Journal of Medicine* 344, 109–113.
8. Jackler R. K., Kaplan M. J. (2004). Ear, nose, and throat. In Tierney L. M., McPhee S. J., Papadakis M. A. (Eds.), *Current medical diagnosis and treatment* (43rd ed., p. 192). New York: Lange Medical Books/McGraw-Hill.
9. Rachelefsky G. S. (1999). National guidelines need to manage rhinitis and prevent complications. *Annals of Allergy, Asthma, and Immunology* 82, 296–305.
10. Sicherer S. H. (1999). Manifestations of food allergy: Evaluation and management. *American Family Physician* 57, 93–102.
11. Sampson H. A. (2002). Peanut allergy. *New England Journal of Medicine* 346, 1294–1299.
12. Sampson H. A. (1998). Fatal food-induced anaphylaxis. *Allergy* 53(Suppl. 46), 125–130.
13. Salvaggio J. E. (1995). The identification of hypersensitivity pneumonitis. *Hospital Practice* 30(5), 57–66.
14. Janeway C. A., Travers P., Walport M., et al. (2001). *Immunobiology* (5th ed., pp. 502–522). New York: Garland.
15. Kamradt T., Mitchison N. A. (2001). Advances in immunology: Tolerance and autoimmunity. *New England Journal of Medicine* 344, 655–664.
16. Davidson A., Diamond B. (2001). Autoimmune disease. *New England Journal of Medicine* 345, 340–350.
17. Ebringer A., Wilson C. (2000). HLA molecules, bacteria, and autoimmunity. *Journal of Molecular Microbiology* 49, 305–311.
18. Cutolo M., Sulli A., Seriolo S., et al. (1995). Estrogens, the immune response and autoimmunity. *Clinical and Experimental Rheumatology* 13, 217–226.
19. Wucherfennig K. W. (2001). Mechanisms of induction of autoimmunity by infectious agents. *Journal of Clinical Investigation* 108, 1097–1104.
20. Albert L. J., Inman R. D. (1999). Molecular mimicry and autoimmunity. *New England Journal of Medicine* 341, 2068–2074.
21. Llewelyn M., Cohen J. (2001). Superantigens antagonist peptides. *Critical Care* 5, 53–55.
22. Ronco C., Chiaramonte S., Remuzzi G. (2005). Transplantation tolerance. *Contributions to Nephrology* 146, 95–104.
23. Lin H., Kauffman M., McBride M. A., et al. (1998). Center-specific graft and patient survival rate. *Journal of the American Medical Association* 280, 1153–1160.
24. Saveigh M. H., Turka L. A. (1998). The role of T-cell costimulatory activation pathways in transplant rejection. *New England Journal of Medicine* 338, 1813–1821.
25. Vogelsang G. B., Lee L., Bensen-Kennedy D. M. (2003). Pathogenesis and treatment of graft-versus-host disease after bone marrow transplant. *Annual Review of Medicine* 54, 29–52.
26. Crawford J. M. (2005). The liver and biliary tract. In Kumar V., Abbas A. K., Fausto N. (Eds.), *Robbins and Cotran pathologic basis of disease* (7th ed., pp. 919–920). Philadelphia: Elsevier Saunders.
27. Shyur S., Hill H. R. (1996). Recent advances in the genetics of primary immunodeficiency syndromes. *Journal of Pediatrics* 129, 8–24.
28. Buckley R. H. (2000). Primary immunodeficiency diseases due to defects in lymphocytes. *New England Journal of Medicine* 343, 1313–1324.

29. Buckley R. (2004). T-, B-, and NK-cell systems. In Behrman R. E., Kliegman R. M., Jenson H. B. (Eds.), *Nelson textbook of pediatrics* (17th ed., pp. 683–700). Philadelphia: Elsevier Saunders.

30. Candotti F., Notarangelo L., Visconti R., et al. (2001). Molecular aspects of primary immunodeficiencies: Lessons from cytokine and other signaling pathways. *Journal of Clinical Investigation* 109, 1261–1269.

31. Sorensen R. U., Moore C. (2000). Antibody deficiency syndromes. *Pediatric Clinics of North America* 47, 1225–1252.

32. Ten R. M. (1998). Primary immunodeficiencies. *Mayo Clinic Proceedings* 73, 865–872.

33. Elder M. E. (2000). T-cell immunodeficiencies. *Pediatric Clinics of North America* 47, 1253–1274.

34. Buckley R. H. (2002). Primary cellular immunodeficiency. *Journal of Allergy and Clinical Immunology* 109, 747–757.

35. Quinn, T. C. (2003). World AIDS day: Reflections on the pandemic. *The Hopkins HIV Report* 15(1), 12–14.

36. Joint United Nations Programme on HIV/AIDS (UNAIDS). (2002). AIDS epidemic update, December 2002. [On-line]. Available: www.unaids.org/worldaidsday/2002/press/Epiupdate.html.

37. Electronic reference from the Centers for Disease Control and Prevention. (2002). [On-line]. Available: www.CDC.gov/stats. Retrieved June 23, 2003.

38. Colpin H. (1999). Prevention of HIV transmission through behavioral changes and sexual means. In Armstrong D., Cohen J. (Eds.), *Infectious diseases* (Section 5, Chapter 2, pp. 1–4). London: Harcourt.

39. Centers for Disease Control and Prevention. (2001). Update: U.S. Public Health Service guidelines for the management of occupational exposures to HBV, HCV, and HIV and recommendations for post exposure prophylaxis. *MMWR Morbidity and Mortality Weekly Report* 50(RR-11), 1–43.

40. Hirschel B. (1999). Primary HIV infection. In Armstrong D., Cohen J. (Eds.), *Infectious diseases* (Section 5, Chapter 8, pp. 1–4). London: Harcourt.

41. Centers for Disease Control and Prevention. (1992). 1993 Revised classification system for HIV infection and expanded surveillance case definition for AIDS among adolescents and adults. *MMWR Morbidity and Mortality Weekly Report* 41(RR-17), 1–23.

42. Centers for Disease Control and Prevention. (1999). Guidelines for national human immunodeficiency virus case surveillance, including monitoring for human immunodeficiency virus infection and acquired immunodeficiency syndrome. *MMWR Morbidity and Mortality Weekly Report* 48(RR-13), 1–28.

43. Rizzardi G. P., Pantaleo G. (1999). The immunopathogenesis of HIV-1 infection. In Armstrong D., Cohen J. (Eds.), *Infectious diseases* (Section 5, Chapter 6, pp. 1–12). London: Harcourt.

44. Clumeck N., Dewit S. (1999). Prevention of opportunistic infections in the presence of HIV infection. In Armstrong D., Cohen J. (Eds.), *Infectious diseases* (Section 5, Chapter 9). London: Harcourt.

45. Masur H. (1999). *Pneumocystis.* In Dolin R., Masur H., Saag M. S. (Eds.), *AIDS therapy* (pp. 291–306). Philadelphia: Churchill Livingstone.

46. Gordin F. (1999). *Mycobacterium tuberculosis.* In Dolin R., Masur H., Saag M. S. (Eds.), *AIDS therapy* (pp. 359–374). Philadelphia: Churchill Livingstone.

47. Wilcox C. M., Monkemuller K. E. (1999). Gastrointestinal disease. In Dolin R., Masur H., Saag M. S. (Eds.), *AIDS therapy* (pp. 752–765). Philadelphia: Churchill Livingstone.

48. Price R. W. (1999). Neurologic disease. In Dolin R., Masur H., Saag M. S. (Eds.), *AIDS therapy* (pp. 620–638). Philadelphia: Churchill Livingstone.

49. Hall C. D. (1999). JC virus neurologic infection. In Dolin R., Masur H., Saag M. S. (Eds.), *AIDS therapy* (pp. 565–572). Philadelphia: Churchill Livingstone.

50. Anteman K., Chang Y. (2000). Kaposi's sarcoma. *New England Journal of Medicine* 342, 1027–1038.

51. Bonnez W. (1999). Sexually transmitted human papillomavirus infection. In Dolin R., Masur H., Saag M. S. (Eds.), *AIDS therapy* (pp. 530–564). Philadelphia: Churchill Livingstone.

52. Von Ruenn J. H., Mulligan K. (1999). Wasting syndrome. In Dolin R., Masur H., Saag M. S. (Eds.), *AIDS therapy* (pp. 607–619). Philadelphia: Churchill Livingstone.

53. Mulligan K., Kotler D. P. (2003). Metabolic and morphologic complications in HIV disease: What's new? *The PRN Notebook* 8(1), 11–20.

54. Chen D., Misra A., Garg A. (2002). Lipodystrophy in human immunodeficiency virus-infected patients. *Journal of Endocrinology & Medicine* 87, 4845–4856.

55. Brun-Vezinet F., Simon F. (1999). Diagnostic tests for HIV infection. In Armstrong D., Cohen J. (Eds.), *Infectious diseases* (Section 5, Chapter 23, pp. 1–10). London: Harcourt.

56. Centers for Disease Control and Prevention. (2002). Notice to readers: Approval of a new rapid test for HIV antibody. *MMWR Morbidity and Mortality Weekly Report* 51(46), 1051–52.

57. Lucas G. M. (2000). Report from the 38th IDSA: Preserving the immune response to HIV, HAART, and long-term toxicities. *The Hopkins HIV Report* 12(5), 1, 6, 12.

58. U.S. Public Health Service. (2000). *Revised public health service recommendations for human immunodeficiency virus screening of pregnant women.* Washington, DC: Author.

59. Havens P. L. (1999). Pediatric AIDS. In Armstrong D., Cohen J. (Eds.), *Infectious diseases* (Section 5, Chapter 20). London: Harcourt.

60. Boyer P., Dillon M., Navaie M., et al. (1994). Factors predictive of maternal-fetal transmission of HIV-1. *Journal of the American Medical Association* 271, 1925–1930.

61. Connor E. M., Sperling R. S., Gelber R., et al. (1994). Reduction of maternal-infant transmission of human immunodeficiency virus type 1 with zidovudine treatment. *New England Journal of Medicine* 331, 1173–1180.

62. U.S. Public Health Service. (2002). U.S. Public Health Service task force recommendations for the use of antiretroviral drugs in pregnant HIV-1 infected women for maternal health and interventions to reduce perinatal transmission in the United States. *MMWR Morbidity and Mortality Weekly Report* 51(RR-18), 1–40.

63. Guay L., Muskoe P., Fleming T., et al. (1999). Intrapartum and neonatal single-dose nevirapine compared with zidovudine for prevention of mother-to-child transmission of HIV-1 in Kampala, Uganda: HIVNET 012 randomised trial. *Lancet* 354, 795–802.

C h a p t e r *16*

Control of Cardiovascular Function

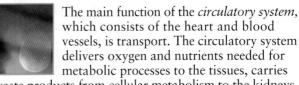 The main function of the *circulatory system*, which consists of the heart and blood vessels, is transport. The circulatory system delivers oxygen and nutrients needed for metabolic processes to the tissues, carries waste products from cellular metabolism to the kidneys and other excretory organs for elimination, and circulates electrolytes and hormones needed to regulate body function. This process of nutrient delivery is carried out with exquisite precision so that the blood flow to each tissue of the body is exactly matched to tissue need.

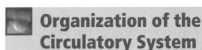 Organization of the Circulatory System

PULMONARY AND SYSTEMIC CIRCULATIONS

The circulatory system can be divided into two parts: the *pulmonary circulation,* which moves blood through the lungs and creates a link with the gas exchange function of the respiratory system, and the *systemic circulation,* which moves blood throughout all the other tissues of the body (Fig. 16-1). The blood that is in the heart and pulmonary circulation is sometimes referred to as the *central circulation* and that outside the central circulation as the *peripheral circulation.*

The pulmonary circulation consists of the right heart, the pulmonary arteries, the pulmonary capillaries, and the pulmonary veins. The large pulmonary vessels are unique in that the pulmonary artery is the only artery that carries deoxygenated venous blood and the pulmonary veins are

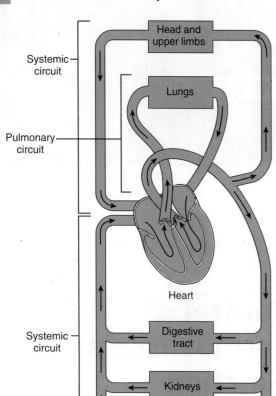

Systemic circuit

Pulmonary circuit

Systemic circuit

Head and upper limbs

Lungs

Heart

Digestive tract

Kidneys

Trunk and lower limbs

FIGURE 16-1 Systemic and pulmonary circulations. The right side of the heart pumps blood to the lungs, and the left side of the heart pumps blood to the systemic circulation.

the only veins that carry oxygenated arterial blood. The systemic circulation consists of the left heart, the aorta and its branches, the capillaries that supply the brain and peripheral tissues, and the systemic venous system and the vena cava. The veins from the lower portion of the body empty into the inferior vena cava and those from the head and upper extremities into the superior vena cava. Blood from both the inferior and superior venae cavae is emptied into the right heart.

Although the pulmonary and systemic systems function similarly, they have some important differences. The pulmonary circulation is the smaller of the two and functions with a much lower pressure. Because the pulmonary circulation is located in the chest near to the heart, it functions as a low-pressure system with a mean arterial pressure of approximately 12 mm Hg. The low pressure of the pulmonary circulation allows blood to move through the lungs more slowly, which is important for gas exchange. Because the systemic circulation must transport blood to distant parts of the body, often against the effects of gravity, it functions as a high-pressure system, with a mean arterial pressure of 90 to 100 mm Hg.

The heart, which propels the blood through the circulation, consists of two pumps in series—the right heart, which propels blood through the lungs, and the left heart, which propels blood to all other tissues of the body. The effective function of the circulatory system requires that the outputs of both sides of the heart pump the same amount of blood over time. If the output of the left heart were to fall below that of the right heart, blood would accumulate in the pulmonary circulation. Likewise, if the right heart were to pump less effectively than the left heart, blood would accumulate in the systemic circulation.

VOLUME AND PRESSURE DISTRIBUTION

Blood flow in the circulatory system depends on a blood volume that is sufficient to fill the blood vessels and a pressure difference across the system that provides the force that is needed to move blood forward. As shown in Figure 16-2, approximately 4% of the blood at any given time is in the left heart, 16% is in the arteries and arterioles, 4% is in the capillaries, 64% is in the venules and veins, and 4% is in the right heart. The arteries and arterioles, which have thick, elastic walls and function as a distribution system, have the highest pressure. The capillaries are small, thin-walled vessels that link the arterial and venous sides of the circulation. They serve as an exchange system where transfer of gases, nutrients, and wastes take place. Because of their small size and large surface area, the capillaries contain the smallest amount of blood. The venules and veins, which contain the largest amount of blood, are thin-walled, distensible vessels that function as a reservoir to collect blood from the capillaries and return it to the right heart.

Blood moves from the arterial to the venous side of the circulation along a pressure difference, moving from an area of higher pressure to one of lower pressure. The

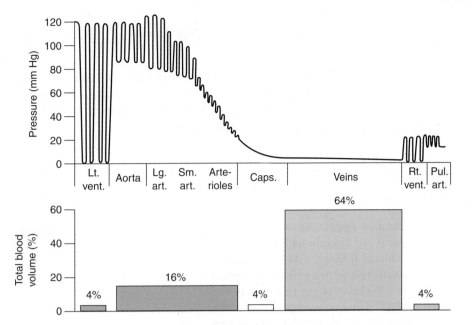

FIGURE 16-2 Pressure and volume distribution in the systemic circulation. The graphs show the inverse relation between internal pressure and volume in different portions of the circulatory system. (From Smith J. J., Kampine J. P. [1990]. *Circulatory physiology: The essentials* [3rd ed.]. Baltimore: Williams & Wilkins.)

pressure distribution in the different parts of the circulation is almost an inverse of the volume distribution (see Fig. 16-2). The pressure in the arterial side of the circulation, which contains only approximately one sixth of the blood volume, is much greater than the pressure on the venous side of the circulation, which contains approximately two thirds of the blood. This pressure and volume distribution is due in large part to the structure and relative elasticity of the arteries and veins. It is the pressure difference between the arterial and venous sides of the circulation (approximately 84 mm Hg) that provides the driving force for flow of blood in the systemic circulation. The pulmonary circulation has a similar arterial-venous pressure difference, albeit of a lesser magnitude, that facilitates blood flow.

Because the pulmonary and systemic circulations are connected and function as a closed system, blood can be shifted from one circulation to the other. In the pulmonary circulation, the blood volume (approximately 450 mL in the adult) can vary from as low as 50% of normal to as high as 200% of normal. An increase in intrathoracic pressure, such as occurs when exhaling against a closed glottis, impedes venous return to the right heart. This can produce a transient shift from the central to the systemic circulation of as much as 250 mL of blood. Body position also affects the distribution of blood volume. In the recumbent position, approximately 25% to 30% of the total blood volume is in the central circulation. On standing, this blood is rapidly displaced to the lower part of the body because of the forces of gravity. Because the volume of the systemic circulation is approximately seven times that of the pulmonary circulation, a shift of blood from one system to the other has a much greater effect in the pulmonary than in the systemic circulation.

In summary, the circulatory system functions as a transport system that circulates nutrients and other materials to the tissues and removes waste products. The circulatory system can be divided into two parts: the systemic and the pulmonary circulation. The heart pumps blood throughout the system, and the blood vessels serve as tubes through which blood flows. The arterial system carries blood from the heart to the tissues, and the veins carry it back to the heart. The cardiovascular system is a closed system with a right and left heart connected in series. The systemic circulation, which is served by the left heart, supplies all the tissues except the lungs, which are served by the right heart and the pulmonary circulation. Blood moves throughout the circulation along a pressure gradient, moving from the high-pressure arterial system to the low-pressure venous system. In the circulatory system, pressure is inversely related to volume. The pressure on the arterial side of the circulation, which contains only approximately one sixth of the blood volume, is much greater than the pressure on the venous side of the circulation, which contains approximately two thirds of the blood.

Principles of Blood Flow

The term *hemodynamics* describes the physics of blood flow as it relates to the circulatory system. Although slightly more complex, these principles are similar to the basic principles that apply to nonbiologic systems, such as household plumbing systems.

Understanding ➡ The Hemodynamics of Blood Flow

The term *hemodynamics* is used to describe factors such as (1) pressure and resistance, (2) vessel radius, (3) cross-sectional area and velocity of flow, and (4) laminar versus turbulent flow that affect blood flow through the blood vessels in the body.

1

Pressure, resistance, and flow. The flow (F) of fluid through a tube, such as blood through a blood vessel, is directly related to a pressure difference $(P_1 - P_2)$ between the two ends of the tube and inversely proportional to the resistance (R) that the fluid encounters as it moves through the tube.

The resistance to flow, in peripheral resistance units (PRU), is determined by the blood vicosity, vessel radius, and whether the vessels are aligned in series or in parallel. In vessels aligned in series, blood travels sequentially from one vessel to another such that the resistance becomes additive (*e.g.*, 2 + 2 + 2 = 6 PRU). In vessels aligned in parallel, such as capillaries, the blood is not confined to a single channel but can travel through each of several parallel channels such that the resistance becomes the reciprocal of the total resistance (*i.e.*, 1/R). As a result, there is no loss of pressure, and the total resistance (*e.g.*, 1/2 + 1/2 + 1/2 = 3/2 PRU) is less than the resistance of any of the channels (*i.e.*, 2) taken separately.

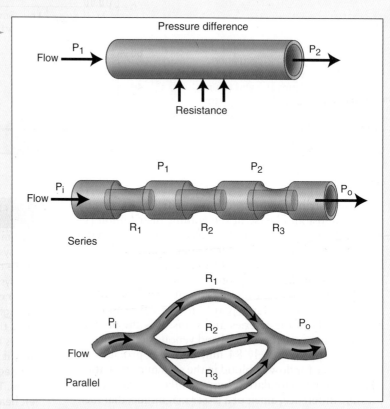

P_i, pressure in; P_o, pressure out.

2

Vessel radius. In addition to pressure and resistance, the rate of blood flow through a vessel is affected by the fourth power of its radius (the radius multiplied by itself four times). Thus, blood flow in vessel B with a radius of 2 mm will be 16 times greater than in vessel A with a radius of 1 mm.

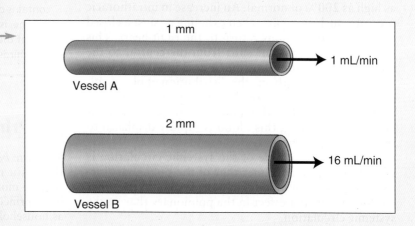

3

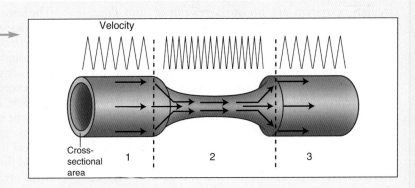

Cross-sectional area and velocity of flow. The velocity or rate of forward movement of the blood is affected by the cross-sectional area of a blood vessel. As the cross-sectional area of a vessel increases (sections 1 and 3), blood must flow laterally as well as forward to fill the increased area. As a result, the mean forward velocity decreases. In contrast, when the cross-sectional area is decreased (section 2), the lateral flow decreases and the mean forward velocity is increased.

4

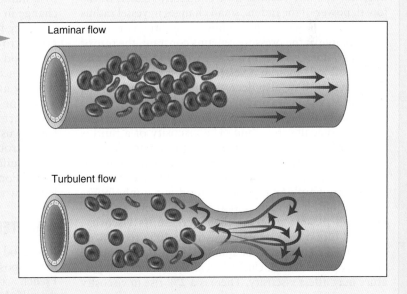

Laminar and turbulent flow. Blood flow is normally laminar, with platelets and blood cells remaining in the center or axis of the bloodstream. Laminar blood flow can be described as layered flow in which a thin layer of plasma adheres to the vessel wall, while the inner layers of blood cells and platelets shear against this motionless layer. This allows each layer to move at a slightly faster velocity, with the greatest velocity occurring in the central part of the bloodstream.

Turbulent blood flow is flow in which the blood elements do not remain confined to a definite lamina or layer, but develop vortices (*i.e.*, a whirlpool effect) that push blood cells and platelets against the wall of the vessel. More pressure is required to force a given flow of blood through the same vessel (or heart valve) when the flow is turbulent rather than laminar. Turbulence can result from an increase in velocity of flow, a decrease in vessel diameter, or low blood viscosity. Turbulence is usually accompanied by vibrations of the fluid and surrounding structures. Some of these vibrations in the cardiovascular system are in the audible frequency range and may be detected as murmurs or bruits.

PRESSURE, RESISTANCE, AND FLOW

The most important factors governing the function of the circulatory system are *pressure, resistance,* and *flow.* Blood flow (F), which is determined by the pressure difference (ΔP) between the two ends of a vessel or group of vessels and the resistance (R) that blood must overcome as it moves through the vessel or vessels, can be expressed by the equation F = P/R. In the circulatory system, blood flow is represented by the cardiac output (CO). Resistance is the opposition to flow caused by friction between the moving blood components and the stationary vessel wall. In the peripheral circulation, the collective resistance of all the vessels in that part of the circulation is referred to as the *peripheral vascular resistance* (PVR) or, sometimes, as the *systemic vascular resistance.*

A helpful equation for understanding factors that affect blood flow ($F = \Delta P \times \pi \times r^4 / 8n \times L \times$ viscosity) was derived by the French physician Poiseuille more than a century ago. It expands the previous equation, F = P/R, by relating flow to several determinants of resistance— vessel radius and blood viscosity. The length (L) of vessels does not usually change and 8n is a constant that does not change. Because flow is directly related to the fourth power of the radius, small changes in vessel radius can produce large changes in flow to an organ or tissue. For example, if the pressure remains constant, the rate of flow is 16 times greater in a vessel with a radius of 2 mm ($2 \times 2 \times 2 \times 2$) than in a vessel with a radius of 1 mm. Resistance to flow also decreases in vessels such as the capillaries, which are arranged in parallel.

Viscosity is the resistance to flow caused by the friction of molecules in a fluid. The viscosity of a fluid is largely related to its thickness. The more particles that are present in a solution, the greater the frictional forces that develop between the molecules. Unlike water that flows through plumbing pipes, blood is a nonhomogeneous liquid. It contains blood cells, platelets, fat globules, and plasma proteins that increase its viscosity. The red blood cells, which constitute 40% to 45% of the formed elements of the blood, largely determine the viscosity of the blood. Under special conditions, temperature may affect viscosity. There is a 2% rise in viscosity for each 1°C decrease in body temperature, a fact that helps explain the sluggish blood flow seen in persons with hypothermia.

Velocity is a distance measurement; it refers to the speed or linear movement with time (centimeters per second) with which blood flows through a vessel. *Flow* is a volume measurement (milliliters per second); it is determined by the cross-sectional area of a vessel and the velocity of flow. When the flow through a given segment of the circulatory system is constant—as it must be for continuous flow— the velocity is inversely proportional to the cross-sectional area of the vessel (*i.e.,* the smaller the cross-sectional area, the greater the velocity of flow). This phenomenon can be compared with cars moving from a two-lane to a single-lane section of a highway. To keep traffic moving at its original pace, cars would have to double their speed in the single-lane section of the highway. So it is with flow in the circulatory system.

The linear velocity of blood flow in the circulatory system varies widely from 30 to 35 cm/second in the aorta to 0.2 to 0.3 mm/second in the capillaries. This is because even though each individual capillary is very small, the total cross-sectional area of all the systemic capillaries greatly exceeds the cross-sectional area of other parts of the circulation. As a result of this large surface area, the slower movement of blood allows ample time for exchange of nutrients, gases, and metabolites between the tissues and the blood.

Blood flow normally is *laminar,* with the blood components arranged in layers so that the plasma is adjacent to the smooth, slippery endothelial surface of the blood vessel, and the blood elements, including the platelets, are in the center or *axis* of the bloodstream. This arrangement reduces friction by allowing the blood layers to slide smoothly over one another, with the axial layer having the most rapid rate of flow.

Under certain conditions, blood flow switches from laminar to turbulent flow. Turbulent flow can be caused by a number of factors, including high velocity of flow, change in vessel diameter, and low blood viscosity. The tendency for turbulence to occur increases in direct proportion to the velocity of flow. Low blood viscosity allows the blood to move faster and accounts for the transient occurrence of heart murmurs in some persons who are severely anemic. Turbulent flow may predispose to clot formation as platelets and other coagulation factors come in contact with the endothelial lining of the vessel. Turbulence is usually accompanied by vibrations of the blood and surrounding structures. Some of these vibrations are in the audible frequency and can be heard using a stethoscope. For example, a heart murmur results from turbulent flow through a diseased heart valve.

WALL TENSION, RADIUS, AND PRESSURE

In a blood vessel, *wall tension* is the force in the vessel wall that opposes the distending pressure inside the vessel. The French astronomer and mathematician Pierre de Laplace described the relationship between wall tension, pressure, and the radius of a vessel or sphere more than 200 years ago. This relationship, which has come to be known as the *Laplace law,* can be expressed by the equation, P = T/r, in which *T* is the wall tension, *P* is the intraluminal pressure, and *r* is the vessel radius (Fig. 16-3A). Accordingly, the internal pressure expands the vessel until it is exactly balanced by the tension in the vessel wall. The smaller the radius, the greater the pressure needed to balance the wall tension. The Laplace law can also be used to express the effect of the radius on wall tension ($T = P \times r$). This correlation can be compared with a partially inflated balloon (see Fig. 16-3B). Because the pressure is equal throughout, the tension in the part of the balloon with the smaller radius is less than the tension in the section

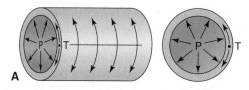

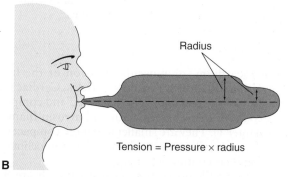

Tension = Pressure × radius

FIGURE 16-3 The Laplace law relates pressure (P), tension (T), and radius in a cylindrical blood vessel. (**A**) The pressure expanding the vessel is equal to the wall tension divided by the vessel radius. (**B**) Effect of the radius of a cylinder on tension. In a balloon, the tension in the wall is proportional to the radius because the pressure is the same everywhere inside the balloon. The tension is lower in the portion of the balloon with the smaller radius. (From Rhoades R. A., Tanner G. A. [1996]. *Medical physiology* [p. 627]. Boston: Little, Brown.)

with the larger radius. The same holds true for an arterial aneurysm in which the tension and risk of rupture increase as the aneurysm grows in size (see Chapter 17).

The Laplace law was later expanded to include wall thickness (T = P × r/wall thickness). Wall tension is inversely related to wall thickness, such that the thicker the vessel wall, the lower the tension, and vice versa. In hypertension, arterial vessel walls hypertrophy and become thicker, thereby reducing the tension and minimizing wall stress. The Laplace law can also be applied to the pressure required to maintain the patency of small blood vessels. Provided that the thickness of a vessel wall remains constant, it takes more pressure to overcome wall tension and keep a vessel open as its radius decreases in size. The critical closing pressure refers to the point at which vessels collapse so that blood can no longer flow through them. For example, in circulatory shock there is a decrease in blood volume and vessel radii, along with a drop in blood pressure. As a result, many of the small vessels collapse as blood pressure drops to the point where it can no longer overcome the wall tension. The collapse of peripheral veins often makes it difficult to insert venous lines that are needed for fluid and blood replacement.

DISTENTION AND COMPLIANCE

Compliance refers to the total quantity of blood that can be stored in a given portion of the circulation for each millimeter rise in pressure. Compliance reflects the

distensibility of the blood vessel. The distensibility of the aorta and large arteries allows them to accommodate the pulsatile output of the heart. The most distensible of all vessels are the veins, which can increase their volume with only slight changes in pressure, allowing them to function as a reservoir for storing large quantities of blood that can be returned to the circulation when it is needed. The compliance of a vein is approximately 24 times that of its corresponding artery, because it is 8 times as distensible and has a volume 3 times as great.

In summary, blood flow is controlled by many of the same mechanisms that control fluid flow in nonbiologic systems. It is influenced by vessel length, pressure differences, vessel radius, blood viscosity, cross-sectional area, and wall tension. The rate of flow is directly related to the pressure difference between the two ends of the vessel and the vessel radius and inversely related to vessel length and blood viscosity. The cross-sectional area of a vessel influences the velocity of flow; as the cross-sectional area decreases, the velocity is increased, and vice versa. Laminar blood flow is flow in which there is layering of blood components in the center of the bloodstream. This reduces frictional forces and prevents clotting factors from coming in contact with the vessel wall. In contrast to laminar flow, turbulent flow is disordered flow, in which the blood moves crosswise and lengthwise in blood vessels. The relation between wall tension, transmural pressure, and radius is described by the Laplace law, which states the pressure needed to overcome wall tension becomes greater as the radius decreases. Wall tension is also affected by wall thickness; it increases as the wall becomes thinner and decreases as the wall becomes thicker.

The Heart as a Pump

The heart is a four-chambered muscular pump approximately the size of a man's fist that beats an average of 70 times each minute, 24 hours each day, 365 days each year for a lifetime. In 1 day, this pump moves more than 1800 gallons of blood throughout the body, and the work performed by the heart over a lifetime would lift 30 tons to a height of 30,000 ft.

FUNCTIONAL ANATOMY OF THE HEART

The heart is located between the lungs in the mediastinal space of the intrathoracic cavity in a loose-fitting sac called the *pericardium*. It is suspended by the great vessels, with its broader side (*i.e.*, base) facing upward and its tip (*i.e.*, apex) pointing downward, forward, and to the left (Fig. 16-4).

The wall of the heart is composed of an outer epicardium, which lines the pericardial cavity; the myocardium or muscle layer; and the smooth endocardium, which lines the chambers of the heart (Fig. 16-5). A fibrous skeleton supports the valvular structures of the heart. The interatrial and interventricular septa divide the heart into a right and a left pump, each composed of two muscular chambers: a thin-walled atrium, which serves as a reservoir for blood coming into the heart, and a thick-walled ventricle, which pumps blood out of the heart. The increased thickness of the left ventricular wall results from the additional work this ventricle is required to perform.

Pericardium

The pericardium forms a fibrous covering around the heart, holding it in a fixed position in the thorax and providing physical protection and a barrier to infection. The pericardium consists of a tough outer fibrous layer and a thin inner serous layer. The outer fibrous layer is attached to the great vessels that enter and leave the heart, the sternum, and the diaphragm. The fibrous pericardium is highly resistant to distention; it prevents acute dilatation of the heart chambers and exerts a restraining effect on the left

ventricle. The inner serous layer consists of a visceral layer and a parietal layer. The visceral layer, also known as the visceral pericardium or *epicardium*, covers the entire heart and great vessels and then folds over to form the parietal layer that lines the fibrous pericardium (see Fig. 16-5). Between the visceral and parietal layers is the *pericardial cavity*, a potential space that contains 30 to 50 mL of serous fluid. This fluid acts as a lubricant to minimize friction as the heart contracts and relaxes.

Myocardium

The myocardium, or muscular portion of the heart, forms the walls of the atria and ventricles. Cardiac muscle cells, like skeletal muscle, are striated and composed of *sarcomeres* that contain actin and myosin filaments (see Chapter 1). They are smaller and more compact than skeletal muscle cells and contain many large mitochondria, reflecting their continuous energy needs.

The contractile properties of cardiac muscle are similar to those of skeletal muscle, except the contractions are involuntary and the duration of contraction is much longer. Unlike the orderly longitudinal arrangement of skeletal muscle fibers, cardiac muscle cells are arranged as an interconnecting latticework, with their fibers dividing, recombining, and then dividing again (Fig. 16-6A). The fibers are separated from neighboring cardiac muscle cells by dense structures called *intercalated disks*. The intercalated disks, which are unique to cardiac muscle, contain gap junctions that serve as low-resistance pathways for passage of ions and electrical impulses from one cardiac cell to another (see Fig. 16-6B). Thus, the myocardium behaves as a single unit, or *syncytium*, rather than as a group of isolated units, as does skeletal muscle. When one myocardial cell becomes excited, the impulse travels rapidly so the heart can beat as a unit.

As in skeletal muscle, cardiac muscle contraction involves actin and myosin filaments, which interact and slide along one another during muscle contraction. However, compared with skeletal muscle cells, cardiac muscle cells have less well-defined sarcoplasmic reticulum for storing calcium, and the distance from the cell membrane to the myofibrils is shorter. Because less calcium can be stored in the muscle cells, cardiac muscle relies more heavily than skeletal muscle on an influx of extracellular calcium ions for contraction. A number of important proteins regulate actin-myosin binding. These include tropomyosin and the troponin complex (see Chapter 1). The troponin complex consists of three subunits (troponin T, troponin I, and troponin C) that regulate calcium-mediated contraction in striated muscle. In clinical practice, the measurement of myocardial forms of troponin T and troponin I is used in the diagnosis of myocardial infarction (see Chapter 18).

Endocardium

The endocardium is a thin, three-layered membrane that lines the heart and covers the valves. The innermost layer consists of smooth endothelial cells supported by a thin

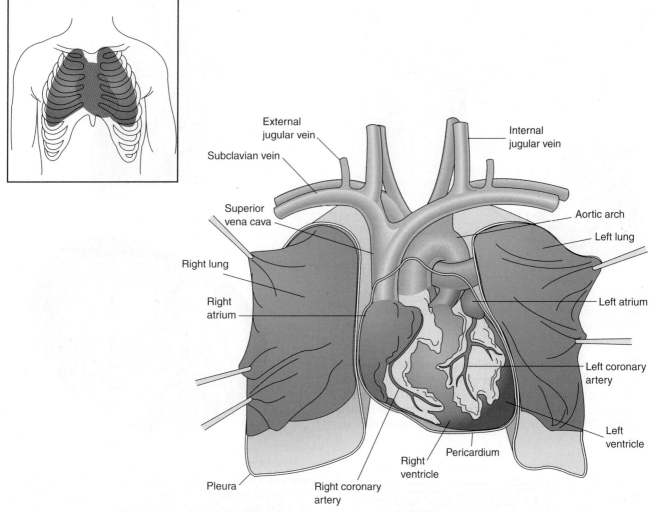

FIGURE 16-4 Anterior view of the heart and great vessels and their relationship to the lungs and skeletal structures of the chest cage (*upper left box*). Note that the lungs, which normally fold over part of the heart's anterior, have been pulled back.

layer of connective tissue. The endothelial lining of the endocardium is continuous with the lining of the blood vessels that enter and leave the heart. The middle layer consists of dense connective tissue with elastic fibers. The outer layer, composed of irregularly arranged connective tissue cells, contains blood vessels and branches of the conduction system and is continuous with the myocardium.

Heart Valves and Fibrous Skeleton

An important structural feature of the heart is its fibrous skeleton, which consists of four interconnecting valve rings and surrounding connective tissue (Fig. 16-7). The fibrous skeleton separates the atria and ventricles and forms a rigid support for attachment of the valves and insertion of the cardiac muscle (Fig. 16-7). The tops of the valve rings are attached to the muscle tissue of the atria, pulmonary trunks, aorta, and valve rings. The bottoms are attached to the ventricular walls. For the heart to function effectively, blood must flow in one direction only, moving

forward through the chambers of the right heart to the lungs and then through the chambers of the left heart to the systemic circulation (Fig. 16-8). This unidirectional flow is provided by the heart's two atrioventricular (*i.e.*, tricuspid and mitral) valves and two semilunar (*i.e.*, pulmonic and aortic) valves.

The atrioventricular (AV) valves control the flow of blood between the atria and the ventricles (Fig. 16-9). The thin edges of the AV valves form cusps, two on the left side of the heart (*i.e.*, bicuspid or *mitral valve*) and three on the right side (*i.e.*, *tricuspid valve*). The AV valves are supported by the papillary muscles, which project from the wall of the ventricles, and the chordae tendineae, which attach to the valve. Contraction of the papillary muscles at the onset of systole ensures closure by producing tension on the leaflets of the AV valves before the full force of ventricular contraction pushes against them. The chordae tendineae are cordlike structures that support the AV valves and prevent them from everting into the atria during systole.

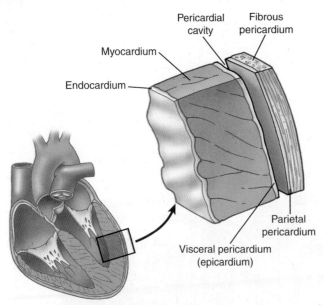

FIGURE 16-5 Layers of the heart, showing the visceral peri-cardium, pericardial cavity, parietal pericardium, fibrous peri-cardium, myocardium, and endocardium.

The *aortic* and *pulmonic* valves control the movement of blood out of the ventricles (Fig. 16-10). Because of their half-moon shape, they often are referred to as the *semilunar valves*. The semilunar valves have three teacup-shaped leaflets. These cuplike structures collect the *retrograde*, or

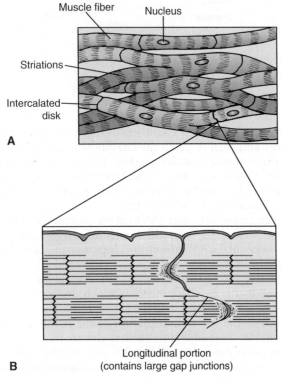

FIGURE 16-6 (**A**) Cardiac muscle fibers, showing the branching structure. (**B**) Area indicated where cell junctions lie in the intercalated disks.

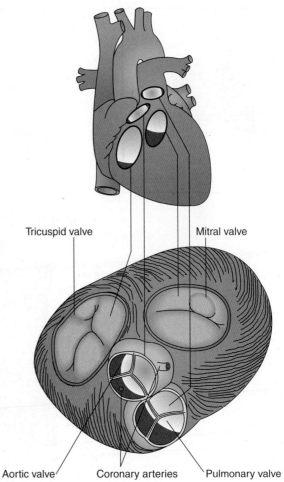

FIGURE 16-7 Fibrous skeleton of the heart, which forms the four interconnecting valve rings and support for attachment of the valves and insertion of cardiac muscle.

backward, flow of blood that occurs toward the end of systole, enhancing closure. For the development of a per-fect seal along the free edges of the semilunar valves, each valve cusp must have a triangular shape, which is facili-tated by a nodular thickening at the apex of each leaflet (see Fig. 16-10). The openings for the coronary arteries are located in the aorta just above the aortic valve.

There are no valves at the atrial sites (*i.e.,* venae cavae and pulmonary veins) where blood enters the heart. This means that excess blood is pushed back into the veins when the atria become distended. For example, the jugu-lar veins typically become prominent in severe right-sided heart failure, whereas normally they are flat or collapsed. Likewise, the pulmonary venous system becomes con-gested when outflow from the left atrium is impeded.

CARDIAC CONDUCTION SYSTEM

Heart muscle is unique among other muscles in that it is capable of generating and rapidly conducting its own action potentials (*i.e.,* electrical impulses). These action potentials result in excitation of muscle fibers throughout the myocardium. Impulse formation and conduction result

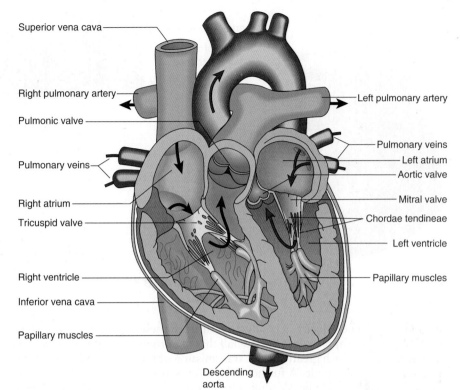

Superior vena cava

Right pulmonary artery

Pulmonic valve

Pulmonary veins

Right atrium

Tricuspid valve

Right ventricle

Inferior vena cava

Papillary muscles

Left pulmonary artery

Pulmonary veins

Left atrium

Aortic valve

Mitral valve

Chordae tendineae

Left ventricle

Papillary muscles

Descending aorta

FIGURE 16-8 Valvular structures of the heart. *Arrows* show the course of blood flow through the heart chambers. The atrioventricular valves are in an open position, and the semilunar valves are closed. There are no valves to control the flow of blood at the inflow channels (*i.e.,* vena cava and pulmonary veins) to the heart. (Modified from Smeltzer S. C., Bare B. G. [2004]. *Brunner and Suddarth's textbook of medical-surgical nursing* [10th ed., p. 648]. Philadelphia: Lippincott Williams & Wilkins.)

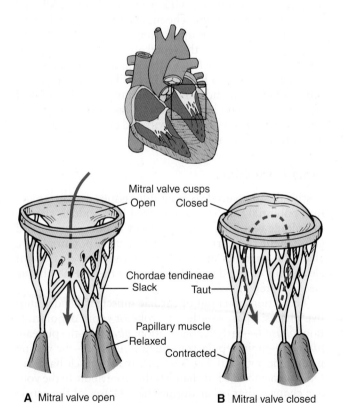

Mitral valve cusps
Open   Closed

Chordae tendineae
Slack   Taut

Papillary muscle
Relaxed   Contracted

A Mitral valve open

B Mitral valve closed

FIGURE 16-9 The mitral valve, showing the papillary muscles and chordae tendineae. (**A**) The open mitral valve with relaxed papillary muscles and slack chordae tendineae. (**B**) The closed mitral valve with contracted papillary muscles and taut chordae tendineae, which prevent the valve cusps from everting into the atrium.

in weak electrical currents that spread through the entire body. When electrodes are applied to various positions on the body and connected to an electrocardiograph machine, an electrocardiogram (ECG) can be recorded.

In certain areas of the heart, the myocardial cells have been modified to form the specialized cells of the conduction system (Fig. 16-11). Although most myocardial cells are capable of initiating and conducting impulses, it is this specialized conduction system that maintains the pumping efficiency of the heart. Specialized pacemaker cells generate impulses at a faster rate than do other types of heart tissue, and the conduction tissue transmits impulses at a faster rate than do other types of heart tissue. Because of these properties, the conduction system usually controls the rhythm of the heart.

The conduction system consists of the sinoatrial node (SA node), where the rhythmic impulse is generated; the internodal pathways, which conduct the impulse from the SA node to the atrioventricular (AV) node; the AV node, in which the impulse from the atria is delayed before passing to the ventricles; the AV bundle, which conducts the impulse from the atria to the ventricles; and the left and right bundles of the Purkinje system, which conduct the cardiac impulses to all parts of the ventricles.

The *SA node* has the fastest intrinsic rate of firing (60 to 100 beats per minute) and is normally the pacemaker of the heart. The heart essentially has two conduction systems: one that controls atrial activity and one that controls ventricular activity. The *AV node* connects the two conduction systems and provides one-way conduction between the atria and ventricles. Within the AV node, atrial fibers connect with very small junctional fibers of

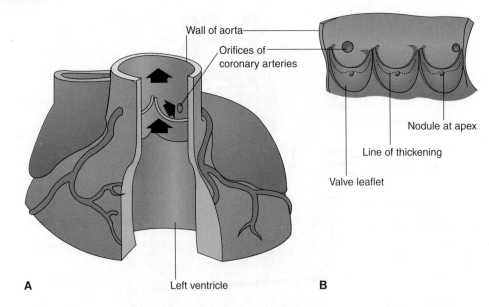

Wall of aorta

Orifices of
coronary arteries

Nodule at apex

Line of thickening

Valve leaflet

A

Left ventricle

B

FIGURE 16-10 Diagram of the aortic valve. (**A**) The position of the aortic valve at the base of the ascending aorta is indicated. (**B**) The appearance of the three leaflets of the aortic valve when the aorta is cut open and spread out, flat. (From Cormack D. H. [1987]. *Ham's histology* [9th ed.]. Philadelphia: J. B. Lippincott.)

the node itself. The velocity of conduction through these fibers is very slow (approximately one-half that of normal cardiac muscle), which greatly delays transmission of the impulse into the AV node. A further delay occurs as the impulse travels through the AV node into the transitional fibers and into the AV bundle, also called the *bundle of His.* This delay provides a mechanical advantage whereby the atria complete their ejection of blood before ventricular contraction begins. Under normal circumstances, the AV node provides the only connection between the two conduction systems. The atria and ventricles would beat independently of each other if the transmission of impulses through the AV node were blocked.

The Purkinje fibers lead from the AV node through the AV bundle into the ventricles, where they divide to form the *right* and *left bundle branches* that straddle the interventricular septum. The main trunk of the left bundle branch extends for approximately 1 to 2 cm before fanning out as it enters the septal area and divides further into two segments: the *left posterior* and *anterior fascicles.* The Purkinje system has very large fibers that allow for rapid conduction and almost simultaneous excitation of the entire right and left ventricles. This rapid rate of conduction is necessary for the swift and efficient ejection of blood from the heart.

Action Potentials

A stimulus delivered to excitable tissues evokes an action potential that is characterized by a sudden change in voltage resulting from transient depolarization and subsequent repolarization. These action potentials are electrical currents involving the movement or flow of electrically charged ions at the level of the cell membrane (see Chapter 1).

The action potential of cardiac muscle is divided into five phases: *phase 0*—the upstroke or rapid depolarization; *phase 1*—early repolarization; *phase 2*—the plateau; *phase 3*—rapid repolarization; and *phase 4*—the resting membrane potential (Fig. 16-12). Cardiac muscle has three types of membrane ion channels that contribute to the voltage changes that occur during these phases of the action potential. They are the (1) fast sodium channels, (2) slow calcium-sodium channels, and (3) potassium channels. During *phase 0* in atrial and ventricular muscle and in the Purkinje system, opening of the fast sodium channels for a few ten-thousandths of a second is responsible for the spikelike onset of the action potential. The point at

---

⚡ KEY CONCEPTS

Cardiac Conduction System

➤ The cardiac conduction system consists of the SA node, which functions as the pacemaker of the heart; the AV node, which connects the atrial and ventricular conduction systems; and the AV bundle and large Purkinje fibers, which provide for rapid depolarization of the ventricles.

➤ Cardiac action potentials are controlled by three types of ion channels—the fast sodium channels, which are responsible for the spikelike onset of the action potential; the slower calcium-sodium channels, which are responsible for the plateau; and the potassium channels, which are responsible for the repolarization phase and return of the membrane to the resting potential.

➤ There are two types of cardiac action potentials: the fast response, which occurs in atrial and ventricular muscle cells and the Purkinje conduction system and uses the fast sodium channels; and the slow response of the SA and AV nodes, which uses the slow calcium channels.

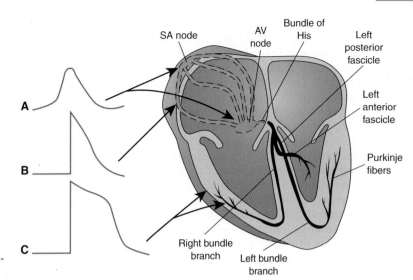

FIGURE 16-11 Conduction system of the heart and action potentials. (**A**) Action potential of sinoatrial (SA) and atrioventricular (AV) nodes; (**B**) atrial muscle action potential; (**C**) action potential of ventricular muscle and Purkinje fibers.

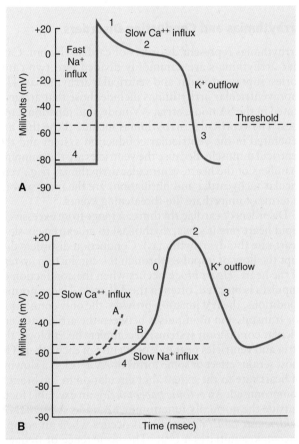

FIGURE 16-12 Changes in action potential recorded from a fast response in cardiac muscle cell (**A**) and from a slow response recorded in the sinoatrial and atrioventricular nodes (**B**). The phases of the action potential are identified by numbers: phase 4, resting membrane potential; phase 0, depolarization; phase 1, brief period of repolarization; phase 2, plateau; phase 3, repolarization. The slow response is characterized by a slow, spontaneous rise in the phase 4 membrane potential to threshold levels; it has a lesser amplitude and shorter duration than the fast response. Increased automaticity occurs when the rate of phase 4 depolarization is increased.

which the sodium gates open is called the *depolarization threshold*. When the cell has reached this threshold, a rapid influx of sodium ions to the interior of the membrane causes the membrane potential to shift from a resting membrane potential of approximately −90 mV to +20 mV.

Phase 1 occurs at the peak of the action potential and signifies inactivation of the fast sodium channels with an abrupt decrease in sodium permeability. *Phase 2* represents the plateau of the action potential. It is caused primarily by the slower opening of the calcium-sodium channels, which lasts for a few tenths of a second. Calcium ions entering the muscle during this phase of the action potential play a key role in the contractile process of the cardiac muscle fibers. These unique features of the phase 2 plateau cause the action potential of cardiac muscle to last 3 to 15 times longer than that of skeletal muscle and cause a corresponding increased period of contraction.

Phase 3 reflects final rapid repolarization and begins with the downslope of the action potential. During the phase 3 repolarization period, the slow channels close and the influx of calcium and sodium ceases. There is a sharp rise in potassium permeability, contributing to the rapid outward movement of potassium during this phase and facilitating the reestablishment of the resting membrane potential (−90 mV). At the conclusion of phase 3, distribution of sodium and potassium returns to the normal resting state. *Phase 4* is the resting membrane potential. During phase 4, the sodium-potassium pump is activated, transporting sodium out of the cell and moving potassium back into the cell.

There are two main types of action potentials in the heart—the slow response and the fast response. The *slow response*, which is initiated by the slow calcium-sodium channels, is found in the SA node, which is the natural pacemaker of the heart, and the conduction fibers of the AV node (see Fig. 16-12). The *fast response*, which is characterized by the opening of the fast sodium channels, occurs in the normal myocardial cells of the atria, the ventricles, and the Purkinje fibers. The fast-response cardiac cells do not normally initiate cardiac action potentials.

Instead, these impulses originate in the specialized slow-response cells of the SA node and are conducted to the fast-response myocardial cells in the atria and ventricles, where they effect a change in membrane potential to the threshold level. On reaching threshold, the voltage-dependent sodium channels open to initiate the rapid upstroke of the phase 1 action potential. The amplitude and the rate of rise of phase 1 are important to the conduction velocity of the fast response.

The hallmark of the pacemaker cells in the SA and AV nodes is a spontaneous phase 4 depolarization. The membrane permeability of these cells allows a slow inward leak of current to occur through the slow channels during phase 4. This leak continues until the threshold for firing is reached, at which point the cell spontaneously depolarizes. The rate of pacemaker cell discharge varies with the resting membrane potential and the slope of phase 4 depolarization (see Fig. 16-12). Catecholamines (*i.e.,* epinephrine and norepinephrine) increase the heart rate by increasing the slope or rate of phase 4 depolarization. Acetylcholine, which is released during vagal stimulation of the heart, slows the heart rate by decreasing the slope of phase 4.

Absolute and Relative Refractory Periods

The pumping action of the heart requires alternating contraction and relaxation. There is a period in the action potential curve during which no stimuli can generate another action potential (Fig. 16-13). This period, which is known as the *absolute refractory period,* includes phases 0, 1, 2, and part of phase 3. During this time, the cell cannot depolarize again under any circumstances. In skeletal muscle, the refractory period is very short compared with the duration of contraction, such that a second contraction can be initiated before the first is over, resulting in a summated tetanized contraction. In cardiac muscle, the absolute refractory period is almost as long as the contraction and a second contraction cannot be stimulated until the first is over. The longer length of the absolute refractory period of cardiac muscle is important in maintaining the alternating contraction and relaxation that is essential to the pumping action of the heart and for the prevention of fatal arrhythmias. When repolarization has returned the membrane potential to below the threshold potential, but not to the resting membrane potential, the cell is capable of responding to a greater-than-normal stimulus. This condition is referred to as the *relative refractory period.* After the relative refractory period there is a short period, called the *supernormal excitatory period,* during which a weak stimulus can evoke a response. It is during this period that many cardiac arrhythmias develop.

Arrhythmias and Conduction Disorders

Arrhythmias represent disorders of cardiac rhythm. Cardiac arrhythmias are commonly divided into two categories: supraventricular and ventricular arrhythmias. The supraventricular arrhythmias include those that are generated in the SA node, atria, AV node, and junctional tissues. The ventricular arrhythmias include those that are generated in the ventricular conduction system and the ventricular muscle. Because the ventricles are the pumping chambers of the heart, ventricular arrhythmias (*e.g.,* ventricular tachycardia and fibrillation) are the most serious in terms of immediate life-threatening events.

Disorders of cardiac rhythm can range from excessively rapid heart rate (tachyarrhythmias) to an extremely slow heart rate (bradyarrhythmias). Conduction disorders disrupt the flow of impulses through the conduction system of the heart. *Heart block* occurs when the conduction of impulses is blocked, often in the AV node. Under normal conditions, the AV junction provides the only connection for transmission of impulses between the atrial and ventricular conduction systems; in complete heart block, the atria and ventricles beat independently of each other. The most serious effect of some forms of AV block is a slowing of heart rate to the extent that circulation to the brain is compromised. An *ectopic pacemaker* is an excitable focus outside the normally functioning SA node. A *premature ventricular contraction* (PVC) occurs when an ectopic pacemaker initiates a beat. The occurrence of frequent PVCs in the diseased heart predisposes one to the development of other, more serious arrhythmias, including ventricular tachycardia and ventricular fibrillation.

Fibrillation is the result of disorganized current flow within the atria (atrial fibrillation) or ventricle (ventricular fibrillation). Fibrillation interrupts the normal contraction of the atria or ventricles. In ventricular fibrillation, the ventricle quivers but does not contract. When the ventricle does not contract, there is no cardiac output,

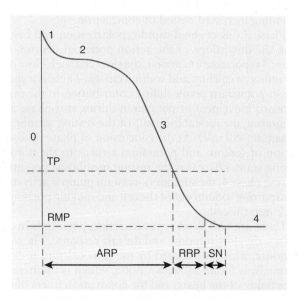

FIGURE 16-13 Diagram of an action potential of a ventricular muscle cell, showing the threshold potential (TP), resting membrane potential (RMP), absolute refractory period (ARP), relative refractory period (RRP), and supernormal (SN) period.

and there are no palpable or audible pulses. Ventricular fibrillation is a fatal event unless treated with immediate defibrillation.

Electrocardiography

The ECG is a recording of the electrical activity of the heart. The electrical currents generated by the heart spread through the body to the skin, where they can be sensed by appropriately placed electrodes, amplified, and viewed on an oscilloscope or chart recorder. The deflection points of an ECG are designated by the letters P, Q, R, S, and T. Figure 16-14 depicts the electrical activity of the conduction system on an ECG tracing. The P wave represents the SA node and atrial depolarization; the QRS complex (*i.e.,* beginning of the Q wave to the end of the S wave) depicts ventricular depolarization; and the T wave portrays ventricular repolarization. The isoelectric line between the P wave and the Q wave represents depolarization of the AV node, bundle branches, and Purkinje system (see Fig. 16-14). Atrial repolarization occurs during ventricular depolarization and is hidden in the QRS complex.

The horizontal axis of the ECG measures time in seconds, and the vertical axis measures the amplitude of the impulse in millivolts (mV). Each heavy vertical line represents 0.2 second, and each thin line represents 0.04 second (see Fig. 16-14). The widths of ECG complexes are commonly referred to in terms of duration of time. On the vertical axis, each heavy horizontal line represents 0.5 mV. The connections of the ECG are arranged such that an

upright deflection indicates a positive potential and a downward deflection indicates a negative potential.

The ECG records the potential difference in charge between two electrodes as the depolarization and repolarization waves move through the heart and are conducted to the skin surface. The shape of the recorder tracing is determined by the direction in which the impulse spreads through the heart muscle in relation to electrode placement. A depolarization wave that moves toward the recording electrode registers as a positive, or upward, deflection. Conversely, if the impulse moves away from the recording electrode, the deflection is downward, or negative. When there is no flow of charge between electrodes, the potential is zero, and a straight line is recorded at the baseline of the chart.

Conventionally, 12 leads are recorded for a diagnostic ECG, each providing a unique view of the electrical forces of the heart from a different position on the body's surface. Six limb leads view the electrical forces as they pass through the heart on the frontal or vertical plane. The electrodes for the limb leads are attached to the four extremities or representative areas on the body near the shoulders and lower chest or abdomen. Chest electrodes provide a view of the electrical forces as they pass through the heart on the horizontal plane. They are moved to different positions on the chest, including the right and left sternal borders and the left anterior surface. The right lower extremity lead is used as a ground electrode. When indicated, additional electrodes may be applied to other areas of the body, such as the back or right anterior chest.

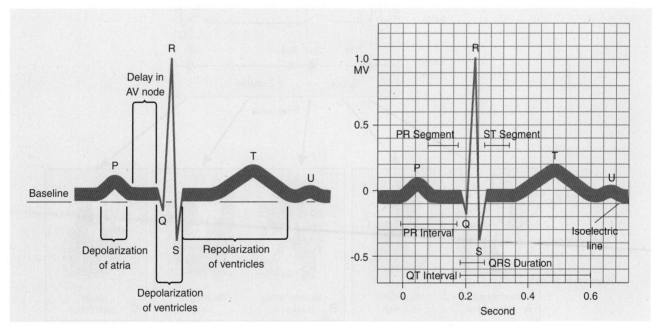

FIGURE 16-14 Diagram of the electrocardiogram (lead II) and representative depolarization and repolarization of the atria and ventricles. The P wave represents atrial depolarization, the QRS complex ventricular depolarization, and the T wave ventricular repolarization. Atrial repolarization occurs during ventricular depolarization and is hidden under the QRS complex.

CARDIAC CYCLE

The term *cardiac cycle* is used to describe the rhythmic pumping action of the heart. The cardiac cycle is divided into two parts: *systole*, the period during which the ventricles are contracting, and *diastole*, the period during which the ventricles are relaxed and filling with blood. Simultaneous changes occur in atrial pressure, ventricular pressure, aortic or pulmonary artery pressure, ventricular volume, the ECG, and heart sounds during the cardiac cycle (Fig. 16-15).

Ventricular Systole and Diastole

Ventricular systole is divided into two periods: the isovolumetric contraction period and the ejection period.

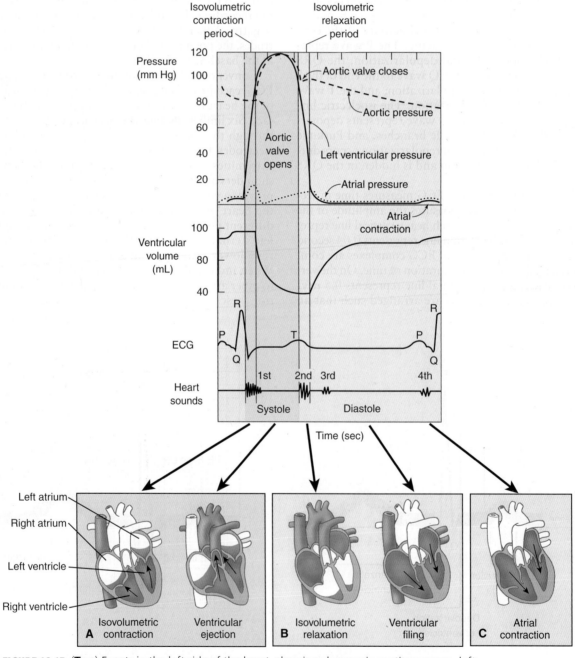

FIGURE 16-15 (Top) Events in the left side of the heart, showing changes in aortic pressure, left ventricular pressure, atrial pressure, left ventricular volume, the electrocardiogram (ECG), and heart sounds during the cardiac cycle. **(Bottom)** Position of the atrioventricular and semilunar valves during **(A)** isovolumetric contraction and ventricular ejection, **(B)** isovolumetric relaxation and ventricular filling, and **(C)** atrial contraction.

The *isovolumetric contraction period,* which begins with the closure of the AV valves and occurrence of the first heart sound, heralds the onset of systole. Immediately after closure of the AV valves, there is an additional 0.02 to 0.03 second during which the semilunar outlet (pulmonic and aortic) valves remain closed. During this period, the ventricular volume remains the same while the ventricles contract, producing an abrupt increase in pressure. The ventricles continue to contract until left ventricular pressure is slightly higher than aortic pressure, and right ventricular pressure is higher than pulmonary artery pressure. At this point, the semilunar valves open, signaling the onset of the *ejection period.* Approximately 60% of the stroke volume is ejected during the first quarter of systole, and the remaining 40% is ejected during the next two quarters of systole. Little blood is ejected from the heart during the last quarter of systole, although the ventricle remains contracted. At the end of systole, the ventricles relax, causing a precipitous fall in intraventricular pressures. As this occurs, blood from the large arteries flows back toward the ventricles, causing the aortic and pulmonic valves to snap shut—an event that is marked by the second heart sound.

The aortic pressure reflects changes in the ejection of blood from the left ventricle. There is a rise in pressure and stretching of the elastic fibers in the aorta as blood is ejected into the aorta at the onset of the ejection period. The aortic pressure continues to rise and then begins to fall during the last quarter of systole as blood flows out of the aorta into the peripheral vessels. The incisura, or notch, in the aortic pressure tracing represents closure of the aortic valve. The aorta is highly elastic and as such stretches during systole to accommodate the blood that is being ejected from the left heart during systole. During diastole, recoil of the elastic fibers in the aorta serves to maintain the arterial pressure.

Diastole is marked by ventricular relaxation and filling. After closure of the semilunar valves, the ventricles continue to relax for another 0.03 to 0.06 second. During this time, which is called the *isovolumetric relaxation period,* ventricular volume remains the same but ventricular pressure drops until it becomes less than atrial pressure. As this happens, the AV valves open, and the blood that has been accumulating in the atria during systole flows into the ventricles. Most of ventricular filling occurs during the first third of diastole, which is called the *rapid filling period.* During the middle third of diastole, inflow into the ventricles is almost at a standstill. The last third of diastole is marked by atrial contraction, which gives an additional thrust to ventricular filling. When audible, the third heart sound is heard during the rapid filling period of diastole as blood flows into a distended or noncompliant ventricle. A fourth heart sound, when present, occurs during the last third of diastole as the atria contract.

During diastole, the ventricles increase their volume to approximately 120 mL (*i.e.,* the *end-diastolic volume*), and at the end of systole, approximately 50 mL of blood (*i.e.,* the *end-systolic volume*) remains in the ventricles.

The difference between the end-diastolic and end-systolic volumes (approximately 70 mL) is called the *stroke volume.* The *ejection fraction,* which is the stroke volume divided by the end-diastolic volume, represents the fraction or percentage of the diastolic volume that is ejected from the heart during systole.

Atrial Filling and Contraction

Because there are no valves between the junctions of the central veins (*i.e.,* venae cavae and pulmonary veins) and the atria, atrial filling occurs during both systole and diastole. During normal quiet breathing, right atrial pressure usually varies between −2 and +2 mm Hg. It is this low atrial pressure that maintains the movement of blood from the systemic veins into the right atrium and from the pulmonary veins into the left atrium.

Right atrial pressure is regulated by a balance between the ability of the right ventricle to move blood out of the right heart and the pressures that move blood from the venous circulation into the right atrium (venous return). When the heart pumps strongly, right atrial pressure is decreased and atrial filling is enhanced. Right atrial pressure is also affected by changes in intrathoracic pressure. It is decreased during inspiration when intrathoracic pressure becomes more negative, and it is increased during coughing or forced expiration when intrathoracic pressure becomes more positive. Venous return is a reflection of the amount of blood in the systemic circulation that is available for return to the right heart and the forces that move blood back to the right heart. Venous return is increased when the blood volume is expanded or when right atrial pressure falls and is decreased in hypovolemic shock or when right atrial pressure rises.

Although the main function of the atria is to store blood as it enters the heart, these chambers also act as pumps that aid in ventricular filling. Atrial contraction occurs during the last third of diastole. Atrial contraction becomes more important during periods of increased activity when the diastolic filling time is decreased because of an increase in heart rate or when heart disease impairs ventricular filling. In these two situations, the cardiac output would fall drastically were it not for the action of the atria. It has been estimated that atrial contraction can contribute as much as 30% to cardiac reserve during periods of increased need, while having little or no effect on cardiac output during rest.

REGULATION OF CARDIAC PERFORMANCE

The efficiency and work of the heart as a pump often is measured in terms of *cardiac output* or the amount of blood the heart pumps each minute. The cardiac output (CO) is the product of the *stroke volume* (SV) and the *heart rate* (HR) and can be expressed by the equation: $CO = SV \times HR$. The cardiac output varies with body size and the metabolic needs of the tissues. It increases with physical activity and decreases during rest and sleep. The average cardiac output in normal adults ranges from 3.5 to 8.0 L/minute. In the highly trained athlete, this value can increase to levels as high as 32 L/minute during maximum exercise.

The *cardiac reserve* refers to the maximum percentage of increase in cardiac output that can be achieved above the normal resting level. The normal young adult has a cardiac reserve of approximately 300% to 400%. The heart's ability to increase its output according to body needs mainly depends on four factors: the *preload*, or ventricular filling; the *afterload*, or resistance to ejection of blood from the heart; *cardiac contractility*; and the *heart rate*. Cardiac performance is influenced by the work demands of the heart and the ability of the coronary circulation to meet its metabolic needs.

Preload

The preload represents the volume work of the heart. It is called the *preload* because it is the work imposed on the heart before the contraction begins. Preload represents the amount of blood that the heart must pump with each beat and is largely determined by the venous return to the heart and the accompanying stretch of the muscle fibers.

The increased force of contraction that accompanies an increase in ventricular end-diastolic volume is referred to as the *Frank-Starling mechanism* or Starling law of the heart (Fig. 16-16). The anatomic arrangement of the actin and myosin filaments in the myocardial muscle fibers is such that the tension or force of contraction is greatest when the muscle fibers are stretched just before the heart begins to contract. The maximum force of contraction and cardiac output is achieved when venous return produces an increase in left ventricular end-diastolic filling (*i.e.*, preload) such that the muscle fibers are stretched about two and one-half times their normal resting length. When the muscle fibers are stretched to this degree, there is optimal overlap of the actin and myosin filaments needed for maximal contraction.

The Frank-Starling mechanism allows the heart to adjust its pumping ability to accommodate various levels of venous return. Cardiac output is less when decreased filling causes excessive overlap of the actin and myosin filaments or when excessive filling causes the filaments to be pulled too far apart.

Afterload

The afterload is the pressure or tension work of the heart; it is the pressure that the heart must generate to move blood into the aorta. It is called the *afterload* because it is the work presented to the heart after the contraction has commenced. The systemic arterial blood pressure is the main source of afterload work on the left heart and the pulmonary arterial pressure is the main source of afterload work for the right heart. The afterload work of the left ventricle is also increased with narrowing (*i.e.*, stenosis) of the aortic valve. For example, in the late stages of aortic stenosis, the left ventricle may need to generate systolic pressures as great as 300 mm Hg to move blood through the diseased valve.

Cardiac Contractility

Cardiac contractility refers to the ability of the heart to change its force of contraction without changing its resting (*i.e.*, diastolic) length. The contractile state of the myocardial muscle is determined by biochemical and biophysical properties that govern the actin and myosin interactions in the myocardial cells. It is strongly influenced by the number of calcium ions that are available to participate in the contractile process.

An *inotropic* influence is one that modifies the contractile state of the myocardium independent of the Frank-Starling mechanism. For instance, sympathetic stimulation produces a positive inotropic effect by increasing the calcium that is available for interaction between the actin and myosin filaments. Hypoxia exerts a negative inotropic effect by interfering with the generation of adenosine triphosphate (ATP), which is needed for muscle contraction.

Heart Rate

The heart rate influences cardiac output and the work of the heart by determining the frequency with which the ventricle contracts and blood is ejected from the heart. Heart rate also determines the time spent in diastolic filling. Although systole and the ejection period remain fairly

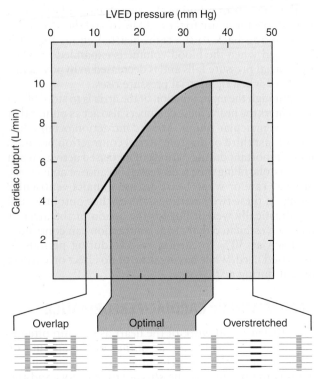

FIGURE 16-16 Starling ventricular function curve in normal heart. An increase in left ventricular end-diastolic (LVED) pressure produces an increase in cardiac output by means of the Frank-Starling mechanism. The maximum (optimal) force of contraction and increased stroke volume are achieved when diastolic filling causes the muscle fibers to be stretched about 2.5 times their resting length.

constant across heart rates, the time spent in diastole and filling of the ventricles becomes shorter as the heart rate increases. This leads to a decrease in stroke volume and, at high heart rates, may produce a decrease in cardiac output. One of the dangers of ventricular tachycardia is a reduction in cardiac output because the heart does not have time to fill adequately.

In summary, the heart is a four-chambered muscular pump that lies in the pericardial sac within the mediastinal space of the intrathoracic cavity. The wall of the heart is composed of an outer epicardium, which lines the pericardial cavity; a fibrous skeleton; the myocardium, or muscle layer; and the smooth endocardium, which lines the chambers of the heart. The four heart valves control the direction of blood flow.

The specialized cells of the heart's conduction system control the rhythmic contraction and relaxation of the heart. The SA node has the fastest inherent rate of impulse generation and acts as the pacemaker of the heart. Impulses from the SA node travel through the atria to the AV node and then to the AV bundle and the ventricular Purkinje system. The AV node provides the only connection between the atrial and ventricular conduction systems. The action potential of cardiac muscle is controlled by the (1) fast sodium channels, (2) slow calcium-sodium channels, and (3) potassium channels. Opening of the fast sodium channels is responsible for the rapid spikelike onset of the ventricular action potential; the slower-opening calcium-sodium channels for the plateau of the action potential; and potassium channels for repolarization and return to the resting membrane potential. The absolute refractory period, which represents the time during which a normal cardiac impulse cannot re-excite an already excited area of cardiac muscle, is important in preventing disorders of cardiac rhythm that would disrupt the normal pumping ability of the heart. Disorders of the cardiac conduction system include arrhythmias and conduction defects. Ventricular arrhythmias are generally more serious than atrial arrhythmias because they afford the potential for disrupting the pumping ability of the heart.

The cardiac cycle describes the pumping action of the heart. It is divided into two parts: systole, during which the ventricles contract and blood is ejected from the heart, and diastole, during which the ventricles are relaxed and blood is filling the heart. The stroke volume (approximately 70 mL) represents the difference between the end-diastolic volume (approximately 120 mL) and the end-systolic volume (approximately 50 mL). Atrial contraction occurs during the last third of diastole. Although the main function of the atria is to store blood as it enters the heart, atrial contraction acts to increase cardiac output during periods of increased activity when the filling time is reduced or in disease conditions in which ventricular filling is impaired.

The heart's ability to increase its output according to body needs depends on the preload, or filling of the ventricles (*i.e.*, end-diastolic volume); the afterload, or resistance to ejection of blood from the heart; cardiac contractility, which is determined by the interaction of the actin and myosin filaments of cardiac muscle fibers; and the heart rate, which determines the frequency with which blood is ejected from the heart. The maximum force of cardiac contraction occurs when an increase in preload stretches muscle fibers of the heart to approximately two and one-half times their resting length (*i.e.*, Frank-Starling mechanism).

Blood Vessels and the Peripheral Circulation

The vascular system functions in the delivery of oxygen and nutrients and removal of wastes from the tissues. It consists of arteries and arterioles, the capillaries, and the venules and veins. Blood vessels are dynamic structures that constrict and relax to adjust blood pressure and flow to meet the varying needs of the many different tissue types and organ systems. Structures such as the heart, brain, liver, and kidneys require a large and continuous flow to carry out their vital functions. In other tissues, such as the skin and skeletal muscle, the need for blood flow varies with the level of function. For example, there is a need for increased blood flow to the skin during fever and for increased skeletal muscle blood flow during exercise.

BLOOD VESSELS

All blood vessels, except the capillaries, have walls composed of three layers, or coats, called *tunicae* (Fig. 16-17). The *tunica intima*, or inner layer, consists of a thin layer of *endothelial cells* that lie adjacent to the blood, a thin layer of subendothelial connective tissue, and an *internal elastic membrane* that joins with the media. The endothelial cells of the intima layer perform a number of functions, including maintenance of a nonthrombogenic surface for blood flow and modulation of vascular reactivity through secretion of vasoconstrictor and vasodilator substances (to be discussed). The *tunica media*, or middle layer, is largely a smooth muscle layer that constricts to regulate and control the diameter of the vessel. The *tunica externa* or *tunica adventitia* is the outermost covering of the vessel. It is usually separated from the tunica media by an inconspicuous *external elastic membrane*. The tunica adventitia is composed of fibrous and connective tissues that support the vessel. It contains blood vessels (vasa vasorum) that supply nutrients to the outer part of the vessel and branches of the sympathetic nervous system that assist in the control of vessel tone. The layers of the different types of blood vessels vary with vessel function. For example, the tunica adventitia of muscle arteries is relatively

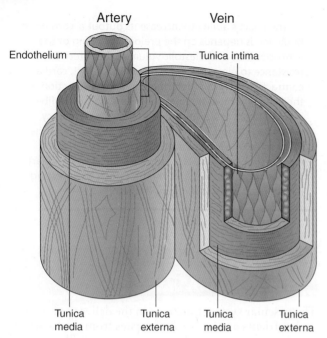

FIGURE 16-17 Medium-sized artery and vein, showing the relative thicknesses of the three layers.

thick and is separated from the tunica media by a recognizable external elastic membrane.

Although vascular smooth muscle contains actin and myosin filaments, these contractile filaments are not arranged in striations as they are in skeletal and cardiac muscle. The smooth muscle fibers are instead linked together in a strong, cable-like system that generates a circular pull as it contracts. In addition, smooth muscle has less well-developed sarcoplasmic reticulum for storing intracellular calcium than do skeletal and cardiac muscle, and it has very few fast sodium channels. Instead, depolarization of smooth muscle relies largely on extracellular calcium, which enters through calcium channels in the muscle membrane. These channels respond to changes in membrane potential or receptor-activated responses to chemical mediators such as norepinephrine. Sympathetic nervous system control of vascular smooth muscle tone occurs by way of receptor-activated channels. In general, α-adrenergic receptors are excitatory and produce vasoconstriction, and β-adrenergic receptors are inhibitory and produce vasodilatation. Calcium-channel–blocking drugs cause vasodilation by blocking calcium entry through the calcium channels.

ARTERIAL SYSTEM

The arterial system consists of the large and medium-sized arteries and the arterioles. Arteries are thick-walled vessels with large amounts of elastic fibers. The elasticity of these vessels allows them to stretch during cardiac systole, when the heart contracts and blood is ejected into the circulation, and to recoil during diastole, when the heart relaxes. The arterioles, which are predominantly smooth muscle, serve as resistance vessels for the circu-

latory system. They act as control valves through which blood is released as it moves into the capillaries. Changes in the activity of sympathetic fibers that innervate these vessels cause them to constrict or relax as needed to maintain blood pressure. The regulation of arterial blood pressure is discussed further in Chapter 17.

Aortic Pressure Pulse

The delivery of blood to the tissues of the body depends on pressure pulsations or waves of pressure that are generated by the intermittent ejection of blood from the left ventricle into the distensible aorta and large arteries of the arterial system. The aortic pressure pulse represents the energy that is transmitted from molecule to molecule along the length of the vessel (Fig. 16-18). In the aorta, this pressure pulse is transmitted at a velocity of 4 to 6 m/second, which is approximately 20 times faster than the flow of blood. Therefore, the pressure pulse has no direct relation to blood flow and could occur if there was no flow at all. When taking a pulse, it is the pressure pulses that are felt, and it is the pressure pulses that produce the Korotkoff sounds heard during blood pressure measurement. The tip or maximum deflection of the pressure pulsation coincides with the systolic blood pressure, and the minimum point of deflection coincides with the diastolic pressure.

Both the pressure values and the conformation of the pressure wave change as the wave moves though the peripheral arteries (see Fig. 16-18). As the pressure wave moves out through the aorta into the arteries, it

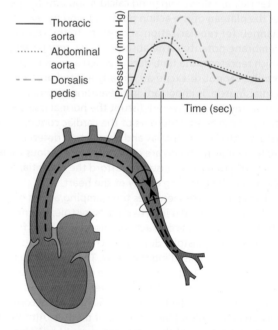

FIGURE 16-18 Amplification of the arterial pressure wave as it moves forward in the peripheral arteries. This amplification occurs as a forward-moving pressure wave merges with a backward-moving reflected pressure wave. (**Inset**) The amplitude of the pressure pulse increases in the thoracic aorta, abdominal aorta, and dorsalis pedis.

changes as it collides with reflected waves from the periphery. This is why the systolic pressure is higher in the medium-sized arteries than in the aorta even though the diastolic pressure is lower. After its initial amplification, the pressure pulse becomes smaller and smaller as it moves through the smaller arteries and arterioles, until it disappears almost entirely in the capillaries. This allows for continuous, rather than pulsatile, flow in the capillary beds.

Although the pressure pulses usually are not transmitted to the capillaries, there are situations in which this does occur. For example, injury to a finger or other area of the body often results in a throbbing sensation. In this case, extreme dilatation of the small vessels in the injured area produces a reduction in the dampening of the pressure pulse. Capillary pulsations also occur in conditions that cause exaggeration of aortic pressure pulses, such as aortic regurgitation (see Chapter 18).

VENOUS SYSTEM

The veins and venules are thin-walled, distensible, and collapsible vessels. The venules collect blood from the capillaries, and the veins transport blood back to the heart. The veins are capable of enlarging and storing large quantities of blood, which can be made available to the circulation as needed. Even though the veins are thin walled, they are muscular. This allows them to contract or expand to accommodate varying amounts of blood. Veins are innervated by the sympathetic nervous system. When blood is lost from the circulation, the veins constrict as a means of transferring blood to the arterial circulation.

The venous system is a low-pressure system, and when a person is in the upright position, blood flow in the venous system must oppose the effects of gravity. Valves in the veins of extremities prevent retrograde flow (Fig. 16-19), and with the help of skeletal muscles that surround and intermittently compress the veins in a milking manner, blood is moved forward to the heart. Their pressure ranges from approximately 10 mm Hg at the end of the venules to approximately 0 mm Hg at the entrance of the vena cava into the heart. There are no valves in the abdominal or thoracic veins, and blood flow in these veins is heavily influenced by the pressure in the abdominal and thoracic cavities, respectively.

LYMPHATIC SYSTEM

The lymphatic system, commonly called the *lymphatics,* serves almost all body tissues, except cartilage, bone, epithelial tissue, and tissues of the central nervous system. However, most of these tissues have prelymphatic channels that eventually flow into areas supplied by the lymphatics. Lymph is derived from interstitial fluids that flow through the lymph channels. It contains plasma proteins and other osmotically active particles that rely on the lymphatics for movement back into the circulatory system. The lymphatic system is also the main route for absorption of nutrients, particularly fats, from the gastrointestinal tract.

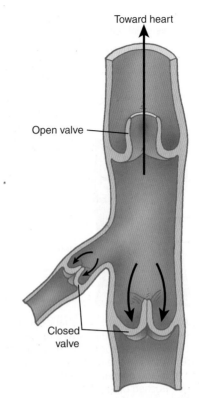

FIGURE 16-19 Portion of a femoral vein opened, to show the valves. The direction of flow is upward. Backward flow closes the valve.

The lymphatic system is made up of vessels similar to those of the circulatory system. These vessels commonly travel along with an arteriole or venule or with its companion artery and vein. The terminal lymphatic vessels are made up of a single layer of connective tissue with an endothelial lining and resemble blood capillaries. The lymphatic vessels lack tight junctions and are loosely anchored to the surrounding tissues by fine filaments (Fig. 16-20). The loose junctions permit the entry of large particles, and the filaments hold the vessels open under conditions of edema, when the pressure of the surrounding tissues would otherwise cause them to collapse. The lymph capillaries drain into larger lymph vessels that ultimately empty into the right and left thoracic ducts (Fig. 16-21). The thoracic ducts empty into the circulation at the junctions of the subclavian and internal jugular veins.

Although the divisions are not as distinct as in the circulatory system, the larger lymph vessels show evidence of having intimal, medial, and adventitial layers similar to those of blood vessels. Contraction of the smooth muscle in the medial layer of the larger collecting lymph channels assists in propelling lymph fluid toward the thorax. External compression of the lymph channels by active and passive movements of body parts also aid in forward propulsion of lymph fluid. The rate of flow through the lymphatic system by way of all of the various lymph channels, approximately 120 mL/hour, is determined by the interstitial fluid pressure and the activity of lymph pumps.

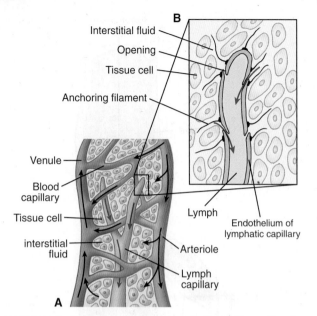

FIGURE 16-20 (**A**) Location of the lymphatic capillary. Blood from the arterial side of the capillary bed moves into the interstitial spaces and is reabsorbed in the venous side of the capillary bed. (**B**) Details of the lymphatic capillary with its anchoring filaments and overlapping edges that serve as valves and can be pushed open, allowing the inflow of interstitial fluid and its suspended particles.

THE MICROCIRCULATION AND LOCAL CONTROL OF BLOOD FLOW

The capillaries, venules, and arterioles of the circulatory system are collectively referred to as the *microcirculation*. It is here that the exchange of gases, nutrients, and metabolites takes place between the tissues and the circulating blood. The lymphatic system represents an accessory system that removes excess fluid, proteins, and large particles from the interstitial spaces and returns them to the circulation. Because of their size, these particles cannot be reabsorbed into the capillaries.

Capillaries

Capillaries are microscopic, single-cell–thick vessels that connect the arterial and venous segments of the circulation. In each person, there are approximately 10 billion capillaries, with a total surface area of 500 to 700 m².

The capillary wall is composed of a single layer of endothelial cells surrounded by a basement membrane or basal lamina (Fig. 16-22). Intercellular junctions join the capillary endothelial cells; these are called the *capillary pores*. Lipid-soluble materials diffuse directly through the capillary cell membrane. Water and water-soluble materials leave and enter the capillary through the capillary pores. The size of the capillary pores varies with cap-

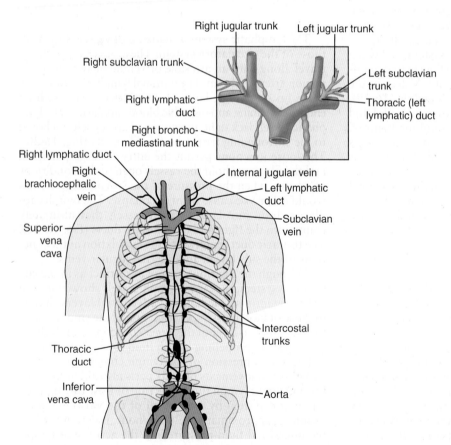

FIGURE 16-21 Lymphatic system, showing the thoracic duct and position of the left and right lymphatic ducts (**inset**).

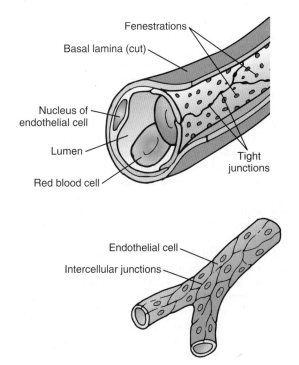

FIGURE 16-22 Endothelial cells and intercellular junctions in a section of capillary.

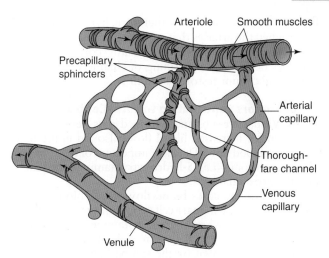

FIGURE 16-23 Capillary bed. Precapillary sphincters control the flow of blood through the capillary network. Thoroughfare channels (i.e., arteriovenous shunts) allow blood to move directly from the arteriole into the venule without moving through nutrient channels of the capillary.

illary function. In the brain, the endothelial cells are joined by tight junctions that form the blood-brain barrier. This prevents substances that would alter neural excitability from leaving the capillary. In organs that process blood contents, such as the liver, capillaries have large pores so that substances can pass easily through the capillary wall. In the kidneys, the glomerular capillaries have small openings called *fenestrations* that pass directly through the middle of the endothelial cells. Fenestrated capillary walls are consistent with the filtration function of the glomerulus.

Blood enters the microcirculation through an arteriole, passes through the capillaries, and leaves by way of a small venule. The metarterioles serve as thoroughfare channels that link arterioles and capillaries (Fig. 16-23). Small cuffs of smooth muscle, the precapillary sphincters, are positioned at the arterial end of the capillary. The smooth muscle tone of the arterioles, venules, and precapillary sphincters controls blood flow through the capillary bed. Depending on venous pressure, blood flows through the capillary channels when the precapillary sphincters are open.

Blood flow through capillary channels, designed for exchange of nutrients and metabolites, is called *nutrient flow*. In some parts of the microcirculation, blood flow bypasses the capillary bed, moving through a connection called an *arteriovenous shunt,* which directly connects an arteriole and a venule. This type of blood flow is called *non-nutrient flow* because it does not allow for nutrient exchange. Non-nutrient channels are common in the skin and are important in terms of heat exchange and temperature regulation.

Autoregulation

Tissue blood flow is regulated on a minute-to-minute basis in relation to tissue needs and on a longer-term basis through the development of collateral circulation. Neural mechanisms regulate the cardiac output and blood pressure needed to support these local mechanisms.

Local control of blood flow is governed largely by the nutritional needs of the tissue. For example, blood flow to organs such as the heart, brain, and kidneys remains relatively constant, although blood pressure may vary throughout a range of 60 to 180 mm Hg. The ability of the tissues to regulate their own blood flow throughout a wide range of pressures is called *autoregulation*. Autoregulation of blood flow is mediated by alterations in blood vessel tone caused by changes in flow through the vessel or by local tissue factors, such as lack of oxygen or accumulation of tissue metabolites (*i.e.,* potassium, lactic acid, or adenosine, which is a breakdown product of ATP). Local control is particularly important in tissues such as skeletal muscle, which has blood flow requirements that vary according to the level of activity.

An increase in local blood flow is called *hyperemia*. The ability of tissues to increase blood flow in situations of increased activity, such as exercise, is called *functional hyperemia*. When the blood supply to an area has been occluded and then restored, local blood flow through the tissues increases within seconds to restore the metabolic equilibrium of the tissues. This increased flow is called *reactive hyperemia*. The transient redness seen on an arm after leaning on a hard surface is an example of reactive hyperemia. Local control mechanisms rely on a continuous flow from the main arteries; therefore, hyperemia cannot occur when the arteries that supply the capillary beds are narrowed. For example, if a major coronary artery becomes occluded, the opening of channels supplied by that vessel cannot restore blood flow.

Tissue Factors Contributing to Local Control of Blood Flow.
Vasoactive substances, formed in tissues in response to a need for increased blood flow, also aid in the local control of blood flow. The most important of these are histamine, serotonin (*i.e.*, 5-hydroxytryptamine), the kinins, and the prostaglandins.

Histamine increases blood flow. Most blood vessels contain histamine in mast cells and non-mast cell stores; when these tissues are injured, histamine is released. In certain tissues, such as skeletal muscle, the activity of the mast cells is mediated by the sympathetic nervous system; when sympathetic control is withdrawn, the mast cells release histamine. Vasodilatation then results from increased histamine and the withdrawal of vasoconstrictor activity.

Serotonin is liberated from aggregating platelets during the clotting process; it causes vasoconstriction and plays a major role in the control of bleeding. Serotonin is found in brain and lung tissues, and there is some speculation that it may be involved in the vascular spasm associated with some allergic pulmonary reactions and migraine headaches.

The *kinins* (*i.e.*, kallidins and bradykinin) are liberated from the globulin kininogen, which is present in body fluids. The kinins cause relaxation of arteriolar smooth muscle, increase capillary permeability, and constrict the venules. In exocrine glands, the formation of kinins contributes to the vasodilatation needed for glandular secretion.

Prostaglandins are synthesized from constituents of the cell membrane (*i.e.*, the long-chain fatty acid *arachidonic acid*). Tissue injury incites the release of arachidonic acid from the cell membrane, which initiates prostaglandin synthesis. There are several prostaglandins (*e.g.*, E_2, F_2, D_2), which are subgrouped according to their solubility; some produce vasoconstriction and some produce vasodilatation. As a rule of thumb, those in the E group are vasodilators, and those in the F group are vasoconstrictors. The adrenal glucocorticoid hormones produce an antiinflammatory response by blocking the release of arachidonic acid, preventing prostaglandin synthesis.

Endothelial Control of Vasodilatation and Vasoconstriction.
The *endothelium*, which lies between the blood and the vascular smooth muscle, serves as a physical barrier for vasoactive substances that circulate in the blood. Once thought to be nothing more than a single layer of cells that lines blood vessels, it is now known that the endothelium plays an active role in controlling vascular function. In capillaries, which are composed of a single layer of endothelial cells, the endothelium is active in transporting cell nutrients and wastes. In addition to its function in capillary transport, the vascular endothelium removes vasoactive agents such as norepinephrine from the blood, and it produces enzymes that convert precursor molecules to active products (*e.g.*, angiotensin I to angiotensin II in lung vessels).

One of the important functions of the endothelial cells in the small arteries and arterioles is to synthesize and release factors that control vessel dilatation. Of particular importance was the discovery, first reported in the early 1980s, that the intact endothelium was able to produce a factor that caused relaxation of vascular smooth muscle. This factor was originally named *endothelium-derived relaxing factor* and is now known to be *nitric oxide*. Many other cell types produce nitric oxide. In these tissues, nitric oxide has other functions, including modulation of nerve activity in the nervous system.

The normal endothelium maintains a continuous release of nitric oxide, which is formed from L-arginine through the action of an enzyme called *nitric oxide synthase* (Fig. 16-24). The production of nitric oxide can be stimulated by a variety of stimuli, including acetylcholine, bradykinin, histamine, and thrombin. *Shear stress* on the endothelium, resulting from an increase in blood flow or blood pressure, also stimulates nitric oxide production and vessel relaxation. Nitric oxide also inhibits platelet aggregation and secretion of platelet contents, many of which cause vasoconstriction. The fact that nitric oxide is released into the vessel lumen (to inactivate platelets) and away from the lumen (to relax smooth muscle) suggests that it protects against both thrombosis and vasoconstriction. Nitroglycerin, which is used in treatment of angina, produces its effects by releasing nitric oxide in vascular smooth muscle.

The endothelium also produces a number of vasoconstrictor substances, including *angiotensin II,* vasoconstrictor prostaglandins, and a family of peptides called *endothelins*. There are at least three endothelins. Endothelin-1, made by endothelial cells, is the most potent endogenous vasoconstrictor known. Receptors for endothelins also have been identified.

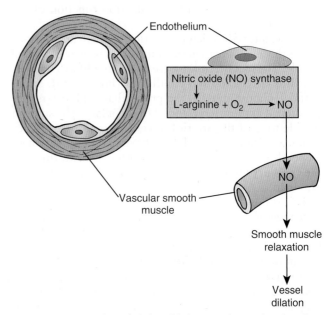

FIGURE 16-24 Function of nitric oxide in smooth muscle relaxation.

Collateral Circulation

Collateral circulation is a mechanism for the long-term regulation of local blood flow. In the heart and other vital structures, anastomotic channels exist between some of the smaller arteries. These channels permit perfusion of an area by more than one artery. When one artery becomes occluded, these anastomotic channels increase in size, allowing blood from a patent artery to perfuse the area supplied by the occluded vessel. For example, persons with extensive obstruction of a coronary blood vessel may rely on collateral circulation to meet the oxygen needs of the myocardial tissue normally supplied by that vessel. As with other long-term compensatory mechanisms, the recruitment of collateral circulation is most efficient when obstruction to flow is gradual, rather than sudden.

In summary, the walls of all blood vessels, except the capillaries, are composed of three layers: the tunica externa, tunica media, and tunica intima. The layers of the vessel vary with its function. Arteries are thick-walled vessels with large amounts of elastic fibers. The walls of the arterioles, which control blood pressure, have large amounts of smooth muscle. Veins are thin-walled, distensible, and collapsible vessels. Venous flow is designed to return blood to the heart. It is a low-pressure system and relies on venous valves and the action of muscle pumps to offset the effects of gravity. Capillaries are single-cell–thick vessels designed for the exchange of gases, nutrients, and waste materials.

The delivery of blood to the tissues of the body depends on pressure pulses that are generated by the intermittent ejection of blood from the left ventricle into the distensible aorta and large arteries of the arterial system. The combination of distensibility of the arteries and their resistance to flow reduces the pressure pulsations; therefore, blood flow is almost constant by the time blood reaches the capillaries. Two major factors affect the pressure pulsations: (1) the stroke volume output of the heart, and (2) the compliance of the arterial system into which the blood is ejected. A large stroke volume or a decrease in arterial compliance produces an increase in pulse pressure.

The mechanisms that control blood flow are designed to ensure adequate delivery of blood to the capillaries in the microcirculation, where the exchange of cellular nutrients and wastes occurs. Local control is governed largely by the needs of the tissues and is regulated by local tissue factors such as lack of oxygen and the accumulation of metabolites. Hyperemia is a local increase in blood flow that occurs after a temporary occlusion of blood flow. It is a compensatory mechanism that decreases the oxygen debt of the deprived tissues. Collateral circulation is a mechanism for long-term regulation of local blood flow that involves the development of collateral vessels.

Autonomic Nervous System Control of Circulatory Function

The neural control of the circulatory system occurs primarily through the *sympathetic* and *parasympathetic* divisions of the autonomic nervous system (ANS). The ANS contributes to the control of cardiovascular function through modulation of cardiac (*i.e.,* heart rate and cardiac contractility) and vascular (*i.e.,* peripheral vascular resistance) function.

The neural control centers for the integration and modulation of cardiac function and blood pressure are located bilaterally in the medulla oblongata. The medullary cardiovascular neurons are grouped into three distinct pools that lead to sympathetic innervation of the heart and blood vessels and parasympathetic innervation of the heart. The first two, which control sympathetic-mediated acceleration of heart rate and blood vessel tone, are called the *vasomotor center*. The third, which controls parasympathetic-mediated slowing of heart rate, is called the *cardioinhibitory center*. These brain stem centers receive information from many areas of the nervous system, including the hypothalamus. The arterial baroreceptors and chemoreceptors provide the medullary cardiovascular center with continuous information regarding changes in blood pressure (see Chapter 17).

AUTONOMIC REGULATION OF CARDIAC FUNCTION

The heart is innervated by the parasympathetic and sympathetic nervous systems. Parasympathetic innervation of the heart is transmitted through the *vagus nerve*. The parasympathetic outflow to the heart originates from the vagal nucleus in the medulla. The axons of these neurons pass to the heart in the cardiac branches of the vagus nerve. The effect of vagal stimulation on heart function is largely limited to heart rate, with increased vagal activity producing a slowing of the heart rate. Sympathetic outflow to the heart and blood vessels arises from neurons located in the reticular formation of the brain stem. The axons of these neurons exit the thoracic segments of the spinal cord to synapse with the postganglionic neurons that innervate the heart. Cardiac sympathetic fibers are widely distributed to the SA and AV nodes and the myocardium. Increased sympathetic activity produces an increase in the heart rate and the velocity and force of cardiac contraction.

AUTONOMIC REGULATION OF VASCULAR FUNCTION

The sympathetic nervous system serves as the final common pathway for controlling the smooth muscle tone of the blood vessels. Most of the sympathetic preganglionic fibers that control vessel function originate in the vasomotor center of the brain stem, travel down the spinal cord, and exit in the thoracic and lumbar (T1 to L2) segments. The sympathetic neurons that supply the blood vessels maintain them in a state of tonic activity, so that even under resting conditions, the blood vessels are partially constricted. Vessel constriction and relaxation are accomplished by altering this basal input. Increasing sympathetic activity causes constriction of some vessels, such as those of the skin, the gastrointestinal tract, and the kidneys. Blood vessels in skeletal muscle are supplied by both vasoconstrictor and vasodilator fibers. Activation of sympathetic vasodilator fibers causes vessel relaxation and provides the muscles with increased blood flow during exercise. Although the parasympathetic nervous system contributes to the regulation of heart function, it has little or no control over blood vessels.

AUTONOMIC NEUROTRANSMITTERS

The actions of the ANS are mediated by chemical neurotransmitters. *Acetylcholine* is the postganglionic neurotransmitter for parasympathetic neurons and *norepinephrine* is the main neurotransmitter for postganglionic sympathetic neurons. Sympathetic neurons also respond to epinephrine, which is released into the bloodstream by the adrenal medulla. The neurotransmitter *dopamine* can also act as a neurotransmitter for some sympathetic neurons. The synthesis, release, and inactivation of the autonomic neurotransmitters are discussed in Chapter 33.

In summary, the neural control centers for the regulation of cardiac function and blood pressure are located in the reticular formation of the lower pons and medulla of the brain stem, where the integration and modulation of ANS responses occur. These brain stem centers receive information from many areas of the nervous system, including the hypothalamus. Both the parasympathetic and sympathetic nervous systems innervate the heart. The parasympathetic nervous system functions in regulating heart rate through the vagus nerve, with increased vagal activity producing a slowing of heart rate. The sympathetic nervous system has an excitatory influence on heart rate and contractility, and it serves as the final common pathway for controlling the smooth muscle tone of the blood vessels.

Review Exercises

Use the Frank-Starling ventricular function curve depicted in Figure 16-16 to explain the changes in cardiac output that occur with changes in respiratory effort.

A. What happens to cardiac output during increased inspiratory effort, in which a marked decrease in intrathoracic pressure produces an increase in venous return to the right heart?

B. What happens to cardiac output during increased expiratory effort, in which a marked increase in intrathoracic pressure produces a decrease in venous return to the right heart?

C. Given these changes in cardiac output that occur during increased respiratory effort, what would you propose as one of the functions of the Frank-Starling curve?

Visit the Porth: Essentials of Pathophysiology: Concepts of Altered Health States web site (http://thePoint.LWW.com/PorthEssentials) for links to chapter-related resources on the Internet, all-new exclusive animations, chapter review questions, and more!

BIBLIOGRAPHY

Berne R. M., Levy M. N. (2000). *Principles of physiology* (3rd ed., pp. 201–275). St. Louis: C. V. Mosby.

Berne R. M., Levy M. N. (2001). *Cardiovascular physiology* (8th ed.). St. Louis: C. V. Mosby.

Feletou M., Vanhoutte P. M. (1999). The alternative: EDHF. *Journal of Molecular and Cellular Cardiology* 31, 15–22.

Ganong W. F. (2005). *Review of medical physiology* (22nd ed., pp. 493–601). Stamford, CT: Appleton & Lange.

Guyton A. C., Hall J. E. (2006). *Medical physiology* (11th ed., pp. 161–245). Philadelphia: Elsevier Saunders.

Rhoades R. A., Tanner G. A. (2003). *Medical physiology* (pp. 207–301). Boston: Little, Brown.

Ross M. H., Kay G. I., Pawlina W. (2003). *Histology: A text and atlas* (4th ed.). Philadelphia: Lippincott Williams & Wilkins.

Smith J. J., Kampine J. P. (1989). *Circulatory physiology* (3rd ed.). Baltimore: Williams & Wilkins.

Vanhoutte P. M. (1999). How to assess endothelial function in human blood vessels. *Journal of Hypertension* 17, 1047–1058.

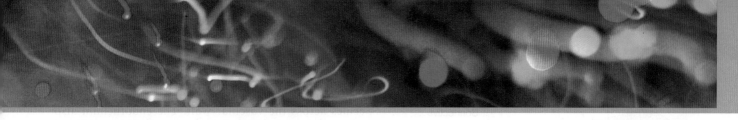

Chapter *17*

Disorders of Blood Flow and Blood Pressure

Disorders of the blood vessels are directly or indirectly responsible for many diseases of the human body. Arterial diseases, such as stroke and coronary heart disease, are responsible for more morbidity and mortality than any other type of disease. Hypertension, or elevation of the arterial blood pressure, is probably the most common of all health problems in adults and is the leading risk factor for cardiovascular disorders. Although disorders of veins are less common, they also cause clinically significant problems. The discussion in this chapter is organized into four parts: blood vessel structure and function, disorders of the arterial circulation, disorders of the arterial blood pressure, and disorders of the venous circulation.

Blood Vessel Structure and Function

Although the heart is the center of the cardiovascular system, it is the blood vessels that carry blood throughout the body. The major constituents of the walls of blood vessels are the endothelial cells, smooth muscle cells, and supporting connective tissue elements (*e.g.,* elastic and collagen fibers).[1,2]

The walls of all blood vessels, except the very smallest, are composed of three distinct layers or coats, called *tunica* (Fig. 17-1). The outermost layer of a vessel, called the *tunica externa* or *tunica adventitia,* is composed primarily of loosely woven collagen fibers that protect the blood vessel and anchor it to the surrounding structures. The tunica externa is infiltrated with nerve fibers and, in larger vessels, a system of tiny blood vessels called the *vasa vasorum.* The middle layer, the *tunica media,* is composed mainly of circularly arranged smooth muscle cells and sheets of elastin. Larger arteries have an external elastic lamina that separates the tunica media from the tunica externa. The innermost layer, the *tunica intima,* consists

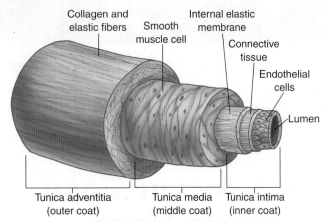

Collagen and elastic fibers
Smooth muscle cell
Internal elastic membrane
Connective tissue
Endothelial cells
Lumen

Tunica adventitia (outer coat)   Tunica media (middle coat)   Tunica intima (inner coat)

FIGURE 17-1 Diagram of a typical artery showing the tunica intima, tunica media, and tunica adventitia (tunica externa).

of a single layer of flattened endothelial cells with minimal underlying subendothelial connective tissue. Beneath the subendothelial tissue is an internal elastic lamina that is especially well developed in muscular arteries.

As the main cellular component of the blood vessel wall, the endothelial and smooth muscle cells play an important role in the pathogenesis of many blood vessel diseases.

ENDOTHELIAL CELLS

Endothelial cells form a continuous lining for the entire vascular system called the *endothelium*. Once thought to be nothing more than a lining for blood vessels, it is now known that the endothelium is a versatile, multifunctional tissue that plays an active role in controlling

vascular function[1,2] (Table 17-1). As a semipermeable membrane, the endothelium controls the transfer of molecules across the vascular wall. The endothelium also plays a role in the control of platelet adhesion and blood clotting; modulation of blood flow and vascular resistance; metabolism of hormones; regulation of immune and inflammatory reactions; and elaboration of factors that influence the growth of other cell types, particularly the smooth muscle cells.

Structurally intact endothelial cells respond to various abnormal stimuli by adjusting their usual functions and by expressing newly acquired functions.[1] The term *endothelial dysfunction* describes several types of potentially reversible changes in endothelial function that occur in response to environmental stimuli. Inducers of endothelial dysfunction include cytokines and bacterial products that cause inflammation; hemodynamic stresses and lipid products that are critical to the pathogenesis of atherosclerosis; viruses and complement components; and hypoxia. Dysfunctional endothelial cells, in turn, produce other cytokines, growth factors, procoagulant or anticoagulant substances, and a variety of other biologically active products. They also influence the reactivity of underlying smooth muscle cells through production of both relaxing factors (*e.g.*, nitric oxide [NO]) or contracting factors (*e.g.*, endothelins).

VASCULAR SMOOTH MUSCLE CELLS

Vascular smooth muscle cells, which form the predominant cellular layer in the tunica media, produce vasoconstriction or dilation of blood vessels. A network of vasomotor nerves of the sympathetic component of the autonomic nervous system supplies the smooth muscle in the blood vessels. These nerves are responsible for vaso-

TABLE 17-1	**Endothelial Cell Properties and Functions**
Major Properties	**Associated Functions/Factors**
Maintenance of a selective permeability barrier	Controls the transfer of small and large molecules across the vessel wall
Regulation of thrombosis	Elaboration of prothrombogenic molecules (von Willebrand factor, plasminogen activator) and antithrombotic molecules (prostacyclin, heparin-like molecules, plasminogen activator)
Modulation of blood flow and vascular reactivity	Elaboration of vasodilators (nitric oxide, prostacyclin) and vasoconstrictors (endothelins, angiotensin-converting enzyme)
Regulation of cell growth, particularly smooth muscle cells	Production of growth-stimulating factors (platelet-derived growth factor, hematopoietic colony-stimulating factor) and growth-inhibiting factors (heparin, transforming growth factor-β)
Regulation of inflammatory/immune responses	Expression of adhesion molecules that regulate leukocyte migration and release of inflammatory and immune system mediators (e.g., interleukins, interferons)
Maintenance of the extracellular matrix	Synthesis of collagen, laminin, proteoglycans
Involvement in lipoprotein metabolism	Oxidation of VLDL, LDL, cholesterol

Data from Schoen F. J. (2005). Blood vessels. In Kumar V., Abbas A. K., Fausto N. (Eds.), *Robbins and Cotran pathologic basis of disease* (7th ed., p. 514). Philadelphia: Elsevier Saunders; and Ross M. H., Kaye G. L., Pawlina W. (2003). *Histology: A text and atlas* (4th ed., p. 332). Philadelphia: Lippincott Williams & Wilkins.

constriction of the vessel walls. Because they do not enter the tunica media of the blood vessel, the nerves do not synapse directly on the smooth muscle cells. Instead, they release the neurotransmitter norepinephrine, which diffuses into the media and acts on the nearby smooth muscle. The resulting impulses are propagated along the smooth muscle cells through their gap junctions, causing contraction of the entire muscle cell layer and thus reducing the radius of the vessel lumen.

Vascular smooth muscle cells also synthesize collagen, elastin, and other components of the extracellular matrix; elaborate growth factors and cytokines; and after vascular injury migrate into the intima and proliferate. Thus, smooth muscle cells are important in both normal vascular repair as well as pathologic processes such as atherosclerosis. The migratory and proliferative activities of vascular smooth muscle cells are stimulated by growth promoters and inhibitors. Promoters include platelet-derived growth factor, thrombin, fibroblast growth factor, and cytokines such as interferon-gamma and interleukin-1. Inhibitors include NO. Other regulators include the renin-angiotensin system (angiotensin II) and the catecholamines.

In summary, the main cellular components of blood vessels are the endothelial cells, which form the endothelium that lines the entire vascular system, and vascular smooth muscle cells, which form the predominant cellular layer in the tunica media. The endothelium controls the transfer of molecules across the vascular wall, plays a role in platelet adhesion and blood clotting, and functions in the modulation of blood flow and vascular resistance. It also participates in the metabolism of hormones, regulation of immune and inflammatory reactions, and elaboration of factors that influence the growth of other cell types, particularly the smooth muscle cells. Vascular smooth muscle produces vasoconstriction or dilatation of blood vessels. It also synthesizes collagen, elastin, and other components of the extracellular matrix that are important in both normal vascular repair as well as pathologic processes such as atherosclerosis.

Disorders of the Arterial Circulation

The arterial system distributes blood to all the tissues in the body. There are three types of arteries: large arteries, including the aorta and its distal branches; medium-sized arteries, such as the coronary and renal arteries; and small arteries and arterioles that pass through the tissues. Each of these different types of arteries tends to be affected by different disease processes. The discussion in this section focuses on hyperlipidemia and atherosclerosis, vasculitides, arterial disease of the extremities, and arterial aneurysms.

 KEY CONCEPTS

Disorders of the Arterial Circulation

➤ The arterial system delivers oxygen and nutrients to the tissues. Disorders of the arterial circulation produce ischemia owing to narrowing of blood vessels, thrombus formation associated with platelet adhesion, and weakening of the vessel wall.

➤ Atherosclerosis is a progressive disease characterized by the formation of fibrofatty plaques in the intima of large and medium-sized arteries, producing a decrease in blood flow due to a narrowing of the vessel lumen.

➤ The vasculitides, which produce inflammation of the vessel wall, represent a common pathway for vessel and tissue injury in a number of diseases.

➤ Aneurysms represent an abnormal localized dilatation of an artery due to a weakness in the vessel wall. As the aneurysm increases in size, the tension in the wall of the vessel increases, predisposing it to rupture.

HYPERLIPIDEMIA AND ATHEROSCLEROSIS

Hyperlipidemia with its associated risk for the development of atherosclerosis is a major cause of cardiovascular disease. According to the American Heart Association, an estimated 37.7 million Americans have high serum cholesterol levels that could contribute to a heart attack, stroke, or other cardiovascular event associated with atherosclerosis.[3]

Hyperlipidemia

Because lipids, namely cholesterol and triglycerides, are insoluble in plasma, they are encapsulated by special fat-carrying proteins called *lipoproteins* for transport in the blood. There are five types of lipoproteins, classified by their densities as measured by ultracentrifugation: chylomicrons, very–low-density lipoprotein (VLDL), intermediate-density lipoprotein (IDL), low-density lipoprotein (LDL), and high-density lipoprotein (HDL). VLDL carries large amounts of triglycerides that have a lower density than cholesterol. LDL is the main carrier of cholesterol, whereas HDL is about 50% protein and carries less cholesterol (Fig. 17-2).

Each type of lipoprotein consists of a large molecular complex of lipids combined with proteins called *apoproteins*.[4,5] The lipoprotein macromolecule is made up of a hydrophobic core of insoluble cholesterol esters and triglycerides, surrounded by a hydrophilic outer layer of soluble phospholipids, nonesterified cholesterol, and apoproteins (Fig. 17-3). The apoproteins control the

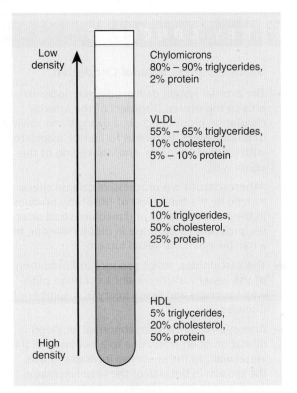

FIGURE 17-2 Lipoproteins are named based on their protein content, which is measured as density. Because fats are less dense than proteins, as the proportion of triglycerides decreases, the density increases.

interactions and ultimate metabolic fate of the lipoproteins. Some of the apoproteins activate the lipolytic enzymes that facilitate the removal of lipids from the lipoproteins; others serve as a reactive site that cellular receptors can recognize and use in the endocytosis and metabolism of the lipoproteins.

There are two sites of lipoprotein synthesis: the small intestine and the liver (Fig. 17-4). The chylomicrons, which

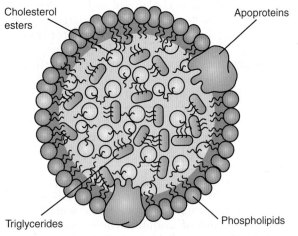

FIGURE 17-3 General structure of a lipoprotein. The cholesterol esters and triglycerides are located in the hydrophobic core of the macromolecule, surrounded by phospholipids and apoproteins.

are the largest of the lipoprotein molecules, are synthesized in the wall of the small intestine. They are involved in the transport of dietary (exogenous) triglycerides and cholesterol that have been absorbed from the gastrointestinal tract. Chylomicrons transfer their triglycerides to skeletal muscle tissue, where they are used for energy, and to adipose tissue, where they are stored. The remnant cholesterol-containing chylomicron particles are then taken up by the liver, and the cholesterol is used in the synthesis of VLDL or excreted in the bile.

The liver synthesizes and releases VLDL and HDL. The VLDLs, which contain large amounts of triglycerides and lesser amounts of cholesterol esters, provide the primary pathway for transport of the endogenous triglycerides produced in the liver to adipose and skeletal muscle tissue, where the triglycerides are removed. The resulting IDL fragments are reduced in triglyceride content and enriched in cholesterol. They are converted to LDL cholesterol in the vascular compartment or returned to the liver, where they are recycled to form VLDL.

LDL cholesterol, sometimes called the *bad cholesterol*, is the main carrier of cholesterol. The IDLs are the main source of LDL cholesterol. Blood levels of LDL cholesterol are controlled by the release of LDL cholesterol from IDLs and its subsequent removal from the blood. Approximately 70% of LDL is removed by way of an LDL receptor–dependent pathway and the rest is metabolized by a non–LDL receptor pathway.[1] Although LDL receptors are widely distributed, approximately 75% are located on hepatocytes; thus, the liver plays an extremely important role in LDL metabolism. Receptor-mediated removal involves the binding of LDL to a cell surface receptor; movement into the cell by endocytosis; and enzymatic degradation of the LDL molecule, resulting in the release of cholesterol into the cell cytoplasm. The released cholesterol not only is used by the cell for membrane synthesis, but takes part in cholesterol homeostasis by a sophisticated system of feedback mechanisms that regulate cholesterol production and synthesis of cell surface receptors. Thus, hepatocytes can control their intracellular cholesterol levels by increasing or decreasing cholesterol synthesis and by adding or removing cell surface LDL receptors.

The non–LDL receptor pathway involves ingestion by phagocytic monocytes and macrophages. These scavenger cells have receptors that bind LDL that has been oxidized or chemically modified. The amount of LDL cholesterol that is removed by the "scavenger pathway" is directly related to blood cholesterol levels. When there is a decrease in LDL receptors or when LDL cholesterol levels exceed receptor availability, the amount of LDL cholesterol that is removed by scavenger cells is greatly increased. The uptake of LDL cholesterol by macrophages in the arterial wall can result in the accumulation of insoluble cholesterol esters, the formation of foam cells, and the development of atherosclerosis.

High-density lipoprotein cholesterol, which is often referred to as the good cholesterol, is synthesized in the liver. It participates in the reverse transport of cholesterol—that is, carrying cholesterol from the peripheral tissues back to the liver. Epidemiologic studies show an inverse relation between HDL levels and the development of athero-

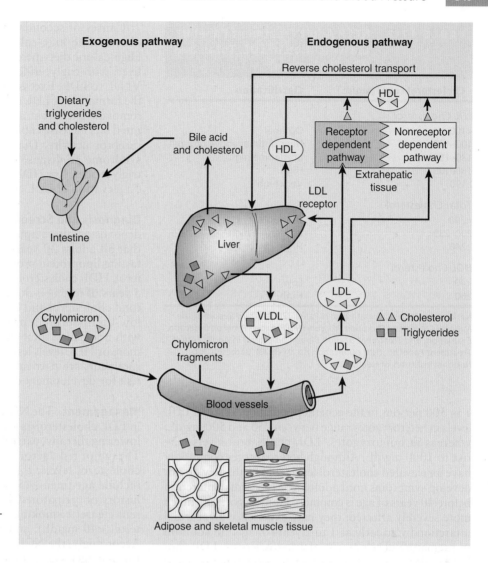

FIGURE 17-4 Schematic representation of the exogenous and endogenous pathways for triglyceride and cholesterol transport.

sclerosis.[6] It is thought that HDL, which is low in cholesterol and rich in surface phospholipids, facilitates the clearance of cholesterol from atheromatous plaques and transports it to the liver, where it may be excreted rather than reused in the formation of VLDL. The mechanism whereby HDL takes up cholesterol from peripheral cells has recently been elucidated. A lipid transporter (adenosine triphosphate [ATP]–binding cassette transporter A class 1, or ABCA1) promotes the movement of cholesterol from peripheral cells to the lipid-poor HDL cholesterol.[7] Defects in this system (resulting from mutations in the ABCA1 transporter) are responsible for Tangier disease, which is characterized by accelerated atherosclerosis and little or no HDL cholesterol. It has been observed that regular exercise and moderate alcohol consumption increase HDL cholesterol levels. Smoking and the metabolic syndrome (see Chapter 32), which are in themselves risk factors for atherosclerosis, are associated with decreased levels of HDL cholesterol.[1,7]

Hypercholesterolemia. The Third Report of the National Cholesterol Education Program (NCEP) Expert Panel on Detection, Evaluation, and Treatment of High Blood Cholesterol in Adults provides a classification system for hyperlipidemia that describes optimal to very high levels of LDL cholesterol, desirable to high levels of total cholesterol, and low and high levels of HDL cholesterol[8] (Table 17-2). Hypercholesterolemia can be classified as primary, in which the hypercholesterolemia develops independent of other causes, and secondary, in which it is associated with other health problems and behaviors.

Many types of primary hypercholesterolemia have a genetic basis. There may be a defective synthesis of the apoproteins, a lack of receptors, defective receptors, or defects in the handling of cholesterol in the cell that are genetically determined.[4,9] For example, the LDL receptor is deficient or defective in the genetic disorder known as *familial hypercholesterolemia*. This autosomal dominant type of hyperlipoproteinemia results from a mutation in the gene specifying the receptor for LDL. Because most of the circulating cholesterol is removed by receptor-dependent mechanisms, blood cholesterol levels are markedly elevated in persons with this disorder. The disorder is probably one of the most common of all mendelian disorders; the frequency of heterozygotes is

TABLE 17-2	**NCEP Adult Treatment Panel III Classification of LDL, Total, and HDL Cholesterol**
Cholesterol Level (mg/dL)	**Classification**
LDL Cholesterol	
<100	Optimal
100–129	Near optimal/above optimal
130–159	Borderline high
160–189	High
≥190	Very high
Total Cholesterol	
<200	Desirable
200–239	Borderline high
≥240	High
HDL Cholesterol	
<40	Low
≥60	High

National Institutes of Health Expert Panel. (2001). *Third Report of the National Cholesterol Education Program (NCEP) Expert Panel on Detection, Evaluation, and Treatment of High Blood Cholesterol in Adults (Adult Treatment Panel III)*. (NIH publication no. 01-3670). Bethesda, MD: National Institutes of Health.

1 in 500 persons in the general population.[9] Plasma LDL levels in heterozygotes range between 250 and 500 mg/dL, whereas in homozygotes, LDL cholesterol levels may rise to 1000 mg/dL. Although heterozygotes commonly have an elevated cholesterol level from birth, they do not develop symptoms until adult life. Myocardial infarction before 40 years of age is common. Homozygotes are much more severely affected; they may experience myocardial infarction by as early as 1 to 2 years of age.[4] In addition to premature development of atherosclerosis, LDL cholesterol deposits, called *xanthomas*, form in the skin and tendons (Fig. 17-5).

Causes of secondary hyperlipoproteinemia include obesity with high-calorie intake and diabetes mellitus. High-calorie diets increase the production of VLDL by the liver, with triglyceride elevation and high conversion of VLDL to LDL. Excess cholesterol in the diet may reduce the formation of LDL receptors and thereby decrease LDL removal. Diets that are high in triglycerides and saturated fats increase cholesterol synthesis and suppress LDL receptor activity. Diabetes mellitus and the metabolic syndrome predispose to dyslipidemia with elevation of triglycerides, low HDL cholesterol, and minimal or modest elevation of LDL cholesterol.[6,8]

Diagnosis and Screening. Diagnosis of hyperlipidemia depends on blood lipid studies. The NCEP recommends that all adults 20 years of age and older should have a fasting lipoprotein profile (total cholesterol, LDL cholesterol, HDL cholesterol, and triglycerides) done once every 5 years. If testing is done in the nonfasting state, only the total cholesterol and HDL are considered useful. A follow-up lipoprotein profile should be done on persons with nonfasting total cholesterol levels of 200 mg/dL or more or HDL levels less than 40 mg/dL. Lipoprotein measurements are particularly important in persons at high risk for development of coronary heart disease (CHD).

Management. The NCEP continues to identify reduction in LDL cholesterol as the primary target for cholesterol-lowering therapy, particularly in people at risk for CHD. The major risk factors for CHD, exclusive of high LDL cholesterol levels, that modify LDL cholesterol goals include age (men ≥45 years; women ≥55 years), family history of premature CHD in a first-degree relative, current cigarette smoking, hypertension, low HDL cholesterol (<40 mg/dL), and diabetes mellitus (Chart 17-1). Accordingly, the NCEP has updated the 2001 guidelines for management of LDL cholesterol based on risk factors.[10] The updated guidelines recommend that persons

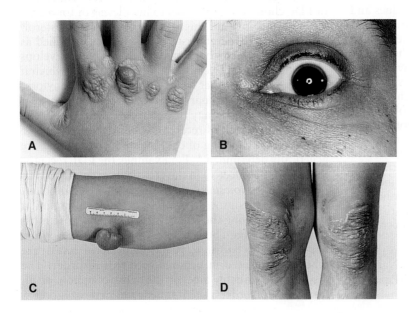

FIGURE 17-5 Xanthomas in the skin and tendons (**A, C, D**). Arcus lipoides represents the deposition of lipids in the peripheral cornea (**B**). (From Gotlieb A. I. [2005]. Blood vessels. In Rubin E., Gorstein F., Rubin R., et al. [Eds.], *Rubin's pathology: Clinicopathologic foundations of medicine* [4th ed., p. 499]. Philadelphia: Lippincott Williams & Wilkins.)

Risk Factors in Coronary Heart Disease Other Than Low-Density Lipoproteins

Positive Risk Factors

Age
  Men: ≥45 years
  Women: ≥55 years or premature menopause without estrogen replacement therapy
Family history of premature coronary heart disease (definite myocardial infarction or sudden death before 55 years of age in father or other male first-degree relative, or before 65 years of age in mother or other female first-degree relative)
Current cigarette smoking
Hypertension (≥140/90 mm Hg* or on antihypertensive medication)
Low HDL cholesterol (<40 mg/dL*)
Diabetes mellitus

Negative Risk Factor

High HDL cholesterol (≥60 mg/dL)

HDL, high-density lipoprotein.
*Confirmed by measurements on several occasions.
Modified from National Institutes of Health Expert Panel (2001). *Third Report of the National Cholesterol Education Program (NCEP) Expert Panel on Detection, Evaluation, and Treatment of High Blood Cholesterol in Adults (Adult Treatment Panel III).* NIH publication no. 01-3670, Bethesda, MD: National Institutes of Health.

with zero or no major risk factors have an LDL cholesterol goal of 160 mg/dL or less; persons with two or more of the major risk factors, a goal of less than 130 mg/dL; persons with *high risk* factors (*i.e.*, those with CHD, other forms of atherosclerotic disease, or diabetes), a goal of less than 100 mg/dL; and persons with *very high risk* factors (*i.e.*, those with acute coronary syndromes [see Chapter 18] or CHD with other risk factors), an LDL cholesterol goal of less than 70 mg/dL.[8,10] The guidelines also recommend that persons with a greater than 20% 10-year risk of experiencing myocardial infarction or coronary death, as determined by the risk assessment tool developed from the Framingham Heart Study data, should have an LDL cholesterol goal of less than 100 mg/dL.*

The management of hypercholesterolemia focuses on dietary and therapeutic lifestyle changes; when these are unsuccessful, pharmacologic treatment may be necessary. Therapeutic lifestyle changes include an increased emphasis on physical activity, dietary measures to reduce LDL cholesterol levels, smoking cessation, and weight reduc-

*To calculate a risk score, see www.nhlbi.nih.gov/guidelines/cholesterol.

tion for people who are overweight. Three dietary elements affect cholesterol and its lipoprotein fractions: (1) excess calories, (2) saturated fats, and (3) cholesterol. Excess calories consistently lower HDL and less consistently elevate LDL. Saturated fats in the diet can strongly influence cholesterol levels. Each 1% of saturated fat relative to caloric intake increases the cholesterol level an average of 2.8 mg/dL.[11] Depending on individual differences, it raises VLDL and LDL cholesterol. Dietary cholesterol tends to increase LDL cholesterol. On average, each 100 mg of ingested cholesterol raises the serum cholesterol 8 to 10 mg/dL.[11]

Lipid-lowering drugs ultimately work by affecting cholesterol production, decreasing cholesterol absorption from the intestine, decreasing intravascular conversion of VLDL and IDL to LDL, or removing cholesterol from the bloodstream. Drugs that act directly to decrease cholesterol levels also have the beneficial effect of further lowering cholesterol levels by stimulating the production of additional LDL receptors. Unless lipid levels are severely elevated, it is recommended that a minimum of 3 months of intensive diet therapy be undertaken before drug therapy is considered.[8]

Five types of medications are available for treating hypercholesterolemia: HMG-CoA reductase inhibitors, bile acid–binding resins, cholesterol absorption inhibitor agents, niacin and its congeners, and fibric acid derivatives.[6] 3-Hydroxy-3-methyl-glutaryl coenzyme A (HMG-CoA) reductase is a key enzyme in the cholesterol biosynthesis pathway. The statins (*e.g.*, atorvastatin, rosuvastatin, fluvastatin, lovastatin, pravastatin, simvastatin), which are inhibitors of HMG-CoA reductase, can reduce or block the hepatic synthesis of cholesterol and are the cornerstone of LDL cholesterol–reducing therapy. Statins also reduce triglyceride levels. The bile acid–binding resins (*e.g.*, cholestyramine, colestipol, and colesevelam) bind and sequester cholesterol-containing bile acids in the intestine and prevent the reabsorption of cholesterol by the chylomicrons. The cholesterol absorption inhibitor (ezetimibe) was recently approved by the U.S. Food and Drug Administration.[6] Nicotinic acid, a niacin congener, blocks the synthesis and release of VLDL by the liver, thereby lowering not only VLDL levels but IDL and LDL cholesterol levels. It also increases HDL cholesterol concentrations up to 30%. The fibric acid derivatives (fenofibrate and gemfibrozil) decrease the hepatic synthesis of VLDL from chylomicron fragments and inhibit the intravascular lipolysis of VLDL and IDL. The resulting decrease in triglycerides and increase in HDL cholesterol with these agents are especially important in the treatment of the metabolic syndrome.[6]

Atherosclerosis

Atherosclerosis is a type of arteriosclerosis or hardening of the arteries. The term *atherosclerosis*, which comes from the Greek words *atheros* (meaning "gruel" or "paste") and *sclerosis* (meaning "hardness"), denotes the formation of fibrofatty lesions in the intimal lining of large and medium-sized arteries such as the aorta and its branches, the coronary arteries, and the large vessels that supply the brain (Fig. 17-6).

Atherosclerotic Lesions. The lesions associated with atherosclerosis are of three types: the fatty streak, the fibrous atheromatous plaque, and the complicated lesion. The latter two are responsible for the clinically significant manifestations of the disorder. *Fatty streaks* are thin, flat, yellow intimal discolorations that progressively enlarge by becoming thicker and slightly elevated as they grow in length. Fatty streaks are present in children, often in the first year of life.[1,4] This occurs regardless of geographic

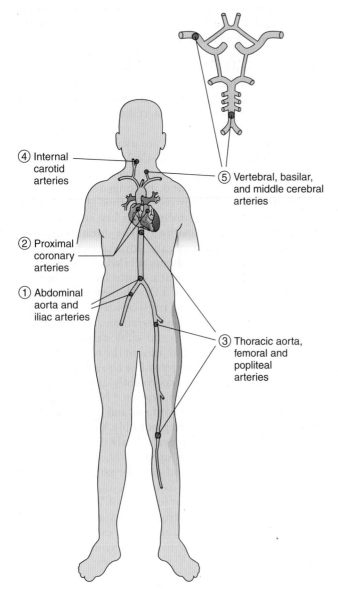

④ Internal carotid arteries

⑤ Vertebral, basilar, and middle cerebral arteries

② Proximal coronary arteries

① Abdominal aorta and iliac arteries

③ Thoracic aorta, femoral and popliteal arteries

FIGURE 17-6 Sites of severe atherosclerosis in order of frequency. (From Gotlieb A. I. [2005]. Blood vessels. In Rubin E., Gorstein F., Rubin R., et al. [Eds.], *Rubin's pathology: Clinicopathologic foundations of medicine* [4th ed., p. 491]. Philadelphia: Lippincott Williams & Wilkins.)

setting, gender, or race. They increase in number until about age 20 years, and then they remain static or regress. There is controversy about whether fatty streaks, in themselves, are precursors of atherosclerotic lesions.

The *fibrous atheromatous plaque* is the basic lesion of clinical atherosclerosis. It is characterized by the accumulation of intracellular and extracellular lipids, proliferation of vascular smooth muscle cells, and formation of scar tissue. The lesion begins as a gray to pearly white, elevated thickening of the vessel intima with a core of extracellular lipid (mainly cholesterol, which usually is complexed to proteins) covered by a fibrous cap of connective tissue and smooth muscle (Fig. 17-7). As the lesions increase in size, they encroach on the lumen of the artery and eventually may occlude the vessel or predispose to thrombus formation, causing a reduction of blood flow. The more advanced and *complicated lesions* are characterized by hemorrhage, ulceration, and scar tissue deposits. Thrombosis is the most important complication of atherosclerosis. It is caused by slow and turbulent blood flow in the region of the plaque and ulceration of the plaque.

Epidemiology and Risk Factors. Although the cause or causes of atherosclerosis have not been determined with certainty, epidemiologic studies have identified predisposing risk factors, which are listed in Chart 17-1.[1,4,8] Some of these are constitutional and cannot be changed, and others are affected by lifestyle and potentially controllable. The major risk factor, hypercholesterolemia, has both a constitutional and lifestyle component.

Nonlipid risk factors, such as increasing age, family history of premature CHD, and male sex, are constitutional and cannot be changed. The tendency to the development of atherosclerosis appears to run in families. Persons who come from families with a strong history of heart disease or stroke due to atherosclerosis are at greater risk for developing atherosclerosis than are those with a negative family history. Several genetically determined alterations in lipoprotein and cholesterol metabolism have been identified, and it seems likely that others will be identified in the future.[9] The incidence of atherosclerosis increases with age. Other factors being equal, men are at greater risk for developing CHD than are premenopausal women, probably because of the protective effects of natural estrogens. After menopause, the incidence of atherosclerosis-related diseases in women increases, and by the seventh to eighth decade of life, the frequency of myocardial infarction in the two sexes tends to equalize.[1]

The major risk factors that are, to a large extent, affected by a change in behavior (traditional cardiovascular risk factors) include hyperlipidemia, hypertension, cigarette smoking, and type 2 diabetes. These risk factors can often be modified or controlled by a change in diet, exercise, health care practices, or medications. The presence of hyperlipidemia is the strongest risk factor for persons younger than 45 years of age. Both primary and secondary hyperlipidemia increase the risk. Hypertension produces mechanical stress on the vessel endothe-

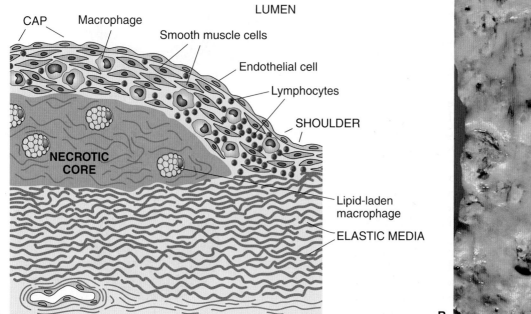

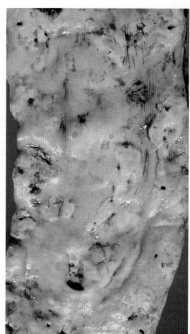

FIGURE 17-7 Fibrofatty plaque of atherosclerosis. (**A**) In this fully developed fibrous plaque, the core contains lipid-filled macrophages and necrotic smooth muscle cell debris. The "fibrous" cap is composed largely of smooth muscle cells, which produce collagen, small amounts of elastin, and glycosaminoglycans. Also shown are infiltrating macrophages and lymphocytes. Note that the endothelium over the surface of the fibrous cap frequently appears intact. (**B**) The aorta shows discrete raised, tan plaques. Focal plaque ulcerations are also evident. (From Gotlieb A. I. [2005]. Blood vessels. In Rubin E., Gorstein F., Rubin R., et al. [Eds.], *Rubin's pathology: Clinico-pathologic foundations of medicine* [4th ed., p. 487]. Philadelphia: Lippincott Williams & Wilkins.)

lium. It is a major risk factor for atherosclerosis at all ages and may be as important or more important than hypercholesterolemia after age 45 years. Both systolic and diastolic pressures are important. Cigarette smoking is a well-established risk factor in men and is thought to account for the relatively recent increase in the incidence and severity of atherosclerosis in women. One hypothesis is that components of cigarette smoke may be toxic, causing damage to the endothelial lining of blood vessels. Endothelial dysfunction may also be worsened by cigarette smoke, which is why cessation of smoking by high-risk individuals often is followed within a few years by reduced risk of ischemic heart disease. Diabetes mellitus (type 2) induces hypercholesterolemia and increases the predisposition to atherosclerosis (see Chapter 32).

However, not all atherothrombotic vascular disease can be explained by the established genetic and environmental risk factors. Other, so-called nontraditional cardiovascular risk factors include serum homocysteine, serum lipoprotein (a), C-reactive protein (CRP), and infectious agents.[1,4]

Homocysteine is derived from the metabolism of dietary methionine, an amino acid that is abundant in animal protein. The normal metabolism of homocysteine requires adequate levels of folate, vitamins B_6 and B_{12}, and riboflavin. There is growing evidence that increased plasma levels of homocysteine are an independent and dose-related risk factor for development of atherosclerosis. Homocysteine inhibits elements of the anticoagulant cascade and is associated with endothelial damage, which is thought to be an important first step in the development of atherosclerosis.[12] Factors tending to increase plasma levels of homocysteine include lower serum levels of folate and vitamins B_6 and B_{12}, genetic defects in homocysteine metabolism, renal impairment, malignancies, increasing age, male sex, and menopause.[12]

Lipoprotein (a) is similar to LDL in composition and is considered an independent risk factor for the development of premature CHD in men. Lipoprotein (a) can cause atherosclerosis by binding to macrophages through a high-affinity receptor that promotes foam cell formation and the deposition of cholesterol in atherosclerotic plaques.

Considerable interest in the role of inflammation in the etiology of atherosclerosis has emerged over the last few years.[13] CRP, which is a serum marker for systemic inflammation (see Chapter 14), is now considered a major risk factor marker.[14,15] Although the pathophysiologic role of CRP in atherosclerosis has not yet been defined, measurement of high-sensitivity CRP (hs-CRP) may be a better predictor of cardiovascular risk than lipid measurement alone.[15] Indeed, approximately 50% of patients with myocardial infarction have a normal serum LDL level.[14] In the Heart Protection Study, statin therapy decreased cardiovascular complications even in patients with a normal LDL.[16] This was thought to be due to the anti-inflammatory effects of these agents.

There is also interest in the possible connection between infectious agents (*Chlamydia pneumoniae,* herpesvirus hominis, cytomegalovirus) and the development of vascular disease. The presence of these organisms in atheromatous lesions has been demonstrated by immunocytochemistry, but no cause-and-effect relationship has been established. The organisms may play a role in atherosclerotic development by initiating and enhancing the inflammatory response.[17]

Of recent interest is the role of endothelial dysfunction as a key variable in the pathogenesis of atherosclerosis and its complications. Endothelial function reflects a balance between factors such as NO, which promotes vasodilatation and inhibits inflammation and vascular smooth muscle proliferation, and endothelium-derived contracting factors, which increase shear stress and promote the development of atherosclerosis. Current evidence suggests that endothelial status is not determined solely by individual risk factors such as lipids, hypertension, and smoking but by an integrated index of all atherogenic and atherosclerotic risk factors present in an individual, including known as well as yet-unknown variables and genetic predisposition.

Pathogenesis. Although the risk factors associated with atherosclerosis have been identified through epidemiologic studies, many unanswered questions remain regarding the mechanisms by which these risk factors contribute to the development of atherosclerosis. The vascular endothelial layer, which consists of a single layer of cells with cell-to-cell attachments, normally serves as a selective barrier that protects the subendothelial layers by interacting with blood cells and other blood components. One hypothesis of plaque formation suggests that injury to the endothelial vessel layer is the initiating factor in the development of atherosclerosis[1,4] (Fig. 17-8). A number of factors are regarded as possible injurious agents, including products associated with smoking, immune mechanisms, and mechanical stress, such as that associated with hypertension. The fact that atherosclerotic lesions tend to form where vessels branch or where there is turbulent flow suggests that hemodynamic factors also play a role (see Fig. 17-6). Hyperlipidemia, particularly LDL with its high cholesterol content, is also believed to play an active role in the pathogenesis of the atherosclerotic lesion. Interactions between the endothelial layer of the vessel wall and white blood cells, particularly the macrophages (blood monocytes), normally occur throughout life; these interactions increase when blood cholesterol levels are elevated. One of the earliest responses to elevated cholesterol levels is the attachment of monocytes to the endothelium. The monocytes have been observed to move through the cell-to-cell attachments of the endothelial layer into the subendothelial spaces, where they are transformed into macrophages.

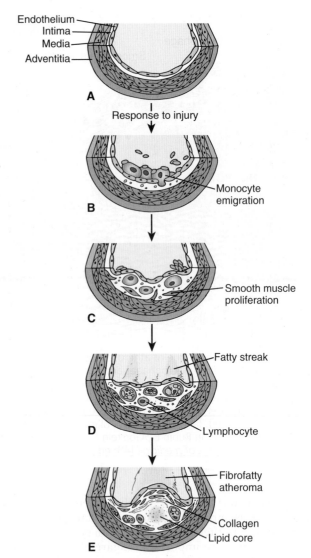

FIGURE 17-8 Response to injury hypothesis: (**A**) normal; (**B**) endothelial dysfunction (*e.g.,* increased permeability and leukocyte adhesion) with monocyte emigration and platelet adhesion; (**C**) smooth muscle cell emigration from the media into the intima; (**D**) macrophage engulfment of lipid and accumulation of lipids in the intima; (**E**) smooth muscle proliferation, collagen and other extracellular matrix deposition, and development of atheromatous plaque with a lipid core. (Modified from Kumar V., Cotran R. S., Robbins S. L. [2003]. *Robbins basic pathology* [7th ed., p. 335]. Philadelphia: W. B. Saunders, with permission from Elsevier Science.)

Activated macrophages release free radicals that oxidize LDL. Oxidized LDL is toxic to the endothelium, causing endothelial cell loss and exposure of the subendothelial tissue to blood components. This leads to platelet adhesion and aggregation and fibrin deposition. Platelets and activated macrophages release various factors that contribute to the proliferation of smooth muscle cells and deposition of extracellular matrix in the lesions[1,4] (see Fig. 17-7). Activated macrophages also ingest oxidized LDL to become foam cells, which are present in all stages of atherosclerotic plaque formation. Lipids released from necrotic foam cells accumulate to form the lipid core of what are termed *unstable plaques*. Unstable plaques typically have features of endothelial erosion (plaque erosion) and fissuring (plaque fissuring) or the presence of fresh thrombosis. They are characterized histologically by a large central lipid core, inflammatory infiltrate, and a thin fibrous cap. These "vulnerable plaques" are at risk of rupture (plaque rupture), normally at the shoulder of the plaque, where the fibrous cap is thinnest (because of the presence of local inflammatory cells and mediators that degrade the cap) and the mechanical stress is highest[18] (see Fig. 17-7A).

Clinical Manifestations. The clinical manifestations of atherosclerosis depend on the vessels involved and the extent of vessel obstruction. Atherosclerotic lesions produce their effects through narrowing of the vessel and production of ischemia; sudden vessel obstruction caused by plaque hemorrhage or rupture; thrombosis and formation of emboli resulting from damage to the vessel endothelium; and aneurysm formation caused by weakening of the vessel wall.[1] In larger vessels, such as the aorta, the important complications are those of thrombus formation and weakening of the vessel wall. In medium-sized arteries such as the coronary and cerebral arteries, ischemia and infarction caused by vessel occlusion are more common.

THE VASCULITIDES

The vasculitides are a group of vascular disorders that cause inflammatory injury and necrosis of the blood vessel wall (vasculitis). The vasculitides, which are a common pathway for tissue and organ involvement in many different disease conditions, involve the endothelial cells and smooth muscle cells of the arterial wall.[1,4,19] Vessels of any type (arteries, veins, and capillaries) in virtually any organ can be affected. Because they may affect veins and capillaries, the terms *vasculitis*, *angiitis*, and *arteritis* often are used interchangeably. Vasculitis may result from direct injury to the vessel, infectious agents, or immune processes, or may be secondary to other disease states such as systemic lupus erythematosus. Physical agents such as cold (*i.e.*, frostbite), irradiation (*i.e.*, sunburn), mechanical injury, and toxins may secondarily cause vessel damage, often leading to necrosis of the vessels.

The vasculitides are commonly classified based on etiology, pathologic findings, and prognosis. One classification system divides the conditions into three groups: (1) small vessel, (2) medium-sized vessel, and (3) large vessel vasculitides[1,4] (Table 17-3). The small vessel (arterioles, venules, and capillaries) vasculitides are involved in a number of different diseases, most of which are mediated by type III immune complex hypersensitivity reactions (see Chapter 15). They commonly involve the skin and are often a complication of an underlying disease

TABLE 17-3	Classification of the Vasculitides	
Group	**Examples**	**Characteristics**
Small vessel vasculitis	Microscopic polyangiitis	Necrotizing vasculitis with few or no immune deposits affecting medium and small blood vessels, including capillaries, venules, arterioles; necrotizing glomerulonephritis and involvement of the pulmonary capillaries is common
	Wegener granulomatosis	Granulomatous inflammation involving the respiratory tract and necrotizing vasculitis affecting capillaries, venules, arterioles, and arteries; necrotizing glomerulonephritis is common
Medium-sized vessel vasculitis	Polyarteritis nodosa	Necrotizing inflammation of medium-sized or small arteries without vasculitis in arteries, capillaries, or venules; usually associated with underlying disease or environmental agents
	Kawasaki disease	Involves large, medium-sized, and small arteries (frequently the coronaries) and is associated with mucocutaneous lymph node syndrome; usually occurs in small children
	Thromboangiitis obliterans	Segmental, thrombosing, acute and chronic inflammation of the medium-sized and small arteries, principally the tibial and radial arteries but sometimes extending to the veins and nerves of the extremities; occurs almost exclusively in men who are heavy smokers
Large vessel vasculitis	Giant cell (temporal) arteritis	Granulomatous inflammation of aorta and its major branches with predilection for extracranial vessels of the carotid artery; infiltration of vessel wall with giant cells and mononuclear cells; usually occurs in people older than 50 years of age and is often associated with polymyalgia rheumatica
	Takayasu arteritis	Granulomatous inflammation of the aorta and its branches; usually occurs in people younger than 50 years of age

(*e.g.,* vasculitis associated with neoplasms or connective tissue disease) and exposure to environmental agents (*e.g.,* serum sickness and urticarial vasculitis).

Medium-sized vessel vasculitides produce necrotizing damage to medium-sized muscular arteries of major organ systems. This group includes polyarteritis nodosa, Kawasaki disease (discussed in Chapter 18), and thromboangiitis obliterans (discussed in the section on Arterial Disease of the Extremities). Polyarteritis nodosa is an uncommon, acute multisystem inflammatory disease of small and medium-sized blood vessels of the kidney, liver, intestine, peripheral nerves, skin, and muscle. The usual course of the disease is progressive with various signs and symptoms according to the pattern of organ involvement. Most cases were fatal before corticosteroid and immunosuppressant agents became available for use in treatment of the disorder.[4]

Large vessel vasculitides involve large elastic arteries; they commonly are called *giant cell arterides* because they involve infiltration of the vessel wall with giant cells and mononuclear cells. Giant cell (temporal) arteritis, the most common of the large vessel vasculitides, is an acute and chronic inflammation of large to small arteries. It mainly affects arteries of the head—especially the temporal arteries—but may include the vertebral and ophthalmic arteries. About half of persons with the disease have accompanying pain and stiffness of the shoulder and hip (polymyalgia rheumatica; see Chapter 43). The most common clinical presentation is headache and tenderness over the superficial temporal artery. Diagnosis is by biopsy of the artery. Diagnosis followed by treatment with corticosteroid drugs is important because involvement of the ophthalmic artery can cause blindness.[1,4]

ARTERIAL DISEASE OF THE EXTREMITIES

In many respects, the disorders that affect arteries in the extremities are the same as those affecting the coronary and cerebral arteries in that they produce ischemia, pain, impaired function, and in some cases infarction and tissue necrosis. This section focuses on peripheral arterial disease, thromboangiitis obliterans, and Raynaud disease and phenomenon.

Peripheral Arterial Disease

Atherosclerosis is an important cause of peripheral arterial disease and is seen most commonly in the vessels of the lower extremities. The condition is sometimes referred to as *arteriosclerosis obliterans.* The superficial femoral and popliteal arteries are the most commonly affected vessels. When lesions develop in the lower leg and foot, the tibial, common peroneal, or pedal vessels are the arteries most commonly affected. The disease is seen most commonly in men in their seventh and eighth decades.[20] The risk factors for this disorder are the same as those for atherosclerosis. Cigarette smoking contributes to the progress of the atherosclerosis of the lower extremities and to the development of symptoms of ischemia.[21] Persons with diabetes mellitus experience more extensive and rapidly progressive vascular disease than do individuals without diabetes.

As with atherosclerosis in other locations, the signs and symptoms of vessel occlusion are gradual. Usually, there is at least a 50% narrowing of the vessel before symptoms of ischemia arise. The primary symptom of chronic obstructive arterial disease is *intermittent claudication* or pain with walking.[20,22] Typically, persons with the disorder report calf pain caused by ischemia of the gastrocnemius muscle, which has the highest oxygen consumption of any muscle group in the leg during walking. Some persons may report a vague aching feeling or numbness, rather than pain. Other signs of ischemia include atrophic changes and thinning of the skin and subcutaneous tissues of the lower leg and diminution in the size of the leg muscles. The foot often is cool, and the popliteal and pedal pulses are weak or absent. Limb color blanches with elevation of the leg because of the effects of gravity on perfusion pressure and becomes deep red when the leg is in the dependent position because of an autoregulatory increase in blood flow and a gravitational increase in perfusion pressure.

When blood flow is reduced to the extent that it no longer meets the minimal needs of resting muscle and nerves, ischemic pain at rest, ulceration, and gangrene develop. As tissue necrosis develops, there typically is severe pain in the region of skin breakdown, which is worse at night with limb elevation and is reduced with standing.[20]

Diagnostic methods include inspection of the limbs for signs of chronic low-grade ischemia, such as subcutaneous atrophy, brittle toenails, hair loss, pallor, coolness, or dependent rubor. Palpation of the femoral, popliteal, posterior tibial, and dorsalis pedis pulses allows for an estimation of the level and degree of obstruction. Blood pressures may be taken at various levels on the leg to determine the level of obstruction. A Doppler ultrasonographic stethoscope may be used for detecting pulses and measuring blood pressure. Ultrasound imaging, radionuclide imaging, and contrast angiography also may be used as diagnostic methods.[20,22]

Treatment includes measures directed at protection of the affected tissues and preservation of functional capacity. Walking (slowly) to the point of claudication usually is encouraged because it increases collateral circulation. Avoidance of injury is important because tissues of extremities affected by atherosclerosis are easily injured and slow to heal. It is important to address other cardiovascular risk factors, including smoking cessation, hypertension, lipid lowering, and diabetes. Antiplatelet agents and other medications (*e.g.,* angiotensin-converting enzyme inhibitors) may also be of value.[22] Surgery (*e.g.,* femoropopliteal bypass grafting using a section of saphenous vein) may be indicated in severe cases. In persons with diabetes, the peroneal arteries between the knees and ankles commonly are involved, making revascularization difficult. Thromboendarterectomy with removal of the occluding core of atherosclerotic tissue may be done if the section of diseased vessel is short. Percutaneous transluminal angioplasty, in which a balloon catheter is inserted into the area of stenosis and the balloon inflated to increase vessel diameter, is another form of treatment.[20–22]

Thromboangiitis Obliterans

Thromboangiitis obliterans (Buerger disease) is a vasculitis affecting the medium-sized arteries, usually the plantar and digital vessels in the foot and lower leg. Arteries in the arm and hand also may be affected. Although primarily an arterial disorder, the inflammatory process often extends to involve adjacent veins and nerves. Usually it is a disease of men between the ages of 25 and 40 years who are heavy cigarette smokers, but it can occur in women. The pathogenesis of the disorder remains uncertain; although cigarette smoking and, in some instances, tobacco chewing seem to be involved. It has been suggested that the tobacco may trigger an immune response in susceptible persons or it may unmask a clotting defect, either of which could incite an inflammatory reaction of the vessel wall.[23]

Pain is the predominant symptom of the disorder. It usually is related to distal arterial ischemia. During the early stages of the disease, there is intermittent claudication in the arch of the foot and the digits. In severe cases, pain is present even when the person is at rest. The impaired circulation increases sensitivity to cold. The peripheral pulses are diminished or absent, and there are changes in the color of the extremity. In moderately advanced cases, the extremity becomes cyanotic when the person assumes a dependent position, and the digits may turn reddish-blue even when in a nondependent position. With lack of blood flow, the skin assumes a thin, shiny look, and hair growth and skin nutrition suffer. Chronic ischemia causes thick, malformed nails. If the disease continues to progress, tissues eventually ulcerate, and gangrenous changes arise that may necessitate amputation.

Diagnostic methods are similar to those for atherosclerotic disease of the lower extremities. It is essential that the person stop smoking cigarettes or using tobacco. Other treatment measures are of secondary importance and focus on methods for producing vasodilatation and preventing tissue injury. Sympathectomy may be done to alleviate the vasospastic manifestations of the disease.

Raynaud Disease and Phenomenon

Raynaud phenomenon is a functional disorder caused by intense vasospasm of the arteries and arterioles in the fingers and, less often, the toes. The disorder is divided into two types: the primary type, called *Raynaud disease*, occurs without demonstrable cause, and the secondary type, called *Raynaud phenomenon*, is associated with other disease states or known causes of vasospasm.[24–26]

Vasospasm implies an excessive vasoconstrictor response to stimuli that normally produce only moderate vasoconstriction. In contrast to other regional circulations that are supplied by vasodilator and vasoconstrictor fibers, the cutaneous vessels of the fingers and toes are innervated only by sympathetic vasoconstrictor fibers. In these vessels, vasodilatation depends on withdrawal of sympathetic stimulation. Cooling of specific body parts, such as the head, neck, and trunk, produces a sympathetic-mediated reduction in digital blood flow, as does emotional stress.

Raynaud disease is usually seen in otherwise healthy young women. It often is precipitated by exposure to cold or by strong emotions and usually is limited to the fingers. It also follows a more benign course than Raynaud phenomenon, seldom causing tissue necrosis. The cause of vasospasm in primary Raynaud disease is unknown. Hyperreactivity of the sympathetic nervous system has been suggested as a contributing cause. Raynaud phenomenon is associated with previous vessel injury, such as frostbite, occupational trauma associated with the use of heavy vibrating tools, collagen diseases, neurologic disorders, and chronic arterial occlusive disorders. Another occupation-related cause is the exposure to alternating hot and cold temperatures, such as that experienced by butchers and food preparers. Raynaud phenomenon often is the first symptom of collagen diseases. It occurs in persons with scleroderma or systemic lupus erythematosus.

In Raynaud disease and Raynaud phenomenon, ischemia caused by vasospasm causes changes in skin color that progress from pallor to cyanosis, a sensation of cold, and changes in sensory perception, such as numbness and tingling. The color changes usually are first noticed in the tips of the fingers, later moving into one or more of the distal phalanges (Fig. 17-9). After the ischemic episode, there is a period of hyperemia with intense redness, throbbing, and paresthesia. The period of hyperemia is followed by a return to normal color. Although all of the fingers usually are affected symmetrically, the involvement may affect only one or two digits. In some cases, only a portion of the digit is affected.

In severe, progressive cases usually associated with Raynaud phenomenon, trophic changes may develop. The nails may become brittle, and the skin over the tips of the affected fingers may thicken. Nutritional impairment of these structures may give rise to arthritis. Ulceration and superficial gangrene of the fingers, although infrequent, may occur.

The initial diagnosis is based on a history of vasospastic attacks supported by other evidence of the disorder.

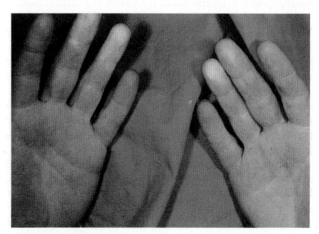

FIGURE 17-9 Raynaud phenomenon. The tips of the fingers show marked pallor. (From Gotlieb A. I. [2005]. Blood vessels. In Rubin E., Gorstein F., Rubin R., et al. [Eds.], *Rubin's pathology: Clinicopathologic foundations of medicine* [4th ed., p. 504]. Philadelphia: Lippincott Williams & Wilkins.)

Immersion of the hand in cold water may be used to initiate an attack as an aid to diagnosis. Laser-Doppler velocimetry may be used to quantify digital blood flow during changes in temperature. Serial computed thermography (finger skin temperature) also may be a useful tool in diagnosing the extent of disease. Raynaud disease is differentiated from Raynaud phenomenon by excluding secondary disorders known to cause vasospasm.

Treatment measures are directed toward eliminating factors that cause vasospasm and protecting the digits from trauma during an ischemic episode. Abstinence from smoking and protection from cold are priorities. Avoidance of emotional stress is another important factor in controlling the disorder because anxiety and stress may precipitate a vascular spasm in predisposed persons. Vasoconstrictor medications, such as the decongestants contained in allergy and cold preparations, should be avoided. Drugs with a vasodilating action (*e.g.,* calcium channel blockers and α-adrenergic receptor–blocking agents) may be indicated, particularly if episodes are frequent. Surgical interruption of sympathetic nerve pathways (sympathectomy) may be used for persons with severe symptoms.

ANEURYSMS AND DISSECTIONS

An *aneurysm* is an abnormal localized dilatation of a blood vessel. Aneurysms can occur in different types of arterial vessels, but they are most common in the aorta. Once initiated, the aneurysm grows larger as the tension in the vessel wall increases. As an aneurysm increases in diameter, the tension in the wall of the vessel increases in direct proportion to its increased size. If untreated, the aneurysm may rupture because of the increased tension. Even an unruptured aneurysm can cause damage by exerting pressure on adjacent structures.

Aneurysms can assume several forms and may be classified according to their cause, location, and anatomic features (Fig. 17-10). A *berry aneurysm* consists of a small, spherical dilatation of the vessel at a bifurcation.[1,4] This type of aneurysm usually is found in the circle of Willis in the cerebral circulation. A *fusiform aneurysm* involves the entire circumference of the vessel and is characterized by a gradual and progressive dilatation of the vessel. A *saccular aneurysm* extends over part of the circumference of the vessel and appears saclike. An *aortic dissection* is a false aneurysm resulting from a tear in the intimal layer of the vessel that allows blood to enter the vessel wall, dissecting its layers to create a blood-filled cavity.

The two most common causes of aortic aneurysms are atherosclerosis and degeneration of the vessel media. However, any vessel can be affected by a wide variety of conditions that weaken the vessel wall, including congenital defects, trauma, and infections. Infection of a major artery that weakens its wall gives rise to mycotic aneurysms. They can originate from embolization or arrest of a septic embolus at some point in a vessel, usually the complication of infective endocarditis; as an extension of an adjacent suppurative process; or from circulating organisms that infect the arterial wall. In the past, syphilis was a common cause of thoracic aortic aneurysms.

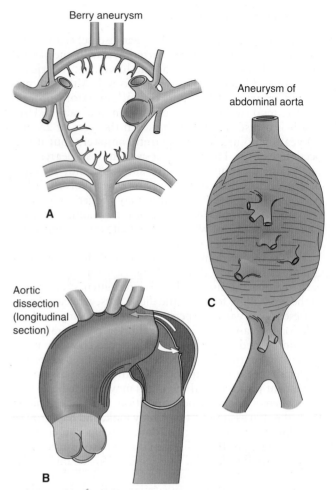

FIGURE 17-10 Three forms of aneurysm: (**A**) berry aneurysm in the circle of Willis, (**B**) aortic dissection and (**C**) fusiform-type aneurysm of the abdominal aorta.

Atherosclerosis, the most frequent etiology of aneurysms, causes arterial thinning through destruction of the vessel media that occurs secondary to plaque formation in the media. Atherosclerotic aneurysms occur most frequently in the abdominal aorta, but the common iliac artery, the aortic arch, and the descending aorta can be involved.

Abdominal Aortic Aneurysms

Abdominal aortic aneurysms usually develop after age 50 years and occur more often in men than women.[1,4] Population-based studies suggest that as many as 9% of persons older than 65 years have unsuspected and asymptomatic abdominal aortic aneurysms and that ruptured abdominal aortic aneurysms cause at least 15,000 deaths each year in the United States.[27]

Atherosclerosis is the major cause of abdominal aortic aneurysms. Although abdominal aortic aneurysms invariably occur in the context of atherosclerosis, other factors may contribute. Half of the persons with aortic aneurysms have hypertension.[4] Genetic factors may also play a role. For example, Marfan syndrome (discussed in Chapter 4) and other genetic defects in a connective tissue component can produce aneurysms and dissection.

Abdominal aortic aneurysms are located most commonly below the level of the renal artery (>90%) and involve the bifurcation of the aorta and proximal end of the common iliac arteries.[1,4] They can involve any part of the vessel circumference (saccular) or extend to involve the entire circumference (fusiform).

Clinical Features. Most abdominal aneurysms are asymptomatic. Because an aneurysm is of arterial origin, a pulsating mass may provide the first evidence of the disorder. The mass may be discovered during a routine physical examination or the affected person may complain of its presence. Calcification, which frequently exists on the wall of the aneurysm, may be detected during abdominal radiologic examination. Pain may be present and varies from mild mid-abdominal or lumbar discomfort to severe abdominal and back pain. As the aneurysm expands, it may compress the lumbar nerve roots, causing lower back pain that radiates to the posterior aspects of the legs. The aneurysm may extend to and impinge on the renal, iliac, mesenteric, or vertebral arteries that supply the spinal cord. An abdominal aneurysm also may cause erosion of vertebrae. Stasis of blood favors thrombus formation along the wall of the vessel (Fig. 17-11), and peripheral emboli may develop, causing symptomatic arterial insufficiency.

Diagnostic methods include the use of ultrasound imaging, echocardiography, computed tomographic (CT) scans, and magnetic resonance imaging (MRI). Surgical repair, in which the involved section of the aorta is replaced with a synthetic graft of woven Dacron, frequently is the treatment of choice.[27]

Aortic Dissection

Aortic dissection is an acute, life-threatening condition. It involves hemorrhage into the vessel wall with longitudinal tearing or separation (*i.e.,* dissection) of the vessel wall to form a blood-filled channel. Aortic dissections are caused by conditions that weaken or cause degenerative changes in the elastic and smooth muscle of the layers of the aorta. Unlike atherosclerotic aneurysms, aortic dissection often occurs without evidence of previous vessel dilatation.

Aortic dissection occurs principally in two groups of persons. The first group, which accounts for about 90% of cases, includes men in the 40- to 60-year-old age group with an antecedent history of hypertension.[1] The second group usually includes younger persons and is associated with connective tissue diseases, such as Marfan syndrome. Other factors that predispose to aortic dissection are congenital defects of the aortic valve (*i.e.,* bicuspid or unicuspid valve structures) and aortic coarctation.

Aortic dissection can originate anywhere along the length of the aorta. Two thirds of dissections involve

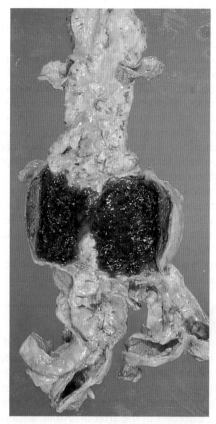

FIGURE 17-11 Atherosclerotic aneurysm of the abdominal aorta. The aneurysm has been opened longitudinally to reveal a large thrombus in the lumen. The aorta and common iliac arteries display complicated lesions of atherosclerosis. (From Gotlieb A. I. [2005]. Blood vessels. In Rubin E., Gorstein F., Rubin R., et al. [Eds.], *Rubin's pathology: Clinicopathologic foundations of medicine* [4th ed., p. 511]. Philadelphia: Lippincott Williams & Wilkins.)

the ascending aorta.[4,28] The second most common site is the thoracic aorta just distal to the origin of the subclavian artery. When the ascending aorta is involved, expansion of the wall of the aorta may impair closure of the aortic valve. There also is the risk of aortic rupture, with blood moving into the pericardium and compressing the heart. Although the length of dissection varies, it is possible for the abdominal aorta to be involved with progression into the renal, iliac, or femoral arteries.

Clinical Features. A major symptom of an aortic dissection is the abrupt presence of excruciating pain, described as "tearing" or "ripping." The location of the pain may point to the site of dissection.[4] Pain associated with dissection of the ascending aorta frequently is located in the anterior chest, and pain associated with dissection of the descending aorta often is located in the back. In the early stages, blood pressure typically is moderately or markedly elevated. Later, the blood pressure and the pulse rate become unobtainable in one or both arms as the dissection disrupts arterial flow to the arms. Syncope, hemiplegia, or paralysis of the lower extremities may occur because of occlusion of blood vessels that supply the brain or spinal cord. Heart failure may develop when the aortic valve is involved.

Diagnosis of aortic dissection is based on history and physical examination. Aortic angiography, trans-esophageal echocardiography, CT scans, and MRI studies aid in the diagnosis. The treatment may be medical or surgical. Aortic dissection is a life-threatening emergency; persons with a probable diagnosis are stabilized medically even before the diagnosis is confirmed. Two important factors that participate in propagating the dissection are high blood pressure and the steepness of the pulse wave. Without intervention, these forces continue to cause extension of the dissection. Thus, medical treatment focuses on control of hypertension and the use of drugs that lessen the force of systolic blood ejection from the heart. Surgical intervention may be indicated when there is a threat of rupture or compromise of major aortic branches.

In summary, the arterial system distributes blood to all the tissues of the body, and lesions of the arterial system exert their effects through ischemia or impaired blood flow. Hyperlipidemia, with elevated cholesterol levels, plays a major role in the development of atherosclerotic disorders of the arterial system. Because cholesterol and triglycerides are insoluble in plasma, they are transported as lipoproteins. Elevated blood levels of LDLs, which carry large amounts of cholesterol, are a major risk factor for atherosclerosis. The HDLs, which are protective, remove cholesterol from the tissues and carry it back to the liver for disposal. LDL receptors play a major role in removing cholesterol from the blood; persons with reduced numbers of LDL receptors are at particularly high risk for the development of atherosclerosis.

Atherosclerosis affects large and medium-sized arteries, such as the coronary and cerebral arteries. It has an insidious onset, and its lesions usually are far advanced before symptoms appear. Along with hyper-cholesterolemia, risk factors associated with the development of atherosclerosis include heredity, sex, and age, which are constitutional and cannot be controlled; other factors include hypertension, smoking, and type 2 diabetes, which can often be modified or controlled by a change in diet, exercise, health care practices, or medications.

The vasculitides are a group of vascular disorders characterized by inflammation and necrosis of blood vessels in various tissues and organs. They can be caused by injury, infectious agents, or immune processes, or occur secondary to disease conditions, such as systemic lupus erythematosus. Arterial disorders of the extremities include atherosclerotic occlusive disease, thromboangiitis obliterans, and Raynaud disease or phenomenon, caused by vessel spasm. These disorders produce ischemia,

pain, impaired function, and in some cases infarction and tissue necrosis.

Aneurysms are localized areas of vessel dilation caused by weakness of the arterial wall. Abdominal aortic aneurysms are the most common type of aneurysm. They are characterized by gradual and progressive enlargement of the abdominal aorta. The most serious consequence of abdominal aneurysms is rupture. Aortic dissection is an acute, life-threatening condition. It involves hemorrhage into the vessel wall with longitudinal tearing (dissection) of the vessel wall to form a blood-filled channel.

Disorders of Arterial Blood Pressure

The arterial blood pressure reflects the rhythmic ejection of blood from the left ventricle into the aorta. It rises as the left ventricle contracts and falls as it relaxes. In healthy adults, the highest pressure, called the *systolic pressure*, is ideally less than 120 mm Hg and the lowest pressure, called the *diastolic pressure*, is less than 80 mm Hg (Fig. 17-12). The difference between the systolic and diastolic pressure (approximately 40 mm Hg) is the *pulse pressure*. The pulse pressure reflects the pulsatile nature of arterial blood flow. It rises when the stroke volume is increased and falls when the resistance to outflow is decreased. The *mean arterial pressure* (approximately 90 to 100 mm Hg) represents the average pressure in the

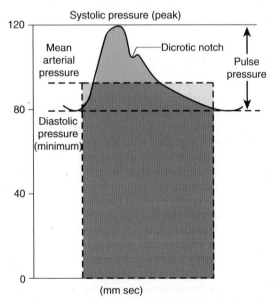

FIGURE 17-12 Intra-arterial pressure tracing made from the brachial artery. Pulse pressure is the difference between systolic and diastolic pressures. The *darker area* represents the mean arterial pressure, which can be calculated by using the formula of mean arterial pressure = diastolic pressure + pulse pressure/3.

arterial system during ventricular contraction and relaxation and is a good indicator of tissue perfusion.

The systolic and diastolic components of blood pressure are determined by the cardiac output and the peripheral vascular resistance and can be expressed as the product of the two (blood pressure = cardiac output × peripheral vascular resistance). The cardiac output is the product of the stroke volume (amount of blood ejected from the heart with each beat) and the heart rate. The peripheral vascular resistance reflects changes in the radius of the arterioles as well as the viscosity or thickness of the blood. The arterioles often are referred to as the *resistance vessels* because they can selectively constrict or relax to control the resistance to outflow of blood into the capillaries. The body maintains its blood pressure by adjusting the cardiac output to compensate for changes in peripheral vascular resistance, and it changes the peripheral vascular resistance to compensate for changes in cardiac output.

In hypertension and disease conditions that affect blood pressure, changes in blood pressure usually are described in terms of systolic, diastolic, pulse pressure, and mean arterial pressures. These pressures are influenced by the stroke volume, the rapidity with which blood is ejected from the heart, the elastic properties of the aorta and large arteries and their ability to accept various amounts of blood as it is ejected from the heart, and the properties of the resistance blood vessels that control the runoff of blood into the smaller vessels and capillaries that connect the arterial and venous circulations.

MECHANISMS OF BLOOD PRESSURE REGULATION

Although different tissues in the body are able to regulate their own blood flow, it is necessary for the arterial pressure to remain relatively constant as blood flow shifts from one area of the body to another. The method by which the arterial pressure is regulated depends on whether short-term or long-term adaptation is needed[29] (Fig. 17-13).

Short-Term Regulation

The mechanisms for short-term regulation of blood pressure, those occurring over minutes or hours, are intended to correct temporary imbalances in blood pressure, such as occur during physical exercise and changes in body position. These mechanisms also are responsible for maintenance of blood pressure at survival levels during life-threatening situations. The short-term regulation of blood

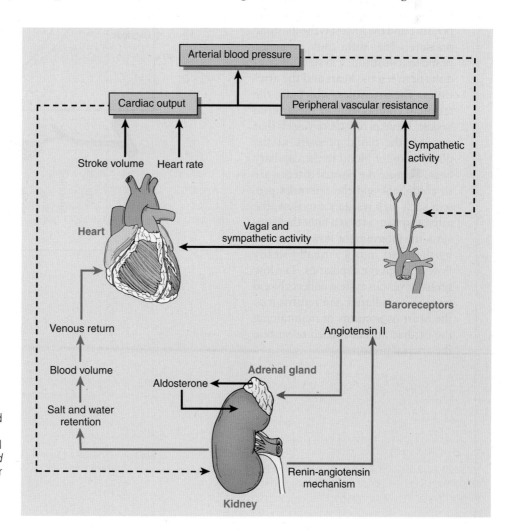

FIGURE 17-13 Mechanisms of blood pressure regulation. The *solid lines* represent the mechanisms for renal and baroreceptor control of blood pressure through changes in cardiac output and peripheral vascular resistance. The *dashed lines* represent the stimulus for regulation of blood pressure by the baroreceptors and the kidneys.

Understanding ➤ Determinants of Blood Pressure

The arterial blood pressure, which is the force that moves blood through the arterial system, reflects the intermittent contraction and relaxation of the left ventricle. It is determined by (1) the properties of the arterial system and the factors that maintain (2) the systolic and (3) the diastolic components of the blood pressure. These factors include the blood volume, elastic properties of the blood vessels, cardiac output, and peripheral vascular resistance.

1

Arterial blood pressure. The arterial blood pressure represents the force that distributes blood to the capillaries throughout the body. The highest arterial pressure is the systolic pressure and the lowest is the diastolic pressure. The aorta and its major branches constitute a system of conduits between the heart and the arterioles. The arterioles, which are the terminal components of the arterial system, serve as resistance vessels that regulate the blood pressure at the distribution of blood to the capillary beds. Because the normal arteries are so compliant and the arterioles present such high resistance to flow, the arterial system acts as a filter that converts the intermittent flow generated by the heart into a virtually steady flow through the capillaries. The low pressure venous system collects blood from the capillaries and returns it to the heart as a means of maintaining the cardiac output needed to sustain the arterial pressure.

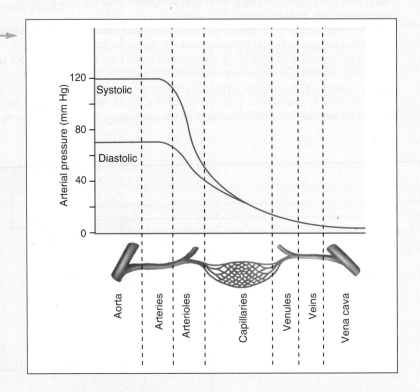

2

Systolic pressure. The systolic blood pressure reflects the amount of blood (stroke volume) that is ejected from the heart with each beat, the rate and force with which it is ejected, and the elasticity or compliance of the aorta and large arteries. The blood that is ejected from the heart during systole does not move directly through the circulation. Instead, a substantial fraction of the stroke volume is stored in large arteries. Because the walls of these vessels are elastic, they can be stretched to accommodate a large volume of blood without an appreciable change in pressure. The systolic pressure often increases with aging as the aorta and large arteries lose their elasticity and become more rigid.

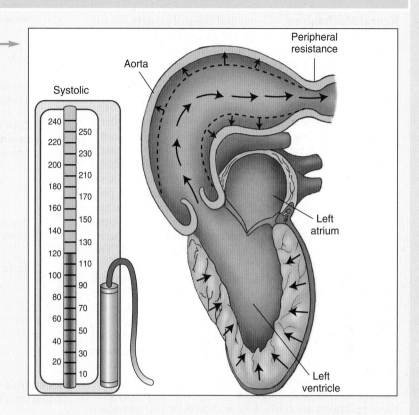

3

Diastolic pressure. The diastolic blood pressure reflects the closure of the aortic valve, the energy that has been stored in the elastic fibers of the large arteries during systole, and the resistance to flow through arterioles into the capillaries. Closure of the aortic valve at the onset of diastole and recoil of the elastic fibers in the aorta and large arteries continue to drive the blood forward, even though the heart is not pumping. These effects, largely restricted to the elastic vessels, convert the discontinuous systolic flow in the ascending aorta into a continuous flow in the peripheral arteries.

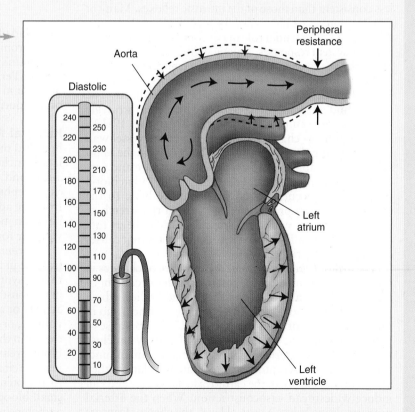

pressure relies mainly on neural and hormonal mechanisms, the most rapid of which are the neural mechanisms.

Neural Mechanisms. The neural control centers for the regulation of blood pressure are located in the reticular formation of the lower pons and medulla of the brain where integration and modulation of autonomic nervous system (ANS) responses occur. This area of the brain contains the vasomotor and cardiac control centers and is often collectively referred to as the *cardiovascular center*. The cardiovascular center transmits parasympathetic impulses to the heart through the vagus nerve and transmits sympathetic impulses to the heart and blood vessels through the spinal cord and peripheral sympathetic nerves. Vagal stimulation of the heart produces a slowing of the heart rate, whereas sympathetic stimulation produces an increase in heart rate and cardiac contractility. Blood vessels are selectively innervated by the sympathetic nervous system, with increased sympathetic activity producing constriction of the resistance vessels and decreased activity producing relaxation of the vessels.

The ANS control of blood pressure is mediated through intrinsic circulatory reflexes, extrinsic reflexes, and higher neural control centers. The intrinsic reflexes, including the *baroreceptor-* and *chemoreceptor-mediated reflexes,* are located in the circulatory system and are essential for rapid and short-term regulation of blood pressure. The sensors for extrinsic reflexes are found outside the circulation. They include blood pressure responses associated with factors such as pain and cold. The neural pathways for these reactions are more diffuse, and their responses are less consistent than those of the intrinsic reflexes. Many of these responses are channeled through the hypothalamus, which plays an essential role in the control of sympathetic nervous system responses. Among higher-center responses are those due to changes in mood and emotion.

The *baroreceptors* are pressure-sensitive receptors located in the walls of blood vessels and the heart. The carotid and aortic baroreceptors are located in strategic positions between the heart and the brain (Fig. 17-14). They respond to changes in the stretch of the vessel wall by sending impulses to cardiovascular centers in the brain stem to effect appropriate changes in heart rate and vascular smooth muscle tone. For example, the fall in blood pressure that occurs on moving from the lying to the standing position produces a decrease in the stretch of the baroreceptors with a resultant increase in heart rate and sympathetically induced vasoconstriction that causes an increase in peripheral vascular resistance.

The *arterial chemoreceptors* are sensitive to changes in the oxygen, carbon dioxide, and hydrogen ion content of the blood. They are located in the carotid bodies, which lie in the bifurcation of the two common carotids, and in the aortic bodies of the aorta (see Fig. 17-14). Because of their location, these chemoreceptors are always in close contact with the arterial blood. Although the main function of the chemoreceptors is to regulate ventilation, they also communicate with the cardiovascular center and can induce widespread vasoconstriction. When the arterial pressure drops below a critical level, the chemoreceptors are stimulated because of a diminished oxygen supply and

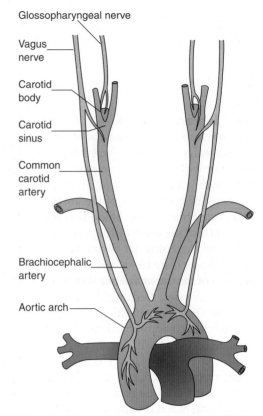

FIGURE 17-14 Location and innervation of the aortic arch and carotid sinus baroreceptors and carotid body chemoreceptors.

a buildup of carbon dioxide and hydrogen ions. In persons with chronic lung disease, systemic and pulmonary hypertension may develop because of hypoxemia (see Chapter 22). Persons with sleep apnea also may experience an increase in blood pressure because of the hypoxia that occurs during the apneic periods.

Humoral Mechanisms. A number of hormones and humoral mechanisms contribute to blood pressure regulation, including the *renin-angiotensin-aldosterone mechanism* and *vasopressin.* Other humoral substances such as epinephrine, a sympathetic neurotransmitter released from the adrenal gland, have the effect of directly stimulating an increase in heart rate, cardiac contractility, and vascular tone.

The *renin-angiotensin-aldosterone* system plays a central role in blood pressure regulation. Renin is an enzyme that is synthesized, stored, and released by the kidneys in response to an increase in sympathetic nervous system activity or a decrease in blood pressure, extracellular fluid volume, or extracellular sodium concentration. Most of the renin that is released leaves the kidney and enters the bloodstream, where it acts enzymatically to convert an inactive circulating plasma protein called *angiotensinogen* to angiotensin I (Fig. 17-15). Angiotensin I travels to the small blood vessels of the lung, where it is converted to angiotensin II by the angiotensin-converting enzyme that is present in the endothelium of the lung vessels.

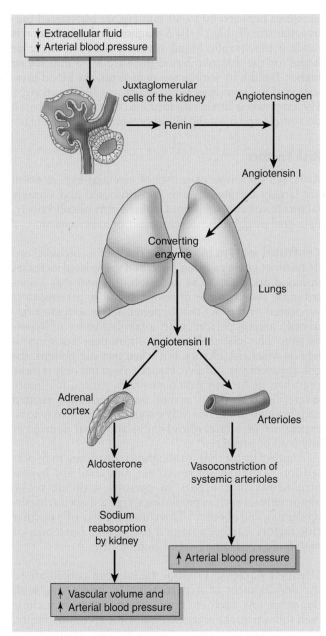

FIGURE 17-15 Control of blood pressure by the renin-angiotensin-aldosterone system. Renin enzymatically converts the plasma protein angiotensinogen to angiotensin I; angiotensin-converting enzyme in the lung converts angiotensin I to angiotensin II; and angiotensin II produces vasoconstriction and increases salt and water retention through direct action on the kidney and through increased aldosterone secretion by the adrenal cortex.

Angiotensin II functions in both the short-term and long-term regulation of blood pressure. It is a strong vasoconstrictor, particularly of arterioles and to a lesser extent of veins. The vasoconstrictor response produces an increase in peripheral vascular resistance (and blood pressure) and functions in the short-term regulation of blood pressure. A second major function of angiotensin II,

stimulation of aldosterone secretion from the adrenal gland, contributes to the long-term regulation of blood pressure by increasing sodium and water retention by the kidney. It also acts directly on the kidney to decrease the elimination of sodium and water.

Vasopressin, also known as antidiuretic hormone (ADH), is released from the posterior pituitary gland in response to decreases in blood volume and blood pressure, an increase in the osmolality of body fluids, and other stimuli (discussed in Chapter 6). Vasopressin has a direct vasoconstrictor effect on blood vessels, particularly those of the splanchnic circulation that supplies the abdominal viscera. However, long-term increases in vasopressin cannot maintain volume expansion or hypertension, and vasopressin does not enhance hypertension produced by sodium-retaining hormones or other vasoconstricting substances. It has been suggested that vasopressin plays a permissive role in hypertension through its fluid-retaining properties or as a neurotransmitter that serves to modify ANS function.

Long-Term Regulation

Long-term mechanisms, which are responsible for the daily, weekly, and monthly regulation of blood pressure, are largely vested in the kidneys and their role in regulation of extracellular fluid volume.[29] These mechanisms function largely by regulating the blood pressure around an equilibrium point, which represents the normal pressure for a given individual. Accordingly, when the body contains too much extracellular fluid, the arterial pressure rises and the rate at which water (*i.e., pressure diuresis*) and sodium (*i.e., pressure natriuresis*) are excreted by the kidney is increased.[29] When blood pressure returns to its equilibrium point, water and sodium excretion return to normal. A fall in blood pressure due to a decrease in extracellular fluid volume has the opposite effect. In persons with hypertension, renal control mechanisms are often altered such that the equilibrium point for blood pressure regulation is maintained at a higher level of sodium and water elimination.

There are several ways that extracellular fluid volume serves to regulate blood pressure. One is through a direct effect on cardiac output and renal blood flow; another is indirect, resulting from autoregulation of blood flow and its effect on peripheral vascular resistance. Autoregulatory mechanisms function in distributing blood flow to the various tissues of the body according to their metabolic needs (see Chapter 16). When the blood flow to a specific tissue bed is excessive, local blood vessels constrict, and when the flow is deficient, the local vessels dilate. In situations of increased blood volume and cardiac output, all of the tissues of the body are exposed to the same increase in flow. This results in a generalized constriction of arterioles and an increase in the peripheral vascular resistance.

The role that the kidneys play in blood pressure regulation is emphasized by the fact that many hypertension medications produce their blood pressure–lowering effects by increasing sodium and water elimination.

ESSENTIAL HYPERTENSION

Hypertension, or high blood pressure, is probably the most common of all health problems in adults and is the leading risk factor for cardiovascular disorders. It affects approximately 50 million individuals in the United States and approximately 1 billion worldwide.[30] Hypertension is more common in younger men compared with younger women, in blacks compared with whites, in persons from lower socioeconomic groups, and in older persons. Men have higher blood pressures than women up until the time of menopause, at which point women quickly lose their protection. The prevalence of hypertension increases with age. Recent data from the Framingham Study suggest that persons who are normotensive at age 55 years have a 90% lifetime risk of developing hypertension.[31] Thus, the problem of hypertension can be expected to become even greater with the aging of the "baby boomer" population.

Hypertension commonly is divided into the categories of primary and secondary hypertension. In primary, or *essential*, hypertension, the chronic elevation of blood pressure occurs without evidence of other disease. Primary hypertension accounts for 90% to 95% of hypertension. In secondary hypertension, the elevation of blood pressure results from some other disorder, such as kidney disease.

The seventh report of the Joint National Committee on Detection, Evaluation, and Treatment of High Blood Pressure (JNC-7) of the National Institutes of Health was published in 2003.[30] According to the JNC-7 recommendations, a systolic pressure of less than 120 mm Hg and diastolic pressure less than 80 mm Hg are normal and systolic pressures between 120 to 139 mm Hg or diastolic pressures between 80 to 89 mm Hg are considered prehypertensive (Table 17-4). A diagnosis of hypertension is made if the systolic blood pressure is 140 mm Hg or higher or the diastolic blood pressure is 90 mm Hg or higher. For adults with diabetes mellitus, the blood pressure goal has been lowered to less than 130/80 mm Hg.[32] Hypertension is further divided into stages 1 and 2 based on systolic and diastolic blood pressure measurements.

Risk Factors

Although the cause or causes of essential hypertension are largely unknown, both constitutional and lifestyle factors have been implicated, either singly or collectively, in contributing to the development of hypertension.

Constitutional Factors. These risk factors include family history of hypertension, race, and age-related increases in blood pressure.[33] The inclusion of heredity as a contributing factor in the development of hypertension is supported by the fact that hypertension is seen most frequently among persons with a family history of hypertension. The inherited predisposition does not seem to rely on other risk factors, but when they are present, the risk apparently is additive. Hypertension not only is more prevalent in African Americans than whites, it is more severe, tends to occur earlier, and often is not treated early enough or aggressively enough. Blacks also tend to experience greater cardiovascular and renal damage at any level of pressure.[34]

Another factor that is thought to contribute to hypertension is the insulin resistance and resultant hyperinsulinemia that occurs in persons with metabolic abnormalities such as prediabetes, type 2 diabetes, hyperlipidemias, and obesity.[35] This clustering of cardiovascular risk factors has been named the *insulin resistance* or *metabolic syndrome*[36] (see Chapter 32).

Lifestyle Factors. Lifestyle factors can contribute to the development of hypertension by interacting with the other risk factors. These lifestyle factors include high sodium intake, excessive calorie intake and obesity, physical inactivity, and excessive alcohol consumption. Oral contraceptive drugs also may increase blood pressure in predisposed women. Although stress can raise blood pressure acutely, there is less evidence linking it to chronic elevations in blood pressure. Dietary fats and cholesterol are independent risk factors for cardiovascular disease, but there is no evidence that they raise blood pressure. Smoking, although not identified as a primary risk factor in hypertension, is an independent risk factor in CHD and should be avoided. Sleep apnea, with its attendant periods of hypoxia, has recently been added to the list of risk factors for hypertension.

Increased sodium intake has long been implicated as an etiologic factor in the development of hypertension.[30,37,38] Just how increased sodium intake contributes to the development of hypertension is still unclear. It may be that sodium produces an expansion of the extracellular fluid volume, increases the sensitivity of cardiovascular or

---

⏻ KEY CONCEPTS

Hypertension

→ Essential hypertension is characterized by a chronic elevation in blood pressure that occurs without evidence of other disease, and secondary hypertension by an elevation of blood pressure that results from some other disorder, such as kidney disease.

→ The pathogenesis of essential hypertension is thought to reside with the kidney and its role regulating vascular volume through salt and water elimination; the renin-angiotensin-aldosterone system through its effects on blood vessel tone, regulation of renal blood flow, and salt metabolism; and the sympathetic nervous system, which regulates the tone of the resistance vessels.

→ Uncontrolled hypertension increases the work demands on the heart, resulting in left ventricular hypertrophy and heart failure, and on the vessels of the arterial system, leading to atherosclerosis, kidney disease, and stroke.

TABLE 17-4	Classification of Blood Pressure for Adults	
Blood Pressure Classification	Systolic Blood Pressure (mm Hg)	Diastolic Blood Pressure (mm Hg)
Normal	<120	and <80
Prehypertensive	120–139	or 80–89
Stage 1 hypertension	140–159	or 90–99
Stage 2 hypertension	≥160	or ≥100

Modified from National Heart, Lung, and Blood Institute (2003): *The seventh report of the National Committee on Detection, Evaluation, and Treatment of High Blood Pressure.* NIH publication no. 03–5233. Bethesda, MD: NIH.

renal mechanisms to sympathetic nervous system stimuli, or exerts its effects through some other mechanisms such as the renin-angiotensin-aldosterone system.

Excessive weight commonly is associated with hypertension.[39] It has been suggested that fat distribution might be a more critical indicator of hypertension risk than actual overweight (see Chapter 8). The waist-to-hip ratio commonly is used to differentiate central or upper body obesity (*i.e.,* fat cell deposits in the abdomen) from peripheral or lower body obesity (*i.e.,* fat cell deposits in the buttocks and legs).

Regular alcohol consumption can play a role in the development of hypertension. The effect is seen with different types of alcoholic beverages, in men and women, and in a variety of ethnic groups.[40] Systolic pressure is usually more markedly affected than diastolic pressure. Blood pressure may improve or return to normal when alcohol consumption is decreased or eliminated.

Oral contraceptives cause a mild increase in blood pressure in many women and overt hypertension in approximately 5%.[41] Various contraceptive drugs contain different amounts and combinations of estrogen and progestational agents, and these differences may contribute to the occurrence of hypertension in some women but not others. Fortunately, the hypertension associated with oral contraceptives usually disappears after use of the drug has been discontinued, although it may take as long as 6 months for this to happen. However, in some women, the blood pressure may not return to normal; they may be at risk for hypertension. The risk of hypertension-associated cardiovascular complications is found primarily in women older than 35 years of age and in those who smoke.[30]

Manifestations

Essential hypertension is typically an asymptomatic disorder. When symptoms do occur, they usually are related to the long-term effects of hypertension on the organ systems of the body, including the kidneys, heart, eyes, and blood vessels. The 2003 JNC-7 report uses the term *target-organ damage* to describe the heart, brain, peripheral vascular, kidney, and retinal complications associated with hypertension[30] (Chart 17-2). The excess morbidity and mortality related to hypertension is progressive over the entire range of elevated systolic and diastolic pressures. Target-organ damage varies markedly among persons with similar levels of hypertension.

Hypertension is a major risk factor for atherosclerosis; it predisposes to all major atherosclerotic cardiovascular disorders, including heart failure, stroke, coronary artery disease, and peripheral artery disease. The risk of coronary artery disease and stroke depends to a great extent on other risk factors such as obesity, smoking, and elevated cholesterol levels. Cerebrovascular complications are more closely related to systolic than diastolic hypertension. The incidence of these complications is greatly reduced by antihypertensive therapy.

Hypertension increases the workload of the left ventricle by increasing the pressure against which the heart must pump as it ejects blood into the systemic circulation. As the workload of the heart increases, the left ventricular wall hypertrophies to compensate for the increased pressure work.[42] The prevalence of left ventricular hypertrophy increases with age and is highest in persons with blood pressures over 160/95 mm Hg. Despite its adaptive advantage, left ventricular hypertrophy is a major risk factor for ischemic heart disease, cardiac arrhythmias, sudden death, and congestive heart failure. Hypertensive left ventricular hypertrophy usually regresses with therapy. Regression is most closely related to systolic pressure reduction and does not appear to reflect the particular type of medication used.

CHART 17-2

Target Organ Damage

Heart
- Left ventricular hypertrophy
- Angina or prior myocardial infarction
- Prior coronary revascularization
- Heart failure

Brain
- Stroke or transient ischemic attack

Chronic kidney disease

Peripheral vascular disease

Retinopathy

National Heart, Lung, and Blood Institute. (2003): *The seventh report of the National Committee on Detection, Evaluation, and Treatment of High Blood Pressure.* NIH publication no. 03–5233. Bethesda, MD: NIH.

Hypertension also can lead to nephrosclerosis, a common cause of renal insufficiency (see Chapter 24). Hypertensive kidney disease is more common in blacks than whites. Hypertension also plays an important role in accelerating the course of other types of kidney disease, particularly diabetic nephropathy.[32]

Diagnosis and Treatment

Unlike disorders of organ structure that are diagnosed by methods such as x-rays and tissue examination, hypertension and other blood pressure disorders are determined by repeated blood pressure measurement. Laboratory tests, x-ray films, and other diagnostic tests usually are done to exclude secondary hypertension and determine the presence or extent of target-organ disease.

Blood pressure measurements that are used in the diagnosis and follow-up treatment of hypertension are usually obtained by the auscultatory method, which uses a sphygmomanometer and a stethoscope (automated systems may be used for self-monitoring of blood pressure in persons with hypertension). Accuracy of the measurements requires that persons taking the pressure are adequately trained in blood pressure measurement, the equipment is properly maintained and calibrated, and the cuff bladder is appropriate for the arm size.[43] The width of the bladder should be at least 40% of arm circumference and the length at least 80% of arm circumference. Undercuffing (using a cuff with a bladder that is too small) can cause an overestimation of blood pressure.[44] This is because a cuff that is too small results in an uneven distribution of pressure across the arm, such that a greater cuff pressure is needed to occlude blood flow. Likewise, overcuffing (using a cuff with a bladder that is too large) can cause an underestimation of blood pressure.

The JNC-7 report emphasizes that obtaining one elevated blood pressure reading should not constitute the diagnosis of hypertension. The diagnosis of hypertension in a person who is not taking antihypertensive medications should be based on the average of at least two or more blood pressure readings taken at each of two or more visits after an initial screening visit.[30] Blood pressure measurements should be taken when the person is relaxed and has rested for at least 5 minutes and has not smoked or ingested caffeine within 30 minutes. Because blood pressure in many individuals is highly variable, blood pressure should be measured on different occasions over a period of several months before a diagnosis of hypertension is made unless the pressure is extremely elevated or associated with symptoms.

The main objective for treatment of essential hypertension is to achieve and maintain arterial blood pressure of less than 140/90 mm Hg, with the goal of preventing morbidity and mortality. For persons with secondary hypertension, efforts are made to correct or control the disease condition causing the hypertension. Antihypertensive medications and other measures supplement the treatment for the underlying disease. The JNC-7 report contains a treatment algorithm for hypertension that includes lifestyle modification and, when necessary, guidelines for the use of pharmacologic agents to achieve and maintain systolic pressure below 140 mm Hg and diastolic pressure below 90 mm Hg.[30]

Lifestyle Modification. Lifestyle modification has been shown to reduce blood pressure, enhance antihypertensive drug therapy, and prevent cardiovascular risk. Major lifestyle modifications shown to lower blood pressure include weight reduction in persons who are overweight or obese, regular physical activity, adoption of the Dietary Approaches to Stop Hypertension (DASH) eating plan, reduction of dietary sodium intake, and moderation of alcohol intake[30] (Table 17-5).

Pharmacologic Treatment. The decision to initiate pharmacologic treatment is based on the severity of the hypertension, the presence of target-organ disease, and

TABLE 17-5	Lifestyle Modifications to Manage Hypertension[*][†]	
Modification	**Recommendation**	**Approximate Systolic Blood Pressure Reduction (mm HG)**
Weight reduction	Maintain normal body weight (BMI, 18.5–24.9 kg/m^2)	5–20 mm Hg/10 kg weight loss
Adopt DASH eating plan	Consume a diet rich in fruits, vegetables, and low-fat diary products with a reduced content of saturated and total fat	8–14 mm Hg
Dietary sodium reduction	Reduce dietary sodium intake to no more than 100 mmol per day (2.4 g sodium or 6 g sodium chloride)	2–8 mm Hg
Physical activity	Engage in regular aerobic physical activity such as brisk walking (at least 30 minutes per day, most days of the week)	4–9 mm Hg
Moderation of alcohol consumption	Limit consumption to no more than 2 drinks (1 oz or 30 mL ethanol; e.g., 24 oz beer, 10 oz wine, or 3 oz 80-proof whiskey) per day in most men and 1 drink per day in women and lighter-weight persons	2–4 mm Hg

DASH, Dietary Approaches to Stop Hypertension; BMI, body mass index.
[*]For overall cardiovascular reduction, stop smoking.
[†]The effects of implementing these modifications is dose and time dependent, and could be greater for some individuals.
From National Heart, Lung, and Blood Institute. (2003): *The seventh report of the National Committee on Detection, Evaluation, and Treatment of High Blood Pressure.* NIH publication no. 03–5233. Bethesda, MD: NIH.

the existence of other conditions and risk factors. Drug selection is based on the stage of hypertension. Among the drugs used in the treatment of hypertension are diuretics, β-adrenergic receptor blockers, angiotensin-converting enzyme (ACE) inhibitors or angiotensin II receptor blockers, the calcium channel blockers, central α$_2$-adrenergic agonists, α$_1$-adrenergic receptor blockers, and vasodilators.

The physiologic mechanisms whereby the different antihypertension drugs produce a reduction in blood pressure differ among agents. Diuretics lower blood pressure initially by decreasing vascular volume (by suppressing renal reabsorption of sodium and increasing sodium and water excretion) and cardiac output. With continued therapy, a reduction in peripheral resistance becomes a major mechanism of blood pressure reduction. The β-adrenergic blockers are effective in treating hypertension because they decrease heart rate, cardiac output, and renin release by the kidney. The ACE inhibitors act by inhibiting the conversion of angiotensin I to angiotensin II, thus decreasing angiotensin II levels and reducing its effect on vasoconstriction, aldosterone levels, intrarenal blood flow, and glomerular filtration rate. The calcium channel blockers decrease peripheral vascular resistance by inhibiting the movement of calcium into arterial smooth muscle cells. The centrally acting α$_2$-adrenergic agonists act in a negative-feedback manner to decrease sympathetic outflow from the central nervous system. The α$_1$-adrenergic receptor antagonists block α$_1$ receptors on vascular smooth muscle, causing vasodilatation and a reduction in peripheral vascular resistance. The direct-acting smooth muscle vasodilators promote a decrease in peripheral vascular resistance by producing relaxation of vascular smooth muscle, particularly of the arterioles.

Pharmacologic treatment of hypertension usually follows a stepwise approach.[30] It is usually initiated with a low dose of a single drug. The dose is slowly increased at a schedule dependent on the person's age, needs, and desired response. If the response to the initial drug is not adequate, one of three approaches can be used: the dose can be increased if the initial dose was below the maximum recommended; a drug with a different mode of action can be added; or the initial drug can be discontinued and another substituted. Combining drugs with different modes of action often allows smaller doses to be used to achieve blood pressure control, while minimizing the dose-dependent side effects from any one drug.

Systolic Hypertension

Essential hypertension may be classified as systolic/diastolic hypertension in which both the systolic and diastolic pressures are elevated; as diastolic hypertension in which the diastolic pressure is selectively elevated; or as systolic hypertension in which the systolic pressure is selectively elevated. The JNC-7 report defined systolic hypertension as a systolic pressure of 140 mm Hg or greater and a diastolic pressure of less than 90 mm Hg, indicating a need for increased recognition and control of isolated systolic hypertension.[30] Historically, diastolic hypertension was thought to confer a greater risk for cardiovascular events than systolic hypertension.[30] However, there is mounting evidence that elevated systolic blood pressure is at least as important, if not more so, than diastolic hypertension.[45]

There are two aspects of systolic hypertension that confer increased risk of cardiovascular events—one is the actual elevation in systolic pressure and the other is the disproportionate rise in pulse pressure. Elevated pressures during systole favor the development of left ventricular hypertrophy, increased myocardial oxygen demands, and eventual left heart failure. At the same time, the absolute or relative lowering of diastolic pressure is a limiting factor in coronary perfusion because coronary perfusion is greatest during diastole. Elevated pulse pressures produce greater stretch of arteries, causing damage to the elastic elements of the vessel and thus predisposing to aneurysms and development of the endothelial cell damage that leads to atherosclerosis and thrombosis.

SECONDARY HYPERTENSION

Only 5% to 10% of hypertensive cases are classified as secondary hypertension (*i.e.*, hypertension due to another disease condition). Unlike essential hypertension, many of the conditions causing secondary hypertension can be corrected or cured by surgery or specific medical treatment. Secondary hypertension tends to be seen more commonly in persons younger than 30 years and those older than 50 years of age.[46] Among the most common causes of secondary hypertension are kidney disease (*i.e.*, renovascular hypertension), adrenocortical disorders, pheochromocytoma, and coarctation of the aorta. Cocaine and cocaine-like substances also can cause significant hypertension.

Renal Hypertension

With the dominant role that the kidney assumes in blood pressure regulation, it is not surprising that the largest single cause of secondary hypertension is renal disease. Hypertension is present in more than 80% of patients with chronic renal failure and is a major factor associated with their increased cardiovascular risk. Most acute kidney disorders result in decreased urine formation, retention of sodium and water, and hypertension. This includes acute glomerulonephritis, acute renal failure, and acute urinary tract obstruction. Hypertension also is common among persons with chronic pyelonephritis, polycystic kidney disease, diabetic nephropathy, and end-stage renal disease, regardless of cause.

Renovascular hypertension refers to hypertension caused by reduced renal blood flow and activation of the renin-angiotensin-aldosterone mechanism. It is the most common cause of secondary hypertension, accounting for 1% to 2% of all cases of hypertension.[47] The reduced renal blood flow that occurs with renovascular disease causes the affected kidney to release excessive amounts of renin, increasing circulating levels of angiotensin II. Angiotensin II, in turn, acts as a vasoconstrictor to increase peripheral vascular resistance and as a stimulus for increasing aldosterone levels and sodium retention by the kidney. One or both of the kidneys may be affected. Manifestations of renovascular hypertension include hypokalemia (caused by increased aldosterone levels), the presence of an abdominal bruit, and duration of hypertension of less than 1 year (to help distinguish renovascular hypertension from essential hypertension).

Diagnostic tests for renovascular hypertension may include studies to assess overall kidney function, physiologic studies to assess the renin-angiotensin system, perfusion studies to assess renal blood flow, and imaging studies to identify renal artery stenosis.[47] The goal of treatment is to control the blood pressure and stabilize renal function. Angioplasty or revascularization has been shown to be an effective long-term treatment for the disorder. ACE inhibitors may be used in medical management of renal stenosis. Because renal blood flow depends on increased blood pressure generated by the angiotensin-aldosterone system, these agents must be used with caution.

Disorders of Adrenocorticosteroid Hormones

Excess production of aldosterone caused by adrenocortical hyperplasia or adenoma (primary hyperaldosteronism) and excess levels of glucocorticoid (Cushing disease or syndrome) tend to raise the blood pressure (see Chapter 31). These hormones produce hypertension through increased sodium and water retention by the kidney. For persons with primary hyperaldosteronism, a sodium-restricted diet often produces a reduction in blood pressure. Because aldosterone acts on the distal renal tubule to increase sodium absorption in exchange for potassium elimination in the urine, persons with hyperaldosteronism usually have decreased potassium levels. Potassium-sparing diuretics, such as spironolactone, which is an aldosterone antagonist, often are used in the treatment of the disorder.

Pheochromocytoma

A pheochromocytoma is a tumor of chromaffin tissue, which contains sympathetic nerve cells. The tumor is most commonly located in the adrenal medulla but can arise in other sites, such as sympathetic ganglia, where there is chromaffin tissue.[48] Although only 0.1% to 0.5% of persons with hypertension have an underlying pheochromocytoma, the disorder can cause serious hypertensive crises. Eight percent to 10% of the tumors are malignant.

Like adrenal medullary cells, the tumor cells of a pheochromocytoma produce and secrete the catecholamines epinephrine and norepinephrine. The hypertension that develops is the result of a massive release of these catecholamines. Their release may be paroxysmal rather than continuous, causing periodic episodes of headache, excessive sweating, and palpitations. Headache is the most common symptom and can be quite severe. Nervousness, tremor, facial pallor, weakness, fatigue, and weight loss occur less frequently. Marked

variability in blood pressure between episodes is typical. Some persons with pheochromocytoma have paroxysmal episodes of hypertension, sometimes to dangerously high levels; others may have sustained hypertension; and some may even be normotensive.

Diagnostic methods include urinary and blood assays for catecholamines and their metabolites and CT and MRI imaging studies to locate tumors and possible metastases. Surgical removal of the tumor or tumors is the treatment of choice.

Coarctation of the Aorta

Coarctation of the aorta represents a narrowing of the aorta just distal to the origin of the subclavian arteries[49] (see Chapter 18). The ejection of a large stroke volume into a narrowed aorta results in an increase in systolic blood pressure and blood flow to the upper part of the body. Blood pressure in the lower extremities may be normal, although it frequently is low. It has been suggested that the increase in cardiac output and maintenance of the pressure to the lower part of the body is achieved through the renin-angiotensin-aldosterone mechanism in response to a decrease in renal blood flow.

Coarctation of the aorta should be considered as a cause of secondary hypertension in young people with an elevation in blood pressure. Because the aortic capacity is diminished in coarctation of the aorta, there usually is a marked increase in pressure (measured in the arms) during exercise, when the stroke volume and heart rate are exaggerated. Pulse pressure in the legs almost always is narrowed, and the femoral pulses are weak. It is important that blood pressure be measured in both arms and one leg when coarctation of the aorta is suspected. A pressure in the arms 20 mm Hg or more higher than in the legs suggests coarctation of the aorta. Surgical correction of the defect is the treatment of choice and is most effective when done at a young age.

Malignant Hypertension

A small number of persons with secondary hypertension develop an accelerated and potentially fatal form of the disease: malignant hypertension.[50] This usually is a disease of young persons, particularly young African-American men, women with hypertension of pregnancy, and persons with renal and collagen diseases.

Malignant hypertension is characterized by sudden marked elevations in blood pressure (diastolic values >120 mm Hg), renal disorders, vascular changes, and retinopathy. There may be intense arterial spasm of the cerebral arteries with hypertensive encephalopathy. Cerebral vasoconstriction probably is an exaggerated homeostatic response designed to protect the brain from excesses of blood pressure and flow. The regulatory mechanisms often are insufficient to protect the capillaries, and cerebral edema frequently develops. As it advances, papilledema (*i.e.,* swelling of the optic nerve at its point of entrance into the eye) ensues, giving evidence of the effects of pressure on the optic nerve and retinal vessels. The patient may have headache, restlessness, confusion, stupor, motor and sensory deficits, and visual disturbances. In severe cases, convulsions and coma follow.

The complications associated with a hypertensive crisis demand immediate and rigorous medical treatment in an intensive care unit with continuous monitoring of arterial blood pressure. With proper therapy, the death rate from this cause can be markedly reduced, as can the potential for additional episodes. Because chronic hypertension is associated with autoregulatory changes in cerebral blood flow, care is taken to avoid excessively rapid decreases in blood pressure, which can lead to cerebral hypoperfusion and brain injury.

HYPERTENSION IN SPECIAL POPULATIONS

 Hypertension During Pregnancy

Hypertensive disorders complicate about 10% of all pregnancies. Of these, approximately one third are caused by chronic hypertension and two thirds are due to preeclampsia. After embolism, they are the second leading cause of maternal mortality in the United States, accounting for almost 15% of such deaths. They also contribute to stillbirths and neonatal morbidity and mortality. The incidence of hypertensive disorders of pregnancy increases with maternal age and is greater in African-American than Caucasian women.[51]

Classification. The National Institutes of Health Working Group Report on High Blood Pressure in Pregnancy published a revised classification system for high blood pressure in pregnancy that included preeclampsia-eclampsia, preeclampsia superimposed on chronic hypertension, chronic hypertension, and gestational hypertension[52] (Table 17-6).

Preeclampsia-eclampsia is a pregnancy-specific syndrome. It is determined by an increased blood pressure (gestational blood pressure elevation [systolic pressure >140 mm Hg or diastolic pressure >90 mm Hg]) accompanied by proteinuria (excretion of ≥0.3 g protein in 24

hours) developing after the 20th week of gestation. The presence of systolic pressure of 160 mm Hg or more or diastolic pressure of 110 mm Hg or more; proteinuria (≥2.0 g/24 hours); increased serum creatinine (>1.2 mg/dL); platelet counts of less than 100,000 cells/mm³; elevated liver enzymes; persistent headache or cerebral or visual disturbances; and persistent epigastric pain serve to increase the certainty of the diagnosis.[52] Preeclampsia may occur in women who already are hypertensive, in which case the prognosis for the mother and fetus tends to be worse than for either condition alone.[52] Eclampsia is the occurrence, in a woman with preeclampsia, of seizures that cannot be attributed to other causes.

Preeclampsia occurs primarily during first pregnancies and during subsequent pregnancies in women with multiple fetuses, diabetes mellitus, or coexisting renal disease. It is associated with a condition called a *hydatidiform mole* (*i.e.,* abnormal pregnancy caused by a pathologic ovum, resulting in a mass of cysts). Women with chronic hypertension who become pregnant have an increased risk of preeclampsia and adverse neonatal outcomes, particularly when associated with proteinuria early in pregnancy.

Pregnancy-induced hypertension is thought to involve a decrease in placental blood flow, leading to the release of toxic mediators that alter the function of endothelial cells in blood vessels throughout the body, including those of the kidney, brain, liver, and heart.[51] Endothelial cell changes result in signs and symptoms of preeclampsia and, in more severe cases, of intravascular clotting and hypoperfusion of vital organs. There is risk for development of disseminated intravascular coagulation (see Chapter 10), cerebral hemorrhage, hepatic failure, and acute renal failure. Thrombocytopenia is the most common hematologic complication of preeclampsia. Platelet counts less than 100,000/mm³ signal serious disease. The cause of thrombocytopenia has been ascribed to platelet deposition at the site of endothelial injury. The renal changes that occur with preeclampsia include a decrease in glomerular filtration rate and renal blood flow. Sodium excretion may be impaired, although this is variable. Edema may or may not be present. Some of the most severe forms of preeclampsia occur in the absence of edema. Even when there is extensive edema, the plasma volume usually is

TABLE 17-6	Classification of High Blood Pressure in Pregnancy
Classification	**Description**
Gestational hypertension	Blood pressure elevation (systolic >140 and diastolic >90 mm Hg), without proteinuria, that is detected for the first time during midpregnancy and returns to normal by 12 weeks postpartum.
Chronic hypertension	Blood pressure ≥140 mm Hg systolic or ≥90 mm Hg diastolic that is present and observable before the 20th week of pregnancy. Hypertension that is diagnosed for the first time during pregnancy and does not resolve after pregnancy also is classified as chronic hypertension.
Preeclampsia–eclampsia	Pregnancy-specific syndrome of blood pressure elevation (blood pressure >140 mm Hg systolic or >90 mm Hg diastolic) that occurs after the first 20 weeks of pregnancy and is accompanied by proteinuria (urinary excretion of ≥0.3 g protein in a 24-hour specimen).
Preeclampsia superimposed on chronic hypertension	Chronic hypertension (blood pressure ≥140 mm Hg systolic or ≥90 mm Hg diastolic prior to 20th week of pregnancy) with superimposed proteinuria and with or without signs of the preeclampsia syndrome.

Developed using information from National Institutes of Health. 2000: *Working group report on high blood pressure in pregnancy.* NIH publication no. 00–3029. Bethesda, MD: Author. Available: www.nhlbi.nih.gov/health/prof/heart/hbp/hbp_preg.htm)

lower than that seen in normal pregnancy. Liver damage, when it occurs, may range from mild hepatocellular necrosis with elevation of liver enzymes to the more ominous hemolysis, elevated liver function tests, and low platelet count (HELLP) syndrome that is associated with significant maternal mortality. Eclampsia, the convulsive stage of preeclampsia, is a significant cause of maternal mortality. The pathogenesis of eclampsia remains unclear and has been attributed to both increased coagulability and fibrin deposition in the cerebral vessels.

Chronic hypertension is considered as hypertension that is unrelated to the pregnancy. It is defined as a history of high blood pressure before pregnancy, identification of hypertension before 20 weeks of pregnancy, and hypertension that persists after pregnancy.[52] In women with chronic hypertension, blood pressure often decreases in early pregnancy and increases during the last trimester (3 months) of pregnancy, resembling preeclampsia. Women with chronic hypertension are at increased risk for the development of preeclampsia.

Gestational hypertension represents a blood pressure elevation without proteinuria that is detected for the first time after mid-pregnancy. It includes women with preeclampsia syndrome who have not yet manifested proteinuria, as well as women who do not have the syndrome. The final determination that a woman does not have the preeclampsia syndrome is made only postpartum. If preeclampsia has not developed and blood pressure has returned to normal by 12 weeks postpartum, the condition is considered to be gestational hypertension.[52] If blood pressure elevation persists, a diagnosis of chronic hypertension is made.

Diagnosis and Treatment. Early prenatal care is important in the detection of high blood pressure during pregnancy. It is recommended that all pregnant women, including those with hypertension, refrain from alcohol and tobacco use. Sodium restriction usually is not recommended during pregnancy because pregnant women with hypertension tend to have lower plasma volumes than do normotensive pregnant women and because the severity of hypertension may reflect the degree of volume contraction. The exception is women with preexisting hypertension who have been following a sodium-restricted diet.

In women with preeclampsia, delivery of the fetus is curative. The timing of delivery becomes a difficult decision in preterm pregnancies because the welfare of both the mother and the infant must be taken into account. Bed rest is a traditional therapy. Antihypertensive medications, when required, must be carefully chosen because of their potential effects on uteroplacental blood flow and on the fetus. For example, the ACE inhibitors can cause injury and even death of the fetus when given during the second and third trimesters of pregnancy.

 Hypertension in Children

Blood pressure is known to increase from infancy to late adolescence. The average systolic pressure at 1 day of age is approximately 70 mm Hg and increases to approximately 85 mm Hg at 1 month of age.[53] Systolic blood pressure continues to increase with physical growth to about 120 mm Hg at the end of adolescence. During the preschool years, blood pressure begins to follow a pattern that tends to be maintained as the child grows older. This pattern continues into adolescence and adulthood, suggesting that the roots of essential hypertension have their origin early in life. A familial influence on blood pressure often can be identified early in life. Children of parents with high blood pressure tend to have higher blood pressures than do children with normotensive parents.

Blood pressure norms for children are based on age, height, and gender-specific percentiles[54] (Table 17-7). The National High Blood Pressure Education Program (NHBPEP) first published its recommendations in 1977. The fourth Task Force report (published in 2004) recommended classification of blood pressure (systolic or diastolic) for age, height, and gender into four categories: normal (less than the 90th percentile), high normal (between the 90th to 95th percentiles), stage 1 hypertension (between the 95th to 99th percentiles plus 5 mm Hg), and stage 2 hypertension (greater than the 99th percentile plus 5 mm Hg). The height percentile is determined by using the newly revised Centers for Disease Control and Prevention (CDC) growth charts.[55] As with the JNC-7 report, high normal is now considered as "prehypertensive" and is an indication for lifestyle modification. Children and adolescents with hypertension should be evaluated for target-organ damage.[54]

Secondary hypertension is the most common form of high blood pressure in infants and children. In later childhood and adolescence, essential hypertension is more common. Approximately 75% to 80% of secondary hypertension in children is caused by kidney abnormalities.[56] Coarctation of the aorta is another cause of hypertension in children and adolescents. Endocrine causes of hypertension, such as pheochromocytoma and adrenal cortical disorders, are rare. Hypertension in infants is associated most commonly with high umbilical catheterization and renal artery obstruction caused by thrombosis.[56] Most cases of essential hypertension are associated with obesity or a family history of hypertension.

A number of drugs of abuse, therapeutic agents, and toxins also may increase blood pressure. Alcohol should be considered as a risk factor in adolescents. Oral contraceptives may be a cause of hypertension in adolescent girls. The nephrotoxicity of the drug cyclosporine, an immunosuppressant used in transplant therapy, may cause hypertension in children (and adults) after bone marrow, heart, kidney, or liver transplantation. The coadministration of corticosteroid drugs appears to increase the incidence of hypertension.

Diagnosis and Treatment. The NHBPEP Task Force recommended that children 3 years of age through adolescence should have their blood pressure taken once each year. The auscultatory method using a cuff that is an appropriate size for the child's upper arm is recommended.[54] Repeated measurements over time, rather than a single isolated determination, are required to establish consistent and significant observations. Children with

TABLE 17-7	The 90th and 95th Percentiles of Systolic and Diastolic Blood Pressure for Boys and Girls 1 to 16 Years of Age by Percentiles for Height							
		Height Percentile for Boys				**Height Percentile for Girls**			
Blood Pressure Percentile	**Age (yrs)**	**5th**	**25th**	**75th**	**95th**	**5th**	**25th**	**75th**	**95th**
Systolic Pressure									
90th	1	94	97	100	103	97	98	101	103
95th		98	101	104	106	100	102	105	107
90th	3	100	103	107	109	100	102	104	106
95th		104	107	110	113	104	105	108	110
90th	6	105	108	111	113	104	106	109	111
95th		109	112	115	117	108	110	113	115
90th	10	111	114	117	119	112	114	116	118
95th		115	117	121	123	116	117	120	122
90th	13	117	120	124	126	117	119	122	124
95th		121	124	128	130	121	123	126	128
90th	16	125	128	131	134	121	123	126	128
95th		129	132	135	137	125	127	130	132
Diastolic Pressure									
90th	1	49	51	53	54	52	53	55	56
95th		54	55	58	58	56	57	59	60
90th	3	59	60	62	63	61	62	64	65
95th		63	64	66	67	65	66	68	69
90th	6	68	69	71	72	68	69	70	72
95th		72	73	75	76	72	73	74	76
90th	10	73	74	76	78	73	73	75	76
95th		77	79	81	82	77	77	79	80
90th	13	75	76	78	79	76	76	78	79
95th		79	80	82	83	80	80	82	83
90th	16	78	79	81	82	78	79	81	82
95th		82	83	85	87	82	83	85	86

*The height percentile is determined by using the newly revised CDC growth charts. Blood pressure levels are based on new data from the 1999–2000 National Health and Nutritional Examination Survey (NHANES) that have been added to the childhood BP database.
From the National High Blood Pressure Education Program Working Group on High Blood Pressure in Children and Adults. (2004). Fourth report on the Diagnosis, Evaluation, and Treatment of High Blood Pressure in Children and Adolescents. *Pediatrics* 114, 555–576. [On-line]. Available: www.pediatrics.org/cgi/content/full/114/2/S2/555.

high blood pressure should be referred for medical evaluation and treatment as indicated. Treatment includes nonpharmacologic methods and, if necessary, pharmacologic therapy.

Hypertension in the Elderly

The prevalence of hypertension increases with advancing age to the extent that half of the people 60 to 69 years of age and approximately three fourths of the people 70 years of age and older are affected.[30] The age-related rise in systolic blood pressure is primarily responsible for the increase in hypertension that occurs with increasing age.

Among the aging processes that contribute to an increase in blood pressure are a stiffening of the large arteries, particularly the aorta; decreased baroreceptor sensitivity; increased peripheral vascular resistance; and decreased renal blood flow. Systolic blood pressure rises almost linearly between 30 and 84 years of age, whereas diastolic pressure rises until 50 years of age and then levels off or decreases.[57] This rise in systolic pressure is thought to be related to increased stiffness of the large arteries. With aging, the elastin fibers in the walls of the arteries are gradually replaced by collagen fibers that render the vessels stiffer and less compliant. Differences in the central and peripheral arteries relate to the fact that the larger vessels contain more elastin, whereas the peripheral resistance vessels have more smooth muscle and less elastin. Because of increased wall stiffness, the aorta and large arteries are less able to buffer the increase in systolic pressure that occurs as blood is ejected from the left heart, and they are less able to store the energy needed to maintain the diastolic pressure. As a result, the systolic pressure increases, the diastolic pressure remains unchanged or actually decreases, and the pulse pressure or difference between the systolic pressure and diastolic pressure widens.

Isolated systolic hypertension (systolic pressure ≥140 mm Hg and diastolic pressure <90 mm Hg) is recognized as an important risk factor for cardiovascular morbidity and mortality in older persons.[30] The treatment of hypertension in the elderly has beneficial effects in terms of reducing the incidence of cardiovascular events such as stroke. Studies have shown a reduction in stroke, CHD, and congestive heart failure in persons who were treated for hypertension compared with those who were not.[58,59]

Diagnosis and Treatment. The recommendations for measurement of blood pressure in the elderly are similar to those for the rest of the population.[60] Blood pressure variability is particularly prevalent among older persons, so it is especially important to obtain multiple measurements on different occasions to establish a diagnosis of hypertension. The effects of food, position, and other environmental factors also are exaggerated in older persons. Although sitting has been the standard position for blood pressure measurement, it is recommended that blood pressures also be taken in the supine and standing positions in the elderly. In some elderly persons with hypertension, a silent interval, called the *auscultatory gap*, may occur between the end of the first and beginning of the third phases of the Korotkoff sounds, providing the potential for underestimating the systolic pressure, sometimes by as much as 50 mm Hg. Because the gap occurs only with auscultation, it is recommended that a preliminary determination of systolic blood pressure be made by palpation and the cuff be inflated 30 mm Hg above this value for auscultatory measurement of blood pressure. In some older persons, the indirect measurement using a blood pressure cuff and the Korotkoff sounds has been shown to give falsely elevated readings compared with the direct intra-arterial method. This is because excessive cuff pressure is needed to compress the rigid vessels of some older persons. Pseudohypertension should be suspected in older persons with hypertension in whom the radial or brachial artery remains palpable but pulseless at higher cuff pressures.

The JNC-7 recommendations for treating hypertension in the elderly are similar to those for the general population.[30] However, blood pressure should be reduced slowly and cautiously. When possible, appropriate lifestyle modification measures should be tried first. Antihypertensive medications should be prescribed carefully because the older person may have impaired baroreflex sensitivity and renal function. Usually, medications are initiated at smaller doses, and doses are increased more gradually than for younger adults. There is also the danger of adverse drug interactions in older persons, who may be taking multiple medications, including over-the-counter drugs.

ORTHOSTATIC HYPOTENSION

Orthostatic or postural hypotension is an abnormal drop in blood pressure on assumption of the standing position. After the assumption of the upright posture from the supine position, approximately 500 to 700 mL of blood is momentarily shifted to the lower part of the body, with an accompanying decrease in central blood volume and arterial pressure.[61] Normally, this decrease in blood pressure is transient, lasting through several cardiac cycles, because the baroreceptors located in the thorax and carotid sinus area sense the decreased pressure and initiate reflex constriction of the veins and arterioles and an increase

in heart rate, which brings the blood pressure back to normal. Within a few minutes of a change to the standing position, blood levels of antidiuretic hormone and sympathetic neuromediators increase as a secondary means of ensuring maintenance of normal blood pressure in the standing position. Muscle movement in the lower extremities also aids venous return to the heart by pumping blood out of the legs.

When the standing position is assumed in the absence of normal circulatory reflexes or blood volume, blood pools in the lower part of the body; cardiac output falls, blood pressure drops, and blood flow to the brain is inadequate (Fig. 17-16). Dizziness, syncope (*i.e.*, fainting), or both may occur. Although there is no firm agreement on the definition of orthostatic hypotension, many author-

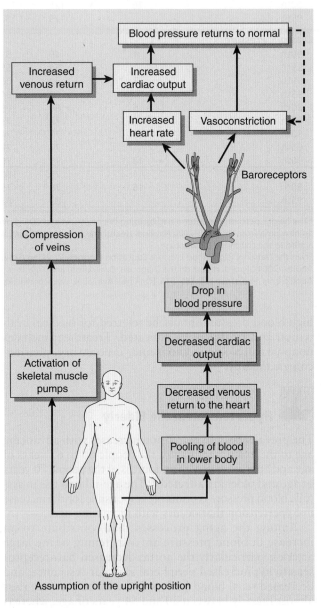

FIGURE 17-16 Mechanisms of blood control on immediate assumption of the upright position.

ities consider a drop in systolic pressure of 20 mm Hg or more or a drop in diastolic pressure of 10 mm Hg or more as diagnostic of the condition.[62] Some authorities regard the presence of orthostatic symptoms (*e.g.,* dizziness, syncope) as being more relevant than the numeric decrease in blood pressure.[63]

Causes

A wide variety of conditions, acute and chronic, are associated with orthostatic hypotension. These include reduced blood volume, drug-induced hypotension, altered vascular responses associated with aging, bed rest, and autonomic nervous system dysfunction.

Reduced Blood Volume. Orthostatic hypotension often is an early sign of reduced blood volume or fluid deficit. When blood volume is decreased, the vascular compartment is only partially filled; although cardiac output may be adequate when a person is in the recumbent position, it often decreases to the point of causing weakness and fainting when the person assumes the standing position. Common causes of orthostatic hypotension related to hypovolemia are excessive use of diuretics, excessive diaphoresis, loss of gastrointestinal fluids through vomiting and diarrhea, and loss of fluid volume associated with prolonged bed rest.

Drug-Induced Hypotension. Antihypertensive drugs and psychotropic drugs are a common cause of chronic orthostatic hypotension. In most cases, the orthostatic hypotension is well tolerated. If postural hypotension is severe enough to cause light-headedness or dizziness, it is recommended that the dosage of the drug be reduced or a different drug be used.

Aging. Weakness and dizziness on standing are common complaints of elderly persons. Although orthostatic tolerance is well maintained in the healthy elderly, after age 70 years there is an increasing tendency toward instability of the arterial pressure and postural hypotension. Although orthostatic hypotension may be either systolic or diastolic, that associated with aging seems more often to be systolic.[61] Several deficiencies in the circulatory response may predispose to this problem in the elderly, including diminished ability to produce an adequate increase in the heart rate, ventricular stroke volume, or peripheral vascular resistance; decreased function of the skeletal muscle pumps; and decreased blood volume. Because cerebral blood flow primarily depends on systolic pressure, patients with impaired cerebral circulation may experience symptoms of weakness, ataxia, dizziness, and syncope when their arterial pressure falls even slightly. This may happen in older persons who are immobilized for brief periods or whose blood volume is decreased owing to inadequate fluid intake or overzealous use of diuretics.

Postprandial (after meal) blood pressure often decreases in elderly persons.[64] The greatest postprandial changes occur after a high-carbohydrate meal. Although the mechanism responsible for these changes is not fully understood, it is thought to result from changes in baroreflex sensitivity and increased splanchnic blood flow mediated by insulin and vasoactive gastrointestinal hormones.

Bed Rest and Immobility. Prolonged bed rest promotes a reduction in plasma volume, a decrease in venous tone, failure of peripheral vasoconstriction, and weakness of the skeletal muscles that support the veins and assist in returning blood to the heart. Physical deconditioning follows even short periods of bed rest. After 3 to 4 days, the blood volume is decreased. Loss of vascular and skeletal muscle tone is less predictable but probably becomes maximal after approximately 2 weeks of bed rest. Orthostatic intolerance is a recognized problem of space flight, a potential risk after reentry into the earth's gravitational field.

Disorders of Autonomic Nervous System Function. The sympathetic nervous system plays an essential role in adjustment to the upright position. Sympathetic stimulation increases heart rate and cardiac contractility and causes constriction of peripheral veins and arterioles. Orthostatic hypotension caused by altered autonomic function is common in peripheral neuropathies associated with diabetes mellitus, after injury or disease of the spinal cord, or as the result of a cerebral vascular accident in which sympathetic outflow from the brain stem is disrupted. The American Autonomic Society and the American Academy of Neurology have distinguished three forms of primary ANS dysfunction: (1) pure autonomic failure, defined as a sporadic, idiopathic cause of persistent orthostatic hypotension and other manifestations of autonomic failure such as urinary retention, impotence, or decreased sweating; (2) Parkinson disease with autonomic failure; and (3) multiple-system atrophy (Shy-Drager syndrome).[65] The Shy-Drager syndrome usually develops in middle to late life and manifests as orthostatic hypotension associated with uncoordinated movements, urinary incontinence, constipation, and other signs of neurologic deficits referable to the corticospinal, extrapyramidal, corticobulbar, and cerebellar systems.

Diagnosis and Treatment

Orthostatic hypotension can be assessed with the auscultatory method of blood pressure measurement. A reading should be made when the patient is supine, immediately after assumption of the seated or upright position, and 2 to 3 minutes after assumption of the standing position. A tilt table also can be used for this purpose. With a tilt table, the recumbent patient can be moved to a head-up position without voluntary movement when the table is tilted. The tilt table also has the advantage of rapidly and safely returning persons with a profound postural drop in blood pressure to the horizontal position. Persons with a drop in blood pressure to orthostatic levels should be evaluated to determine the cause and seriousness of the condition. A history should be taken to elicit information about symptoms, particularly dizziness and history of syncope and falls; medical conditions, particularly those such as diabetes mellitus that predispose to orthostatic hypotension; use of prescription and over-the-counter drugs; and symptoms of ANS dysfunction, such as impotence or bladder dysfunction. A physical examination should document blood pressure in both arms and the heart rate while the patient is in the supine, sitting, and standing positions and should note the occurrence of symptoms. Noninvasive, 24-hour ambulatory blood pressure monitoring may be used to determine blood pressure responses to other stimuli of daily life, such as food ingestion and exertion.

The treatment of orthostatic hypotension usually is directed at alleviating the cause or, if this is not possible, toward helping people learn ways to cope with the disorder. Medications that predispose to postural hypotension should be avoided. Other measures include preventing or correcting the fluid deficit and avoidance of situations that encourage excessive vasodilatation (*e.g.*, drinking alcohol, exercising vigorously in a warm environment). Measures designed to help persons prevent symptomatic orthostatic drops in blood pressure include gradual ambulation (*i.e.*, sitting on the edge of the bed for several minutes and moving the legs to initiate skeletal muscle pump function before standing). Elastic support hose or an abdominal support garment may help prevent pooling of blood in the lower extremities and abdomen.

Pharmacologic treatment may be used when non-pharmacologic methods are unsuccessful. A number of types of drugs can be used for this purpose.[62] Mineralocorticoids can be used to reduce sodium and water loss. Vasopressin-2 receptor agonists (desmopressin as a nasal spray) may be used to reduce nocturnal polyuria. Sympathomimetic drugs that act directly on the resistance vessels or on the capacitance vessels may be used. Many of these agents have undesirable side effects.

In summary, the arterial blood pressure reflects the alternating contraction and relaxation of the left heart. The systolic pressure denotes the peak pressure that occurs during ventricular contraction, and the diastolic pressure denotes the lowest point that occurs during relaxation. The level to which the arterial pressure rises during systole and falls during diastole is determined by the cardiac output (stroke volume × heart rate) and the peripheral vascular resistance.

Hypertension (systolic pressure ≥140 mm Hg or diastolic pressure ≥90 mm Hg) is one of the most common cardiovascular disorders. It may occur as a primary disorder (*i.e.*, essential hypertension) or as a symptom of some other disease (*i.e.*, secondary hypertension). The incidence of essential hypertension increases with age; the condition is seen more frequently among African Americans, and is linked to a family history of high blood pressure, obesity, and increased sodium intake. Causes of secondary hypertension include renal disorders and adrenocortical disorders, such as hyperaldosteronism and Cushing disease, which increase sodium and water retention; pheochromocytomas, which increase catecholamine levels; and coarctation of the aorta, which produces a decrease in leg blood pressures and compensatory increase in arm pressures.

Uncontrolled hypertension increases the risk of heart disease, renal complications, retinopathy, and stroke. Treatment of essential hypertension focuses on non-pharmacologic methods such as weight reduction, reduction of sodium intake, regular physical activity, and modification of alcohol intake. Among the drugs used in the treatment of hypertension are diuretics, adrenergic inhibitors, vasodilators, ACE inhibitors, and calcium channel blockers.

Hypertension among special populations includes hypertension that occurs during pregnancy, hypertension in children, and hypertension in the elderly. Hypertension that occurs during pregnancy can be divided into four categories: chronic hypertension, preeclampsia-eclampsia, chronic hypertension with superimposed preeclampsia-eclampsia, and gestational hypertension. Secondary hypertension is the most common form of high blood pressure in infants and children. In later childhood and adolescence, essential hypertension is more common. Isolated systolic hypertension, the most common type of hypertension in the elderly, represents the effects of aging on the distensibility of the aorta and its ability to stretch and accommodate blood being ejected from the left heart during systole.

Orthostatic hypotension is an abnormal decrease in systolic or diastolic blood pressure that occurs on assumption of the upright position. Dizziness, syncope (*i.e.*, fainting), or both may occur. Among the factors that contribute to its occurrence are decreased fluid volume, medications, aging, defective functioning of the ANS, and the effects of immobility. Treatment includes correcting the reversible causes and assisting the person to compensate for the disorder to prevent falls and injuries.

Disorders of the Venous Circulation

Veins are low-pressure, thin-walled vessels that rely on the ancillary action of skeletal muscle pumps and changes in abdominal and intrathoracic pressure to return blood to the heart. Unlike the arterial system, the venous system is equipped with valves that prevent retrograde flow of blood. Although its structure enables the venous system to serve as a storage area for blood, it also renders the system susceptible to problems related to stasis and venous insufficiency. This section focuses on three common problems of the venous system: varicose veins, venous insufficiency, and venous thrombosis.

VENOUS CIRCULATION OF THE LOWER EXTREMITIES

The venous system in the legs consists of two components: the superficial veins (*i.e.*, saphenous vein and its tributaries) and the deep venous channels (Fig. 17-17). Perforating or communicating veins connect these two

merge with the larger deep veins and where two veins meet. The number of venous valves differs somewhat from one person to another, as does the structural competence, factors that may help to explain the familial predisposition to development of varicose veins.

The action of the leg muscles assists in moving venous blood from the lower extremities back to the heart. When a person walks, the action of the leg muscles serves to increase flow in the deep venous channels and return venous blood to the heart (Fig. 17-18). The function of this so-called muscle pump, located in the gastrocnemius and soleus muscles of the lower extremities, can be compared with the pumping action of the heart.[66] During muscle contraction, which is similar to systole, valves in the communicating channels close to prevent backward flow of blood into the superficial system, as blood in the deep veins is moved forward by the action of the contracting muscles. During muscle relaxation, which is similar to diastole, the communicating valves open, allowing blood from the superficial veins to move into the deep veins.

VARICOSE VEINS

Varicose, or dilated, tortuous veins of the lower extremities are common and often lead to secondary problems of venous insufficiency (see Fig. 17-17). Varicose veins are classified as primary or secondary. Primary varicose veins originate in the superficial saphenous veins, and secondary varicose veins result from impaired flow in the deep venous channels. Approximately 80% to 90%

systems. Blood from the skin and subcutaneous tissues in the leg collects in the superficial veins and is then transported across the communicating veins into the deeper venous channels for return to the heart. Venous valves prevent the retrograde flow of blood and play an important role in the function of the venous system (see Chapter 16, Fig. 16-19). Although these valves are irregularly located along the length of the veins, they almost always are found at junctions where the communicating veins

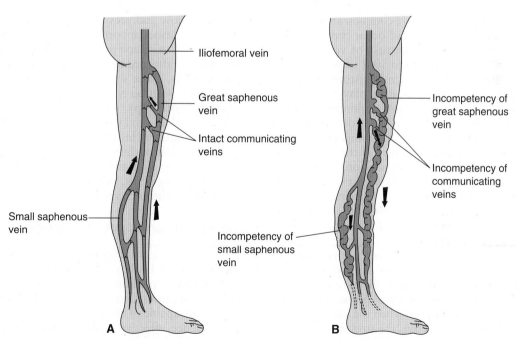

FIGURE 17-17 Superficial and deep venous channels of the leg. (**A**) Normal venous structures and flow patterns. (**B**) Varicosities in the superficial venous system are the result of incompetent valves in the communicating veins. The *arrows* in both views indicate the direction of blood flow. (Modified from Abramson D. I. [1974]. *Vascular disorders of the extremities* [2nd ed.]. Philadelphia: J. B. Lippincott.)

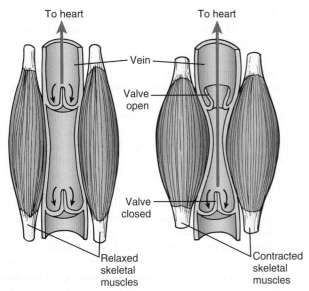

FIGURE 17-18 The skeletal muscle pumps and their function in promoting blood flow in the deep and superficial calf vessels of the leg.

of venous blood from the lower extremities is transported through the deep channels. The development of secondary varicose veins becomes inevitable when flow in these deep channels is impaired or blocked. The most common cause of secondary varicose veins is deep vein thrombosis (DVT). Other causes include congenital or acquired arteriovenous fistulas, congenital venous malformations, and pressure on the abdominal veins caused by pregnancy or a tumor.

Primary varicose veins are more common after 50 years of age and in obese persons, and occur more often in women than men, probably because of venous stasis caused by pregnancy.[4] More than 50% of persons with primary varicose veins have a family history of the disorder, suggesting that heredity may play a role. Prolonged standing and increased intra-abdominal pressure are important contributing factors in the development of primary varicose veins. One of the most important factors in the elevation of venous pressure is the hydrostatic effect associated with the standing position. When a person is in the erect position, the full weight of the venous columns of blood is transmitted to the leg veins. The effects of gravity are compounded in persons who stand for long periods without using their leg muscles to assist in pumping blood back to the heart.

Because there are no valves in the inferior vena cava or common iliac veins, blood in the abdominal veins must be supported by the valves located in the external iliac or femoral veins. When intra-abdominal pressure increases, as it does during pregnancy, or when the valves in these two veins are absent or defective, the stress on the saphenofemoral junction is increased. Lifting also increases intra-abdominal pressure and decreases flow of blood through the abdominal veins. Occupations that require repeated heavy lifting predispose to development of varicose veins.

Prolonged exposure to increased pressure causes the venous valves to become incompetent so they no longer close properly. When this happens, the reflux of blood causes further venous enlargement, pulling the valve leaflets apart and causing more valvular incompetence in sections of adjacent distal veins. Another consideration in the development of varicose veins is the fact that the superficial veins have only subcutaneous fat and superficial fascia for support, but the deep venous channels are supported by muscle, bone, and connective tissue. Obesity reduces the support provided by the superficial fascia and tissues, increasing the risk for development of varicose veins.

The signs and symptoms associated with primary varicose veins vary. Most women with superficial varicose veins complain of their unsightly appearance. In many cases, aching in the lower extremities and edema, especially after long periods of standing, may occur. The edema usually subsides at night when the legs are elevated. When the communicating veins are incompetent, symptoms are more common.

After the venous channels have been repeatedly stretched and the valves rendered incompetent, little can be done to restore normal venous tone and function. Ideally, measures should be taken to prevent the development and progression of varicose veins. These measures center on avoiding activities, such as continued standing, that produce prolonged elevation of venous pressure.

The diagnosis of varicose veins often can be made by physical inspection. The Doppler ultrasonographic flow probe also may be used to assess the flow in the large vessels. Angiographic studies using a radiopaque contrast medium also are used to assess venous function.

Treatment measures for varicose veins focus on improving venous flow and preventing tissue injury. When correctly fitted, elastic support stockings or leggings compress the superficial veins and prevent distention. The most precise control is afforded by prescription stockings measured to fit properly. These stockings should be applied before the standing position is assumed, when the leg veins are empty. Sclerotherapy, which often is used in the treatment of small residual varicosities, involves the injection of a sclerosing agent into the collapsed superficial veins to produce fibrosis of the vessel lumen. Surgical treatment consists of removing the varicosities and the incompetent perforating veins, but it is limited to persons with patent deep venous channels.

CHRONIC VENOUS INSUFFICIENCY

The term *venous insufficiency* refers to the physiologic consequences of DVT, valvular incompetence, or a combination of both conditions. The most common cause is DVT, which causes deformity of the valve leaflets, rendering them incapable of closure. In the presence of valvular incompetence, effective unidirectional flow of blood and emptying of the deep veins cannot occur. The muscle pumps also are ineffective, often driving blood in retrograde directions. Secondary failure of the communicating and superficial veins subjects the subcutaneous tissues to high pressures.

With venous insufficiency, there are signs and symptoms associated with impaired blood flow. In contrast to the ischemia caused by arterial insufficiency, venous insufficiency leads to tissue congestion, edema, and eventual impairment of tissue nutrition.[66,67] The edema is exacerbated by long periods of standing. Necrosis of subcutaneous fat deposits occurs, followed by skin atrophy. Brown pigmentation of the skin caused by hemosiderin deposits resulting from the breakdown of red blood cells is common. Secondary lymphatic insufficiency occurs, with progressive sclerosis of the lymph channels in the face of increased demand for clearance of interstitial fluid.

In advanced venous insufficiency, impaired tissue nutrition causes stasis dermatitis and the development of stasis or venous ulcers[4] (Fig. 17-19). Stasis dermatitis is characterized by the presence of thin, shiny, bluish-brown, irregularly pigmented desquamative skin that lacks the support of the underlying subcutaneous tissues. Minor injury leads to relatively painless ulcerations that are difficult to heal. The lower part of the leg is particularly prone to development of stasis dermatitis and venous ulcers. Most lesions are located medially over the ankle and lower leg, with the highest frequency just above the medial malleolus. Persons with long-standing venous insufficiency may experience stiffening of the ankle joint and loss of muscle mass and strength.

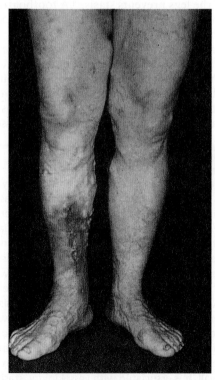

FIGURE 17-19 Varicose veins of the legs. Severe varicosities of the superficial leg veins have led to stasis dermatitis and secondary ulcerations. (From Gotlieb A. I. [2005]. Blood vessels. In Rubin E., Gorstein F., Rubin R., et al. [Eds.], *Rubin's pathology: Clinicopathologic foundations of medicine* [4th ed., p. 514]. Philadelphia: Lippincott Williams & Wilkins.)

VENOUS THROMBOSIS

The term *venous thrombosis*, or *thrombophlebitis*, describes the presence of thrombus in a vein and the accompanying inflammatory response in the vessel wall. Thrombi can develop in the superficial or the deep veins, most commonly those of the lower extremities. DVT of the lower extremity is a serious disorder, complicated by pulmonary embolism (see Chapter 22), recurrent episodes of DVT, and development of chronic venous insufficiency.[68]

In 1846, Rudolph Virchow described the triad that has come to be associated with venous thrombosis: stasis of blood, vessel wall injury, and increased blood coagulability.[69] This triad still applies, with all thrombotic risk factors, whether systemic or molecular, influencing one of the three mechanisms (Chart 17-3). A history of previous thromboembolism remains one of the strongest risk factors for subsequent venous thrombosis in high-risk situations, such as surgery.[70]

Stasis of blood occurs with immobility of an extremity or the entire body. Bed rest and immobilization are associated with decreased blood flow, venous pooling in the lower extremities, and increased risk of DVT. Prolonged bed rest or immobility caused by a hip or pelvic fracture, ventilatory support, and spinal cord injury all contribute to the development of DVT. The risk of DVT is increased in situations of impaired cardiac function. This may account for the relatively high incidence in persons with acute myocardial infarction and congestive heart failure. Elderly persons are more susceptible than younger persons, probably because disorders that produce venous stasis occur more frequently in older persons. Extended airplane travel poses a particular threat in persons predisposed to DVT because of prolonged sitting and increased blood viscosity caused by dehydration.[71]

Trauma and surgery usually result in reduced physical activity, injury to vessels, and release of procoagulant substances from the tissues. Persons who undergo major surgical procedures are particularly at risk for DVT. Certain surgical procedures, such as total hip replacement, are associated with higher incidences of thromboembolic complications. Venous catheters, which cause injury to the vessel endothelium, are another risk factor for venous thrombosis.

Increased blood coagulability can result from inherited or acquired disorders of the coagulation system, cancer, use of oral contraceptive agents, and the postpartum state.[68,70] Inherited disorders that predispose to venous thrombosis include deficiencies in antithrombin III, protein C, protein S, or plasminogen, or factor V Leiden mutation (see Chapter 10). Acquired causes of the hypercoagulability state include hyperhomocysteinemia, the antiphospholipid syndrome, and the production of procoagulation factors by cancer cells. The use of oral contraceptives also increases coagulability and predisposes to venous thrombosis, particularly in women with a previous history or family history of venous thrombosis.[72] The postpartum state is associated with increased levels of fibrinogen, prothrombin, and other coagulation factors.

CHART 17-3

Risk Factors Associated With Venous Thrombosis*

Venous Stasis

Bed rest
Immobility
Spinal cord injury
Acute myocardial infarction
Congestive heart failure
Shock
Venous obstruction

Hyperreactivity of Blood Coagulation

Stress and trauma
Pregnancy
Childbirth
Oral contraceptive use
Dehydration
Cancer

Vascular Trauma

Indwelling venous catheters
Surgery
Massive trauma or infection
Fractured hip
Orthopedic surgery

*Many of these disorders involve more than one mechanism.

Clinical Features

Manifestations. Many persons with venous thrombosis are asymptomatic, probably because the vein is not totally occluded or because of collateral circulation. When present, the most common signs and symptoms of venous thrombosis are those related to the inflammatory process: pain, swelling, and deep muscle tenderness. Fever, general malaise, and an elevated white blood cell count and sedimentation rate are accompanying indications of inflammation. There may be tenderness and pain along the vein. Swelling may vary from minimal to maximal. As much as 50% of persons with DVT are asymptomatic.

The site of thrombus formation determines the location of the physical findings. The most common site is in the venous sinuses in the soleus muscle and posterior tibial and peroneal veins. Swelling in these cases involves the foot and ankle, although it may be slight or absent. Calf pain and tenderness are common. Femoral vein thrombosis with calf thrombosis produces pain and tenderness in the distal thigh and popliteal area. Thrombi in ileofemoral veins produce the most profound manifestations, with swelling, pain, and tenderness of the entire extremity. With DVT in the calf veins, active dorsiflexion produces calf pain (*i.e.*, Homans sign).

Prevention, Diagnosis, and Treatment. Whenever possible, venous thrombosis should be prevented in preference to being treated. Early ambulation after childbirth and surgery is one measure that decreases the risk of thrombus formation. Exercising the legs and wearing support stockings improve venous flow. A further precautionary measure is to avoid assuming body positions that favor venous pooling. Antiembolism stockings of the proper fit and length should be used routinely in persons at risk for DVT. Another strategy used for immobile persons at risk for development of DVT is a sequential pneumatic compression device.[73] This consists of a plastic sleeve that encircles the legs and provides alternating periods of compression on the lower extremity. When properly used, these devices enhance venous emptying to augment flow and reduce stasis. Prophylactic anticoagulation often is used in persons who are at high risk for the development of venous thrombi.

The risk of pulmonary embolism emphasizes the need for early detection and treatment of DVT. Several tests are useful for this purpose, including ascending venography, ultrasonography, and plasma D-dimer levels (measurement of the breakdown products of fibrin from the blood clot).[73,74]

The goals of treatment for DVT are to prevent formation of additional thrombi, prevent extension and embolization of existing thrombi, and minimize venous valve damage. Anticoagulation therapy is used to treat and prevent venous thrombosis. A 15- to 20-degree elevation of the legs prevents stasis.[74] A footboard enables the person to perform leg exercises (ankle flexion and extension) while in bed.

Surgical removal of the thrombus may be undertaken in selected cases. Surgical interruption of the vena cava may be done in persons at high risk for experiencing pulmonary emboli. This procedure involves ligating the vena cava with a suture or clamp or creating a filter-like insertion to prevent large clots from moving through the vessel.

In summary, the storage function of the venous system renders it susceptible to venous insufficiency, stasis, and thrombus formation. Varicose veins occur with prolonged distention and stretching of the superficial veins owing to venous insufficiency. Varicosities can arise because of defects in the superficial veins (*i.e.*, primary varicose veins) or because of impaired blood flow in the deep venous channels (*i.e.*, secondary varicose veins). Venous insufficiency reflects chronic venous stasis resulting from valvular incompetence. It is associated with stasis dermatitis and stasis or venous ulcers. Venous thrombosis describes the presence of thrombus in a vein and the accompanying inflammatory response in the vessel wall. It is associated with vessel injury, stasis of venous flow, and hypercoagulability states. Thrombi can develop in the superficial or the deep veins (*i.e.*, DVT). Thrombus formation in deep veins is a precursor to venous insufficiency and embolus formation.

Review Exercises

The Third Report of the NCEP Expert Panel on Detection, Evaluation, and Treatment of High Cholesterol in Adults recommends that a person's HDL should be above 40 mg/dL.

A. Explain the role of HDL in the prevention of atherosclerosis.

A 55-year-old male executive presents in the clinic for his regular check-up. He was diagnosed with hypertension 5 years ago and has been taking a diuretic and a β-adrenergic blocker to control his blood pressure. His blood pressure is currently being maintained at about 135/70 mm Hg. His total cholesterol level is 180 mg/dL and his HDL cholesterol is 30 mg/dL. He is otherwise well. He is a non-smoker. He has recently read in the media about "inflammation" and the heart and expresses concern about his risk for coronary heart disease.

A. Use the risk assessment tool based on the Framingham Heart Study (www.nhlbi.nih.gov/guidelines/cholesterol/) to calculate this man's 10-year risk for experiencing myocardial infarction and coronary death.

A 34-year-old, otherwise healthy woman complains of episodes lasting several hours in which her fingers become pale and numb. This is followed by a period during which the fingers become red, throbbing, and painful.

A. What do you think is causing this woman's problem?
B. She relates that the episodes often occur when her fingers become cold or when she becomes upset. Explain the possible underlying mechanisms.
C. What types of measures could be used to treat this woman?

Mr. Young, a 47-year-old African American and an executive in a law firm, had his blood pressure taken at a screening program and has been told his pressure was 142/90 mm Hg. His father and older brother have hypertension and his paternal grandparents had a history of stroke and myocardial infarction. Mr. Young enjoys salty foods and routinely uses a salt shaker to add salt to meals his wife prepares, drinks about four beers while watching television in the evening, and gained 15 pounds in the past year. Although his family has encouraged him to engage in physical activities with them, he states he is either too busy or too tired.

A. According to JNC-7 guidelines, into what category does Mr. Young's blood pressure fall?
B. What are his risk factors for hypertension?
C. Explain why an increased salt intake might contribute to an increase in blood pressure.
D. What lifestyle changes would you suggest that Mr. Young make? Explain the rationale for your suggestions.

A 36-year-old woman enters the clinic complaining of headache and not feeling well. Her blood pressure is 175/90 mm Hg. Her renal test results are abnormal, and follow-up tests confirm that she has a stricture of the left renal artery.

A. Would her hypertension be classified as primary or secondary?
B. Explain the physiologic mechanisms underlying her blood pressure elevation.

A 75-year-old woman residing in an extended care facility has multiple health problems, including diabetes, hypertension, and heart failure. Lately she has been feeling dizzy when she stands up, and she has almost fallen on several occasions. Her family is concerned and wants to know why this is happening and what they can do to prevent her from falling and breaking her hip.

A. How would you go about assessing this woman for orthostatic hypotension?
B. What are the causes of orthostatic hypotension in the elderly?
C. How might this woman's medical conditions and their treatment contribute to her orthostatic hypotension?
D. The woman tells you that she feels particularly dizzy after she has eaten, yet the staff insist that she sit up and socialize with the other residents even though she would rather lie down and rest until the dizziness goes away. Explain the possible reason for her dizziness and what measures might be used to counteract the dizziness.

E. The woman recently had an episode of vomiting and diarrhea on an extremely hot day. She told her family that she was so dizzy she was sure she would fall. Explain why her dizziness was more severe under these conditions and what might be done to alleviate the situation.

Visit the Porth: Essentials of Pathophysiology: Concepts of Altered Health States web site (http://thePoint.LWW.com/PorthEssentials) for links to chapter-related resources on the Internet, all-new exclusive animations, chapter review questions, and more!

REFERENCES

1. Schoen F. J. (2005). Blood vessels. In Kumar V., Abbas A. K., Fausto N. (Eds.), *Robbins and Cotran pathologic basis of disease* (7th ed., pp. 511–541). Philadelphia: Elsevier Saunders.
2. Ross M. H., Kaye G. L., Pawlina W. (2003). *Histology: A text and atlas* (4th ed., pp. 326–342). Philadelphia: Lippincott Williams & Wilkins.
3. American Heart Association. (2005). Cholesterol statistics for professionals. [On-line]. Available: www.americanheart.org/cholesterol.
4. Gotlieb A. I. (2005). Blood vessels. In Rubin E., Gorstein F., Rubin R., et al. (Eds.), *Rubin's pathology: Clinicopathologic foundations of medicine* (4th ed., pp. 473–519). Philadelphia: Lippincott Williams & Wilkins.
5. Beisiegel U. (1998). Lipoprotein metabolism. *European Heart Journal* 19(Suppl. A), A20–A23.
6. Kreisberg R. A., Oberman A. (2003). Medical management of hyperlipidemia/dyslipidemia. *Journal of Clinical Endocrinology and Metabolism* 88, 2445–2461.
7. Oram J. F. (2002). ATP-binding cassette transporter A1 and cholesterol trafficking. *Current Opinions in Lipidology* 13, 373–381.
8. National Institutes of Health Expert Panel. (2001). *Third report of the National Cholesterol Education Program (NCEP) Expert Panel on Detection, Evaluation, and Treatment of High Blood Cholesterol in Adults (Adult Treatment Panel III).* NIH publication no. 01-3670. Bethesda, MD: National Institutes of Health.
9. Nabel E. G. (2003). Genomic medicine—cardiovascular disease. *New England Journal of Medicine* 349, 60–72.
10. Grundy S. M., Cleeman J. I., Merz C. N., et al. (2004). Implications of recent clinical trials for the National Cholesterol Education Program (NCEP) Adult Treatment Panel III guidelines. *Circulation* 110, 227–239. [On-line]. Available: http://www.circulationaha.org.
11. AHA Dietary Guidelines. (2000). Revision 2000: A statement for healthcare professionals from the Nutrition Committee of the American Heart Association. *Circulation* 102, 2284–2299.
12. Splaver A., Lamas G., Hennekens C. H. (2004). Homocysteine and cardiovascular disease: Biological mechanisms, observational epidemiology, and the need for randomized trials. *American Heart Journal* 148, 34–40.
13. Libby P., Ridker P. M., Maseri A. (2003). Inflammation and atherosclerosis. *Circulation* 105, 1135–1143.
14. Ridker P. M. (2003). Clinical application of C-reactive protein for cardiovascular disease detection and prevention. *Circulation* 107, 363–369.
15. Sinatra S. T. (2003). Is cholesterol lowering with statins the gold standard for treating patients with cardiovascular risk and disease? *Southern Medical Journal* 96, 220–223.
16. Heart Protection Study Collaborative Group. (2002). MRC/BHF Heart Protection Study of cholesterol lowering with simvastatin in 20,536 high-risk individuals: A randomised placebo-controlled trial. *Lancet* 360, 7–22.
17. Fong I. W. (2000). Emerging relations between infectious diseases and coronary artery disease and atherosclerosis. *Canadian Medical Association Journal* 163, 49–56.
18. Maseri A., Fuster V. (2003). Is there a vulnerable plaque? *Circulation* 107, 2068–2071.
19. Gross W. L., Trabandt A., Reinhold-Keller E. (2000). Diagnosis and evaluation of vasculitis. *Rheumatology* 39, 245–252.
20. Bartholomew J. R., Gray B. H. (1999). Large artery occlusive disease. *Rheumatic Disease Clinics of North America* 25, 669–686.
21. Lu J. T., Creager M. A. (2004). The relationship of cigarette smoking to peripheral artery disease. *Reviews in Cardiovascular Medicine* 5(4), 189–193.
22. Burns P., Gough S., Bradbury A. W. (2003). The management of peripheral artery disease in primary care. *British Medical Journal* 326, 584–588.
23. Olin J. W. (2000). Thromboangiitis obliterans (Buerger's disease). *New England Journal of Medicine* 343, 864–869.
24. Belch J. (1997). Raynaud's phenomenon. *Cardiovascular Research* 33, 25–30.
25. Pope J. (2003). Raynaud's phenomenon. *Clinical Evidence Concise* 9, 254–255.
26. Ho M., Belch J. (1998). Raynaud's phenomenon: State of the art. *Scandinavian Journal of Rheumatology* 27, 319–322.
27. Thompson R. W. (2002). Detection and management of small aortic aneurysms. *New England Journal of Medicine* 346, 1484–1486.
28. Coady M. A., Rizzo J. A., Goldstein L. J., et al. (1999). Natural history, pathogenesis, and etiology of thoracic aortic aneurysms and dissections. *Cardiology Clinics of North America* 17, 615–635.
29. Guyton A. C., Hall J. E. (2006). *Textbook of medical physiology* (11th ed., pp. 216–245). Philadelphia: Elsevier Saunders.
30. National Heart, Lung, and Blood Institute. (2003). *The seventh report of the Joint National Committee on Detection, Evaluation, and Treatment of High Blood Pressure.* NIH publication no. 03-5233. Bethesda, MD: National Institutes of Health.
31. Vassan R. S., Larson M. G., Leip E. P., et al. (2001). Assessment of frequency of progression to hypertension in non-hypertensive participants in the Framingham Heart Study: A cohort study. *Lancet* 358, 1682–1686.
32. American Diabetes Association. (2005). Summary of revisions for the 2005 clinical practice recommendations. *Diabetes Care* 28(Suppl. 1), 1.
33. Staessen J. A., Wang J., Bianchi G., et al. (2003). Essential hypertension. *Lancet* 361, 1629–1641.
34. Grim C. E., Henry J. P., Myers H. (1995). High blood pressure in blacks: Salt, slavery, survival, stress, and racism. In Laragh J. H., Brenner B. M. (Eds.), *Hypertension: Pathophysiology, diagnosis, and management* (pp. 171–207). New York: Raven Press.
35. Ward K. D., Sparrow D., Landsberg L. (1996). Influence of insulin, sympathetic nervous system activity, and obesity on blood pressure: The Normative Aging Study. *Journal of Hypertension* 14, 301–306.
36. Steinberg H. O. (2003). Insulin resistance and hypertension. In Izzo J. L., Black H. R. (Eds.), *Hypertension primer* (3rd ed., pp. 131–132). Dallas: American Heart Association.

37. Kotchen T. A., McCarron D. A. (1998). Dietary electrolytes and blood pressure: A statement for healthcare professionals from the American Heart Association Nutrition Committee. *Circulation* 98, 613–617.

38. Sacks F. M., Svetkey L. P., Vollmer W. M., et al. (2001). Effects on blood pressure of reduced sodium and the Dietary Approaches to Stop Hypertension (DASH) diet. *New England Journal of Medicine* 344, 3–10.

39. Haffner S. M. (2003). Obesity, body fat distribution, and insulin resistance: Clinical relevance. In Izzo J. L., Black H. R. (Eds.), *Hypertension primer* (3rd ed., pp. 286–288). Dallas: American Heart Association.

40. Fuchs F. D., Chambless L. E., Whelton P. K., et al. (2001). Alcohol consumption and the incidence of hypertension. *Hypertension* 37, 1242–1250.

41. Kaplan N. M. (1995). The treatment of hypertension in women. *Archives of Internal Medicine* 155, 563–567.

42. Frohlich E. D. (2003). Pathogenesis of hypertensive left ventricular hypertrophy and diastolic dysfunction. In Izzo J. L., Black H. R. (Eds.), *Hypertension primer* (3rd ed., pp. 175–177). Dallas: American Heart Association.

43. Grim C. E., Grim C. M. (2001). Accurate and reliable blood pressure measurement in the clinic and home: The key to hypertension control. In Hollenberg N. (Ed.), *Hypertension: Mechanisms and management* (3rd ed., pp. 315–324). Philadelphia: Current Medicine.

44. O'Brien E. (1996). Review: A century of confusion; which bladder for accurate blood pressure measurement? *Journal of Human Hypertension* 10, 565–572.

45. Black H. R., Kuller L. H., O'Rourke M. F., et al. (1999). The first report of the Systolic and Pulse Pressure (SYPP) working group. *Journal of Hypertension* 17(Suppl. 5), S3–S14.

46. Onusko E. (2003). Diagnosing secondary hypertension. *American Family Physician* 67, 67–74.

47. Safian R. D., Textor S. C. (2001). Renal-artery stenosis. *New England Journal of Medicine* 344, 431–442.

48. Venkata C., Ram S., Fierro-Carrion G. A. (1995). Pheochromocytoma. *Seminars in Nephrology* 15, 126–137.

49. Roa P. S. (1995). Coarctation of the aorta. *Seminars in Nephrology* 15, 87–105.

50. Vidt D. G. (2003). Treatment of hypertensive emergencies and urgencies. In Izzo J. L., Black H. R. (Eds.), *Hypertension primer* (3rd ed., pp. 462–455). Dallas: American Heart Association.

51. Chames M. C., Sibal B. M. (2001, April 2). When chronic hypertension complicates pregnancy. *Contemporary OB/GYN Archive*. [On-line]. Available: http://ahgyn.pdf.net/public.htm. Accessed May 14, 2001.

52. Gifford R. W., Jr. (Chair). (2000). *National High Blood Pressure Working Group report on high blood pressure in pregnancy*. NIH publication no. 00-3029. Bethesda, MD: National Institutes of Health.

53. Bartosh S. M., Aronson A. J. (1999). Childhood hypertension. *Pediatric Clinics of North America* 46, 235–251.

54. National High Blood Pressure Education Program Working Group on High Blood Pressure in Children and Adolescents. (2004). The fourth report on the diagnosis, evaluation, and treatment of high blood pressure in children and adolescents. *Pediatrics* 114, 555–576.

55. National Center for Health Statistics. (2000). 2000 CDC growth charts. [On-line]. Available: www.cdc.gov/growthcharts.

56. Behrman R. E., Kliegman R. M., Arvin A. M. (2004). Systemic hypertension. In Behrman R. E., Kliegman R. M., Jenson H. B. (Eds.), *Nelson textbook of pediatrics* (17th ed., pp. 1592–1598). Philadelphia: Elsevier Saunders.

57. Franklin S. S., Larson M. G., Khan S. A., et al. (2001). Does the relation of blood pressure to coronary heart disease risk change with aging? *Circulation* 103, 1245–1250.

58. Basile J. N. (2003). Treatment of elderly hypertensive: Systolic hypertension. In Izzo J. L., Black H. R. (Eds.), *Hypertension primer* (3rd ed., pp. 446–449). Dallas: American Heart Association.

59. Staessen J. A., Gasowski J., Wang J. G., et al. (2000). Risks of untreated and treated isolated systolic hypertension in the elderly: Meta-analysis of outcome trials. *Lancet* 355, 865–872.

60. Dickerson L. M., Gibson M. V. (2005). Management of hypertension in older persons. *American Family Physician* 71, 469–476.

61. Smith J. J., Porth C. J. M. (1990). Age and the response to orthostatic stress. In Smith J. J. (Ed.), *Circulatory response to the upright posture* (pp. 121–138). Boca Raton, FL: CRC Press.

62. Mathias C. J., Kimber J. R. (1999). Postural hypotension: Causes, clinical features, investigation, and management. *Annual Review of Medicine* 50, 317–336.

63. Kochar M. S. (1990). Orthostatic hypotension. In Smith J. J. (Ed.), *Circulatory response to the upright posture* (pp. 170–179). Boca Raton, FL: CRC Press.

64. Potter J. F., Heseltine D., Matthews J., et al. (1989). Effects of meal composition on the postprandial blood pressure, catecholamine and insulin changes in elderly subjects. *Clinical Science* 77, 265–272.

65. American Autonomic Society and American Academy of Neurologists. (1996). Consensus statement of the definition of orthostatic hypotension, pure autonomic failure, and multiple system atrophy. *Neurology* 46, 1470.

66. Alguire P. C., Mathes B. M. (1997). Chronic venous insufficiency and venous ulceration. *Journal of General Internal Medicine* 12, 374–383.

67. de Araujo T., Valencia I., Federman D. G., et al. (2003). Managing the patient with venous ulcers. *Annals of Internal Medicine* 138, 326–334.

68. Lopez J. A., Kearon C., Lee A. Y. Y. (2004). Deep venous thrombosis. *Hematology (American Society of Hematology Educational Program)*, 439–456.

69. Virchow R. (1846). Weinere Untersuchungen uber die Verstropfung der Lungenrarterie und ihre Folgen. *Beitrage zur Experimentelle Pathologie und Physiologie* 2, 21.

70. Ginsberg J. S. (1996). Management of venous thromboembolism. *New England Journal of Medicine* 335, 1816–1828.

71. Schurr J. H., Machin S. J., Bailey-King S., et al. (2001). Frequency and prevention of symptomless deep-vein thrombosis in long-haul flights. *Lancet* 357, 1485–1489.

72. Vandebrouchke J. P., Bloemenkamp K. W. M., Helmerhorst F. M., et al. (2001). Oral contraceptives and risk of venous thrombosis. *New England Journal of Medicine* 335, 108–114.

73. Messina L. M., Pak L., Tierney L. M. (2004). Blood vessels and lymphatics. In Tierney L. M., McPhee S., Papadakis M. A. (Eds.), *Current medical diagnosis and treatment* (43rd ed., pp. 452–454). New York: Lange Medical Books/McGraw-Hill.

74. Ramzi D. W., Leeper K. V. (2004). DVT and pulmonary embolism: Part I. Diagnosis. *American Family Physician* 69, 2829–2836.

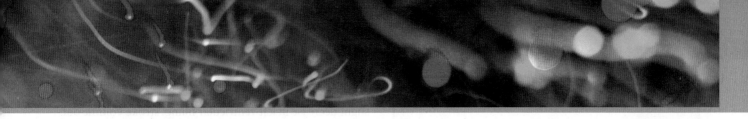

Chapter 18

Disorders of Cardiac Function

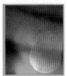 Heart disease remains a leading cause of death and disability in the United States and throughout the world. Currently, it is the number one cause of death in the United States. It is also the leading cause of permanent disability in the U.S. labor force.[1]

In an attempt to focus on common heart problems that affect persons in all age groups, this chapter is organized into five sections: disorders of the pericardium, coronary heart disease, myocardial and endocardial disorders, valvular heart disease, and heart disease in infants and children.

Disorders of the Pericardium

The pericardium is a double-walled fibroserous sac that isolates the heart from other thoracic structures, maintains its position in the thorax, and prevents it from overfilling. The two layers of the pericardium are separated by a thin layer of serous fluid, which prevents frictional forces from developing as the inner visceral layer comes in contact with the outer parietal layer of the fibrous pericardium. Although the fibrous tissue in the pericardium allows for moderate changes in cardiac size, it cannot stretch rapidly enough to accommodate rapid dilatation of the heart or accumulation of pericardial fluid without increasing pericardial and intracardiac pressures.

The pericardium is subject to many of the same pathologic processes (*e.g.*, congenital disorders, infections, trauma, immune mechanisms, and neoplastic disease) that affect other structures of the body. Pericardial disorders frequently are associated with or result from another disease in the heart or the surrounding structures.

PERICARDIAL EFFUSION

Pericardial effusion refers to the accumulation of fluid in the pericardial cavity. It may develop as the result of injury, inflammation, or increased capillary filtration

ing right atrial and ventricular filling. This causes the interventricular septum to bulge to the left, producing a slight decrease in left ventricular filling, stroke volume output, and systolic blood pressure. In cardiac tamponade, the left ventricle is compressed from within by movement of the interventricular septum and from without by fluid in the pericardium (Fig. 18-1). This produces a marked decrease in left ventricular filling and stroke volume output, and an exaggerated fall in systolic blood pressure, often within a beat of the beginning of inspiration.

The echocardiogram is a rapid, accurate, and widely used method of evaluating pericardial effusion. Aspiration and laboratory evaluation of the pericardial fluid may be used to identify the causative agent. Cardiac catheterization may be used to determine the hemodynamic effects of pericardial effusion and cardiac tamponade. Pericardiocentesis or removal of fluid from the pericardial sac, often with a needle inserted through the chest wall, may be an emergency lifesaving measure in severe cardiac tamponade. Surgical treatment may be required for traumatic lesions of the heart.

pressures. Its major threat is compression of the heart chambers. The amount of fluid, the rapidity with which it accumulates, and the elasticity of the pericardium determine the effect the effusion has on cardiac function. Small pericardial effusions may produce no symptoms or abnormal clinical findings. Even a large effusion that develops slowly may cause few or no symptoms, provided the pericardium is able to stretch and avoid compressing the heart. However, a sudden accumulation of even 200 mL may raise intracardiac pressure to levels that seriously limit venous return to the heart. Symptoms of cardiac compression also may occur with relatively small accumulations of fluid when the pericardium has become thickened by scar tissue or neoplastic infiltrations.

Cardiac tamponade is a life-threatening, slow or rapid compression of the heart due to the accumulation of fluid, pus, or blood in the pericardial sac.[2,3] It can occur as the result of conditions such as trauma, cardiac surgery, cancer, uremia, or cardiac rupture due to myocardial infarction. The seriousness of cardiac tamponade results from increased intracardiac pressure, a progressive decline in ventricular diastolic filling, and a resultant reduction in stroke volume and cardiac output. The severity of the condition depends on the amount of fluid that is present and the rate at which it accumulated. A rapid accumulation of fluid results in an elevation of central venous pressure, jugular venous distention, a decline in venous return to the heart, a decrease in cardiac output despite an increase in heart rate, a fall in systolic blood pressure, and signs of circulatory shock.

A key diagnostic finding in cardiac tamponade is *pulsus paradoxus*, commonly defined as a 10 mm Hg or more fall in the systolic blood pressure during normal breathing.[2,3] Normally, the decrease in intrathoracic pressure that occurs during inspiration accelerates venous flow, increas-

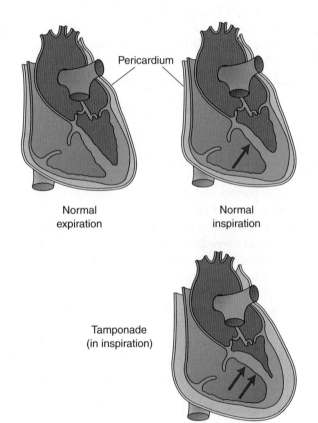

FIGURE 18-1 Effects of respiration and cardiac tamponade on ventricular filling and cardiac output. During inspiration, venous flow into the right heart increases, causing the interventricular septum to bulge into the left ventricle. This produces a decrease in left ventricular volume, with a subsequent decrease in stroke volume output. In cardiac tamponade, the fluid in the pericardial sac produces further compression of the left ventricle, causing an exaggeration of the normal inspiratory decrease in stroke volume and systolic blood pressure.

PERICARDITIS

Pericarditis represents an inflammatory process of the pericardium.[2,4] It can result from a number of diverse causes. Most forms of pericarditis occur as the result of other systemic or cardiac diseases. Primary pericarditis is unusual and usually of viral origin. Most cases of pericarditis evoke an acute inflammatory process. Exceptions are tuberculosis and fungal infections, which often produce a chronic pericarditis.

Acute Pericarditis

Acute pericarditis can be classified according to cause (*e.g.,* infections, trauma) or the nature of the exudate (*e.g.,* serous, fibrinous, purulent, hemorrhagic). Like other inflammatory conditions, acute pericarditis often is associated with increased capillary permeability. The capillaries that supply the serous pericardium become permeable, allowing plasma proteins, including fibrinogen, to leave the capillaries and enter the pericardial space. This results in an exudate that varies in type and amount according to the causative agent. Acute pericarditis frequently is associated with a fibrinous (fibrin-containing) exudate (Fig. 18-2), which heals by resolution or progresses to deposition of scar tissue and formation of adhesions between the layers of the serous pericardium.

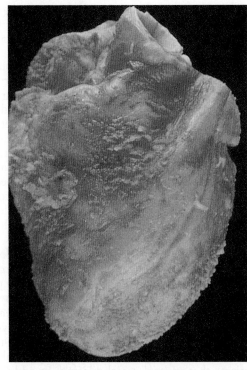

FIGURE 18-2 Fibrinous pericarditis. The heart of a patient who died in uremia displays a shaggy, fibrinous exudate covering the visceral pericardium. (From Saffitz J. E., Steinburger C., Jr. [2005]. The heart. In Rubin E., Gorstein F., Rubin R., et al. [Eds.], *Rubin's pathology: Clinicopathologic foundations of medicine* [4th ed., p. 577]. Philadelphia: Lippincott Williams & Wilkins.)

Viral infection (especially infections with the coxsackie-viruses and echoviruses, but also influenza, Epstein-Barr, varicella, hepatitis, mumps, and human immunodeficiency [HIV] viruses) is the most common cause of acute pericarditis. Acute viral pericarditis is seen more frequently in men than in women and often is preceded by a pro-dromal phase during which fever, malaise, and other flu-like symptoms are present. In some cases, a well-defined infection elsewhere in the body, such as an upper respiratory tract infection, precedes the onset of pericarditis and is the primary site of infection. Although the acute symptoms usually subside in several weeks, easy fatigability often continues for several months. In many cases the condition is self-limited, resolving in 2 to 6 weeks, but in other cases it may persist and produce recurrent subacute or chronic disease.

Other causes of acute pericarditis are rheumatic fever, the postpericardiotomy syndrome, post-traumatic pericarditis, metabolic disorders (*e.g.,* uremia, myxedema), and pericarditis associated with connective tissue diseases (*e.g.,* systemic lupus erythematosus, rheumatoid arthritis). With the increased use of open heart surgery in the treatment of various heart disorders, the postpericardiotomy syndrome has become a commonly recognized form of pericarditis. Pericarditis with effusion is a common complication in persons with renal failure, including those being treated with hemodialysis. Irradiation may initiate a subacute pericarditis, with an onset usually within the first year of therapy. It is most commonly associated with high doses of radiation delivered to areas near the heart.

The manifestations of acute pericarditis include a triad of chest pain, pericardial friction rub, and electrocardiographic (ECG) changes. The clinical findings may vary according to the causative agent. Nearly all persons with acute pericarditis have chest pain. The pain usually is abrupt in onset, occurs in the precordial area, and is described as sharp. It may radiate to the neck, back, abdomen, or side. It typically is worse with deep breathing, coughing, swallowing, and positional changes because of changes in venous return and cardiac filling. Many persons seek relief by sitting up and leaning forward. Only a small portion of the pericardium, the outer layer of the lower parietal pericardium below the fifth and sixth intercostal spaces, is sensitive to pain. This means that pericardial pain probably results from inflammation of the surrounding structures, particularly the pleura.

Diagnosis of acute pericarditis is based on clinical manifestations, ECG, chest radiography, and echocardiography. A pericardial friction rub (heard through a stethoscope), which is often described as "leathery" or "close to the ear," results from the rubbing and friction between the inflamed pericardial surfaces.[4] Treatment depends on the cause. When infection is present, antibiotics specific for the causative agent usually are prescribed. Aspirin and other nonsteroidal anti-inflammatory drugs (NSAIDs) may be given to minimize the inflammatory response and the accompanying undesirable effects.

Chronic Pericarditis With Effusion

Chronic pericarditis with effusion is characterized by an increase in inflammatory exudate that continues beyond the acute period. In some cases, the exudate persists for several years. In most cases of chronic pericarditis, no specific pathogen can be identified. The process commonly is associated with other forms of heart disease, such as rheumatic fever, congenital heart lesions, or hypertensive heart disease. Systemic diseases, such as lupus erythematosus, rheumatoid arthritis, scleroderma, and myxedema, also are causes of chronic pericarditis, as are metabolic disturbances associated with acute and chronic renal failure. Unlike acute pericarditis, the signs and symptoms of chronic pericarditis often are minimal, with the condition being detected on a routine chest x-ray film. As the condition progresses, the fluid may accumulate and compress the adjacent cardiac structures and impair cardiac filling.

Constrictive Pericarditis

In constrictive pericarditis, fibrous scar tissue develops between the visceral and parietal layers of the serous pericardium. In time, the scar tissue contracts and interferes with diastolic filling of the heart, at which point cardiac output and cardiac reserve become fixed. Ascites is a prominent early finding and may be accompanied by pedal edema, dyspnea on exertion, and fatigue. The jugular veins also are distended. Kussmaul sign is an inspiratory distention of the jugular veins caused by the inability of the right atrium, encased in its rigid pericardium, to accommodate the increase in venous return that occurs with inspiration. In chronic constrictive pericarditis, surgical removal or resection of the pericardium (*i.e.,* pericardiectomy) is often the treatment of choice.

In summary, disorders of the pericardium include pericardial effusion, cardiac tamponade, and pericarditis. The major threat of pericardial disease is compression of the heart chambers. Pericardial effusion refers to the presence of an exudate in the pericardial cavity, and the condition can be acute or chronic. It can increase intracardiac pressure, compress the heart, and interfere with venous return to the heart. The amount of exudate, the rapidity with which it accumulates, and the elasticity of the pericardium determine the effect the effusion has on cardiac function. Cardiac tamponade is a life-threatening cardiac compression resulting from excess fluid in the pericardial sac. Acute pericarditis is characterized by chest pain, ECG changes, and a friction rub. Among its causes are infections, uremia, rheumatic fever, connective tissue diseases, and myocardial infarction. Chronic pericarditis with effusion is characterized by an increase in inflammatory exudate that continues beyond the acute period. In constrictive pericarditis, scar tissue develops between the visceral and parietal layers of the serous pericardium. In time, the scar tissue contracts and interferes with cardiac filling.

Coronary Heart Disease

The term *coronary heart disease* (CHD) describes heart disease due to impaired coronary blood flow, usually the result of atherosclerosis. Diseases of the coronary arteries can cause angina, myocardial infarction or heart attack, cardiac arrhythmias, conduction defects, heart failure, and sudden death.

CORONARY CIRCULATION

There are two main coronary arteries, the left and the right, which arise from the coronary sinus just above the aortic valve (Fig. 18-3). The left coronary artery extends for approximately 3.5 cm as the *left main coronary artery* and then divides into the left anterior descending and circumflex branches. The *left anterior descending artery* passes down through the groove between the two ventricles, giving off diagonal branches, which supply the left ventricle, and perforating branches, which supply the anterior portion of the interventricular septum and the anterior papillary muscle of the left ventricle. The *circumflex branch* of the left coronary artery passes to the left and moves posteriorly in the groove that separates the left atrium and ventricle, giving off branches that supply the left lateral wall of the left ventricle. The *right coronary artery* lies in the right atrioventricular (AV) groove, and its branches supply the right ventricle. The right coronary artery usually moves to the back of the heart, where it forms the *posterior descending artery,* which supplies the posterior portion of the heart, interventricular septum, sinoatrial (SA) and AV nodes, and posterior papillary muscle.

The large epicardial coronary arteries lie on the surface of the heart, with the smaller intramyocardial coronary arteries branching off and penetrating the myocardium before merging with a network or plexus of subendocardial vessels. Although there are no connections between the large coronary arteries, there are anastomotic channels that join the small arteries (Fig. 18-4). With gradual occlusion of the larger vessels, the smaller collateral vessels increase in size and provide alternative channels for blood flow. One of the reasons CHD does not produce symptoms until it is far advanced is that the collateral channels develop at the same time the atherosclerotic changes are occurring.

Blood flow in the coronary arteries is controlled largely by physical, neural, and metabolic factors. The coronary arteries have their origin in the aortic sinuses at the proximal part of the ascending aorta. Thus, the main force responsible for perfusion of the myocardium is aortic pressure, which is generated by the heart itself. Myocardial blood flow, in turn, is largely regulated by the metabolic activity of the myocardium and autoregulatory mechanisms that control vessel dilation. In addition to generating the aortic pressure that moves blood through the coronary vessels, the contracting heart muscle influences its own blood supply by compressing the intramyocardial and subendocardial blood vessels during systole.[5] The autonomic nervous system exerts its effects on coro-

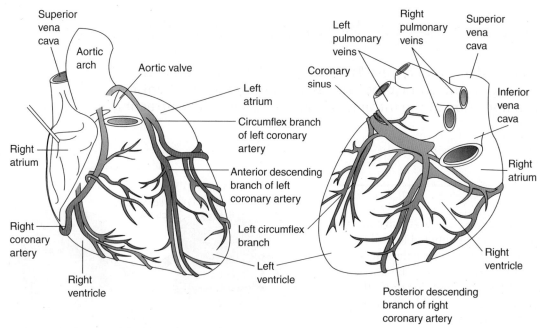

FIGURE 18-3 Coronary arteries and some of the coronary sinus veins.

nary blood flow through changes in heart rate, cardiac contractility, and blood pressure.

Blood flow usually is regulated by the need of the cardiac muscle for oxygen. Even under normal resting conditions, the heart extracts and uses 60% to 80% of oxygen in blood flowing through the coronary arteries,

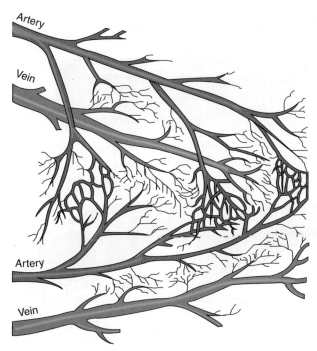

FIGURE 18-4 Anastomoses of the smaller coronary arterial vessels. (From Guyton A. C., Hall J. E. [1996]. *Textbook of medical physiology* [9th ed., p. 260]. Philadelphia: W. B. Saunders.)

compared with the 25% to 30% extracted by skeletal muscle.[5] Because there is little oxygen reserve in the blood, the coronary arteries must increase their flow to meet the metabolic needs of the myocardium during periods of increased activity. Numerous substances act as mediators for the vasodilatation that accompanies increased cardiac work. These substances, which include potassium ions, lactic acid, carbon dioxide, and adenosine, are released from working myocardial cells. Of these substances, adenosine has the greatest vasodilator action and is perhaps the critical mediator of local metabolic regulation.[5,6]

The endothelial cells that line blood vessels, including the coronaries, normally form a barrier between the blood and the arterial wall, and they have antithrombogenic properties that inhibit platelet aggregation and clot formation (see Chapter 17). They also synthesize several substances called *endothelium-derived relaxing factors* that induced relaxation of the smooth muscle in the vessel wall. The most important of these is *nitric oxide*.[6] The endothelium also is the source of *endothelium-derived contracting factors,* the best known of which are the endothelins.

PATHOGENESIS OF CORONARY HEART DISEASE

Atherosclerosis (discussed in Chapter 17) is by far the most common cause of CHD, and atherosclerotic plaque disruption the most frequent cause of myocardial infarction and sudden cardiac death. More than 90% of persons with CHD have coronary atherosclerosis.[7] Atherosclerosis can affect one or all three of the major coronary arteries and their branches. Clinically significant lesions may be located anywhere in these vessels, but tend to predominate in the first several centimeters of the left anterior descending and

Understanding ➤ Myocardial Blood Flow

Blood flow in the coronary vessels that supply the myocardium is influenced by (1) the aortic pressure, (2) autoregulatory mechanisms, and (3) compression of the intramyocardial vessels by the contracting heart muscle.

1

Aortic pressure. The two main coronary arteries that supply blood flow to the myocardium arise in the sinuses behind the two cusps of the aortic valve. Because of their location, the pressure and flow of blood in the coronary arteries reflects that of the aorta. During systole, when the aortic valve is open, the velocity of blood flow and position of the valve cusps cause the blood to move rapidly past the coronary artery inlets, and during diastole, when the aortic valve is closed, blood flow and the aortic pressure is transmitted directly into the coronary arteries.

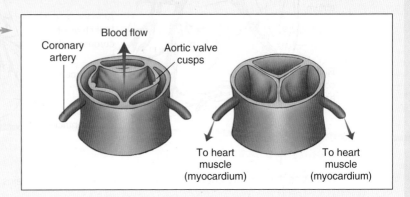

2

Autoregulatory mechanisms. The heart normally extracts 60% to 80% of the oxygen in the blood delivered to it, leaving little in reserve. Accordingly, oxygen delivery during periods of increased metabolic demand depends on autoregulatory mechanisms that regulate blood flow through a change in vessel tone. During increased metabolic demand, vasodilatation produces an increase in blood flow; during decreased demand, vasoconstriction or return of vessel tone to normal produces a reduction in flow. The mechanisms that link the metabolic activity of the heart to changes in vessel tone result from vasoactive mediators released from myocardial cells and the vascular endothelium.

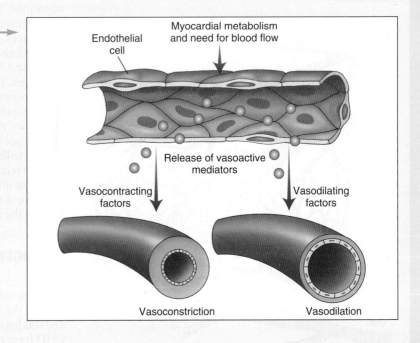

3

Vessel compression. The large coronary arteries lie on the epicardial surface of the heart, with smaller intramyocardial vessels branching off and moving through the myocardium before merging with a plexus of vessels that supply the subendocardial muscle with blood. During systole, the contracting cardiac muscle has a squeezing effect on the intramyocardial vessels, while at the same time producing an increase in intraventricular pressure that pushes against and compresses the subendocardial vessels. As a result, blood flow to the subendocardial muscle is greatest during diastole. Because the time spent in diastole becomes shortened as the heart rate increases, myocardial blood flow can be greatly reduced during sustained periods of tachycardia.

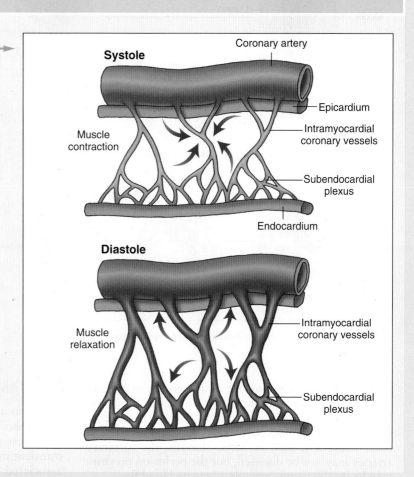

left circumflex or the entire length of the right coronary artery.[7] Sometimes the major secondary branches also are involved.

There are two types of atherosclerotic lesions: the fixed or stable plaque, which obstructs blood flow, and the unstable or vulnerable plaque, which can rupture and cause platelet adhesion and thrombus formation. The fixed or stable plaque is commonly implicated in stable angina and the unstable plaque in unstable angina and myocardial infarction. There are three major determinants of plaque vulnerability to rupture: (1) the size of the lipid-rich core and the stability and thickness of its fibrous cap, (2) the presence of inflammation with plaque degradation, (3) and the lack of smooth muscle cells with impaired healing and plaque stabilization[7-9] (Fig. 18-5). Plaques with a thin fibrous cap overlaying a large lipid core are at high risk for rupture.

There are two types of thrombi formed as a result of plaque disruption—white platelet-containing thrombi and red fibrin-containing thrombi. The thrombi in unstable angina have been characterized as grayish-white and presumably platelet rich.[10] Red thrombi, which develop with

vessel occlusion in myocardial infarction, are rich in fibrin and red blood cells superimposed on the platelet component and extended by the stasis of blood flow.

Coronary heart disease is commonly divided into two types of disorders: chronic ischemic heart disease and the acute coronary syndromes (Fig. 18-6). There are three types of chronic ischemic heart disease: chronic stable angina, silent myocardial ischemia, and variant or vasospastic angina. The acute coronary syndromes represent the spectrum of ischemic coronary disease ranging from unstable angina through myocardial infarction.

CHRONIC ISCHEMIC HEART DISEASE

Ischemic heart disease is a generic term used to describe a group of closely related syndromes resulting from myocardial ischemia—an imbalance between the blood supply and the demands of the heart for oxygenated blood. Limitations in coronary blood flow most commonly are the result of atherosclerosis, with vasospasm and thrombosis as contributing factors. The metabolic demands of the heart are increased with everyday activities

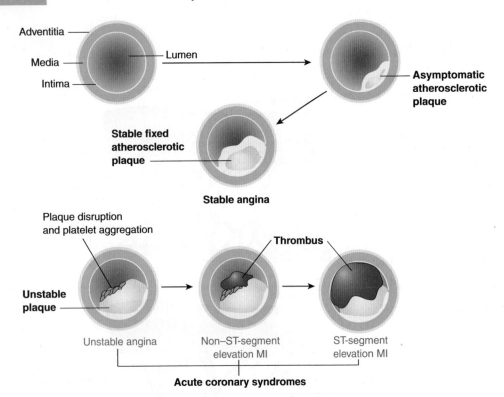

FIGURE 18-5 Atherosclerotic plaque: stable fixed atherosclerotic plaque in stable angina and the unstable plaque with plaque disruption and platelet aggregation in the acute coronary syndromes.

such as mental stress, exercise, and exposure to cold. In certain disease states such as thyrotoxicosis, the metabolic demands may be so excessive that the blood flow may be inadequate despite normal coronary arteries. In other situations, such as aortic stenosis, the coronary arteries may not be diseased, but the perfusion pressure may be insufficient to provide adequate blood flow.

Stable Angina

The term *angina* is derived from a Latin word meaning "to choke." Angina pectoris is a symptomatic paroxysmal chest pain or pressure sensation associated with transient myocardial ischemia. Chronic stable angina is associated with a fixed coronary obstruction that produces a disparity between coronary blood flow and the metabolic demands of the myocardium. Stable angina is the initial manifestation of ischemic heart disease in approximately half of persons with CHD.[11] Although most persons with stable angina have atherosclerotic heart disease, angina does not develop in a considerable number of persons with advanced coronary atherosclerosis. This probably is because of their sedentary lifestyle, the development of adequate collateral circulation, or the inability of these persons to perceive pain.

Stable angina usually is precipitated by situations that increase the work demands of the heart, such as physical exertion, exposure to cold, and emotional stress. The pain typically is described as a constricting, squeezing, or suffocating sensation. It usually is steady, increasing in intensity only at the onset and end of the attack. The pain of angina commonly is located in the precordial or substernal area of the chest; it is similar to myocardial infarction in that it may radiate to the left shoulder, jaw, arm, or other areas of the chest (Fig. 18-7). In some persons, the arm or shoulder pain may be confused with arthritis; in others, epigastric pain is confused with indigestion. Angina commonly is categorized according to whether it occurs with exercise or during rest, is of new onset, or is of increasing severity.

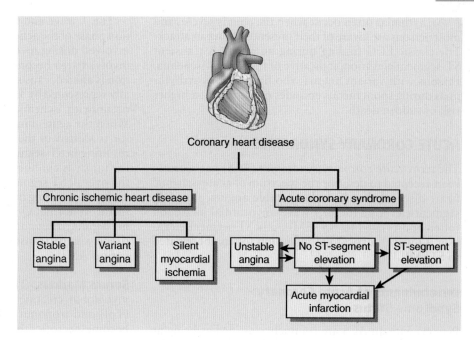

FIGURE 18-6 Types of coronary heart disease.

Typically, chronic stable angina is provoked by exertion or emotional stress and relieved within minutes by rest or the use of nitroglycerin. Angina that occurs at rest, is of new onset, or is increasing in intensity or duration denotes an increased risk for myocardial infarction and should be evaluated using the criteria for acute coronary syndromes (discussed later).

Silent Myocardial Ischemia

Silent myocardial ischemia occurs in the absence of anginal pain. Silent myocardial ischemia affects three populations—persons who are asymptomatic without other evidence of CHD, persons who have had a myocardial infarct and continue to have episodes of silent ischemia, and persons with angina who also have episodes of silent ischemia.[12] The reason for the painless episodes of ischemia is unclear. The episodes may be shorter and involve less myocardial tissue than those producing pain. Another explanation is that persons with silent angina have defects in pain threshold or pain transmission, or autonomic neuropathy with sensory denervation. There is evidence of an increased incidence of silent myocardial ischemia in persons with diabetes mellitus, probably the result of autonomic neuropathy, which is a common complication of diabetes.[13]

Variant or Vasospastic Angina

The syndrome of variant angina or *Prinzmetal angina* was first described by Prinzmetal and associates in 1959.[14] Subsequent evidence indicated variant angina is caused by spasms of the coronary arteries; hence, the condition is referred to as *vasospastic angina*. In most instances, the spasms occur in the presence of coronary artery stenosis; however, variant angina has occurred in the absence of visible disease. Unlike stable angina that occurs with exertion or stress, variant angina usually occurs during rest or with minimal exercise and frequently occurs nocturnally (between midnight and 8 AM).[12] The mechanism of coronary vasospasm is uncertain. It has been suggested that it may result from hyperactive sympathetic nervous system responses, from a defect in the handling of calcium in vascular smooth muscle, from disturbances in the production and release of endothelium-derived relaxing factors (*e.g.*, nitric oxide), or from an imbalance between endothelium-derived relaxing and contracting factors.

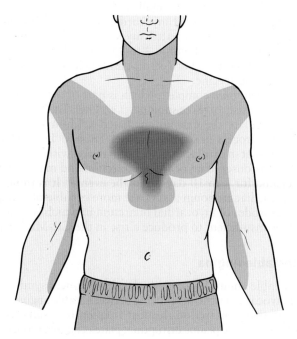

FIGURE 18-7 Areas of pain due to angina.

Arrhythmias often occur when the pain is severe, and most persons are aware of their presence during an attack. The classic ECG finding during an attack is transient ST-segment elevation, indicative of transmural ischemia. Persons with variant angina who have serious arrhythmias during spontaneous episodes of pain are at a higher risk of sudden death.

ACUTE CORONARY SYNDROMES

The term *acute coronary syndromes* (ACS) has recently been accepted to describe the spectrum of acute ischemic heart diseases that include unstable angina, non–ST-segment elevation (non–Q-wave) myocardial infarction (often abbreviated to NSTEMI), and ST-segment elevation (Q-wave) myocardial infarction (often abbreviated to STEMI).[15,16]

Determinants of Acute Coronary Syndrome Status

Persons with an ACS are routinely classified as being at low or high risk for acute myocardial infarction (AMI) based on presenting characteristics, ECG variables, serum cardiac markers, and the timing of presentation.

Electrocardiographic Changes. The classic ECG changes that occur with ACS involve T-wave inversion, ST-segment depression or elevation, and development of an abnormal Q wave[17] (Fig. 18-8). These changes vary considerably depending on the duration of the ischemic event (acute versus evolving), its extent (subendocardial versus transmural), and its location (anterior versus inferior posterior). Because these changes usually occur over time and are seen on the ECG leads that view the involved area of the myocardium, provision for continuous and 12-lead ECG monitoring is usually indicated.

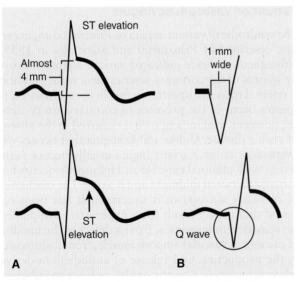

FIGURE 18-8 Illustration of an ECG tracing showing ST-segment elevation (**A**) and Q wave in acute coronary syndromes (**B**).

The T wave and ST segment on the ECG (repolarization phase of the action potential) are usually the first to be involved during myocardial ischemia and injury. As the involved area becomes ischemic, myocardial repolarization is altered, causing changes in the T wave. This is usually represented by T-wave inversion. ST-segment changes occur with ischemia that produces myocardial injury. When the acute injury is transmural, the overall ST vector is shifted in the direction of the outer epicardium, resulting in ST-segment elevation[17] (see Fig. 18-8). When the injury is confined primarily to the subendocardium, the overall ST segment shifts toward the inner ventricular layer, resulting in an overall depression of the ST segment. Abnormal Q waves, which develop when there is no depolarizing current conduction from the necrotic tissue, signify transmural infarction or ST-segment elevation AMI.

Serum Markers. The serum markers for AMI include myoglobin, creatine kinase MB (CK-MB), and troponin I (TnI) and troponin T (TnT).[18] As the myocardial cells become necrotic, their intracellular enzymes and other components begin to diffuse into the surrounding interstitium and then into the blood. The rate at which the serum markers appear in the blood depends on their intracellular location, their molecular weight, and local blood flow. For example, they may appear at an earlier than predicted time because of return of blood flow in patients who have undergone successful reperfusion therapy.

Creatine kinase is an intracellular enzyme found in muscle cells. CK exceeds normal ranges within 4 to 8 hours of myocardial injury and declines to normal within 2 to 3 days.[18] There are three isoenzymes of CK, with the MB isoenzyme being highly specific for injury to myocardial tissue. *Myoglobin* is an oxygen-carrying protein, similar to hemoglobin, that is normally present in cardiac and skeletal muscle. It is a small molecule that is released quickly from infarcted myocardial tissue and becomes elevated within 1 hour after myocardial cell death, with peak levels reached within 4 to 8 hours.[18] Because myoglobin is present in both cardiac and skeletal muscle, it is not cardiac specific.

The *troponin* complex, which is part of the actin filament, consists of three subunits (*i.e.,* TnC, TnT, and TnI) that regulate the calcium-mediated actin-myosin contractile process in striated muscle. TnI and TnT, which are present in cardiac muscle, begin to rise within 3 hours after the onset of myocardial infarction and may remain elevated for 7 to 10 days after the event.[18] It is thought that cardiac troponin assays are more capable of detecting episodes of myocardial infarction in which cell damage is insufficient to produce a rise in the CK-MB level.

Unstable Angina

Unstable angina is considered to be a clinical syndrome of myocardial ischemia ranging between stable angina and myocardial infarction. It most frequently results from atherosclerotic plaque disruption, platelet aggregation, and secondary hemostasis. Coronary vasoconstriction may also play a role. Unstable angina may occur as a primary disorder (*i.e.*, progression of variant or stable angina); as a secondary disorder due to a noncoronary condition (*e.g.*, anemia, infection, cocaine use); or as a postinfarction angina that develops within 2 weeks of an AMI.[15] Cocaine can induce myocardial ischemia through increased myocardial oxygen demand or decreased oxygen supply from coronary artery spasm or thrombosis, and can cause unstable angina and myocardial infarction.[19]

In contrast to stable angina, the pain associated with unstable angina has a more persistent and severe course and is characterized by at least one of three features: (1) it occurs at rest (or with minimal exertion) and usually lasts more than 20 minutes (if not interrupted by nitroglycerin); (2) it is severe and described as frank pain of new onset (*i.e.*, within 1 month); and (3) it occurs with a pattern that is more severe, prolonged, or frequent than previously experienced.[15]

The differential diagnosis of unstable angina and non–ST-segment AMI is based on pain severity and presenting symptoms, heart rate and blood pressure stability, ECG findings, and serum cardiac markers. Guidelines developed by the American College of Cardiology and American Heart Association (ACC/AHA) Task Force on Practice Guidelines for Management of Patients with Unstable Angina and non–ST-segment AMI indicate that the two conditions are similar but of different severity.[20] They differ primarily in whether the ischemia is severe enough to cause sufficient myocardial damage to release detectable quantities of serum cardiac markers. Persons who have no evidence of serum markers for myocardial damage are considered to have unstable angina, whereas a diagnosis of non–ST-segment AMI is indicated if a serum marker of myocardial injury is present.

Acute Myocardial Infarction

Acute myocardial infarction, also known as a *heart attack*, is characterized by the ischemic death of myocardial tissue. The area of infarction is determined by the coronary artery that is affected and by its distribution of blood flow.

The onset of AMI usually is abrupt, with pain as the significant symptom. The pain typically is severe and crushing, often described as being constricting, suffocating, or like "someone sitting on my chest." The pain usually is substernal, radiating to the left arm, neck, or jaw, although it may be experienced in other areas of the chest. Unlike that of angina, the pain associated with AMI is more prolonged and not relieved by rest or nitroglycerin, and narcotics frequently are required. Women often experience atypical ischemic-type chest discomfort, whereas the elderly may complain of shortness of breath more frequently than chest pain.[20]

Gastrointestinal complaints are common. There may be a sensation of epigastric distress; nausea and vomiting may occur. These symptoms are thought to be related to the severity of the pain and vagal stimulation. The epigastric distress may be mistaken for indigestion, and the patient may seek relief with antacids or other home remedies, which only delays getting medical attention.

Complaints of fatigue and weakness, especially of the arms and legs, are common. Pain and sympathetic stimulation combine to give rise to tachycardia, anxiety, restlessness, and feelings of impending doom. The skin often is pale, cool, and moist. Impairment of myocardial function may lead to hypotension and shock.

Sudden death from AMI is death that occurs within 1 hour of symptom onset. It usually is attributed to fatal arrhythmias, which may occur without evidence of infarction. Early hospitalization after onset of symptoms greatly improves the chances of averting sudden death because appropriate resuscitation facilities are immediately available when the ventricular arrhythmia occurs.

Pathologic Changes. The extent of the infarct depends on the location and extent of occlusion, amount of heart tissue supplied by the vessel, duration of the occlusion, metabolic needs of the affected tissue, extent of collateral circulation, and other factors such as heart rate, blood pressure, and cardiac rhythm. An infarct may involve the endocardium, myocardium, epicardium, or a combination of these. *Transmural infarcts* (ST-segment elevation AMI) involve the full thickness of the ventricular wall and most commonly occur when there is obstruction of a single artery. *Subendocardial infarcts* (non–ST-segment elevation AMI) involve the inner one third to one half of the ventricular wall and occur more frequently in the presence of severely narrowed but still patent arteries. Most infarcts are transmural, involving the free wall of the left ventricle and the interventricular septum (Fig. 18-9).

Although gross tissue changes are not apparent for hours after onset of an AMI, the ischemic area ceases to function within a matter of minutes, and irreversible

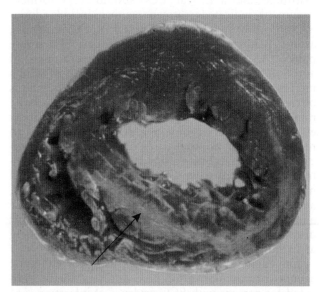

FIGURE 18-9 Acute myocardial infarct. A cross section of the ventricles of a man who died a few days after the onset of severe chest pain shows a transmural infarct in the posterior and septal regions of the left ventricle. The necrotic myocardium is soft, yellowish, and sharply demarcated. (From Rubin E., Farber J. L. [1999]. *Pathology,* [3rd ed., p. 558]. Philadelphia: Lippincott Williams & Wilkins.)

damage to cells occurs in approximately 40 minutes. Irreversible myocardial cell death (necrosis) occurs after 20 to 40 minutes of severe ischemia.[7] The term *reperfusion* refers to reestablishment of blood flow through use of thrombolytic therapy or revascularization procedures. Early reperfusion (within 15 to 20 minutes) after onset of ischemia can prevent necrosis. Reperfusion after a longer interval can salvage some of the myocardial cells that would have died owing to longer periods of ischemia. It also may prevent microvascular injury that occurs over a longer period. Even though much of the viable myocardium existing at the time of reperfusion ultimately recovers, critical abnormalities in biochemical function may persist, causing impaired ventricular function. The recovering area of the heart is often referred to as a *stunned myocardium.* Because myocardial function is lost before cell death occurs, a stunned myocardium may not be capable of sustaining life, and persons with large areas of dysfunctional myocardium may require life support until the stunned regions regain their function.[10]

Diagnosis and Treatment. Diagnosis of AMI is based on presenting signs and symptoms, ECG changes, and serum cardiac markers. ECG changes may not be present immediately after the onset of symptoms, except as arrhythmias. The occurrence of arrhythmias and conduction defects depends on the areas of the heart and conduction pathways that are included in the infarct.

The treatment of ACS depends on the extent of ischemia or infarction. Because the specific diagnosis of AMI often is difficult to make at the time of entry into the health care system, the immediate management of all cases of ACS in general is the same. ECG monitoring should be instituted, and a 12-lead ECG should be performed. Commonly indicated treatment regimens include administration of oxygen by nasal prongs, analgesic agents, aspirin, β-adrenergic blockers, and nitrates.[20] The severe pain of AMI gives rise to anxiety and recruitment of autonomic nervous system responses, both of which increase the work demands of the heart. Morphine is often given intravenously for pain relief because it has a rapid onset of action. Aspirin is given for its antiplatelet effects. β-Adrenergic–blocking drugs may be used to reduce sympathetic stimulation of the heart after myocardial infarction. These drugs decrease myocardial contractility and cardiac workload, alter resting myocardial membrane potentials and decrease arrhythmia frequency, and may aid in redistributing coronary artery blood flow and improving myocardial blood flow. Antiarrhythmic drugs may be given to prevent or treat life-threatening arrhythmias that often occur with AMI.

Immediate reperfusion therapy, using thrombolytic agents or revascularization procedures, is usually indicated for persons with ECG evidence of infarction (*i.e.,* ST-segment elevation AMI). Thrombolytic drugs dissolve blood and platelet clots and are used to reduce mortality and limit infarct size. These agents interact with plasminogen to generate plasmin, which lyses fibrin clots and digests clotting factors V and VIII, prothrombin, and fibrinogen (see Chapter 10). The best results

occur if treatment is initiated within 60 to 90 minutes of symptom onset.[20] The magnitude of benefit declines after this period, but it is possible that some benefit can be achieved for up to 12 hours after the onset of pain. The person must be a low-risk candidate for complications caused by bleeding.

Revascularization interventions include percutaneous coronary intervention and coronary artery bypass surgery. These interventions are increasingly being used on an emergency basis as a primary intervention to relieve coronary artery obstruction caused by atherosclerotic lesions. *Percutaneous coronary intervention* (PCI) includes percutaneous transluminal coronary angioplasty (PTCA), stent implantation, atherectomy, and thrombectomy.[21] *Balloon PTCA* involves dilatation of a vessel containing a stenotic atherosclerotic plaque with an inflatable balloon (Fig. 18-10). The procedure is done under local anesthesia in the cardiac catheterization laboratory. Implantation of coronary stents (fenestrated, stainless steel tubes) reduces the occurrence of restenosis after PTCA.[21] A relatively new approach to the prevention of coronary restenosis after balloon angioplasty and stent placement is the use of localized intracoronary radiation. The procedure, also known as *brachytherapy,* is credited with inhibiting cell proliferation and vascular lesion formation and preventing constrictive arterial remodeling. The radiation source can be impregnated into stents, or the radiation can be delivered by a radiation catheter containing a sealed source of radiation (radioactive seeds, wire, or ribbon) that is inserted into the treatment site, after which the catheter is removed.[22,23] Drug-eluting stents are also an important new development in the prevention of coro-

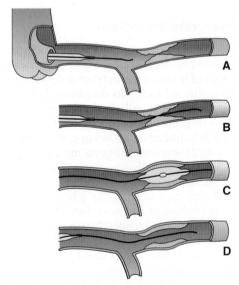

FIGURE 18-10 (A) Percutaneous transluminal coronary angioplasty (PTCA) dilation catheter and guidewire exiting the guiding catheter. **(B)** Guidewire advanced across the stenosis. **(C)** Dilation catheter advanced across the stenosis and inflated. **(D)** Dilation catheter pulled back to assess luminal diameter. (Reprinted with permission of Advanced Cardiovascular Systems [ACS], Inc., Santa Clara, CA.)

nary restenosis. These stents contain a slow-release drug (sirolimus or paclitaxel) that decreases the intimal hyperplasia causing restenosis.

Coronary artery bypass grafting (CABG) may be the treatment of choice for people with significant CHD who do not respond to medical treatment and who are not suitable candidates for PCI. It may also be indicated as a treatment for AMI, in which case the surgery should be done within 4 to 6 hours of symptom onset if possible. The procedure involves revascularization of the affected myocardium by placing a saphenous vein graft between the aorta and the affected coronary artery distal to the site of occlusion, or by using the internal mammary artery to revascularize the left anterior descending artery or its branches (Fig. 18-11). One to five distal anastomoses commonly are done.

Myocardial Postinfarction Recovery Period. After a myocardial infarction, there usually are three zones of tissue damage: a zone of myocardial tissue that becomes necrotic because of an absolute lack of blood flow; a surrounding zone of injured cells, some of which will recover; and an outer zone in which cells are ischemic and can be salvaged if blood flow can be reestablished (Fig. 18-12).

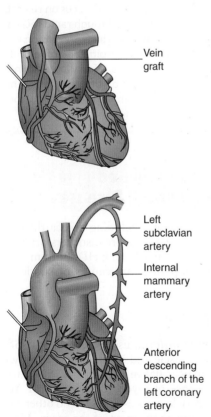

FIGURE 18-11 Coronary artery revascularization. (**Top**) Saphenous vein bypass graft. The vein segment is sutured to the ascending aorta and the right coronary artery at a point distal to the occluding lesion. (**Bottom**) Mammary artery bypass. The mammary artery is anastomosed to the anterior descending left coronary artery, bypassing the obstructing lesion.

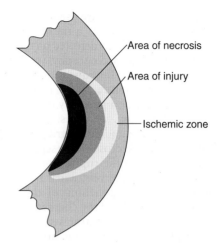

FIGURE 18-12 Areas of tissue damage after myocardial infarction.

The boundaries of these zones may change with time after the infarction and with the success of treatment measures to reestablish blood flow. The progression of ischemic necrosis usually begins in the subendocardial area of the heart and extends through the myocardium to involve progressively more of the transmural thickness of the ischemic zone.

Myocardial cells that undergo necrosis are gradually replaced with scar tissue. An acute inflammatory response develops in the area of necrosis approximately 2 to 3 days after infarction. Thereafter, macrophages begin removing the necrotic tissue; the damaged area is gradually replaced with an ingrowth of highly vascularized granulation tissue, which gradually becomes less vascular and more fibrous.[7] At approximately 4 to 7 days, the center of the infarcted area is soft and yellow; if rupture of the ventricle, interventricular septum, or valve structures occurs, it usually happens at this time. Replacement of the necrotic myocardial tissue usually is complete by the seventh week.

The stages of recovery from AMI are closely related to the size of the infarct and the changes that have taken place in the infarcted area. Fibrous scar tissue lacks the contractile, elastic, and conductive properties of normal myocardial cells; the residual effects and complications are determined essentially by the extent and location of the injury. Among the complications of AMI are sudden death, heart failure and cardiogenic shock, pericarditis and Dressler syndrome, thromboemboli, rupture of the heart, and ventricular aneurysms.

Pericarditis may complicate the course of AMI. Acute pericarditis usually appears on the second or third day after infarction and tends to be associated with large transmural infarctions. Pericarditis developing later (2 to 10 weeks) after AMI may represent *Dressler syndrome*, which is thought to be a hypersensitivity response to tissue necrosis. Thromboemboli are a potential complication of AMI, arising as venous thrombi or occasionally as clots from the wall of the ventricle. Immobility and impaired cardiac function contribute to stasis of blood in the venous system. Elastic stockings, active and passive leg exercises, as well as heparin are usually included in the postinfarction treatment plan as a means of preventing thrombus formation. If a clot is detected on the wall of the ventricle (usually by echocardiography), treatment with anticoagulants is indicated. Infrequent but dreaded complications of AMI are rupture of the myocardium, the interventricular septum, or a papillary muscle. Complete rupture of the myocardium, which usually occurs 3 to 7 days after AMI, when the injured ventricular tissue is soft and weak, often is fatal. Necrosis of the septal wall or papillary muscle may lead to the rupture of either of these structures, with worsening of ventricular performance.

An aneurysm is an outpouching of the ventricular wall. Scar tissue does not have the characteristics of normal myocardial tissue; when a large section of ventricular muscle is replaced by scar tissue, an aneurysm may develop (Fig. 18-13). This section of the myocardium does not contract with the rest of the ventricle during systole. Instead, it diminishes the pumping efficiency of the heart and increases the work of the left ventricle, predisposing the patient to heart failure. Ischemia in the surrounding area predisposes the patient to development of arrhythmias, and stasis of blood in the aneurysm can lead to thrombus formation. Surgical resection may be performed to improve ventricular function.

In summary, CHD is a disorder of impaired coronary blood flow, usually caused by atherosclerosis. Myocardial ischemia occurs when there is a disparity between coronary blood flow and the metabolic needs of the heart. Ischemia can be present as chronic ischemic heart disease and as an ACS. Diagnostic methods for CHD include ECG methods, exercise stress testing, nuclear imaging studies, and angiographic studies in the cardiac catheterization laboratory.

The chronic ischemic heart diseases include chronic stable angina, variant angina, and silent myocardial ischemia. Chronic stable angina is associated with a fixed atherosclerotic obstruction and pain that is precipitated by increased work demands on the heart and relieved by rest. Silent myocardial ischemia occurs without symptoms. Variant angina results from spasms of the coronary arteries.

The acute coronary syndromes result from unstable atherosclerotic plaques, platelet aggregation, and thrombus formation. They include unstable angina and AMI. Unstable angina is an accelerated form of angina in which the pain occurs more frequently, is more severe, and lasts longer than in chronic stable angina. AMI refers to the ischemic death of myocardial tissue associated with obstructed blood flow in the coronary arteries due to plaque disruption and occlusion of blood flow. The complications of AMI include potentially fatal arrhythmias, heart failure and cardiogenic shock, pericarditis, thromboembolic disease, rupture of cardiac structures, and ventricular aneurysms. Diagnostic methods include ECG monitoring and assessment of serum cardiac marker levels. Treatment goals focus on reestablishment of myocardial blood flow through rapid recanalization of the occluded coronary artery, prevention of clot extension through use of aspirin and other antiplatelet and antithrombotic agents, alleviation of pain, measures such as administration of oxygen to increase the oxygen saturation of hemoglobin, and the use of vasodilators to reduce the work demands of the heart.

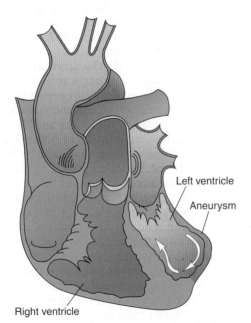

FIGURE 18-13 Paradoxical movement of a ventricular aneurysm during systole.

 Myocardial and Endocardial Diseases

Myocardial diseases, including myocarditis and the primary cardiomyopathies, are disorders originating in the myocardium, but not from CHD. Both myocarditis and the cardiomyopathies are causes of sudden death and heart failure.

MYOCARDITIS

The term *myocarditis* is used to describe an inflammation of the heart muscle and conduction system without evidence of myocardial infarction.[24] Viruses are the most important cause of myocarditis in North America and Europe. Coxsackieviruses A and B and other enteroviruses probably account for most of the cases. Myocarditis is a frequent pathologic cardiac finding in persons with acquired immunodeficiency syndrome (AIDS), although it is unclear whether it is due to HIV or to a secondary infection. Other causes of myocarditis are radiation therapy, hypersensitivity reactions, or exposure to chemical or physical agents that induce acute myocardial necrosis and secondary inflammatory changes.

Myocardial injury due to infectious agents is thought to result from necrosis caused by direct invasion of the offending organism, toxic effects of exotoxins or endotoxins produced by a systemic pathogen, or destruction of cardiac tissue by immunologic mechanisms initiated by the infectious agent. The immunologic response may be directed at foreign antigens of the infectious agent that share molecular characteristics with those of the host cardiac myocytes (*i.e.*, molecular mimicry; see Chapter 15), providing a continuous stimulus for the immune response even after the infectious agent has been cleared from the body.

The *manifestations* of myocarditis vary from an absence of symptoms to profound heart failure or sudden death. When viral myocarditis occurs in children or young adults, it often is asymptomatic. Acute symptomatic myocarditis typically manifests as a flulike syndrome with malaise, low-grade fever, and tachycardia that is more pronounced than would be expected for the level of fever present. There commonly is a history of an upper respiratory tract or gastrointestinal tract infection, followed by a latent period of several days. In approximately one half of the cases, myocarditis is transient, and symptoms subside within 1 to 2 months. In other cases, fulminant heart failure and life-threatening arrhythmias develop, causing sudden death. Still others progress to subacute and chronic disease.

The *diagnosis* of myocarditis can be suggested by clinical manifestations. The ECG changes of acute myocarditis include conduction disturbances such as ventricular arrhythmias, AV junctional block, ST-segment elevation, T-wave inversion, and transient Q waves. Serum creatinine kinase often is elevated. Troponin T or troponin I, or both, may be elevated, providing evidence of myocardial cell damage. Confirmation of active myocarditis requires endomyocardial biopsy.

Treatment measures focus on symptom management and prevention of myocardial damage. Bed rest is necessary, and activity restriction must be maintained until fever and cardiac symptoms subside to decrease the myocardial workload. Specific antimicrobial therapy is indicated when an infectious agent has been identified. The use of corticosteroids and immunosuppressant drugs such as azathioprine and cyclosporine remains controversial. Although treatment of myocarditis is successful in many persons, some progress to congestive heart failure and can expect only a limited life span. For these persons, heart transplantation becomes an alternative.

CARDIOMYOPATHIES

The cardiomyopathies are a group of disorders that affect the heart muscle. They can develop as primary or secondary disorders.[25] The primary cardiomyopathies, which include dilated, hypertrophic, restrictive (Fig. 18-14), and peripartum cardiomyopathy, are heart muscle diseases of unknown origin. Secondary cardiomyopathies

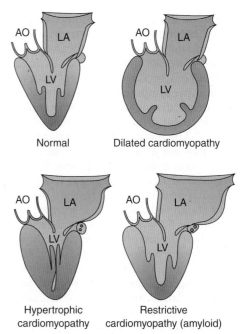

FIGURE 18-14 The various types of cardiomyopathies compared with the normal heart. (From Roberts W. C., Ferrans V. J. [1975]. Pathologic anatomy of the cardiomyopathies. *Human pathology* 6, 289, with permission from Elsevier Science.)

are conditions in which the cardiac abnormality results from another cardiovascular disease, such as myocardial infarction.

Dilated Cardiomyopathies

Dilated cardiomyopathies are characterized by progressive cardiac hypertrophy and dilatation and impaired pumping ability of one or both ventricles. Although all four chambers of the heart are affected, the ventricles are more dilated than the atria. Because of the wall thinning that accompanies dilatation, the thickness of the ventricular wall often is less than would be expected for the amount of hypertrophy present.[26] Mural thrombi are common and may be a source of thromboemboli. The cardiac valves are intrinsically normal. Microscopically, there is evidence of scarring and atrophy of myocardial cells.

Dilated cardiomyopathy may result from a number of different myocardial insults, including infectious myocarditis, alcohol and other toxic agents, metabolic influences, neuromuscular diseases, and immunologic disorders. Genetic influences have been documented in some cases. One study found that 20% of affected persons have first-degree relatives with myocardial dysfunction.[27] These disorders can be inherited in an autosomal dominant, autosomal recessive, or X-linked pattern. High alcohol consumption is another cause of cardiomyopathy. It accounts for 3.8% of all cardiomyopathy cases and is reported to be the second leading cause of a dilated cardiomyopathy.[28] Often the cause is unknown; these cases are appropriately designated as *idiopathic dilated cardiomyopathy.*

The most common initial manifestations of dilated cardiomyopathy are those related to heart failure. There is a profound reduction in the left ventricular ejection fraction (*i.e.*, ratio of stroke volume to end-diastolic volume) to 40% or less, compared with a normal value of approximately 67%. After symptoms have developed, the course of the disorder is distinguished by worsening of heart failure, development of mural thrombi, and ventricular arrhythmias.[29] The most striking symptoms of dilated cardiomyopathy are dyspnea on exertion, paroxysmal nocturnal dyspnea, orthopnea, weakness, fatigue, ascites, and peripheral edema. On physical examination, an enlarged apical beat with the presence of a third and fourth heart sound and a murmur associated with regurgitation of one or both AV valves frequently are found. The systolic blood pressure is normal or low, and the peripheral pulses often are of low amplitude. Pulsus alternans, in which the pulse regularly alternates between weaker and stronger volume, may be present. Sinus tachycardia, atrial fibrillation, and complex ventricular arrhythmias leading to sudden cardiac death are common.

The treatment of dilated cardiomyopathy is directed toward relieving the symptoms of heart failure and reducing the workload of the heart. Digoxin, diuretics, angiotensin-converting enzyme inhibitors, aldosterone antagonists (*e.g.*, spironolactone), and β-blocker drugs are used to improve myocardial contractility and decrease left ventricular filling pressures. Avoiding myocardial depressants, including alcohol, and pacing rest with asymptomatic levels of exercise or activity is imperative. Proper electrolyte balance and implantable cardioverter-defibrillators are effective in controlling recurrent ventricular arrhythmias associated with dilated cardiomyopathy. Chronic anticoagulation with warfarin is also warranted for patients with a very low ejection fraction because of the high risk of thromboemboli. In persons with severe heart failure that is refractory to treatment, cardiac transplantation may be considered.

Hypertrophic Cardiomyopathies

Hypertrophic cardiomyopathy is characterized by an abnormality that involves excessive ventricular growth or hypertrophy.[30–32] Although the hypertrophy may be symmetric, the involvement of the ventricular septum often is disproportionate, producing intermittent left ventricular outflow obstruction (Fig. 18-15A). Synonyms for this disorder include *idiopathic hypertrophic subaortic stenosis* and *asymmetric septal hypertrophy*.

Symptomatic hypertrophic cardiomyopathy commonly is a disease of young adulthood and is the most common cause of sudden cardiac death in the young.[30] The cause of the disorder is unknown, although it often is of familial origin, with the disorder being inherited as an autosomal dominant trait. Molecular studies of the genetic alterations responsible for hypertrophic cardiomyopathy suggest that the disease is caused by mutation in 1 of 10 genes encoding the proteins of the cardiac sarcomeres (*i.e.*, muscle fibers).[31] Three of the mutant genes predominate: the β-myosin heavy chain, cardiac troponin T, and myosin-binding protein C. The other genes account for a minority of cases. The prognosis of persons with different myosin mutations varies greatly; some mutations are relatively benign, whereas others are associated with premature death.

A distinctive microscopic finding in hypertrophic cardiomyopathy is myofibril disarray (see Fig. 18-15B). Instead of the normal parallel arrangement of myofibrils,

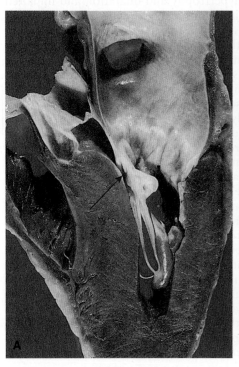 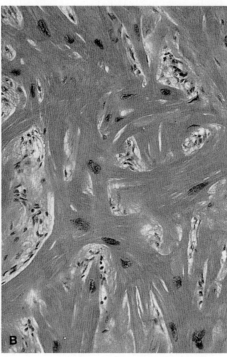

FIGURE 18-15 Hypertrophic cardiomyopathy. (**A**) The heart has been opened to show striking asymmetric left ventricular hypertrophy. The interventricular septum is thicker than the free wall of the ventricle and impinges on the outflow tract (*arrow*). (**B**) A section of the myocardium shows myocardial fiber disarray characterized by oblique and often perpendicular orientation of adjacent hypertrophic myocytes. (From Saffitz J. E., [2005]. The heart. In Rubin E., Gorstein F., Rubin R., et al. [Eds.], *Rubin's pathology: Clinicopathologic foundations of medicine* [4th ed., p. 572]. Philadelphia: Lippincott Williams & Wilkins.)

the myofibrils branch off at random angles, sometimes at right angles to an adjacent fiber with which they connect. Small bundles of fibers may course haphazardly through normally arranged muscle fibers.[7,32] These disordered fibers may produce abnormal movements of the ventricles, with uncoordinated contraction and impaired relaxation. Arrhythmias and premature sudden death are common with this disorder.

The manifestations of hypertrophic cardiomyopathy are variable; for reasons that are unclear, some persons with the disorder remain stable for many years and gradually acquire more symptoms as the disease progresses, but others experience sudden cardiac death as first evidence of the disease.[30,31] Atrial fibrillation is a common precursor to sudden death in those who die of arrhythmias. Dyspnea is the most common symptom associated with a gradual elevation in left ventricular diastolic pressure resulting from impaired ventricular filling and increased wall stiffness due to ventricular hypertrophy. Because of the obstruction to outflow from the left ventricle, increasingly greater levels of ventricular pressure are needed to eject blood into the aorta, limiting cardiac output. Chest pain, fatigue, and syncope are common and worsen during exertion.

Diagnosis of hypertrophic cardiomyopathy is usually based on history and physical examination. It may be first suspected because of a heart murmur (occasionally discovered during sports preparation examination), positive family history, or ECG findings.[31] Clinical diagnosis is usually established through echocardiography. Screening of first-degree relatives should be encouraged once a diagnosis is made. However, not all people harboring the gene express the clinical features of the gene mutation, such as echocardiographic evidence of left ventricular hypertrophy. For example, it is not unusual for children younger than 13 years of age to carry the gene without evidence of left ventricular hypertrophy. This is because substantial left ventricular remodeling with spontaneous appearance of hypertrophic cardiomyopathy occurs with the accelerated rate of growth during adolescence, and morphologic expression of the gene is usually completed by about 17 to 18 years of age.[31]

The treatment of hypertrophic cardiomyopathy includes medical and surgical management. The goal of medical management is to decrease the risk of sudden death and relieve the symptoms associated with the disorder. Drugs that block the β-adrenergic receptors may be used in persons with chest pain, arrhythmias, or dyspnea.[31,33] These drugs reduce the heart rate and improve myocardial function by allowing more time for ventricular filling and reducing ventricular stiffness. The calcium channel–blocking drug verapamil may be used as an alternative to the β-adrenergic blockers. Increased calcium uptake and intracellular calcium content are associated with an increased contractile state, a characteristic finding in patients with hypertrophic cardiomyopathy. Most persons with hypertrophic cardiomyopathy should undergo a risk stratification assessment using echocardiography, 24- to 48-hour Holter ECGs, and exercise testing. An implantable cardioverter-defibrillator

may be used in persons at high risk for developing lethal arrhythmias.[31]

Surgical treatment may be used if severe symptoms persist despite medical treatment. It involves incision of the septum (*i.e.*, myotomy) with or without the removal of part of the tissue (*i.e.*, myectomy). It is accompanied by all the risks of open heart surgery.

Restrictive Cardiomyopathies

Of the three categories of cardiomyopathies, the restrictive type is the least common in Western countries. With this form of cardiomyopathy, ventricular filling is restricted because of excessive rigidity of the ventricular walls, although the contractile properties of the heart remain relatively normal. The condition is endemic in parts of Africa, India, South and Central America, and Asia.[32] Outside the tropics, the most common causes of restrictive cardiomyopathy are endocardial infiltrations such as amyloidosis. Amyloid infiltrations of the heart are common in the elderly. The idiopathic form of the disorder may have a familial origin.

Symptoms of restrictive cardiomyopathy include dyspnea, paroxysmal nocturnal dyspnea, orthopnea, peripheral edema, ascites, fatigue, and weakness. The manifestations of restrictive cardiomyopathy resemble those of constrictive pericarditis. In the advanced form of the disease, all the signs of heart failure are present except cardiomegaly.

 ## Peripartum Cardiomyopathy

Peripartum cardiomyopathy refers to left ventricular dysfunction developing in the last month before delivery to 5 months postpartum. The condition is relatively rare, with an estimated incidence of 1 per 3000 to 4000 live births.[34] Risk factors for peripartum cardiomyopathy include advanced maternal age, African-American race, multifetal pregnancies, preeclampsia, and gestational hypertension.[34] The reported mortality rate ranges from 18% to 56%. Survivors may not recover completely and may require heart transplantation.

The cause of peripartum cardiomyopathy is uncertain. A number of causes have been proposed, including myocarditis, an abnormal immune response to pregnancy, maladaptive response to the hemodynamic stresses of pregnancy, or prolonged inhibition of contractions in premature labor. There is stronger evidence for myocarditis as a cause than for other purported etiologies.[35]

The signs and symptoms resemble those of dilated cardiomyopathy. Because many women experience dyspnea, fatigue, and pedal edema during the last month of normal pregnancy, the symptoms may be ignored and the diagnosis delayed. The diagnosis is based on echocardiography studies, ECG, and other tests of cardiac function. Treatment methods are similar to those used in dilated cardiomyopathy.

There are two possible outcomes of peripartum cardiomyopathy. In approximately one half of cases, the heart returns to normal within 6 months, and the chances for long-term survival are good. In these women, heart failure returns only during subsequent pregnancies. In the other half of cases, the dilated cardiomyopathy persists, and the prognosis is poor and death is probable if another pregnancy occurs. In women with cardiomyopathy from documented viral myocarditis, the likelihood of recurrence is low.

DISORDERS AFFECTING THE ENDOCARDIUM

Infective Endocarditis

Infective endocarditis is a relatively uncommon, life-threatening infection of the endocardial surface of the heart, including the heart valves. It is characterized by colonization or invasion of the heart valves and the mural endocardium by a microbial agent, leading to the formation of bulky, friable vegetations and destruction of underlying cardiac tissues.[7] Because bacteria are the most frequent infecting organisms, the condition may be referred to as *bacterial endocarditis*. Despite important advances in antimicrobial therapy and improved ability to diagnose and treat complications, infective endocarditis continues to produce substantial morbidity and mortality.

Etiology and Pathogenesis. Two factors contribute to the development of infective endocarditis: a damaged endocardial surface and a portal of entry by which the organism gains access to the circulatory system. The presence of valvular disease, prosthetic heart valves, or congenital heart defects provides an environment conducive to bacterial growth.[7,36,37] In persons with preexisting valvular or endocardial defects, simple gum massage or an innocuous oral lesion may afford the pathogenic bacteria access to the bloodstream. Transient bacteremia may also emerge in the course of seemingly minor health problems, such as an upper respiratory tract infection, a skin lesion, or a dental procedure.

Although infective endocarditis usually occurs in persons with preexisting heart lesions, it also can develop in normal hearts of intravenous drug abusers. The mode of infection is a contaminated drug solution or a needle contaminated with skin flora. Intravenous drug abuse is the most common source of right-sided (tricuspid) lesions. Although staphylococcal infections are common, intravenous drug users may be infected with unusual organisms, such as gram-negative bacilli, yeasts, and fungi. In hospitalized patients, infective endocarditis may arise as a complication of infected intravascular or urinary tract catheters. Infective endocarditis also may complicate prosthetic heart valve replacement. It can develop as an early infection that follows surgery or as a later infection resulting from the long-term presence of the prosthesis.

Depending on the duration of the disease, presenting manifestations, and complications, cases of infective endocarditis can be classified as acute, subacute, or chronic. Acute infective endocarditis is typically caused by *Staphylococcus aureus*,[36] which produces a rapidly progressive and destructive form of the disease. Subacute endocarditis is usually caused by less virulent organisms such as *Streptococcus viridans*, coagulase-negative staphylococci, enterococci, and other gram-negative bacilli.[36]

Both subacute and acute forms of infective endocarditis involve the formation of intracardiac vegetative lesions that have local and systemic effects. The vegetative lesion that is characteristic of infective endocarditis consists of a collection of infectious organisms and cellular debris enmeshed in the fibrin strands of clotted blood. The infectious loci continuously release bacteria into the bloodstream and are a source of persistent bacteremia. These lesions may be singular or multiple, may grow to be as large as several centimeters, and usually are found loosely attached to the free edges of the valve surface[32] (Fig. 18-16). As the lesions grow, they cause valve destruction, leading to valvular regurgitation, abscesses of the valve ring with heart block, and valve perforation. The loose organization of these lesions permits the organisms and fragments of the lesions to form emboli and travel in the bloodstream. The fragments may lodge in small blood vessels, causing small hemorrhages, abscesses, and infarction of tissue. The bacteremia also can initiate immune responses thought to be responsible for the skin manifestations, arthritis, glomerulonephritis, and other immune disorders associated with the condition.

Clinical Course. The clinical course of infective endocarditis is determined by the extent of heart damage, the type of organism involved, site of infection (*i.e.*, right or left side of the heart), and whether embolization from the site of infection occurs. Destruction of infected heart valves is common with certain organisms, such as *S. aureus*. Peripheral embolization can lead to metastatic infections and abscess formation; these are particularly serious when they affect organs such as the brain and kidneys. In right-sided endocarditis, which usually involves the tricuspid valve, septic emboli travel to the lung, causing infarction and lung abscesses.

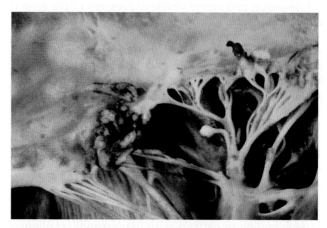

FIGURE 18-16 Bacterial endocarditis. The mitral valve shows destructive vegetations, which have eroded through the free margin of the valve leaflet. (From Rubin E., Farber J. L. [Eds.]. [1999]. *Pathology* [3rd ed., p. 572]. Philadelphia: Lippincott Williams & Wilkins.)

The signs and symptoms of infective endocarditis include fever and signs of systemic infection, change in the character of an existing heart murmur, and evidence of embolic distribution of the vegetative lesions. In the acute form, the fever usually is spiking and accompanied by chills. In the subacute form, the fever usually is low grade, of gradual onset, and frequently accompanied by other systemic signs of inflammation, such as anorexia, malaise, and lethargy. Small petechial hemorrhages frequently result when emboli lodge in the small vessels of the skin, nail beds, and mucous membranes. Splinter hemorrhages (*i.e.*, dark red lines) under the nails of the fingers and toes are common. Cough, dyspnea, arthralgia or arthritis, diarrhea, and abdominal or flank pain may occur as the result of systemic emboli.

Diagnosis and Treatment. The blood culture is the most definitive diagnostic procedure and is essential to guide treatment. The optimal time to obtain cultures is during a chill, just before a temperature rise. Positive cultures usually are obtainable for infections caused by gram-positive cocci, but cultures may fail to identify gram-negative organisms or fungi. The echocardiogram is useful in detecting underlying valvular disease. Transesophageal echocardiography is rapid and noninvasive, and has proved useful for detecting vegetations. Other diagnostic criteria include a predisposing heart condition; fever; vascular phenomena such as emboli, mycotic aneurysm, or intracranial hemorrhage; and immunologic phenomena such as glomerulonephritis or rheumatoid factor.

Treatment of infective endocarditis focuses on identifying and eliminating the causative microorganism, minimizing the residual cardiac effects, and treating the pathologic effects of the emboli. Antibiotic therapy is used to eradicate the pathogen. Blood cultures are used to identify the causative organism and determine the most appropriate antibiotic regimen. Surgery may be indicated for moderate to severe heart failure, progressive renal failure, significant emboli, arrhythmias, or left-sided endocarditis. Infected prosthetic valves may need to be replaced.

Of great importance is the prevention of infective endocarditis in persons with prosthetic heart valves, previous bacterial endocarditis, certain congenital heart defects, and other known risk factors.[38] Prevention can be accomplished largely through prophylactic administration of an antibiotic before dental and other procedures that may cause bacteremia.[38]

Rheumatic Heart Disease

Rheumatic fever is an acute, immune-mediated, multisystem inflammatory disease that follows a group A (β-hemolytic) streptococcal (GAS) throat infection. The most serious aspect of rheumatic fever is the development of chronic valvular disorders that produce permanent cardiac dysfunction and sometimes cause fatal heart failure years later. In the United States and other industrialized countries, the incidence of rheumatic fever and prevalence of rheumatic heart disease has markedly declined in the past 40 to 50 years.[39] This decline has been attributed to the introduction of antimicrobial agents for improved treatment of GAS pharyngitis, increased access to medical care, and improved economic standards, along with better and less crowded housing. Unfortunately, rheumatic fever and rheumatic heart disease continue to be major health problems in many underdeveloped countries, where inadequate health care, poor nutrition, and crowded living conditions still prevail.

Rheumatic fever is primarily a disease of school-aged children. The incidence of acute rheumatic fever peaks between 5 and 15 years of age.[7] The disease usually follows an inciting GAS throat infection by 1 to 4 weeks. Rheumatic fever and its cardiac complications can be prevented by antibiotic treatment of the initial GAS throat infection.

Pathogenesis. The pathogenesis of rheumatic fever is unclear. The time frame for development of symptoms in relation to the sore throat and the presence of antibodies to the GAS organism strongly suggests an immunologic origin. Like other immunologic phenomena, rheumatic fever requires an initial sensitizing exposure to the offending streptococcal agent, and the risk of recurrence is high after each subsequent exposure. Although only a small percentage (*e.g.*, 3%) of persons with untreated GAS pharyngitis develop rheumatic fever, the incidence of recurrence with a subsequent untreated infection is substantially greater (about 50%).[39] These observations and more recent studies suggest a familial predisposition to development of the disease.

Clinical Course. Rheumatic fever can manifest as an acute, recurrent, or chronic disorder. The *acute stage* of rheumatic fever includes a history of an initiating streptococcal infection and subsequent involvement of the connective tissue elements of the heart, blood vessels, joints, and subcutaneous tissues. Common to all is a lesion called the *Aschoff body*,[7] which is a localized area of tissue necrosis surrounded by immune cells. The *recurrent phase* usually involves extension of the cardiac effects of the disease. The *chronic phase* of rheumatic fever is characterized by permanent deformity of the heart valves and is a common cause of mitral valve stenosis. Chronic rheumatic heart disease usually does not appear until at least 10 years after the initial attack, sometimes decades later.

Most children with rheumatic fever have a history of sore throat, headache, fever, abdominal pain, nausea, vomiting, swollen glands (usually at the angle of the jaw), and other signs and symptoms of streptococcal infection. Other clinical features associated with an acute episode of rheumatic fever are related to the acute inflammatory process and the structures involved in the disease process. The course of the disease is characterized by a constellation of findings that includes carditis, migratory polyarthritis of the large joints, erythema marginatum, subcutaneous nodules, and Sydenham chorea.[39]

Acute rheumatic carditis, which complicates the acute phase of rheumatic fever, can affect the pericardium, myocardium, or endocardium. Usually all three layers of the heart are involved. Both the pericarditis and myocarditis usually are self-limited manifestations of the acute stage of rheumatic fever. The involvement of the endocardium and valvular structures produces the permanent and disabling effects of rheumatic fever. Although any of the four valves can be involved, the mitral and aortic valves are affected most often. During the acute inflammatory stage of the disease, the valvular structures become red and swollen; small vegetative lesions develop on the valve leaflets. The acute inflammatory changes gradually proceed to development of fibrous scar tissue, which tends to contract and cause deformity of the valve leaflets and shortening of the chordae tendineae. In some cases, the edges or commissures of the valve leaflets fuse together as healing occurs.

The manifestations of acute rheumatic carditis include a heart murmur in a child without a previous history of rheumatic fever, change in the character of a murmur in a person with a previous history of the disease, cardiomegaly or enlargement of the heart, friction rub or other signs of pericarditis, and congestive heart failure in a child without discernible cause.

Although not a cause of permanent disability, *polyarthritis* is the most common finding in rheumatic fever. The arthritis involves the larger joints, particularly the knees, ankles, elbows, and wrists, and almost always is migratory, affecting one joint and then moving to another. In untreated cases, the arthritis lasts approximately 4 weeks. A striking feature of rheumatic arthritis is the dramatic response (usually within 48 hours) to salicylates.

Erythema marginatum lesions are maplike, macular areas most commonly seen on the trunk or inner aspects of the upper arm and thigh. Skin lesions are present only in approximately 10% of patients who have rheumatic fever; they are transitory and disappear during the course of the disease. The *subcutaneous nodules* are 1 to 4 cm in diameter. They are hard, painless, and freely movable and usually overlie the extensor muscles of the wrist, elbow, ankle, and knee joints. Subcutaneous nodules are rare, but when present, they occur most often in persons with carditis.

Chorea (*i.e.,* Sydenham chorea), sometimes called *St. Vitus' dance*, is the major central nervous system manifestation. It is seen most frequently in girls. There typically is an insidious onset of irritability and other behavior problems. The child often is fidgety, cries easily, begins to walk clumsily, and drops things. The choreic movements are spontaneous, rapid, purposeless, jerking movements that interfere with voluntary activities. Facial grimaces are common, and even speech may be affected. The chorea is self-limited, usually running its course within a matter of weeks or months.

Diagnosis and Treatment. The diagnosis of rheumatic fever is based on the Jones criteria, which were initially proposed in 1955 and revised in 1984 and 1992 by a committee of the AHA.[40] The criteria group the signs and symptoms of rheumatic fever into major and minor categories. The presence of two major signs (*i.e.,* cardi-

tis, polyarthritis, chorea, erythema marginatum, and subcutaneous nodules) or one major and two minor signs (*i.e.,* arthralgia, fever, and prolonged PR interval) accompanied by evidence of a preceding GAS infection indicates a high probability of rheumatic fever. The erythrocyte sedimentation rate, C-reactive protein, and white blood cell count commonly are used to confirm recent infection. Echocardiography/Doppler ultrasonography (echo-Doppler) may be used to identify cardiac lesions in persons who do not have typical signs of cardiac involvement during an attack of rheumatic fever.

Treatment of acute rheumatic fever is designed to control the acute inflammatory process and prevent cardiac complications and recurrence of the disease. During the acute phase, antibiotics, anti-inflammatory drugs, and selective restriction of physical activities are prescribed. Penicillin is usually the antibiotic of choice. Salicylates are used to reduce fever and relieve joint pain and swelling. A short course of corticosteroids may be used when the response to salicylates is ineffective. Because of the high risk for recurrence after subsequent GAS throat infections, treatment during the acute phase of the disease is usually followed by secondary prophylaxis using penicillin or an alternative antibiotic.[41] The duration of prophylaxis depends on whether residual valvular disease is present or absent. Usually, prophylaxis is also instituted during dental or other procedures that might provide GAS with access to the bloodstream.

In summary, myocardial disorders represent a diverse group of disorders of myocardial muscle cells, not related to coronary artery disease. Myocarditis is an acute inflammation of cardiac muscle cells, most often of viral origin. Myocardial injury from myocarditis is thought to result from necrosis due to direct invasion of the offending organism, toxic effects of exogenous toxins or endotoxins produced by a systemic pathogen, and destruction of cardiac tissue by immunologic mechanisms initiated by the infectious agent. Although the disease usually is benign and self-limited, it can result in sudden death or chronic heart failure, for which heart transplantation may be considered.

The cardiomyopathies represent disorders of the heart muscle. Cardiomyopathies may manifest as primary or secondary disorders. There are three main types of primary cardiomyopathies: dilated cardiomyopathy, in which fibrosis and atrophy of myocardial cells produces progressive dilatation and impaired pumping ability of the heart; hypertrophic cardiomyopathy, characterized by myocardial hypertrophy, abnormal diastolic filling, and in many cases intermittent left ventricular outflow obstruction; and restrictive cardiomyopathy, in which there is excessive rigidity of the ventricular wall. Peripartum cardiomyopathy occurs during pregnancy. The cause of many of the primary cardiomyopathies is unknown. The disease is suspected when cardiomegaly and heart failure develop in a young, previously healthy person.

Disorders of the endocardium include infective endocarditis and rheumatic fever. Infective endocarditis involves the invasion of the endocardium by pathogens that produce vegetative lesions on the endocardial surface. The loose organization of these lesions permits the organisms and fragments of the lesions to be disseminated throughout the systemic circulation. Two predisposing factors contribute to the development of infective endocarditis: a damaged endocardium and a portal of entry through which the organisms gain access to the bloodstream. Rheumatic fever, which is associated with an antecedent GAS throat infection, is an important cause of heart disease. Its most serious and disabling effects result from involvement of the heart valves. Because there is no single laboratory test, sign, or symptom that is pathognomonic of acute rheumatic fever, the Jones criteria are used to establish the diagnosis during the acute stage of the disease.

KEY CONCEPTS

Valvular Heart Disease

➤ The heart valves determine the direction of blood flow through the heart chambers.

➤ Valvular heart defects exert their effects by obstructing flow of blood (stenotic valve disorder) or allowing backward flow of blood (regurgitant valve disorders).

➤ Stenotic valvular defects produce distention of the heart chamber that empties blood through the diseased valve and impaired filling of the chamber that receives blood that moves through the valve.

➤ Regurgitant valves allow blood to move back through the valve when it should be closed. This produces distention and places increased work demands on the chamber ejecting blood through the diseased valve.

Valvular Heart Disease

The past three decades have brought remarkable advances in the treatment and outlook for people with valvular heart disease. This is undoubtedly due to improved methods for noninvasive monitoring of ventricular function, improvement in prosthetic valves, advances in valve reconstruction procedures, and the development of useful guidelines to improve the timing of surgical interventions.[42,43] Nonetheless, valvular heart disease continues to produce considerable mortality and morbidity.

HEMODYNAMIC DERANGEMENTS

The heart valves consist of thin leaflets of tough, flexible, endothelium-covered fibrous tissue firmly attached at the base to the fibrous valve rings (see Chapter 16). Capillaries and smooth muscle are present at the base of the leaflet but do not extend up into the valve. The leaflets of the heart valves may be injured or become the site of an inflammatory process that can deform their line of closure. Healing of the valve leaflets often is associated with increased collagen content and scarring, causing the leaflets to shorten and become stiffer. The edges or commissures of the valve leaflets can heal together so that the valve does not open or close properly.

Two types of mechanical disruptions occur with valvular heart disease: narrowing of the valve opening so it does not open properly and distortion of the valve so it does not close properly (Fig. 18-17). *Stenosis* refers to a narrowing of the valve orifice and failure of the valve leaflets to open normally. Blood flow through a normal valve can increase by five to seven times the resting volume; consequently, valvular stenosis must be severe before it causes problems. Significant narrowing of the valve orifice increases the resistance to blood flow through the

valve, converting the normally smooth laminar flow to a less efficient turbulent flow. This increases the volume and work of the chamber emptying through the narrowed valve—the left atrium in the case of mitral stenosis and the left ventricle in aortic stenosis. Symptoms usually are noticed first during situations of increased flow, such as exercise. An *incompetent* or *regurgitant valve* permits backward flow to occur when the valve should be closed—flowing back into the left ventricle during diastole when the aortic valve is affected and back into the left atrium during systole when the mitral valve is diseased.

The effect that valvular heart disease has on cardiac function is related to alterations in blood flow across the valve and to the resultant increase in work demands on the heart that the disorder generates. Many valvular heart defects are characterized by heart murmurs resulting from turbulent blood flow through a diseased valve. Disorders in valve flow and heart chamber size for mitral and aortic valve disorders are illustrated in Figure 18-18.

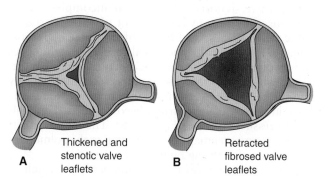

A Thickened and stenotic valve leaflets

B Retracted fibrosed valve leaflets

FIGURE 18-17 Disease of the aortic valve as viewed from the aorta. (**A**) Stenosis of the valve opening. (**B**) An incompetent or regurgitant valve that is unable to close completely.

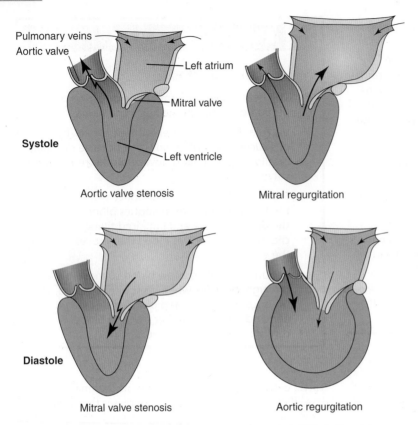

Systole

Pulmonary veins
Aortic valve
Left atrium
Mitral valve
Left ventricle

Aortic valve stenosis

Mitral regurgitation

Diastole

Mitral valve stenosis

Aortic regurgitation

FIGURE 18-18 Alterations in hemodynamic function that accompany aortic stenosis, mitral valve regurgitation, mitral valve stenosis, and aortic valve regurgitation. The *thin arrows* indicate the direction of normal flow and the *thick arrows* the direction of abnormal flow.

MITRAL VALVE DISORDERS

The mitral valve controls the directional flow of blood between the left atrium and the left ventricle. The edges or cusps of the mitral valve are thinner than those of the aortic valve and they are anchored to the papillary muscles by the chordae tendineae, which are attached to the ventricular wall (see Chapter 16, Fig. 16-9). During much of systole, the mitral valve is subjected to the high pressure generated by the left ventricle as it pumps blood into the systemic circulation. During this period of increased pressure, the chordae tendineae prevent the eversion of the valve leaflets into the left atrium.

Mitral Valve Stenosis

Mitral valve stenosis represents the incomplete opening caused by fibrous replacement of valvular tissue, along with stiffness and fusion of the valve apparatus (Fig. 18-19). Typically, the mitral cusps fuse at the edges and involvement of the chordae tendineae causes shortening, which pulls the valvular structures more deeply into the ventricles. As the resistance to flow through the valve increases, the left atrium becomes dilated and left atrial pressure rises (see Fig. 18-18). The increased left atrial pressure eventually is transmitted to the pulmonary venous system, causing pulmonary congestion.

Mitral valve stenosis is most commonly the result of rheumatic fever.[44] Less frequently, the defect is congenital and manifests during infancy or early childhood. Mitral valve stenosis is a continuous, progressive, lifelong dis-

order, consisting of a slow, stable course in the early years and progressive acceleration in later years.

The signs and symptoms of mitral valve stenosis depend on the severity of the obstruction and are related to the elevation in left atrial pressure and pulmonary congestion, decreased cardiac output owing to impaired left ventricular filling, and left atrial enlargement with development of atrial arrhythmias and mural thrombi. The

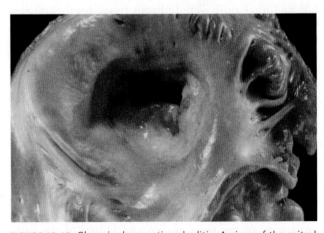

FIGURE 18-19 Chronic rheumatic valvulitis. A view of the mitral valve from the left atrium shows rigid, thickened, and fused leaflets with a narrow orifice, creating the characteristic "fish mouth" appearance of the rheumatic mitral stenosis. (From Rubin E., Farber J. L. [1999]. *Pathology* [3rd ed., p. 570]. Philadelphia: Lippincott Williams & Wilkins.)

normal mitral valve area is 4 to 5 cm². Narrowing of the valve area to less than 2 cm² must occur before mild symptoms begin to develop.[44] The symptoms are those of pulmonary congestion, including nocturnal paroxysmal dyspnea and orthopnea. Palpitations, chest pain, weakness, and fatigue are common complaints. Premature atrial beats, paroxysmal atrial tachycardia, and atrial fibrillation may occur as a result of distention of the left atrium. Atrial fibrillation develops in 30% to 40% of persons with symptomatic mitral stenosis.[44] Together, the fibrillation and distention predispose to mural thrombus formation. The risk of complications due to arterial embolization, particularly stroke, is significantly increased in persons with atrial fibrillation. The murmur of mitral valve stenosis is heard during diastole when blood is flowing through the constricted valve orifice; it is characteristically a low-pitched, rumbling murmur, best heard at the apex of the heart.

Mitral Valve Regurgitation

Mitral valve regurgitation is characterized by incomplete closure of the mitral valve, with the left ventricular stroke volume being divided between the forward stroke volume that moves into the aorta and the regurgitant stroke volume that moves back into the left atrium during systole (see Fig. 18-18). Mitral valve regurgitation can result from many processes. Rheumatic heart disease is associated with a rigid and thickened valve that does not open or close completely. In addition to rheumatic disease, mitral regurgitation can result from rupture of the chordae tendineae or papillary muscles, papillary muscle dysfunction, or stretching of the valve structures due to dilatation of the left ventricle or valve orifice. Mitral valve prolapse is a common cause of mitral valve regurgitation.

The hemodynamic changes that occur with chronic mitral valve regurgitation evolve slowly, allowing for recruitment of compensatory mechanisms. An increase in left ventricular end-diastolic volume permits an increase in total stroke volume, with restoration of forward flow into the aorta. Augmented preload and reduced or normal afterload (provided by unloading the left ventricle into the left atrium) facilitates ejection of blood into the aorta. At the same time, a gradual increase in left atrial size allows for accommodation of the regurgitant volume at a lower filling pressure.

The increased volume work associated with mitral regurgitation is relatively well tolerated, and many persons with the disorder remain asymptomatic for many years, with the average interval of 16 years from diagnosis to onset of symptoms.[45] The degree of left ventricular enlargement reflects the severity of regurgitation. As the disorder progresses, left ventricular function becomes impaired, the forward (aortic) stroke volume decreases, and the left atrial pressure increases, with the subsequent development of pulmonary congestion. Mitral regurgitation, like mitral stenosis, predisposes to atrial fibrillation. A characteristic feature of mitral valve regurgitation is an enlarged left ventricle, a hyperdynamic left ventricular impulse, and a pansystolic (throughout systole) heart murmur.

Mitral Valve Prolapse

Sometimes referred to as the *floppy mitral valve syndrome*, mitral valve prolapse occurs in 2.4% to 7% of the general population.[46] The disorder is seen more frequently in women than in men and may have a familial basis. Although the cause of the disorder usually is unknown, it has been associated with Marfan syndrome, osteogenesis imperfecta, and other connective tissue disorders and with cardiac, hematologic, neuroendocrine, metabolic, and psychological disorders.

Pathologic findings in persons with mitral valve prolapse include a myxedematous (mucinous) degeneration of mitral valve leaflets that causes them to become enlarged and floppy so that they prolapse or balloon back into the left atrium during systole (Fig. 18-20). Secondary fibrotic changes reflect the stresses and injury that the ballooning movements impose on the valve. Certain forms of mitral valve prolapse may arise from disorders of the myocardium that result in abnormal movement of the ventricular wall or papillary muscle; this places undue stress on the mitral valve.

Most persons with mitral valve prolapse are asymptomatic and the disorder is discovered during a routine physical examination. A minority of persons have chest pain mimicking angina, dyspnea, fatigue, anxiety, palpitations, and light-headedness. Unlike angina, the chest pain often is prolonged, ill defined, and not associated with exercise or exertion. The pain has been attributed to ischemia resulting from traction of the prolapsing valve leaflets. The anxiety, palpitations, and arrhythmias may result from abnormal autonomic nervous system function that commonly accompanies the disorder. Rare cases of sudden death have been reported for persons with mitral valve prolapse, mainly those with a family history of similar occurrences.

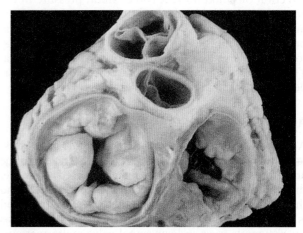

FIGURE 18-20 Mitral valve prolapse. A view of the mitral valve from the left atrium shows redundant and deformed leaflets that billow into the left atrial cavity. (From Saffitz J. E., Steinburger C., Jr. [2005]. The heart. In Rubin E., Gorstein F., Rubin R., et al. [Eds.], *Rubin's pathology: Clinicopathologic foundations of medicine* [4th ed., p. 563]. Philadelphia: Lippincott Williams & Wilkins.)

The disorder is characterized by a spectrum of auscultatory findings, ranging from a silent form to one or more mid-systolic clicks followed by a late systolic murmur. Various abnormal ECG changes can occur. Arrhythmias may be brought out by exercise stress testing or detected on 24-hour ECG monitoring. Echocardiographic studies have become a method for the diagnosis of mitral valve prolapse, and the availability of this technique undoubtedly has contributed to increased recognition of the problem, particularly in its asymptomatic form.

The treatment of mitral valve prolapse focuses on the relief of symptoms and the prevention of complications.[43,46] Persons with palpitations and mild tachyarrhythmias or increased adrenergic symptoms and those with chest discomfort, anxiety, and fatigue often respond to therapy with the β-adrenergic–blocking drugs. In many cases, the cessation of stimulants such as caffeine, alcohol, and cigarettes may be sufficient to control symptoms. Infective endocarditis is an uncommon complication in persons with a murmur; antibiotic prophylaxis usually is recommended before dental or surgical procedures associated with bacteremia.

AORTIC VALVE DISORDERS

The aortic valve is located between the aorta and left ventricle. The aortic valve has three cusps and sometimes is referred to as the *aortic semilunar valve* because its leaflets are crescent or moon shaped (see Chapter 16, Fig. 16-10). The aortic valve has no chordae tendineae. Although their structures are similar, the cusps of the aortic valve are thicker than those of the mitral valve. The middle layer of the aortic valve is thickened near the middle, where the three leaflets meet, ensuring a tight seal.

An important aspect of the aortic valve is the location of the orifices for the two main coronary arteries, which are located behind the valve and at right angles to the direction of blood flow. It is the lateral pressure in the aorta that propels blood into the coronary arteries. During the ejection phase of the cardiac cycle, the lateral pressure is diminished by conversion of potential energy to kinetic energy as blood moves forward into the aorta. This process is grossly exaggerated in aortic stenosis because of the high flow velocities.

Aortic Valve Stenosis

Aortic valve stenosis is characterized by increased resistance to ejection of blood from the left ventricle into the aorta (see Fig. 18-18). Because of the increased resistance, the work demands on the left ventricle are increased, and the volume of blood ejected into the systemic circulation is decreased. The most common causes of aortic stenosis are rheumatic fever and congenital valve malformations. Congenital malformations may result in unicuspid, bicuspid, or misshaped valve leaflets. In elderly persons, stenosis may be related to degenerative atherosclerotic changes of the valve leaflets. Approximately 25% of persons older than 65 and 35% of those older than 70 years of age have echocardiographic evidence of sclerosis, with

10% to 20% progressing to hemodynamically significant aortic stenosis in 10 to 15 years.[47]

The progression of aortic stenosis varies widely among individuals. The progression may be more rapid in persons with degenerative calcific disease than in those with congenital or rheumatic disease. The aortic valve opening must be reduced to approximately one-fourth its normal size before critical changes in cardiac function occur.[48] Significant obstruction to aortic outflow causes a decrease in stroke volume, along with a reduction in systolic blood pressure and pulse pressure. Because of the narrowed valve opening, it takes longer for the heart to eject blood; the heart rate often is slow, and the pulse is of low amplitude. There is a soft, absent, or paradoxically split S_2 sound and a harsh systolic ejection murmur that is heard best along the left sternal border.

Persons with aortic stenosis tend to be asymptomatic for many years despite severe obstruction. Eventually, symptoms of angina, syncope, and heart failure develop. Angina occurs in approximately two thirds of persons with advanced aortic stenosis and is similar to that observed in CHD. Syncope (fainting) is most commonly due to the reduced cerebral circulation that occurs during exertion when the arterial pressure declines consequent to vasodilatation in the presence of a fixed cardiac output. Exertional hypotension may cause "graying out" spells or dizziness on exercise.[44] Dyspnea, marked fatigability, peripheral cyanosis, and other signs of low-output heart failure usually are not prominent until late in the course of the disease.

Aortic Valve Regurgitation

Aortic regurgitation is the result of an incompetent aortic valve that allows blood to flow back to the left ventricle during diastole (see Fig. 18-18). As a result, the left ventricle must increase its stroke volume to include blood entering from the lungs as well as that leaking back through the regurgitant valve. This defect may result from conditions that cause scarring of the valve leaflets or from enlargement of the valve orifice to the extent that the valve leaflets no longer meet. Rheumatic fever ranks first on the list of causes of aortic regurgitation; failure of a prosthetic valve is another cause.

Chronic aortic regurgitation, which usually has a gradual onset, represents a condition of combined left ventricular volume and pressure overload. As the valve deformity increases, regurgitant flow into the left ventricle increases, diastolic blood pressure falls, and the left ventricle progressively enlarges. Hemodynamically, the increase in left ventricular volume results in the ejection of a large stroke volume that usually is adequate to maintain the forward cardiac output until late in the course of the disease. Most persons remain asymptomatic during this compensated phase, which may last decades. The only sign for many years may be a soft systolic aortic murmur.

As the disease progresses, signs and symptoms of left ventricular failure begin to appear. These include exertional dyspnea, orthopnea, and paroxysmal nocturnal dyspnea. In aortic regurgitation, failure of aortic valve closure during diastole causes an abnormal drop in diastolic pressure. Because coronary blood flow is greatest during diastole, the drop in diastolic pressure produces a decrease in coronary perfusion. Although angina is rare, it may occur when the heart rate increases or the diastolic pressure falls to low levels. Persons with severe aortic regurgitation often complain of an uncomfortable awareness of heartbeat, particularly when lying down, and chest discomfort due to pounding of the heart against the chest wall. Tachycardia, occurring with emotional stress or exertion, may produce palpitations, head pounding, and premature ventricular contractions.

The major physical findings relate to the widening of the arterial pulse pressure. The pulse has a rapid rise and fall, with an elevated systolic pressure and low diastolic pressure caused by the large stroke volume and rapid diastolic runoff of blood back into the left ventricle. Korotkoff sounds may persist to zero, even though intra-arterial pressure rarely falls below 30 mm Hg.[44] The large stroke volume and wide pulse pressure may result in prominent carotid pulsations in the neck, throbbing peripheral pulses, and a left ventricular impulse that causes the chest to move with each beat. The turbulence of flow across the aortic valve during diastole produces a high-pitched or blowing sound.

DIAGNOSIS AND TREATMENT

Valvular defects usually are detected through cardiac auscultation (*i.e.*, heart sounds). Diagnosis is aided by phonocardiography, echocardiography, and cardiac catheterization. A phonocardiogram (a permanent recording of the heart sounds) is obtained by placing a high-fidelity microphone on the chest wall over the heart while a recording is made. An ECG tracing usually is made simultaneously for timing purposes.

The treatment of valvular defects consists of medical management of heart failure and associated problems and surgical intervention to repair or replace the defective valve. Surgical valve repair or replacement depends on the valve that is involved and the extent of deformity. Valvular replacement with a prosthetic device or a homograft usually is reserved for severe disease because the ideal substitute valve has not as yet been developed. Percutaneous balloon valvuloplasty involves the opening of a stenotic valve by guiding an inflated balloon through the valve orifice. The procedure is done in the cardiac catheterization laboratory and involves the insertion of a balloon catheter into the heart through a peripheral blood vessel.

In summary, dysfunction of the heart valves can result from a number of disorders, including congenital defects, trauma, ischemic heart disease, degenerative changes, and inflammation. Rheumatic fever is a common cause. Valvular heart disease produces its effects through disturbances of blood flow. A stenotic valvular defect is one that causes a decrease in blood flow through a valve, resulting in impaired emptying and increased work demands on the heart chamber that empties blood across the diseased valve. A regurgitant valvular defect permits the blood flow to continue when the valve is closed. Valvular heart disorders produce blood flow turbulence and often are detected through cardiac auscultation.

Heart Disease in Infants and Children

Heart disease in infants and children encompasses both congenital and acquired disorders. About 36,000 infants are born each year with a congenital heart defect, and 25% of these have defects that are severe enough to cause death within the first year if not corrected.[1] Premature infants have a higher incidence of congenital heart defects, most commonly patent ductus arteriosus and atrial septal defects. Advances in diagnostic methods and surgical treatment have greatly increased the long-term survival and outcomes for children born with congenital heart defects. This section of the chapter provides a discussion of the fetal and perinatal circulations; congenital heart disorders, and Kawasaki disease, an acquired heart disorder of young children.

FETAL AND PERINATAL CIRCULATION

The fetal circulation is different anatomically and physiologically from the postnatal circulation. Before birth, oxygenation of blood occurs through the placenta. The fetus is maintained in a low-oxygen state (PO_2 to 30 to 35 mm Hg and 60% to 70% saturation).[49–52] To compensate, fetal cardiac output is higher than at any other time in life (400 to 500 mL/kg/minute). Also, the pulmonary vessels in the fetus are markedly constricted because of the fluid-filled lungs and the heightened hypoxic stimulus for vasoconstriction that is present in the fetus. As a result, blood flow through the lungs is less than at any other time in life.

In the fetus, blood enters the circulation through the umbilical vein and returns to the placenta by way of the two umbilical arteries (Fig. 18-21). A vessel called the *ductus venosum* allows blood from the umbilical vein to bypass the hepatic circulation and pass directly into the inferior vena cava. From the inferior vena cava, blood flows into the right atrium and then moves through the foramen ovale into the left atrium. It then passes into the left ventricle and is ejected into the ascending aorta to perfuse the head and upper extremities. In this way, the best-oxygenated blood from the placenta is used to perfuse the brain. At the same time, venous blood from the head and upper extremities returns to the right side of the heart by way of the superior vena cava, moves into the right ventricle, and is ejected into the pulmonary artery. Because of the very high pulmonary vascular resistance, blood ejected into the pulmonary artery gets diverted

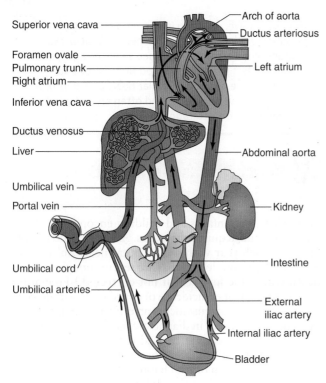

Superior vena cava
Foramen ovale
Pulmonary trunk
Right atrium
Inferior vena cava
Ductus venosus
Liver
Umbilical vein
Portal vein
Umbilical cord
Umbilical arteries

Arch of aorta
Ductus arteriosus
Left atrium
Abdominal aorta
Kidney
Intestine
External iliac artery
Internal iliac artery
Bladder

FIGURE 18-21 Fetal circulation.

through the ductus arteriosus into the descending aorta. This blood perfuses the lower extremities and is returned to the placenta by way of the umbilical arteries.

At birth, the infant takes its first breath and switches from placental to pulmonary oxygenation of the blood. The pressure in the pulmonary circulation and the right side of the heart fall as fetal lung fluid is replaced by air and as lung expansion decreases the pressure transmitted to the pulmonary blood vessels. With lung inflation, the alveolar oxygen tension increases, causing reversal of the hypoxemia-induced pulmonary vasoconstriction of the fetal circulation. Cord clamping and removal of the low-resistance placental circulation produce an increase in systemic vascular resistance and a resultant increase in left ventricular pressure. The resultant decrease in right atrial pressure and increase in left atrial pressure produce closure of the foramen ovale. Reversal of the fetal hypoxemic state also produces constriction of ductal smooth muscle, contributing to closure of the ductus arteriosus. The foramen ovale and the ductus arteriosus normally close within the first day of life, effectively separating the pulmonary and systemic circulations.

After the initial precipitous fall in pulmonary vascular resistance, a more gradual decrease in pulmonary vascular resistance is related to regression of smooth muscle in the medial layer of the pulmonary arteries. During the first 2 to 9 weeks of life, gradual thinning of the smooth muscle layer results in further decreases in pulmonary vascular resistance. By the time a healthy, term infant is several weeks old, the pulmonary vascular resistance has fallen to adult levels. Several factors, including prema-

turity, alveolar hypoxia, lung disease, and congenital heart defects, may affect postnatal pulmonary vascular development.[51] Much of the development of the smooth muscle layer in the pulmonary arterioles occurs during the latter part of gestation; as a result, infants who are born prematurely have less medial smooth muscle. These infants follow the same pattern of smooth muscle regression, but because less muscle exists, the smooth muscle layer may regress in a shorter period. The pulmonary vascular smooth muscle in premature infants also may be less responsive to the hypoxic stimulus for vasoconstriction. For these reasons, a premature infant may demonstrate a larger decrease in pulmonary vascular resistance and resultant increase in shunting of blood from the aorta through the ductus arteriosus to the pulmonary artery within hours of birth.

Hypoxia may also delay or prevent the normal decrease in pulmonary vascular resistance that occurs during the first weeks of life. During this period, the pulmonary arteries remain highly reactive and can constrict in response to hypoxia, acidosis, hyperinflation of the alveoli, and hypothermia. Alveolar hypoxia is one of the most potent stimuli of pulmonary vasoconstriction and pulmonary hypertension in the neonate.

CONGENITAL HEART DEFECTS

The major development of the fetal heart occurs between the fourth and seventh weeks of gestation, and most congenital heart defects arise during this time. The development of the heart may be altered by environmental, genetic, and chromosomal influences. Most congenital heart defects are thought to be multifactorial in origin, resulting from an interaction between a genetic predisposition to develop a heart defect and environmental influences. Infants born to parents with congenital heart defects or with siblings who have congenital heart defects are at higher risk. A number of chromosomal abnormalities are associated with congenital heart diseases, most prominently Down syndrome and Turner syndrome (see Chapter 4). Other intrauterine factors such as maternal diabetes, congenital rubella, maternal alcohol ingestion, and treatment with anticonvulsant drugs are also associated with congenital heart disorders.

Ultrasound technology now allows examination of fetal development and function in utero.[49,52] Diagnostic images of the fetal heart can be obtained as early as 16 weeks of gestation. Echocardiography of the fetus allows for differentiation among heart defects. Among the disorders that can be diagnosed with certainty by fetal echocardiography are hypoplastic left heart syndrome, aortic valve stenosis, hypertrophic cardiomyopathy, pulmonic valve stenosis, AV septal defect, and transposition of the great arteries.[52]

Congenital heart diseases are commonly classified according to their anatomic defects (atrial septal or ventricular septal defects), the hemodynamic alterations caused by the anatomic defects (left-to-right or right-to-left shunts), and their effect on tissue oxygenation (cyanotic or noncyanotic defects).[52,53]

Shunting and Cyanotic Disorders

Shunting of blood refers to the diverting of blood flow from one system to the other—from the arterial to the venous system (*i.e.*, left-to-right shunt) or from the venous to the arterial system (*i.e.*, right-to-left shunt). The shunting of blood in congenital heart defects is determined by the presence of an abnormal opening between the right and left circulations and the degree of resistance to flow through the opening. The shunting of blood can affect both the oxygen content of the blood and the volume of blood being delivered to the vessels in the pulmonary circulation.

A *right-to-left* shunt results in unoxygenated blood moving from the right side of the heart into the left side of the heart and then being ejected into the systemic circulation. Cyanosis develops when sufficient unoxygenated blood mixes with oxygenated blood in the left side of the heart. Children with right-to-left shunts are considered to have a cyanotic heart defect, regardless of whether they have recognizable cyanosis. In a *left-to-right* shunt, blood intended for ejection into the systemic circulation is recirculated through the right side of the heart and back through the lungs; this increased volume distends the right side of the heart and pulmonary circulation and increases the workload placed on the right ventricle. Children with left-to-right shunts are considered to have a noncyanotic heart defect even though they are cyanotic for other reasons, such as low cardiac output.

Congenital heart defects manifest with numerous signs and symptoms. Some defects, such as patent ductus arteriosus and small ventricular septal defects, close spontaneously, and in other, less severe defects, there are no signs and symptoms. The disorder typically is discovered during a routine health examination. Pulmonary congestion, heart failure, and decreased peripheral perfusion are the major concerns in children with more severe defects. Such defects often cause problems shortly after birth or early in infancy. The child may exhibit cyanosis, respiratory difficulty, and fatigability and is likely to have difficulty with feeding and failure to thrive. A generalized cyanosis that persists longer than 3 hours after birth suggests congenital heart disease. One technique for evaluating the cyanosis consists of administering 100% oxygen for 10 minutes. If the infant "pinks up," the cyanosis probably was caused by a respiratory problem and not a heart defect. Because infant cyanosis may appear as duskiness, it is important to assess the color of the mucous membranes, tongue, and lips.

The manifestations and treatment of heart failure in the infant and young child are similar to those in the adult, but the infant's small size and limited physical reserve make the manifestations more serious and treatment more difficult (see Chapter 19). The treatment plan usually includes supportive therapy designed to help the infant compensate for the limitations in cardiac reserve and to prevent complications. Surgical intervention often is required for severe defects; it may be done in the early weeks of life or, conditions permitting, delayed until the child is older.

Most children with structural congenital heart disease and those who have had corrective surgery are at risk for the development of infectious endocarditis. These children should receive prophylactic antibiotic therapy during periods of increased risk of bacteremia.

Types of Defects

Congenital heart defects can affect almost any of the cardiac structures or central blood vessels. Defects include communication between heart chambers, interrupted development of the heart chambers or valve structures, malposition of heart chambers and great vessels, and altered closure of fetal communication channels. The particular defect reflects the embryo's stage of development at the time it occurred. Some congenital heart disorders, such as tetralogy of Fallot, involve several defects. The development of the heart is simultaneous and sequential; a heart defect may reflect the multiple developmental events that were occurring simultaneously or sequentially. At least 35 types of defects have been identified, the most common being patent ductus arteriosus (6% to 8%), atrial septal defects (6% to 8%), and ventricular septal defects (20% to 30%).[49]

Patent Ductus Arteriosus. Patent ductus arteriosus results from persistence of the fetal ductus beyond the prenatal period.[51] In fetal life, the ductus arteriosus is the vital link by which blood from the right side of the heart bypasses the lungs and enters the systemic circulation (Fig. 18-22G). After birth, this passage no longer is needed, and it usually closes during the first 24 to 72 hours. The physiologic stimulus and mechanisms associated with permanent closure of the ductus are not entirely known, but the fact that infant hypoxia predisposes to a delayed closure suggests that the increase in arterial oxygen levels that occurs immediately after birth plays a role. Additional factors that contribute to closure are a fall in endogenous levels of prostaglandins and adenosine and the release of vasoactive substances. After constriction, the lumen of the ductus becomes permanently sealed with fibrous tissue within 2 to 3 weeks. Ductal closure may be delayed or prevented in very premature infants, probably as a result of a combination of factors, including decreased medial smooth muscle in the ductus wall, a decreased vasoconstriction response to oxygen, and increased circulating levels of prostaglandins, which have a vasodilating effect. Ductal closure also may be delayed in infants with congenital heart defects that produce a decrease in oxygen tension.

As is true of other heart and circulatory defects, patency of the ductus arteriosus may vary; the size of the opening may be small, medium, or large. After the infant's pulmonary vascular resistance falls, the patent ductus arteriosus provides for a continuous runoff of aortic blood into the pulmonary artery, causing a decrease in aortic diastolic and mean arterial pressure and a widening of the pulse pressure. With a large patent ductus, the runoff is continuous, resulting in increased pulmonary blood flow, pulmonary congestion, and increased resistance

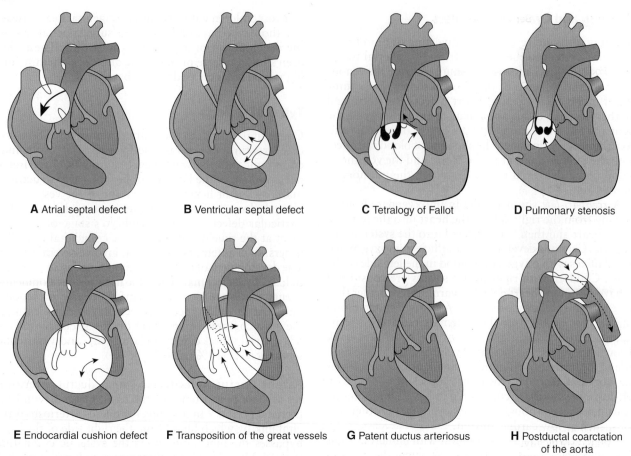

A Atrial septal defect   **B** Ventricular septal defect   **C** Tetralogy of Fallot   **D** Pulmonary stenosis

E Endocardial cushion defect   **F** Transposition of the great vessels   **G** Patent ductus arteriosus   **H** Postductal coarctation of the aorta

FIGURE 18-22 Congenital heart defects. (**A**) Atrial septal defect. Blood is shunted from left to right. (**B**) Ventricular septal defect. Blood is usually shunted from left to right. (**C**) Tetralogy of Fallot. This involves a ventricular septal defect, dextroposition of the aorta, right ventricular outflow obstruction, and right ventricular hypertrophy. Blood is shunted from right to left. (**D**) Pulmonary stenosis, with decreased pulmonary blood flow and right ventricular hypertrophy. (**E**) Endocardial cushion defects. Blood flows between the chambers of the heart. (**F**) Transposition of the great vessels. The pulmonary artery is attached to the left side of the heart and the aorta to the right side. (**G**) Patent ductus arteriosus. The high-pressure blood of the aorta is shunted back to the pulmonary artery. (**H**) Postductal coarctation of the aorta.

against which the right side of the heart must pump. Increased pulmonary venous return and increased work demands may lead to left ventricular failure.

Patent ductus arteriosus can be treated either pharmacologically or surgically. Drugs that inhibit prostaglandin synthesis (*e.g.*, indomethacin) may be used to induce closure of a patent ductus arteriosus.

Atrial Septal Defects. In atrial septal defects, a hole in the atrial septum persists as a result of improper septal formation (see Fig. 18-22A). Partitioning of the atria takes place during the fourth and fifth weeks of development and occurs in two stages, beginning with the formation of a thin, crescent-shaped membrane called the *septum primum* followed by the development of a second membrane called the *septum secundum*. As the septum secundum develops, it gradually overlaps an opening in the upper part of the septum primum, forming an oval opening with a flap-type valve called the *foramen ovale*

(Fig. 18-23). The foramen ovale, which closes shortly after birth, allows blood from the umbilical vein to pass directly into the left heart, bypassing the lungs.

Atrial septal defects may be single or multiple and vary from a small, asymptomatic opening to a large, symptomatic opening. Most atrial septal defects are small and are discovered inadvertently during a routine physical examination.[55] In the case of an isolated septal defect large enough to allow shunting, the flow of blood usually is from the left side to the right side of the heart because of the more compliant right ventricle and because the pulmonary vascular resistance is lower than the systemic vascular resistance. This produces right ventricular volume overload and increased pulmonary blood flow.

Young children with atrial septal defects are usually asymptomatic but experience symptoms later in life, usually during adolescence when the changes in pulmonary vasculature may reverse the direction of flow through the defect and create a right-to-left shunt with development

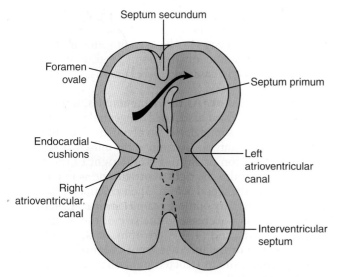

FIGURE 18-23 Development of the endocardial cushions, right and left atrioventricular canals, interventricular septum, and septum primum and septum secundum of the foramen ovale. Note that blood from the right atrium flows through the foramen ovale to the left atrium.

of cyanosis. Adolescents and young adults may experience atrial fibrillation or atrial flutter and palpitations because of atrial dilatation. Symptomatic defects are usually treated surgically. Because spontaneous closure occurs in some children, surgical treatment usually is delayed until the child is of school age.[52]

Ventricular Septal Defects. A ventricular septal defect is an opening in the ventricular septum that results from an imperfect separation of the ventricles during early fetal development (see Fig. 18-22B). Ventricular septal defects are the most common form of congenital heart defect, accounting for 20% to 30% of congenital heart disorders.[49] Ventricular septal defect may be the only cardiac defect, or it may be one of multiple cardiac anomalies.

The ventricular septum originates from two sources: the interventricular groove of the folded tubular heart that gives rise to the muscular part of the septum, and the endocardial cushions that extend to form the membranous portion of the septum (see Fig. 18-23). The upper membranous portion of the septum is the last area to close, and it is here that most defects occur.

Depending on the size of the opening, the signs and symptoms of a ventricular septal defect may range from an asymptomatic murmur to congestive heart failure. If the defect is small, it allows a small shunt and small increases in pulmonary blood flow. These defects produce few symptoms, and approximately one third close spontaneously.[49,52] With medium-sized defects, a larger shunt occurs, producing a larger increase in pulmonary blood flow (i.e., twice as much blood may pass through the pulmonary circulation as through the systemic circulation). The increased pulmonary flow most often occurs under relatively low pressure. Most of the children with

such defects are asymptomatic and have a low risk for development of pulmonary vascular disease.

Children with large defects have an increase in pulmonary blood flow. Because the defect is nonrestrictive, the pressure in the left and right sides of the heart is equalized, and blood is shunted from the left side of the heart into the pulmonary artery under high pressures that are sufficient to produce pulmonary hypertension. In these children, left-to-right shunting through the ventricular defect is lessened when pulmonary and systemic circulations offer equal resistance to flow. The child's symptoms improve during this time. As the child's pulmonary vascular resistance increases further, a right-to-left shunt develops, and the child demonstrates cyanosis. This reversal of the direction of shunt flow is called *Eisenmenger syndrome.*

Most infants with a ventricular septal defect are asymptomatic during early infancy because the higher pulmonary vascular resistance prevents shunting from occurring. After an infant's pulmonary vascular resistance falls and a shunt develops, a characteristic systolic murmur develops. The infant with a large, uncomplicated ventricular septal defect usually is asymptomatic until pulmonary vascular resistance begins to fall at approximately 4 to 25 weeks of age. At this point, the mother reports that the infant breathes more rapidly and shows signs of cyanosis (due to right-to-left shunting), feeds poorly, and is diaphoretic (*i.e.*, signs of congestive heart failure).

The treatment of a ventricular septal defect depends on the size of the defect and accompanying hemodynamic derangements. Children with small or medium-sized defects are followed closely in the hope that the defect will close spontaneously. Prophylactic antibiotic therapy is given during periods of increased risk for bacteremia. Cardiac catheterization may be performed in children with medium-sized or large defects who become symptomatic to document the location of the lesion, identify any associated heart defects, and determine the pulmonary vascular resistance. Congestive heart failure is treated medically. Surgical intervention is required for infants who do not respond to medical management.

Endocardial Cushion Defects. The endocardial cushions form the AV canals, the upper part of the ventricular septum, and the lower part of the atrial septum. Endocardial cushion defects are responsible for approximately 5% of all congenital heart defects. As much as 50% of children with Down syndrome have endocardial cushion defects.[49]

Because endocardial cushions contribute to multiple aspects of heart development, several variations with this type of defect are possible. The terms most commonly used to categorize endocardial cushion defects are *partial* and *complete AV canal defects*. In partial AV canal defects, the two AV valve rings are complete and separate. The most common type of partial AV canal defect is an ostium primum defect, with a cleft in the mitral valve. In complete canal defect, there is a common AV valve (tricuspid and mitral) orifice along with defects in both the atrial and ventricular septal tissue. Many variations of these two forms of endocardial cushion defect are possible (see Fig. 18-22E). The Ebstein anomaly is a defect in endocardial cushion development characterized by displacement of tricuspid valvular tissue into the ventricle. The displaced tricuspid leaflets are attached directly to the right ventricular endocardial surface or to shortened or malformed chordae tendineae.

The direction and magnitude of a shunt in a child with endocardial cushion defects are determined by the combination of defects and the child's pulmonary and systemic vascular resistance. The hemodynamic effects of an isolated ostium primum defect are those of the previously described atrial septal defect. These children are largely asymptomatic during childhood. If a ventricular septal defect is present, pulmonary blood flow is increased after pulmonary vascular resistance falls. Many children with ventricular septal defects have effort intolerance, easy fatigability, and recurrent infections, particularly when the shunt is large. The larger the defect, the greater is the shunt and the higher is the pressure in the pulmonary vascular system.

With complete AV canal defects, congestive heart failure and intercurrent pulmonary infections appear early in infancy. There is left-to-right shunting and transatrial and transventricular mixing of blood. Pulmonary hypertension and increased pulmonary vascular resistance are common. Cyanosis develops with progressive shunting.

The treatment for endocardial cushion defects is determined by the severity of the defect. With an atrial septal defect, surgical repair usually is planned on an elective basis before the child enters school. Palliative or corrective surgery is required in infants with complete AV canal defects who have congestive heart failure and do not respond to medical treatment. Total surgical repair of complete AV canal defects can be accomplished with low operative risk.

Pulmonary Stenosis. Pulmonary stenosis may occur as an isolated valvular lesion or in conjunction with more complex defects, such as tetralogy of Fallot. In isolated valvular defects, the pulmonary cusps may be absent or malformed, or they may remain fused at their commissural edges; often there are coexisting abnormalities.

Pulmonary valvular defects usually cause some impairment of pulmonary blood flow and increase the workload imposed on the right side of the heart (see Fig. 18-22D). Most children with pulmonic valve stenosis have mild to moderate stenosis that does not increase in severity. These children are largely asymptomatic. Severe defects are manifested by marked impairment of pulmonary blood flow that begins during infancy and is likely to become more severe as the child grows. Cyanosis develops in approximately one third of children younger than 2 years of age.[51] The ductus arteriosus may provide the vital accessory route for perfusing the lungs in infants with severe stenosis. When pulmonary stenosis is extreme, increased pressures in the right side of the heart may delay closure of the foramen ovale.

Treatment measures designed to maintain the patency of the ductus arteriosus may be used as a palliative mea-

sure to maintain or increase pulmonary blood flow in infants with severe pulmonary stenosis. Transcatheter balloon valvuloplasty may be used in some infants with moderate degrees of obstruction. Surgical valvotomy may be required in cases of severe stenosis.

Tetralogy of Fallot. As the name implies, tetralogy of Fallot consists of four associated congenital heart defects: (1) a ventricular septal defect involving the membranous septum and the anterior portion of the muscular septum; (2) dextroposition or shifting to the right of the aorta, so that it overrides the right ventricle and is in communication with the septal defect; (3) obstruction or narrowing of the pulmonary outflow channel, including pulmonic valve stenosis, a decrease in the size of the pulmonary trunk, or both; and (4) hypertrophy of the right ventricle because of the increased work required to pump blood through the obstructed pulmonary channels[49,52] (see Fig. 18-22C).

Most children with tetralogy of Fallot display some degree of cyanosis—hence the term *blue babies*. The cyanosis develops as the result of decreased pulmonary blood flow and because the right-to-left shunt causes mixing of unoxygenated blood with the oxygenated blood, which is ejected into the peripheral circulation. Hypercyanotic attacks ("tet spells") may occur during the first months of life. With the hypercyanotic spell, the infant becomes acutely cyanotic, hyperpneic, irritable, and diaphoretic. Later in the spell, the infant becomes limp and may lose consciousness. These spells typically occur in the morning during activities such crying, feeding, or defecation that increase the infant's oxygen requirements. Crying and defecating may further increase pulmonary vascular resistance, thereby increasing right-to-left shunting and decreasing pulmonary blood flow. Placing the infant in the knee-chest position increases systemic vascular resistance, which increases pulmonary blood flow and decreases right-to-left shunting. During a hypercyanotic spell, toddlers and older children may spontaneously assume the squatting position, which functions like the knee-chest position to relieve the spell.[51]

Total surgical correction is ultimately advised for all children with tetralogy of Fallot. Early definitive repair, even in infancy, is currently advocated in most centers that are experienced in intracardiac surgery in infants.[52]

Transposition of the Great Vessels. In complete transposition of the great vessels, the aorta originates in the right ventricle, and the pulmonary artery originates in the left ventricle (see Fig. 18-22F). The defect is more common in infants whose mothers have diabetes, and in boys. In infants born with this defect, survival depends on communication between the right and left sides of the heart in the form of a patent ductus arteriosus or septal defect. Prostaglandin E_1 may be administered in an effort to maintain the patency of the ductus arteriosus. Balloon atrial septostomy may be done to increase the blood flow between the two sides of the heart. In this procedure, a balloon-tipped catheter is inserted into the heart through the vena cava and then passed through the foramen ovale into the left atrium. The balloon is then inflated and brought back through the foramen ovale, enlarging the opening as it goes.

Corrective surgery is essential for long-term survival.[49] An arterial switch procedure may be done. This procedure, which corrects the relation of the systemic and pulmonary blood flows, is preferably performed in the first 2 to 3 weeks of life, before postnatal reduction in pulmonary vascular resistance. An atrial (venous) switch procedure is performed on older children. Both of these procedures reverse the blood flow at the atrial level by the surgical formation of intra-atrial baffles. The atrial switch procedures have a much higher long-term morbidity and are done when conditions prevent performance of the arterial switch procedure.

Coarctation of the Aorta. Coarctation of the aorta is a localized narrowing of the aorta, proximal (preductal or coarctation of infancy) or distal (postductal) to the ductus (see Fig. 18-22H). Approximately 98% of coarctations are postductal. The anomaly occurs twice as often in boys as in girls.

Coarctation of the aorta may be a feature of Turner syndrome (see Chapter 4). The classic sign of postductal coarctation of the aorta is a disparity in pulsations and blood pressures in the arms and legs. The femoral, popliteal, and dorsalis pedis pulsations are weak or delayed compared with the bounding pulses of the arms and carotid vessels. The systolic blood pressure in the legs obtained by the cuff method normally is 10 to 20 mm Hg higher than in the arms.[49] In coarctation, the pressure is lower and may be difficult to obtain. The differential in blood pressure is common in children older than 1 year of age, approximately 90% of whom have hypertension in the upper extremities greater than the 95th percentile for age (see Chapter 17).

Children with significant coarctation should be treated surgically; the optimal age for surgery is 2 to 4 years. If untreated, most persons with coarctation of the aorta die between 20 and 40 years of age. The common serious complications are related to the hypertensive state. In some centers, balloon valvoplasty has been used for treatment of unoperated coarctation. This method is still being developed and ongoing clinical trials are needed to determine its long-term effectiveness and possible complications.[49]

KAWASAKI DISEASE

Kawasaki disease, also known as *mucocutaneous lymph node syndrome,* is an acute febrile disease of young children. First described in Japan in 1967 by Dr. Tomisaku Kawasaki, the disease affects the skin, brain, eyes, joints, liver, lymph nodes, and heart.[55,56] The disease can produce aneurysmal disease of the coronary arteries and is the most common cause of acquired heart disease in young children. Although first reported in Japanese children, the disease affects children of many races, occurs worldwide, and is increasing in frequency.

The disease is characterized by a vasculitis (*i.e.,* inflammation of the blood vessels) that begins in the small vessels (*i.e.,* arterioles, venules, and capillaries) and progresses to involve some of the larger arteries, such as the coronaries. The cause of Kawasaki disease is unknown, but it is thought to be of immunologic origin. It has been hypothesized that some unknown antigen, possibly a common infectious agent, triggers the immune response in a genetically predisposed child.

Clinical Course

The course of the disease is triphasic and includes an acute febrile phase that lasts approximately 7 to 14 days; a subacute phase that follows the acute phase and lasts from days 10 through 24; and a convalescent phase that follows the subacute stage and continues until the signs of the acute-phase inflammatory response have subsided and the signs of the illness have disappeared.

The *acute phase* begins with an abrupt onset of fever, followed by bilateral conjunctivitis, usually without exudates; erythema of the oral and pharyngeal mucosa with "strawberry tongue" and dry, fissured lips; redness and swelling of the hands and feet; rash of various forms; and enlarged cervical lymph nodes. The fever typically is high, reaching 40°C (104°F) or more, has an erratic spiking pattern, is unresponsive to antibiotics, and persists for 5 or more days.[55] The conjunctivitis begins shortly after the onset of fever, persists throughout the febrile course of the disease, and may last as long as 3 to 5 weeks.

The *subacute phase* begins when the fever breaks and lasts until all signs of the disease have disappeared. During the subacute phase, desquamation (*i.e.,* peeling) of the skin of the fingers and toe tips begins and progresses to involve the entire surface of the palms and soles. Patchy peeling of skin areas other than the hands and feet may occur in some children. The *convalescent stage* persists from the complete resolution of symptoms until all signs of inflammation have disappeared. This usually takes approximately 8 weeks.

In addition to the major manifestations that occur during the acute stage of the illness, there are several associated, less specific characteristics of the disease, including arthritis, urethritis and pyuria, gastrointestinal manifestations (*e.g.,* diarrhea, abdominal pain), hepatitis, and hydrops of the gallbladder. Arthritis or arthralgia occurs in approximately 30% of children with the disease, characterized by symmetric joint swelling that involves large and small joints. Central nervous system involvement occurs in almost all children and is characterized by pronounced irritability and lability of mood.

Cardiac involvement is the most important manifestation of Kawasaki disease. Coronary vasculitis develops in between 10% and 40% of children within the first 2 weeks of the illness, manifested by dilatation and aneurysm formation in the coronary arteries, as seen on two-dimensional echocardiography. The manifestations of coronary artery involvement include signs and symptoms of myocardial ischemia or, rarely, overt myocardial infarction or rupture of the aneurysm. Pericarditis, myocarditis, endocarditis, heart failure, and arrhythmias also may develop.

Diagnosis and Treatment

As with rheumatic fever, the diagnosis of Kawasaki disease is based on clinical findings because no specific laboratory test for the disease exists. The AHA Council on Cardiovascular Disease in the Young, Committee on Rheumatic Fever, Endocarditis, and Kawasaki Disease has established guidelines for diagnosis of the disease.[57] According to these guidelines, a diagnosis of Kawasaki disease is confirmed by the presence of a fever that lasts 5 or more days without another more reasonable explanation and by at least four of the following five acute-stage manifestations of the disease: changes in the extremities (an acute erythema and edema of the hands, followed by membranous desquamation of fingertips during the convalescent period); skin eruption involving the trunk and extremities; bilateral, painless bulbar conjunctival hyperemia without exudate; changes in the lips and oral cavity (*e.g.*, erythema and cracking of the lips, strawberry tongue, diffuse congestion of the oral and pharyngeal mucosae); and cervical lymphadenopathy (≥1.5 cm in diameter). Chest radiographs, ECG tests, and two-dimensional echocardiography are used to detect coronary artery involvement and follow its progress. Coronary angiography may be used to determine the extent of coronary artery involvement.

Intravenous gamma globulin and aspirin are considered the best therapy for prevention of coronary artery abnormalities in children with Kawasaki disease.[56] During the acute phase of the illness, aspirin usually is given in larger doses and for its anti-inflammatory and antipyretic effects. After the fever is controlled, the aspirin dose is lowered, and the drug is given for its anti–platelet-aggregating effects.

In summary, congenital heart defects arise during fetal heart development, which occurs during weeks 4 through 7 after conception, and reflect the stage of development at the time the causative event occurred. Several factors contribute to the development of congenital heart defects, including genetic and chromosomal influences, viruses, and environmental agents such as drugs and radiation. The cause of the defect often is unknown.

Congenital heart defects may produce no effects, or they may markedly affect cardiac function. The defects may produce shunting of blood from the right to the left side of the heart or from the left to the right side of the heart. Left-to-right shunts typically increase the volume of the right side of the heart and pulmonary circulation, and right-to-left shunts transfer unoxygenated blood from the right side of the heart to the left side, diluting the oxygen content of blood that is being ejected into the systemic circulation and causing cyanosis. The direction and degree of shunt depend on the size of the defect that connects the two sides of the heart and the difference in resistance between the two sides of the circulation. Congenital heart defects often are classified as defects that produce cyanosis and those that produce little or no cyanosis. Depending on the severity of the defect, congenital heart defects may be treated medically or surgically. Medical and surgical treatment often is indicated in children with severe defects.

Kawasaki disease is an acute febrile disease of young children that affects the skin, brain, eyes, joints, liver, lymph nodes, and heart. The disease can produce aneurysmal disease of the coronary arteries and is the most common cause of acquired heart disease in young children.

Review Exercises

A 40-year-old man presents in the emergency department complaining of substernal chest pain that is also felt in his left shoulder. He is short of breath and nauseated. His blood pressure is 148/90 mm Hg and his heart rate is 110 beats per minute. His ECG shows an ST-segment elevation with T-wave inversion. He is given aspirin, morphine, and oxygen. Blood tests reveal elevated CK-MB and troponin I.

A. What is the probable cause of the man's symptoms?
B. Explain the origin of the left arm pain, nausea, and increased heart rate.
C. What is the significance of the ST-segment changes and elevation in CK-MB and troponin I?
D. Relate the actions of aspirin, morphine, and oxygen to the treatment of this man's condition.

A 50-year-old woman presents with complaints of paroxysmal nocturnal dyspnea and orthopnea, palpitations, and fatigue. An echocardiogram demonstrates a thickened, immobile mitral valve with anterior and posterior leaflets moving together; slow early diastolic filling of the ventricle; and left atrial enlargement.

A. What is the probable cause of this woman's symptoms?
B. Explain the pathologic significance of the slow early diastolic filling, distended left atrium, and palpitations.
C. Given the echocardiographic data, what type of cardiac murmur would you expect to find in this woman?
D. Which circulation (systemic or pulmonary) would you expect to be affected as this woman's disorder progresses?

A 4-month-old male infant is brought into the pediatric clinic by his mother. She reports that she noted over the past several weeks that the baby's lips and mouth and his fingernails and toenails have taken on a bluish-gray color. She also states that he seems to tire easily and that even nursing seems to wear him out. Lately, he has had several spells where he has suddenly turned blue, has had difficulty breathing, and been very irritable. During one of these spells, he turned limp and seemed to pass out for a short time. An echocardiogram reveals a thickening of the right ventricular wall with overriding of the aorta, a large subaortic ventricular septal defect, and a narrowing of the pulmonary outflow with stenosis of the pulmonary valve.

A. What is this infant's probable diagnosis?
B. Describe the shunting of blood that occurs with this disorder and its relationship to the development of cyanosis.
C. The mother is instructed regarding the placement of the infant in the knee-chest position when he has one of the spells in which he becomes blue and irritable. How does this position help to relieve the cyanosis and impaired oxygenation of tissues?
D. The surgical creation of a shunt between the aorta and pulmonary artery may be performed as a palliative procedure for infants with marked hypoplasia of the pulmonary artery, with corrective surgery performed later in childhood. Explain how this procedure increases blood flow to the lungs.

Visit the Porth: Essentials of Pathophysiology: Concepts of Altered Health States web site (http://thePoint.LWW.com/PorthEssentials) for links to chapter-related resources on the Internet, all-new exclusive animations, chapter review questions, and more!

REFERENCES

1. American Heart Association. (2005). *Heart diseases and stroke statistics—2005 update.* Dallas: Author.
2. LeWinter M. M., Kabani S. (2005). Pericardial diseases. In Zipes D. P., Libby P., Bonow R. O., et al. (Eds.), *Braunwald's heart disease: A textbook of cardiovascular medicine* (7th ed., pp. 1757–1780). Philadelphia: Elsevier Saunders.
3. Spodick D. H. (2003). Acute cardiac tamponade. *New England Journal of Medicine* 349, 684–690.
4. Krishan K. G., Walling A. D. (2002). Diagnosing pericarditis. *American Family Physician* 66, 1695–1702.
5. Guyton A., Hall J. E. (2006). *Textbook of medical physiology* (11th ed., pp. 199–200, 249–257, 277). Philadelphia: Elsevier Saunders.
6. Kern M. J. (2005). Coronary blood flow and myocardial ischemia. In Zipes D. P., Libby P., Bonow R. O., et al. (Eds.), *Braunwald's heart disease: A textbook of cardiovascular medicine* (7th ed., pp. 1103–1128). Philadelphia: Elsevier Saunders.
7. Schoen F. J. (2005). The heart. In Kumar V., Abbas A. K., Fausto N. (Eds.), *Robbins and Cotran pathologic basis of disease* (7th ed., pp. 555–617). Philadelphia: Elsevier Saunders.
8. Forrester J. S. (2000). Role of plaque rupture in acute coronary syndromes. *American Journal of Cardiology* 86(Suppl.) 15J–23J.
9. Yeghiazarians Y., Braunstein J. B., Askari A., et al. (2000). Unstable angina pectoris. *New England Journal of Medicine* 342, 101–114.
10. Ambrose J. A., Dangas G. (2000). Unstable angina: Current concepts of pathogenesis and treatment. *Archives of Internal Medicine* 160, 25–35.
11. Gibbons R. J., Abrams J., Chatterjee K., et al., Members of the Committee to Update the 1999 Guidelines. (2002). ACC/AHA 2002 guideline update for the management of patients with chronic stable angina: A report of the American College of Cardiology/American Heart Association Task Force on Practice Guidelines. [On-line]. Available: www.acc.org/clinical/guidelines/stable/stable.pdf.
12. Morrow D. A., Gersh B. J., Braunwald E. (2005). Chronic coronary artery disease. In Zipes D. P., Libby P., Bonow R. O., et al. (Eds.), *Braunwald's heart disease: A textbook of cardiovascular medicine* (7th ed., pp. 1757–1780). Philadelphia: Elsevier Saunders.
13. Chiariello M., Indolfi C. (1996). Silent myocardial ischemia in patients with diabetes mellitus. *Circulation* 93, 2089–2091.
14. Prinzmetal M., Kennamer R., Merliss R., et al. (1959). A variant form of angina pectoris. *American Journal of Medicine* 27, 375–388.
15. Cannon C. C., Braunwald E. (2005). Unstable angina and non-ST elevation myocardial infarction. In Zipes D. P., Libby P., Bonow R. O., et al. (Eds.), *Braunwald's heart disease: A textbook of cardiovascular medicine* (7th ed., pp. 1243–1279). Philadelphia: Elsevier Saunders.
16. Braunwald E., Antman E. M., Beasley J. W., et al., Committee Members. (2002). ACC/AHA guideline update for the management of patients with unstable angina and non-ST-segment elevation myocardial infarction—2002: Executive summary and recommendations. *Circulation* 106, 1893–1900.
17. Mirvis D. M., Goldberger A. L. (2005). Electrocardiography. In Zipes D. P., Libby P., Bonow R. O., et al. (Eds.), *Braunwald's heart disease: A textbook of cardiovascular medicine* (7th ed., pp. 107–148). Philadelphia: Elsevier Saunders.
18. Antman E. M., Braunwald E. (2005). ST-segment elevation myocardial infarction: Pathology, pathophysiology, and clinical features. In Zipes D. P., Libby P., Bonow R. O., et al. (Eds.), *Braunwald's heart disease: A textbook of cardiovascular medicine* (7th ed., pp. 1141–1166). Philadelphia: Elsevier Saunders.
19. Kloner R. A., Rezkalla S. H. (2003). Cocaine and the heart. *New England Journal of Medicine* 348, 487–488.
20. Ryan T. J., Antman E. M., Brooks N. H., et al., Committee Members. (1999). 1999 Update: ACC/AHA guidelines for the management of acute myocardial infarction: Executive summary and recommendation. A report of the American College of Cardiology/American Heart Association Task Force on Practice Guidelines (Committee on Management of Acute Myocardial Infarction). *Journal of the American College of Cardiology* 28, 1328–1428.

21. Popma J. J., Kuntz R. E., Baim D. S. (2005). Percutaneous coronary and valvular intervention In Zipes D. P., Libby P., Bonow R. O., et al. (Eds.), *Braunwald's heart disease: A textbook of cardiovascular medicine* (7th ed., pp. 1367–1397). Philadelphia: Elsevier Saunders.

22. Shepard R., Eisenberg M. J. (2001). Intracoronary radiotherapy for restenosis. *New England Journal of Medicine 344*, 295–296.

23. Sapirstein W., Zuckerman B., Dillard J. (2001). FDA approval of coronary-artery brachytherapy. *New England Journal of Medicine 344*, 297–298.

24. Feldman A. M., McNamara D. (2000). Myocarditis. *New England Journal of Medicine 343*, 1388–1398.

25. Wyne J., Braunwald E. (2005). The cardiomyopathies. In Zipes D. P., Libby P., Bonow R. O., et al. (Eds.), *Braunwald's heart disease: A textbook of cardiovascular medicine* (7th ed., pp. 1659–1696). Philadelphia: Elsevier Saunders.

26. Dec G. W., Fuster V. (1994). Idiopathic dilated cardiomyopathy. *New England Journal of Medicine 331*, 1564–1575.

27. Mohan S., Parker M., Wehbi M., et al. (2002). Idiopathic dilated cardiomyopathy: A common but mystifying cause of heart failure. *Cleveland Clinic Journal of Medicine 69*, 481–487.

28. Manolio T. A., Baughman K. I., Rodeheffer R., et al. (1992). Prevalence and etiology of idiopathic dilated cardiomyopathy (Summary of the National Heart, Lung, and Blood Institute Workshop). *American Journal of Cardiology 69*, 1458.

29. Piano M. R. (2002). Alcoholic cardiomyopathy. *Chest 121*, 1638–1650.

30. Roberts R., Sigwart U. (2001). New concepts in hypertrophic cardiomyopathies, Part I and Part II. *Circulation 104*, 2113–2116, 2249–2252.

31. Maron B. J. (2002). Hypertrophic cardiomyopathy. *Journal of the American Medical Association 287*, 1308–1320.

32. Saffitz J. E, Steinburger C., Jr. (2005). The heart. In Rubin E., Gorstein F., Rubin R., et al. (Eds.), *Rubin's pathology: Clinicopathologic foundations of medicine* (4th ed., pp. 521–580). Philadelphia: Lippincott Williams & Wilkins.

33. Golledge P., Knight C. J. (2001). Current management of hypertrophic cardiomyopathy. *Hospital Medicine 62*(2), 79–82.

34. Pearson G. D., Veille J., Rahimtoola S., et al. (2000). Peripartum cardiomyopathy: National Heart, Lung, and Blood Institute and Office of Rare Diseases (National Institutes of Health) Workshop recommendations and review. *Journal of the American Medical Association 283*, 83–88.

35. Felker G. M., Jaeger C. J., Kodas E., et al. (2000). Myocarditis and long-term survival in peripartum cardiomyopathy. *American Heart Journal 140*, 785–791.

36. Karchmer A. W. (2005). Infective endocarditis. In Zipes D. P., Libby P., Bonow R. O., et al. (Eds.), *Braunwald's heart disease: A textbook of cardiovascular medicine* (7th ed., pp. 1633–1655). Philadelphia: Elsevier Saunders.

37. Mylonakis E., Calderwood S. B. (2001). Infective endocarditis in adults. *New England Journal of Medicine 345*, 1318–1330.

38. American Heart Association Advisory and Coordinating Committee. (1998). Diagnosis and management of infective endocarditis and its complications. *Circulation 98*, 2936–2948.

39. Ad Hoc Committee to Revise Jones Criteria (Modified) of the Council on Rheumatic Fever and Congenital Heart Disease of the American Heart Association. (1984). Jones criteria (revised) for guidance in the diagnosis of rheumatic fever. *Circulation 69*, 203A–208A.

40. Dajani A. (2005). Rheumatic fever. In Zipes D. P., Libby P., Bonow R. O., et al. (Eds.), *Braunwald's heart disease: A textbook of cardiovascular medicine* (7th ed., pp. 2093–2100). Philadelphia: Elsevier Saunders.

41. Dajani A., Taubert K., Ferrieri P., et al., Committee Members. (1995). Treatment of acute streptococcal pharyngitis and prevention of rheumatic fever: A statement for health professionals. [On-line]. Available: www.americanheart.org/Scientific/statements.

42. Bonow R. O., Carabello B., deLeon A. D., Jr., et al., Committee on Management of Patients with Valvular Heart Disease. (1998). Guideline for the management of patients with valvular heart disease: Executive summary. A report of the American College of Cardiology/American Heart Association Task Force on Guidelines. *Circulation 98*, 1949–1984.

43. Carabello B. A., Crawford F. A. (1997). Valvular heart disease. *New England Journal of Medicine 337*, 32–41.

44. Bonow R. O., Braunwald E. (2005). Valvular heart disease. In Zipes D. P., Libby P., Bonow R. O., et al. (Eds.), *Braunwald's heart disease: A textbook of cardiovascular medicine* (7th ed., pp. 1553–1632). Philadelphia: Elsevier Saunders.

45. Otto C. M. (2001). Evaluation and management of chronic mitral regurgitation. *New England Journal of Medicine 345*, 740–746.

46. Playford D., Weyman A. E. (2001). Mitral valve prolapse: Time for a fresh look. *Reviews in Cardiovascular Medicine 2*, 73–76.

47. Brashore T. M., Granger C. B. (2006). Heart. In Tierney L. M., McPhee S. J., Papadakis M. A. (Eds.), *Current medical diagnosis and treatment* (45th ed., pp. 325–339). New York: Lange Medical Books/McGraw-Hill.

48. Carbello B. A. (2002). Aortic stenosis. *New England Journal of Medicine 346*, 677–682.

49. Bernstein D. (2004). The cardiovascular system. In Behrman R. E., Kliegman R. M., Jenson H. B. (Eds.), *Nelson textbook of pediatrics* (17th ed., pp. 1475–1554). Philadelphia: Elsevier Saunders.

50. Moore K. L., Persaud T. V. N. (2003). *The developing human* (7th ed., pp. 329–377). Philadelphia: Elsevier Saunders.

51. Hazinski M. F. (1999). *Manual of pediatric critical care* (pp. 84–91, 220–268). St. Louis: Mosby.

52. Webb G. D., Smallhorn J.F., Therrien J., et al. (2005). Congenital heart disease. In Zipes D. P., Libby P., Bonow R. O., et al. (Eds.), *Braunwald's heart disease: A textbook of cardiovascular medicine* (7th ed., pp. 1489–1552). Philadelphia: Elsevier Saunders.

53. Nouri S. (1997). Congenital heart defects: Cyanotic and acyanotic. *Pediatric Annals 26*, 92–98.

54. Driscoll D. J. (1999). Left-to-right shunt lesions. *Pediatric Clinics of North America 46*, 355–368.

55. Rowley A. H., Schulman S. T. (2004). Kawasaki disease. In Behrman R. E., Kliegman R. M., Jenson H. B. (Eds.), *Nelson textbook of pediatrics* (17th ed., pp. 823–826). Philadelphia: Elsevier Saunders.

56. Lueng D. Y. M., Meissner H. C. (2001). The many faces of Kawasaki syndrome. *Hospital Practice 35*(1), 77–94.

57. Council on Cardiovascular Disease in the Young, Committee on Rheumatic Fever, Endocarditis, and Kawasaki Disease, American Heart Association. (2001). Diagnostic guidelines for Kawasaki disease. *Circulation 103*, 335–336.

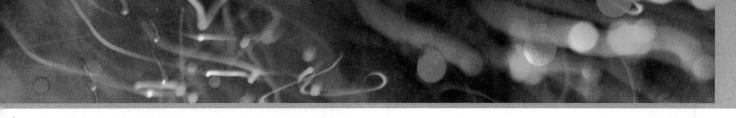

Chapter *19*

Heart Failure and Circulatory Shock

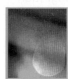

Adequate perfusion of body tissues depends on the pumping ability of the heart, a vascular system that transports blood to the cells and back to the heart, sufficient blood to fill the circulatory system, and tissues that are able to extract and use oxygen and nutrients from the blood. Impaired pumping ability of the heart and circulatory shock are separate conditions that reflect failure of the circulatory system. Both conditions exhibit common compensatory mechanisms even though they differ in terms of pathogenesis and causes.

Heart Failure

Heart failure affects an estimated 5 million Americans, with approximately 550,000 new cases diagnosed each year.[1] Although morbidity and mortality rates from other cardiovascular diseases have decreased over the past several decades, the incidence of heart failure is increasing at an alarming rate. This change undoubtedly reflects improved treatment methods and increased survival from other forms of heart disease. Despite advances in treatment, 80% of men and 79% of women younger than 65 years of age who have heart failure will die within 8 years.[1]

PHYSIOLOGY OF HEART FAILURE

The term *heart failure* denotes the failure of the heart as a pump. The heart has the amazing capacity to adjust its pumping ability to meet the varying needs of the body. During sleep, its output declines, and during exercise, it increases markedly. The ability to increase cardiac output during increased activity is called the *cardiac reserve*. For example, competitive swimmers and long-distance runners have large cardiac reserves. During exercise, the cardiac output of these athletes rapidly increases to as much as five to six times their resting level. In sharp contrast to healthy athletes, persons with heart failure often use their cardiac reserve at rest. For them, just climbing

KEY CONCEPTS

Heart Failure

➤ The function of the heart is to move deoxygenated blood from the venous system through the right heart into the pulmonary circulation and to move the oxygenated blood from the pulmonary circulation through the left heart into the arterial system.

➤ To function effectively, the right and left hearts must maintain an equal output.

➤ Right heart failure represents failure of the right heart to pump blood forward into the pulmonary circulation; blood backs up in the systemic circulation, causing peripheral edema and congestion of the abdominal organs.

➤ Left heart failure represents failure of the left heart to move blood from the pulmonary circulation into the systemic circulation; blood backs up in the pulmonary circulation.

a flight of stairs may cause shortness of breath because they have exceeded their cardiac reserve.

The pathophysiology of heart failure involves an interaction between two factors: a decrease in pumping ability of the heart with a consequent decrease in the cardiac reserve, and the adaptive mechanisms that serve to maintain the cardiac output while also contributing to the progression of heart failure.

Cardiac Output

The cardiac output is the amount of blood the heart pumps each minute. It reflects how often the heart beats each minute (heart rate) and how much blood the heart pumps with each beat (stroke volume) and can be expressed as the product of the heart rate and stroke volume. The heart rate is regulated by a balance between the activity of the sympathetic nervous system, which produces an increase in heart rate, and the parasympathetic nervous system, which slows it down. The stroke volume is a function of preload, afterload, and cardiac contractility.

Preload and Afterload. The work that the heart performs consists mainly of ejecting blood that has returned to the ventricles during diastole into the pulmonary or systemic circulations. It is determined largely by the loading conditions or what is called the *preload* and *afterload*.

Preload reflects the loading condition of the heart at the end of diastole just before the onset of systole. It is the volume of blood stretching the heart muscle at the end of diastole (end-diastolic volume) and is determined mainly by the venous return to the heart. *Afterload* represents the force that the contracting heart must generate to eject blood from the filled heart. The main components of afterload are the systemic (peripheral) vascular resis-

tance and ventricular wall tension. When the systemic vascular resistance is elevated, as with arterial hypertension, an increased intraventricular pressure must be generated first to open the aortic valve and then to move blood out of the heart and into the systemic circulation.

Cardiac Contractility. Cardiac contractility refers to the mechanical performance of the heart—the ability of the contractile elements (actin and myosin filaments) of the heart muscle to interact and shorten against a load. Contractility increases cardiac output independent of preload filling and muscle stretch.

An *inotropic influence* is one that increases cardiac contractility. Sympathetic stimulation increases the strength of cardiac contraction (*i.e.*, positive inotropic action), and hypoxia and ischemia decrease contractility (*i.e.*, negative inotropic effect). The drug digitalis, which is classified as an inotropic agent, increases cardiac contractility such that the heart is able to eject more blood at any level of preload filling.

Adaptive Mechanisms

In heart failure, the cardiac reserve is largely maintained through compensatory or adaptive responses such as the Frank-Starling mechanism; activation of neurohumoral influences such as the sympathetic nervous system, the renin-angiotensin-aldosterone mechanism, natriuretic peptides, and locally produced vasoactive substances; and myocardial hypertrophy and remodeling (Fig. 19-1). The first two of these adaptations occur rapidly over minutes to hours of myocardial dysfunction and may be adequate to maintain the overall pumping performance of the heart at relatively normal levels. Myocardial hypertrophy and remodeling occur slowly over weeks to months, and play an important role in the long-term adaptation to hemodynamic overload. In the failing heart, early decreases in cardiac function may go unnoticed because these compensatory mechanisms maintain the cardiac output. This is called *compensated heart failure*. However, these mechanisms contribute not only to the adaptation of the failing heart but to the pathophysiologic process of the eventual heart failure.

Frank-Starling Mechanism. The Frank-Starling mechanism describes the process whereby the heart increases its stroke volume through an increase in ventricular end-diastolic volume (Fig. 19-2). With increased diastolic filling, there is increased stretching of the myocardial fibers, more optimal approximation of the actin and myosin filaments, and a resultant increase in the force of the next contraction (see Chapter 16).

In heart failure, a decrease in cardiac output and renal blood flow leads to increased salt and water retention, a resultant increase in vascular volume and venous return to the heart, and an increase in ventricular end-diastolic volume. Within limits, as preload and ventricular end-diastolic volume increase, there is a resultant increase in cardiac output. Although this may preserve the resting cardiac output, the resulting chronic elevation of left

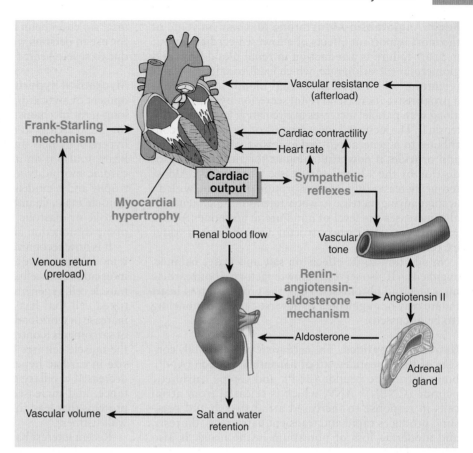

FIGURE 19-1 Compensatory mechanisms in heart failure. The Frank-Starling mechanism, sympathetic reflexes, renin-angiotensin-aldosterone mechanism, and myocardial hypertrophy function in maintaining cardiac output for the failing heart.

ventricular end-diastolic pressure is eventually transmitted to the atria and to the pulmonary circulation, causing pulmonary congestion (see Fig. 19-2).

An important determinant of myocardial energy consumption is ventricular wall tension. Overfilling of the ventricle produces a decrease in wall thickness and an increase in wall tension. Because increased wall tension increases myocardial oxygen requirements, it can produce ischemia and further impairment of cardiac function. The use of diuretics in persons with heart failure helps to reduce vascular volume and ventricular filling, thereby unloading the heart and reducing ventricular wall tension.

Sympathetic Nervous System Activity. Stimulation of the sympathetic nervous system plays an important role in the compensatory response to decreased cardiac output and to the pathogenesis of heart failure.[2,3] Both cardiac sympathetic tone and catecholamine (epinephrine and norepinephrine) levels are elevated during the late stages of most forms of heart failure. By direct stimulation of heart rate and cardiac contractility and by regulation of vascular tone, the sympathetic nervous system helps to maintain perfusion of the various organs, particularly the heart and brain. In persons who progress to more severe heart failure, blood is diverted to the more critical cerebral and coronary circulations.

The negative aspects of increased sympathetic activity include an increase in peripheral vascular resistance and the afterload against which the heart must pump. Excessive sympathetic stimulation also may result in decreased blood flow to the skin, muscle, kidneys, and abdominal organs. The catecholamines also may contribute to the high rate of sudden death by promoting arrhythmias.

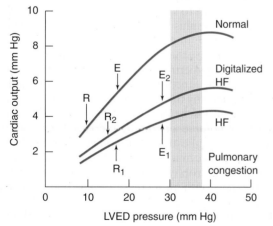

FIGURE 19-2 Frank-Starling curves. R, resting; E, exercise; LVED, left ventricular end-diastolic; HF, heart failure. (From Iseri L. T., Benvenuti D. J. [1983]. Pathogenesis and management of congestive heart failure—revisited. *American Heart Journal* 105 [2], 346.)

Renin-Angiotensin-Aldosterone Mechanism. One of the most important effects of a lowered cardiac output in heart failure is a reduction in renal blood flow and glomerular filtration rate, which leads to salt and water retention.[4] With decreased renal blood flow, there is a progressive increase in renin secretion by the kidneys along with parallel increases in circulating levels of angiotensin II. The increased concentration of angiotensin II contributes to a generalized and excessive vasoconstriction and provides a powerful stimulus for aldosterone production by the adrenal cortex (see Chapter 17). Aldosterone increases tubular reabsorption of sodium, with an accompanying increase in water retention. Angiotensin II also increases the level of antidiuretic hormone (ADH), which serves as a vasoconstrictor and inhibitor of water excretion.

In addition to its effects on salt and water balance, angiotensin II also serves as growth factor for both cardiac myocytes and fibroblasts. Thus, the progression of heart failure may be augmented by adverse cardiac remodeling (to be discussed).

Natriuretic Peptides. The natriuretic peptide family consists of three peptides: atrial natriuretic peptide (ANP), brain natriuretic peptide (BNP), and C-type natriuretic peptide (CNP).[5,6] ANP, which is released from atrial cells in response to increased atrial stretch and pressure, produces rapid and transient natriuresis, diuresis, and moderate loss of potassium in the urine. It also inhibits aldosterone and renin secretion, acts as an antagonist to angiotensin II, and inhibits the release of norepinephrine from presynaptic nerve terminals. BNP, so named because it was originally found in extracts of porcine brain, is stored mainly in the ventricular cells and is responsive to increased ventricular filling pressures. BNP has cardiovascular effects similar to those of ANP. The role of CNP, which is found primarily in vascular tissue, has not yet been clarified.

Circulating levels of both ANP and BNP are reportedly elevated in persons with heart failure. The concentrations are correlated with the extent of ventricular dysfunction, increasing up to 30-fold in persons with advanced heart disease.[5] Reliable assays of BNP are now available and are used clinically in the diagnosis and follow-up care of persons with heart failure. Human BNP, synthesized by recombinant deoxyribonucleic acid (DNA) technology, is now available for treatment of persons with acutely decompensated heart failure (to be discussed).

Endothelin. The endothelins, released from the endothelial cells throughout the circulation, are potent vasoconstrictors. Other actions of the endothelins include induction of vascular smooth muscle cell proliferation and myocyte hypertrophy. Thus far, four endothelin peptides (endothelin-1 [ET-1], ET-2, ET-3, and ET-4) have been identified.[7] There are at least two types of endothelin receptors—type A and type B.[2,7] Plasma ET-1 levels correlate directly with pulmonary vascular resistance, and it is thought that the peptide may play a role in mediating pulmonary hypertension in persons with heart fail-

ure.[2] An endothelin receptor antagonist is now available for use in persons with pulmonary arterial hypertension due to severe heart failure.

Myocardial Hypertrophy and Remodeling. The development of myocardial hypertrophy is one of the principal long-term mechanisms by which the heart compensates for an increase in workload.[2,3] Although ventricular hypertrophy may improve the work performance of the heart, it also is an important risk factor for subsequent cardiac morbidity and mortality. Inappropriate hypertrophy and remodeling can result in changes in structure (muscle mass, chamber dilation) and function (impaired systolic or diastolic function) that often lead to further pump dysfunction and hemodynamic overload.

It is now recognized that myocardial hypertrophy and remodeling involve a series of complex events at both the molecular and cellular levels. The cardiac myocyte, or muscle cell, is generally considered a terminally differentiated cell that has lost its ability to divide. Thus, an increase in workload is met with an increased production of sarcomeres (contractile elements) and mitochondria in the muscle cell (see Chapter 1). The increased myocyte size in cardiac hypertrophy is usually accompanied by decreased capillary density, increased intercapillary distance, and increased synthesis of extracellular matrix proteins that lead to myocardial fibrosis and ventricular wall stiffness.[8]

Recent interest has focused on the type of hypertrophy that develops in persons with heart failure. At the cellular level, cardiac muscle cells respond to stimuli from stress placed on the ventricular wall by pressure and volume overload with the initiation of several different processes that lead to hypertrophy. These include stimuli that produce a *symmetric hypertrophy* with a proportionate increase in muscle length and width, as occurs in athletes; *concentric hypertrophy* with an increase in wall thickness, as occurs in hypertension due to pressure overload; and *eccentric hypertrophy* with a disproportionate increase in muscle length, as occurs in dilated cardiomyopathy due to volume overload[2] (Fig. 19-3). When the primary stimulus for hypertrophy is *pressure overload*, the increase in wall stress leads to parallel replication of sarcomeres, thickening of the individual myocytes, and concentric hypertrophy. Concentric hypertrophy may preserve systolic function for a period, but eventually the work performed by the ventricle exceeds its blood supply, predisposing to ischemia. When the primary stimulus is *ventricular volume overload*, increased diastolic wall stress leads to replication of sarcomeres in series, elongation of the cardiac muscle cells, and eccentric hypertrophy. Eccentric hypertrophy leads to a decrease in ventricular wall thickness with an increase in diastolic volume and wall tension.

The stimuli for hypertrophy and remodeling are thought to reflect not only the mechanical stress placed on the myocytes, but growth signals provided by the release of substances such as angiotensin II, ANP, and ET-1. It is hoped that further research into the signals that cause specific features of inappropriate myocar-

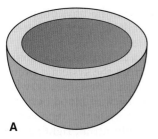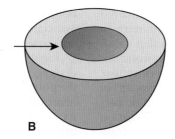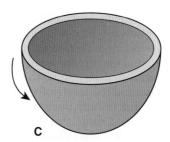

FIGURE 19-3 Different types of myocardial hypertrophy: (**A**) normal symmetric hypertrophy with proportionate increases in myocardial wall thickness and length; (**B**) concentric hypertrophy with a disproportionate increase in wall thickness; and (**C**) eccentric hypertrophy with a disproportionate decrease in wall thickness and ventricular dilatation.

dial hypertrophy and remodeling will lead to the identification of targets whose actions can be interrupted or modified.

HEART FAILURE

Heart failure occurs when the pumping ability of the heart becomes impaired. Heart failure may be caused by a variety of conditions, including acute myocardial infarction, hypertension, or degenerative conditions of the heart muscle known collectively as *cardiomyopathies*. It also may occur because of excessive work demands, such as occur with hypermetabolic states, or with volume overload, such as occurs with renal failure. Either of these states may exceed the work capacity of even a healthy heart. In persons with asymptomatic heart disease, heart failure may be precipitated by an unrelated illness or stress. Table 19-1 lists major causes of heart failure.

Types of Heart Failure

Heart failure may be described as high-output or low-output failure, systolic or diastolic failure, and as right-sided or left-sided failure.

High-Output Versus Low-Output Failure. High- and low-output heart failure are described in terms of cardiac output. *High-output failure* is an uncommon type of heart failure that is caused by an excessive need for cardiac output. With high-output failure, the function of the heart may be supranormal but inadequate owing to excessive metabolic needs. Causes of high-output failure include severe anemia, thyrotoxicosis, conditions that cause arteriovenous shunting, and Paget disease. High-output failure tends to be specifically treatable. *Low-output failure* is caused by disorders that impair the pumping ability of the heart, such as ischemic heart disease and cardiomyopathy.

Systolic Versus Diastolic Failure. A functional classification separates the pathophysiology of heart failure into systolic dysfunction and diastolic dysfunction. With systolic dysfunction, there is impaired ejection of blood from the heart during systole; with diastolic dysfunction, there is impaired filling of the ventricles during diastole. Many persons with heart failure fall into an intermediate category, with combined elements of both systolic failure and diastolic failure.

Systolic dysfunction involves a decrease in cardiac contractility and ejection fraction. It commonly results from conditions that impair the contractile performance of the heart (*e.g.*, ischemic heart disease and cardiomyopathy), produce a volume overload (*e.g.*, valvular insufficiency and anemia), or generate a pressure overload (*e.g.*, hypertension and valvular stenosis) on the heart. A normal heart ejects approximately 65% of the blood that is present in the ventricle at the end of diastole when it contracts. This is called the *ejection fraction*. In systolic heart failure, the ejection fraction declines progressively with increasing degrees of myocardial dysfunction. In very severe forms of heart failure, the ejection fraction may drop to a single-digit percentage. With a decrease in ejection fraction, there is a resultant increase in diastolic volume, ventricular dilation, and ventricular wall tension and a rise in ventricular end-diastolic pressure. The symptoms of persons with systolic dysfunction result mainly from reductions in ejection fraction and cardiac output.

Diastolic dysfunction, which reportedly accounts for approximately 40% of all cases of heart failure, is characterized by a smaller ventricular chamber size, ventricular hypertrophy, and poor ventricular compliance

TABLE 19-1	Causes of Heart Failure
Impaired Cardiac Function	**Excess Work Demands**
Myocardial Disease	**Increased Pressure Work**
Cardiomyopathies	Systemic hypertension
Myocarditis	Pulmonary hypertension
Coronary insufficiency	Coarctation of the aorta
Myocardial infarction	
Valvular Heart Disease	**Increased Volume Work**
Stenotic valvular disease	Arteriovenous shunt
Regurgitant valvular disease	Excessive administration of intravenous fluids
Congenital Heart Defects	**Increased Perfusion Work**
	Thyrotoxicosis
	Anemia
Constrictive Pericarditis	

(*i.e.*, ability to stretch during filling).[9] Because of impaired filling, congestive symptoms tend to predominate in diastolic dysfunction. Among the conditions that cause diastolic dysfunction are those that restrict diastolic filling (*e.g.*, mitral stenosis), those that increase ventricular wall thickness and reduce chamber size (*e.g.*, myocardial hypertrophy due to lung disease and hypertrophic cardiomyopathy), and those that delay diastolic relaxation (*e.g.*, aging, ischemic heart disease). Aging often is accompanied by a delay in relaxation of the heart during diastole; diastolic filling begins while the ventricle is still stiff and resistant to stretching to accept an increase in volume.[10] A similar delay occurs with myocardial ischemia, resulting from a lack of energy to break the rigor bonds that form between the actin and myosin filaments of the contracting cardiac muscle. Because tachycardia produces a decrease in diastolic filling time, persons with diastolic dysfunction often become symptomatic during activities and situations that increase heart rate.

Right-Sided Versus Left-Sided Heart Failure. Heart failure also can be classified according to the side of the heart (right or left) that is affected. An important feature of the circulatory system is that the right and left ventricles act as two pumps that are connected in series. To function effectively, the right and left ventricles must maintain equal outputs. Although the initial event that leads to heart failure may be primarily right sided or left sided in origin, long-term heart failure usually involves both sides. To understand the physiologic mechanisms associated with heart failure, right- and left-sided failure are considered separately.

Right-sided heart failure impairs the ability to move deoxygenated blood from the systemic circulation into the pulmonary circulation. Consequently, when the right heart fails, a damming back of blood occurs, leading to its accumulation in the systemic venous system. This causes an increase in right atrial, right ventricular end-diastolic, and systemic venous pressures. A major effect of right-sided heart failure is the development of peripheral edema (Fig. 19-4). Because of the effects of gravity, the edema is most pronounced in the dependent parts of the body—in the lower extremities when the person is in the upright position and in the area over the sacrum when the person is supine. The accumulation of edema fluid is evidenced by a gain in weight (*i.e.*, 1 pint of accumulated fluid results in a 1-lb weight gain). Daily measurement of weight can be used as a means of assessing fluid accumulation in a patient with chronic heart failure.

Right-sided heart failure also produces congestion of the viscera. As venous distention progresses, blood backs up in the hepatic veins that drain into the inferior vena cava and the liver becomes engorged. This may cause hepatomegaly and right upper quadrant pain. In severe and prolonged right-sided failure, liver function is impaired and hepatic cells may die. Congestion of the portal circulation also may lead to engorgement of the spleen and the development of ascites. Congestion of the gastro-

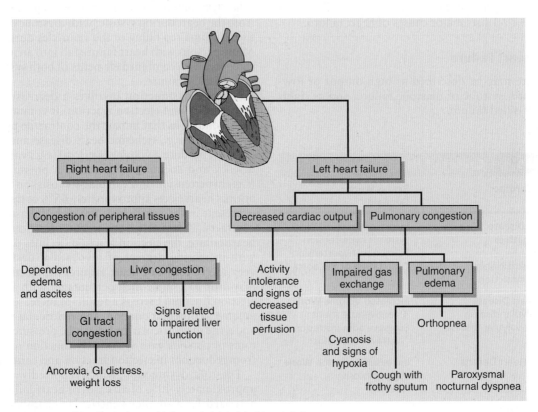

FIGURE 19-4 Manifestations of left- and right-sided heart failure.

intestinal tract may interfere with digestion and absorption of nutrients, causing anorexia and abdominal discomfort. The jugular veins, which are above the level of the heart, are normally collapsed in the standing position or when sitting with the head at higher than a 30-degree angle. In severe right-sided failure, the external jugular veins become distended and can be visualized when the person is sitting up or standing.

The causes of right-sided heart failure include conditions that weaken the heart muscle or restrict blood flow into the lungs. Stenosis or regurgitation of the tricuspid or pulmonic valves, right ventricular infarction, cardiomyopathy, and persistent left-sided failure are common causes. Acute or chronic pulmonary disease, such as severe pneumonia, pulmonary embolus, or pulmonary hypertension, can cause right heart failure, referred to as *cor pulmonale*.

Left-sided heart failure impairs the pumping of blood from the low-pressure pulmonary circulation into the high-pressure arterial side of the systemic circulation. With impairment of left heart function, there is a decrease in cardiac output; an increase in left atrial and left ventricular end-diastolic pressures; and congestion in the pulmonary circulation (see Fig. 19-4). When the pulmonary capillary filtration pressure (normally approximately 10 mm Hg) exceeds the capillary osmotic pressure (normally approximately 25 mm Hg), there is a shift of intravascular fluid into the interstitium of the lung, and pulmonary edema develops (Fig. 19-5). An episode of pulmonary edema often occurs at night, after the person has been reclining for some time and the gravitational forces have been removed from the circulatory system. It is then that the edema fluid that had been sequestered in the lower extremities during the day is returned to the vascular compartment and redistributed to the pulmonary circulation.

The most common causes of left-sided heart failure are acute myocardial infarction and cardiomyopathy. Left-sided heart failure and pulmonary congestion can develop very rapidly in persons with acute myocardial infarction. Even when the infarcted area is small, there may be a surrounding area of ischemic tissue. This may result in a large area of nonpumping ventricle and the rapid onset of pulmonary edema. Another cause of left heart failure is valvular defects such as mitral regurgitation and aortic stenosis or regurgitation. These valvular defects increase the work of the left heart and eventually lead to heart failure unless the valve is repaired or replaced.

Manifestations of Heart Failure

The manifestations of heart failure depend on the extent and type of cardiac dysfunction (*e.g.,* systolic versus diastolic) that is present and the rapidity with which it develops. A person with previously stable compensated heart failure may develop signs of heart failure for the first time when the condition has advanced to a critical point, such as with a progressive increase in pulmonary hypertension in a person with mitral valve regurgitation. Overt heart failure also may be precipitated by conditions such as infec-

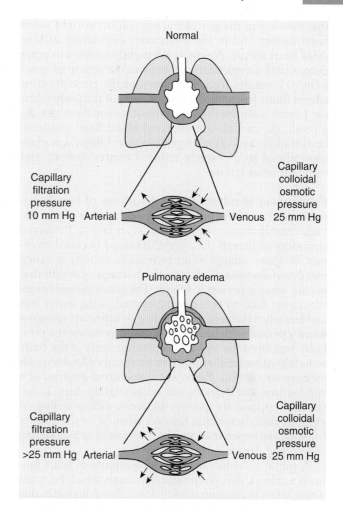

FIGURE 19-5 Mechanism of respiratory symptoms in left-sided heart failure. In the normal exchange of fluid in the pulmonary capillaries (**top**), the capillary filtration pressure that moves fluid out of the capillary into the lung is less than the capillary colloidal osmotic pressure that pulls fluid back into the capillary. Development of pulmonary edema (**bottom**) occurs when the capillary filtration pressure exceeds the capillary colloidal osmotic pressure that pulls fluid back into the capillary.

tion, emotional stress, uncontrolled hypertension, administration of fluid overload, or inappropriate reduction in therapy. Many persons with serious underlying heart disease, regardless of whether they have previously experienced heart failure, may be relatively asymptomatic as long as they carefully adhere to their treatment regimen.

The manifestations of heart failure reflect the physiologic effects of the impaired pumping ability of the heart, decreased renal blood flow, and activation of the sympathetic compensatory mechanisms. The signs and symptoms include fluid retention and edema, shortness of breath and other respiratory manifestations, fatigue and limited exercise tolerance, cachexia and malnutrition, and cyanosis.

Fluid Retention and Edema. Many of the manifestations of heart failure result from fluid retention by the kidneys and the resultant increases in capillary pressure that develop in the peripheral circulation in right-sided heart failure and in the pulmonary circulation in left-sided heart failure. *Nocturia* is a nightly increase in urine output that occurs relatively early in the course of heart failure. It results from the return to the circulation of edema fluids from the dependent parts of the body when the person assumes the supine position for the night. As a result, the cardiac output, renal blood flow, glomerular filtration, and urine output increase. Oliguria is a late sign related to a severely reduced cardiac output and resultant renal failure.

Respiratory Manifestations. Shortness of breath due to congestion of the pulmonary circulation is one of the major manifestations of left-sided heart failure. Perceived shortness of breath (*i.e.*, breathlessness) is called *dyspnea*. Dyspnea related to an increase in activity is called *exertional dyspnea*. *Orthopnea* is shortness of breath that occurs when a person is supine. The gravitational forces that cause fluid to become sequestered in the lower legs and feet when the person is standing or sitting are removed when a person with heart failure assumes the supine position; fluid from the legs and dependent parts of the body is mobilized and redistributed to an already distended pulmonary circulation. *Paroxysmal nocturnal dyspnea* is a sudden attack of dyspnea that occurs during sleep. It disrupts sleep, and the person awakens with a feeling of extreme suffocation that resolves when he or she sits up. Initially, the experience may be interpreted as awakening from a bad dream.

A subtle and often overlooked symptom of heart failure is a chronic dry, nonproductive cough, which becomes worse when the person is lying down. Bronchospasm due to congestion of the bronchial mucosa may cause wheezing and difficulty in breathing. This condition is sometimes referred to as *cardiac asthma*.

Cheyne-Stokes respiration, also known as *periodic breathing*, is characterized by a slow waxing and waning of respiration. The person breathes deeply for a period when the arterial carbon dioxide pressure (PCO_2) is high and then slightly or not all when the PCO_2 falls. In persons with left-sided heart failure, the condition is thought to be caused by a prolongation of the heart-to-brain circulation, particularly in persons with hypertension and associated cerebral vascular disease. Cheyne-Stokes breathing may contribute to daytime sleepiness, and occasionally the person awakens at night with dyspnea precipitated by Cheyne-Stokes breathing.

Fatigue and Limited Exercise Tolerance. Fatigue and limb weakness often accompany diminished output from the left ventricle. Cardiac fatigue is different from general fatigue in that it usually is not present in the morning but appears and progresses as activity increases during the day. In acute or severe left-sided failure, cardiac output may fall to levels that are insufficient for providing the brain with adequate oxygen, and there are indications of mental confusion and disturbed behavior. Confusion, impairment of memory, anxiety, restlessness, and insomnia are common in elderly persons with advanced heart failure, particularly in those with cerebral atherosclerosis. These very symptoms may confuse the diagnosis of heart failure in the elderly because of the myriad other causes of fatigue.

Cachexia and Malnutrition. Cardiac cachexia is a condition of malnutrition and tissue wasting that occurs in persons with end-stage heart failure. A number of factors probably contribute to its development, including the fatigue and depression that interfere with food intake, the congestion of the liver and gastrointestinal structures that impairs digestion and absorption and produces feelings of fullness, and the circulating toxins and mediators released from poorly perfused tissues that impair appetite and contribute to tissue wasting.

Cyanosis. Cyanosis is the bluish discoloration of the skin and mucous membranes caused by excess desaturated hemoglobin in the blood; it often is a late sign of heart failure. Central cyanosis is caused by impaired oxygenation of the arterial blood, such as occurs with pulmonary congestion. Peripheral cyanosis is caused by conditions such as low-output failure that cause delivery of poorly oxygenated blood to the peripheral tissues or by conditions that cause excessive removal of oxygen from the blood. Central cyanosis is best monitored in the lips and mucous membranes because these areas are not subject to conditions such as cold that cause peripheral cyanosis.

Diagnosis and Treatment

Diagnosis. Diagnostic methods in heart failure are directed toward establishing the cause of the disorder and determining the extent of the dysfunction.[11] Because heart failure represents the failure of the heart as a pump and can occur in the course of a number of heart diseases or other systemic disorders, the diagnosis of heart failure often is based on signs and symptoms related to the failing heart itself, such as shortness of breath and fatigue. The functional classification of the New York Heart Association (NYHA) is one guide to classifying the extent of dysfunction (Table 19-2).

The diagnostic methods include history and physical examination, laboratory studies, electrocardiography, chest radiography, and echocardiography. The history should include information related to dyspnea, cough, nocturia, generalized fatigue, and other signs and symptoms of heart failure. A complete physical examination includes assessment of heart rate, heart sounds, and blood pressure, examination of jugular veins for venous congestion, auscultation of lungs for signs of pulmonary congestion, and examination of the lower extremities for edema. Pulse oximetry can be used to measure the percentage of hemoglobin oxygen saturation.

Laboratory tests are used in the diagnosis of anemia and electrolyte imbalances and to detect signs of chronic liver congestion. Measurements of BNP are increasingly being used to confirm the diagnosis of heart failure; to evaluate the severity of left ventricular compromise and to estimate the prognosis and predict future cardiac events,

TABLE 19-2	New York Heart Association Functional Classification of Patients With Heart Disease
Classification	**Characteristics**
Class I	Patients with cardiac disease but without the resulting limitations in physical activity. Ordinary activity does not cause undue fatigue, palpitation, dyspnea, or anginal pain.
Class II	Patients with heart disease resulting in slight limitations of physical activity. They are comfortable at rest. Ordinary physical activity results in fatigue, palpitation, dyspnea, or anginal pain.
Class III	Patients with cardiac disease resulting in marked limitation of physical activity. They are comfortable at rest. Less than ordinary physical activity causes fatigue, palpitation, dyspnea, or anginal pain.
Class IV	Patients with cardiac disease resulting in inability to carry on any physical activity without discomfort. The symptoms of cardiac insufficiency or of the anginal syndrome may be present even at rest. If any physical activity is undertaken, discomfort increases.

(From Criteria Committee of the New York Heart Association. [1964]. *Diseases of the heart and blood vessels: Nomenclature and criteria for diagnosis* [6th ed., pp. 112–113]. Boston: Little, Brown)

such as sudden death; and to evaluate the effectiveness of treatment.[12,13]

Echocardiography plays a key role in assessing the anatomic and functional abnormalities in heart failure, which include the size and function of cardiac valves, the motion of both ventricles, and the ventricular ejection fraction.[14] Electrocardiographic findings may indicate atrial or ventricular hypertrophy, underlying disorders of cardiac rhythm, or conduction abnormalities such as right or left bundle branch block. Radionuclide angiography and cardiac catheterization are other diagnostic tests used to detect the underlying causes of heart failure. Chest radiographs provide information about the size and shape of the heart and pulmonary vasculature. They also can be used to determine the relative severity of the failure by revealing if pulmonary edema is predominantly vascular, interstitial, or advanced to the alveolar and bronchial stages.

Treatment. The goals of treatment for heart failure are directed toward relieving the symptoms and improving the quality of life, with a long-term goal of slowing, halting, or reversing the cardiac dysfunction.[3,13,15] Treatment measures include correction of reversible causes such as anemia or thyrotoxicosis, surgical repair of a ventricular defect or an improperly functioning valve, pharmacologic and nonpharmacologic control of afterload stresses such as hypertension, modification of activities and lifestyle to a level consistent with the functional limitations of a

reduced cardiac reserve, and the use of medications to improve cardiac function and limit excessive compensatory mechanisms. Restriction of salt intake and diuretic therapy facilitate the excretion of edema fluid. Counseling, health teaching, and ongoing evaluation programs help persons with heart failure to manage and cope with their treatment regimen.

In severe heart failure, restriction of activity, including bed rest if necessary, often facilitates temporary recompensation of cardiac function. However, there is no convincing evidence that continued bed rest is of benefit. Carefully designed and managed exercise programs for patients with heart failure are well tolerated and beneficial to patients with stable NYHA class I to III heart failure.[16]

Pharmacologic Treatment. Once heart failure is moderate to severe, polypharmacy becomes a management standard and often includes diuretics, digoxin, angiotensin-converting enzyme (ACE) inhibitors, and β-adrenergic blocking agents.[17] The choice of pharmacologic agents is determined by problems caused by the disorder (*i.e.*, systolic or diastolic dysfunction) and those brought about by activation of compensatory mechanisms (*e.g.*, excess fluid retention, inappropriate activation of sympathetic mechanisms).

Diuretics are among the most frequently prescribed medications for heart failure. They promote the excretion of edema fluid and help to sustain cardiac output and tissue perfusion by reducing preload and allowing the heart to operate at a more optimal part of the Frank-Starling curve. *Digitalis* drugs are inotropic agents that improve cardiac function by increasing the force and strength of ventricular contraction. They also produce a decrease in sinoatrial node activity and conduction through the atrioventricular node, thus slowing heart rate and increasing diastolic filling time. Although not a diuretic, digitalis promotes urine output by improving cardiac output and renal blood flow. The *ACE inhibitors*, which prevent the conversion of angiotensin I to angiotensin II, have been effectively used in the treatment of heart failure. In heart failure, renin activity frequently is elevated because of decreased renal blood flow. The net result is an increase in angiotensin II, which causes vasoconstriction and increased aldosterone production with a subsequent increase in salt and water retention by the kidney. Both mechanisms increase the workload of the heart. The newer angiotensin II receptor blockers have the advantage of not causing a cough, which is a troublesome side effect of the ACE inhibitors for many persons.

β-Adrenergic blocking agents are used to decrease left ventricular dysfunction associated with activation of the sympathetic nervous system. Chronic elevation of norepinephrine levels has been shown to cause cardiac muscle cell death and progressive left ventricular dysfunction, and is associated with poor prognosis in heart failure. The β-adrenergic blocking agents also decrease the risk of serious cardiac arrhythmias in persons with heart failure.

A new agent, a recombinant form of human B-type natriuretic peptide (nesiritide), has recently been approved for treatment of acute and decompensated heart failure.[18]

The drug, which has the same structure as the endogenous natriuretic peptide, is a potent vasodilator that reduces ventricular filling pressures and improves cardiac output. Because it must be given intravenously in a closely supervised clinical setting, it is usually reserved for patients with severe heart failure who do not respond to other forms of therapy.

ACUTE PULMONARY EDEMA

Acute pulmonary edema is the most dramatic symptom of left heart failure. It is a life-threatening condition in which capillary fluid moves into the alveoli. The accumulated fluid in the alveoli and respiratory airways causes lung stiffness, makes lung expansion more difficult, and impairs the gas exchange function of the lung. With the decreased ability of the lungs to oxygenate the blood, the hemoglobin leaves the pulmonary circulation without being fully oxygenated, resulting in shortness of breath and cyanosis.

Acute pulmonary edema usually is a terrifying experience. The person usually is seen sitting and gasping for air, in obvious apprehension. The pulse is rapid, the skin is moist and cool, and the lips and nail beds are cyanotic. As the lung edema worsens and the oxygen supply to the brain drops, confusion and stupor appear. Dyspnea and air hunger are accompanied by a cough productive of frothy (resembling beaten egg whites) and often blood-tinged sputum—the effect of air mixing with serum albumin and red blood cells that have moved into the alveoli. The movement of air through the alveolar fluid produces fine crepitant sounds called *crackles*, which can be heard through a stethoscope placed on the chest. As fluid moves into the larger airways, the breathing becomes louder. The crackles heard earlier become louder and coarser.

Treatment of acute pulmonary edema is directed toward reducing the fluid volume in the pulmonary circulation. This can be accomplished by reducing the amount of blood that the right heart delivers to the lungs or by improving the work performance of the left heart. Several measures can decrease the blood volume in the pulmonary circulation; the seriousness of the pulmonary edema determines which are used. One of the simplest measures to relieve orthopnea is assumption of the seated position. For many persons, sitting up or standing is almost instinctive and may be sufficient to relieve the symptoms associated with mild accumulation of fluid.

Measures to improve left heart performance focus on decreasing the preload by reducing the filling pressure of the left ventricle and on reducing the afterload against which the left heart must pump. This can be accomplished through the use of diuretics, vasodilator drugs, treatment of arrhythmias that impair cardiac function, and improvement of the contractile properties of the left ventricle with digitalis. Rapid digitalization can be accomplished with intravenous administration of the drug. Although its mechanisms of action are unclear, morphine sulfate usually is the drug of choice in acute pulmonary edema. Morphine relieves anxiety and depresses the pulmonary reflexes that cause spasm of the pulmonary vessels. It also increases venous pooling by vasodilatation. Oxygen therapy, usually delivered by face mask, increases the oxygen content of the blood and helps relieve anxiety. Noninvasive pressure-support ventilation may be used to improve oxygenation and prevent carbon dioxide retention while pharmacologic interventions take effect.

CARDIOGENIC SHOCK

Cardiogenic shock implies failure of the heart to pump blood adequately. Cardiogenic shock can occur relatively quickly because of the damage to the heart that occurs during myocardial infarction; ineffective pumping caused by cardiac arrhythmias; mechanical defects that may occur as a complication of myocardial infarction, such as ventricular septal defect; ventricular aneurysm; acute disruption of valvular function; or problems associated with open heart surgery. Cardiogenic shock also may ensue as an end-stage condition of coronary artery disease or cardiomyopathy.

The most common cause of cardiogenic shock is myocardial infarction. Most patients who die of cardiogenic shock have lost at least 40% of the contracting muscle of the left ventricle because of a recent infarct or a combination of recent and old infarcts.[19] Cardiogenic shock can follow other types of shock associated with inadequate coronary blood flow, or it can develop because substances released from ischemic tissues impair cardiac function. One such substance, myocardial depressant factor, is thought to be released into the circulation during severe shock. Myocardial depressant factor produces reversible (although often severe) myocardial depression, ventricular dilation, and decreased left ventricular ejection fraction and diastolic pressure.[19]

In all cases of cardiogenic shock, there is failure to eject blood from the heart, hypotension, and inadequate cardiac output. Increased systemic vascular resistance often contributes to the deterioration of cardiac function by increasing afterload or the resistance to ventricular systole. The filling pressure, or preload of the heart, also is increased as blood returning to the heart is added to blood that previously was returned but not pumped forward, resulting in an increase in end-systolic ventricular volume. Increased resistance to ventricular systole (*i.e.*, afterload) combined with the decreased myocardial contractility causes the increased end-systolic ventricular volume and preload, which further complicate cardiac status.

The signs and symptoms of cardiogenic shock are consistent with those of extreme heart failure. The lips, nail beds, and skin are cyanotic because of stagnation of blood flow and increased extraction of oxygen from the hemoglobin as it passes through the capillary bed. The central venous and pulmonary capillary pressures rise as a result of volume overload caused by the pumping failure of the heart.

Treatment of cardiogenic shock requires a precarious balance between improving cardiac output, reducing the workload and oxygen needs of the myocardium, and preserving coronary perfusion. Fluid volume must be regulated within a level that maintains the filling pressure (*i.e.,* venous return) of the heart and maximum use of the Frank-Starling mechanism without causing pulmonary congestion.

Pharmacologic treatment includes the use of vasodilators such as nitroprusside and nitroglycerin. Nitroprusside causes arterial and venous dilatation, producing a decrease in venous return to the heart, with a reduction in arterial resistance against which the left heart must pump. Nitroglycerin focuses its effects on the venous vascular beds until, at high doses, it begins to dilate the arterial beds as well. The arterial pressure is maintained by an increased ventricular stroke volume ejected against a lowered systemic vascular resistance; this allows blood to be redistributed from the pulmonary vascular bed to the systemic circulation. Catecholamines increase cardiac contractility but must be used with caution because they also produce vasoconstriction and increase cardiac workload by increasing the afterload.

The intra-aortic balloon pump provides a means of increasing aortic diastolic pressure and enhances coronary and peripheral blood flow without increasing systolic pressure and the afterload, against which the left ventricle must pump.[20] The device, which pumps in synchrony with the heart, consists of a 10-inch-long balloon that is inserted through a catheter into the descending aorta (Fig. 19-6). The balloon is positioned so that the distal tip lies approximately 1 inch from the aortic arch. The balloon is filled with helium and is timed to inflate during ventricular diastole and deflate just before ventricular systole. Diastolic inflation creates a pressure wave in the ascending aorta that increases coronary artery flow and a less intense wave in the lower aorta that enhances organ perfusion. The sudden balloon deflation at the onset of systole lowers the resistance to ejection of blood from the left ventricle; thereby increasing the heart's pumping efficiency and decreasing myocardial oxygen consumption.

MECHANICAL SUPPORT AND HEART TRANSPLANTATION

Refractory heart failure reflects a deterioration in cardiac function that is unresponsive to medical or surgical interventions. With improved methods of treatment, more people are reaching a point where a cure is unachievable and death is imminent without mechanical support or heart transplantation.

Since the early 1960s, significant progress has been made in improving the efficacy of *ventricular assist devices* (VADs), which are mechanical pumps used to support ventricular function.[21] VADs are used to decrease the workload of the myocardium while maintaining cardiac output and systemic arterial pressure. This decreases the workload on the ventricle and allows it to rest and recover. Most VADs require an invasive open chest procedure for implantation. They may be used in patients who fail or have difficulty being weaned from cardiopulmonary bypass after cardiac surgery; those who develop cardiogenic shock after myocardial infarction; those with end-stage cardiomyopathy; and those who are awaiting cardiac transplantation. VADs can be used to support the function of the left ventricle, right ventricle, or both.

Heart transplantation remains the treatment of choice for end-stage cardiac failure. The number of successful heart transplantations has declined recently, with over 2600 procedures performed per year.[1] Patients with heart transplants who are treated with triple-immunosuppressant therapy have a 5-year survival rate of 75% in men to 62% in women.[22] Despite the overall success of heart transplantation, donor availability and complications from infection, rejection, and immunosuppression drug therapy remain problems.

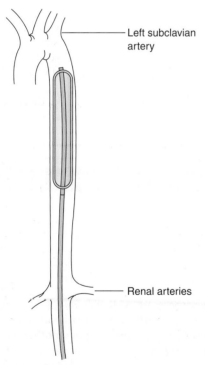

Left subclavian artery

Renal arteries

FIGURE 19-6 Aortic balloon pump. The balloon inflates during diastole, producing a pressure wave in the ascending aorta that improves coronary perfusion and a lesser wave in the descending aorta that improves blood flow in the peripheral circulation; it deflates during systole, producing a decrease in afterload or resistance to outflow of blood from the left ventricle. (From Hudak C. M., Gallo B. M. [1994]. *Critical care nursing* [6th ed.]. Philadelphia: J. B. Lippincott.)

In summary, heart failure occurs when the heart fails to pump sufficient blood to meet the metabolic needs of body tissues. The physiology of heart failure reflects an interplay between a decrease in cardiac output that accompanies impaired function of the failing heart and the compensatory mechanisms designed to preserve the cardiac reserve. Adaptive mechanisms include the Frank-Starling mechanism, sympathetic nervous system activation, the renin-angiotensin-aldosterone mechanism, natriuretic peptides, endothelins, and myocardial hypertrophy and remodeling. In the failing heart, early decreases in cardiac function may go unnoticed because these compensatory mechanisms maintain the cardiac output. This is called *compensated heart failure.* Unfortunately, the mechanisms were not intended for long-term use, and in severe and prolonged decompensated heart failure, the compensatory mechanisms no longer are effective, and instead contribute to the progression of cardiac heart failure.

Heart failure may be described as high-output or low-output failure, systolic or diastolic failure, and right-sided or left-sided failure. With high-output failure, the function of the heart may be supranormal but inadequate because of excessive metabolic demands. With low-output failure, the function of the heart is inadequate because of disorders that impair the pumping ability of the heart. With systolic dysfunction, there is impaired ejection of blood from the heart during systole; with diastolic dysfunction, there is impaired filling of the heart during diastole. Right-sided failure is characterized by congestion in the peripheral circulation, and left-sided failure by congestion in the pulmonary circulation.

The manifestations of heart failure include edema, nocturia, fatigue and impaired exercise tolerance, cyanosis, signs of increased sympathetic nervous system activity, and impaired gastrointestinal function and malnutrition. In right-sided failure, there is dependent edema of the lower parts of the body, engorgement of the liver, and ascites. In left-sided failure, there is pulmonary congestion with shortness of breath and a chronic nonproductive cough.

The diagnostic methods in heart failure are directed toward establishing the cause and extent of the disorder. Treatment is directed toward correcting the cause whenever possible, improving cardiac function, maintaining the fluid volume within a compensatory level, and developing an activity pattern consistent with individual limitations in cardiac reserve. Among the medications used in the treatment of heart failure are diuretics, digoxin, ACE inhibitors, and β-adrenergic blockers.

Acute pulmonary edema is a life-threatening condition in which the accumulation of fluid in the interstitium of the lung and alveoli interferes with lung expansion and gas exchange. It is characterized by extreme breathlessness, crackles, frothy sputum, cyanosis, and signs of hypoxemia. In cardiogenic shock, there is failure to eject blood from the heart, hypotension, inadequate cardiac output, and impaired perfusion of peripheral tissues. Mechanical support devices, including the intra-aortic balloon pump (for acute failure) and the VAD, sustain life in persons with severe heart failure. Heart transplantation remains the treatment of choice for many persons with end-stage heart failure.

Circulatory Failure (Shock)

The functions of the circulatory system are to perfuse body tissues and supply them with oxygen. Whereas heart failure results from impaired ability of the heart as a pump, circulatory shock results from a failure of the blood vessels to supply the peripheral tissues and organs of the body with an adequate blood supply. As with heart failure, circulatory shock is not a specific disease but can occur in the course of many life-threatening traumatic or disease states.

Adequate perfusion of body tissues depends on the pumping ability of the heart, a vascular system that transports blood to the cells and back to the heart, sufficient blood to fill the vascular system, and tissues that are able to use and extract oxygen and nutrients from the blood. As with heart failure, circulatory shock produces compensatory physiologic responses that eventually decompensate into various shock states if the condition is not properly treated in a timely manner.

TYPES OF SHOCK

Circulatory shock is used to describe a critical decrease in tissue perfusion caused by a loss or redistribution of intravascular fluid. It can be classified as hypovolemic, obstructive, or distributive. These three main types of shock are summarized in Chart 19-1. Cardiogenic shock, which results from failure of the heart as a pump, was discussed earlier in the chapter.

Hypovolemic Shock

Hypovolemic shock is characterized by diminished blood volume such that there is inadequate filling of the vascular compartment (Fig. 19-7). It occurs when there is an

---

CHART 19-1

Classification of Circulatory Shock

Hypovolemic

Loss of whole blood
Loss of plasma
Loss of extracellular fluid

Obstructive

Inability of the heart to fill properly (cardiac tamponade)
Obstruction to outflow from the heart (pulmonary embolus, cardiac myxoma, pneumothorax, or dissecting aneurysm)

Distributive

Loss of sympathetic vasomotor tone
Presence of vasodilating substances in the blood (anaphylactic shock)
Presence of inflammatory mediators (septic shock) in the systemic circulation

Hypovolemic shock, which has been the most widely studied type of shock, is often used as a prototype for discussing the manifestations of shock. Because the characteristics of shock change at different degrees of severity, it is commonly divided into three major stages: (1) the nonprogressive stage, in which the normal compensatory mechanisms prevent large changes in circulatory function; (2) the progressive stage, in which the shock becomes progressively worse; and (3) the irreversible stage, in which the shock has progressed to such an extent that all known forms of therapy are insufficient to save the person's life.[23] Approximately 10% blood volume can be removed without changing the cardiovascular function, but the loss of greater amounts usually diminishes cardiac output first and later blood pressure.[23] The average blood donor loses a pint of blood without experiencing adverse effects.

Without compensatory mechanisms to maintain the cardiac output and blood pressure, the loss of vascular volume would result in a rapid progression from the initial to the progressive and irreversible stages of shock. The most immediate of the compensatory mechanisms are the sympathetic-mediated responses designed to maintain cardiac output and blood pressure (Fig. 19-8). Within seconds after the onset of hemorrhage or the loss of blood volume, tachycardia, increased cardiac contractility, vasoconstriction, and other signs of sympathetic and adrenal medullary activity appear. The sympathetic vasoconstrictor response also mobilizes blood that has been stored in the venous side of the circulation as a means of increasing venous return to the heart. There is considerable capacity for blood storage in the large veins of the abdomen and liver. Approximately 350 mL of blood that can be mobilized in shock is stored in the liver.[23]

Compensatory mechanisms designed to restore blood volume include absorption of fluid from the interstitial spaces, conservation of salt and water by the kidneys, and thirst. Extracellular fluid is distributed between the interstitial spaces and the vascular compartment. When there is a loss of vascular volume, capillary pressures decrease, and water is drawn into the vascular compartment from the interstitial spaces. The maintenance of vascular volume is further enhanced by renal mechanisms that conserve fluid. A decrease in renal blood flow and glomerular filtration rate results in activation of the renin-angiotensin-aldosterone mechanism, which produces an increase in sodium reabsorption by the kidney. The decrease in blood volume also stimulates centers in the hypothalamus that regulate ADH release and thirst. ADH, also known as *vasopressin*, constricts the peripheral arteries and veins and greatly increases water retention by the kidneys. Although the mechanism for ADH release is more sensitive to changes in serum osmolality, a decrease of 10% to 15% in blood volume serves as a strong stimulus for ADH secretion.[24]

As hypovolemic shock progresses, vasoconstriction of the blood vessels that supply the skin, skeletal muscles, kidneys, and abdominal organs becomes more severe, with a resultant decrease in blood flow and conversion to anaerobic metabolism with lactic acid formation. Without sufficient energy production, normal cell function cannot

acute loss of 15% to 20% of the circulating blood volume. The decrease may be caused by an external loss of whole blood (*e.g.*, hemorrhage), plasma (*e.g.*, severe burns), or extracellular fluid (*e.g.*, gastrointestinal fluids lost in vomiting or diarrhea). Hypovolemic shock also can result from an internal hemorrhage or from third-space losses, when extracellular fluid is shifted from the vascular compartment to the interstitial space or compartment.

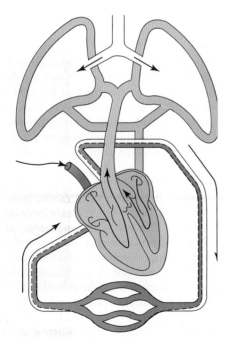

FIGURE 19-7 Hypovolemic shock is caused by diminished blood volume with decreased filling of the circulatory system.

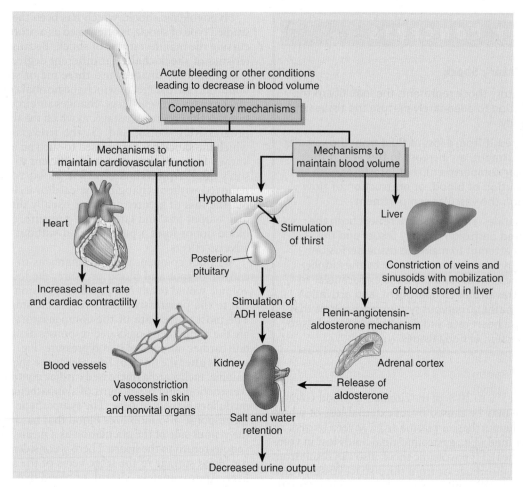

FIGURE 19-8 Compensatory mechanisms used to maintain circulatory function and blood volume in hypovolemic shock.

be maintained, and the activity of the sodium-potassium membrane pump is impaired. Consequently, sodium chloride accumulates in cells and potassium is lost from cells. The cells then swell, and their membranes become more permeable. Depression of mitochondrial activity and rupture of lysosomal membranes with release of lysosomal enzymes cause further damage of intracellular structures. This is followed by cell death and the release of intracellular contents into the extracellular spaces, producing changes in the microcirculation that reduce the chance of recovery.

Manifestations. The signs and symptoms of hypovolemic shock depend on shock stage and are closely related to low peripheral blood flow and excessive sympathetic stimulation. They include thirst, an increase in heart rate, cool and clammy skin, a decrease in arterial blood pressure, and a decrease in urine output. Laboratory tests of hemoglobin and hematocrit provide information regarding the severity of blood loss or hemoconcentration due to dehydration. Serum lactate and arterial pH provide information about the severity of acidosis.

An increase in heart rate is often an early sign of shock. As shock progresses, the pulse becomes weak and thready, indicating vasoconstriction and a reduction in filling of the vascular compartment. Although the arterial blood pressure is decreased in moderate to severe shock, it may be relatively normal during the early stages of shock. This is because compensatory mechanisms tend to preserve blood pressure until shock is relatively far advanced.

Decreased intravascular volume results in decreased venous return to the heart and a decrease in central venous pressure. When shock becomes severe, the peripheral veins collapse, making it difficult to insert peripheral venous lines. Sympathetic stimulation also leads to intense vasoconstriction of the skin vessels and activation of the sweat glands. As a result, the skin is cool and moist. When shock is caused by hemorrhage, the loss of red blood cells leaves the skin and mucous membranes looking pale.

Urine output decreases very quickly in hypovolemic and other forms of shock. Compensatory mechanisms decrease renal blood flow as a means of diverting blood flow to the heart and brain. Oliguria of 20 mL/hour or less indicates severe shock and inadequate renal perfusion. Continuous measurement of urine output is essential for assessing the circulatory status of the person in shock.

Restlessness and apprehension are common behaviors in early shock. As the shock progresses and blood flow to the brain decreases, restlessness is replaced by apathy and stupor. If shock is unchecked, the apathy progresses to coma. Coma caused by blood loss alone and not related to head injury or other factors is an unfavorable sign.

Treatment. The treatment of hypovolemic shock is directed toward correcting or controlling the underlying cause and improving tissue perfusion. Persons who have sustained blood loss are commonly placed in supine position with the legs elevated to maximize cerebral blood flow. Oxygen is administered to persons with signs of hypoxemia. Because subcutaneous administration is unpredictable, pain medications usually are administered intravenously. Frequent measurements of heart rate and cardiac rhythm, blood pressure, and urine flow are used to assess the severity of circulatory compromise and to monitor treatment.

In hypovolemic shock, the goal of treatment is to restore vascular volume. This can be accomplished through intravenous administration of fluids and blood. The crystalloids (*e.g.,* isotonic saline) are readily available for emergencies and mass casualties. They often are effective, at least temporarily, when given in adequate doses. Blood or blood products (packed or frozen red cells) are administered based on hematocrit and hemodynamic findings.

Vasoactive drugs (*e.g.,* adrenergic agents) are agents capable of constricting or dilating blood vessels. As a general rule, the adrenergic drugs are not used as a primary form of therapy in shock. Simple blood pressure elevation produced by vasopressor drugs has little effect on the underlying cause of shock and in many cases may be detrimental. These agents are given only when hypotension persists after volume deficits have been corrected. Dopamine, which produces a more favorable array of α- and β-receptor actions than many of the other adrenergic drugs, may be used in the treatment of severe and prolonged shock. When given in low doses, it is thought to increase blood flow to the kidneys, liver, and other abdominal organs while maintaining vasoconstriction of less vital structures, such as the skin and skeletal muscles. In severe shock, higher doses may be needed to maintain blood pressure. After dopamine administration exceeds this low-dose range, it has vasoconstrictive effects on blood flow to the kidneys and abdominal organs that are similar to those of epinephrine.

Obstructive Shock

The term *obstructive shock* is used to describe the circulatory shock that occurs with mechanical obstruction of blood flow through the central circulation (great veins, heart, or lungs; Fig. 19-9). Obstructive shock may be caused by a number of conditions, including dissecting aortic aneurysm, cardiac tamponade, pneumothorax,

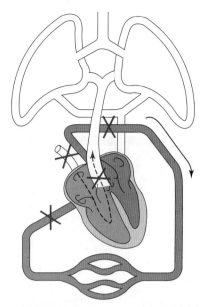

FIGURE 19-9 Obstructive shock is caused by mechanical impediment to flow of blood through the central circulation (great veins, heart, and pulmonary circulation).

atrial myxoma, or evisceration of abdominal contents into the thoracic cavity because of a ruptured hemidiaphragm. The most frequent cause of obstructive shock is pulmonary embolism.

The primary physiologic results of obstructive shock are elevated right heart pressure and impaired venous return to the heart. The signs of right heart failure are seen, including elevation of central venous pressure and jugular venous distention. Treatment modalities focus on correcting the cause of the disorder, frequently with surgical interventions such as pulmonary embolectomy, pericardiocentesis (*i.e.,* removal of fluid from the pericardial sac) for cardiac tamponade, or the insertion of a chest tube for correction of a tension pneumothorax or hemothorax. In select cases of pulmonary embolus, thrombolytic drugs may be used to dissolve the clots causing the obstruction.

Distributive Shock

Distributive or vasodilatory shock is characterized by loss of blood vessel tone, enlargement of the vascular compartment, and displacement of the vascular volume away from the heart and central circulation.[25] With distributive shock, sometimes called *normovolemic shock*, the capacity of the vascular compartment expands to the extent that a normal volume of blood does not fill the circulatory system (Fig. 19-10). Loss of vessel tone has two main causes: a decrease in the sympathetic control of vasomotor tone or the presence of vasodilator substances in the blood. It can also occur as a complication of vessel damage resulting from prolonged and severe hypotension due to irreversible or late-phase hemorrhagic shock.[25] There are three shock states that share the basic circulatory pattern

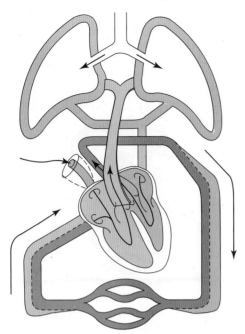

FIGURE 19-10 Distributive shock is caused by enlargement of the vascular compartment and displacement of blood away from the heart and central circulation.

of distributive shock: neurogenic shock, anaphylactic shock, and septic shock.

Neurogenic Shock. Neurogenic shock describes shock caused by decreased sympathetic control of blood vessel tone due to a defect in the vasomotor center in the brain stem or the sympathetic outflow to the blood vessels. Output from the vasomotor center can be interrupted by brain injury, the depressant action of drugs, general anesthesia, hypoxia, or lack of glucose (*e.g.,* insulin reaction). Fainting due to emotional causes is a transient form of neurogenic shock. Spinal anesthesia or spinal cord injury above the mid-thoracic region can interrupt the transmission of outflow from the vasomotor center. The term *spinal shock* is used to describe the neurogenic shock that occurs in persons with spinal cord injury. Many general anesthetic agents can cause a neurogenic shock–like reaction, especially during induction, because of interference with sympathetic nervous system function. In contrast to hypovolemic shock, the heart rate in neurogenic shock often is slower than normal, and the skin is dry and warm. This type of distributive shock is rare and usually transitory.

Anaphylactic Shock. Anaphylaxis is a clinical syndrome that represents the most severe systemic allergic reaction.[26,27] It results from an immunologically mediated reaction in which vasodilator substances such as histamine are released into the blood (see Chapter 15). These substances cause vasodilatation of arterioles and venules along with a marked increase in capillary permeability. The vascular response in anaphylaxis is often accompanied by life-threatening laryngeal edema and bron-

chospasm, circulatory collapse, contraction of gastro-intestinal and uterine smooth muscle, and urticaria (hives) or angioedema.

Among the most frequent causes of anaphylactic shock are reactions to drugs, such as penicillin; foods, such as nuts and shellfish; and insect venoms. The most common cause is stings from insects of the order Hymenoptera (*i.e.,* bees, wasps, and fire ants). Latex allergy has caused life-threatening anaphylaxis in a growing segment of the population. Health care workers and others who are exposed to latex are developing latex sensitivities that range from mild urticaria, contact dermatitis, and mild respiratory distress to anaphylactic shock.[28] Children with spina bifida also are at extreme risk for this increasingly serious allergy.

The onset of anaphylaxis depends on the sensitivity of the person and the rate and quantity of antigen exposure. Anaphylactic shock often develops suddenly; death can occur within a matter of minutes unless appropriate medical intervention is promptly instituted. Signs and symptoms associated with impending anaphylactic shock include abdominal cramps; apprehension; burning and warm sensation of the skin, itching, and urticaria; and coughing, choking, wheezing, chest tightness, and difficulty in breathing. After blood begins to pool peripherally, there is a precipitous drop in blood pressure and the pulse becomes so weak that it is difficult to detect. Life-threatening airway obstruction may ensue as a result of laryngeal edema or bronchial spasm.

Treatment includes immediate discontinuance of the inciting agent or institution of measures to decrease its absorption (*e.g.,* application of ice to a bee sting); close monitoring of cardiovascular and respiratory function; and maintenance of adequate respiratory gas exchange, cardiac output, and tissue perfusion. Epinephrine constricts the blood vessels and relaxes the smooth muscle in the bronchioles; it usually is the first drug to be given to a patient believed to be experiencing an anaphylactic reaction. Other treatment measures include the administration of oxygen, antihistaminic drugs, and corticosteroids. Resuscitation measures may be required.

The prevention of anaphylactic shock is preferable to treatment. Once a person has been sensitized to an antigen, the risk of repeated anaphylactic reactions with subsequent exposure is high. All health care providers should question patients regarding previous drug reactions and inform patients as to the name of the medication they are to receive before it is administered or prescribed. Persons with known hypersensitivities should carry some form of medical identification to alert medical personnel if they become unconscious or unable to relate this information. Persons who are at risk for anaphylaxis should be provided with emergency medications (*e.g.,* epinephrine autoinjector) and instructed in procedures to follow in case they are inadvertently exposed to the offending antigen.

Sepsis and Septic Shock. Septic shock, which is the most common type of vasodilatory shock, is associated with severe infection and the release of inflammatory mediators into the systemic circulation.[25] It is associated most frequently with gram-negative bacteremia, although it can be caused by gram-positive bacilli and other microorganisms such as fungi, which carry an even greater risk of mortality.[29] Unlike other types of shock, septic shock commonly is associated with pathologic complications, such as pulmonary insufficiency, disseminated intravascular coagulation, and multiple organ dysfunction syndrome.

Severe sepsis accompanied by acute organ dysfunction is a frequently occurring condition in critically ill patients, affecting approximately 750,000 Americans annually and causing more than 200,000 deaths.[30,31] The growing incidence has been attributed to an increased awareness of the diagnosis, increased numbers of immunocompromised patients, increased use of invasive procedures, increased number of resistant organisms, and an increased number of elderly patients.[32] Despite advances in treatment methods, the mortality rate remains approximately 40%.[33]

Septic shock has been described in the context of what has been termed the *systemic inflammatory response syndrome* (SIRS). The common clinical manifestations of sepsis include alterations in body temperature (fever or hypothermia), tachypnea or hyperventilation, tachycardia, increase or decrease in white blood cell count, altered blood pressure, and alterations in mental status. Although usually associated with infection, the SIRS can be initiated by noninfectious disorders such as acute trauma and pancreatitis.[29]

Mechanisms. The mechanisms of sepsis and SIRS are thought to be related to mediators of the inflammatory response.[29–33] Even though the immune system and the inflammatory response are designed to overcome infection and eliminate bacterial breakdown products, the unregulated release of inflammatory mediators or cytokines (see Chapter 14) may elicit toxic reactions, resulting in the potentially fatal sepsis syndrome. The most widely investigated cytokines have been tumor necrosis factor-α (TNF-α), interleukin-1, and interleukin-8, which usually are proinflammatory, and interleukin-6 and interleukin-10, which tend to be anti-inflammatory. A trigger such as a microbial toxin stimulates the release of TNF-α and interleukin-1, which in turn promote endothelial cell–leukocyte adhesion, release of cell-damaging proteases and prostaglandins, and activation of the clotting cascade. The prostaglandins, thromboxane A_2 (a vasoconstrictor), prostacyclin (a vasodilator), and prostaglandin E_2, participate in the generation of fever, tachycardia, ventilation–perfusion abnormalities, and lactic acidosis. Interleukin-8, a neutrophil chemotaxin, may have a particularly important role in perpetuating tissue inflammation. Interleukin-6 and interleukin-10, which have anti-inflammatory actions and perhaps are counter-regulatory, augment the acute-phase response and consequent generation of additional proinflammatory mediators.[34]

In addition to inducing the release of inflammatory mediators, the sepsis-producing endotoxins may induce tissue damage by directly activating pathways such as the coagulation and complement cascades, by causing vessel injury, or by triggering the release of vasodilating prostaglandins.[34] Thus, the processes that result in the sepsis syndrome are complex consequences of microbial products that profoundly dysregulate the release of inflammatory mediators and disrupt the regulation of several important inflammatory and coagulation pathways.

Manifestations. Septic shock typically manifests with fever, vasodilatation, and warm, flushed skin. Mild hyperventilation, respiratory alkalosis, and abrupt changes in personality and behavior due to reduced cerebral blood flow may be the earliest signs and symptoms of septic shock. These manifestations, which are thought to be a primary response to the bacteremia, commonly precede the usual signs and symptoms of sepsis by several hours or days. Unlike other forms of shock (*i.e.*, cardiogenic, hypovolemic, and obstructive) that are characterized by a compensatory increase in systemic vascular resistance, septic shock often presents with hypovolemia and decreased blood pressure because of arterial and venous dilatation and leakage of plasma into the interstitial spaces.

Treatment. The treatment of sepsis and septic shock focuses on the control of the causative agent and support of the circulation. The administration of antibiotics that are specific for the infectious agent is essential.[35] The cardiovascular status of the patient must be supported to maintain oxygen delivery to the cells. Swift and aggressive fluid administration is needed to compensate for third spacing, and equally aggressive use of vasopressor agents is needed to counteract the vasodilatation caused by endotoxins.

Among the more recent advances in the treatment of sepsis are the use of intensive insulin therapy for hyperglycemia[31] and the administration of recombinant human activated protein C.[35,36] The protective mechanism of insulin in sepsis is unknown. The phagocytic function of neutrophils is impaired in hyperglycemia, suggesting that this may be one of the reasons for insulin's efficacy. In addition, insulin also prevents apoptotic cell death by numerous stimuli, suggesting a second reason. Recombinant human activated protein C, a naturally occurring anticoagulant that acts by inactivating coagulation factors Va and VIII (see Chapter 10), is the first anti-inflammatory agent that has proved effective in the treatment of sepsis.[36] Along with its anticoagulant actions, activated protein C has direct anti-inflammatory properties, including blocking the production of cytokines by monocytes and blocking cell adhesion. Activated protein C also has antiapoptotic actions that may contribute to its effectiveness.

COMPLICATIONS OF SHOCK

Wiggers, a noted circulatory physiologist, stated, "Shock not only stops the machine, but it wrecks the machinery."[37] Many body systems are wrecked by severe shock. Five major complications of severe shock are shock lung, acute renal failure, gastrointestinal ulceration, disseminated intravascular coagulation, and multiple organ dysfunction syndrome. The complications of shock are serious and often fatal.

Acute Respiratory Distress Syndrome

Acute respiratory distress syndrome (ARDS) is a potentially lethal form of respiratory failure that can follow severe shock (see Chapter 22). Its mortality rate remains greater than 50% despite advances in mechanical ventilation.[38]

The symptoms of ARDS usually do not develop until 24 to 48 hours after the initial trauma; in some instances, they occur later. The respiratory rate and effort of breathing increase. Arterial blood gas analysis establishes the presence of profound hypoxemia with hypercapnia, resulting from impaired matching of ventilation and perfusion and from the greatly reduced diffusion of blood gases across the thickened alveolar membranes.

The exact cause of ARDS is unknown, although neutrophils are thought to play a key role in its pathogenesis. A cytokine-mediated activation and accumulation of neutrophils in the pulmonary vasculature and subsequent endothelial injury are thought to cause leakage of fluid and plasma proteins into the interstitium and alveolar spaces.[38,39] The fluid leakage impairs gas exchange and makes the lung stiffer and more difficult to inflate. Abnormalities in the production, composition, and function of surfactant may contribute to alveolar collapse and gas exchange abnormalities.[39]

Interventions for ARDS focus on increasing the oxygen concentration in the inspired air and supporting ventilation mechanically to optimize gas exchange while avoiding oxygen toxicity and preventing further lung injury. Despite the delivery of high levels of oxygen using high-pressure mechanical ventilatory support and positive end-expiratory pressure, many persons with ARDS remain hypoxic, often with a fatal outcome.

Acute Renal Failure

The renal tubules are particularly vulnerable to ischemia, and acute renal failure is one important late cause of death in severe shock. Sepsis and trauma account for most cases of acute renal failure. The endotoxins implicated in septic shock are powerful vasoconstrictors that are capable of activating the sympathetic nervous system and causing intravascular clotting. They have been shown to trigger all the separate physiologic mechanisms that contribute to the onset of acute renal failure. The degree of renal damage is related to the severity and duration of shock. The renal lesion most frequently seen after severe shock is acute tubular necrosis. Acute tubular necrosis usually is reversible, although return to normal renal function may require weeks or months (see Chapter 25). Continuous monitoring of urine output during shock provides a means of assessing renal blood flow. Frequent monitoring of serum creatinine and blood urea nitrogen levels also provides valuable information regarding renal status.

Gastrointestinal Complications

The gastrointestinal tract is particularly vulnerable to ischemia because of the changes in distribution of blood flow to its mucosal surface. In shock, there is widespread constriction of blood vessels that supply the gastrointestinal tract, causing a redistribution of blood flow that severely diminishes mucosal perfusion. Superficial mucosal lesions of the stomach and duodenum can develop within hours of severe trauma, sepsis, or burn.

Bleeding is a common symptom of gastrointestinal ulceration caused by shock. Hemorrhage has its onset usually within 2 to 10 days after the original insult and often begins without warning. Poor perfusion in the gastrointestinal tract has also been credited with allowing intestinal bacteria to enter the bloodstream, thereby contributing to the development of sepsis and shock.[40]

Histamine type 2 receptor antagonists, proton pump inhibitors, or sucralfate may be given prophylactically to prevent gastrointestinal ulcerations caused by shock.[40] Nasogastric tubes, when attached to intermittent suction, also help to diminish the accumulation of acid in the stomach.

Disseminated Intravascular Coagulation

Disseminated intravascular coagulation (DIC) is characterized by widespread activation of the coagulation system with resultant formation of fibrin clots and thrombotic occlusion of small and mid-sized vessels (see Chapter 10). The systemic formation of fibrin results from increased generation of thrombin, the simultaneous suppression of physiologic anticoagulation mechanisms, and the delayed removal of fibrin as a consequence of impaired fibrinolysis. Clinically overt DIC is reported to occur in as much as 30% to 50% of persons with sepsis and septic shock.[41] As with other systemic inflammatory responses, the derangement of coagulation and fibrinolysis is thought to be effected by inflammatory mediators.

The contribution of DIC to morbidity and mortality in sepsis depends on the underlying clinical condition and the intensity of the coagulation disorder. Depletion of the platelets and coagulation factors increases the risk of bleeding. Deposition of fibrin in the vasculature of organs contributes to ischemic damage and organ failure. In a large number of clinical trials, the occurrence of DIC appeared to be associated with an unfavorable outcome and was an independent predictor of mortality.[41] However, it remains uncertain whether DIC was a predictor of unfavorable outcome or merely a marker of the seriousness of the underlying condition causing the DIC.

The management of sepsis-induced DIC focuses on treatment of the underlying disorder and measures to interrupt the coagulation process. Treatment options include anticoagulation therapy and administration of platelets and plasma. The use of antithrombin III, a coagulation inhibitor, is under investigation. Other therapeutic options, aimed at interrupting the intrinsic coagulation pathway at the point where tissue factor complexes with factor VIIa, also are being investigated.[41]

Multiple Organ Dysfunction Syndrome

Multiple organ dysfunction syndrome (MODS) represents the presence of altered organ function in an acutely ill patient such that homeostasis cannot be maintained without intervention. As the name implies, MODS commonly affects multiple organ systems, including the kidneys, lungs, liver, brain, and heart. MODS is a particularly life-threatening complication of shock, especially septic shock. It has been reported as the most frequent cause of death in the noncoronary intensive care unit. Mortality rates vary from 30% to 100%, depending on the number of organs involved.[42] Mortality rates increase with the number of organs failing. A high mortality rate is associated with failure of the brain, liver, kidney, and lung. The pathogenesis of MODS is not clearly understood, and current management therefore is primarily supportive. Major risk factors for the development of MODS are sepsis, shock, prolonged periods of hypotension, hepatic dysfunction, trauma, infarcted bowel, advanced age, and alcohol abuse.[42] Interventions for multiple organ failure are focused on support of the affected organs.

In summary, circulatory shock is an acute emergency in which body tissues are deprived of oxygen and cellular nutrients or are unable to use these materials in their metabolic processes. Circulatory shock may develop because there is not enough blood in the circulatory system (i.e., hypovolemic shock), blood flow or venous return is obstructed (i.e., obstructive shock), or the size of the vascular compartment is enlarged causing inadequate filling (i.e., distributive shock). Three types of shock share the basic circulatory pattern of distributive shock: neurogenic shock, anaphylactic shock, and septic shock. Septic shock, which is the most common of these three types, is associated with a severe, overwhelming infection and has a mortality rate of approximately 40%.

The manifestations of hypovolemic shock, which serves as a prototype for circulatory shock, are related to low peripheral blood flow and excessive sympathetic stimulation. The low peripheral blood flow produces thirst; intense vasoconstriction of blood vessels, producing a pale and cool skin; decreased arterial and venous pressures along with a compensatory increase in heart rate; and decreased renal blood flow and urine output. The intense vasoconstriction that serves to maintain blood flow to the heart and brain causes a decrease in tissue perfusion, impaired cellular metabolism, liberation of lactic acid, and, eventually, cell death. Whether the shock is irreversible or the patient survives is determined largely by changes that occur at the cellular level.

The complications of shock result from the deprivation of blood flow to vital organs or systems, such as the lungs, kidneys, gastrointestinal tract, and blood coagulation system. ARDS produces lung changes that occur with shock. It is characterized by changes in the permeability of the alveolar-capillary membrane with the development of interstitial edema and severe hypoxia that does not respond to oxygen therapy. The renal tubules are particularly vulnerable to ischemia, and acute renal failure is an important complication of shock. Gastrointestinal ischemia may lead to gastrointestinal bleeding and increased permeability to the intestinal bacteria, which cause further sepsis and shock. DIC is characterized by formation of small clots in the circulation. It is thought to be caused by inappropriate activation of the coagulation cascade because of toxins or other products released as a result of the shock state. Multiple organ failure, perhaps the most ominous complication of shock, rapidly depletes the body's ability to compensate and recover from a shock state.

Circulatory Failure in Children and the Elderly

HEART FAILURE IN INFANTS AND CHILDREN

As in adults, heart failure in infants and children results from the inability of the heart to maintain the cardiac output required to sustain metabolic demands.[43–45] Congenital heart defects are the most common cause of heart failure during childhood. Surgical correction of congenital heart defects may cause heart failure as a result of intraoperative manipulation of the heart and resection of heart tissue, with subsequent alterations in pressure, flow, and resistance. Usually, the heart failure that results is acute and resolves after the effects of the surgical procedure have subsided. Chronic heart failure occasionally is observed in children with severe chronic anemia, inflammatory heart disease, end-stage congenital heart disease, or cardiomyopathy. Inflammatory heart disorders (e.g., myocarditis, rheumatic fever, bacterial endocarditis, Kawasaki disease), cardiomyopathy, and congenital heart disorders are discussed in Chapter 18.

Manifestations

Many of the signs and symptoms of heart failure in infants and children are similar to those in adults. They include fatigue, effort intolerance, cough, anorexia, and abdominal pain. A subtle sign of cardiorespiratory distress in infants and children is a change in disposition or responsiveness, including irritability or lethargy. Sympathetic stimulation produces peripheral vasoconstriction and diaphoresis. Decreased renal blood flow often results in a urine output of less than 0.5 to 1 mL/kg/hour, despite adequate fluid intake.[44] When right ventricular function is impaired, systemic venous congestion develops. Hepatomegaly due to liver congestion often is one of the first signs of systemic venous congestion in infants and children. However, dependent edema or ascites rarely is seen unless the central venous pressure is extremely high. Because of their short, fat necks, jugular venous distention is difficult to detect in infants; it is not a reliable sign until the child is of school age or older.

Most commonly, children with heart failure develop interstitial edema rather than alveolar pulmonary edema. This reduces lung compliance and increases the work of breathing, causing tachypnea and increased respiratory effort. Older children display use of accessory muscles (*i.e.,* scapular and sternocleidomastoid). Head bobbing and nasal flaring may be observed in infants. Signs of respiratory distress often are the first and most noticeable indication of heart failure in infants and young children. Pulmonary congestion may be mistaken for bronchiolitis or lower respiratory tract infection. The infant or young child with respiratory distress often grunts with expiration. This grunting effort (essentially, exhaling against a closed glottis) is an instinctive effort to increase end-expiratory pressures and prevent collapse of small airways and the development of atelectasis. Respiratory crackles are uncommon in infants and usually suggest development of a respiratory tract infection. Wheezes may be heard, particularly if there is a large left-to-right shunt.

Infants with heart failure often have increased respiratory problems during feeding.[43,45] The history is one of prolonged feeding with excessive respiratory effort and fatigue. Weight gain is slow owing to high energy requirements and low calorie intake. Other frequent manifestations of heart failure in infants are excessive sweating (due to increased sympathetic tone), particularly over the head and neck, and repeated lower respiratory tract infections. Peripheral perfusion usually is poor, with cool extremities; tachycardia is common (resting heart rate >150 beats per minute); and respiratory rate is increased (resting rate >50 breaths per minute).[44]

Diagnosis and Treatment

Diagnosis of heart failure in infants and children is based on symptomatology, chest radiographic films, electrocardiographic findings, echocardiographic techniques to assess cardiac structures and ventricular function (*i.e.,* end-systolic and end-diastolic diameters), arterial blood gases to determine intracardiac shunting and ventilation–perfusion inequalities, and other laboratory studies to determine anemia and electrolyte imbalances.

Treatment of heart failure in infants and children includes measures aimed at improving cardiac function and eliminating excess intravascular fluid. Oxygen delivery must be supported and oxygen demands controlled or minimized. Whenever possible, the cause of the disorder is corrected (*e.g.,* medical treatment of sepsis and anemia, surgical correction of congenital heart defects). With congenital anomalies that are amenable to surgery, medical treatment often is needed for a time before surgery and usually is continued in the immediate postoperative period. For many children, only medical management can be provided.

Medical management of heart failure in infants and children is similar to that in the adult, although it is tailored to the special developmental needs of the child. Inotropic agents, such as digitalis, often are used to increase cardiac contractility. Diuretics may be given to reduce preload, and vasodilating drugs may be used to manipulate the afterload. Drug doses must be carefully tailored to control for the child's weight and conditions such as reduced renal function. Daily weighing and accurate measurement of intake and output are imperative during acute episodes of failure.

Most children feel better in the semiupright position. An infant seat is useful for infants with chronic heart failure. Activity restrictions usually are designed to allow children to be as active as possible within the limitations of their heart disease. Infants with heart failure often have problems feeding. Small, frequent feedings usually are more successful than larger, less frequent feedings. Severely ill infants may lack sufficient strength to suck and may need to be tube fed.

The treatment of heart failure in children should be designed to allow optimal physical and psychosocial development. It requires the full involvement of the parents, who often are the primary care providers; therefore, parent education and support are essential.

HEART FAILURE IN THE ELDERLY

Heart failure is one of the most common causes of disability in the elderly and is the most frequent hospital discharge diagnosis for the elderly. More than 75% of patients with heart failure are older than 65 years of age. Among the factors that have contributed to the increased numbers of older people with heart failure are the improved therapies for ischemic and hypertensive heart disease.[46] Thus, persons who would have died from acute myocardial disease 20 years ago are now surviving, but with residual left ventricular dysfunction. Similarly, improved blood pressure control has led to a 60% decline in stroke mortality rates, yet these same people remain at risk for heart failure as a complication of hypertension. Also, advances in treatment of other diseases have contributed indirectly to the rising prevalence of heart failure in the older population.

Coronary heart disease, hypertension, and valvular heart disease (particularly aortic stenosis and mitral regurgitation) are common causes of heart failure in older adults.[46,47] Although the pathophysiology of heart failure is similar in younger and older persons, elderly persons tend to develop cardiac failure when confronted with stresses that would not produce failure in younger persons. There are several changes associated with cardiovascular aging that tend to impair the ability to respond to stress.[46] First, reduced responsiveness to β-adrenergic stimulation limits the heart's capacity to maximally increase heart rate and contractility. Second, increased vascular stiffness results in an increased resistance to left ventricular ejection (afterload) and contributes to the development of systolic hypertension in the elderly. Third, in addition to increased vascular stiffness, the heart itself becomes stiffer and less compliant with age. The changes in diastolic stiffness result in important alterations in diastolic filling and atrial function. A reduction in ventricular filling not only affects cardiac output, but produces an elevation in diastolic pressure that is transmitted back to the left atrium, where it stretches the muscle wall and predisposes to atrial ectopic beats and atrial fibrillation.

Manifestations

The manifestations of heart failure in the elderly often are masked by other disease conditions.[47,48] Nocturia is an early symptom but may be caused by other conditions, such as prostatic hypertrophy. Dyspnea on exertion may result from lung disease, lack of exercise, and deconditioning. Lower extremity edema commonly is caused by venous insufficiency.

Among the acute manifestations of heart failure in the elderly are increasing lethargy and confusion, probably the result of impaired cerebral perfusion. Activity intolerance is common. Instead of dyspnea, the prominent sign may be restlessness. Impaired perfusion of the gastrointestinal tract is a common cause of anorexia and profound loss of lean body mass. Loss of lean body mass may be masked by edema.

The elderly also maintain a precarious balance between the managed symptom state and acute symptom exacerbation. During the managed symptom state, they are relatively symptom free while adhering to their treatment regimen. Acute symptom exacerbation, often requiring emergency medical treatment, can be precipitated by seemingly minor conditions such as poor compliance with sodium restriction, infection, or stress. Failure to seek medical care promptly is a common cause of progressive acceleration of symptoms.

Diagnosis and Treatment

The diagnosis of heart failure in the elderly is based on the history, physical examination, chest radiograph, and electrocardiographic findings.[47] However, the presenting symptoms of heart failure often are difficult to evaluate. Symptoms of dyspnea on exertion are often attributed to a sign of "getting older" or deconditioning from other diseases. Ankle edema is not unusual in the elderly because of decreased skin turgor, and the elderly tend to be more sedentary with the legs kept in a dependent position.

Treatment of heart failure in the elderly involves many of the same methods as in younger persons. Activities are restricted to a level that is commensurate with the cardiac reserve. Seldom is bed rest recommended or advised. Bed rest causes rapid deconditioning of skeletal muscles and increases the risk of complications, such as orthostatic hypotension and thromboemboli. Instead, carefully prescribed exercise programs can help to maintain activity tolerance. Even walking around a room usually is preferable to continuous bed rest. Sodium restriction usually is indicated.

Age- and disease-related changes increase the likelihood of adverse drug reactions and drug interactions. Drug dosages and the number of drugs that are prescribed should be kept to a minimum. Compliance with

drug regimens often is difficult; the simpler the regimen, the more likely it is that the older person will comply. In general, the treatment plan for elderly persons with heart failure must be put in the context of the person's overall needs. An improvement in the quality of life may take precedence over increasing the length of survival.

In summary, the mechanisms of heart failure in children and the elderly are similar to those in adults. However, the causes and manifestations may differ because of age. In children, heart failure is seen most commonly during infancy and immediately after heart surgery. It can be caused by congenital and acquired heart defects and is characterized by fatigue, effort intolerance, cough, anorexia, abdominal pain, and impaired growth. Treatment of heart failure in children includes correction of the underlying cause whenever possible. For congenital anomalies that are amenable to surgery, medical treatment often is needed for a time before surgery and usually is continued in the immediate postoperative period. For many children, only medical management can be provided.

In the elderly, age-related changes in cardiovascular functioning contribute to heart failure but are not in themselves sufficient to cause heart failure. The manifestations of heart failure often are different and superimposed on other disease conditions; therefore, heart failure often is more difficult to diagnose in the elderly than in younger persons. Because the elderly are more susceptible to adverse drug reactions and have more problems with compliance, the number of drugs that are prescribed is kept to a minimum, and the drug regimen is kept as simple as possible.

Review Exercises

A 75-year-old woman with long-standing hypertension and angina due to coronary heart disease presents with ankle edema, nocturia, increased shortness of breath with activity, and a chronic nonproductive cough. Her blood pressure is 170/80 mm Hg and her heart rate 92 beats per minute. Electrocardiographic and chest x-ray reports indicate the presence of left ventricular hypertrophy.

A. Relate the presence of uncontrolled hypertension and coronary artery disease to the development of heart failure in this woman.

B. Explain the significance of left ventricular hypertrophy as a compensatory mechanism and as a pathologic mechanism in the progression of heart failure

C. Use Figure 19-2 to explain this woman's symptoms, including shortness of breath and nonproductive cough.

A 26-year-old man is admitted to the emergency department with excessive blood loss after an automobile injury. He is alert and anxious, his skin is cool and moist, his heart rate is 135 beats per minute, and his blood pressure 100/85 mm Hg. He is receiving intravenous fluids, which were started at the scene of the accident by an emergency medical technician. He has been typed and cross-matched for blood transfusions, and a urinary catheter has been inserted to monitor his urine output. His urine output has been less than 10 mL since admission, and his blood pressure has dropped to 85/70 mm Hg. Efforts to control his bleeding have been unsuccessful, and he is being prepared for emergency surgery.

A. Use information regarding the compensatory mechanisms in circulatory shock to explain this man's presenting symptoms, including urine output.

B. Explain why a loss of up to 25% of blood volume can occur and a person can still have a blood pressure that is within a normal or near-normal range.

C. The treatment of hypovolemic shock is usually directed at maintaining the circulatory volume through fluid resuscitation rather than maintaining the blood pressure through the use of vasoactive medications. Explain.

Visit the Porth: Essentials of Pathophysiology: Concepts of Altered Health States web site (http://thePoint.LWW.com/PorthEssentials) for links to chapter-related resources on the Internet, all-new exclusive animations, chapter review questions, and more!

REFERENCES

1. American Heart Association. (2005). *Heart disease and stroke statistics—2005 update.* Dallas: Author.
2. Colucci W. C., Braunwald E. (2005). Pathophysiology of heart failure. In Zipes D. P., Libby P., Bonow R. O. (Eds.), *Braunwald's heart disease: A textbook of cardiovascular medicine* (7th ed., pp. 509–538). Philadelphia: Elsevier Saunders.
3. Jessup M., Brozena S. (2003). Heart failure. *New England Journal of Medicine* 348, 2007–2018.
4. Weber K. T. (2001). Aldosterone in congestive heart failure. *New England Journal of Medicine* 345, 1689–1697.
5. Levin E. R., Gardner D. G., Samson W. K. (1998). Natriuretic peptides. *New England Journal of Medicine* 339, 321–328.
6. Baughman K. L. (2002). B-type natriuretic peptide: A window to the heart. *New England Journal of Medicine* 347, 158–159.
7. Spieker L. E., Lüscher T. F. (2003). Will endothelin receptor antagonists have a role in heart failure? *Medical Clinics of North America* 87, 259–474.
8. Schoen F. J. (2005). The heart. In Kumar V., Abbas A. K., Fausto N. (Eds.), *Robbins and Cotran pathologic basis of disease* (7th ed., pp. 560–563). Philadelphia: Elsevier Saunders.
9. Angeja B. G., Grossman W. (2003). Evaluation and management of diastolic heart failure. *Circulation* 107, 659–663.
10. Tresch D. D., McGough M. F. (1995). Heart failure with normal systolic function: A common disorder in older people. *Journal of the American Geriatric Society* 49, 1035–1042.
11. Shamsham F., Mitchell J. (2000). Essentials of the diagnosis of heart failure. *American Family Physician* 61, 1319–1328.
12. Maisel A. S., Krishnaswamy P., Nowak R. M., et al. (2002). Rapid measurement of B-type natriuretic peptide in the emergency diagnosis of heart failure. *New England Journal of Medicine* 347, 161–167.
13. Hunt S. A. (Chair). (2001). ACC/AHA guidelines for the evaluation and management of chronic heart failure in the adult: Executive summary. *Circulation* 104, 2996–3007.
14. Vitarelli A., Gheorghiade M. (2000). Transthoracic and transesophageal echocardiogram in the hemodynamic assessment of patients with CHF. *American Journal of Cardiology* 86, 366–406.
15. Parker W. R., Anderson A. S. (2001). Slowing the progression of CHF. *Postgraduate Medicine* 109(3), 36–45.
16. Piña H. L. (Chair Writing Group). (2003). Exercise and heart failure: A statement from the American Heart Association Committee on Exercise, Rehabilitation, and Prevention. *Circulation* 107, 1210–1225.
17. Stanek, B. (2000). Optimizing management of patients with advanced heart failure: The importance of preventing progression. *Drugs and Aging* 16, 87–106.
18. Young J. B. (2001). New therapeutic choices in management of acute heart failure. *Reviews in Cardiovascular Medicine* 2(Suppl. 2), S19–S24.
19. Hollenberg S. M., Kavinsky C. J., Parrillo J. E. (1999). Cardiogenic shock. *Annals of Internal Medicine* 131, 47–59.
20. Bristow M. R., Lowes B. D. (2005). Management of heart failure. In Zipes D. P., Libby P., Bonow R. O. (Eds.), *Braunwald's heart disease: A textbook of cardiovascular medicine* (7th ed., pp. 603–624). Philadelphia: Elsevier Saunders.
21. Mussivand T. (1999). Mechanical circulatory devices for the treatment of heart failure. *Journal of Cardiac Surgery* 14, 218–228.
22. Hunt S. A., Kouretas P. C., Balsam L. G., et. al. (2005). Heart transplantation. In Zipes D. P., Libby P., Bonow R. O. (Eds.), *Braunwald's heart disease: A textbook of cardiovascular medicine* (7th ed., pp. 641–650). Philadelphia: Elsevier Saunders.
23. Guyton A. C., Hall J. E. (2006). *Textbook of medical physiology* (11th ed., pp. 270–281). Philadelphia: Elsevier Saunders.
24. Berne R. M., Levy M. N. (2000). *Principles of physiology* (3rd ed., pp. 437–443). St. Louis: Mosby.
25. Landry D. W., Oliver J. A. (2001). The pathogenesis of vasodilatory shock. *New England Journal of Medicine* 345, 588–595.
26. Bochner B. S., Lichtenstein L. M. (1991). Anaphylaxis. *New England Journal of Medicine* 324, 1785–1790.
27. Ellis A. K., Day J. H. (2003). Diagnosis and management of anaphylaxis. *Canadian Medical Association Journal* 169, 307–312.
28. Stankiewicz J., Ruta W., Gorski P. (1995). Latex allergy. *International Journal of Occupational Medicine and Environmental Health* 8, 139–148.

29. Parrillo J. E. (1995). Pathogenetic mechanisms of septic shock. *New England Journal of Medicine* 328, 1471–1477.
30. Sommers M. S. (2003). The cellular basis of septic shock. *Critical Care Nursing Clinics of North America* 15, 13–25.
31. Hotchkiss R. S., Karl I. E. (2003). The pathogenesis and treatment of sepsis. *New England Journal of Medicine* 348, 138–150.
32. Balk R. A. (2000). Severe sepsis and septic shock. *Critical Care Clinics* 16, 179–191.
33. Carcillo J. A., Cunnin R. E. (1997). Septic shock. *Critical Care Clinics* 13, 553–574.
34. Wheeler A. P., Bernard G. R. (1999). Treating patients with severe sepsis. *New England Journal of Medicine* 340, 207–214.
35. Ahrens T. (2003). Severe sepsis management: Are we doing enough? *Critical Care Nurse* (Suppl. 5), 2–15.
36. Matthay M. A. (2001). Severe sepsis: A new treatment with both anticoagulant and anti-inflammatory properties. *New England Journal of Medicine* 344, 759–762.
37. Smith J. J., Kampine J. P. (1980). *Circulatory physiology* (p. 298). Baltimore: Williams & Wilkins.
38. Fein A. M., Calalang-Colucci M. G. (2000). Acute lung injury and acute respiratory distress syndrome in sepsis and septic shock. *Critical Care Clinics* 4, 289–317.
39. Ware L. B., Mattay M. A. (2000). The acute respiratory distress syndrome. *New England Journal of Medicine* 342, 1334–1349.
40. Fink M. (1991). Gastrointestinal mucosal injury in experimental models of shock, trauma and sepsis. *Critical Care Medicine* 19, 627–641.
41. Levi M., Ten Cate H. T. (1999). Disseminated intravascular coagulation. *New England Journal of Medicine* 341, 586–592.
42. Balk R. A. (2000). Pathogenesis and management of multiple organ dysfunction or failure in acute sepsis and septic shock. *Critical Care Clinics* 16, 337–352.
43. Bernstein D. (2004). Heart failure. In Behrman R. E., Kliegman R. M., Jenson H. B. (Eds.), *Nelson textbook of pediatrics* (17th ed., pp. 1582–1587). Philadelphia: Elsevier Saunders.
44. Kay J. D., Colan S. D., Graham T. P. (2001). Congestive heart failure in pediatric patients. *American Heart Journal* 142, 923–928.
45. Hazinski F. H. (1992). *Nursing care of the critically ill child* (2nd ed., pp. 156–170). St. Louis: C. V. Mosby.
46. Rich M. W. (1997). Epidemiology, pathophysiology, and etiology of congestive heart failure in older adults. *Journal of the American Geriatrics Society* 45, 968–974.
47. Schwartz J. B., Zipes D. P. (2005). Cardiovascular disease in the elderly. In Zipes D. P., Libby P., Bonow R. O. (Eds.), *Braunwald's heart disease: A textbook of cardiovascular medicine* (7th ed., pp. 1925–1950). Philadelphia: Elsevier Saunders.
48. Abdelhafiz A. H. (2002). Heart failure in older people: Causes, diagnosis, and treatment. *Age and Aging* 31, 29–36.

UNIT VI
Respiratory Function

Chapter *20*

Control of Respiratory Function

The respiratory system supplies the body with oxygen and rids the body of carbon dioxide. Respiration can be divided into three parts: ventilation, or the movement of air between the atmosphere and the respiratory portion of the lungs; perfusion, or the flow of blood through the lungs; and diffusion, or the transfer of gases between the air-filled spaces in the lungs and the blood. The nervous system controls the movement of the respiratory muscles and adjusts the rate of breathing so that it matches the needs of the body during various levels of activity. The content in this chapter focuses on the structure and function of the respiratory system as it relates to these aspects of respiration. The function of the red blood cell in the transport of oxygen is discussed in Chapter 11.

 Structural Organization of the Respiratory System

The respiratory system consists of the air passages and the lungs. Functionally, the respiratory system can be divided into two parts: the *conducting airways,* through which air moves as it passes between the atmosphere and the lungs, and the *respiratory tissues* of the lungs, where gas exchange takes place. The process of moving air into and out of the lungs is referred to as *ventilation* and the process of gas exchange as *diffusion.*

THE CONDUCTING AIRWAYS

The conducting airways consist of the nasal passages, mouth and pharynx, larynx, trachea, bronchi, and bronchioles (Fig. 20-1). The air we breathe is warmed, filtered,

poorly differentiated basal cells (that possibly serve as stem cells for replacement of other cell types). In addition, some less common cell types are interspersed in different parts of the airways. The epithelial layer gradually becomes thinner as it moves from the pseudostratified epithelium of the bronchi to cuboidal epithelium of the bronchioles and then to squamous epithelium of the alveoli.

The mucus produced by the epithelial cells in the conducting airways forms a layer called the *mucociliary blanket* that protects the respiratory system by entrapping dust, bacteria, and other foreign particles that enter the airways. The cilia, which constantly are in motion, move the mucociliary blanket with its entrapped particles in an escalator-like fashion toward the oropharynx, from which it is expectorated or swallowed. The function of cilia in clearing the lower airways and alveoli is optimal at normal oxygen levels and is impaired in situations of low and high oxygen levels. It is also impaired by drying conditions, such as breathing heated but unhumidified indoor air during the winter months. Cigarette smoking slows down or paralyzes the motility of the cilia. This slowing allows the residue from tobacco smoke, dust, and other particles to accumulate in the lungs, decreasing the efficiency of this pulmonary defense system. As discussed in Chapter 22, these changes are thought to contribute to the development of chronic bronchitis and emphysema.

The air in the conducting airways is kept moist by water contained in the mucous layer. Moisture is added to the air as it moves through the conducting airways. (As water mixes with air, it is called *water vapor*.) The capacity of the air to contain water vapor without condensation increases as the temperature rises. Thus, the air in the alveoli, which is maintained at body temperature, usually contains considerably more water vapor than the atmospheric-temperature air that we breathe. The difference between the water vapor contained in the

and moistened as it moves through these structures. Heat is transferred to the air from the blood flowing through the walls of the respiratory passages; the mucociliary blanket removes foreign materials; and water from the mucous membranes is used to moisten the air.

The wall of conducting airways consists of three major components: a mucosal lining that is composed of epithelial and connective tissue, an underlying smooth muscle layer, and a supporting connective tissue layer (Fig. 20-2). The pseudostratified epithelial lining of the airways contains a mosaic of mucus-secreting gland cells, ciliated cells with hairlike projection, serous glands that secrete a watery fluid containing antibacterial enzymes, and the

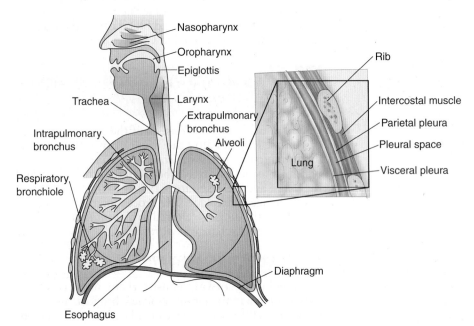

FIGURE 20-1 Structures of the respiratory system. The structures of the pleura are shown in the inset.

BRONCHUS   BRONCHIOLE   ALVEOLUS

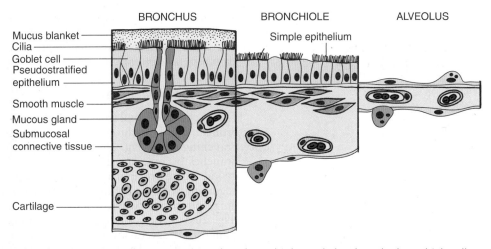

Mucus blanket
Cilia
Goblet cell
Pseudostratified epithelium
Smooth muscle
Mucous gland
Submucosal connective tissue
Cartilage

Simple epithelium

FIGURE 20-2 Airway wall structure: bronchus, bronchiole, and alveolus. The bronchial wall contains pseudostratified epithelium, smooth muscle cells, mucous glands, connective tissue, and cartilage. In smaller bronchioles, a simple epithelium is found, cartilage is absent, and the wall is thinner. The alveolar wall is designed for gas exchange, rather than structural support. (From Weibel E. R., Taylor R. C. [1988]. Design and structure of the human lung. In Fishman A. P. [ed.]. *Pulmonary diseases and disorders* [Vol. 1., p. 14]. New York: McGraw-Hill. Reproduced with permission of the McGraw-Hill Companies.)

air we breathe and that found in the alveoli is drawn from the moist surface of the mucous membranes that line the conducting airways and is a source of insensible water loss (see Chapter 6). Under normal conditions, approximately 1 pint of water is used each day to humidify the air we breathe. During fever, the water vapor in the lungs increases, causing more water to be lost through the respiratory tract. In addition, fever usually is accompanied by an increase in respiratory rate so that more air passes through the airways, withdrawing moisture from its mucosal surface. As a result, respiratory secretions thicken, preventing free movement of the cilia and impairing the protective function of the mucociliary defense system. This is particularly true in persons whose water intake is inadequate.

Nasopharyngeal Airways

The nose is the preferred route for the entrance of air into the respiratory tract during normal breathing. As air passes through the nasal passages, it is filtered, warmed, and humidified. The outer nasal passages are lined with coarse hairs, which filter and trap dust and other large particles from the air. The upper portion of the nasal cavity is lined with a mucous membrane that contains a rich network of small blood vessels; this portion of the nasal cavity supplies warmth and moisture to the air we breathe.

The mouth serves as an alternative airway when the nasal passages are plugged or when there is a need for the exchange of large amounts of air, as occurs during exercise. The oropharynx extends posteriorly from the soft palate to the epiglottis. The oropharynx is the only opening between the nose and mouth and the lungs. Both swallowed food on its way to the esophagus and air on its way to the larynx pass through it. Obstruction of the oropharynx leads to immediate cessation of ventilation. Neural control of the tongue and pharyngeal muscles may be impaired in coma and certain types of neurologic disease. In these conditions, the tongue falls back into the pharynx and obstructs the airway, particularly if the person is lying on his or her back. Swelling of the pharyngeal structures caused by injury, infection, or severe allergic reaction also predisposes a person to airway obstruction, as does the presence of a foreign body.

Laryngotracheal Airways

The larynx connects the oropharynx with the trachea. The walls of the larynx are supported by rigid cartilaginous structures that prevent collapse during inspiration. The functions of the larynx can be divided into two categories: those associated with speech and those associated with protecting the lungs from substances other than air. The larynx is located in a strategic position between the upper airways and the lungs and sometimes is referred to as the "watchdog of the lungs."

The cavity of the larynx is divided into two pairs of two-by-two folds of mucous membrane stretching from front to back with an opening in the midline (Fig. 20-3). The upper pair of folds, called the *vestibular folds*, has a protective function. The lower pair of folds has cord-like margins; they are termed the *vocal folds* because their vibrations are required for making vocal sounds. The true vocal folds and the elongated opening between them is called the *glottis*. A complex set of muscles controls the opening and closing of the glottis. Speech involves the intermittent release of expired air and opening and closing of the glottis. The epiglottis, which is located above the vocal folds, is a large, leaf-shaped piece of cartilage that is covered with epithelium. During swallowing, the free

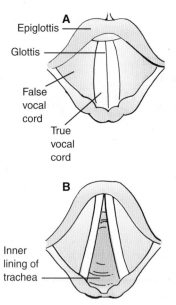

FIGURE 20-3 Epiglottis and vocal cords viewed from above with (**A**) glottis closed and (**B**) glottis open.

edges of the epiglottis move downward to cover the larynx, thus routing liquids and foods into the esophagus.

In addition to opening and closing the glottis for speech, the vocal folds of the larynx can perform a sphincter function in closing off the airways. When confronted with substances other than air, the laryngeal muscles contract and close off the airway. At the same time, the cough reflex is initiated as a means of removing a foreign substance from the airway. If the swallowing mechanism is partially or totally paralyzed, food and fluids can enter the airways instead of the esophagus when a

person attempts to swallow. These substances are not easily removed; and when they are pulled into the lungs, they can cause a serious inflammatory condition called *aspiration pneumonia.*

Tracheobronchial Tree

The tracheobronchial tree, which consists of the trachea, bronchi, and bronchioles, can be viewed as a system of branching tubes (Fig. 20-4). It is similar to a tree whose branches become smaller and more numerous as they divide. There are approximately 23 levels of branching, beginning with the conducting airways and ending with the respiratory airways, where gas exchange takes place (Fig. 20-5). The walls of the tracheobronchial tree are composed of several layers: an inner mucosal layer, a submucosal layer, and an outer adventitial layer. These layers vary at different levels of the tracheobronchial tree.

The trachea, or windpipe, is a continuous tube that connects the larynx and the major bronchi of the lungs (see Fig. 20-4). The walls of the trachea are supported by horseshoe- or C-shaped rings of hyaline cartilage, which prevent it from collapsing when the pressure in the thorax becomes negative. The open part of the C-shaped ring, which abuts the esophagus, is connected by smooth muscle. Since this portion of the trachea is not rigid, the esophagus can expand anteriorly as swallowed food passes through it.

The trachea divides into two branches, forming the right and left main or primary bronchi. Between the main bronchi is a keel-like ridge called the *carina.* The mucosa of the carina is highly sensitive; violent coughing is initiated when a foreign object (*e.g.,* suction catheter) makes contact with it. The structure of the primary bronchi is similar to that of the trachea in that these airways are lined with a mucosal surface and supported by cartilagi-

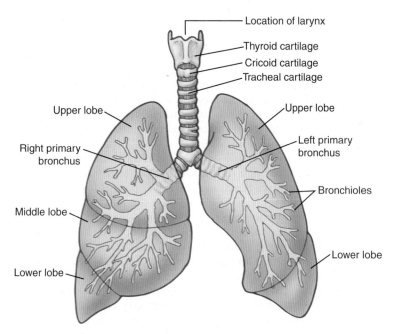

FIGURE 20-4 Larynx, trachea, and bronchial tree (anterior view).

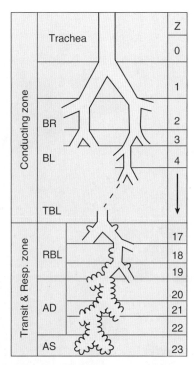

FIGURE 20-5 Idealization of the human airways. The first 16 generations of branching (Z) make up the conducting airways, and the last seven constitute the respiratory zone (or transitional and respiratory zone). BR, bronchus; BL, bronchiole; TBL, terminal bronchiole; RBL, respiratory bronchiole; AD, alveolar ducts; AS, alveolar sacs. (From Weibel E. R. [1962]. *Morphometry of the human lung* [p. 111]. Berlin: Springer-Verlag.)

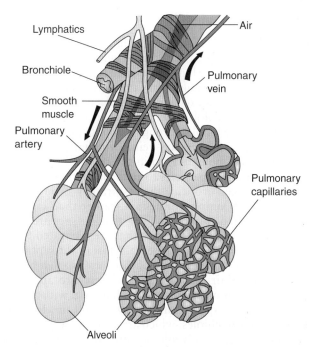

FIGURE 20-6 Lobule of the lung, showing the bronchial smooth muscle fibers, pulmonary blood vessels, and lymphatics.

nous rings. Each primary bronchus, accompanied by the pulmonary arteries, veins, and lymph vessels, enters the lung through a slit called the *hilus*.

Each primary bronchus divides into secondary or lobular bronchi that supply each of the lobes of the lung—three in the right lung and two in the left. The right middle lobe bronchus is of relatively small diameter and length and sometimes bends sharply near its bifurcation. It is surrounded by a collar of lymph nodes that drain the middle and the lower lobe and is particularly subject to obstruction. The secondary bronchi, in turn, divide to form the segmental bronchi, which supply the bronchopulmonary segments of the lung. These segments are identified according to their location in the lung (*e.g.*, the apical segment of the right upper lobe) and are the smallest named units in the lung. Lung lesions such as atelectasis and pneumonia often are localized to a particular bronchopulmonary segment. The structure of the secondary and segmental bronchi is similar to that of the primary bronchi, except the cartilage "C"-shaped rings are replaced by irregular plates of hyaline cartilage that completely surround the lumina of the bronchi and there are two layers of smooth muscle spiraling in opposite direction (Fig. 20-6).

The segmental bronchi continue to branch, forming smaller bronchi, until they become the terminal bronchioles, the smallest of the conducting airways. As these

bronchi branch and become smaller, their wall structure changes. The cartilage gradually decreases and there is an increase in smooth muscle and elastic tissue (with respect to the thickness of the wall). By the time the bronchioles are reached, there is no cartilage present and their walls are composed mainly of smooth muscle and elastic fibers. Bronchospasm, or contraction of these muscles, causes narrowing of the bronchioles and impairs air flow. The elastic fibers, which radiate from the adventitia of the bronchial wall and connect with elastic fibers arising from other parts of the bronchial tree, exert tension on the bronchial walls; by pulling uniformly in all directions, they help maintain airway patency.

THE LUNGS AND RESPIRATORY AIRWAYS

The lungs are soft, spongy, cone-shaped organs located side by side in the chest cavity (see Fig. 20-1). They are separated from each other by the *mediastinum* (*i.e.*, the space between the lungs) and its contents—the heart, blood vessels, lymph nodes, nerve fibers, thymus gland, and esophagus. The upper part of the lung, which lies against the top of the thoracic cavity, is called the *apex*, and the lower part, which lies against the diaphragm, is called the *base*. The lungs are divided into lobes: three in the right lung and two in the left (see Fig. 20-4).

The lungs are the functional structures of the respiratory system. In addition to their gas exchange function, they inactivate vasoactive substances such as bradykinin; they convert angiotensin I to angiotensin II; and they serve as a reservoir for blood storage. Heparin-producing cells are particularly abundant in the capillaries of the lung, where small clots may be trapped.

Respiratory Lobules

The gas exchange function of the lung takes place in the lobules of the lungs. Each lobule, which is the smallest functional unit of the lung, is supplied by a terminal bronchiole, an arteriole, pulmonary capillaries, and a venule (see Fig. 20-6). Gas exchange takes place in the terminal respiratory bronchioles and the alveolar ducts and sacs. Blood enters the lobules through a pulmonary artery and exits through a pulmonary vein. Lymphatic structures surround the lobule and aid in the removal of plasma proteins and other particles from the interstitial spaces.

Unlike larger bronchi, the respiratory bronchioles are lined with simple epithelium, rather than ciliated pseudostratified epithelium. The alveolar sacs are cup-shaped, thin-walled structures that are separated from each other by thin alveolar septa. Most of the septa are occupied by a single network of capillaries so that blood is exposed to air on both sides. There are approximately 300 million alveoli in the adult lung, with a total surface area of approximately 50 to 100 m². In contrast to the bronchioles, which are tubes with their own separate walls, the alveoli are interconnecting spaces that have no separate walls (Fig. 20-7). As a result of this arrangement, there is a continual mixing of air in the alveolar structures.

The alveolar structures are composed of two types of cells: type I alveolar cells and type II alveolar cells (Fig. 20-8). The type I alveolar cells are flat squamous epithelial cells across which gas exchange takes place. The type II alveolar cells produce surfactant, a lipoprotein substance that decreases the surface tension in the alveoli. The alveoli also contain alveolar macrophages, which are responsible for the removal of offending substances from the alveolar epithelium.

Lung Circulation

The lungs are provided with a dual blood supply: the pulmonary and bronchial circulations. The pulmonary circulation arises from the pulmonary artery and provides for the gas exchange function of the lungs. Deoxygenated blood leaves the right heart through the pulmonary artery, which divides into a left pulmonary artery that enters the left lung and a right pulmonary artery that enters the right lung. Return of oxygenated blood to the heart occurs by way of the pulmonary veins, which empty into the left atrium. This is the only part of the circulation where arteries carry unoxygenated blood and veins carry oxygenated blood.

The bronchial circulation distributes blood to the conducting airways and supporting structures of the lung. The bronchial circulation has a secondary function of warming and humidifying incoming air as it moves through the conducting airways. The bronchial arteries arise from the thoracic aorta and enter the lungs with the major bronchi, dividing and subdividing along with the bronchi as they move out into the lung, supplying them and other lung structures with oxygen. The blood from the capillaries in the bronchial circulation drains into the

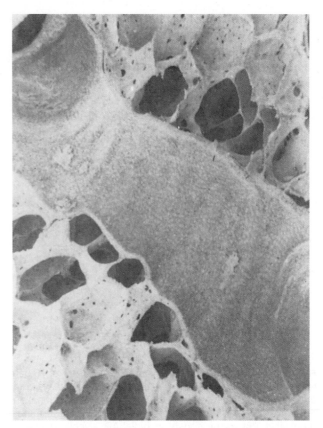

FIGURE 20-7 Close-up of a cross section of a small bronchus and surrounding alveoli. (Courtesy of Janice A. Nowell, University of California, Santa Cruz.)

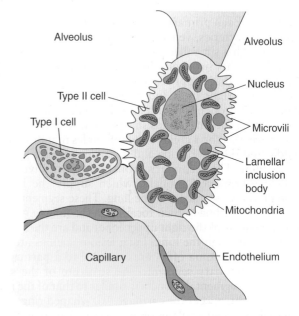

FIGURE 20-8 Schematic drawing of the two types of alveolar cells and their relation to alveoli and capillaries. Alveoli type I cells comprise most of the alveolar surface. Alveolar type II cells are located in the corner between two adjacent alveoli. Also shown are endothelial cells that line the pulmonary capillaries. (From Rhoades R.A., Tanner G.A. [2003]. *Medical physiology* [2nd ed., p. 329]. Philadelphia: Lippincott Williams & Wilkins.)

bronchial veins, with blood from the larger bronchial veins emptying into the vena cava. The blood from the smaller bronchial veins empties into the pulmonary veins. Because the bronchial circulation does not participate in gas exchange, this blood is unoxygenated. As a result, it dilutes the oxygenated blood returning to the left side of the heart by way of the pulmonary veins.

The bronchial blood vessels are the only ones that undergo angiogenesis (formation of new vessels) and develop collateral circulation when vessels in the pulmonary circulation are obstructed, as in pulmonary embolism. The development of new blood vessels helps to keep lung tissue alive until the pulmonary circulation can be restored.

PLEURA

A thin, transparent, double-layered serous membrane, called the *pleura*, lines the thoracic cavity and encases the lungs. The outer parietal layer lies adjacent to the chest wall, and the inner visceral layer adheres to the outer surface of the lung (see Fig. 20-1). The parietal pleura lines the pulmonary cavities and adheres to the thoracic wall, the mediastinum, and the diaphragm. The visceral pleura closely covers the lung and is adherent to all its surfaces. It is continuous with the parietal pleura at the hilum of the lung, where the major bronchus and pulmonary vessels enter and leave the lung. A thin film of serous fluid separates the two pleural layers, allowing the two layers to glide over each other and yet hold together, so there is no separation between the lungs and the chest wall. The pleural cavity is a potential space in which serous fluid or inflammatory exudate can accumulate. The term *pleural effusion* is used to describe an abnormal collection of fluid or exudate in the pleural cavity.

In summary, the respiratory system consists of the air passages and the lungs, where gas exchange takes place. Functionally and structurally, the air passages of the respiratory system can be divided into two parts: the conducting airways, through which air moves as it passes into and out of the lungs, and the respiratory tissues, where gas exchange actually takes place. The conducting airways include the nasal passages, mouth and nasopharynx, larynx, and tracheobronchial tree. Air is warmed, filtered, and humidified as it passes through these structures.

The lungs are the functional structures of the respiratory system. In addition to their gas exchange function, they inactivate vasoactive substances such as bradykinin; they convert angiotensin I to angiotensin II; and they serve as a reservoir for blood. The lobules, which are the functional units of the lung, consist of the respiratory bronchioles, alveoli, and pulmonary capillaries. It is here that gas exchange takes place. Oxygen from the alveoli diffuses across the alveolar-capillary membrane into the blood, and carbon dioxide from the blood diffuses into the alveoli.

The lungs are provided with a dual blood supply: the pulmonary circulation provides for the gas exchange function of the lungs, and the bronchial circulation distributes blood to the conducting airways and supporting structures of the lung. The lungs are encased in a thin, transparent, double-layered serous membrane called the *pleura*.

Exchange of Gases Between the Atmosphere and the Lungs

BASIC PROPERTIES OF GASES

The air we breathe is made up of a mixture of gases, mainly nitrogen and oxygen. These gases exert a combined pressure called the *atmospheric pressure*. The pressure at sea level is defined as 1 atmosphere, which is equal to 760 millimeters of mercury (mm Hg) or 14.7 pounds per square inch (PSI). When measuring respiratory pressures, atmospheric pressure is assigned a value of 0. This means that a respiratory pressure of +15 mm Hg is 15 mm Hg above atmospheric pressure, and a respiratory pressure of −15 mm Hg is 15 mm Hg less than atmospheric pressure. Respiratory pressures often are expressed in centimeters of water (cm H_2O) because of the small pressures involved (1 mm Hg = 1.35 cm H_2O pressure).

The pressure exerted by a single gas in a mixture is called the *partial pressure*. The capital letter "P" followed by the chemical symbol of the gas (*e.g.*, PO_2) is used to denote its partial pressure. The law of partial pressures states that the total pressure of a mixture of gases, as in the atmosphere, is equal to the sum of the partial pressures of the different gases in the mixture. If the concentration of oxygen at 760 mm Hg (1 atmosphere) is 20%, its partial pressure is 152 mm Hg (760 × 0.20).

Water vapor is different from other types of gases; its partial pressure is affected by temperature but not atmospheric pressure. The relative humidity refers to the percentage of moisture in the air compared with the amount that the air can hold without causing condensation (100% saturation). Warm air holds more moisture than cold air. This is the reason that precipitation in the form of rain or snow commonly occurs when the relative humidity is high and there is a sudden drop in atmospheric temperature. The air in the alveoli, which is 100% saturated at normal body temperature, has a water vapor pressure of 47 mm Hg. The water vapor pressure must be included in the sum of the total pressure of the gases in the alveoli (*i.e.*, the total pressure of the other gases in the alveoli is 760 − 47 = 713 mm Hg).

Air moves between the atmosphere and the lungs because of a pressure difference. According to the laws of physics, the pressure of a gas varies inversely with the volume of its container, provided the temperature remains constant. If equal amounts of a gas are placed in two different-size containers, the pressure of the gas in the smaller container will be greater than the pressure in the larger container. The movement of gases is always from the container with the greater pressure to the one with the lesser pressure. The chest cavity can be viewed as a volume container. During inspiration, the size of the chest cavity increases and air moves into the lungs; during expiration, air moves out as the size of the chest cavity decreases.

VENTILATION AND THE MECHANICS OF BREATHING

Ventilation is concerned with the movement of gases into and out of the lungs. It relies on a system of open airways and the respiratory pressures created as the movements of the respiratory muscles change the size of the chest cage. The degree to which the lungs inflate and deflate depends on the respiratory pressures inflating the lung, compliance of the lungs, and airway resistance.

Respiratory Pressures

The pressure inside the airways and alveoli of the lungs is called the *intrapulmonary pressure* or *alveolar pressure*. The gases in this area of the lungs are in communication with atmospheric pressure (Fig. 20-9). When the glottis is open and air is not moving into or out of the lungs, as occurs just before inspiration or expiration, the intrapulmonary pressure is zero or equal to atmospheric pressure.

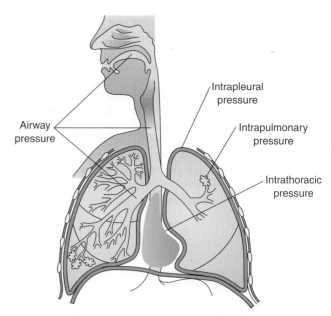

FIGURE 20-9 Partitioning of respiratory pressures.

The pressure in the pleural cavity is called the *intrapleural pressure*. The intrapleural pressure is always negative in relation to alveolar pressure in the normally inflated lung, approximately −4 mm Hg between breaths when the glottis is open and the alveolar spaces are open to the atmosphere. The lungs and the chest wall have elastic properties, each pulling in the opposite direction. If removed from the chest, the lungs would contract to a smaller size, and the chest wall, if freed from the lungs, would expand. The opposing forces of the chest wall and lungs create a pull against the visceral and parietal layers of the pleura, causing the pressure in the pleural cavity to become negative. During inspiration, the elastic recoil of the lungs increases, causing intrapleural pressure to become more negative than during expiration. Without the negative intrapleural pressure holding the lungs against the chest wall, their elastic recoil properties would cause them to collapse. Although the intrapleural pressure of the inflated lung is always negative in relation to alveolar pressure, it may become positive in relation to atmospheric pressure (*e.g.*, during forced expiration and coughing).

The *intrathoracic pressure* is the pressure in the thoracic cavity. It is essentially equal to intrapleural pressure and is the pressure to which the lungs, heart, and great vessels are exposed. Forced expiration against a closed glottis (Valsalva maneuver) compresses the air in the thoracic cavity and produces marked increases in intrathoracic and intrapleural pressures.

The Chest Cage and Respiratory Muscles

The lungs and major airways share the chest cavity with the heart, great vessels, and esophagus. The chest cavity is a closed compartment bounded on the top by the neck muscles and at the bottom by the diaphragm. The outer

KEY CONCEPTS

Ventilation and Gas Exchange

➤ Ventilation refers to the movement of gases into and out of the lungs through a system of open airways and along a pressure gradient resulting from a change in chest volume.

➤ During inspiration, air is drawn into the lungs as the respiratory muscles expand the chest cavity; during expiration, air moves out of the lungs as the chest muscles recoil and the chest cavity becomes smaller.

➤ The ease with which air is moved into and out of the lung depends on the resistance of the airways, which is inversely related to the fourth power of the airway radius, and lung compliance, or the ease with which the lungs can be inflated.

➤ The minute volume, which is determined by the metabolic needs of the body, is the amount of air that is exchanged each minute. It is the product of the tidal volume or amount of air that is exchanged with each breath multiplied by the respiratory rate.

walls of the chest cavity are formed by 12 pairs of ribs, the sternum, the thoracic vertebrae, and the intercostal muscles that lie between the ribs. Mechanically, ventilation or the act of breathing depends on the fact that the chest cavity is a closed compartment whose only opening to the exterior is the trachea.

Ventilation consists of inspiration and expiration. During *inspiration*, the size of the chest cavity increases, the intrathoracic pressure becomes more negative, and air is drawn into the lungs. *Expiration* occurs as the elastic components of the chest wall and lung structures that were stretched during inspiration recoil, causing the size of the chest cavity to decrease and the pressure in the chest cavity to increase (Fig. 20-10).

The diaphragm is the principal muscle of inspiration. When the diaphragm contracts, the abdominal contents are forced downward and the chest expands from top to bottom (see Fig. 20-10). During normal levels of inspiration, the diaphragm moves approximately 1 cm, but this can be increased to 10 cm on forced inspiration. The diaphragm is innervated by the phrenic nerve roots, which arise from the cervical level of the spinal cord, mainly from C4 but also from C3 and C5. Paralysis of one side of the diaphragm causes the chest to move up on that side rather than down during inspiration because of the negative pressure in the chest. This is called *paradoxical movement*.

The external intercostal muscles, which also aid in inspiration, connect to the adjacent ribs and slope downward and forward (Fig. 20-11). When they contract, they raise the ribs and rotate them slightly so that the sternum is pushed forward; this enlarges the chest from side to side and from front to back. The intercostal muscles receive their innervation from nerves that exit the central nervous system at the thoracic level of the spinal cord. Paralysis of these muscles usually does not have a serious effect on respiration because of the effectiveness of the diaphragm.

The accessory muscles of inspiration include the scalene muscles and the sternocleidomastoid muscles. The scalene muscles elevate the first two ribs, and the sternocleidomastoid muscles raise the sternum to increase the size of the chest cavity. These muscles contribute little to quiet breathing but contract vigorously during exercise. For the accessory muscles to assist in ventilation, they must be stabilized in some way. For example, persons with bronchial asthma often brace their arms against a firm object during an attack as a means of stabilizing their shoulders so that the attached accessory muscles can exert their full effect on ventilation. The head commonly is bent backward so that the scalene and sternocleidomastoid muscles can elevate the ribs more effectively. Other muscles that play a minor role in inspiration are the alae nasi, which produce flaring of the nostrils during obstructed breathing.

Expiration is largely passive. It occurs as the elastic components of the chest wall and lung structures that were stretched during inspiration recoil, causing air to leave the lungs as the intrathoracic pressure increases. When needed, the abdominal and the internal intercostal muscles can be used to increase expiratory effort (see Fig. 20-11). The increase in intra-abdominal pressure that accompanies the forceful contraction of the abdominal muscles pushes the diaphragm upward and results in an increase in intrathoracic pressure. The internal intercostal muscles move inward, which pulls the chest downward, increasing expiratory effort.

Lung Compliance

Lung compliance refers to the ease with which the lungs can be inflated. Compliance can be appreciated by comparing the ease of blowing up a new balloon that is stiff and noncompliant with one that has been previously blown up and stretched. Specifically, lung compliance is a measure of the change in lung volume that occurs with a change in intrapulmonary pressure. The normal compliance of both lungs in the average adult is approximately 200 mL/cm H_2O. This means that every time the intrapulmonary pressure increases by 1 cm/H_2O, the lung volume expands by 200 mL. It would take more pressure to move the same amount of air into a noncompliant lung.

Lung compliance is determined by the elastin and collagen fibers of the lung, its water content, and surface

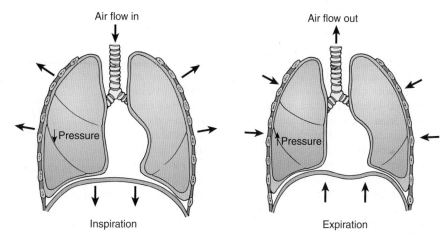

FIGURE 20-10 Movement of the diaphragm and changes in chest volume and pressure during inspiration and expiration. During inspiration, contraction of the diaphragm and expansion of the chest cavity produce a decrease in intrathoracic pressure, causing air to move into the lungs. During expiration, relaxation of the diaphragm and chest cavity produces an increase in intrathoracic pressure, causing air to move out of the lungs.

Air flow in

Air flow out

↓Pressure

Pressure

Inspiration

Expiration

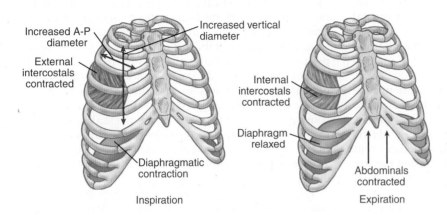

FIGURE 20-11 Expansion and contraction of the chest cage during expiration and inspiration, demonstrating especially diaphragmatic contraction, elevation of the rib cage, and function of the external and internal intercostals.

tension. It also depends on the compliance of the thoracic cage. It is diminished by conditions that reduce the natural elasticity of the lung; block the bronchi or smaller airways; increase the surface tension of the fluid film in the alveoli, or impair the flexibility of the thoracic cage.

Changes in Elastin/Collagen Composition of Lung Tissue. Lung tissue is made up of elastin and collagen fibers. The elastin fibers are easily stretched and increase the ease of lung inflation, whereas the collagen fibers resist stretching and make lung inflation more difficult. In lung diseases such as interstitial lung disease and pulmonary fibrosis, the lungs become stiff and noncompliant as the elastin fibers are replaced with scar tissue. Pulmonary congestion and edema produce a reversible decrease in pulmonary compliance.

Elastic recoil describes the ability of the elastic components of the lung to recoil to their original position after having been stretched. Overstretching of the elastic components, as occurs with emphysema, causes the elastic components of the lung to lose their recoil, making the lung easier to inflate but more difficult to deflate because of its inability to recoil.

Surface Tension. An important factor in lung compliance is the *surface tension* in the alveoli. The alveoli are lined with a thin film of liquid, and it is at the interface between this liquid film and the alveolar air that surface tension develops. This is because the forces that hold the liquid film molecules together are stronger than those that hold the air molecules together. In the alveoli, excess surface tension causes the liquid film to contract, making lung inflation more difficult.

The pressure in the alveoli (which are modeled as spheres with open airways projecting from them) can be predicted using Laplace law (pressure = 2 × surface tension/radius). If the surface tension were equal throughout the lungs, the alveoli with the smallest radii would have the greatest pressure, and this would cause them to empty into the larger alveoli (Fig. 20-12). This does not occur because special surface tension–lowering molecules, called *surfactant,* line the inner surface of the alveoli.

Surfactant is a complex mixture of lipoproteins (largely phospholipids) and small amounts of carbohydrates that is synthesized in type II alveolar cells. The surfactant molecule has two ends: a hydrophobic (water-insoluble) tail and a hydrophilic (water-soluble) head (Fig. 20-13). The hydrophilic head of the surfactant molecule attaches to the liquid molecules and the hydrophobic tail to the gas molecules, interrupting the intermolecular forces that are responsible for creating the surface tension.

Surfactant exerts four important effects on lung inflation: (1) it lowers the surface tension; (2) it increases lung compliance and ease of inflation; (3) it provides for stability and more even inflation of the alveoli; and (4) it assists in preventing pulmonary edema by keeping the alveoli dry. Without surfactant, lung inflation would be extremely difficult, requiring an intrapleural pressure of –20 to –30 mm Hg, compared with the –3 to –5 mm Hg pressure that normally is needed. The surfactant molecules are more densely packed in the small alveoli than in larger alveoli, where the density of the molecules is less. Therefore, surfactant reduces the surface tension more effectively in the small alveoli, which have the greatest tendency to collapse, providing for stability and more even distribution of ventilation. Surfactant also helps to keep the alveoli dry and prevent pulmonary edema. This is because water is pulled out of the pulmonary capillaries

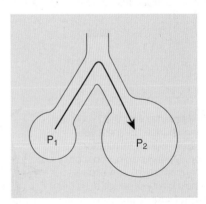

FIGURE 20-12 Law of Laplace (P = 2T/r; P = pressure, T = tension, r = radius). The effect of the radius on the pressure and movement of gases in the alveolar structures is depicted. Air moves from P_1 with a small radius and higher pressure to P_2 with its larger radius and lower pressure.

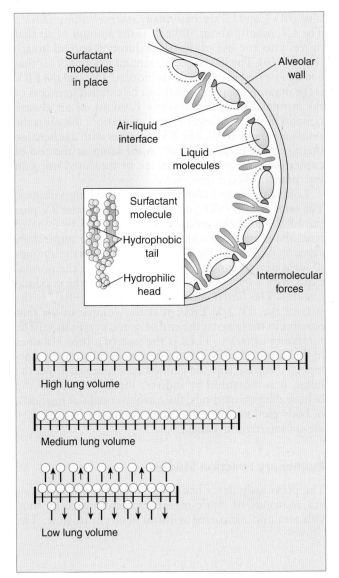

Airway Resistance

The volume of air that moves into and out of the air exchange portion of the lungs is directly related to the pressure difference between the lungs and the atmosphere and inversely related to the resistance that the air encounters as it moves through the airways. The effects of airway resistance on airflow can be illustrated using *Poiseuille law*. According to Poiseuille law, the resistance to flow is inversely related to the fourth power of the radius ($R = 1/r^4$). If the radius is reduced by one half, the resistance increases 16-fold ($2 \times 2 \times 2 \times 2 = 16$). Because the resistance of the airways is inversely proportional to the fourth power of the radius, small changes in airway caliber, such as those caused by pulmonary secretions or bronchospasm, can produce a marked increase in airway resistance.

Airway resistance is also affected by lung volumes, being less during inspiration than during expiration. This is because elastic-type fibers connect the outside of the airways to the surrounding lung tissues. As a result, these airways are pulled open as the lungs expand during inspiration, and they become narrower as the lungs deflate during expiration (Fig. 20-14). This is one of the reasons that persons with conditions that increase airway resistance, such as bronchial asthma, usually have less difficulty during inspiration than during expiration.

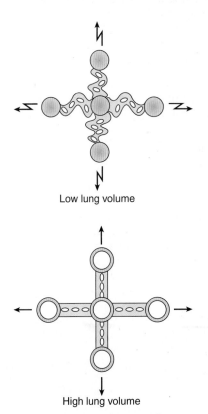

Low lung volume

High lung volume

FIGURE 20-14 Interaction of tissue forces on airways during low and high lung volumes. At low lung volumes, the tissue forces promote folding or collapsing and place less tension on the airways, which become smaller; during high lung volumes, the tissue forces stretch and pull the airways open.

FIGURE 20-13 (**Top**) Alveolar wall depicting surface tension resulting from the intramolecular forces in the air–liquid film interface; the surfactant molecule with its hydrophobic tail and hydrophilic head; and its function in reducing surface tension by disrupting the intermolecular forces. (**Bottom**) The concentration of surfactant molecules at high, medium, and low lung volumes.

into the alveoli when increased surface tension causes the alveoli to contract.

The type II alveolar cells that produce surfactant do not begin to mature until the 26th to 28th week of gestation; consequently, many premature infants have difficulty producing sufficient amounts of surfactant. This can lead to alveolar collapse and severe respiratory distress. This condition, called *infant respiratory distress syndrome*, is the single most common cause of respiratory disease in premature infants. Surfactant dysfunction also is possible in the adult. This usually occurs as the result of severe injury or infection and can contribute to the development of a condition called *acute respiratory distress syndrome* (see Chapter 22).

Airway Compression. Airflow through the collapsible airways in the lungs depends on the distending airway (intrapulmonary) pressures that hold the airways open and the external (intrapleural or intrathoracic) pressures that surround and compress the airways. The difference between these two pressures (airway pressure minus intrathoracic pressure) is called the *transpulmonary pressure*. For airflow to occur, the distending pressure inside the airways must be greater than the compressing pressure outside the airways (Fig. 20-15).

During forced expiration, the transpulmonary pressure is decreased because of a disproportionate increase in the intrathoracic pressure compared with airway pressure. The resistance that air encounters as it moves out of the lungs causes a further drop in airway pressure. If this drop in airway pressure is sufficiently great, the surrounding intrathoracic pressure will compress the collapsible airways (*i.e.*, those that lack cartilaginous support), causing airflow to be interrupted and air to be trapped in the alveoli (see Fig. 20-15). Although this type of airway compression usually is seen only during forced expiration in persons with normal respiratory function, it may occur during normal breathing in persons with lung disease. For example, in conditions that increase airway resistance, such as chronic obstructive pulmonary disease (COPD), the pressure drop along the smaller airways is magnified, and an increase in intra-airway pressure is needed to maintain airway patency (see Chapter 22). Measures such as pursed-lip breathing increase airway pressure and improve expiratory flow rates in persons with COPD.

LUNG VOLUMES

Lung volumes, or the amount of air exchanged during ventilation, can be subdivided into three components: (1) the tidal volume (TV), (2) the inspiratory reserve vol-

ume (IRV), and (3) the expiratory reserve volume (ERV). The TV, usually about 500 mL, is the amount of air that moves into and out of the lungs during a normal breath (Fig. 20-16). The IRV is the maximum amount of air that can be inspired in excess of the normal TV, and the ERV is the maximum amount that can be exhaled in excess of the normal TV. Approximately 1200 mL of air always remains in the lungs after forced expiration; this air is the *residual volume* (RV). The RV increases with age because there is more trapping of air in the lungs at the end of expiration. The lung volumes can be measured using an instrument called a *spirometer*.

Lung capacities include two or more lung volumes. The *vital capacity* (VC) equals the IRV plus the TV plus the ERV and is the amount of air that can be exhaled from the point of maximal inspiration. The *inspiratory capacity* (IC) equals the TV plus the IRV. It is the amount of air a person can breathe in beginning at the normal expiratory level and distending the lungs to the maximal amount. The *functional residual capacity* (FRC) is the sum of the RV and ERV; it is the volume of air that remains in the lungs at the end of normal expiration. The *total lung capacity* (TLC) is the sum of all the volumes in the lungs. The RV cannot be measured with the spirometer because this air cannot be expressed from the lungs. It is measured by indirect methods, such as the helium dilution methods, the nitrogen washout methods, or body plethysmography. Lung volumes and capacities are summarized in Table 20-1.

Pulmonary Function Studies

The previously described lung volumes and capacities are anatomic or static measures, determined by lung volumes and measured without relation to time. The

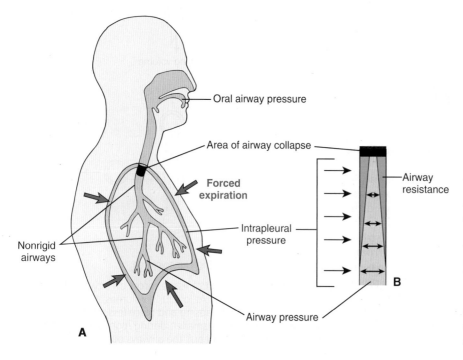

FIGURE 20-15 Mechanism that limits maximal expiratory flow rate. (**A**) Airway patency and airflow in the nonrigid airways of the lungs rely on a transpulmonary pressure gradient in which airway pressure is greater than intrapleural pressure. (**B**) Airway resistance normally produces a drop in airway pressure as air moves out of the lungs. The increased intrapleural pressure that occurs with forced expiration produces airway collapse in the nonrigid airways at the point where intrapleural pressure exceeds airway pressure.

FIGURE 20-16 Tracings of respiratory volumes (**left**) and lung capacities (**right**) as they would appear if made using a spirometer. The tidal volume (*yellow*) represents the amount inhaled and exhaled during normal breathing; the inspiratory reserve volume (*pink*), the maximal amount of air in excess of the tidal volume that can be forcefully inhaled; the maximal expiratory reserve (*blue*), the maximal amount of air that can be exhaled in excess of the tidal volume; and the residual volume (*green*), the air that continues to remain in the lung after maximal expiratory effort. The inspiratory capacity represents the sum of the inspiratory reserve volume and the tidal volume; the functional residual capacity, the sum of the maximal expiratory reserve and residual volumes; and the total lung capacity, the sum of all the volumes.

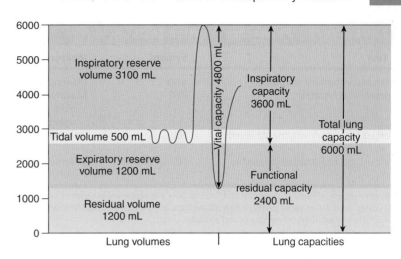

spirometer also is used to measure dynamic lung function (*i.e.*, ventilation with respect to time); these tests often are used in assessing pulmonary function (Table 20-2). The *maximum voluntary ventilation* measures the volume of air that a person can move into and out of the lungs during maximum effort lasting for a specific period of time. This measurement usually is converted to liters per minute. Two other useful tests are the *forced vital capacity* (FVC) and the *forced expiratory volume* (FEV). The FVC involves full inspiration to total lung capacity followed by forceful maximal expiration. Obstruction of airways produces an FVC that is lower than that observed with more slowly performed vital capacity measurements. The FEV is the expiratory volume achieved in a given time period. The $FEV_{1.0}$ is the forced expiratory volume that can be exhaled in 1 second. The $FEV_{1.0}$ frequently is expressed as a percentage of the FVC. The $FEV_{1.0}$ and FVC are used in the diagnosis of obstructive lung disorders.

EFFICIENCY AND THE WORK OF BREATHING

The *minute volume*, or total ventilation, is the amount of air that is exchanged in 1 minute. It is determined by the metabolic needs of the body. The minute volume is equal to the TV multiplied by the respiratory rate. During normal activity it is about 6000 mL (500 mL TV × respiratory rate of 12 breaths per minute). The efficiency of breathing is determined by matching the TV and respiratory rate in a manner that provides an optimal minute volume while minimizing the work of breathing.

The work of breathing is determined by the amount of effort required to move air through the conducting airways and by the ease of lung expansion or compliance. Expansion of the lungs is difficult for persons with stiff and noncompliant lungs; they usually find it easier to breathe if they keep their TV low and breathe at a more rapid rate (*e.g.*, 300 × 20 = 6000 mL) to achieve their minute volume and meet their oxygen needs. In contrast,

TABLE 20-1	Lung Volumes and Capacities	
Volume	**Symbol**	**Measurement**
Tidal volume (about 500 mL at rest)	TV	Amount of air that moves into and out of the lungs with each breath
Inspiratory reserve volume (about 3000 mL)	IRV	Maximum amount of air that can be inhaled from the point of maximal expiration
Expiratory reserve volume (about 1200 mL)	ERV	Maximum volume of air that can be exhaled from the resting end-expiratory level
Residual volume (about 1200 mL)	RV	Volume of air remaining in the lungs after maximal expiration. This volume cannot be measured with the spirometer; it is measured indirectly using methods such as the helium dilution method, the nitrogen washout technique, or body plethysmography.
Functional residual capacity (about 2400 mL)	FRC	Volume of air remaining in the lungs at end-expiration (sum of RV and ERV)
Inspiratory capacity (about 3600 mL)	IC	Sum of IRV and TV
Vital capacity (about 4800 mL)	VC	Maximal amount of air that can be exhaled from the point of maximal inspiration
Total lung capacity (about 6000 mL)	TLC	Total amount of air that the lungs can hold; it is the sum of all the volume components after maximal inspiration. This value is about 20% to 25% less in females than in males.

TABLE 20-2	Pulmonary Function Tests	
Test	**Symbol**	**Measurement***
Maximal voluntary ventilation	MVV	Maximum amount of air that can be breathed in a given time
Forced vital capacity	FVC	Maximum amount of air that can be rapidly and forcefully exhaled from the lungs after full inspiration. The expired volume is plotted against time.
Forced expiratory volume achieved in 1 second	$FEV_{1.0}$	Volume of air expired in the first second of FVC
Percentage of forced vital capacity	$FEV_{1.0}/FVC\%$	Volume of air expired in the first second, expressed as a percentage of FVC

*By convention, all the lung volumes and rates of flow are expressed in terms of body temperature and pressure and saturated with water vapor (BTPS), which allows for a comparison of the pulmonary function data from laboratories with different ambient temperatures and altitudes.

persons with obstructive airway disease usually find it less difficult to inflate their lungs but expend more energy in moving air through the airways. As a result, these persons tend to take deeper breaths and breathe at a slower rate (*e.g.*, $600 \times 10 = 6000$ mL) to achieve their oxygen needs.

In summary, the movement of air between the atmosphere and the lungs follows the laws of physics as they relate to gases. The air in the alveoli contains a mixture of gases, including nitrogen, oxygen, carbon dioxide, and water vapor. With the exception of water vapor, each gas exerts a pressure that is determined by the atmospheric pressure and the concentration of the gas in the mixture. Water vapor pressure is affected by temperature but not atmospheric pressure. Air moves into the lungs along a pressure gradient. The pressure inside the airways and alveoli of the lungs is called *intrapulmonary* (or *alveolar*) *pressure;* the pressure in the pleural cavity is called *intrapleural pressure;* and the pressure in the thoracic cavity is called *intrathoracic pressure.*

Breathing is the movement of gases between the atmosphere and the lungs. It requires a system of open airways and pressure changes resulting from the action of the respiratory muscles in changing the volume of the chest cage. The diaphragm is the principal muscle of inspiration, assisted by the external intercostal muscles. The scalene and sternocleidomastoid muscles elevate the ribs and act as accessory muscles for inspiration. Expiration is largely passive, aided by the elastic recoil of the respiratory muscles that were stretched during inspiration. When needed, the abdominal and internal intercostal muscles can be used to increase expiratory effort.

Lung compliance describes the ease with which the lungs can be inflated. It reflects the elasticity of the lung tissue and the surface tension in the alveoli. Surfactant molecules, produced by type II alveolar cells, reduce the surface tension in the lungs, thereby increasing lung compliance. Airway resistance refers to the impediment to flow that the air encounters as it moves through the airways. The minute volume, which is determined by the metabolic needs of the body, is the amount of air that is exchanged in 1 minute (*i.e.*, respiratory rate × TV). The efficiency and work of breathing are determined by factors such as impaired lung compliance and airway diseases that increase the work involved in maintaining the minute volume. Lung volumes and lung capacities can be measured using a spirometer. Pulmonary function studies are used to assess ventilation with respect to time.

Exchange and Transport of Gases

The primary functions of the lungs are oxygenation of the blood and removal of carbon dioxide. Pulmonary gas exchange is conventionally divided into three processes: (1) ventilation or the flow of gases into and out of the alveoli of the lungs, (2) perfusion or flow of blood in the adjacent pulmonary capillaries, and (3) diffusion or transfer of gases between the alveoli and the pulmonary capillaries. The efficiency of gas exchange requires that alveolar ventilation occur adjacent to perfused pulmonary capillaries.

VENTILATION

Ventilation refers to the exchange of gases in the respiratory system. There are two types of ventilation: pulmonary and alveolar. *Pulmonary ventilation* refers to the total exchange of gases between the atmosphere and the lungs. *Alveolar ventilation* is the exchange of gases within the gas exchange portion of the lungs. Ventilation requires a system of open airways and a pressure difference that moves air into and out of the lungs. It is affected by body position and lung volume as well as by disease conditions that affect the heart and respiratory system.

Distribution of Ventilation

The distribution of ventilation between the base (bottom) and apex (top) of the lung varies with body position and reflects the effects of gravity on intrapleural pressure and lung compliance. Compliance reflects the change in volume that occurs with a change in intrapleural pressure. It is less in fully expanded alveoli, which have difficulty accommodating more air, and greater in alveoli that are less inflated and can more easily expand to accommodate more air. In the seated or standing position, gravity exerts a downward pull on the lung, causing intrapleural pressure at the apex of the lung to become more negative. As a result, the alveoli at the apex of the lung are more fully expanded and less compliant than those at the base of the lung. The same holds true for lung expansion in the dependent portions of the lung in the supine or lateral position. In the supine position, ventilation in the lowermost (posterior) parts of the lung exceeds that in the uppermost (anterior) parts. In the lateral position (i.e., lying on the side), the dependent lung is better ventilated.

The distribution of ventilation also is affected by lung volumes. During full inspiration (high lung volumes) in the seated or standing position, the airways are pulled open and air moves into the more compliant portions of the lower lung. At low lung volumes, the opposite occurs. At functional residual capacity, the intrapleural pressure at the base of the lung exceeds airway pressure, compressing the airways so that ventilation is greatly reduced. In contrast, the airways in the apex of the lung remain open, and this area of the lung is well ventilated.

PERFUSION

The term *perfusion* is used to describe the flow of blood through the pulmonary capillary bed. The primary functions of the pulmonary circulation are to perfuse or provide blood flow to the gas exchange portion of the lung and to facilitate gas exchange. The pulmonary circulation serves several important functions in addition to gas exchange. It filters all the blood that moves from the right to the left side of the circulation; it removes most of the thromboemboli that might form; and it serves as a reservoir of blood for the left side of the heart.

The gas exchange function of the lungs requires a continuous flow of blood through the respiratory portion of the lungs. Deoxygenated blood enters the lung through the pulmonary artery, which has its origin in the right side of the heart and enters the lung at the hilus, along with the primary bronchus. The pulmonary arteries branch in a manner similar to that of the airways. The small pulmonary arteries accompany the bronchi as they move down the lobules and branch to supply the capillary network that surrounds the alveoli (see Fig. 20-6). The oxygenated capillary blood is collected in the small pulmonary veins of the lobules, and then it moves to the larger veins to be collected in the four large pulmonary veins that empty into the left atrium.

Distribution of Blood Flow

As with ventilation, the distribution of pulmonary blood flow is affected by body position and gravity. In the upright position, the distance of the upper apices of the lung above the level of the heart may exceed the perfusion capabilities of the mean pulmonary arterial pressure (approximately 12 mm Hg); therefore, blood flow in the upper part of the lungs is less than that in the base or bottom part of the lungs. In the supine position, the lungs and the heart are at the same level, and blood flow to the apices and base of the lungs becomes more uniform. In this position, blood flow to the posterior or dependent portions (e.g., bottom of the lung when lying on the side) exceeds flow in the anterior or nondependent portions of the lungs. In persons with left-sided heart failure, congestion develops in the dependent portions of the lungs exposed to increased blood flow.

Effects of Hypoxia

The blood vessels in the pulmonary circulation undergo marked vasoconstriction when they are exposed to hypoxia. When alveolar oxygen levels drop below 60 mm Hg, marked vasoconstriction may occur, and at very low oxygen levels, the local flow may be almost abolished. In regional hypoxia, as occurs with a localized airway obstruction (e.g., atelectasis), vasoconstriction is localized to a specific region of the lung. In this situation, vasoconstriction has the effect of directing blood flow away from the hypoxic regions of the lungs.

Generalized hypoxia causes vasoconstriction throughout all of the vessels of the lung. Generalized vasoconstriction occurs when the partial pressure of oxygen is decreased at high altitudes, or it can occur in persons with chronic hypoxia caused by lung disease. Prolonged hypoxia can lead to pulmonary hypertension and increased workload on the right heart. A low blood pH also produces vasoconstriction, especially when alveolar hypoxia is present (e.g., during circulatory shock).

DIFFUSION

Diffusion refers to the movement of gases in the alveoli and across the alveolar-capillary membrane. Diffusion of gases in the lung is affected by: (1) the difference in the pressure of gas across the membrane, (2) the surface area that is available for diffusion, (3) the thickness of the alveolar-capillary membrane through which the gas must pass, and (4) the characteristics of the gas. Administration of high concentrations of oxygen increases the pressure difference between the two sides of the membrane and increases the diffusion of the gas. Diseases that destroy lung tissue and the surface area for diffusion and those that increase the thickness of the alveolar-capillary membrane adversely influence the diffusing capacity of the lungs. For example, the removal of one lung reduces the diffusing capacity by one half. The thickness of the alveolar-capillary membrane and the distance for diffusion are increased in persons with pulmonary edema or pneumonia. The characteristics of the gas and its molecular weight and solubility constitute the diffusion coefficient and determine how rapidly the gas diffuses through the respiratory membranes. For example, carbon dioxide diffuses 20 times more rapidly than oxygen because of its greater solubility in the respiratory membranes.

MATCHING OF VENTILATION AND PERFUSION

The gas exchange properties of the lung depend on the matching of ventilation and perfusion, ensuring that equal amounts of air and blood are entering the respiratory portion of the lungs (Fig. 20-17). There are two factors that may interfere with the matching of ventilation and perfusion: (1) dead air space, and (2) shunt.

Dead Air Space

Dead space refers to the air that must be moved with each breath but does not participate in gas exchange. The movement of air through dead space contributes to the work of breathing but not to gas exchange. There are two types of dead space: that contained in the conducting airways, called the *anatomic dead space*, and that contained in the respiratory portion of the lung, called the *alveolar dead space*. The volume of anatomic airway dead space is fixed at approximately 150 to 200 mL, depending on body size. It constitutes air contained in the nose, pharynx, trachea, and bronchi. The creation of an opening in the trachea to facilitate ventilation (tracheostomy) decreases anatomic dead space ventilation because air does not have to move through the nasal and oral airways. Alveolar dead space, normally about 5 to 10 mL, constitutes alveolar air that does not participate in gas exchange. When alveoli are ventilated but deprived of blood flow, they do not contribute to gas exchange and thereby constitute alveolar dead space.

The *physiologic dead space* includes the anatomic dead space plus alveolar dead space. In persons with normal respiratory function, physiologic dead space is about the same as anatomic dead space. Only in lung disease does physiologic dead space increase.

Shunt

Shunt refers to blood that moves from the right to the left side of the circulation without being oxygenated. There are two types of shunts: physiologic and anatomic. In a *physiologic shunt*, there is mismatching of ventilation and perfusion, resulting in insufficient ventilation to provide the oxygen needed to oxygenate the blood flowing through the alveolar capillaries. Physiologic shunting of blood usually results from destructive lung disease that impairs ventilation or from heart failure that interferes with movement of blood through sections of the lungs. In an *anatomic shunt*, blood moves from the venous to the arterial side of the circulation without moving through the lungs. Anatomic intracardiac shunting of blood caused by congenital heart defects is discussed in Chapter 18.

Mismatching of Ventilation and Perfusion

Mismatching of ventilation and perfusion occurs when there is perfusion without ventilation or ventilation without perfusion (see Fig. 20-17). Perfusion without ventilation (shunt) results in a low ventilation–perfusion ratio. This is the type of situation that occurs when there is incomplete expansion of the lung, such as in atelectasis (see Chapter 22). Ventilation without perfusion (dead air space) results in a high ventilation–perfusion ratio. An example of this type of situation is pulmonary embolism, when a blood clot obstructs flow (see Chapter 22). The PO_2 in the arterial blood leaving the pulmonary circula-

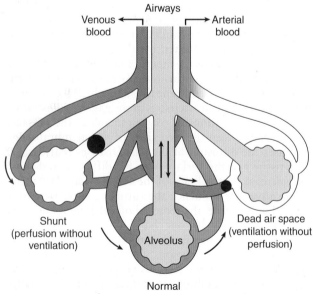

FIGURE 20-17 Matching of ventilation and perfusion. (**Center**) Normal matching of ventilation and perfusion; (**left**) perfusion without ventilation (*i.e.,* shunt); (**right**) ventilation without perfusion (*i.e.,* dead air space).

KEY CONCEPTS

Matching of Ventilation and Perfusion

➤ Exchange of gases between the air in the alveoli and the blood in pulmonary capillaries requires a matching of ventilation and perfusion.

➤ Dead air space refers to air that is moved with each breath but is not ventilated. Anatomic dead space is that contained in the conducting airways that normally do not participate in gas exchange. Alveolar dead space results from alveoli that are ventilated but not perfused.

➤ Shunt refers to blood that moves from the right to the left side of the circulation without being oxygenated. With an anatomic shunt, blood moves from the venous to the arterial side of the circulation without going through the lungs. Physiologic shunting results from blood moving through unventilated parts of the lung.

tion reflects the mixing of blood from areas of shunt and dead air space.

OXYGEN AND CARBON DIOXIDE TRANSPORT

The lungs enable inhaled air to come in contact with blood flowing through the pulmonary capillaries so that exchange of gases between the external environment and the internal environment of the body can occur. The lungs restore the oxygen content of the arterial blood and remove carbon dioxide from the venous blood.

The blood carries oxygen and carbon dioxide as dissolved gases and in combination with hemoglobin. Carbon dioxide also is converted to bicarbonate and transported in that form (see Chapter 6). In the clinical setting, blood gas measurements are used to determine the partial pressure of the dissolved oxygen (PO_2) and carbon dioxide (PCO_2) in the blood. Arterial blood usually is used for measuring blood gases. Venous blood is not used because venous levels of oxygen and carbon dioxide reflect the metabolic demands of the tissues, rather than the gas exchange function of the lungs. The PO_2 of arterial blood normally is greater than 80 mm Hg, and the PCO_2 is in the range of 35 to 45 mm Hg. Normally, the arterial blood gases are the same or nearly the same as the partial pressure of the gases in the alveoli. The arterial PO_2 often is written PaO_2, and the alveolar PO_2 as PAO_2, with the same types of designations being used for PCO_2. This text uses PO_2 and PCO_2 to designate both arterial and alveolar levels of the gases.

The PO_2 and PCO_2 in the blood reflect the partial pressure of the gas in the alveoli, increasing as the alveolar pressure increases and decreasing as the pressure decreases. The effect of alveolar pressures on dissolved gases in the blood can be compared with the dissolved carbon dioxide in a capped bottle of a carbonated drink. In the case of the carbonated drink, carbon dioxide is added under increased pressure as a means of increasing the amount of carbon dioxide that can be dissolved. When the bottle cap is removed and the pressure reduced, tiny bubbles can be seen as the carbon dioxide moves from the dissolved to the gaseous state.

Oxygen Transport

Oxygen is transported in two forms: (1) in chemical combination with hemoglobin, and (2) in the dissolved state. Hemoglobin carries about 98% to 99% of oxygen in the blood and is the main transporter of oxygen. The remaining 1% to 2% of the oxygen is carried in the dissolved state. Only dissolved oxygen that is not bound to hemoglobin can pass through the capillary wall, diffuse through the cell membrane, and make itself available for use in cell metabolism. The oxygen content of the blood (measured in milliliters per 100 milliliters of blood) includes the oxygen carried by hemoglobin and the dissolved form of the gas.

Hemoglobin Transport. Hemoglobin is a highly efficient carrier of oxygen. Hemoglobin with bound oxygen is called *oxyhemoglobin,* and when oxygen is removed, it is called *deoxygenated* or *reduced hemoglobin.* Each gram of hemoglobin carries approximately 1.34 mL of oxygen when it is fully saturated. This means that a person with 14 g/100 mL hemoglobin carries 18.8 mL of oxygen per milliliter of blood when the hemoglobin is completely saturated (100 mL = 1 deciliter [dL]). In the lungs, oxygen moves across the alveolar-capillary membrane, through the plasma, and into the red blood cell, where it forms a loose and reversible bond with the hemoglobin molecule. In normal lungs, this process is rapid, so that even with a fast heart rate, the hemoglobin is almost completely saturated with oxygen during the short time it spends in the pulmonary capillaries.

The oxygenated hemoglobin is transported in the arterial blood to the peripheral capillaries, where the oxygen is released and made available to the tissues for use in cell metabolism. As the oxygen moves out of the capillaries in response to the needs of the tissues, the hemoglobin saturation, which usually is approximately 95% to 97% as the blood leaves the left side of the heart, drops to approximately 75% as the mixed venous blood returns to the right side of the heart.

Dissolved Oxygen. The PO_2 represents the level of dissolved oxygen in plasma. The amount of gas that can be dissolved in a liquid depends on the solubility of the gas and its partial pressure. The solubility of oxygen in plasma is fixed and very small. For every 1 mm Hg of PO_2 present in the alveoli, 0.003 mL of oxygen becomes dissolved in 100 mL of plasma. This means that at a normal alveolar PO_2 of 100 mm Hg, the blood carries only 0.3 mL of dissolved oxygen in each 100 mL of plasma. This amount is very small compared with the amount that can be carried in an equal amount of blood when oxygen is attached to hemoglobin. Although the amount of oxygen carried in plasma under normal conditions is small, it can become a lifesaving mode of transport in carbon monoxide poisoning, when most of the hemoglobin sites are occupied by carbon monoxide and are unavailable for transport of oxygen. The use of a hyperbaric chamber, in which 100% oxygen can be administered at high atmospheric pressures, increases the amount of oxygen that can be carried in the dissolved state.

Oxygen-Hemoglobin Dissociation Curve. The relation between the oxygen carried in combination with hemoglobin and the PO_2 of the blood can be described using the *oxygen-hemoglobin dissociation curve,* which is shown in Figure 20-18. The x axis of the graph depicts the PO_2 of the dissolved oxygen; the left y axis, hemoglobin saturation; and the right y axis, the oxygen content. The PO_2 reflects the partial pressure of the gas in the lung and can vary from 60 mm Hg under hypoxic conditions to greater than 100 mm Hg in hyperoxic conditions such as breathing oxygen-enriched air. The hemoglobin saturation reflects the percentage of hemoglobin that is saturated with oxygen. The saturation of arterial blood is normally 97% to 98% rather than 100% because of

Understanding ➤ Oxygen Transport

All body tissues rely on oxygen (O_2) that is transported in the blood to meet their metabolic needs. Oxygen is carried in two forms: dissolved and bound to hemoglobin. About 98% of O_2 is carried by hemoglobin and the remaining 2% is carried in the dissolved state. Dissolved oxygen is the only form that diffuses across cell membranes and produces a partial pressure (PO_2), which, in turn, drives diffusion. The transport of O_2 involves (1) transfer from the alveoli to the pulmonary capillaries in the lung; (2) hemoglobin binding and transport; and (3) the dissociation from hemoglobin in the tissue capillaries.

1

Alveoli-to-capillary transfer. In the lung, O_2 moves from the alveoli to the pulmonary capillaries as a dissolved gas. Its movement occurs along a concentration gradient, moving from the alveoli, where the partial pressure of PO_2 is about 100 mm Hg, to the venous end of the pulmonary capillaries with their lesser O_2 concentration and lower PO_2. The dissolved O_2 moves rapidly between the alveoli and the pulmonary capillaries, such that the PO_2 at the arterial end of the capillary is almost if not the same as that in the alveoli.

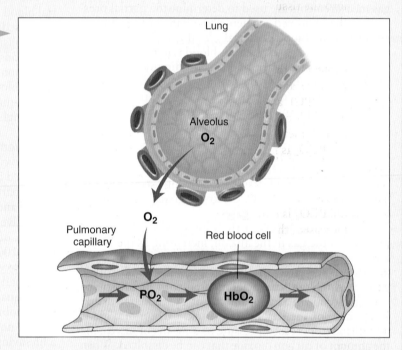

2

Hemoglobin binding and transport. Oxygen, which is relatively insoluble in plasma, relies on hemoglobin for transport in the blood. Once oxygen has diffused into the pulmonary capillary, it moves rapidly into the red blood cells and reversibly binds to hemoglobin to form HbO_2. The hemoglobin molecule contains four heme units, each capable of attaching an oxygen molecule. Hemoglobin is 100% saturated when all four units are occupied and is usually about 97% saturated in the systemic arterial blood. The capacity of the blood to carry O_2 is dependent both on hemoglobin levels and the ability of the lungs to oxygenate the hemoglobin.

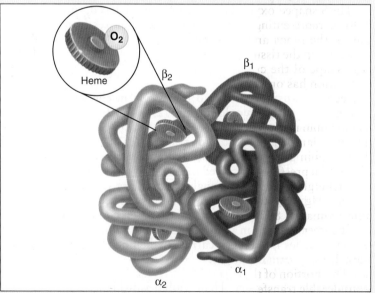

3

Oxygen dissociation in the tissues.
The dissociation or release of O_2 from hemoglobin occurs in the tissue capillaries where the PO_2 is less than that of the arterial blood. As oxygen dissociates from hemoglobin, it dissolves in the plasma and then moves into the tissues where the PO_2 is less than that in the capillaries. The affinity of hemoglobin for O_2 is influenced by the carbon dioxide (PCO_2) content of the blood and its pH temperature, and 2,3-diphosphoglycerate (2,3-DPG), a byproduct of glycolysis in red blood cells. Under conditions of high metabolic demand, in which the PCO_2 is increased and the pH is decreased, the binding affinity of hemoglobin is decreased, and during decreased metabolic demand, when the PCO_2 is decreased and the pH is increased, the affinity is increased.

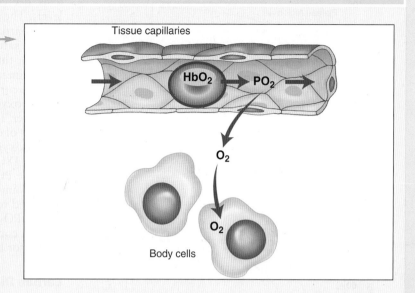

the dilution with unoxygenated blood that occurs in the left heart.

The S-shaped oxygen dissociation curve has a flat top portion representing binding of oxygen by the hemoglobin in the lungs and a steep portion representing its release into the tissue capillaries (see Fig. 20-18A). The "S" shape of the curve reflects the effect that oxygen saturation has on the conformation of the hemoglobin molecule and its affinity for oxygen. At approximately 100 mm Hg PO_2, a plateau occurs, at which point the hemoglobin is approximately 98% saturated. Increasing the alveolar PO_2 above this level does not increase the hemoglobin saturation. Even at high altitudes, when the partial pressure of oxygen is considerably decreased, the hemoglobin remains relatively well saturated. At 60 mm Hg PO_2, for example, the hemoglobin is still approximately 89% saturated.

The steep portion of the dissociation curve—between 60 and 40 mm Hg—represents the removal of oxygen from hemoglobin as it moves through the tissue capillaries. This portion of the curve reflects the fact that there is considerable transfer of oxygen from hemoglobin to the tissues with only a small drop in PO_2, thereby ensuring

an adequate concentration gradient for movement of oxygen from the capillary to the tissues. The tissues normally remove approximately 5 mL of oxygen per 100 mL of blood, with the hemoglobin of mixed venous blood being approximately 75% saturated as it returns to the right side of the heart. At hemoglobin saturation levels below 75%, the rate at which oxygen is released from hemoglobin is determined largely by tissue uptake.

Hemoglobin can be regarded as a buffer system that regulates the delivery of oxygen to the tissues. To function as a buffer system, the affinity of hemoglobin for oxygen must change with the metabolic needs of the tissues. This change is represented by a shift to the right or left in the dissociation curve (see Fig. 20-18B). A shift to the right indicates that the tissue PO_2 is greater for any given level of hemoglobin saturation and represents reduced affinity of hemoglobin for oxygen. It usually is caused by conditions such as fever or acidosis or by an increase in PCO_2, which reflects increased tissue metabolism. High altitude and conditions such as pulmonary insufficiency, heart failure, and severe anemia also cause the oxygen dissociation curve to shift to the right. A shift to the left on the oxygen dissociation curve represents an increased affinity

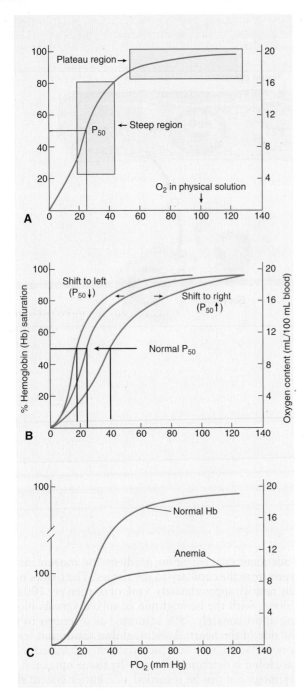

FIGURE 20-18 Oxygen-hemoglobin dissociation curve (**A**) Left boxed area represents the steep portion of the curve where oxygen is released from hemoglobin (Hb) to the tissues, and the top boxed area the plateau of the curve where oxygen is loaded onto hemoglobin in the lung. P_{50} is the partial pressure of oxygen required to saturate 50% of hemoglobin with oxygen. (**B**) The effect of body temperature, arterial PCO_2, and pH on hemoglobin affinity for oxygen as indicated by a shift in the curve and position of the P_{50}. A shift of the curve to the right due to an increase in temperature, PCO_2, or decreased pH favors release of oxygen to the tissues. A decrease in temperature, PCO_2, or increase in pH shifts the curve to the left. (**C**) Effect of anemia on the oxygen-carrying capacity of blood. The hemoglobin can be completely saturated, but the oxygen content of the blood is reduced. (Adapted from Rhoades R. A., Tanner G. A. [1996]. *Medical physiology.* Boston: Little, Brown.)

of hemoglobin for oxygen and occurs in situations associated with a decrease in tissue metabolism, such as alkalosis, decreased body temperature, and decreased PCO_2 levels. The degree of shift can be determined by the P_{50}, or the partial pressure of oxygen that is needed to achieve a 50% saturation of hemoglobin. Returning to Figure 20-18B, the dissociation curve on the left has a P_{50} of approximately 20 mm Hg; the normal curve, a P_{50} of 26; and the curve on the right, a P_{50} of 39 mm Hg.

The oxygen content of the blood (measured in milliliters per 100 milliliters of blood) represents the total amount of oxygen carried in the blood, including the dissolved oxygen and that carried by the hemoglobin (see Fig. 20-18C). It is the oxygen content of the blood rather than the PO_2 or hemoglobin saturation that determines the amount of oxygen that is carried in the blood and delivered to the tissues. An anemic person may have a normal PO_2 and hemoglobin saturation level but decreased oxygen content because of the lower amount of hemoglobin for binding oxygen.

Carbon Dioxide Transport

Carbon dioxide is transported in the blood in three forms: as dissolved carbon dioxide (10%), attached to hemoglobin (30%), and as bicarbonate (60%). Acid-base balance is influenced by the amount of dissolved carbon dioxide and the bicarbonate level in the blood (see Chapter 6).

As carbon dioxide is formed during the metabolic process, it diffuses out of cells into the tissue spaces and then into the capillaries. The amount of dissolved carbon dioxide that can be carried in plasma is determined by the partial pressure of the gas and its solubility coefficient (0.03 mL/100 mL/1 mm Hg PCO_2). Carbon dioxide is 20 times more soluble in plasma than oxygen. Thus, the dissolved state plays a greater role in transport of carbon dioxide compared with oxygen.

Most of the carbon dioxide diffuses into the red blood cells, where it forms carbonic acid or combines with hemoglobin. Carbonic acid (H_2CO_3) is formed when carbon dioxide combines with water ($CO_2 + H_2O = H^+ + HCO_3^-$). The process is catalyzed by an enzyme called *carbonic anhydrase*, which greatly increases the rate of the reaction. Carbonic acid readily ionizes to form a bicarbonate (HCO_3^-) and a hydrogen (H^+) ion. The hydrogen ion that is generated combines with the hemoglobin, which is a powerful acid-base buffer, and the bicarbonate ion diffuses into plasma in exchange for a chloride ion.

In addition to the carbonic anhydrase–mediated reaction with water, carbon dioxide reacts directly with hemoglobin to form *carbaminohemoglobin*. The combination of carbon dioxide with hemoglobin is a reversible reaction involving a loose bond that allows transport of carbon dioxide from tissues to the lungs, where it is released into the alveoli for exchange with the external environment. The release of oxygen from hemoglobin in the tissues enhances the binding of carbon dioxide to hemoglobin; in the lungs, the combining of oxygen with hemoglobin displaces carbon dioxide. The binding of carbon dioxide to hemoglobin is determined by the acidic nature of hemoglobin. Binding with carbon dioxide causes the hemoglobin to become a stronger acid. In the lungs, the highly acidic hemoglobin has a lesser tendency to form carbaminohemoglobin, and carbon dioxide is released from hemoglobin into the alveoli. In the tissues, the release of oxygen from hemoglobin causes hemoglobin to become less acid, thereby increasing its ability to combine with carbon dioxide and form carbaminohemoglobin.

In summary, the primary functions of the lungs are oxygenation of the blood and removal of carbon dioxide. Pulmonary gas exchange is conventionally divided into three processes: ventilation, or the flow of gases into the alveoli of the lungs; perfusion, or movement of blood through the adjacent pulmonary capillaries; and diffusion, or transfer of gases between the alveoli and the pulmonary capillaries.

Ventilation is the movement of air between the atmosphere and the lungs. Pulmonary ventilation refers to the total exchange of gases between the atmosphere and the lungs, and alveolar ventilation refers to ventilation in the gas exchange portion of the lungs. The distribution of alveolar ventilation and pulmonary capillary blood flow varies with lung volume and body position. In the upright position and at high lung volumes, ventilation is greatest in the lower parts of the lungs. The upright position also produces a decrease in blood flow to the upper parts of the lung, resulting from the distance above the level of the heart and the low mean arterial pressure in the pulmonary circulation.

The diffusion of gases in the lungs is influenced by four factors: the surface area available for diffusion; the thickness of the alveolar-capillary membrane, through which the gases diffuse; the differences in the partial pressure of the gas on either side of the membrane; and the characteristics of the gas. The efficiency of gas exchange requires matching of ventilation and perfusion so that equal amounts of air and blood enter the respiratory portion of the lungs. Two factors—dead air space and shunt—interfere with matching of ventilation and perfusion and do not contribute to gas exchange. Dead air space occurs when areas of the lungs are ventilated but not perfused. Shunt is the condition under which areas of the lungs are perfused but not ventilated.

The blood transports oxygen to the cells and returns carbon dioxide to the lungs. Oxygen is transported in two forms: in chemical combination with hemoglobin and physically dissolved in plasma (PO_2). Hemoglobin is an efficient carrier of oxygen, and approximately 98% to 99% of oxygen is transported in this manner. Carbon dioxide is carried in three forms: carbaminohemoglobin (30%), dissolved carbon dioxide (10%), and bicarbonate (60%).

Control of Breathing

Unlike the heart, which has inherent rhythmic properties and can beat independently of the nervous system, the muscles that control respiration require continuous input from the nervous system. Movement of the diaphragm, intercostal muscles, sternocleidomastoid, and other accessory muscles that control ventilation is integrated by neurons located in the pons and medulla. These neurons are collectively referred to as the *respiratory center* (Fig. 20-19).

RESPIRATORY CENTER

The respiratory center consists of two dense, bilateral aggregates of respiratory neurons involved in initiating inspiration and expiration and incorporating afferent impulses into motor responses of the respiratory muscles. The first, or dorsal, group of neurons in the respiratory center is concerned primarily with inspiration. These neurons control the activity of the phrenic nerves that innervate the diaphragm and drive the second, or ventral, group of respiratory neurons. They are thought to integrate sensory input from the lungs and airways into the ventilatory response. The second group of neurons, which contains inspiratory and expiratory neurons, controls the spinal motor neurons of the intercostal and abdominal muscles.

The pacemaker properties of the respiratory center result from the cycling of the two groups of respiratory neurons: the *pneumotaxic center* in the upper pons and the *apneustic center* in the lower pons. These two groups of neurons contribute to the function of the respiratory center in the medulla. The apneustic center has an excitatory effect on inspiration, tending to prolong inspiration. The pneumotaxic center switches inspiration off, assisting in the control of respiratory rate and inspiratory volume. Brain injury, which damages the connections between the pneumotaxic and apneustic centers, results in an irregular breathing pattern consisting of prolonged inspiratory gasps interrupted by expiratory efforts.

Axons from the neurons in the respiratory center cross in the midline and descend in the ventrolateral columns of the spinal cord. The tracts that control expiration and inspiration are spatially separated in the cord, as are the tracts that transmit specialized reflexes (*i.e.*, coughing and hiccuping) and voluntary control of ventilation. Only at the level of the spinal cord are the respiratory impulses integrated to produce a reflex response.

REGULATION OF BREATHING

The control of breathing has automatic and voluntary components. The automatic regulation of ventilation is controlled by input from two types of sensors or receptors: chemoreceptors and lung receptors. Chemoreceptors monitor blood levels of oxygen, carbon dioxide, and pH and adjust ventilation to meet the changing metabolic needs of the body. Lung receptors monitor breathing patterns and lung function.

Voluntary regulation of ventilation integrates breathing with voluntary acts such as speaking, blowing, and singing. These acts, which are initiated by the motor and premotor cortex, cause a temporary suspension of automatic breathing. The automatic and voluntary components of respiration are regulated by afferent impulses that are transmitted to the respiratory center from a number

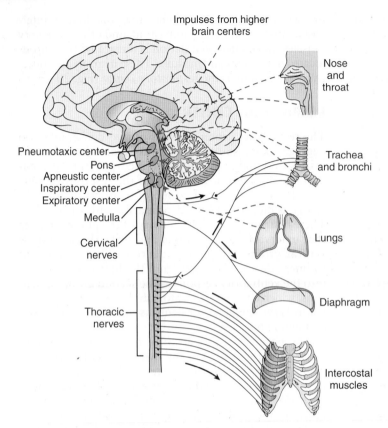

Impulses from higher
brain centers

Nose
and
throat

Pneumotaxic center
Pons
Apneustic center
Inspiratory center
Expiratory center

Trachea
and bronchi

Medulla

Cervical
nerves

Lungs

Thoracic
nerves

Diaphragm

Intercostal
muscles

FIGURE 20-19 Schematic representation of activity in the respiratory center. Impulses traveling over afferent neurons (*dashed lines*) communicate with central neurons, which activate efferent neurons that supply the muscles of respiration. Respiratory movements can be altered by a variety of stimuli.

of sources. Afferent input from higher brain centers is evidenced by the fact that a person can consciously alter the depth and rate of respiration. Fever, pain, and emotion exert their influence through lower brain centers. Vagal afferents from sensory receptors in the lungs and airways are integrated in the dorsal area of the respiratory center.

Chemoreceptors

Tissue needs for oxygen and the removal of carbon dioxide are regulated by chemoreceptors that monitor blood levels of these gases. Input from these sensors is transmitted to the respiratory center, and ventilation is adjusted to maintain the arterial blood gases within a normal range.

There are two types of chemoreceptors: central and peripheral. The most important chemoreceptors for sensing changes in blood carbon dioxide content are the *central chemoreceptors*. These receptors are located in chemosensitive regions near the respiratory center in the medulla and are bathed in cerebrospinal fluid (CSF). Although the central chemoreceptors monitor carbon dioxide levels, the actual stimulus for these receptors is provided by hydrogen ions in the CSF. The CSF is separated from the blood by the blood-brain barrier, which permits free diffusion of carbon dioxide but not bicarbonate or hydrogen ions. The carbon dioxide combines rapidly with water to form carbonic acid, which dissociates into hydrogen and bicarbonate ions. The carbon dioxide content in the blood regulates ventilation through its effect on the pH of the extracellular fluid of the brain.

The central chemoreceptors are extremely sensitive to short-term changes in carbon dioxide. An increase in carbon dioxide levels produces an increase in ventilation that reaches its peak within a minute or so and then declines if the carbon dioxide level remains elevated. Thus, persons with chronically elevated levels of carbon dioxide no longer have a response to this stimulus for increased ventilation but rely on the stimulus provided by a decrease in blood oxygen levels.

The *peripheral chemoreceptors* are located in the carotid and aortic bodies, which are found at the bifurcation of the common carotid arteries and in the arch of the aorta, respectively. These chemoreceptors monitor arterial blood oxygen levels. Although the peripheral chemoreceptors also monitor carbon dioxide, they play a much more important role in monitoring oxygen levels. These receptors exert little control over ventilation until the PO_2 has dropped below 60 mm Hg. Thus, hypoxia is the main stimulus for ventilation in persons with chronically elevated levels of carbon dioxide. If these patients are given oxygen therapy at a level sufficient to increase the PO_2 above that needed to stimulate the peripheral chemoreceptors, their ventilation may be seriously depressed.

Lung Receptors

Lung and chest wall receptors monitor the status of breathing in terms of airway resistance and lung expansion. There are three types of lung receptors: stretch, irritant, and juxtacapillary receptors.

Stretch receptors are located in the smooth muscle layers of the conducting airways. They respond to changes in pressure in the walls of the airways. When the lungs are inflated, these receptors inhibit inspiration and promote expiration. They are important in establishing breathing patterns and minimizing the work of breathing by adjusting respiratory rate and TV to accommodate changes in lung compliance and airway resistance.

The *irritant receptors* are located between the airway epithelial cells. They are stimulated by noxious gases, cigarette smoke, inhaled dust, and cold air. Stimulation of the irritant receptors leads to airway constriction and a pattern of rapid, shallow breathing. This pattern of breathing probably protects respiratory tissues from the damaging effects of toxic inhalants. It also is thought that the mechanical stimulation of these receptors may ensure more uniform lung expansion by initiating periodic sighing and yawning. It is possible that these receptors are involved in the bronchoconstriction response that occurs in some persons with bronchial asthma.

The *juxtacapillary* or *J receptors* are located in the alveolar wall, close to the pulmonary capillaries. It is thought that these receptors sense lung congestion. These receptors may be responsible for the rapid, shallow breathing that occurs with pulmonary edema, pulmonary embolism, and pneumonia.

COUGH REFLEX

Coughing is a neurally mediated reflex that protects the lungs from the accumulation of secretions and from entry of irritating and destructive substances. It is one of the primary defense mechanisms of the respiratory tract. The cough reflex is initiated by receptors located in the tracheobronchial wall; these receptors are extremely sensitive to irritating substances and to the presence of excess secretions. Afferent impulses from these receptors are transmitted through the vagus to the medullary center, which integrates the cough response.

Coughing itself requires the rapid inspiration of a large volume of air (usually about 2.5 L), followed by rapid closure of the glottis and forceful contraction of the abdominal and expiratory muscles. As these muscles contract, intrathoracic pressures are elevated to levels of 100 mm Hg or more. The rapid opening of the glottis at this point leads to an explosive expulsion of air.

Many conditions can interfere with the cough reflex and its protective function. The reflex is impaired in persons whose abdominal or respiratory muscles are weak. This problem can be caused by disease conditions that lead to muscle weakness or paralysis, by prolonged inactivity, or as an outcome of surgery involving these muscles. Bed rest interferes with expansion of the chest and limits the amount of air that can be taken into the lungs in preparation for coughing, making the cough weak and ineffective. Disease conditions that prevent effective closure of the glottis and laryngeal muscles interfere with production of the marked increase in intrathoracic pressure that is needed for effective coughing. For example, the presence of a nasogastric tube may prevent closure of the upper airway structures and may fatigue the recep-

tors for the cough reflex that are located in the area. The cough reflex also is impaired when there is depressed function of the medullary centers in the brain that integrate the cough reflex. Interruption of the central integration aspect of the cough reflex can arise as the result of disease of this part of the brain or the action of drugs that depress the cough center.

Although the cough reflex is a protective mechanism, frequent and prolonged coughing can be exhausting and painful and can have undesirable effects on the cardiovascular and respiratory systems and on the elastic tissues of the lungs. This is particularly true in young children and elderly persons.

In summary, the respiratory system requires continuous input from the nervous system. Movement of the diaphragm, intercostal muscles, and other respiratory muscles is controlled by neurons of the respiratory center located in the pons and medulla. The control of breathing has automatic and voluntary components. Voluntary respiratory control is needed for integrating breathing and actions such as speaking, blowing, and singing. These acts, which are initiated by the motor and premotor cortex, cause temporary suspension of automatic breathing.

The automatic regulation of ventilation is controlled by two types of receptors: lung receptors, which protect respiratory structures, and chemoreceptors, which monitor the gas exchange function of the lungs by sensing changes in blood levels of carbon dioxide, oxygen, and pH. There are three types of lung receptors: stretch receptors, which monitor lung inflation; irritant receptors, which protect against the damaging effects of toxic inhalants; and J receptors, which are thought to sense lung congestion. There are two groups of chemoreceptors: central and peripheral. The central chemoreceptors are the most important in sensing changes in carbon dioxide levels, and the peripheral chemoreceptors function in sensing arterial blood oxygen levels.

The cough reflex protects the lungs from the accumulation of secretions and from the entry of irritating and destructive substances; it is one of the primary defense mechanisms of the respiratory tract.

Review Exercises

Use the solubility coefficient for oxygen and the oxygen dissociation curve depicted in Figure 20-18 to answer the following questions:

A. What is the hemoglobin saturation at a high altitude in which the barometric pressure is 500 mm Hg (consider oxygen to represent 21% of the total gases)?

B. It is usually recommended that the hemoglobin saturation of persons with chronic lung disease be maintained at about 89% when they are receiving supplemental low-flow oxygen. What would their PO_2 be at this level of hemoglobin saturation, and what is the rationale for keeping the PO_2 at this level?

C. What is the oxygen content of a person with a hemoglobin level of 6 g/dL who is breathing room air?

D. What is the oxygen content of a person with carbon monoxide poisoning who is receiving 100% oxygen at 3 atmospheres pressure in a hyperbaric chamber? Consider that most of the person's hemoglobin is saturated with carbon monoxide.

Visit the Porth: Essentials of Pathophysiology: Concepts of Altered Health States web site (http://thePoint.LWW.com/PorthEssentials) for links to chapter-related resources on the Internet, all-new exclusive animations, chapter review questions, and more!

BIBLIOGRAPHY

Berne R. M., Levy M. N. (2000). *Principles of physiology* (3rd ed., pp. 302–352). St. Louis: C. V. Mosby.

Crapo R. O. (1994). Pulmonary function testing. *New England Journal of Medicine* 331, 25–30.

Fishman A. P. (1980). *Assessment of pulmonary function.* New York: McGraw-Hill.

Ganong W. F. (2005). *Review of medical physiology* (22nd ed., pp. 647–697). New York: Lange Medical Books/McGraw-Hill.

Gartner L. P., Hiatt J. L. (2001). *Color textbook of histology* (2nd ed., pp. 343–364). Philadelphia: W. B. Saunders.

Guyton A., Hall J. E. (2006). *Textbook of medical physiology* (11th ed., pp. 471–523). Philadelphia: Elsevier Saunders.

Moore K. L., Dalley A. F. (2003). *Clinically oriented anatomy* (5th ed., pp. 241–252). Philadelphia: Lippincott Williams & Wilkins.

Rhoades R. A., Tanner G. A. (2003). *Medical physiology* (2nd ed., pp. 309–375). Philadelphia: Lippincott Williams & Wilkins.

Ross M. H. (2003). *Histology: A text and atlas* (4th ed., pp. 568–590). Philadelphia: Lippincott Williams & Wilkins.

West J. B. (2004). *Respiratory physiology: The essentials* (7th ed.). Philadelphia: Lippincott Williams & Wilkins.

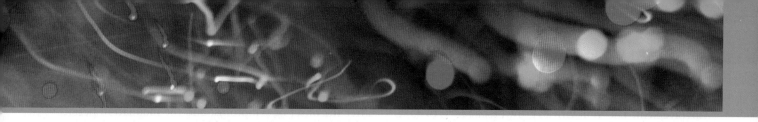

Chapter 21

Respiratory Tract Infections, Neoplasia, and Childhood Disorders

 Respiratory illnesses represent one of the more common reasons for visits to the physician, admission to the hospital, and forced inactivity among all age groups. The common cold, although not usually serious, results in missed work and school days. Pneumonia is the sixth leading cause of death in the United States, particularly among the elderly and those with compromised immune function. Tuberculosis remains one of the deadliest diseases in the world. In addition to microbial pathogens, cigarette smoking contributes significantly to disorders of the respiratory tract, including lung cancer. The content in this chapter is divided into three sections: respiratory tract infections, cancer of the lung, and respiratory disorders in children.

Respiratory Tract Infections

Respiratory tract infections can involve the upper respiratory tract (*i.e.*, nose, oropharynx, and larynx), the lower respiratory tract (*i.e.*, lower airways and lungs), or the upper and lower airways. The discussion in this section of the chapter focuses on the common cold, rhinosinusitis, influenza, pneumonia, tuberculosis, and fungal infections of the lung. Acute respiratory infections in children are discussed in the last section of the chapter.

The respiratory tract is susceptible to infectious processes caused by many different types of microorganisms. For the most part, the signs and symptoms of respiratory tract infections depend on the function of the structure involved, the severity of the infectious process, and the person's age and general health status.

Viruses are the most frequent cause of respiratory tract infections. They can cause infections ranging from a self-limited cold to life-threatening pneumonia. Moreover, viral infections can damage bronchial epithelium, obstruct airways, and lead to secondary bacterial infections. Each viral species has its own pattern of respiratory tract involvement. The rhinoviruses grow best at 33°C to 35°C and remain strictly confined to the upper respiratory tract.[1] The influenza viruses can infect both the upper and lower respiratory tracts. Measles and chickenpox viruses "pass through" the respiratory tract and do not cause respiratory symptoms until secondary viremic spread has occurred. Other microorganisms, such as bacteria (*e.g.*, pneumococci, staphylococci), mycobacteria (*e.g.*, *Mycobacterium tuberculosis*), fungi (*e.g.*, histoplasmosis, coccidioidomycosis, blastomycosis), and opportunistic organisms (*e.g.*, *Pneumocystis carinii*), also produce infections of the lung, many of which produce significant morbidity and mortality.

THE COMMON COLD

The common cold is a viral infection of the upper respiratory tract. It occurs more frequently than any other respiratory tract infection. Most adults have two to four colds per year; the average school child may have up to 10 per year.[2] The condition usually begins with a feeling of dryness and stuffiness affecting mainly the nasopharynx; it is accompanied by excessive production of nasal secretions and lacrimation, or tearing of the eyes. Usually, the secretions remain clear and watery. The mucous membranes of the upper respiratory tract become reddened, swollen, and bathed in secretions. Involvement of the pharynx and larynx causes sore throat and hoarseness. The affected person may experience headache and generalized malaise. In severe cases, there may be chills, fever, and exhaustion. The disease process is usually self-limited, lasting approximately 7 days.

Initially thought to be caused by either a single "cold virus" or a group of them, the common cold is now recognized to be associated with a number of viruses.[3] The most common of these are the rhinoviruses, parainfluenza viruses, respiratory syncytial virus, coronaviruses, and adenoviruses. The season of the year, age, and prior exposure are important factors in the type of virus causing the infection and the type of symptoms that occurs. For example, outbreaks of colds due to the rhinoviruses are most common in early fall and late spring; those due to the respiratory syncytial virus peak in the winter and spring months; and infections due to the adenoviruses and coronaviruses are more frequent during the winter and spring months. Infections resulting from the respiratory syncytial virus and parainfluenza viruses are most common and severe in children younger than 3 years of age. The rhinoviruses are the most common cause of colds in persons between 5 and 40 years of age. There are over 100 serotypes of rhinovirus.[3,4] Although people acquire lifetime immunity to an individual serotype, it would take a long time to become immune to all serotypes.

The "cold viruses" are rapidly spread from person to person. Children are the major reservoir of cold viruses, often acquiring a new virus from another child in school or day care. The fingers are the greatest source of spread, and the nasal mucosa and conjunctival surface of the eyes are the most common portals of entry of the virus. The most highly contagious period is during the first 3 days after the onset of symptoms, and the incubation period is approximately 5 days. Cold viruses have been found to survive for more than 5 hours on the skin and hard surfaces, such as plastic countertops.[3,4] Aerosol spread of colds through coughing and sneezing is much less important than the spread by fingers picking up the virus from contaminated surfaces and carrying it to the nasal membranes and eyes.[5] This suggests that careful attention to hand washing is one of the most important preventive measures for avoiding the common cold.

Because the common cold is an acute and self-limited illness in persons who are otherwise healthy, symptomatic treatment with rest and antipyretic drugs is usually all that is needed. Antibiotics are ineffective against viral infections and are not recommended. Efforts to develop vaccines against the cold viruses have been largely unsuccessful, mainly because of the number of viruses involved and their large array of serotypes.

RHINOSINUSITIS

The term *rhinosinusitis* is a more accurate term for what is commonly called *sinusitis*, because the mucous membranes of the nose and paranasal sinuses are contiguous and subject to the same conditions.[6] The paranasal sinuses are air-filled extensions of the respiratory part of the nasal cavities into the frontal, ethmoid, sphenoid, and maxilla bones (Fig. 21-1). The sinuses, which are named for the bones in which they are found, are connected by narrow openings or *ostia* with the superior, middle, and inferior nasal turbinates of the nasal cavity.[6,7] The mucosal lining of the paranasal sinuses, like that of the nasal passages, has numerous ciliated and columnar cells whose cilia help move fluid and microorganisms out of the sinuses and into the nasal cavity. The lower oxygen content in the sinuses facilitates the growth of organisms, impairs local defenses, and alters the function of immune cells.

The most common causes of rhinosinusitis are conditions that obstruct the narrow ostia that drain the sinuses. Most commonly, rhinosinusitis develops when upper respiratory tract infection or allergic rhinitis (discussed in Chapter 15) narrows the ostia and obstructs the flow of mucus. Nasal polyps also can obstruct the sinus opening and facilitate sinus infection. Barotrauma caused by changes in barometric pressure, as occurs in airline pilots and flight attendants, may lead to impaired sinus ventilation and clearance of secretions. Swimming, diving, and abuse of nasal decongestants are other causes of sinus irritation and impaired drainage.

Clinical Features

Rhinosinusitis can be classified as acute, subacute, or chronic.[6-8] Acute rhinosinusitis may be of viral, bacterial, or mixed viral-bacterial origin and may last from 5 to 7 days in the case of acute viral rhinosinusitis and up to 4 weeks in the case of acute bacterial rhinosinusitis. Recurrent acute rhinosinusitis is defined as four or more

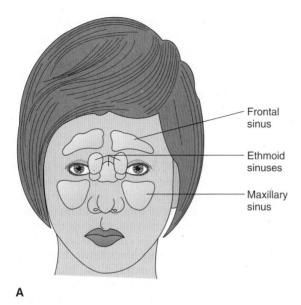

Frontal sinus

Ethmoid sinuses

Maxillary sinus

A

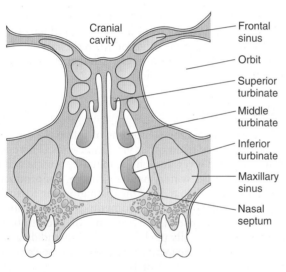

Cranial cavity

Frontal sinus

Orbit

Superior turbinate

Middle turbinate

Inferior turbinate

Maxillary sinus

Nasal septum

B

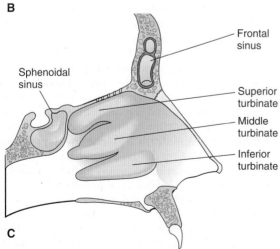

Sphenoidal sinus

Frontal sinus

Superior turbinate

Middle turbinate

Inferior turbinate

C

FIGURE 21-1 Paranasal sinuses. (**A**) Frontal view; (**B**) cross section of nasal cavity, anterior view; (**C**) lateral wall, left nasal cavity. (Courtesy of Carole Russell Hilmer, C.M.I.)

episodes of acute disease within a 12-month period. Subacute rhinosinusitis lasts from 4 weeks to less than 12 weeks, whereas chronic rhinosinusitis lasts beyond 12 weeks.

Acute bacterial rhinosinusitis most commonly results from infection with *Haemophilus influenzae* or *Streptococcus pneumoniae*.[6–8] In chronic rhinosinusitis, anaerobic organisms, including species of *Peptostreptococcus*, *Fusobacterium*, and *Prevotella*, tend to predominate, alone or in combination with aerobes such as the *Streptococcus* species or *Staphylococcus aureus*. In immunocompromised persons, such as those with human immunodeficiency virus (HIV) infection, the sinuses may become infected with gram-negative species and opportunistic fungi. In this group, particularly those with leukopenia, the disease may have a fulminant and even fatal course.

Potential complications of bacterial sinusitis include local extension to the sinus bones, infection of the intracranial cavity, and the spread of infection to the central nervous system, resulting in meningitis or brain abscess.

Manifestations. The symptoms of acute rhinosinusitis often are difficult to differentiate from those of the common cold and allergic rhinitis. They include facial pain, headache, purulent nasal discharge, decreased sense of smell, and fever. A history of a preceding common cold and the presence of purulent rhinitis, pain on bending, unilateral maxillary pain, and pain in the teeth are common findings with involvement of the maxillary sinuses. The symptoms of acute viral rhinosinusitis usually resolve within 5 to 7 days without medical treatment. Acute bacterial rhinosinusitis is suggested by symptoms that worsen after 5 to 7 days or persist beyond 10 days, or symptoms that are out of proportion to those usually associated with a viral upper respiratory tract infection.[9]

In persons with chronic rhinosinusitis, the only symptoms may be those such as nasal obstruction, a sense of fullness in the ears, postnasal drip, hoarseness, chronic cough, loss of taste and smell, or unpleasant breath. Sinus pain often is absent; instead, the person may complain of a headache that is dull and constant. Persons with chronic rhinosinusitis may have superimposed bouts of acute rhinosinusitis. The epithelial changes that occur during acute and subacute forms of rhinosinusitis usually are reversible, but the mucosal changes that occur with chronic rhinosinusitis often are irreversible.

Diagnosis and Treatment. The diagnosis of rhinosinusitis usually is based on symptom history and a physical examination that includes inspection of the nose and throat. Headache due to sinusitis needs to be differentiated from other types of headache. Sinusitis headache usually is exaggerated by bending forward, coughing, or sneezing. Physical examination findings in acute bacterial sinusitis include turbinate edema, nasal crusts, purulence of the nasal cavity, and failure of transillumination of the maxillary sinuses. Transillumination is done in a completely darkened room by placing a flashlight against the skin overlying the infraorbital rim, directing the light inferiorly, having the person open his or her mouth, and observing the hard palate for light transmission.[9] Sinus radiographs and computed tomography (CT) scans may be used. CT scans usually are reserved for diagnosis of chronic rhinosinusitis or to exclude complications.

Treatment of rhinosinusitis includes appropriate antibiotic therapy. The duration of antibiotic therapy is longer for chronic rhinosinusitis than for acute rhinosinusitis. In addition to antibiotic therapy, the treatment of acute rhinosinusitis includes measures to promote adequate drainage by reducing nasal congestion. Oral and topical decongestants may be used for this purpose. The use of intranasal decongestants should be limited to 3 to 5 days to prevent rebound vasodilatation.[8] The use of antihistamines is controversial, particularly for acute rhinosinusitis, because they can dry up secretions and thereby decrease drainage. Mucolytic agents such as guaifenesin may be used to thin secretions. Topical corticosteroids may be used to decrease inflammation in persons with allergic rhinitis or rhinosinusitis. Nonpharmacologic measures include saline nasal sprays and steam inhalations.

Surgical intervention directed at correcting obstruction of the ostiomeatal openings may be indicated in persons with chronic rhinosinusitis that is resistant to other forms of therapy. Indications for surgical intervention include obstructive nasal polyps and obstructive nasal deformities.

INFLUENZA

Influenza is a viral infection that can affect the upper and lower respiratory tracts. Until the advent of acquired immunodeficiency syndrome (AIDS), it was the last uncontrolled pandemic killer of humans. In the United States, approximately 36,000 persons die each year of influenza-related illness during nonpandemic years.[10] Rates of infection are highest among children, but rates of serious illness and death are highest among persons who are 65 years of age or older.

There are three types of influenza viruses that cause disease in humans: types A, B, and C. Type A affects humans, pigs, horses, and birds and is the major cause of epidemics and pandemics. The influenza viruses are further divided into subtypes based on two surface glycoproteins: hemagglutinin (HA) and neuroaminidase (NA).[10,11] Hemagglutinin is an attachment protein that allows the virus to enter epithelial cells in the respiratory tract, and NA facilitates viral replication and release from the cell. Host antibodies to HA or NA prevent or ameliorate infection with the influenza virus. Contagion results from the ability of the influenza A virus to develop new HA and NA subtypes (e.g., H1, H2, H3, N1, N2, N3) against which the population is not protected. An *antigenic shift,* which involves a major change in either antigen, may lead to epidemic or pandemic infection. Influenza B and C viruses do not exhibit antigenic shift, probably because few related viruses exist in animals.

As with many viral respiratory tract infections, influenza is more contagious than bacterial respiratory tract infections. Transmission is by aerosol or direct contact. Inhalation of as few as three infective particles can transmit the infection.[12] Young children are most likely to become infected and also to spread the infection. The incubation period for influenza is 1 to 4 days, with 2 days being the average. Persons become infectious starting 1 day before their symptoms begin and remain infectious through approximately 5 days after illness onset.[10] Children can be infectious for greater than 10 days, and young children can shed virus for up to 6 days before their illness onset. Severely immunocompromised persons can shed virus for weeks or months.

Pathogenesis

The influenza viruses can cause three types of infections: an uncomplicated upper respiratory infection (rhinotracheitis), viral pneumonia, and a respiratory viral infection followed by a bacterial infection. Influenza initially establishes upper airway infection. In doing this, the virus first targets and kills mucous-secreting, ciliated, and other epithelial cells, leaving gaping holes between the underlying basal cells and allowing extracellular fluid to escape. This is the reason for the "runny nose" that is characteristic of this phase of the infection. If the virus spreads to the lower respiratory tract, the infection can cause severe shedding of bronchial and alveolar cells down to a single-cell–thick basal layer. In addition to compromising the natural defenses of the respiratory tract, influenza infection promotes bacterial adhesion to epithelial cells. Pneumonia may result from a viral pathogenesis or from a secondary bacterial infection.

Clinical Features

In the early stages, the symptoms of influenza often are indistinguishable from other viral infections. There is an abrupt onset of fever and chills, malaise, muscle aching, headache, profuse, watery nasal discharge, nonproductive cough, and sore throat.[10,13] One distinguishing feature of influenza is the rapid onset, sometimes within minutes, of profound malaise. The symptoms of uncomplicated rhinotracheitis usually peak by days 3 to 5 and disappear by days 7 to 10. The symptoms above can be caused by any strain of influenza A or B. Influenza C causes symptoms similar to those of the common cold.

Viral pneumonia occurs as a complication of influenza most frequently in the elderly or in persons with cardiopulmonary disease, but has been reported in pregnant women and in healthy, immunocompetent people. It typically develops within 1 day after onset of symptoms and is characterized by rapid progression of fever, tachypnea, tachycardia, cyanosis, and hypotension.[14,15] The clinical course of influenza pneumonia progresses rapidly. It can cause hypoxemia and death within a few days of onset. Survivors often develop diffuse pulmonary fibrosis.[15]

Secondary complications typically include sinusitis, otitis media, bronchitis, and bacterial pneumonia. Reye syndrome (fatty liver with encephalitis) is a rare complication of influenza, particularly in young children.[15] It is most commonly associated with aspirin use during a viral infection such as influenza. Persons who develop secondary bacterial pneumonia usually report that they were beginning to feel better when they experienced a return of fever, shaking chills, pleuritic chest pain, and productive cough. The most common causes of secondary bacterial pneumonia are *S. pneumoniae, S. aureus, H. influenzae,* and *Moraxella catarrhalis.* Influenza-related deaths, particularly in the elderly, can result from pneumonia as well as exacerbations of cardiopulmonary conditions and other disease.

Diagnosis and Treatment. The appropriate treatment of people with influenza depends on accurate and timely diagnosis. Early diagnosis can reduce the inappropriate use of antibiotics and provide the opportunity for use of an antiviral drug. Rapid diagnostic tests, which are available for use in outpatient settings, allow health care providers to diagnose influenza more accurately, consider treatment options more carefully, and monitor influenza type and its prevalence in their community.[16]

The goals of treatment for influenza are designed to limit the infection to the upper respiratory tract. The symptomatic approach for treatment of uncomplicated influenza rhinotracheitis focuses on rest, keeping warm, and drinking large amounts of liquids. Antipyretic and cough medications can also be used. Rest decreases the oxygen requirements of the body and reduces the respiratory rate and the chance of spreading the virus from the upper to lower respiratory tract. Keeping warm helps maintain the respiratory epithelium at a core body temperature of 37°C (or higher if fever is present), thereby inhibiting viral replication, which is optimal at 35°C. Drinking large amounts of liquids ensures that the function of the epithelial lining of the respiratory tract is not further compromised by dehydration. Antiviral medications may be indicated in some persons. Antibacterial antibiotics should be reserved for bacterial complications. The use of aspirin to treat fever should be avoided in children.

Four antiviral drugs are available for treatment of influenza: amantadine, rimantadine, zanamivir, and oseltamivir.[17,18] The first-generation antiviral drugs amantadine and rimantadine are similarly effective against influenza A but not influenza B. These agents inhibit the uncoating of viral ribonucleic acid (RNA) in the host cells and prevent its replication. Both drugs are effective in prevention of influenza A in high-risk groups and in treatment of persons who acquire the disease. Unfortunately, resistance to the drugs develops rapidly and strains that are resistant to amantadine also are resistant to rimantadine. The second-generation antiviral drugs zanamivir and oseltamivir are inhibitors of NA, the viral glycoprotein that is necessary for viral replication and release. These drugs, which result in less resistance than amantadine and rimantadine, have been approved for treatment of acute uncomplicated influenza infection and are effective against both influenza A and B viruses. Zanamivir is administered intranasally and oseltamivir is administered orally. Zanamivir can cause bronchospasm and is not recommended for persons with asthma or chronic obstructive lung disease. To be effective, the antiviral drugs should be initiated within 30 hours after onset of symptoms.

Influenza Immunization

Because influenza is so highly contagious, prevention relies primarily on immunization.[19] Currently, there are two types of influenza vaccines available: the trivalent inactivated influenza vaccine (TIIV), which was developed in the 1940s, and the live, attenuated influenza vaccine (LAIV), which was approved for use in 2003.[20] The formulation of the vaccines must be changed yearly in response to antigenic changes in the influenza virus. The Centers for Disease Control and Prevention (CDC) Advisory Committee on Immunization Practices (ACIP) annually updates its recommendations for the composition of the vaccine.

The TIIV, which is administered by injection, has become the mainstay for prevention of influenza. It has proven to be inexpensive and effective in reducing illness caused by influenza.

Immunization is recommended for members of high-risk groups who, because of their age or underlying health problems, are unable to cope well with the infection and often require medical attention, including hospitalization. Immunization is also recommended for persons who can transmit the infection to high-risk groups (*e.g.,* health care workers and caregivers). Because the TIIV is an inactivated vaccine, it is thought to be safe during pregnancy.[10] The effectiveness of the influenza vaccine in preventing and lessening the effects of influenza infection depend primarily on the age and immunocompetence of the recipient and the match between the virus strains included in the vaccine and those that circulate during the influenza season.[10,19] When there is a good match, the vaccine is effective in preventing the illness in approximately 70% to 90% of healthy persons younger than 65 years of age.[10,19]

The LAIV, which is administered intranasally, has been approved for use in healthy persons 5 to 49 years of age.[20] The LAIVs are in use in Russia and have been in development in the United States since the 1960s. The LAIVs are cold-adapted viruses that replicate efficiently in the 25°C temperature of the nasopharynx, inducing protective immunity against viruses included in the vaccine, but replicate inefficiently at the 38°C to 39°C temperature of the lower airways.

PNEUMONIAS

The term *pneumonia* describes inflammation of parenchymal structures of the lung, such as the alveoli and the bronchioles. Although antibiotics have significantly reduced the mortality rate from pneumonias, these diseases remain the sixth leading cause of death in the United States and are an important immediate cause of death in the elderly and persons with debilitating diseases.[21] Etiologic agents include infectious and noninfectious agents. Although much less common than infectious pneumonia, inhalation of irritating fumes or aspiration of gastric contents can result in severe pneumonia.

Classification

Pneumonias can be classified according the type of agent (typical or atypical) causing the infection, distribution of the infection (lobar pneumonia or bronchopneumonia), and setting (community or hospital) in which it occurs.

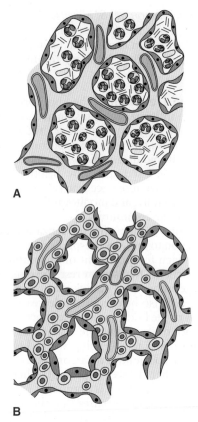

FIGURE 21-2 Location of inflammatory processes in (**A**) typical and (**B**) atypical forms of pneumonia.

KEY CONCEPTS

Pneumonias

➡ Pneumonias are respiratory disorders involving inflammation of the lung structures, such as the alveoli and bronchioles.

➡ Pneumonia can be caused by infectious agents, such as bacteria and viruses, and noninfectious agents, such as gastric secretions that are aspirated into the lungs.

➡ The development of pneumonia is facilitated by an exceedingly virulent organism, large inoculum, and impaired host defenses.

➡ Pneumonias caused by infectious agents commonly are classified according to the source of infection (community- vs. hospital-acquired) and according to the immune status of the host (pneumonia in the immunocompromised person).

Typical pneumonias result from infection by bacteria that multiply extracellularly in the alveoli and cause inflammation and exudation of fluid into the air-filled spaces of the alveoli (Fig. 21-2). *Atypical pneumonias* are caused by viral and mycoplasma infections that involve the alveolar septum and interstitium of the lung. They produce less striking symptoms and physical findings than bacterial pneumonia; there is a lack of alveolar infiltration and purulent sputum, leukocytosis, and lobar consolidation on the radiograph.[21] Acute bacterial pneumonias can be classified as lobar pneumonia or bronchopneumonia, based on their anatomic pattern of distribution.[22] In general, *lobar pneumonia* refers to consolidation of a part or all of a lung lobe, and *bronchopneumonia* signifies a patchy consolidation involving more than one lobe (Fig. 21-3).

Because of the overlap in symptomatology and changing spectrum of infectious organisms involved, pneumonias are increasingly being classified according to the setting (community-acquired or hospital-acquired) in which they occur. Persons with compromised immune function constitute a special concern in both categories.

Community-Acquired Pneumonia. The term *community-acquired pneumonia* is used to describe infections from organisms found in the community rather than in the hospital or nursing home. It is defined as an infection that begins outside the hospital or is diagnosed within 48 hours after admission to the hospital in a person who has not resided in a long-term care facility for 14 days or more before admission.[23] Community-acquired pneumonia may be further categorized according to risk of mortality and need for hospitalization based on age, presence of coexisting disease, and severity of illness as determined by physical examination, laboratory, and radiologic findings.[24]

Community-acquired pneumonias may be either bacterial or viral. The most common cause of community-acquired pneumonia is *S. pneumoniae*.[21] Other common pathogens include *H. influenzae*, *S. aureus*, and gram-negative bacilli. Less common agents are *M. catarrhalis*,

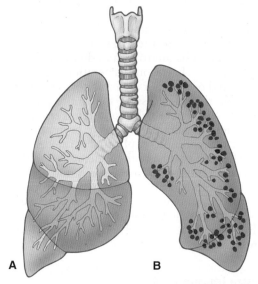

FIGURE 21-3 Distribution of lung involvement in (**A**) lobar pneumonia and (**B**) bronchopneumonia.

Klebsiella pneumoniae, and *Neisseria meningitidis.* *Legionella* species, *Mycoplasma pneumoniae,* and *Chlamydia pneumoniae* (strain TWAR), sometimes called *atypical agents,* account for 20% to 40% of all cases.[25] Common viral causes of community-acquired pneumonia include the influenza virus, respiratory syncytial virus, adenovirus, and parainfluenza virus.

The methods used in the diagnosis of community-acquired pneumonia depend on age, coexisting health problems, and the severity of illness. In persons younger than 65 years of age and without coexisting disease, the diagnosis usually is based on history and physical examination, chest radiographs, and knowledge of the microorganisms currently causing infections in the community. Sputum specimens may be obtained for staining procedures and culture. Blood cultures may be done for persons requiring hospitalization.

Hospital-Acquired Pneumonia. Hospital-acquired, or nosocomial, pneumonia is defined as a lower respiratory tract infection that was not present or incubating on admission to the hospital. Usually, infections occurring 48 hours or more after admission are considered hospital acquired.[23,26] Hospital-acquired pneumonia is the second most common cause of hospital-acquired infection and has a mortality rate of 20% to 50%.[26] Persons requiring mechanical ventilation are particularly at risk, as are those with compromised immune function, chronic lung disease, and airway instrumentation, such as endotracheal intubation or tracheotomy.

Ninety percent of infections are bacterial. The organisms are those present in the hospital environment and include *Pseudomonas aeruginosa,* *S. aureus,* *Enterobacter* species, *Klebsiella* species, *Escherichia coli,* and *Serratia.* The organisms that are responsible for hospital-acquired pneumonias are different from those responsible for community-acquired pneumonia, and many of them have acquired antibiotic resistance and are more difficult to treat.

Pneumonia in Immunocompromised Persons. Pneumonia in immunocompromised persons remains a major source of morbidity and mortality. The term *immuno-* *compromised host* usually is applied to persons with a variety of underlying defects in host defenses. It includes persons with primary and acquired immunodeficiency states, those who have undergone bone marrow or organ transplantation, persons with solid organ or hematologic cancers, and those on corticosteroid and other immunosuppressant drugs.[27]

Although almost all types of microorganisms can cause pulmonary infection in immunocompromised persons, certain types of immunologic defects tend to favor certain types of infections. Defects in humoral immunity predispose to bacterial infections against which antibodies play an important role; defects in cellular immunity predispose to infections with viruses, fungi, mycobacteria, and protozoa. Neutropenia and impaired granulocyte function, as occur with leukemia, chemotherapy, and bone marrow metaplasia, predispose to infections caused by *S. aureus,* *Aspergillus,* gram-negative bacilli, and *Candida.* The time course of infection often provides a hint to the type of agent involved. A fulminant pneumonia usually is caused by bacterial infection, but an insidious onset probably heralds viral, fungal, protozoal, or mycobacterial infection.

Acute Bacterial (Typical) Pneumonias

Bacterial pneumonias remain an important cause of morbidity and mortality, particularly among the elderly. Most bacteria that cause bacterial pneumonia are normal inhabitants of the oropharynx or nasopharynx and reach the alveoli by aspiration of secretions. Other routes of infection include inhalation of microorganisms in the environment. Normally, these organisms do not cause infection because of the small number that are inhaled or aspirated and because the respiratory tract's defense mechanisms prevent them from entering the distal airways[21] (Table 21-1). Loss of the cough reflex, damage to the ciliated endothelium that lines the respiratory tract, and impaired immune defenses predispose to colonization and infection of the lower respiratory system. Bacterial adherence also plays a role in colonization of the lower airways. The epithelial cells of critically and chronically ill persons are more receptive to binding microorganisms that cause pneumonia. Other clinical risk factors favoring colonization of

TABLE 21-1	Respiratory Defense Mechanisms and Conditions That Impair Their Effectiveness	
Defense Mechanism	**Function**	**Factors That Impair Effectiveness**
Glottic and cough reflexes	Protect against aspiration into tracheobronchial tree	Loss of cough reflex due to stroke or neural lesion, neuromuscular disease, abdominal or chest surgery, depression of the cough reflex due to sedation or anesthesia, presence of a nasogastric tube (tends to cause adaptation of afferent receptors)
Mucociliary blanket	Removes secretions, microorganisms, and particles from the respiratory tract	Smoking, viral diseases, chilling, inhalation of irritating gases
Phagocytic and bactericidal action of alveolar macrophages	Removes microorganisms and foreign particles from the lung	Tobacco smoke, chilling, alcohol, oxygen intoxication
Immune defenses (IgA and IgG and cell-mediated immunity)	Destroys microorganisms	Congenital and acquired immunodeficiency states

the tracheobronchial tree include antibiotic therapy that alters the normal bacterial flora, diabetes, smoking, chronic bronchitis, and viral infection.

Bacterial pneumonias are usually classified according to etiologic agent. This is because the clinical and morphologic features, and thus the therapeutic implications, often vary with the causative agent. The discussion in this section focuses on two types of bacterial pneumonia: *S. pneumoniae* pneumonia and Legionnaires disease.

***S. pneumoniae* Pneumonia.** *S. pneumoniae* (pneumococcus) remains the most common cause of bacterial pneumonia. *S. pneumoniae* are gram-positive diplococci, possessing a capsule of polysaccharide. There are 90 serologically distinct types of *S. pneumoniae* based on the antigenic properties of their capsular polysaccharides. The virulence of the pneumococcus is a function of its capsule, which prevents or delays digestion by phagocytes. The polysaccharide is an antigen that primarily elicits a B-cell response with antibody production. In the absence of antibody, clearance of the pneumococci from the body relies on the reticuloendothelial system, with the macrophages in the spleen playing a major role in elimination of the organism.[28] This, along with the spleen's role in antibody production, increases the risk of pneumococcal bacteremia in persons who are anatomically or functionally asplenic, such as children with sickle cell disease. The initial step in the pathogenesis of pneumococcal infection is the attachment and colonization of the organism in the nasopharynx. Colonization does not equate with signs of infection. Perfectly healthy people can be colonized without evidence of infection; the spread of particular strains of pneumococci, particularly antibiotic-resistant strains, is largely by healthy colonized individuals.

The signs and symptoms of pneumococcal pneumonia vary widely, depending on the age and health of the infected person. In previously healthy persons, the onset usually is sudden and is characterized by malaise, severe shaking chill, and fever. The temperature may go as high as 106°F. During the initial or congestive stage, coughing brings up watery sputum, and breath sounds are limited, with fine crackles. As the disease progresses, the character of the sputum changes; it may be blood tinged or rust colored to purulent. Pleuritic pain, a sharp pain that is more severe with respiratory movements, is common. With antibiotic therapy, fever usually subsides in approximately 48 to 72 hours, and recovery is uneventful. Elderly persons are less likely to experience marked elevations in temperature; in these persons, the only sign of pneumonia may be a loss of appetite and deterioration in mental status.

Treatment includes the use of antibiotics that are effective against *S. pneumoniae*. In the past, *S. pneumoniae* was uniformly susceptible to penicillin. However, penicillin-resistant and multidrug-resistant strains have been emerging in the United States and other countries.[24,25,28]

Pneumococcal pneumonia can be prevented through immunization. A 23-valent pneumococcal vaccine, composed of antigens from 23 types of *S. pneumoniae* capsular polysaccharides, is used.[29] The vaccine is recommended for persons 65 years of age or older and persons aged 2 to 65 years with chronic illnesses, immunocompromised persons 2 years of age or older, for residents in special environments or social settings in which the risk for invasive pneumococcal disease is increased, and for residents of nursing homes and long-term care facilities. Because their immune system is immature, the antibody response to most pneumococcal capsular polysaccharides usually is poor or inconsistent in children younger than 2 years of age. A 7-valent pneumococcal polysaccharide-protein conjugate vaccine (Prevnar) is now available for use in infants and children.[30]

Legionnaires Disease. Legionnaires disease is a form of bronchopneumonia caused by a gram-negative rod, *Legionella pneumophila*. It ranks among the three or four most common causes of community-acquired pneumonia.[31] The organism frequently is found in water, particularly in warm, standing water. Although healthy persons can contract the infection, the risk is greatest among smokers, persons with chronic diseases, and those with impaired cell-mediated immunity.[21]

Symptoms of the disease typically begin approximately 2 to 10 days after infection, with malaise, weakness, lethargy, fever, and dry cough. Other manifestations include disturbances of central nervous system function, gastrointestinal tract involvement, arthralgias, and elevation in body temperature, sometimes to more than 104°F. The presence of pneumonia along with diarrhea, hyponatremia, and confusion is characteristic of *Legionella* pneumonia. The disease causes consolidation of lung tissues and impairs gas exchange.

Diagnosis is based on clinical manifestations, radiologic studies, and specialized laboratory tests to detect the presence of the organism. Of these, the *Legionella* urinary antigen test is a relatively inexpensive, rapid test that detects antigens of *L. pneumophila* in the urine.[31] The urine test usually is easier to obtain because people with legionellosis often have a nonproductive cough and the results remain positive for weeks despite antibiotic therapy.

Treatment consists of administration of antibiotics that are known to be effective against *L. pneumophila*. Delay in instituting antibiotic therapy significantly increases mortality rates; therefore, antibiotics known to be effective against *L. pneumophila* should be included in the treatment regimen for severe community-acquired pneumonia.

Primary Atypical Pneumonias

The primary atypical pneumonias are characterized by patchy inflammatory changes in the lungs, largely confined to the alveolar septa and pulmonary interstitium. The term *atypical pneumonia* denotes a lack of lung consolidation, production of moderate amounts of sputum, moderate elevation of white blood cell count, and lack of alveolar exudate.[22] These pneumonias are caused by a variety of agents, the most common being *Mycoplasma pneumoniae*. Mycoplasma infections are particularly common among children and young adults. Other etiologic agents include viruses (*e.g.*, influenza virus, respiratory syncytial viruses, adenoviruses, rhinoviruses, and the rubeola [measles] and varicella [chickenpox] viruses) and *Chlamydia pneumoniae*. In some cases, the cause is unknown.

The clinical course among persons with atypical pneumonias varies widely from a mild infection that masquerades as a chest cold to a more serious and even fatal outcome (*e.g.*, chickenpox pneumonia). The symptoms may remain confined to chills and fever, headache, and muscle aches and pains. Cough, when present, is characteristically dry, hacking, and nonproductive. The diagnosis is usually made based on history, physical findings, and chest radiographs.

The sporadic form of atypical pneumonia is usually mild with a low mortality rate. It may, however, assume epidemic proportions with intensified severity and greater mortality as in the influenza pandemics of 1915 and 1918. The agents that cause atypical pneumonias damage the respiratory tract epithelium and impair respiratory tract defenses, thereby predisposing to secondary bacterial infections.

TUBERCULOSIS

Pulmonary tuberculosis is the world's foremost cause of death from a single infectious agent, causing 26% of avoidable deaths in developing countries.[32,33] It is more common among foreign-born persons from countries with a high incidence of tuberculosis and among residents of high-risk congregate settings such as correctional facilities, drug treatment facilities, and homeless shelters. There is increased occurrence of tuberculosis among HIV-positive individuals. Worldwide, it is one of the leading causes of morbidity and mortality among people with HIV infection. Outbreaks of a drug-resistant form of tuberculosis have occurred, complicating the selection of drugs and affecting the duration of treatment.

Tuberculosis is an infectious disease caused by the mycobacterium, *M. tuberculosis hominis* (human tuberculosis). The mycobacteria are slender, rod-shaped, aerobic bacteria that do not form spores. They are similar to other bacterial organisms except for an outer waxy capsule that makes them more resistant to destruction; the organism can persist in old necrotic and calcified lesions and remain capable of reinitiating growth. The waxy coat also causes the organism to retain red dye when treated with acid in acid-fast staining.[33,34] Thus, the mycobacteria are often referred to as *acid-fast bacilli*. Although *M. tuberculosis* can infect practically any organ of the body, the lungs are most frequently involved.

Tuberculosis is an airborne infection spread by minute, invisible particles called *droplet nuclei* that are harbored in the respiratory secretions of persons with active tuberculosis. Coughing, sneezing, and talking all create respiratory droplets; these droplets evaporate, leaving the organisms (droplet nuclei), which remain suspended in the air and are circulated by air currents. Thus, living under crowded and confined conditions increases the risk for spread of the disease.

Pathogenesis

The pathogenesis of tuberculosis in a previously unexposed immunocompetent person is centered on the development of a cell-mediated immune response that confers resistance to the organism and development of hypersensitivity to the tubercular antigens[33,34] (see Chapter 15). The pathologic manifestations of tuberculosis, such as caseating granuloma and cavitation, are the result of the hypersensitivity reaction that the bacillus evokes, rather than its inherent destructive capabilities.

Macrophages are the primary cell infected with *M. tuberculosis*. Inhaled droplet nuclei pass down the bronchial tree without settling on the epithelium and are deposited in the alveoli. Soon after entering the lung, the bacilli are surrounded and engulfed by macrophages. Although the macrophages that first ingest *M. tuberculosis* cannot kill the organisms, they initiate a cell-mediated immune response that eventually contains the infection. As the tubercle bacilli multiply, the infected macrophages degrade the mycobacteria and present their antigens to T lymphocytes. The sensitized T lymphocytes, in turn, stimulate the macrophages to increase their concentration of lytic enzymes and ability to kill the mycobacteria. When released, these lytic enzymes also damage lung tissue. The development of a population of activated T lymphocytes and the related development of activated macrophages capable of ingesting and destroying the bacilli constitute the cell-mediated immune response, a process that takes about 3 to 6 weeks to become effective.

In persons with intact cell-mediated immunity, the cell-mediated immune response results in the development of a gray-white, circumscribed granulomatous lesion, called a *Ghon focus*, that contains the tubercle bacilli, modified macrophages, and other immune cells.[34] It is usually located in the subpleural area of the upper segments of

---

> ### 🔄 KEY CONCEPTS
>
> **Tuberculosis**
>
> ➤ Tuberculosis is an infectious disease caused by *Mycobacterium tuberculosis*, a rod-shaped aerobic bacterium that is resistant to destruction and can persist in necrotic and calcified lesions for prolonged periods and remain capable of reinstating growth.
>
> ➤ The organism is spread by inhaling the mycobacterium-containing droplet nuclei that circulate in the air.
>
> ➤ The cell-mediated response plays a dominant role in walling off the tubercle bacilli and preventing the development of active tuberculosis. People with impaired cell-mediated immunity are more likely to experience active tuberculosis when infected.
>
> ➤ A positive tuberculin skin test results from a cell-mediated immune response and implies that a person has been infected with *M. tuberculosis* and has mounted a cell-mediated immune response. It does not mean that the person has active tuberculosis.

the lower lobes or in the lower segments of the upper lobe. When the number of organisms is high, the hypersensitivity reaction produces significant tissue necrosis, causing the central portion of the Ghon focus to undergo soft, caseous (cheeselike) necrosis. During this same period, tubercle bacilli, free or inside macrophages, drain along the lymph channels to the tracheobronchial lymph nodes of the affected lung and there evoke the formation of caseous granulomas. The combination of the primary lung lesion and lymph node granulomas is called *Ghon complex* (Fig. 21-4).

Primary Tuberculosis

Primary tuberculosis is a form of the disease that develops in previously unexposed, and therefore unsensitized persons. It typically is initiated as a result of inhaling droplet nuclei that contain the tubercle bacillus[33,34] (Fig. 21-5). Primary tuberculosis usually is clinically and radiologically silent. Most people with primary tuberculosis go on to develop *latent infection* in which T lymphocytes and macrophages surround the organism in granulomas that limit their spread. Individuals with latent tuberculosis do not have active disease and cannot transmit the organism to others.[35]

In approximately 5% of newly infected people, the immune response is inadequate; these people go on to

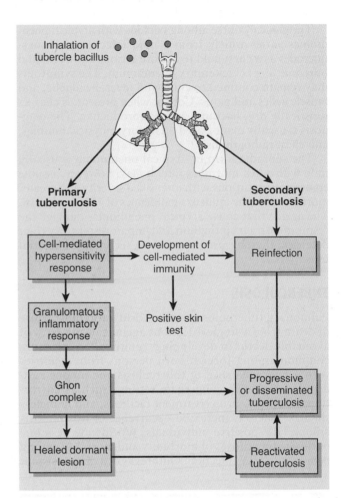

FIGURE 21-5 Pathogenesis of tuberculosis infection.

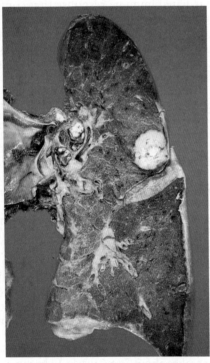

FIGURE 21-4 Primary tuberculosis. A healed Ghon complex is represented by a subpleural nodule and involved hilar lymph nodes. (From Travis W. D., Beasley M. B., Rubin E. [2005]. The respiratory system. In Rubin E., Gorstein F., Rubin R., et al. [Eds.], *Rubin's pathology: Clinicopathologic foundations of medicine* [4th ed., p. 597]. Philadelphia: Lippincott Williams & Wilkins.)

develop progressive primary tuberculosis with continued destruction of lung tissue and spread to multiple sites in the lung.[33] People with HIV infection and others with disorders of cell-mediated immunity are more likely to develop progressive tuberculosis if they become infected. In those who develop progressive disease, the symptoms are usually insidious and nonspecific, with fever, weight loss, fatigue, and night sweats. Sometimes the onset of symptoms is abrupt, with high fever, pleuritis, and lymphadenitis. As the disease spreads, the organism gains access to the sputum, allowing the person to infect others.

In rare instances, tuberculosis may erode into a blood vessel, giving rise to hematogenic dissemination. *Miliary tuberculosis* describes minute lesions, resembling millet seeds, resulting from this type of dissemination that can involve almost any organ, particularly the brain, meninges, liver, kidney, and bone marrow.

Secondary Tuberculosis

Secondary tuberculosis represents either reinfection from inhaled droplet nuclei or reactivation of a previously healed primary lesion (see Fig. 21-5). It often occurs in situations of impaired host defenses. Secondary tuberculosis is classically localized in the apex of the upper lobes of one or both lungs, probably because the higher oxygen content in the apices favors the growth of the bacteria.[33] Because of the preexistence of a cell-mediated immune response, the bacilli elicit a prompt and marked tissue response that tends to wall off the infection. As a result, involvement of the regional lymph nodes is less prominent than in primary tuberculosis. Instead, cavitation occurs readily as the bacteria are disseminated along the airways, and erosion into the airways is a common source of infection. The cavities may coalesce to a size of up to 3 to 10 cm in diameter[34] (Fig. 21-6). Pleural effusion and tuberculous empyema are common as the disease progresses.

Persons with secondary tuberculosis commonly present with cough (which may be erroneously attributed to smoking or a cold), low-grade fevers, night sweats, easy fatigability, anorexia, and weight loss. The cough initially is dry but later becomes productive with purulent and sometimes blood-tinged sputum. Dyspnea and orthopnea develop as the disease advances. Untreated secondary tuberculosis is a wasting disease that is eventually fatal.

Diagnosis and Treatment

Diagnosis. The most frequently used screening methods for pulmonary tuberculosis are the tuberculin skin tests and chest radiographic studies. The tuberculin skin test measures delayed hypersensitivity (*i.e.,* cell-mediated, type IV) that follows exposure to the tubercle bacillus. Persons who become tuberculin positive usually remain so for the remainder of their lives. A positive reaction to the skin test does not mean that a person has active tuberculosis, only that there has been exposure to the bacillus and that cell-mediated immunity to the organism has developed. False-positive and false-negative skin test reactions can occur. False-positive reactions often result from cross-reactions with other mycobacteria, such as *M. avium-intracellulare* complex.[36] Because the hyper-

sensitivity response to the tuberculin test depends on cell-mediated immunity, a false-negative test result can occur because of immunodeficiency states that result from HIV infection, immunosuppressive therapy, lymphoreticular malignancies, or aging. This is called *anergy.* In the immunocompromised person, a negative tuberculin test result can mean that the person has a true lack of exposure to tuberculosis or is unable to mount an immune response to the test. Because of the problem with anergy in persons with HIV infection and other immunocompromised states, the use of control tests is recommended. Three antigens that can be used for control testing are *Candida,* mumps virus, and tetanus toxoid. Most healthy, immunocompetent persons have been exposed to these antigens and will display a positive response to these control tests.[36]

A two-step testing procedure, which uses a "boosting" phenomenon, may be used to increase the reaction to a subsequent tuberculin test in persons who have been infected with tuberculosis.[36] If the first test result of the two-step procedure is negative, a second test is administered 1 week later. If the second test result is negative, the person is considered to be uninfected or anergic. If the second test result is positive, it is assumed to have occurred because of a boosted response. The boosted effect can last for 1 year or longer. Use of the two-step test procedure for employee health or institutional screening can reduce the likelihood that a boosted response in a subsequent test will not be interpreted as a recent infection.

Diagnosis of active pulmonary tuberculosis requires identification of the organism in respiratory tract secretions. Bacteriologic studies (*i.e.,* acid-fast stain and cultures) of early sputum specimens, gastric aspirations, or bronchial washings obtained during fiberoptic bronchoscopy may be used. The polymerase chain reaction (PCR) allows rapid detection of *M. tuberculosis* and its differentiation from other mycobacteria (see Chapter 21). Genotyping can be done to identify different strains of *M. tuberculosis.* It can be used to evaluate second episodes of tuberculosis to determine whether the second episode was due to relapse or reinfection. Genotyping also permits the evaluation of isolates with different patterns of drug susceptibility.[37] In addition, genotyping is useful in investigating outbreaks of infection and determining sites and patterns of *M. tuberculosis* transmission in communities.

Treatment. The primary drugs used in the treatment of tuberculosis are isoniazid (INH), rifampin, pyrazinamide, ethambutol, and streptomycin.[38] The tubercle bacillus is an aerobic organism that multiplies slowly and remains relatively dormant in oxygen-poor caseous material. It undergoes a high rate of mutation and tends to acquire resistance to any one drug. For this reason, multidrug regimens are used for treating persons with active tuberculosis.

Two groups meet the criteria established for the use of antimycobacterial therapy for tuberculosis: (1) persons with an active form of the disease, and (2) those who have had contact with cases of active tuberculosis and who are at risk for the development of active tuberculosis. Tuberculosis is an unusual disease in that chemotherapy is required for a relatively long time. Short-course programs

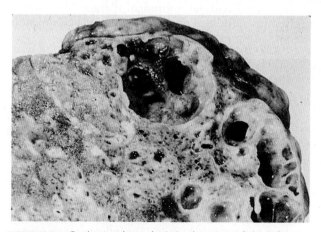

FIGURE 21-6 Cavitary tuberculosis in the apex of the left upper lobe of the lung. (From Travis W. D., Beasley M. B., Rubin E. [2005]. The respiratory system. In Rubin E., Gorstein F., Rubin R., et al. [Eds.], *Rubin's pathology: Clinicopathologic foundations of medicine* [4th ed., p. 598]. Philadelphia: Lippincott Williams & Wilkins.)

of therapy (usually 6 to 12 months) have replaced the earlier 18- to 24-month multidrug regimens. Treatment may need to be prolonged in persons with HIV infection and in those with drug-resistant strains of *M. tuberculosis*. Drug susceptibility tests are used to guide treatment in drug-resistant forms of the disease.

Outbreaks of multidrug-resistant tuberculosis have posed a problem for the prophylactic treatment of exposed persons, including health care workers.[39] Most exposed persons who have contracted active multidrug-resistant tuberculosis were infected with the HIV virus; the fatality rate among these persons is high. Various treatment protocols are recommended, depending on the type of resistant strain that is identified.

FUNGAL INFECTIONS

Fungal infections are commonly classified as superficial, subcutaneous, deep-seated, and opportunistic pathogenic fungi. The superficial and subcutaneous fungi almost always limit their infections to the skin and subcutaneous tissues. Opportunistic fungi are organisms of low virulence (*e.g., Candida* species) that cause localized or systemic infections in people who are immunocompromised, such as those with HIV infection.

The deep-seated fungal infections are caused by highly virulent dimorphic fungi, with the ability to invade deeply into tissues and cause systemic disease. They include *Histoplasma capsulatum, Coccidioides immitis*, and *Blastomyces dermatitidis*. Isolated, self-limited pulmonary involvement is commonly seen in people with normal immune function, whereas immunocompromised people often present with disseminated disease. In HIV-infected persons in endemic areas, coccidioidomycosis is now a common opportunistic infection.

Each of the dimorphic fungi has a typical geographic distribution. *H. capsulatum*, which is the etiologic agent in histoplasmosis, is endemic along the major river valleys of the Midwest—the Ohio, the Mississippi, and the Missouri.[40,41] The organism grows in soil and other areas that have been enriched with bird excreta: old chicken houses, pigeon lofts, barns, and trees where birds roost. The infection is acquired by inhaling the fungal spores that are released when the dirt or dust from the infected areas is disturbed. *C. immitis*, which causes coccidioidomycosis, is most prevalent in the southwestern United States, principally in California, Arizona, and Texas.[42,43] Because of its prevalence in the San Joaquin Valley, the disease is sometimes referred to as *San Joaquin fever* or *valley fever*. *C. immitis* lives in soil and can establish new sites in the soil. Events such as dust storms and digging for construction have been associated with increased incidence of the disease. *B. capsulatum*, the agent causing blastomycosis, is most commonly found in the southern and north central United States, especially in areas bordering the Mississippi and Ohio River basins and the Great Lakes.[44]

Clinical Features

The signs and symptoms of the fungal infections commonly resemble those of tuberculosis. Depending on the host's resistance and immunocompetence, the diseases usually take one of three forms: (1) an acute primary disease, (2) a chronic (cavitary) pulmonary disease, or (3) a disseminated infection. The primary pulmonary lesions consist of nodules containing aggregates of macrophages with engulfed microorganisms. Similar nodules develop in the regional lymph nodes. There is a striking similarity to the primary lesions of tuberculosis. The clinical manifestations consist of a mild, self-limited flulike syndrome.

In the vulnerable host, chronic cavitary lesions develop, with a predilection for the upper lobe, resembling the secondary form of tuberculosis. The most common manifestations are productive cough, fever, night sweats, and weight loss.

Disseminated disease most often develops as an acute and fulminating infection in the very old or the very young or in persons with compromised immune function. Although the macrophages of the reticuloendothelial system can remove the fungi from the bloodstream, they are unable to destroy them. Characteristically, this form of the disease presents with a high fever, generalized lymph node enlargement, hepatosplenomegaly, muscle wasting, anemia, leukopenia, and thrombocytopenia. There may be hoarseness, ulcerations of the mouth and tongue, nausea, vomiting, diarrhea, and abdominal pain. Often, meningitis becomes a dominant feature of the disease. Persons with blastomycosis may experience cutaneous infections that induce pseudoepitheliomatous hyperplasia, which may be mistaken for squamous cell carcinoma.

Skin tests similar to the tuberculin test can be used to detect exposure to *Histoplasma* and *Coccidioides*. There is no reliable skin test for *Blastomyces*. The diagnosis of acute infection is usually made by direct visualization of the organism in tissue sections or sputum culture. Serologic tests that detect antibodies against the specific fungi are available, but lack sensitivity and specificity.

Treatment depends on the severity of infection. Persons without associated risk factors such as HIV infection or without specific evidence of progressive disease usually can be treated without antifungal therapy. The oral or intravenous antifungal drugs are used in the treatment of persons with progressive disease.

In summary, respiratory infections are the most common cause of respiratory illness. They include the common cold, rhinosinusitis, influenza, the pneumonias, tuberculosis, and fungal infections. The common cold occurs more frequently than any other respiratory infection. The fingers are the usual source of transmission, and the most common portals of entry are the nasal mucosa and the conjunctiva of the eye. Rhinosinusitis refers to acute, subacute, or chronic infection of the nasal mucosa and paranasal sinuses. The influenza virus is one of the most important causes of upper respiratory tract infections. There are three types of influenza viruses: types A, B, and C. Type A is further divided into subtypes based on two surface antigens, HA and NA. Epidemics occur through mutations or antigenic shifts in HA and NA that allow the virus to escape most host antibodies.

Pneumonia describes an infection of the parenchymal tissues of the lung, such as the alveoli and bronchioles. Loss of the cough reflex, damage to the ciliated endothelium that lines the respiratory tract, or impaired immune defenses predispose to development of pneumonia. Pneumonia is being increasingly classified as community-acquired (infections that occur outside the hospital) and hospital-acquired (infections that result from organisms in the hospital environment). Persons with compromised immune function constitute a special concern in both categories. The most common cause of community-acquired pneumonia is *S. pneumoniae*. Legionnaires disease is a form of bronchopneumonia caused by the gram-negative bacillus *L. pneumophila*. Viral or atypical pneumonia can occur as a primary infection, such as that caused by influenza virus, or as a complication of other viral infections, such as measles or chickenpox. Viral and atypical pneumonias involve the interstitium of the lung and often masquerade as a chest cold.

Tuberculosis is a chronic respiratory infection caused by *M. tuberculosis,* which is spread by minute, invisible particles called *droplet nuclei.* Tuberculosis is a particular threat among HIV-infected persons, persons from countries with a high incidence of tuberculosis, and residents of high-risk congregate settings such as correctional facilities, drug treatment facilities, and homeless shelters. The tubercle bacillus incites a distinctive chronic inflammatory response referred to as *granulomatous inflammation.* The destructiveness of the disease results from the cell-mediated immune response that the bacillus evokes rather than its inherent destructive capabilities. The treatment of tuberculosis, which has been complicated by outbreaks of drug-resistant forms of the disease, requires multidrug regimens taken over a relatively long period of time.

Infections caused by the fungi *H. capsulatum* (histoplasmosis), *C. immitis* (coccidioidomycosis), and *B. dermatitidis* (blastomycosis) produce pulmonary manifestations that resemble tuberculosis. These infections are common but seldom serious unless they produce progressive destruction of lung tissue or the infection disseminates to organs and tissues outside the lungs.

 Cancer of the Lung

Lung cancer is the leading cause of cancer deaths among men and women in the United States. In 2004, it was responsible for the deaths of approximately 93,000 men and 80,500 women.[45] The increase in lung cancer incidence and deaths over the past 50 years has coincided closely with the increase in cigarette smoking over the same period. Between 1980 and 1998, lung cancer mor-

tality rates decreased for persons younger than 55 years and increased for those older than 65 years, reflecting generational patterns in smoking prevalence.[46,47] Because lung cancer often is far advanced before it is discovered, the prognosis is generally poor. The overall 5-year survival rate is 13% to 15%, a dismal statistic that has not changed since the late 1960s.

With regard to carcinogenic influences, there is strong evidence that smoking is to a large extent responsible for the genetic changes that convert normal bronchial cells to cancer cells. Other influences may act in concert with smoking or may by themselves be responsible for some lung cancers. For example, there is increased incidence of lung cancer in asbestos workers and workers exposed to dusts containing arsenic, chromium, nickel, and vinyl chloride.

Most primary lung tumors (about 95%) arise from the bronchial epithelium (bronchogenic carcinoma). The remaining 5% are a miscellaneous group that includes bronchial carcinoid tumors (neuroendocrine tumors), bronchial gland tumors, fibrosarcomas, and lymphomas. The lung is also a frequent site of metastasis from cancers in other parts of the body.

BRONCHOGENIC CARCINOMA

Bronchogenic carcinomas are aggressive, locally invasive, and widely metastatic tumors that arise from the epithelial lining of the major bronchi. These tumors begin as small mucosal lesions that may follow one of several patterns of growth. They may form intraluminal masses that invade the bronchial mucosa and infiltrate the peribronchial connective tissue, or they may form large, bulky masses that extend into the adjacent lung tissue. Some large tumors undergo central necrosis and acquire local areas of hemorrhage, whereas some invade the pleural cavity and chest wall and spread to adjacent intrathoracic structures.[21] All forms of bronchiogenic carcinomas, especially small-cell lung carcinoma, have the capacity to synthesize bioactive products and produce paraneoplastic syndromes (to be discussed).

Bronchogenic carcinomas can be subdivided into four major categories: squamous cell lung carcinoma (25% to 40%), adenocarcinoma (25% to 40%), small-cell carcinoma (20% to 25%), and large-cell carcinoma (10% to 15%).[21] For purposes of staging and treatment, bronchogenic cancers are commonly identified as small-cell lung cancer (SCLC) or non–small-cell lung cancer (NSCLC). The main reason for this classification is that most SCLCs have metastasized by the time of diagnosis and hence are not amenable to cancer surgery. They are usually best treated with chemotherapy, with or without radiation.

Small-Cell Lung Cancers

Small-cell lung cancers are characterized by a distinctive cell type—small, round to oval cells that are approximately the size of a lymphocyte.[21] The cells grow in clusters that exhibit neither glandular nor squamous organization.

This type of lung cancer has the strongest association with cigarette smoking and is rarely observed in someone who has not smoked.[47] The SCLCs are highly malignant, tend to infiltrate widely, disseminate early in their course, and rarely are resectable. About 70% have detectable metastases at the time of diagnosis.[48] Brain metastases are particularly common with SCLC and may provide the first evidence of the tumor. Without treatment, one half of persons with SCLC die within 12 to 15 weeks.

Non–Small-Cell Lung Cancers

The NSCLCs include squamous cell carcinomas, adenocarcinomas, and large-cell carcinomas. *Squamous cell carcinoma* is found most commonly in men and is closely correlated with a smoking history. Squamous cell carcinoma tends to originate in the central bronchi as an intraluminal growth and is thus more amenable to early detection through cytologic examination of the sputum than other forms of lung cancer. It tends to spread centrally into major bronchi and hilar lymph nodes and disseminates outside the thorax later than other types of bronchogenic cancers.

Currently, *adenocarcinoma* is the most common type of lung cancer found in North America.[22] Its association with cigarette smoking is weaker than for squamous cell carcinoma. It is the most common type of lung cancer in women and nonsmokers. Adenocarcinomas can have their origin in either the bronchiolar or alveolar tissues of the lung. These tumors tend to be located more peripherally than squamous cell sarcomas and sometimes are associated with areas of scarring (Fig. 21-7). The scars may be due to old infarcts, metallic foreign bodies, wounds, and

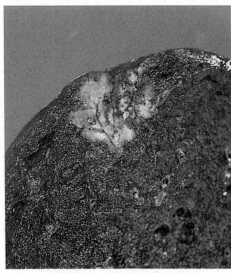

FIGURE 21-7 Adenocarcinoma of the lung. A peripheral tumor in the upper right lobe of the lung has an irregular border and a tan or gray cut surface. (From Travis W. D., Beasley M. B., Rubin E. [2005]. The respiratory system. In Rubin E., Gorstein F., Rubin R., et al. [Eds.], *Rubin's pathology: Clinicopathologic foundations of medicine* [4th ed., p. 649]. Philadelphia: Lippincott Williams & Wilkins.)

granulomatous infections such as tuberculosis. In general, adenocarcinomas have a poorer stage-for-stage prognosis compared with squamous cell carcinomas.

Large-cell carcinomas have large polygonal cells. They constitute a group of neoplasms that are highly anaplastic and difficult to categorize as squamous or adenocarcinoma. They tend to occur in the periphery of the lung, invading subsegmental bronchi and larger airways. They have a poor prognosis because of their tendency to spread to distant sites early in their course.

Clinical Features

Manifestations. The manifestations of lung cancer are extremely variable, depending on the location of the tumor, the presence of distant metastasis, and the occurrence of paraneoplastic syndromes. Often the malignancy develops insidiously, giving little or no warning of its presence. Because its symptoms are similar to those associated with smoking and chronic bronchitis, they often are disregarded.

The manifestations of lung cancer can be divided into three categories: those due to involvement of the lung and adjacent structures, the effects of local spread and metastasis, and the nonmetastatic paraneoplastic manifestations involving endocrine, neurologic, and connective tissue function. As with other cancers, lung cancer also causes nonspecific symptoms such as anorexia and weight loss.

Many of the manifestations of lung cancers result from local irritation and obstruction of the airways and from invasion of the mediastinum and pleural space. The earliest symptoms usually are chronic cough, shortness of breath, and wheezing because of airway irritation and obstruction. Hemoptysis (*i.e.*, blood in the sputum) occurs when the lesion erodes blood vessels. Pain receptors in the chest are limited to the parietal pleura, mediastinum, larger blood vessels, and peribronchial afferent vagal fibers. Dull, intermittent, poorly localized retrosternal pain is common in tumors that involve the mediastinum. Pain becomes persistent, localized, and more severe when the disease invades the pleura.

Tumors that invade the mediastinum may cause hoarseness because of the involvement of the recurrent laryngeal nerve and cause difficulty in swallowing because of compression of the esophagus. An uncommon complication called the *superior vena cava syndrome* can occur in some persons with mediastinal involvement. Interruption of blood flow in this vessel usually results from compression by the tumor or involved lymph nodes. The disorder can interfere with venous drainage from the head, neck, and chest wall. The outcome is determined by the speed with which the disorder develops and the adequacy of the collateral circulation.

Tumors adjacent to the visceral pleura often insidiously produce pleural effusion. This effusion can compress the lung and cause atelectasis and dyspnea. It is less likely to cause fever, pleural friction rub, or pain than pleural effusion resulting from other causes.

Metastatic spread occurs by way of lymph channels and the vascular system. Metastases already exist in 50%

of patients presenting with evidence of lung cancer and develop eventually in 90% of patients. The most common sites of metastases are the brain, bone, and liver.

All varieties of bronchogenic carcinomas, especially SCLCs, have the capacity to synthesize bioactive products and produce paraneoplastic syndromes (see Chapter 5). These syndromes include hypercalcemia from secretion of parathyroid-like peptide, Cushing syndrome from adrenocorticotropic hormone (ACTH) secretion, inappropriate secretion of antidiuretic hormone (ADH), neuromuscular syndromes (*e.g.*, Eaton-Lambert syndrome), and hematologic disorders (*e.g.*, migratory thrombophlebitis, nonbacterial endocarditis, disseminated intravascular coagulation). Manifestations of the paraneoplastic syndrome may precede the onset of other signs of lung cancer and may lead to discovery of an occult tumor. Hypercalcemia is seen most often in persons with squamous cell carcinoma, hematologic syndromes in persons with adenocarcinomas, and the remaining syndromes in persons with SCLCs. Neurologic or muscular symptoms can develop 6 months to 4 years before the lung tumor is detected. One of the more common of these problems is weakness and wasting of the proximal muscles of the pelvic and shoulder girdles, with decreased deep tendon reflexes but without sensory changes.

Diagnosis and Treatment. The diagnosis of lung cancer is based on a careful history and physical examination and other tests such as chest radiography, bronchoscopy, cytologic studies (Papanicolaou [Pap] test) of the sputum or bronchial washings, percutaneous needle biopsy of lung tissue, and scalene lymph node biopsy.[46] CT scans, magnetic resonance imaging (MRI) studies, and ultrasonography are used to locate lesions and evaluate the extent of the disease. Positron emission tomography (PET) is a noninvasive alternative for identifying metastatic lesions in the mediastinum or distant sites. Persons with SCLC should also have a CT scan or MRI of the brain for detection of metastasis.

Treatment methods for NSCLC include surgery, radiation therapy, and chemotherapy.[46] These treatments may be used singly or in combination. Surgery is used for the removal of small, localized NSCLC tumors. It can involve a lobectomy, pneumonectomy, or segmental resection of the lung. Radiation therapy can be used as a definitive or main treatment modality, as part of a combined treatment plan, or for palliation of symptoms. Because of the frequency of metastases, chemotherapy often is used in treating lung cancer. Combination chemotherapy, which uses a regimen of several drugs, usually is used. New targeted treatments are under development with the goal of increasing survival and ultimately providing a cure for this type of cancer.

Therapy for SCLC is based on chemotherapy and radiation therapy.[46,48,49] Because SCLC may metastasize to the brain, prophylactic cranial irradiation is often indicated. Advances in the use of combination chemotherapy, along with thoracic irradiation, have improved the outlook for persons with SCLC. In persons who achieve a complete remission from SCLC, the brain is the most frequent site of relapse. About half of such persons develop clinical metastases within 3 years. Newer combination chemotherapy regimens and targeted therapies are being developed in hopes of providing treatment alternatives that increase survival and produce fewer treatment liabilities.

In summary, cancer of the lung is a leading cause of death among men and women in the United States. The increased death rate from lung cancer has coincided with an increase in cigarette smoking. Industrial hazards, such as exposure to asbestos, increase the risk for development of lung cancer. Because lung cancer develops insidiously, it often is far advanced before it is diagnosed; a fact that helps explain the poor 5-year survival rate.

Bronchogenic carcinoma, which accounts for 95% of all primary lung cancers, can be subdivided into SCLC and NSCLCs (squamous cell carcinoma, adenocarcinoma, large-cell carcinoma). The manifestations of lung cancer can be attributed to the involvement of the lung and adjacent structures, the effects of local spread and metastasis, and paraneoplastic syndromes involving endocrine, neurologic, and hematologic dysfunction. As with other cancers, lung cancer causes nonspecific symptoms such as anorexia and weight loss. Treatment methods for lung cancer include surgery, irradiation, and chemotherapy.

 Respiratory Disorders in Children

Acute respiratory disease is a common cause of illness in infancy and childhood. The etiology and course of these disorders are influenced by a number of factors, including the age of the child, immaturity of the respiratory system, preexisting medical problems, and season of the year. This section focuses on (1) lung development, with an emphasis on the developmental basis for lung disorders in children; (2) respiratory disorders in the neonate; and (3) respiratory infections in children. A discussion of bronchial asthma in children and cystic fibrosis is included in Chapter 22.

LUNG DEVELOPMENT

Although other body systems are physiologically ready for extrauterine life as early as 25 weeks of gestation, the lungs require much longer. Immaturity of the respiratory system is a major cause of morbidity and mortality in infants born prematurely. Even at birth, the lungs are not fully mature, and additional growth and maturation continue well into childhood.

Lung development may be divided into five stages: the embryonic, glandular, canicular, saccular, and alveolar periods.[50] The first three phases are devoted to development of the conducting airways, and the last two phases are devoted to development of the gas exchange portion of the lung. By the 25th to 28th weeks of gestation, sufficient terminal air sacs are present to permit survival. It is also during this period that the type II alveolar cells, which produce surfactant, begin to function. Lung development is incomplete at birth; an infant is born with only one eighth to one sixth the adult number of alveoli. Alveoli continue to be formed during early childhood, reaching the adult number of approximately 300 million alveoli by 5 to 6 years of age.[50]

Ventilation in the Neonate

Effective ventilation requires coordinated interaction between the muscles of the upper airways, including those of the pharynx and larynx, the diaphragm, and the intercostal muscles of the chest wall. In the infant, the diaphragm inserts more horizontally than in the adult. As a result, contraction of the diaphragm tends to draw the lower ribs inward, especially if the infant is placed in the horizontal position. The intercostal muscles, which normally lift the ribs during inspiration, are not fully developed in the infant.[51] Instead, they function largely to stabilize the chest. Under circumstances such as crying, the intercostal muscles of the neonate function together with the diaphragm to splint the chest wall and prevent its collapse.

The chest wall of the neonate is highly compliant. A striking characteristic of neonatal breathing is the paradoxical inward movement of the upper chest during inspiration, especially during active sleep. Normally, the infant's lungs also are compliant, which is advantageous to the infant with its compliant chest cage because it takes only small changes in inspiratory pressure to inflate a compliant lung. However, with respiratory disorders that decrease lung compliance, the diaphragm must generate more negative pressure; as a result, the compliant chest wall structures are sucked inward. *Retractions* are abnormal inward movements of the chest wall during inspiration; they may occur intercostally (between the ribs), in the substernal or epigastric area, and in the supraclavicular spaces (Fig. 21-8).

Airway Resistance

Normal lung inflation requires uninterrupted movement of air through the extrathoracic airways (*i.e.,* nose, pharynx, larynx, and upper trachea) and intrathoracic airways (*i.e.,* bronchi and bronchioles). The neonate (0 to 4 weeks of age) breathes predominantly through the nose and does not adapt well to mouth breathing. Any obstruction of the nose or nasopharynx may increase upper airway resistance and increase the work of breathing.

The airways of the infant and small child are much smaller than those of the adult. Because airflow is directly related to the fourth power of the radius, relatively small amounts of mucus secretion, edema, or airway constriction can produce marked changes in airflow. *Nasal flaring* is a method that infants use to take in more air. This method of breathing increases the size of the nares and decreases the resistance of the small airways.

Normally, the extrathoracic airways in the infant narrow during inspiration and widen during expiration, and the intrathoracic airways widen during inspiration and narrow during expiration. This occurs because the pressure inside the extrathoracic airways reflects the intrapleural pressures that are generated during breathing, whereas the pressure outside the airways is similar to atmospheric pressure. Thus, during inspiration, the pressure inside becomes more negative, causing the airways to narrow, and during expiration it becomes more positive, causing them to widen. In contrast to the extrathoracic airways, the pressure outside the intrathoracic airways is equal to the intrapleural pressure. These airways widen during inspiration as the surrounding intrapleural pressure becomes more negative and pulls them open, and they narrow during expiration as the surrounding pressure becomes more positive.

Lung Volumes and Gas Exchange

The functional residual capacity, which is the air left in the lungs at the end of normal expiration, plays an important role in gas exchange in the infant. In the infant, the functional residual capacity represents a higher lung volume than in the older child or adult. This higher end-expiratory volume results from a more rapid respiratory rate, which leaves less time for expiration. However, the increased residual volume is important to the neonate because it holds the airways open throughout all phases of respiration; it favors the reabsorption of intrapulmonary fluids; and it maintains more uniform lung expansion and enhances gas exchange. During sleep, the tone of the upper airway muscles is reduced, so that the time spent in expiration is shorter and the intercostal activity that stabilizes the chest wall is less; this produces a lower end-expiratory volume and less optimal gas exchange during active sleep.[52]

Control of Ventilation

Fetal blood oxygen (PO_2) levels normally range from 25 to 30 mm Hg, and carbon dioxide (PCO_2) levels range

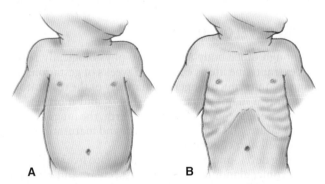

FIGURE 21-8 (**A**) Normal inspiratory appearance of the chest during unobstructed breathing. (**B**) Sternal and intercostal retraction during obstructed breathing in the neonate.

from 45 to 50 mm Hg, independent of any respiratory movements. Switching to oxygen derived from the aerated lung at birth causes an immediate increase in PO_2 to approximately 50 mm Hg; within a few hours, it increases to approximately 70 mm Hg.[53] These levels, which greatly exceed fetal levels, cause the chemoreceptors (see Chapter 20) to become silent for several days. Although the infant's PO_2 may fluctuate during this critical time, the chemoreceptors do not respond appropriately. It is not until several days after birth that the chemoreceptors "reset" their PO_2 threshold; only then do they contribute to the control of breathing. However, the response seems to be biphasic, with an initial hyperventilation followed by a decreased respiratory rate and even apnea. In normal neonates, particularly in preterm infants, breathing patterns and respiratory reflexes depend on the arousal state.[52] Periodic breathing and apnea are characteristic of premature infants and reflect patterns of fetal breathing. The fact that they occur with sleep and disappear during wakefulness underscores the importance of arousal.

ALTERATIONS IN BREATHING PATTERNS

Most respiratory disorders in infants produce a decrease in lung compliance (restrictive lung disorders) or an increase in airway resistance manifested by changes in breathing patterns, rib cage distortion (retractions), audible sounds, and use of accessory muscles.[53]

Children with restrictive lung disorders, such as pulmonary edema or respiratory distress syndrome, breathe at faster rates, and their respiratory excursions are shallow. *Grunting* is an audible noise emitted during expiration. An expiratory grunt is common as the child tries to raise the end-expiratory pressure and thus prolong the period of oxygen and carbon dioxide exchange across the alveolar capillary membrane.

Increased airway resistance can occur in either the extrathoracic or intrathoracic airways. When the obstruction is in the extrathoracic airways, inspiration is more prolonged than expiration. *Nasal flaring* (enlargement of the nares) helps reduce the nasal resistance and maintain airway patency. It can be a sign of increased work of breathing and is a significant finding in an infant. *Inspiratory retractions*, or pulling in of the soft tissue surrounding the cartilaginous and bony thorax, is often observed with airway obstruction in infants and small children (see Fig. 21-8). In conditions such as croup, the pressures distal to the point of obstruction must become more negative to overcome the resistance; this causes collapse of the distal airways, and the increased turbulence of air moving through the obstructed airways produces an audible crowing sound during inspiration called *stridor*.

When the obstruction is in the intrathoracic airways, as occurs with bronchiolitis and bronchial asthma, expiration is prolonged and the child makes use of the accessory expiratory muscles (abdominals). Rib cage retractions may also be present. Intrapleural pressure becomes more positive during expiration because of air trapping; this causes collapse of intrathoracic airways and produces an audible wheezing or whistling sound during expiration.

RESPIRATORY DISORDERS IN THE NEONATE

The neonatal period is one of transition from placental dependency to air breathing. This transition requires functioning of the surfactant system, conditioning of the respiratory muscles, and establishment of parallel pulmonary and systemic circulations. Respiratory disorders develop in infants who are born prematurely or who have other problems that impair this transition. Among the respiratory disorders of the neonate are the respiratory distress syndrome, bronchopulmonary dysplasia, and persistent fetal circulation (*i.e.*, delayed closure of the ductus arteriosus and foramen ovale).

Respiratory Distress Syndrome

Respiratory distress syndrome (RDS), also known as *hyaline membrane disease*, is one of the most common causes of respiratory disease in premature infants.[54,55] In these infants, pulmonary immaturity, together with surfactant deficiency, lead to alveolar collapse (Fig. 21-9). The type II

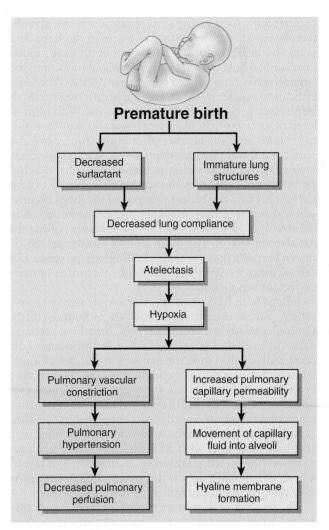

FIGURE 21-9 Pathogenesis of respiratory distress syndrome (RSD) in the infant.

alveolar cells that produce surfactant do not begin to mature until approximately the 25th to 28th weeks of gestation; consequently, many premature infants are born with poorly functioning type II alveolar cells and have difficulty producing sufficient amounts of surfactant. The incidence of RDS is higher among preterm male infants, white infants, infants of diabetic mothers, and those subjected to asphyxia, cold stress, precipitous deliveries, and delivery by cesarean section (when performed before the 38th week of gestation).

Surfactant synthesis is influenced by several hormones, including insulin and cortisol. Insulin tends to inhibit surfactant production; this explains why infants of insulin-dependent diabetic mothers are at increased risk for development of RDS. Cortisol can accelerate maturation of type II cells and formation of surfactant. The reason that premature infants born by cesarean section presumably are at greater risk for development of RDS is because they are not subjected to the stress of vaginal delivery, which is thought to increase the infants' cortisol levels. These observations have led to administration of corticosteroid drugs before delivery to mothers with infants at high risk for development of RDS.[54]

Surfactant reduces the surface tension in the alveoli, thereby equalizing the retractive forces in the large and small alveoli and reducing the amount of pressure needed to inflate and hold the alveoli open. Without surfactant, the large alveoli remain inflated while the small alveoli become difficult to inflate. At birth, the first breath requires high inspiratory pressures to expand the lungs. With normal levels of surfactant, the lungs retain up to 40% of the residual volume after the first breath, and subsequent breaths require far lower inspiratory pressures. With a surfactant deficiency, the lungs collapse between breaths, making the infant work as hard with each successive breath as with the first breath. The airless portions of the lungs become stiff and noncompliant. A hyaline membrane forms inside the alveoli as protein- and fibrin-rich fluids are pulled into the alveolar spaces. The fibrin-hyaline membrane constitutes a barrier to gas exchange, leading to hypoxemia and carbon dioxide retention, a condition that further impairs surfactant production.

Infants with RDS present with multiple signs of respiratory distress, usually within the first 24 hours of birth. Central cyanosis is a prominent sign. Breathing becomes more difficult, and retractions occur as the infant's soft chest wall is pulled in as the diaphragm descends. Grunting sounds occur during expiration. As the tidal volume drops because of atelectasis, the respiration rate increases (usually to 60 to 120 breaths/minute) in an effort to maintain normal minute ventilation. Fatigue may develop rapidly because of the increased work of breathing. The stiff lung of infants with RDS also increases resistance to blood flow in the pulmonary circulation. As a result, a hemodynamically significant patent ductus arteriosus may develop in infants with RDS (see Chapter 18).

The basic principles of treatment for infants with suspected RDS focus on the provision of supportive care, including gentle handling and minimal disturbance.[54] An isolette (incubator) or radiant warmer is used to prevent hypothermia and increased oxygen consumption. Con-tinuous cardiorespiratory monitoring is needed. Monitoring of blood glucose and prevention of hypoglycemia are also recommended. Oxygen levels can be assessed through an arterial line (umbilical) or by a transcutaneous oxygen sensor. Treatment includes administration of supplemental oxygen, continuous positive airway pressure through nasal prongs, and often assisted mechanical ventilation.

Exogenous surfactant therapy is used to prevent and treat RDS.[54,55] The surfactants are suspended in saline and administered into the airways, usually through an endotracheal tube. The treatment often is initiated soon after birth in infants who are at high risk for RDS.

Bronchopulmonary Dysplasia

Bronchopulmonary dysplasia (BPD) is a chronic lung disease that develops in premature infants who were treated with mechanical ventilation, mainly for RDS.[54–57] The condition is considered to be present if the neonate is oxygen dependent at 36 weeks after gestation. The disorder is thought to be a response of the premature lung to early injury. High inspired oxygen concentration and injury from positive-pressure ventilation (i.e., barotrauma) have been implicated. Newer therapies such as administration of surfactants, high-frequency ventilation, and prenatal or postnatal administration of corticosteroids may have altered the severity of BPD, but the condition remains a major health problem.[56,57]

Bronchopulmonary dysplasia is characterized by chronic respiratory distress, persistent hypoxemia when breathing room air, reduced lung compliance, increased airway resistance, and severe expiratory flow limitation. There is a mismatching of ventilation and perfusion with development of hypoxemia and hypercapnia. Pulmonary vascular resistance may be increased and pulmonary hypertension and cor pulmonale (i.e., right heart failure associated with lung disease) may develop. The infant with BPD may have tachycardia, shallow breathing, chest retractions, cough, barrel chest, and poor weight gain. In infants with right heart failure, tachycardia, tachypnea, hepatomegaly, and periorbital edema develop. Clubbing of the fingers occurs in children with severe disease.

The treatment of BPD includes mechanical ventilation and administration of adequate oxygenation. Weaning from ventilation is accomplished gradually, and some infants may require ventilation at home. Rapid lung growth occurs during the first year of life, and lung function usually improves. Adequate nutrition is essential for recovery of infants with BPD.

Most adolescents and young adults who had severe BPD during infancy have some degree of pulmonary dysfunction, consisting of airway obstruction, airway hyperreactivity, or hyperinflation.

RESPIRATORY INFECTIONS IN CHILDREN

In children, respiratory tract infections are common, and although they are troublesome, they usually are not serious. Frequent infections occur because the immune system of infants and small children has not been exposed to many common pathogens; consequently, they tend to contract infections with each new exposure.[55,58] Although most of these infections are not serious, the small size of an infant or child's airways tends to foster impaired airflow and obstruction. For example, an infection that causes only sore throat and hoarseness in an adult may result in serious airway obstruction in a small child.

Upper Airway Infections

Acute upper airway infections are important in infants and small children. They include croup (laryngotracheobronchitis) and epiglottitis. Croup is the more common one, and it usually is benign and self-limited. Epiglottitis is a rapidly progressive and life-threatening condition. The site of involvement is illustrated in Figure 21-10, and the characteristics of both infections are described in Table 21-2.

Obstruction of the upper airways because of infection tends to exert its greatest effect during the inspiratory phase of respiration. Movement of air through an obstructed upper airway, particularly the vocal cords in the larynx, causes stridor.[59] Impairment of the expiratory phase of respiration also can occur, causing wheezing. With mild to moderate obstruction, inspiratory stridor is more prominent than expiratory wheezing because the airways tend to dilate with expiration. When the swelling and obstruction become severe, the airways no longer can dilate during expiration, and both stridor and wheezing occur.

Cartilaginous support of the trachea and the larynx is poorly developed in infants and small children. These structures are soft and tend to collapse when the airway is obstructed and the child cries, causing the inspiratory pressures to become more negative. When this happens, the stridor and inspiratory effort are increased. The phenomenon of airway collapse in the small child is analogous to what happens when a thick beverage, such as a milkshake, is drunk through a soft paper or plastic straw. The straw collapses when the negative pressure produced

by the sucking effort exceeds the flow of liquid through the straw.

Viral Croup. Croup is characterized by inspiratory stridor, hoarseness, and a barking cough. The British use the term *croup* to describe the cry of the crow or raven, and this is undoubtedly how the term originated.

Viral croup, more appropriately called *acute laryngotracheobronchitis*, is a viral infection that affects the larynx, trachea, and bronchi. The parainfluenza viruses account for approximately 75% all cases; the remaining 25% are caused by adenoviruses, respiratory syncytial virus, influenza A and B viruses, and measles virus.[59–62] Viral croup usually is seen in children 3 months to 5 years of age. The condition may affect the entire laryngotracheal tree, but because the subglottic area is the narrowest part of the respiratory tree in this age group, the obstruction usually is greatest in this area. For example, the subglottic airway in the 1- to 2-year-old child is approximately 6.5 mm in diameter, and 1 mm of edema can reduce the cross-sectional area by 50%.[59]

Although the respiratory manifestations of croup often appear suddenly, they usually are preceded by upper respiratory infections that cause rhinorrhea (*i.e.*, runny nose), coryza (*i.e.*, common cold), hoarseness, and a low-grade fever. In most children, the manifestation of croup advances only to stridor and slight dyspnea before they begin to recover. The symptoms usually subside when the child is exposed to moist air. For example, letting the bathroom shower run and then taking the child into the bathroom often brings prompt and dramatic relief of symptoms. Exposure to cold air also seems to relieve the airway spasm; often, the severe symptoms are relieved simply because the child is exposed to cold air on the way to the hospital emergency department.

Airway obstruction may progress in some children. As obstruction increases, the stridor becomes continuous and is associated with nasal flaring with substernal and intercostal retractions. Agitation and crying aggravate the signs and symptoms, and the child prefers to sit up or be held upright. In the cyanotic, pale, or obstructed child, any manipulation of the pharynx, including use of a tongue depressor, can cause cardiorespiratory arrest and should be done only in a medical setting that has the facilities for emergency airway management.

Treatment of viral croup is based on symptoms. Children with mild croup, as indicated by a barking cough and no stridor, usually require only supportive care with oral hydration and minimal handling. A humidifier or mist therapy may be used. Children with stridor at rest require additional interventions. Nebulized racemic epinephrine (L-epinephrine and D-epinephrine) is commonly used because of its rapid onset of action. Corticosteroids may be used to decrease the edema of the laryngeal mucosa through their anti-inflammatory action. Children with progressive stridor, severe stridor at rest, respiratory distress, hypoxia, cyanosis, or depressed mental status should be hospitalized.[58]

Spasmodic Croup. Spasmodic croup manifests with symptoms similar to those of acute viral croup. Because the child is afebrile and lacks other manifestations of the

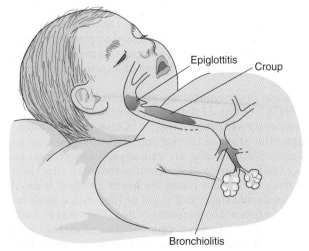

FIGURE 21-10 Location of airway obstruction in epiglottitis, acute laryngotracheobronchitis (croup), and bronchiolitis. (Courtesy of Carole Russell Hilmer, C.M.I.)

TABLE 21-2 Characteristics of Epiglottitis, Croup, and Bronchiolitis in Small Children

Characteristics	Epiglottitis	Croup	Bronchiolitis
Common causative agent	*Haemophilus influenzae* type B bacterium	Mainly parainfluenza virus	Respiratory syncytial virus
Most commonly affected age group	2–7 years (peak 3–5 years)	3 months to 5 years	Less than 2 years (most severe in infants younger than 6 months)
Onset and preceding history	Sudden onset	Usually follows symptoms of a cold	Preceded by stuffy nose and other signs
Prominent features	Child appears very sick and toxic Sits with mouth open and chin thrust forward Low-pitched stridor, difficulty swallowing, fever, drooling, anxiety *Danger of airway obstruction and asphyxia*	Stridor and a wet, barking cough Usually occurs at night Relieved by exposure to cold or moist air	Breathlessness, rapid, shallow breathing, wheezing, cough, and retractions of lower ribs and sternum during inspiration
Usual treatment	Hospitalization Intubation or tracheotomy Treatment with appropriate antibiotic	Hydration Mist tent or vaporizer Administration of oxygen Nebulized epinephrine	Supportive treatment, administration of oxygen and hydration

viral prodrome, it is thought that it may have an allergic origin. Spasmodic croup characteristically occurs at night and tends to recur with respiratory tract infections. The episode usually lasts several hours and may recur several nights in a row.

Most children with spasmodic croup can be effectively managed at home. An environment of high humidification (*i.e.*, cold-water room humidifier or taking the child into a bathroom with a warm, running shower) lessens irritation and prevents drying of secretions.

Epiglottitis. Acute epiglottitis is a dramatic, potentially fatal condition that is characterized by inflammatory edema of the supraglottic area, including the epiglottis and pharyngeal structures (see Fig. 21-10), and that comes on suddenly, bringing danger of airway obstruction and asphyxia.[59,60] In the past, the *H. influenzae* type B bacterium was the most commonly identified etiology. It is seen less commonly since the widespread use of immunization against *H. influenzae* type B. Therefore, other agents such as *Streptococcus pyogenes*, *S. pneumoniae*, and *S. aureus* now represent the most common cause of pediatric epiglottitis.[59]

The child appears pale, toxic, and lethargic and assumes a distinctive position—sitting up with the mouth open and the chin thrust forward. There is difficulty in swallowing, a muffled voice, drooling, fever, and extreme anxiety. Moderate to severe respiratory distress is evident. There is inspiratory and sometimes expiratory stridor, flaring of the nares, and inspiratory retractions of the suprasternal notch and supraclavicular and intercostal spaces. Within a matter of hours, epiglottitis may progress to complete obstruction of the airway and death unless adequate treatment is instituted. Epiglottitis is a medical emergency and immediate establishment of an airway by endotracheal tube or tracheotomy usually is needed. If

epiglottitis is suspected, the child should never be forced to lie down because this causes the epiglottis to fall backward and may lead to complete airway obstruction. Examination of the throat with a tongue blade or other instrument may cause cardiopulmonary arrest and should be done only by medical personnel experienced in intubation of small children. It also is unwise to attempt any procedure, such as drawing blood, that would heighten the child's anxiety because this also could precipitate airway spasm and cause death. Recovery from epiglottitis usually is rapid and uneventful after an adequate airway has been established and appropriate antibiotic therapy has been initiated.

Lower Airway Infections

Lower airway infections produce air trapping with prolonged expiration. Wheezing results from bronchospasm, mucosal inflammation, and edema. The child presents with increased expiratory effort, increased respiratory rate, and wheezing. If the infection is severe, there also are marked intercostal retractions and signs of impending respiratory failure.

Acute bronchiolitis is a viral infection of the lower airways (see Fig. 21-10), most commonly caused by the respiratory syncytial virus.[62,63] Other viruses, such as parainfluenza 3 virus and some adenoviruses, as well as mycoplasmas, also are causative. The infection produces inflammatory obstruction of the small airways and necrosis of the cells lining the lower airways. It usually occurs during the first 2 years of life, with a peak incidence between 3 to 6 months of age. The source of infection usually is a family member with a minor respiratory illness. Older children and adults tolerate bronchiolar edema much better than infants and do not manifest the clinical picture of bronchiolitis. Because the resistance to airflow in a tube is related to the fourth power of the radius, even minor swelling of bronchioles in an infant can produce profound changes in airflow.

Most affected infants in whom bronchiolitis develops have a history of a mild upper respiratory tract infection. These symptoms usually last several days and may be accompanied by fever and diminished appetite. There is then a gradual development of respiratory distress, characterized by a wheezy cough, dyspnea, and irritability. The infant usually is able to take in sufficient air but has trouble exhaling it. Air becomes trapped in the lung distal to the site of obstruction and interferes with gas exchange. Hypoxemia and, in severe cases, hypercapnia may develop. Airway obstruction may produce air trapping and hyperinflation of the lungs or collapse of the alveoli. Infants with acute bronchiolitis have a typical appearance, marked by breathlessness with rapid respirations, a distressing cough, and retractions of the lower ribs and sternum. Crying and feeding exaggerate these signs. Wheezing and rales may or may not be present, depending on the degree of airway obstruction. In infants with severe airway obstruction, wheezing decreases as the airflow diminishes. Usually, the most critical phase of the disease is the first 48 to 72 hours. Cyanosis, pallor, listlessness, and sudden diminution or absence of breath sounds indicate impending respiratory failure. The characteristics of bronchiolitis are described in Table 21-2.

Infants with respiratory distress usually are hospitalized. Treatment is supportive and includes administration of humidified oxygen to relieve hypoxia. Elevation of the head facilitates respiratory movements and avoids airway compression. Handling is kept at a minimum to avoid tiring. Because the infection is viral, antibiotics are not effective and are given only for a secondary bacterial infection. Dehydration may occur as the result of increased insensible water losses because of the rapid respiratory rate and feeding difficulties, and measures to ensure adequate hydration are needed. Recovery usually begins after the first 48 to 72 hours and usually is rapid and complete.

Signs of Impending Respiratory Failure

Respiratory problems of infants and small children often begin suddenly, and recovery usually is rapid and complete. Children are at risk for the development of airway obstruction and respiratory failure resulting from obstructive disorders or lung infection. The child with epiglottitis is at risk for airway obstruction. The child with bronchiolitis is at risk for respiratory failure resulting from impaired gas exchange. Children with impending respiratory failure due to airway or lung disease have rapid breathing, exaggerated use of the accessory muscles, retractions that are more pronounced in the child than in the adult because of a more compliant chest, nasal flaring, and grunting during expiration.[64] The signs and symptoms of impending respiratory failure are listed in Chart 21-1.

Respiratory failure can result from central nervous system conditions such as narcotic overdose or brain tumor that cause a decreased ventilatory drive and hypoventilation.

CHART 21-1

Signs of Respiratory Distress and Impending Respiratory Failure in the Infant and Small Child

Severe increase in respiratory effort, including severe retractions or grunting, decreased chest movement

Cyanosis that is not relieved by administration of oxygen (40%)

Heart rate of 150 per minute or greater and increasing

Bradycardia

Very rapid breathing (rate 60 per minute in the newborn to 6 months or above 30 per minute in children 6 months to 2 years)

Very depressed breathing (rate 20 per minute or below)

Retractions of the supraclavicular area, sternum, epigastrium, and intercostal spaces

Extreme anxiety and agitation

Fatigue

Decreased level of consciousness

In summary, although other body systems are physiologically ready for extrauterine life as early as 25 weeks of gestation, the lungs take longer. It is also during this period that type II alveolar cells, which produce surfactant, begin to function. Lung development is incomplete at birth; an infant is born with only one-eighth to one-sixth the adult number of alveoli. Alveoli continue to be formed during early childhood, reaching the adult number of 300 million alveoli by 5 to 6 years of age.

Most lung diseases in infants and children produce a decrease in lung compliance with manifestations of restrictive lung disease. They breathe at faster rates and their respiratory excursions are shallow. An *expiratory grunt* is common as the child tries to raise the functional residual capacity by closing the glottis at the end of expiration. *Nasal flaring* helps reduce the nasal resistance and maintain airway patency. *Inspiratory retractions,* or pulling in of the soft tissue surrounding the cartilaginous and bony thorax, is often observed with airway obstruction in infants and small children. Obstruction of the extrathoracic airways often produces turbulence of airflow and an audible inspiratory crowing sound called *stridor,* and obstruction of the intrathoracic airways produces an audible expiratory wheezing or whistling sound.

The neonatal period is one of transition from placental dependence to air breathing. Respiratory disorders develop in infants who are born prematurely or have other problems that impair this transition. RDS is one of the most common causes of respiratory disease in premature infants. In these infants, pulmonary immaturity, together with surfactant deficiency, lead to decreased lung compliance, atelectasis, hypoxia, decreased pulmonary perfusion, and formation of a hyaline membrane. BPD is a chronic pulmonary disease that develops in premature infants who were treated with mechanical ventilation.

Acute respiratory infections are the most common cause of illness in infancy and childhood. Because of the small size of the airway of infants and children, infections that may cause only a sore throat and hoarseness in the adult may produce serious obstruction in the child. Among the respiratory tract infections that affect small children are croup, epiglottitis, and bronchiolitis. Croup or acute laryngotracheobronchitis is a viral infection that affects the larynx, trachea, and bronchi. Epiglottitis is a life-threatening supraglottic infection that may cause airway obstruction and asphyxia. Acute bronchiolitis is a viral infection of the lower airways, most commonly caused by the respiratory syncytial virus.

Review Exercises

It is influenza season, and although you had a flu shot last year, you have not had one this year. Imagine yourself experiencing the abrupt onset of fever, chills, malaise, muscle aching, and nasal stuffiness.

A. Which of these symptoms would lead you to believe you are coming down with the flu?
B. Because you have to miss class, you decide to go to the student health center and obtain an antibiotic. After being seen by the health professional, you are told that antibiotics are ineffective against the influenza virus, and you are instructed not to attend classes but instead go home, take acetaminophen for your fever, go to bed and stay warm, and drink a lot of fluid. Explain the rationale for each of these recommendations.
C. Explain why last year's flu shot did not protect you during this year's flu season. There is current concern about the possibility of an influenza pandemic such as occurred during the 1917–1918 season. What is the rationale for this concern?

A nurse working in an extended care facility finds out that the tuberculin skin test she had is positive. The test she had done a year ago was negative.

A. Explain what this means in terms of recency of exposure to *M. tuberculosis*. Does she have tuberculosis?

Bacterial (*e.g., Streptococcus pneumoniae*) pneumonia is commonly manifested by a cough productive of sputum, whereas with atypical (*e.g., Mycoplasma pneumoniae*) pneumonia, the cough is usually nonproductive or absent.

A. Explain.

A 4-month-old infant is admitted to the pediatric intensive care unit with a diagnosis of bronchiolitis. The infant is tachypneic, with wheezing, nasal flaring, and retractions of the lower sternum and intercostal spaces during inspiration.

A. What is the usual pathogen in bronchiolitis? Would this infection be treated with an antibiotic?
B. Explain the physiologic mechanism involved in the retraction of the lower sternum and intercostal spaces during inspiration.
C. What would be the signs of impending respiratory failure in this infant?

Visit the Porth: Essentials of Pathophysiology: Concepts of Altered Health States web site (http://thePoint.LWW.com/PorthEssentials) for links to chapter-related resources on the Internet, all-new exclusive animations, chapter review questions, and more!

REFERENCES

1. McAdam A. J., Sharpe A. H. (2005). Infectious diseases. In Kumar V., Abbas A. K., Fausto N. (Eds.), *Robbins and Cotran pathologic basis of disease* (7th ed., p. 353). Philadelphia: Elsevier Saunders.
2. Kirkpatrick G. L. (1996). The common cold. *Primary Care* 23, 657–673.
3. Heikkinen T., Järvinsen A. (2003). The common cold. *Lancet* 361, 51–59.
4. Greenberg S. B. (2003). Respiratory consequences of rhinovirus infection. *Archives of Internal Medicine* 163, 278–284.
5. Goldman D. A. (2000). Transmission of viral respiratory tract infections in the home. *Pediatric Infectious Disease Journal* 19, S97–S10.
6. Osguthorpe J. D. (2001). Adult rhinosinusitis: Diagnosis and management. *American Family Physician* 63, 69–76.
7. Dykewicz M. S. (2003). Rhinitis and sinusitis. *Journal of Allergy and Clinical Immunology* 111, S520–S539.
8. Winstead W. (2003). Rhinosinusitis. *Primary Care in Clinical Office Practice* 30, 137–154.

9. Piccirillo J. F. (2004). Acute bacterial sinusitis. *New England Journal of Medicine* 351, 902–910.

10. Advisory Committee on Immunization Practices. (2003). Prevention and control of influenza: Recommendations of the Advisory Committee on Immunization Practices (ACIP). *MMWR Morbidity and Mortality Weekly Report* 52(RR-8), 1–20.

11. Moorman J. P. (2003). Viral characteristics of influenza. *Southern Medical Journal* 96, 758–761.

12. Musher D. M. (2003). How contagious are common respiratory infections? *New England Journal of Medicine* 348, 1256–1266.

13. Shorman M., Moorman J. P. (2003). Clinical manifestations and diagnosis of influenza. *Southern Medical Journal* 96, 737–739.

14. Olshaker J. S. (2003). Influenza. *Emergency Medicine Clinics of North America* 21, 353–361.

15. Khater F., Moorman J. P. (2003). Complications of influenza. *Southern Medical Journal* 96, 740–743.

16. Montal N. J. (2003). An office-based approach to influenza: Clinical diagnosis and laboratory testing. *American Family Physician* 67, 111–118.

17. Stiver G. (2003). The treatment of influenza with antiviral drugs. *Canadian Medical Association Journal* 168, 49–57.

18. Myers J. W. (2003). Influenza therapy. *Southern Medical Journal* 96, 744–749.

19. Palese P., Garcia-Sastre A. (2002). Influenza vaccines: Present and future. *Journal of Clinical Investigation* 110, 9–13.

20. Advisory Committee on Immunization Practices. (2003). Using live attenuated influenza vaccine for prevention and control of influenza. *MMWR Morbidity and Mortality Weekly Report* 52 (RR-13), 1–8.

21. Maitra A., Kumar V. (2003). The lung and upper respiratory tract. In Kumar V., Cotran R. S., Robbins S. L. (Eds.), *Robbins basic pathology* (7th ed., pp. 478–495). Philadelphia: Elsevier Saunders.

22. Travis W. D., Beasley M. B., Rubin E. (2005). The respiratory system. In Rubin E., Gorstein F., Rubin R., et al. (Eds.), *Rubin's pathology: Clinicopathologic foundations of medicine* (4th ed., pp. 592–599). Philadelphia: Lippincott Williams & Wilkins.

23. Chestnutt M. S., Prendergast T. J. (2004). Lung. In Tierney L. M., McPhee S. J., Papadakis M. A. (Eds.), *Current medical diagnosis and treatment* (43rd ed., pp. 241–259). New York: Lange Medical Books/McGraw-Hill.

24. Neiderman M. S., Mandell L. A., Co-chairs. (2001). American Thoracic Society guidelines for the initial management of adults with community-acquired pneumonia. *American Journal of Respiratory and Critical Care Medicine* 163, 1730–1754.

25. Halm E. A., Teirstein A. S. (2002). Management of community-acquired pneumonia. *New England Journal of Medicine* 347, 2039–2045.

26. McEachen R., Campbell G. D. (1998). Hospital-acquired pneumonia: Epidemiology, etiology, and treatment. *Infectious Disease Clinics of North America* 12, 761–779.

27. Collin B. A., Ramphal R. (1998). Pneumonia in the compromised host including cancer patients and transplant patients. *Infectious Disease Clinics of North America* 12, 781–801.

28. Catterall J. R. (1999). *Streptococcus pneumoniae*. *Thorax* 54, 929–937.

29. Centers for Disease Control and Prevention. (1996). Prevention of pneumococcal disease: Recommendations of the Advisory Committee on Immunization Practices (ACIP). *MMWR Morbidity and Mortality Weekly Report* 46(RR-8), 1–24.

30. Centers for Disease Control and Prevention. (2000). Preventing pneumococcal disease among infants and small children: Recommendations of the Advisory Committee on Immunization

Practices (ACIP). *MMWR Morbidity and Mortality Weekly Report* 46(RR-9), 1–38.

31. Stout J. E., Yu V. C. (1997). Legionellosis. *New England Journal of Medicine* 337, 682–688.

32. American Lung Association Research and Scientific Affairs Epidemiology and Statistics Unit. (2003). Trends in tuberculosis morbidity and mortality. [On-line]. Available: www. lungusa.org.

33. McAdam A. J., Sharpe A. H. (2005). Infectious diseases. In Kumar V., Cotran R. S., Robbins S. L. (Eds.), *Robbins basic pathology* (7th ed., pp. 381–386). Philadelphia: Elsevier Saunders.

34. Schwartz D., Genta D. M., Connor D. H. (2005). Infectious and parasitic diseases. In Rubin E., Gorstein F., Rubin R., et al. (Eds.), *Rubin's pathology: Clinicopathologic foundations of medicine* (4th ed., pp. 421–427). Philadelphia: Lippincott Williams & Wilkins.

35. Jasmer R. M., Nahid P., Hopewell P. C. (2002). Latent tuberculosis infection. *New England Journal of Medicine* 347, 1860–1866.

36. American Thoracic Society and Centers for Disease Control and Prevention. (2000). Diagnostic standards and classification of tuberculosis in adults and children. *American Review of Respiratory Disease* 161, 1376–1395.

37. Barnes P. F., Cave M. D. (2003). Molecular epidemiology of tuberculosis. *New England Journal of Medicine* 349, 1149–1156.

38. American Thoracic Society, Centers for Disease Control and Prevention, and Infectious Diseases Society of America. (2003). Treatment of tuberculosis. *MMWR Morbidity and Mortality Weekly Report* 52(RR-11), 1–14.

39. Spiegler P., Ilowitz J. (1999). Multiple-drug-resistant tuberculosis: Parts 1 and 2. *Emergency Medicine* 31, 10–23.

40. Wheat L. J., Kauffman C. A. (2003). Histoplasmosis. *Infectious Disease Clinics of North America* 17, 1–19.

41. Hamill R. J. (2003). Infectious disease: Mycotic. In Tierney L. M., McPhee S. J., Papadakis M. A. (Eds.), *Current medical diagnosis and treatment* (42nd ed., pp. 1482–1494). New York: Lange Medical Books/McGraw-Hill.

42. Galgiani J. N. (1999). Coccidioidomycosis: A regional disease of national importance. *Annals of Internal Medicine* 130, 293–300.

43. Chiller T. M., Galgiani J. N., Stevens D. A. (2003). Coccidioidomycosis. *Infectious Disease Clinics of North America* 17, 41–57.

44. Bradsher R. W., Chapman S. W., Pappas P. G. (2003). Blastomycosis. *Infectious Disease Clinics of North America* 17, 21–40.

45. American Cancer Society. (2004). Lung cancer: Overview. [On-line]. Available: www.cancer.org

46. Thomas C. R., Williams T. E., Cobos E., et al. (2001). Lung cancer. In Lenhard R. E., Osteen R. T., Gansler T. (Eds.), *The American Cancer Society's clinical oncology* (pp. 269–295). Atlanta: American Cancer Society.

47. Hurria A. (2003). Management of lung cancer in older adults. *CA: A Cancer Journal for Clinicians* 53, 325–341.

48. Oklund S. H., Jett J. R. (2002). Small cell lung cancer: Current therapy and promising new regimens. *Oncologist* 7, 234–238.

49. Walker S. (2003). Updates in small cell lung cancer treatment. *Clinical Journal of Oncology Nursing* 7, 563–568.

50. Moore K., Persaud T. V. N. (2003). *The developing human* (6th ed., pp. 242–253). Philadelphia: Elsevier Saunders.

51. Haddad G. G., Fontán J. J. P. (2004). Development of the respiratory system. In Behrman R. E., Kliegman R. M., Jenson H. L. (Eds.), *Nelson textbook of pediatrics* (17th ed., pp. 1357–1362). Philadelphia: Elsevier Saunders.

52. Oski F. A. (Ed.). (1994). *Principles and practices of pediatrics* (2nd ed., pp. 336–339, 365–370). Philadelphia: J. B. Lippincott.

53. Fontán J. J. P., Haddad G. G. (2004). Respiratory pathophysiology. In Behrman R. E., Kliegman R. M., Jenson H. L. (Eds.), *Nelson textbook of pediatrics* (17th ed., pp. 1362–1367). Philadelphia: Elsevier Saunders.

54. Stoll B. J., Kliegman R. M. (2004). The fetus and neonatal infant. In Behrman R. E., Kliegman R. M., Jenson H. L. (Eds.), *Nelson textbook of pediatrics* (17th ed., pp. 573–583). Philadelphia: Elsevier Saunders.

55. Crocetti M., Barone M. A. (2004). In F. A. Oski (Ed.), *Oski's essential pediatrics* (2nd ed., pp. 33–55, 377–380). Philadelphia: Lippincott Williams & Wilkins.

56. McColley S. A. (1998). Bronchopulmonary dysplasia. *Pediatric Clinics of North America* 45, 573–585.

57. Jobe A. H., Bancalari E. (2001). Bronchopulmonary dysplasia. *American Journal of Respiratory and Critical Care* 163, 1723–1729.

58. Roosevelt G. E. (2004). Acute inflammatory upper airway obstruction. In Behrman R. E., Kiegman R. M., Jenson H. L. (Eds.), *Nelson textbook of pediatrics* (17th ed., pp. 1405–1409). Philadelphia: Elsevier Saunders.

59. Klassen T. P. (1999). Croup: A current perspective. *Pediatric Clinics of North American* 46, 1167–1177.

60. Knutson D., Aring A. (2004). Viral croup. *American Family Physician* 69, 535–542.

61. Wright R. B., Pomerantz W. J., Luria J. W. (2002). New approaches to respiratory infections in children. *Emergency Medicine Clinics of North America* 20, 93–111.

62. Rotta A. T., Wiryawan B. (2003). Respiratory emergencies in children. *Respiratory Care* 48, 248–258.

63. Steiner R. W. P, (2004). Treating acute bronchiolitis associated with RSV. *American Family Physician* 69, 325–330.

64. Frankel L. R. (2004). Respiratory distress and failure. In Behrman R. E., Kliegman R. M., Jenson H. L. (Eds.), *Nelson textbook of pediatrics* (17th ed., pp. 301–306). Philadelphia: Elsevier Saunders.

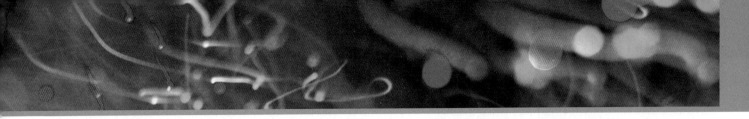

C h a p t e r *22*

Disorders of Ventilation and Gas Exchange

The major function of the lungs is to oxygenate and remove carbon dioxide from the blood as a means of supporting the metabolic functions of body cells. The gas exchange function of the lungs depends on a system of open airways, expansion of the lungs, an adequate area for gas diffusion, and blood flow that carries the gases to the rest of the body. The content in this chapter focuses on disorders of lung inflation, obstructive airway disorders, interstitial lung disease, pulmonary vascular disorders, and respiratory failure.

Disorders of Lung Inflation

Air entering through the airways inflates the lung, and the negative pressure in the pleural cavity keeps the lung from collapsing. Disorders of lung inflation are caused by conditions that produce lung compression or collapse. There can be compression of the lung by an accumulation of fluid in the intrapleural space, complete collapse of an entire lung as in pneumothorax, or collapse of a segment of the lung as in atelectasis.

DISORDERS OF THE PLEURA

The pleura is a thin, double-layered serous membrane that encases the lungs (Fig. 22-1). The outer *parietal layer* lines the thoracic wall and superior aspect of the diaphragm. It continues around the heart and between the lungs, forming the lateral walls of the mediastinum. The inner *visceral layer* covers the lung and is adherent to all its surfaces. It provides the lung with a slippery surface, enabling it to move freely on the parietal pleura. The pleural cavity or space between the two layers contains a thin layer of serous fluid, which lubricates the pleural surfaces and allows the pleurae to slide smoothly over each other during breathing movements. The pressure in the pleural cavity, which is negative in relation to atmospheric pressure,

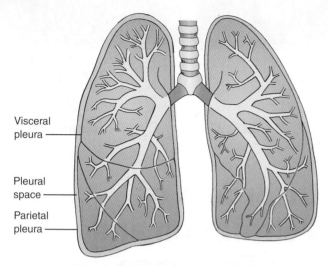

Visceral pleura

Pleural space

Parietal pleura

FIGURE 22-1 The relationship between the parietal and visceral pleurae and the pleural space, which is the site of fluid accumulation in pleural effusions.

holds the lungs against the chest wall and keeps them from collapsing (see Chapter 20). Disorders of the pleura include pleuritic chest pain, pleural effusion, and pneumothorax.

Pleuritic Chest Pain

Chest pain caused by respiratory diseases usually originates from involvement of the parietal pleura. Causes include primary pleural disorders, such as neoplasms or inflammatory disorders affecting the pleura, or pulmonary disorders that extend to the pleural surface, such as pneumonia. Most commonly the pain is abrupt in onset, such that the person experiencing it can cite almost to the minute when the pain started. It usually is unilateral and tends to be localized to the lower and lateral part of the chest. When the part of the pleura that covers the diaphragm is irritated, the pain may be referred to the shoulder. The pain is usually made worse by chest movements such as deep breathing and coughing that accentuate pressure changes in the pleural cavity and increase movement of the inflamed or injured pleural surfaces. Because deep breathing is painful, tidal volumes usually are kept small, and breathing becomes more rapid. Reflex splinting of the chest muscles may occur, causing a lesser respiratory excursion on the affected side.

It is important to differentiate pleural pain from pain produced by other conditions, such as musculoskeletal strain of chest muscles, bronchial irritation, and myocardial disease. Musculoskeletal pain may occur as the result of frequent, forceful coughing. This type of pain usually is bilateral and located in the inferior portions of the rib cage, where the abdominal muscles insert into the anterior rib cage. It is made worse by movements associated with contraction of the abdominal muscles. The pain associated with irritation of the bronchi usually is substernal and dull, rather than sharp. It is made worse with coughing but is not affected by deep breathing. Myocardial pain, which is discussed in Chapter 18, usually is located

in the substernal area and is not affected by respiratory movements.

Pleural Effusion

Pleural effusion refers to an abnormal collection of fluid in the pleural cavity. The fluid may be a transudate, exudate, purulent drainage (empyema), chyle, or blood. Normally, only a thin layer (<10 to 20 mL) of serous fluid separates the visceral and parietal layers of the pleural cavity. Like fluid developing in other transcellular spaces in the body, pleural effusion occurs when the rate of fluid formation exceeds the rate of its removal (see Chapter 6). Five mechanisms have been linked to the abnormal collection of fluid in the pleural cavity: (1) increased capillary pressure, as in congestive heart failure; (2) increased capillary permeability, which occurs with inflammatory conditions; (3) decreased colloidal osmotic pressure, such as the hypoalbuminemia occurring with liver disease and nephrosis; (4) increased negative intrapleural pressure, which develops with atelectasis; and (5) impaired lymphatic drainage of the pleural space, which results from obstructive processes such as mediastinal carcinoma.

The accumulation of a serous transudate (clear fluid) in the pleural cavity often is referred to as *hydrothorax*. The condition may be unilateral or bilateral. The most common cause of hydrothorax is congestive heart failure.[1] Other causes are renal failure, nephrosis, liver failure, and malignancy. An *exudate* is a pleural fluid that has a specific gravity greater than 1.020 and, often, inflammatory cells. Conditions that produce exudative pleural effusions are infections, pulmonary infarction, malignancies, rheumatoid arthritis, and lupus erythematosus.

Empyema refers to purulent drainage (pus) in the pleural cavity. It is caused by direct infection of the pleural space from an adjacent bacterial pneumonia, rupture of a lung abscess into the pleural space, invasion from a subdiaphragmatic infection, or infection associated with trauma.

Chylothorax represents the effusion of lymph in the thoracic cavity.[2] Chyle, a milky fluid containing chylomicrons (fat-carrying lipoproteins), is found in the lymph fluid originating in the gastrointestinal tract. Chylothorax can result from trauma, inflammation, or malignant infiltration of the thoracic duct that transports chyle to the central circulation (see Chapter 16, Fig. 16-21). It also can occur as a complication of intrathoracic surgical procedures and use of the great veins for total parenteral nutrition and hemodynamic monitoring.

Hemothorax is the presence of blood in the pleural cavity. Bleeding may arise from chest injury, a complication of chest surgery, malignancies, or rupture of a great vessel such as an aortic aneurysm. It is usually diagnosed by the presence of blood in the pleural fluid. Hemothorax usually requires drainage, and if the bleeding continues, surgery to control the bleeding may be required.

The manifestations of pleural effusion vary with the cause. Hemothorax may be accompanied by signs of blood loss and empyema by fever and other signs of inflammation. Fluid in the pleural cavity acts as a space-occupying mass; it causes a decrease in lung expansion on the affected side that is proportional to the amount of fluid that is present. The effusion may cause a shift in the mediastinal structures toward the opposite side of the chest with a decrease in lung volume on that side as well as the side with the pneumothorax. Characteristic signs of pleural effusion are dullness or flatness to percussion and diminished breath sounds. Dyspnea, the most common symptom, occurs when fluid compresses the lung, resulting in decreased ventilation. Pleuritic pain usually occurs only when inflammation is present, although constant discomfort may be felt with large effusions. Mild hypoxemia may occur and usually is corrected with supplemental oxygen.

Diagnosis of pleural effusion is based on chest radiographs, chest ultrasonography, and computed tomography (CT) scans. Thoracentesis is the aspiration of fluid from the pleural space. It can be used to obtain a sample of pleural fluid for diagnosis, or it can be used for therapeutic purposes. The treatment of pleural effusion is directed at the cause of the disorder. With large effusions, thoracentesis may be used to remove fluid from the intrapleural space and allow for reexpansion of the lung. A palliative method used for treatment of pleural effusions caused by a malignancy is the injection of a sclerosing agent into the pleural cavity. This method of treatment causes obliteration of the pleural space and prevents the reaccumulation of fluid. Open surgical drainage may be necessary in cases of continued effusion.

Pneumothorax

Normally, the pleural cavity is free of air and contains only a thin layer of fluid. When air enters the pleural cavity, it is called *pneumothorax*. Pneumothorax causes partial or complete collapse of the affected lung. Pneumothorax can occur without an obvious cause or injury (*i.e.,* spontaneous pneumothorax) or as a result of direct injury to the chest wall or major airways (*i.e.,* traumatic pneumothorax). Tension pneumothorax describes a life-threatening condition of excessive pressure in the pleural cavity.

Spontaneous Pneumothorax. Spontaneous pneumothorax occurs when an air-filled bleb, or blister, on the lung surface ruptures. Rupture of these blebs allows atmospheric air from the airways to enter the pleural cavity (Fig. 22-2). Because alveolar pressure normally is greater than pleural pressure, air flows from the alveoli into the pleural space, causing the involved portion of the lung to collapse as a result of its own recoil. Air continues to flow into the pleural space until a pressure gradient no longer exists or until the decline in lung size causes the leak to seal. Spontaneous pneumothoraces can be divided into primary and secondary pneumothoraces.[3] Primary spontaneous pneumothorax occurs in otherwise healthy persons. Secondary spontaneous pneumothorax occurs in persons with underlying lung disease.

In primary spontaneous pneumothorax, the air-filled bleb that ruptures is usually on the top of the lung. The condition is seen most often in tall boys and young men between 10 and 30 years of age.[3] It has been suggested that the difference in pleural pressure from the top to the

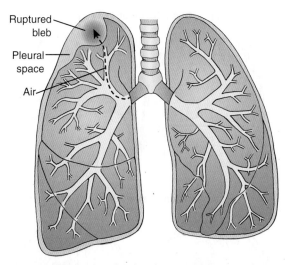

FIGURE 22-2 Mechanism for development of spontaneous pneumothorax in which an air-filled bleb on the surface of the lung ruptures, allowing atmospheric air to enter the pleural space.

bottom of the lung is greater in tall persons and that this difference in pressure may contribute to the development of blebs. Another factor that has been associated with primary spontaneous pneumothorax is smoking. Disease of the small airways related to smoking probably contributes to the condition.

Secondary spontaneous pneumothoraces usually are more serious because they occur in persons with lung disease. They are associated with many different types of lung conditions that cause trapping of gases and destruction of lung tissue, including asthma, tuberculosis, cystic fibrosis, sarcoidosis, bronchogenic carcinoma, and metastatic pleural diseases. The most common cause of secondary spontaneous pneumothorax is emphysema.

Traumatic Pneumothorax. Traumatic pneumothorax may be caused by penetrating or nonpenetrating chest injuries. Fractured or dislocated ribs that penetrate the pleura are the most common cause of pneumothorax from nonpenetrating chest injuries. Hemothorax often accompanies these injuries. Pneumothorax also may accompany fracture of the trachea or major bronchus or rupture of the esophagus. Persons with pneumothorax caused by chest trauma frequently have other complications and may require chest surgery. Medical procedures such as transthoracic needle aspirations, intubation, and positive-pressure ventilation occasionally may cause pneumothorax. Traumatic pneumothorax also can occur as a complication of cardiopulmonary resuscitation.

Tension Pneumothorax. Tension pneumothorax occurs when the intrapleural pressure exceeds atmospheric pressure. It is a life-threatening condition and occurs when injury to the chest or respiratory structures permits air to enter but not leave the pleural space (Fig. 22-3). This results in a rapid increase in pressure in the chest with a compression atelectasis of the unaffected lung, a shift in the mediastinum to the opposite side of the chest, and compression of the vena cava with impairment of venous return

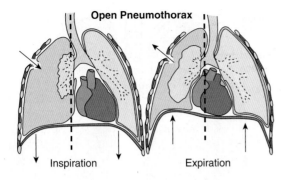

Open Pneumothorax

Inspiration   Expiration

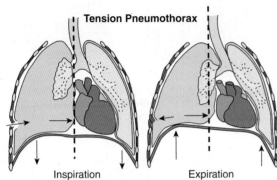

Tension Pneumothorax

Inspiration   Expiration

FIGURE 22-3 Open or communicating pneumothorax (**top**) and tension pneumothorax (**bottom**). In an open pneumothorax, air enters the chest during inspiration and exits during expiration. There may be slight inflation of the affected lung because of a decrease in pressure as air moves out of the chest. In tension pneumothorax, air can enter but not leave the chest. As the pressure in the chest increases, the heart and great vessels are compressed and the mediastinal structures are shifted toward the opposite side of the chest. The trachea is pushed from its normal midline position toward the opposite side of the chest, and the unaffected lung is compressed.

to the heart.[4] Although tension pneumothorax can develop in persons with spontaneous pneumothoraces, it is seen most often in persons with traumatic pneumothoraces.

With tension pneumothorax, the structures in the mediastinal space shift toward the opposite side of the chest (see Fig. 22-3). When this occurs, the position of the trachea, normally located in the midline of the neck, deviates with the mediastinum. There may be distention of the neck veins, subcutaneous emphysema (*i.e.*, air bubbles in the subcutaneous tissues of the chest and neck), and clinical signs of shock.

Clinical Features. The manifestations of pneumothorax depend on its size and the integrity of the underlying lung. In spontaneous pneumothorax, manifestations of the disorder include development of ipsilateral (same side) chest pain in an otherwise healthy person. There is an almost immediate increase in respiratory rate, often accompanied by dyspnea that occurs as a result of the activation of receptors that monitor lung volume. Heart rate is increased. Asymmetry of chest movement may occur because of the air trapped in the pleural cavity on the affected side. Percussion of the chest produces a more

hyperresonant sound, and breath sounds are decreased or absent over the area of the pneumothorax.

Hypoxemia usually develops immediately after a large pneumothorax, followed by vasoconstriction of the blood vessels in the affected lung, causing the blood flow to shift to the unaffected lung. In persons with primary spontaneous pneumothorax, this mechanism usually returns oxygen saturation to normal within 24 hours. Hypoxemia usually is more serious in persons with underlying lung disease in whom secondary spontaneous pneumothorax develops. In these persons, the hypoxemia caused by the partial or total loss of lung function can be life threatening.

Diagnosis of pneumothorax can be confirmed by chest radiograph or CT scan. Blood gas analysis may be done to determine the effect of the condition on blood oxygen levels. Treatment varies with the cause and extent of the disorder. Even without treatment, air in the pleural space usually reabsorbs after the pleural leak seals. In small spontaneous pneumothoraces, the air usually reabsorbs, and observation and follow-up chest radiographs are all that is required. Supplemental oxygen may be used to increase the rate at which the air is reabsorbed. In larger pneumothoraces, the air is removed by needle aspiration or a closed drainage system used with or without an aspiration pump. This type of drainage system uses a one-way valve or a tube submerged in water to allow air to exit the pleural space and prevent it from re-entering the chest. In traumatic pneumothoraces, surgical closure of the chest wall defect, ruptured airway, or perforated esophagus may be required.

Emergency treatment of tension pneumothorax involves the prompt insertion of a large-bore needle or chest tube into the affected side of the chest along with one-way valve drainage or continuous chest suction to aid in lung expansion. Sucking chest wounds, which allow air to pass in and out of the chest cavity, should be treated by promptly covering the area with an airtight covering. Chest tubes are inserted as soon as possible.

ATELECTASIS

Atelectasis refers to the incomplete expansion of a lung or portion of a lung. It can be caused by airway obstruction, lung compression such as occurs in pneumothorax or pleural effusion, or the increased recoil of the lung caused by inadequate pulmonary surfactant (see Chapter 20).

Atelectasis is caused most commonly by airway obstruction (Fig. 22-4). Obstruction can be caused by a mucus plug in the airway or by external compression by fluid, tumor mass, exudate, or other matter in the area surrounding the airway. A small segment of lung or an entire lung lobe may be involved in obstructive atelectasis. Complete obstruction of an airway is followed by the absorption of air from the dependent alveoli and collapse of that portion of the lung. The danger of obstructive atelectasis increases after surgery. Anesthesia, pain, administration of narcotics, and immobility tend to promote retention of viscid bronchial secretions and thus airway obstruction.

Another cause of atelectasis is compression of lung tissue. It occurs when the pleural cavity is partially or com-

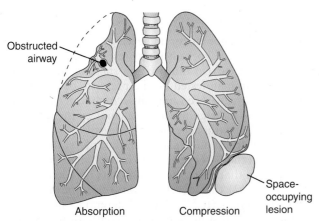

Obstructed airway

Absorption   Compression

Space-occupying lesion

FIGURE 22-4 Atelectasis caused by airway obstruction and absorption of air from the involved lung area (**left**) and by compression of lung tissue (**right**).

pletely filled with fluid, exudate, blood, a tumor mass, or air. It is observed most commonly in persons with pleural effusion from congestive heart failure or cancer. In compression atelectasis, the mediastinum shifts away from the affected lung.

The clinical manifestations of atelectasis include tachypnea, tachycardia, dyspnea, cyanosis, signs of hypoxemia, diminished chest expansion, absence of breath sounds, and intercostal retractions. Fever and other signs of infection may develop. Both chest expansion and breath sounds are decreased on the affected side. There may be intercostal retraction (pulling in of the intercostal spaces) over the involved area during inspiration. If the collapsed area is large, the mediastinum and trachea shift to the affected side. Signs of respiratory distress are proportional to the extent of lung collapse.

The diagnosis of atelectasis is based on signs and symptoms. Chest radiographs are used to confirm the diagnosis. CT scans may be used to show the exact location of the obstruction. Treatment depends on the cause and extent of lung involvement. It is directed at reducing the airway obstruction or lung compression and at reinflating the collapsed area of the lung. Ambulation and body positions that favor increased lung expansion are used when appropriate. Administration of oxygen may be needed to treat the hypoxemia. Bronchoscopy may be used as a diagnostic and treatment method.

In summary, lung inflation depends on a negative intrapleural pressure and unobstructed intrapulmonary airways. Disorders of the pleura include pleuritic chest pain, pleural effusion, and pneumothorax. Pain is commonly associated with conditions that produce inflammation of the pleura. Characteristically, it is unilateral, abrupt in onset, and exaggerated by respiratory movements. Pleural effusion refers to the abnormal accumulation of fluid in the pleural cavity. The fluid may be a transudate (*i.e.*, hydrothorax), exudate (*i.e.*, empyema),

blood (*i.e.*, hemothorax), or chyle (*i.e.*, chylothorax). Pneumothorax refers to an accumulation of air in the pleural cavity with the partial or complete collapse of the lung. It can result from rupture of an air-filled bleb on the lung surface or from penetrating or nonpenetrating injuries. A tension pneumothorax is a life-threatening event in which air progressively accumulates in the thorax, collapsing the lung on the injured side and progressively shifting the mediastinum to the opposite side of the thorax, producing severe cardiorespiratory impairment.

Atelectasis refers to an incomplete expansion of the lung. In adults, atelectasis usually results from airway obstruction caused by a mucus plug or external compression by fluid, tumor mass, exudate, or other matter in the area surrounding the airway.

Obstructive Airway Disorders

Obstructive airway diseases are caused by disorders that increase the resistance to airflow. Bronchial asthma represents a reversible form of airway disease caused by narrowing of airways due to bronchospasm, inflammation, and increased airway secretions. Chronic obstructive airway disease can be caused by a variety of airway diseases, including chronic bronchitis, emphysema, bronchiectasis, and cystic fibrosis.

PHYSIOLOGY OF AIRWAY DISEASE

Air moves through the upper airways (*i.e.*, trachea and major bronchi) into the lower or pulmonary airways (*i.e.*, bronchi and alveoli), which are located in the lung. In the pulmonary airways, the cartilaginous layer that provides support for the trachea and major bronchi gradually disappears and is replaced with crisscrossing strips of smooth muscle (see Chapter 20). The contraction and relaxation of the smooth muscle layer, which is innervated by the autonomic nervous system (ANS), controls the diameter of the pulmonary airways and consequent resistance to airflow. Parasympathetic stimulation, through the vagus nerve and cholinergic receptors, produces bronchoconstriction, and sympathetic stimulation, through β_2-adrenergic receptors, increases bronchodilation. Normally, a slight vagal-mediated bronchoconstrictor tone predominates. When there is need for increased airflow, as during exercise, the vagal-mediated bronchoconstrictor tone is inhibited, and the bronchodilator effects of the sympathetic nervous system are increased. Bronchial smooth muscle also responds to inflammatory mediators, such as histamine, that act directly on smooth muscle cells to produce bronchoconstriction.

BRONCHIAL ASTHMA

Bronchial asthma is a chronic disorder of the airways that causes episodes of airway obstruction, bronchial hyperresponsiveness, and airway inflammation that usually

KEY CONCEPTS

Airway Disorders

→ Airway disorders affect the movement of gases into and out of the lung. They involve bronchial smooth muscle tone, mucosal injury, and obstruction due to secretions.

→ The tone of the bronchial smooth muscles surrounding the airways determines airway radius, and the presence or absence of airway secretions influences airway patency.

→ Bronchial smooth muscle is innervated by the autonomic nervous system—the parasympathetic nervous system, via the vagus nerve, produces bronchoconstriction and the sympathetic nervous system produces bronchodilation.

→ Inflammatory mediators that are released in response to environmental irritants, immune responses, and infectious agents increase airway responsiveness by producing bronchospasm, increasing mucus secretion, and producing injury to the mucosal lining of the airways.

are reversible.[5,6] According to 2001 data, an estimated 20.3 million Americans have been diagnosed with asthma.[5] Although the prevalence rates for asthma have increased over the past several decades, the mortality rate and hospitalizations due to asthma have plateaued during the last few years, indicating a higher level of disease management.

The National Heart, Lung, and Blood Institute's Second Expert Panel on the Management of Asthma defined bronchial asthma as "a chronic inflammatory disorder of the airways in which many cells and cellular elements play a role, in particular, mast cells, eosinophils, T lymphocytes, and epithelial cells."[6] This inflammatory process produces recurrent episodes of airway obstruction, characterized by wheezing, breathlessness, chest tightness, and a cough that often is worse at night and in the early morning. These episodes, which usually are reversible either spontaneously or with treatment, also cause an associated increase in bronchial responsiveness to a variety of stimuli.[6]

In susceptible persons, an asthma attack can be triggered by a variety of stimuli that do not normally cause symptoms. Typically, asthma has been categorized into extrinsic asthma (initiated by a type I hypersensitivity [atopic] response to an extrinsic antigen) and intrinsic asthma (initiated by diverse nonimmune mechanisms, including respiratory tract infections, exercise, ingestion of aspirin, emotional upset, and exposure to bronchial irritants such as cigarette smoke).[7] Although this distinction is useful from a pathophysiologic point of view, it is less useful clinically because many persons with asthma manifest overlapping characteristics of both extrinsic and intrinsic asthma.

Pathogenesis

The common denominator underlying all forms of asthma is an exaggerated hypersensitivity response to a variety of stimuli. Most current information suggests that airway inflammation manifested by the presence of inflammatory cells (particularly eosinophils, lymphocytes, and mast cells) and by damage to the bronchial epithelium contributes to the pathogenesis of the disease.

Recent interest has focused on the role of the T lymphocytes in the pathogenesis of bronchial asthma. It is now known that there are two subsets of T helper cells (T_H1 and T_H2) that develop from the same precursor CD4+ T lymphocyte.[7] T_H1 cells differentiate in response to microbes and stimulate the differentiation of B cells into immunoglobulin M (IgM)- and IgG-producing plasma cells, whereas T_H2 cells respond to allergens and helminths (intestinal parasites) by stimulating differentiation of B cells into IgE-producing plasma cells, acting as growth factors for mast cells, and recruiting and activating eosinophils (see Chapter 15, Fig. 15-1). It appears that in persons with allergic asthma, T-cell differentiation is skewed toward T_H2 cells. Although the molecular basis for this preferential differentiation is unclear, it seems likely that both genetic and environmental factors play a role.

Extrinsic (Atopic) Asthma. Extrinsic or atopic asthma is typically initiated by a type I hypersensitivity reaction induced by exposure to an extrinsic antigen or allergen.[7–10] It usually has its onset in childhood or adolescence and is seen in persons with a family history of atopic allergy (see Chapter 15). Candidate genes for predisposition to atopy and airway hyperresponsiveness are currently subjects for intensive research and include genes involved in antigen presentation, T-cell activation, regulation of cytokine production or function, and receptors for bronchodilating substances.[7]

Persons with atopic asthma often have other allergic disorders, such as hay fever, hives, and eczema. Attacks are related to exposure to specific allergens. Among airborne allergens implicated in perennial (year-round) asthma are house dust mite allergens, cockroach allergens, animal danders, and the fungus *Alternaria*.

The mechanisms of response to antigens in atopic asthma can be described in terms of the early- and the late-phase responses[7] (Fig. 22-5). Recall that IgE-mediated hypersensitivity responses (discussed in Chapter 15) involve an initial antigen (allergen) sensitization, which leads to the production of presensitized IgE-coated mast cells. The symptoms of the *acute response*, which usually develop within 10 to 20 minutes, are caused by the release of chemical mediators from the presensitized mast cells. In the case of airborne antigens, the reaction occurs when antigen binds to previously sensitized mast cells on the mucosal surface of the airways (Fig. 22-6). Mediator release results in the infiltration of inflammatory cells and opening of the mucosal intercellular junctions and increased access of antigen to the more prevalent submucosal mast cells. In addition, there is bronchospasm

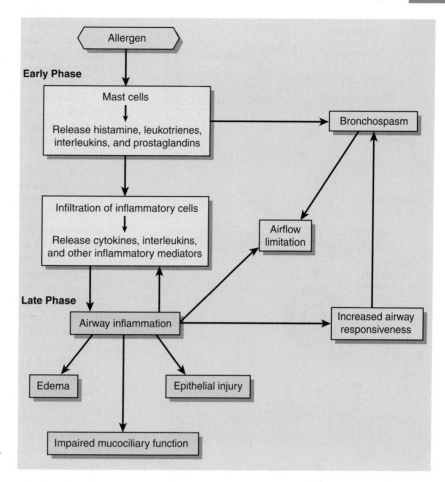

FIGURE 22-5 Mechanisms of early- and late-phase IgE-mediated bronchospasm.

caused by direct stimulation of parasympathetic receptors, mucosal edema caused by increased vascular permeability, and increased mucus secretions.

The *late-phase response* develops 4 to 8 hours after exposure to an asthmatic trigger.[7] The late-phase response involves inflammation and increased airway responsiveness that prolong the asthma attack and set into motion a vicious cycle of exacerbations. Typically, the response reaches a maximum within a few hours and may last for days or even weeks. An initial trigger in the late-phase response causes the release of inflammatory mediators from mast cells, macrophages, and epithelial cells. These substances induce the migration and activation of other inflammatory cells (*e.g.*, basophils, eosinophils, neutrophils), which then produce epithelial cell injury, changes in mucociliary function and reduced clearance of respiratory tract secretions, increased vascular permeability and edema, and continued bronchospasm and heightened airway responsiveness (see Fig. 22-6). Responsiveness to cholinergic mediators often is increased, suggesting changes in parasympathetic control of airway function. Chronic inflammation can lead to airway remodeling, with more permanent changes in airway resistance.[6]

Intrinsic (Nonatopic) Asthma. Intrinsic or nonatopic asthma triggers include respiratory tract infections, exer-cise, hyperventilation, cold air, exercise, drugs and chemicals, hormonal changes and emotional upsets, airborne pollutants, and gastroesophageal reflux.

Respiratory tract infections, especially those caused by viruses, may produce their effects by causing epithelial damage and stimulating the production of IgE antibodies directed toward the viral antigens. In addition to precipitating an asthmatic attack, viral respiratory infections increase airway responsiveness to other asthma triggers that may persist for weeks beyond the original infection.

Exercise-induced asthma occurs in 40% to 90% of persons with bronchial asthma.[11] The cause of exercise-induced asthma is unclear. It has been suggested that during exercise, bronchospasm may be caused by the loss of heat and water from the tracheobronchial tree because of the need for conditioning (*i.e.*, warming and humidification) of large volumes of air. The response is commonly exaggerated when the person exercises in a cold environment.

Inhaled irritants, such as tobacco smoke and strong odors, are thought to induce bronchospasm by way of irritant receptors and a vagal reflex. Exposure to parental smoking has been reported to increase asthma severity in children.[12] High doses of irritant gases such as sulfur dioxide, nitrogen dioxide, and ozone may induce inflammatory

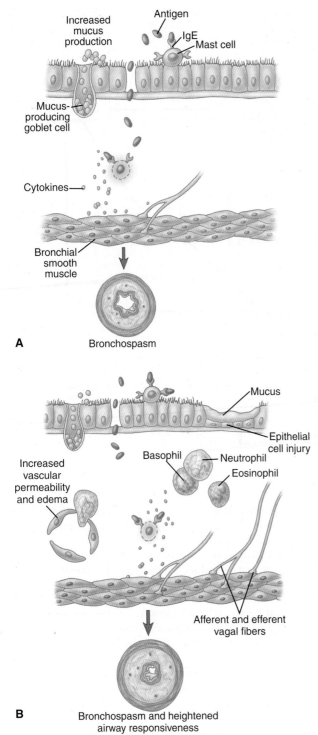

A

- Increased mucus production
- Antigen
- IgE
- Mast cell
- Mucus-producing goblet cell
- Cytokines
- Bronchial smooth muscle
- Bronchospasm

B

- Mucus
- Epithelial cell injury
- Basophil
- Neutrophil
- Eosinophil
- Increased vascular permeability and edema
- Afferent and efferent vagal fibers
- Bronchospasm and heightened airway responsiveness

FIGURE 22-6 Pathogenesis of bronchial asthma. (**A**) The immediate or early-phase response triggered by an IgE-mediated release of mediators from sensitized mast cells. The release of chemical mediators results in increased mucous production, opening of mucosal intercellular junctions with exposure of submucosal mast cells to antigen, and bronchospasm. (**B**) The late-phase response involves epithelial cell injury with decreased mucociliary function and accumulation of mucus; release of inflammatory mediators with recruitment of neutophils, eosinophils, and basophils; increased vascular permeability and edema; and increased airway responsiveness and bronchospasm.

exacerbations of airway responsiveness (*e.g.*, smog-related asthma). Occupational asthma is stimulated by fumes and gases (*e.g.*, epoxy resins, plastics, toluene), organic and chemical dusts (*i.e.*, wood, cotton, platinum), and other chemicals (*e.g.*, formaldehyde) in the workplace.[13]

There is a small group of persons with the clinical triad of asthma, chronic rhinosinusitis with nasal polyps, and precipitation of asthma and rhinitis attacks in response to aspirin and other nonsteroidal anti-inflammatory drugs (NSAIDs).[14,15] The mechanism of the hypersensitivity reaction is complex and not fully understood, but most evidence points toward an abnormality in arachidonic acid (AA) metabolism (see Chapter 14). Cyclooxygenase (COX), the rate-limiting enzyme in AA metabolism, exists in two main forms: COX-1 and COX-2. COX-1 is responsible for the synthesis of protective prostaglandins and COX-2 for the synthesis of mediators of inflammation and bronchoconstriction. It has been hypothesized that in persons with aspirin-induced asthma, the inhibition of COX-1 shunts the metabolism of AA away from the production of protective prostaglandins and toward the generation of COX-2 and other mediators of inflammation and bronchoconstriction.[15] Avoidance of aspirin and all NSAIDs is a necessary part of the treatment program. An addition to the list of chemicals that can provoke an asthmatic attack is the sulfites used in food processing and as preservatives added to beer, wine, and fresh vegetables.

Both emotional factors and changes in hormone levels are thought to contribute to an increase in asthma symptoms. Emotional factors produce bronchospasm by way of vagal pathways. They can act as a bronchospastic trigger, or they can increase airway responsiveness to other triggers through noninflammatory mechanisms. The role of sex hormones in asthma is unclear, although there is much circumstantial evidence to suggest they may be important. As much as 40% of women with asthma report a premenstrual increase in asthma symptoms.[16] Female sex hormones have a regulatory role in β_2-adrenergic function, and it has been suggested that abnormal regulation may be a possible mechanism for premenstrual asthma.[16]

Symptoms of gastroesophageal reflux are common in both adults and children with asthma, suggesting that reflux of gastric secretions may act as a bronchospastic trigger. Reflux during sleep is thought to contribute to nocturnal asthma.[6]

Clinical Features

Persons with asthma exhibit a wide range of signs and symptoms, from episodic wheezing and feelings of chest tightness to an acute, immobilizing attack. The attacks differ from person to person, and between attacks many persons are symptom free. Attacks may occur spontaneously or in response to various triggers, respiratory infections, emotional stress, or weather changes. Asthma is often worse at night. Nocturnal asthma attacks usually occur at approximately 4 AM because of the occurrence of the late response to allergens inhaled during the evening and because of circadian variations in bronchial reactivity.[17]

During an asthmatic attack, the airways narrow because of bronchospasm, edema of the bronchial mucosa, and mucus plugging. Expiration becomes prolonged because of progressive airway obstruction. The amount of air that can be forcibly expired in 1 second (forced expiratory volume [$FEV_{1.0}$]) and the peak expiratory flow rate (PEF), measured in liters per second, are decreased. With a prolonged attack, air becomes trapped behind the occluded and narrowed airways, causing hyperinflation of the lungs and an increase in the residual volume (RV). As a result, more energy is needed to overcome the tension already present in the lungs, and the accessory muscles (*i.e.*, sternocleidomastoid muscles) are used to maintain ventilation and gas exchange. This causes dyspnea and fatigue. Because air is trapped in the alveoli and inspiration is occurring at higher residual lung volumes, the cough becomes less effective. As the condition progresses, the effectiveness of alveolar ventilation declines, and mismatching of ventilation and perfusion occurs, causing hypoxemia and hypercapnia. Pulmonary vascular resistance may increase as a result of the hypoxemia and hyperinflation, leading to a rise in pulmonary artery pressure and increased work demands on the right heart.

Manifestations. The physical signs of bronchial asthma vary with the severity of the attack. A mild attack may produce a feeling of chest tightness, a slight increase in respiratory rate with prolonged expiration, and mild wheezing. A cough may accompany the wheezing. More severe attacks are associated with use of the accessory muscles, distant breath sounds caused by air trapping, and loud wheezing. Fatigue develops as the attack progresses, the skin becomes moist, and anxiety and apprehension are obvious. Dyspnea may be severe, and often the person is able to speak only one or two words before taking a breath. At the point at which airflow is markedly decreased, breath sounds become inaudible with diminished wheezing, and the cough becomes ineffective despite being repetitive and hacking.[6] This point often marks the onset of respiratory failure.

Diagnosis and Treatment. The diagnosis of asthma is based on a careful history and physical examination, laboratory findings, and pulmonary function studies. Spirometry provides a means for measuring the PEF, $FEV_{1.0}$, forced vital capacity (FVC), and other indices of lung function (see Chapter 20). The level of airway responsiveness can be measured by inhalation challenge tests using methacholine (a cholinergic agonist), histamine, or exposure to a nonpharmacologic agent such as cold air. The Expert Panel of the National Education and Prevention Program of the National Heart, Lung, and Blood Institute has developed an asthma severity classification system intended for use in directing asthma treatment and identifying persons at high risk for the development of life-threatening asthma attacks[6] (Table 22-1).

Small, inexpensive, portable meters that measure PEF are available. Although not intended for use in diagnosis of asthma, they can be used in clinics and physicians' offices and in the home by persons with asthma to provide frequent measures of flow rates. A *person's best performance* (personal best) is established from readings taken throughout several weeks and is used as a reference to indicate changes in respiratory function.[6] Day-night (circadian) variations in asthma symptoms and PEF variability can be used to indicate the severity of bronchial hyperreactivity. For example, a fall in the PEF to levels below 50% of the predicted value during an acute asthmatic attack indicates a severe exacerbation and the need for emergency department treatment.[6]

TABLE 22-1	Classification of Asthma Severity		
	Symptoms	**Nighttime Symptoms**	**Lung Function**
Mild intermittent	Symptoms ≤2 times a week Asymptomatic and normal PEF between exacerbations Exacerbations brief (from a few hours to a few days); intensity may vary	≤2 times a month	$FEV_{1.0}$ or PEF ≥80% predicted PEF variability <20%
Mild persistent	Symptoms >2 times a week but <1 time a day Exacerbations may affect activity	>2 times a month	$FEV_{1.0}$ or PEF ≥80% predicted PEF variability 20%–30%
Moderate persistent	Daily symptoms Daily use of inhaled short-acting β_2-agonist Exacerbations affect activity Exacerbations ≥2 times a week; may last days	>1 time a week	$FEV_{1.0}$ or PEF >60%–<80% predicted PEF variability >30%
Severe persistent	Continual symptoms Limited physical activity Frequent exacerbations	Frequent	$FEV_{1.0}$ or PEF ≤60% predicted PEF variability >30%

$FEV_{1.0}$, forced expiratory volume in 1 second; PEF, peak expiratory flow rate.
Adapted from National Education and Prevention Program. (1997). *Expert Panel report 2: Guidelines for the diagnosis and management of asthma.* National Institutes of Health publication no. 97-4051. Bethesda, MD: National Institutes of Health.

The treatment of bronchial asthma focuses on control of factors contributing to asthma severity and pharmacologic treatment.[6] Measures to control factors contributing to asthma severity are aimed at prevention of exposure to allergens and factors that increase asthma symptoms and precipitate asthma exacerbations.

Pharmacologic treatment is used to prevent or treat reversible airway obstruction and airway hyperresponsiveness caused by the inflammatory process. The Expert Panel recommends a stepwise approach to pharmacologic therapy based on frequency and severity of disease symptoms.[6] The medications used in the treatment of asthma include those with bronchodilator and anti-inflammatory actions. They are categorized into two general categories: quick-relief medications and long-term–control medications.

The *quick-relief medications* include the short-acting β_2-adrenergic agonists, anticholinergic agents, and systemic corticosteroids. The short-acting β_2-adrenergic agonists relax bronchial smooth muscle and provide prompt relief of symptoms, usually within 30 minutes. They are administered by inhalation (*i.e.,* metered-dose inhaler [MDI] or nebulizer). The short-acting β_2-agonists are used for treating acute attacks of asthma but are not recommended for daily use because of concern over safety.[6] Ipratropium is an inhaled anticholinergic agent that blocks the parasympathetic pathways that cause bronchoconstriction. A short course of corticosteroids administered orally or parenterally may be used for treating the inflammatory reaction associated with the late-phase response.

The *long-term medications* are taken on a daily basis to achieve and maintain control of persistent asthma symptoms. They include anti-inflammatory agents, long-acting bronchodilators, and leukotriene modifiers. The corticosteroids are considered the most effective anti-inflammatory agents for use in long-term treatment of asthma. Inhaled corticosteroids that are administered by MDI usually are preferred because of minimal systemic absorption and disruption of hypothalamic-pituitary-adrenal function. In severe cases, oral or parenterally administered corticosteroids may be necessary.

The long-acting β_2-agonists, which are available in inhalation or oral forms, act by relaxing bronchial smooth muscle. These agents have a duration of action of at least 12 hours and should not be used to treat acute symptoms or exacerbations.[6] The anti-inflammatory agents sodium cromolyn and nedocromil are also used to prevent an asthmatic attack. These agents act by stabilizing mast cells, thereby preventing release of the inflammatory mediators that cause an asthmatic attack. They are used prophylactically to prevent early and late responses. A newer group of drugs called the *leukotriene modifiers* have become available for use in the treatment of asthma. The leukotrienes are potent biochemical mediators released from mast cells that cause bronchoconstriction, increased mucus secretion, and attraction and activation of inflammatory cells in the airways of people with asthma (see Chapter 14, Fig. 14-3). A particular advantage of the leukotriene modifiers is that they are taken orally.

Severe Asthma

Severe or refractory asthma represents a subgroup (probably less than 5%) of persons with asthma who have more troublesome disease as evidenced by high medication requirements to maintain good disease control or persistent symptoms despite high medication use.[18,19] These persons are at increased risk for fatal or near-fatal asthmatic attacks.

Fatal and near-fatal asthmatic attacks, although uncommon, have increased in frequency over the past several decades. Most asthma deaths have occurred outside the hospital. Persons at highest risk are those with previous exacerbations resulting in respiratory failure, respiratory acidosis, and the need for intubation. Although the cause of death during an acute asthmatic attack is largely unknown, both cardiac dysrhythmias and asphyxia due to severe airway obstruction have been implicated. It has been suggested that an underestimation of the severity of the attack may be a contributing factor. Deterioration often occurs rapidly during an acute attack, and underestimation of its severity may lead to a life-threatening delay in seeking medical attention. Frequent and repetitive use of β_2-agonist inhalers (more than twice in a month) far in excess of the recommended doses may temporarily blunt symptoms and mask the severity of the condition. It has been suggested that persons who have fatal or near-fatal asthmatic attacks may have impaired perception of dyspnea and its severity.[20] Thus, they may not realize the severity of their condition and may not take the appropriate measures in terms of securing appropriate emergency treatment. Lack of access to medical care is another risk factor associated with asthma-related death. Distance, as in rural areas, or lack of financial resources, as in the uninsured or underinsured, may limit access to emergency care.

Bronchial Asthma in Children

Asthma is a leading cause of chronic illness in children and is responsible for a significant number of lost school days. It is the most frequent admitting diagnosis in children's hospitals. According to statistics collected by the United States Center for Health Statistics in 1998, 8.65 million children (12.1%) were reported to have physician- or health care professional–diagnosed asthma at some time during childhood.[21] Although childhood asthma may have its onset at any age, 80% of children are symptomatic by 6 years of age.[21,22] Asthma is more prevalent in African-American than white children, and results in more frequent disability and more frequent hospitalizations in African-American children.[22]

As with adults, asthma in children commonly is associated with an IgE-related reaction. It has been suggested that IgE directed against respiratory viruses in particular may be important in the pathogenesis of wheezing illnesses in infants (*i.e.,* bronchiolitis), which often precedes the onset of asthma. The respiratory syncytial virus and parainfluenza viruses are the most commonly involved.[23] Other contributing factors include exposure to environmental allergens such as pet dander, dust mite antigens, and cockroach allergens. Exposure to environmental tobacco smoke also may contribute to asthma in children. Of particular concern is the effect of in utero exposure to maternal smoking on lung function in infants and children.[24]

The signs and symptoms of asthma in infants and small children vary with the stage and the severity of an attack. Because airway patency decreases at night, many children have acute signs of asthma at this time. Often, previously well infants and children develop what may seem to be a cold with rhinorrhea, rapidly followed by irritability, a tight and nonproductive cough, wheezing, tachypnea, dyspnea with prolonged expiration, and use of accessory muscles of respiration. Cyanosis, hyperinflation of the chest, and tachycardia indicate increasing severity of the attack. Wheezing may be absent in children with extreme respiratory distress. The symptoms may progress rapidly and require emergency department treatment or hospitalization.

The Expert Panel of the National Heart, Lung, and Blood Institute's National Asthma Education Program has developed guidelines for management of asthma in infants and children younger than 5 years of age and for adults and children older than 5 years of age.[6,25] As with adults and older children, the Expert Panel recommends a stepwise approach to diagnosing and managing asthma in infants and children younger than 5 years of age. The anti-inflammatory agents cromolyn and nedocromil are recommended as an initial therapy for mild to moderate persistent asthma in infants and children. Inhaled short-acting β_2-agonists may be used for mild intermittent symptoms or exacerbations. More severe symptoms may require the use of inhaled corticosteroids. Systemic corticosteroids may be required during an episode of severe disease. Growth velocity should be monitored in children and adolescents receiving long-term corticosteroid therapy by any route because these drugs may suppress growth.[6]

Special delivery systems for administration of inhalation medications are available for infants and small children, including nebulizers with face masks and spacers/holding chambers for use with an MDI. For children younger than 2 years of age, nebulizer therapy usually is preferred. Children between 3 and 5 years of age may begin using an MDI with a spacer/holding chamber. The child's caregiver should be carefully instructed in the appropriate use of these devices.

The Expert Panel recommends that adolescents (and younger children when appropriate) be directly involved in developing their asthma management plans.[6] Active participation in physical activities, exercise, and sports should be encouraged.

CHRONIC OBSTRUCTIVE PULMONARY DISEASE

Chronic obstructive pulmonary disease (COPD) denotes a group of respiratory disorders characterized by chronic and recurrent obstruction of airflow in the pulmonary airways.[26–28] The airflow obstruction is usually progressive, may be accompanied by airway hyperresponsive-

ness, and may be partially reversible. COPD affects over 11 million Americans and now represents the fourth leading cause of death in the United States, accounting for over 100,000 deaths annually.[29] The death rate from COPD is increasing rapidly, especially among older men.

The most common cause of COPD is smoking.[26–28] Thus, the disease is largely preventable. Unfortunately, clinical findings are almost always absent during the early stages of COPD, and by the time symptoms appear, the disease usually is far advanced. For smokers with early signs of airway disease, there is hope that early recognition, combined with appropriate treatment and smoking cessation, may prevent or delay the usually relentless progression of the disease.

The term *chronic obstructive pulmonary disease* encompasses two types of obstructive airway disease: *emphysema*, with enlargement of air spaces and destruction of lung tissue, and *chronic obstructive bronchitis*, with obstruction of small airways. Persons with COPD often have overlapping features of both disorders.

The mechanisms involved in the pathogenesis of COPD usually are multiple and include inflammation and fibrosis of the bronchial wall, hypertrophy of the submucosal glands and hypersecretion of mucus, and loss of alveolar tissue and elastic lung fibers[26] (Fig. 22-7). Inflammation and fibrosis of the bronchial wall, along with excess mucus secretion, obstruct airflow and cause mismatching of ventilation and perfusion. Destruction of alveolar tissue decreases the surface area for gas exchange, and the loss of elastic fibers impairs the expiratory flow rate, increases air trapping, and predisposes to airway collapse.

Emphysema

Emphysema is characterized by a loss of lung elasticity and abnormal enlargement of the air spaces distal to the terminal bronchioles, with destruction of the alveolar

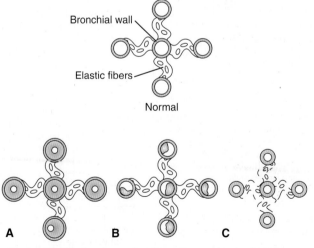

FIGURE 22-7 Mechanisms of airflow obstruction in chronic obstructive lung disease. (**Top**) Normal bronchial airway with elastic fibers that provide traction and hold the airway open. (**Bottom**) Obstruction of the airway caused by (**A**) hypertrophy of the bronchial wall, (**B**) inflammation and hypersecretion of mucus, and (**C**) loss of elastic fibers that hold the airway open.

walls and capillary beds. Enlargement of the alveolar air spaces leads to hyperinflation of the lungs and produces an increase in total lung capacity (TLC). Two of the recognized causes of emphysema are smoking, which incites lung injury, and an inherited deficiency of α_1-*antitrypsin*, an antiprotease enzyme that protects the lung from injury. Genetic factors other than an inherited α_1-antitrypsin deficiency also may play a role in smokers who develop COPD at an early age.[30]

Emphysema is thought to result from the breakdown of elastin and other alveolar wall components by enzymes, called *proteases*, that digest proteins. These proteases, particularly elastase, are released from polymorphonuclear leukocytes (*i.e.*, neutrophils), alveolar macrophages, and other inflammatory cells.[26] Normally, the lung is protected by antiprotease enzymes, including α_1-antitrypsin. Cigarette smoke and other irritants stimulate the movement of inflammatory cells into the lungs, resulting in increased release of elastase and other proteases. In smokers in whom COPD develops, antiprotease production and release may be inadequate to neutralize the excess protease production such that the process of elastic tissue destruction goes unchecked (Fig. 22-8).

A hereditary deficiency in α_1-antitrypsin accounts for approximately 1% of all cases of COPD and is more common in young persons with emphysema.[26] An α_1-antitrypsin deficiency is inherited as an autosomal recessive disorder. It is most common in persons of Scandinavian descent and is rare in Jews, blacks, and Japanese.[30] Homozygotes who carry two defective genes have only about 15% to 20% of the normal plasma concentration

of α_1-antitrypsin. Almost all persons who have emphysema before the age of 40 years have an α_1-antitrypsin deficiency. Smoking and repeated respiratory tract infections, which also decrease α_1-antitrypsin levels, contribute to the risk of emphysema in persons with an α_1-antitrypsin deficiency. Laboratory methods are available for measuring α_1-antitrypsin levels. A recombinant human α_1-antitrypsin is available for replacement therapy in persons with a hereditary deficiency of the enzyme.

There are two commonly recognized types of emphysema: centriacinar and panacinar (Fig. 22-9). The centriacinar type affects the bronchioles in the central part of the respiratory lobule, with initial preservation of the alveolar ducts and sacs[30] (Fig. 22-10). It is the most common type of emphysema and is seen predominantly in male smokers. The panacinar type produces initial involvement of the peripheral alveoli and later extends to involve the more central bronchioles. This type of emphysema is more common in persons with α_1-antitrypsin deficiency. It also is found in smokers in association with centrilobular emphysema. In such cases, panacinar changes are commonly seen in the lower parts of the lung and centriacinar changes in the upper parts of the lung.

Chronic Bronchitis

Chronic bronchitis represents airway obstruction of the major and small airways. The condition is seen most commonly in middle-aged men and is associated with chronic irritation from smoking and recurrent infections. A clinical diagnosis of chronic bronchitis requires the history of a chronic productive cough for at least 3 consecutive months in at least 2 consecutive years.[27] Typically, the cough has been present for many years, with a gradual increase in acute exacerbations that produce frankly purulent sputum.

The earliest feature of chronic bronchitis is hypersecretion of mucus in the large airways, associated with hypertrophy of the submucosal glands in the trachea and bronchi.[30] Although mucus hypersecretion in the large airways is the cause of sputum overproduction, it is now thought that accompanying changes in the small airways (small bronchi and bronchioles) are physiologically important in the airway obstruction that develops in chronic

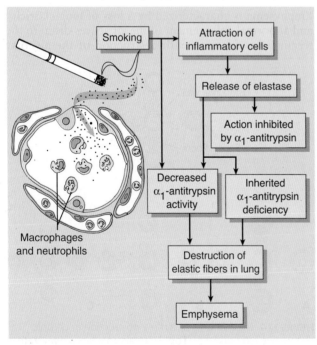

FIGURE 22-8 Protease (elastase)-antiprotease (antitrypsin) mechanisms of emphysema. The effects of smoking and an inherited α_1-antitrypsin deficiency on the destruction of elastic fibers in the lung and development of emphysema.

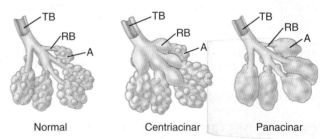

FIGURE 22-9 Centriacinar and panacinar emphysema. In centriacinar emphysema, the destruction is confined to the terminal (TB) and respiratory bronchioles (RB). In panacinar emphysema, the peripheral alveoli (A) are also involved. (Adapted from West J. B. [1997]. *Pulmonary pathophysiology* [5th ed., p. 53]. Philadelphia: Lippincott-Raven.)

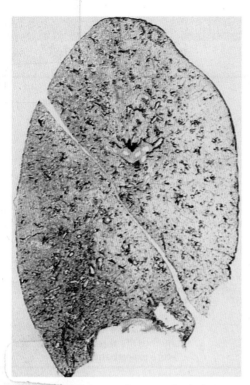

FIGURE 22-10 Centrilobular emphysema. A whole mount of the left lung of a smoker with mild emphysema shows enlarged air spaces scattered throughout both lobes, which represent destruction of terminal bronchioles in the central part of the pulmonary lobule. These abnormal spaces are surrounded by intact pulmonary parenchyma. (From Travis W. D., Beasley M. B., Rubin E. [2005]. The respiratory system. In Rubin E., Gorstein F., Rubin R., et al. [Eds.], *Rubin's pathology: Clinicopathologic foundations of medicine* [4th ed., p. 618]. Philadelphia: Lippincott Williams & Wilkins.)

bronchitis.[7] Histologically, these changes include a marked increase in goblet cells and excess mucus production with plugging of the airway lumen, inflammatory infiltration, and fibrosis of the bronchiolar wall. It is thought that both the submucosal hypertrophy in the larger airways and the increase in goblet cells in the smaller airways are protective metaplastic reactions against tobacco smoke and other pollutants. Viral and bacterial infections are common in persons with chronic bronchitis and are thought to be a result rather than a cause of the problem. Although infections are not responsible for initiating the problem, they are probably important in maintaining it and may be critical in producing acute exacerbations.[7]

Clinical Features

The mnemonics "pink puffer" and "blue bloater" have been used to differentiate the clinical manifestations of emphysema and chronic obstructive bronchitis.[1] The important features of these forms of COPD are described in Table 22-2. In practice, differentiation between the two types is often difficult because persons with COPD usually have some degree of both emphysema and chronic bronchitis.

A major difference between the pink puffers and the blue bloaters is the respiratory responsiveness to hypoxic stimuli. With pulmonary emphysema, there is a proportionate loss of ventilation and perfusion area in the lung. These persons are pink puffers, or fighters able to overventilate and thus maintain relatively normal blood gas levels until late in the disease. Chronic obstructive bronchitis is characterized by excessive bronchial secretions and airway obstruction that causes mismatching of ventilation and perfusion. Thus, persons with chronic bronchitis are unable to compensate by increasing their ventilation; instead, hypoxemia and cyanosis develop. These are the blue bloaters, or nonfighters.

Persons with emphysema have marked dyspnea and struggle to maintain normal blood gas levels with increased ventilatory effort, including prominent use of the accessory muscles. The seated position, which stabilizes chest structures and allows for maximum chest expansion and use of accessory muscles, is preferred. With loss of lung elasticity and hyperinflation of the lungs, the airways often collapse during expiration because pressure in surrounding lung tissues exceeds airway pressure. Air becomes trapped in lungs, producing an increase in the anteroposterior dimensions of the chest, the so-called *barrel chest* that is typical of persons with emphysema (Fig. 22-11). Expiration often is accomplished through pursed lips. Pursed-lip ("puffer") breathing, which increases the resistance to the outflow of air, helps to prevent airway collapse by increasing airway pressure. The work of breathing is greatly increased in persons with emphysema, and eating often is difficult. As a result, there often is considerable weight loss.

Chronic bronchitis is characterized by shortness of breath with a progressive decrease in exercise tolerance. As the disease progresses, breathing becomes increasingly more labored, even at rest. The expiratory phase of respiration is prolonged, and expiratory wheezes and crackles can be heard on auscultation. In contrast to persons with emphysema, those with chronic obstructive bronchitis are unable to maintain normal blood gases by increasing their breathing effort. Hypoxemia, hypercapnia, and cyanosis develop, reflecting an imbalance between ventilation and perfusion. Hypoxemia causes reflex vasoconstriction of the pulmonary vessels and further impairment of gas exchange in the lung. Hypoxemia also stimulates red blood cell production, causing polycythemia. As a result, persons with chronic bronchitis develop pulmonary hypertension and, eventually, right-sided heart failure (*i.e.*, cor pulmonale) with peripheral edema ("bloater").

Persons with combined forms of COPD characteristically seek medical attention in the fifth or sixth decade of life, complaining of cough, sputum production, and shortness of breath. The symptoms typically have existed to some extent for 10 years or longer. The productive cough usually occurs in the morning. Dyspnea becomes more severe as the disease progresses. Frequent exacerbations of infection and respiratory insufficiency are common, causing absence from work and eventual disability. The late stages of COPD are characterized by pulmonary hypertension, cor pulmonale (to be discussed),

TABLE 22-2 Characteristics of Emphysema and Chronic Bronchitis

Characteristic	Type A Pulmonary Emphysema ("Pink Puffers")	Type B Chronic Bronchitis ("Blue Bloaters")
Smoking history	Usual	Usual
Clinical features		
Barrel chest (hyperinflation of the lungs)	Often dramatic	May be present
Weight loss	May be severe in advanced disease	Infrequent
Shortness of breath	May be absent early in disease	Predominant early symptom, insidious in onset, exertional
Decreased breath sounds	Characteristic	Variable
Wheezing	Usually absent	Variable
Rhonchi	Usually absent or minimal	Often prominent
Sputum	May be absent or may develop late in the course	Frequent early manifestation, frequent infections, abundant purulent sputum
Cyanosis	Often absent, even late in the disease when there is low PO_2	Often dramatic
Blood gases	Relatively normal until late in the disease process	Hypercapnia may be present Hypoxemia may be present
Cor pulmonale	Only in advanced cases	Frequent Peripheral edema
Polycythemia	Only in advanced cases	Frequent
Prognosis	Slowly debilitating disease	Numerous life-threatening episodes due to acute exacerbations

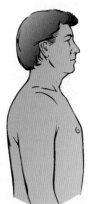
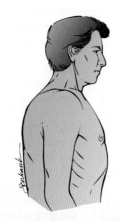
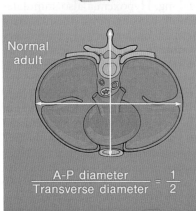
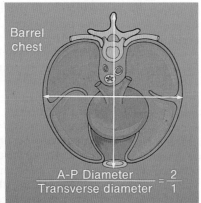

$$\frac{\text{A-P diameter}}{\text{Transverse diameter}} = \frac{1}{2}$$

$$\frac{\text{A-P Diameter}}{\text{Transverse diameter}} = \frac{2}{1}$$

FIGURE 22-11 Characteristics of normal chest wall and chest wall in emphysema. The normal chest wall and its cross-section are illustrated on the left. The barrel-shaped chest of emphysema and its cross-section are illustrated on the right. (From Smeltzer S. C., Bare B. G. [2004]. *Medical-surgical nursing* [10th ed., p. 572]. Philadelphia: Lippincott Williams & Wilkins.)

recurrent respiratory infections, and chronic respiratory failure. Death usually occurs during an exacerbation of illness associated with infection and respiratory failure.

Diagnosis and Treatment. The diagnosis of COPD is based on a careful history and physical examination, pulmonary function studies, chest radiographs, and laboratory tests. Airway obstruction prolongs the expiratory phase of respiration and affords the potential for impaired gas exchange because of mismatching of ventilation and perfusion. The FVC is the amount of air that can be forcibly exhaled after maximal inspiration. In an adult with normal respiratory function, this should be achieved in 4 to 6 seconds. In patients with chronic lung disease, the time required for FVC is increased, the $FEV_{1.0}$ is decreased, and the ratio of $FEV_{1.0}$ to FVC is decreased. In severe disease, the FVC is markedly reduced. Lung volume measurements reveal a marked increase in RV, an increase in TLC, and elevation of the RV to TLC ratio. These and other measurements of expiratory flow are determined by spirometry and are used in the diagnosis of COPD (see Chapter 20, Fig. 20-16). Other diagnostic measures become important as the disease advances. Measures of exercise tolerance, nutritional status, hemoglobin saturation, and arterial blood gases can be used to assess the overall impact of COPD on health status and to direct treatment.

The treatment of COPD depends on the stage of the disease and often requires an interdisciplinary approach. Smoking cessation is the only measure that slows the progression of the disease. Persons in more advanced stages of the disease often require measures to maintain and improve physical and psychosocial functioning, pharmacologic interventions, and oxygen therapy. Respiratory tract infections can prove life threatening to persons with severe COPD. A person with COPD should avoid exposure to others with known respiratory tract infections. Immunization for influenza and pneumococcal infections decreases the likelihood of their occurrence.

The pharmacologic treatment of COPD includes the use of bronchodilators, including inhaled adrenergic and anticholinergic agents.[26–28] Inhaled β_2-adrenergic agonists have been the mainstay of treatment for COPD for many years. The anticholinergic drugs (*e.g.*, ipratropium), which are administered by inhalation, produce bronchodilation by blocking parasympathetic cholinergic receptors that induce contraction of bronchial smooth muscle. They also reduce the volume of sputum without altering its viscosity. Inhalers that combine an anticholinergic drug with a β_2-adrenergic agonist are available. Oral theophylline, a bronchodilator, may be used in treatment of persons who fail to respond to inhaled bronchodilators. The long-acting theophylline preparations may be used to reduce overnight declines in respiratory function.

Oxygen therapy is prescribed for selected persons with significant hypoxemia (arterial $PO_2 \leq 55$ mm Hg or hemoglobin saturation $\leq 88\%$).[31] The use of continuous low-flow oxygen decreases dyspnea, helps to prevent pulmonary hypertension, and improves neuropsychological function and activity tolerance. Portable oxygen administration units, which allow mobility and the performance of activities of daily living, usually are used. The overall goal of oxygen therapy is to maintain a hemoglobin oxygen saturation of at least 90%, representing an arterial PO_2 of approximately 60 mm Hg (see Chapter 20, Fig. 20-18). Because the ventilatory drive associated with hypoxic stimulation of the peripheral chemoreceptors does not occur until the arterial PO_2 has been reduced to about 60 mm Hg or less, the oxygen flow rate usually is titrated to provide an arterial PO_2 of 60 to 65 mm Hg. Increasing the arterial PO_2 above that level tends to depress ventilation, which can lead to carbon dioxide retention.

BRONCHIECTASIS

Bronchiectasis is an uncommon type of COPD characterized by a permanent dilatation of the bronchi and bronchioles caused by destruction of the muscle and elastic supporting tissue resulting from a vicious cycle of infection and inflammation.[32] It is not a primary disease but occurs secondary to persistent infection or obstruction.[7] In the past, bronchiectasis often followed a necrotizing bacterial pneumonia that frequently complicated measles, pertussis, or influenza. Tuberculosis was also commonly associated with bronchiectasis. Thus, with the advent of antibiotics that more effectively treat respiratory infections such as tuberculosis and immunizations against pertussis and measles, there has been a marked decrease in the prevalence of bronchiectasis.

Pathogenesis

Two processes are critical to the pathogenesis of bronchiectasis: obstruction and chronic persistent infection.[7] Regardless of which may come first, both cause damage to the bronchial walls, leading to weakening and dilatation. On gross examination, bronchial dilatation is classified as saccular, cylindrical, or varicose. Saccular bronchiectasis involves the proximal third to fourth generation of bronchi[30] (see Chapter 20, Fig. 20-5). These bronchi become severely dilated and end blindly in dilated sacs with collapse and fibrosis of more distal lung tissue (Fig. 22-12). Cylindrical bronchiectasis involves uniform and moderate dilatation of the sixth to eighth generations of airways. It is a milder form of disease than saccular bronchiectasis and leads to fewer symptoms. Varicose bronchiectasis involves the second through eighth branchings of bronchi and results in bronchi that resemble varicose veins. Bronchiolar obliteration is not as severe and symptoms are variable.

Bronchiectasis can present in either of two forms: a local obstructive process involving a lobe or segment of a lung or a diffuse process involving much of both lungs.[32] *Localized bronchiectasis* is most commonly caused by conditions such as tumors, foreign bodies, and mucus plugs that produce atelectasis and infection due to obstructed drainage of bronchial secretions. It can affect any area of the lung, the area being determined by the site

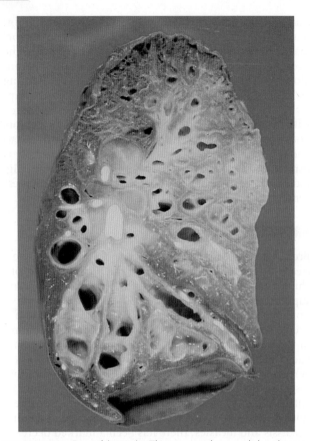

FIGURE 22-12 Bronchiectasis. The resected upper lobe shows widely dilated bronchi, with thickening of the bronchial walls and collapse and fibrosis of the pulmonary parenchyma. (From Travis W. D., Beasley M. B., Rubin E. [2005]. The respiratory system. In Rubin E., Gorstein F., Rubin R., et al. [Eds.], *Rubin's pathology: Clinicopathologic foundations of medicine* [4th ed., p. 591]. Philadelphia: Lippincott Williams & Wilkins.)

of obstruction or infection. *Generalized bronchiectasis* usually is bilateral and most commonly affects the lower lobes. It is due largely to inherited impairments of host mechanisms or acquired disorders that permit introduction of infectious organisms into the airways. They include inherited conditions such as cystic fibrosis, in which airway obstruction is caused by impairment of normal mucociliary function; congenital and acquired immunodeficiency states, which predispose to respiratory tract infections; lung infection (*e.g.*, tuberculosis, fungal infections, lung abscess); and exposure to toxic gases that cause airway obstruction.

Clinical Features

Bronchiectasis is associated with a number of abnormalities that profoundly affect respiratory function, including atelectasis, obstruction of the smaller airways, and diffuse bronchitis. Affected persons have recurrent bronchopulmonary infection; coughing; production of copious amounts of foul-smelling, purulent sputum; and hemoptysis. Weight loss and anemia are common.

The manifestations of bronchiectasis are similar to those seen in chronic bronchitis and emphysema. As in the latter two conditions, chronic bronchial obstruction leads to marked dyspnea and cyanosis. Clubbing of the fingers, which is not usually seen in other types of obstructive lung disease, is common in moderate to advanced bronchiectasis.

Diagnosis is based on history and imaging studies. The condition often is evident on chest radiographs. High-resolution CT scanning of the chest allows for definitive diagnosis. Accuracy of diagnosis is important because interventional bronchoscopy or surgery may be palliative or curative in some of the more obstructive forms of the disease.

Treatment consists of early recognition and treatment of infection along with regular postural drainage and chest physical therapy. Persons with this disorder benefit from many of the rehabilitation and treatment measures used for chronic bronchitis and emphysema.

 CYSTIC FIBROSIS

Cystic fibrosis (CF), which is the major cause of severe chronic respiratory disease in children, is an autosomal recessive disorder involving fluid secretion in the exocrine glands in the epithelial lining of the respiratory, gastrointestinal, and reproductive tracts.[32–36] In addition to chronic respiratory disease, CF is manifested by pancreatic exocrine deficiency and elevation of sodium chloride in the sweat. Nasal polyps, sinus infections, pancreatitis, and cholelithiasis also are common. Excessive loss of sodium in the sweat predisposes young children to salt depletion episodes. Most boys with CF have congenital bilateral absence of the vas deferens with azoospermia.

The disease affects approximately 30,000 children and adults in the United States, and more than 10 million persons are asymptomatic carriers of the defective gene.[33] The gene is rare in African blacks and Asians. Homozygotes (*i.e.*, persons with two defective genes) have all or substantially all of the clinical symptoms of the disease, compared with heterozygotes, who are carriers of the disease but have no recognizable symptoms.

Pathogenesis

Cystic fibrosis is caused by mutations in a single gene on the long arm of chromosome 7 that encodes for the cystic fibrosis transmembrane regulator (CFTR), which functions as a chloride (Cl^-) channel in epithelial cell membranes. Mutations in the CFTR render the epithelial membrane relatively impermeable to the chloride ion (Fig. 22-13).

The impact on transport function is relatively tissue specific. In the sweat glands, the concentration of sodium (Na^+) and Cl^- secreted into the lumen of the gland remains unaffected, whereas the reabsorption of Cl^- through the CFTR and accompanying reabsorption of Na^+ in the ducts of the gland fails to occur. This accounts for the high concentration of NaCl in the sweat of persons with CF.[35] In the normal airway epithelium, Cl^- is secreted into the airway lumen through the CFTR. In CF, the

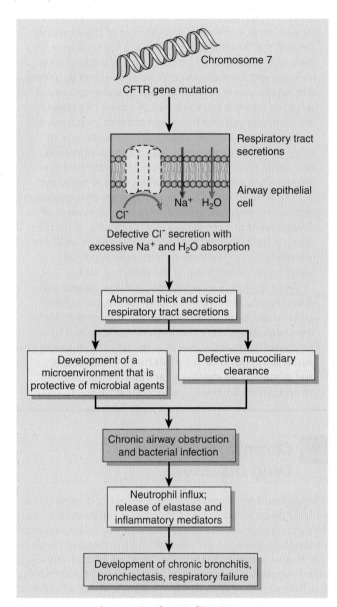

FIGURE 22-13 Pathogenesis of cystic fibrosis.

and bronchitis are the initial lung manifestations, but after months and years, structural changes in the bronchial wall lead to bronchiectasis. In addition to airway obstruction, the basic genetic defect that occurs with CF predisposes to chronic infection with a surprisingly small number of organisms, the most common being *Pseudomonas aeruginosa, Staphylococcus aureus, and Burkholderia cepacia*, that rarely affect the lungs of other individuals.[35] Soon after birth, initial infection with bacterial pathogens occurs and is associated with an excessive neutrophilic inflammatory response that appears to occur independent of infection. There is evidence that the CF airway epithelial cells or surface liquids provide a favorable environment for harboring these organisms. *P. aeruginosa*, in particular, has a propensity to undergo mucoid transformation in this environment.[35] The complex polysaccharide produced by these organisms provides a hypoxic environment and generates a biofilm that protects *P. aeruginosa* against antimicrobial agents.

Pancreatic function is abnormal in approximately 80% to 90% of persons with CF.[35] Steatorrhea, diarrhea, and abdominal pain and discomfort are common. In the newborn, meconium ileus may cause intestinal obstruction. The degree of pancreatic involvement is highly variable. In some children, the defect is relatively mild, and in others the involvement is severe and impairs intestinal absorption. In addition to exocrine pancreatic insufficiency, hyperglycemia may occur, especially after 10 years of age, when approximately 8% of persons with CF develop diabetes mellitus.[35]

Diagnosis and Treatment. Early diagnosis and treatment are important in delaying the onset and severity of chronic illness in children with CF. Diagnosis is based on the presence of respiratory and gastrointestinal manifestations typical of CF, a history of CF in a sibling, or a positive newborn screening test. Confirmatory laboratory tests include the sweat test, assessment of bioelectrical properties of respiratory epithelia by measurement of transepithelial potential differences in the nasal membrane, and genetic tests for CFTR gene mutations.[35] The *sweat test*, using pilocarpine iontophoresis to collect the sweat and chemical analysis of its chloride content, remains the standard approach to diagnosis. Newborns with CF have elevated blood levels of immunoreactive trypsinogen, presumably because of secretory obstruction in the pancreas. *Newborn screening* consists of a test for determination of immunoreactive trypsinogen. The test can be done on blood spots collected for routine newborn screening tests.

At present there are no approved treatments for correcting the genetic defects in CF or to reverse the ion transport abnormalities associated with the dysfunctional CFTR. Thus, treatment measures are directed toward slowing the progression of secondary organ dysfunction and sequelae such as chronic lung infection and pancreatic insufficiency. They include the use of antibiotics to prevent and manage infections; the use of chest physical therapy (chest percussion and postural drainage) and mucolytic agents to prevent airway obstruction; and pancreatic enzyme replacement and nutritional therapy. Routine

impaired transport of Cl⁻ ultimately leads to a series of secondary events that includes increased absorption of Na⁺ and water from the airway lumen. This lowers the water content of the mucociliary blanket coating the respiratory epithelium, causing it to become more viscid. The resulting dehydration of the mucus layer leads to defective mucociliary action and accumulation of viscid secretions that obstruct the airways and predispose to recurrent pulmonary infections. Similar transport abnormalities and pathophysiologic events take place in the pancreatic and biliary ducts (and in the vas deferens).

Clinical Features

Respiratory manifestations of CF are caused by an accumulation of viscid mucus in the bronchi, impaired mucociliary clearance, and lung infections. Chronic bronchiolitis

laboratory evaluations are crucial for assessing pulmonary function and response to therapeutic interventions. These studies include radiologic examinations, pulmonary function testing, and microbiologic cultures of respiratory secretions.

The abnormal viscosity of airway secretions is attributed largely to the presence of polymorphonuclear white blood cells and their degradation products. A purified recombinant human deoxyribonuclease (rhDNase), an enzyme that breaks down these products, has been developed.[32,36] Clinical trials have shown that the drug, which is administered by inhalation, can improve pulmonary symptoms and reduce the frequency of respiratory exacerbations. Although many persons benefit from the therapy, the drug is costly, and recommendations for its use are evolving.

Up to 90% of patients with CF have complete loss of exocrine pancreas function and inadequate digestion of fats and proteins. They require diet adjustment, pancreatic enzyme replacement, and supplemental vitamins and minerals. Pancreatic enzyme dosage and product are individualized for each patient. Enteric-coated, pH-sensitive enzyme microspheres are available.

Progress of the disease is variable. Improved medical management has led to longer survival. Currently, the median age for survival of people with CF has increased to 35.1 years.[32] Current hopes reside in research that would make gene therapy a feasible alternative for persons with the disease.

In summary, obstructive ventilatory disorders are characterized by airway obstruction and limitation in expiratory airflow. Bronchial asthma is a chronic inflammatory disorder of the airways, characterized by airway hypersensitivity and episodic attacks of airway narrowing. An asthmatic attack can be triggered by a variety of stimuli. Typically, asthma has been categorized into extrinsic (initiated by a type I hypersensitivity [atopic] response to an extrinsic antigen) and intrinsic (initiated by diverse nonimmune mechanisms, including respiratory tract infections, exercise, ingestion of aspirin, emotional upset, and exposure to bronchial irritants such as cigarette smoke). There are two types of response in persons with atopic asthma: the acute or early-phase response and the late-phase response. The acute response results in immediate bronchoconstriction on exposure to an inhaled antigen and usually subsides within 90 minutes. The late-phase response usually develops 4 to 8 hours after exposure to an asthmatic trigger; it involves inflammation and increased airway responsiveness that prolong the attack and cause a vicious cycle of exacerbations.

Chronic obstructive pulmonary disease describes a group of conditions characterized by obstruction to airflow in the lungs. Among the conditions associated with COPD are emphysema, chronic bronchitis, and bronchiectasis. Emphysema is characterized by a loss of lung elastic-

ity; abnormal, permanent enlargement of the air spaces distal to the terminal bronchioles; and hyperinflation of the lungs. Chronic bronchitis is caused by inflammation of major and small airways and is characterized by edema and hyperplasia of submucosal glands and excess mucus secretion into the bronchial tree. A history of a chronic productive cough that has persisted for at least 3 months and for at least 2 consecutive years in the absence of other disease is necessary for the diagnosis of chronic bronchitis. Emphysema and chronic bronchitis are manifested by the eventual mismatching of ventilation and perfusion. As the condition advances, signs of respiratory distress and impaired gas exchange become evident, with development of hypercapnia and hypoxemia. Bronchiectasis is a form of COPD that is characterized by an abnormal dilatation of the large bronchi associated with infection and destruction of the bronchial walls.

Cystic fibrosis is an autosomal recessive genetic disorder manifested by chronic lung disease, pancreatic exocrine deficiency, and elevation of sodium chloride in the sweat. Respiratory manifestations are caused by an accumulation of viscid mucus in the bronchi, impaired mucociliary clearance, lung infections, bronchiectasis, and dilatation. Mucus plugs can result in the total obstruction of an airway, causing atelectasis.

Chronic Interstitial Lung Diseases

The diffuse interstitial lung diseases are a diverse group of lung disorders that produce similar inflammatory and fibrotic changes in the interstitium or interalveolar septa of the lung. Because the interstitial lung diseases result in a stiff and noncompliant lung, they are commonly classified as restrictive lung disorders. In contrast to obstructive lung diseases, the lungs are stiff and difficult to expand, despite normal functioning airways.

KEY CONCEPTS

Interstitial or Restrictive Lung Diseases

➤ Interstitial lung diseases result from inflammatory conditions that affect the interalveolar structures of the lung and produce lung fibrosis and a stiff lung.

➤ A stiff and noncompliant lung is difficult to inflate, increasing the work of breathing and causing decreased exercise tolerance due to hypoxemia.

➤ Because of the increased effort needed for lung expansion, persons with interstitial lung disease tend to take small but more frequent breaths.

The interstitial lung diseases may be acute or insidious in onset; they may be rapidly progressive, slowly progressive, or static in their course. They include hypersensitivity pneumonitis (see Chapter 15), lung diseases caused by exposure to toxic drugs (*e.g.*, the cancer drug bleomycin and the antiarrhythmic drug amiodarone) and radiation, sarcoidosis, and occupational lung diseases, including the pneumoconioses that are caused by the inhalation of inorganic dusts such as silica, coal dust, and asbestos. Some of the most common interstitial lung diseases are caused by exposure to inhaled dust and particles. In many cases, no specific cause can be found.[37–39] Examples of interstitial lung diseases and their causes are listed in Chart 22-1.

PATHOGENESIS

Current theory suggests that most interstitial lung diseases, regardless of the causes, have a common pathogenesis. It is thought that these disorders are initiated by some type of injury to the alveolar epithelium, followed by an inflammatory process that involves the alveoli and interstitium of the lung. An accumulation of inflammatory and immune cells causes continued damage of lung tissue and the replacement of normal, functioning lung tissue with fibrous scar tissue.

CLINICAL FEATURES

Persons with interstitial lung diseases experience dyspnea, tachypnea, and eventual cyanosis, without evidence of wheezing or signs of airway obstruction. Usually there is an insidious onset of breathlessness that initially occurs during exercise and may progress to the point that the person is totally incapacitated. A nonproductive cough may develop, particularly with continued exposure to the inhaled irritant. Typically, a person with a restrictive lung disease breathes with a pattern of rapid, shallow respirations. This tachypneic pattern of breathing, in which the respiratory rate is increased and the tidal volume is decreased, reduces the work of breathing because it takes less work to move air through the airways at an increased rate than it does to stretch a stiff lung to accommodate a larger tidal volume.

Although resting arterial blood gases usually are normal early in the course of the disease, arterial PO_2 levels may fall during exercise, and in cases of advanced disease, hypoxemia often is present even at rest. In the late stages of the disease, hypercapnia and respiratory acidosis develop. Clubbing of the fingers and toes may develop because of chronic hypoxemia.

The diagnosis of interstitial lung disease requires a careful personal and family history, with particular emphasis on exposure to environmental, occupational, and other injurious agents. Chest radiographs may be used as an initial diagnostic method, and serial chest films often are used to follow the progress of the disease. A biopsy specimen for histologic study and culture may be obtained by surgical incision or bronchoscopy using a fiberoptic bronchoscope. Gallium lung scans often are used to detect and quantify the chronic alveolitis that occurs in interstitial lung disease. Gallium does not localize in normal lung tissue, but uptake of the radionuclide is increased in interstitial lung disease and other diffuse lung diseases.

The treatment goals for persons with interstitial lung disease focus on identifying and removing the injurious agent, suppressing the inflammatory response, preventing progression of the disease, and providing supportive therapy for persons with advanced disease. In general, the treatment measures vary with the type of lung disease. Corticosteroid drugs frequently are used to suppress the inflammatory response. Many of the supportive treatment measures used in the late stages of the disease, such as oxygen therapy and measures to prevent infection, are similar to those discussed for persons with COPD.

CHART 22-1

Causes of Interstitial Lung Diseases*

Occupational and Environmental Inhalants

Inorganic dusts
  Asbestosis
  Silicosis
  Coal miner's pneumoconiosis
Organic dusts
  Hypersensitivity pneumonitis
Gases and fumes
  Ammonia, phosgene, sulfur dioxide

Drugs and Therapeutic Agents

Cancer chemotherapeutic agents
  Busulfan
  Bleomycin
  Methotrexate
Ionizing radiation

Immunologic Lung Disease

Sarcoidosis
Collagen vascular diseases
  Systemic lupus erythematosus
  Rheumatoid arthritis
  Scleroderma
  Dermatomyositis-polymyositis

Miscellaneous

Postacute respiratory distress syndrome
Idiopathic pulmonary fibrosis

*This list is not intended to be inclusive.

In summary, the interstitial lung diseases are characterized by fibrosis and decreased compliance of the lung. They include the occupational lung diseases, lung diseases caused by toxic drugs and radiation, and lung diseases of unknown origin, such as sarcoidosis. These disorders are thought to result from an inflammatory process that begins in the alveoli and extends to involve the interstitial tissues of the lung. Unlike COPD, which affects the airways, interstitial lung diseases affect the supporting collagen and elastic tissues that lie between the airways and blood vessels. These lung diseases decrease lung volumes, reduce the diffusing capacity of the lung, and cause various degrees of hypoxia. Because lung compliance is reduced, persons with this form of lung disease have a rapid, shallow breathing pattern.

Pulmonary Vascular Disorders

As blood moves through the lung, blood oxygen levels are raised and carbon dioxide is removed. These processes depend on the matching of ventilation (*i.e.*, gas exchange) and perfusion (*i.e.*, blood flow). This section discusses three major disorders of the pulmonary circulation: pulmonary embolism, pulmonary hypertension, and acute respiratory distress syndrome. Pulmonary edema, another major problem of the pulmonary circulation, is discussed in Chapter 19.

PULMONARY EMBOLISM

Pulmonary embolism develops when a blood-borne substance lodges in a branch of the pulmonary artery and obstructs the flow.[40–42] The embolism may consist of a thrombus (Fig. 22-14), air that has accidentally been injected during intravenous infusion, fat that has been mobilized from the bone marrow after a fracture or from a traumatized fat depot (see Chapter 42), or amniotic fluid that has entered the maternal circulation after rupture of the membranes at the time of delivery.

Almost all pulmonary thromboemboli arise from a deep vein thrombosis (DVT) in the lower extremities (see Chapter 17). The presence of thrombosis in the deep veins of the legs or pelvis often is unsuspected until embolism occurs. The effects of emboli on the pulmonary circulation are related to mechanical obstruction of the pulmonary circulation by the blood clot and associated reflex vasoconstriction. Obstruction of pulmonary blood flow also causes reflex bronchoconstriction in the affected area of the lung, wasted ventilation and impaired gas exchange, and loss of alveolar surfactant. Pulmonary hypertension and right heart failure may develop when there is massive vasoconstriction because of a large embolus. Although small areas of infarction may occur, frank pulmonary infarction is uncommon.

Among the physiologic factors that contribute to DVT are venous stasis, venous endothelial injury, and hypercoagulability states. Venous stasis and venous endothelial injury can result from prolonged bed rest, trauma, surgery, childbirth, fractures of the hip and femur, myocardial infarction and congestive heart failure, and spinal cord injury. Persons undergoing orthopedic surgery and gynecologic cancer surgery are at particular risk, as are

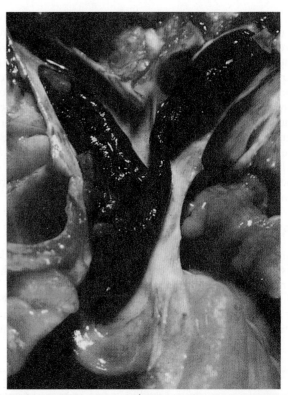

FIGURE 22-14 Pulmonary embolism. The main pulmonary artery and its bifurcation have opened to reveal a large saddle embolus. (From McManus B. M., Allard M. F., Yanagawa B. [2005]. Hemodynamic disorders. In Rubin E., Gorstein F., Rubin R., et al. [Eds.], *Rubin's pathology: Clinicopathologic foundations of medicine* [4th ed., p. 291]. Philadelphia: Lippincott Williams & Wilkins.)

bedridden patients in an intensive care unit. Cancer cells can produce thrombin and synthesize procoagulation factors, increasing the risk of thromboembolism. Use of oral contraceptives, pregnancy, and hormone replacement therapy are thought to increase the resistance to endogenous anticoagulants. The risk of pulmonary embolism among users of oral contraceptives is approximately three times the risk of nonusers.[40] Women who smoke are at particular risk.

Clinical Features

Manifestations. The manifestations of pulmonary embolism depend on the size and location of the obstruction. Chest pain, dyspnea, and increased respiratory rate are the most frequent signs and symptoms of pulmonary embolism. Pulmonary infarction often causes pleuritic pain that changes with respiration; it is more severe on inspiration and less severe on expiration. Moderate hypoxemia without carbon dioxide retention occurs as a result of impaired gas exchange. Small emboli that become lodged in the peripheral branches of the pulmonary artery may exert little effect and go unrecognized. However, repeated small emboli often result in a gradual reduction in the size of the pulmonary capillary bed, resulting in pulmonary hypertension. Moderate-size emboli often present with breathlessness accompanied by pleuritic pain, apprehension, slight fever, rapid and shallow breathing, and cough productive of blood-streaked sputum. Persons with massive emboli usually present with sudden collapse, crushing substernal chest pain, shock, and sometimes loss of consciousness. The pulse is rapid and weak, the blood pressure is low, the neck veins are distended, and the skin is cyanotic and diaphoretic. Massive pulmonary emboli often are fatal.

Diagnosis and Treatment. The diagnosis of pulmonary embolism is based on clinical signs and symptoms, blood gas determinations, venous thrombosis studies, D-dimer testing, lung scans, helical CT scans of the chest, and, in selected cases, pulmonary angiography.[41,42] Laboratory studies and radiologic films are useful in ruling out other conditions that might give rise to similar symptoms. Because emboli can cause an increase in pulmonary vascular resistance, the electrocardiogram (ECG) may be used to detect signs of right heart strain. There has been recent interest in combining several noninvasive methods (lower limb compression ultrasonography, D-dimer measurements, and clinical assessment measures) as a means of establishing a diagnosis of pulmonary embolism.

Because almost all pulmonary emboli originate from DVT, venous studies such as *lower limb compression ultrasonography, impedance plethysmography,* and *contrast venography* often are used as initial diagnostic procedures. *D-dimer testing* involves the measurement of plasma D-dimer, a degradation product of coagulation factors that have been activated as the result of a thromboembolic event. The *ventilation-perfusion scan* uses radiolabeled albumin, which is injected intravenously, and a radiolabeled gas, which is inhaled. A scintillation (gamma) camera is used to scan the various lung segments for blood flow and distribution of the radiolabeled gas. *Helical (spiral) CT angiography* requires administration of an intravenous radiocontrast media. It is sensitive for the detection of emboli in the proximal pulmonary arteries and provides another method of diagnosis. *Pulmonary angiography* involves the passage of a venous catheter through the right heart and into the pulmonary artery under fluoroscopy. Although it remains the most accurate method of diagnosis, it is an invasive procedure; therefore, its use is reserved for selected cases. An embolectomy sometimes is performed during this procedure.

The treatment goals for pulmonary emboli focus on preventing DVT and the development of thromboemboli, protecting the lungs from exposure to thromboemboli when they occur, and in the case of large and life-threatening pulmonary emboli, sustaining life and restoring pulmonary blood flow. Thrombolytic therapy using streptokinase, urokinase, or recombinant tissue plasminogen activator may be indicated in persons with multiple or large emboli. Thrombolytic therapy is followed by administration of heparin and then warfarin. Restoration of blood flow in persons with life-threatening pulmonary emboli can be accomplished through the surgical removal of the embolus or emboli.

Prevention. Prevention focuses on identification of persons at risk, avoidance of venous stasis and hypercoagulability states, and early detection of venous thrombosis. For patients at risk, graded compression elastic stockings and intermittent pneumatic compression (IPC) boots can be used to prevent venous stasis. Both of these devices are safe and practical ways to prevent venous thrombosis. IPC boots provide intermittent inflation of air-filled sleeves that prevent venous stasis. Some devices produce sequential gradient compression that moves blood upward in the leg.

Pharmacologic prophylaxis involves the use of anticoagulant drugs (see Chapter 10). Anticoagulant therapy may be used to decrease the likelihood of DVT, thromboembolism, and fatal pulmonary embolism after major surgical procedures. Low–molecular-weight heparin, which can be administered subcutaneously on an outpatient basis, often is used. Warfarin, an oral anticoagulation drug, may be used for persons with long-term risk of developing thromboemboli.

PULMONARY HYPERTENSION

The pulmonary circulation is a low-pressure system designed to accommodate varying amounts of blood delivered to the right heart and to facilitate gas exchange. The main pulmonary artery and major branches are relatively thin-walled, compliant vessels. The distal pulmonary arterioles also are thin walled and have the capacity to dilate, collapse, or constrict, depending on the presence of vasoactive substances released from the endothelial cells of the vessel, neurohumoral influences, flow velocity, oxygen tension, and alveolar ventilation.

The term *pulmonary hypertension* describes the elevation of pressure in the pulmonary arterial system. The normal mean pulmonary artery pressure is approximately 15 mm Hg (*e.g.,* 28 mm Hg systolic/8 mm Hg diastolic). Pulmonary hypertension is defined as a sustained elevation of the mean pulmonary artery pressure to more than 25 mm Hg at rest or to more 30 mm Hg with exercise.[43] Pulmonary hypertension can be caused by an elevation in left atrial pressure, increased pulmonary blood flow, or increased pulmonary vascular resistance. Because of the increased pressure in the pulmonary circulation, pulmonary hypertension increases the workload of the right heart. Although pulmonary hypertension can develop as a primary disorder, most cases develop secondary to some other condition.

Secondary Pulmonary Hypertension

Secondary pulmonary hypertension refers to an increase in pulmonary pressures associated with other disease conditions, usually cardiac or pulmonary. Secondary causes, or mechanisms, of pulmonary hypertension can be divided into four major categories: (1) elevation of pulmonary venous pressure, (2) increased pulmonary blood flow, (3) pulmonary vascular obstruction, and (4) hypoxemia.[44] Often more than one factor, such as COPD, heart failure, and sleep apnea, contributes to the elevation in pulmonary pressures.

Elevation of pulmonary venous pressure is common in conditions such as mitral valve stenosis and left ventricular heart failure, in which an elevated left atrial pressure is transmitted to the pulmonary circulation. Continued increases in left atrial pressure can lead to medial hypertrophy and intimal thickening of the small pulmonary arteries, causing sustained hypertension. *Increased pulmonary blood flow* results from increased flow through left-to-right shunts in congenital heart diseases such as atrial or ventricular septal defects and patent ductus arteriosus. If the high-flow state is allowed to continue, morphologic changes occur in the pulmonary vessels, leading to sustained pulmonary hypertension. The pulmonary vascular changes that occur with congenital heart disorders are discussed in Chapter 18. *Obstruction of pulmonary blood vessels* is most commonly the result of pulmonary emboli. Once initiated, the pulmonary hypertension that develops is self-perpetuating because of hypertrophy and proliferation of vascular smooth muscle.

Hypoxemia is another common cause of pulmonary hypertension. Unlike the vessels in the systemic circulation, most of which dilate in response to hypoxemia and hypercapnia, the pulmonary vessels constrict. The stimulus for constriction is thought to originate in the air spaces near the smaller branches of the pulmonary arteries. In situations in which certain regions of the lung are hypoventilated, the response is adaptive in that it diverts blood flow away from the poorly ventilated areas to more adequately ventilated portions of the lung. However, this effect becomes less beneficial as more and more areas of the lung become poorly ventilated. Pulmonary hypertension is a common problem in persons with advanced COPD. It also may develop at high altitudes in persons with normal lungs. Persons who experience marked hypoxemia during sleep (*i.e.,* those with sleep apnea) may also experience marked elevations in pulmonary arterial pressure.

The signs and symptoms of secondary pulmonary hypertension reflect not only the underlying cause, but the effect that the elevated pressure has on right heart function and oxygen transport. Dyspnea and fatigue are common. Peripheral edema, ascites, and signs of right heart failure (cor pulmonale, to be discussed) develop as the condition progresses.

Diagnosis is based on radiographic findings, echocardiography, and Doppler ultrasonography. Precise measurement of pulmonary pressures can be obtained only through right heart cardiac catheterization. Treatment measures are directed toward the underlying disorder. Vasodilator therapy may be indicated for some persons.

Primary Pulmonary Hypertension

Primary pulmonary hypertension is a relatively rare and rapidly progressive form of pulmonary hypertension that often leads to right ventricular failure and death within a few years. Estimates of incidence range from one to two cases per million people in the general population.[45] The disease can occur at any age, and familial occurrences have been reported. Persons with the disorder usually have a steadily progressive downhill course, with death occur-

ring in 3 to 4 years. Overall, the 5-year survival rate of untreated primary pulmonary hypertension is approximately 20%.[45]

Primary pulmonary hypertension is thought to be associated with a number of factors, including an autosomal dominant genetic predisposition along with an exogenous trigger. Triggers include low oxygen levels that occur at high altitudes, exposure to certain drugs, human immunodeficiency virus infection, and autoimmune disorders. Studies of a rare familial form of the disease point to a mutation in the transforming growth factor-β (TGF-β) superfamily of receptors as being responsible for the vascular thickening.[46] Mutations in these receptors are thought to prevent TGF-β and related molecules from exerting an inhibitory effect on smooth muscle and endothelial cell proliferation. A potent endogenous peptide, endothelin-1, is also thought to have a role in pulmonary hypertension.[47] Endothelin-1 acts on two receptors, endothelin-A and endothelin-B receptors. Activation of endothelin-B receptors causes vasodilatation, and activation of endothelin-A receptors results in vasoconstriction and smooth muscle growth.

Primary pulmonary hypertension is characterized by endothelial damage, coagulation abnormalities, and marked intimal fibrosis leading to obliteration or obstruction of the pulmonary arteries and arterioles. Most of the manifestations of the disorder are attributable to increased work demands on the right heart and a decrease in cardiac output. Symptoms are the same as those for secondary hypertension. The most obvious are dyspnea and fatigue that is out of proportion to other signs of the person's well-being.

Treatment consists of measures to improve right heart function to reduce fatigue and peripheral edema. Supplemental oxygen may used to increase exercise tolerance. The calcium channel blockers may be effective early in the course of the disease, but offer little relief in advanced stages. More advanced disease has been managed with epoprostenol, a prostacyclin that has potent pulmonary vasodilator effects.[45,47] Because of its short half-life (3 to 5 minutes), the drug must be administered by continuous infusion through an indwelling catheter with an automatic ambulatory pump. Properties of the drug other than its vasodilating effects include inhibition of platelet aggregation and beneficial vascular remodeling effects. This agent often improves symptoms, sometimes dramatically, in persons who have not responded to other vasodilators. Bosentan, an oral endothelin antagonist, has proved to be effective in treating moderate to severe primary pulmonary hypertension and may become the treatment of choice for all stages of the disease.[47]

Cor Pulmonale

The term *cor pulmonale* refers to right heart failure resulting from primary lung disease and long-standing primary or secondary pulmonary hypertension. It involves hypertrophy and the eventual failure of the right ventricle. The manifestations of cor pulmonale include the signs and symptoms of the primary lung disease and the signs of right-sided heart failure (see Chapter 19). Signs of right-sided heart failure include venous congestion, peripheral edema, shortness of breath, and a productive cough, which becomes worse during periods of worsening failure. Plethora (*i.e.*, redness) and cyanosis and warm, moist skin may result from the compensatory polycythemia and desaturation of arterial blood that accompany chronic lung disease. Drowsiness and altered consciousness may occur as the result of carbon dioxide retention. Management of cor pulmonale focuses on the treatment of the lung disease and the heart failure. Low-flow oxygen therapy may be used to reduce the pulmonary hypertension and polycythemia associated with severe hypoxemia caused by chronic lung disease.

ACUTE RESPIRATORY DISTRESS SYNDROME

Acute respiratory distress syndrome (ARDS), first described in 1967, is a devastating syndrome of acute lung injury. Initially called the *adult respiratory distress syndrome*, it is now called the *acute respiratory distress syndrome* because it also affects children. ARDS affects approximately 150,000 to 200,000 persons each year; at least 50% to 60% of these persons die, despite the most sophisticated intensive care.[48–50] The disorder is the final common pathway through which many serious localized and systemic disorders produce diffuse injury to the alveolar-capillary membrane.

Acute respiratory distress syndrome may result from a number of conditions, including aspiration of gastric contents, major trauma (with or without fat emboli), sepsis secondary to pulmonary or nonpulmonary infections, acute pancreatitis, hematologic disorders, metabolic events, and reactions to drugs and toxins[48–50] (Chart 22-2).

Although a number of conditions may lead to ARDS, they all produce similar pathologic lung changes that include diffuse epithelial cell injury with increased per-

---

CHART 22-2

Conditions in Which ARDS Can Develop*

Aspiration

Near drowning
Aspiration of gastric contents

Drugs, Toxins, Therapeutic Agents

Heroin
Inhaled gases (*e.g.*, smoke, ammonia)
Oxygen
Radiation

Infections

Gram-negative septicemia
Other bacterial infections
Viral infections

Trauma and Shock

Burns
Fat embolism
Chest trauma

---

*This list is not intended to be inclusive.

---

meability of the alveolar-capillary membrane (Fig. 22-15). The increased permeability permits fluid, protein, and blood cells to move out of the vascular compartment into the interstitium and alveoli of the lung. Alveolar cell damage leads to accumulation of edema fluid, surfactant inactivation, and formation of a hyaline membrane that is impervious to gas exchange. As the disease progresses,

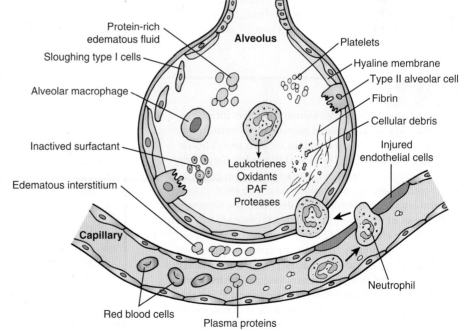

FIGURE 22-15 The mechanism of lung changes in ARDS. Injury and increased permeability of the alveolar capillary membrane allow fluid, protein, cellular debris, platelets, and blood cells to move out of the vascular compartment and enter the interstitium and alveoli. Activated neutrophils release a variety of products including toxic oxygen species (*e.g.*, oxidants), phospholipid products (*e.g.*, leukotrienes), proteolytic enzymes (proteases), and platelet-activating factor (PAF) that damage alveolar cells, inactivate surfactant, and lead to formation of a hyaline membrane.

Labels in figure: Protein-rich edematous fluid; Sloughing type I cells; Alveolar macrophage; Inactived surfactant; Edematous interstitium; Alveolus; Platelets; Hyaline membrane; Type II alveolar cell; Fibrin; Cellular debris; Injured endothelial cells; Leukotrienes Oxidants PAF Proteases; Neutrophil; Capillary; Red blood cells; Plasma proteins

the work of breathing becomes greatly increased as the lung stiffens and becomes more difficult to inflate. There is increased intrapulmonary shunting of blood, impaired gas exchange, and profound hypoxia. Gas exchange is further compromised by alveolar collapse resulting from abnormalities in surfactant production. When injury to the alveolar epithelium is severe, disorganized epithelial repair may lead to fibrosis.

The pathogenesis of ARDS is unclear. Neutrophils accumulate early in the course of the disorder and are thought to play a role in its pathogenesis. Activated neutrophils synthesize and release a variety of products, including proteolytic enzymes, toxic oxygen species, and phospholipid products, that increase the inflammatory response and cause injury to the capillary endothelium and alveolar epithelium.

Clinically, ARDS is marked by a rapid onset, usually within 12 to 18 hours of the initiating event, of respiratory distress, an increase in respiratory rate, and signs of respiratory failure. Chest radiography shows diffuse bilateral consolidation of the lung tissue. Marked hypoxemia occurs that is refractory to treatment with supplemental oxygen therapy. Many persons with ARDS demonstrate multiple organ failure, particularly involving the kidneys and gastrointestinal, central nervous, and cardiovascular systems.

The treatment goals in ARDS are to supply oxygen to vital organs and provide supportive care until the condition causing the pathologic process has been reversed and the lungs have had a chance to heal. Assisted ventilation using high concentrations of oxygen may be required to overcome the hypoxia. Positive end-expiratory pressure breathing, which increases the pressure in the airways during expiration, may be used to assist in reinflating the collapsed areas of the lung and to improve the matching of ventilation and perfusion.

Most survivors of ARDS are left with some pulmonary symptoms (cough, dyspnea, sputum production) that may improve over time. Mild abnormalities of oxygenation, diffusing capacity, and lung mechanics persist in some individuals.

In summary, pulmonary vascular disorders include pulmonary embolism and pulmonary hypertension. Pulmonary embolism develops when a blood-borne substance lodges in a branch of the pulmonary artery and obstructs blood flow. The embolus can consist of a thrombus, air, fat, or amniotic fluid. The most common form is a thromboembolus arising from the deep venous channels of the lower extremities. Pulmonary hypertension is the elevation of pulmonary arterial pressure. It can occur secondary to cardiac or pulmonary diseases that produce elevated left atrial pressure, increased pulmonary blood flow, pulmonary vascular obstruction, or hypoxemia. Primary pulmonary hypertension is a relatively rare and rapidly progressive form of pulmonary

hypertension. The term *cor pulmonale* describes right heart failure caused by primary pulmonary disease and long-standing pulmonary hypertension.

Acute respiratory distress syndrome is a devastating syndrome of acute lung injury resulting from a number of serious localized and systemic disorders that damage the alveolar-capillary membrane of the lung. It results in interstitial lung edema; an increase in surface tension caused by inactivation of surfactant; collapse of the alveolar structures; a stiff and noncompliant lung that is difficult to inflate; and impaired diffusion of the respiratory gases with severe hypoxia that is resistant to oxygen therapy.

Respiratory Failure

Respiratory failure is a condition in which the respiratory system fails in one or both of its gas exchange functions (*i.e.*, oxygenation of or elimination of carbon dioxide from the mixed venous blood).[51,52] It may occur in previously healthy persons as the result of acute disease or trauma involving the respiratory system, or it may develop in the course of a chronic neuromuscular or respiratory disease.

The common result of respiratory failure is *hypoxemia*, or a low level of oxygen in the blood, and *hypercapnia* (sometimes referred to as *hypercarbia*), or excess carbon dioxide in the blood. The abbreviation PO_2 often is used to indicate the partial pressure of oxygen in arterial

---

KEY CONCEPTS

Disorders of Blood Gases in Respiratory Failure

➤ Respiratory failure represents failure of the lungs adequately to oxygenate the blood (hypoxemia) and prevent carbon dioxide retention (hypercarbia.)

➤ Hypoxemia results from decreased concentration of oxygen in the inspired air, airway diseases that impair ventilation, respiratory disorders that impair ventilation or perfusion, and cardiovascular disorders that impair movement of blood through the respiratory portions of the lung.

➤ Carbon dioxide retention is characteristic of conditions that produce hypoventilation.

➤ Conditions such as acute respiratory distress syndrome that impede the diffusion of gases in the lung impair the oxygenation of blood but do not interfere with the elimination of carbon dioxide.

blood, and the abbreviation PCO_2, the partial pressure of carbon dioxide.

CAUSES

Respiratory failure is not a specific disease, but the result of a number of conditions that impair ventilation, compromise the matching of ventilation and perfusion, or impair gas diffusion. The causes of respiratory failure are summarized in Chart 22-3.

Hypoventilation

Hypoventilation or ventilatory failure occurs when the volume of "fresh" air moving into and out of the lung is significantly reduced. It is commonly caused by conditions outside the lung such as depression of the respiratory center (*e.g.*, drug overdose, high-flow oxygen therapy in persons with advanced COPD), diseases of the nerves supplying the respiratory muscles (*e.g.*, Guillain-Barré syndrome), disorders of the respiratory muscles (*e.g.*, muscular dystrophy), or thoracic cage disorders (*e.g.*, severe scoliosis or crushed chest). (Other causes of hypoventilation are discussed later in the section on Hypercapnia.)

Hypoventilation has two important effects on arterial blood gases. First, it almost always causes an increase in PCO_2. The rise in PCO_2 is directly related to the level of ventilation; reducing the ventilation by one half causes a doubling of the PCO_2. Thus, the PCO_2 level is a good diagnostic measure for hypoventilation.[51] Second, hypoxemia that is caused by hypoventilation can be readily abolished by increasing the oxygen content of the inspired air.

Ventilation-Perfusion Mismatching

The mismatching of ventilation and perfusion occurs when areas of the lung are ventilated but not perfused or when areas are perfused but not ventilated. Usually the hypoxemia seen in situations of ventilation-perfusion mismatching is more severe in relation to hypercapnia than that seen in hypoventilation. Severe mismatching of ventilation and perfusion often is seen in persons with advanced COPD. These disorders contribute to the retention of carbon dioxide by reducing the effective alveolar ventilation, even when total ventilation is maintained. This occurs because a region of the lung is not perfused and gas exchange cannot take place or because an area of the lung is not being ventilated. Maintaining a high ventilation rate effectively prevents hypercapnia but also increases the work of breathing.

The hypoxemia associated with ventilation-perfusion disorders often is exaggerated by conditions such as hypoventilation and decreased cardiac output. For example, sedation can cause hypoventilation in persons with severe COPD, resulting in further impairment of ventilation. Likewise, a decrease in cardiac output because of myocardial infarction can exaggerate the ventilation-perfusion impairment in a person with mild pulmonary edema.

The beneficial effect of oxygen administration on PO_2 levels in ventilation-perfusion disorders depends on the degree of mismatching that is present. Because oxygen administration increases the diffusion gradient in ventilated portions of the lung, it usually is effective in raising arterial PO_2 levels. However, it may also decrease the respiratory drive and produce an increase in PCO_2.

Impaired Diffusion

Impaired diffusion describes a condition in which gas exchange between the alveolar air and pulmonary blood is impeded because of an increase in the distance for diffusion or a decrease in the permeability of the respiratory membranes to the movement of gases. It most commonly occurs in conditions such as interstitial lung disease, ARDS, pulmonary edema, and pneumonia.

Conditions that impair diffusion may produce severe hypoxemia but no hypercapnia because of increased ventilation. Hypoxemia resulting from impaired diffusion can be partially or completely corrected by the administration of high concentrations of oxygen. In this case, the high concentration of oxygen serves to overcome the resistance to diffusion by establishing a large alveolar-to-capillary diffusion gradient.

MANIFESTATIONS

Respiratory failure is manifested by varying degrees of hypoxemia and hypercapnia. There is no absolute definition of the levels of PO_2 and PCO_2 that indicate respira-

---

CHART 22-3

Causes of Respiratory Failure*

Impaired Ventilation

Upper airway obstruction
 Infection (*e.g.*, epiglottitis)
 Foreign body
 Laryngospasm
 Tumors
Weakness or paralysis of respiratory muscles
 Brain injury
 Drug overdose
 Guillain-Barré syndrome
 Muscular dystrophy
 Spinal cord injury
Chest wall injury

Impaired Matching of Ventilation and Perfusion

Chronic obstructive pulmonary disease
Restrictive lung disease
Severe pneumonia
Atelectasis

Impaired Diffusion

Pulmonary edema
Acute respiratory distress syndrome

---

*This list is not intended to be inclusive.

tory failure. Respiratory failure is conventionally defined by an arterial PO_2 of less than 60 mm Hg, an arterial PCO_2 of more than 50 mm Hg, or both.[51] It is important to emphasize that these cut-off values are not rigid, but simply serve as a general guide in combination with history and physical assessment information.

Hypoxemia

The signs and symptoms of acute hypoxemia can be grouped into two categories: those resulting from impaired function of vital centers and those resulting from activation of compensatory mechanisms. Mild hypoxemia produces few manifestations. There may be slight impairment of mental performance and visual acuity and sometimes hyperventilation. More pronounced hypoxemia may produce personality changes, restlessness, agitated or combative behavior, uncoordinated muscle movements, euphoria, impaired judgment, delirium, and, eventually, stupor and coma. Recruitment of sympathetic nervous system compensatory mechanisms produces an increase in heart rate, peripheral vasoconstriction, diaphoresis, and a mild increase in blood pressure. Profound acute hypoxemia can cause convulsions, retinal hemorrhages, and permanent brain damage. Hypotension and bradycardia often are preterminal events in persons with hypoxemia, indicating the failure of compensatory mechanisms.

In conditions of chronic hypoxemia, the manifestations may be insidious in onset and attributed to other causes, particularly in chronic lung disease. Decreased sensory function, such as impaired vision or fewer complaints of pain, may be an early sign of worsening hypoxemia. This is probably because the involved sensory neurons have the same need for high levels of oxygen as do other parts of the nervous system. Pulmonary hypertension is common because of associated alveolar hypoxia.

Cyanosis refers to the bluish discoloration of the skin and mucous membranes that results from an excessive concentration of reduced or deoxygenated hemoglobin in the small blood vessels. It usually is most marked in the lips, nail beds, ears, and cheeks. The degree of cyanosis is modified by the amount of cutaneous pigment, skin thickness, and the state of the cutaneous capillaries. Cyanosis is more difficult to distinguish in persons with dark skin and in areas of the body with increased skin thickness.

Although cyanosis may be evident in persons with respiratory failure, it often is a late sign. A concentration of approximately 5 g/dL of deoxygenated hemoglobin is required in the circulating blood for cyanosis.[53] It is the absolute quantity (gm/dL) of reduced hemoglobin rather than the relative quantity (%) of reduced hemoglobin that is important in producing cyanosis. Persons with anemia and low hemoglobin levels are less likely to exhibit cyanosis (because they have less hemoglobin to deoxygenate), even though they may be relatively hypoxic because of their decreased ability to transport oxygen, than persons who have high hemoglobin concentrations. Someone with a high hemoglobin level because of polycythemia may be cyanotic without being hypoxic.

Cyanosis can be divided into two types: central or peripheral. *Central cyanosis* is evident in the tongue and lips. It is caused by an increased amount of deoxygenated hemoglobin or an abnormal hemoglobin derivative in the arterial blood. *Peripheral cyanosis* occurs in the extremities and on the tip of the nose or ears. It is caused by slowing of blood flow to an area of the body, with increased extraction of oxygen from the blood. It results from vasoconstriction and diminished peripheral blood flow, as occurs with cold exposure, shock, congestive heart failure, and peripheral vascular disease.

Diagnosis. The diagnosis of hypoxemia is based on clinical observation and diagnostic measures of oxygen levels. The analysis of arterial blood gases provides a direct measure of the oxygen content of the blood and is a good indicator of the lungs' ability to oxygenate the blood. Noninvasive measurements of arterial oxygen saturation of hemoglobin can be obtained using an instrument called the *pulse oximeter*. The pulse oximeter uses light-emitting diodes and combines plethysmography (*i.e.,* changes in light absorbance and vasodilatation) with spectrophotometry.[54,55] Spectrophotometry uses a red-wavelength light that passes through oxygenated hemoglobin and is absorbed by deoxygenated hemoglobin and an infrared-wavelength light that is absorbed by oxygenated hemoglobin and passes through deoxygenated hemoglobin. Sensors that can be placed on the ear, finger, toe, or forehead are available. These methods, although not as accurate as the invasive methods, provide a means for continuous monitoring of oxygen levels and are useful indicators of respiratory and circulatory status. Pulse oximeters do not measure hemoglobin levels and the oxygen-carrying capacity of blood nor can they distinguish between oxygen-carrying hemoglobin and carbon monoxide–carrying hemoglobin. In addition, the pulse oximeter cannot detect elevated levels of methemoglobin.

Hypercapnia

Hypercapnia refers to an increase in the CO_2 content of the arterial blood.[56] The respiratory center, which is located in the brain stem, controls the activity of the muscles of respiration and plays a critical role in the regulation of ventilation and elimination of CO_2 (see Chapter 20). The activity of the respiratory center is regulated by chemoreceptors that monitor changes in the chemical composition of the blood. The most important chemoreceptors in terms of the minute-by-minute control of ventilation are the central chemoreceptors that respond to changes in the hydrogen ion (H^+) concentration of the cerebrospinal fluid. Although the blood-brain barrier is impermeable to H^+ ions, CO_2 crosses it with ease. The CO_2, in turn, reacts with water to form carbonic acid, which dissociates to form H^+ and bicarbonate (HCO_3^-) ions. When the CO_2 content of the blood rises, CO_2 crosses the blood-brain barrier, liberating H^+ ions that stimulate the central chemoreceptors. Stimulation of the respiratory center is greatest during the first 1 to 2 days that PCO_2 levels are elevated, but it gradually declines over the next 1 to 2 days.[56] Part of this decline results from renal compensatory mechanisms that readjust the blood pH by increasing blood HCO_3^- levels.

An important cause of carbon dioxide retention in respiratory failure is the injudicious use of oxygen therapy. In persons with respiratory problems that cause chronic hypoxia and hypercapnia, the peripheral chemoreceptors become the driving force for ventilation. These chemoreceptors, which are located in the bifurcation of the common carotid arteries and in the aortic arch, respond to a decrease in arterial PO_2. Administration of high-flow oxygen to these persons can abolish the input from these peripheral receptors, causing a decrease in alveolar ventilation and a further rise in PCO_2 levels.

Manifestations. Hypercapnia affects a number of body functions, including renal function, neural function, cardiovascular function, and acid-base balance. Elevated levels of PCO_2 produce a decrease in pH and respiratory acidosis (see Chapter 6). The kidneys normally compensate for an increase in PCO_2 by increasing bicarbonate reabsorption. As long as the pH is in an acceptable range, the main complications of hypercapnia are those resulting from the accompanying hypoxia. Because the body adapts to chronic increases in blood levels of carbon dioxide, persons with chronic hypercapnia may not have symptoms until the PCO_2 becomes markedly elevated.

Carbon dioxide has a direct vasodilating effect on many blood vessels and a sedative effect on the nervous system. In acute respiratory failure, elevated PCO_2 levels greatly increase cerebral blood flow, causing headache, increased cerebrospinal fluid pressure, and sometimes papilledema. There is headache due to dilatation of the cerebral vessels; the conjunctivae are hyperemic; and the skin is warm and flushed. Hypercapnia has nervous system effects similar to those of an anesthetic—hence the term *carbon dioxide narcosis*. There is progressive somnolence, disorientation, and, if the condition is untreated, coma. Mild to moderate increases in blood pressure are common. Air hunger and rapid breathing occur when alveolar PCO_2 levels rise to approximately 60 to 75 mm Hg; as PCO_2 levels reach 80 to 100 mm Hg, the person becomes lethargic and sometimes semicomatose. Anesthesia and death can result when PCO_2 levels reach 100 to 150 mm Hg.[53]

Diagnosis. The diagnosis of hypercapnia is based on physiologic manifestations, arterial blood gas levels, and arterial pH. At the end of exhalation, arterial PCO_2 measurements approximate alveolar carbon dioxide measurements. Therefore, samples of exhaled carbon dioxide, measured at the end of exhalation, can be used as estimates of alveolar carbon dioxide, and because arterial and alveolar carbon dioxide levels are similar, as estimates of arterial PCO_2. Methods for monitoring samples of expired gas from an oral airway or endotracheal tube are available and are sometimes used for monitoring patients during weaning from a ventilator or cardiopulmonary resuscitation.

TREATMENT OF RESPIRATORY FAILURE

The treatment of respiratory failure focuses on correcting the problem causing impaired gas exchange when possible and on relieving the hypoxemia and hypercapnia. A number of treatment modalities are available, including the establishment of an airway, use of bronchodilating drugs, and antibiotics for respiratory infections. Controlled oxygen therapy and mechanical ventilation are used in treating blood gas abnormalities associated with respiratory failure.

Hypoxemia is usually treated with oxygen therapy. Oxygen may be delivered by nasal cannula or mask. It also may be administered directly into an endotracheal or tracheostomy tube in persons who are being ventilated. A high-flow administration system is one in which the flow rate and reserve capacity are sufficient to provide all the inspired air.[55] A low-flow oxygen system delivers less than the total inspired air.[55] The oxygen should be humidified as it is being administered. The concentration of oxygen that is being administered (usually determined by the flow rate) is based on the PO_2. The rate must be carefully monitored in persons with chronic lung disease because increases in PO_2 above 60 mm Hg are likely to depress the ventilatory drive. There also is the danger of oxygen toxicity with high concentrations of oxygen. Continuous breathing of oxygen at high concentrations can lead to diffuse parenchymal lung injury. Persons with healthy lungs begin to experience respiratory symptoms such as cough, sore throat, substernal distress, nasal congestion, and painful inspiration after breathing pure oxygen for 24 hours.[51]

Therapy for hypercapnia is directed at decreasing the work of breathing and improving the ventilation-perfusion balance. Intermittent rest therapy, such as nocturnal negative-pressure ventilation, applied to hypercapnic patients with COPD or chest wall disease may be effective in increasing the strength and endurance of the respiratory muscles and improving the PCO_2. Respiratory muscle retraining aimed at improving the respiratory muscles, their endurance, or both has been used to improve exercise tolerance and diminish the likelihood of respiratory fatigue.

When alveolar ventilation is inadequate to maintain PO_2 or PCO_2 levels because of respiratory or neurologic failure, mechanical ventilation may be lifesaving. Usually a nasotracheal, orotracheal, or tracheotomy tube is inserted into the trachea to provide the patient with the airway needed for mechanical ventilation. There has been recent interest in noninvasive forms of mechanical ventilation that use a face mask to deliver positive-pressure ventilation.[57]

In summary, the lungs enable inhaled air to come in proximity to the blood flowing through the pulmonary capillaries, so that the exchange of gases between the internal environment of the body and the external environment can take place. Respiratory failure is a condition in which the lungs fail to oxygenate the blood adequately and prevent carbon dioxide retention. It can result from a number of conditions that impair ventilation, compromise the matching of ventilation and perfusion, or impair gas diffusion and may arise acutely in persons with previously healthy lungs, or it may be superimposed on chronic lung disease. Respiratory failure is defined as a PO_2 of less than 60 mm Hg, a PCO_2 of more than 50 mm Hg, or both.

Hypoxia refers to an acute or chronic reduction in tissue oxygenation. Acute hypoxia incites sympathetic nervous system responses such as tachycardia and produces symptoms that are similar to those of alcohol intoxication. In conditions of chronic hypoxia, the manifestations may be insidious in onset and attributed to other causes, particularly in chronic lung disease. The development of cyanosis requires a concentration of 5 g/dL of deoxygenated hemoglobin. Hypercapnia refers to an increase in carbon dioxide levels. The manifestations of hypercapnia consist of those associated with dilatation of blood vessels, including those in the brain, and depression of the central nervous system (*e.g.*, carbon dioxide narcosis).

Review Exercises

A 30-year-old man is brought to the emergency department with a knife wound to the chest. On visual inspection, the asymmetry of chest movement during inspiration, displacement of the trachea, and absence of breath sounds on the side the wound are noted. His neck veins are distended and his pulse is rapid and thready. A rapid diagnosis of tension pneumothorax is made.

A. Explain the observed respiratory and cardiovascular function in terms of the impaired lung expansion and air that has entered the chest as a result of the injury.
B. What type of emergent treatment is necessary to save this man's life?

A 10-year-old boy who is having an acute asthmatic attack is brought to the emergency department by his parents. The boy is observed to be sitting up and struggling to breathe. His breathing is accompanied by use of the accessory muscles, a weak cough, and audible wheezing sounds. His pulse is rapid and weak and both heart and breath sounds are distant on auscultation. His parents relate that his asthma began to worsen after he developed a "cold" and now he does not even get relief from his "albuterol" inhaler.

A. Explain the changes in physiologic function underlying this boy's signs and symptoms.

B. What is the most probable reason for the progression of this boy's asthma in terms of the early- and late-phase responses?
C. The boy is treated with a systemic corticosteroid, and an inhaled anticholinergic agent and β_2-adrenergic agonist, and then transferred to the intensive care unit. Explain the action of each of these medications in terms of relieving this boy's symptoms.

A 62-year-old man with an 8-year history of chronic bronchitis reports to his health care provider with complaints of increasing shortness of breath, ankle swelling, and a feeling of fullness in his upper abdomen.

The expiratory phase of his respirations is prolonged and expiratory wheezes and crackles are heard on auscultation. His blood pressure is 160/90 mm Hg, his red blood cell count is $6.0 \times 10^6/\mu l$ (normal 4.2 to $5.4 \times 10^6/\mu l$), his hematocrit is 65% (normal male value 40% to 50%), his arterial PO_2 is 55 mm Hg, and his O_2 saturation, which is 85% while he is resting, drops to 55% during walking exercise.

A. Explain the physiologic mechanisms responsible for his edema, hypertension, and elevated red blood cell count.
B. His arterial PO_2 and O_2 saturation indicate that he is a candidate for continuous low-flow oxygen. Explain the benefits of this treatment in terms of his activity tolerance, blood pressure, and red blood cell count.
C. Explain why the oxygen flow rate for persons with COPD is normally titrated to maintain the arterial PO_2 between 60 to 65 mm Hg.

An 18 year-old female is admitted to the emergency room with a suspected drug overdose. Her respiratory rate is slow (4 to 6 times/minute) and shallow. Arterial blood gases reveal a PCO_2 of 80 mm Hg and a PO_2 of 60 mm Hg.

A. What is the cause of this woman's high PCO_2 and low PO_2?
B. Hypoventilation almost always causes an increase in PCO_2. Explain.
C. Even though her PO_2 increases to 90 mm Hg with institution of oxygen therapy, her PCO_2 remains elevated. Explain.

REFERENCES

1. Chestnut M. S., Prendergast T. J. (2004). Lung. In Tierney L. M., McPhee S. J., Papadakis M. A. (Eds.), *Current medical diagnosis and treatment* (43rd ed., pp. 294–299). New York: Lange Medical Books/McGraw-Hill.

2. Romero S. (2000). Nontraumatic chylothorax. *Current Opinion in Pulmonary Medicine* 6, 287–291.

3. Sahn S. A., Heffner J. E. (2000). Spontaneous pneumothorax. *New England Journal of Medicine* 342, 868–874.

4. Light R. W. (1995). Diseases of the pleura, mediastinum, chest wall, and diaphragm. In George R. B., Light R. W., Matthay M. A., et al. (Eds.), *Chest medicine* (3rd ed., pp. 501–520). Baltimore: Williams & Wilkins.

5. American Lung Association. (2003). *American Lung Association fact sheet: Asthma in adults.* [On-line]. Available: http://lungusa.org/data. Accessed May 10, 2005.

6. National Asthma Education and Prevention Program. (1997, 2002). *Expert Panel report 2: Guidelines for the diagnosis and management of asthma,* and *Guidelines for the diagnosis and management of asthma—Update on selected topics 2002.* Bethesda, MD: National Institutes of Health, National Heart, Lung, and Blood Institute. [On-line]. Available: www.nhlbi.nih.gov/guidelines/asthma.

7. Husain A. N., Kumar V. (2005). The lung. In Kumar V., Abbas A. K., Fausto N. (Eds.), *Robbins and Cotran pathologic basis of disease* (7th ed., pp. 711–772). Philadelphia: Elsevier Saunders.

8. Fireman P. (2003). Understanding asthma pathophysiology. *Allergy and Asthma Proceedings* 24(2), 79–83.

9. Busse W. W., Lemanske R. F. (2001). Asthma. *New England Journal of Medicine* 344, 350–362.

10. Jarjour N. N., Kelly E. A. B. (2002). Pathogenesis of asthma. *Medical Clinics of North America* 86, 925–936.

11. McFadden E. R., Gilbert I. A. (1994). Exercise-induced asthma. *New England Journal of Medicine* 330, 1362–1366.

12. Young S., LeSouef P. N., Geelhoed G. C., et al. (1991). The influence of a family history of asthma and parental smoking on airway responsiveness in early infancy. *New England Journal of Medicine* 324, 1168–1173.

13. Chan-Yeung M., Malo J. (1995). Occupational asthma. *New England Journal of Medicine* 333, 107–112.

14. Babu K. S., Salvi S. S. (2000). Aspirin and asthma. *Chest* 118, 1470–1476.

15. Hamad A. M., Sutcliffe A. M., Knox A. J. (2004). Aspirin-induced asthma: Clinical aspects, pathogenesis and management. *Drugs* 64, 2417–2432.

16. Tan K. S., McFarlane L. C., Lipworth B. J. (1997). Loss of normal cyclical B_2 adrenoreceptor regulation and increased premenstrual responsiveness to adenosine monophosphate in stable female asthmatic patients. *Thorax* 52, 608–611.

17. Dubuske D. M. (1994). Asthma: Diagnosis and management of nocturnal symptoms. *Comprehensive Therapy* 20, 628–639.

18. Wenzel S. (Chair). (2000). Proceedings of the ATS workshop on refractory asthma. *American Journal of Respiratory and Critical Care Medicine* 162, 2341–2351.

19. Papiris S., Kotanidou A., Malagari K., et al. (2002). Clinical review: Severe asthma. *Critical Care* 6, 30–44.

20. Magadle R., Berar-Yanay N., Weiner P. (2002). The risk of hospitalization and near-fatal and fatal asthma in relation to the perception of dyspnea. *Chest* 121, 329–333.

21. Lui A. H., Spahn J. D., Leung D. Y. M. (2004). Childhood asthma. In Behrman R. E., Kliegman R. M., Jenson H. B. (Eds.), *Nelson textbook of pediatrics* (17th ed., pp. 760–774). Philadelphia: Elsevier Saunders.

22. Kemp J. P., Kemp J. A. (2001). Management of asthma in children. *American Family Physician* 63, 1341–1348.

23. Gern J. E., Lemanske R. F. (2003). Infectious triggers of pediatric asthma. *Pediatric Clinics of North America* 50, 555–575.

24. Gilliland F. D., Berhane K., McConnell R., et al. (2000). Maternal smoking during pregnancy, environmental tobacco smoke exposure and childhood lung function. *Thorax* 55, 271–276.

25. Szefler S. J. (2003). Identifying the child in need of asthma therapy. *Pediatric Clinics of North America* 50, 577–591.

26. Barnes P. J. (2000). Chronic obstructive pulmonary disease. *New England Journal of Medicine* 343, 269–280.

27. Calverley P. M. A., Walker P. (2003). Chronic obstructive pulmonary disease. *Lancet* 362, 1053–1061.

28. Pawels R. A., Buist A. S., Calverley P. M. A., et al. (2003). Global strategy for the diagnosis, management, and prevention of chronic obstructive pulmonary disease: NHLBI/WHO Global Initiative for Chronic Obstructive Lung Disease (GOLD) Workshop update. [On-line]. Available: www.goldcopd.com.

29. American Lung Association. (2003). *Trends in chronic bronchitis and emphysema: Morbidity and mortality.* [On-line]. Available: http://lungusa.org/data.

30. Travis W. D., Beasley M. B., Rubin E. (2005). The respiratory system. In Rubin E., Gorstein F., Rubin R., et al. (Eds.), *Rubin's pathology: Clinicopathologic foundations of medicine* (4th ed., pp. 583–658). Philadelphia: Lippincott Williams & Wilkins.

31. Sutherland E. R., Cherniak R. M. (2004). Management of chronic obstructive pulmonary disease. *New England Journal of Medicine* 350, 2689–2697.

32. Ratjen F. (2003). Cystic fibrosis. *Lancet* 361, 681–689.

33. Cystic Fibrosis Foundation. (2005). *Facts about cystic fibrosis.* [On-line]. Available: www.cff.org.

34. Maitra A., Kumar V. (2005). Diseases of infancy and childhood. In Kumar V., Abbas A. K., Fausto N. (Eds.), *Robbins and Cotran pathologic basis of disease* (7th ed., pp. 489–495). Philadelphia: Elsevier Saunders.

35. Boat T. F. (2004). Cystic fibrosis. In Behrman R. E., Kliegman R. M., Jenson H. B. (Eds.), *Nelson textbook of pediatrics* (17th ed., pp. 1437–1450). Philadelphia: Elsevier Saunders.

36. Gibsen R. L., Burns J. L., Ramsey B. W. (2003). Pathophysiology and management of pulmonary infections in cystic fibrosis. *American Journal of Respiratory and Critical Care* 168, 918–951.

37. Gross F. H. Y. (2002). Overview of pulmonary fibrosis. *Chest* 122(6 Suppl.), 334S–335S.

38. Gross T. J., Hunninghake G. W. (2001). Idiopathic pulmonary fibrosis. *New England Journal of Medicine* 345, 517–525.

39. Khalil N., O'Connor R. (2004). Idiopathic pulmonary fibrosis: Current understanding of the pathogenesis and the status of treatment. *Canadian Medical Association Journal* 171, 153–160.

40. Goldhaber S. Z. (1998). Pulmonary embolism. *New England Journal of Medicine* 339, 93–104.

41. Kearon C. (2003). Diagnosis of pulmonary embolism. *Canadian Medical Association Journal* 168, 183–194.

42. Olin J. W. (2002). Pulmonary embolism. *Reviews in Cardiovascular Medicine* 3(Suppl. 2), S68–S75.

43. Farber H. W., Loscalzo J. (2004). Pulmonary arterial hypertension. *New England Journal of Medicine* 351, 1655–1665.

44. Richardi M. J., Rubenfire M. (1999). How to manage secondary pulmonary hypertension. *Postgraduate Medicine* 105, 183–190.

45. Rubin L. J. (1997). Primary pulmonary hypertension. *New England Journal of Medicine* 336, 111–117.

46. Newman J. H., Wheeler I., Barst R. J., et al. (2001). Mutations in the gene for bone morphogenic protein receptor II as a cause of primary pulmonary hypertension in large kindred. *New England Journal of Medicine* 345, 319–324.

47. Hoeper M. M., Galiè N., Simmoneau G., et al. (2002). New treatments for pulmonary arterial hypertension. *American Journal of Respiratory and Critical Care Medicine* 165, 1209–1216.

48. Ware L. B., Matthay M. A. (2000). The acute respiratory distress syndrome. *New England Journal of Medicine* 342, 1334–1348.
49. Mortellitti M. P., Manning H. L. (2002). Acute respiratory distress syndrome. *American Family Physician* 65, 1823–1830.
50. Udobi K., Childs E., Touther K. (2003). Acute respiratory distress syndrome. *American Family Physician* 67, 315–322.
51. West J. B. (2001). *Pulmonary physiology and pathophysiology.* Philadelphia: Lippincott Williams & Wilkins.
52. Roussos C., Koutsoukou A. (2003). Respiratory failure. *European Respiratory Journal* 22(Suppl. 47), 3s–14s.
53. Guyton A. C., Hall J. E. (2000). *Textbook of medical physiology* (10th ed., pp. 477–478, 491–492, 804). Philadelphia: W. B. Saunders.

54. St. John R. E., Thomson P. D. (1999). Noninvasive respiratory monitoring. *Critical Care Nursing Clinics of North America* 11, 423–434.
55. Grap M. J. (2002). Pulse oximetry. *Critical Care Nurse* 22(3), 69–74.
56. Weinberger S. E., Schwartzstein R. M., Weiss J. W. (1989). Hypercapnia. *New England Journal of Medicine* 321, 1223–1230.
57. American Thoracic Society. (2001). International consensus conference in intensive care medicine: Noninvasive positive pressure ventilation in acute respiratory failure. *American Journal of Respiratory and Critical Care Medicine* 163, 283–291.

C h a p t e r *23*

Control of Kidney Function

It is no exaggeration to say that the composition of the blood is determined not so much by what the mouth takes in as by what the kidneys keep.

—HOMER SMITH,
From Fish to Philosopher

 The kidneys are remarkable organs. Each is smaller than a person's fist, but in a single day the two organs process approximately 1700 L of blood and combine its waste products into approximately 1.5 L of urine. As part of their function, the kidneys filter physiologically essential substances, such as sodium and potassium ions, from the blood and selectively reabsorb those substances that are needed to maintain the normal composition of internal body fluids. Substances that are not needed for this purpose or are present in excess pass into the urine. The kidneys also have endocrine functions. The renin-angiotensin-aldosterone mechanism participates in the regulation of blood pressure and the maintenance of circulating blood volume, and erythropoietin stimulates red blood cell production.

Kidney Structure and Function

GROSS STRUCTURE AND LOCATION

The kidneys are paired, bean-shaped organs that lie outside the peritoneal cavity in the back of the upper abdomen, one on each side of the vertebral column at the level of the 12th thoracic to 3rd lumbar vertebrae (Fig. 23-1). The right kidney normally is situated lower than the left, presumably because of the position of the liver. In the adult, each kidney is approximately 10 to 12 cm long, 5 to 6 cm wide, and 2.5 cm deep and weighs approximately 113 to 170 g. The medial border of the kidney is indented by a deep fissure called the *hilus*. It is here that blood vessels and nerves enter and leave the kidney. The ureters, which connect the kidneys with the bladder, also enter the kidney at the hilus.

The kidney is a multilobular structure, composed of up to 18 lobes. Each lobule is composed of nephrons, which are the functional units of the kidney. Each nephron has a glomerulus that filters the blood and a system of tubular structures that selectively reabsorb material from the filtrate back into the blood and secrete materials from the blood into the filtrate as urine is being formed.

On longitudinal section, a kidney can be divided into an outer cortex and an inner medulla (Fig. 23-2). The cortex, which is reddish-brown, contains the glomeruli and convoluted tubules of the nephron and blood vessels. The medulla consists of light-colored, cone-shaped masses—the renal pyramids—that are divided by the columns of the cortex (*i.e.*, columns of Bertin) that extend into the medulla. Each pyramid, topped by a region of cortex, forms a lobe of the kidney. The apices of the pyramids form the papillae, which are perforated by the openings of the collecting ducts. The renal pelvis is a wide, funnel-shaped structure at the upper end of the ureter. It is made up of the calices or cuplike structures that drain the upper and lower halves of the kidney.

The kidney is ensheathed in a fibrous external capsule and surrounded by a mass of fatty connective tissue, especially at its ends and borders. The adipose tissue protects the kidney from mechanical blows and assists, together with the attached blood vessels and fascia, in holding the kidney in place. Although the kidneys are relatively well protected, they may be bruised by blows to the loin or by compression between the lower ribs and the ilium. Because the kidneys are outside the peritoneal cavity, injury and rupture do not produce the same threat of peritoneal involvement as rupture of organs such as the liver or spleen.

Each kidney is supplied by a single renal artery that arises on either side of the aorta. As the renal artery approaches the kidney, it divides into five segmental arteries that enter the hilus of the kidney. In the kidney, each segmental artery subdivides and branches several times. The smallest branches, the intralobular arteries, give rise to the afferent arterioles that supply the glomeruli (Fig. 23-3). Although nearly all the blood flow to the kidneys passes through the cortex, less than 10% is directed to the medulla and only approximately 1% goes to the papillae. Under conditions of decreased perfusion or increased sympathetic nervous system stimulation, blood flow is redistributed away from the cortex toward the medulla. This redistribution of blood flow decreases glomerular filtration while maintaining the urine-concentrating ability of the kidneys, a factor that is important during conditions such as shock.

THE NEPHRON

Each kidney is composed of more than 1 million tiny, closely packed functional units called *nephrons* (Fig. 23-4). Each nephron consists of a glomerulus, where blood is filtered, and a tubular component. Here, water, electrolytes, and other substances needed to maintain the constancy of the internal environment are reabsorbed into the bloodstream while other unneeded materials are secreted into the tubular filtrate for elimination.

The nephron is supplied by two capillary systems, the glomerulus and the peritubular capillary network (see Fig. 23-4). The glomerulus is a unique, high-pressure capillary filtration system located between two arterioles—the afferent and the efferent arterioles—that selectively dilate or constrict to regulate glomerular capillary pressure. The peritubular capillary network is a low-pressure reabsorptive system that originates from the efferent arteriole. These capillaries surround all portions of the tubules, an arrangement that permits rapid movement of solutes and water between the fluid in the tubular lumen and the blood in the capillaries. The peritubular capillaries rejoin

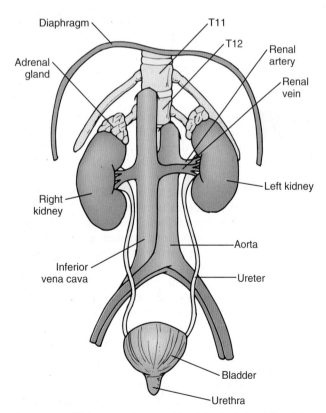

FIGURE 23-1 Kidneys, ureters, and bladder (note that the right kidney is usually lower than the left).

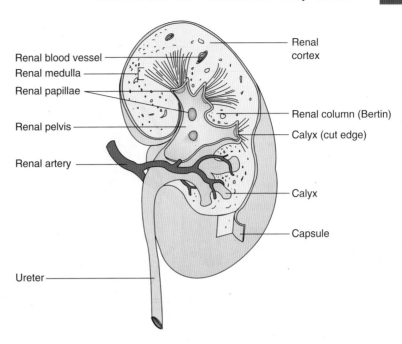

FIGURE 23-2 Internal structure of the kidney.

to form the venous channels by which blood leaves the kidneys and empties into the inferior vena cava.

The Glomerulus

The glomerulus consists of a compact tuft of capillaries encased in a thin, double-walled capsule, called *Bowman's capsule*. Blood flows into the glomerular capillaries from the afferent arteriole and flows out of the glomerular capillaries into the efferent arteriole, which leads into the peritubular capillaries. Fluid and particles from the blood are filtered through the capillary membrane into a fluid-filled space in Bowman's capsule, called *Bowman's space*. The mass of capillaries and its surrounding epithelial capsule are collectively referred to as the *renal corpuscle* (Fig.

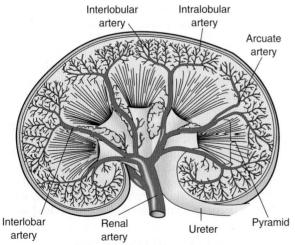

FIGURE 23-3 Simplified illustration of the arterial supply of the kidney. (From Cormack D. H. [1987]. *Ham's histology* [9th ed.]. Philadelphia: J. B. Lippincott.)

23-5A). The glomerular capillary membrane is composed of three layers: the capillary endothelial layer, the basement membrane, and the single-celled capsular epithelial layer (see Fig. 23-5B). The endothelial layer lines the glomerulus and interfaces with blood as it moves through the capillary. This layer contains many small perforations, called *fenestrations*.

The epithelial layer that covers the glomerulus is continuous with the epithelium that lines Bowman's capsule. The cells of the epithelial layer have unusual, octopus-like structures that possess a large number of extensions, or *foot processes* (*i.e.*, podocytes), that are embedded in the basement membrane. These foot processes form *slit pores* through which the glomerular filtrate passes. The *basement membrane* consists of a homogeneous acellular meshwork of collagen fibers, glycoproteins, and mucopolysaccharides (see Fig. 23-5C). Because the endothelial and the epithelial layers of the glomerular capillary have porous structures, the basement membrane determines the permeability of the glomerular capillary membrane. The spaces between the fibers that make up the basement membrane represent the pores of a filter and determine the size-dependent permeability barrier of the glomerulus. The size of the pores in the basement membrane normally prevents red blood cells and plasma proteins from passing through the glomerular membrane into the filtrate. There is evidence that the epithelium plays a major role in producing the basement membrane components, and it is probable that the epithelial cells are active in forming new basement membrane material throughout life. Alterations in the structure and function of the glomerular basement membrane are responsible for the leakage of proteins and blood cells into the filtrate that occurs in many forms of glomerular disease.

Another important component of the glomerulus is the *mesangium*. In some areas, the capillary endothelium and the basement membrane do not completely surround each

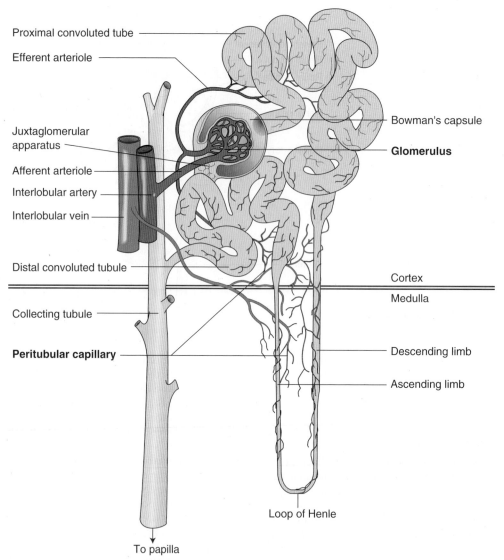

Proximal convoluted tube

Efferent arteriole

Juxtaglomerular apparatus

Afferent arteriole

Interlobular artery

Interlobular vein

Distal convoluted tubule

Collecting tubule

Peritubular capillary

Bowman's capsule

Glomerulus

Cortex

Medulla

Descending limb

Ascending limb

Loop of Henle

To papilla

FIGURE 23-4 Nephron, showing the glomerular and tubular structures along with the blood supply.

KEY CONCEPTS

The Nephron

➡ The nephron, which contains a glomerulus and tubular structures, is the functional unit of the kidney.

➡ Each nephron is closely associated with two capillary beds: the glomerulus, where water-soluble nutrients, wastes, and other small particles are filtered from the blood, and the peritubular capillaries that surround the tubular structures.

➡ Tubular structures process the glomerular (urine) filtrate, selectively reabsorbing substances from the tubular fluid into the peritubular capillaries and secreting substances from the peritubular capillaries into the urine filtrate.

capillary. Instead, the mesangial cells, which lie between the capillary tufts, provide support for the glomerulus in these areas (see Fig. 23-5B). The mesangial cells produce an intercellular substance similar to that of the basement membrane. This substance covers the endothelial cells where they are not covered by basement membrane. The mesangial cells possess (or can develop) phagocytic properties and remove macromolecular materials that enter the intercapillary spaces. Mesangial cells also exhibit contractile properties in response to neurohumoral substances and are thought to contribute to the regulation of blood flow through the glomerulus. In normal glomeruli, the mesangial area is narrow and contains only a small number of cells. Mesangial hyperplasia and increased mesangial matrix occur in a number of glomerular diseases.

Tubular Components of the Nephron

The nephron tubule is divided into four segments: a highly coiled segment called the *proximal convoluted tubule*, which drains Bowman's capsule; a thin, looped structure

categories. Approximately 85% of the nephrons originate in the superficial part of the cortex and are called *cortical nephrons*. They have short, thick loops of Henle that penetrate only a short distance into the medulla. The remaining 15% are called *juxtamedullary nephrons*. They originate deeper in the cortex and have longer and thinner loops of Henle that penetrate the entire length of the medulla. The juxtamedullary nephrons are largely concerned with urine concentration.

The proximal tubule is a highly coiled structure that dips toward the renal pelvis to become the descending limb of the loop of Henle. The ascending loop of Henle returns to the region of the renal corpuscle, where it becomes the distal tubule. The distal convoluted tubule, which begins at the juxtaglomerular complex, is divided into two segments: the *diluting segment* and the *late distal tubule*. The late distal tubule fuses with the collecting tubule. Like the distal tubule, the collecting duct is divided into two segments: the *cortical collecting tubule* and the *inner medullary collecting tubule*.

Throughout its course, the tubule is composed of a single layer of epithelial cells resting on a basement membrane. The structure of the epithelial cells varies with tubular function. The cells of the proximal tubule have a fine villous structure that increases the surface area for reabsorption; they also are rich in mitochondria, which support active transport processes. The epithelial layer of the thin segment of the loop of Henle has few mitochondria, indicating minimal metabolic activity and passive reabsorptive function.

URINE FORMATION

Urine formation involves the filtration of blood by the glomerulus to form an *ultrafiltrate of plasma* and the tubular reabsorption of electrolytes and nutrients needed to maintain the constancy of the internal environment while eliminating waste materials.

Glomerular Filtration

Urine formation begins with the filtration of fluid through the glomerular capillaries into Bowman's space. The movement of fluid through the glomerular capillaries is determined by the same factors (*i.e.,* capillary filtration pressure, colloidal osmotic pressure, and capillary permeability) that affect fluid movement through other capillaries in the body (see Chapter 6). The glomerular filtrate has a chemical composition similar to plasma, but it contains almost no proteins because large molecules do not readily cross the glomerular wall. Approximately 125 mL of filtrate is formed each minute. This is called the *glomerular filtration rate* (GFR). The GFR can vary from a few milliliters per minute to as high as 200 mL/minute.

The location of the glomerulus between two arterioles allows for maintenance of a high-pressure filtration system. The capillary filtration pressure (approximately 60 mm Hg) in the glomerulus is approximately two to three times higher than that of other capillary beds in the body. The filtration pressure and the GFR are regulated by the constriction and relaxation of the afferent and

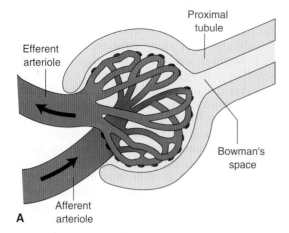
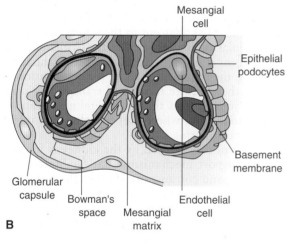
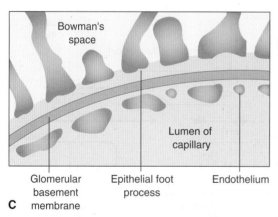

FIGURE 23-5 Renal corpuscle. (**A**) Structures of the glomerulus. (**B**) Position of the mesangial cells in relation to the capillary loops and Bowman's capsule. (**C**) Cross-section of the glomerular membrane, showing the position of the endothelium, basement membrane, and epithelial foot processes.

called the *loop of Henle*; a distal coiled portion called the *distal convoluted tubule*; and a final segment called the *collecting tubule*, which joins with several tubules to collect the filtrate (see Fig. 23-4). The filtrate passes through each of these segments before reaching the pelvis of the kidney. Nephrons can be roughly grouped into two

efferent arterioles. Constriction of the efferent arteriole increases resistance to outflow from the glomeruli and increases the glomerular pressure and the GFR. Constriction of the afferent arteriole causes a reduction in the renal blood flow, glomerular filtration pressure, and GFR. The afferent and the efferent arterioles are innervated by the sympathetic nervous system and also are sensitive to vasoactive hormones, such as angiotensin II. During periods of strong sympathetic stimulation, such as occurs during shock, constriction of the afferent arteriole causes a marked decrease in renal blood flow and thus glomerular filtration pressure. Consequently, urine output can fall almost to zero.

Tubular Reabsorption and Secretion

From Bowman's capsule, the glomerular filtrate moves into the tubular segments of the nephron. In its movement through the lumen of the tubular segments, the glomerular filtrate is changed considerably by the tubular transport of water and solutes. Tubular transport can result in reabsorption of substances from the tubular fluid into the blood or secretion of substances from the blood into the tubular fluid (Fig. 23-6). Segments of the renal tubule are adapted to reabsorb or secrete specific substances, using particular modes of transport.

The basic mechanisms of transport across the tubular epithelial cell membrane are similar to those of other cell

membranes in the body and include active and passive transport mechanisms (see Chapter 1). Water and urea are passively absorbed along concentration gradients. Sodium, potassium, chloride, calcium, and phosphate ions, as well as urate, glucose, and amino acids are reabsorbed using primary or secondary active transport mechanisms for movement across the tubular membrane. Some substances, such as hydrogen, potassium, and urate ions, are secreted into the tubular fluids. Under normal conditions, only approximately 1 mL of the 125 mL of glomerular filtrate that is formed each minute is excreted in the urine. The other 124 mL is reabsorbed in the tubules.

Renal tubular cells have two membrane surfaces through which substances must pass as they are reabsorbed from the tubular fluid. The side of the cell that is in contact with the tubular lumen and tubular filtrate is called the *luminal membrane* (Fig. 23-7). The outside membrane that lies adjacent to the interstitial fluid and the peritubular capillaries is called the *basolateral membrane*. In most cases, substances move from the tubular filtrate into the tubular cell along a concentration gradient, but they require facilitated transport or carrier systems to move across the basolateral membrane into the interstitial fluid, where they are absorbed into the peritubular capillaries.

The bulk of energy used by the kidney is for active sodium transport mechanisms that facilitate sodium reabsorption and cotransport of other electrolytes and substances such as glucose and amino acids. This is called *secondary active transport* or *cotransport* (see Fig. 23-7). Secondary active transport depends on the energy-

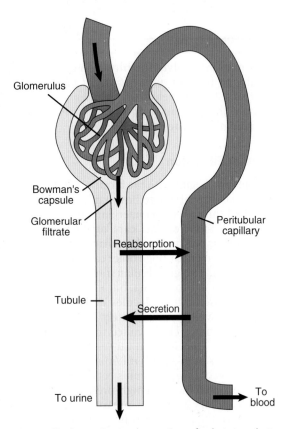

FIGURE 23-6 Reabsorption and secretion of substances between the renal tubules and peritubular capillaries.

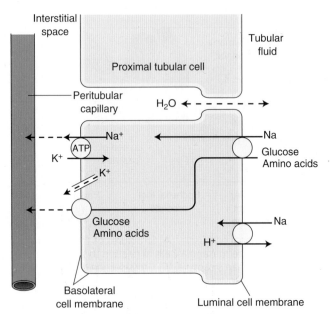

FIGURE 23-7 Mechanism for secondary active transport or cotransport of glucose and amino acids in the proximal tubule. The energy-dependent sodium-potassium pump on the basolateral surface of the cell maintains a low intracellular gradient that facilitates the downhill movement of sodium and glucose or amino acids (cotransport) from the tubular lumen into the tubular cell and then into the peritubular capillary.

dependent sodium-potassium adenosine triphosphatase (ATPase) pump on the basolateral side of renal tubular cells. The pump maintains a low intracellular sodium concentration that facilitates the downhill (*i.e.,* from a higher to lower concentration) movement of sodium from the filtrate across the luminal membrane. Cotransport uses a carrier system in which the downhill movement of one substance such as sodium is coupled to the uphill movement (*i.e.,* from a lower to higher concentration) of another substance such as glucose or an amino acid. A few substances, such as hydrogen, are secreted into the tubule using countertransport, in which the movement of one substance, such as sodium, enables the movement of a second substance in the opposite direction.

Proximal Tubule. Approximately 65% of all reabsorptive and secretory processes that occur in the tubular system take place in the proximal tubule. There is almost complete reabsorption of nutritionally important substances, such as glucose, amino acids, lactate, and water-soluble vitamins. Electrolytes, such as sodium, potassium, chloride, and bicarbonate, are 65% to 80% reabsorbed. As these solutes move into the tubular cells, their concentration in the tubular lumen decreases, providing a concentration gradient for the osmotic reabsorption of water and urea. The proximal tubule is highly permeable to water, and the osmotic movement of water follows solute movement.

Many substances, such as glucose, are freely filtered in the glomerulus and reabsorbed by energy-dependent cotransport carrier mechanisms. The maximum amount of substance that these transport systems can reabsorb per unit time is called the *transport maximum*. The transport maximum is related to the number of carrier proteins that are available for transport and usually is sufficient to ensure that all of a filtered substance such as glucose can be reabsorbed, rather than being eliminated in the urine. The plasma level at which the substance appears in the urine is called the *renal threshold* (Fig. 23-8). Under some circumstances, the amount of substance filtered in the glomerulus exceeds the transport maximum. For example, when the blood glucose level is elevated in uncontrolled diabetes mellitus, the amount that is filtered in the glomerulus often exceeds the transport maximum (approximately 320 mg/minute), and glucose spills into the urine.

The Loop of Henle. The loop of Henle plays an important role in controlling the concentration of the urine. It does this by establishing a high concentration of osmotically active particles in the interstitium surrounding the medullary collecting tubules where the antidiuretic hormone exerts its effects (to be discussed).

The loop of Henle is divided into three segments: the thin descending segment, the thin ascending segment, and thick ascending segment. The loop of Henle, taken as a whole, always reabsorbs more sodium and chloride than water. This is in contrast to the proximal tubule, which reabsorbs sodium and water in equal proportions. The thin descending limb is highly permeable to water and

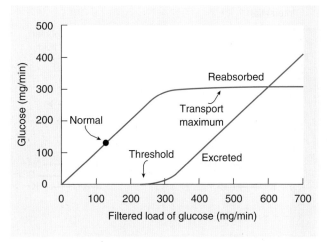

FIGURE 23-8 Relations among the filtered load (plasma concentration of glucose × GFR) of glucose, the rate of glucose reabsorption by the renal tubules, and the rate of glucose excretion in the urine. The *transport maximum* is the maximum rate at which glucose can be reabsorbed from the tubules. The *threshold* for glucose refers to the filtered load of glucose at which glucose first begins to appear in the urine. (From Guyton A., Hall J. E. [1996]. *Textbook of medical physiology* [9th ed., p. 335]. Philadelphia: W. B. Saunders, with permission from Elsevier Science.)

moderately permeable to urea, sodium, and other ions. As the urine filtrate moves down the descending limb, water moves out of the filtrate into the surrounding interstitium. Thus, the osmolality of the filtrate reaches its highest point at the elbow of the loop of Henle. In contrast to the descending limb, the ascending limb of the loop of Henle is impermeable to water. In this segment, solutes are reabsorbed, but water cannot follow and remains in the filtrate; as a result, the tubular filtrate becomes more and more dilute, often reaching an osmolality of 100 mOsm/kg of H_2O as it enters the distal convoluted tubule, compared with the 285 mOsm/kg of H_2O in plasma. This allows for excretion of free water from the body. For this reason, it is often called the *diluting segment.*

The thick segment of the loop of Henle begins in the ascending limb where the epithelial cells become thickened. As with the thin ascending limb, this segment is impermeable to water. The thick segment contains a $Na^+/K^+/2Cl^-$ cotransport system. This system involves the cotransport of a positively charged sodium and a positively charged potassium ion accompanied by two negatively charged chloride ions (Fig. 23-9). The gradient for the operation of this cotransport system is provided by the basolateral sodium-potassium pump, which maintains a low intracellular sodium concentration. Approximately 20% to 25% of the filtered load of sodium, potassium, and chloride is reabsorbed in the thick loop of Henle. Movement of these ions out of the tubule leads to the development of a transmembrane potential that favors the passive reabsorption of small divalent cations such as calcium and magnesium. The so-called *loop diuretics* (*e.g.,* furosemide [Lasix]) exert their effects at this site in the kidney.

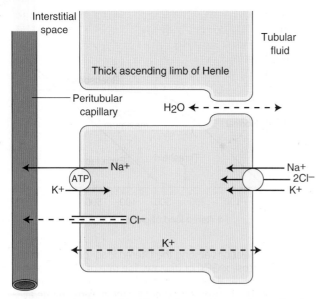

FIGURE 23-9 Sodium, chloride, and potassium reabsorption in the thick segment of the loop of Henle.

Distal and Collecting Tubules. Like the thick ascending loop of Henle, the distal convoluted tubule is relatively impermeable to water, and reabsorption of sodium chloride from this segment further dilutes the tubular fluid. Sodium reabsorption occurs through a sodium and chloride cotransport mechanism. Approximately 10% of filtered sodium chloride is reabsorbed in this section of the tubule. Unlike the thick ascending loop of Henle, neither calcium nor magnesium is passively absorbed in this segment of the tubule. Instead, calcium ions are actively reabsorbed in a process that is largely regulated by parathyroid hormone and possibly by vitamin D. The thiazide diuretics exert their action by inhibiting sodium chloride reabsorption in this segment of the renal tubules.

The late distal tubule and the cortical collecting tubule constitute the site where aldosterone exerts its action on sodium and potassium reabsorption. Although responsible for only 2% to 5% of sodium chloride reabsorption, this site is largely responsible for determining the final sodium concentration of the urine. The late distal tubule with the cortical collecting tubule also is the major site for regulation of potassium excretion by the kidney. When the body is confronted with a potassium excess, as occurs with a diet high in potassium content, the amount of potassium secreted at this site may exceed the amount filtered in the glomerulus.

The mechanism for sodium reabsorption and potassium secretion in this section of the nephron is distinct from other tubular segments. This tubular segment is composed of two types of cells, the *intercalated cells*, where potassium is reabsorbed and hydrogen is secreted, and the *principal cells*, where aldosterone exerts its action. The secretion of hydrogen ions into the tubular fluid by the intercalated cells is accompanied by the reabsorption of bicarbonate ions. The intercalated cells can also reabsorb potassium ions. The principal cells reabsorb sodium and facilitate the movement of potassium into the urine

filtrate. Under the influence of aldosterone, sodium moves from the urine filtrate into principal cells; from there it moves into the surrounding interstitial fluid and peritubular capillaries. Potassium moves from the peritubular capillaries into the principal cells and then into the urine filtrate.

Regulation of Urine Concentration

The ability of the kidney to respond to changes in the osmolality of the extracellular fluids by producing either a concentrated or dilute urine depends on the establishment of a high concentration of osmotically active particles (approximately 1200 mOsm/kg of H_2O) in the interstitium of the kidney medulla and the action of antidiuretic hormone (ADH) in regulating the water permeability of the surrounding medullary collecting tubules.

In approximately one fifth of the juxtamedullary nephrons, the loops of Henle and special hairpin-shaped capillaries called the *vasa recta* descend into the medullary portion of the kidney, forming a countercurrent system that controls water and solute movement so that water is kept out of the area surrounding the tubule and solutes are retained. The term *countercurrent* refers to a flow of fluids in opposite directions in adjacent structures. In this case, there is an exchange of solutes between the adjacent descending and ascending loops of Henle and between the ascending and descending sections of the vasa recta. Because of these exchange processes, a high concentration of osmotically active particles (approximately 1200 mOsm/kg of H_2O) collects in the interstitium of the kidney medulla. The presence of these osmotically active particles in the interstitium surrounding the medullary collecting tubules facilitates the ADH-mediated reabsorption of water.

Antidiuretic hormone assists in maintenance of the extracellular fluid volume by controlling the permeability of the medullary collecting tubules. Osmoreceptors in the hypothalamus sense an increase in osmolality of extracellular fluids and stimulate the release of ADH from the posterior pituitary gland (see Chapter 6). In exerting its effect, ADH, also known as *vasopressin*, binds to receptors on the basolateral side of the tubular cells. Binding of ADH to the vasopressin receptors causes water channels, known as *aquaporin-2 channels*, to move into the luminal side of the tubular cell membrane, producing a marked increase in water permeability. At the basolateral side of the membrane, water exits the tubular cell into the hyperosmotic interstitium of the medullary area, where it enters the peritubular capillaries for return to the vascular system. The aquaporin-2 channels are thought to have a critical role in inherited and acquired disorders of water reabsorption by the kidney (*e.g.*, diabetes insipidus).

REGULATION OF RENAL BLOOD FLOW

In the adult, the kidneys are perfused with 1000 to 1300 mL of blood per minute, or 20% to 25% of the cardiac output. This large blood flow is mainly needed to ensure a sufficient GFR for the removal of waste products from the blood, rather than for the metabolic needs of the kidney. Neural, humoral, and autoregulatory feedback mechanisms normally keep blood flow and GFR constant despite changes in arterial blood pressure.

Neural and Humoral Control Mechanisms

The kidney is richly innervated by the sympathetic nervous system. Increased sympathetic activity causes constriction of the afferent and efferent arterioles, producing a decrease in renal blood flow. Intense sympathetic stimulation such as occurs in shock and trauma can produce marked decreases in renal blood flow and GFR, even to the extent of causing blood flow to cease altogether.

Several humoral substances, including angiotensin II, ADH, and the endothelins, produce vasoconstriction of renal vessels. The endothelins are a group of peptides released from damaged endothelial cells in the kidney and other tissues. Although not thought to be important regulators of renal blood flow during everyday activities, endothelin I may play a role in reduction of blood flow in conditions such as postischemic acute renal failure (see Chapter 25). Other substances such as dopamine, nitric oxide, and prostaglandins E_2 and I_2 produce vasodilatation. Nitric oxide, a vasodilator produced by the vascular endothelium, appears to be important in preventing excessive vasoconstriction of renal blood vessels and allowing normal excretion of sodium and water. Prostaglandins are a group of mediators of cell function that are produced locally and exert their effects locally. Although prostaglandins do not appear to be of major importance in regulating renal blood flow and GFR under normal conditions, they may protect the kidneys against the vasoconstricting effects of sympathetic stimulation and angiotensin II. Salicylates and the nonsteroidal anti-inflammatory drugs (NSAIDs) that inhibit prostaglandin synthesis may produce a reduction in renal blood flow and GFR under certain conditions.

Autoregulatory Mechanisms

The constancy of renal blood flow is maintained by a process called *autoregulation* (see Chapter 16). Normally, autoregulation of blood flow is designed to maintain blood flow at a level consistent with the metabolic needs of the tissues. In the kidney, autoregulation of blood flow also must allow for precise regulation of water and solute secretion. For autoregulation to occur, the resistance to blood flow through the kidneys must be varied in direct proportion to the arterial pressure. The exact mechanisms responsible for the intrarenal regulation of blood flow are unclear. One of the proposed mechanisms involves a direct effect on renal vascular smooth muscle that causes the blood vessels to relax when there is an increase in blood pressure, and to constrict when there is a decrease in pressure. A second proposed mechanism involves feedback regulation by the juxtaglomerular complex.

The Juxtaglomerular Complex

The juxtaglomerular complex is thought to represent a feedback control system that links changes in the GFR with renal blood flow. The juxtaglomerular complex is located at the site where the distal tubule extends back to the glomerulus and then passes between the afferent and efferent arteriole (Fig. 23-10). The distal tubular site that is nearest the glomerulus is characterized by densely nucleated cells called the *macula densa*.

In the adjacent afferent arteriole, the smooth muscle cells of the media are modified as special secretory cells called *juxtaglomerular cells*. These cells contain granules of inactive renin, an enzyme that functions in the conversion of angiotensinogen to angiotensin. Renin functions by way of angiotensin II to produce vasoconstriction of the efferent arteriole as a means of preventing serious decreases in the glomerular filtration rate (see Chapter 16). Angiotensin II also increases sodium reabsorption indirectly by stimulating aldosterone secretion from the adrenal gland and directly by increasing sodium reabsorption in the proximal tubule.

Because of its location between the afferent and efferent arteriole, the juxtaglomerular complex is thought to play an essential feedback role in linking the level of arterial blood pressure and renal blood flow to the GFR and the composition of the distal tubular fluid. The juxtaglomerular complex monitors the arterial blood pressure by sensing the stretch of the afferent arteriole, and it monitors the concentration of sodium chloride in the tubular filtrate as it passes through the macula densa. This information is then used in determining how much renin should be released to keep the arterial blood pressure within its normal range and maintain a relatively constant GFR.

ELIMINATION FUNCTIONS OF THE KIDNEY

The functions of the kidney focus on elimination of water, waste products, excess electrolytes, and unwanted substances from the blood. As renal function declines, there

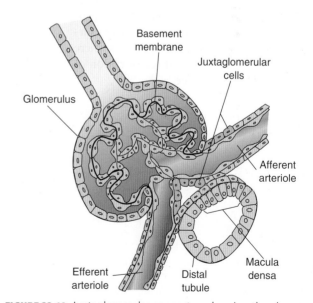

FIGURE 23-10 Juxtaglomerular apparatus, showing the close contact of the distal tubule with the afferent arteriole, the macula densa, and the juxtaglomerular cells.

Understanding ➤ How the Kidney Concentrates Urine

The osmolarity of body fluids relies heavily on the ability of the kidney to produce dilute or concentrated urine. Urine concentration is dependent upon three factors: (1) the osmolarity of interstitial fluids in the urine-concentrating part of the kidney, (2) the antidiuretic hormone (ADH), and (3) the action of ADH on the cells in the collecting tubules of the kidney.

1

Osmolarity. In approximately one fifth of the juxtamedullary nephrons, the loops of Henle and special hairpin-shaped capillaries called the *vasa recta* descend into the medullary portion of the kidney to form a countercurrent system—a set of parallel passages in which the contents flow in opposite directions. The countercurrent design serves to increase the osmolarity in this part of the kidney by promoting the exchange of solutes between the adjacent descending and ascending loops of Henle and between the descending and ascending sections of the vasa recta. Because of these exchange processes, a high concentration of osmotically active particles (approximately 1200 mOsm/kg of H_2O) collects in the interstitium surrounding the collecting tubules where the ADH-mediated reabsorption of water takes place.

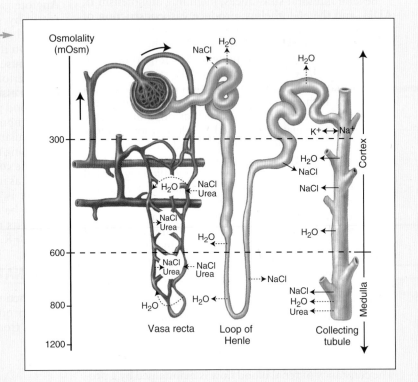

2

Antidiuretic hormone. ADH, which regulates the ability of the kidneys to concentrate urine, is synthesized by neurons in the hypothalamus and transported down their axons to the posterior pituitary gland and then released into the circulation. One of the main stimuli for synthesis and release of ADH is an increase in serum osmolarity. ADH release is also controlled by cardiovascular reflexes that respond to changes in blood pressure and/or blood volume.

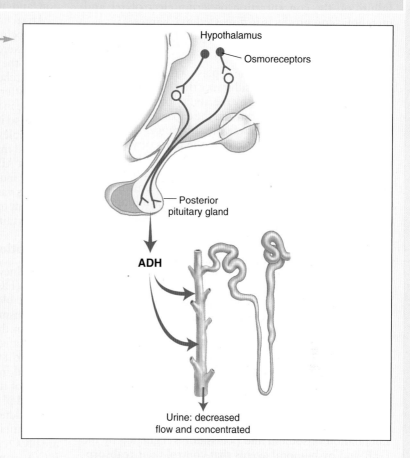

3

Action of ADH. ADH, also known as vasopressin, acts at the level of the collecting tubule to increase water absorption. It exerts its action by binding to vasopressin receptors on the basolateral membrane of the tubular cell. Binding of ADH to the vasopressin receptors causes water channels (*aquaporin-2 channels*) to move into the luminal side of the cell membrane, which is normally impermeable to water. Insertion of the channels allows water from the tubular fluid to move into the tubular cell and then out into the surrounding hyperosmotic interstitial fluid on the basolateral side of the cell, and from there it moves into the peritubular capillaries for return to the circulatory system. Thus, when ADH is present, the water that moved from the blood into the urine filtrate in the glomeruli is returned to the circulatory system, and when ADH is absent, the water is excreted in the urine.

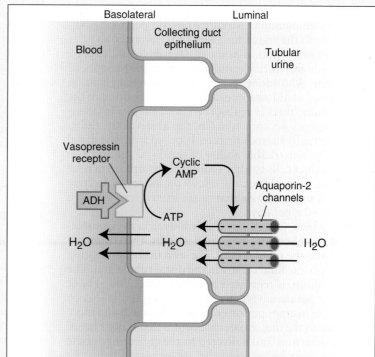

is an increase in serum levels of substances such urea, creatinine, phosphate, and potassium. The effect of renal failure on the concentration of serum electrolytes and metabolic end products is discussed in Chapter 25.

Renal Clearance

Renal clearance is the volume of plasma that is completely cleared each minute of any substance that finds its way into the urine. It is determined by the ability of the substance to be filtered in the glomeruli and the capacity of the renal tubules to reabsorb or secrete the substance. Every substance has its own clearance rate, the units of which are expressed as the volume of plasma that is cleared per unit time. It can be determined by measuring the amount of a substance that is excreted in the urine (*i.e.*, urine concentration × urine flow rate in milliliters per minute) and dividing by its plasma concentration. Inulin, a large polysaccharide, is freely filtered in the glomeruli and neither reabsorbed nor secreted by the tubular cells. After intravenous injection, the amount that appears in the urine is equal to the amount that is filtered in the glomeruli (*i.e.*, the clearance rate is equal to the GFR). Because of these properties, inulin can be used as a laboratory measure of the GFR. Some substances, such as urea, are freely filtered in the glomeruli, but the volume that is cleared from the plasma is less than the GFR, indicating that at least some of the substance is being reabsorbed. At normal plasma levels, glucose has a clearance of zero because it is reabsorbed in the tubules and none appears in the urine.

Regulation of Sodium and Potassium Elimination

Elimination of sodium and potassium is regulated by the GFR and by humoral agents that control their reabsorption. Aldosterone functions in the regulation of sodium and potassium elimination. Atrial natriuretic peptide (ANP) contributes to the regulation of sodium elimination.

Sodium reabsorption in the distal tubule and collecting duct is highly variable and depends on the presence of aldosterone, a hormone secreted by the adrenal gland. In the presence of aldosterone, almost all the sodium in the distal tubular fluid is reabsorbed, and the urine essentially becomes sodium free. In the absence of aldosterone, virtually no sodium is reabsorbed from the distal tubule. The remarkable ability of the distal tubular and collecting duct cells to alter sodium reabsorption in relation to changes in aldosterone allows the kidneys to excrete urine with sodium levels that range from a few tenths of a gram to 40 g per day.

Like sodium, potassium is freely filtered in the glomerulus, but unlike sodium, potassium is reabsorbed from and secreted into the tubular fluid. The secretion of potassium into the tubular fluid occurs in the distal tubule and, like that of sodium, is regulated by aldosterone. Only about 70 mEq of potassium is delivered to the distal tubule each day, but the average person consumes this much and more potassium in the diet. Excess potassium that is not filtered in the glomerulus and delivered to the collecting tubule therefore must be secreted (*i.e.*, transported from the blood) into the tubular fluid for elimination from the body. In the absence of aldosterone (as in Addison disease; see

Chapter 31), potassium secretion becomes minimal. In these circumstances, potassium reabsorption exceeds secretion, and blood levels of potassium increase.

Atrial natriuretic peptide, discovered in 1981, is a hormone believed to have an important role in salt and water excretion by the kidney. It is synthesized in muscle cells of the atria of the heart and released when the atria are stretched. The actions of ANP include vasodilatation of the afferent and efferent arterioles, which results in an increase in renal blood flow and glomerular filtration rate. ANP also inhibits sodium reabsorption from the collecting tubules through its inhibition of aldosterone secretion and through direct action on the tubular cells. It also inhibits ADH release from the posterior pituitary gland, thereby increasing excretion of water by the kidneys. ANP also has vasodilator properties. Whether these effects are sufficient to produce long-term changes in blood pressure is uncertain.

Regulation of pH

The kidneys regulate body pH by conserving base bicarbonate (HCO_3^-) and eliminating hydrogen ions (H^+). Neither the blood buffer systems nor the respiratory control mechanisms for carbon dioxide elimination can eliminate H^+ from the body. This is accomplished by the kidneys. The average North American diet results in the liberation of 40 to 80 mmol of H^+ each day. Virtually all the H^+ excreted in the urine is secreted into the tubular fluid by means of tubular secretory mechanisms. The lowest tubular fluid pH that can be achieved is 4.4 to 4.5. The ability of the kidneys to excrete H^+ depends on buffers in the urine that combine with the H^+. The three major urine buffers are HCO_3^-, phosphate (HPO_4^-), and ammonia (NH_3). The HCO_3^- ions, which are present in the urine filtrate, combine with H^+ ions that have been secreted into the tubular fluid; this results in the formation of carbon dioxide and water. The carbon dioxide is then absorbed into the tubular cells, and bicarbonate is regenerated. The HPO_4^- ion is a metabolic end product that is filtered into the tubular fluid; it combines with a secreted H^+ ion and is not reabsorbed. Ammonia is synthesized in tubular cells by deamination of the amino acid glutamine; it diffuses into the tubular fluid and combines with the H^+ ion. An important aspect of this buffer system is that the deamination process increases when the body's H^+ ion concentration remains elevated for 1 to 2 days. These mechanisms for pH regulation are described more fully in Chapter 6.

pH-Dependent Elimination of Organic Ions

The proximal tubule actively secretes large amounts of different organic anions. Foreign anions (*e.g.*, salicylates, penicillin) and endogenously produced anions (*e.g.*, bile acids, uric acid) are actively secreted into the tubular fluid. Most of the anions that are secreted use the same transport system, allowing the kidneys to rid the body of many different drugs and environmental agents. Because the same transport system is shared by different anions, there is competition for transport such that elevated levels of one substance tend to inhibit the secretion of other anions. The proximal tubules also possess an active transport system for organic cations that is analogous to that for organic ions.

Uric Acid Elimination

Uric acid is a product of purine metabolism (see Chapter 43). Excessively high blood levels (*i.e.*, hyperuricemia) can cause gout, and excessive levels in the urine can cause kidney stones. Uric acid is freely filtered in the glomerulus and is both reabsorbed from and secreted into the proximal tubules. Uric acid is one of the anions that use the previously described anion transport system in the proximal tubule. Tubular reabsorption normally exceeds secretion, and the net effect is removal of uric acid from the urine filtrate. Although the rate of reabsorption exceeds secretion, the secretory process is homeostatically controlled to maintain a constant plasma level. Many persons with elevated uric acid levels secrete less uric acid than do persons with normal uric acid levels.

Uric acid uses the same transport systems as other anions, such as aspirin, sulfinpyrazone, and probenecid. Small doses of aspirin compete with uric acid for secretion into the tubular fluid and reduce uric acid secretion, and large doses compete with uric acid for reabsorption and increase uric acid excretion in the urine. Because of its effect on uric acid secretion, aspirin is not recommended for treatment of gouty arthritis. Thiazide and loop diuretics (*i.e.*, furosemide and ethacrynic acid) also can cause hyperuricemia and gouty arthritis, presumably through a decrease in extracellular fluid volume and enhanced uric acid reabsorption.

Urea Elimination

Urea is an end product of protein metabolism. The normal adult produces 25 to 30 g/day; the quantity rises when a high-protein diet is consumed, when there is excessive tissue breakdown, or in the presence of gastrointestinal bleeding. With gastrointestinal bleeding, the blood proteins are broken down to form ammonia in the intestine; the ammonia is then absorbed into the portal circulation and converted to urea by the liver before being released into the bloodstream. The kidneys, in their role as regulators of blood urea nitrogen (BUN) levels, filter urea in the glomeruli and then reabsorb it in the tubules. This enables maintenance of a normal BUN, which is in the range of 8 to 20 mg/dL. During periods of dehydration, the blood volume and GFR drop, and BUN levels increase. The renal tubules are permeable to urea, which means that the longer the tubular fluid remains in the kidneys, the greater is the reabsorption of urea into the blood. Only small amounts of urea are reabsorbed into the blood when the GFR is high, but relatively large amounts of urea are returned to the blood when the GFR is reduced.

Drug Elimination

Many drugs are eliminated in the urine. These drugs are selectively filtered in the glomerulus and reabsorbed or secreted into the tubular fluid. Only drugs that are not bound to plasma proteins are filtered in the glomerulus and therefore able to be eliminated by the kidneys. Many drugs are weak acids or weak bases and are present in the renal tubular fluid partly as water-soluble ions and partly as nonionized lipid-soluble molecules. The nonionized lipid-soluble form of a drug diffuses more readily through the lipid membrane of the tubular cells and then back into the bloodstream. The water-soluble ionized form remains in the urine filtrate. The ratio of ionized to nonionized drug depends on the pH of the urine. For example, aspirin is highly ionized in alkaline urine and in this form is rapidly excreted in the urine, while it is largely nonionized in acid urine and is reabsorbed, rather than excreted. Acidification or alkalinization of the urine may be used to increase the elimination of drugs, particularly in situations of drug overdose.

ENDOCRINE FUNCTIONS OF THE KIDNEY

In addition to their function in regulating body fluids and electrolytes, the kidneys function as an endocrine organ in that they produce chemical mediators that travel through the blood to distant sites where they exert their actions. The kidneys participate in control of blood pressure by way of the renin-angiotensin-aldosterone mechanism, in calcium metabolism by activating vitamin D, and in regulating red blood cell production through the synthesis of erythropoietin.

The Renin-Angiotensin-Aldosterone Mechanism

The renin-angiotensin-aldosterone mechanism plays an important part in the short- and long-term regulation of blood pressure (see Chapter 17). Renin is synthesized and stored in the juxtaglomerular cells of the kidney. This enzyme is released in response to a decrease in renal blood flow or a change in the composition of the distal tubular fluid, or as the result of sympathetic nervous system stimulation. Most of the renin that is released leaves the kidney and enters the bloodstream, where it acts enzymatically to convert an inactive circulating plasma protein called *angiotensinogen* to angiotensin I. Angiotensin I, in turn, travels to the small blood vessels of the lung, where it is converted to angiotensin II by the angiotensin-converting enzyme that is present in the endothelium of the lung vessels. Angiotensin II is a potent vasoconstrictor, and it acts directly on the kidneys to decrease salt and water excretion.

KEY CONCEPTS

Endocrine Functions of the Kidney

- Long-term regulation of blood pressure is facilitated through the kidney's activation of the renin-angiotensin system and regulation of sodium and water balance.

- The activation of vitamin D, which is important for intestinal absorption of calcium, occurs in the kidney.

- The kidney synthesizes erythropoietin, which stimulates bone marrow production of red blood cells.

Both mechanisms have relatively short periods of action. Angiotensin II also stimulates aldosterone secretion by the adrenal gland. Aldosterone, in turn, acts on the distal tubule to increase sodium reabsorption and exerts a longer-term effect on the maintenance of blood pressure. Renin also functions through angiotensin II to produce constriction of the efferent arteriole as a means of preventing a serious decrease in glomerular filtration pressure.

Erythropoietin

Erythropoietin is a polypeptide hormone that regulates the differentiation of red blood cells in the bone marrow (see Chapter 11). Between 89% and 95% of erythropoietin is formed in the kidneys. The synthesis of erythropoietin is stimulated by tissue hypoxia, which may be brought about by anemia, residence at high altitudes, or impaired oxygenation of tissues caused by cardiac or pulmonary disease. Persons with end-stage kidney disease often are anemic because of an inability of the kidneys to produce erythropoietin. This anemia usually is managed by the administration of epoetin alfa, a synthetic form of erythropoietin produced through deoxyribonucleic acid (DNA) technology, to stimulate erythropoiesis.

Vitamin D

Activation of vitamin D occurs in the kidneys. Vitamin D increases calcium absorption from the gastrointestinal tract and helps to regulate calcium deposition in bone. It also has a weak stimulatory effect on renal calcium absorption. Although vitamin D is not synthesized and released from an endocrine gland, it often is considered a hormone because of its pathway of molecular activation and mechanism of action.

It exists in several forms: natural vitamin D (cholecalciferol), which results from ultraviolet irradiation of the skin, and synthetic vitamin D (ergocalciferol), which is derived from irradiation of ergosterol. The active form of vitamin D is 1,25-dihydroxycholecalciferol. Cholecalciferol and ergocalciferol must undergo chemical transformation to become active: first to 25-hydroxycholecalciferol in the liver and then to 1,25-dihydroxycholecalciferol in the kidneys. Persons with end-stage renal disease are unable to transform vitamin D to its active form and must rely on pharmacologic preparations of the active vitamin (calcitriol) for maintaining mineralization of their bones.

In summary, the kidneys perform excretory and endocrine functions. In the process of excreting wastes, the kidneys filter the blood and then selectively reabsorb those materials that are needed to maintain a stable internal environment. The kidneys rid the body of metabolic wastes, regulate fluid volume, control the concentration of electrolytes, assist in maintaining acid-base balance, and aid in the regulation of blood pressure.

The kidneys selectively eliminate water, waste products, excess electrolytes, and other substances that are not needed to maintain the constancy of the internal environment. Renal clearance is the volume of plasma that is completely cleared each minute of any substance that finds its way into the urine. It is determined by the ability of the substance to be filtered in the glomeruli and the capacity of the renal tubules to reabsorb or secrete the substance. The GFR is the amount of filtrate that is formed each minute as blood moves through the glomeruli. It is regulated by the arterial blood pressure and renal blood flow in the normally functioning kidney. The juxtaglomerular complex is thought to represent a feedback control system that links changes in the GFR with renal blood flow.

In addition to their function in regulating body fluids and electrolytes, the kidneys function as an endocrine organ in that they produce chemical mediators that travel through the blood to distant sites where they exert their actions. The kidneys participate in control of blood pressure by way of the renin-angiotensin-aldosterone mechanism, in calcium metabolism by activating vitamin D, and in regulating red blood cell production through the synthesis of erythropoietin.

Tests of Renal Function

The functions of the kidney are to filter the blood and selectively reabsorb those substances that are needed to maintain the constancy of body fluids and excrete metabolic wastes. Laboratory tests of the urine and blood can provide valuable information about kidney disease and the adequacy of renal function.

URINE TESTS

Urine is a clear, amber-colored fluid that is approximately 95% water and 5% dissolved solids. The kidneys normally produce approximately 1.5 L of urine each day. Normal urine contains metabolic wastes and few or no plasma proteins, blood cells, or glucose molecules. Urine tests can be performed on a single urine specimen or on a 24-hour urine specimen. First-voided morning specimens are useful for qualitative protein and specific gravity testing. A freshly voided specimen is most reliable. Urine specimens that have been left standing may contain lysed red blood cells, disintegrating *casts,* and rapidly multiplying bacteria.

Casts are molds of the distal nephron lumen. A gel-like substance called *Tamm-Horsfall mucoprotein,* which is formed in the tubular epithelium, is the major protein constituent of urinary casts. Casts composed of this gel but devoid of cells are called *hyaline casts.* These casts develop when the protein concentration of the urine is high (as in nephrotic syndrome), urine osmolality is high, and urine pH is low. The inclusion of granules or cells in the matrix of the protein gel leads to the formation of various other types of casts.

Because of the glomerular capillary filtration barrier, less than 150 mg of protein is excreted in the urine during 24 hours in a healthy person. Qualitative and quantitative tests to determine urinary protein content are important tools to assess the extent of glomerular disease. pH-Sensitive reagent strips are used to test for the presence of proteins, whereas immunoassay methods are used to test for microalbuminuria (30 to 300 mg albumin/ 24 hours).

The *specific gravity* (or osmolality) of urine varies with its concentration of solutes. Urine specific gravity provides a valuable index of the hydration status and functional ability of the kidneys. Healthy kidneys can produce concentrated urine with a specific gravity of 1.030 to 1.040. During periods of marked hydration, the specific gravity can approach 1.000. With the loss of nephrons and diminished renal function, there is a loss of renal concentrating ability, and the urine specific gravity may fall to levels of 1.006 to 1.010 (usual range is 1.010 to 1.025 with normal fluid intake). These low levels are particularly significant if they occur during periods that follow a decrease in water intake (*e.g.*, during the first urine specimen on arising in the morning). The ability to concentrate urine also depends on the availability of and renal response to ADH. The urine specific gravity is decreased when ADH levels are decreased, such as in diabetes insipidus, and it is increased when ADH levels are inappropriately elevated, such as in the syndrome of inappropriate ADH secretion.

GLOMERULAR FILTRATION RATE

The GFR provides a gauge of renal function. It can be measured clinically by collecting timed samples of blood and urine. *Creatinine*, a product of creatine metabolism by the muscle, is filtered by the kidneys but not reabsorbed in the renal tubule. Creatinine levels in the blood and urine can be used to measure GFR. The clearance rate for creatinine is the amount that is completely cleared by the kidneys in 1 minute. The formula is expressed as $C = UV/P$, in which C is the clearance rate (mL/minute), U is the urine concentration (mg/dL), V is the urine volume excreted (mL/minute or 24 hours), and P is plasma concentration (mg/dL).

Normal creatinine clearance is 115 to 125 mL/minute. This value is corrected for body surface area, which reflects the muscle mass where creatinine metabolism takes place. The test may be done on a 24-hour basis, with blood being drawn when the urine collection is completed. In another method, two 1-hour urine specimens are collected, and a blood sample is drawn in between.

BLOOD TESTS

Blood tests can provide valuable information about the kidneys' ability to remove metabolic wastes from the blood and maintain normal electrolyte and pH composition of the blood. Normal blood values are listed in Table 23-1. Serum levels of potassium, phosphate, BUN, and creatinine increase in renal failure. Serum pH, calcium, and bicarbonate levels decrease in renal failure. The effect of renal failure on the concentration of serum electrolytes and metabolic end products is discussed in Chapter 25.

TABLE 23-1	**Normal Blood Chemistry Levels**
Substance	**Normal Value***
Blood urea nitrogen	8.0–20.0 mg/dL (2.9–7.1 mmol/L)
Creatinine	0.6–1.2 mg/dL (50–100 µmol/L)
Sodium	135–145 mEq/L (135–148 mmol/L)
Chloride	98–106 mEq/L (98–106 mmol/L)
Potassium	3.5–5 mEq/L (3.5–5 mmol/L)
Carbon dioxide (CO₂ content)	24–29 mEq/L (24–29 mmol/L)
Calcium	8.5–10.5 mg/dL (2.1–2.6 mmol/L)
Phosphate	2.5–4.5 mg/dL (0.77–1.45 mmol/L)
Uric acid	1.4–7.4 mg/dL (0.154–0.42 mmol/L)
pH	7.35–7.45

*Values may vary among laboratories, depending on the method of analysis used.

Serum Creatinine

Serum creatinine levels reflect the glomerular filtration rate. Because these measurements are easily obtained and relatively inexpensive, they often are used as a screening measure of renal function. Creatinine is a product of creatine metabolism in muscles; its formation and release are relatively constant and proportional to the amount of muscle mass present. Creatinine is freely filtered in the glomeruli, is not reabsorbed from the tubules into the blood, and is only minimally secreted into the tubules from the blood; therefore, its blood values depend closely on the GFR. The normal creatinine value is approximately 0.6 mg/dL of blood for a woman with a small frame, approximately 1.0 mg/dL of blood for a normal adult man, and approximately 1.2 mg/dL of blood for a muscular man. A normal serum creatinine level usually indicates normal renal function. In addition to its use in calculating the GFR, the serum creatinine level is used in estimating the functional capacity of the kidneys (Fig. 23-11). If the serum creatinine value doubles, the GFR—and renal function—probably has fallen to one half of its normal state. A rise in the serum creatinine level to three times its normal value suggests that there is a 75% loss of renal function, and with creatinine values of 10 mg/dL or more, it can be assumed that approximately 90% of renal function has been lost. Serum creatinine levels provide a less accurate estimate of GFR

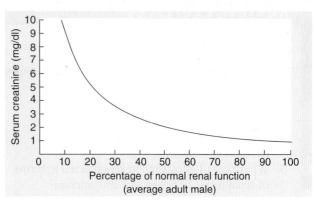

FIGURE 23-11 Relation between the percentage of renal function and serum creatinine levels.

in elderly persons because of a decrease in creatinine production due to a decrease in muscle mass. Therefore, the prediction of GFR using serum creatinine levels is often adjusted for age and weight (see Chapter 25).

Blood Urea Nitrogen

Urea is formed in the liver as a byproduct of protein metabolism and is eliminated entirely by the kidneys. Therefore, BUN is related to the GFR but, unlike creatinine, also is influenced by protein intake, gastrointestinal bleeding, and hydration status. Increased protein intake and gastrointestinal bleeding produce an increase in urea because of protein metabolism. In gastrointestinal bleeding, the blood is broken down by the intestinal flora, and the nitrogenous waste is absorbed into the portal vein and transported to the liver, where it is converted to urea. During dehydration, elevated BUN levels result from increased concentration. Approximately two thirds of renal function must be lost before a significant rise in the BUN level occurs.

The BUN is less specific for renal insufficiency than creatinine, but the *BUN–creatinine ratio* may provide useful diagnostic information. The ratio normally is approximately 10:1. Ratios greater than 15:1 represent prerenal conditions, such as congestive heart failure and upper gastrointestinal tract bleeding, that produce an increase in BUN but not in creatinine. A ratio of less than 10:1 occurs in persons with liver disease and in those who receive a low-protein diet or chronic dialysis because BUN is more readily dialyzable than creatinine.

In summary, urinalysis and blood tests that measure levels of byproducts of metabolism and electrolytes provide information about renal function. Serum creatinine reflects the GFR and can be used as an estimate of renal function. Measurements of BUN, which is formed in liver as a byproduct of protein metabolism and eliminated almost entirely by the kidney, are also a measure of renal function.

Review Exercises

A 60-year-old woman with a diagnosis of hypertension is being treated with a thiazide diuretic.

A. What diuretic effect would you expect the woman to have based on the percentage of sodium reaching the site where the diuretic exerted its action?

B. What type of effects might be expected in terms of renal losses of potassium and calcium?

A 54-year-old man, seen by his physician for elevated blood pressure, was found to have a serum creatinine of 2.5 mg/dL. He complains that he has been urinating more frequently than usual, and the lab report for his first morning urine specimen reveals a dilute urine with a specific gravity of 1.010.

A. Explain the elevation of serum creatinine in terms of renal function.

B. Explain the inability of persons with early renal failure to produce a concentrated urine as evidenced by the frequency of urination and the low specific gravity of his first morning urine specimen.

A 10-year-old boy with bed-wetting was placed on an ADH nasal spray at bedtime as a means of treating the disorder.

A. Explain the rationale for the use of ADH treatment on urine output.

Visit the Porth: Essentials of Pathophysiology: Concepts of Altered Health States web site (http://thePoint.LWW.com/PorthEssentials) for links to chapter-related resources on the Internet, all-new exclusive animations, chapter review questions, and more!

B I B L I O G R A P H Y

Berne R. M., Levy M. N. (2000). *Principles of physiology* (3rd ed., pp. 408–432). Philadelphia: Mosby.

Ganong W. F. (2005). *Review of medical physiology* (22nd ed., pp. 699–730). New York: Lange Medical Books/McGraw-Hill.

Gartner L. P., Hiatt J. L. (2001). *Color textbook of histology* (2nd ed., pp. 435–456). Philadelphia: W. B. Saunders.

Guyton A. C., Hall J. E. (2006). *Textbook of medical physiology* (11th ed., pp. 307–382). Philadelphia: Elsevier Saunders.

Koeppen B. M., Stanton B. A. (1997). *Renal physiology* (2nd ed.). St. Louis: Mosby.

Price C. P., Finney H. (2000). Developments in the assessment of glomerular filtration rate. *Clinica Chimica Acta* 297, 55–66.

Rahn K. H., Heidenreich S., Bruckner D. (1999). How to assess glomerular function and damage in humans. *Journal of Hypertension* 17, 309–317.

Rhoades R. A., Tanner G. A. (2003). *Medical physiology* (2nd ed., pp. 377–402). Boston: Little, Brown.

Ross G. I., Pawlina W. (2003). *Histology: A text and atlas* (4th ed., pp. 604–624). Philadelphia: Lippincott Williams & Wilkins.

Schrier R. W. (2003). *Renal and electrolyte disorders* (6th ed.). Philadelphia: Lippincott Williams & Wilkins.

Smith H. (1953). *From fish to philosopher* (p. 4). Boston: Little, Brown.

Vander A. J. (1995). *Renal physiology* (5th ed.). New York: McGraw-Hill.

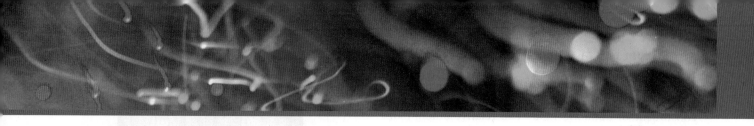

Chapter 24

Disorders of Renal Function

 More than 20 million North Americans or 1 in 9 adults have chronic kidney disease.[1] Kidney and urologic diseases continue to be major causes of work loss, physician visits, and hospitalizations among men and women. Each year, kidney stones account for 1 million physician office visits and 300,000 hospitalizations, and urinary tract infections result in nearly 9.1 million office visits and 1.8 million hospitalizations.[1]

The kidneys are subject to many of the same types of disorders that affect other body structures, including developmental defects, infections, altered immune responses, and neoplasms. Although many forms of kidney disease originate in the kidneys, others develop secondary to disorders such as hypertension, diabetes mellitus, and systemic lupus erythematosus (SLE). The content in this chapter focuses on congenital disorders of the kidneys, obstructive disorders, urinary tract infections (UTIs), disorders of glomerular function, tubulo-interstitial disorders, and neoplasms of the kidneys. Acute and chronic renal failure are discussed in Chapter 25, and the effects of other disease conditions, such as hypertension, shock, and diabetes mellitus, are discussed in other sections of the book.

Congenital Disorders of the Kidneys

Some abnormality of the kidneys and ureters is seen in approximately 3% to 4% of newborn infants.[2] Anomalies in shape and position are the most common. Less common are disorders involving a decrease in renal mass (*e.g.*, agenesis, hypogenesis) or a change in renal structure (*e.g.*, renal cysts). Many fetal anomalies can be detected before birth by ultrasonography. In the normal fetus, the kidneys can be visualized as early as 12 weeks.

AGENESIS AND HYPOPLASIA

The kidneys begin to develop early in the fifth week of gestation and start to function approximately 3 weeks later. Formation of urine begins in the 9th to 12th weeks of gestation; by the 32nd week, fetal production of urine reaches approximately 28 mL/hour.[3] Urine is the main constituent of amniotic fluid. The relative amount of amniotic fluid can provide information about the status of fetal renal function. In pregnancies that involve infants with nonfunctional kidneys or outflow obstruction of urine from the kidneys, the amount of amniotic fluid is small—a condition called *oligohydramnios*. The condition causes compression of the developing fetus and is often associated with impaired development of fetal structures.[2]

The term *dysgenesis* refers to a failure of an organ to develop normally. *Agenesis* is the complete failure of an organ to develop. Total agenesis of both kidneys is incompatible with extrauterine life. Infants are stillborn or die shortly after birth of pulmonary hypoplasia. Newborns with renal agenesis often have characteristic facial features, termed *Potter syndrome*.[4–6] The eyes are widely separated and have epicanthic folds, the ears are low set, the nose is broad and flat, the chin is receding, and limb defects often are present.[4] Other causes of neonatal renal failure with the Potter phenotype include cystic renal dysplasia, obstructive uropathy, and autosomal recessive polycystic disease. Unilateral agenesis is an uncommon anomaly that is compatible with life if no other abnormality is present. The opposite kidney usually is enlarged as a result of compensatory hypertrophy.

In *renal hypoplasia*, the kidneys do not develop to normal size. Like agenesis, hypoplasia more commonly affects only one kidney. When both kidneys are affected, there is progressive development of renal failure. It has been suggested that true hypoplasia is extremely rare; most cases probably represent acquired scarring due to vascular, infectious, or other kidney diseases rather than an underlying developmental failure.[5,6]

ALTERATIONS IN KIDNEY POSITION AND FORM

The development of the kidneys during embryonic life can result in kidneys that lie outside their normal position, usually just above the pelvic brim or within the pelvis. Because of the abnormal position, kinking of the ureters and obstruction of urine flow may occur.

One of the most common alterations in kidney form is an abnormality called a *horseshoe kidney*. This abnormality occurs in approximately 1 of every 500 to 1000 persons.[4,5] In this disorder, the upper or lower poles of the two kidneys are fused, producing a horseshoe-shaped structure that is continuous along the midline of the body anterior to the great vessels. Most horseshoe kidneys are fused at the lower pole[6] (Fig. 24-1). The condition usually does not cause problems unless there is an associated defect in the renal pelvis or other urinary structures that obstructs urine flow.

CYSTIC DISEASE OF THE KIDNEY

Renal cysts are fluid-filled sacs or segments of a dilated nephron. The cysts may be single or multiple and can vary in size from microscopic to several centimeters in diameter. There are four basic types of renal cystic disease: sim-

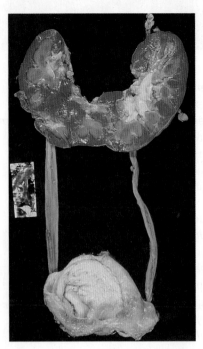

FIGURE 24-1 Horseshoe kidney. The kidneys are fused at the lower poles. (From Jennette J. C. [2005]. The kidney. In Rubin E., Gorstein F., Rubin R., et al. [Eds.], *Rubin's pathology: Clinicopathologic foundations of medicine* [4th ed., p. 831]. Philadelphia: Lippincott Williams & Wilkins.)

ple kidney cysts, acquired cystic disease, medullary sponge kidney, and polycystic kidney disease. Although some types of cysts are not congenital, they are included in this section for convenience.

Renal cystic disease is thought to result from tubular obstructions that increase intratubular pressure or from changes in the basement membrane of the renal tubules that predispose to cystic dilatation. After a cyst begins to form, continued fluid accumulation contributes to its persistent growth. Renal cystic diseases probably exert their effects by compressing renal blood vessels, producing degeneration of functional renal tissue and obstructing tubular flow.

Simple and Acquired Renal Cysts

Simple cysts are a common disorder of the kidney. The cysts may be single or multiple, unilateral or bilateral, and usually are less than 1 cm in diameter, although they may grow larger. Most simple cysts do not produce signs or symptoms or compromise renal function. When symptomatic, they may cause flank pain, hematuria, infection, and hypertension related to ischemia-produced stimulation of the renin-angiotensin system. They are most common in older persons. Even though the cysts are benign, they may be confused clinically with renal cell carcinoma.

An acquired form of renal cystic disease occurs in persons with end-stage renal failure who have undergone prolonged dialysis treatment. The cysts, which measure 0.2 to 2 cm in diameter, are thought to develop as a result of tubular obstruction.[5] Although the condition is largely asymptomatic, the cysts may bleed, causing hematuria. Tumors, usually adenomas but occasionally adenosarcomas, may develop in the walls of these cysts.

Medullary Cystic Disease

There are two major types of cystic disease that involve the medullary portion of the kidney—medullary sponge kidney and nephronophthisis–medullary cystic disease complex.[5,6] *Medullary sponge kidney* is characterized by small (<5 mm in diameter), multiple cystic dilatations of the collecting ducts of the medulla. The disorder does not cause progressive renal failure; it does, however, produce urinary stasis and predisposes to kidney infections and kidney stones. The disease usually is asymptomatic in young adults. Symptomatic disease usually develops between the ages of 30 and 60 years, when affected persons begin to have flank pain, dysuria, hematuria, and "gravel" in the urine as a result of stone formation in the cysts.[6]

Nephronophthisis–medullary cystic disease complex is a group of related diseases characterized by renal medullary cysts, sclerotic kidneys, and renal failure. Approximately 85% of cases have a hereditary basis. Symptoms usually develop during childhood, and the disorder accounts for 10% to 20% of renal failure in children. Polyuria, polydipsia, and enuresis (bed-wetting), which are early manifestations of the disorder, reflect impaired ability of the kidneys to concentrate urine.[5,6]

Autosomal Dominant Polycystic Kidney Disease

The most common form of renal cystic disease is autosomal dominant polycystic kidney disease, which is the result of a hereditary trait. It is one of the most common hereditary diseases in the United States, affecting more than 600,000 Americans.[1] There is also an autosomal recessive form of the disease. Autosomal recessive polycystic disease is rare and usually presents during infancy with severe renal dysfunction, accompanied by signs of impaired lung development and variable degrees of liver fibrosis and portal hypertension. Approximately 75% of infants die in the perinatal period, often because the large kidneys compromise expansion of the lungs.[6]

Genetics and Pathogenesis. Autosomal dominant polycystic kidney disease (ADPKD), also called *adult polycystic kidney disease,* is a systemic disorder that primarily affects the kidneys. The disease, which is inherited as an autosomal trait, results in the formation of fluid-filled cysts in both kidneys with the threat of progression to chronic renal failure. Other manifestations of the disease include hypertension, cardiovascular abnormalities, cerebral aneurysms, and cyst formation in other organs such as the liver and pancreas.

Two mutant genes have been implicated in most cases of the disorder.[5–8] A polycystic kidney disease gene called *PKD1,* located on chromosome 16, is responsible for approximately 85% of cases. It encodes a large membrane protein called *polycystin 1* that has domains similar to proteins involved in cell-to-cell and cell-to-extracellular

matrix interactions. A second gene, called *PKD2* and located on chromosome 4, encodes for a product called *polycystin 2,* which is an integral membrane protein that is similar to certain calcium and sodium channel proteins as well as a portion of polycystin 1. Although the two mutations produce almost identical disease phenotypes, disease progression is typically more rapid in people with ADPKD type 1 disease than with ADPKD type 2 disease.[7,8]

The link between the genetic defect in the polycystin proteins and the formation of the fluid-filled cysts in the kidney has not been fully established. It is thought that the membrane proteins may play a role in extracellular matrix interactions that are important in tubular epithelial cell growth and differentiation. Accordingly, it is hypothesized that cysts develop as the result of an abnormality in tubular cell differentiation, increased transepithelial fluid secretion, and formation of an abnormal extracellular matrix that allows the cysts to grow and separate from adjacent tubules. Progression of the disease is characterized by tubular dilatation with cyst formation interspersed among normally functioning nephrons. As the fluid accumulates, the cysts gradually increase in size, with some becoming as large as 5 cm in diameter.[5,6] The kidneys of persons with polycystic kidney disease eventually become enlarged because of the presence of multiple cysts (Fig. 24-2).

Cysts also may be found in the liver and, less commonly, the pancreas and spleen. Mitral valve prolapse and other valvular heart diseases occur in 20% to 25% of persons, but are largely asymptomatic. Most persons with polycystic disease also have colonic diverticula. One of the most devastating extrarenal manifestations is a weakness in the walls of the cerebral arteries that can lead to aneurysm formation. Approximately 20% of persons with polycystic kidney disease have an associated aneurysm, and subarachnoid hemorrhage is a frequent cause of death.[6]

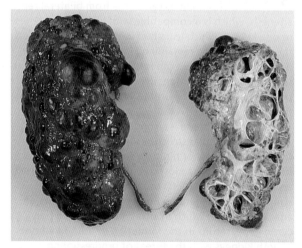

FIGURE 24-2 Adult polycystic disease. The kidney is enlarged, and the parenchyma is almost entirely replaced by cysts of varying size. (From Jennette J. C. [2005]. The kidney. In Rubin E., Gorstein F., Rubin R., et al. [Eds.], *Rubin's pathology: Clinicopathologic foundations of medicine* [4th ed., p. 833]. Philadelphia: Lippincott Williams & Wilkins.)

Manifestations. The manifestations of ADPKD include pain from the enlarging cysts that may reach debilitating levels, episodes of gross hematuria from bleeding into a cyst, infected cysts from ascending UTIs, and hypertension resulting from compression of intrarenal blood vessels with activation of the renin-angiotensin mechanism.[9,10] Renal colic caused by kidney stones occurs in about 20% of persons with ADPKD.[10] The progress of the disease is slow, and end-stage renal disease is uncommon before 40 years of age.

Diagnosis and Treatment. Ultrasonography usually is the preferred technique for diagnosis of symptomatic patients and for screening asymptomatic family members.[9] The ability to detect cysts increases with age; 80% to 90% of affected persons older than age 20 years have detectable cysts. Computed tomography (CT) scanning may be used for detection of small cysts. Genetic linkage studies are now available for diagnosis of ADPKD, but are usually reserved for cases where radiographic imaging is negative and a definitive diagnosis is essential, such as screening family members for potential kidney donation.[9]

The treatment of ADPKD is largely supportive and aimed at delaying the progression of the disease. Control of hypertension and prevention of ascending urinary tract infections is important. Pain is a common complaint of persons with ADPKD, and a systematic approach is needed to differentiate the etiology of the pain and define an approach for management.[10] Dialysis and kidney transplantation are reserved for those who progress to end-stage renal disease.

In summary, approximately 10% of infants are born with potentially significant malformations of the urinary system. These abnormalities can range from bilateral renal agenesis, which is incompatible with life, to hypogenesis of one kidney, which usually causes no problems unless the function of the remaining kidney is impaired. The developmental process can result in kidneys that lie outside their normal position. Because of the abnormal position, kinking of the ureters and obstruction of urine flow can occur.

Renal cystic disease is a condition in which there is dilatation of tubular structures with cyst formation. Cysts may be single or multiple and they may be inherited or acquired. The most common form of renal cystic disease is ADPKD. ADPKD usually does not become symptomatic until later in life, often after 40 years of age. The disease, which involves mutations in a polycystin gene, results in the formation of fluid-filled cysts in both kidneys with the threat of progression to chronic renal failure. Other manifestations of the disease include hypertension, cardiovascular abnormalities, cerebral aneurysms, and cysts in other organs such as the liver and pancreas.

Obstructive Disorders

Urinary obstruction can occur in persons of any age and can involve any level of the urinary tract from the urethra to the renal pelvis (Fig. 24-3). The conditions that cause urinary tract obstruction include developmental defects, calculi (*i.e.*, stones), pregnancy, benign prostatic hyperplasia, scar tissue resulting from infection and inflammation, tumors, and neurologic disorders such as spinal cord injury. The causes of urinary tract obstruction are summarized in Table 24-1.

Obstructive uropathy is usually classified according to site, degree, and duration of obstruction. Lower urinary tract obstructions are located below the ureterovesical junction and are bilateral. Upper urinary tract obstructions are located above the ureterovesical junction and are usually unilateral. The condition causing the obstruction can cause complete or partial occlusion of urine outflow. When the obstruction is of short duration (*e.g.*, less than a few days), it is said to be acute and is usually caused by conditions such as renal calculi. An obstruction that develops slowly and is longer lasting is said to be chronic and is usually caused by conditions such as congenital ureterovesical abnormalities. Bilateral acute urinary tract obstruction causes acute renal failure. Because many causes of acute obstruction are reversible, prompt recognition is important. If left untreated, an obstructed kidney undergoes atrophy, and in the case of bilateral obstruction, chronic renal failure occurs.

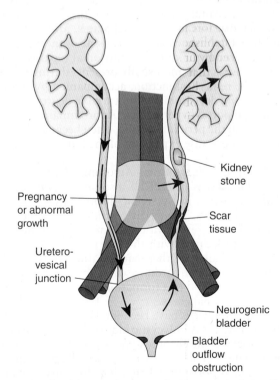

FIGURE 24-3 Locations and causes of urinary tract obstruction.

TABLE 24-1	Causes of Urinary Tract Obstruction
Level of Obstruction	**Cause**
Renal pelvis	Renal calculi
	Papillary necrosis
Ureter	Renal calculi
	Pregnancy
	Tumors that compress the ureter
	Ureteral stricture
	Congenital disorders of the ureterovesical junction and ureteropelvic junction strictures
Bladder and urethra	Bladder cancer
	Neurogenic bladder
	Bladder stones
	Prostatic hyperplasia or cancer
	Urethral strictures
	Congenital urethral defects

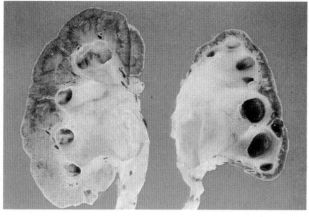

FIGURE 24-4 Hydronephrosis. Bilateral urinary tract obstruction has led to conspicuous dilatation of the ureters, pelves, and calices. The kidney on the right shows severe cortical atrophy. (From Jennette J. C. [2005]. The kidney. In Rubin E., Gorstein F., Rubin R., et al. [Eds.], *Rubin's pathology: Clinicopathologic foundations of medicine* [4th ed., p. 877]. Philadelphia: Lippincott Williams & Wilkins.)

HYDRONEPHROSIS

The most damaging effects of urinary obstruction are stasis of urine, which predisposes to infection and stone formation, and unrelieved obstruction of urine outflow, which leads to dilatation of the renal pelvis and calices with progressive atrophy of the kidney and predisposition to hydronephrosis. Acute obstructions that are of short duration and those that cause partial occlusion of urine flow are less likely to have damaging effects than are those that cause complete obstruction and persist for a longer time.

Stagnation of urine predisposes to infection, which may spread throughout the urinary tract. When present, urinary calculi serve as foreign bodies and contribute to the infection. Once established, the infection is difficult to treat. It often is caused by urea-splitting organisms (*e.g., Proteus,* staphylococci) that increase ammonia production and cause the urine to become alkaline.[11] Recurrent infections superimposed on obstructive lesions predispose to renal inflammation, scarring, and chronic pyelonephritis.

In severe partial or complete obstruction, the impediment to the outflow of urine causes dilatation of the renal pelvis and calices associated with progressive atrophy of the kidney. Even with complete obstruction, glomerular filtration continues for some time. Because of the continued filtration, the calices and pelvis of the affected kidney become dilated, often markedly so. The high pressure in the renal pelvis is transmitted back through the collecting ducts into the kidney, compressing renal vasculature and causing renal atrophy. Initially, the functional alterations are largely tubular, manifested primarily by impaired urine-concentrating ability. Only later does the glomerular filtration rate begin to diminish.

Hydronephrosis refers to urine-filled dilatation of the renal pelvis and calices associated with progressive atrophy of the kidney due to obstruction of the outflow of urine. The kidney eventually is destroyed and appears as a thin-walled shell that is filled with fluid (Fig. 24-4). The degree of hydronephrosis depends on the duration, degree, and site of obstruction. Bilateral hydronephrosis occurs only when the obstruction is below the level of the ureters. If the obstruction occurs at the level of the ureters or above, hydronephrosis is unilateral.

Clinical Features

The manifestations of urinary obstruction depend on the site of obstruction, the cause, and the rapidity with which the condition develops. Most commonly, the person has pain, signs and symptoms of UTI, and manifestations of renal dysfunction, such as an impaired ability to concentrate urine. Unilateral obstruction may remain silent for long periods because the unaffected kidney can maintain adequate renal function. In bilateral partial obstruction, the first manifestation is the inability to concentrate urine. Complete bilateral obstruction results in oliguria and anuria and is incompatible with survival unless the obstruction is removed.

Pain, which often is the factor that causes a person to seek medical attention, is the result of distention of the bladder, collecting system, or renal capsule. Its severity is related most closely to the rate rather than the degree of distention. Pain most often occurs with acute obstruction, in which the distention of urinary structures is rapid. This is in contrast to chronic obstruction, in which distention is gradual and may not cause pain. Instead, gradual obstruction may produce only vague abdominal or back discomfort. When pain occurs, it is related to the site of obstruction. Obstruction of the renal pelvis or upper ureter causes pain and tenderness over the flank area. With lower levels of obstruction, the pain may radiate to the testes in the male or the labia in the female. With partial obstruction, particularly of the ureteropelvic junction, pain may occur during periods of high fluid intake, when a high rate of urine flow causes an acute distention of the renal pelvis. Because of its visceral innervation, ureteral obstruction may produce reflex impairment of gastrointestinal tract peristalsis and motility with abdominal distention and, in severe cases, paralytic ileus.

Hypertension is an occasional complication of urinary tract obstruction. It is more common in cases of unilateral obstruction in which renin secretion is enhanced, probably secondary to impaired renal blood flow. In these circumstances, removal of the obstruction often leads to a reduction in blood pressure.

RENAL CALCULI

The most common cause of upper urinary tract obstruction is urinary calculi or urolithiasis. Although urinary calculi can form in any part of the urinary tract, most develop in the kidneys. Renal calculi (nephrolithiasis) are the third most common disorder of the urinary tract, exceeded only by UTIs and disorders of the prostate.[12]

Kidney stones are crystalline structures made of materials the kidneys normally excrete in the urine. The etiology of urinary stone formation is complex and not all aspects are well understood. It is thought to encompass a number of factors, including increases in blood and urinary levels of stone components and interactions among the components; anatomic changes in urinary tract structures; metabolic and endocrine influences; dietary and intestinal absorption factors; and UTI. Adding to the mystery of stone formation is the fact that although both kidneys are exposed to the same urinary constituents, kidney stones tend to form in only one kidney. Three major theories are used to explain stone formation: the saturation theory, the matrix theory, and the inhibitor deficiency theory.[5,12–14] One or more of these theories may apply to stone formation in the same person.

Kidney stones require a nidus, or nucleus, to form and a urinary environment that supports continued precipitation of stone components to grow. The *saturation theory* states that the risk of stone formation is increased when the urine is supersaturated with stone components (*e.g.*, calcium salts, uric acid, magnesium ammonium phosphate, cystine). Supersaturation depends on urinary pH, solute concentration, ionic strength, and complexation. The greater the concentration of two ions, the more likely they are to precipitate. Complexation is influenced by the availability of specific ions. For example, sodium complexes with oxalate, decreasing its free ionic form.

The *matrix theory* proposes that organic materials, such as mucopolysaccharides derived from the epithelial cells that line the tubules, act as a nidus for stone formation. This theory is based on the observation that organic matrix materials can be found in all layers of kidney stones. It is not known whether the matrix material contributes to the initiation of stone formation or the material is merely entrapped as the stone forms.

The *inhibitor theory* suggests that persons who have a deficiency of substances that inhibit stone formation in their urine are at increased risk for stone formation. Among the substances known to inhibit calcium stone formation is urinary citrate, which forms a complex with calcium and inhibits early- and late-stage crystal formation and propagation.[14] Citrate is a normal byproduct of the citric acid cycle in renal cells; metabolic stimuli that consume this product (as with metabolic acidosis due to fasting, hypokalemia, or hypomagnesemia) reduce the excretion of citrate in the urine. Citrate supplementation (potassium citrate) may be used in the treatment of some forms of hypocitraturic kidney stones.[12] A number of urinary glycoproteins have also been identified as inhibitors of calcium oxalate stone formation, including nephrocalcin, Tamm-Horsfall mucoprotein, and uropontin.[6,13,14] The physiologic role of these inhibitors is the subject of intense investigation, with the hope that better understanding of their role will lead to new therapeutic strategies.

Types of Stones

There are four basic types of kidney stones: calcium stones (*i.e.*, oxalate or phosphate), magnesium ammonium phosphate stones, uric acid stones, and cystine stones. The causes and treatment measures for each of these types of renal stones are described in Table 24-2. Most kidney stones (70% to 80%) are calcium stones—calcium oxalate, calcium phosphate, or a combination of the two materials. Calcium stones usually are associated with increased concentrations of calcium in the blood and urine. Excessive bone resorption caused by immobility, bone disease, hyperparathyroidism, and renal tubular acidosis all are contributing conditions. High oxalate concentrations in the blood and urine predispose to formation of calcium oxalate stones.

Magnesium ammonium phosphate stones, also called *struvite stones*, form only in alkaline urine and in the presence of bacteria that possess an enzyme called *urease*, which splits the urea in the urine into ammonia and carbon dioxide. The ammonia that is formed takes up a hydrogen ion to become an ammonium ion, increasing the pH of the urine so that it becomes more alkaline. Because phosphate

---

⨎ **KEY CONCEPTS**

Kidney Stones

➤ Kidney stones are crystalline structures that form from components of the urine.

➤ Stones require a nidus to form and a urinary environment that supports continued crystallization of stone components.

➤ Stone formation is influenced by the concentration of stone components in the urine, the ability of the stone components to complex and form stones, and the presence of substances that inhibit stone formation.

TABLE 24-2	Composition, Contributing Factors, and Treatment of Kidney Stones	
Type of Stone	**Contributing Factors**	**Treatment**
Calcium (oxalate and phosphate)	Hypercalcemia and hypercalciuria	Treatment of underlying conditions
	Immobilization	Increased fluid intake
		Thiazide diuretics
	Hyperparathyroidism	
	Vitamin D intoxication	
	Diffuse bone disease	
	Milk-alkali syndrome	
	Renal tubular acidosis	
	Hyperoxaluria	Dietary restriction of foods high in oxalate
	Intestinal bypass surgery	
Magnesium ammonium phosphate (struvite)	Urea-splitting urinary tract infections	Treatment of urinary tract infection
		Acidification of the urine
		Increased fluid intake
Uric acid (urate)	Formed in acid urine with pH of approximately 5.5	Increased fluid intake
	Gout	Allopurinol for hyperuricosuria
	High-purine diet	Alkalinization of urine
Cystine	Cystinuria (inherited disorder of amino acid metabolism)	Increased fluid intake
		Alkalinization of urine

levels are increased in alkaline urine and because magnesium always is present in the urine, struvite stones form. These stones enlarge as the bacterial count grows, and they can increase in size until they fill an entire renal pelvis (Fig. 24-5). Because of their shape, they often are called *staghorn stones*. Staghorn stones almost always are associated with UTIs and persistently alkaline urine. Because these stones act as a foreign body, treatment of the infection often is difficult. Struvite stones usually are too large to be passed and require lithotripsy or surgical removal.

Uric acid stones develop in conditions of gout and high concentrations of uric acid in the urine. Hyperuricosuria also may contribute to calcium stone formation by providing nuclei for calcium oxalate stone formation. Unlike radiopaque calcium stones, uric acid stones are not visible on x-ray films. Uric acid stones form most readily in urine with a pH of 5.1 to 5.9.[14] Thus, these stones can be treated by raising the urinary pH to 6 to 6.5 with potassium alkali salts.

Cystine stones are rare. They are seen in cystinuria, which results from a genetic defect in renal transport of cystine. These stones resemble struvite stones except that infection is unlikely to be present.

Clinical Features

Manifestations. One of the major manifestations of kidney stones is pain. Depending on location, there are two types of pain associated with kidney stones: renal colic and noncolicky renal pain.[15] *Renal colic* is the term used to describe the colicky pain that accompanies stretching of the collecting system or ureter. The symptoms of renal colic are caused by stones 1 to 5 mm in diameter that can move into the ureter and obstruct flow. Classic ureteral colic is manifested by acute, intermittent, and excruciating pain in the flank and upper outer quadrant of the abdomen on the affected side. The pain may

radiate to the lower abdominal quadrant, bladder area, perineum, or scrotum in the male. The skin may be cool and clammy, and nausea and vomiting are common. Noncolicky pain is caused by stones that produce distention of the renal calices or renal pelvis. The pain usually

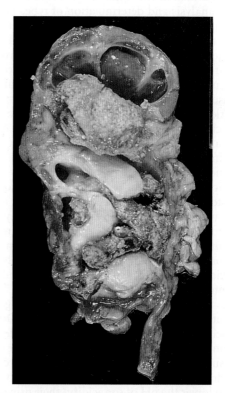

FIGURE 24-5 Staghorn stones. The kidney shows hydronephrosis and stones that are casts of the dilated calices. (From Jennette J. C. [2005]. The kidney. In Rubin E., Gorstein F., Rubin R., et al. [Eds.], *Rubin's pathology: Clinicopathologic foundations of medicine* [4th ed., p. 877]. Philadelphia: Lippincott Williams & Wilkins.)

is a dull, deep ache in the flank or back that can vary in intensity from mild to severe. The pain is often exaggerated by drinking large amounts of fluid.

Diagnosis and Treatment. Persons with kidney stones often present with acute renal colic, and the diagnosis is based on symptomatology and diagnostic tests, which include urinalysis, plain film radiography, intravenous pyelography, and abdominal ultrasonography. Urinalysis provides information related to hematuria, infection, the presence of stone-forming crystals, and urine pH. At least 90% of stones are radiopaque and readily visible on a plain radiograph of the abdomen. Intravenous pyelography uses an intravenously injected contrast medium that is filtered in the glomeruli to visualize the collecting system and the ureters of the kidneys. Abdominal ultrasonography is highly sensitive to hydronephrosis, which may be a manifestation of ureteral obstruction. Retrograde urography and CT scanning also may be used. A new imaging technique called *nuclear scintigraphy* uses bisphosphonate markers as a means of imaging stones.[12] The method has been credited with identifying stones that are too small to be detected by other methods.

Treatment of acute renal colic usually is supportive. Pain relief may be needed during acute phases of obstruction, and antibiotic therapy may be necessary to treat urinary infections. Most stones that are less than 5 mm in diameter pass spontaneously. All urine should be strained during an attack in the hope of retrieving the stone for chemical analysis and determination of type. This information, along with a careful history and laboratory tests, provides the basis for long-term preventive measures.

A major goal of treatment in persons who have passed kidney stones or have had them removed is to prevent their recurrence. Prevention requires investigation into the cause of stone formation using urine tests, blood chemistries, and stone analysis. Underlying disease conditions, such as hyperparathyroidism, are treated. Adequate fluid intake reduces the concentration of stone-forming crystals in the urine and needs to be encouraged. Depending on the type of stone that is formed, dietary changes, medications, or both may be used to alter the concentration of stone-forming elements in the urine. For example, persons who form calcium oxalate stones may need to decrease their intake of foods that are high in oxalate (*e.g.,* spinach, Swiss chard, chocolate). Calcium supplementation with calcium salts such as calcium carbonate and calcium phosphate also may be used to bind oxalate in the intestine and decrease its absorption. Thiazide diuretics lower urinary calcium by increasing tubular reabsorption so that less remains in the urine. Drugs that bind calcium in the gut (*e.g.,* cellulose phosphate) may be used to inhibit calcium absorption and urinary excretion.

Measures to change the pH of the urine also can influence kidney stone formation. In persons who lose the ability to lower the pH of (or acidify) their urine, there is an increase in the divalent and trivalent forms of urine phosphate that combine with calcium to form calcium phosphate stones. The formation of uric acid stones is increased in acid urine; stone formation can be reduced by raising the pH of urine to 6.0 to 6.5 with potassium alkali (*e.g.,* potassium citrate) salts. Table 24-2 summarizes measures for preventing the recurrence of different types of kidney stones.

In some cases, stone removal may be necessary. Several methods, including ureteroscopic removal and extracorporeal lithotripsy, are available for removing kidney stones. Ureteroscopic removal involves the passage of an instrument through the urethra into the bladder and then into the ureter. *Extracorporeal shock-wave lithotripsy* uses acoustic shock waves to break up the stones so they can be passed in the urine. All these procedures eliminate the need for an open surgical procedure. Open stone surgery may be required to remove large calculi or those that are resistant to other forms of removal.

In summary, obstruction of urine flow can occur at any level of the urinary tract. Among the causes of urinary tract obstruction are developmental defects, pregnancy, infection and inflammation, kidney stones, neurologic defects, and prostatic hypertrophy. Depending on the location (upper or lower urinary tract), degree (partial or complete), and duration (acute or chronic), urinary obstructive disorders produce stasis of urine, predisposing to infection and calculi formation and the development of increased pressure within the kidney, which interferes with renal blood flow, destroys kidney tissue, and predisposes to hydronephrosis.

Kidney stones are a major cause of upper urinary tract obstruction. There are four types of kidney stones: calcium (*i.e.,* oxalate and phosphate) stones, which are associated with increased serum calcium levels; magnesium ammonium phosphate (*i.e.,* struvite) stones, which are associated with UTIs; uric acid stones, which are related to elevated uric acid levels; and cystine stones, which are seen in cystinuria. A major goal of treatment for persons who have passed kidney stones or have had them removed is to identify stone composition and prevent their recurrence. Treatment measures depend on stone type and include adequate fluid intake to prevent urine saturation, dietary modification to decrease intake of stone-forming constituents, treatment of UTI, measures to change urine pH, and the use of thiazide diuretics to decrease the calcium concentration in urine.

Urinary Tract Infections

Urinary tract infections are the second most common type of bacterial infection seen by health care providers, respiratory tract infections being the first.[1] UTIs can include several distinct entities, including asymptomatic bacteriuria, symptomatic infections, lower UTIs such as cystitis, and upper UTIs such as pyelonephritis. Because of their ability to cause renal damage, upper UTIs are considered more serious than lower UTIs.

ETIOLOGIC FACTORS

Most uncomplicated UTIs are caused by *Escherichia coli*. Other uropathic pathogens include *Staphylococcus saprophyticus* in uncomplicated UTIs, and both non–*E. coli* gram-negative rods (*Proteus mirabilis, Klebsiella pneumoniae, Enterobacter, Pseudomonas,* and *Serratia*) and gram-positive cocci (*Staphylococcus aureus,* group B *Streptococcus*) in complicated UTIs.[16–18] Most commonly, UTIs are caused by bacteria that enter through the urethra. Bacteria can also enter through the bloodstream, usually in immunocompromised persons and neonates. Although the distal portion of the urethra often contains pathogens, the urine formed in the kidneys and found in the bladder normally is sterile or free of bacteria. This is because of the *washout phenomenon,* in which urine from the bladder normally washes bacteria out of the urethra. When a UTI occurs, the bacteria that have colonized the urethra, vagina, or perianal area are often responsible.

There is an increased risk of UTI in persons with urinary obstruction and reflux; in people with neurogenic disorders that impair bladder emptying; in women who are sexually active, especially if they use a diaphragm or spermicide for contraception; in postmenopausal women; in men with diseases of the prostate; and in elderly persons. Instrumentation and urinary catheterization are the most common predisposing factors for nosocomial UTIs. UTIs are also more common in women with diabetes than in women without the disease. People with diabetes are also at increased risk of complications associated with UTIs, including pyelonephritis, and they are more susceptible to fungal infections (particularly, *Candida* species) and infections with gram-negative pathogens other than *E. coli,* both of which are accompanied by increased severity and unusual manifestations.[19]

Host-Agent Interactions

Because certain people tend to be predisposed to development of UTIs, considerable interest has been focused on *host-agent interactions* that increase the risk of UTI.

Host Defenses. In the development of a UTI, host defenses are matched against the virulence of the pathogen. The host defenses of the bladder have several components, including the washout phenomenon, in which bacteria are removed from the bladder and urethra during voiding; the protective mucin layer that lines the bladder and protects against bacterial invasion; and local immune responses. In the ureters, peristaltic movements facilitate the movement of urine from the renal pelvis through the ureters and into the bladder. Immune mechanisms, particularly secretory immunoglobulin A (IgA), appear to provide an important antibacterial defense. Phagocytic blood cells further assist in the removal of bacteria from the urinary tract.

There has been a growing appreciation of the protective function of the bladder's mucin layer.[18] It is thought that the epithelial cells that line the bladder synthesize protective substances that subsequently become incorporated into the mucin layer that adheres to the bladder wall. One theory proposes that the mucin layer acts by binding water, which then constitutes a protective barrier between the bacteria and the bladder epithelium. Elderly and postmenopausal women produce less mucin than younger women, suggesting that estrogen may play a role in mucin production in women.

Other important host factors include the normal flora of the periurethral area in women and prostate secretions in men. In women, the normal flora of the periurethral area consisting of organisms such as *Lactobacillus* provide defense against the colonization of uropathic bacteria. Alterations in the periurethral environment, such as occur with a decrease in estrogen levels during menopause or with the use of antibiotics, can damage the protective periurethral flora, allowing uropathogens to colonize and enter the urinary tract. In men, the prostatic fluid has antimicrobial properties that protect the urethra from colonization.

Pathogen Virulence. Not all bacteria are capable of infecting the urinary tract. Of the many strains of *E. coli* and other uropathogens, only those with adherence properties are able to infect the urinary tract. These bacteria have fine protein filaments called *pili or fimbriae* that help them adhere to receptors on the lining of urinary tract structures.[18] Among the factors that contribute to bacterial virulence, the type of *pili* that the bacteria possess may be the most important. Bacteria with certain types of *pili* are associated primarily with cystitis, and those with other types are associated with a high incidence of pyelonephritis. The bacteria associated with pyelonephritis are thought to have *pili* that bind to carbohydrates that are specific to the surfaces of epithelial cells in the upper urinary tract.

Obstruction and Reflux

Obstruction and reflux are important contributing factors in the development of UTIs. Any microorganisms that enter the bladder normally are washed out during voiding. When outflow is obstructed, urine remains in the bladder and acts as a medium for microbial growth;

the microorganisms in the contaminated urine can then ascend along the ureters to infect the kidneys. The presence of residual urine correlates closely with bacteriuria and with its recurrence after treatment. Another aspect of bladder outflow obstruction and bladder distention is increased intravesicular pressure, which compresses blood vessels in the bladder wall, leading to a decrease in the mucosal defenses of the bladder.

In UTIs associated with stasis of urine flow, the obstruction may be anatomic or functional. Anatomic obstructions include urinary tract stones, prostatic hyperplasia, pregnancy, and malformations of the ureterovesical junction. Functional obstructions include neurogenic bladder, infrequent voiding, detrusor (bladder) muscle instability, and constipation.

Reflux occurs when urine from the urethra moves into the bladder (*i.e.,* urethrovesical reflux) or from the bladder into the ureters (*i.e.,* vesicoureteral reflux). In women, *urethrovesical reflux* can occur during activities such as coughing or squatting, in which an increase in intra-abdominal pressure causes the urine to be squeezed into the urethra and then to flow back into the bladder as the pressure decreases. This also can happen when voiding is abruptly interrupted. Because the urethral orifice frequently is contaminated with bacteria, the reflux mechanism may cause bacteria to be drawn back into the bladder.

A second type of reflux mechanism, *vesicoureteral reflux,* occurs at the level of the bladder and ureter. Normally, the distal portion of the ureter courses between the muscle layer and the mucosal surface of the bladder wall, forming a flap. The flap is compressed against the bladder wall during micturition, preventing urine from being forced into the ureter (Fig. 24-6). In persons with vesicoureteral reflux, the ureter enters the bladder at an approximate right angle such that urine is forced into the ureter during micturition. It is seen most commonly in children with UTIs and is believed to result from congenital defects in length, diameter, muscle structure, or innervation of the submucosal segment of the ureter. Vesicoureteral reflux also is seen in adults with obstruction to bladder outflow, primarily due to increased bladder volume and pressure.

Catheter-Induced Infection

Urinary catheters are tubes made of latex or plastic. They are inserted through the urethra into the bladder for the purpose of draining urine. They are a source of urethral irritation and provide a means for entry of microorganisms into the urinary tract.

Catheter-associated bacteriuria remains the most frequent cause of gram-negative septicemia in hospitalized patients. Studies have shown that bacteria adhere to the surface of the catheter and initiate the growth of a biofilm that then covers the surface of the catheter.[18] The biofilm tends to protect the bacteria from the action of antibiotics and makes treatment difficult. A closed drainage system (*i.e.,* closed to air and other sources of contamination) and careful attention to perineal hygiene (*i.e.,* cleaning the area around the urethral meatus) help to prevent

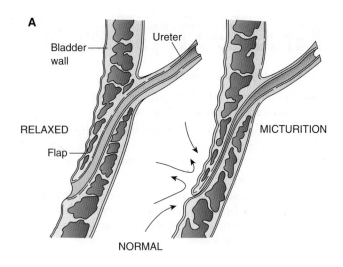

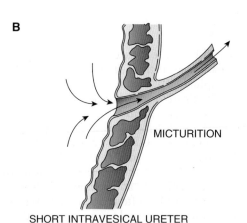

FIGURE 24-6 Anatomic features of the bladder in pyelonephritis caused by vesicoureteral reflux. (**A**) In the normal bladder, the distal portion of the intravesical ureter courses between the mucosa and the muscularis of the bladder. A mucosal flap is thus formed. On micturition, the elevated intravesicular pressure compresses the flap against the bladder wall, thereby occluding the lumen. (**B**) Persons with a congenitally short intravesical ureter have no mucosal flap because the entry of the ureter into the bladder approaches a right angle. Thus, micturition forces urine into the ureter. (From Jennette J. C. [2005]. The kidney. In Rubin E., Gorstein F., Rubin R., et al. [Eds.], *Rubin's pathology: Clinicopathologic foundations of medicine* [4th ed., p. 870]. Philadelphia: Lippincott Williams & Wilkins; courtesy of Dmitri Karetnikov, artist.)

infections in persons who require an indwelling catheter. Careful hand washing and early detection and treatment of UTIs also are essential.

CLINICAL FEATURES

Manifestations

The manifestations of UTI depend on whether the infection involves the lower (bladder) or upper (kidney) urinary tract and whether the infection is acute or chronic.

The majority of UTIs are acute uncomplicated bladder infections that occur in women. Upper UTIs affect the parenchyma and pelvis of the kidney (pyelonephritis, to be discussed). They are less common and occur more frequently in children and adults with urinary tract obstructions or other predisposing conditions such as diabetes.

An acute episode of cystitis (bladder infection) is characterized by frequency and urgency of urination (sometimes as often as every 20 minutes), burning and pain on urination (*i.e.,* dysuria), and lower abdominal or back discomfort. Occasionally the urine is cloudy and foul smelling. In adults, fever and other signs of infection usually are absent. If there are no complications, the symptoms disappear within 48 hours of treatment. The symptoms of cystitis also may represent urethritis caused by *Chlamydia trachomatis, Neisseria gonorrhoeae,* or herpes simplex virus, or vaginitis attributable to *Trichomonas vaginalis* or *Candida* species (see Chapter 40).

Diagnosis and Treatment

The diagnosis of UTI usually is based on symptoms and on examination of the urine for the presence of microorganisms. When necessary, x-ray films, ultrasonography, and CT and renal scans are used to identify contributing factors, such as obstruction.

Microscopic urine tests are used to establish the presence of bacteria and blood cells in the urine.[18] A commonly accepted criterion for diagnosis of a UTI is the presence of 10^5 or more bacteria per milliliter of urine.[18] Colonization usually is defined as the multiplication of microorganisms in or on a host without apparent evidence of invasiveness or tissue injury. Pyuria (the presence of less than five to eight leukocytes per high-power field) indicates a host response to infection rather than asymptomatic bacterial colonization. A Gram stain may be done to determine the type of organism that is present (gram positive or gram negative).

Chemical screening (urine dipstick) for markers of infection may provide useful information but is less sensitive than microscopic analysis. A urine culture confirms the presence of pathogenic bacteria in urine specimens, allows for their identification, and permits the determination of their sensitivity to specific antibiotics.

The treatment of UTI is based on the type of infection that is present (lower or upper UTI), the pathogen causing the infection, and the presence of contributing host-agent factors. Other considerations include whether the infection is acute, recurrent, or chronic.

Most acute lower UTIs, which occur mainly in women and are generally caused by *E. coli,* are treated successfully with a short course of antimicrobial therapy.[20] Forcing fluids may relieve signs and symptoms, and this approach is used as an adjunct to antimicrobial treatment. Because there is risk of permanent kidney damage with upper UTIs, these infections are treated more aggressively.

Recurrent lower UTIs are those that return after treatment. They are due either to bacterial persistence or reinfection. Bacterial persistence usually is curable by removal of the infectious source (*e.g.,* urinary catheter or infected bladder stones). Reinfection is managed principally through education regarding pathogen transmission and prevention measures. Cranberry juice or blueberry juice has been suggested as a preventive measure for persons with frequent UTIs.[21,22] Studies suggest that these juices reduce bacterial adherence to the epithelial lining of the urinary tract.[22] Because of their mechanism of action, these juices are used more appropriately in prevention rather than treatment of an established UTI.

Chronic UTIs are more difficult to treat. Because they often are associated with obstructive uropathy or reflux flow of urine, diagnostic tests usually are performed to detect such abnormalities. When possible, the condition causing the reflux flow or obstruction is corrected. Most persons with recurrent UTIs are treated with antimicrobial agents for 10 to 14 days in doses sufficient to maintain high urine levels of the drug, and they are examined for obstruction or other causes of infection. Men in particular should be investigated for obstructive disorders or a prostatic focus of infection.

INFECTIONS IN SPECIAL POPULATIONS

Urinary tract infections affect persons of all ages. In infants, they occur more often in boys than in girls. UTIs occur more frequently in women because of the shorter length of the urethra and because the vaginal vestibule can be easily contaminated with fecal flora. Approximately half of all adult women have at least one UTI during their lifetime.[23] In men, the longer length of the urethra and the antibacterial properties of the prostatic fluid provide some protection from ascending UTIs until approximately 50 years of age. After this age, prostatic hypertrophy becomes more common, and with it may come obstruction and increased risk of UTI (see Chapter 38).

Urinary Tract Infections in Women

In women, the urethra is short and close to the vagina and rectum, offering little protection against entry of microorganisms into the bladder. There is a peak incidence of these infections in the 15- to 24-year-old age group, suggesting that hormonal and anatomic changes associated with puberty and sexual activity contribute to UTIs.

The role of sexual activity in the development of urethritis and cystitis is controversial. The well-documented "honeymoon cystitis" suggests that sexual activity may contribute to such infections in susceptible women. The anterior urethra usually is colonized with bacteria; urethral massage or sexual intercourse can force these bacteria back into the bladder. Using a diaphragm and spermicide enhances the susceptibility to infection.[23,24] A nonpharmacologic approach to the treatment of frequent UTIs associated with sexual intercourse is to increase fluid intake before intercourse and to void soon after intercourse. This procedure uses the washout phenomenon to remove bacteria from the bladder.

Pregnant women are at increased risk for UTIs. Normal changes in the functioning of the urinary tract that occur during pregnancy predispose to UTIs.[25] These changes involve the collecting system of the kidneys and include dilatation of the renal calices, pelves, and ureters that begins during the first trimester and becomes most pronounced during the third trimester. This dilatation of the upper urinary system is accompanied by a reduction in the peristaltic activity of the ureters that is thought to result from the muscle-relaxing effects of progesterone-like hormones and mechanical obstruction from the enlarging uterus. In addition to the changes in the kidneys and ureters, the bladder becomes displaced from its pelvic position to a more abdominal position, producing further changes in ureteral position.

Asymptomatic UTIs are common, with a prevalence rate of 10% in pregnant women. The complications of asymptomatic UTIs during pregnancy include persistent bacteriuria, acute and chronic pyelonephritis, toxemia of pregnancy, and premature delivery. Evidence suggests that few women become bacteriuric during pregnancy. Rather, it appears that symptomatic UTIs during pregnancy reflect preexisting asymptomatic bacteriuria, and that changes occurring during pregnancy simply permit the prior urinary colonization to lead to symptomatic infection and invasion of the kidneys.[25] Because bacteriuria may occur as an asymptomatic condition in pregnant women, the American College of Obstetrics and Gynecology recommends that a urine culture be obtained at the first prenatal visit.[26] A repeat culture should be obtained during the third trimester. Women with bacteriuria should be followed closely, and infections should be properly treated to prevent complications. The choice of antimicrobial agent should address the common infecting organisms and should be safe for the mother and fetus.

Urinary Tract Infections in Children

Urinary tract infections occur in as many as 3% to 5% of female and 1% of male children.[4,27] In girls, the first diagnosis is made by age 5 years, with peaks during infancy and toilet training. In boys, most UTIs occur during the first year of life; they are more common in uncircumcised than in circumcised boys. Children who are at increased risk for bacteriuria or symptomatic UTIs are premature infants discharged from neonatal intensive care units; children with systemic or immunologic disease; children with urinary tract abnormalities such as neurogenic bladder or vesicoureteral reflux; children with a family history of UTI; and girls younger than 5 years of age with a history of UTI.[4,27]

UTIs in children frequently involve the upper urinary tract (pyelonephritis). In children in whom renal development is not complete, pyelonephritis can lead to renal scarring and permanent kidney damage. It has been reported that more than 75% of children younger than 5 years of age with febrile UTIs have pyelonephritis, and that renal scarring occurs in 27% to 64% of children with pyelonephritis.[28] Most UTIs that lead to scarring

and diminished kidney growth occur in children younger than 4 years, especially infants younger than 1 year of age. The incidence of scarring is greatest in children with gross vesicoureteral reflux or obstruction, in children with recurrent UTIs, and those with a delay in treatment.

Unlike adults, children frequently do not present with the typical signs of a UTI.[28] Many neonates with UTIs have bacteremia and may show signs and symptoms of septicemia, including fever, hypothermia, apneic spells, poor skin perfusion, abdominal distention, diarrhea, vomiting, lethargy, and irritability. Older infants may present with feeding problems, failure to thrive, diarrhea, vomiting, fever, and foul-smelling urine. Toddlers often present with abdominal pain, vomiting, diarrhea, abnormal voiding patterns, foul-smelling urine, fever, and poor growth. In older children with lower UTIs, the classic features—enuresis, frequency, dysuria, and suprapubic discomfort—are more common. Fever is a common sign of UTI in children, and the possibility of UTI should be considered in children with unexplained fever.

Diagnosis is based on a careful history of voiding patterns and symptomatology; physical examination to determine fever, hypertension, abdominal or suprapubic tenderness, and other manifestations of UTI; and urinalysis to determine bacteriuria, pyuria, proteinuria, and hematuria. A positive urine culture that is obtained correctly is essential for the diagnosis. Additional diagnostic methods may be needed to determine the cause of the disorder. Vesicoureteral reflux is the most commonly associated abnormality in UTIs, and reflux nephropathy is an important cause of end-stage renal disease in children and adolescents. Children with a relatively uncomplicated first UTI may turn out to have significant reflux. Therefore, even a single documented UTI in a child requires careful diagnosis. Urinary symptoms in the absence of bacteriuria suggest vaginitis, urethritis, sexual molestation, the use of irritating bubble baths, pinworms, or viral cystitis. In adolescent girls, a history of dysuria and vaginal discharge makes vaginitis or vulvitis a consideration.

The approach to treatment is based on the clinical severity of the infection, the site of infection (*i.e.,* lower vs. upper urinary tract), the risk of sepsis, and the presence of structural abnormalities. The immediate treatment of infants and young children is essential. Most infants with symptomatic UTIs and many children with clinical evidence of acute upper UTIs require hospitalization and intravenous antibiotic therapy. Follow-up is essential for children with febrile UTIs to ensure resolution of the infection. Follow-up urine cultures often are done at the end of treatment. Imaging studies often are recommended for children after first UTIs to detect renal scarring, vesicoureteral reflux, or other abnormalities.[28]

Urinary Tract Infections in the Elderly

Urinary tract infections are relatively common in elderly persons.[29] It is the second most common form of infection, after respiratory tract infections, among otherwise healthy community-dwelling elderly. It is particularly prevalent in elderly persons living in nursing homes or extended-care facilities.

Most of these infections follow invasion of the urinary tract by the ascending route. Several factors predispose elderly persons to UTIs: immobility resulting in poor bladder emptying, bladder outflow obstruction caused by prostatic hyperplasia or kidney stones, bladder ischemia caused by urine retention, senile vaginitis, constipation, and diminished bactericidal activity of urine and prostatic secretions. Added to these risks are other health problems that necessitate instrumentation of the urinary tract. UTIs develop in 1% of ambulatory patients after a single catheterization and within 3 to 4 days in essentially all patients with indwelling catheters.[29]

Elderly persons with bacteriuria have varying symptoms, ranging from the absence of symptoms to the presence of typical UTI symptoms. Even when symptoms of lower UTIs are present, they may be difficult to interpret because elderly persons without UTIs commonly experience urgency, frequency, and incontinence. Alternatively, elderly persons may have vague symptoms such as anorexia, fatigue, weakness, or change in mental status. Even with more serious upper UTIs (*e.g.*, pyelonephritis), the classic signs of infection such as fever, chills, flank pain, and tenderness may be altered or absent in elderly persons. Sometime no symptoms occur until the infection is far advanced.

In summary, UTI is the second most common type of bacterial infection seen by health care professionals. Infections can range from simple bacteriuria to severe kidney infections that cause irreversible kidney damage. Predisposition to infection is determined by host defenses and pathogen virulence. Host defenses include the washout phenomenon associated with voiding, the protective mucin lining of the bladder, and local immune defenses. Pathogen virulence is enhanced by the presence of pili that facilitate adherence to structures in the urinary tract.

Most UTIs ascend from the urethra and bladder. A number of factors interact in determining the predisposition to the development of UTIs, including urinary tract obstruction, urine stasis and reflux, pregnancy-induced changes in urinary tract function, age-related changes in the urinary tract, changes in the protective mechanisms of the bladder and ureters, impaired immune function, and virulence of the pathogen. Urinary tract catheters and urinary instrumentation contribute to the incidence of UTIs. Early diagnosis and treatment of UTI are essential to preventing permanent kidney damage.

Disorders of Glomerular Function

The glomeruli are tufts of capillaries that lie between the afferent and efferent arterioles of the nephron. They are arranged in lobules and supported by a stalk consisting of mesangial cells and a basement membrane–like extracellular matrix (Fig. 24-7). The glomerular membrane is composed of three layers: an endothelial layer lining the capillary, a basement membrane, and a layer of epithelial cells forming the outer surface of the capillary and lining Bowman capsule (see Chapter 23, Fig. 23-5). The epithelial cells are attached to the basement membrane by discrete cytoplasmic extensions, the foot processes (*i.e.*, podocytes). In the glomeruli, blood is filtered, and the urine filtrate formed. The glomerular membrane is selectively permeable. It allows water, electrolytes, and dissolved particles, such as glucose and amino acids, to leave the capillary and enter Bowman space and it prevents larger particles, such as plasma proteins and blood cells, from leaving the blood.

Glomerulonephritis, an inflammatory process that involves glomerular structures, is the leading cause of chronic renal failure in the United States. There are many causes of glomerular disease. The disease may occur as a primary condition in which the glomerular abnormality is the only disease present, or it may occur as a secondary

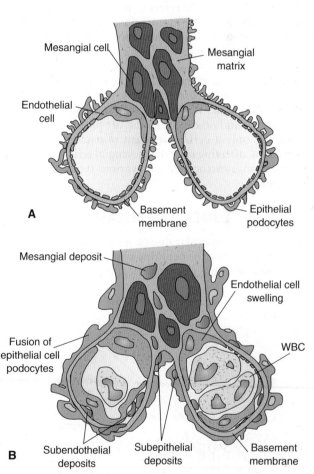

FIGURE 24-7 Schematic representation of glomerulus. (**A**) Normal; (**B**) localization of immune deposits (mesangial, subendothelial, subepithelial) and changes in glomerular architecture associated with injury. (From Whitley K., Keane W. F., Vernier R. L. [1984]. Acute glomerulonephritis: A clinical overview. *Medical Clinics of North America* 68, 263.)

condition in which the glomerular abnormality results from another disease, such as diabetes mellitus or SLE.

PATHOGENESIS

Although little is known about the causative agents or triggering events that produce glomerular disease, most cases of primary and many cases of secondary glomerular disease probably have an immune origin.[5,6,30,31] Two types of immune mechanisms have been implicated in the development of glomerular disease: injury resulting from antibodies reacting with fixed glomerular antigens, and injury resulting from circulating antigen–antibody complexes that become trapped in the glomerular membrane (Fig. 24-8). Antigens responsible for development of the immune response may be of endogenous origin, such as deoxyribonucleic acid (DNA) in SLE, or they may be of exogenous origin, such as streptococcal membrane antigens in poststreptococcal glomerulonephritis. Frequently, the source of the antigen is unknown.

The cellular changes that occur with glomerular disease include proliferative, sclerotic, and membranous changes. The term *proliferative* refers to an increase in the cellular components of the glomerulus, regardless of origin; *sclerotic* to an increase in the noncellular components of the glomerulus, primarily collagen; and *membranous* to an increase in the thickness of the glomerular capillary wall, often caused by immune complex deposition. Glomerular changes can be *diffuse,* involving all glomeruli and all parts of the glomeruli; *focal,* in which only some glomeruli are affected and others are essentially normal; *segmental,* involving only a certain segment of each glomeruli; or *mesangial,* affecting only the mesangial cells. Figure 24-8 shows changes associated with various types of glomerular disease.

TYPES OF GLOMERULAR DISEASE

The types of glomerular disease generally fall into one of several categories: the nephritic syndromes, the nephrotic syndrome, chronic glomerulonephritis, and glomerular lesions associated with other systemic diseases. The nephritic syndromes produce a proliferative inflammatory response, whereas the nephrotic syndrome produces increased permeability of the glomerulus. Because most glomerular disorders can produce mixed nephritic and nephrotic syndromes, a definitive diagnosis often requires renal biopsy, although clinical and laboratory data may provide presumptive evidence of a specific disease.

Nephritic Syndromes

The nephritic syndromes are characterized by hematuria with red cell casts, a diminished glomerular filtration rate (GFR), azotemia (presence of nitrogenous wastes in the blood), oliguria, and hypertension. They are caused by diseases that provoke a proliferative inflammatory response of the endothelial, mesangial, or epithelial cells of the glomeruli. The inflammatory process damages the capillary wall, permitting red blood cells to escape into the urine and producing hemodynamic changes that decrease the GFR. Glomerular disorders that are manifest by the nephritic syndromes include acute proliferative glomerulonephritis, rapidly progressive glomerulonephritis, and IgA nephropathy.

Acute Proliferative Glomerulonephritis. The most commonly recognized form of acute glomerulonephritis is diffuse proliferative glomerulonephritis, which follows infections caused by strains of group A β-hemolytic streptococci. Diffuse proliferative glomerulonephritis also may occur after infections by other organisms, including staphylococci and a number of viral agents, such as those responsible for mumps, measles, and chickenpox. With this type of glomerulonephritis, the inflammatory response is caused by an immune reaction that occurs when circulating immune complexes become entrapped in the glomerular membrane. Proliferation of the endothelial cells that line the glomerular capillary (i.e., endocapillary form of the disease) and the mesangial cells lying between the endothelium and the epithelium follows (see Fig. 24-7). The capillary membrane swells and becomes per-

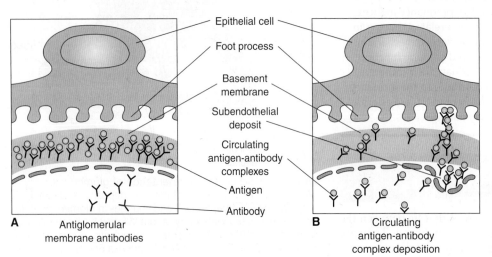

A Antiglomerular membrane antibodies

B Circulating antigen-antibody complex deposition

Epithelial cell
Foot process
Basement membrane
Subendothelial deposit
Circulating antigen-antibody complexes
Antigen
Antibody

FIGURE 24-8 Immune mechanisms of glomerular disease. (**A**) Antiglomerular membrane antibodies leave the circulation and interact with antigens that are present in the basement membrane of the glomerulus. (**B**) Antigen–antibody complexes circulating in the blood become trapped as they are filtered in the glomerulus.

KEY CONCEPTS

Glomerular Disease

➤ Glomerular disorders affect the glomerular capillary membrane structures that filter materials from the blood.

➤ Nephritic syndromes are caused by diseases that produce proliferative inflammatory responses that decrease the permeability of the glomerular capillary membrane.

➤ The nephrotic syndrome is caused by disorders that increase the permeability of the glomerular capillary membrane, causing massive loss of protein in the urine.

meable to plasma proteins and blood cells. Although the disease is seen primarily in children, adults of any age also can be affected.

The classic case of poststreptococcal glomerulonephritis follows a streptococcal infection by approximately 7 to 12 days—the time needed for the development of antibodies.[30] Oliguria, which develops as the GFR decreases, is one of the first symptoms. Proteinuria and hematuria follow because of increased glomerular capillary wall permeability. The blood is degraded by materials in the urine, and cola-colored urine may be the first sign of the disorder. Sodium and water retention gives rise to edema, particularly of the face and hands, and hypertension. Important laboratory findings include an elevated streptococcal exoenzyme (antistreptolysin O) titer, a decline in C3 complement (see Chapter 13), and cryoglobulins (i.e., large immune complexes) in the serum.

Treatment for acute poststreptococcal glomerulonephritis is largely symptomatic. The acute symptoms usually begin to subside in approximately 10 days to 2 weeks, although in some children the proteinuria may persist for several months. The immediate prognosis is favorable and approximately 95% of children recover spontaneously.[5] The outlook for adults is less favorable; approximately 60% recover completely. In the remainder of cases, the lesions eventually resolve, but there may be permanent kidney damage.

Rapidly Progressive Glomerulonephritis. Rapidly progressive glomerulonephritis is a clinical syndrome characterized by signs of severe glomerular injury that does not have a specific cause. As its name indicates, this type of glomerulonephritis is rapidly progressive, often within a matter of months. Rapidly proliferative glomerulonephritis may be caused by a number of immunologic disorders, some systemic and others restricted to the kidney. Among the diseases associated with this form of glomerulonephritis are immune complex disorders such as SLE, the small vessel vasculitides (e.g., microscopic polyangiitis), and an immune disorder condition called *Goodpasture syndrome.*

Goodpasture syndrome, which is caused by antibodies to the glomerular basement membrane (GBM), accounts for approximately 5% of cases of rapidly progressive glomerulonephritis. It is a relatively rare disease and is associated with a triad of pulmonary hemorrhage, iron-deficiency anemia, and glomerulonephritis. All of these manifestations result from anti-GBM antibody deposition in the lungs and glomeruli. The cause of the disorder is unknown, although influenza infection and exposure to hydrocarbon solvent (found in paints and dyes) have been implicated in some persons, as have various drugs and cancers. Treatment includes plasmapheresis to remove circulating anti-GBM antibodies and immunosuppressive therapy (i.e., corticosteroids and cyclophosphamide) to inhibit antibody production.

IgA Nephropathy. IgA nephropathy (i.e., Buerger disease) is a primary glomerulonephritis characterized by the deposition of IgA-containing immune complexes in the mesangium of the glomerulus. The cause of the disorder is unknown. Some, but not all persons with the disorder have elevated serum IgA levels. Recent studies have focused on potential abnormalities of the IgA molecule as a factor in the pathogenesis of the disorder.[32]

The clinical onset of IgA nephropathy is usually in the second and third decades of life.[32] The disease occurs much more commonly in men than women and is the most common cause of glomerular nephritis in Asians. Early in the disease, many persons with the disorder have no obvious symptoms and are unaware of the problem. In these persons, IgA nephropathy is suspected during routine screening or examination for another condition. In other persons the disorder presents with gross hematuria that is preceded by upper respiratory tract infection, gastrointestinal tract symptoms, or a flulike illness. The hematuria usually lasts for 2 to 6 days. Approximately one half of the persons with gross hematuria have a single episode; the remainder has gradual progression of glomerular disease with recurrent episodes of hematuria and mild proteinuria. Progression usually is slow, extending over several decades.

There is no satisfactory treatment for IgA nephropathy. The role of immunosuppressive drugs such as steroids and cytotoxic drugs is not clear. There has been recent interest in the use of omega-3 fatty acids (fish oil) in delaying the progression of the disease. Research suggests that the daily use of fish oil in the diet may retard the progress of the disease, particularly in persons with mildly impaired renal function.[32]

Nephrotic Syndrome

The nephrotic syndrome is not a specific glomerular disease but a constellation of clinical findings that result from increased glomerular permeability to the plasma proteins (Fig. 24-9). The glomerular derangements that occur with nephrosis can develop as a primary disorder or secondary to changes caused by systemic diseases such as diabetes mellitus, amyloidosis, and SLE. Among the primary glomerular lesions leading to nephrotic syndrome

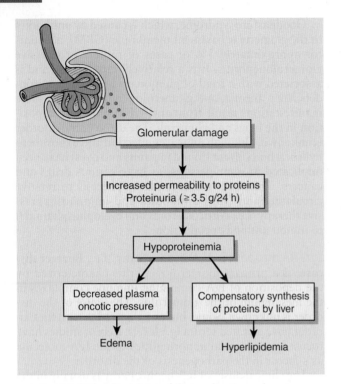

FIGURE 24-9 Pathophysiology of the nephrotic syndrome.

are membranous glomerulonephritis, minimal change disease (lipoid nephrosis), and focal segmental glomerulosclerosis. The relative frequency of these causes varies with age. In children younger than 15 years of age, nephrotic syndrome almost always is caused by primary idiopathic glomerular disease, whereas in adults it often is a secondary disorder.[5,33]

The nephrotic syndrome is characterized by massive proteinuria (>3.5 g/day) and lipiduria (*e.g.*, free fat, oval bodies, fatty casts), along with an associated hypoalbuminemia (<3 g/dL), generalized edema, and hyperlipidemia (cholesterol >300 mg/dL).[6,34–36] The initiating event in the development of nephrosis is a derangement in the glomerular membrane that causes increased permeability to plasma proteins. The glomerular membrane acts as a size and charge barrier through which the glomerular filtrate must pass. Any increased permeability allows protein to escape from the plasma into the glomerular filtrate.

Generalized edema, which is a hallmark of nephrosis, results from salt and water retention and a decrease in plasma colloidal osmotic (oncotic) pressure due to loss of albumin in the urine.[5] The sodium and water retention appears to be due to several factors, including a compensatory increase in aldosterone, stimulation of the sympathetic nervous system, and a reduction in secretion of natriuretic factors. Initially, the edema presents in dependent parts of the body such as the lower extremities, but becomes more generalized as the disease progresses. Dyspnea due to pulmonary edema, pleural effusions, and diaphragmatic compromise due to ascites can develop in persons with nephrotic syndrome.

Although the largest proportion of plasma protein loss is in albumin, globulins also are lost. As a result, persons with nephrosis are particularly vulnerable to infections, particularly those caused by staphylococci and pneumococci.[5] This decreased resistance to infection probably is related to loss of both immunoglobulins and complement proteins in the urine. Many binding proteins also are lost in the urine. Consequently, the plasma levels of many ions (iron, copper, zinc), hormones (thyroid and sex hormones), and drugs may be low. Many drugs require protein binding for transport. Hypoalbuminemia reduces the available protein binding sites, thereby producing the potential for drug overdose due to increased amounts of unbound or free (active) drug.[34]

Thrombotic complications also have evolved as a risk in persons with nephrotic syndrome.[33] These disorders reflect a disruption in the function of the coagulation system brought about by a loss of coagulation and anticoagulation factors. Renal vein thrombosis, once thought to be a cause of the disorder, is more likely a consequence of the hypercoagulable state.[5] Other thrombotic complications include deep vein thrombosis and pulmonary emboli.

The hyperlipidemia that occurs in persons with nephrosis is characterized by elevated levels of triglycerides and low-density lipoproteins (LDL). Levels of high-density lipoproteins (HDL) usually are normal. It is thought that these abnormalities are related, at least in part, to increased synthesis of lipoproteins in the liver secondary to a compensatory increase in albumin production.[33] Because of the elevated LDL levels, persons with nephrotic syndrome are at increased risk for development of atherosclerosis.

Membranous Glomerulonephritis. Membranous glomerulonephritis is the most common cause of primary nephrosis in adults, most commonly in their sixth or seventh decade. The disorders are caused by diffuse thickening of the GBM due to deposition of immune complexes. The disorder may be idiopathic or associated with a number of disorders, including autoimmune diseases such as SLE, infections such as chronic hepatitis B, metabolic disorders such as diabetes mellitus and thyroiditis, and use of certain drugs such as gold, penicillamine, and captopril.[5] Because of the presence of immunoglobulins and complement in the subendothelial deposits, it is thought that the disease represents a chronic antigen–antibody complex–mediated disorder.

The disorder is treated with corticosteroids. Cytotoxic drugs may be added to the treatment regimen. The progress of the disease is variable; approximately one half of persons sustain a slow but progressive loss of renal function.

Minimal Change Disease (Lipoid Nephrosis). Minimal change disease is characterized by diffuse loss (through fusion) of the foot processes from the epithelial layer of the glomerular membrane. The peak incidence is between 2 and 6 years of age. The cause of minimal change nephrosis is unknown; however, children in whom the disease develops often have a history of recent upper respiratory infections or of receiving routine immunizations.[5]

Although minimal change disease does not progress to renal failure, it can cause significant complications, including predisposition to infection with gram-positive organisms, a tendency toward thromboembolic events, hyperlipidemia, and protein malnutrition. There usually is a dramatic response to corticosteroid therapy.[5,33]

Focal Segmental Glomerulosclerosis. Focal segmental glomerulosclerosis is characterized by sclerosis (*i.e.*, increased collagen deposition) of some but not all glomeruli, and in the affected glomeruli, only a portion of the glomerular tuft is involved.[5] Although focal segmental sclerosis often is an idiopathic syndrome, it may be associated with reduced oxygen in the blood (*e.g.*, sickle cell disease and cyanotic congenital heart disease), human immunodeficiency virus (HIV) infection, or intravenous drug abuse, or it may be a secondary event reflecting glomerular scarring due to other forms of glomerulonephritis or reflux nephropathy.[5,6] The presence of hypertension and decreased renal function distinguishes focal sclerosis from minimal change disease. The disorder usually is treated with corticosteroids. Most persons with the disorder progress to end-stage renal disease within 5 to 10 years.

Chronic Glomerulonephritis

Chronic glomerulonephritis represents the chronic phase of a number of specific types of glomerulonephritis.[5] Some forms of glomerulonephritis (*e.g.*, poststreptococcal glomerulonephritis) undergo complete resolution, whereas others progress at variable rates to chronic glomerulonephritis. Some persons who present with chronic glomerulonephritis have no history of glomerular disease. These cases may represent the end result of relatively asymptomatic forms of glomerulonephritis. Histologically, the condition is characterized by small kidneys with sclerosed glomeruli. In most cases, chronic glomerulonephritis develops insidiously and slowly progresses to end-stage renal disease over a period of years (see Chapter 25).

Glomerular Lesions Associated With Systemic Disease

Many immunologic, metabolic, or hereditary systemic diseases are associated with glomerular injury. In some diseases, such as SLE and diabetes mellitus, the glomerular involvement may be a major clinical manifestation. The glomerular lesions associated with diabetes mellitus and hypertension are discussed in this chapter.

Diabetic Glomerulosclerosis. Diabetic nephropathy, or kidney disease, is a major complication of diabetes mellitus. It affects approximately 30% of persons with type 1 diabetes and accounts for 20% of deaths in patients with diabetes younger than 40 years of age.[5]

The glomerulus is the most commonly affected structure in diabetic nephropathy. The morphologic changes in the glomeruli include capillary basement thickening, diffuse mesangial sclerosis, and nodular glomerulosclerosis.

Widespread thickening of the glomerular capillary basement membrane occurs in almost all persons with diabetes and can occur without evidence of proteinuria.[5] This is followed by a diffuse expansion of the mesangial matrix and development of nodular sclerotic lesions, accompanied by deteriorating renal function and increasing proteinuria.[5] In nodular glomerulosclerosis, also known as *intracapillary sclerosis* or *Kimmelstiel-Wilson syndrome,* there is nodular deposition of hyaline in the mesangial portion of the glomerulus. As the sclerotic process progresses in the diffuse and nodular forms of glomerulosclerosis, there is complete obliteration of the glomerulus, with impairment of renal function.

Although the mechanisms of glomerular change in diabetes are uncertain, they are thought to represent enhanced or defective synthesis of the GBM and mesangial matrix with an inappropriate incorporation of glucose into the noncellular components of these glomerular structures. Alternatively, hemodynamic changes that occur secondary to elevated blood glucose levels may contribute to the initiation and progression of diabetic glomerulosclerosis. It has been hypothesized that elevations in blood glucose produce an increase in GFR and glomerular intracapillary pressure that leads to an enlargement of glomerular capillary pores by a mechanism that is at least partly mediated by angiotensin II. This enlargement impairs the size-selective function of the membrane so that the protein content of the glomerular filtrate increases, which in turn requires increased endocytosis of protein by the tubular endothelial cells, a process that ultimately leads to nephron destruction and progressive deterioration of renal function.[37,38]

The clinical manifestations of diabetic glomerulosclerosis are closely linked to those of diabetes. The increased GFR that occurs in persons with early alterations in renal function is associated with *microalbuminuria,* defined as urinary albumin excretion greater than 30 mg/24 hours and no more than 300 mg/24 hours.[38] Microalbuminuria is an important predictor of future diabetic nephropathies.[5] In many cases, these early changes in glomerular function can be reversed by careful control of blood glucose levels (see Chapter 32). Inhibition of angiotensin by angiotensin-converting enzyme inhibitors (*e.g.*, captopril) has been shown to have a beneficial effect, possibly by reversing increased glomerular pressure.[6] Hypertension and cigarette smoking have been implicated in the progression of diabetic nephropathy. Thus, control of high blood pressure and smoking cessation are recommended as primary and secondary prevention strategies in persons with diabetes.

Hypertensive Glomerular Disease. Hypertension can be viewed as both a cause and an effect of kidney disease. Most persons with advanced kidney disease have hypertension, and many persons with long-standing hypertension eventually sustain changes in kidney function. Renal failure and azotemia occur in 1% to 5% of persons with long-standing hypertension (see Chapter 17). Hypertension is associated with a number of changes in glomerular structures, including sclerotic changes. As the glomerular vascular structures thicken and perfusion diminishes, blood supply to the nephron decreases, causing the kidneys to lose some of their ability to concentrate the urine. This may be evidenced by nocturia. Blood urea nitrogen levels also may become elevated, particularly during periods of water deprivation. Proteinuria may occur as a result of changes in glomerular structure.

> **In summary,** diseases of the glomerulus disrupt glomerular filtration and alter the permeability of the glomerular capillary membrane to plasma proteins and blood cells. *Glomerulonephritis* is a term used to describe a group of diseases that result in inflammation and injury of the glomerulus. Glomerulonephritis may occur as a primary condition in which the glomerular abnormality is the only disease present, or it may occur as a secondary condition in which the glomerular abnormality results from another disease, such as diabetes mellitus or SLE. Almost all types of primary glomerulonephritis are caused by immune mechanisms.
>
> Glomerular diseases have been grouped into two categories: the nephritic and the nephrotic syndromes. The nephritic syndromes evoke an inflammatory response in the glomeruli and are characterized by hematuria with red cell casts in the urine, a diminished GFR, azotemia, oliguria, and hypertension. The nephrotic syndrome affects the integrity of the glomerular capillary membrane and is characterized by massive proteinuria, hypoalbuminemia, generalized edema, lipiduria, and hyperlipidemia. Both conditions can lead to progressive loss of glomerular function and eventual development of end-stage renal disease.
>
> Among the secondary causes of glomerular kidney disease are diabetes and hypertension. Kidney disease is a major complication of diabetes mellitus and is thought to be related to hemodynamic changes associated with a defective synthesis of glomerular structures secondary to increased blood glucose levels. Hypertension is closely linked with kidney disease, and kidney disease can be a cause or effect of elevated blood pressure.

Tubulointerstitial Disorders

Several disorders affect renal tubular structures, including the proximal and distal tubules. Most of these disorders also affect the interstitial tissue that surrounds the tubules. These disorders, sometimes referred to as *tubulointerstitial disorders,* include acute tubular necrosis (see Chapter 25), pyelonephritis, and the effects of drugs and toxins.

Tubulointerstitial renal diseases may be divided into acute and chronic disorders. The acute disorders are characterized by their sudden onset and by signs and symptoms of interstitial edema; they include acute pyelonephritis and acute hypersensitivity reaction to drugs. The chronic disorders produce interstitial fibrosis, atrophy, and mononuclear infiltrates; most persons are asymptomatic until late

in the course of the disease. In the early stages, tubulointerstitial diseases commonly are manifested by fluid and electrolyte imbalances that reflect subtle changes in tubular function. These manifestations can include inability to concentrate urine, as evidenced by polyuria and nocturia; interference with acidification of urine, resulting in metabolic acidosis; and diminished tubular reabsorption of sodium and other substances.[5]

PYELONEPHRITIS

Pyelonephritis refers to an inflammation affecting the tubules, interstitium, and renal pelvis. It occurs in two forms. Acute pyelonephritis is caused by bacterial infection. Chronic pyelonephritis is a more complex disorder involving not only bacterial infection but other factors such as reflux.

Acute Pyelonephritis

Acute pyelonephritis represents a patchy interstitial infectious inflammatory process, with abscess formation and tubular necrosis. Gram-negative bacteria, including *E. coli, Proteus, Klebsiella, Enterobacter,* and *Pseudomonas,* are the most common causative agents.[5,39] Gram-positive bacteria are less commonly seen, but include *Enterococcus faecalis* and *S. aureus.* The infection usually ascends from the lower urinary tract, with the exception of *S. aureus,* which is usually spread through the bloodstream. Factors that contribute to the development of acute pyelonephritis are catheterization and urinary instrumentation, vesicoureteral reflux, pregnancy, and neurogenic bladder. A second, less frequent and more serious type of acute pyelonephritis, called *necrotizing pyelonephritis,* is characterized by necrosis of the renal papillae. It is particularly common in persons with diabetes and may also be a complication of acute pyelonephritis when there is significant urinary tract obstruction.

The onset of acute pyelonephritis typically is abrupt, with chills, fever, headache, back pain, tenderness over the costovertebral angle, and general malaise. It usually is accompanied by symptoms of bladder irritation, such as dysuria, frequency, and urgency. Pyuria occurs but is not diagnostic because it also occurs in lower UTIs. The development of necrotizing papillitis is associated with a much poorer prognosis. These persons have evidence of overwhelming sepsis with frequent development of renal failure.

Acute pyelonephritis is treated with appropriate antimicrobial drugs. Unless obstruction or other complications occur, the symptoms usually disappear within several days. Hospitalization during initial treatment may be necessary. Depending on the cause, recurrent infections are possible.

Chronic Pyelonephritis

Chronic pyelonephritis represents a progressive process. There is scarring and deformation of the renal calices and pelvis[6] (Fig. 24-10). The disorder appears to involve a bacterial infection superimposed on obstructive abnor-

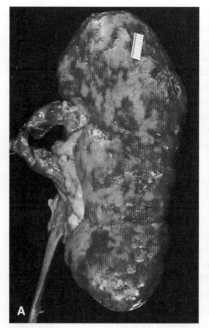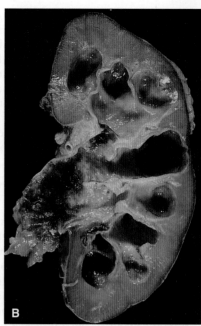

FIGURE 24-10 Chronic pyelonephritis. (**A**) The cortical surface contains many irregular, depressed scars (reddish areas). (**B**) There is marked dilatation of calices caused by inflammatory destruction of papillae, with atrophy and scarring of the overlying cortex. (From Jennette J. C. [2005]. The kidney. In Rubin E., Gorstein F., Rubin R., et al. [Eds.], *Rubin's pathology: Clinicopathologic foundations of medicine* [4th ed., p. 873]. Philadelphia: Lippincott Williams & Wilkins.)

malities or vesicoureteral reflux. Chronic obstructive pyelonephritis is associated with recurrent bouts of inflammation and scarring, which eventually lead to chronic pyelonephritis. Reflux, which is the most common cause of chronic pyelonephritis, results from superimposition of infection on congenital vesicoureteral reflux or intrarenal reflux. Reflux may be unilateral with involvement of a single kidney, or bilateral, leading to scarring and atrophy of both kidneys with the eventual development of chronic renal insufficiency.

Chronic pyelonephritis may cause many of the same symptoms as acute pyelonephritis, or its onset may be insidious. Loss of tubular function and of the ability to concentrate urine give rise to polyuria and nocturia, and mild proteinuria is common. Severe hypertension often is a contributing factor in the progress of the disease. Chronic pyelonephritis is a significant cause of renal failure. It is thought to be responsible for 10% to 20% of all cases of end-stage renal disease.[5]

DRUG-RELATED NEPHROPATHIES

Drug-related nephropathies involve functional or structural changes in the kidneys that occur after exposure to a drug. The kidneys are exposed to a high rate of delivery of any substance in the blood because of their large blood flow and high filtration pressure. The kidneys also are active in the metabolic transformation of drugs and therefore are exposed to a number of toxic metabolites. The tolerance to drugs varies with age and depends on renal function, state of hydration, blood pressure, and the pH of the urine. Because of a decrease in physiologic function, elderly persons are particularly susceptible to kidney damage caused by drugs and toxins. The dangers of nephrotoxicity are increased when two or more drugs capable of producing kidney damage are given at the same time.

Drugs and toxic substances can damage the kidneys by causing a decrease in renal blood flow; obstructing urine flow; directly damaging tubulointerstitial structures; or by producing hypersensitivity reactions.[40] Some drugs such as diuretics, radiocontrast media, immunosuppressive drugs (cyclosporine and tacrolimus), and the nonsteroidal antiinflammatory drugs (NSAIDs) can cause acute prerenal failure by decreasing renal blood flow (see Chapter 25). Persons at risk are those who already have compromised renal blood flow. Other drugs such as sulfonamides and vitamin C (due to oxalate crystals) can form crystals that cause kidney damage by obstructing urine flow in the tubules.

Acute drug-related hypersensitivity reactions produce tubulointerstitial nephritis, with damage to the tubules and interstitium. This condition was observed initially in persons who were sensitive to the sulfonamide drugs; currently, it is observed most often with the use of methicillin and other synthetic antibiotics, and with the use of furosemide and the thiazide diuretics in persons sensitive to these drugs. The condition begins approximately 15 days (range, 2 to 40 days) after exposure to the drug.[5] At the onset, there is fever, eosinophilia, hematuria, mild proteinuria, and in approximately one fourth of cases, a rash. In approximately 50% of cases, signs and symptoms of acute renal failure develop.[5] Withdrawal of the drug commonly is followed by complete recovery, but there may be permanent damage in some persons, usually in older persons.

Chronic analgesic nephritis, which is associated with analgesic abuse, causes interstitial nephritis with renal papillary necrosis.[5] When first observed, it was attributed to phenacetin, a then-common ingredient of over-the-counter medications containing aspirin, phenacetin, and caffeine. Although phenacetin is no longer contained in these preparations, it has been suggested that other ingredients, such as aspirin, acetaminophen, and NSAIDs, also may contribute to the disorder. How much analgesic it takes to produce papillary necrosis is unknown. The deleterious effects of aspirin and the NSAIDs on the kidney are thought to result from their ability to inhibit the vasodilatory effects of prostaglandin, predisposing to ischemia of the renal papillae. Persons who are particularly at risk are the elderly because of age-related changes in renal function, persons who are dehydrated or have a decrease in blood volume, and persons with preexisting kidney disease or renal insufficiency.

In summary, tubulointerstitial diseases affect the tubules and the surrounding interstitium of the kidneys. These disorders include pyelonephritis and the effects of drugs and toxins. Pyelonephritis, or infection of the kidney and kidney pelvis, can occur as an acute or a chronic condition. Acute pyelonephritis typically is caused by ascending bladder infections or infections that come from the bloodstream; it usually is successfully treated with appropriate antimicrobial drugs. Chronic pyelonephritis is a progressive disease that produces scarring and deformation of the renal calices and pelvis. Drug-induced impairment of tubulointerstitial structure and function usually is the result of direct toxic injury, decreased blood flow, or hypersensitivity reactions. Analgesic nephropathy is a chronic form of tubulo-interstitial nephritis due to aspirin and NSAID abuse. These compounds induce their effects by inhibiting the vasodilatory effects of prostaglandins, predisposing to ischemia of the papillary structures of the kidney.

Neoplasms

There are two major groups of renal neoplasms: embryonic kidney tumors (*i.e.*, Wilms tumor), which occur during childhood, and adult kidney cancers.

WILMS TUMOR

Wilms tumor (*i.e.*, nephroblastoma) is one of the most common primary neoplasms of young children. The median age at time of diagnosis of unilateral Wilms tumor is approximately 3 to 5 years.[41,42] Classically the tumor is composed of all three embryonic cell types: blastemic, stromal, and epithelial. An important feature of Wilms tumor is its association with other congenital anomalies, the most frequent being those affecting genitourinary structures. Several chromosomal abnormalities have been associated with Wilms tumor. Deletions involving at least two loci on chromosome 11 have been found in approximately 20% of children with Wilms tumor.[41]

Wilms tumor usually is a solitary mass that occurs in any part of the kidney. It usually is sharply demarcated and variably encapsulated (Fig. 24-11). The tumors grow to a large size, distorting kidney structure. The

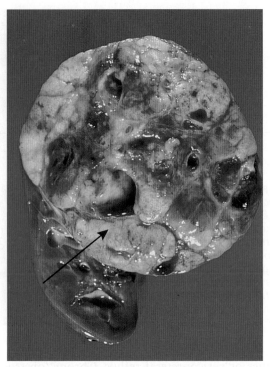

FIGURE 24-11 Wilms tumor. A cross-section of a pale tan neoplasm (arrow) attached to a residual portion of the kidney. (From Jennette J. C. [2005]. The kidney. In Rubin E., Gorstein F., Rubin R., et al. [Eds.], *Rubin's pathology: Clinicopathologic foundations of medicine* [4th ed., p. 882]. Philadelphia: Lippincott Williams & Wilkins.)

tumors usually are staged using the Wilms Tumor Study Group classification.[41] Stage I tumors are limited to the kidney and can be excised with the capsular surface intact. Stage II tumors extend into the kidney but can be excised. In stage III, extension of the tumor is confined to the abdomen, and in stage IV, hematogenous metastasis most commonly involves the lung. Bilateral kidney involvement occurs in 5% to 10% of cases.

The common presenting signs are a large, asymptomatic abdominal mass and hypertension. The tumor is often discovered inadvertently and it is not uncommon for the mother to discover it while bathing the child. Some children may present with abdominal pain, vomiting, or both. Microscopic and gross hematuria is present in 10% to 25% of children. CT scans are used to confirm the diagnosis.

Treatment involves surgery, chemotherapy, and sometimes radiation therapy. Long-term survival rates have increased to greater than 80% with an aggressive treatment plan.[41,42]

ADULT KIDNEY CANCER

Adult kidney cancer accounts for 2% to 3% of all new cancers. Men are affected about twice as often as women, and the mean age at time of diagnosis is about 60 years.[43] The increased use of imaging procedures such as ultrasonography, CT scanning, and magnetic resonance imaging (MRI) has contributed significantly to earlier diagnosis and more accurate staging of kidney cancers.[44]

Renal cell carcinoma originates in the renal cortex and accounts for approximately 80% to 85% of kidney tumors, with transitional or squamous cell cancers of the renal pelvis accounting for most of the remaining cancers.[5] The cause of renal cell carcinoma remains unclear. It occurs most often in older persons in the sixth to seventh decade. Men are affected twice as frequently as women. Some of these tumors may occur as a result of chronic irritation associated with kidney stones. Epidemiologic evidence suggests a correlation between smoking and kidney cancer. Obesity also is a risk factor, particularly in women.[5] Additional risk factors include occupational exposure to petroleum products, heavy metals, and asbestos. The risk of renal cell carcinoma also is increased in persons with acquired cystic kidney disease associated with chronic renal insufficiency. Most cases of renal cell carcinoma occur without a recognizable hereditary pattern.

Kidney cancer is largely a silent disorder during its early stages, and symptoms usually denote advanced disease. Presenting features include hematuria, costovertebral pain, presence of a palpable flank mass, polycythemia, and fever. Hematuria, which occurs in 70% to 90% of cases, is the most reliable sign. It is, however, intermittent and may be microscopic; as a result, the tumor may reach considerable size before it is detected. In approximately one third of cases, metastases are present at the time of diagnosis.

Kidney cancer is suspected when there are findings of hematuria and a renal mass. Ultrasonography, CT scanning, excretory urography, and renal angiography are used to confirm the diagnosis. MRI with intravenous gadolinium may be used when involvement of the inferior vena cava is suspected.

Surgery (radical nephrectomy with lymph node dissection) is the treatment of choice for all resectable tumors. Nephron-sparing surgery may be done when both kidneys are involved or when the contralateral kidney is threatened by an associated disease such as hypertension or diabetes mellitus. Single-agent and combination chemotherapy have been used with limited success. Immunotherapy involving interferon-alfa and interleukin-2 has been used with some success. The 5-year survival rate for stage I disease ranges from 65% to 85%; 45% to 80% for stage II disease; 15% to 35% for stage III disease; and 0% to 10% for stage IV disease.[44]

In summary, there are two major groups of renal neoplasms: embryonic kidney tumors (*i.e.,* Wilms tumor) that occur during childhood and adult renal cell carcinomas. Wilms tumor is the most common malignant tumor of children. The most common presenting signs are a large abdominal mass and hypertension. Treatment is surgery, chemotherapy, and sometimes radiation therapy. The long-term survival rate for children with Wilms tumor is greater than 80% with an aggressive plan of treatment.

Adult kidney cancers account for 2% to 3% of all new cancers. Renal cell carcinoma is the most frequent type of kidney cancer. These tumors are characterized by a lack of early warning signs, diverse clinical manifestations, and resistance to chemotherapy and radiation therapy. Because of the lack of early warning signs, the tumors often are far advanced at the time of diagnosis. Diagnostic methods include ultrasonography and CT scans. The treatment of choice is surgical resection.

Review Exercises

A 6-year-old boy is diagnosed with glomerulonephritis secondary to a streptococcal throat infection. He had been diagnosed with nephrotic syndrome several months ago. At this time the following manifestations are noted: a decrease in urine output, increasing lethargy, hyperventilation, and generalized edema. Trace amounts of protein are detected in his urine. Blood analysis reveals the following: pH = 7.30, HCO_3^- = 18 mEq/L, hematocrit (Hct) = 29%, Na = 132 mEq/L, K = 5.6 mEq/L, blood urea nitrogen (BUN) = 62 mg/dL, creatinine = 4.1 mg/dL, albumin = 2 g/dL.

A. What is the probable pathologic mechanism(s) underlying of this boy's glomerular disease?
B. Use the laboratory values in Appendix A to interpret his laboratory values. Which are significant, and why?
C. Is he progressing to uremia? How can you tell?

A 26-year-old woman makes an appointment with her health care provider complaining of urinary frequency, urgency, and burning. She reports that her urine is cloudy and smells abnormal. Her urine is cultured and she is given a prescription for antibiotics.

A. What is the most likely cause of the woman's symptoms?
B. What microorganism is most likely responsible for the infection?
C. What factors may have predisposed to this disorder?
D. What could this woman do to prevent future infection?

Visit the Porth: Essentials of Pathophysiology: Concepts of Altered Health States web site (http://thePoint.LWW.com/PorthEssentials) for links to chapter-related resources on the Internet, all-new exclusive animations, chapter review questions, and more!

REFERENCES

1. National Kidney Foundation. (2005). *Fact sheets: The problem of kidney and urologic diseases.* [On-line]. Available: www.kidney.org.

2. Moore K. L., Persaud T. V. N. (2003). *The developing human: Clinically oriented embryology* (7th ed., pp. 288–296). Philadelphia: Elsevier Saunders.

3. Stewart C. L., Jose P. A. (1991). Transitional nephrology. *Urologic Clinics of North America* 18, 143–149.

4. Elder J. S. (2004). Urologic disorders in infants and children. In Behrman R. E., Kliegman R. M., Jenson H. B. (Eds.), *Nelson textbook of pediatrics* (17th ed., pp. 1783–1789). Philadelphia: Elsevier Saunders.

5. Alpers C. E. (2005). The kidney. In Kumar V., Abbas A. K., Fausto N. (Eds.), *Robbins and Cotran pathologic basis of disease* (7th ed., pp. 995–1021). Philadelphia: Elsevier Saunders.

6. Jennette J. C. (2005). The kidney. In Rubin E., Gorstein F., Rubin R., et al. (Eds.), *Rubin's pathology: Clinicopathologic foundations of medicine* (4th ed., pp. 827–884). Philadelphia: Lippincott Williams & Wilkins.

7. Wilson P. D. (2004). Polycystic kidney disease. *New England Journal of Medicine* 350, 151–164.

8. Peters D. J. M., Breuning M. H. (2001). Autosomal dominant polycystic kidney disease: Modification of disease progression. *Lancet* 358, 1439–1444.

9. Martinez J. R., Grantham J. J. (1995). Polycystic kidney disease: Etiology, pathogenesis, and treatment. *Disease-a-Month* 41, 696–765.

10. Bajwa Z. H., Gupta S., Warfield C. A., et al. (2001). Pain management in polycystic kidney disease. *Kidney International* 60, 1631–1644.

11. Tanagho E. A. (2004). Urinary obstruction and stasis. In Tanagho E. A., McAninch J. W. (Eds.), *Smith's general urology* (16th ed., p. 175). New York: Lange Medical Books/McGraw-Hill.

12. Stoller M. L. (2004). Urinary stone disease. In Tanagho E. A., McAninch J. W. (Eds.), *Smith's general urology* (16th ed., pp. 256–290). New York: Lange Medical Books/McGraw-Hill.

13. Parmur M. S. (2004). Kidney stones. *British Medical Journal* 329, 1420–1424.

14. Morton A. R., Iliescu E. A., Wilson J. W. L. (2002). Nephrology: I. Investigation and treatment of recurrent kidney stones. *Canadian Medical Association Journal* 166, 213–218.

15. Portis A. J., Sundram C. P. (2001). Diagnosis and initial management of kidney stones. *American Family Physician* 63, 1329–1338.

16. Stamm W. E. (2002). Scientific and clinical challenges in the management of urinary tract infections. *American Journal of Medicine* 113(1A), 1S–4S.

17. Ronald A. (2002). The etiology of urinary tract infections: Traditional and emerging pathogens. *American Journal of Medicine* 113(1A), 14S–19S.

18. Nguyen H. T. (2004). Bacterial infections of the genitourinary tract. In Tanagho E. A., McAninch J. W. (Eds.), *Smith's general urology* (16th ed., pp. 203–227). New York: Lange Medical Books/McGraw-Hill.

19. Stapleton A. (2002). Urinary tract infections in patients with diabetes. *American Journal of Medicine* 113(1A), 80S–84S.

20. Nicolle L. E. (2002). Urinary tract infections: Traditional pharmacologic therapies. *American Journal of Medicine* 113(1A), 35S–44S.

21. Lynch D. M. (2004). Cranberry juice for prevention of urinary tract infection. *American Family Physician* 70, 2175–2177.

22. Ofek I., Goldhar J., Zafriri D., et al. (1991). Anti-*Escherichia coli* adhesin activity of cranberry and blueberry juices. *New England Journal of Medicine* 324, 1599.

23. Fihn S. D. (2003). Acute uncomplicated urinary tract infections in women. *New England Journal of Medicine* 349, 259–266.

24. Hooton T. M., Scholes D., Hughes J. P., et al. (1996). A prospective study of risk factors for symptomatic urinary tract infections in young women. *New England Journal of Medicine* 335, 468–474.

25. Delzell J. E., Lefevre M. L. (2000). Urinary tract infections during pregnancy. *American Family Physician* 61, 713–721.

26. American College of Obstetricians and Gynecologists. (1998). *Antimicrobial therapy for obstetric patients* (pp. 8–10). ACOG Educational Bulletin no. 245. Washington, DC: Author.

27. Shortliffe L. M., McCue J. D. (2002). Urinary tract infections at the age extremes: Pediatrics and geriatrics. *American Journal of Medicine* 113(1A), 55S–66S.

28. Shaw K. N., Gorelick M. H. (1999). Urinary tract infections in children. *Pediatric Clinics of North America* 46, 1111–1122.

29. Mouton C. P., Pierce B., Espino D. V. (2001). Common infections in older adults. *American Family Physician* 63, 257–268.

30. Hricik D. E., Chung-Park M., Sedor J. R. (1998). Glomerulonephritis. *New England Journal of Medicine* 339, 888–899.

31. Glassock R. J. (2003). The glomerulopathies. In Shrier R. W. (Ed.), *Renal and electrolyte disorders* (6th ed., pp. 633–670). Philadelphia: Lippincott Williams & Wilkins.

32. Donadio J. V., Grande J. P. (2002). IgA nephropathy. *New England Journal of Medicine* 347, 738–748.

33. Eddy A. A., Symons J. M. (2003). Nephrotic syndrome in childhood. *Lancet* 362, 629–639.

34. Vincenti F. G., Amend W. J. C. (2004). Diagnosis of medical renal diseases. In Tanagho E. A., McAninch J. W. (Eds.), *Smith's general urology* (16th ed., pp. 527–537). New York: Lange Medical Books/McGraw-Hill.

35. Orth S. R., Ritz E. (1998). The nephrotic syndrome. *New England Journal of Medicine* 339, 1202–1211.

36. Kaysen G. A. (2003). Proteinuria and the nephrotic syndrome. In Shrier R. W. (Ed.), *Renal and electrolyte disorders* (6th ed., pp. 580–622). Philadelphia: Lippincott Williams & Wilkins.

37. Remuzzi G., Bertani T. (1998). Pathophysiology of progressive nephropathies. *New England Journal of Medicine* 339, 1448–1455.

38. Parving H.-H., Østerby R., Ritz E. (2000). Diabetic nephropathy. In Brenner B. M. (Ed.), *Brenner and Rector's the kidney* (6th ed., pp. 1731–1753). Philadelphia: W. B. Saunders.

39. Kalyanakrishnan R., Scheid E. C. (2005). Diagnosis and management of acute pyelonephritis in adults. *American Family Physician* 71, 933–942.

40. Guo S., Nzerue C. (2002). How to prevent, recognize, and treat drug-induced nephrotoxicity. *Cleveland Clinic Journal of Medicine* 69, 289–297.

41. Jaffe N., Huff V. (2004). Neoplasms of the kidney. In Behrman R. E., Kliegman R. M., Jenson H. B. (Eds.), *Nelson textbook of pediatrics* (17th ed., pp. 1711–1714). Philadelphia: Elsevier Saunders.

42. Marcus K. C. (2001). Pediatric solid tumors. In Lenhard R. E., Osteen R. T., Gansler T. (Eds.), *The American Cancer Society's clinical oncology* (pp. 588–590). Atlanta: American Cancer Society.

43. Bostwick D. G. (2001). Renal cell carcinoma. In Lenhard R. E., Osteen R. T., Gansler T. (Eds.), *The American Cancer Society's clinical oncology* (pp. 415–419). Atlanta: American Cancer Society.

44. Chow W. H., Devesa S. S., Warren J. L., et. al. (1999). Rising incidence of renal cell cancer in the United States. *Journal of the American Medical Association* 281, 1628–1631.

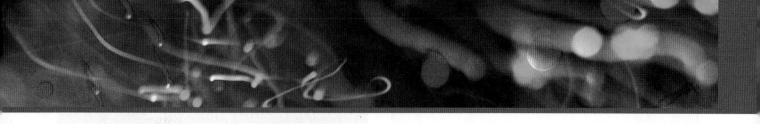

Chapter 25

Renal Failure

 Renal failure is a condition in which the kidneys fail to remove metabolic end products from the blood and regulate the fluid, electrolyte, and pH balance of the extracellular fluids. The underlying cause may be renal disease, systemic disease, or urinary tract disorders of nonrenal origin. Renal failure can occur as an acute or a chronic disorder. Acute renal failure is abrupt in onset and often is reversible if recognized early and treated appropriately. In contrast, chronic renal failure is the end result of irreparable damage to the kidneys. It develops slowly, usually over the course of a number of years.

Acute Renal Failure

Acute renal failure represents a rapid decline in renal function sufficient to increase blood levels of nitrogenous wastes and impair fluid and electrolyte balance. It is a common threat to seriously ill persons in intensive care units, with a mortality rate ranging from 40% to 75%.[1] Although treatment methods such as dialysis and renal replacement methods are effective in correcting life-threatening fluid and electrolyte disorders, the mortality rate from acute renal failure has not changed substantially since the 1960s. This probably is because acute renal failure is seen more often in older persons than before, and because it frequently is superimposed on other life-threatening conditions such as trauma, shock, and sepsis.

The most common indicator of acute renal failure is *azotemia*, an accumulation of nitrogenous wastes (urea nitrogen, uric acid, and creatinine) in the blood. In acute renal failure the glomerular filtration rate (GFR) is decreased. As a result, excretion of nitrogenous wastes is reduced and fluid and electrolyte balance cannot be maintained.

TYPES OF ACUTE RENAL FAILURE

Acute renal failure can be caused by several types of conditions, including a decrease in blood flow without ischemic injury; ischemic, toxic, or obstructive tubular injury; and obstruction of urinary tract outflow. The causes of acute renal failure commonly are categorized

KEY CONCEPTS

Acute Renal Failure

➤ Acute renal failure is caused by conditions that produce an acute shutdown in renal function.

➤ It can result from decreased blood flow to the kidney (prerenal failure), disorders that interfere with the elimination of urine from the kidney (postrenal failure), or disorders that disrupt the structures in the kidney (intrinsic or intrarenal failure).

➤ Acute renal failure, although it causes an accumulation of products normally cleared by the kidney, is a reversible process if the factors causing the condition can be corrected.

CHART 25-1

Causes of Acute Renal Failure

Prerenal

Hypovolemia
  Hemorrhage
  Dehydration
  Excessive loss of gastrointestinal tract fluids
  Excessive loss of fluid due to burn injury
Decreased vascular filling
  Anaphylactic shock
  Septic shock
Heart failure and cardiogenic shock
Decreased renal perfusion due to vasoactive mediators, drugs, diagnostic agents

Postrenal

Bilateral ureteral obstruction
Bladder outlet obstruction

Intrinsic or Intrarenal

Acute tubular necrosis
  Prolonged renal ischemia
  Exposure to nephrotoxic drugs, heavy metals, and organic solvents
  Intratubular obstruction resulting from hemoglobinuria, myoglobinuria, myeloma light chains, or uric acid casts
  Acute renal disease (acute glomerulonephritis, pyelonephritis)

as prerenal, intrinsic, and postrenal[1-4] (Fig. 25-1). Collectively, prerenal and intrinsic causes account for 90% to 95% of cases of acute renal failure.[1] Causes of renal failure within these categories are summarized in Chart 25-1.

Prerenal Failure

Prerenal failure, the most common form of acute renal failure, is characterized by a marked decrease in renal blood flow. It is reversible if the cause of the decreased renal blood flow can be identified and corrected before kidney damage occurs.

Normally, the kidneys receive 20% to 25% of the cardiac output.[5] This large blood supply is required to remove metabolic wastes and regulate body fluids and electrolytes. Fortunately, the normal kidney can tolerate relatively large reductions in blood flow before renal damage occurs. As renal blood flow is reduced, the GFR drops, the amount

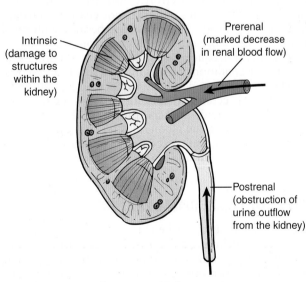

FIGURE 25-1 Types of acute renal failure.

of sodium and other substances that is filtered by the glomeruli is reduced, and the need for energy-dependent mechanisms to reabsorb these substance is reduced (see Chapter 23). As the GFR and urine output approach zero, oxygen consumption by the kidney approximates that required to keep renal tubular cells alive.[5] When blood flow falls below this level, which is about 20% of normal, ischemic changes occur. Because of their high metabolic rate, the tubular epithelial cells are most vulnerable to ischemic injury. Improperly treated, prolonged renal hypoperfusion can lead to ischemic tubular necrosis with significant morbidity and mortality.

Causes of prerenal failure include profound depletion of vascular volume (*e.g.,* hemorrhage, loss of extracellular fluid volume), impaired perfusion due to heart failure and cardiogenic shock, and decreased vascular filling because of increased vascular capacity (*e.g.,* anaphylaxis or sepsis). Elderly persons are particularly at risk because of their predisposition to hypovolemia and their high prevalence of renal vascular disorders.

Some vasoactive mediators, drugs, and diagnostic agents produce intense intrarenal vasoconstriction, causing glomerular hypoperfusion and prerenal failure. Examples include bacterial endotoxins, radiocontrast agents such as those used for cardiac catheterization, cyclosporine (an immunosuppressant drug used to prevent transplant rejection), amphotericin B (an antifungal agent), epinephrine, and high doses of dopamine. Many of these agents also cause acute tubular necrosis (discussed later). In addition, several commonly used classes of drugs impair renal adaptive mechanisms and can convert compensated renal hypoperfusion into prerenal failure. Angiotensin-converting enzyme (ACE) inhibitors reduce the effects of renin on renal blood flow; when combined with diuretics, they may cause prerenal failure in persons with decreased blood flow due to large-vessel or small-vessel renal vascular disease. Prostaglandins have a vasodilatory effect on renal blood vessels. Nonsteroidal anti-inflammatory drugs (NSAIDs) reduce renal blood flow through inhibition of prostaglandin synthesis. In some persons with diminished renal perfusion, NSAIDs can precipitate prerenal failure.

Acute renal failure is manifested by a sharp decrease in urine output and a disproportionate elevation of blood urea nitrogen (BUN) in relation to serum creatinine levels (ratio greater than 15:1 to 20:1, compared with a normal value of approximately 10:1).[1] The kidney normally responds to a decrease in the GFR with a decrease in urine output. Thus, an early sign of prerenal failure is a sharp decrease in urine output. BUN levels also depend on the GFR. A low GFR allows more time for small particles such as urea to be reabsorbed into the blood. Creatinine, which is larger and nondiffusible, remains in the tubular fluid, and the total amount of creatinine that is filtered, although small, is excreted in the urine.

Postrenal Failure

Postrenal failure results from obstruction of urine outflow from the kidneys. The obstruction can occur in the ureter (*i.e.*, calculi and strictures), bladder (*i.e.*, tumors or neurogenic bladder), or urethra (*i.e.*, prostatic hyperplasia). Prostatic hyperplasia is the most common underlying problem (see Chapter 38). Because the outflow from both ureters must be occluded to produce renal failure, obstruction of bladder outflow rarely causes acute renal failure unless one of the kidneys already is damaged or a person has only one kidney. The treatment of acute postrenal failure consists of treating the underlying cause of obstruction so that urine flow can be reestablished before permanent nephron damage occurs.

Intrinsic Renal Failure

Intrinsic or intrarenal renal failure results from conditions that cause damage to structures within the kidney—glomerular, tubular, or interstitial. The major causes of intrarenal failure are ischemia associated with prerenal failure, toxic insult to the tubular structures of the nephron, and intratubular obstruction. Injury to the tubules (acute tubular necrosis) is most common and often is ischemic or toxic in origin. Acute glomerulonephritis and acute pyelonephritis also are intrarenal causes of acute renal failure.

Acute Tubular Necrosis. Acute tubular necrosis (ATN) is characterized by destruction of tubular epithelial cells with acute suppression of renal function[6] (Fig. 25-2). ATN can be caused by a variety of conditions, including

acute tubular damage due to ischemia, the nephrotoxic effects of drugs, intratubular obstruction, and toxins from a massive infection. Tubular epithelial cells are particularly sensitive to ischemia and also are vulnerable to toxins. The tubular injury that occurs in ATN frequently is reversible. The process depends on the recovery of the injured cells, removal of the necrotic cells and intratubular casts, and regeneration of renal cells to restore the normal continuity of the tubular epithelium. If, however, the ischemia is severe enough to cause cortical necrosis, irreversible damage occurs.

Ischemic ATN occurs most frequently in persons who have major surgery, severe hypovolemia, overwhelming sepsis, trauma, and burns.[3] Sepsis produces ischemia by provoking a combination of systemic vasodilatation and intrarenal hypoperfusion. In addition, sepsis results in the generation of toxins that sensitize renal tubular cells to the damaging effects of ischemia. ATN complicating trauma and burns frequently is multifactorial in origin and due to the combined effects of hypovolemia and myoglobinuria or other toxins released from damaged tissue.

Nephrotoxic ATN complicates the administration of or exposure to many structurally diverse drugs and other toxic agents. Nephrotoxic agents cause renal injury by inducing varying combinations of renal vasoconstriction, direct tubular damage, or intratubular obstruction. The kidney is particularly vulnerable to nephrotoxic injury

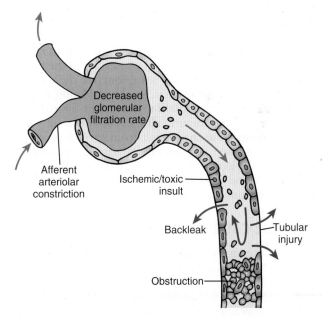

FIGURE 25-2 Pathogenesis of acute tubular necrosis. Sloughing and necrosis of tubular epithelial cells lead to obstruction and increased intraluminal pressure, which reduces glomerular filtration. Afferent arteriolar vasoconstriction, caused in part by tubuloglomerular feedback, results in decreased glomerular capillary filtration pressure. Tubular injury and increased intraluminal pressure cause fluid to move from the tubular lumen into the interstitium (backleak). (Modified from Jennette J. C. [2005]. The kidney. In Rubin E., Gorstein F., Rubin R., et al. [Eds.], *Rubin's pathology: Clinicopathologic foundations of medicine* [4th ed., p. 868]. Philadelphia: Lippincott Williams & Wilkins.)

because of its rich blood supply and ability to concentrate toxins to high levels in the medullary portion of the kidney. In addition, the kidney is an important site for metabolic processes that transform relatively harmless agents into toxic metabolites. Pharmacologic agents that are directly toxic to the renal tubule include the aminoglycoside antibiotics, cancer chemotherapeutic drugs such as cisplatin, and the radiocontrast agents. Several factors predispose to aminoglycoside nephrotoxicity, including a decrease in the GFR, preexisting renal disease, hypovolemia, and concurrent administration of other drugs that have a nephrotoxic effect. Cisplatin accumulates in proximal tubule cells, inducing mitochondrial injury and inhibition of adenosine triphosphate (ATP) formation and solute transport. Radiocontrast media–induced nephrotoxicity is thought to result from direct tubular toxicity and renal ischemia.[7] The risk of renal damage caused by radiocontrast media is greatest in elderly persons, in persons with diabetes mellitus, and in persons who, for various reasons, are susceptible to kidney disease. Heavy metals (*e.g.,* lead, mercury) and organic solvents (*e.g.,* carbon tetrachloride, ethylene glycol) are other nephrotoxic agents.

The presence of myoglobin, hemoglobin, uric acid, myeloma light chains, or excess uric acid in the urine is the most frequent cause of ATN due to intratubular obstruction. Both myeloma cast nephropathy and acute urate nephropathy usually are seen in the setting of widespread malignancy or massive tumor destruction by therapeutic agents.[3] Hemoglobinuria results from blood transfusion reactions and other hemolytic crises. Skeletal and cardiac muscles contain myoglobin, which accounts for their rubiginous color. Myoglobin corresponds to hemoglobin in function, serving as an oxygen reservoir in the muscle fibers. Myoglobin normally is not found in the serum or urine. It has a low molecular weight of 17,000 daltons; if it escapes into the circulation, it is rapidly filtered in the glomerulus. Myoglobinuria most commonly results from muscle trauma, but may result from extreme exertion, hyperthermia, sepsis, prolonged seizures, potassium or phosphate depletion, and alcoholism or drug abuse. Both myoglobin and hemoglobin discolor the urine, which may range from the color of tea to red, brown, or black.

CLINICAL COURSE

The clinical course of ATN can be divided into three phases: the onset or initiating phase, the maintenance phase, and the recovery or convalescent phase.[3] The *onset* or *initiating phase*, which lasts hours or days, is the time from the onset of the precipitating event (*e.g.,* ischemic phase of prerenal failure or toxin exposure) until tubular injury occurs.

The *maintenance phase* of ATN is characterized by a marked decrease in the GFR, causing sudden retention of endogenous metabolites, such as urea, potassium, sulfate, and creatinine, that normally are cleared by the kidneys. The urine output usually is lowest at this point. Fluid retention gives rise to edema, water intoxication, and pulmonary congestion. If the period of oliguria is prolonged, hypertension frequently develops, and with it signs of

uremia. When untreated, the neurologic manifestations of uremia progress from neuromuscular irritability to seizures, somnolence, coma, and death. Hyperkalemia usually is asymptomatic until serum levels of potassium rise above 6 to 6.5 mEq/L, at which point characteristic electrocardiographic changes and symptoms of muscle weakness are seen.

Formerly, most patients with ATN were oliguric. During the past several decades, a nonoliguric form of ATN has become increasingly prevalent. Persons with nonoliguric failure have higher levels of glomerular filtration and excrete more nitrogenous waste, water, and electrolytes in their urine than persons with acute oliguric renal failure. Abnormalities in blood chemistry levels usually are milder and cause fewer complications. The decrease in oliguric ATN probably reflects new approaches to the treatment of poor cardiac performance and circulatory failure that focus on vigorous plasma volume expansion and the selective use of dopamine and other drugs to improve renal blood flow. Dopamine has renal vasodilator properties and inhibits sodium reabsorption in the proximal tubule, thereby decreasing the work demands on the nephron.

The *recovery phase* is the period during which repair of renal tissue takes place. Its onset usually is heralded by a gradual increase in urine output and a fall in serum creatinine, indicating that the nephrons have recovered to the point where urine excretion is possible. Diuresis often occurs before renal function has fully returned to normal. Consequently, BUN and serum creatinine, potassium, and phosphate levels may remain elevated or continue to rise even though urine output is increased. In some cases, the diuresis may result from impaired nephron function and may cause excessive loss of water and electrolytes. Eventually, renal tubular function is restored with improvement in concentrating ability. At about the same time, the BUN and creatinine begin to return to normal. In some cases, however, mild to moderate kidney damage persists.

DIAGNOSIS AND TREATMENT

Given the high morbidity and mortality rates associated with acute renal failure, attention should be focused on prevention and early diagnosis. This includes assessment measures to identify persons at risk for development of acute renal failure, including those with preexisting renal insufficiency and diabetes. These persons are particularly at risk for development of acute renal failure due to nephrotoxic drugs (*e.g.,* aminoglycosides, radiocontrast agents) or drugs, such as the NSAIDs, that alter intrarenal hemodynamics. Elderly persons are susceptible to all forms of acute renal failure because of the effects of aging on renal reserve.

Careful observation of urine output is essential for persons at risk for development of acute renal failure. Urine tests that measure urine osmolality, urinary sodium concentration, and fractional excretion of sodium help differentiate prerenal azotemia, in which the reabsorptive capacity of the tubular cells is maintained, from tubular necrosis, in which these functions are lost. One of the earliest manifestations of tubular damage is the inability to concentrate the urine.

Further diagnostic information that can be obtained from the urinalysis includes evidence of proteinuria, hemoglobinuria, and casts or crystals in the urine. Blood tests for BUN and creatinine provide information regarding the ability to remove nitrogenous wastes from the blood. It also is important to exclude urinary obstruction.

A major concern in the treatment of acute renal failure is identifying and correcting the cause (*e.g.*, improving renal perfusion, discontinuing nephrotoxic drugs). Fluids are carefully regulated in an effort to maintain normal fluid volume and electrolyte concentrations. Adequate caloric intake is needed to prevent the breakdown of body proteins, which increases nitrogenous wastes. Parenteral hyperalimentation may be used for this purpose. Because secondary infections are a major cause of death in persons with acute renal failure, constant effort is needed to prevent and treat such infections.

Intermittent hemodialysis or continuous renal replacement therapy (CRRT) may be indicated when nitrogenous wastes and the water and electrolyte balance cannot be kept under control by other means. Venovenous or arteriovenous CRRT has emerged as a method for treating acute renal failure in patients too hemodynamically unstable to tolerate hemodialysis.[8] An associated advantage of the continuous renal replacement therapies is the ability to administer nutritional support. The disadvantages are the need for prolonged anticoagulation and continuous sophisticated monitoring.

In summary, acute renal failure represents an acute and usually reversible suppression of kidney function. It is a common threat to seriously ill persons in intensive care units, with a mortality rate of 40% to 75%. Acute renal failure is characterized by an accumulation of nitrogenous wastes in the blood (*i.e.*, azotemia) and alterations in body fluids and electrolytes. Acute renal failure is classified as prerenal, intrinsic or intrarenal, or postrenal in origin. Prerenal failure is caused by decreased blood flow to the kidneys; postrenal failure by obstruction to urine output; and intrinsic renal failure by disorders in the kidney itself. ATN, due to ischemia or nephrotoxic agents, is a common cause of acute intrinsic renal failure. ATN typically progresses through three phases: the initiation phase, during which tubular injury is induced; the maintenance phase, during which the GFR falls, nitrogenous wastes accumulate, and urine output decreases; and the recovery or reparative phase, during which the GFR, urine output, and blood levels of nitrogenous wastes return to normal.

Because of the high morbidity and mortality rates associated with acute renal failure, identification of persons at risk is important to clinical decision making. Acute renal failure often is reversible, making early identification and correction of the underlying cause (*e.g.*, improving renal perfusion, discontinuing nephrotoxic drugs) important. Treatment includes the judicious administration of fluids and dialysis or CRRT.

Chronic Renal Failure

Unlike acute renal failure, chronic renal failure represents progressive and irreversible destruction of kidney structures. As recently as 1965, many patients with chronic renal failure progressed to the final stages of the disease and then died. The high mortality rate was associated with limitations in the treatment of renal disease and with the tremendous cost of ongoing treatment. In 1972, federal support for dialysis and transplantation was made available through a Medicare entitlement program.[9]

Chronic renal failure can result from a number of conditions that cause permanent loss of nephrons, including diabetes, hypertension, glomerulonephritis, and polycystic kidney disease.[10,11] Diabetic kidney disease is the largest single cause of kidney failure in the United States.[10]

STAGES OF PROGRESSION

Regardless of cause, chronic renal failure results in loss of renal cells with progressive deterioration of glomerular filtration, tubular reabsorptive capacity, and endocrine functions of the kidneys.[12] All forms of renal failure are characterized by a reduction in the GFR, reflecting a corresponding reduction in the number of functional nephrons. The rate of nephron destruction differs from case to case, ranging from several months to many years.

The progression of chronic renal failure usually occurs in four stages: diminished renal reserve, renal insufficiency,

---

KEY CONCEPTS

Chronic Renal Failure

➤ Chronic renal failure represents the end result of conditions that greatly reduce kidney function by destroying renal nephrons and producing a marked decrease in the glomerular filtration rate (GFR).

➤ Signs of renal failure begin to appear as renal function moves from renal insufficiency (GFR 50% to 20% normal), to renal failure (20% to 5% normal), to end-stage renal disease (<5% normal). When the GFR decreases to less than 5% of normal, dialysis or kidney transplantation is necessary for survival.

➤ The manifestations of chronic renal failure represent the inability of the kidney to perform its normal functions in terms of regulating fluid and electrolyte balance, controlling blood pressure through fluid volume and the renin-angiotensin system, eliminating nitrogenous and other waste products, governing the red blood cell count through erythropoietin synthesis, and directing parathyroid and skeletal function through phosphate elimination and activation of vitamin D.

renal failure, and end-stage renal disease (ESRD).[12] Typically, the signs and symptoms of chronic renal failure occur gradually and do not become evident until the disease is far advanced. This is because of the amazing compensatory ability of the kidneys. As kidney structures are destroyed, the remaining nephrons undergo structural and functional hypertrophy, each increasing its function as a means of compensating for those that have been lost (Fig. 25-3). It is only when the few remaining nephrons are destroyed that the manifestations of renal failure become evident.

Diminished Renal Reserve

The GFR is considered the best measure of overall function of the kidney. The normal level of GFR varies with age, sex, and body size. The normal GFR for young healthy adults is approximately 120 to 130 mL/minute (1.73 mL/minute per mm^2).[10] Diminished renal reserve occurs when the GFR drops to approximately 50% of normal. At this point, the serum BUN and creatinine levels still are normal, and no symptoms of impaired renal function are evident. This is supported by the fact that many persons

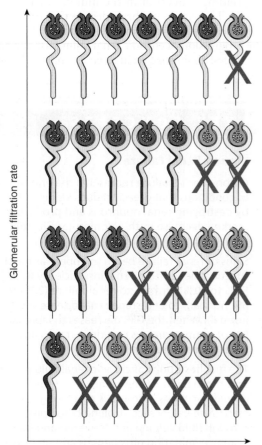

FIGURE 25-3 Relation of renal function and nephron mass. Each kidney contains about 1 million nephrons. A proportional relation exists between the number of nephrons affected by disease and the resulting glomerular filtration rate.

(y-axis label: Glomerular filtration rate; x-axis label: Number of functioning nephrons)

survive an entire lifetime with only one kidney. Because of the diminished reserve, the risk for development of azotemia increases with an additional renal insult, such as that due to nephrotoxic drugs.

Renal Insufficiency

Renal insufficiency represents a reduction in the GFR to 20% to 50% of normal. The kidneys initially have tremendous adaptive capabilities. As nephrons are destroyed, the remaining nephrons undergo changes to compensate for those that are lost. In the process, each of the remaining nephrons must filter more solute particles from the blood. Because the solute particles are osmotically active, they cause additional water to be lost in the urine. Thus, one of the earliest signs of renal insufficiency is *isosthenuria*, or polyuria with urine that is almost isotonic with plasma.[12] It is during this stage that azotemia, anemia, and hypertension also begin to appear.

Conservative treatment during this stage includes measures to retard deterioration of renal function and assist the body in managing the effects of impaired function. Urinary tract infections should be treated promptly and potentially nephrotoxic medications should be avoided. Blood pressure control is important, as is control of blood sugar in persons with diabetes. Smoking cessation is recommended, particularly in persons with diabetic nephropathy.[13] Because the kidneys have difficulty eliminating the waste products of protein metabolism, a restricted-protein diet usually produces fewer uremic symptoms and slows progression of renal failure. The few remaining nephrons that constitute the functional reserve of the kidneys can be easily disrupted, after which renal failure progresses rapidly.

Renal Failure and End-Stage Renal Disease

Renal failure develops when the GFR is less than 20% to 25% of normal.[12] At this point, the kidneys can no longer regulate the volume and solute composition of the extracellular fluids, and edema, metabolic acidosis, and hyperkalemia begin to appear. Overt uremia may ensue with neurologic, gastrointestinal, and cardiovascular manifestations.

End-stage renal disease (ESRD) occurs when the GFR is less than 5% of normal. Histologic findings of an end-stage kidney include a reduction in renal capillaries and scarring in the glomeruli. Atrophy and fibrosis are evident in the tubules. The mass of the kidneys usually is reduced. At this final stage of renal failure, treatment with dialysis or transplantation becomes necessary for survival.

The National Kidney Foundation Practice Guidelines, published in 2003, define renal failure "as either (1) a GFR of less than 15 mL/min per 1.73 m^2, which is accompanied by most signs and symptoms of uremia, or (2) a need to start renal replacement therapy (dialysis or transplantation)."[10] These guidelines point out that ESRD is an administrative term in the United States, indicating that a person requires treatment with dialysis or transplantation, which is a condition for payment of health care by the Medicare ESRD program.[10]

CLINICAL MANIFESTATIONS

The manifestations of chronic renal failure include an accumulation of nitrogenous wastes; alterations in water, electrolyte and acid-base balance; mineral and skeletal disorders; anemia and coagulation disorders; hypertension and alterations in cardiovascular function; gastrointestinal disorders; neurologic complications; disorders of skin integrity; and immunologic disorders[13] (Fig. 25-4). There currently are four target populations that comprise the entire population of persons with chronic renal failure: persons with chronic renal insufficiency who are managed medically, those with renal failure being treated with hemodialysis, those being treated with peritoneal dialysis, and renal transplant recipients. The manifestations of renal failure are determined largely by the extent of renal function that is present, coexisting disease conditions, and the type of renal replacement therapy that the person is receiving.

Accumulation of Nitrogenous Wastes

Azotemia, or the accumulation of nitrogenous wastes in the blood, is an early sign of renal failure, usually occurring before other symptoms become evident. Urea is one of the first nitrogenous wastes to accumulate in the blood, and the BUN level becomes increasingly elevated as renal failure progresses. The normal concentration of urea in the plasma is approximately 20 mg/dL. In renal failure, this level may rise to as high as 800 mg/dL. Creatinine, a byproduct of muscle metabolism, is freely filtered in the glomerulus and is not reabsorbed in the renal tubules. Creatinine is produced at a relatively constant rate and any creatinine that is filtered in the glomerulus is lost in the urine rather than being reabsorbed into the blood. Thus, serum creatinine can be used as an indirect method for assessing the GFR and the extent of renal damage that has occurred in renal failure (see Chapter 23).

Uremia, which literally means "urine in the blood," is the term used to describe the clinical manifestations of renal failure. Few symptoms of uremia appear until at least two thirds of the nephrons have been destroyed. Uremia differs from azotemia, which merely indicates the accumulation of nitrogenous wastes in the blood and can occur without symptoms. The uremic state includes signs and symptoms of altered fluid, electrolyte, and acid-base balance; impaired regulatory functions of the kidney (*e.g.,* hypertension, anemia, osteodystrophy); and the effects of uremia on body function (*e.g.,* uremic encephalopathy, peripheral neuropathy, pruritus). The symptoms at the onset of the uremic state (*e.g.,* weakness, fatigue, nausea, apathy) often are subtle. More severe symptoms include extreme weakness, frequent vomiting, lethargy, and confusion. Without treatment, coma and death follow.

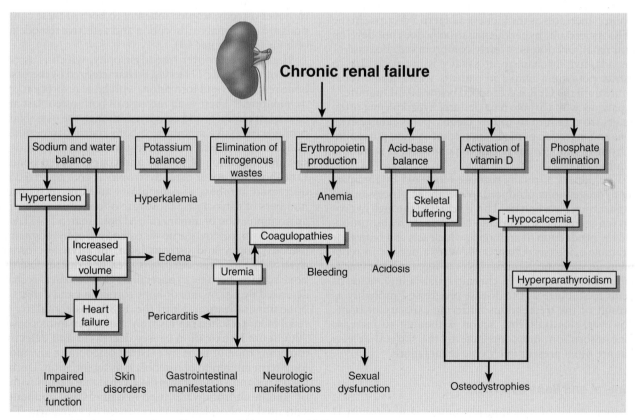

FIGURE 25-4 Mechanisms and manifestations of chronic renal failure.

Disorders of Water, Electrolyte, and Acid-Base Balance

The kidneys function in the regulation of extracellular fluid volume. They do this by either eliminating or conserving sodium and water. Chronic renal failure can produce dehydration or fluid overload, depending on the pathologic process of the renal disease. In addition to volume regulation, the ability of the kidneys to concentrate the urine is diminished. In renal failure, the specific gravity of the urine becomes fixed (1.008 to 1.012) and varies little from voiding to voiding. Polyuria and nocturia are common.

As renal function declines further, the ability to regulate sodium excretion is reduced. The kidneys normally tolerate large variations in sodium intake while maintaining normal serum sodium levels. In chronic renal failure, they lose the ability to regulate sodium excretion. There is impaired ability to adjust to a sudden reduction in sodium intake and poor tolerance of an acute sodium overload. Volume depletion with an accompanying decrease in the GFR can occur with a restricted sodium intake or excess sodium loss caused by diarrhea or vomiting. Salt wasting is a common problem in advanced renal failure because of impaired tubular reabsorption of sodium. Increasing sodium intake in persons with chronic renal failure often improves the GFR and whatever renal function remains. In persons with associated hypertension, the possibility of increasing blood pressure or production of congestive heart failure often excludes supplemental sodium intake.

Approximately 90% of potassium excretion is through the kidneys. In renal failure, potassium excretion by each nephron increases as the kidneys adapt to a decrease in the GFR. As a result, hyperkalemia usually does not develop until renal function is severely compromised. Because of this adaptive mechanism, it usually is not necessary to restrict potassium intake in patients with chronic renal failure until the GFR has dropped below 10 mL/minute.[13] In patients with chronic renal failure, hyperkalemia often results from failure to follow dietary potassium restrictions and ingestion of medications that contain potassium or from an endogenous release of potassium, as in trauma or infection.

The kidneys normally regulate blood pH by eliminating hydrogen ions produced in metabolic processes and regenerating bicarbonate. This is achieved through hydrogen ion secretion, sodium and bicarbonate reabsorption, and the production of ammonia, which acts as a buffer for titratable acids (see Chapter 6). With a decline in renal function, these mechanisms become impaired and metabolic acidosis results. In chronic renal failure, acidosis seems to stabilize as the disease progresses, probably as a result of the tremendous buffering capacity of bone. However, this buffering action is thought to increase bone resorption and contribute to the skeletal defects that are often present in chronic renal failure.

Mineral and Bone Disorders

Abnormalities of calcium, phosphate, and vitamin D metabolism occur early in the course of chronic renal failure.[14] The regulation of serum phosphate levels requires a daily urinary excretion of an amount equal to that ingested in the diet. With deteriorating renal function, phosphate excretion is impaired, and as a result, serum phosphate levels rise. At the same time, serum calcium levels, which are inversely regulated in relation to serum phosphate levels, fall (see Chapter 6). The drop in serum calcium, in turn, stimulates parathyroid hormone (PTH) release, with a resultant increase in calcium resorption from bone. Many people with ESRD develop a secondary hyperparathyroidism, the result of chronic stimulation of the parathyroid glands. Although serum calcium levels are maintained through increased PTH function, this adjustment is accomplished at the expense of the skeletal system and other body organs.

Vitamin D synthesis also is impaired in renal failure. The kidneys regulate vitamin D activity by converting the inactive form of vitamin D [25(OH) vitamin D_3] to its active form (1,25-OH_2 vitamin D_3). Decreased levels of active vitamin D lead to a decrease in intestinal absorption of calcium with a resultant increase in PTH levels. Vitamin D also regulates osteoblast differentiation, thereby affecting bone matrix formation and mineralization.

The term *renal osteodystrophy* is used to describe the skeletal complications of ESRD.[13,14] Several factors are thought to contribute to the development of renal osteodystrophy, including elevated serum phosphate levels, decreased serum calcium levels, impaired renal activation of vitamin D, and hyperparathyroidism. The skeletal changes that occur with renal failure have been divided into two major types of disorders: high-turnover and low-turnover osteodystrophy. Inherent to both of these conditions are abnormal reabsorption and defective remodeling of bone (see Chapter 43).

High–bone-turnover osteodystrophy, which is associated with elevated PTH levels, is characterized by increased bone resorption and formation, with bone resorption predominating.[13] There is an increase in both osteoblast and osteoclast numbers and activity. Although the osteoblasts produce excessive amounts of bone matrix, mineralization fails to keep pace, and there is a decrease in bone density and formation of porous and coarse-fibered bone.[15] Low–bone-turnover osteodystrophy is characterized by decreased numbers of osteoblasts and low or reduced numbers of osteoclasts, a low rate of bone turnover, and an accumulation of unmineralized bone matrix.[14,15] There are two forms of low-turnover osteodystrophy: adynamic osteodystrophy and osteomalacia. In *adynamic osteodystrophy,* bone remodeling is greatly reduced, and the bone surfaces become hypocellular. *Osteomalacia* is characterized by a slow rate of bone formation and defects in bone mineralization. Until the 1980s, osteomalacia in renal failure resulted mainly from aluminum intoxication. Aluminum intoxication causes decreased and defective mineralization of bone by existing osteoblasts and more long-term inhibition of osteoblast differentiation. During the 1970s and 1980s, it was discovered that accumulation of aluminum from water used in dialysis and aluminum salts used in phosphate binders caused osteomalacia. This discovery led to a change in the composition of dialysis solutions and substitution of calcium carbonate for aluminum salts in phosphate binders. As a result, the incidence of osteomalacia in persons with ESRD has declined.

The symptoms of renal osteodystrophy, which occur late in the disease, include bone tenderness and muscle weakness. Proximal muscle weakness in the lower extremities is common, making it difficult to get out of a chair or climb stairs.[14] Fractures are more common with low-turnover osteomalacia and adynamic renal bone disease.

Early treatment of hyperphosphatemia and hypocalcemia is important to prevent or slow long-term skeletal complications.[16] Milk products and other foods with a high phosphorus content are restricted in the diet. Phosphate-binding antacids may be prescribed to decrease absorption of phosphate from the gastrointestinal tract. Calcium-containing phosphate binders can lead to hypercalcemia, thus worsening soft tissue calcification, especially in persons on vitamin D therapy. Aluminum-containing antacids can contribute to the development of osteomalacia and other complications. To avoid these side effects, an aluminum- and calcium-free binder (sevelamer), which is resistant to digestive degradation and not absorbed, has been developed. Activated forms of vitamin D and calcium supplements often are used to facilitate intestinal absorption of calcium, increase serum calcium levels, and prevent parathyroid gland overactivity.[17]

Hematologic Disorders

Chronic anemia is the most profound hematologic alteration that accompanies renal failure. The kidneys are the primary site for the production of the hormone *erythropoietin*, which controls red blood cell production. In renal failure, erythropoietin production usually is insufficient to stimulate adequate red blood cell production by the bone marrow. The accumulation of uremic toxins further suppresses red cell production in the bone marrow, and the cells that are produced have a shortened life span. Iron is essential for erythropoiesis. Many persons on maintenance hemodialysis also are iron deficient because of blood sampling and accidental loss of blood during dialysis. Other causes of iron deficiency include factors such as anorexia and dietary restrictions that limit iron intake.

When untreated, anemia causes or contributes to weakness, fatigue, depression, insomnia, and decreased cognitive function. There is increasing concern regarding the physiologic effects of anemia on cardiovascular function. The anemia of renal failure produces a decrease in blood viscosity and a compensatory increase in heart rate. The decreased blood viscosity also exacerbates peripheral vasodilatation and contributes to decreased vascular resistance. Cardiac output increases in a compensatory fashion to maintain tissue perfusion. Echocardiographic studies after initiation of chronic dialysis have shown ventricular dilatation with compensatory left ventricular hypertrophy.[18] Anemia also limits myocardial oxygen supply, particularly in persons with coronary heart disease, leading to angina pectoris and other ischemic events. Thus, anemia, when coupled with hypertension, may be a major

contributing factor to the development of left ventricular dysfunction and congestive heart failure in persons with ESRD.

A remarkable advance in medical management of ESRD occurred with the availability of recombinant human erythropoietin (rhEPO). Secondary benefits of treating anemia with rhEPO, previously attributed to the correction of uremia, include improvement in appetite, energy level, sexual function, skin color, and hair and nail growth, and reduced cold intolerance. Worsening of hypertension and seizures has occurred when the hematocrit was raised too suddenly; therefore, frequent measurements of hematocrit are necessary. Because iron deficiency is common among persons with chronic renal failure, iron supplementation may also be needed.

Bleeding disorders are manifested by epistaxis, menorrhagia, gastrointestinal bleeding, and bruising of the skin and subcutaneous tissues. Although platelet production often is normal in ESRD, platelet function is impaired. Coagulative function improves with dialysis but does not completely normalize, suggesting that uremia contributes to the problem. Anemia may accentuate the problem by changing the position of the platelets with respect to the vessel wall. Normally the red cells occupy the center of the bloodstream and the platelets are in the skimming layer along the endothelial surface. In anemia, the platelets become dispersed, impairing the platelet–endothelial cell adherence needed to initiate hemostasis.[19]

Cardiovascular Disorders

Cardiovascular disease is the major cause of death in patients with ESRD. The overall mortality rate from cardiovascular disease for people with renal failure is 30 times that of the general population.[20] Coexisting conditions that have been identified as contributing to the burden of cardiovascular disease include hypertension, anemia, diabetes mellitus, dyslipidemia, and coagulopathies.

Hypertension commonly is an early manifestation of chronic renal failure. The mechanisms that produce hypertension in ESRD are multifactorial; they include an increased vascular volume, elevation of peripheral vascular resistance, decreased levels of renal vasodilator prostaglandins, and increased activity of the renin-angiotensin system.[21] Early identification and aggressive treatment of hypertension has been shown to slow the rate of renal impairment in many types of renal disease. Treatment involves salt and water restriction and the use of antihypertensive medications to control blood pressure. Many persons with renal insufficiency need to take several antihypertensive medications to control blood pressure.

The spectrum of cardiovascular disease includes left ventricular hypertrophy and ischemic heart disease. Congestive heart failure and pulmonary edema tend to occur in the late stages of renal failure. People with renal failure tend to have an increased prevalence of left ventricular dysfunction, both with a depressed left ventricular ejection fraction, as in systolic dysfunction, as well as impaired ventricular filling, as in diastolic failure[22] (see Chapter 19). There are multiple factors that lead to development of left ventricular dysfunction, including extracellular fluid overload, shunting of blood through an arteriovenous fistula for dialysis, and anemia. These abnormalities, coupled with the hypertension that often is present, cause increased myocardial work and oxygen demand, with eventual development of heart failure.

Pericarditis occurs in approximately 20% of persons receiving chronic dialysis.[23] It can result from metabolic toxins associated with the uremic state or from dialysis. The manifestations of uremic pericarditis resemble those of viral pericarditis, with all its complications, including cardiac tamponade (see Chapter 18).

Gastrointestinal Disorders

Anorexia, nausea, and vomiting are common in patients with uremia, along with a metallic taste in the mouth that further depresses the appetite. Early-morning nausea is common. Ulceration and bleeding of the gastrointestinal mucosa may develop, and hiccups are common. A possible cause of nausea and vomiting is the decomposition of urea by intestinal flora, resulting in a high concentration of ammonia. PTH increases gastric acid secretion and contributes to gastrointestinal problems. Nausea and vomiting often improve with restriction of dietary protein and initiation of dialysis, and disappear after kidney transplantation.

Disorders of Neural Function

Many persons with chronic renal failure have alterations in peripheral and central nervous system function. Peripheral neuropathy, or involvement of the peripheral nerves, affects the lower limbs more frequently than the upper limbs. It is symmetric and affects both sensory and motor function. Neuropathy is caused by atrophy and demyelination of nerve fibers, possibly due to uremic toxins. Restless legs syndrome is a manifestation of peripheral nerve involvement and can be seen in as many as two thirds of patients on dialysis. This syndrome is characterized by creeping, prickling, and itching sensations that typically are more intense at rest. Temporary relief is obtained by moving the legs. A burning sensation of the feet, which may be followed by muscle weakness and atrophy, is a frequent manifestation of uremia.

The central nervous system disturbances in uremia are similar to those caused by other metabolic and toxic disorders. Sometimes referred to as *uremic encephalopathy,* the condition is poorly understood and may result, at least in part, from an excess of toxic organic acids that alter neural function. Electrolyte abnormalities, such as sodium shifts, also may contribute. The manifestations are more closely related to the progress of the uremic disorder than to the level of the metabolic end products. Reduction in alertness is one of the earliest and most significant indications of uremic encephalopathy. This often is followed by an inability to fix attention, loss of recent memory, and perceptual errors in identifying persons and objects. Delirium and coma occur late in the course; seizures are the preterminal event.

Disorders of motor function commonly accompany the neurologic manifestations of uremic encephalopathy. During the early stages, there often is difficulty in performing fine movements of the extremities; the gait becomes unsteady and clumsy, with tremulousness of movement. Asterixis (dorsiflexion movements of the hands and feet) typically occurs as the disease progresses. It can be elicited by having the person hyperextend his or her arms at the elbow and wrist with the fingers spread apart. If asterixis is present, this position causes side-to-side flapping movements of the fingers.

Altered Immune Function

Infection is a common complication and cause of hospitalization and death in persons with chronic renal failure. Immunologic abnormalities decrease the efficiency of the immune response to infection. All aspects of inflammation and immune function may be affected adversely by the high levels of urea and metabolic wastes, including a decrease in granulocyte count, impaired humoral and cell-mediated immunity, and defective phagocyte function. The acute inflammatory response and delayed-type hypersensitivity response are impaired. Although persons with ESRD have normal humoral responses to vaccines, a more aggressive immunization program may be needed. Skin and mucosal barriers to infection also may be defective. In persons who are maintained on dialysis, vascular access devices are common portals of entry for pathogens. Many persons with ESRD fail to mount a fever with infection, making the diagnosis more difficult.

Disorders of Skin Integrity

Skin manifestations are common in persons with renal failure. The skin often is pale owing to anemia and may have a sallow, yellow-brown hue. The skin and mucous membranes often are dry, and subcutaneous bruising is common. Skin dryness is caused by a reduction in perspiration owing to the decreased size of sweat glands and the diminished activity of oil glands. Pruritus is common; it results from the high serum phosphate levels and the development of phosphate crystals that occur with hyperparathyroidism. Severe scratching and repeated needle sticks, especially with hemodialysis, break the skin integrity and increase the risk for infection. In the advanced stages of untreated renal failure, urea crystals may precipitate on the skin as a result of the high urea concentration in body fluids. The fingernails may become thin and brittle, with a dark band just behind the leading edge of the nail, followed by a white band. This appearance is known as *Terry's nails.*

Sexual Dysfunction

The cause of sexual dysfunction in men and women with chronic renal failure is unclear. The cause probably is multifactorial and may result from high levels of uremic toxins, neuropathy, altered endocrine function, psychological factors, and medications (*e.g.,* antihypertensive drugs). Alterations in physiologic sexual responses, reproductive ability, and libido are common.

Approximately 50% of men with ESRD complain of erectile disfunction.[24] Derangements of the pituitary and gonadal hormones, such as decreases in testosterone levels and increases in prolactin and luteinizing hormone levels, are common and cause erectile difficulties and decreased spermatocyte counts. Loss of libido may result from chronic anemia and decreased testosterone levels. Several drugs, such as exogenous testosterone and bromocriptine, have been used in an attempt to return hormone levels to normal.

Impaired sexual function in women is manifested by abnormal levels of progesterone, luteinizing hormone, and prolactin. Hypofertility, menstrual abnormalities, decreased vaginal lubrication, and various orgasmic problems have been described.[13] Amenorrhea is common among women who are on dialysis therapy.

Elimination of Drugs

The kidneys are responsible for the elimination of many drugs and their metabolites. Renal failure and its treatment can interfere with the absorption, distribution, and elimination of drugs. The administration of large quantities of phosphate-binding antacids to control hyperphosphatemia and hypocalcemia in patients with advanced renal failure interferes with the absorption of some drugs. Many drugs are bound to plasma proteins, such as albumin, for transport in the body; the unbound portion of the drug is available to act at the various receptor sites and is free to be metabolized. A decrease in plasma proteins, particularly albumin, that occurs in many persons with renal failure results in less protein-bound drug and greater amounts of free drug.

In the process of metabolism, some drugs form intermediate metabolites that are toxic if not eliminated. Some pathways of drug metabolism, such as hydrolysis, are slowed with uremia. In persons with diabetes, for example, insulin requirements may be reduced as renal function deteriorates. Decreased elimination by the kidneys allows drugs or their metabolites to accumulate in the body and requires that drug dosages be adjusted accordingly. Some drugs contain unwanted nitrogen, sodium, potassium, and magnesium and must be avoided in patients with renal failure. Penicillin, for example, contains potassium. Nitrofurantoin and ammonium chloride add to the body's nitrogen pool. Many antacids contain magnesium, which is eliminated by the kidney. Because of problems with drug dosing and elimination, persons with renal failure should be cautioned against the use of over-the-counter remedies.

TREATMENT

During the past several decades, an increasing number of persons have required renal replacement therapy with dialysis or transplantation. The growing volume is largely attributable to the improvement in treatment and more liberal policies regarding who is treated.

Medical Management

Chronic renal failure can be treated by conservative management of renal insufficiency and by renal replacement therapy with dialysis or transplantation. Conservative treatment consists of measures to prevent or retard deterioration in remaining renal function and to assist the body in compensating for the existing impairment. Interventions that have been shown significantly to retard the progression of chronic renal insufficiency include dietary protein restriction and blood pressure normalization. Various interventions are used to compensate for reduced renal function and correct the resulting anemia, hypocalcemia, and acidosis. These interventions often are used in conjunction with dialysis therapy for patients with ESRD.

Dialysis and Transplantation

Dialysis or renal replacement therapy is indicated when advanced uremia or serious electrolyte imbalances are present. The choice between dialysis and transplantation is dictated by age, related health problems, donor availability, and personal preference. Although transplantation often is the treatment preference, dialysis plays a critical role as a treatment method for ESRD. It is life sustaining for persons who are not candidates for transplantation or who are awaiting transplantation. There are two broad categories of dialysis: hemodialysis and peritoneal dialysis.

Hemodialysis. The basic principles of hemodialysis have remained unchanged over the years, although new technology has improved the efficiency and speed of dialysis.[25] A hemodialysis system, or artificial kidney, consists of three parts: a blood compartment, a dialysis fluid compartment, and a semipermeable membrane that separates the two compartments. There are several types of dialyzers; all incorporate these parts, and all function in a similar manner.

The dialysis membrane is semipermeable, permitting all molecules except blood cells and plasma proteins to move freely in both directions—from the blood into the dialyzing solution and from the dialyzing solution into the blood. The direction of flow is determined by the concentration of the substances contained in the two solutions. The waste products and excess electrolytes in the blood normally diffuse into the dialyzing solution. If there is a need to replace or add substances, such as bicarbonate, to the blood, these can be added to the dialyzing solution (Fig. 25-5).

During dialysis, blood moves from an artery through the tubing and blood chamber in the dialysis machine and then back into the body through a vein. Access to the vascular system is accomplished through an external arteriovenous shunt (*i.e.,* tubing implanted into an artery and a vein) or, more commonly, through an internal arteriovenous fistula (*i.e.,* anastomosis of a vein to an artery, usually in the forearm). Heparin is used to prevent clotting during the dialysis treatment; it can be administered continuously or intermittently. Most persons receive dialysis

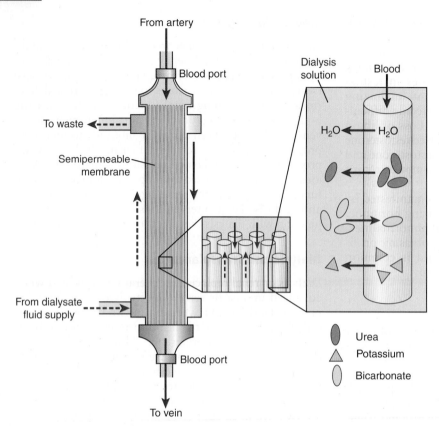

FIGURE 25-5 Schematic diagram of a hemodialysis system. The blood compartment and dialysis solution compartment are separated by a semipermeable membrane. This membrane is porous enough to allow all the constituents, except the plasma proteins and blood cells, to diffuse between the two compartments.

three times each week for 3 to 4 hours. Many dialysis centers provide the option for patients to learn how to perform hemodialysis at home.

Peritoneal Dialysis. Peritoneal dialysis was introduced in the mid-1970s. Improvements in technology and the ability to deliver adequate dialysis resulted in improved outcomes and the acceptance of peritoneal dialysis as a renal replacement therapy.

The same principles of diffusion, osmosis, and ultrafiltration that apply to hemodialysis apply to peritoneal dialysis. The thin serous membrane of the peritoneal cavity serves as the dialyzing membrane. A Silastic catheter is surgically implanted in the peritoneal cavity below the umbilicus to provide access (Fig. 25-6). The dialysis process involves instilling a sterile dialyzing solution (usually 2 L) through the catheter over a period of approximately 10 minutes. The solution then is allowed to remain, or dwell, in the peritoneal cavity for a prescribed amount of time, during which the metabolic end products and extracellular fluid diffuse into the dialysis solution. At the end of the dwell time, the dialysis fluid is drained out of the peritoneal cavity by gravity into a sterile bag. In contrast to hemodialysis, which uses pressure to push water through the dialyzing membrane, peritoneal dialysis uses the osmotic effect of the glucose contained in the dialyzing solution. Commercial dialysis solution is available in 1.5%, 2.5%, and 4.25% dextrose concentrations. Solutions with higher dextrose levels increase osmosis,

causing more fluid to be removed from the body. Peritoneal dialysis can be performed at home or in a center, by an automated or manual system, and on an intermittent or continuous basis—all with variations in the number of exchanges and in dwell time. Individual preference,

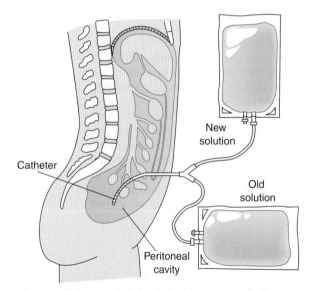

FIGURE 25-6 Peritoneal dialysis. A semipermeable membrane, richly supplied with small blood vessels, lines the peritoneal cavity. With dialysate dwelling in the peritoneal cavity, waste products diffuse from the network of blood cells into the dialysate.

manual ability, lifestyle, knowledge of the procedure, and physiologic response to treatment are used to determine the dialysis schedule.

Transplantation. Greatly improved success rates have made kidney transplantation the treatment of choice for many patients with chronic renal failure. The availability of donor organs continues to limit the number of transplantations performed each year. Donor organs are obtained from cadavers and living related donors (*e.g.*, parent, sibling). Transplants from living nonrelated donors (*e.g.*, spouse) have been used in cases of suitable ABO blood types and tissue compatibility. The success of transplantation depends primarily on the degree of histocompatibility, adequate organ preservation, and immunologic management.[26]

Dietary Management

A major component in the treatment of chronic renal failure is dietary management.[27] The goal of dietary treatment is to provide optimum nutrition while maintaining tolerable levels of metabolic wastes. The specific diet prescription depends on the type and severity of renal disease and on the dialysis modality. Because of the severe restrictions placed on food and fluid intake, these diets may be complicated and unappetizing.

Restriction of dietary proteins may decrease the progress of renal impairment in persons with advanced renal disease. Proteins are broken down to form nitrogenous wastes, and reducing the amount of protein in the diet usually lowers the BUN and reduces symptoms. Moreover, a high-protein diet is high in phosphates and inorganic acids. Considerable controversy exists over the degree of restriction needed. If the diet is too low in protein, protein malnutrition can occur, with a loss of strength, muscle mass, and body weight.

With renal failure, adequate calories in the form of carbohydrates and fat are required to meet energy needs. This is particularly important when the protein content of the diet is severely restricted. If sufficient calories are not available, the limited protein in the diet goes into energy production, or proteins from body tissues are used for energy purposes.

When the GFR falls to extremely low levels in ESRD or in patients undergoing hemodialysis therapy, dietary restriction of potassium becomes mandatory. Using salt substitutes that contain potassium or ingesting fruits, fruit juices, chocolate, or other high-potassium foods can cause hyperkalemia.

The sodium and fluid restrictions depend on the kidneys' ability to excrete sodium and water and must be individually determined. Renal disease of glomerular origin is more likely to contribute to sodium retention, whereas tubular dysfunction causes salt wasting. Fluid intake in excess of what the kidneys can excrete causes circulatory overload, edema, and water intoxication. Thirst is a common problem among patients on hemodialysis, often resulting in large weight gains between treatments.

Inadequate intake, on the other hand, causes volume depletion and hypotension and can cause further decreases in the already compromised GFR.

In summary, chronic renal failure results from the destructive effects of many forms of renal disease. Regardless of the cause, the consequences of nephron destruction in ESRD are alterations in the filtration, reabsorption, and endocrine functions of the kidneys. The progression of chronic renal failure usually occurs in four stages: diminished renal reserve, renal insufficiency, renal failure, and ESRD. Renal insufficiency represents a reduction in the GFR to approximately 20% to 50% of normal; renal failure, a reduction to less than 20% to 25% of normal; and ESRD, a decrease in GFR to less than 5% of normal.

End-stage renal disease affects almost every body system. It causes an accumulation of nitrogenous wastes, alters sodium and water excretion, and alters regulation of body levels of potassium, phosphate, calcium, and magnesium. It also causes skeletal problems, anemia, cardiovascular disorders, neurologic disturbances, gastrointestinal dysfunction, and discomforting skin changes.

The treatment of ESRD can be divided into two types: conservative management of renal insufficiency and renal replacement therapy with dialysis or transplantation. Conservative treatment consists of measures to prevent or retard deterioration in remaining renal function and to assist the body in compensating for the existing impairment. Activated vitamin D can be used to increase calcium absorption and control secondary hyperparathyroidism. Recombinant human erythropoietin is used to treat the profound anemia that occurs in persons with ESRD.

Renal Failure in Children and Elderly Persons

Although the spectrum of renal disease among children and elderly persons is similar to that of adults, several unique issues affecting these groups warrant further discussion.

CHRONIC RENAL FAILURE IN CHILDREN

The true incidence of chronic renal failure in infants and children is unknown. Available data suggest that 1% to 2% of patients with chronic renal failure are in the pediatric age range.[28] The causes of chronic renal failure in children include congenital malformations, inherited disorders, acquired diseases, and metabolic syndromes. The underlying cause correlates closely with the age of the child. In children younger than 5 years of age, chronic renal failure is commonly the result of congenital malformations such as renal dysplasia or obstructive uropathy.[29] After 5 years of age, acquired diseases (*e.g.,* glomerulonephritis) and inherited disorders (*e.g.,* familial juvenile nephrophthisis) predominate. Chronic renal failure related to metabolic disorders, such as hyperoxaluria, and inherited disorders, such as polycystic kidney disease, may present throughout childhood.[29]

The manifestations of chronic renal failure in children are quite varied and depend on the underlying disease condition. Features of renal disease that are marked during childhood include severe growth impairment, delayed sexual maturation, bone abnormalities, and development of psychosocial problems. Critical growth periods occur during the first 2 years of life and during adolescence. Physical growth and cognitive development occur at a slower rate as consequences of renal disease, especially among children with congenital kidney diseases.[30] Puberty usually occurs at a later age in children with renal failure, partly because of endocrine abnormalities. Renal osteodystrophy is more common and extensive in children than in adults because of the presence of open epiphyses. As a result, metaphyseal fractures, bone pain, impaired bone growth, short stature, and osteitis fibrosa cystica (a condition in which cysts develop in the bone) occur with greater frequency. Some hereditary renal diseases, such as medullary cystic disease, have patterns of skeletal involvement that further complicate the problems of renal osteodystrophy. Factors related to impaired growth include deficient nutrition, anemia, renal osteodystrophy, chronic acidosis, and cases of nephrotic syndrome that require high-dose corticosteroid therapy.

Success of treatment in children with renal failure depends on the level of bone maturation at the initiation of therapy. Nutrition is believed to be the most important determinant during infancy. During childhood, growth hormone is important, and gonadotropic hormones become important during puberty. Parental heights provide a means of assessing growth potential (see Chapter 31). For many children, catch-up growth is important because a growth deficit frequently is established during the first months of life. Recombinant human growth hormone therapy has been used to improve growth in children with ESRD.[31] Success of treatment depends on the level of bone maturation at the initiation of therapy.

All forms of renal replacement therapy can be safely and reliably used for children. Children typically are treated with continuous ambulatory peritoneal dialysis (CAPD) or transplantation to optimize growth and development.[28] Renal transplantation is considered the best alternative for children.[32] Early transplantation in young children is regarded as the best way to promote physical growth, improve cognitive function, and foster psychosocial development. Immunosuppressive therapy in children is similar to that used in adults. All of these immunosuppressive agents have side effects, including increased risk of infection. Corticosteroids, which have been the mainstay of chronic immunosuppressive therapy for decades, carry the risk of hypertension, orthopedic complications (especially aseptic necrosis), cataracts, and growth retardation.

CHRONIC RENAL FAILURE IN ELDERLY PERSONS

Since the mid-1980s, there have been increasing numbers of elderly persons accepted to ESRD programs. In 2000, 19.8% of persons being treated for ESRD were 65 to 74 years of age, and 14.7% were older than 75 years of age.[33] Among elderly persons, the presentation and course of renal failure may be altered because of age-related changes in the kidneys and concurrent medical conditions.

Normal aging is associated with a decline in the GFR and reduced regulation of renal function under stressful conditions.[34] This reduction in GFR makes elderly persons more susceptible to the detrimental effects of nephrotoxic drugs, such as radiographic contrast compounds. The reduction in GFR related to aging is not accompanied by a parallel rise in the serum creatinine level because the serum creatinine level, which results from muscle metabolism, is significantly reduced in elderly persons owing to diminished muscle mass and other age-related changes. Evaluation of renal function in elderly persons should include a measurement of creatinine clearance along with the serum creatinine level.

The prevalence of chronic disease affecting the cerebrovascular, cardiovascular, and skeletal systems is higher in this age group. Because of concurrent disease, the presenting symptoms of renal disease in elderly persons may be less typical than those observed in younger adults. For example, congestive heart failure and hypertension may be the dominant clinical features with the onset of acute glomerulonephritis, whereas oliguria and discolored urine more often are the first signs in younger adults. The course of renal failure may be more complicated in older patients with numerous chronic diseases.

Treatment options for chronic renal failure in elderly patients include hemodialysis, peritoneal dialysis, and transplantation. Neither hemodialysis nor peritoneal dialysis has proven to be superior in the elderly. The mode of renal replacement therapy should be individualized, taking into account underlying medical and psychosocial factors. Age alone should not preclude renal transplantation.[35] With increasing experience, many transplantation centers have increased the age for acceptance on transplant waiting lists. Reluctance to provide transplantation as an alternative may have been due, at least in part, to the scarcity of available organs and the view that younger persons are more likely to benefit for a longer time.[35] The general reduction in T-cell function that occurs with aging has been suggested as a beneficial effect that increases transplant graft survival.

In summary, available data suggest that 1% to 2% of patients with chronic renal failure are in the pediatric age range. The causes of renal failure include congenital malformations (*e.g.,* renal dysplasia and obstructive uropathy), inherited disorders (*e.g.,* polycystic kidney disease), acquired diseases (*e.g.,* glomerulonephritis), and metabolic syndromes (*e.g.,* hyperoxaluria). Problems associated with renal failure in children include growth impairment, delay in sexual maturation, and more extensive bone abnormalities than in adults. Although all forms of renal replacement therapy can be safely and reliably used for children, CAPD or transplantation optimizes growth and development.

Adults 65 years of age and older account for close to one half of the new cases of ESRD each year. Normal aging is associated with a decline in the GFR, which makes elderly persons more susceptible to the detrimental effects of nephrotoxic drugs and other conditions that compromise renal function. Treatment options for chronic renal failure in elderly patients are similar to those for younger persons.

Review Exercises

A 55-year-old man with diabetes and coronary heart disease, who underwent cardiac catheterization with use of radiocontrast agent 2 days ago, is admitted to the emergency department with a flulike syndrome, including chills, nausea, vomiting, abdominal pain, fatigue, and pulmonary congestion. His serum creatinine is elevated and he has protein in his urine. He is admitted to the intensive care unit with a tentative diagnosis of acute renal failure due to radiocontrast nephropathy.

A. Radiocontrast agents are thought to exert their effects through decreased renal perfusion and through direct toxic effects on renal tubular structures. Explain how each of these phenomena contributes to the development of acute renal failure.

B. Explain the elevated serum creatinine, proteinuria, and presence of pulmonary congestion.

Chronic renal failure is accompanied by hyperphosphatemia, hypocalcemia, impaired activation of vitamin D, hyperparathyroidism, and skeletal complications.

A. Explain the impaired activation of vitamin D and its consequences for calcium and phosphate homeostasis, parathyroid function, and mineralization of bone in persons with renal failure.

B. Explain the possible complications of the administration of activated forms of vitamin D on parathyroid function and calcium and phosphate homeostasis (*e.g.,* calcium × phosphate product).

Visit the Porth: Essentials of Pathophysiology: Concepts of Altered Health States web site (http://thePoint.LWW.com/PorthEssentials) for links to chapter-related resources on the Internet, all-new exclusive animations, chapter review questions, and more!

REFERENCES

1. Singri N., Ahya S. N., Levin M. L. (2003). Acute renal failure. *Journal of the American Medical Association* 289, 747–751.
2. Edelstein C. L., Schrier R. W. (2003). Acute renal failure: Pathogenesis, diagnosis, and management. In Schrier R. W. (Ed.), *Renal and electrolyte disorders* (6th ed., pp. 401–455). Philadelphia: Lippincott Williams & Wilkins.
3. Brady H. R., Brenner B. M., Clarkson M. R., et al. (2000). Acute renal failure. In Brenner B. M. (Ed.), *Brenner and Rector's the kidney* (6th ed., pp. 1201–1247). Philadelphia: W. B. Saunders.
4. Abernethy V. E., Lieberthal W. (2002). Acute renal failure in the critically ill patient. *Critical Care Clinics* 18, 203–222.
5. Guyton A., Hall J. E. (2006). *Textbook of medical physiology* (11th ed., pp. 308–325, 343–347). Philadelphia: Elsevier Saunders.
6. Jennette J. C. (2005). The kidney. In Rubin E., Gorstein F., Rubin R., et al. (Eds.), *Rubin's pathology: Clinicopathologic foundations of medicine* (4th ed., pp. 867–869). Philadelphia: Lippincott Williams & Wilkins.
7. Gerlach A. T., Pickworth K. K. (2000). Contrast medium-induced nephrotoxicity: Pathophysiology and prevention. *Pharmacotherapy* 20, 540–548.
8. Forni L. G., Hilton P. J. (1997). Continuous hemofiltration in the treatment of acute renal failure. *New England Journal of Medicine* 336, 1303–1309.
9. Rettig R. A. (1996). The social contract and the treatment of permanent renal failure. *Journal of the American Medical Association* 274, 1123–1126.
10. Levey A. S., Coresh J., Balk E., et al. (2003). National Kidney Foundation practice guidelines for chronic kidney disease: Evaluation, classification, and stratification. *Annals of Internal Medicine* 139, 137–147.
11. Yu H. T. (2003). Progression of chronic renal failure. *Archives of Internal Medicine* 163, 1417–1429.
12. Alpers C. E. (2005). The kidney. In Kumar V., Abbas A. K., Fausto N. (Eds.), *Robbins and Cotran pathologic basis of disease* (7th ed., pp. 993–996). Philadelphia: Elsevier Saunders.
13. Skorecki K., Green J., Brenner B. M. (2001). Chronic renal failure. In Braunwald E., Fauci A. S., Kasper D. L., et al. (Eds.), *Harrison's principles of internal medicine* (15th ed., pp. 1551–1572). New York: McGraw-Hill.
14. Llach F., Bover J. (2000). Renal osteodystrophies. In Brenner B. M. (Ed.), *Brenner and Rector's the kidney* (6th ed., pp. 2103–2135). Philadelphia: W. B. Saunders.
15. Elder G. (2002). Pathophysiology and recent advances in the management of renal osteodystrophy. *Journal of Bone and Mineral Research* 17, 2094–2105.
16. Albaaj F., Hutchison A. J. (2003). Hyperphosphatemia in renal failure. *Drugs* 63, 577–596.
17. Drüeke T. B. (2001). Control of secondary hyperthyroidism by vitamin D derivatives. *American Journal of Kidney Diseases* 37(1 Suppl. 2), S58–S61.
18. Tong E. M., Nissenson A. R. (2001). Erythropoietin and anemia. *Seminars in Nephrology* 21, 190–203.
19. Eberst M. E., Berkowitz L. R. (1993). Hemostasis in renal disease: Pathophysiology and management. *American Journal of Medicine* 96, 168–179.

20. National Kidney Foundation Task Force on Cardiovascular Disease. (1998). Controlling the epidemic of cardiovascular disease in chronic renal disease. *American Journal of Kidney Diseases* 32, 853–906.

21. Preston R. A., Singer I., Epstein M. (1996). Renal parenchymal hypertension. *Archives of Internal Medicine* 156, 602–611.

22. Al-Ahmad A., Sarnak M. J., Salem D. N., Konstam M. A. (2001). Cause and management of heart failure in patients with chronic renal disease. *Seminars in Nephrology* 21, 3–12.

23. Gunukula S., Spodick D. H. (2001). Pericardial disease in renal failure. *Seminars in Nephrology* 21, 52–56.

24. Palmer B. (1999). Sexual dysfunction in uremia. *Journal of the American Society of Nephrology* 10, 1381–1388.

25. Daelemans R. A., D'Haese P. C., BeBroe M. E. (2001). Dialysis. *Seminars in Nephrology* 21, 204–212.

26. Ramanathan V., Goral S., Helderman J. H. (2001). Renal transplantation. *Seminars in Nephrology* 21, 213–219.

27. National Kidney Foundation. (2000). *Clinical practice guidelines for nutrition in chronic renal failure.* [On-line]. Available: http://kidney.org/professionals/doqi/doqi/doqi_nut.html.

28. Chan J. C. M., Williams D. M., Roth K. S. (2002). Kidney failure in infants and children. *Pediatrics in Review* 23(2), 47–60.

29. Vogt B. A., Avner E. D. (2004). Renal failure. In Behrman R. E., Kliegman R. M., Jensen H. B. (Eds.), *Nelson textbook of pediatrics* (17th ed., pp. 1767–1775). Philadelphia: Elsevier Saunders.

30. Hanna J. D., Krieg R. J., Scheinman J. I., et al. (1996). Effects of uremia on growth in children. *Seminars in Nephrology* 16, 230–241.

31. Haffner D., Schaffer F., Nissel R., et al. (Study Group for Growth Hormone Treatment in Chronic Renal Failure). (2000). Effect of growth hormone treatment on the adult height of children with chronic renal failure. *New England Journal of Medicine* 343, 923–930.

32. Urizar R. E. (2004). Renal transplantation. In Behrman R. E., Kliegman R. M., Jensen H. B. (Eds.), *Nelson textbook of pediatrics* (17th ed., pp. 1775–1782). Philadelphia: Elsevier Saunders.

33. National Kidney Foundation. (2003). *End stage renal disease.* [On-line]. Available: http://www.kidney.org/newsroom/fsitem.cfm.

34. Choudhury D., Raj D. S. D., Palmer B., et al. (2000). Effect of aging on renal function and disease. In Brenner B. M. (Ed.), *Brenner and Rector's the kidney* (6th ed., pp. 2187–2210). Philadelphia: W. B. Saunders.

35. Davison A. M. (1998). Renal disease in the elderly. *Nephron* 80, 6–16.

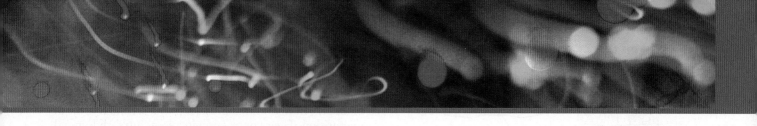

C h a p t e r 26

Disorders of Urine Elimination

 Although the kidneys control the formation of urine and regulate the composition of body fluids, it is the bladder that stores urine and controls its elimination from the body. Alterations in the storage and expulsion functions of the bladder can result in incontinence, with its accompanying social and hygienic problems, or obstruction of urinary flow, which has deleterious effects on ureteral and, ultimately, renal function. The discussion in this chapter focuses on normal control of urine elimination, urinary obstruction and stasis, neurogenic bladder, incontinence, and bladder cancer. Bladder infections are discussed in Chapter 24.

Control of Urine Elimination

The bladder, also known as the *urinary vesicle*, is a freely movable organ located behind the pelvic bone in men and in front of the vagina in women. It consists of two parts: the fundus, or body, and the neck, or posterior urethra. In the man, the urethra continues anteriorly through the penis. Urine passes from the kidneys to the bladder through the ureters, which are 4 to 5 mm in diameter and approximately 30 cm long. The ureters enter the bladder bilaterally at a location toward its base and close to the urethra (Fig. 26-1). The triangular area that is bounded by the ureters and the urethra is called the *trigone*. There are no valves at the ureteral openings, but as the pressure of the urine in the bladder rises, the ends of the ureters are compressed against the bladder wall to prevent the backflow of urine.

BLADDER STRUCTURE

The bladder is composed of four layers. The first is an outer serosal layer, which covers the upper surface and is continuous with the peritoneum. The second is a network of smooth muscle fibers called the *detrusor muscle*. The third is a submucosal layer of loose connective tissue, and the fourth is an inner mucosal lining of transitional epithelium.

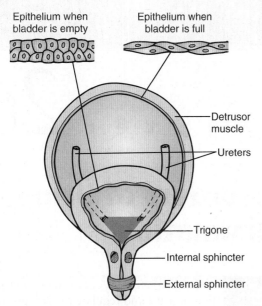

Epithelium when bladder is empty

Epithelium when bladder is full

Detrusor muscle

Ureters

Trigone

Internal sphincter

External sphincter

FIGURE 26-1 Diagram of the full and empty bladder, showing the detrusor muscle, ureters, trigone area, and urethral orifice. Note the flattening of epithelial cells when the bladder is full and the wall is stretched.

The tonicity of the urine often is quite different from that of the blood, and the transitional epithelial lining of the bladder acts as an effective barrier to prevent the passage of water between the bladder contents and the blood. The inner layers of the bladder form smooth folds, or rugae. As the bladder expands during filling, these rugae spread out to form a single layer without disrupting the integrity of the epithelial lining.

KEY CONCEPTS

Bladder Function

➤ The storage and emptying of urine involve both involuntary (autonomic nervous system) and voluntary (somatic nervous system) control.

➤ The parasympathetic nervous system promotes bladder emptying. It produces contraction of the smooth muscle of the bladder wall and relaxation of the internal sphincter.

➤ The sympathetic nervous system promotes bladder filling. It produces relaxation of the smooth muscle of the bladder wall and contraction of the internal sphincter.

➤ The striated muscles in the external sphincter and pelvic floor, which are innervated by the somatic nervous system, provide for the voluntary control of urination and maintenance of continence.

The detrusor muscle is the muscle of micturition (passage of urine). When it contracts, urine is expelled from the bladder. The abdominal muscles play a secondary role in micturition. Their contraction increases intra-abdominal pressure, which further increases intravesicular pressure.

Muscles in the bladder neck, sometimes referred to as the *internal sphincter,* are a continuation of the detrusor muscle. They run down obliquely behind the proximal urethra, forming the posterior urethra in men and the entire urethra in women. When the bladder is relaxed, these circular smooth muscle fibers act as a sphincter. When the detrusor muscle contracts, the sphincter is pulled open by the changes that occur in bladder shape. In the woman, the urethra (2.5 to 3.5 cm) is shorter than in the man (16.5 to 18.5 cm), and usually affords less resistance to urine outflow.

Another muscle important to bladder function is the *external sphincter,* a circular muscle composed of striated muscle fibers that surrounds the urethra distal to the base of the bladder. The external sphincter operates as a reserve mechanism to stop micturition when it is occurring and to maintain continence in the face of unusually high bladder pressure. The skeletal muscle of the pelvic floor also contributes to the support of the bladder and the maintenance of continence.

NEURAL CONTROL OF BLADDER FUNCTION

The control of bladder emptying (also referred to as micturition, urination, or voiding) is unique in that it involves both involuntary autonomic nervous system (ANS) reflexes and some voluntary control. The excitatory input to the bladder that causes bladder emptying is controlled by the parasympathetic nervous system. The sympathetic nervous system relaxes the bladder smooth muscle. There are three main levels of neurologic control for bladder function: the spinal cord reflex centers, the micturition center in the pons, and the cortical and subcortical centers.

Spinal Cord Centers

The centers for reflex control of micturition are located in the sacral (S2 through S4) and thoracolumbar (T11 through L1) segments of the spinal cord[1-4] (Fig. 26-2). The parasympathetic lower motor neurons (LMNs) for the detrusor muscle of the bladder are located in the sacral segments of the spinal cord; their axons travel to the bladder by way of the *pelvic nerve.* LMNs for the external sphincter also are located in the sacral segments of the spinal cord. These LMNs receive their control from the motor cortex by way of the corticospinal tract and send impulses to the external sphincter through the *pudendal nerve.* The bladder neck and trigone area of the bladder, because of their different embryonic origin, receive sympathetic outflow from the thoracolumbar (T11 to L2) segments of the spinal cord. The seminal vesicles, ampulla of the vas, and vas deferens in the male also receive sympathetic innervation from the thoracolumbar segments of the cord.

The afferent or sensory input from the bladder and urethra is carried to the spinal cord by way of fibers

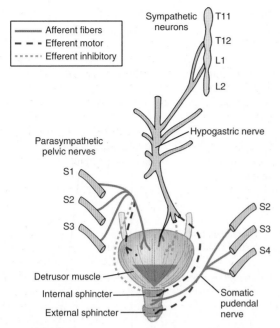

FIGURE 26-2 Nerve supply to the bladder and the urethra.

that travel with the parasympathetic (pelvic), somatic (pudendal), and sympathetic (hypogastric) nerves. The pelvic nerve carries sensory fibers from the stretch receptors in the bladder wall; the pudendal nerve carries sensory fibers from the external sphincter and pelvic muscles; and the hypogastric nerve carries sensory fibers from the trigone area.[3]

Pontine Micturition Center

The immediate coordination of the normal micturition reflex occurs in the micturition center in the pons, facilitated by descending input from the forebrain and ascending input from the reflex centers in the spinal cord[1,2] (Fig. 26-3). This center is thought to coordinate the activity of the detrusor muscle and the external sphincter. As bladder filling occurs, ascending spinal afferents relay this information to the micturition center, which also receives important descending information from the forebrain concerning behavioral cues for bladder emptying. Descending pathways from the pontine micturition center produce coordinated inhibition or relaxation of the external sphincter. Interruption of pontine control of micturition, as in spinal cord injury, results in uninhibited spinal reflex–controlled contraction of the bladder without relaxation of the external sphincter, a condition known as *detrusor-sphincter dyssynergia.*

Cortical and Subcortical Centers

Cortical brain centers enable inhibition of the micturition center in the pons and conscious control of urination. Neural influences from the subcortical centers in the basal ganglia, which are conveyed by extrapyramidal pathways, modulate the contractile response. They modify and delay the detrusor contractile response during filling and then modulate the expulsive activity of the bladder to facilitate complete emptying.

Neuromediator Control of Bladder Function

The ANS and its neuromediators play a central role in micturition. Parasympathetic innervation of the bladder is mediated by the neurotransmitter acetylcholine. Two types of cholinergic receptors affect various aspects of micturition: nicotinic and muscarinic. *Nicotinic* (N) receptors are found in the synapses between the preganglionic and postganglionic neurons of the sympathetic and the parasympathetic system, as well as in the neuromuscular end plates of the striated muscle fibers of the external sphincter and pelvic muscles. *Muscarinic* (M) receptors are found in the postganglionic parasympathetic endings of the detrusor muscle. Several subtypes of M receptors have been identified. The M_2 and M_3 receptors appear predominantly to mediate detrusor contraction and internal sphincter contraction. The M_3 receptor also mediates salivary secretion and bowel activity.[5] The identification of receptor subtypes has facilitated the development of medications that selectively target bladder structures while minimizing other, undesired effects.

Although sympathetic innervation is not essential to the act of micturition, it allows the bladder to store a large volume without the involuntary escape of urine—a mechanism that is consistent with the fight-or-flight function subserved by the sympathetic nervous system. The bladder is supplied with α_1- and β_2-adrenergic receptors. The β_2-adrenergic receptors are found in the detrusor muscle; they produce relaxation of the detrusor muscle, increasing the bladder volume at which the micturition reflex is triggered. The α_1-adrenergic receptors are found in the trigone area, including the intramural ureteral musculature, bladder neck, and internal sphincter. The activation of α_1 receptors produces contraction of these muscles. Sympathetic activity ceases when the micturition reflex is activated. During male ejaculation, which is mediated by the sympathetic nervous system, the musculature of the trigone area and that of the bladder neck and prostatic urethra contracts and prevents the backflow of seminal fluid into the bladder.

Micturition and Maintenance of Continence

Micturition involves both sensory and motor functions associated with bladder emptying. When the bladder is distended to 150 to 250 mL in the adult, the sensation of fullness is transmitted to the spinal cord and then to the cerebral cortex, allowing for conscious inhibition of the micturition reflex.[4] During the act of micturition, the detrusor muscle of the bladder fundus and bladder neck contract down on the urine; the ureteral orifices are forced shut; the bladder neck is widened and shortened as it is pulled up by the globular muscles in the bladder fundus; the resistance of the internal sphincter in the bladder neck is decreased; and the external sphincter relaxes as urine moves out of the bladder.

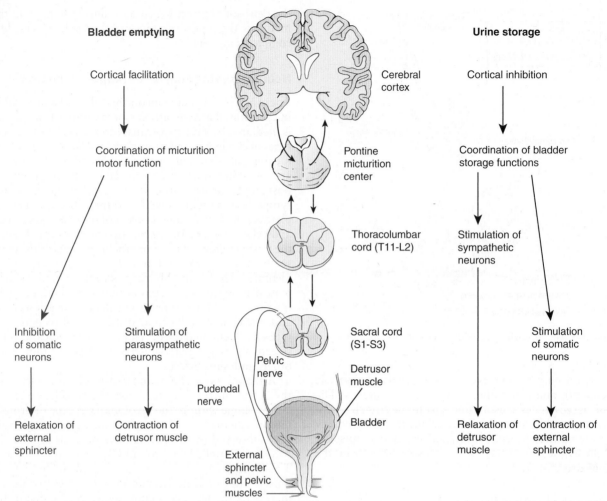

FIGURE 26-3 Pathways and central nervous system centers involved in the control of bladder emptying (**left**) and storage (**right**) functions.

To maintain continence, or retention of urine, the bladder must function as a low-pressure storage system; the pressure in the bladder must remain lower than urethral pressure. To ensure that this condition is met, the increase in intravesicular pressure that accompanies bladder filling is almost imperceptible. An increase in bladder volume from 10 to 400 mL may be accompanied by only a 5 cm H_2O increase in pressure.[1] Sustained elevations in intravesicular pressures (>40 to 50 cm H_2O) often are associated with vesicoureteral reflux (*i.e.,* backflow of urine from the bladder into the ureter) and the development of ureteral dilatation (see Chapter 24). Although the pressure in the bladder is maintained at low levels, sphincter pressure remains high (45 to 65 cm H_2O) as a means of preventing loss of urine as the bladder fills.

Continence in Children

In infants and young children, micturition is an involuntary act that is triggered by a spinal cord reflex; when the bladder fills to a given capacity, the detrusor muscle contracts and the external sphincter relaxes. As the child grows, the bladder gradually enlarges with an increase in capacity. The average bladder capacity (in ounces) is equal to the age (in years) + 2 of the child. This formula applies up to ages 12 to 14 years. As the bladder grows and increases in capacity, the tone of the external sphincter muscle increases. Toilet training begins at about 2 to 3 years of age when the child becomes conscious of the need to urinate. Conscious control of bladder function depends on (1) normal bladder growth, (2) myelination of the ascending afferents that signal awareness of bladder filling, (3) development of cortical control and descending communication with the sacral micturition center, (4) ability to consciously tighten the external sphincter to prevent incontinence, and (5) motivation of the child to stay dry. Girls typically achieve continence before boys and bowel control is typically achieved before bladder control. By 5 years of age, 90% to 95% of children are continent during the day and 80% to 85% are continent at night.[6]

EVALUATION OF BLADDER FUNCTION

Bladder function can be assessed by a number of methods.[7] Reports or observations of frequency, hesitancy, straining to void, and a weak or interrupted stream are suggestive of outflow obstruction. Palpation and percussion provide information about bladder distention.

Postvoid residual (PVR) urine volume provides information about bladder emptying. It can be estimated by abdominal palpation and percussion. Catheterization and ultrasonography can be used to obtain specific measurements of PVR. A PVR value of less than 50 mL is considered adequate bladder emptying, and more than 200 mL indicates inadequate bladder emptying.[8]

Pelvic examination is used in women to assess perineal skin condition, perivaginal muscle tone, genital atrophy, pelvic prolapse (e.g., cystocele, rectocele, uterine prolapse), pelvic mass, or other conditions that may impair bladder function. Bimanual examination (i.e., pelvic and abdominal palpation) can be used to assess PVR volume. Rectal examination is used to test for perineal sensation, sphincter tone, fecal impaction, and rectal mass. It is used to assess the contour of the prostate in men.

Urine tests provide information about kidney function and urinary tract infections. The presence of bacteriuria or pyuria suggests urinary tract infection and the possibility of urinary tract obstruction. Blood tests (i.e., blood urea nitrogen and creatinine) provide information about renal function.

Bladder structures can be visualized indirectly by taking x-ray films of the abdomen and by using excretory urography, which involves the use of a radiopaque dye, computed tomographic (CT) scanning, magnetic resonance imaging (MRI), or ultrasonography. Cystoscopy enables direct visualization of the urethra, bladder, and ureteral orifices. The ultrasound bladder scan provides a noninvasive method for estimating bladder volume. Urodynamic studies may be used to study bladder function and voiding problems.

In summary, although the kidneys function in the formation of urine and the regulation of body fluids, it is the bladder that stores and controls the elimination of urine. Micturition is a function of the peripheral ANS, subject to facilitation or inhibition from higher neurologic centers. The parasympathetic nervous system controls the motor function of the bladder detrusor muscle and the tone of the internal sphincter; its cell bodies are located in the sacral spinal cord and communicate with the bladder through the pelvic nerve. Efferent sympathetic control originates at the level of segments T11 through L1 of the spinal cord and produces relaxation of the detrusor muscle and contraction of the internal sphincter. Skeletal muscle found in the external sphincter and the pelvic muscles that support the bladder are supplied by the pudendal nerve, which exits the spinal cord at the level of segments S2 through S4. The micturition center in the brain stem coordinates the action of the detrusor muscle and the external sphincter, whereas cortical centers permit conscious control of micturition.

Bladder function can be evaluated using urodynamic studies that measure bladder, urethral, and abdominal pressures; urine flow characteristics; and skeletal muscle activity of the external sphincter.

Alterations in Bladder Function

Alterations in bladder function include urinary obstruction with retention or stasis of urine and urinary incontinence with involuntary loss of urine. Although the two conditions have almost opposite effects on urination, they can have similar causes. Both can result from structural changes in the bladder, urethra, or surrounding organs or from impairment of neurologic control of bladder function.

URINARY OBSTRUCTION AND STASIS

In lower urinary tract obstruction, urine is produced normally by the kidneys but is retained in the bladder. Obstructions can be classified according to their location (bladder neck, urethra, or external urethral meatus), cause (congenital or acquired), degree (partial or complete), and duration (acute or chronic).[9] Because it has the potential to produce vesicoureteral reflux and cause kidney damage, urinary obstruction is a serious disorder.

Congenital narrowing of the external meatus (i.e., meatal stenosis) is more common in boys, and obstructive disorders of the posterior urethra are more common in girls. Another common cause of congenital obstruction is the damage to sacral nerves that occurs in spina bifida and meningomyelocele.

The acquired causes of lower urinary tract obstruction and stasis are numerous. In men, the most important cause of urinary obstruction is external compression of the urethra caused by the enlargement of the prostate gland. Gonorrhea and other sexually transmitted diseases contribute to the incidence of infection-produced urethral strictures. Bladder tumors and secondary invasion of the bladder by tumors arising in structures that surround the urethra can compress the bladder neck or urethra and cause obstruction. Constipation and fecal impaction can compress the urethra and produce urethral obstruction. This can be a particular problem in elderly persons.

The body compensates for the obstruction of urine outflow with mechanisms designed to prevent urine retention. These mechanisms can be divided into two stages: a compensatory stage and a decompensatory stage.[9] The degree to which these changes occur and their effect on bladder structure and urinary function depend on the extent of the obstruction, the rapidity with which it occurs,

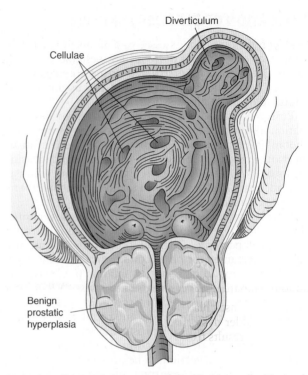

FIGURE 26-4 Destructive changes of the bladder wall with development of diverticula caused by benign prostatic hyperplasia.

and the presence of other contributing factors, such as neurologic impairment and infection.

During the early stage of obstruction, the bladder begins to hypertrophy and becomes hypersensitive to afferent stimuli arising from bladder filling. The ability to suppress urination is diminished, and bladder contractions can become so strong that they virtually produces bladder spasm. There is urgency, sometimes to the point of incontinence, and frequency during the day and at night.

With continuation and progression of the obstruction, compensatory changes begin to occur. There is further hypertrophy of the bladder muscle, the thickness of the bladder wall may double, and the pressure generated by detrusor contraction can increase from a normal 20 to 40 cm H_2O to 50 to 100 cm H_2O to overcome the resistance from the obstruction. As the force needed to expel urine from the bladder increases, compensatory mechanisms may become ineffective, causing detrusor muscle fatigue to occur before complete emptying can be accomplished. After a few minutes, voiding can again be initiated and completed, accounting for the frequency of urination.

The inner bladder surface forms smooth folds. With continued outflow obstruction, this smooth surface is replaced with coarsely woven structures (*i.e.*, hypertrophied smooth muscle fibers) called *trabeculae*. Small pockets of mucosal tissue, called *cellules*, commonly develop between the trabecular ridges. These pockets form diverticula when they extend between the actual fibers of the bladder muscle (Fig. 26-4). Because the diverticula have no muscle, they are unable to contract and expel their urine into the bladder, and secondary infections caused by stasis are common.

Along with hypertrophy of the bladder wall, there is hypertrophy of the trigone area and the interureteric ridge, which is located between the two ureters. This causes back-pressure on the ureters, the development of hydroureters (*i.e.*, dilated, urine-filled ureters), and, eventually, kidney damage. Stasis of urine predisposes to urinary tract infections.

When compensatory mechanisms no longer are effective, signs of decompensation begin to occur. The period of detrusor muscle contraction becomes too short to expel the urine completely, and residual urine remains in the bladder. At this point, the symptoms of obstruction—frequency of urination, hesitancy, need to strain to initiate urination, a weak and small stream, and termination of the stream before the bladder is completely emptied—become pronounced. With progressive decompensation, the bladder may become severely overstretched with a residual urine volume of 1000 to 3000 mL.[9] At this point, it loses its power of contraction and overflow incontinence occurs. The signs of urine retention are summarized in Chart 26-1.

The immediate treatment of lower urinary obstruction and stasis is directed toward relief of bladder distention. This usually is accomplished through urinary catheterization (discussed later in this chapter). Long-term treatment is directed toward correcting the problem causing the obstruction.

NEUROGENIC BLADDER DISORDERS

The urinary bladder is unique in that it is probably the only autonomically innervated visceral organ that is under CNS control. The neural control of bladder function can be interrupted at the level of the peripheral nerves that connect the bladder to the micturition center in the spinal cord, at the ascending and descending tracts in the spinal

CHART 26-1

Signs of Outflow Obstruction and Urine Retention

Bladder distention
Hesitancy
Straining when initiating urination
Small and weak stream
Frequency
Feeling of incomplete bladder emptying
Overflow incontinence

cord, the pontine micturition center, or the cortical centers that are involved in the voluntary control of micturition.[10,11] Neurogenic disorders of bladder function commonly are manifested in one of two ways: failure to store urine (spastic bladder dysfunction) or failure to empty (flaccid bladder dysfunction).[10] Spastic bladder dysfunction usually results from neurologic lesions located above the level of the sacral micturition reflexes, whereas flaccid bladder dysfunction results from lesions at the level of sacral reflexes or the peripheral nerves that innervate the bladder. In addition to disorders of detrusor muscle function, disruption of micturition occurs when the neurologic control of external sphincter function is disrupted. Some disorders, such as stroke and Parkinson disease, may affect both the storage and emptying functions of the bladder. Table 26-1 describes the characteristics of neurogenic bladder according to the level of the lesion.

Spastic Bladder: Failure to Store Urine

Failure to store urine results from conditions that cause reflex bladder spasm and a decrease in bladder volume. It commonly is caused by conditions that produce partial or extensive neural damage above the micturition reflex center in the sacral cord (see Fig. 26-3). As a result, bladder function is regulated by segmental reflexes, without control from higher brain centers. The degree of bladder spasticity and dysfunction depends on the level and extent of neurologic dysfunction. Usually both the ANS neurons controlling bladder function and the somatic neurons controlling the function of the striated muscles in the external sphincter are affected. In some cases, there is a detrusor-sphincter dyssynergia with uncoordinated contraction and relaxation of the detrusor and external sphincter muscles. The most common causes of spastic bladder dysfunction are spinal cord lesions such as spinal cord injury, herniated intervertebral disk, vascular lesions, tumors, and myelitis. Other neurologic conditions that affect voiding are stroke, multiple sclerosis, and brain tumors.

Bladder Dysfunction Caused by Spinal Cord Injury. One of the most common types of spinal cord lesions is spinal cord injury (see Chapter 35). The immediate and early effects of spinal cord injury on bladder function are quite different from those that follow recovery from the initial injury. During the period immediately after spinal cord injury, a state of spinal shock develops, during which all the reflexes, including the micturition reflex, are depressed. During this stage, the bladder becomes atonic and cannot contract. Catheterization is necessary to prevent injury to urinary structures associated with overdistention of the bladder. Aseptic intermittent catheterization is the preferred method of catheterization. Depression of reflexes lasts from a few weeks to 6 months (usually 2 to 3 months), after which the spinal reflexes return and become hyperactive.

After the acute stage of spinal cord injury, the micturition response changes from a long-tract reflex to a segmental reflex. Because the sacral reflex arc remains intact,

TABLE 26-1 Types and Characteristics of Neurogenic Bladder

Level of Lesion	Change in Bladder Function	Common Causes
Sensory cortex, motor cortex, or corticospinal tract	Loss of ability to perceive bladder filling; low-volume, physiologically normal micturition that occurs suddenly and is difficult to inhibit	Stroke and advanced age
Basal ganglia or extrapyramidal tract	Detrusor contractions are elicited suddenly, without warning, and are difficult to control; bladder contraction is shorter than normal and does not produce full bladder emptying	Parkinson disease
Pontine micturition center or communicating tracts in the spinal cord	Storage reflexes are provoked during filling, and external sphincter responses are heightened; uninhibited bladder contractions occur at a lower volume than normal and do not continue until the bladder is emptied; antagonistic activity occurs between the detrusor muscle and the external sphincter	Spinal cord injury
Sacral cord or nerve roots	Areflexic bladder fills but does not contract; loss of external sphincter tone occurs when the lesion affects the α-adrenergic motor neurons or pudendal nerve	Injury to sacral cord or spinal roots
Pelvic nerve	Increased filling and impaired sphincter control cause increased intravesicular pressure	Radical pelvic surgery
Autonomic peripheral sensory pathways	Bladder overfilling occurs owing to a loss of ability to perceive bladder filling	Diabetic neuropathies, multiple sclerosis

stimuli generated by bladder stretch receptors during filling produce frequent spontaneous contractions of the detrusor muscle. This creates a small, hyperactive bladder subject to high-pressure and short-duration uninhibited bladder contractions. Voiding is interrupted, involuntary, or incomplete. Dilation of the internal sphincter and spasticity of the external sphincter and perineal muscles innervated by upper motoneurons occur, producing resistance to bladder emptying. Hypertrophy of the trigone develops, often leading to vesicoureteral reflux and renal damage.

Spastic bladder due to spinal cord injuries at the cervical level is often accompanied by a condition known as autonomic dysreflexia (see Chapter 35). Because the injury interrupts the CNS control of sympathetic reflexes in the spinal cord, severe hypertension, bradycardia, and sweating can be triggered by insertion of a catheter or mild overdistention of the bladder.

Uninhibited Neurogenic Bladder. A mild form of reflex neurogenic bladder, sometimes called *uninhibited bladder,* can develop after a stroke, during the early stages of multiple sclerosis, or as a result of lesions located in inhibitory centers of the cortex or the pyramidal tract. With this type of disorder, the sacral reflex arc and sensation are retained, the urine stream is normal, and there is no residual urine. Bladder capacity is diminished, however, because of increased detrusor muscle tone and spasticity.

Detrusor-Sphincter Dyssynergia. Effective bladder emptying requires the integrated activity of the detrusor muscle and the external bladder sphincter. Lesions that affect the micturition center in the pons or impair communication between this center and spinal cord centers interrupt the coordinated activity of the detrusor muscle and the external sphincter. This is called *detrusor-sphincter dyssynergia.* Instead of relaxing during micturition, the external sphincter becomes more constricted. This condition can lead to elevated intravesicular pressures, vesicoureteral reflux, and kidney damage.

Treatment. Among the methods used to treat spastic bladder are the administration of anticholinergic medications to decrease bladder hyperactivity and urinary catheterization to produce bladder emptying. A sphincterotomy (surgical resection of the external sphincter) or implantable urethral stent may be used to decrease outflow resistance in a person who cannot be managed with medications and catheterization procedures. An alternative to surgical resection of the external sphincter is the injection of botulinum-A toxin to produce paralysis of the striated muscles in the external sphincter. The effects of the injection last from 3 to 9 months, after which the injection must be repeated.[10]

Flaccid Bladder: Failure to Empty Urine

Failure to empty the bladder can be due to flaccid bladder dysfunction, peripheral neuropathies that interrupt afferent or efferent communication between the bladder and the spinal cord, or conditions that prevent relaxation of the external sphincter (see Fig. 26-3).

Flaccid Bladder Dysfunction. Detrusor muscle areflexia, or flaccid neurogenic bladder, occurs when there is injury to the micturition center of the sacral cord, the cauda equina, or the sacral roots that supply the bladder.[11] Atony of the detrusor muscle and loss of the perception of bladder fullness permit the overstretching of the detrusor muscle that contributes to weak and ineffective bladder contractions. External sphincter tone and perineal muscle tone are diminished. Voluntary urination does not occur, but fairly efficient emptying usually can be achieved by increased intra-abdominal pressure or manual suprapubic pressure. Among the causes of flaccid neurogenic bladder are trauma, tumors, and congenital anomalies (*e.g.*, spina bifida, meningomyelocele).

Bladder Dysfunction Caused by Peripheral Neuropathies. In addition to CNS lesions and conditions that disrupt bladder function, disorders of the peripheral (pelvic, pudendal, and hypogastric) neurons that supply the bladder can occur. These neuropathies can selectively interrupt sensory or motor pathways for the bladder or involve both pathways.

Bladder atony and dysfunction is a frequent complication of diabetes mellitus.[12,13] The disorder initially affects the sensory axons of the urinary bladder without involvement of the pudendal nerve. This leads to large residual volumes after micturition, sometimes complicated by infection. There frequently is a need for straining, accompanied by hesitation, weakness of the stream, dribbling, and a sensation of incomplete bladder emptying.[13] The chief complications are vesicoureteral reflux and ascending urinary tract infection. Because persons with diabetes are already at risk for development of glomerular disease, reflux can have serious effects on kidney function. Treatment consists of client education, including the need for frequent voiding (*e.g.*, every 3 to 4 hours while awake), use of abdominal compression to effect more complete bladder emptying, and intermittent catheterization when necessary.[12]

Nonrelaxing External Sphincter

Another condition that affects micturition and bladder function is the nonrelaxing external sphincter. This condition usually is related to a delay in maturation, developmental regression, psychomotor disorders, or locally irritative lesions. Inadequate relaxation of the external sphincter can be the result of anxiety or depression. Any local irritation can produce spasms of the sphincter by means of afferent sensory input from the pudendal nerve; included are vaginitis, perineal inflammation, and inflammation or irritation of the urethra. In men, chronic prostatitis contributes to the impaired relaxation of the external sphincter.

Treatment

The goals of treatment for flaccid bladder disorders focus on preventing bladder overdistention, urinary tract infections, and potentially life-threatening renal damage, and reducing the undesirable social and psychological effects of the disorder. The methods used in treatment of neurogenic bladder disorders are individualized based on the type of neurologic lesion that is involved; information obtained through the health history, including fluid intake; report or observation of voiding patterns; presence of other health problems; urodynamic studies when indicated; and the ability of the person to participate in the treatment. Treatment methods include catheterization, bladder training, pharmacologic manipulation of bladder function, and surgery.

URINARY INCONTINENCE

The Urinary Incontinence Guideline Panel defines urinary incontinence as an involuntary loss of urine that is sufficient to be a problem.[8] This panel was convened by the Agency for Health Care Policy and Research in 1992 and again in 1996 for the purpose of developing specific guidelines to improve the care of persons with urinary incontinence.[8]

Urinary incontinence affects approximately 13 million Americans. Many body functions decline with age, and incontinence, although not a normal accompaniment of the aging process, is seen with increased frequency in elderly persons.[8] For elderly persons living in the community, the prevalence of incontinence ranges from 15% to 35%,[14,15] with women being affected twice as often as men.[14] The increase in health problems often seen in elderly persons probably contributes to the greater frequency of incontinence. Despite the prevalence of incontinence, most affected persons do not seek help for it, primarily because of embarrassment or because they are not aware that help is available.

Incontinence can be caused by a number of conditions. It can occur without the person's knowledge; at other times, the person may be aware of the condition but be unable to prevent it. The Urinary Incontinence Guideline Panel has identified four main types of incontinence: stress incontinence, urge incontinence, overflow incontinence, and mixed incontinence, which is a combination of stress and urge incontinence.[8] Recently, the term *overactive bladder* has been designated as a term to replace *urge incontinence*.[14] Table 26-2 summarizes the characteristics of stress incontinence, urge incontinence/overactive bladder, and overflow incontinence.

Incontinence may occur as a transient and correctable phenomenon, or it may not be totally correctable and occur with various degrees of frequency. Among the transient causes of urinary incontinence are confusional states; medications that alter bladder function or perception of bladder filling and the need to urinate; diuretics and conditions that increase bladder filling; restricted mobility; and stool impaction.[16]

Stress Incontinence

Stress incontinence is the involuntary loss of urine during coughing, laughing, sneezing, or lifting that increases intra-abdominal pressure. With severe urinary stress incontinence, any strain or increase in bladder pressure leads to urinary leakage. It is usually the result of pelvic floor weakness and poor support of the vesicourethral sphincter. The angle between the bladder and the posterior proximal urethrovesical (PVU) junction is important to continence[17] (Fig. 26-5). In women, loss of muscle tone associated with normal aging, childbirth, or surgical procedures can cause weakness of the pelvic floor muscles and result in stress incontinence by obliterating the critical PUV angle. When this angle is lost, any activity that causes downward pressure on the bladder is sufficient to allow the urine to escape involuntarily.

Another cause of stress incontinence is intrinsic urethral deficiency, which may result from congenital sphincter weakness, as occurs with meningomyelocele. It also may be

---

KEY CONCEPTS

Incontinence

➤ Incontinence represents the involuntary loss of urine due to increased bladder pressures (overactive bladder with urge incontinence or overflow incontinence) or decreased ability of the vesicourethral sphincter to prevent the escape of urine (stress incontinence).

➤ Overactive bladder with urge incontinence is caused by neurogenic or myogenic disorders that result in hyperactive bladder contractions.

➤ Overflow incontinence results from overfilling of the bladder with escape of urine.

➤ Stress incontinence is caused by the decreased ability of the vesicourethral sphincter to prevent the escape of urine during activities, such as lifting and coughing, that raise bladder pressure above the sphincter closing pressure.

TABLE 26-2	Types and Characteristics of Urinary Incontinence
Type	**Characteristics**
Stress	Involuntary loss of urine associated with activities, such as coughing, that increase intra-abdominal pressure
Overactive bladder/ urge incontinence	Urgency and frequency associated with hyperactivity of the detrusor muscle; may or may not involve involuntary loss of urine
Overflow	Involuntary loss of urine when intravesicular pressure exceeds maximal urethral pressure in the absence of detrusor activity

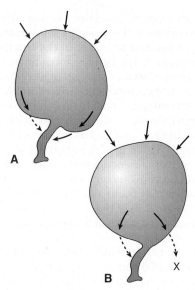

FIGURE 26-5 Importance of the posterior urethrovesical (PU-V) angle to the continence mechanism. (**A**) In the presence of the normal PU-V angle, sudden changes in intro-abdominal pressure are transmitted optimally (indicated by the *arrows* with dotted lines) to all sides of the proximal urethra. In this way, intraurethral pressure is maintained higher than the simultaneously elevated intravesicular pressure. This prevents loss of urine with sudden stress. (**B**) Loss of the PU-V angle results in displacement of the vesicle neck to the most dependent portion of the bladder, preventing the equal transmission of sudden increases in intra-abdominal pressure to the lumen of the proximal urethra. Thus, the pressure in the region of the vesicle neck rises considerably more than the intraurethral pressure just beyond it, and stress incontinence occurs. (Green, J. T., Jr. [1968]. *Obstetrical and Gynecological Survey* 23, 603. Reprinted with permission)

acquired as a result of trauma, irradiation, or sacral cord lesion. Stress incontinence in men may result from a congenital defect or from trauma or surgery to the bladder outlet, as occurs with prostatectomy. Neurologic dysfunction, as occurs with impaired sympathetic innervation of the bladder neck, impaired pelvic nerve innervation to the internal sphincter, or impaired pudendal nerve innervation to the external sphincter, may also be a contributing factor.

Urge Incontinence/Overactive Bladder

The Urinary Incontinence Guideline Panel has defined urge incontinence as the involuntary loss of urine associated with a strong desire to void (urgency).[8] To expand the number and types of patients eligible for clinical trials, the U.S. Food and Drug Administration adopted the term *overactive bladder* to describe a clinical syndrome that can include urgency, frequency, dysuria, and nocturia as well as urge incontinence.[8] Although overactive bladder often is associated with urge incontinence, it can occur without incontinence.[18]

Although some cases of overactive bladder result from specific conditions such as acute or chronic urinary tract infections, in many cases the cause is unknown. Regard-

less of the primary cause of overactive bladder, two types of mechanisms are thought to contribute to its symptomatology: those involving CNS control of bladder sensation and emptying (neurogenic), and those involving the smooth muscle of the bladder itself (myogenic).[18]

The CNS functions as an on-off switching circuit for voluntary control of bladder function. Therefore, neurologic damage to central inhibitory pathways or sensitization of peripheral afferent terminals in the bladder may trigger bladder overactivity owing to uncontrolled voiding reflexes. Neurogenic causes of overactive bladder include stroke, Parkinson disease, and multiple sclerosis. Other neurogenic causes of overactive bladder include increased peripheral afferent activity or increased peripheral sensitivity to efferent impulses.

Myogenic causes of overactive bladder are thought to be due to spontaneous elevations in bladder pressure arising from changes in the properties of the smooth muscle of the bladder itself. One example is overactive bladder associated with bladder outlet obstruction. It is hypothesized that the sustained increase in intravesicular pressure that occurs with the outlet obstruction causes a partial destruction of the efferent nerve endings that control bladder excitability.[18] The result is urgency and frequency of urination due to spontaneous bladder contractions resulting from detrusor muscle hyperexcitability. Disorders of detrusor muscle structure and excitability also can occur as the result of the aging process or disease conditions such as diabetes mellitus. Overactive bladder symptoms usually are exaggerated by incomplete bladder emptying.

In persons with overactive bladder, urge incontinence may occur because the interval between knowing the bladder needs to be emptied and being able to stop it from emptying may be less than the time needed to reach the lavatory. Musculoskeletal disorders, such as arthritis and joint instability, also may prevent an otherwise continent person from reaching the toilet in time. Drugs such as hypnotics, tranquilizers, and sedatives can interfere with the conscious inhibition of voiding, leading to urge incontinence. Diuretics, particularly in elderly persons, increase the flow of urine and may contribute to incontinence, particularly in persons with diminished bladder capacity and in those who have difficulty reaching the toilet.

Treatment methods for overactive bladder include the use of behavioral methods and pharmacologic agents. Behavioral methods include fluid management, modification of voiding frequency, and bladder retraining.[18,19] Bladder retraining and biofeedback techniques seek to reestablish cortical control over bladder function by having the person ignore urgency and respond only to cortical signals during waking hours. An anticholinergic medication (e.g., tolterodine and extended-release oxybutynin) may be used to inhibit detrusor muscle hyperactivity and thereby increase overall bladder capacity.[18–20]

Overflow Incontinence

Overflow incontinence is an involuntary loss of urine that occurs when intravesicular pressure exceeds the maximal urethral pressure because of bladder distention in the absence of detrusor activity. It can occur with retention of urine owing to nervous system lesions or obstruction of the bladder neck. With this type of incontinence, the bladder is distended and small amounts of urine are passed, particularly at night. In men, one of the most common causes of obstructive incontinence is enlargement of the prostate gland. Another cause that commonly is overlooked is fecal impaction (*i.e.*, dry, hard feces in the rectum). When a large bolus of stool forms in the rectum, it can push against the urethra and block the flow of urine.

The Standardization Sub-Committee of the International Continence Committee recommends that the term *overflow incontinence* should no longer be used, indicating that the term is confusing and lacking definition.[21] Instead, it suggests that more specific terms such as *reduced urethral function* or *overactivity/low bladder compliance* be used.

Other Causes of Incontinence

Another cause of incontinence is decreased bladder compliance or distensibility. This abnormal bladder condition may result from radiation therapy, radical pelvic surgery, or interstitial cystitis. Many persons with this disorder have severe urgency related to bladder hypersensitivity that results in loss of bladder elasticity, such that any small increase in bladder volume or detrusor function causes a sharp rise in bladder pressure and severe urgency.

Incontinence also may be caused by factors outside the lower urinary tract, such as the inability to locate, reach, or receive assistance in reaching an appropriate place to void.[14] This may be a particular problem for elderly persons, who may have problems with mobility and manual dexterity or find themselves in unfamiliar surroundings. It occurs when a person cannot find or reach the bathroom or manipulate clothing quickly enough. Failing vision may contribute to the problem. Embarrassment in front of other persons at having to use the bathroom, particularly if the timing seems inappropriate, may cause a person to delay emptying the bladder and may lead to incontinence.

Treatment with drugs such as diuretics may cause the bladder to fill more rapidly than usual, making it difficult to reach the bathroom in time if there are problems with mobility or if a bathroom is not readily available. Night sedation may cause a person to sleep through the signal that normally would waken a person so he or she could get up and empty the bladder and avoid wetting the bed.

Diagnosis and Treatment

Urinary incontinence is a frequent and major health problem. It increases social isolation, frequently leads to institutionalization of elderly persons, and predisposes to infections and skin breakdown.

Urinary incontinence is not a single disease but a symptom with many possible causes. As a symptom, it requires full investigation to establish its cause. This usually is accomplished through a careful history, physical examination, blood tests, and urinalysis. A voiding record (*i.e.*, diary) may be used to determine the frequency, timing, amount of voiding, and other factors associated with the incontinence. Because many drugs affect bladder func-

tion, a full drug history is essential. Estimation of PVR volume is recommended for all persons with incontinence. Provocative stress testing, such as having a person relax and then cough vigorously, may be done when stress incontinence is suspected. Urodynamic studies may be needed to provide information about urinary pressures and urine flow rates.

Treatment or management depends on the type of incontinence, accompanying health problems, and the person's age. Exercises to strengthen the pelvic muscles and surgical correction of pelvic relaxation disorders often are used for women with stress incontinence. The α-adrenergic agonist drugs, such as pseudoephedrine, increase sympathetic relaxation of the detrusor muscle and internal sphincter tone and may be used in treating stress incontinence.[5]

Noncatheter devices to obstruct urine flow or collect urine as it is passed may be used when urine flow cannot be controlled. Indwelling catheters, although a solution to the problem of urinary incontinence, usually are considered only after all other treatment methods have failed. In some types of incontinence, such as that associated with spinal cord injury or meningomyelocele, self-catheterization provides the means for controlling urine elimination.

Surgical intervention may be considered when other treatment methods have proved ineffective. Three types of surgical procedures are used: procedures that increase outlet resistance, surgeries that decrease detrusor muscle instability, and operations that remove outflow obstruction to reduce overflow incontinence and detrusor muscle instability.[8] A minimally invasive procedure for the treatment of stress incontinence is periurethral injection of a bulking agent (glutaraldehyde cross-linked bovine collagen or carbon-coated beads). Both of these agents typically require multiple treatment sessions to achieve cure.[14]

Surgically implanted artificial sphincters are available for use in men and women. These devices consist of an inflatable cuff that surrounds the proximal urethra. The cuff is connected by tubing to an implanted fluid reservoir and an inflation bulb.

Special Needs of Elderly Persons

Urinary incontinence is a common problem in elderly persons. An estimated 15% to 30% of community-dwelling elders and 50% of institutionalized elders have severe urinary incontinence.[22] The economic and social costs of incontinence are staggering, with over $3 billion spent annually for managing incontinence in nursing homes alone.[23]

Many factors contribute to incontinence in elderly persons, a number of which can be altered. More than half of normal elderly persons experience nocturia. The overall capacity of the bladder is reduced, as is the urethral closing pressure.[15] Detrusor muscle function also tends to decline with aging so there is a trend toward a reduction in the strength of bladder contraction and impairment in emptying that leads to larger PVR volumes.[2,15] It has been proposed that many of these changes are due to degenerative detrusor muscle changes rather than neurologic changes, as was once thought. The combination of involuntary detrusor contraction (detrusor hyperactivity) leading to urge incontinence along with impaired contractile function results in incomplete bladder emptying. Pelvic relaxation disorders are also more frequent in older than in younger women, and prostatic hyperplasia is more common in older than in younger men.

Furthermore, advancing age often results in restricted mobility, an increasing number of medications being taken, comorbid illness, infection, and stool impaction, all of which can precipitate urinary incontinence.[15,24] Many elderly persons have difficulty getting to the toilet in time. This can be caused by arthritis that makes walking or removing clothing difficult or by failing vision that makes trips to the bathroom precarious, especially in new and unfamiliar surroundings.

Medication prescribed for other health problems may prevent a healthy bladder from functioning normally.[15,22,24] Potent, fast-acting diuretics are known for their ability to cause urge incontinence. Psychoactive drugs, such as tranquilizers and sedatives, may diminish normal attention to bladder clues. Impaired thirst or limited access to fluids predisposes to constipation with urethral obstruction and overflow incontinence and to concentrated and infected urine, which increases bladder excitability.

Treatment may involve changes in the physical environment so that the older person can reach the bathroom more easily or remove clothing more quickly. Habit training with regularly scheduled toileting—usually every 2 to 4 hours—often is effective. Many elderly persons who void on a regular schedule can gradually increase the interval between toileting while improving their ability to suppress bladder instability. The treatment plan may require dietary changes to prevent constipation or a plan to promote adequate fluid intake to ensure adequate bladder filling and prevent urinary stasis and symptomatic urinary tract infections.

In summary, alterations in bladder function include urinary obstruction with retention of urine, neurogenic bladder, and urinary incontinence with involuntary loss of urine. Urine retention occurs when the outflow of urine from the bladder is obstructed because of urethral obstruction or impaired bladder innervation. Urethral obstruction causes bladder irritability, detrusor muscle hypertrophy, trabeculation and the formation of diverticula, development of hydroureters, and, eventually, renal failure.

Neurogenic bladder is caused by interruption in the innervation of the bladder. It can result in spastic bladder dysfunction caused by failure of the bladder to fill or flaccid bladder dysfunction caused by failure of the bladder to empty. Spastic bladder dysfunction usually results from neurologic lesions that are above the level of the sacral micturition reflex center; flaccid bladder dysfunction results from lesions at the level of the sacral micturition reflexes or peripheral innervation of the bladder. A third type of neurogenic disorder involves a nonrelaxing external sphincter.

Urinary incontinence is the involuntary loss of urine in amounts sufficient to be a problem. It may manifest as stress incontinence, in which the loss of urine occurs as a result of coughing, sneezing, laughing, or lifting; overactive bladder, characterized by frequency and urgency associated with hyperactive bladder contractions; or overflow incontinence, which results when intravesicular pressure exceeds the maximal urethral pressure because of bladder distention. Other causes of incontinence include a small, contracted bladder or external environmental conditions that make it difficult to access proper toileting facilities.

The treatment of urinary obstruction, neurogenic bladder, and incontinence requires careful diagnosis to determine the cause and contributing factors. Treatment methods include correction of the underlying cause, such as obstruction due to prostatic hyperplasia; pharmacologic methods to improve bladder and external sphincter tone; behavior methods that focus on bladder and habit training; exercises to improve pelvic floor function; and the use of catheters and urine collection devices.

Cancer of the Bladder

Bladder cancer is the most frequent form of urinary tract cancer in the United States, accounting for an estimated 63,210 new cases and 13,180 deaths in 2005.[25] It is three times more common in men than women and has an average age of onset of 65 years. Its incidence is higher in whites than African Americans.[26]

Approximately 90% of bladder cancers are derived from the epithelial cells that line the bladder.[27] These tumors can range from low-grade noninvasive tumors to high-grade tumors that invade the bladder wall and metastasize frequently. The low-grade tumors, which may recur after resection, have an excellent prognosis, with only a small number progressing to higher-grade tumors.[28,29] The high-grade tumors tend to have greater invasive and metastatic potential.

Although the cause of bladder cancer is unknown, evidence suggests that its origin is related to local influences, such as carcinogens that are excreted in the urine and stored in the bladder. These include the breakdown products of aromatic amines used in the dye industry, and products used in the manufacture of rubber, textiles, paint, chemicals, and petroleum.[29] Smoking also deserves attention[28,29]; 50% of bladder cancers in men and 31% in women are associated with cigarette smoking.[27] Chronic bladder infections and bladder stones also increase the risk of bladder cancer. Bladder cancer is more frequent among persons harboring the parasite *Schistosoma haematobium* in their bladders.[27] The parasite is endemic in Egypt and Sudan. It is not known whether the parasite excretes a carcinogen or produces its effects through irritation of the manifestations bladder.

MANIFESTATIONS

The most common sign of bladder cancer is painless hematuria.[26,28,29] Gross hematuria is a presenting sign in 75% of persons with the disease, and microscopic hematuria is present in most others. Frequency, urgency, and dysuria occasionally accompany the hematuria. Because hematuria often is intermittent, the diagnosis may be delayed. Periodic urine cytology is recommended for all persons who are at high risk for the development of bladder cancer because of exposure to urinary tract carcinogens. Ureteral invasion leading to bacterial and obstructive renal disease and dissemination of the cancer are potential complications and ultimate causes of death. The prognosis depends on the histologic grade of the cancer and the stage of the disease at the time of diagnosis.

DIAGNOSIS AND TREATMENT

Diagnostic methods include cytologic studies, excretory urography, cystoscopy, and biopsy. Ultrasonography, CT scans, and MRI are used as aids for staging the tumor. Cytologic studies performed on biopsy tissues or cells obtained from bladder washings may be used to detect the presence of malignant cells.

The treatment of bladder cancer depends on the extent of the lesion and the health of the patient. Endoscopic resection usually is done for diagnostic purposes and may be used as a treatment for superficial lesions. Diathermy (*i.e.*, electrocautery) may be used to remove the tumors. Segmental surgical resection may be used for removing a large single lesion. When the tumor is invasive, cystectomy with resection of the pelvic lymph nodes frequently is the treatment of choice. In men, the prostate and seminal vesicles often are removed as well. Until the 1980s, most men who underwent radical cystectomy became impotent. Newer surgical approaches designed to preserve erectile function now are being used. Cystectomy requires urinary diversion with creation of an alternative reservoir, usually fashioned from the ileum (*e.g.*, an ileal loop), that is designed to collect the urine. Traditionally, the ileostomy reservoir drains urine continuously into an external collecting device. External-beam irradiation is an alternative to radical cystectomy in some patients with deeply infiltrating bladder cancer.

Although a number of chemotherapeutic drugs have been used in the treatment of bladder cancer, no chemotherapeutic regimens for the disease have been established. Perhaps of more importance is the increasing use of intravesicular chemotherapy, in which the cytotoxic drug is instilled directly into the bladder, thereby avoiding the side effects of systemic therapy. These drugs can be instilled prophylactically after surgical resection of all demonstrable tumor or therapeutically in the presence of residual disease. The intervesicular administration of bacillus Calmette-Guérin (BCG) vaccine, a strain of *Mycobacterium bovis* that formerly was used to protect against tuberculosis, causes a significant reduction in the rate of relapse and prolongs the relapse-free interval in persons with cancer in situ.[26] Bacillus Calmette-Guérin is thought to act as a nonspecific stimulator of cell-mediated immunity. It is not known whether the effects of BCG are immunologic or include a component of direct toxicity.

In summary, cancer of the bladder is the most common urinary tract cancer in the United States. Bladder cancers fall into two major groups: low-grade noninvasive tumors and high-grade invasive tumors that are associated with metastasis and a worse prognosis. Although the cause of cancer of the bladder is unknown, evidence suggests that carcinogens excreted in the urine may play a role. Microscopic and gross, painless hematuria are the most frequent presenting signs of bladder cancer. The methods used in treatment of bladder cancer depend on the cytologic grade of the tumor and the lesion's degree of invasiveness. The methods include surgical removal of the tumor, radiation therapy, and chemotherapy. In many cases, chemotherapeutic or immunotherapeutic agents can be instilled directly into the bladder, thereby avoiding the side effects of systemic therapy.

Review Exercises

A 23-year-old man is recovering after the acute phase of a cervical (C6) spinal cord injury with complete loss of motor and sensory function below the level of injury. He is now experiencing spastic bladder contractions with involuntary and incomplete urination. Urodynamic studies reveal spastic contraction of the external sphincter with urine retention and high bladder pressures.

A. Explain the reason for the involuntary urination and incomplete emptying of the bladder despite high bladder pressures.
B. What are possible problems associated with overdistention and high pressure in the bladder?

A 66-year-old woman complains of leakage of urine during coughing, sneezing, laughing, or squatting down.

A. Explain the source of this woman's problem.
B. One of the recommended treatments for stress incontinence is Kegel's exercises, which focus on strengthening the muscles of the pelvic floor. Explain how these exercises contribute to control of urine leakage in women with stress incontinence.

REFERENCES

1. Kandel E. R., Schwartz J. H., Jessel T. M. (2000). *Principles of neural science* (4th ed.). New York: McGraw-Hill.
2. Fowler C. J. (1999). Neurological disorders of micturition and their treatment. *Brain* 122, 1213–1231.
3. Guyton A. C., Hall J. E. (2000). *Textbook of medical physiology* (10th ed., pp. 364–367). Philadelphia: W. B. Saunders.
4. Rhoades R. A., Tanner G. A. (2003). *Medical physiology* (2nd ed., pp. 423–424). Philadelphia: Lippincott Williams & Wilkins.
5. Dmochowski R. R., Appell R. A. (2000). Advances in pharmacologic management of overactive bladder. *Urology* 56(Suppl. 6A), 41–49.
6. Elder J. S. (2004). Voiding dysfunction. In Behrman R. E., Kliegman R. M., Jenson H. B. (Eds.), *Nelson textbook of pediatrics* (17th ed., pp. 1808–1809). Philadelphia: Elsevier Saunders.
7. Tanagho E. A. (2004). Urodynamic studies. In Tanagho E. A., McAninch J. W. (Eds.), *Smith's general urology* (16th ed., pp. 453–472). New York: Lange Medical Books/McGraw-Hill.
8. Agency for Health Care Policy and Research (AHCPR), Public Health Service, U.S. Department of Heath and Human Services. (1996). *Urinary incontinence in adults: Acute and chronic management.* Clinical practice guideline. AHCPR publication no. 96-0682. Washington, DC: U.S. Government Printing Office.
9. Tanagho E. A. (2004). Urinary obstruction and stasis. In Tanagho E. A., McAninch J. W. (Eds.), *Smith's general urology* (16th ed., pp. 175–187). New York: Lange Medical Books/McGraw-Hill.
10. Elliott D. S., Boone T. B. (2000). Recent advances in management of neurogenic bladder. *Urology* 56(Suppl. 6A), 76–81.
11. Tanagho E. A., Lue T. F. (2004). Neuropathic bladder disorders. In Tanagho E. A., McAninch J. W. (Eds.), *Smith's general urology* (16th ed., pp. 435–452). New York: Lange Medical Books/McGraw-Hill.
12. Sasaki K., Yoshimura N., Chancellor M. B. (2003). Implication of diabetes mellitus in urology. *Urological Clinics of North America* 30, 1–12.
13. Vinik A. I., Maser R. E., Mitchell B. D., et al. (2003). Diabetic autonomic neuropathy. *Diabetes Care* 26, 1553–1579.
14. Culligan P. J., Heit M. (2000). Urinary incontinence in women: Evaluation and management. *American Family Physician* 62, 2433–2452.
15. Klausner A. P., Vapnek J. M. (2003). Urinary incontinence in the geriatric population. *Mount Sinai Journal of Medicine* 70, 54–61.
16. Gray M., Burns S. M. (1996). Continence management. *Critical Care Clinics of North America* 8, 29–38.
17. Tanagho E. A. (2004). Urinary incontinence. In Tanagho E. A., McAninch J. W. (Eds.), *Smith's general urology* (16th ed., pp. 473–491). New York: Lange Medical Books/McGraw-Hill.
18. Dmochowski R. R., Appell R. A. (2000). Advancements in pharmacologic management of overactive bladder. *Urology* 56(Suppl. 6A), 41–49.
19. Wein A. J. (2001). Putting overactive bladder into clinical perspective. *Patient Care for the Nurse Practitioner* (Spring Suppl.), 1–5.
20. Roberts R. R. (2001). Current management strategies for overactive bladder. *Patient Care for the Nurse Practitioner* (Spring Suppl.), 22–30.
21. Abrams P., Cardozo L., Fall M., et al. (2003). The standardization of terminology in lower urinary tract function: Report of the standardization sub-committee of the International Continence Society. *Urology* 61, 37–49
22. Lee S. Y., Phanumus D., Fields S. D. (2000). Urinary incontinence: A primary guide to managing acute and chronic symptoms in older adults. *Geriatrics* 55(11), 65–71.
23. Weiss B. D. (1998). Diagnostic evaluation of urinary incontinence in geriatric patients. *American Family Physician* 57, 2675–2684, 2688–2690.
24. Dubeau C. E. (2002). The continuum of urinary incontinence in an aging population. *Geriatrics* 57(Suppl. 1), 12–17.
25. American Cancer Society (2005). *Bladder cancer: Overview.* [On-line]. Available: www3.cancer.org/cancerinfo.
26. Grossfeld G. D., Carroll P. (2004). Urothelial carcinoma: Cancers of the bladder, ureter, and renal pelvis. In Tanagho E. A., McAninch J. W. (Eds.), *Smith's general urology* (16th ed., pp. 324–345). New York: Lange Medical Books/McGraw-Hill.
27. Epstein J. I. (2005). The lower urinary tract and male genitourinary system. In Kumar V., Abbas A. K., Fausto N. (Eds.), *Robbins and Cotran pathologic basis of disease* (7th ed., pp. 1028–1033). Philadelphia: Elsevier Saunders.
28. Lee R., Droller M. J. (2000). The natural history of bladder cancer. *Urologic Clinics of North America* 27, 1–13.
29. Murphy G. P. (2001). Urologic and male genital cancer. In Lenhard R. E., Osteen R. T., Gansler T. (Eds.), *Clinical oncology* (pp. 408–415). Atlanta: American Cancer Society.

Gastrointestinal and Hepatobiliary Function

Chapter 27

Structure and Function of the Gastrointestinal System

Structurally, the gastrointestinal tract is a long, hollow tube with its lumen inside the body and its wall acting as an interface between the internal and external environments. The wall does not normally allow harmful agents to enter the body, nor does it permit body fluids and other materials to escape. The process of digestion and absorption of nutrients requires an intact and healthy epithelial lining that can resist the effects of its own digestive secretions. The process also involves movement of materials through the gastrointestinal tract at a rate that facilitates absorption, and it requires the presence of enzymes for the digestion and absorption of nutrients.

As a matter of semantics, the gastrointestinal tract also is referred to as the *digestive tract*, the *alimentary canal*, and, at times, the *gut*. The intestinal portion also may be called the *bowel*. For the purposes of this text, the salivary glands, the liver, and the pancreas, which produce secretions that aid in digestion, are considered *accessory organs*.

Structure and Organization of the Gastrointestinal Tract

In the digestive tract, food and other materials move slowly along its length as they are systematically broken down into ions and molecules that can be absorbed into the body. In the large intestine, unabsorbed nutrients and wastes are collected for later elimination. Although the gastrointestinal tract is located inside the body, it is a long, hollow tube, the lumen (*i.e.,* hollow center) of which is an extension of the external environment. Nutrients do not become part of the internal environment until they have passed through the intestinal wall and have entered the blood or lymph channels.

For simplicity and understanding, the digestive system can be divided into four parts (Fig. 27-1). The upper part—the mouth, esophagus, and stomach—acts as an intake source and receptacle through which food passes and in which initial digestive processes take place. The middle portion consists of the small intestine—the duodenum, jejunum, and ileum. Most digestive and absorptive processes occur in the small intestine. The lower segment—the cecum, colon, and rectum—serves as a storage channel

for the efficient elimination of waste. The fourth part consists of the accessory organs—the salivary glands, liver, and pancreas. These structures produce digestive secretions that help dismantle foods and regulate the use and storage of nutrients. The discussion in this chapter focuses on the first three parts of the gastrointestinal tract. The liver and pancreas are discussed in Chapter 29.

UPPER GASTROINTESTINAL TRACT

The mouth forms the entryway into the gastrointestinal tract for food; it contains the teeth, used in the mastication of food, and the tongue and other structures needed to direct food toward the pharyngeal structures and the esophagus.

Esophagus

The esophagus is a tube that connects the oropharynx with the stomach. The esophagus begins at the lower end of the pharynx. It is a muscular, collapsible tube, approximately 25 cm (10 in) long that lies behind the trachea. The muscular walls of the upper third of the esophagus are skeletal-type striated muscle; these muscle fibers are gradually replaced by smooth muscle fibers until, at the lower third of the esophagus, the muscle layer is entirely smooth muscle.

The esophagus functions primarily as a conduit for passage of food from the pharynx to the stomach, and the structures of its walls are designed for this purpose: the smooth muscle layers provide the peristaltic movements needed to move food along its length, and the epithelial layer secretes mucus, which protects its surface and aids in lubricating food. There are sphincters at either end of the esophagus: an upper esophageal sphincter and a lower esophageal sphincter. The upper esophageal, or pharyngoesophageal, sphincter consists of a circular layer of striated muscle. The lower esophageal, or gastroesophageal, sphincter is an area approximately 3 cm above the junction with the stomach. The circular muscle in this area normally remains tonically contracted, creating a zone of high pressure that serves to prevent reflux of gastric contents into the esophagus. During swallowing, there is "receptive relaxation" of the lower esophageal sphincter, which allows easy propulsion of the esophageal contents into the stomach. The lower esophageal sphincter passes through an opening, or hiatus, in the diaphragm as it joins with the stomach, which is located in the abdomen. The portion of the diaphragm that surrounds the lower esophageal sphincter helps to maintain the zone of high pressure needed to prevent reflux of stomach contents into the esophagus.

Stomach

The stomach is a pouchlike structure that lies in the upper part of the abdomen and serves as a food storage reservoir during the early stages of digestion. Although the residual volume of the stomach is only approximately

KEY CONCEPTS

Structure and Function of the Gastrointestinal Tract

➤ The gastrointestinal tract is a long, hollow tube that extends from the mouth to the anus; food and fluids that enter the gastrointestinal tract do not become part of the internal environment until they have been broken down and absorbed into the blood or lymph channels.

➤ The wall of the gastrointestinal tract is essentially a five-layered tube: an inner mucosal layer; a supporting submucosal layer of connective tissue; a layer of circular and longitudinal smooth muscle that functions to propel its contents in a proximal-to-distal direction; and an outer, two-layered peritoneum that prevents friction between the continuously moving segments of the intestine.

➤ The nutrients contained in ingested foods and fluids must be broken down into molecules that can be absorbed across the wall of the intestine. Gastric acids and pepsin from the stomach begin the digestive process: bile from the liver, digestive enzymes from the pancreas, and brush border enzymes break down carbohydrates, fats, and proteins into molecules that can be absorbed from the intestine.

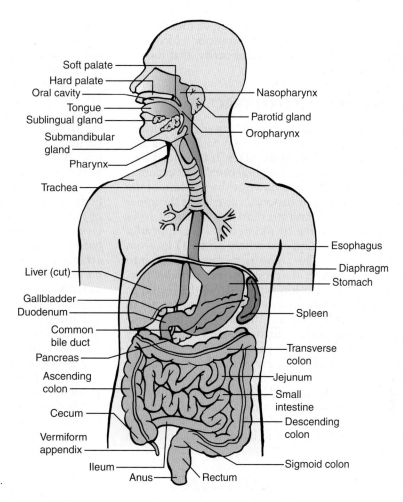

FIGURE 27-1 The digestive system.

50 mL, it can increase to almost 1000 mL before the intra-luminal pressure begins to rise. The esophagus opens into the stomach through an opening called the *cardiac orifice*, so named because of its proximity to the heart. The part of the stomach that lies above and to the left of the cardiac orifice is called the *fundus*, the central portion is called the *body*, the orifice encircled by a ringlike muscle that opens into the small intestine is called the *pylorus*, and the portion between the body and pylorus is called the *antrum* (Fig. 27-2). The presence of a true pyloric sphincter is a matter of controversy. Regardless of whether an actual sphincter exists, contractions of the smooth muscle in the pyloric area control the rate of gastric emptying.

MIDDLE GASTROINTESTINAL TRACT

The small intestine, which forms the middle portion of the digestive tract, consists of three subdivisions: the duodenum, the jejunum, and the ileum. The duodenum, which is approximately 22 cm (10 in) long, connects the stomach to the jejunum and contains the opening for the common bile duct and the main pancreatic duct. Bile and pancreatic juices enter the intestine through these

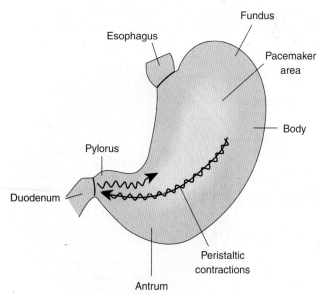

FIGURE 27-2 Structures of the stomach, showing the pacemaker area and the direction of chyme movement resulting from peristaltic contractions.

ducts. It is in the jejunum and ileum, which together are approximately 7 m (23 ft) long and must be folded onto themselves to fit into the abdominal cavity, that food is digested and absorbed.

LOWER GASTROINTESTINAL TRACT

The large intestine, which forms the lower gastrointestinal tract, is approximately 1.5 m (4.5 to 5 ft) long and 6 to 7 cm (2.4 to 2.7 in) in diameter. It is divided into the cecum, colon, rectum, and anal canal. The cecum is a blind pouch that projects down at the junction of the ileum and the colon. The ileocecal valve lies at the upper border of the cecum and prevents the return of feces from the cecum into the small intestine. The appendix arises from the cecum approximately 2.5 cm (1 in) from the ileocecal valve. The colon is further divided into ascending, transverse, descending, and sigmoid portions. The ascending colon extends from the cecum to the undersurface of the liver, where it turns abruptly to form the right colic (hepatic) flexure. The transverse colon crosses the upper half of the abdominal cavity from right to left and then curves sharply downward beneath the lower end of the spleen, forming the left colic (splenic) flexure. The descending colon extends from the colic flexure to the sigmoid colon. The rectum extends from the sigmoid colon to the anus. The anal canal passes between the two medial borders of the levator ani muscles. Powerful sphincter muscles guard against fecal incontinence.

GASTROINTESTINAL WALL STRUCTURE

The digestive tract is essentially a five-layered tube (Fig. 27-3). The inner luminal layer, or *mucosal layer*, is so named because its cells produce mucus that lubricates and protects the inner surface of the alimentary canal. The epithelial cells in this layer have a rapid turnover rate and are replaced every 4 to 5 days. Approximately 250 g of these cells are shed each day in the stool. Because of the regenerative capabilities of the mucosal layer, injury to this layer of tissue heals rapidly without leaving scar tissue. The *submucosal layer* consists of connective tissue. This layer contains blood vessels, nerves, and structures responsible for secreting digestive enzymes. The third and fourth layers, the *circular* and *longitudinal muscle layers*, facilitate movement of the contents of the gastrointestinal tract. The outer layer, the *peritoneum*, is loosely attached to the outer wall of the intestine.

The peritoneum is the largest serous membrane in the body, having a surface area approximately equal to that of the skin. The peritoneum consists of two continuous layers—the parietal and the visceral peritoneum. The *parietal peritoneum* comes in contact with and is loosely attached to the abdominal wall, whereas the *visceral peritoneum* covers the viscera such as the stomach and intestines. A thin layer of serous fluid separates the parietal and visceral peritoneum, forming a potential space called the *peritoneal cavity*. The serous fluid forms a moist and slippery surface that prevents friction between the continuously moving abdominal structures. In certain pathologic states, the amount of fluid in the potential space of the peritoneal cavity is increased, causing a condition called *ascites*.

The jejunum and ileum are suspended by a double-layered fold of peritoneum called the *mesentery* (Fig. 27-4). The mesentery contains the blood vessels, nerves, and lymphatic vessels that supply the intestinal wall. The mesentery is gathered in folds that attach to the dorsal abdominal wall along a short line of insertion, giving a fan-shaped appearance, with the intestines at the edge.

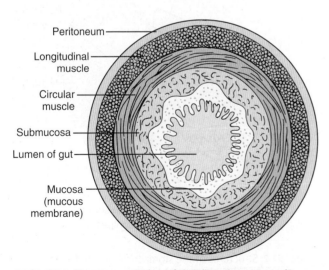

FIGURE 27-3 Transverse section of the digestive system. (From Thomson J. S. [1977]. *Core textbook of anatomy.* Philadelphia: J. B. Lippincott.)

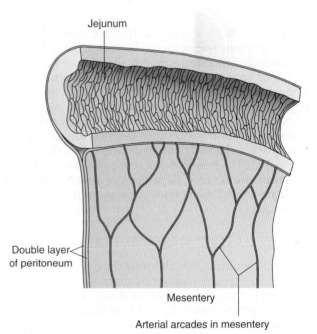

FIGURE 27-4 The attachment of the mesentery to the small bowel. (From Thomson J. S. [1977]. *Core textbook of anatomy.* Philadelphia: J. B. Lippincott.)

A filmy, double fold of peritoneal membrane called the *greater omentum* extends from the stomach to cover the transverse colon and folds of the intestine (Fig. 27-5). The greater omentum protects the intestines from cold. It always contains some fat, which in obese persons can be a considerable amount. The omentum also controls the spread of infection from gastrointestinal contents. In the case of infection, the omentum adheres to the inflamed area so that the infection is less likely to enter the peritoneal cavity. The lesser omentum extends between the transverse fissure of the liver and the lesser curvature of the stomach.

In summary, the gastrointestinal tract is a long, hollow tube, the lumen of which is an extension of the external environment. The digestive tract can be divided into four parts: an upper part, consisting of the mouth, esophagus, and stomach; a middle part, consisting of the small intestine; a lower part, consisting of the cecum, colon, and rectum; and the accessory organs, consisting of the salivary glands, the liver, and the pancreas. Throughout its length, except for the mouth, throat, and upper esophagus, the gastrointestinal tract is composed of five layers: an inner mucosal layer, a submucosal layer, a layer of circular smooth muscle fibers, a layer of longitudinal smooth muscle fibers, and an outer serosal layer that forms the peritoneum and is continuous with the mesentery.

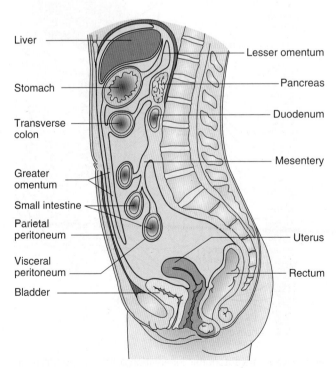

FIGURE 27-5 Reflections of the peritoneum as seen in sagittal section.

Innervation and Motility

The motility of the gastrointestinal tract propels food products and fluids along its length, from mouth to anus, in a manner that facilitates digestion and absorption. Except in the pharynx and upper third of the esophagus, smooth muscle provides the contractile force for gastrointestinal motility (the actions of smooth muscle are discussed in Chapter 1). The rhythmic movements of the digestive tract are self-perpetuating, much like the activity of the heart, and are influenced by local, humoral (*i.e.*, blood-borne), and neural influences. The ability to initiate impulses is a property of the smooth muscle itself. Impulses are conducted from one muscle fiber to another.

The smooth muscle movements of the gastrointestinal tract are tonic and rhythmic. The *tonic movements* are continuous movements that last for minutes or even hours. Tonic contractions occur at sphincters. The *rhythmic movements* consist of intermittent contractions that are responsible for mixing and moving food along the digestive tract. *Peristaltic movements* are rhythmic propulsive movements that occur when the smooth muscle layer constricts, forming a contractile band that forces the intraluminal contents forward. During peristalsis, the segment that lies distal to, or ahead of, the contracted portion relaxes, and the contents move forward with ease. Normal peristalsis always moves in the direction from the mouth toward the anus.

INNERVATION

Gastrointestinal function is controlled by the *enteric nervous system,* which lies entirely within the wall of the gastrointestinal tract, and by the parasympathetic and sympathetic divisions of the autonomic nervous system (ANS).

Enteric Nervous System

The intramural neurons (*i.e.*, those contained within the wall of the gastrointestinal tract) consist of two networks: the myenteric and submucosal plexuses. Both plexuses are aggregates of ganglionic cells that extend along the length of the gastrointestinal wall. The myenteric (Auerbach) plexus is located between the circular muscle and longitudinal muscle layers, and the submucosal (Meissner) plexus between the mucosal layer and the circular muscle layers (Fig. 27-6). The activity of the neurons in the myenteric and submucosal plexuses is regulated by local influences, input from the ANS, and by interconnecting fibers that transmit information between the two plexuses.

The myenteric plexus consists mainly of a linear chain of interconnecting neurons that extend the full length of the gastrointestinal tract. Because it extends all the way down the intestinal wall and because it lies between the two muscle layers, it is concerned mainly with motility along the length of the gut. The submucosal plexus, which lies between the mucosal and circular muscle layers of

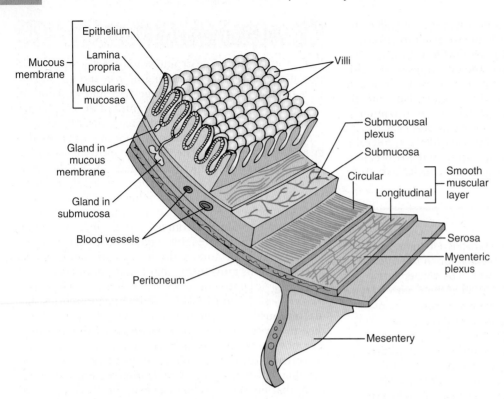

FIGURE 27-6 Diagram of the four main layers of the wall of the digestive tract: mucosa, submucosa, muscular, and serosa (below the diaphragm).

the intestinal wall, is mainly concerned with controlling the function of each segment of the intestinal tract. It integrates signals received from the mucosal layer into local control of motility, intestinal secretions, and absorption of nutrients.

Intramural plexus neurons also communicate with receptors in the mucosal and muscle layers. Mechanoreceptors monitor the stretch and distention of the gastrointestinal tract wall, and chemoreceptors monitor the chemical composition (*i.e.*, osmolality, pH, and digestive products of protein and fat metabolism) of its contents. These receptors can communicate directly with ganglionic cells in the intramural plexuses or with visceral afferent fibers that influence ANS control of gastrointestinal function.

Autonomic Nervous System

The gastrointestinal tract is innervated by both the sympathetic and parasympathetic nervous systems. Parasympathetic innervation to the stomach, small intestine, cecum, ascending colon, and transverse colon occurs by way of the vagus nerve (Fig. 27-7). The remainder of the colon is innervated by parasympathetic fibers that exit the sacral segments of the spinal cord by way of the pelvic nerve. Preganglionic parasympathetic fibers can synapse with intramural plexus neurons, or they can act directly on intestinal smooth muscle. Most parasympathetic fibers are excitatory. Numerous vagovagal reflexes influence motility and secretions of the digestive tract.

Sympathetic innervation of the gastrointestinal tract occurs through the thoracic chain of sympathetic ganglia and the celiac, superior mesenteric, and inferior mesen-

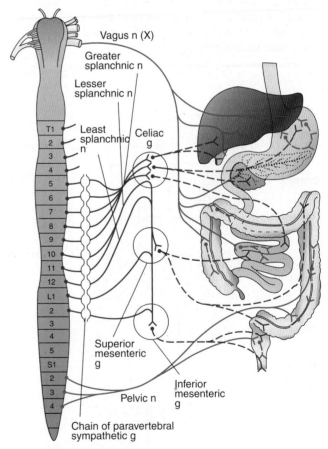

FIGURE 27-7 The autonomic innervation of the gastrointestinal tract (g, ganglion; n, nerve). *Blue* represents parasympathetic fibers and *red*, sympathetic fibers.

teric ganglia. Sympathetic control of gastrointestinal function is largely mediated by altering the activity of neurons in the intramural plexuses. The sympathetic nervous system exerts several effects on gastrointestinal function. It controls mucus secretion by the mucosal glands, reduces motility by inhibiting the activity of intramural plexus neurons, enhances sphincter function, and increases the vascular smooth muscle tone of the blood vessels that supply the gastrointestinal tract. The sympathetic fibers that supply the lower esophageal, pyloric, and internal and external anal sphincters are largely excitatory, but their role in controlling these sphincters is poorly understood.

SWALLOWING AND ESOPHAGEAL MOTILITY

The movement of foods and fluids in the gastrointestinal tract begins with chewing, in the case of solid foods, and swallowing. Chewing begins the digestive process; it breaks the food into particles of a size that can be swallowed, lubricates it by mixing it with saliva, and mixes starch-containing food with salivary amylase. Although chewing usually is considered a voluntary act, it can be carried out involuntarily by a person who has lost the function of the cerebral cortex.

The swallowing reflex is a rigidly ordered sequence of events that results in the propulsion of food from the mouth to the stomach through the esophagus. Although swallowing is initiated as a voluntary activity, it becomes involuntary as food or fluid reaches the pharynx. Sensory impulses for the reflex begin at tactile receptors in the pharynx and esophagus and are integrated with the motor components of the response in an area of the reticular formation of the medulla and lower pons called the *swallowing center*. The motor impulses for the oral and pharyngeal phases of swallowing are carried in the trigeminal (V), glossopharyngeal (IX), vagus (X), and hypoglossal (XII) cranial nerves, and impulses for the esophageal phase are carried by the vagus nerve. Diseases that disrupt these brain centers or their cranial nerves disrupt the coordination of swallowing and predispose an individual to food and fluid lodging in the trachea and bronchi, leading to risk of asphyxiation or aspiration pneumonia.

Swallowing consists of three phases: an oral, or voluntary phase; a pharyngeal phase; and an esophageal phase. During the *oral phase,* the bolus is collected at the back of the mouth so the tongue can lift the food upward until it touches the posterior wall of the pharynx. At this point, the *pharyngeal phase* of swallowing is initiated. The soft palate is pulled upward, the palatopharyngeal folds are pulled together so that food does not enter the nasopharynx, the vocal cords are pulled together, and the epiglottis is moved so that it covers the larynx. Respiration is inhibited, and the bolus is moved backward into the esophagus by constrictive movements of the pharynx. Although the striated muscles of the pharynx are involved in the second stage of swallowing, it is an involuntary stage.

The third phase of swallowing is the *esophageal stage.* As food enters the esophagus and stretches its walls, local and central nervous system reflexes that initiate peristalsis are triggered. There are two types of peristalsis: primary and secondary. Primary peristalsis is controlled by the swallowing center in the brain stem and begins when food enters the esophagus. Secondary peristalsis is partially mediated by smooth muscle fibers in the esophagus and occurs when primary peristalsis is inadequate to move food through the esophagus. Peristalsis begins at the site of distention and moves downward. Before the peristaltic wave reaches the stomach, the lower esophageal sphincter relaxes to allow the bolus of food to enter the stomach. The pressure in the lower esophageal sphincter normally is greater than that in the stomach, an important factor in preventing the reflux of gastric contents.

GASTRIC MOTILITY

The stomach serves as a reservoir for ingested solids and liquids. Motility of the stomach results in the churning and grinding of solid foods and regulates the emptying of the gastric contents, or chyme, into the duodenum. Peristaltic mixing and churning contractions begin in a pacemaker area in the middle of the stomach and move toward the antrum (see Fig. 27-2). They occur at a frequency of three to five contractions per minute, each with a duration of 2 to 20 seconds. As the peristaltic wave approaches the antrum, it speeds up, and the entire terminal 5 to 10 cm of the antrum contracts, occluding the pyloric opening. Contraction of the antrum reverses the movement of the chyme, returning the larger particles to the body of the stomach for further churning and kneading. Because the pylorus is contracted during antral contraction, the gastric contents are emptied into the duodenum between contractions.

Although the pylorus does not contain a true anatomic sphincter, it does function as a physiologic sphincter to prevent the backflow of gastric contents and allow them to flow into the duodenum at a rate commensurate with the ability of the duodenum to accept them. This is important because the regurgitation of bile salts and duodenal contents can damage the mucosal surface of the antrum and lead to gastric ulcers. Likewise, the duodenal mucosa can be damaged by the rapid influx of highly acidic gastric contents.

Like other parts of the gastrointestinal tract, the stomach is richly innervated by the enteric nervous system and its connections with the sympathetic and parasympathetic nervous systems. Axons from the intramural plexuses innervate the smooth muscles and glands of the stomach. Parasympathetic innervation is provided by the vagus nerve and sympathetic innervation by the celiac ganglia. The emptying of the stomach is regulated by hormonal and neural mechanisms. The hormones cholecystokinin and gastric inhibitory peptide, which are thought to control gastric emptying, are released in response to the pH and the osmolar and fatty acid composition of the chyme. Both local and central circuitry are involved in the neural control of gastric emptying. Afferent receptor fibers synapse with the neurons in the intramural plexus or trigger intrinsic reflexes through vagal or sympathetic pathways that participate in extrinsic reflexes.

Disorders of gastric motility can occur when the rate is too slow or too fast. A rate that is too slow leads to gastric retention. It can be caused by obstruction or gastric atony. Gastric atony can occur as a complication of visceral neuropathies in diabetes mellitus. Surgical procedures that disrupt vagal activity also can result in gastric atony. Abnormally fast emptying occurs in the dumping syndrome, which is a consequence of certain types of gastric operations. This condition is characterized by the rapid dumping of highly acidic and hyperosmotic gastric secretions into the duodenum and jejunum.

SMALL INTESTINAL MOTILITY

The small intestine is the major site for the digestion and absorption of food; its movements are mixing and propulsive. Regular peristaltic movements begin in the duodenum near the entry sites of the common duct and the main hepatic duct. A series of local pacemakers maintains the frequency of intestinal contraction. The peristaltic movements (approximately 12 per minute in the jejunum) become less frequent as they move further from the pylorus, becoming approximately 9 per minute in the ileum.

The peristaltic contractions produce segmentation waves and propulsive movements of the small intestine. With segmentation waves, slow contractions of circular muscle occlude the lumen and drive the contents forward and backward. Most of the contractions that produce segmentation waves are local events involving only 1 to 4 cm at a time. They function mainly to mix the chyme with the digestive enzymes from the pancreas and to ensure adequate exposure of all parts of the chyme to the mucosal surface of the intestine, where absorption takes place. The frequency of segmenting activity increases after a meal, presumably stimulated by receptors in the stomach and intestine.

Propulsive movements occur with synchronized activity in a section 10 to 20 cm long. They are accomplished by contraction of the proximal portion of the intestine with the sequential relaxation of its distal, or anal, portion. After material has been propelled to the ileocecal junction by peristaltic movement, stretching of the distal ileum produces a local reflex that relaxes the sphincter and allows fluid to squirt into the cecum.

Motility disturbances of the small bowel are common, and auscultation of the abdomen can be used to assess bowel activity. Inflammatory changes increase motility. In many instances, it is not certain whether changes in motility occur because of inflammation or are due to the effects of toxins and unabsorbed materials. Delayed passage of materials in the small intestine also can be a problem. Transient interruption of intestinal motility often occurs after gastrointestinal surgery. Intubation with suction often is required to remove the accumulating intestinal contents and gases until activity is resumed.

COLONIC MOTILITY

The storage function of the colon dictates that movements in this section of the gut are different from those in the small intestine. Movements in the colon are of two types.

First are the segmental mixing movements, called *haustrations*, so named because they occur within sacculations called *haustra*. These movements produce a local digging-type action, which ensures that all portions of the fecal mass are exposed to the intestinal surface. Second are the propulsive mass movements, in which a large segment of the colon ($\geq$20 cm) contracts as a unit, moving the fecal contents forward as a unit. Mass movements last approximately 30 seconds, followed by a 2- to 3-minute period of relaxation, after which another contraction occurs. A series of mass movements lasts only for 10 to 30 minutes and may occur only several times a day. Defecation normally is initiated by the mass movements.

DEFECATION

Defecation is controlled by the action of two sphincters, the internal and external anal sphincters. The internal sphincter is a several–centimeters-long circular thickening of smooth muscle that lies inside the anus. The external sphincter, which is composed of striated voluntary muscle, surrounds the internal sphincter. Defecation is controlled by defecation reflexes. One of these reflexes is the intrinsic myenteric reflex mediated by the local enteric nervous system. It is initiated by distention of the rectal wall, with initiation of reflex peristaltic waves that spread through the descending colon, sigmoid colon, and rectum. A second defecation reflex, the parasympathetic reflex, is integrated at the level of the sacral cord. When the nerve endings in the rectum are stimulated, signals are transmitted first to the sacral cord and then reflexly back to the descending colon, sigmoid colon, rectum, and anus by way of the pelvic nerves (Fig. 27-8). These impulses greatly increase peristaltic movements as well as relax the internal sphincter.

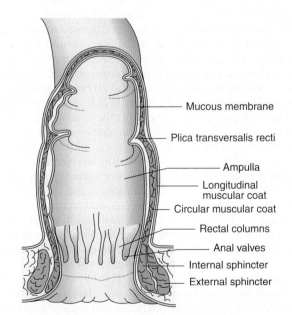

Mucous membrane

Plica transversalis recti

Ampulla

Longitudinal muscular coat

Circular muscular coat

Rectal columns

Anal valves

Internal sphincter

External sphincter

FIGURE 27-8 Interior of the rectum and anal canal.

To prevent involuntary defecation from occurring, the external anal sphincter, which is supplied by nerve fibers in the pudendal nerve, is under the conscious control of the cortex. As afferent impulses arrive at the sacral cord, signaling the presence of a distended rectum, messages are transmitted to the cortex. If defecation is inappropriate, the cortex initiates impulses that constrict the external sphincter and inhibit efferent parasympathetic activity. Normally, the afferent impulses in this reflex loop fatigue easily, and the urge to defecate soon ceases. At a more convenient time, contraction of the abdominal muscles compresses the contents in the large bowel, reinitiating afferent impulses to the cord.

In summary, motility of the gastrointestinal tract propels food products and fluids along its length from mouth to anus. Although the activity of gastrointestinal smooth muscle is self-propagating and can continue without input from the nervous system, its rate and strength of contractions are regulated by a network of intramural neurons that receive input from the ANS and local receptors that monitor wall stretch and the chemical composition of luminal contents. Parasympathetic innervation occurs by means of the vagus nerve and nerve fibers from sacral segments of the spinal cord; it increases gastrointestinal motility. Sympathetic activity occurs by way of thoracolumbar output from the spinal cord, its paravertebral ganglia, and the celiac, superior mesenteric, and inferior mesenteric ganglia. Sympathetic stimulation enhances sphincter function and reduces motility by inhibiting the activity of intramural plexus neurons.

Hormonal and Secretory Function

Each day, approximately 7000 mL of fluid is secreted into the gastrointestinal tract (Table 27-1). Approximately 50 to 200 mL of this fluid leaves the body in the stool; the remainder is reabsorbed in the small and large intestines.

TABLE 27-1	**Secretions of the Gastrointestinal Tract**
Secretions	**Amount Daily (mL)**
Salivary	1200
Gastric	2000
Pancreatic	1200
Biliary	700
Intestinal	2000
Total	7100

These secretions are mainly water and have sodium and potassium concentrations similar to those of extracellular fluid. Because water and electrolytes for digestive tract secretions are derived from the extracellular fluid compartment, excessive secretion or impaired absorption can lead to extracellular fluid deficit.

The secretory activity of the gut is influenced by local, humoral, and neural influences. Neural control of gastrointestinal secretory activity is mediated through the ANS. Secretory activity, like motility, is increased with parasympathetic stimulation and inhibited with sympathetic activity. Many of the local influences, including pH, osmolality, and chyme, consistently act as stimuli for neural and humoral mechanisms.

GASTROINTESTINAL HORMONES

The gastrointestinal tract is the largest endocrine organ in the body. It produces hormones that act locally, pass into the general circulation for distribution to more distant sites, and interact with the central nervous system through the enteric and autonomic nervous systems. Among the hormones produced by the gastrointestinal tract are gastrin, ghrelin, secretin, cholecystokinin, and the incretin hormones (glucagon-like peptide-1 [GLP-1] and glucose-dependent insulinotropic polypeptide). These hormones influence appetite, gastrointestinal motility, enzyme activity, electrolyte levels, and secretion and actions of hormones such as growth hormone, insulin, and glucagon. The actions of many of these hormones overlap; two or more gastrointestinal hormones may affect the same process in the same direction, or they may inhibit each other. The gastrointestinal tract hormones and their functions are summarized in Table 27-2.

The stomach is the source of two gastrointestinal hormones: gastrin and ghrelin. *Gastrin* is produced by G cells in the antrum of the stomach. The primary function of gastrin is the stimulation of gastric acid secretion. Gastrin also has a trophic, or growth-producing, effect on the mucosa of the small intestine, colon, and oxyntic (acid-secreting) gland area of the stomach. Removal of the tissue that produces gastrin results in atrophy of these structures. This atrophy can be reversed by the administration of exogenous gastrin. *Ghrelin* is a newly discovered peptide hormone produced by endocrine cells in the mucosal layer of the fundus of the stomach. It displays potent growth hormone–releasing activity and has a stimulatory effect on food intake and digestive function, while reducing energy expenditure. The isolation of this hormone has led to new insights into the gut-brain regulation of growth hormone secretion and energy balance.

The intestine is the source of secretin, cholecystokinin, and incretin hormones. *Secretin,* which is secreted by S cells in the mucosa of the duodenum and jejunum, inhibits gastric acid secretion. The entry of an acidic chyme into the intestine stimulates the release of secretin, which inhibits the release of gastrin. Secretin also stimulates the pancreas to secrete large quantities of fluid with a high bicarbonate concentration and low chloride

TABLE 27-2   Selected Gastrointestinal Hormones and Their Actions

Hormone	Site of Secretion	Stimulus for Secretion	Action
Cholecystokinin	Duodenum, jejunum	Products of protein digestion and long-chain fatty acids	Stimulates contraction of gall-bladder and secretion of pancreatic enzymes; slows gastric emptying; inhibits food intake
Gastrin	Antrum of stomach, duodenum	Vagal stimulation; epinephrine; neutral amino acids; calcium-containing foods such as milk; alcohol Secretion inhibited by acid content of stomach antrum (pH < 2.5)	Stimulates secretion of gastric acid and pepsinogen; increases gastric blood flow; stimulates gastric smooth muscle contractions; stimulates growth of gastric and intestinal mucosal cells
Ghrelin	Fundus of stomach	Nutritional (fasting) and hormonal (decreased levels of growth hormone)	Stimulates secretion of growth hormone; acts as an appetite-stimulating signal from stomach when an increase in metabolic efficiency is necessary
Glucagon-like peptide-1	Distal small intestine	High-carbohydrate meal	Augments insulin release; suppresses glucagon release; slows gastric emptying; decreases appetite and body weight
Glucose-dependent insulinotropic polypeptide	Small intestine, mainly jejunum	High-carbohydrate meal	Augments insulin release
Secretin	Duodenum	Acid pH or chyme entering duodenum (pH < 3.0)	Stimulates secretion of bicarbonate-containing fluids by pancreas and liver

concentration. The primary function of *cholecystokinin*, secreted by I cells in the intestinal mucosa, is the stimulation of pancreatic enzyme secretion. It potentiates the action of secretin, increasing the pancreatic bicarbonate response to low circulating levels of secretin, it stimulates biliary secretion of fluid and bicarbonate, and it regulates gallbladder contraction and gastric emptying. Cholecystokinin has also been shown to inhibit food intake and to be an important mediator for the control of meal size.

Several gut-derived hormones have been identified as having what is termed an *incretin* effect, meaning that they increase insulin release after an oral glucose load. This suggests that gut-derived factors can stimulate insulin secretion after a predominantly carbohydrate meal. The two hormones that account for about 90% of the incretin effect are GLP-1, which is released from L cells in the distal small bowel, and glucose-dependent insulinotropic polypeptide (GIP; previously known as *gastric inhibitory polypeptide*), which is released by K cells in the upper gut (mainly the jejunum). Because increased levels of both GLP-1 and GIP can lower blood glucose levels by augmenting insulin release in a glucose-dependent manner (*i.e.*, at low blood glucose levels no further insulin is secreted, thus minimizing the risk of hypoglycemia), these factors have been targeted as possible antidiabetic drugs. Moreover, GLP-1 can exert other metabolically beneficial effects, including suppressing glucagon release, slowing gastric emptying, augmenting net glucose clearance, and decreasing appetite and body weight.

GASTROINTESTINAL SECRETIONS

Salivary Secretions

Saliva is secreted by the salivary glands. The salivary glands consist of the parotid, submaxillary, sublingual, and buccal glands. Saliva has three functions. The first is protection and lubrication. Saliva is rich in mucus, which protects the oral mucosa and coats the food as it passes through the mouth, pharynx, and esophagus. The sublingual and buccal glands produce only mucus-type secretions. The second function of saliva is its protective antimicrobial action. The saliva cleans the mouth and contains the enzyme lysozyme, which has an antibacterial action. Third, saliva contains ptyalin and amylase, which initiate the digestion of dietary starches. Secretions from the salivary glands are primarily regulated by the ANS. Parasympathetic stimulation increases flow, and sympathetic stimulation decreases flow. The dry mouth that accompanies anxiety attests to the effects of sympathetic activity on salivary secretions.

Mumps, or parotitis, is an infection of the parotid glands. Although most of us associate mumps with the contagious viral form of the disease, inflammation of the parotid glands can occur in the seriously ill person who does not receive adequate oral hygiene and who is unable to take fluids orally. Potassium iodide increases the secretory activity of the salivary glands, including the parotid glands. In a small percentage of persons, parotid swelling may occur in the course of treatment with this drug.

Gastric Secretions

In addition to mucus-secreting cells that line the entire surface of the stomach, the stomach mucosa has two types of glands: oxyntic (or gastric) glands and pyloric glands. The *oxyntic glands* are located in the proximal 80% (body and fundus) of the stomach. They secrete hydrochloric acid, pepsinogen, intrinsic factor, and mucus. The *pyloric glands* are located in the distal 20%, or antrum, of the stomach. The pyloric glands secrete mainly mucus, some pepsinogen, and the hormone gastrin.

The oxyntic gland area of the stomach is composed of glands and pits (Fig. 27-9). The surface area and gastric pits are lined with mucus-producing epithelial cells. The bases of the gastric pits contain the parietal (or oxyntic) cells, which secrete hydrochloric acid and intrinsic factor, and the chief (peptic) cells, which secrete large quantities of pepsinogen. There are approximately 1 billion parietal cells in the stomach; together they produce and secrete approximately 20 mEq of hydrochloric acid in several hundred milliliters of gastric juice each hour. Gastric intrinsic factor, which is produced by the parietal cells, is necessary for the absorption of vitamin B_{12} (see Chapter 11). The pepsinogen that is secreted by the chief cells is rapidly converted to pepsin when exposed to the low pH of the gastric juices.

One of the important characteristics of the gastric mucosa is resistance to the highly acidic secretions that it produces. When the gastric mucosa is damaged by aspirin, nonsteroidal anti-inflammatory drugs (NSAIDs), ethyl alcohol, or bile salts, this resistance is disrupted, and hydrogen ions move into the mucosal cells. As the hydrogen ions accumulate in the mucosal cells, intracellular pH decreases, enzymatic reactions become impaired, and cellular structures are disrupted. The result is local ischemia and tissue necrosis. The mucosal surface is further protected by prostaglandins.

Parasympathetic stimulation (through the vagus nerve) and gastrin increase gastric secretions. Histamine also increases gastric acid secretions. The relation of gastric acid secretion to peptic ulcers is discussed in Chapter 28.

Intestinal Secretions

The small intestine secretes digestive juices and receives secretions from the liver and pancreas (see Chapter 29). An extensive array of mucus-producing glands, called *Brunner glands*, is concentrated at the site where the contents from the stomach and secretions from the liver and pancreas enter the duodenum. These glands secrete large amounts of alkaline mucus that protect the duodenum from the acid content in the gastric chyme and from the action of the digestive enzymes. The activity of Brunner glands is strongly influenced by ANS activity. For example, sympathetic stimulation causes a marked decrease in mucus production, leaving this area more susceptible to irritation.

In addition to mucus, the intestinal mucosa produces two other types of secretions. The first is a serous fluid (pH 6.5 to 7.5) secreted by specialized cells (*i.e.*, crypts of Lieberkühn) in the intestinal mucosal layer. This fluid, which is produced at the rate of 2000 mL/day, acts as a vehicle for absorption. The second type of secretion consists of surface enzymes that aid absorption. These enzymes are the peptidases, or enzymes that separate amino acids, and the disaccharidases, or enzymes that split sugars.

The large intestine usually secretes only mucus. ANS activity strongly influences mucus production in the bowel, as in other parts of the digestive tract. During intense parasympathetic stimulation, mucus secretion may increase to the point that the stool contains large amounts of obvious mucus. Although the bowel normally does not secrete water or electrolytes, these substances are lost

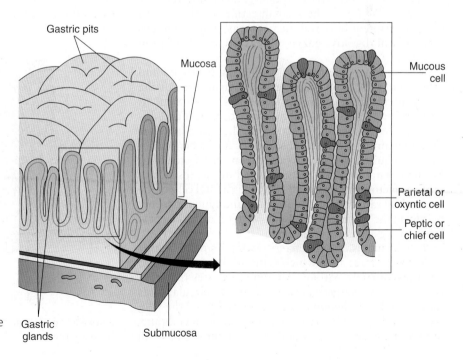

FIGURE 27-9 Gastric pit from body of the stomach.

Gastric pits

Mucosa

Mucous cell

Gastric glands

Submucosa

Parietal or oxyntic cell

Peptic or chief cell

in large quantities when the bowel becomes irritated or inflamed.

In summary, the secretions of the gastrointestinal tract include saliva, gastric juices, bile, and pancreatic and intestinal secretions. Each day, more than 7000 mL of fluid is secreted into the digestive tract; all but 50 to 200 mL of this fluid is reabsorbed. Water, derived from the extracellular fluid compartment, is the major component of gastrointestinal tract secretions. Neural, humoral, and local mechanisms contribute to the control of these secretions. The parasympathetic nervous system increases secretion, and sympathetic activity exerts an inhibitory effect. In addition to secreting fluids containing digestive enzymes, the gastrointestinal tract produces and secretes hormones, such as gastrin, secretin, and cholecystokinin, that contribute to the control of gastrointestinal function.

Digestion and Absorption

Digestion is the process of dismantling foods into their constituent parts. Digestion requires hydrolysis, enzyme cleavage, and fat emulsification. Hydrolysis is the breakdown of a compound that involves a chemical reaction with water. The importance of hydrolysis to digestion is evidenced by the amount of water (7 to 8 L) that is secreted into the gastrointestinal tract daily. The intestinal mucosa is impermeable to most large molecules. Most proteins, fats, and carbohydrates must be broken down into smaller particles before they can be absorbed. Although some digestion of carbohydrates and proteins begins in the stomach, digestion takes place mainly in the small intestine. The breakdown of fats to free fatty acids and monoglycerides takes place entirely in the small intestine. The liver, with its production of bile, and the pancreas, which supplies a number of digestive enzymes, play important roles in digestion.

Absorption is the process of moving nutrients and other materials from the external environment of the gastrointestinal tract into the internal environment. Absorption is accomplished by active transport and diffusion. The absorptive function of the large intestine focuses mainly on water reabsorption. A number of substances require a specific carrier or transport system. For example, vitamin B_{12} is not absorbed in the absence of intrinsic factor, which is secreted by the parietal cells of the stomach. Transport of amino acids and glucose occurs mainly in the presence of sodium. Water is absorbed passively along an osmotic gradient.

The distinguishing characteristic of the small intestine is its large surface area, which in the adult is estimated to be approximately 250 m². Anatomic features that contribute to this enlarged surface area are the circular folds that extend into the lumen of the intestine and the villi, which are finger-like projections of mucous membrane, numbering as many as 25,000, that line the entire small

intestine (Fig. 27-10). Each villus is equipped with an arrangement of blood vessels for the absorption of fluid and dissolved material into the portal blood and a central lacteal for absorption into the lymph (Fig. 27-11). Fats rely largely on the lymphatics for absorption.

Each villus is covered with cells called *enterocytes* that contribute to the absorptive and digestive functions of the small bowel, and goblet cells that provide mucus. The crypts of Lieberkühn are glandular structures that open into the spaces between the villi. The enterocytes have a life span of approximately 4 to 5 days; their replacement cells differentiate from progenitor cells located in the area of the crypts. The maturing enterocytes migrate up the villus and eventually are extruded from the tip.

The enterocytes secrete enzymes that aid in the digestion of carbohydrates and proteins. These enzymes are called *brush border enzymes* because they adhere to the border of the villus structures. In this way they have access to the carbohydrates and protein molecules as they come in contact with the absorptive surface of the intestine. This mechanism of secretion places the enzymes where they are needed and eliminates the need to produce enough enzymes to mix with the entire contents that fill the lumen of the small bowel. The digested molecules diffuse through the membrane or are actively transported across the mucosal surface to enter the blood or, in the case of fatty acids, the lacteal. These molecules are then transported through the portal vein or lymphatics into the systemic circulation.

CARBOHYDRATES

Carbohydrates must be broken down into monosaccharides, or single sugars, before they can be absorbed from the small intestine. The average daily intake of carbohydrate in the American diet is approximately 350 to 400 g. Starch makes up approximately 50% of this total, sucrose (*i.e.*, table sugar) approximately 30%, lactose

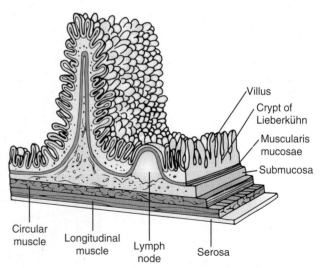

FIGURE 27-10 The mucous membrane of the small intestine. Note the numerous villi on a circular fold.

Villus

Crypt of Lieberkühn

Muscularis mucosae

Submucosa

Circular muscle

Longitudinal muscle

Lymph node

Serosa

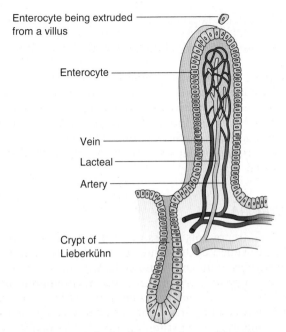

Enterocyte being extruded
from a villus

Enterocyte

Vein

Lacteal

Artery

Crypt of
Lieberkühn

FIGURE 27-11 A single villus from the small intestine.

(*i.e.,* milk sugar) approximately 6%, and maltose approximately 1.5%.

Digestion of starch begins in the mouth with the action of amylase. Pancreatic secretions also contain an amylase. Amylase breaks down starch into several disaccharides, including maltose, isomaltose, and α-dextrins. The brush border enzymes convert the disaccharides into monosaccharides that can be absorbed (Table 27-3). Sucrose yields glucose and fructose, lactose is converted to glucose and galactose, and maltose is converted to two glucose molecules. When the disaccharides are not broken down to monosaccharides, they cannot be absorbed but remain as osmotically active particles in the contents of the digestive system, causing diarrhea. For example, persons with a lactase deficiency experience diarrhea when they drink milk or eat dairy products that contain lactose.

Fructose is transported across the intestinal mucosa by facilitated diffusion, which does not require energy expenditure. In this case, fructose moves along a concentration gradient. Glucose and galactose are transported by way of a sodium-dependent carrier system that uses adenosine triphosphate (ATP) and the Na^+/K^+-ATPase pump as an energy source (Fig. 27-12). Water absorption from the intestine is linked to absorption of osmotically active particles, such as glucose and sodium. It follows that an important consideration in facilitating the transport of water across the intestine (and decreasing diarrhea) after temporary disruption in bowel function is to include sodium and glucose in the fluids that are ingested.

FATS

The average adult eats approximately 60 to 100 g of fat daily, principally as triglycerides containing long-chain fatty acids. These triglycerides are broken down by pancreatic lipase. Bile salts act as a carrier system for the fatty acids and fat-soluble vitamins A, D, E, and K by forming micelles, which transport these substances to the surface of intestinal villi, where they are absorbed by the lacteal. The major site of fat absorption is the upper jejunum. Medium-chain triglycerides, with 6 to 10 carbon atoms in their structures, are better absorbed than longer-chain fatty acids because they are more completely broken down by pancreatic lipase and they form micelles more easily. Because they are easily absorbed, medium-chain triglycerides often are used in the treatment of persons with malabsorption syndrome. The absorption of vitamins A, D, E, and K, which are fat-soluble vitamins, requires the presence of bile salts.

Fat that is not absorbed in the intestine is excreted in the stool. *Steatorrhea* is the term used to describe fatty stools. It usually indicates that there is 20 g or more of fat in a 24-hour stool sample. Normally, a chemical test is done on a 72-hour stool collection, during which time the diet is restricted to 80 to 100 g of fat per day.

PROTEINS

Proteins from the diet must be broken down into amino acids to be absorbed. Protein digestion begins in the stomach with the action of pepsin. Pepsinogen, the enzyme precursor of pepsin, is secreted by the chief cells in response to a meal and acid pH. Acid in the stomach is required for the conversion of pepsinogen to pepsin. Pepsin is inactivated when it enters the intestine by the alkaline pH.

Proteins are broken down further by pancreatic enzymes, such as trypsin, chymotrypsin, carboxypeptidase, and elastase. As with pepsin, the pancreatic enzymes are secreted as precursor molecules. Trypsinogen, which lacks enzymatic activity, is activated by an enzyme located on the brush border cells of the duodenal enterocytes. Activated trypsin activates additional trypsinogen molecules

TABLE 27-3	**Enzymes Used in Digestion of Carbohydrates**	
Dietary Carbohydrates	**Enzyme**	**Monosaccharides Produced**
Lactose	Lactase	Glucose and galactose
Sucrose	Sucrase	Fructose and glucose
Starch	Amylase	Maltose, isomaltose, and α-dextrins
Maltose and maltotriose	Maltase	Glucose and glucose
α-Dextrins	α-Dextrimase	Glucose and glucose

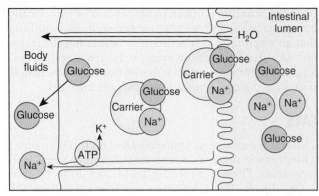

FIGURE 27-12 The hypothetical sodium-dependent transport system for glucose. Both sodium and glucose must attach to the transport carrier before either can be transported into the cell. The concentration of glucose builds up in the intestinal cell until a diffusion gradient develops, causing glucose to move into the body fluids. Sodium is transported out of the cell by the energy-dependent Na^+/K^+-ATPase pump. This creates the gradient needed to operate the transport system. Water is passively absorbed along a concentration gradient generated by the absorption of solutes. (ATP, adenosine triphosphate.)

and other pancreatic precursor proteolytic enzymes. The amino acids are liberated intramurally or on the surface of the villi by brush border enzymes that degrade proteins into peptides that are one, two, or three amino acids long. Similar to glucose, many amino acids are transported across the mucosal membrane in a sodium-linked process that uses the Na^+/K^+-ATPase pump as an energy source.

In summary, the digestion and absorption of foodstuffs take place in the small intestine. Digestion is the process of dismantling foods into their constituent parts. Digestion requires hydrolysis, enzyme cleavage, and fat emulsification. Proteins, fats, carbohydrates, and other components of the diet are broken down into molecules that can be transported from the intestinal lumen into the body fluids. Absorption is the process of moving nutrients and other materials from the external environment of the gastrointestinal tract into the internal environment. Brush border enzymes break carbohydrates into monosaccharides that can be transported across the intestine into the bloodstream. The digestion of proteins begins in the stomach with the action of pepsin and is further facilitated in the intestine by the pancreatic enzymes, such as trypsin, chymotrypsin, carboxypeptidase, and elastase. The absorption of glucose and amino acids is facilitated by a sodium-dependent transport system. Fat in the diet is broken down by pancreatic lipase into triglycerides containing medium- and long-chain fatty acids. Bile salts form micelles that transport these substances to the surface of intestinal villi, where they are absorbed.

 ## Anorexia, Nausea, and Vomiting

Anorexia, nausea, and vomiting are physiologic responses that are common to many gastrointestinal disorders. These responses are protective to the extent that they signal the presence of disease and, in the case of vomiting, remove noxious agents from the gastrointestinal tract. They also can contribute to impaired intake or loss of fluids and nutrients.

ANOREXIA

Anorexia represents a loss of appetite. Several factors influence appetite. One is hunger, which is stimulated by contractions of the empty stomach. Appetite or the desire for food intake is regulated by the hypothalamus and other associated centers in the brain (see Chapter 8). Smell plays an important role, as evidenced by the fact that appetite can be stimulated or suppressed by the smell of food. Loss of appetite is associated with emotional factors, such as fear, depression, frustration, and anxiety. Many drugs and disease states cause anorexia. For example, in uremia the accumulation of nitrogenous wastes in the blood contributes to the development of anorexia. Anorexia often is a forerunner of nausea, and most conditions that cause nausea and vomiting also produce anorexia.

NAUSEA

Nausea is an ill-defined and unpleasant subjective sensation. It is the conscious sensation resulting from stimulation of the medullary vomiting center that often precedes or accompanies vomiting. Nausea usually is preceded by anorexia, and stimuli such as foods and drugs that cause anorexia in small doses usually produce nausea when given in larger doses. A common cause of nausea is distention of the duodenum or upper small intestinal tract. Nausea frequently is accompanied by ANS manifestations such as watery salivation and vasoconstriction with pallor, sweating, and tachycardia. Nausea may function as an early warning signal of a pathologic process.

VOMITING

Vomiting, or emesis, is the sudden and forceful oral expulsion of the contents of the stomach. It usually is preceded by nausea. The contents that are vomited are called *vomitus*. Vomiting, as a basic physiologic protective mechanism, limits the possibility of damage from ingested noxious agents by emptying the contents of the stomach and portions of the small intestine. Nausea and vomiting may represent a total-body response to drug therapy, including overdosage, cumulative effects, toxicity, and side effects.

Vomiting involves two functionally distinct medullary centers: the vomiting center and the chemoreceptor trigger zone. The act of vomiting is integrated by the vomiting center, which is located in the dorsal portion of the reticular formation of the medulla near the sensory nuclei of the vagus. The chemoreceptor trigger zone is located in a small area on the floor of the fourth ventricle, where it is exposed to both blood and cerebrospinal fluid. It is thought to mediate the emetic effects of blood-borne drugs and toxins.

The act of vomiting consists of taking a deep breath, closing the airways, and producing a strong, forceful contraction of the diaphragm and abdominal muscles along with relaxation of the gastroesophageal sphincter. Respiration ceases during the act of vomiting. Vomiting may be accompanied by dizziness, light-headedness, decrease in blood pressure, and bradycardia.

The vomiting center receives input from the gastrointestinal tract and other organs; from the cerebral cortex; from the vestibular apparatus, which is responsible for motion sickness; and from the chemoreceptor trigger zone, which is activated by many drugs and endogenous and exogenous toxins. Hypoxia exerts a direct effect on the vomiting center, producing nausea and vomiting. This direct effect probably accounts for the vomiting that occurs during periods of decreased cardiac output, shock, environmental hypoxia, and brain ischemia caused by increased intracranial pressure. Inflammation of any of the intra-abdominal organs, including the liver, gallbladder, or urinary tract, can cause vomiting because of the stimulation of the visceral afferent pathways that communicate with the vomiting center. Distention or irritation of the gastrointestinal tract also causes vomiting through the stimulation of visceral afferent neurons.

Several neurotransmitters and receptor subtypes are implicated as neuromediators in nausea and vomiting. Dopamine, serotonin, and opioid receptors are found in the gastrointestinal tract and in the vomiting and chemoreceptor trigger zone. Dopamine antagonists, such as prochlorperazine, depress vomiting caused by stimulation of the chemoreceptor trigger zone. Serotonin is believed to be involved in the nausea and emesis associated with cancer chemotherapy and radiation therapy. Serotonin antagonists (*e.g.*, granisetron and ondansetron) are effective in treating the nausea and vomiting associated with these stimuli. Motion sickness appears to be a central nervous system (CNS) response to vestibular stimuli. Norepinephrine and acetylcholine receptors are located in the vestibular center. The acetylcholine receptors are thought to mediate the impulses responsible for exciting the vomiting center; norepinephrine receptors may have a stabilizing influence that resists motion sickness. Many of the motion sickness drugs (*e.g.*, dimenhydrinate) have a strong CNS anticholinergic effect and act on the receptors in the vomiting center and areas related to the vestibular system.

In summary, the signs and symptoms of many gastrointestinal tract disorders are manifested by anorexia, nausea, and vomiting. Anorexia, or loss of appetite, may occur alone or may accompany nausea and vomiting. Nausea, which is an ill-defined, unpleasant sensation, signals the stimulation of the medullary vomiting center. It often precedes vomiting and frequently is accompanied by autonomic responses, such as salivation and vasoconstriction with pallor, sweating, and tachycardia. The act of vomiting, which is integrated by the vomiting center, involves the forceful oral expulsion of the gastric contents. It is a basic physiologic mechanism that rids the gastrointestinal tract of noxious agents.

Review Exercises

Persons receiving chemotherapeutic agents, which interfere with mitosis of cancer cells as well as the cells of other rapidly proliferating tissues in the body, often experience disorders such as ulcerations in the mucosal tissues of the mouth and other parts of the gastrointestinal tract. These disorders are resolved once the chemotherapy treatment has been completed.

A. Explain.

People with gastroesophageal reflux (movement of gastric contents into the esophagus) often complain of heartburn that worsens as the pressure in the stomach increases.

A. Use information on hormonal control of gastric emptying to explain why eating a meal that is high in fat content often exaggerates the problem.

Infections of the gastrointestinal tract, such as the "gastrointestinal flu," often cause profound diarrhea.

A. Describe the neural mechanisms involved in the increase in gastrointestinal motility that produces the diarrhea.

People with lactase deficiency often experience bloating and diarrhea.

A. Explain.

Visit the Porth: Essentials of Pathophysiology: Concepts of Altered Health States web site (http://thePoint.LWW.com/PorthEssentials) for links to chapter-related resources on the Internet, all-new exclusive animations, chapter review questions, and more!

BIBLIOGRAPHY

Berne R. M., Levy M. N. (2000). *Principles of physiology* (3rd ed., pp. 354–400). St. Louis: Mosby.

Deacon C. F. (2004). Therapeutic strategies based on glucagon-like peptide 1. *Diabetes* 53, 2181–2189.

Gershon M. D. (1999). The enteric nervous system: A second brain. *Hospital Practice* 34(7), 31–52.

Guyton A. C., Hall J. E. (2006). *Textbook of medical physiology* (11th ed., pp. 771–825). Philadelphia: Elsevier Saunders.

Inul A., Asakawa A., Bowers C. Y., et al. (2004). Ghrelin, appetite, and gastric motility: The emerging role of the stomach as an endocrine organ. *FASEB Journal* 18, 439–456.

Johnson L. R. (2001). *Gastrointestinal physiology* (6th ed.). St. Louis: C. V. Mosby.

Moran T. H., Kinzig K. P. (2004). Gastrointestinal satiety signals: II. Cholecystokinin. *American Journal of Physiology: Gastrointestinal and Liver Physiology* 286, G183–G188.

Rhoades R. A., Tanner G. A. (2003). Medical physiology (2nd ed., pp. 449–489). Philadelphia: Lippincott Williams & Wilkins.

St.-Pierre D. H., Wang L., Tache Y. (2003). Ghrelin: A novel player in the gut-brain regulation of growth hormone and energy balance. *News in Physiological Sciences* 18, 242–246.

Toft-Nielson M. B., Damholt M. B., Madsbad S., et al. (2001). Determinants of impaired secretion of glucagon-like peptide-1 in type 2 diabetic patients. *Journal of Clinical Endocrinology and Metabolism* 86, 3717–3723.

Chapter 28

Disorders of Gastrointestinal Function

 Gastrointestinal disorders are not cited as the leading cause of death in the United States, nor do they receive the same publicity as heart disease and cancer. However, according to government reports, digestive diseases rank third in the total economic burden of illness, resulting in considerable human suffering, personal expenditures for treatment, lost working hours, and a drain on the nation's economy. It has been estimated that 60 to 70 million people in the United States have a digestive disease and more than 10 million (13%) of all hospitalization are for digestive disorders.[1] Even more important is the fact that proper nutrition or a change in health practices could prevent or minimize many of these disorders.

Disorders of the Esophagus

The esophagus is a tube that connects the oropharynx with the stomach. It lies posterior to the trachea and larynx and extends through the mediastinum, intersecting the diaphragm at the level of the T11 or T12 vertebra.[2] The esophagus functions primarily as a conduit for passage of food from the pharynx to the stomach, and the structures of its walls are designed for this purpose: the smooth muscle layers provide the peristaltic movements needed to move food along its length, and the epithelial layer secretes mucus, which protects its surface and aids in lubricating food. There are sphincters at either end of the esophagus: an upper esophageal, or pharyngoesophageal, sphincter that prevents reflux into the pharynx from the esophagus and a lower esophageal, or gastroesophageal, sphincter that prevents reflux into the esophagus from the stomach. The lower esophageal sphincter passes through an opening, or hiatus, in the diaphragm as it joins with the stomach, which is located in the abdomen. As the esophagus passes through the hiatus it is reinforced by fibers of the diaphragm. Development of an abnormal gap around

605

the wall of the esophagus can lead to herniation of stomach into the thoracic cage, a condition known as hiatal hernia.[2]

DYSPHAGIA

The act of swallowing depends on the coordinated action of the tongue and pharynx. These structures are innervated by cranial nerves V, IX, X, and XII. *Dysphagia* refers to difficulty in swallowing. If swallowing is painful, it is referred to as *odynophagia*. Dysphagia can result from altered nerve function or from disorders that produce narrowing of the esophagus. Lesions of the central nervous system (CNS), such as a stroke, often involve the cranial nerves that control swallowing. Cancer of the esophagus and strictures resulting from scarring can reduce the size of the esophageal lumen and make swallowing difficult. Scleroderma, an autoimmune disease that causes fibrous replacement of tissues in the muscularis layer of the gastrointestinal tract, is another important cause of dysphagia.[3] Persons with dysphagia usually complain of choking, coughing, or an abnormal sensation of food sticking in the back of the throat or upper chest when they swallow.

In a condition called *achalasia,* the lower esophageal sphincter fails to relax; food that has been swallowed has difficulty passing into the stomach, and the esophagus above the lower esophageal sphincter becomes enlarged. One or several meals may lodge in the esophagus and pass slowly into the stomach over time. There is danger of aspiration of esophageal contents into the lungs when the person lies down.

ESOPHAGEAL DIVERTICULUM

A diverticulum of the esophagus is an outpouching of the esophageal wall caused by a weakness of the muscularis layer. An esophageal diverticulum tends to retain food. Complaints that the food stops before it reaches the stomach are common, as are reports of gurgling, belching, coughing, and foul-smelling breath. The trapped food may cause esophagitis and ulceration. Because the condition usually is progressive, correction of the defect requires surgical intervention.

GASTROESOPHAGEAL REFLUX DISEASE

The term *reflux* refers to backward or return movement. In the context of gastroesophageal reflux, it refers to the backward movement of gastric contents into the esophagus, a condition that causes heartburn. It probably is the most common disorder originating in the gastrointestinal tract. Most persons experience heartburn occasionally as a result of reflux. Such symptoms usually occur soon after eating, are short lived, and seldom cause more serious problems. However, for some persons, persistent heartburn can represent gastroesophageal reflux disease with esophagitis.

The lower esophageal sphincter regulates the flow of food from the esophagus into the stomach. Both internal and external mechanisms function in maintaining the antireflux function of the lower esophageal sphincter.[4,5] Relaxation of the lower esophageal sphincter is a brain stem reflex that is mediated by the vagus nerve in response to a number of afferent stimuli. Transient relaxation with reflux is common after meals. Gastric distention and meals high in fat increase the frequency of relaxation. Normally, refluxed material is returned to the stomach by secondary peristaltic waves in the esophagus and swallowed saliva neutralizes and washes away the refluxed acid.

Gastroesophageal reflux disease is thought to be associated with a weak or incompetent lower esophageal sphincter that allows reflux to occur, exposing the esophagus to the irritant effects of the refluxate and decreasing clearance of the refluxed acid from the esophagus after it has occurred (Fig. 28-1). Reflux esophagitis involves mucosal injury to the esophagus, hyperemia, and inflammation. Esophageal mucosal injury is related to the destructive nature of the refluxate and the amount of time it is in contact with mucosa. Acidic gastric fluids (pH <4.0) are particularly damaging.

There is controversy regarding the importance of hiatal hernia in the pathogenesis of reflux disease. Small hiatal hernias are common and considered to be of no significance in asymptomatic people. However, in cases of severe erosive esophagitis where gastroesophageal reflux and a large hiatal hernia coexist, the hernia may retard esophageal acid clearance and contribute to the disorder.[2]

The most frequent symptom of gastroesophageal reflux is heartburn. It frequently is severe, occurring 30 to 60 minutes after eating. It often is made worse by bending at the waist and recumbency and usually is relieved by sitting upright. The severity of heartburn is not indicative of the extent of mucosal injury; only a small percentage of

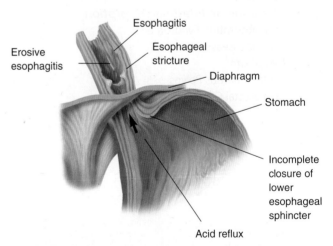

FIGURE 28-1 Gastroesophageal junction and site of gastroesophageal reflux. (From Springhouse. [2004]. *Atlas of pathophysiology* [p. 171]. Springhouse, PA: Springhouse.)

people who complain of heartburn have mucosal injury. Often, the heartburn occurs during the night. Antacids give prompt, although transient relief. Other symptoms include belching and chest pain. The pain usually is located in the epigastric or retrosternal area and often radiates to the throat, shoulder, or back. Because of its location, the pain may be confused with angina. The reflux of gastric contents also may produce respiratory symptoms such as wheezing, chronic cough, and hoarseness. There is considerable evidence linking gastroesophageal reflux with bronchial asthma.[6] The proposed mechanisms of reflux-associated asthma and chronic cough include micro-aspiration and macroaspiration, laryngeal injury, and vagal-mediated bronchospasm.

Complications can result from persistent reflux, which produces a cycle of mucosal damage that causes hyperemia, edema, and erosion of the luminal surface. These complications include strictures and a condition called *Barrett esophagus*.[7] Strictures are caused by a combination of scar tissue, spasm, and edema. They produce narrowing of the esophagus and cause dysphagia when the lumen becomes sufficiently constricted. Barrett esophagus is characterized by a reparative process in which the squamous mucosa that normally lines the esophagus gradually is replaced by columnar epithelium resembling that in the stomach or intestines.[7] It is associated with increased risk for development of esophageal cancer.

Diagnosis of gastroesophageal reflux depends on a history of reflux symptomatology and selective use of diagnostic methods, including radiographic studies using a contrast medium such as barium, esophagoscopy, and 24-hour ambulatory esophageal pH monitoring.[8]

The treatment of gastroesophageal reflux usually focuses on conservative measures. These measures include avoidance of positions and conditions that increase gastric reflux.[8] Avoidance of large meals and foods that reduce lower esophageal sphincter tone (*e.g.*, caffeine, fats, chocolate), alcohol, and smoking is recommended. It is recommended that meals be eaten sitting up and that the recumbent position be avoided for several hours after a meal. Bending for long periods should be avoided, because it tends to increase intra-abdominal pressure and cause gastric reflux. Sleeping with the head elevated helps to prevent reflux during the night. Weight loss usually is recommended in overweight people.

Antacids or a combination of antacids and alginic acid also are recommended for mild disease. Alginic acid foams when it comes in contact with gastric acid; if reflux occurs, the foam rather than acid rises into the esophagus. Histamine-2 receptor (H_2)–blocking agents, which inhibit gastric acid production, often are recommended when additional treatment is needed. The proton pump inhibitors act by inhibiting the gastric proton pump, which regulates the final pathway for acid secretion. These agents may be used for persons who continue to have daytime symptoms, recurrent strictures, or large esophageal ulcerations. Surgical treatment may be indicated in some people.

Gastroesophageal Reflux in Children

Gastroesophageal reflux is a common problem in infants and children. The small reservoir capacity of an infant's esophagus coupled with frequent spontaneous reductions in sphincter pressure contribute to reflux. At least one episode of regurgitation per day occurs in as many as half of infants aged 0 to 3 months. By 6 months of age it becomes less frequent, and it abates by 2 years of age as the child assumes a more upright posture and eats solid foods.[9,10] Although many infants have minor degrees of reflux, complications occur in 1 of every 300 to 500 children.[9] The condition occurs more frequently in children with cerebral palsy, Down syndrome, and other neurologic disorders.

In most cases, infants with simple reflux are thriving and healthy, and symptoms resolve between 9 and 24 months of age. Pathologic reflux is classified into three categories: (1) regurgitation and malnutrition, (2) esophagitis, and (3) respiratory problems. Symptoms of esophagitis include evidence of pain when swallowing, hematemesis, anemia due to esophageal bleeding, heartburn, irritability, and sudden or inconsolable crying. Parents often report feeding problems in their infants.[9] These infants often are irritable and demonstrate early satiety. Sometimes the problems progress to actual resistance to feeding. Tilting of the head to one side and arching of the back may be noted in children with severe reflux. The head positioning is thought to represent an attempt to protect the airway or reduce the pain-associated reflux. Sometimes regurgitation is associated with dental caries and recurrent otalgia. The ear pain is thought to result from referral from the vagus nerve in the esophagus to the ear. A variety of respiratory symptoms are caused by damage to the respiratory mucosa when gastric reflux enters the esophagus. Reflux may cause laryngospasm, apnea, and bradycardia. A relationship between reflux and acute life-threatening events or sudden infant death syndrome has been proposed. However, the association remains controversial and the linkage may be coincidental.[9]

Diagnosis of gastroesophageal reflux in infants and children often is based on parental and clinical observations. The diagnosis may be confirmed by esophageal pH probe studies or barium fluoroscopic esophagography. In severe cases, esophagoscopy may be used to demonstrate reflux and obtain a biopsy.

Various treatment methods are available for infants and children with gastroesophageal reflux. Small, frequent feedings are recommended because of the association between gastric volume and transient relaxation of the esophagus. Thickening an infant's feedings with cereal tends to decrease the volume of reflux, decrease crying and energy expenditure, and increase the calorie density of the formula.[9,10] In infants, positioning on the left side seems to decrease reflux. In older infants and children, raising the head of the bed and keeping the child upright may help. Medications usually are not added to the treatment regimen until pathologic reflux has been documented by diagnostic testing. Antacids are the most commonly used antireflux therapy and are readily available as over-the-counter preparations. H_2 receptor antagonists and proton pump inhibitors may be used in children with persistent reflux. Promotility agents may be used in selected cases.

CANCER OF THE ESOPHAGUS

Carcinoma of the esophagus accounts for approximately 6% of all gastrointestinal cancers. This disease is more common in older persons, with a mean age at diagnosis of 67 years. It is more frequent in men than women and is the seventh leading cause of cancer death among men, particularly black men.[2,11]

There are two types of esophageal cancers: squamous cell carcinoma and adenocarcinoma. Most squamous cell esophageal carcinomas are attributable to alcohol and tobacco use. Worldwide, squamous cell carcinomas constitute 90% of esophageal cancers, but in the United States there has been an exponential increase in adenocarcinomas associated with Barrett esophagus.[2] Endoscopic surveillance in people with Barrett esophagus provides the means for detecting adenocarcinoma at an earlier stage, when it is most amenable to curative surgical resection.[11] Although adenocarcinomas are usually found in the distal esophagus and may invade the adjacent upper part of the stomach, squamous cell carcinomas usually occur in the middle and lower third of the esophagus.[11]

Dysphagia is by far the most frequent complaint of persons with esophageal cancer. It is apparent first with ingestion of bulky food, later with soft food, and finally with liquids. Unfortunately, it is a late manifestation of the disease. Weight loss, anorexia, fatigue, and pain on swallowing also may occur.

Treatment of esophageal cancer depends on tumor stage. Surgical resection provides a means of cure when done in early disease and palliation when done in late disease. Radiation may be used as an alternative to surgery. Chemotherapy may be used before surgery to decrease the size of the tumor, or it may be used along with irradiation and surgery in an effort to increase survival.[11]

The prognosis for persons with cancer of the esophagus, although poor, has improved. Even with modern forms of therapy, however, the long-term survival is limited because, in many cases, the disease has already metastasized by the time the diagnosis is made.

> **In summary,** the esophagus is a tube that connects the oropharynx with the stomach; it functions primarily as a conduit for passage of food from the pharynx to the stomach. Dysphagia refers to difficulty in swallowing; it can result from altered nerve function or from disorders that produce narrowing of the esophagus. A diverticulum of the esophagus is an outpouching of the esophageal wall caused by a weakness of the muscularis layer.

> Gastroesophageal reflux refers to the backward movement of gastric contents into the esophagus, a condition that causes heartburn. Although most persons experience occasional esophageal reflux and heartburn, persistent reflux can cause esophagitis. Complications can result from persistent reflux, which produces a cycle of mucosal damage that causes hyperemia, edema, and erosion of the luminal surface. Persistent reflux can result in Barrett esophagus, a condition associated with increased risk for development of esophageal cancer. Gastroesophageal reflux is a common problem in infants and children. Reflux commonly corrects itself with age, and symptoms abate in most children by 2 years of age. Although many infants have minor degrees of reflux, some infants and small children have significant reflux that interferes with feeding, causes esophagitis, and results in respiratory symptoms and other complications.

> Carcinoma of the esophagus, which accounts for 6% of all gastrointestinal cancers, is more common in older persons (mean age, 67 years) and is more frequent in men than women. There are two types of esophageal cancer: squamous cell carcinomas and adenocarcinomas. Most squamous cell carcinomas are attributable to alcohol and tobacco use, whereas adenocarcinomas are more closely linked to esophageal reflux and Barrett esophagus.

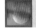

Disorders of the Stomach

The stomach is a reservoir for contents entering the digestive tract. It lies in the upper abdomen, anterior to the pancreas, splenic vessels, and left kidney. Anteriorly, the stomach is bounded by the anterior abdominal wall and the left inferior lobe of the liver. While in the stomach, food is churned and mixed with hydrochloric acid and pepsin before being released into the small intestine. Normally, the mucosal surface of the stomach provides a barrier that protects it from the hydrochloric acid and pepsin contained in gastric secretions. Disorders of the stomach include gastritis, peptic ulcer, and gastric carcinoma.

GASTRIC MUCOSAL BARRIER

The stomach lining usually is impermeable to the acid it secretes, a property that allows the stomach to contain acid and pepsin without having its wall digested. Several factors contribute to the protection of the gastric mucosa, including an impermeable epithelial cell surface covering, mechanisms for the selective transport of hydrogen and bicarbonate ions, and the characteristics of gastric mucus.[2,12] These mechanisms are collectively referred to as the *gastric mucosal barrier*.

The gastric epithelial cells are connected by tight junctions that prevent acid penetration, and they are covered with an impermeable hydrophobic lipid layer that prevents diffusion of ionized water-soluble molecules. Aspirin,

KEY CONCEPTS

Disruption of the Gastric Mucosa and Ulcer Development

➤ The stomach is protected by tight cellular junctions, a protective mucus layer, and prostaglandins that serve as chemical messengers to protect the stomach lining by improving blood flow, increasing bicarbonate secretion, and enhancing mucus production.

➤ Two of the major causes of gastric irritation and ulcer formation are aspirin or nonsteroidal anti-inflammatory drugs (NSAIDs) and infection with *Helicobacter pylori*.

➤ Aspirin and NSAIDs exert their destructive effects by damaging epithelial cells, impairing mucus production, and inhibiting prostaglandin synthesis.

➤ *H. pylori* is an infectious agent that thrives in the acid environment of the stomach and disrupts the mucosal barrier that protects the stomach from the harmful effects of its digestive enzymes.

which is nonionized and lipid soluble in acid solutions, rapidly diffuses across this lipid layer, increasing mucosal permeability and damaging epithelial cells. Gastric irritation and occult bleeding due to gastric irritation occur in a significant number of persons who take aspirin on a regular basis.[13] Alcohol, which also is lipid soluble, disrupts the mucosal barrier; when aspirin and alcohol are taken in combination, as they often are, there is increased risk of gastric irritation. Bile acids also attack the lipid components of the mucosal barrier and afford the potential for gastric irritation when there is reflux of duodenal contents into the stomach.

Normally, the secretion of hydrochloric acid by the parietal cells of the stomach is accompanied by secretion of bicarbonate ions (HCO_3^-). For every hydrogen ion (H^+) that is secreted, an HCO_3^- is produced, and as long as HCO_3^- production is equal to H^+ secretion, mucosal injury does not occur. Changes in gastric blood flow, as in shock, tend to decrease HCO_3^- production. This is particularly true in situations in which decreased blood flow is accompanied by acidosis. Prostaglandins, chemical messengers derived from cell membrane lipids, play an important role in protecting the gastrointestinal mucosa from injury. The prostaglandins probably exert their effect through improved blood flow, increased bicarbonate ion secretion, and enhanced mucus production. Aspirin and the nonsteroidal anti-inflammatory drugs (NSAIDs) inhibit both HCO_3^- secretion and prostaglandin synthesis, accounting in large part for their ability to produce gastric irritation.

GASTRITIS

Gastritis refers to inflammation of the gastric mucosa. There are many causes of gastritis, most of which can be grouped under the headings of acute and chronic gastritis.

Acute Gastritis

Acute gastritis refers to a transient inflammation of the gastric mucosa. It is most commonly associated with local irritants such as bacterial endotoxins, alcohol, and aspirin. Depending on the severity of the disorder, the mucosal response may vary from moderate edema and hyperemia to hemorrhagic erosion of the gastric mucosa.

The complaints of persons with acute gastritis vary. Persons with aspirin-related gastritis can be totally unaware of the condition or may complain only of heartburn or sour stomach. Gastritis associated with excessive alcohol consumption is a different situation; it often causes transient gastric distress, which may lead to vomiting and, in more severe situations, to bleeding and hematemesis. Gastritis caused by the toxins of infectious organisms, such as the staphylococcal enterotoxins, usually has an abrupt and violent onset, with gastric distress and vomiting ensuing approximately 5 hours after the ingestion of a contaminated food source. Acute gastritis usually is a self-limiting disorder, with complete regeneration and healing occurring within several days.

Chronic Gastritis

Chronic gastritis is a separate entity from acute gastritis. It is characterized by the absence of grossly visible erosions and the presence of chronic inflammatory changes leading eventually to atrophy of the glandular epithelium of the stomach. There are three major types of chronic gastritis: *Helicobacter pylori* gastritis, autoimmune gastritis, and chemical gastropathy.[14]

Helicobacter pylori **Gastritis.** *H. pylori* gastritis is a chronic inflammatory disease of the antrum and body of the stomach. It is the most common type of chronic nonerosive gastritis in the United States. In addition to chronic gastritis, this organism plays a critical role in other gastric and duodenal diseases, including peptic ulcer disease, gastric adenocarcinoma, and low-grade B-cell gastric lymphoma.[2,15–16] *H. pylori* are small, curved, gram-negative rods (protobacteria) that can colonize the mucus-secreting epithelial cells of the stomach[2,14–16] (Fig. 28-2). Circumstantial evidence suggests that the mode of transmission of *H. pylori* is primarily person-to-person. *H. pylori* have multiple flagella, which allow them to move through the mucous layer of the stomach, and they secrete urease, which enables them to produce sufficient ammonia to buffer the acidity of their immediate environment. These properties help to explain why the organism is able to survive in the acidic environment of the stomach. *H. pylori* produce enzymes and toxins that can interfere with the mucosal protection against injury from gastric acid, produce intense inflammation, and elicit an immune

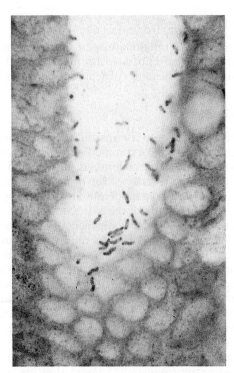

FIGURE 28-2 Infective gastritis. *H. pylori* appears on silver staining as small, curved rods on the surface of the gastric mucosa. (From Rubin E., Palazzo J. P. [2005]. The gastrointestinal tract. In Rubin E., Gorstein F., Rubin R., et al. [Eds.], *Rubin's pathology: Clinicopathologic foundations of medicine* [4th ed., p. 678]. Philadelphia: Lippincott Williams & Wilkins.)

response. There is increased production of proinflammatory cytokines that serve to recruit and activate neutrophils. Several *H. pylori* proteins are immunogenic and evoke an intense immune response in the mucosa. Both T and B cells can be seen in the chronic gastritis caused by *H. pylori*. Although the role of T and B cells in causing epithelial injury has not established, T-cell driven activation of B cells may be involved in the pathogenesis of gastric lymphomas.[2]

Methods for establishing the presence of *H. pylori* infection include a serologic test for antibodies, fecal bacterial detection, a urea breath test, and endoscopic biopsy for urease testing. The breath test is based on the generation of ammonia by bacterial urease. The serologic test can establish that a person has been infected with *H. pylori,* but it cannot determine how recently the infection occurred.

The goal for *H. pylori* treatment is the complete elimination of the organism. Current treatment consists of combination therapy that includes two or more antibiotics and a proton pump inhibitor or bismuth.[15,16] *H. pylori* mutate rapidly to develop antibiotic-resistant strains. The combination of two or more antimicrobial agents increases the rates of cure and reduces the risk of developing resistant strains. The proton pump inhibitors have direct antimicrobial properties against *H. pylori*, and by raising the intragastric pH they suppress bacterial growth and optimize antibiotic efficacy. Bismuth also has a direct antibacterial effect against *H. pylori*.

Autoimmune Gastritis. Autoimmune gastritis is the least common form of chronic gastritis. It typically involves the fundus and the body of the stomach and is associated with pernicious anemia. Most persons with the disorder have circulating antibodies to parietal cells and intrinsic factor, and hence this form of chronic gastritis is considered to be of autoimmune origin. Autoimmune destruction of the parietal cells leads to hypochlorhydria or achlorhydria, a high intragastric pH, and hypergastrinemia. Pernicious anemia is a megaloblastic anemia that is caused by malabsorption of vitamin B_{12} due to a deficiency of intrinsic factor (see Chapter 11). This type of chronic gastritis frequently is associated with other autoimmune disorders such as Hashimoto thyroiditis and Addison disease. Persons with autoimmune gastritis have a significant risk of developing gastric carcinoma.[2]

Chemical Gastropathy. Chemical gastropathy is a chronic gastric injury resulting from reflux of alkaline duodenal contents, pancreatic secretions, and bile into the stomach. It is most commonly seen in persons who have had gastroduodenostomy or gastrojejunostomy surgery. A milder form may occur in persons with gastric ulcer, gallbladder disease, or various motility disorders of the distal stomach.

ULCER DISEASE

Peptic Ulcer

Peptic ulcer is a term used to describe a group of ulcerative disorders that occur in areas of the upper gastrointestinal tract that are exposed to acid-pepsin secretions. The most common forms of peptic ulcer are duodenal and gastric ulcers. Peptic ulcer disease, with its remissions and exacerbations, represents a chronic health problem. Duodenal ulcers occur five times more commonly than gastric ulcers. Ulcers in the duodenum occur at any age and frequently are seen in early adulthood. Gastric ulcers tend to affect the older age group, with a peak incidence between 55 and 70 years of age. Both types of ulcers affect men three to four times more frequently than women.

A peptic ulcer can affect one or all layers of the stomach or duodenum (Fig. 28-3). The ulcer may penetrate only the mucosal surface, or it may extend into the smooth muscle layers. Occasionally, an ulcer penetrates the outer wall of the stomach or duodenum. Spontaneous remissions and exacerbations are common. Healing of the muscularis layer involves replacement with scar tissue; although the mucosal layers that cover the scarred muscle layer regenerate, the regeneration often is less than perfect, which contributes to repeated episodes of ulceration.

Since the early 1980s, there has been a radical shift in thinking regarding the cause of peptic ulcer. No longer is peptic ulcer thought to result from a genetic predisposition, stress, or dietary indiscretions. Most cases of peptic ulcer are caused by *H. pylori* infection.[16,17] The second most common cause of peptic ulcer is aspirin and other NSAIDs.[2] Aspirin appears to be the most ulcerogenic of the NSAIDs. In contrast to peptic ulcer from other causes,

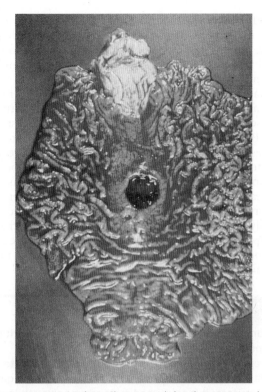

FIGURE 28-3 Gastric ulcer. The stomach has been opened to reveal a sharply demarcated, deep peptic ulcer on the lesser curvature. (From Rubin E., Palazzo J. P. [2005]. The gastrointestinal tract. In Rubin E., Gorstein F., Rubin R., et al. [Eds.], *Rubin's pathology: Clinicopathologic foundations of medicine* [4th ed., p. 683]. Philadelphia: Lippincott Williams & Wilkins.)

NSAID-induced gastric injury often is without symptoms, and life-threatening complications can occur without warning.

Manifestations. The clinical manifestations of uncomplicated peptic ulcer center around discomfort and pain. The pain, which is described as burning, gnawing, or cramplike, usually is rhythmic and frequently occurs when the stomach is empty—between meals and at 1 or 2 o'clock in the morning. The pain usually is located over a small area near the midline in the epigastrium near the xiphoid, and may radiate below the costal margins, into the back, or, rarely, to the right shoulder. Superficial and deep epigastric tenderness and voluntary muscle guarding may occur with more extensive lesions. An additional characteristic of ulcer pain is periodicity. The pain tends to recur at intervals of weeks or months. During an exacerbation, it occurs daily for a period of several weeks and then remits until the next recurrence. Characteristically, the pain is relieved by food or antacids.

The complications of peptic ulcer include hemorrhage, obstruction, and perforation. Hemorrhage is caused by bleeding from granulation tissue or from erosion of an ulcer into an artery or vein. Bleeding may be sudden, severe, and without warning, or it may be insidious, producing only occult blood in the stool. Acute hemorrhage is evidenced by the sudden onset of weakness, dizziness, thirst, cold, moist skin, the desire to defecate, and the passage of loose, tarry, or even red stools and coffee-ground emesis. Signs of circulatory shock develop depending on the amount of blood lost.

Obstruction is caused by edema, spasm, or contraction of scar tissue and interference with the free passage of gastric contents through the pylorus or adjacent areas. There is a feeling of epigastric fullness and heaviness after meals. With severe obstruction, there is vomiting of undigested food.

Perforation occurs when an ulcer erodes through all the layers of the stomach or duodenum wall. With perforation, gastrointestinal contents enter the peritoneum and cause peritonitis, or penetrate adjacent structures such as the pancreas. Radiation of the pain into the back, severe night distress, and inadequate pain relief from eating foods or taking antacids in persons with a long history of peptic ulcer may signify perforation. Peritonitis is discussed as a separate topic near the end of this chapter.

Diagnosis and Treatment. Diagnostic procedures for peptic ulcer include laboratory tests, radiologic imaging, and endoscopic examination. Laboratory findings of hypochromic anemia and occult blood in the stools indicate bleeding. Endoscopy (*i.e.*, gastroscopy and duodenoscopy) can be used to visualize the ulcer area and obtain biopsy specimens to test for *H. pylori* and exclude malignant disease. X-ray studies with a contrast medium such as barium are used to detect the presence of an ulcer crater and to exclude gastric carcinoma.

The treatment of peptic ulcer has changed dramatically over the past several years, and now aims to eradicate the cause and produce a permanent cure for the disease. Pharmacologic treatment focuses on eradication of *H. pylori* when infection is present, relieving ulcer symptoms, and healing the ulcer crater. With current therapies aimed at neutralization of gastric acid, inhibition of gastric acid (H_2 antagonists and proton pump inhibitors), and promotion of mucosal protection, most ulcers heal within a matter of weeks. When surgery is needed, it usually is performed using minimally invasive methods.

Zollinger-Ellison Syndrome

The Zollinger-Ellison syndrome is a rare condition caused by a gastrin-secreting tumor (gastrinoma). In persons with this disorder, gastric acid secretion reaches such levels that ulceration becomes inevitable.[17] The tumors may be single or multiple; although most tumors are located in the pancreas, a few develop in the submucosa of the stomach or duodenum. Over two thirds of gastrinomas are malignant.[17] The increased gastric secretions cause symptoms related to peptic ulcer. Diarrhea may result from hypersecretion or from the inactivation of intestinal lipase and impaired fat digestion that occurs with a decrease in intestinal pH.

Hypergastrinemia may also occur in an autosomal dominant disorder called the *multiple endocrine neoplasia type 1* (MEN 1) syndrome, which is characterized by hyperthyroidism and multiple endocrine neoplasms. The diagnosis of the Zollinger-Ellison syndrome is based on elevated serum gastrin and basal gastric acid levels and elimination of the MEN 1 syndrome as a cause of the disorder. Proton pump inhibitors are used to control gastric acid secretion. Computed tomography (CT), abdominal ultrasonography, and selective angiography are used to localize the tumor and determine if metastatic disease is present. Surgical removal is indicated when the tumor is malignant and has not metastasized.

Stress Ulcers

A stress ulcer, sometimes called *Curling ulcer*, refers to gastrointestinal ulcerations that develop in relation to major physiologic stress.[2] Persons at high risk for development of stress ulcers include those with large–surface-area burns, trauma, sepsis, acute respiratory distress syndrome, severe liver failure, and major surgical procedures. These lesions occur most often in the fundus of the stomach and proximal duodenum and are thought to result from ischemia, tissue acidosis, and bile salts entering the stomach in critically ill persons with decreased gastrointestinal tract motility.[2,18] Another form of stress ulcer, called *Cushing ulcer*, consists of gastric, duodenal, and esophageal ulcers arising in persons with intracranial injury, operations, or tumors. They are thought to be caused by hypersecretion of gastric acid resulting from stimulation of vagal nuclei by increased intracranial pressure.

Persons admitted to hospital intensive care units are at particular risk for development of stress ulcers. They usually are manifested by painless upper gastrointestinal tract bleeding. Monitoring and maintaining the gastric pH at 3.5 or higher helps to prevent the development of stress ulcers. H_2 receptor antagonists, proton pump inhibitors, and sucralfate are used in the prevention and treatment of stress ulcers.

CANCER OF THE STOMACH

Stomach cancer is the second most common cancer worldwide. However, its incidence varies widely, being particularly high in Japan, central Europe, the Scandinavian countries, South and Central America, the countries of the former Soviet Union, China, and Korea. In the United States, it accounts for about 2.5% of all cancer deaths.[2]

Among the factors that increase the risk of gastric cancer are a genetic predisposition, carcinogenic factors in the diet (*e.g.,* N-nitroso compounds and benzopyrene found in smoked and preserved foods), autoimmune gastritis, and gastric adenomas or polyps. The incidence of stomach cancer in the United States has decreased fourfold since 1930, presumably because of improved storage of food and decreased consumption of salted, smoked, and preserved foods.[2,14] Infection with *H. pylori* appears to serve as a cofactor in some types of gastric carcinomas.

Between 50% and 60% of gastric cancers occur in the pyloric region or adjacent to the antrum. Compared with a benign ulcer, which has smooth margins and is concentrically shaped, gastric cancers tend to be larger, are irregularly shaped, and have irregular margins.

Unfortunately, stomach cancers often are asymptomatic until late in their course. Symptoms, when they do occur, usually are vague and include indigestion, anorexia, weight loss, vague epigastric pain, vomiting, and an abdominal mass.

Diagnosis of gastric cancer is accomplished by means of a variety of techniques, including barium x-ray studies, endoscopic studies with biopsy, and cytologic studies (*e.g.,* Papanicolaou smear) of gastric secretions. Cytologic studies can prove particularly useful as routine screening tests for persons with atrophic gastritis or gastric polyps. CT and endoscopic ultrasonography often are used to delineate the spread of a diagnosed stomach cancer.

Surgery in the form of radical subtotal gastrectomy usually is the treatment of choice, with or without chemotherapy or radiation. The prognosis for stomach cancer depends on the depth of invasion and extent of nodal and distant metastasis at the time of diagnosis.[2]

In summary, disorders of the stomach include gastritis, peptic ulcer, and cancer of the stomach. Gastritis refers to inflammation of the gastric mucosa. Acute gastritis refers to a transient inflammation of the gastric mucosa; it is associated most commonly with local irritants such as bacterial endotoxins, caffeine, alcohol, and aspirin. Chronic gastritis is characterized by the absence of grossly visible erosions and the presence of chronic inflammatory changes leading eventually to atrophy of the glandular epithelium of the stomach. There are three main types of chronic gastritis: *H. pylori* gastritis, autoimmune gastritis, and chemical gastropathy. Chronic gastritis increases the risk of stomach cancer.

Peptic ulcer is a term used to describe a group of ulcerative disorders that occur in areas of the upper gastrointestinal tract that are exposed to acid-pepsin secretions, most commonly the duodenum and stomach. There are two main causes of peptic ulcer: *H. pylori* infection and aspirin or NSAID use. The treatment of peptic ulcer focuses on eradication of *H. pylori*, avoidance of gastric irritation from NSAIDs, and conventional pharmacologic treatment directed at symptom relief and ulcer healing.

The Zollinger-Ellison syndrome is a rare condition caused by a gastrin-secreting tumor, in which gastric acid secretion reaches such levels that ulceration becomes inevitable. Stress ulcers, also called *Curling ulcers*, occur in relation to major physiologic stresses such as burns and trauma and are thought to result from ischemia, tissue acidosis, and bile salts entering the stomach in critically ill persons with decreased gastrointestinal tract motility. Another form of stress ulcer, Cushing ulcers, occurs in persons with intracranial trauma or surgery and is thought to be caused by hypersecretion of gastric acid resulting from stimulation of vagal nuclei by increased intracranial pressure.

Although the incidence of stomach cancer has decreased during the past six decades in the United States, it remains the second most common cancer worldwide. Among the factors thought to predispose to the development of stomach cancer are *H. pylori* infection, carcinogenic factors in the diet (*e.g., N*-nitroso compounds and benzopyrene found in smoked and preserved foods), chronic gastritis, and gastric adenomas. Because there are few early symptoms with this form of cancer, the disease often is far advanced at the time of diagnosis.

Disorders of the Small and Large Intestines

There are many similarities in conditions that disrupt the integrity and function of the small and large intestine. The walls of the small and large intestines consist of five layers (see Chapter 27, Fig. 27-3): an outer serosal layer; a muscularis layer, which is divided into a layer of circular and a layer of longitudinal muscle fibers; a submucosal layer; and an inner mucosal layer, which lines the lumen of the intestine. Among the conditions that cause altered intestinal function are irritable bowel disease, inflammatory bowel disease, infectious colitis, diverticulitis, appendicitis, alterations in bowel motility (*i.e.,* diarrhea, constipation, and bowel obstruction), malabsorption syndrome, and cancer of the colon and rectum.

IRRITABLE BOWEL SYNDROME

The term *irritable bowel syndrome* is used to describe a functional gastrointestinal disorder characterized by a variable combination of chronic and recurrent intestinal symptoms not explained by structural or biochemical abnormalities. There is evidence to suggest that 10% to 20% of people in Western countries have the disorder, although most do not seek medical attention.[19]

Irritable bowel disease is characterized by persistent or recurrent symptoms of abdominal pain, altered bowel function, and varying complaints of flatulence, bloating, nausea and anorexia, constipation or diarrhea, and anxiety or depression. A hallmark of irritable bowel syndrome is abdominal pain that is relieved by defecation and associated with a change in consistency or frequency of stools. Abdominal pain usually is intermittent, cramping, and in the lower abdomen. It does not usually occur at night or interfere with sleep. The condition is believed to result from dysregulation of intestinal motor and sensory functions modulated by the CNS.[19,20] Persons with irritable bowel syndrome tend to experience increased motility and abnormal intestinal contractions in response to psychological and physiologic stress. Although changes in intestinal activity are normal responses to stress, these responses appear to be exaggerated in persons with irritable bowel syndrome. Women tend to be affected more often than men. Menarche often is associated with onset of the disorder. Women frequently notice an exacerbation of symptoms during the premenstrual period, suggesting a hormonal component.

Diagnosis of irritable bowel disease is usually based on signs and symptoms of abdominal pain or discomfort, bloating, constipation, diarrhea, or alternating constipation and diarrhea. A commonly used set of diagnostic criteria require continuous or recurrent symptoms of at least 12 weeks' duration (which may be nonconsecutive) of abdominal discomfort or pain in the preceding 12 months with two of three accompanying features: relief with defecation, onset associated with a change in bowel frequency, or onset associated with a change in form (appearance) of stool.[21] Other symptoms that support the diagnosis of irritable bowel syndrome include abnormal stool frequency (more than three times per day or less than three times per week), abnormal stool form (lumpy/hard or loose/watery), abnormal stool passage (straining, urgency, or feeling of incomplete evacuation), passage of mucus, and bloating or a feeling of abdominal distention.[21] A history of lactose intolerance should be considered because intolerance to lactose and other sugars may be a precipitating factor in some persons. The acute onset of symptoms raises the likelihood of organic disease, as do weight loss, anemia, fever, occult blood in the stool, nighttime symptoms, or signs and symptoms of malabsorption. These signs and symptoms require additional investigation.

The treatment of irritable bowel syndrome focuses on methods of stress management, particularly those related to symptom production. Reassurance is important. Usually, no special diet is indicated, although adequate fiber intake usually is recommended. Avoidance of offending dietary substances such as fatty and gas-producing foods, alcohol, and caffeine-containing beverages may be beneficial. Various pharmacologic agents, including antispasmodic and anticholinergic drugs, have been used with varying success in treatment of the disorder.

INFLAMMATORY BOWEL DISEASE

The term *inflammatory bowel disease* is used to designate two related inflammatory intestinal disorders: Crohn disease and ulcerative colitis. Even though the two diseases differ sufficiently to be distinguishable, they have many features in common. Both diseases produce inflammation of the bowel, both lack confirming evidence of a proven causative agent, both have a pattern of familial occurrence, and both can be accompanied by systemic manifestations.[22] The distinguishing characteristics of Crohn disease and ulcerative colitis are summarized in Table 28-1.

A number of systemic manifestations have been identified in persons with Crohn disease and ulcerative colitis. These include axial arthritis affecting the spine and sacroiliac joints and oligoarticular arthritis affecting the large joints of the arms and legs; inflammatory conditions of the eye, usually uveitis; skin lesions, especially erythema nodosum; stomatitis; and autoimmune anemia, hypercoagulability of blood, and sclerosing cholangitis. Occasionally, these systemic manifestations may

TABLE 28-1	Differentiating Characteristics of Crohn Disease and Ulcerative Colitis	
Characteristic	**Crohn Disease**	**Ulcerative Colitis**
Types of inflammation	Granulomatous	Ulcerative and exudative
Level of involvement	Primarily submucosal	Primarily mucosal
Extent of involvement	Skip lesions	Continuous
Areas of involvement	Primarily ileum, secondarily colon	Primarily rectum and left colon
Diarrhea	Common	Common
Rectal bleeding	Rare	Common
Fistulas	Common	Rare
Strictures	Common	Rare
Perianal abscesses	Common	Rare
Development of cancer	Uncommon	Relatively common

herald the recurrence of intestinal disease. In children, growth retardation may occur, particularly if the symptoms are prolonged and nutrient intake has been poor.

The causes of Crohn disease and ulcerative colitis are largely unknown. One of the common beliefs is that genetic factors predispose to some form of autoimmune reaction, possibly triggered by a relatively innocuous environmental agent such as a dietary antigen or microbial agent. The sites affected by inflammatory bowel disease, the distal ileum and the colon, are awash with bacteria. Although it is unlikely that inflammatory bowel disease is caused by microbes, it seems more likely that microbes may provide the antigenic trigger for an unregulated immune response. Interestingly, smoking tobacco has the opposite effect on the two forms of inflammatory bowel disease. It predisposes to development of Crohn disease, yet is associated with a reduced incidence of ulcerative colitis. Smoking also increases the likelihood of disease exaggeration and need for surgery in people with Crohn disease.[22]

A genetic basis of inflammatory bowel disease has long been suspected. Approximately 15% of persons with inflammatory bowel disease have affected first-degree relatives.[23] Both Crohn disease and ulcerative colitis have been linked to specific major histocompatibility class II (human leukocyte antigen [HLA]) alleles. Ulcerative colitis has been associated with HLA-D2 and Crohn disease with HLA-DR1 and HLA-DQw5 alleles, suggesting that the two diseases are genetically distinct.[2] A family history of inflammatory bowel disease is more common in Crohn disease than in ulcerative colitis. A putative susceptibility locus for Crohn disease has been mapped to chromosome 16.[23,24] Other susceptibility loci may located on chromosomes 3, 7, and 12.

Crohn Disease

Crohn disease is a recurrent, granulomatous type of inflammatory response that can affect any area of the gastrointestinal tract from the mouth to the anus. It most commonly affects the proximal portion of the colon and, less often, the terminal ileum. It is a slowly progressive, relentless, and often disabling disease. The disease usually

strikes people in their twenties or thirties, with women being affected slightly more often than men.

A characteristic feature of Crohn disease is the sharply demarcated, granulomatous lesions that are surrounded by normal-appearing mucosal tissue. When the lesions are multiple, they often are referred to as *skip lesions* because they are interspersed between what appear to be normal segments of the bowel. All the layers of the bowel are involved, with the submucosal layer affected to the greatest extent. The surface of the inflamed bowel usually has a characteristic "cobblestone" appearance resulting from the fissures and crevices that develop and that are surrounded by areas of submucosal edema[2,14] (Fig. 28-4). There usually is a relative sparing of the smooth muscle layers of the bowel, with marked inflammatory and fibrotic changes of the submucosal layer. Eventually, the bowel wall often becomes thick and inflexible; its appearance has been likened to a lead pipe or rubber hose. The adjacent mesentery may become inflamed, and the regional lymph nodes and channels may become enlarged.

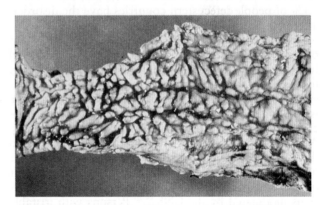

FIGURE 28-4 Crohn disease. The mucosal surface of the colon displays a "cobblestone" appearance owing to the presence of linear ulcerations and edema and inflammation of the intervening tissue. (From Rubin E., Palazzo J. P. [2005]. The gastrointestinal tract. In Rubin E., Gorstein F., Rubin R., et al. [Eds.], *Rubin's pathology: Clinicopathologic foundations of medicine* [4th ed., p. 714]. Philadelphia: Lippincott Williams & Wilkins.)

The clinical course of Crohn disease is variable; often, there are periods of exacerbations and remissions, with symptoms being related to the location of the lesions. The principal symptoms include intermittent diarrhea, colicky pain (usually in the lower right quadrant), weight loss, fluid and electrolyte disorders, malaise, and low-grade fever.[25] Because Crohn disease affects the submucosal layer to a greater extent than the mucosal layer, there is less bloody diarrhea than with ulcerative colitis. Ulceration of the perianal skin is common, largely because of the severity of the diarrhea. The absorptive surface of the intestine may be disrupted; nutritional deficiencies may occur, related to the specific segment of the intestine that is involved. When Crohn disease occurs in childhood, one of its major manifestations may be retardation of growth and physical development.

Complications of Crohn disease include fistula formation, abdominal abscess formation, and intestinal obstruction. Fistulas are tubelike passages that form connections between different sites in the gastrointestinal tract. They also may develop between other sites, including the bladder, vagina, urethra, and skin. Perineal fistulas that originate in the ileum are relatively common. Fistulas between segments of the gastrointestinal tract may lead to malabsorption, syndromes of bacterial overgrowth, and diarrhea. They also can become infected and cause abscess formation.

Diagnosis and Treatment. The diagnosis of Crohn disease requires a thorough history and physical examination. Sigmoidoscopy is used for direct visualization of the affected areas and to obtain biopsies. Measures are taken to exclude infectious agents as the cause of the disorder. This usually is accomplished by the use of stool cultures and examination of fresh stool specimens for ova and parasites. In persons suspected of having Crohn disease, radiographic contrast studies provide a means for determining the extent of involvement of the small bowel and establishing the presence and nature of fistulas. CT scans may be used to detect an inflammatory mass or abscess.

Treatment methods focus on terminating the inflammatory response and promoting healing, maintaining adequate nutrition, and preventing and treating complications. Nutritional deficiencies are common in Crohn disease because of diarrhea, steatorrhea (fatty stools), and other malabsorption problems. A nutritious diet that is high in calories, vitamins, and proteins is recommended. Elemental diets, which are nutritionally balanced but residue free and bulk free, may be given during the acute phase of the illness. These diets are largely absorbed in the jejunum and allow the inflamed bowel to rest. Total parenteral nutrition (i.e., parenteral hyperalimentation), which is administered intravenously, may be needed when food cannot be absorbed from the intestine.

Several medications have been successful in suppressing the inflammatory reaction, including the corticosteroids, sulfasalazine, metronidazole, 6-mercaptopurine, and cyclosporine. Sulfasalazine is a topically active agent that has a variety of anti-inflammatory effects. The beneficial effects of sulfasalazine are attributable to one compo-

nent of the drug, 5-aminosalicylic acid (5-ASA). Agents containing 5-ASA affect multiple sites in the arachidonic acid pathway critical to the pathogenesis of inflammation. Metronidazole is an antibiotic used to treat bacterial overgrowth in the small intestine. Immunosuppressive drugs such as cyclosporine and azathioprine or its active derivative, 6-mercaptopurine, also may be used. Infliximab, a monoclonal antibody that targets tumor necrosis factor-α (TNF-α), a mediator of the inflammatory response that is known to be important in granulomatous inflammatory processes such as Crohn disease, may be used for treatment of cases that do not respond to standard therapies.[23] Surgical resection of damaged bowel, drainage of abscesses, or repair of fistula tracts may be necessary.

Ulcerative Colitis

Ulcerative colitis is a nonspecific inflammatory condition of the colon. The disease is more common in the United States and Western countries. The disease may arise at any age, with a peak incidence between 20 and 25 years.[2] Unlike Crohn disease, which can affect various sites in the gastrointestinal tract, ulcerative colitis is confined to the rectum and colon. The disease usually begins in the rectum and spreads proximally, affecting primarily the mucosal layer, although it can extend into the submucosal layer. The length of proximal extension varies. It may involve the rectum alone (ulcerative proctitis), the rectum and sigmoid colon (proctosigmoiditis), or the entire colon (pancolitis). The inflammatory process tends to be confluent and continuous instead of skipping areas, as it does in Crohn disease.

Characteristic of the disease are the lesions that form in the crypts of Lieberkühn in the base of the mucosal layer (see Chapter 27, Fig. 27-10). The inflammatory process leads to the formation of pinpoint mucosal hemorrhages, which in time suppurate and develop into *crypt abscesses*. These inflammatory lesions may become necrotic and ulcerate. Although the ulcerations usually are superficial, they often extend, causing large denuded areas (Fig. 28-5). As a result of the inflammatory process, the mucosal layer often develops tonguelike projections that resemble polyps and therefore are called *pseudopolyps*. The bowel wall thickens in response to repeated episodes of colitis.

Diarrhea, which is the characteristic manifestation of ulcerative colitis, varies according to the severity of the disease. There may be up to 30 to 40 bowel movements a day. Because ulcerative colitis affects the mucosal layer of the bowel, the stools typically contain blood and mucus. Nocturnal diarrhea usually occurs when daytime symptoms are severe. There may be mild abdominal cramping and fecal incontinence. Anorexia, weakness, and fatigability are common.

Ulcerative colitis usually follows a course of remissions and exacerbations. The severity of the disease varies from mild to fulminating. Accordingly, the disease has been divided into three types: mild chronic, chronic intermittent, and acute fulminating. The most common form of the disease is the mild chronic, in which bleeding and diarrhea

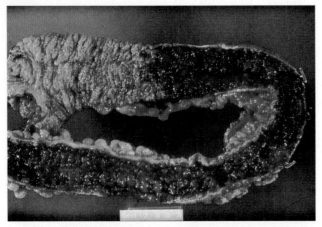

FIGURE 28-5 Ulcerative colitis. Prominent erythema and ulceration of the colon begin in the ascending colon and are most severe in the rectosigmoid area. (From Rubin E., Palazzo J. P. [2005]. The gastrointestinal tract. In Rubin E., Gorstein F., Rubin R., et al. [Eds.], *Rubin's pathology: Clinicopathologic foundations of medicine* [4th ed., p. 716]. Philadelphia: Lippincott Williams & Wilkins.)

are mild and systemic signs are minimal or absent. This form of the disease usually can be managed conservatively. The chronic intermittent form continues after the initial attack. Compared with the milder form, more of the colon surface usually is involved with the chronic intermittent form, and there are more systemic signs and complications. In approximately 15% of affected persons, the disease assumes a more fulminant course, involves the entire colon, and manifests with severe, bloody diarrhea, fever, and acute abdominal pain. These persons are at risk for development of toxic megacolon, which is characterized by dilatation of the colon and signs of systemic toxicity. It results from extension of the inflammatory response, with involvement of neural and vascular components of the bowel. Contributing factors include use of laxatives, narcotics, and anticholinergic drugs and the presence of hypokalemia.

Cancer of the colon is one of the feared complications of ulcerative colitis. The risk for development of cancer among persons who have had pancolitis for 10 years or more is 20 to 30 times that of the general population.[2,14]

Diagnosis and Treatment. Diagnosis of ulcerative colitis is based on history and physical examination. The diagnosis usually is confirmed by proctosigmoidoscopy.

Treatment depends on the extent of the disease and severity of symptoms. It includes measures to control the acute manifestations of the disease and prevent recurrence. Some people with mild to moderate symptoms are able to control their symptoms simply by avoiding caffeine, lactose (milk), highly spiced foods, and gas-forming foods. Fiber supplements may be used to decrease diarrhea and rectal symptoms.

The medications used in treatment of ulcerative colitis are similar to those used in the treatment of Crohn disease.[25] The corticosteroids are used selectively to lessen the acute inflammatory response. Many of these medications can be administered rectally by suppository or enema. Immunosuppressant drugs, such as cyclosporine, may be used to treat persons with severe colitis. Surgical treatment (*i.e.*, removal of the rectum and entire colon) with the creation of an ileostomy or ileoanal anastomosis may be required for those persons with ulcerative colitis who do not respond to conservative methods of treatment.

INFECTIOUS ENTEROCOLITIS

A number of microbial agents can infect the intestine, including viruses, bacteria, and protozoa. Most infections are spread by oral-fecal route, often through contaminated water or food.

Viral Infection

Most viral infections affect the superficial epithelium of the small intestine, destroying these cells and disrupting their absorptive function. Repopulation of the small intestine villi with immature enterocytes and preservation of crypt secretory cells leads to net secretion of water and electrolytes compounded by incomplete absorption of nutrients and osmotic diarrhea. Symptomatic disease is caused by several distinct viruses, including the rotavirus, which most commonly affects children 6 to 24 months of age; caliciviruses, previously referred to as the Norwalk family of viruses, which are responsible for most cases of nonbacterial gastroenteritis in older children and adults; and adenoviruses, which are another common cause of diarrhea in children.[14]

Rotavirus. Worldwide, rotavirus is estimated to cause more than 125 million cases of diarrhea in children younger than 5 years of age. In the United States, the disease causes 3 million cases of diarrhea, 50,000 hospitalizations, and 20 to 40 deaths.[26] The disease tends to be most severe in children 3 to 24 months of age. Infants younger than 3 months of age are relatively protected by transplacental antibodies and possibly by breast-feeding. The virus is spread through a fecal-oral route and outbreaks are common in children in day care centers. The virus is shed before and for days after clinical illness.

Rotavirus infection typically begins after an incubation period of less than 24 hours, with mild to moderate fever and vomiting, followed by onset of frequent, watery stools. The fever and vomiting usually disappear on about the second day, but the diarrhea continues for 5 to 7 days. Dehydration may develop rapidly, particularly in infants. Treatment is largely supportive. Avoiding and treating dehydration are the main goals.[26]

Bacterial Infection

Bacterial infections exert their effects through the ingestion of organisms that proliferate in the gut lumen and elaborate an enterotoxin or that invade and destroy the epithelial cells of the intestine. The pathogenic effects of bacterial infections depend on the ability of the organism to adhere to the mucosal epithelial cells, elaborate enterotoxins, and invade the epithelial cells of the intestinal mucosa. Some forms of food poisoning result from the ingestion of preformed bacterial toxins, one of the major offenders being the toxins of *Staphylococcus aureus.*

In general, bacterial infections produce more severe effects than viral infections. The complications of bacterial enterocolitis result from massive fluid loss or destruction of intestinal mucosa and include dehydration, sepsis, and perforation. Two particularly serious forms of bacterial enterocolitis are those caused by *Clostridium difficile* and *Escherichia coli* O157:H7.

Clostridium difficile Colitis.

C. difficile colitis, sometimes called *antibiotic-associated colitis,* usually occurs in persons without a history of enteric disease after a course of antibiotic therapy.[2,27] *C. difficile* is a gram-positive, spore-forming bacillus that is part of the normal flora in 1% to 3% of humans.[27] The spores are resistant to the acid environment of the stomach and convert to vegetative forms in the colon. Treatment with broad-spectrum antibiotics predisposes to disruption of the normal protective bacterial flora of the colon, leading to colonization by *C. difficile* along with the release of toxins that cause mucosal damage and inflammation. Almost any antibiotic may cause *C. difficile* colitis, but broad-spectrum antibiotics with activity against gram-negative enteric bacteria are the most frequent agents. After antibiotic therapy has made the bowel susceptible to infection, colonization by *C. difficile* occurs by the oral-fecal route. *C. difficile* infection usually is acquired in the hospital, where the organism is commonly encountered.

In general, *C. difficile* is noninvasive. Development of *C. difficile* colitis and diarrhea requires an alteration in the normal gut flora, acquisition and germination of the spores, overgrowth of *C. difficile,* and toxin production. The toxins bind to the intestinal mucosa, causing hemorrhage, inflammation, and necrosis. The toxins also interfere with protein synthesis, attract inflammatory cells, increase capillary permeability, and stimulate intestinal peristalsis. The infection commonly manifests with diarrhea that is mild to moderate and sometimes is accompanied by lower abdominal cramping. Typically, symptoms begin within 1 to 2 weeks after an antibiotic treatment has been started, although presentation varies from 1 day to 6 weeks.[27] In most cases, systemic manifestations are absent, and the symptoms subside after the antibiotic has been discontinued.

Diagnostic findings include a history of antibiotic use and laboratory tests that confirm the presence of *C. difficile* toxins in the stool. Treatment includes the immediate discontinuation of antibiotic therapy. Specific treatment aimed at eradicating *C. difficile* is used when symptoms are severe or persistent.

A more severe form of colitis, *pseudomembranous colitis,* is characterized by an adherent inflammatory membrane overlying the areas of mucosal injury.[2] It is a life-threatening form of the disease. Persons with the disease are acutely ill, with lethargy, fever, tachycardia, abdominal pain and distention, and dehydration. The smooth muscle tone of the colon may be lost, resulting in toxic dilatation of the colon. Prompt therapy is needed to prevent perforation of the bowel.

Escherichia coli O157:H7 Infection.

E. coli O157:H7 is now recognized as an important cause of epidemic and sporadic colitis.[28] *E. coli* O157:H7 is a strain of *E. coli* found in feces and contaminated milk of healthy dairy and beef cattle, but it also has been found in contaminated pork, poultry, and lamb. Infection usually is by food-borne transmission, often by ingesting undercooked hamburger. The organism also can be transferred to nonmeat products such as fruits and vegetables. Person-to-person transmission may occur, particularly in nursing homes, day care settings, and hospitals. The very young and the very old are particularly at risk for the infection and its complications.

The infection may cause no symptoms or cause a variety of manifestations, including acute, nonbloody diarrhea, hemorrhagic colitis, hemolytic-uremic syndrome, and thrombotic thrombocytopenic purpura. The infection often presents with abdominal cramping and watery diarrhea and subsequently may progress to bloody diarrhea. The diarrhea commonly lasts 3 to 7 days or longer, with 10 to 12 diarrheal episodes per day. Fever occurs in up to one third of the cases.

An important aspect of the disease is the production of toxins and the ability to produce toxemia. Two complications of the infection, hemolytic-uremic syndrome and thrombotic thrombocytopenic purpura, reflect the effects of toxins. Hemolytic-uremic syndrome is characterized by hemolytic anemia, thrombocytopenia, and renal failure. It occurs predominantly in infants and young children and is the most common cause of acute renal failure in children.[28] It has a mortality rate of 5% to 10%, and one third of the survivors are left with permanent disability. Thrombotic thrombocytopenic purpura is manifested by thrombocytopenia, renal failure, fever, and neurologic manifestations. It often is regarded as the severe end of the disease that leads to hemolytic-uremic syndrome plus neurologic problems.

No specific therapy is available for *E. coli* O157:H7 infection. Treatment is largely symptomatic and directed toward treating the effects of complications. Antibiotics have not proved useful and may even be harmful, extending the duration of bloody diarrhea. Because of the seriousness of the infection and its complications, education of the public about techniques for decreasing primary transmission of the infection from animal sources is important. Undercooked meats and unpasteurized milk are sources of transmission. The U.S. Food and Drug Administration recommends a minimal internal temperature of 155°F for cooked hamburger. Food handlers and consumers should be aware of the proper methods for handling uncooked meat to prevent cross-contamination of other foods. Particular attention should be paid to hygiene in day care centers and nursing homes, where the spread of infection to the very young and very old may result in severe complications.[28]

DIVERTICULAR DISEASE

Diverticulosis is a condition in which the mucosal layer of the colon herniates through the muscularis layer.[29] There are often multiple diverticula, most of which occur in the sigmoid colon (Fig. 28-6). Diverticular disease is common in Western society, affecting approximately 5% to 10% of the population older than 45 years of age and almost 80% of those older than 85 years.[29] Although the disorder is prevalent in the developed countries of the world, it is almost nonexistent in many African nations and underdeveloped countries. This suggests that dietary factors (*e.g.,* lack of fiber content), a decrease in physical activity, and poor bowel habits (*e.g.,* neglecting the urge to defecate), along with the effects of aging, contribute to the development of the disease.

In the colon, the longitudinal muscle does not form a continuous layer, as it does in the small bowel. Instead, there are three separate longitudinal bands of muscle called the *teniae coli.* In a manner similar to the small intestine, bands of circular muscle constrict the large intestine. At each of these constrictive points (approximately every 2.5 cm), the circular muscle contracts, sometimes constricting the lumen of the bowel so that it is almost occluded (see Fig. 28-6). The combined contraction of the circular muscle and the lack of a continuous longitudinal muscle layer normally causes the intestine to bulge outward into pouches called *haustra.* Diverticula develop between the longitudinal muscle bands of the haustra, in the area where the blood vessels pierce the circular muscle layer to bring blood to the mucosal layer. An increase in intraluminal pressure in the haustra provides the force for creating these herniations. The increase in pressure is thought to be related to the volume of the colonic contents. The scantier the contents, the more vigorous are the contractions and the greater is the pressure in the haustra.

Most persons with diverticular disease remain asymptomatic. The disease often is found when x-ray studies are done for other purposes. When symptoms do occur, they often are attributed to other causes. Ill-defined lower abdominal discomfort, a change in bowel habits (*e.g.,* diarrhea, constipation), bloating, and flatulence are common.

Diverticulitis is a complication of diverticulosis in which there is inflammation and gross or microscopic perforation of the diverticulum. One of the most common complaints of diverticulitis is pain in the lower left quadrant, accom-

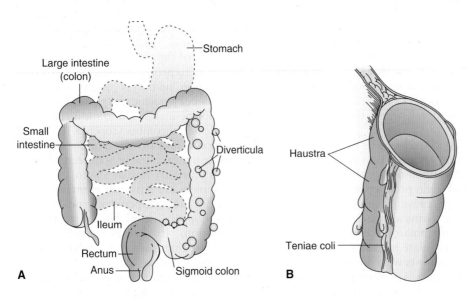

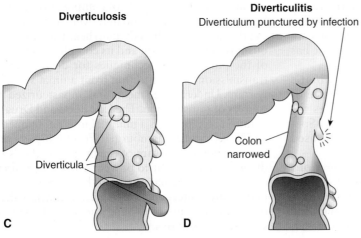

FIGURE 28-6 (**A**) Location of diverticula in the sigmoid colon. (**B**) A portion of the sigmoid colon, showing the haustra and teniae coli. (**C**) Diverticulosis. (**D**) Diverticulitis. (From National Digestive Diseases Information Clearinghouse. [1989]. *Clearinghouse fact sheet: Diverticulosis and diverticulitis.* NIH publication no. 90-1163. Washington, DC: U.S. Department of Health and Human Services.)

panied by nausea and vomiting, tenderness in the lower left quadrant, a slight fever, and an elevated white blood cell count. These symptoms usually last for several days, unless complications occur, and usually are caused by localized inflammation of the diverticula with perforation and development of a small, localized abscess. Complications include perforation with peritonitis, hemorrhage, and bowel obstruction. Fistulas can form, usually involving the bladder (*i.e.,* vesicosigmoid fistula) but sometimes involving the skin, perianal area, or small bowel.

The diagnosis of diverticular disease is based on history and presenting clinical manifestations. The disease may be confirmed by barium enema x-ray studies, CT scans, and ultrasonographic studies. CT scans are the safest and most cost-effective method.[29] Because of the risk of peritonitis, barium enema studies should be avoided in persons who are suspected of having acute diverticulitis. Flat abdominal radiographs may be used to detect complications associated with acute diverticulitis.

The usual treatment for diverticular disease is aimed at preventing symptoms and complications. This includes increasing the bulk in the diet and bowel retraining so that the person has at least one bowel movement each day. The increased bulk promotes regular defecation and increases colonic contents and colon diameter, thereby decreasing intraluminal pressure. Acute diverticulitis is treated by withholding solid food and administering a broad-spectrum antibiotic. Surgical treatment is reserved for complications.

APPENDICITIS

Acute appendicitis is extremely common. It is seen most frequently in the 5- to 30-year-old age group, but can occur at any age. The appendix becomes inflamed, swollen, and gangrenous, and it eventually perforates if not treated. Although the cause of appendicitis is unknown, it is thought to be related to intraluminal obstruction with a fecalith (*i.e.,* hard piece of stool) or to twisting.

Appendicitis usually has an abrupt onset, with pain referred to the epigastric or periumbilical area. This pain is caused by stretching of the appendix during the early inflammatory process. At approximately the same time that the pain appears, there are one or two episodes of nausea. Initially, the pain is vague, but over a period of 2 to 12 hours, it gradually increases and may become colicky. When the inflammatory process has extended to involve the serosal layer of the appendix and the peritoneum, the pain becomes localized to the lower right quadrant. There usually is an elevation in temperature and a white blood cell count. Palpation of the abdomen usually reveals a deep tenderness in the lower right quadrant, which is confined to a small area approximately the size of the fingertip. Rebound tenderness, which is pain that occurs when pressure is applied to the area and then released, and spasm of the overlying abdominal muscles are common.

Diagnosis is usually based on history and findings on physical examination. Ultrasonography or CT may be used to confirm the diagnosis.[30] Treatment consists of surgical removal of the appendix. Complications include peri-

tonitis, localized periappendiceal abscess formation, and septicemia.

ALTERATIONS IN INTESTINAL MOTILITY

The movement of contents through the gastrointestinal tract is controlled by neurons located in the submucosal and myenteric plexuses of the gut (see Chapter 27). The axons from the cell bodies in the myenteric plexus innervate the circular and longitudinal smooth muscle layers of the gut. These neurons receive impulses from local receptors located in the mucosal and muscle layers of the gut and extrinsic input from the parasympathetic and sympathetic nervous systems. As a general rule, the parasympathetic nervous system tends to increase the motility of the bowel, whereas sympathetic stimulation tends to slow its activity.

The colon has sphincters at both ends: the ileocecal sphincter, which separates it from the small intestine, and the anal sphincter, which prevents the movement of feces to the outside of the body. The colon acts as a reservoir for fecal material. Normally, approximately 400 mL of water, 55 mEq of sodium, 30 mEq of chloride, and 15 mEq of bicarbonate are absorbed each day in the colon. At the same time, approximately 5 mEq of potassium is secreted into the lumen of the colon. The amount of water and electrolytes that remains in the stool reflects the absorption or secretion that occurs in the colon. The average adult ingesting a typical American diet evacuates approximately 200 to 300 g of stool each day.

Diarrhea

The usual definition of *diarrhea* is excessively frequent passage of stools. Diarrhea can be acute or chronic. Diarrhea is considered to be chronic when the symptoms persist

KEY CONCEPTS

Alterations in Intestinal Motility

- The enteric nervous system that is incorporated into the wall of the gut controls the basic motility of the gastrointestinal tract, with input from the autonomic nervous system.

- Local irritation and the composition and constituents of gastrointestinal contents influence motility through the submucosal afferent neurons of the enteric nervous system. Gastrointestinal wall distention, chemical irritants, osmotic gradients, and bacterial toxins exert many of their effects on gastrointestinal motility through these afferent pathways.

- Autonomic influences generated by factors such as medications, trauma, and emotional experiences interact with the enteric nervous system to alter gastrointestinal motility.

for 3 weeks in children or adults and 4 weeks in infants. In developing countries, diarrhea is a common cause of mortality among children younger than 5 years of age, with an estimated two million deaths annually.[31] Even though diarrheal diseases are less prevalent in the United States than in other countries, they place a burden on the health care system. Approximately 1.5 million children are seen in outpatient clinics and 220,000 are hospitalized each year for acute gastroenteritis.[31]

The complaint of diarrhea is a general one and can be related to a number of pathologic and nonpathologic factors. Diarrhea can be acute or chronic and can be caused by infectious organisms, food intolerance, drugs, or intestinal disease. Acute diarrheas that last less than 4 days are predominantly caused by infectious agents and follow a self-limited course.[32] Chronic diarrheas are those that persist for longer than 3 to 4 weeks. They often are caused by conditions such as inflammatory bowel disease, irritable bowel syndrome, malabsorption syndrome, endocrine disorders (hyperthyroidism, diabetic autonomic neuropathy), or radiation colitis.

Diarrhea commonly is divided into two types, large volume and small volume, based on the characteristics of the diarrheal stool. Large-volume diarrhea results from an increase in the water content of the stool, and small-volume diarrhea results from an increase in the propulsive activity of the bowel. Some of the common causes of small- and large-volume diarrhea are summarized in Chart 28-1. Often, diarrhea is a combination of these two types.

CHART 28-1

Causes of Large- and Small-Volume Diarrhea

Large-Volume Diarrhea

Osmotic diarrhea
   Saline cathartics
   Lactase deficiency
Secretory diarrhea
   Acute infectious diarrhea
   Failure to absorb bile salts
   Fat malabsorption
   Chronic laxative abuse
   Carcinoid syndrome
   Zollinger-Ellison syndrome
   Fecal impaction

Small-Volume Diarrhea

Inflammatory bowel disease
   Crohn disease
   Ulcerative colitis
Infectious disease
   Shigellosis
   Salmonellosis
Irritable colon

Large-Volume Diarrhea. Large-volume diarrhea can be classified as secretory or osmotic, according to the cause of the increased water content in the feces. Water is pulled into the colon along an osmotic gradient (*i.e.,* osmotic diarrhea) or is secreted into the bowel by the mucosal cells (*i.e.,* secretory diarrhea). The large-volume form of diarrhea usually is a painless, watery type without blood or pus in the stools.

In osmotic diarrhea, water is pulled into the bowel by the hyperosmotic nature of its contents. It occurs when osmotically active particles are not absorbed. In persons with lactase deficiency, the lactose in milk cannot be broken down and absorbed. Magnesium salts, which are contained in milk of magnesia and many antacids, are poorly absorbed and cause diarrhea when taken in sufficient quantities. Another cause of osmotic diarrhea is decreased transit time, which interferes with absorption. Osmotic diarrhea usually disappears with fasting.

Secretory diarrhea occurs when the secretory processes of the bowel are increased. Most acute infectious diarrheas are of this type. Enteric organisms cause diarrhea by several ways. Some are noninvasive but secrete toxins that stimulate fluid secretion (*e.g., Vibrio cholerae,* pathogenic *E. coli,* and rotavirus).[33,34] Others (*e.g., Shigella, Salmonella, Yersinia,* and *Campylobacter*) invade and destroy intestinal epithelial cells, thereby altering fluid transport so that secretory activity continues while absorption activity is halted.[33] Secretory diarrhea also occurs when excess bile acids remain in the intestinal contents as they enter the colon. This can occur with disease processes of the ileum because bile salts are absorbed there, or it may be caused by bacterial overgrowth in the small bowel, which interferes with bile absorption.

Small-Volume Diarrhea. Small-volume diarrhea commonly is associated with acute or chronic inflammation or intrinsic disease of the colon, such as ulcerative colitis or Crohn disease. Small-volume diarrhea usually is evidenced by frequency and urgency and colicky abdominal pain. It commonly is accompanied by tenesmus (*i.e.,* painful straining at stool), fecal soiling of clothing, and awakening during the night with the urge to defecate.

Diagnosis and Treatment. The diagnosis of diarrhea is based on complaints of frequent stools and a history of accompanying factors such as concurrent illnesses, medication use, and exposure to potential intestinal pathogens. If the onset of diarrhea is related to travel outside the United States, the possibility of traveler's diarrhea must be considered.

Although most acute forms of diarrhea are self-limited and require no treatment, diarrhea can be particularly serious in infants and small children, persons with other illnesses, and the elderly. Thus, the replacement of fluids and electrolytes is considered to be a primary therapeutic goal in the treatment of diarrhea. Oral replacement therapy (ORT) can be used in situations of uncomplicated diarrhea that can be treated at home. First applied to the treatment of diarrhea in developing countries, ORT can be regarded as a case of reverse technology, in which the protocols originally implemented in these countries have changed health care practices in industrialized countries as well.[31] Complete ORT solutions contain carbohydrate, sodium, potassium, chloride, and base to replace that lost in the diarrheal stool.[31,35] Commonly used beverages such as apple juice and cola drinks, which have increased osmolarity because of their high carbohydrate and low electrolyte content, are not recommended. The effectiveness of ORT is based on the coupled transport of sodium and glucose or other actively transported small organic molecules. ORT can be particularly effective in treating dehydration associated with diarrheal diseases in infants and small children. Bottled ORT solutions are available but can be costly, particularly in cases where large amounts of replacement fluids are needed. Less expensive premeasured packets and recipes for preparing replacement solutions are available.

Evidence suggests that feeding should be continued during diarrheal illness, particularly in children.[31] It is recommended that children who require rehydration therapy because of diarrhea be fed an age-appropriate diet. Starch and simple proteins are thought to provide cotransport molecules with little osmotic activity, increasing fluid and electrolyte absorption by intestinal cells.[31,35] Although there is little agreement on which foods are best, fatty foods and foods high in simple sugars are best avoided.

Drugs used in the treatment of diarrhea include diphenoxylate and loperamide, which are opium-like drugs. These drugs decrease gastrointestinal motility and stimulate water and electrolyte absorption. Adsorbents, such as kaolin and pectin, available in many over-the-counter preparations, adsorb irritants and toxins from the bowel. Diarrheal medications should not be used in persons with bloody diarrhea, high fever, or signs of toxicity for fear of worsening the disease. Antibiotics are reserved for persons with identified enteric pathogens.

Constipation

Constipation can be defined as the infrequent passage of stools. The difficulty with this definition arises from the many individual variations of function that are normal. What is considered normal for one person (*e.g.*, two or three bowel movements per week) may be considered evidence of constipation by another. The problem increases with age; there is a sharp rise in health care visits for constipation after 65 years of age.

Constipation can occur as a primary problem or as a problem associated with another disease condition. Some common causes of constipation are failure to respond to the urge to defecate, inadequate fiber in the diet, inadequate fluid intake, weakness of the abdominal muscles, inactivity and bed rest, pregnancy, and hemorrhoids. Diseases associated with chronic constipation include neurologic diseases such as spinal cord injury, Parkinson disease, and multiple sclerosis; endocrine disorders such as hypothyroidism; and obstructive lesions in the gastrointestinal tract. Drugs such as narcotics, anticholinergic agents, calcium channel blockers, diuretics, calcium (antacids and supplements), iron supplements, and aluminum antacids

tend to cause constipation. Elderly people with long-standing constipation may develop dilatation of the rectum, colon, or both. This condition allows large amounts of stool to accumulate with little or no sensation. Constipation, in the context of a change in bowel habits, may be a sign of colorectal cancer.

Diagnosis of constipation usually is based on a history of infrequent stools, straining with defecation, the passing of hard and lumpy stools, or the sense of incomplete evacuation with defecation.[36] Constipation as a sign of another disease condition should be ruled out. The treatment of constipation usually is directed toward relieving the cause. A conscious effort should be made to respond to the defecation urge. A time should be set aside after a meal, when mass movements in the colon are most likely to occur, for a bowel movement. Adequate fluid intake and bulk in the diet should be encouraged. Moderate exercise is essential, and persons on bed rest benefit from passive and active exercises. Laxatives and enemas should be used judiciously. They should not be used on a regular basis to treat simple constipation because they interfere with the defecation reflex and actually may damage the rectal mucosa.

Intestinal Obstruction

Intestinal obstruction designates an impairment of movement of intestinal contents in a cephalocaudal direction. The causes can be categorized as mechanical or paralytic obstruction. Strangulation (occlusion of blood vessels) with necrosis of the bowel may occur and lead to perforation, peritonitis, and sepsis.

Mechanical obstruction can result from a number of conditions, intrinsic or extrinsic, that encroach on the patency of the bowel lumen (Fig. 28-7). Major inciting causes include external hernia (*i.e.*, inguinal, femoral, or umbilical) and postoperative adhesions. Less common causes are strictures, tumor, foreign bodies, intussusception, and volvulus. Intussusception involves the telescoping of bowel into the adjacent segment. It is the most common cause of intestinal obstruction in children younger than 2 years of age.[37] The most common form is intussusception of the terminal ileum into the right colon, but other areas of the bowel may be involved. In most cases, the cause of the disorder is unknown. The condition can also occur in adults when an intraluminal mass or tumor acts as a traction force and pulls the segment along as it telescopes into the distal segment. Volvulus refers to a complete twisting of the bowel on an axis formed by its mesentery (see Fig. 28-7). Mechanical bowel obstruction may take the form of a simple obstruction, in which there is no alteration in blood flow, or a strangulated obstruction, in which there is impairment of blood flow and necrosis of bowel tissue.

Paralytic, or adynamic, obstruction results from neurogenic or muscular impairment of peristalsis. Paralytic ileus is seen most commonly after abdominal surgery. It also accompanies inflammatory conditions of the abdomen, intestinal ischemia, pelvic fractures, and back injuries. It occurs early in the course of peritonitis and can result from chemical irritation caused by bile, bacterial toxins,

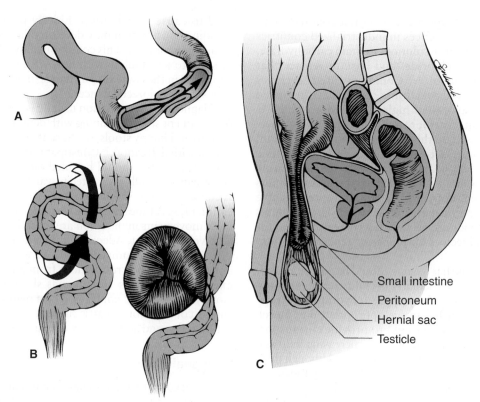

Small intestine
Peritoneum
Hernial sac
Testicle

FIGURE 28-7 Three causes of intestinal obstruction. (**A**) Intussusception with invagination or shortening of the bowel caused by movement of one segment of the bowel into another. (**B**) Volvulus of the sigmoid colon; the twist is counterclockwise in most cases. Note the edematous section of bowel. (**C**) Hernia (inguinal). The sac of the hernia is a continuation of the peritoneum of the abdomen. The hernial contents are intestine, omentum, or other abdominal contents that pass through the hernial opening into the hernial sac. (From Smeltzer S. C., Bare B. G. [2004]. *Brunner and Suddarth's textbook of medical-surgical nursing* [10th ed., p. 1055]. Philadelphia: Lippincott Williams & Wilkins.)

electrolyte imbalances as in hypokalemia, and vascular insufficiency.

The major effects of both types of intestinal obstruction are abdominal distention and loss of fluids and electrolytes (Fig. 28-8). Gases and fluids accumulate in the area; if untreated, the distention resulting from bowel obstruction tends to perpetuate itself by causing atony of the bowel and further distention. Distention is further aggravated by the accumulation of gases. Approximately 70% of these gases are derived from swallowed air. As the process continues, the distention moves proximally (*i.e.,* toward the mouth), involving additional segments of bowel. Either form of obstruction eventually may lead to strangulation (*i.e.,* interruption of blood flow), gangrenous changes, and, ultimately, perforation of the bowel. The increased pressure in the intestine tends to compromise mucosal blood flow, leading to necrosis and movement of blood into the luminal fluids. This promotes rapid growth of bacteria in the obstructed bowel. Anaerobes grow rapidly in this favorable environment and can produce a lethal endotoxin.

The manifestations of intestinal obstruction depend on the degree of obstruction and its duration. With acute obstruction, the onset usually is sudden and dramatic. With chronic conditions, the onset often is more gradual. The cardinal symptoms of intestinal obstruction are pain, absolute constipation, abdominal distention, and vomiting. With mechanical obstruction, the pain is severe and colicky, in contrast with the continuous pain and silent abdomen of paralytic ileus. There also is borborygmus (*i.e.,* rumbling sounds made by propulsion of gas in the intestine); audible, high-pitched peristalsis; and peristaltic rushes. Visible peristalsis may appear along the course of the distended intestine. Extreme restlessness and conscious awareness of intestinal movements are experienced along with weakness, perspiration, and anxiety. Should strangulation occur, the character of the pain shifts from the intermittent colicky pain caused by the hyperperistaltic movements of the intestine to a severe and steady type of pain. Vomiting and fluid and electrolyte disorders occur with both types of obstruction.

Diagnosis of intestinal obstruction usually is based on history and physical findings. Plain film radiography of the abdomen may be used to detect the presence of a gas-filled bowel. CT scans and ultrasonography may also be used to detect the presence of mechanical obstruction. Treat-

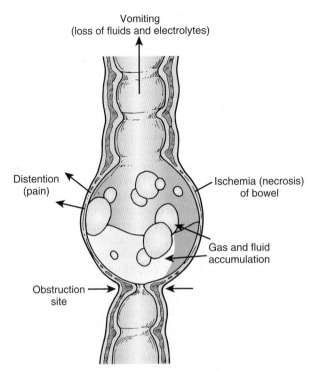

Vomiting
(loss of fluids and electrolytes)

Distention
(pain)

Ischemia (necrosis)
of bowel

Gas and fluid
accumulation

Obstruction
site

FIGURE 28-8 Pathophysiology of intestinal obstruction.

ment depends on the cause and type of obstruction. Most cases of adynamic obstruction respond to decompression of the bowel through nasogastric suction and correction of fluid and electrolyte imbalances. Strangulation and complete bowel obstruction require surgical intervention.

Peritonitis

Peritonitis is an inflammatory response of the serous membrane that lines the abdominal cavity and covers the visceral organs. It can be caused by bacterial invasion or chemical irritation. Most commonly, enteric bacteria enter the peritoneum because of a defect in the wall of one of the abdominal organs. The most common causes of peritonitis are perforated peptic ulcer, ruptured appendix, perforated diverticulum, gangrenous bowel, pelvic inflammatory disease, and gangrenous gallbladder. Other causes are abdominal trauma and wounds. Generalized peritonitis, although no longer the overwhelming problem it once was, can occur as a complication of abdominal surgery.

The peritoneum has several characteristics that increase its vulnerability to or protect it from the effects of peritonitis. One weakness of the peritoneal cavity is that it is a large, unbroken space that favors the dissemination of contaminants. For the same reason, it has a large surface that permits rapid absorption of bacterial toxins into the blood. The peritoneum is particularly well adapted for producing an inflammatory response as a means of controlling infection. It tends, for example, to exude a thick, sticky, and fibrinous substance that adheres to other structures, such as the mesentery and omentum, and that seals

off the perforated viscus and aids in localizing the process. Localization is enhanced by sympathetic stimulation that limits intestinal motility. Although the diminished or absent peristalsis that occurs tends to give rise to associated problems, it does inhibit the movement of contaminants throughout the peritoneal cavity.

One of the most important manifestations of peritonitis is the translocation of extracellular fluid into the peritoneal cavity (through weeping or serous fluid from the inflamed peritoneum) and into the bowel as a result of bowel obstruction. Nausea and vomiting cause further losses of fluid. The fluid loss may encourage development of hypovolemia and shock.

The onset of peritonitis may be acute, as with a ruptured appendix, or it may have a more gradual onset, as occurs in pelvic inflammatory disease. Pain and tenderness are common symptoms. The pain usually is more intense over the inflamed area. The person with peritonitis usually lies still because any movement aggravates the pain. Breathing often is shallow to prevent movement of the abdominal muscles. The abdomen usually is rigid and sometimes described as boardlike because of reflex muscle guarding. Vomiting is common. Fever, an elevated white blood cell count, tachycardia, and hypotension are common. Hiccups may develop because of irritation of the phrenic nerve. Paralytic ileus occurs shortly after the onset of widespread peritonitis and is accompanied by abdominal distention. Peritonitis that progresses and is untreated leads to toxemia and shock.

Treatment measures for peritonitis are directed toward preventing the extension of the inflammatory response, correcting the fluid and electrolyte imbalances that develop, and minimizing the effects of paralytic ileus and abdominal distention. Surgical intervention may be needed to remove an acutely inflamed appendix or close the opening in a perforated peptic ulcer. Oral fluids are forbidden. Nasogastric suction, which entails the insertion of a tube placed through the nose into the stomach or intestine, is used to decompress the bowel and relieve the abdominal distention. Fluid and electrolyte replacement is essential. These fluids are prescribed on the basis of frequent blood chemistry determinations. Antibiotics are given to combat infection. Narcotics often are needed for pain relief.

ALTERATIONS IN INTESTINAL ABSORPTION

Malabsorption is the failure to transport dietary constituents, such as fats, carbohydrates, proteins, vitamins, and minerals, from the lumen of the intestine to the extracellular fluid compartment for transport to the various parts of the body. It can selectively affect a single component, such as vitamin B_{12} or lactose, or its effects can extend to all the substances absorbed in a specific segment of the intestine. When one segment of the intestine is affected, another may compensate. For example, the ileum may compensate for malabsorption in the proximal small intestine by absorbing substantial amounts of fats, carbohydrates, and amino acids. Similarly, the colon, which normally absorbs water, sodium, chloride, and bicarbonate, can compensate for small intestine malabsorption by absorbing additional end products of bacterial carbohydrate metabolism.

The conditions that impair one or more steps involved in digestion and absorption of nutrients can be divided into three broad categories: intraluminal maldigestion, disorders of transepithelial transport, and lymphatic obstruction. Intraluminal maldigestion involves a defect in processing of nutrients in the intestinal lumen. The most common causes are pancreatic insufficiency, hepatobiliary disease, and intraluminal bacterial growth. Disorders of transepithelial transport are caused by mucosal lesions that impair uptake and transport of available intraluminal nutrients across the mucosal surface of the intestine. They include disorders such as celiac disease and Crohn disease. Lymphatic obstruction interferes with the transport of the products of fat digestion to the systemic circulation after they have been absorbed by the intestinal mucosa. The process can be interrupted by congenital defects, neoplasms, trauma, and selected infectious diseases.

Malabsorption Syndrome

Persons with intestinal malabsorption usually have symptoms related to the site of involvement and the dietary constituents that are affected (Table 28-2). Symptoms frequently include diarrhea, steatorrhea, flatulence, bloating, abdominal pain, and cramps. Weakness, muscle wasting, weight loss, and abdominal distention often are present. Weight loss often occurs despite normal or excessive caloric intake. Steatorrheic stools contain excess fat. The fat content causes bulky, yellow-gray, malodorous stools. In a person consuming a diet containing 80 to 100 g of fat each day, excretion of 7 to 9 g of fat indicates steatorrhea.

Along with loss of fat in the stools, there is failure to absorb the fat-soluble vitamins. This can lead to easy bruising and bleeding (*i.e.*, vitamin K deficiency), bone pain, a predisposition to the development of fractures and tetany (*i.e.*, vitamin D and calcium deficiency), macrocytic anemia, and glossitis (*i.e.*, folic acid deficiency). Neuropathy, atrophy of the skin, and peripheral edema may be present.

Celiac Disease

Celiac disease, also known as *celiac sprue* and *gluten-sensitive enteropathy,* is an immune-mediated disorder triggered by ingestion of gluten-containing grains (including wheat, barley, and rye). Until recently, the disorder was considered to be relatively uncommon in the United States, with an estimated prevalence of 1 per 3000 population. However, increased awareness and newer and more accurate serologic tests have led to the realization the condition is much more common, affecting 1 in every 120 to 300 persons in both Europe and North America.[38]

The disease results from an inappropriate T-cell–mediated immune response against ingested α-gliadin (a component of gluten protein) in genetically predisposed people. The genetic component is supported by the approximate 10% prevalence of the disease among first-degree relatives.[38,39] Almost all persons with the disorder share the major histocompatibility complex class II allele HLA-DQ2 or HLA-DQ8.[2,38] Persons with the disease have increased levels of antibodies to a variety of antigens, including transglutaminase, endomysium, and gliadin. The resultant immune response produces an intense inflammatory reaction that results in loss of absorptive villi from the small intestine. When the resulting lesions are extensive, they may impair absorption of macronutrients (*i.e.*, proteins, carbohydrates, fats) and micronutrients (*i.e.*, vitamins and minerals). Small bowel involvement is most prominent in the proximal part of the small intestine, where the exposure to gluten is greatest.

The classic form of celiac disease presents in infancy and manifests as failure to thrive, diarrhea, abdominal distention, and, occasionally, severe malnutrition. Beyond infancy, the manifestations tend to be less dramatic. Older children may present with constitutional short stature and dental enamel defects. Women comprise about 75% of adults with newly diagnosed celiac disease. In adults, gastrointestinal symptoms may manifest as diarrhea, constipation, or other symptoms of malabsorption such as bloating, flatus, or belching.

The diagnosis of celiac disease is based on clinical manifestations and confirmed by serum immunoglobulin A (IgA) antiendomysial antibody tests and intestinal biopsy. The IgA antiendomysial antibody test has been shown to be 85% to 100% sensitive for celiac disease. Usually, additional laboratory tests are done to determine if the disorder has resulted in nutritional disorders such as iron deficiency anemia.

The primary treatment of celiac disease consists of removal of gluten and related proteins from the diet. Gluten is the primary protein in wheat, barley, and rye. Oats, which are nontoxic, may be contaminated with wheat. Many gluten-free types of bread, cereals, cookies, and other products are available. Meats, vegetables, fruits, and dairy products are free of gluten as long as they are not contaminated during processing. Complete exclusion of dietary gluten usually results in rapid and complete healing of the intestinal mucosa.

NEOPLASMS

Epithelial cell tumors of the intestines are a major cause of morbidity and mortality worldwide. The colon, including the rectum, is the site of more primary neoplasms than any other organ in the body.[2] Although the small intestine accounts for approximately 75% of the length of the gastrointestinal tract, it is an uncommon site of benign or malignant tumors.

Adenomatous Polyps

By far the most common types of neoplasms of the intestine are adenomatous polyps. A gastrointestinal polyp can be described as a mass that protrudes into the lumen of gut.[2] Polyps can be subdivided according to their attachment to the bowel wall (sessile [raised mucosal nodules] or pedunculated [attached by a stalk]); their histopatho-

TABLE 28-2   Sites of and Requirements for Absorption of Dietary Constituents and Manifestations of Malabsorption

Dietary Constituent	Site of Absorption	Requirements	Manifestations
Water and electrolytes	Mainly small bowel	Osmotic gradient	Diarrhea Dehydration Cramps
Fat	Upper jejunum	Pancreatic lipase Bile salts Functioning lymphatic channels	Weight loss Steatorrhea Fat-soluble vitamin deficiency
Carbohydrates			
Starch	Small intestine	Amylase Maltase Isomaltase α-dextrins	Diarrhea Flatulence Abdominal discomfort
Sucrose	Small intestine	Sucrase	
Lactose	Small intestine	Lactase	
Maltose	Small intestine	Maltase	
Fructose	Small intestine		
Protein	Small intestine	Pancreatic enzymes (e.g., trypsin, chymotrypsin, elastin)	Loss of muscle mass Weakness Edema
Vitamins			
A	Upper jejunum	Bile salts	Night blindness Dry eyes Corneal irritation
Folic acid	Duodenum and jejunum	Absorptive; may be impaired by some drugs (i.e., anticonvulsants)	Cheilosis Glossitis Megaloblastic anemia
B_{12}	Ileum	Intrinsic factor	Glossitis Neuropathy Megaloblastic anemia
D	Upper jejunum	Bile salts	Bone pain Fractures Tetany
E	Upper jejunum	Bile salts	Uncertain
K	Upper jejunum	Bile salts	Easy bruising and bleeding
Calcium	Duodenum	Vitamin D and parathyroid hormone	Bone pain Fractures Tetany
Iron	Duodenum and jejunum	Normal pH (hydrochloric acid secretion)	Iron-deficiency anemia Glossitis

logic appearance (hyperplastic or adenomatous); and their neoplastic potential (benign or malignant).[2]

Adenomatous polyps (adenomas) are benign neoplasms that arise from the mucosal epithelium of the intestine. They are composed of neoplastic cells that have proliferated in excess of those needed to replace the cells that normally are shed from the mucosal surface (Fig. 28-9). The pathogenesis of adenoma formation involves neoplastic alteration in the replication of the crypt epithelial cells. There may be diminished apoptosis (see Chapter 2), persistence of cell replication, and failure of maturation and differentiation of the cells that migrate to the surface of the crypts.[2] Normally, deoxyribonucleic acid (DNA) synthesis ceases as the cells reach the upper two thirds of the crypts, after which they mature, migrate to the surface, and become senescent. They then become apoptotic and are shed from the surface.[2] Adenomas arise from a disruption in this sequence, such that the epithelial cells retain their proliferative ability throughout the entire length of the crypt. Alterations in cell differentiation can lead to dysplasia and progression to the development of invasive carcinoma.

Most cases of colorectal cancer begin as benign adenomatous colonic polyps. The frequency of polyps increases with age, as does the prevalence of adenomatous polyps.[2] Men and women are equally affected. The peak incidence of adenomatous polyps precedes by some years the peak for colorectal cancer. Programs that provide careful follow-up for persons with adenomatous polyps and removal of all suspect lesions have substantially reduced the incidence of colorectal cancer.[14]

Colorectal Cancer

Colorectal cancer is the third most common cancer in men and women and the second leading cause of cancer death in the United States. In 2005, there were an estimated 147,290 new cases (affecting 73,820 men and

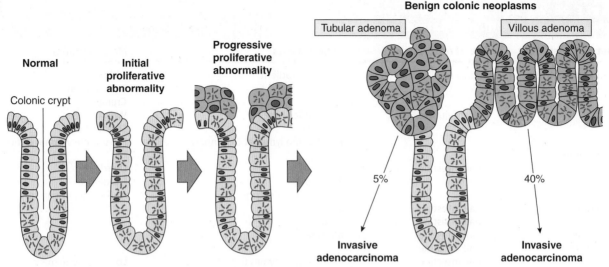

FIGURE 28-9 Histogenesis of adenomatous polyps of the colon. The initial proliferative abnormality of the colonic mucosa, the extension of the mitotic zone in the crypts, leads to accumulation of mucosal cells. The formation of the adenoma may reflect epithelial-mesenchymal interactions. (From Rubin E., Palazzo J. P. [2005]. The gastrointestinal tract. In Rubin E., Gorstein F., Rubin R., et al. [Eds.], *Rubin's pathology: Clinicopathologic foundations of medicine* [4th ed., p. 724]. Philadelphia: Lippincott Williams & Wilkins.)

73,470 women) and 56,290 deaths (of 28,540 men and 27,750 women) from colorectal cancer in the United States.[40] The death rate for colorectal cancer has been steadily declining since the early 1980s. This may due to a decreased number of advanced cases because more of the cases are found earlier, and because treatments have improved.

The cause of cancer of the colon and rectum is largely unknown. Its incidence increases with age, as evidenced by the fact that approximately 90% of persons who develop this form of cancer are older than 50 years of age.[40] Its incidence is increased among persons with a family history of cancer, persons with Crohn disease or ulcerative colitis, and those with familial adenomatous polyposis of the colon. Familial adenomatous polyposis is a rare autosomal dominant trait linked to a mutation in the long arm of chromosome 5. Persons with the disorder develop multiple adenomatous polyps of the colon at an early age.[41] Carcinoma of the colon is inevitable, often by 40 years of age, unless a total colectomy is performed.

Diet also is thought to play a role.[40] Attention has focused on dietary fat intake, refined sugar intake, fiber intake, and the adequacy of such protective micronutrients as vitamins A, C, and E in the diet. It has been hypothesized that a high level of fat in the diet increases the synthesis of bile acids in the liver, which may be converted to potential carcinogens by the bacterial flora in the colon. Bacterial organisms in particular are suspected of converting bile acids to carcinogens; their proliferation is enhanced by a high dietary level of refined sugars. Dietary fiber is thought to increase stool bulk and thereby dilute and remove potential carcinogens. Refined diets often contain reduced amounts of vitamins A, C, and E, which may act as oxygen free radical scavengers.

Several epidemiologic studies suggest that the use of aspirin and other NSAIDs exerts a protective effect against colorectal cancer.[2] An analysis of the incidence of colorectal cancer in the Nurses Health Study showed a decreased incidence of colorectal cancer among women who took four to six aspirin per week.[42] Although the mechanism of action is unknown, it may be related to the inhibition of cyclooxygenase-2 (see Chapter 14). This enzyme is overexpressed in neoplastic epithelium and appears to regulate angiogenesis and apoptosis.[2] There has been recent interest in what has been termed *chemoprevention* or the use of oral agents such as aspirin or other NSAIDs in the prevention of colorectal cancer.[43]

Usually, cancer of the colon and rectum is present for a long time before it produces symptoms. Bleeding is a highly significant early symptom, and commonly is the one that causes persons to seek medical care. Other symptoms include a change in bowel habits, diarrhea or constipation, and sometimes a sense of urgency or incomplete emptying of the bowel. Pain usually is a late symptom.

Screening, Diagnosis, and Treatment. The single most important prognostic indicator of colorectal cancer is the extent (stage) of the tumor at time of diagnosis. Therefore, the challenge is to discover the tumors at their earliest stages. Among the methods used for the detection of colorectal cancers are stool occult blood tests and digital rectal examination, usually done during routine physical examinations; x-ray studies using barium (*e.g.,* barium enema); and flexible sigmoidoscopy and colonoscopy.[40,44] Digital rectal examinations are most helpful in detecting neoplasms of the rectum. Rectal examination should be considered a routine part of a good physical examination. The American Cancer Society recommends that all asymptomatic men and women older than 40 years of age should have a digital rectal examination performed annually as a part of their physical examination, and that those older than 50 years should have an annual stool test for occult blood; or a flexible sigmoidoscopy every 5 years, preferably in addition to yearly stool tests for occult blood; or a double-contrast barium enema every 5 years; or a colonoscopy every 10 years.[40] People with increased risk for colorectal cancer should be screened earlier and more often. Colonoscopy is recommended whenever a screening test is positive.

Almost all cancers of the colon and rectum bleed intermittently, although the amount of blood is small and usually not apparent in the stools. It therefore is feasible to screen for colorectal cancers using commercially prepared tests for occult blood in the stool. Persons with a positive stool occult blood test should be referred to their physicians for further study. Usually, a physical examination, rectal examination, barium enema, and sigmoidoscopy or colonoscopy is done.

Flexible sigmoidoscopy involves examination of the rectum and sigmoid colon with a hollow, lighted tube that is inserted through the rectum. The procedure is performed without sedation and is well tolerated. Polyps can be removed or tissue can be obtained for biopsy during the procedure. Colonoscopy provides a means for direct visualization of the rectum and colon. This method is used for screening persons at high risk for developing cancer of the colon (e.g., those with ulcerative colitis) and for those with symptoms. Colonoscopy also is useful for obtaining a biopsy and for removing polyps. Although this method is one of the most accurate for detecting early colorectal cancers, it is not suitable for mass screening because it is expensive and time consuming and must be done by a person who is highly trained in the use of the instrument.

The only recognized treatment for cancer of the colon and rectum is surgical removal.[44] Preoperative radiation therapy may be used and has in some cases demonstrated increased 5-year survival rates. Postoperative adjuvant chemotherapy may be used. Radiation therapy and chemotherapy also are used as palliative treatment methods.

The prognosis for persons with colorectal cancer depends largely on the extent of bowel involvement and on the presence of metastasis at the time of diagnosis. In general, the disease has spread beyond the range of curative surgery in 25% to 30% of patients.[2]

In summary, disorders of the small and large intestines include irritable bowel syndrome, inflammatory bowel disease, infectious enterocolitis, diverticular disease, disorders of motility (i.e., diarrhea, constipation, and intestinal obstruction), alterations in intestinal absorption, and colorectal cancer. Irritable bowel syndrome is a functional disorder characterized by a variable combination of chronic and recurrent intestinal symptoms not explained by structural or biochemical abnormalities. The term *inflammatory bowel disease* is used to designate two inflammatory conditions: Crohn disease, which affects the small and large bowel, and ulcerative colitis, which affects the colon and rectum. Both are chronic diseases characterized by remissions and exacerbations of diarrhea, weight loss, fluid and electrolyte disorders, and systemic signs of inflammation. Infectious forms of enterocolitis include viral (e.g., rotavirus) and bacterial (e.g., C. difficile and E. coli O157:H7) infections. Diverticular disease includes diverticulosis, which is a condition in which the mucosal layer of the colon herniates through the muscularis layer, and diverticulitis, in which there is inflammation and gross or microscopic perforation of the diverticulum.

Diarrhea and constipation represent disorders of intestinal motility. Diarrhea, characterized by excessively frequent passage of stools, can be divided into large-volume diarrhea, manifested by increased water content in the feces, and small-volume diarrhea, associated with intrinsic bowel disease and frequent passage of small stools. Constipation can be defined as the infrequent passage of stools; it commonly is caused by failure to respond to the urge to defecate, inadequate fiber or fluid intake, weakness of the abdominal muscles, inactivity and bed rest, pregnancy, hemorrhoids, and gastrointestinal disease. Intestinal obstruction designates an impairment of movement of intestinal contents in a cephalocaudal direction as the result of mechanical or paralytic mechanisms. Peritonitis is an inflammatory response of the serous membrane that lines the abdominal cavity and covers the visceral organs. It can be caused by bacterial invasion or chemical irritation resulting from perforation of the viscera or abdominal organs.

Malabsorption results from disorders of the small intestine that impair the absorption of nutrients and other dietary constituents from the intestine. It can involve a single dietary constituent, such as vitamin B_{12}, or extend to involve all of the substances absorbed in a particular part of the small intestine. Colorectal cancer, the second most common fatal cancer, is seen most commonly in persons older than 50 years of age. Most, if not all, cancers of the colon and rectum arise in preexisting adenomatous polyps. Programs that provide careful follow-up for persons with adenomatous polyps and removal of all suspect lesions have substantially reduced the incidence of colorectal cancer.

Review Exercises

A 40-year-old man reports to his health care provider complaining of heartburn that occurs after eating and also wakes him up at night. He is overweight and admits to enjoying fatty foods and lying down on the sofa and watching TV in the evening. He also complains that lately he has been having a cough and some wheezing. A diagnosis of gastroesophageal reflux disease (GERD) was made.

A. Explain the cause of heartburn and why it becomes worse after eating.

B. Persons with GERD are advised to lose weight, avoid eating fatty foods, to remain sitting after eating, and to sleep with their head slightly elevated. Explain the possible relationship between these situations and the occurrence of reflux.

C. Explain the possible relationship between GERD and the respiratory symptoms this man is having.

A 36-year-old woman, who has been taking aspirin for back pain, experiences a sudden episode of tachycardia and feeling faint that is accompanied by the vomiting of coffee-ground emesis and the passing of a tarry stool. She relates that she has not had any signs of a "stomach ulcer" such as pain or heartburn.

A. Relate the mucosal protective effects of prostaglandins to the development of peptic ulcer associated with aspirin or nonsteroidal anti-inflammatory drug (NSAID) use.

B. Explain the apparent suddenness of the bleeding and the fact that the woman did not experience pain as a warning signal

C. Among the results of her initial laboratory tests is an elevated blood urea nitrogen (BUN) level. Explain the reason for the elevated BUN.

A 29-year-old woman has been diagnosed with Crohn disease. Her medical history reveals that she began having symptoms of the disease at age 24 years and that her mother died of complications of the disease at 54 years of age. She complains of diarrhea and chronic cramping abdominal pain.

A. Define the term *inflammatory bowel disease* and compare the pathophysiology and manifestations of Crohn disease and ulcerative colitis.

B. Describe the possible association between genetic and environmental factors in the pathogenesis of Crohn disease.

C. Relate the use of the monoclonal antibody infliximab to the pathogenesis of the inflammatory lesions that occur in Crohn disease.

Visit the Porth: Essentials of Pathophysiology: Concepts of Altered Health States web site (http://thePoint.LWW.com/PorthEssentials) for links to chapter-related resources on the Internet, all-new exclusive animations, chapter review questions, and more!

REFERENCES

1. National Digestive Diseases Information Clearing House (NDDIC). (2004). Digestive disease statistics. [On-line]. Available: http://digestive.niddk.nih.gov/statistics/statistics.htm. Accessed January 14, 2004.
2. Liu C., Crawford J. M. (2005). The gastrointestinal tract. In Kumar V., Abbas A. K., Fausto N. (Eds.), *Robbins and Cotran pathologic basis of disease* (7th ed., pp. 797–875). Philadelphia: Elsevier Saunders.
3. Spieker M. R. (2000). Evaluating dysphagia. *American Family Physician* 61, 3639–3648.
4. Mittal R. K., Balaban D. H. (1997). The esophagogastric junction. *New England Journal of Medicine* 336, 924–931.
5. Orlando R. C. (2002). Pathogenesis of gastroesophageal reflux disease. *Gastroenterology Clinics of North America* 31, S35–S44.
6. Alexander J. A., Hunt L. W., Patel A. M. (1999). Prevalence, pathophysiology, and treatment of patients with asthma and gastroesophageal reflux disease. *Mayo Clinic Proceedings* 75, 1055–1063.
7. Spechler S. J. (2002). Barrett's esophagus. *New England Journal of Medicine* 346, 836–842.
8. Scott M., Gelhot A. R. (1999). Gastroesophageal reflux disease: Diagnosis and management. *American Family Physician* 59, 1161–1169, 1199.
9. Mason D. B. (2000). Gastroesophageal reflux in children. *Nursing Clinics of North America* 35, 15–36.
10. Orenstein S., Peters J., Khan S., et al. (2004). The esophagus. In Behrman R. E., Kliegman R. M., Jenson H. B. (Eds.), *Nelson textbook of pediatrics* (17th ed., pp. 1222–1224). Philadelphia: Elsevier Saunders.
11. Enzinger P. C., Mayer R. J. (2003). Esophageal cancer. *New England Journal of Medicine* 349, 2241–2252.
12. Fromm D. (1987). Mechanisms involved in gastric mucosal resistance to injury. *Annual Review of Medicine* 38, 119.
13. Wolfe M. M., Lichtenstein D. R., Singh G. (1999). Gastrointestinal toxicity of nonsteroidal anti-inflammatory drugs. *New England Journal of Medicine* 340, 1888–1899.
14. Rubin E., Palazzo J. P. (2005). The gastrointestinal tract. In Rubin E., Gorstein F., Rubin R., et al. (Eds.), *Rubin's pathology: Clinicopathologic foundations of medicine* (4th ed., pp. 660–695, 727–746). Philadelphia: Lippincott Williams & Wilkins.
15. Suerbaum S., Michetti P. (2002). *Helicobacter pylori* infections. *New England Journal of Medicine* 347, 1175–1186.
16. Shiotani A., Nurgalieva Z. Z., Yamaoka Y., et al. (2000). *Helicobacter pylori*. *Medical Clinics of North America* 84, 1125–1136.
17. Fass R. (1995). Zollinger-Ellison syndrome: Diagnosis and management. *Hospital Practice*, November 15, 73–80.
18. Konopad E., Noseworthy T. (1988). Stress ulceration: A serious complication in critically ill patients. *Heart and Lung* 17, 339.
19. Viera A. J., Hoag S., Shaughnessy J. (2002). Management of irritable bowel syndrome. *American Family Physician* 66, 1867–1874.

20. Olden K. W. (2003). Irritable bowel syndrome: An overview of diagnosis and pharmacologic treatment. *Cleveland Clinic Journal of Medicine* 70(Suppl. 2), S3–S17.

21. Thompson W. G., Longstreth G. E., Drossman D. A. et al. (Committee on Functional Bowel Disorders and Functional Abdominal Pain, Multinational Working Teams to Develop Diagnostic Criteria for Functional Gastrointestinal Disorders [ROME II], University of Ottawa, Canada). (1999). Functional bowel disorders and functional abdominal pain. *Gut* 45(Suppl. 2), 1143–1147.

22. Bridget S., Lee J. C., Bjarnason I., et al. (2002). In siblings with similar genetic susceptibility for inflammatory bowel disease, smokers tend to develop Crohn's disease and nonsmokers develop ulcerative colitis. *Gut* 51, 21–25.

23. Podolsky D. K. (2002). Inflammatory bowel disease. *New England Journal of Medicine* 347, 417–429.

24. Chinyu S., Lichtenstein G. R. (2002). Recent developments in inflammatory bowel disease. *Medical Clinics of North America* 86, 1497–1523.

25. Hanauer S. B., Present D. H. (2003). The state of the art in the management of inflammatory bowel disease. *Reviews in Gastrointestinal Disorders* 3(2), 81–92.

26. Bass D. M. (2004). Rotavirus and other agents of viral gastroenteritis. In Behrman R. E., Kliegman R. M., Jenson H. B. (Eds.), *Nelson textbook of pediatrics* (17th ed., pp. 1081–1083). Philadelphia: Elsevier Saunders.

27. Mylonakis E., Ryan E. T., Claderswood S. B. (2001). *Clostridium difficile*-associated diarrhea: A review. *Archives of Internal Medicine* 161, 525–533.

28. Greenwald D. A., Brandt L. J. (1997). Recognizing *E. coli* O157:H7 infection. *Hospital Practice* 32, 123–140.

29. Ferzoco L. B., Raptopoulos V., Silen W. (1998). Acute diverticulitis. *New England Journal of Medicine* 338, 1521–1526.

30. Paulson E. K., Kalady M. F., Pappas T. N. (2003). Suspected appendicitis. *New England Journal of Medicine* 348, 236–242.

31. King C. K., Glass R., Brewer J. S., et al. (2003). Managing acute gastroenteritis among children: Oral rehydration, maintenance, and nutritional therapy. *MMWR Morbidity and Mortality Weekly Reviews* 52(RR-16), 1–16.

32. Schiller L. R. (2000). Diarrhea. *Medical Clinics of North America* 84, 1259–1275.

33. Field M., Rao M. C., Chang E. B. (1989). Intestinal electrolyte transport and diarrheal disease (part 2). *New England Journal of Medicine* 321, 879–883.

34. Field M. (2003). Intestinal ion transport and the pathophysiology of diarrhea. *Journal of Clinical Investigation* 111, 931–943.

35. American Academy of Pediatrics, Subcommittee on Acute Gastroenteritis. (1996). Practice parameter: The management of acute gastroenteritis in young children. *Pediatrics* 97 424–435.

36. Lembo A., Camilleri M. (2003). Chronic constipation. *New England Journal of Medicine* 349, 1360–1368.

37. Wyllie R. (2000). Ileus, adhesions, intussusception, and closed-loop obstruction. In Bierman R. E., Kliegman R. M., Jenson H. B. (Eds.), *Nelson textbook of pediatrics* (17th ed., pp. 1241–1243). Philadelphia: Elsevier Saunders.

38. Farrell R. J., Kelly C. (2002). Celiac sprue. *New England Journal of Medicine* 346, 180–188.

39. Garcia-Carega M., Kerner J. A. (2004). Malabsorption disorders. In Bierman R. E., Kliegman R. M., Jenson H. B. (Eds.), *Nelson textbook of pediatrics* (16th ed., pp. 1264–1266). Philadelphia: Elsevier Saunders.

40. American Cancer Society. (2004). Colorectal cancer. [On-line]. Available: http://www.cancer.org.

41. Guttmacher A. E., de la Chapelle A. (2003). Hereditary colorectal cancer. *New England Journal of Medicine* 348, 919–932.

42. Marcus A. J. (1995). Aspirin as prophylaxis against colorectal cancer. *New England Journal of Medicine* 333, 656–657.

43. Pasi J. A., Mayer R. J. (2000). Chemoprevention of colorectal cancer. *New England Journal of Medicine* 342, 1960–1966.

44. Engstrom P. F. (2001). Colorectal cancer. In Lenhard R. E., Osteen R. T., Gansler T. (Eds.), *The American Cancer Society's clinical oncology* (pp. 362–372). Atlanta: American Cancer Society.

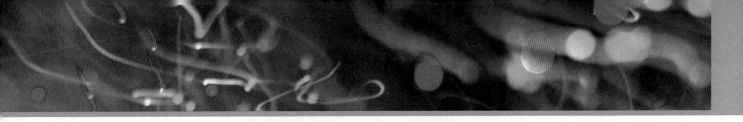

Chapter *29*

Disorders of Hepatobiliary and Exocrine Pancreas Function

 The liver, the gallbladder, and the exocrine pancreas are classified as accessory organs of the gastrointestinal tract. In addition to producing digestive secretions, the liver and the pancreas have other important functions. The endocrine pancreas, for example, supplies the insulin and glucagon needed in cell metabolism, whereas the liver synthesizes glucose, plasma proteins, and blood clotting factors and is responsible for the degradation and elimination of drugs and hormones, among other functions. This chapter focuses on functions and disorders of the liver, the biliary tract and gallbladder, and the exocrine pancreas.

The Liver and Hepatobiliary System

The liver is the largest visceral organ in the body, weighing approximately 1.3 kg (3 lb) in the adult. It is located below the diaphragm and occupies much of the right hypochondrium (Fig. 29-1). The liver is surrounded by a tough fibroelastic capsule called *Glisson capsule*. The falciform ligament, which extends from the peritoneal surface of the anterior abdominal wall between the umbilicus and diaphragm, divides the liver into two lobes, a large right lobe and a small left lobe. There are two additional lobes on the visceral surface of the liver: the caudate and quadrate lobes. Except for the portion that is in the epigastric area, the liver is contained within the rib cage and in healthy persons cannot normally be palpated.

The liver is unique among the abdominal organs in having a dual blood supply—the hepatic artery and the portal vein. Approximately 300 mL of blood per minute enters the liver through the hepatic artery; another 1050 mL/minute enters by way of the valveless

631

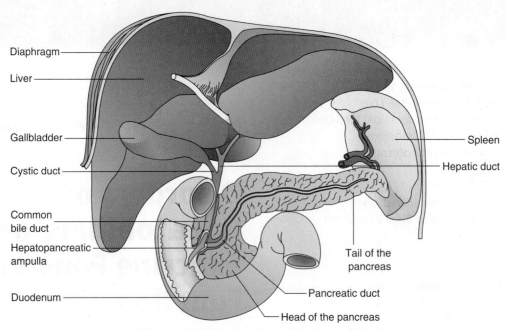

FIGURE 29-1 The liver and biliary system, including the gallbladder and bile ducts.

portal vein, which carries blood from the stomach, the small and the large intestines, the pancreas, and the spleen[1] (Fig. 29-2). Although the blood from the portal vein is incompletely saturated with oxygen, it supplies approximately 60% to 70% of the oxygen needs of the liver. The venous outflow from the liver is carried by the valveless hepatic veins, which empty into the inferior vena cava just below the level of the diaphragm. The pressure difference between the hepatic vein and the portal vein normally is such that the liver stores approximately 450 mL of blood.[1] This blood can be shifted back into the general circulation during periods of hypovolemia and shock. In congestive heart failure, in which the pressure in the vena cava increases, blood backs up and accumulates in the liver.

The *lobules* are the functional units of the liver. Each lobule is a cylindrical structure that measures approximately 0.8 to 2 mm in diameter and several millimeters long. There are approximately 50,000 to 100,000 lobules in the liver.[1] Each lobule is organized around a central vein that empties into the hepatic veins and from there into the vena cava. The terminal bile ducts and small branches of the portal vein and hepatic artery are located at the periphery of the lobule. Plates of hepatic cells radiate centrifugally from the central vein like spokes on a wheel (Fig. 29-3). These hepatic plates are separated by wide, thin-walled channels, called *sinusoids,* that extend from the periphery of the lobule to its central vein. The sinusoids are supplied by blood from the portal vein and hepatic artery. Because the plates of hepatic cells are no more than two layers thick, every cell is exposed to the blood that travels through the sinusoids. Thus, the hepatic cells can remove substances from the blood or can release substances into the blood as it moves through the sinusoids.

The venous sinusoids are lined with two types of cells: the typical endothelial cells and Kupffer cells. *Kupffer*

cells are reticuloendothelial cells that are capable of removing and phagocytizing old and defective blood cells, bacteria, and other foreign material from the portal blood as it flows through the sinusoid. This phagocytic action removes the enteric bacilli and other harmful substances that filter into the blood from the intestine.

The lobules also are supplied by small tubular channels, called *bile canaliculi,* that lie between the cell membranes of adjacent hepatocytes. The bile produced by the hepatocytes flows into the canaliculi and then to the periphery of the lobules, which drain into progressively larger ducts, until it reaches the right and left hepatic ducts. The intrahepatic and extrahepatic bile ducts often are collectively referred to as the *hepatobiliary tree.* These ducts unite to form the common duct (see Fig. 29-1). The common bile duct, which is approximately 10 to 15 cm long, descends and passes behind the pancreas and enters the descending duodenum. The pancreatic duct joins the common bile duct at a short dilated tube called the *hepatopancreatic ampulla* (ampulla of Vater), which empties into the duodenum through the duodenal papilla. Muscle tissue at the junction of the papilla, sometimes called the *sphincter of Oddi,* regulates the flow of bile into the duodenum. When this sphincter is closed, bile moves back into the common duct and gallbladder.

METABOLIC FUNCTIONS OF THE LIVER

The liver is one of the most versatile and active organs in the body. It produces bile; metabolizes hormones and drugs; synthesizes proteins, glucose, and blood clotting factors; stores vitamins and minerals; changes ammonia produced by deamination of amino acids to urea; and converts fatty acids to ketones. In its capacity for metabolizing drugs and hormones, the liver serves as an excre-

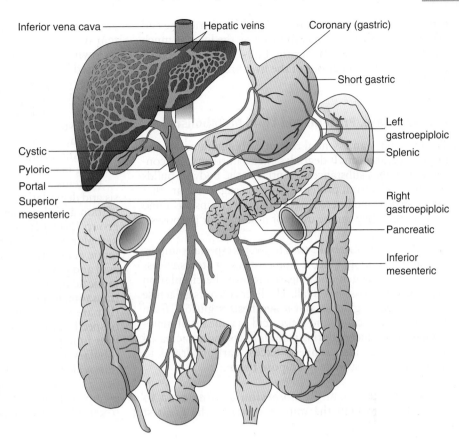

FIGURE 29-2 The portal circulation and veins carrying blood from the gastro-intestinal tract, spleen, and liver that empty into the portal vein. Blood from these veins travels to the liver through the portal vein before moving into the vena cava for return to the heart.

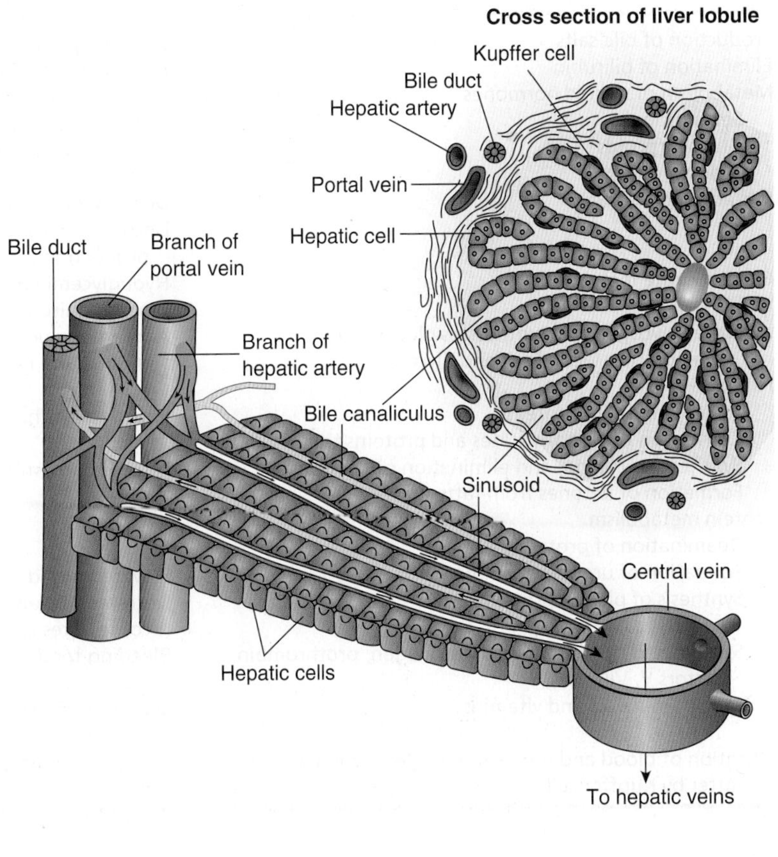

FIGURE 29-3 A section of liver lobule showing the location of the hepatic veins, hepatic cells, liver sinusoids, and branches of the portal vein and hepatic artery.

tory organ. In this respect, the bile, which carries the end products of substances metabolized by the liver, is much like the urine, which carries the body wastes filtered by the kidneys. The functions of the liver are summarized in Table 29-1.

Carbohydrate, Protein, and Lipid Metabolism

The liver plays an essential role in carbohydrate, fat, and protein metabolism. It degrades excess nutrients and converts them into substances essential to the body. It builds carbohydrates from proteins, converts sugars to fats that can be stored, and interchanges chemical groups on amino acids so that they can be used for a number of purposes.

Carbohydrate Metabolism. The liver is especially important in maintaining glucose homeostasis. It stores excess glucose as glycogen and releases it into the circulation when blood glucose levels fall. The liver converts galactose and fructose to glucose and it synthesizes glucose from amino acids, glycerol, and lactic acid as a means of maintaining blood glucose during periods of fasting or increased need. The liver also converts excess carbohydrates to triglycerides for storage in adipose tissue.

Protein Synthesis and Conversion of Ammonia to Urea. Even though the muscle contains the greatest amount of protein, the liver has the greatest rate of protein synthesis per gram of tissue. It produces proteins for its own cellular needs and secretory proteins that are released into the circulation. The most important of these secretory proteins is albumin. Albumin contributes significantly to the plasma colloidal osmotic pressure (see Chapter 6) and to the binding and transport of numerous substances, including some hormones, fatty acids, bilirubin, and other anions. The liver also produces other important proteins, such as fibrinogen and the blood clotting factors.

Proteins are made up of amino acids. Protein synthesis and degradation involves two major reactions: transamination and deamination. In *transamination*, the amino group (NH_2) from an amino acid is transferred to α-ketoglutaric acid (a Krebs cycle keto acid) to form glutamic acid. The transferring amino acid becomes a keto acid and α-ketoglutaric acid becomes an amino acid (glutamic acid). The reaction is fully reversible. The process of transamination is catalyzed by *aminotransferases*, enzymes that are found in high amounts in the liver. Serum levels of specific aminotransferases are used in the assessment of liver function (discussed in the section on Tests of Hepatobiliary Function). Oxidative *deamination* involves the removal of an amino group from an amino acid. This occurs mainly by transamination, in which the amino group of glutamic acid is removed as ammonia, and α-ketoglutaric acid is regenerated. Because ammonia is

TABLE 29-1	**Functions of the Liver and Manifestations of Altered Function**
Function	**Manifestations of Altered Function**
Production of bile salts	Malabsorption of fat and fat-soluble vitamins
Elimination of bilirubin	Elevation in serum bilirubin and jaundice
Metabolism of steroid hormones	
Sex hormones	Disturbances in gonadal function, including gynecomastia in men
Glucocorticoids	Signs of increased cortisol levels (*i.e.,* Cushing syndrome)
Aldosterone	Signs of hyperaldosteronism (*e.g.,* sodium retention and hypokalemia)
Metabolism of drugs	Decreased drug metabolism
	Decreased plasma binding of drugs owing to a decrease in albumin production
Carbohydrate metabolism	Hypoglycemia may develop when glycogenolysis and gluconeogenesis are impaired
Stores glycogen and synthesizes glucose from amino acids, lactic acid, and glycerol	Abnormal glucose tolerance curve may occur because of impaired uptake and release of glucose by the liver
Fat metabolism	
Formation of lipoproteins	Impaired synthesis of lipoproteins
Conversion of carbohydrates and proteins to fat	
Synthesis, recycling, and elimination of cholesterol	Altered cholesterol levels
Formation of ketones from fatty acid	
Protein metabolism	
Deamination of proteins	
Formation of urea from ammonia	Elevated blood ammonia levels
Synthesis of plasma proteins	Decreased levels of plasma proteins, particularly albumin, which contributes to edema formation
Synthesis of clotting factors (fibrinogen, prothrombin, factors V, VII, IX, X)	Bleeding tendency
Storage of minerals and vitamins	Signs of deficiency of fat-soluble and other vitamins that are stored in the liver
Filtration of blood and removal of bacteria and particulate matter by Kupffer cells	Increased exposure of the body to colonic bacteria and other foreign matter

very toxic to body tissues, particularly neurons, it is converted to urea in the liver and then excreted by the kidneys. The goal of amino acid degradation is to produce molecules that can be used to generate energy or be converted to glucose.

Pathways of Lipid Metabolism. Although most body cells can metabolize fat, certain aspects of lipid metabolism occur mainly in the liver. These include the oxidation of fatty acids to supply energy for other body functions; the synthesis of large quantities of cholesterol, phospholipids, and most lipoproteins; and the formation of triglycerides from carbohydrates and proteins. To derive energy from neutral fats (triglycerides), the fat must first be split into glycerol and fatty acids, and then the fatty acids split into acetyl-coenzyme A (acetyl-CoA). Acetyl-CoA can be used by the liver to produce adenosine triphosphate (ATP) or it can be converted to acetoacetic acid and released into the bloodstream and transported to other tissues, where it is used for energy. The acetyl-CoA units from fat metabolism also are used to synthesize cholesterol and bile acids. Cholesterol has several fates in the liver: it can be esterified and stored, it can be exported bound to lipoproteins, or it can be converted to bile acids.

Drug and Hormone Metabolism

By virtue of its many enzyme systems involved in biochemical transformations and modifications, the liver has an important role in the metabolism of many drugs and chemical substances. The liver is particularly important in terms of metabolizing lipid-soluble substances that cannot be directly excreted by the kidneys. Two major types of reactions are involved in the hepatic detoxification and metabolism of drugs and other chemicals: phase 1 reactions, which involve chemical modification or inactivation of a substance, and phase 2 reactions, which involve conversion of lipid-soluble substances to water-soluble derivatives.[2,3] Often, the two types of reactions are linked. Many phase 1 reactants are not soluble and must therefore undergo a subsequent phase 2 reaction to be eliminated. These reactions, which are called *biotransformations,* are important considerations in drug therapy. Because the liver is central to metabolic disposition of virtually all drugs and foreign substances, drug-induced liver toxicity is a potential complication of many medications.

In addition to its role in metabolism of drugs and chemicals, the liver also is responsible for hormone inactivation or modification. Insulin and glucagon are inactivated by proteolysis or deamination. Thyroxine and triiodothyronine are metabolized by reactions involving deiodination. Steroid hormones such as the glucocorticoids are first inactivated by a phase 1 reaction and then converted to a more water-soluble product by a phase 2 reaction.

BILE PRODUCTION AND CHOLESTASIS

The secretion of bile is essential for digestion of dietary fats and absorption of fats and fat-soluble vitamins from the intestine. The liver produces approximately 600 to 1200 mL of yellow-green bile daily.[1] Bile contains water, bile salts, bilirubin, cholesterol, fatty acids, lecithin, and electrolytes. Of these, only bile salts, which are formed from cholesterol, are important in digestion. The other components of bile depend on the secretion of sodium, chloride, bicarbonate, and potassium by the bile ducts.

The liver forms approximately 0.6 g of bile salts daily.[1] Bile salts serve an important function in digestion; they aid in emulsifying dietary fats, and they are necessary for the formation of the micelles that transport fatty acids and fat-soluble vitamins to the surface of the intestinal mucosa for absorption. Approximately 94% of bile salts that enter the intestine are reabsorbed into the portal circulation by an active transport process that takes place in the distal ileum. From the portal circulation, the bile salts pass into the liver, where they are recycled. Normally, bile salts travel this entire circuit approximately 18 times before being expelled in the feces.[1] This system for recirculation of bile is called the *enterohepatic circulation.*

Cholestasis

Cholestasis represents a decrease in bile flow through the intrahepatic canaliculi and a reduction in secretion of water, bilirubin, and bile acids by the hepatocytes. As a result, the materials normally transferred to the bile, including bilirubin, cholesterol, and bile acids, accumulate in the blood.[2,3] The condition may be caused by intrinsic liver disease, in which case it is referred to as *intrahepatic cholestasis,* or by obstruction of the large bile ducts, a condition known as *extrahepatic cholestasis.*

A number of mechanisms are implicated in the pathogenesis of cholestasis. Primary biliary cirrhosis and primary sclerosing cholangitis are caused by disorders of the small intrahepatic canaliculi and bile ducts. In the case of extrahepatic obstruction, such as that caused by conditions such as cholelithiasis, common duct strictures, or obstructing neoplasms, the effects begin with increased pressure in the large bile ducts. Genetic disorders involving the transport of bile into the canaliculi also can result in cholestasis.

The morphologic features of cholestasis depend on the underlying cause. Common to all types of obstructive and hepatocellular cholestasis is the accumulation of bile pigment in the liver. Elongated green-brown plugs of bile are visible in the dilated bile canaliculi. Rupture of the canaliculi leads to extravasation of bile and subsequent degenerative changes in the surrounding hepatocytes. Prolonged obstructive cholestasis leads not only to fatty changes in the hepatocytes but to destruction of the supporting connective tissue, giving rise to bile lakes filled with cellular debris and pigment.[3] Unrelieved obstruction leads to biliary tract fibrosis and ultimately to end-stage biliary cirrhosis.

Pruritus is the most common presenting symptom in persons with cholestasis, probably related to increased bile acids in the blood. Skin xanthomas (focal accumulations of cholesterol) may occur, the result of hyperlipidemia and impaired excretion of cholesterol. A characteristic laboratory finding is an elevated serum alkaline phosphatase level, an enzyme present in the bile duct epithelium and canalicular membrane of hepatocytes. Other manifestations of reduced bile flow relate to intestinal absorption, including nutritional deficiencies of fat-soluble vitamins A, D, K.

Bilirubin Elimination

Bilirubin is the substance that gives bile its color. It is formed from senescent red blood cells. In the process of degradation, the hemoglobin from the red blood cell is broken down to form biliverdin, which is rapidly converted to free bilirubin (Fig. 29-4). Free bilirubin, which is insoluble in plasma, is transported in the blood attached to serum albumin. Even when it is bound to albumin, this bilirubin is still called *free bilirubin*. As it passes through the liver, free bilirubin is released from the albumin carrier molecule and moved into the hepatocytes. Inside the hepatocytes, free bilirubin is converted to conjugated bilirubin, making it soluble in bile. Conjugated bilirubin is secreted as a constituent of bile, and in this form it passes through the bile ducts into the small intestine. In the intestine, approximately one half of the bilirubin is converted into a highly soluble substance called *urobilinogen* by the intestinal flora. Urobilinogen is either absorbed

into the portal circulation or excreted in the feces. Most of the urobilinogen that is absorbed is returned to the liver to be re-excreted into the bile. A small amount of urobilinogen, approximately 5%, is absorbed into the general circulation and then excreted by the kidneys.

Usually, only a small amount of bilirubin is found in the blood; the normal level of total serum bilirubin is 0.1 to 1.2 mg/dL. Laboratory measurements of bilirubin usually include free and conjugated bilirubin as well as the total bilirubin. These are reported as the direct (conjugated) bilirubin and the indirect (unconjugated or free) bilirubin.

Jaundice. Jaundice (*i.e.,* icterus) results from an abnormally high accumulation of bilirubin in the blood, as a result of which there is a yellowish discoloration to the skin and deep tissues. Jaundice becomes evident when the serum bilirubin levels rise above 2 to 2.5 mg/dL.[2,3] Because normal skin has a yellow cast, the early signs of jaundice often are difficult to detect, especially in persons with dark skin. Bilirubin has a special affinity for elastic tissue. The sclera of the eye, which contains a high proportion of elastic fibers, usually is one of the first structures in which jaundice can be detected (Fig. 29-5).

The four major causes of jaundice are excessive destruction of red blood cells, impaired uptake of bilirubin by the liver cells, decreased conjugation of bilirubin, and obstruction of bile flow in the canaliculi of the hepatic lobules or in the intrahepatic or extrahepatic bile ducts. From an anatomic standpoint, jaundice can be categorized as prehepatic, intrahepatic, and posthepatic. Chart 29-1 lists the common causes of prehepatic, hepatic, and posthepatic jaundice.

The major cause of prehepatic jaundice is excessive hemolysis of red blood cells. Hemolytic jaundice occurs when red blood cells are destroyed at a rate in excess of the liver's ability to remove the bilirubin from the blood.

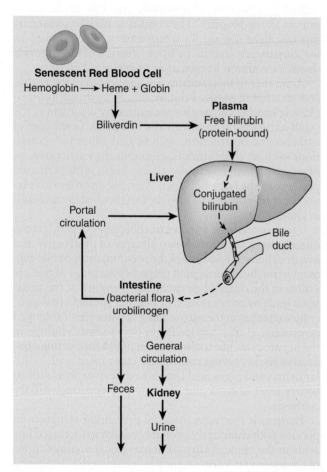

FIGURE 29-4 The process of bilirubin formation, circulation, and elimination.

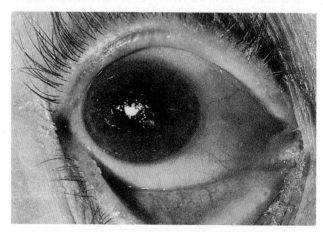

FIGURE 29-5 Jaundice. A patient with hepatic failure displays a yellow sclera. (From Rubin E., Rubin R. [2005]. The liver and biliary system. In Rubin E., Gorstein F., Rubin R., et al. [Eds.], *Rubin's pathophysiology: Clinicopathologic foundations of medicine* [4th ed., p. 747]. Philadelphia: Lippincott Williams & Wilkins.)

Causes of Jaundice

Prehepatic (Excessive Red Blood Cell Destruction)

Hemolytic blood transfusion reaction
Hereditary disorders of the red blood cell
    Sickle cell anemia
    Thalassemia
    Spherocytosis
Acquired hemolytic disorders
Hemolytic disease of the newborn
Autoimmune hemolytic anemias

Intrahepatic

Decreased bilirubin uptake by the liver
Decreased conjugation of bilirubin
Hepatocellular liver damage
    Hepatitis
    Cirrhosis
    Cancer of the liver
Drug-induced cholestasis

Posthepatic (Obstruction of Bile Flow)

Structural disorders of the bile duct
Cholelithiasis
Congenital atresia of the extrahepatic bile ducts
Bile duct obstruction caused by tumors

It may follow a hemolytic blood transfusion reaction or may occur in diseases such as hereditary spherocytosis, in which the red cell membranes are defective, or in hemolytic disease of the newborn (see Chapter 11). Neonatal hyperbilirubinemia results from an increased production of bilirubin in newborn infants and their limited ability to excrete it.[4] Premature infants are at particular risk because their red cells have a shorter life span and higher turnover rate. In prehepatic jaundice, there is mild jaundice, the unconjugated bilirubin is elevated, the stools are of normal color, and there is no bilirubin in the urine.

Intrahepatic or hepatocellular jaundice is caused by disorders that directly affect the ability of the liver to remove bilirubin from the blood or conjugate it so it can be eliminated in the bile. Gilbert disease is inherited as a dominant trait and results in a reduced removal of bilirubin from the blood; the disorder is benign and fairly common. Affected persons have no symptoms other than a slightly elevated serum level of unconjugated bilirubin and mild jaundice. Conjugation of bilirubin is impaired whenever liver cells are damaged, when transport of bilirubin into liver cells becomes deficient, or when the enzymes needed to conjugate the bile are lacking. Liver diseases such as hepatitis and cirrhosis are the most common causes of intrahepatic jaundice. Drugs such as the anesthetic agent halothane, oral contraceptives, estrogen, anabolic steroids, isoniazid, and chlorpromazine may also be implicated in this type of jaundice.

Intrahepatic or hepatocellular jaundice usually interferes with all phases of bilirubin metabolism—uptake, conjugation, and excretion. Conjugated and unconjugated bilirubin levels are both elevated, the urine often is dark because of bilirubin in the urine, and serum alkaline phosphatase levels are slightly elevated. Alkaline phosphatase is produced by the bile duct epithelium and canalicular membranes of hepatocytes and excreted with the bile; when bile flow is obstructed, the blood alkaline phosphatase level becomes elevated.

Posthepatic or obstructive jaundice, also called *cholestatic jaundice,* occurs when bile flow is obstructed between the liver and the intestine, with the obstruction located at any point between the junction of the right or left hepatic duct and the point where the bile duct opens into the intestine. Among the causes are strictures of the bile duct, gallstones, and tumors of the bile duct or the pancreas. Conjugated bilirubin levels usually are elevated, the stools are clay colored because of the lack of bilirubin in the bile, the urine is dark, and serum alkaline phosphatase levels are often markedly elevated. Blood levels of bile acids often are elevated in obstructive jaundice. As the bile acids accumulate in the blood, pruritus develops. A history of pruritus preceding jaundice is common in obstructive jaundice.

TESTS OF HEPATOBILIARY FUNCTION

The history and physical examination, in most instances, provide clues about liver function. Laboratory and other diagnostic tests commonly are used to assess liver function and confirm the diagnosis of liver disease.

Liver function tests, including serum levels of liver enzymes, are used to assess injury to liver cells, the liver's ability to synthesize proteins, and the excretory functions of the liver.[5] Elevated serum enzyme test results usually indicate liver injury earlier than other indicators of liver function. The key enzymes are alanine aminotransferase (ALT) and aspartate aminotransferase (AST), which are present in liver cells. ALT is liver specific, whereas AST is derived from organs other than the liver. In most cases of liver damage, there are parallel rises in ALT and AST. The most dramatic rise is seen in cases of acute hepatocellular injury, as occurs with viral hepatitis, hypoxic or ischemic injury, acute toxic injury, or Reye syndrome.

The liver's synthetic capacity is reflected in measures of serum protein levels and prothrombin time (*i.e.,* synthesis of coagulation factors). Hypoalbuminemia due to depressed synthesis may complicate severe liver disease. Deficiencies of coagulation factor V and vitamin K–dependent factors (II, VII, IX, and X) may also occur.

Serum bilirubin, γ-glutamyltransferase (GGT), and alkaline phosphatase measure hepatic excretory function. Alkaline phosphatase is present in the membranes between liver cells and the bile duct and is released by disorders affecting the bile duct.[5] GGT is thought to function in the transport of amino acids and peptides into liver cells; it is a sensitive indicator of hepatobiliary disease. Measurement of GGT may be helpful in diagnosing alcohol abuse.[5]

Ultrasonography provides information about the size, composition, and blood flow of the liver. It has largely replaced cholangiography in detecting stones in the gallbladder or biliary tree. Computed tomography (CT) scanning provides information similar to that obtained by ultrasonography. Magnetic resonance imaging (MRI) has proved to be useful in some disorders. Selective angiography of the celiac, superior mesenteric, or hepatic artery may be used to visualize the hepatic or portal circulation. A liver biopsy affords a means of examining liver tissue without surgery.

In summary, the hepatobiliary system consists of the liver, gallbladder, and bile ducts. The liver is the largest and, in its functions, one of the most versatile organs in the body. It is located between the gastrointestinal tract and the systemic circulation; venous blood from the intestine flows through the liver before it is returned to the heart. In this way, nutrients can be removed for processing and storage, and bacteria and other foreign matter can be removed by Kupffer's cells before the blood is returned to the systemic circulation.

The liver synthesizes fats, glucose, and plasma proteins. Other important functions of the liver include the deamination and interconversion of amino acids, conversion of ammonia to urea, and the metabolism of drugs and hormones. The liver produces approximately 600 to 1200 mL of yellow-green bile daily. Bile serves as an excretory vehicle for bilirubin, cholesterol, and certain products of organic metabolism and it contains bile salts that are essential for digestion of fats and absorption of fat-soluble vitamins. The liver also removes, conjugates, and secretes bilirubin into the bile. Jaundice occurs when bilirubin accumulates in the blood. It can occur because of excessive red blood cell destruction, failure of the liver to remove and conjugate the bilirubin, or obstructed biliary flow.

Liver function tests, including serum aminotransferase levels, are used to assess injury to liver cells. Serum bilirubin, GGT, and alkaline phosphatase are used as a measure of hepatic excretory function. Ultrasonography, CT scans, and MRI are used to evaluate liver structures. Angiography may be used to visualize the hepatic or portal circulation, and a liver biopsy may be used to obtain tissue specimens for microscopic examination.

Disorders of Hepatic and Biliary Function

The structures of the hepatobiliary system are subject to many of the same pathologic conditions that affect other body systems: injury from drugs and toxins; infection, inflammation, and immune responses; metabolic dis-

orders; and neoplasms. This section focuses on alterations in liver function; viral and autoimmune hepatitis; intrahepatic biliary tract disorders; alcoholic and nonalcoholic fatty liver disease; cirrhosis, portal hypertension, and liver failure; and cancer of the liver.

HEPATITIS

Hepatitis refers to inflammation of the liver. Acute hepatitis can be caused by autoimmune disorders or reactions to drugs and toxins; by infectious disorders such as malaria, infectious mononucleosis, salmonellosis, and amebiasis that cause primary infections of extrahepatic tissues and secondary hepatitis; and by hepatotropic viruses that primarily affect liver cells or hepatocytes.

Chronic hepatitis is defined as "symptomatic, biochemical or serologic evidence of continuing or relapsing hepatic disease of more than 6 months' duration."[2] It is characterized by persistently elevated serum aminotransferase levels and characteristic histologic findings on liver biopsy. Although hepatitis viruses account for many of the cases of chronic hepatitis, there are many other causes, including chronic alcoholism, drug toxicities, and autoimmune disorders.

Viral Hepatitis

Viral hepatitis refers to infections of the liver caused by a group of viruses that have particular affinity for the liver.[2] The known hepatotropic viruses include hepatitis A virus (HAV), hepatitis B virus (HBV), the hepatitis B–associated delta virus (HDV), hepatitis C virus (HCV), and hepatitis E virus (HEV). Although all of these viruses cause acute hepatitis, they differ in the mode of trans-

KEY CONCEPTS

Diseases of the Liver

➡ Diseases of the liver can affect the hepatocytes or the biliary drainage system.

➡ Disorders of hepatocyte function impair the metabolic and synthetic functions of the liver, causing disorders in carbohydrate, protein, and fat metabolism; metabolism and removal of drugs, hormones, toxins, ammonia, and bilirubin from the blood; and the interconversion of amino acids and synthesis of proteins. Elevations in serum aminotransferase levels signal the presence of hepatocyte damage.

➡ Disorders of the biliary drainage system obstruct the flow of bile and interfere with the elimination of bile salts and bilirubin, producing cholestatic liver damage because of the backup of bile into the lobules of the liver. Elevations in bilirubin and alkaline phosphatase signal the presence of cholestatic liver damage.

mission and incubation period; mechanism, degree, and chronicity of liver damage; and ability to evolve to a carrier state. The presence of viral antigens and antigen antibodies can be determined through laboratory tests.

Hepatitis A. Hepatitis A is caused by the small, un-enveloped, ribonucleic acid (RNA)–containing HAV. It usually is a benign, self-limited disease, although it can cause acute fulminant hepatitis and death from liver failure in rare cases. The onset of symptoms usually is abrupt and includes fever, malaise, nausea, anorexia, abdominal discomfort, dark urine, and jaundice. The likelihood of having symptoms is related to age.[6,7] Children younger than 5 years of age often are asymptomatic. The illness in older children and adults usually is symptomatic and jaundice occurs in approximately 90% of cases. Symptoms usually last approximately 2 months but can last longer. HAV does not cause chronic hepatitis or induce a carrier state.

Hepatitis A has a brief incubation period (15 to 45 days) and usually is transmitted by the fecal-oral route.[6,7] The virus replicates in the liver, is excreted in the bile, and shed in the stool. The fecal shedding of HAV occurs up to 2 weeks before the development of symptoms and ends as immunoglobulin M (IgM) levels rise.[2] The disease often occurs sporadically or in epidemics. Drinking contaminated milk or water and eating shellfish from infected waters are fairly common routes of transmission. At special risk are persons traveling abroad who have not previously been exposed to the virus. Because young children are asymptomatic, they play an important role in the spread of the disease. Institutions housing large numbers of persons (usually children) sometimes are stricken with an epidemic of hepatitis A. Oral behavior and lack of toilet training promote viral infection among children attending preschool day care centers, who then carry the virus home to older siblings and parents. Hepatitis A usually is not transmitted by transfusion of blood or plasma derivatives, presumably because its short period of viremia usually coincides with clinical illness, so that the disease is apparent and blood donations are not accepted.

Serologic Diagnosis. Antibodies to HAV (anti-HAV) appear early in the disease and tend to persist in the serum (Fig. 29-6). The IgM antibodies (see Chapter 13) usually appear during the first week of symptomatic disease and begin to decline in a few months. Their presence coincides with a decline in fecal shedding of the virus. Peak levels of IgG antibodies occur after 1 month of illness and may persist for years; they provide long-term protective immunity against reinfection. The presence of IgM anti-HAV is indicative of acute hepatitis A, whereas IgG anti-HAV merely documents past exposure.

Vaccination. A hepatitis A vaccine is available.[8] Vaccination is recommended for international travelers to regions where sanitation is poor and endemic HAV infections are high, children living in communities with high rates of HAV infection, homosexually active men, and users of illicit drugs. Persons with preexisting chronic

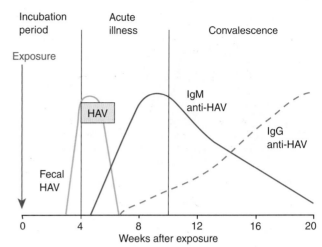

FIGURE 29-6 The sequence of fecal shedding of the hepatitis A virus (HAV), HAV viremia, and HAV antibody (IgM and IgG anti-HAV) changes in hepatitis A.

liver disease also may benefit from immunization. A public health benefit also may be derived from vaccinating persons with increased potential for transmitting the disease (*e.g.,* food handlers). Because the vaccine is of little benefit in prevention of hepatitis in persons with known HAV exposure, immune globulin (IgG) is recommended for these persons.

Hepatitis B. Hepatitis B is caused by a double-stranded deoxyribonucleic acid (DNA) virus (HBV).[2,9] The complete virion, also called a *Dane particle,* consists of an outer envelope and an inner nucleocapsid that contains HBV DNA and DNA polymerase (Fig. 29-7). Hepatitis B can produce acute hepatitis, chronic hepatitis, progression of chronic hepatitis to cirrhosis, fulminant hepatitis with massive hepatic necrosis, and the carrier state. It also participates in the development of hepatitis D.

More than 350 million people worldwide have been infected with HBV.[2,9,10] Seventy-five percent of all chronic carriers live in Asia and the Western Pacific rim. In the United States alone, there are approximately 1.2 million people with chronic HBV infection who are sources of HBV transmission to others.[11] At particular risk of becoming carriers are infants born to hepatitis B–infected mothers. However, since the late 1980s, the incidence of acute hepatitis B has declined steadily, especially among vaccinated children.[11] The decline was much lower among adults, indicating a need for vaccination programs that target high-risk populations.

Hepatitis B has a longer incubation period (4 to 6 weeks) and represents a more serious health problem than hepatitis A. HBV usually is transmitted through inoculation with infected blood or serum. However, the viral antigen can be found in most body secretions and can be spread by oral or sexual contact. In the United States, most persons with hepatitis B acquire the infection as adults or adolescents. The disease is highly prevalent among injecting drug users, persons with multiple sex partners, and men who have sex with men.[12] Health

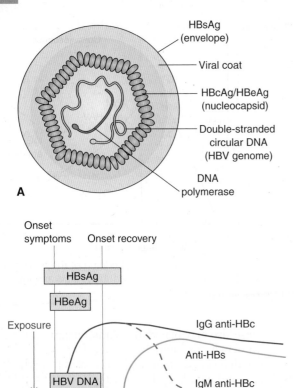

FIGURE 29-7 (A) The hepatitis B virus. **(B)** The sequence of hepatitis B virus (HBV) viral antigens (HBsAg, HBeAg), HBV DNA, and HBV antibody (IgM, IgG, anti-HBc, and anti-HBs) changes in acute resolving hepatitis B.

care workers are at risk owing to blood exposure and accidental needle injuries. Although the virus can be spread through transfusion or administration of blood products, routine screening methods have appreciably reduced transmission through this route. The risk of hepatitis B in infants born to HBV-infected mothers ranges from 10% to 85%, depending on the mother's HBV core antigen (HBeAg) status. Infants who become infected have a 90% risk of becoming chronic carriers, and up to 25% will die of chronic liver disease as adults.[12]

Serologic Diagnosis. Three well-defined antigens are associated with the virus: two core antigens, HBcAg and HBeAg, which are contained in the nucleocapsid, and a third, surface antigen, HBsAg, which is found in the outer envelope of the virus (see Fig. 29-7). These HBV antigens evoke specific antibodies: anti-HBs, anti-HBc, and anti-HBe. These antigens and their antibodies serve as serologic markers for following the course of the disease.

The *HBsAg* is the viral antigen measured most routinely in blood. It is produced in abundance by infected liver cells and released into the serum. HBsAg is the earliest serologic marker to appear; it appears before the onset of symptoms and is an indicator of acute or chronic infection. The HBsAg level begins to decline after the onset of the illness and usually is undetectable in 3 to 6 months.

Persistence beyond 6 months indicates continued viral replication, infectivity, and risk of chronic hepatitis. *Anti-HBs*, the specific antibody to HBsAg, occurs in most individuals after clearance of HBsAg. There often is a delay in appearance of anti-HBs after clearance of HBsAg. During this period of serologic gap, called the *window period*, infectivity has been demonstrated. Development of anti-HBs signals recovery from HBV infection, noninfectivity, and protection from future HBV infection. Anti-HBs is the antibody present in persons who have been successfully immunized for HBV.

The *HBeAg* is thought to be a cleavage product of the viral core antigen; it may be found in the serum as a soluble protein and is an active marker for the disease and shedding of complete virions into the bloodstream. It appears during the incubation period, shortly after the appearance of HBsAg, and is found only in the presence of HBsAg. HBeAg usually disappears before HBsAg. The antibody to HBeAg, *anti-HBe*, begins to appear in the serum at about the time that HBeAg disappears, and its appearance signals the onset of resolution of the acute illness. The clinical usefulness of the antigen and its antibody lies in their predictive value as markers for infectivity.

The *HBcAg* does not circulate in the blood; therefore, it is not a useful marker for the disease. Although the antigen is not found in the blood, its antibodies (anti-HBc) are the first to be detected. They appear toward the end of the incubation period and persist during the acute illness and for several months to years after that. The initial HBcAg antibody is IgM; it serves as a marker for recent infection and is followed in 6 to 18 months by IgG antibodies. These antibodies are not protective and are detectable in the presence of chronic disease.

The presence of viral DNA (HBV DNA) in the serum is the most certain indicator of hepatitis B infection. It is transiently present during the presymptomatic period and for a brief time during the acute illness. The presence of DNA polymerase, the enzyme used in viral replication, usually is transient but may persist for years in persons who are chronic carriers and is an indication of continued infectivity.

Vaccination. Hepatitis B vaccine provides long-term protection against HBV infection.[13] The Centers for Disease Control and Prevention (CDC) recommends vaccination of all children ages 0 to 18 years as a means of preventing HBV transmission.[14] The vaccine also is recommended for all persons who are at high risk for exposure to the virus, including health care workers exposed to blood (required by Occupational Safety and Health Administration regulations). It is recommended that persons with end-stage renal disease be vaccinated before they require hemodialysis and that universal hepatitis B vaccination of teenagers be implemented in communities where injecting drug use, pregnancy among teenagers, and sexually transmitted diseases are common. The CDC also recommends that all pregnant women be routinely tested for HBsAg during an early prenatal visit and that infants born to HBsAg-positive mothers receive appropriate doses of hepatitis immune globulin and hepatitis B vaccine.[12]

Hepatitis C. Hepatitis C is the most common cause of chronic hepatitis, cirrhosis, and hepatocellular cancer in the world. Before 1990, the main route of transmission was through contaminated blood transfusions or blood products. With implementation of HCV testing in blood banks, the risk of HCV infection from blood transfusion is almost nonexistent.[15] There are approximately 3.9 million persons infected with the virus.[15] Most of these people are chronically infected and unaware of their infection because they are not clinically ill. Infected persons serve as a source of infection to others and are at risk for chronic liver disease during the first two or more decades after initial infection.

Formerly known as *non-A, non-B hepatitis*, hepatitis C is caused by a single-stranded RNA virus (HCV) that is distantly related to the viruses that cause yellow fever and dengue fever. There are at least 6 genotypes and more than 50 subtypes of the virus.[15,16] Genotype 1, which is associated with more severe liver disease, accounts for 70% to 75% of cases in the United States. It is likely that the wide diversity of genotypes contributes to the pathogenicity of the virus, allowing it to escape the actions of host immune mechanisms and antiviral medications, and to the difficulties in developing a preventative vaccine.[15,16] Currently, injecting drug use is thought to be the single most important risk factor for HCV infection. There also is concern that transmission of small amounts of blood during tattooing, acupuncture, and body piercing may facilitate the transmission of HCV. Although, the virus may also be transmitted through sexual contact or through vertical transmission from mother to infant, the incidence of such transmission is uncertain.[17] Occupational exposure through incidents such as unintentional needle sticks can result in infection. However, the prevalence of HCV among health care, emergency medical, and public safety workers who are exposed to blood in the workplace is reported to be no greater than in the general public.

The incubation period for HCV infection ranges from 2 to 26 weeks (mean, 6 to 12 weeks).[2] Clinical symptoms with acute hepatitis C tend to be milder than those seen in persons with other types of viral hepatitis. Children and adults who acquire the infection usually are asymptomatic, or have a nonspecific clinical disease characterized by fatigue, malaise, anorexia, and weight loss. Jaundice is uncommon, and only 25% to 30% of symptomatic adults have jaundice.[18] These symptoms usually last for 2 to 12 weeks. Unlike hepatitis A and B viral infections, fulminant hepatic failure is rare and only a few cases have been reported. The most alarming aspects of HCV infection are its high rate of persistence and ability to induce chronic hepatitis and cirrhosis. HCV also increases the risk for development of hepatocellular cancer.

Serologic Diagnosis. Both antibody and HCV RNA tests are available for detecting the presence of hepatitis C infection (Fig. 29-8). Antibody testing has the advantage of being readily available and having a relatively

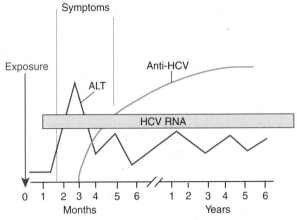

FIGURE 29-8 The sequence of serologic changes in chronic hepatitis C with persistence of hepatitis C virus (HCV) RNA and exacerbations and remissions of clinical symptoms designated by changes in serum alanine aminotransferase (ALT) levels.

lower cost. With newer antibody testing methods, infection often can be detected as early as 6 to 8 weeks after exposure. False-negative results can occur in immunocompromised people and early in the course of the disease before antibodies develop. The HCV RNA tests are highly sensitive and specific, but more costly than antibody tests. HCV RNA is detectable in the blood for 1 to 3 weeks, coincident with elevations in serum aminotransferases. Unlike hepatitis A and B, antibodies to HCV are not protective, but they serve as markers for the disease. At present, there is no vaccine that protects against HCV infection.

Hepatitis D. Hepatitis D virus, or the delta hepatitis agent, is a defective RNA virus. It can cause acute or chronic hepatitis. Infection depends on concomitant infection with hepatitis B, specifically the presence of HBsAg. Acute hepatitis D occurs in two forms: coinfection that occurs simultaneously with acute hepatitis B and as a superinfection in which hepatitis D is imposed on chronic hepatitis B or the hepatitis B carrier state.[19] The delta agent often increases the severity of HBV infection. It can convert mild HBV infection into severe, fulminating hepatitis, cause acute hepatitis in asymptomatic carriers, or increase the tendency for progression to chronic hepatitis and cirrhosis.

The routes of transmission of hepatitis D are similar to those for hepatitis B. In the United States, infection is restricted largely to persons at high risk for HBV infection, particularly injecting drug users and persons receiving clotting factor concentrates. The greatest risk is in HBV carriers; these persons should be informed about the dangers of HDV superinfection.

Hepatitis D is diagnosed by detection of antibody to HDV (anti-HDV) in the serum or HDV RNA in the serum. There is no specific treatment for hepatitis D. Because the infection is linked to hepatitis B, prevention of hepatitis D should begin with prevention of hepatitis B through vaccination.

Hepatitis E. Hepatitis E virus is an unenveloped, single-stranded RNA virus. It is transmitted by the fecal-oral route and causes manifestations of acute hepatitis that are similar to hepatitis A. It does not cause chronic hepatitis or the carrier state. Its distinguishing feature is the high mortality rate (approximately 20%) among pregnant women, owing to the development of fulminant hepatitis. The infection occurs primarily in developing areas such as India, other Southeast Asian countries, parts of Africa, and Mexico. The only reported cases in the United States have been in persons who have recently been in an endemic area.

Clinical Course in Viral Hepatitis

There are two mechanisms of liver injury in viral hepatitis: direct cellular injury and induction of immune responses against the viral-infected hepatocytes. The mechanisms of injury have been most closely studied in HBV. It is thought that the extent of inflammation and necrosis depends on the individual's immune response. Accordingly, a prompt immune response during the acute phase of the infection would be expected to cause cell injury but at the same time eliminate the virus. Thus, people who respond with fewer symptoms and a marginal immune response are less likely to eliminate the virus, and hepatocytes expressing the viral antigens persist, leading to the chronic or carrier state. Fulminant hepatitis would be explained in terms of an accelerated immune response with severe liver necrosis.

The clinical course of viral hepatitis involves a number of syndromes, including acute asymptomatic infection with only serologic evidence of disease; acute symptomatic hepatitis; chronic hepatitis with or without progression to cirrhosis; or fulminating disease (>1% to 3%) with submassive hepatic necrosis and rapid onset of liver failure.[2] Not all hepatotoxic viruses provoke each of the clinical syndromes.

Acute Asymptomatic Viral Hepatitis. Acute asymptomatic viral hepatitis is identified only incidentally by elevated serum aminotransferases or, after the fact, by the presence of antiviral antibodies. Asymptomatic acute infection is seen most commonly in persons infected with HCV.

Acute Symptomatic Viral Hepatitis. The manifestations of *acute symptomatic viral hepatitis* can be divided into three phases: the prodromal or preicteric period, the icterus period, and the convalescent period. The manifestations of the prodromal period vary from abrupt to insidious, with general malaise, myalgia, arthralgia, easy fatigability, and severe anorexia out of proportion to the degree of illness. Gastrointestinal symptoms such as nausea, vomiting, and diarrhea or constipation may occur. Abdominal pain is usually mild and is felt on the right side. Chills and fever may mark an abrupt onset. In persons who smoke, there may be distaste for smoking that parallels the anorexia. Serum levels of AST and ALT show variable increases during the preicteric phase of acute hepatitis and precede a rise in bilirubin that accom-panies the onset of the icterus or jaundice phase of infection. The icterus phase, if it occurs, usually follows the prodromal phase by 5 to 10 days. Jaundice is less likely to occur with HCV infection. The prodromal symptoms may become worse with the onset of jaundice, followed by progressive clinical improvement. Severe pruritus and liver tenderness are common during the icterus period. The convalescent phase is characterized by an increased sense of well-being, return of appetite, and disappearance of jaundice. The acute illness usually subsides gradually over a 2- to 3-week period, with complete clinical recovery by approximately 9 weeks in hepatitis A and 16 weeks in uncomplicated hepatitis B.

Chronic Viral Hepatitis. Chronic viral hepatitis is the principal cause of chronic liver disease, cirrhosis, and hepatocellular cancer in the world and now ranks as the chief reason for liver transplantation in adults.[20] Of the hepatotropic viruses, only three are known to cause chronic hepatitis—HBV, HCV, and HDV.

Chronic hepatitis C accounts for most cases of chronic viral hepatitis. HCV infection becomes chronic in 75% to 80% of cases.[15] Chronic HCV infection often smolders over a period of years, silently destroying liver cells. Most persons with chronic hepatitis C are asymptomatic, and diagnosis usually follows a finding of elevated serum aminotransferase levels, a tender liver, or complaints of fatigue or nonspecific weakness. Because the course of acute hepatitis C often is mild, many persons do not recall the events of the acute infection. Hepatitis B is less likely than hepatitis C to progress to chronic infection. Chronic hepatitis B is characterized by the persistence of HBV DNA and usually by HBeAg in the serum, indicating active viral replication.

The clinical features of chronic viral hepatitis are highly variable and not predictive of outcome. Many persons with chronic viral hepatitis are asymptomatic at the time of diagnosis, and elevated serum aminotransferase levels are the first sign of infection. The most common symptoms are fatigue, malaise, loss of appetite, and occasional bouts of jaundice. Elevation of serum aminotransferase concentrations depends on the level of disease activity.

Chronic viral hepatitis constitutes a carrier state in which the person does not have symptoms but harbors the virus and can therefore transmit the disease. Evidence indicates a carrier state for HBV, HCV, and HDV infection. There is no carrier state for HAV infection. There are two types of carriers: healthy carriers who have few or no ill effects, and those with chronic disease who may or may not have symptoms. Factors that increase the risk of becoming a carrier are age at time of infection and immune status. The carrier state for infections that occur early in life, as in infants of HBV-infected mothers, may be as high as 90% to 95%, compared with 1% to 10% of infected adults.[3] Other persons at high risk for becoming carriers are those with impaired immunity, those who have received multiple transfusions or blood products, those who are on hemodialysis, and drug addicts.

There are no simple and effective treatment methods for chronic viral hepatitis. Persons with chronic hepatitis

B who have evidence of active viral replication may be treated with a course of recombinant interferon alfa-2b.[21] The nucleoside analogs, which directly block replication of the HBV genome (*e.g.*, lamivudine), may be used as a substitute for interferon alfa. Chronic HCV may be treated with a combination of the new pegylated forms of interferon (alfa-2b or alfa-2a) plus ribavirin.[21] Peginterferons were developed by adding a polyethylene glycol (PEG) moiety to an interferon molecule, resulting in a prolonged serum half-life and the ability to administer the compound once weekly rather than three times a week.[22] Ribavirin, a nucleoside analog, may be added to the treatment regimen. Treatment with peginterferon and ribavirin is costly and the side effects, which include flulike symptoms, are almost universal. More serious side effects, which include psychiatric symptoms (depression), thyroid dysfunction, and bone marrow depression, are less common.[22]

Liver transplantation is a treatment option for end-stage liver disease due to viral hepatitis. Liver transplantation has been more successful in persons with hepatitis C than those with hepatitis B. Although the graft often is reinfected, the disease seems to progress more slowly.

Fulminant Hepatitis. Fulminant hepatitis represents the rapid progression from onset of symptoms to hepatic encephalopathy within 2 to 3 weeks.[2] A less rapid course, extending up to 3 months, is called *subfulminant failure.* In the United States viral hepatitis accounts for about 12% of cases of fulminant liver failure, almost all due to HAV and HBV.[2] Drugs and chemical toxicity account for a substantial share of the remainder. Fulminant hepatic failure may present as jaundice, encephalopathy, and other signs of liver failure. Notably missing are evidence of chronic liver disease (to be discussed). The overall mortality rate ranges from 25% to 90% in the absence of liver transplantation.

Autoimmune Hepatitis

Chronic autoimmune hepatitis is a chronic inflammatory liver disease of unknown origin, but it is associated with circulating autoantibodies and high serum gamma globulin levels. Autoimmune hepatitis accounts for only approximately 10% of chronic hepatitis in the United States, a decrease from previously reported rates that probably reflect not a true change in incidence but better methods of detecting hepatitis due to viral pathogens. The pathogenesis of the disorder is one of a genetically predisposed person exposed to an environmental agent that triggers an autoimmune response directed at liver cell antigens.[23] The resulting immune response produces a necrotizing inflammatory response that eventually leads to destruction of liver cells and development of cirrhosis. The factors surrounding the genetic predisposition and the triggering events that lead to the autoimmune response are unclear. Autoimmune hepatitis is mainly a disease of young women, although it can occur at any age and in men or women. Other forms of autoimmune hepatitis are present in persons with rheumatic arthritis, thyroiditis, Sjögren syndrome, and ulcerative colitis.[2]

Clinical presentation is similar to other forms of chronic hepatitis. Manifestations of the disorder cover a spectrum that extends from no apparent symptoms to the signs accompanying liver failure. An acute appearance of clinical illness is common, and a fulminant presentation is possible. In asymptomatic cases, the disorder may be discovered when abnormal serum enzyme levels are discovered during performance of routine screening tests.

The differential diagnosis includes measures to exclude other causes of liver disease, including hepatitis B and C. A characteristic laboratory finding is that of a marked elevation in serum gamma globulins. A biopsy is used to confirm the diagnosis.

Corticosteroid drugs and immunosuppressant drugs are the treatment of choice for this type of hepatitis. Liver transplantation may be the only treatment for end-stage disease.

INTRAHEPATIC BILIARY DISORDERS

Intrahepatic biliary diseases disrupt the flow of bile through the liver, causing cholestasis and biliary cirrhosis. Among the causes of intrahepatic biliary disease are primary biliary cirrhosis, primary sclerosing cholangitis, and secondary biliary cirrhosis.

Primary Biliary Cirrhosis

Primary biliary cirrhosis involves inflammation and scarring of small intrahepatic bile ducts, portal inflammation, and progressive scarring of liver tissue.[24,25] The disease is seen most commonly in women 40 to 60 years of age and accounts for 2% to 5% of cases of cirrhosis. Familial occurrences of the disease are found between parents and children and among siblings. Abnormalities of cell-mediated and humoral immunity suggest an autoimmune mechanism. Antimitochondrial antibodies are found in 98% of persons with the disease, but their role in the pathogenesis of the disease is unclear.[25] Up to 84% of persons with primary biliary cirrhosis have at least one other autoimmune disorder, such as scleroderma, Hashimoto thyroiditis, rheumatoid arthritis, or Sjögren syndrome.

The disorder is characterized by an insidious onset and progressive scarring and destruction of liver tissue. The liver becomes enlarged and takes on a green hue because of the accumulated bile. The earliest symptoms are unexplained pruritus or itching, weight loss, and fatigue, followed by dark urine and pale stools. Jaundice is a late manifestation of the disorder, as are other signs of liver failure. Serum alkaline phosphatase levels are elevated in persons with primary biliary cirrhosis.

Treatment is largely symptomatic. Bile acid–binding drugs are used as a treatment for itching. Some persons have responded to ultraviolet B light, methyltestosterone, cimetidine, phenobarbital, and prednisone. There is no generally accepted treatment for the underlying disease. Clinical trials using ursodiol, a drug that increases bile flow and decreases the toxicity of bile contents, have shown a decreased rate of clinical deterioration with drug treatment.[25] Colchicine, which acts to prevent leukocyte migration and phagocytosis, and methotrexate, a drug with immunosuppressive properties, have had some reported benefit in improving symptoms. However, liver transplantation remains the only treatment for advanced disease. Primary biliary cirrhosis does not recur after liver transplantation if appropriate immunosuppression is used.[24,25]

Primary Sclerosing Cholangitis

Cholangitis involves inflammation of hepatic bile ducts. Primary sclerosing cholangitis is a chronic cholestatic disease of unknown origin that causes destruction and fibrosis of intrahepatic and extrahepatic bile ducts.[26] Bile flow is obstructed (*i.e.*, cholestasis), and the bile retention destroys hepatic structures. The disease commonly is associated with inflammatory bowel disease, occurs more often in men than women, and is seen most commonly in the third to fifth decades of life. Primary sclerosing cholangitis, although much less common than alcoholic cirrhosis, is the fourth leading indication for liver transplantation in adults in the United States.[26]

Most persons with the disorder are initially asymptomatic, with the disorder being detected during routine liver function tests that reveal elevated levels of serum alkaline phosphatase or GGT. Alternatively, some persons present with progressive fatigue, jaundice, and pruritus. The later stages of the disease are characterized by cirrhosis, portal hypertension, and liver failure.[26] Ten-year survival rates range from 50% to 75%. Other than measures aimed at symptom relief, the only treatment is liver transplantation.

Secondary Biliary Cirrhosis

Secondary biliary cirrhosis results from prolonged obstruction of the extrabiliary tree. The most common cause is cholelithiasis. Other causes of secondary biliary cirrhosis are malignant neoplasms of the biliary tree or head of the pancreas and strictures of the common duct caused by previous surgical procedures. Extrahepatic biliary cirrhosis may benefit from surgical procedures designed to relieve the obstruction.

ALCOHOLIC LIVER DISEASE

The spectrum of alcoholic liver disease includes fatty liver disease, alcoholic hepatitis, and cirrhosis. Alcoholic cirrhosis causes 100,000 to 200,000 deaths annually and is the fifth leading cause of death in the United States.[2] Most deaths from alcoholic cirrhosis are attributable to liver failure, bleeding esophageal varices, or kidney failure. It has been estimated that there are 10 million alcoholics in the United States. Only approximately 10% to 15% of alcoholics develop cirrhosis, however, suggesting that other conditions such as genetic and environmental factors contribute to its occurrence.[2]

Although the mechanism by which alcohol exerts its toxic effects on liver structures is somewhat uncertain, the changes that develop can be divided into three stages: fatty changes, alcoholic hepatitis, and cirrhosis.[2,3] *Fatty liver* is characterized by the accumulation of fat in hepa-

tocytes, a condition called *steatosis* (Fig. 29-9). The liver becomes yellow and enlarges owing to excessive fat accumulation. The pathogenesis of fatty liver is not completely understood and can depend on the amount of alcohol consumed, dietary fat content, body stores of fat, hormonal status, and other factors.[27,28] There is evidence that ingestion of large amounts of alcohol can cause fatty liver changes even with an adequate diet. For example, young, nonalcoholic volunteers had fatty liver changes after 2 days of consuming 18 to 24 oz of alcohol, even though adequate carbohydrates, fats, and proteins were included in the diet.[29] The fatty changes that occur with ingestion of alcohol usually do not produce symptoms and are reversible after the alcohol intake has been discontinued.

Alcoholic hepatitis is the intermediate stage between fatty changes and cirrhosis. It often is seen after an abrupt increase in alcohol intake and is common in "spree" drinkers. Alcoholic hepatitis is characterized by inflammation and necrosis of liver cells. This stage usually is characterized by hepatic tenderness, pain, anorexia, nausea, fever, jaundice, ascites, and liver failure, but some individuals may be asymptomatic. The condition is always serious and sometimes fatal. The immediate prognosis correlates with severity of liver cell injury. In some cases, the disease progresses rapidly to liver failure and death. The mortality rate in the acute stage ranges from 10% to 30%.[2] In persons who survive and continue to drink, the acute

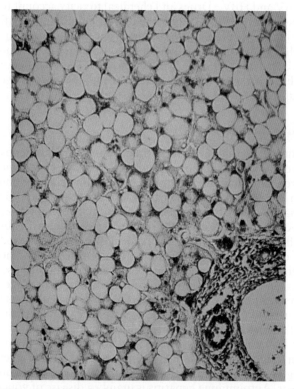

FIGURE 29-9 Alcoholic fatty liver. A photomicrograph shows the cytoplasm of almost all the hepatocytes to be distended by fat, which displaces the nucleus to the periphery. Note the absence of inflammation and fibrosis. (From Rubin E., Farber J. L. [1999]. *Pathology* [3rd ed., p. 791]. Philadelphia: Lippincott Williams & Wilkins.)

phase often is followed by persistent alcoholic hepatitis with progression to cirrhosis in a matter of 1 to 2 years.[2]

Alcoholic cirrhosis is the end result of repeated bouts of drinking-related liver injury and designates the onset of end-stage alcoholic liver disease. The gross appearance of the early cirrhotic liver is one of fine, uniform nodules on its surface. The condition has traditionally been called *micronodular* or *Laennec cirrhosis*. With more advanced cirrhosis, regenerative processes cause the nodules to become larger and more irregular in size and shape. As this happens, the nodules cause the liver to become relobulized through the formation of new portal tracts and venous outflow channels. The nodules may compress the hepatic veins, curtailing blood flow out of the liver and producing portal hypertension, extrahepatic portosystemic shunts, and cholestasis.

NONALCOHOLIC FATTY LIVER DISEASE

The term *nonalcoholic fatty liver disease* (NAFLD) is often used to describe fatty liver disease with its potential for progression to cirrhosis and end-stage liver disease arising from causes other than alcohol.[30,31] The condition can range from simple steatosis to steatohepatitis. Although steatosis alone does not appear to be progressive, approximately 20% of persons with steatohepatitis progress to cirrhosis over a decade.[30] Obesity, type 2 diabetes, the metabolic syndrome (see Chapter 32), and hypertriglyceridemia are coexisting conditions frequently associated with fatty liver disease. The condition is also associated with other nutritional abnormalities, surgical conditions, drugs, and occupational exposure to toxins. Both rapid weight loss and parenteral nutrition may lead to NAFLD. Jejunoileal bypass, a surgical procedure used for weight loss, has largely been abandoned for this reason.

The pathogenesis of nonalcoholic liver disease is thought to involve both hepatic fat accumulation and oxidative stress associated with formation of free radicals. Several factors, presumably resulting from impaired responsiveness to insulin, are thought to lead to the accumulation of fat in the liver of persons with NAFLD. These factors include increased mobilization of fatty acids from fat stores, increased synthesis of triglycerides and very low density lipoproteins by hepatocytes, and decreased clearance of triglyceride-rich lipoproteins by adipose tissue and skeletal muscle. The accumulation of toxic levels of free fatty acids increases the formation of free radicals, with subsequent hepatocytes injury (see Chapter 2).

CIRRHOSIS

Cirrhosis represents the end stage of chronic liver disease in which much of the functional liver tissue has been replaced by fibrous tissue. It is characterized by diffuse fibrosis and conversion of normal liver architecture into structurally abnormal nodules.[2,3] The fibrous tissue replaces normally functioning liver tissue and forms constrictive bands that disrupt flow in the vascular channels and biliary duct systems of the liver. The disruption of vascular channels predisposes to portal hypertension and its complications; obstruction of biliary channels and exposure to the destructive effects of bile stasis; and loss of liver cells, leading to liver failure. Although cirrhosis usually is associated with alcoholism, it can develop in the course of other disorders, including viral hepatitis, toxic reactions to drugs and chemicals, biliary obstruction, and heart failure. Cirrhosis also accompanies metabolic disorders that cause the deposition of minerals in the liver. Two of these disorders are hemochromatosis (*i.e.*, iron deposition) and Wilson disease (*i.e.*, copper deposition).

The manifestations of cirrhosis are variable, ranging from asymptomatic hepatomegaly to hepatic failure. Often there are no symptoms until the disease is far advanced. The most common signs and symptoms of cirrhosis are weight loss (sometimes masked by ascites), weakness, and anorexia. Jaundice, usually not an early sign, is mild at first but increases in severity during the later stages of the disease. Diarrhea frequently is present, although some persons may complain of constipation. There may be abdominal pain because of liver enlargement or stretching of Glisson capsule. This pain is located in the epigastric area or in the upper right quadrant and is described as dull, aching, and causing a sensation of fullness.

The late manifestations of cirrhosis are related to portal hypertension and liver failure. Splenomegaly, ascites, and portosystemic shunts (*i.e.*, esophageal varices, anorectal varices, and caput medusae) result from portal hypertension. Other late complications include bleeding due to decreased clotting factors, thrombocytopenia due to splenomegaly, gynecomastia and a feminizing pattern of pubic hair distribution in men because of testicular atrophy, spider angiomas, palmar erythema, and encephalopathy with asterixis and neurologic signs.

Portal Hypertension

Portal hypertension is characterized by increased resistance to flow in the portal venous system and sustained portal vein pressure above 22 mm Hg (normal, 5 to 10 mm Hg).[3]

 KEY CONCEPTS

Portal Hypertension

→ Venous blood from the gastrointestinal tract empties into the portal vein and travels through the liver before moving into the general venous circulation.

→ Obstruction of blood flow and development of portal hypertension produces an increase in the hydrostatic pressure within the peritoneal capillaries, contributing to the development of ascites, splenic engorgement with sequestration and destruction of blood cells and platelets, and shunting of blood to collateral venous channels causing varicosities of the hemorrhoidal and esophageal veins.

Normally, venous blood returning to the heart from the abdominal organs collects in the portal vein and travels through the liver before entering the vena cava. Portal hypertension can be caused by a variety of conditions that increase resistance to hepatic blood flow, including prehepatic, posthepatic, and intrahepatic obstructions (with *hepatic* referring to the liver lobules rather than the entire liver).[3] *Prehepatic* causes of portal hypertension include portal vein thrombosis and external compression due to cancer or enlarged lymph nodes that produce obstruction of the portal vein before it enters the liver.

Posthepatic obstruction refers to any obstruction to blood flow through the hepatic veins beyond the liver lobules, either within or distal to the liver. It is caused by conditions such as thrombosis of the hepatic veins, veno-occlusive disease, and severe right-sided heart failure that impede the outflow of venous blood from the liver. *Budd-Chiari syndrome* refers to congestive disease of the liver caused by occlusion of the portal veins and their tributaries. The principal cause of the Budd-Chiari syndrome is thrombosis of the hepatic veins, in association with diverse conditions such as polycythemia vera, hypercoagulability states associated with malignant tumors, pregnancy, bacterial infection, metastatic disease of the liver, and trauma. *Hepatic veno-occlusive disease* is a variant of the Budd-Chiari syndrome seen most commonly in persons treated with certain cancer chemotherapeutic drugs, hepatic irradiation, or bone marrow transplantation, possibly because of graft-versus-host disease.[3]

Intrahepatic causes of portal hypertension include conditions that cause obstruction of blood flow within the liver. In alcoholic cirrhosis, which is the major cause of portal hypertension, bands of fibrous tissue and fibrous nodules distort the architecture of the liver and increase the resistance to portal blood flow, which leads to portal hypertension.

Complications of portal hypertension arise from the increased pressure and dilatation of the venous channels behind the obstruction. In addition, collateral channels open that connect the portal circulation with the systemic circulation. The major complications of the increased portal vein pressure and the opening of collateral channels are ascites, splenomegaly, and the formation of portosystemic shunts with bleeding from esophageal varices (Fig. 29-10).

Ascites. Ascites occurs when the amount of fluid in the peritoneal cavity is increased, and is a late-stage manifestation of cirrhosis and portal hypertension.[32] It is not uncommon for persons with advanced cirrhosis to present with an accumulation of 15 L or more of ascitic fluid. Those who gain this much fluid often experience abdominal discomfort, dyspnea, and insomnia, and they may have difficulty walking or living independently.[33]

Although the mechanisms responsible for the development of ascites are not completely understood, several factors seem to contribute to fluid accumulation, including an increase in capillary pressure due to portal hypertension and obstruction of venous flow through the liver, and salt and water retention by the kidney. These disturbances include failure of the liver to metabolize aldosterone, causing an increase in salt and water retention by the kidney. Another likely contributing factor in the pathogenesis of ascites is a decreased colloidal osmotic pressure, which limits reabsorption of fluid from the peritoneal cavity (see Chapter 6).

Treatment of ascites usually focuses on dietary restriction of sodium and administration of diuretics. Water intake also may need to be restricted. Because of the many limitations in sodium restriction, the use of diuretics has become the mainstay of treatment for ascites. Two classes of diuretics are used: the potassium-sparing diuretics (*e.g.,* spironolactone) that act on the distal part of the nephron to inhibit aldosterone-dependent sodium reabsorption, and the loop diuretics (*e.g.,* furosemide) that inhibit sodium chloride reabsorption in the thick ascending loop of Henle. Oral potassium supplements often are given to prevent hypokalemia. The upright position is associated with the activation of the renin-angiotensin-aldosterone system; therefore, bed rest may be recommended for persons with a large amount of ascites.[34]

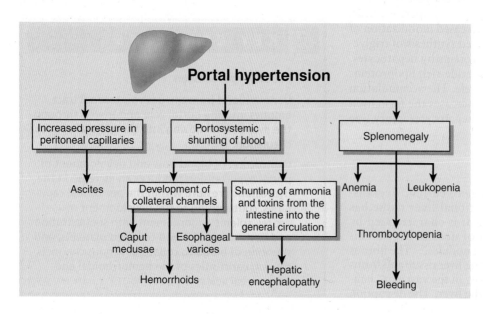

FIGURE 29-10 Mechanisms of disturbed liver function related to portal hypertension.

Large-volume paracentesis (removal of 5 L or more of ascitic fluid) may be done in persons with massive ascites and pulmonary compromise. Because the removal of fluid produces a decrease in vascular volume along with increased plasma renin activity and aldosterone-mediated sodium and water reabsorption by the kidneys, a volume expander such as albumin usually is administered to maintain the effective circulating volume.[20] A transjugular intrahepatic portosystemic shunt may be inserted in persons with refractory ascites (to be discussed).[20]

Spontaneous bacterial peritonitis is a complication in persons with both cirrhosis and ascites. The infection is serious and carries a high mortality rate even when treated with antibiotics. Presumably, the peritoneal fluid becomes seeded with bacteria from the blood or lymph or from passage of bacteria through the bowel wall. Symptoms include fever and abdominal pain. Other manifestations include worsening of hepatic encephalopathy, diarrhea, hypothermia, and shock. It is diagnosed by a neutrophil count of 250/mm^3 or higher and a protein concentration of 1 g/dL or less in the ascitic fluid.[20]

Splenomegaly. The spleen enlarges progressively in portal hypertension because of shunting of blood into the splenic vein. The enlarged spleen can sequester significant numbers of blood elements, often leading to development of a syndrome known as *hypersplenism*. Hypersplenism is characterized by a decrease in the life span and a subsequent decrease in all the formed elements of the blood, leading to anemia, thrombocytopenia, and leukopenia. The decreased life span of the blood elements is thought to result from an increased rate of removal because of the prolonged transit time through the enlarged spleen.

Portosystemic Shunts. With the gradual obstruction of venous blood flow in the liver, the pressure in the portal vein increases, and large collateral channels develop between the portal and systemic veins that supply the lower rectum and esophagus and the umbilical veins of the falciform ligament that attaches to the anterior wall of the abdomen. The collaterals between the inferior and internal iliac veins may give rise to hemorrhoids. In some persons, the fetal umbilical vein is not totally obliterated; it forms a channel on the anterior abdominal wall (Fig. 29-11). Dilated veins around the umbilicus are called *caput medusae*. Portopulmonary shunts also may develop and cause blood to bypass the pulmonary capillaries, interfering with blood oxygenation and producing cyanosis.

Clinically, the most important collateral channels are those connecting the portal and coronary veins that lead to reversal of flow and formation of thin-walled varicosities in the submucosa of the esophagus (Fig. 29-12). These thin-walled *esophageal varices* are subject to rupture, producing massive and sometimes fatal hemorrhage.[35,36] Impaired hepatic synthesis of coagulation factors and decreased platelet levels (*i.e.*, thrombocytopenia) due to splenomegaly may further complicate the control of esophageal bleeding. Esophageal varices develop in approximately 65% of persons with advanced cirrhosis and cause massive hemorrhage and death in approximately half of them.[3]

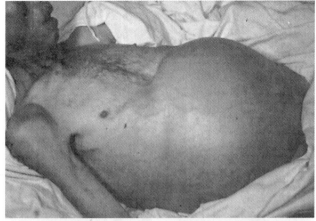
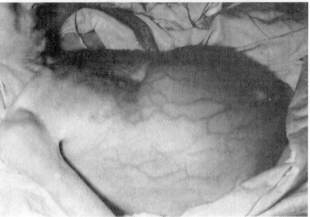

FIGURE 29-11 Collateral abdominal veins on the anterior abdominal wall in a patient with alcoholic liver disease as recorded by black and white photography (**top**) and infrared photography (**bottom**). (From Schiff L. [1982]. *Diseases of the liver.* Philadelphia: J. B. Lippincott.)

Treatment. Treatment of portal hypertension and esophageal varices is directed at prevention of initial hemorrhage, management of acute hemorrhage, and prevention of recurrent variceal hemorrhage. Pharmacologic therapy is used to lower portal venous pressure and prevent initial hemorrhage. β-Adrenergic–blocking drugs (*e.g.*, propranolol) commonly are used for this purpose. These agents reduce portal venous pressure by decreasing splanchnic blood flow and thereby decreasing blood flow in collateral channels. Long-acting nitrates may be used to decrease the risk of variceal rebleeding in people who cannot tolerate β-blockers.

Several methods are used to control acute hemorrhage, including administration of drugs that constrict the splanchnic circulation (*e.g.*, octreotide or vasopressin), balloon tamponade, endoscopic injection sclerotherapy, vessel ligation, and esophageal transection.[36] Balloon tamponade provides compression of the varices and is accomplished through insertion of a tube with inflatable gastric and esophageal balloons. During endoscopic sclerotherapy, the varices are injected with a sclerosing solution that obliterates the vessel lumen.

Prevention of recurrent hemorrhage focuses on lowering portal venous pressure and diverting blood flow away

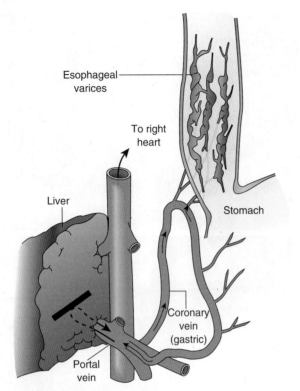

FIGURE 29-12 Obstruction of blood flow in the portal circulation, with portal hypertension and diversion of blood flow to other venous channels, including the gastric and esophageal veins.

from the easily ruptured collateral channels. Two procedures may be used for this purpose: the surgical creation of a portosystemic shunt or a transjugular intrahepatic portosystemic shunt (TIPS). *Surgical portosystemic shunt* procedures involve the creation of an opening between the portal vein and a systemic vein. These shunts have a considerable complication rate, and TIPS has evolved as the preferred treatment for refractory portal hypertension. The TIPS procedure involves insertion of an expandable metal stent between a branch of the hepatic vein and the portal vein using a catheter inserted through the internal jugular vein. A complication that is associated with the creation of a portosystemic shunt is hepatic encephalopathy, which is thought to result when ammonia and other neurotoxic substances from the gut pass directly into the systemic circulation without going through the liver.

LIVER FAILURE

The most severe clinical consequences of liver disease is hepatic failure. It may result from sudden and massive liver destruction, as in fulminant hepatitis, or be the result of progressive damage to the liver as occurs in alcoholic cirrhosis. Whatever the cause, 80% to 90% of hepatic functional capacity must be lost before liver failure occurs.[2] In many cases, the progressive decompensating effects of the disease are hastened by intercurrent conditions such as gastrointestinal bleeding, systemic infection, elec-

trolyte disturbances, or superimposed diseases such as heart failure.

Manifestations

The manifestations of liver failure reflect the various synthesis, storage, metabolic, and elimination functions of the liver (Fig. 29-13). *Fetor hepaticus* refers to a characteristic musty, sweetish odor of the breath in the patient in advanced liver failure, resulting from the metabolic byproducts of the intestinal bacteria.

Hematologic Disorders. Liver failure can cause anemia, thrombocytopenia, coagulation defects, and leukopenia. Anemia may be caused by blood loss, excessive red blood cell destruction, and impaired formation of red blood cells. A folic acid deficiency may lead to severe megaloblastic anemia. Changes in the lipid composition of the red cell membrane increase hemolysis. Because factors V, VII, IX, and X, prothrombin, and fibrinogen are synthesized by the liver, their decline in liver disease contributes to bleeding disorders. Malabsorption of the fat-soluble vitamin K contributes further to the impaired synthesis of these clotting factors. Thrombocytopenia often occurs as the result of splenomegaly. The person with liver failure is subject to purpura, easy bruising, hematuria, and abnormal menstrual bleeding, and is vulnerable to bleeding from the esophagus and other segments of the gastrointestinal tract.

Endocrine Disorders. Endocrine disorders, particularly disturbances in gonadal (sex hormone) function, are common accompaniments of cirrhosis and liver failure. The liver metabolizes the steroid hormones; therefore, these hormones are often elevated in persons with liver failure. A decrease in aldosterone metabolism may contribute to salt and water retention by the kidney, along with a lowering of serum potassium resulting from increased elimination of potassium. Women may have menstrual irregularities (usually amenorrhea), loss of libido, and sterility. Men may experience testicular atrophy, loss of libido, impotence, and development of gynecomastia. These changes may occur as the result of increased androgens in women and excess estrogens in men, and, in alcoholic liver disease, from a direct toxic effect of alcohol on the gonads.[3]

Skin Disorders. Liver failure brings on numerous skin disorders. These lesions, called variously *vascular spiders, telangiectases, spider angiomas,* and *spider nevi,* are seen most often in the upper half of the body. They consist of a central pulsating arteriole from which smaller vessels radiate. Palmar erythema is redness of the palms, probably caused by increased blood flow from higher cardiac output. Clubbing of the fingers may be seen in persons with cirrhosis. Jaundice usually is a late manifestation of liver failure.

Hepatorenal Syndrome. The hepatorenal syndrome refers to a functional renal failure sometimes seen during

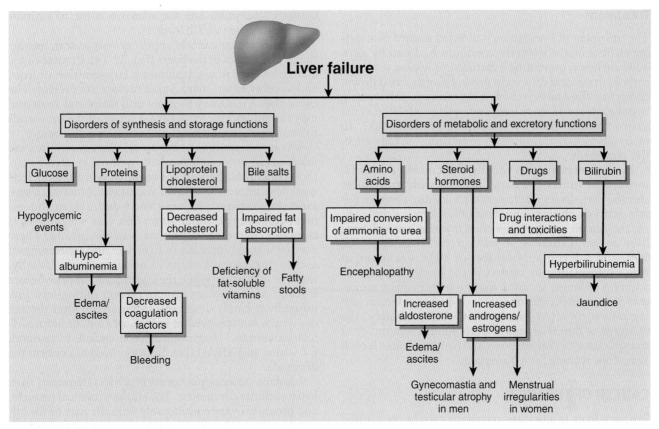

FIGURE 29-13 Alterations in liver function and manifestations of liver failure.

the terminal stages of liver failure with ascites.[37] It is characterized by progressive azotemia, increased serum creatinine levels, and oliguria. Although the basic cause is unknown, a decrease in renal blood flow is believed to play a part. Ultimately, when renal failure is superimposed on liver failure, azotemia and elevated levels of blood ammonia occur; this condition is thought to contribute to hepatic encephalopathy and coma.

Hepatic Encephalopathy. Hepatic encephalopathy refers to the totality of central nervous system (CNS) manifestations of liver failure. It is characterized by neural disturbances ranging from a lack of mental alertness to confusion, coma, and convulsions. A very early sign of hepatic encephalopathy is a flapping tremor called *asterixis*. Various degrees of memory loss may occur, coupled with personality changes such as euphoria, irritability, anxiety, and lack of concern about personal appearance and self. Speech may be impaired, and the patient may be unable to perform certain purposeful movements. The encephalopathy may progress to decerebrate rigidity and then to a terminal deep coma.

Although the cause of hepatic encephalopathy is unclear, the accumulation of neurotoxins, which appear in the blood because the liver has lost its detoxifying capacity, is believed to be a factor. Hepatic encephalopathy develops in approximately 10% of persons with portosystemic shunts.

One of the suspected neurotoxins is ammonia. A particularly important function of the liver is the conversion of ammonia, a byproduct of protein and amino acid metabolism, to urea. The ammonium ion is produced in abundance in the intestinal tract, particularly in the colon, by the bacterial degradation of luminal proteins and amino acids. Normally, these ammonium ions diffuse into the portal blood and are transported to the liver, where they are converted to urea before entering the general circulation. When the blood from the intestine bypasses the liver or the liver is unable to convert ammonia to urea, ammonia moves directly into the general circulation and from there to the cerebral circulation. Hepatic encephalopathy may become worse after a large protein meal or gastrointestinal tract bleeding. Narcotics and tranquilizers are poorly metabolized by the liver, and administration of these drugs may contribute to CNS depression and precipitate hepatic encephalopathy.

A nonabsorbable antibiotic, such as neomycin, may be given to eradicate bacteria from the bowel and thus prevent this cause of ammonia production. Another drug that may be given is lactulose. It is not absorbed from the small intestine but moves directly to the large intestine, where it is catabolized by colonic bacteria to small organic acids that cause production of large, loose stools with a low pH. The low pH favors the conversion of ammonia to ammonium ions, which are not absorbed by the blood. The acid pH also inhibits the degradation of amino acids, proteins, and blood.

Treatment

The treatment of liver failure is directed toward eliminating alcohol intake when the condition is caused by alcoholic cirrhosis; preventing infections; providing sufficient carbohydrates and calories to prevent protein breakdown; correcting fluid and electrolyte imbalances, particularly hypokalemia; and decreasing ammonia production in the gastrointestinal tract by controlling protein intake. In many cases, liver transplantation remains the only effective treatment.

Liver transplantation rapidly is becoming a realistic form of treatment for many persons with irreversible chronic liver disease, fulminant liver failure, primary biliary cirrhosis, chronic active hepatitis, sclerosing cholangitis, and certain metabolic disorders that result in end-stage liver disease. Currently, 1-year survival rates approach 90% and a 3-year survival rate of 80% is achieved at many transplantation centers in the United States.[38] In addition to longer survival, many liver transplant recipients are now experiencing improved quality of life, including return to active employment. Unfortunately, the shortage of donor organs severely limits the number of transplantations that are done, and many persons die each year while waiting for a transplant.

CANCER OF THE LIVER

Primary liver tumors are relatively rare in the United States, accounting for approximately 0.5% to 2% of all cancer deaths.[2] The American Cancer Society estimates that in 2005, 17,550 people in the United States were newly diagnosed with primary liver cancer and 15,420 people died of the disease during the same period.[39] This is in contrast to many other countries, in which primary liver cancer accounts for 20% to 40% of all cancers. The global distribution of primary liver cancer is strongly linked to HBV and HCV infection.

There are two major types of primary liver cancer: hepatocellular carcinoma, which arises from the liver cells and is the common type of liver cancer, and cholangiocarcinoma, which is a primary cancer of bile duct cells.[2] Hepatocellular cancer is one of the few cancers for which an underlying etiology can be identified in most cases, and is unique because it usually occurs in a background of chronic liver disease.[40] Among the factors identified as etiologic agents in liver cancer are chronic viral hepatitis (HBV, HCV, HDV), cirrhosis, long-term exposure to environmental agents such as aflatoxin, and drinking water contaminated with arsenic. Just how these etiologic agents contribute to the development of liver cancer is still unclear. With HBV and HCV, both of which become integrated into the host DNA, repeated cycles of cell death and regeneration afford the potential for development of cancer-producing mutations. Aflatoxins, produced by food spoilage molds in certain areas endemic for hepatocellular carcinoma, are particularly potent carcinogenic agents.[2,41] They are activated by hepatocytes and their products incorporated into the host DNA with the potential for causing cancer-producing mutations. A particularly susceptible site for aflatoxin is the p53 tumor suppressor gene (see Chapter 5).

Hepatocellular cancers appear grossly as soft, hemorrhagic tan masses in the liver[3] (Fig. 29-14). In some cases, a large solitary tumor occupies a large portion of liver, and in other cases, many small tumors are present. The cancer has a tendency to grow into the portal veins and may extend into the vena cava. Cancer of the liver tends to metastasize to the lungs and portal lymph nodes.

The manifestations of hepatocellular cancer often are insidious in onset and masked by those related to cirrhosis or chronic hepatitis. The initial symptoms include weakness, anorexia, weight loss, fatigue, bloating, a sensation of abdominal fullness, and a dull, aching abdominal pain. Ascites, which often obscures weight loss, is common. Jaundice, if present, usually is mild. There may be a rapid increase in liver size and worsening of ascites in persons with preexisting cirrhosis. Usually, the liver is enlarged when these symptoms appear. Serum α-fetoprotein, a serum protein present during fetal life, normally is barely detectable in the serum after the age of 2 years, but it is present in 90% of cases of hepatocellular carcinoma.[2] Diagnostic methods include ultrasound, CT scans, and MRI. Liver biopsy is used to confirm the diagnosis.

Cholangiocarcinoma occurs much less frequently than hepatocellular carcinoma. The etiology, clinical features, and prognosis vary considerably with the part of the biliary tree that is the site of origin. Cholangiocarcinoma is not associated with the same risk factors as hepatocellular carcinoma. Instead, most of the risk factors revolve around long-standing inflammation and injury of the bile duct epithelium. Cholangiocarcinoma often presents with

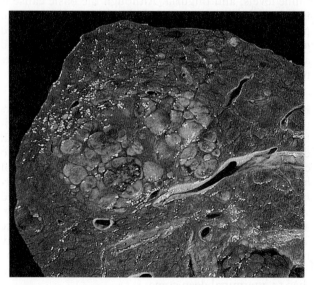

FIGURE 29-14 Hepatocellular carcinoma. Cross-section of a cirrhotic liver shows a poorly circumscribed, nodular area of yellow, partially hemorrhagic carcinoma. (From Rubin E., Rubin R. [2005]. The liver and biliary system. In Rubin E., Gorstein F., Rubin R., et al. [Eds.], *Rubin's pathophysiology: Clinicopathologic foundations of medicine* [4th ed., p. 799]. Philadelphia: Lippincott Williams & Wilkins.)

pain, weight loss, anorexia, and abdominal swelling or awareness of a mass in the right hypochondrium. Tumors affecting the central or distal bile ducts may present with jaundice.

Primary cancers of the liver usually are far advanced at the time of diagnosis; the 5-year survival rate is approximately 7%.[39] The treatment of choice is subtotal hepatectomy, if conditions permit. Chemotherapy and radiation therapy are largely palliative. Although liver transplantation may be an option for people with well-compensated cirrhosis and small tumors, it often is impractical because of the shortage of donor organs.

Metastatic tumors of the liver are much more common than primary tumors. Common sources include colorectal cancer and spread from the breast, lung, or urogenital cancers. In addition, tumors of neuroendocrine origin spread to the liver. It often is difficult to distinguish primary from metastatic tumors with the use of CT scans, MRI, or ultrasonography. Usually the diagnosis is confirmed by biopsy.

In summary, the liver is subject to most of the disease processes that affect other body structures, such as vascular disorders, inflammation, metabolic diseases, toxic injury, and neoplasms. Hepatitis is characterized by inflammation of the liver. Acute viral hepatitis is caused by hepatitis viruses A, B, C, D, and E. Although all these viruses cause acute hepatitis, they differ in terms of mode of transmission, incubation period, mechanism, degree and chronicity of liver damage, and the ability to evolve to a carrier state. HBV, HCV, and HDV have the potential for progression to the carrier state, chronic hepatitis, and hepatocellular carcinoma.

Intrahepatic biliary diseases disrupt the flow of bile through the liver, causing cholestasis and biliary cirrhosis. Among the causes of intrahepatic biliary diseases are primary biliary cirrhosis, primary sclerosing cholangitis, and secondary biliary cirrhosis. Because alcohol competes for use of intracellular cofactors normally needed by the liver for other metabolic processes, it tends to disrupt the metabolic functions of the liver. The spectrum of alcoholic liver disease includes fatty liver disease, alcoholic hepatitis, and cirrhosis.

Cirrhosis represents the end stage of chronic liver disease in which much of the functional liver tissue has been replaced by fibrous tissue. The fibrous tissue replaces normally functioning liver tissue and forms constrictive bands that disrupt flow in the vascular channels and biliary duct systems of the liver. The disruption of vascular channels predisposes to portal hypertension and its complications, loss of liver cells, and eventual liver failure. Portal hypertension is characterized by increased resistance to flow and increased pressure in the portal venous system; the pathologic consequences of the disorder include ascites, the formation of collateral bypass channels (*e.g.*, esophageal varices) from the portosystemic circulation, and splenomegaly. Liver fail-

ure represents the end stage of a number of liver diseases and occurs when less than 10% of liver tissue is functional. The manifestations of liver failure reflect the various functions of the liver, including hematologic disorders, disruption of endocrine function, skin disorders, hepatorenal syndrome, and hepatic encephalopathy.

Cancers of the liver include metastatic and primary neoplasms. Primary hepatic neoplasms are rare and those involving the hepatocytes or liver cells are commonly associated with underlying diseases of the liver such as cirrhosis and chronic hepatitis. Liver cancer usually is far advanced at the time of diagnosis.

Disorders of the Gallbladder and Exocrine Pancreas

DISORDERS OF THE GALLBLADDER AND EXTRAHEPATIC BILE DUCTS

The so-called hepatobiliary system consists of the gallbladder, the left and right hepatic ducts, which come together to form the common hepatic duct, the cystic duct, which extends to the gallbladder, and the common bile duct, which is formed by the union of the common hepatic duct and the cystic duct (Fig. 29-15). The common bile duct descends posterior to the first part of the duodenum, where it comes in contact with the main pancreatic duct. These ducts unite to form the hepatopancreatic ampulla. The circular muscle around the distal end of the bile duct is thickened to form the sphincter of the bile duct.

The gallbladder is a distensible, pear-shaped, muscular sac located on the ventral surface of the liver. It has an outer serous peritoneal layer, a middle smooth muscle layer, and an inner mucosal layer that is continuous with the linings of the bile duct. The function of the gallbladder is to store and concentrate bile. Bile contains bile salts, cholesterol, bilirubin, lecithin, fatty acids, and water and the electrolytes normally found in the plasma. The cholesterol found in bile has no known function; it is assumed to be a byproduct of bile salt formation, and its presence is linked to the excretory function of bile. Normally insoluble in water, cholesterol is rendered soluble by the action of bile salts and lecithin, which combine with it to form micelles. In the gallbladder, water and electrolytes are absorbed from the liver bile, causing the bile to become more concentrated. Because neither lecithin nor bile salts are absorbed in the gallbladder, their concentration increases along with that of cholesterol; in this way, the solubility of cholesterol is maintained.

Entrance of food into the intestine causes the gallbladder to contract and the sphincter of the bile duct to relax, such that bile stored in the gallbladder moves into the duodenum. The stimulus for gallbladder contraction is primarily hormonal. Products of food digestion, particularly lipids, stimulate the release of a gastrointestinal hormone called *cholecystokinin* from the mucosa of the duodenum.

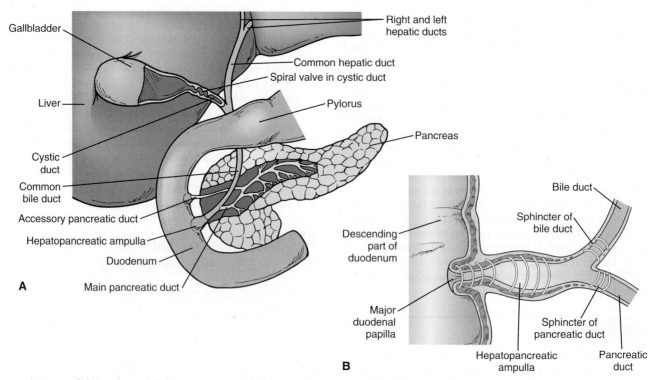

FIGURE 29-15 (**A**) Extrahepatic bile passages, gallbladder, and pancreatic ducts. (**B**) Entry of bile duct and pancreatic duct into the hepatopancreatic ampulla, which opens into the duodenum.

Cholecystokinin provides a strong stimulus for gallbladder contraction. The role of other gastrointestinal hormones in bile release is less clearly understood.

Passage of bile into the intestine is regulated largely by the pressure in the common duct. Normally, the gallbladder regulates this pressure. It collects and stores bile as it relaxes and the pressure in the common bile duct decreases, and it empties bile into the intestine as the gallbladder contracts, producing an increase in common duct pressure. After gallbladder surgery, the pressure in the common duct changes, causing the common duct to dilate. The flow of bile then is regulated by the sphincters in the common duct.

Two common disorders of the biliary system are cholelithiasis (*i.e.*, gallstones) and inflammation of the gallbladder (cholecystitis) or common bile duct (cholangitis). At least 10% of adults have gallstones.[42,43] Approximately twice as many women as men have gallstones, and there is an increased prevalence with age—after 60 years of age, 10% to 15% among men and 20% to 40% among women.[43]

Cholelithiasis

Cholelithiasis or gallstones is caused by precipitation of substances contained in bile, mainly cholesterol and bilirubin. The bile of which gallstones are formed usually is supersaturated with cholesterol or bilirubinate. Approximately 80% of gallstones are composed primarily of cholesterol; the other 20% are black or brown pigment stones consisting of calcium salts with bilirubin.[42] Many stones have a mixed composition. Figure 29-16 shows a gallbladder with numerous cholesterol gallstones.

Three factors contribute to the formation of gallstones: abnormalities in the composition of bile, stasis of bile, and inflammation of the gallbladder. The formation of cholesterol stones is associated with obesity and occurs more frequently in women, especially women who have had multiple pregnancies or who are taking oral contraceptives. All of these factors cause the liver to excrete more cholesterol into the bile. Cholesterol gallstones are extremely common among Native Americans, which suggests that a genetic component may have a role in gallstone formation. Gallbladder sludge (thickened gallbladder mucoprotein with tiny trapped cholesterol crystals) is thought to be a precursor of gallstones. Sludge frequently develops during pregnancy, starvation, and rapid weight loss.[42] Drugs that lower serum cholesterol levels, such as clofibrate, also cause increased cholesterol excretion into the bile. Malabsorption disorders stemming from ileal disease or intestinal bypass surgery, for example, tend to interfere with the absorption of bile salts, which are needed to maintain the solubility of cholesterol. Inflammation of the gallbladder alters the absorptive characteristics of the mucosal layer, allowing excessive absorption of water and bile salts. Pigment stones containing bilirubin are seen in persons with hemolytic disease (*e.g.*, sickle cell disease) and hepatic cirrhosis.

Many persons with gallstones have no symptoms. Gallstones cause symptoms when they obstruct bile flow. Small stones (*e.g.*, <8 mm in diameter) pass into the common duct, producing symptoms of indigestion and bil-

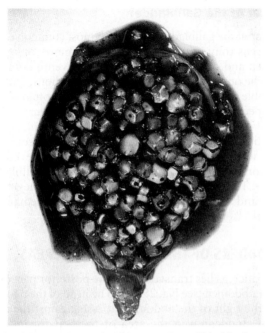

FIGURE 29-16 Cholesterol gallstones. The gallbladder has been opened to reveal numerous yellow cholesterol gallstones (From Rubin E., Rubin R. [2005]. The liver and biliary system. In Rubin E., Gorstein F., Rubin R., et al. [Eds.], *Rubin's pathophysiology: Clinicopathologic foundations of medicine* [4th ed., p. 806]. Philadelphia: Lippincott Williams & Wilkins.)

iary colic. Larger stones are more likely to obstruct flow and cause jaundice. The pain of biliary colic usually is abrupt in onset and increases steadily in intensity until it reaches a climax in 30 to 60 minutes. The upper right quadrant, or epigastric area, is the usual location of the pain, often with referred pain to the back, above the waist, the right shoulder, and the right scapula or the midscapular region. A few persons experience pain on the left side. The pain usually persists for 2 to 8 hours and is followed by soreness in the upper right quadrant.

Acute and Chronic Cholecystitis

The term *cholecystitis* refers to inflammation of the gallbladder. Both acute and chronic cholecystitis are associated with cholelithiasis. Acute cholecystitis may be superimposed on chronic cholecystitis.

Acute Cholecystitis. Acute cholecystitis almost always is associated with complete or partial obstruction of the cystic or common bile ducts. It is believed that the inflammation is caused by chemical irritation from the concentrated bile, along with mucosal swelling and ischemia resulting from venous congestion and lymphatic stasis. The gallbladder usually is markedly distended. Bacterial infections may arise secondary to the ischemia and chemical irritation. The bacteria reach the injured gallbladder through the blood, lymphatics, or bile ducts or from adjacent organs. Among the common pathogens are staphylococci and enterococci. The wall of the gallbladder is most vulnerable to the effects of ischemia, as a result of

which mucosal necrosis and sloughing occur. The process may lead to gangrenous changes and perforation of the gallbladder.

The signs and symptoms of acute cholecystitis vary with the severity of obstruction and inflammation. Pain, initially similar to that of biliary colic, is characteristic of acute cholecystitis. It often is precipitated by a fatty meal and may initiate with complaints of indigestion. It does not, however, subside spontaneously and responds poorly or only temporarily to potent analgesics. When the inflammation progresses to involve the peritoneum, the pain becomes more pronounced in the right upper quadrant. The right subcostal region is tender, and the muscles that surround the area spasm. Approximately 75% of patients have vomiting, and approximately 25% have jaundice.[42] Fever and an abnormally high white blood cell count attest to the presence of inflammation. Total serum bilirubin, aminotransferase, and alkaline phosphatase levels usually are elevated.

Chronic Cholecystitis. Chronic cholecystitis results from repeated episodes of acute cholecystitis or chronic irritation of the gallbladder by stones. It is characterized by varying degrees of chronic inflammation. Gallstones almost always are present. Cholelithiasis with chronic cholecystitis may be associated with acute exacerbations of gallbladder inflammation, common duct stones, pancreatitis, and, rarely, carcinoma of the gallbladder.

The manifestations of chronic cholecystitis are more vague than those of acute cholecystitis. There may be intolerance to fatty foods, belching, and other indications of discomfort. Often, there are episodes of colicky pain with obstruction of biliary flow caused by gallstones. The gallbladder, which in chronic cholecystitis usually contains stones, may be enlarged, shrunken, or of normal size.

Diagnosis and Treatment. The methods used to diagnose gallbladder disease include ultrasonography and cholescintigraphy (nuclear scanning).[43] Ultrasonography is widely used in diagnosing gallbladder disease and has largely replaced the oral cholecystogram in most medical centers. It can detect stones as small as 1 to 2 cm, and its overall accuracy in detecting gallbladder disease is high. In addition to stones, ultrasonography can detect wall thickening, which indicates inflammation. It also can rule out other causes of right upper quadrant pain such as tumors. Cholescintigraphy, also called a *gallbladder scan,* relies on the ability of the liver to extract a rapidly injected radionuclide, technetium-99m, bound to one of several iminodiacetic acids that are excreted into the bile ducts. Serial scanning images are obtained within several minutes of the injection of the tracer and every 10 to 15 minutes during the next hour. The gallbladder scan is highly accurate in detecting acute cholecystitis.

Gallbladder disease usually is treated by removing the gallbladder. The gallbladder stores and concentrates bile, and its removal usually does not interfere with digestion. Laparoscopic cholecystectomy has become the treatment of choice for symptomatic gallbladder disease.[43] The procedure involves insertion of a laparoscope through a small incision near the umbilicus, and surgical instruments are inserted through several stab wounds in the upper abdomen. Although the procedure requires more time than the older open surgical procedure, it usually requires only one night in the hospital. A major advantage of the procedure is that patients can return to work in 1 to 2 weeks, compared with 4 to 6 weeks after open cholecystectomy.

Choledocholithiasis and Cholangitis

Choledocholithiasis refers to stones in the common duct and *cholangitis* to inflammation of the common duct. Common duct stones usually originate in the gallbladder, but can form spontaneously in the common duct. The stones frequently are clinically silent unless there is obstruction.

The manifestations of choledocholithiasis are similar to those of gallstones and acute cholecystitis. There is a history of acute biliary colic and right upper abdominal pain, with chills, fever, and jaundice associated with episodes of abdominal pain. Bilirubinuria and an elevated serum bilirubin are present if the common duct is obstructed.

Complications include acute suppurative cholangitis accompanied by pus in the common duct. It is characterized by the presence of an altered sensorium, lethargy, and septic shock.[42] Acute suppurative cholangitis represents an endoscopic or surgical emergency. Common duct stones also can obstruct the outflow of the pancreatic duct, causing a secondary pancreatitis.

Diagnosis and Treatment. Ultrasonography, CT scans, and radionuclide imaging may be used to demonstrate dilatation of bile ducts and impaired blood flow. Endoscopic ultrasonography and magnetic resonance cholangiography are used for detecting common duct stones. Both percutaneous transhepatic cholangiography (PTC) and endoscopic retrograde cholangiopancreatography (ERCP) provide a direct means for determining the cause, location, and extent of obstruction. PTC involves the injection of dye directly into the biliary tree. It requires the insertion of a thin, flexible needle through a small incision in the skin with advancement into the biliary tree. ERCP involves the passage of an endoscope into the duodenum and the passage of a catheter into the hepatopancreatic ampulla. ERCP can be used to enlarge the opening of the sphincter of the pancreatic duct, which may allow the lodged stone to pass, or an instrument may be inserted into the common duct to remove the stone.

Common duct stones in persons with cholelithiasis usually are treated by stone extraction followed by laparoscopic cholecystectomy. Antibiotic therapy with an agent that penetrates the bile is used to treat the infection. Emergency decompression of the common duct, usually by ERCP, may be necessary for persons who are septic or fail to improve with antibiotic treatment.

Cancer of the Gallbladder

Cancer of the gallbladder is the fifth most common cancer of the gastrointestinal tract. It is slightly more common in women and occurs more often in the seventh decade of life. The onset of symptoms usually is insidious, and they resemble those of cholecystitis; the diagnosis often is made unexpectedly at the time of gallbladder surgery. About 80% to 85% of persons with gallbladder cancer have cholelithiasis.[43] Because of their ability to produce chronic irritation of the gallbladder mucosa, it is believed that gallstones play a role in the development of gallbladder cancer. The tumor is seldom resectable at the time of diagnosis and the mean 5-year survival rate has remained a dismal 1% for many years.[2]

DISORDERS OF THE EXOCRINE PANCREAS

The pancreas lies transversely in the posterior part of the upper abdomen (see Fig. 29-15). The head of the pancreas is at the right of the abdomen; it rests against the curve of the duodenum in the area of the hepatopancreatic ampulla and its entrance into the duodenum. The body of the pancreas lies beneath the stomach. The tail touches the spleen. The pancreas is virtually hidden because of its posterior position; unlike many other organs, it cannot be palpated. Because of the position of the pancreas and its large functional reserve, symptoms from conditions such as cancer of the pancreas do not usually appear until the disorder is far advanced.

The pancreas is both an endocrine and exocrine organ. Its function as an endocrine organ is discussed in Chapter 32. The exocrine pancreas is made up of lobules that consist of acinar cells, which secrete digestive enzymes into a system of microscopic ducts. These ducts empty into the main pancreatic duct, which extends from left to right through the substance of the pancreas. The main pancreatic duct and the bile duct unite to the form hepatopancreatic ampulla, which empties into the duodenum. The sphincter of the pancreatic duct controls the flow of pancreatic secretion into duodenum (see Fig. 29-15).

The pancreatic secretions contain proteolytic enzymes that break down dietary proteins, including trypsin, chymotrypsin, carboxypolypeptidase, ribonuclease, and deoxyribonuclease. The pancreas also secretes pancreatic amylase, which breaks down starch, and lipases, which hydrolyze neutral fats into glycerol and fatty acids. The pancreatic enzymes are secreted in the inactive form and become activated in the intestine. This is important because the enzymes would digest the tissue of the pancreas itself if they were secreted in the active form. The acinar cells secrete a trypsin inhibitor, which prevents trypsin activation. Because trypsin activates other proteolytic enzymes, the trypsin inhibitor prevents subsequent activation of those other enzymes.

Two types of pancreatic disease are discussed in this chapter: acute and chronic pancreatitis and cancer of the pancreas.

Acute Pancreatitis

Acute pancreatitis is a severe, life-threatening disorder associated with the escape of activated pancreatic enzymes into the pancreas and surrounding tissues. These enzymes cause fat necrosis, or autodigestion, of the pancreas and produce fatty deposits in the abdominal cavity with hemorrhage from the necrotic vessels. Although a number of factors are associated with the development of acute pancreatitis, most cases result from gallstones (stones in the common duct) or alcohol abuse.[44–46] In the case of biliary tract obstruction due to gallstones, pancreatic duct obstruction or biliary reflux is believed to activate the enzymes in the pancreatic duct system. The precise mechanisms whereby alcohol exerts its action are largely unknown. Alcohol is known to be a potent stimulator of pancreatic secretions, and it also is known to cause spasm and partial obstruction of the sphincter of the pancreatic duct. Acute pancreatitis also is associated with hyperlipidemia, hyperparathyroidism, infections (particularly viral), abdominal and surgical trauma, and drugs such as steroids and thiazide diuretics.

The onset of acute pancreatitis usually is abrupt and dramatic, and it may follow a heavy meal or an alcoholic binge. The most common initial symptom is severe epigastric and abdominal pain that radiates to the back. The pain is aggravated when the person is lying supine; it is less severe when the person is sitting and leaning forward. Abdominal distention accompanied by hypoactive bowel sounds is common. An important disturbance related to acute pancreatitis is the loss of a large volume of fluid into the retroperitoneal and peripancreatic spaces and the abdominal cavity. Tachycardia, hypotension, cool and clammy skin, and fever often are evident. Signs of hypocalcemia may develop, probably as a result of the precipitation of serum calcium in the areas of fat necrosis. Mild jaundice may appear after the first 24 hours because of biliary obstruction.

Total serum amylase is the test used most frequently in the diagnosis of acute pancreatitis. Serum amylase levels rise within the first 24 hours after onset of symptoms and remain elevated for 48 to 72 hours. Serum lipase levels are also elevated during the first 24 to 48 hours, but remains elevated for 5 to 14 days. Urinary clearance of amylase is increased. Because the serum amylase level may be elevated as a result of other serious illnesses, the urinary level of amylase is often measured. The white blood cell count may be increased, and hyperglycemia and an elevated serum bilirubin level may be present. Plain radiographs of the abdomen may be used for detecting gallstones or abdominal complications. CT scans and dynamic contrast-enhanced CT scanning of the pancreas are used to detect necrosis and fluid accumulation.

Complications include acute respiratory distress syndrome and acute tubular necrosis. Hypocalcemia occurs in approximately 25% of patients. Age older than 55 years, an elevated white blood cell count (>16,000/µL), and elevated levels of blood glucose (>200 mg/dL), serum lactate dehydrogenase (>350 IU/L), and AST (>250 IU/L) at the time of diagnosis are associated with a poorer prognosis, as are a decrease in hematocrit and serum calcium, increased fluid sequestration (>6 L), an arterial oxygen tension less than 60 mm Hg, and a base deficit greater than 4 mEq/L that develop within the first 48 hours.[45]

The treatment consists of measures directed at pain relief, "putting the pancreas to rest," and restoration of lost plasma volume. The person with severe pancreatitis usually requires attention in the intensive care unit. Antibiotic prophylaxis is used to prevent infection of necrotic pancreatic tissue. Meperidine (Demerol) rather than morphine usually is given for pain relief because it causes fewer spasms of the sphincter of the pancreatic duct. Papaverine, nitroglycerin, barbiturates, or anticholinergic drugs may be given as supplements to provide smooth muscle relaxation. Oral foods and fluids are withheld, and gastric suction is instituted to treat distention of the bowel and prevent further stimulation of the secretion of pancreatic enzymes. Intravenous fluids and electrolytes are administered to replace those lost from the circulation and to combat hypotension and shock. Intravenous colloid solutions are given to replace the fluid that has become sequestered in the abdomen and retroperitoneal space. If a pancreatic abscess develops, it must be drained, usually through the flank.

A pseudocyst is a collection of pancreatic fluid in the peritoneal cavity enclosed in a layer of inflammatory tissue. Autodigestion or liquefaction of pancreatic tissue may be the cause. The pseudocyst most often is connected to a pancreatic duct, so that it continues to increase in mass. The symptoms depend on its location; for example, jaundice may occur when a cyst develops near the head of the pancreas, close to the common duct. Pseudocysts may resolve or, if they persist, may require surgical intervention.

Chronic Pancreatitis

Chronic pancreatitis is characterized by progressive destruction of the pancreas. It can be divided into two types: chronic calcifying pancreatitis and chronic obstructive pancreatitis.[47] In chronic calcifying pancreatitis, calcified protein plugs (i.e., calculi) form in the pancreatic ducts. This form is seen most often in alcoholics. Alcohol damages pancreatic cells directly and also increases the concentration of proteins in the pancreatic secretions, which eventually leads to formation of protein plugs.[48] Other causes of chronic pancreatitis are cystic fibrosis and chronic obstructive pancreatitis owing to stenosis of the sphincter of the pancreatic duct. In obstructive pancreatitis, lesions are more prominent in the head of the pancreas. The disease usually is caused by cholelithiasis and sometimes is relieved by removal of the stones.

Chronic pancreatitis is manifested in episodes that are similar, albeit of lesser severity, to those of acute pancreatitis. Patients have persistent, recurring episodes of epigastric and upper left quadrant pain; the attacks often are precipitated by alcohol abuse or overeating. Anorexia, nausea, vomiting, constipation, and flatulence are common. Eventually the disease progresses to the extent that endocrine and exocrine pancreatic functions become deficient. At this point, signs of diabetes mellitus and the malabsorption syndrome (*e.g.*, weight loss, fatty stools [steatorrhea]) become apparent.

Treatment consists of measures to treat coexisting biliary tract disease. A low-fat diet usually is prescribed. The signs of malabsorption may be treated with pancreatic enzymes. When diabetes is present, it is treated with insulin. Alcohol is forbidden because it frequently precipitates attacks. Because of the frequent episodes of pain, narcotic addiction is a potential problem in persons with chronic pancreatitis. Surgical intervention sometimes is needed to relieve the pain and usually focuses on relieving any obstruction that may be present. In advanced cases, a subtotal or total pancreatectomy may be necessary.[48]

Cancer of the Pancreas

Pancreatic cancer is now the fourth leading cause of cancer death in the United States, with more than 28,000 deaths attributed to the neoplasm each year.[49] Considered to be one of the most deadly malignancies, pancreatic cancer is associated with a death-to-incidence ratio of approximately 0.99. The risk of pancreatic cancer increases after the age of 50 years, with most cases occurring between the ages of 60 and 80 years. The incidence and mortality rates for both male and female African Americans are higher than for whites.

The cause of pancreatic cancer is unknown. Smoking appears to be a major risk factor.[49,50] The incidence of pancreatic cancer is twice as high among smokers than nonsmokers. The second most important factor appears to be diet. There appears to be an association of pancreatic cancer with an increasing total calorie intake and a high intake of fat, meat, salt, dehydrated foods, fried foods, refined sugars, soybeans, and nitrosamines. Data from animal studies indicate that nitrosamines and tobacco smoke are carcinogenic in the pancreas. A protective effect has been ascribed to a diet containing dietary fiber, vitamin C, fresh fruits and vegetables, and no preservatives. Diabetes and chronic pancreatitis also are associated with pancreatic cancer, although neither the nature nor the sequence of the possible cause-and-effect relation has been established.[50,51] Genetic alterations appear to play a role. There appears to be an association between pancreatic cancer and certain genetic disorders, including nonpolyposis colon cancer, familial breast cancer with the BRCA2 gene mutation (see Chapter 5), ataxia-telangiectasia syndrome, familial atypical multiple mole–melanoma syndrome, and hereditary pancreatitis.[49] There has been a recent focus on the molecular genetics of pancreatic cancer, and more insights into the genetic mechanisms involved in pancreatic cancer undoubtedly will be forthcoming.

Cancer of the pancreas usually has an insidious onset. Pain, jaundice, and weight loss constitute the classic presentation of the disease. The most common pain is a dull epigastric pain often accompanied by back pain, often worse in the supine position, and relieved by sitting forward. Duodenal obstruction with nausea and vomiting is a late sign.

Cancer of the pancreas can arise anywhere in the pancreas, the frequent focus being the head of the pancreas, followed by the body of the pancreas, and then the tail of the pancreas. On gross examination, pancreatic carcinoma is a poorly demarcated multinodular mass (Fig. 29-17). Because of the proximity of the pancreas to the common duct and the hepatopancreatic ampulla, cancer of the head of the pancreas tends to obstruct bile flow; this causes distention of the gallbladder and jaundice. Jaundice frequently is the presenting symptom of a person with cancer of the head of the pancreas, and it usually is accompanied by complaints of pain and pruritus. Cancer of the body of the pancreas usually impinges on the celiac ganglion, causing pain. The pain usually worsens with ingestion of food or with assumption of the supine position. Cancer of the tail of the pancreas usually has metastasized before symptoms appear.

Ultrasonography and CT scanning are the most frequently used diagnostic methods to confirm the disease. Intravenous and oral contrast–enhanced spiral CT is the preferred method for imaging the pancreas. Percutaneous fine-needle aspiration cytology of the pancreas has been one of the major advances in the diagnosis of pancreatic cancer. Unfortunately, the smaller and more curable tumors are most likely to be missed by this procedure. ERCP may be used for evaluation of persons with suspected pancreatic cancer and obstructive jaundice.

Most cancers of the pancreas have metastasized by the time of diagnosis. Surgical resection of the tumor is done when the tumor is localized, or as a palliative measure. Radiation therapy may be useful when the disease is not resectable but appears to be localized. The use of irradiation and chemotherapy for pancreatic cancer continues to be investigated. Pain control is one of the most important aspects in the management of persons with end-stage pancreatic cancer.

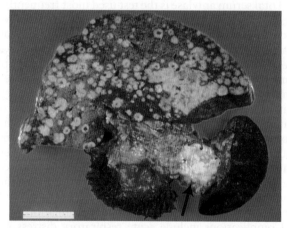

FIGURE 29-17 Carcinoma of the pancreas. An autopsy specimen shows a large tumor in the tail of the pancreas (*arrow*) and extensive metastasis in the liver. (From Rubin E., Rubin R. [2005]. The liver and biliary system. In Rubin E., Gorstein F., Rubin R., et al. [Eds.], *Rubin's pathophysiology: Clinicopathologic foundations of medicine* [4th ed., p. 819]. Philadelphia: Lippincott Williams & Wilkins.)

In summary, the biliary tract serves as a passageway for the delivery of bile from the liver to the intestine. This tract consists of the bile ducts and gallbladder. The most common causes of biliary tract disease are cholelithiasis and cholecystitis. Three factors contribute to the development of cholelithiasis: abnormalities in the composition of bile, stasis of bile, and inflammation of the gallbladder. Cholelithiasis predisposes to obstruction of bile flow, causing biliary colic and acute or chronic cholecystitis. Cancer of the gallbladder, which has a poor 5-year survival rate, occurs in 2% of persons with biliary tract disease.

The pancreas is an endocrine and exocrine organ. Diabetes mellitus is the most common disorder of the endocrine pancreas, and it occurs independently of disease of the exocrine pancreas. The exocrine pancreas produces digestive enzymes that are secreted in an inactive form and transported to the small intestine through the main pancreatic duct, which usually empties into the hepatopancreatic ampulla and then into the duodenum through the sphincter of the pancreatic duct. The most common diseases of the exocrine pancreas are acute and chronic forms of pancreatitis, and cancer. Acute and chronic types of pancreatitis are associated with biliary reflux and chronic alcoholism. Acute pancreatitis is a dramatic and life-threatening disorder in which there is autodigestion of pancreatic tissue. Chronic pancreatitis causes progressive destruction of the endocrine and exocrine pancreas. It is characterized by episodes of pain and epigastric distress that are similar to but less severe than those that occur with acute pancreatitis. Cancer of the pancreas is the fourth leading cause of cancer death in the United States. It usually is far advanced at the time of diagnosis, and the 5-year survival rate is less than 3%.

Review Exercises

A 24-year-old woman reports to her health care professional with complaints of a yellow discoloration of her skin, loss of appetite, and a feeling of upper gastric discomfort. She denies use of intravenous drugs and has not received blood products. She cannot recall eating uncooked shellfish or drinking water that might have been contaminated. She has a daughter who attends day care.

A. What tests could be done to confirm a diagnosis of hepatitis A?

B. What is the most common mode of transmission for hepatitis A? It is suggested that the source might be the day care center that her daughter attends. Explain.

C. What methods could be used to protect other family members from getting the disease?

A 56-year-old man with a history of heavy alcohol consumption and a previous diagnosis of alcoholic cirrhosis and portal hypertension is admitted to the emergency department with acute gastrointestinal bleeding due to a tentative diagnosis of bleeding esophageal varices and signs of circulatory shock.

A. Relate the development of esophageal varices to portal hypertension in persons with cirrhosis of the liver.

B. Many persons with esophageal varices have blood coagulation problems. Explain.

C. What are the possible treatment measures for this man, both in terms of controlling the current bleeding episode and preventing further bleeding episodes?

A 40-year-old woman presents in the emergency department with sudden episode of vomiting and severe right epigastric pain that developed after eating a fatty evening meal. Although there is no evidence of jaundice in her skin, the sclera of her eyes has a yellowish discoloration. Palpation reveals tenderness of the upper right quadrant with muscle splinting and rebound pain. Right upper quadrant abdominal ultrasonography confirms the presence of gallstones. The woman is treated conservatively with pain and antiemetic medications. She is subsequently scheduled for a laparoscopic cholecystectomy.

A. Relate this woman's signs and symptoms to gallstones and their effect on gallbladder function.

B. Explain the initial appearance of jaundice in the eyes as opposed to the skin. Which of the two laboratory tests for bilirubin would you expect to be elevated—direct (conjugated) or indirect (unconjugated or free)?

C. What effect will removal of the gallbladder have on the storage and release of bile into the intestine, particularly as it relates to meals?

REFERENCES

1. Guyton A., Hall J. E. (2000). *Textbook of medical physiology* (10th ed., pp. 781–802). Philadelphia: W. B. Saunders.
2. Crawford J. M. (2005). The liver and biliary tract. In Kumar V., Abbas A. K., Fausto N. (Eds.), *Robbins and Cotran pathologic basis of disease* (7th ed., pp. 877–936). Philadelphia: Elsevier Saunders.
3. Rubin E., Rubin R. (2005). The liver and biliary system. In Rubin E., Gorstein F., Rubin R., et al. (Eds.), *Rubin's pathophysiology: Clinicopathologic foundations of medicine* (4th ed., pp. 741–809). Philadelphia: Lippincott Williams & Wilkins.
4. Denery P. A., Seidman D. S., Stevenson D. K. (2001). Neonatal hyperbilirubinemia. *New England Journal of Medicine* 344, 581–590.
5. Pratt D. S., Kaplan M. M. (2000). Evaluation of abnormal liver-enzyme results in asymptomatic patients. *New England Journal of Medicine* 342, 1266–1271.
6. Marsano L. S. (2003). Hepatitis. *Primary Care* 30, 81–107.
7. Kemmer N. M., Miskovsky E. P. (2000). Hepatitis A. *Infectious Disease Clinics of North America* 14, 605–615.
8. Advisory Committee on Immunization Practices. (1999). Prevention of hepatitis A through active and passive immunization. *MMWR Morbidity and Mortality Weekly Reports* 48 (RR-12), 1–25.
9. Lee W. M. (1997). Hepatitis B virus infection. *New England Journal of Medicine* 337, 1733–1745.
10. Befeler A. S., DiBisceglie A. M. (2000). Hepatitis B. *Infectious Disease Clinics of North America* 14, 617–632.
11. Centers for Disease Control and Prevention. (2003). Incidence of acute hepatitis B—United States, 1990–2002. *MMWR Morbidity and Mortality Weekly Reports* 52, 1252–1254.
12. Advisory Committee on Immunization Practices. (1991). Hepatitis B: A comprehensive strategy for eliminating transmission in the United States through universal childhood vaccination. *MMWR Morbidity and Mortality Weekly Reports* 40(RR-13), 1–25.
13. Lemon S. M., Thomas D. L. (1997). Vaccines to prevent viral hepatitis. *New England Journal of Medicine* 336, 196–203.
14. Advisory Committee on Immunization Practices. (1999). Notice to readers update: Recommendations to prevent hepatitis B transmission—United States. *MMWR Morbidity and Mortality Weekly Report* 48(2), 33–34.
15. National Institutes of Health. (2002). National Institutes of Health Consensus Development Conference Statement: Management of hepatitis C. *Gastroenterology* 123, 476–482.
16. Lauer G. M., Walker R. D. (2001). Hepatitis C infection. *New England Journal of Medicine* 345, 41–52.
17. Liang T. J., Reheman B., Seeff L. B., et al. (2000). Pathogenesis, natural history, treatment, and prevention of hepatitis C. *Annals of Internal Medicine* 132, 296–305.
18. Cheney C. P., Chopra S., Graham C. (2000). Hepatitis C. *Infectious Disease Clinics of North America* 14, 633–659.
19. Hoffnagle J. H. (1989). Type D (delta) hepatitis. *Journal of the American Medical Association* 261, 1321–1325.
20. Friedman S. (2003). Liver, biliary tract and pancreas. In Tierney L. M., McPhee S. J., Papadakis M. A. (Eds.), *Current medical diagnosis and treatment* (42nd ed., pp. 631–641, 644–651, 657–666). New York: Lange Medical Books/McGraw-Hill.
21. Davis G. L. (2002). Update on the management of chronic hepatitis B. *Reviews in Gastroenterological Disorders* 2(3), 10–115.
22. Russo M. W., Zacks S. L., Fried M. W. (2003). Management of newly diagnosed hepatitis C infection. *Cleveland Clinic Journal of Medicine* 70(Suppl. 4), S14–S20.
23. Krawitt E. L. (1996). Autoimmune hepatitis. *New England Journal of Medicine* 334, 897–902.
24. Talwalker J. A. (2003). Primary biliary cirrhosis. *Lancet* 362, 53–61.
25. Kaplan M. M. (1996). Primary biliary cirrhosis. *New England Journal of Medicine* 335, 1570–1580.
26. Lee Y.-M., Kaplan M. M. (1995). Primary sclerosing cholangitis. *New England Journal of Medicine* 332, 924–932.
27. Lieber C. S. (2000). Alcohol: Its metabolism and interaction with nutrients. *Annual Review of Nutrition* 20, 395–430.
28. Alchord J. L. (1995). Alcohol and the liver. *Scientific American Science and Medicine* 2(2), 16–25.
29. Rubin E., Lieber C. S. (1968). Alcohol-induced hepatic injury in non-alcoholic volunteers. *New England Journal of Medicine* 278, 869–876.
30. Angulo P. (2002). Nonalcoholic fatty liver disease. *New England Journal of Medicine* 346, 1221–1231.
31. Yu A. S., Keeffe E. B. (2002). Nonalcoholic fatty liver disease. *Reviews in Gastrointestinal Disorders* 2(1), 11–19.
32. Roberts L. R., Kamath P. S. (1996). Ascites and hepatorenal syndrome: Pathophysiology and management. *Mayo Clinic Proceedings* 71, 874–881.
33. Epstein M. (1995). Renal sodium retention in liver disease. *Hospital Practice* 30(9), 33–41.
34. Garcia N., Sanyal A. J. (2001). Minimizing ascites: Complications of cirrhosis signals clinical deterioration. *Postgraduate Medicine* 109(2), 91–103.
35. Trevillyan J., Carroll P. J. (1997). Management of portal hypertension and esophageal varices in alcoholic cirrhosis. *American Family Physician* 55, 1851–1858.
36. Hegab A. M., Luketic V. A. (2001). Bleeding esophageal varices. *Postgraduate Medicine* 109(2), 75–89.
37. Brigalia A. E., Anania F. A. (2002). Hepatorenal syndrome: Definition, pathophysiology, and intervention. *Critical Care Clinics* 18, 345–373.
38. Weimer R. H., Rakela J., Ishitani M. B., et al. (2003). Recent advances in liver transplantation. *Mayo Clinic Proceedings* 78, 197–210.
39. American Cancer Society. (2005). How many people get liver cancer? [On-line]. Available: www.cancer.org. Updated January 1, 2005.
40. DiBisceglie A. M. (1999). Malignant neoplasms of the liver. In Schiff E. R., Sorrell M. F., Maddrey W. C. (Eds.), *Schiff's diseases of the liver* (8th ed., pp. 1281–1300). Philadelphia: Lippincott Williams & Wilkins.
41. Hamnett R. J. H., Gollan J. L. (2001). Liver cancer. In Lenhard R. E., Osteen R. T., Gansler T. (Eds.), *The American Cancer Society's clinical oncology* (pp. 395–405). Atlanta: American Cancer Society.
42. Crawford J. M. (2003). The biliary tract. In Kumar V., Cotran R. S., Collins T. (Eds.), *Basic pathology* (7th ed., pp. 628–633). Philadelphia: Elsevier Saunders.
43. Vogt D. P. (2002). Gallbladder disease. *Cleveland Clinic Journal of Medicine* 69, 977–984.
44. Steinberg W., Jenner S. (1994). Acute pancreatitis. *New England Journal of Medicine* 330, 1198–1210.
45. Baron T. H., Morgan D. E. (1999). Acute necrotizing pancreatitis. *New England Journal of Medicine* 340, 1412–1417.
46. Cartmell M. T., Kingsnorth A. N. (2000). Acute pancreatitis. *Hospital Medicine* 61, 382–385.
47. Steer M. L., Waxman L., Freeman S. (1995). Chronic pancreatitis. *New England Journal of Medicine* 332, 1482–1490.
48. Isla A. M. (2000). Chronic pancreatitis. *Hospital Medicine* 61, 386–389.
49. Lillemoe K. D. (2000). Pancreatic cancer: State-of-the-art care. *CA: A Cancer Journal for Clinicians* 50, 241–268.
50. Warshaw A. I., Castillo C. F. (1992). Pancreatic carcinoma. *New England Journal of Medicine* 326, 455–465.
51. Wanebo H. J., Vezeridis M. P. (1996). Pancreatic cancer in perspective. *Cancer* 76, 580–587.

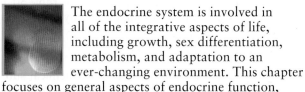

Chapter *30*

Organization and Control of the Endocrine System

 The endocrine system is involved in all of the integrative aspects of life, including growth, sex differentiation, metabolism, and adaptation to an ever-changing environment. This chapter focuses on general aspects of endocrine function, organization of the endocrine system, hormone receptors and hormone actions, and regulation of hormone levels.

The Endocrine System

The endocrine system uses chemical substances called *hormones* as a means of regulating and integrating body functions. The endocrine system participates in the regulation of digestion; use and storage of nutrients; growth and development; electrolyte and water metabolism; and reproductive functions. Although the endocrine system once was thought to consist solely of discrete endocrine glands, it is now known that a number of other tissues release chemical messengers that modulate body processes. The functions of the endocrine system are closely linked with those of the nervous system and the immune system. For example, neurotransmitters such as epinephrine can act as neurotransmitters or as hormones. The functions of the immune system also are closely linked with those of the endocrine system. The immune system responds to foreign agents through chemical messengers (cytokines, such as interleukins, interferons) and complex receptor mechanisms (see Chapter 13). The immune system also is extensively regulated by hormones such as the adrenal corticosteroid hormones.

HORMONES

Hormones generally are thought of as chemical messengers that are transported in body fluids. They are highly specialized organic molecules produced by endocrine organs that exert their action on specific target cells. Hormones do not initiate reactions; they are modulators of systemic and cellular responses. Most hormones are present in body fluids at all times but in greater or lesser amounts, depending on the needs of the body.

A characteristic of hormones is that a single hormone can exert various effects in different tissues or, conversely, a single function can be regulated by several hormones. For example, estradiol, which is produced by the ovary, can act on the ovarian follicles to promote their maturation, on the uterus to stimulate its growth and maintain the cyclic changes in the uterine mucosa, on the mammary gland to stimulate ductal growth, on the hypothalamic-pituitary system to regulate the secretion of gonadotropins and prolactin, and on general metabolic processes to affect adipose tissue distribution. Lipolysis, which is the release of free fatty acids from adipose tissue, is an example of a single function that is regulated by several hormones, including the catecholamines, glucagon, and secretin, but also the cytokine, tumor necrosis factor-alpha (TNFa). Table 30-1 lists the major functions and sources of body hormones.

Paracrine and Autocrine Actions

In the past, hormones were described as chemical substances that were released into the bloodstream and transported to distant target sites, where they exerted their action (Fig. 30-1). Although many hormones travel by

this mechanism, some hormones and hormone-like substances never enter the bloodstream but instead act locally in the vicinity in which they are released. When they act locally on cells other than those that produced the hormone, the action is called *paracrine*. The action of sex steroids on the ovary is a paracrine action. Hormones also can exert an *autocrine* action on the cells from which they were produced. The release of insulin from pancreatic beta cells can inhibit its release from the same cells. *Juxtacrine* refers to a mechanism whereby a chemical messenger that is embedded in, bound to, or associated with the plasma membrane of one cell interacts with a specific receptor in a juxtaposed cell.

Eicosanoids and Retinoids

A group of compounds that have a hormone-like action are the eicosanoids, which are derived from polyunsaturated fatty acids in the cell membrane. Among these, *arachidonic acid* is the most important and abundant precursor of the various eicosanoids. The most important of the eicosanoids are the prostaglandins, leukotrienes, and thromboxanes. These fatty acid derivatives are produced by most body cells, are rapidly cleared from the circulation, and are thought to act mainly by paracrine and autocrine mechanisms. Eicosanoid synthesis often is stimulated in response to hormones, and they serve as mediators of hormone action. Retinoids (*e.g.*, retinoic acid) also are derived from fatty acids and have an important role in regulating nuclear receptor action.

Structural Classification

Hormones have diverse structures, ranging from single amino acids to complex proteins and lipids. Hormones usually are divided into four categories according to their structures: (1) amines and amino acids; (2) peptides, polypeptides, glycoproteins, and proteins; (3) steroids; and (4) fatty acid derivatives (Table 30-2). The first category, the amines, includes norepinephrine and epinephrine, which are derived from a single amino acid (*i.e.*, tyrosine), and the thyroid hormones, which are derived from two iodinated tyrosine amino acid residues. The second category, the peptides, polypeptides, glycoproteins, and proteins, can be as small as thyrotropin-releasing hormone (TRH), which contains three amino acids, and as large and complex as growth hormone (GH) and follicle-stimulating hormone (FSH), which have approximately 200 amino acids. Glycoproteins are large peptide hormones associated with a carbohydrate (*e.g.*, FSH). The third category comprises the steroid hormones, which are derivatives of cholesterol. The fourth category, the fatty acid derivatives, includes the eicosanoids and retinoids.

Synthesis and Transport

The mechanisms for hormone synthesis vary with hormone structure. Protein and peptide hormones are synthesized and stored in granules or vesicles in the cytoplasm of the cell until secretion is required. The lipid-soluble steroid hormones are released as they are synthesized.

KEY CONCEPTS

Hormones

➤ Hormones function as chemical messengers, moving through the blood to distant target sites of action, or acting more locally as paracrine or autocrine messengers that incite more local effects.

➤ Most hormones are present in body fluids at all times but in greater or lesser amounts, depending on the needs of the body.

➤ Hormones exert their actions by interacting with high-affinity receptors, which in turn are linked to one or more effector systems in the cell. Some hormone receptors are located on the surface of the cell and act through second messenger mechanisms, and others are located in the cell, where they modulate the synthesis of enzymes, transport proteins, or structural proteins.

TABLE 30-1   Major Action and Source of Selected Hormones

Source	Hormone	Major Action

Hypothalamus	Releasing and inhibiting hormones
	    Corticotropin-releasing hormone (CRH)
	    Thyrotropin-releasing hormone (TRH)
	    Growth hormone–releasing hormone (GHRH)
	    Gonadotropin-releasing hormone (GnRH)
		Controls the release of pituitary hormones

Anterior pituitary	Growth hormone (GH)	Stimulates growth of bone and muscle, promotes protein synthesis and fat metabolism, decreases carbohydrate metabolism
	Adrenocorticotropic hormone (ACTH)	Stimulates synthesis and secretion of adrenal cortical hormones
	Thyroid-stimulating hormone (TSH)	Stimulates synthesis and secretion of thyroid hormone
	Follicle-stimulating hormone (FSH)	Female: stimulates growth of ovarian follicle, ovulation Male: stimulates sperm production
	Luteinizing hormone (LH)	Female: stimulates development of corpus luteum, release of oocyte, production of estrogen and progesterone Male: stimulates secretion of testosterone, development of interstitial tissue of testes
Posterior pituitary	Antidiuretic hormone (ADH)	Increases water reabsorption by kidney
	Oxytocin	Stimulates contraction of pregnant uterus, milk ejection from breasts after childbirth
Adrenal cortex	Mineralocorticosteroids, mainly aldosterone	Increases sodium absorption, potassium loss by kidney
	Glucocorticoids, mainly cortisol	Affects metabolism of all nutrients; regulates blood glucose levels, affects growth, has anti-inflammatory action, and decreases effects of stress
	Adrenal androgens, mainly dehydroepiandrosterone (DHEA) and androstenedione	Have minimal intrinsic androgenic activity; they are converted to testosterone and dihydrotestosterone in the periphery
Adrenal medulla	Epinephrine Norepinephrine	Serve as neurotransmitters for the sympathetic nervous system
Thyroid (follicular cells)	Thyroid hormones: triiodothyronine (T_3), thyroxine (T_4)	Increase the metabolic rate; increase protein and bone turnover; increase responsiveness to catecholamines; necessary for fetal and infant growth and development
Thyroid C cells	Calcitonin	Lowers blood calcium and phosphate levels
Parathyroid glands	Parathyroid hormone	Regulates serum calcium
Pancreatic islet cells	Insulin	Lowers blood glucose by facilitating glucose transport across cell membranes of muscle, liver, and adipose tissue
	Glucagon	Increases blood glucose concentration by stimulation of glycogenolysis and gluconeogenesis
	Somatostatin	Delays intestinal absorption of glucose
Kidney	1,25-Dihydroxyvitamin D	Stimulates calcium absorption from the intestine
Ovaries	Estrogen	Affects development of female sex organs and secondary sex characteristics
	Progesterone	Influences menstrual cycle; stimulates growth of uterine wall; maintains pregnancy
Testes	Androgens, mainly testosterone	Affect development of male sex organs and secondary sex characteristics; aid in sperm production

Protein and peptide hormones are synthesized in the rough endoplasmic reticulum in a manner similar to the synthesis of other proteins (see Chapter 1). The appropriate amino acid sequence is dictated by messenger ribonucleic acids (RNAs) from the nucleus. Usually, synthesis involves the production of a precursor hormone, which is modified by the addition of peptides or sugar units. These precursor hormones often contain extra peptide units that ensure proper folding of the molecule and insertion of essential linkages. If extra amino acids are present, as in insulin, the precursor hormone is called a *prohormone*. After synthesis and sequestration in the endoplasmic reticulum, the protein and peptide hormones move into the Golgi complex, where they are packaged in granules or vesicles. It is in the Golgi complex that prohormones are converted into hormones.

Steroid hormones are synthesized in the smooth endoplasmic reticulum, and steroid-secreting cells can be identified by their large amounts of smooth endoplasmic reticulum. Certain steroids serve as precursors for the production of other hormones. For example, in the adrenal cortex, progesterone and other steroid intermediates

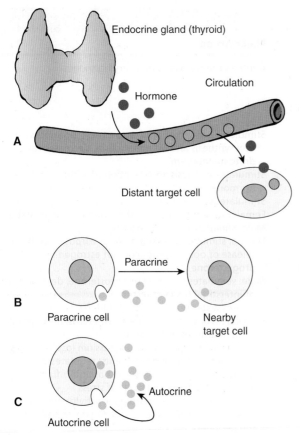

Endocrine gland (thyroid)

Circulation

Hormone

A

Distant target cell

Paracrine

B

Paracrine cell

Nearby
target cell

Autocrine

C

Autocrine cell

FIGURE 30-1 Examples of endocrine (**A**), paracrine (**B**), and autocrine (**C**) secretions.

are enzymatically converted into aldosterone, cortisol, or androgens (see Chapter 31, Fig. 31-10).

Hormones that are released into the bloodstream circulate as either free, unbound molecules or as hormones attached to transport carriers (Fig. 30-2). Peptide hormones and protein hormones usually circulate unbound in the blood. Steroid hormones and thyroid hormone are carried by specific carrier proteins synthesized in the liver. The extent of carrier binding influences the rate at which hormones leave the blood and enter the cells. The half-life of a hormone—the time it takes for the body to reduce the concentration of the hormone by one half—is positively correlated with its percentage of protein binding. Thyroxine, which is more than 99% protein bound, has a half-life of 6 days. Aldosterone, which is only 15% bound, has a half-life of only 25 minutes. Drugs that compete with a hormone for binding with transport carrier molecules increase hormone action by increasing the availability of the active unbound hormone. For example, aspirin competes with thyroid hormone for binding to transport proteins; when the drug is administered to persons with excessive levels of circulating thyroid hormone, such as during thyroid crisis, serious effects may occur due to the dissociation of free hormone from the binding proteins.

Metabolism and Elimination

Metabolism of hormones and their precursors can generate more or less active products or it can degrade them to inactive forms. In some cases, hormones are eliminated in the intact form. Hormones secreted by endocrine cells must be inactivated continuously to prevent their accumulation. Intracellular and extracellular mechanisms participate in the termination of hormone function. Some hormones are enzymatically inactivated at receptor sites where they exert their action. The catecholamines, which have a very short half-life, are degraded by catechol-O-methyltransferase (COMT) and monoamine oxidase (MAO). Because of their short half-life, their production is measured by some of their metabolites. In general, peptide hormones also have a short life span in the circulation. Their major mechanism of degradation is through binding to cell surface receptors, with subsequent uptake and degradation by enzymes in the cell membrane or inside the cell. Steroid hormones are bound to protein

TABLE 30-2	Classes of Hormones Based on Structure		
Amines and Amino Acids	**Peptides, Polypeptides, and Proteins**	**Steroids**	**Fatty Acid Compounds**
Dopamine	Corticotropin-releasing hormone (CRH)	Aldosterone	Eicosanoids
Epinephrine	Growth hormone–releasing hormone (GHRH)	Glucocorticoids	Retinoids
Norepinephrine	Thyrotropin-releasing hormone (TRH)	Estrogens	
Thyroid hormone	Adrenocorticotropic hormone (ACTH)	Testosterone	
	Follicle-stimulating hormone (FSH)	Progesterone	
	Luteinizing hormone (LH)	Androstenedione	
	Thyroid-stimulating hormone (TSH)	1,25-Dihydroxyvitamin D	
	Growth hormone (GH)	Dihydrotestosterone (DHT)	
	Antidiuretic hormone (ADH)	Dehydroepiandrosterone (DHEA)	
	Oxytocin		
	Insulin		
	Glucagon		
	Somatostatin		
	Calcitonin		
	Parathyroid hormone		

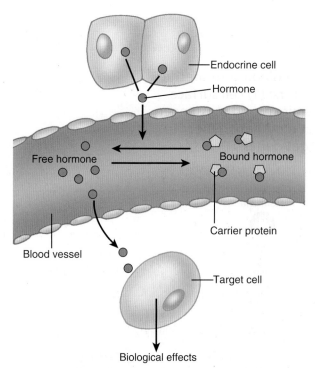

FIGURE 30-2 Relationship of free and carrier-bound hormone.

carriers for transport and are inactive in the bound state. Their activity depends on the availability of transport carriers. Unbound adrenal and gonadal steroid hormones are conjugated in the liver, which renders them inactive, and then excreted in the bile or urine. Thyroid hormones also are transported by carrier molecules. The free hormone is rendered inactive by the removal of amino acids (*i.e.*, deamination) in the tissues, and the hormone is conjugated in the liver and eliminated in the bile.

Mechanisms of Action

Hormones produce their effects through interaction with high-affinity receptors, which in turn are linked to one or more effector systems within the cell. These mechanisms involve many of the cell's metabolic activities, ranging from ion transport at the cell surface to stimulation of nuclear transcription of complex molecules. The rate at which hormones react depends on their mechanism of action. The neurotransmitters, which control the opening of ion channels, have a reaction time of milliseconds. Thyroid hormone, which functions in the control of cell metabolism and synthesis of intracellular signaling molecules, requires days for its full effect to occur.

Receptors. Hormones exert their action by binding to high-affinity receptors located either on the surface or inside the target cells. The function of these receptors is to recognize a specific hormone and translate the hormonal signal into a cellular response. The structure of these receptors varies in a manner that allows target cells to respond to one hormone and not to others. For

example, receptors in the thyroid are specific for thyroid-stimulating hormone, and receptors on the gonads respond to the gonadotropic hormones.

The response of a target cell to a hormone varies with the *number* of receptors present and with the *affinity* of these receptors for hormone binding. A variety of factors influence the number of receptors that are present on target cells and their affinity for hormone binding.

There are approximately 2000 to 100,000 hormone receptor molecules per cell. The number of hormone receptors on a cell may be altered for any of several reasons. Antibodies may destroy or block the receptor proteins. Increased or decreased hormone levels often induce changes in the activity of the genes that regulate receptor synthesis. For example, decreased hormone levels often produce an increase in receptor numbers by means of a process called *up-regulation;* this increases the sensitivity of the body to existing hormone levels. Likewise, sustained levels of excess hormone often bring about a decrease in receptor numbers by *down-regulation,* producing a decrease in hormone sensitivity. In some instances, the reverse effect occurs, and an increase in hormone levels appears to recruit its own receptors, thereby increasing the sensitivity of the cell to the hormone. The process of up-regulation and down-regulation of receptors is regulated largely by inducing or repressing the transcription of receptor genes.

The affinity of receptors for binding hormones also is affected by a number of conditions. For example, the pH of the body fluids plays an important role in the affinity of insulin receptors. In ketoacidosis, a lower pH reduces insulin binding.

Some hormone receptors are located on the surface of the cell and act through second messenger mechanisms, and others are located within the cell, where they modulate the synthesis of enzymes, transport proteins, or structural proteins. The receptors for thyroid hormones, which are found in the nucleus, are thought to be directly associated with controlling the activity of genes located on one or more of the chromosomes. Chart 30-1 lists hormones that act through the two types of receptors.

Surface Receptors. Because of their low solubility in the lipid layer of cell membranes, peptide hormones and catecholamines cannot readily cross the cell membrane. Instead, these hormones interact with surface receptors in a manner that incites the generation of an intracellular signal or message. The intracellular signal system is termed the *second messenger,* and the hormone is considered to be the first messenger. For example, the first messenger glucagon binds to surface receptors on liver cells to incite glycogen breakdown by way of the second messenger system.

The most widely distributed second messenger is cyclic adenosine monophosphate (cAMP). cAMP is formed from cellular adenosine triphosphate (ATP) by the enzyme adenylate cyclase, a membrane-bound enzyme that is located on the inner aspect of the cell membrane. Adenylate cyclase is functionally coupled to various cell surface

Understanding ➤ Hormone Receptors

Hormones bring about their effects on cell activity by binding to specific cell receptors. There are two general types of receptors: (1) cell surface receptors that exert their actions through cytoplasmic second messenger systems, and (2) intracellular nuclear receptors that modulate gene expression by binding to DNA or promotors of target genes.

1

Cell surface receptors. Water-soluble peptide hormones, such as parathyroid hormone and glucagon, which cannot penetrate the lipid layer of the cell plasma membrane, exert their effects through intracellular second messengers. They bind to a portion of a membrane receptor that protrudes through the surface of the cell. This produces a structural change in the receptor molecule itself, causing activation of a hormone-regulated signal system located on the inner aspect of the cell membrane. This system allows the cell to sense extracellular events and pass this information to the intracellular environment. There are several types of cell surface receptors, including G-protein–coupled receptors that mediate the actions of catecholamines, prostaglandins, thyroid-stimulating hormone, and others. Binding of the hormone to the receptor activates a G protein, which in turn acts on an effector such as adenyl cyclase and in that way generate second messengers such as cyclic adenosine monophosphate (cAMP). The second messenger, in turn, activates other enzymes that participate in cellular secretion, gene activation, or other target cell responses.

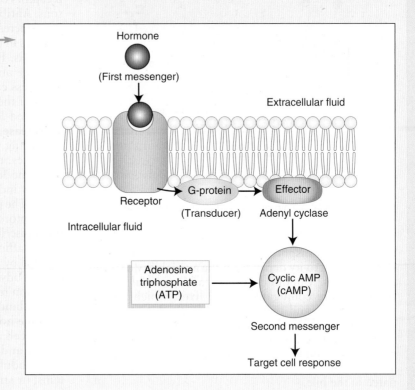

Nuclear receptors. Steroid hormones, vitamin D, thyroid hormones, and other lipid-soluble hormones diffuse across the cell membrane into the cytoplasm of the target cell. Once inside, they bind to an intracellular receptor that is activated by the interaction. The activated hormone–receptor complex then moves to the nucleus, where the hormone binds to a hormone response element (HRE) in the promoters on a target gene or to another transcription factor. Attachment to the HRE results in transcription of a specific messenger RNA (mRNA). The mRNA then moves into the cytoplasm, where the "transcribed message" is translated and used by cytoplasmic ribosomes to produce new cellular proteins or changes in the production of existing proteins. These proteins promote a specific cellular response or, in some cases, the synthesis of a structural protein that is exported from the cell.

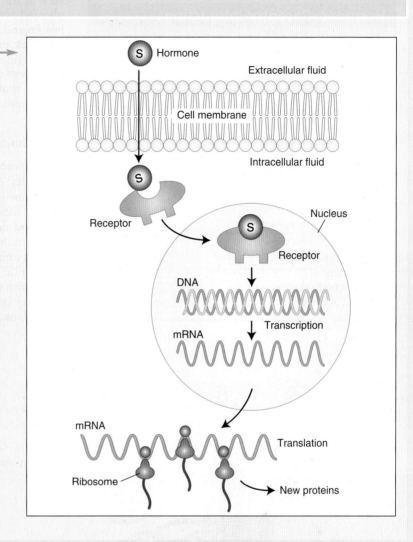

receptors by the regulatory actions of G proteins (see Chapter 1 and Fig. 1-10). A second messenger similar to cAMP is cyclic GMP, derived from guanine triphosphate (GTP). As a result of binding to specific cell receptors, many peptide hormones incite a series of enzymatic reactions that produce an almost immediate increase in cAMP. Some hormones act to decrease cAMP levels and have an opposite effect.

In some cells, the binding of hormones or neurotransmitters to surface receptors acts directly, rather than through a second messenger, to open ion channels in the cell membrane. The influx of ions serves as an intracellular signal to convey the hormonal message to the cell interior. In many instances, the activation of hormone receptors results in the opening of calcium channels. The increasing cytoplasmic concentration of calcium may result in direct activation of calcium-dependent enzymes or calcium–calmodulin complexes with their attendant effects.

Intracellular Receptors. A second type of receptor mechanism is involved in mediating the action of hormones such as the steroid and thyroid hormones. These hormones are lipid soluble and pass freely through the cell membrane. They then attach to intracellular receptors and form a hormone–receptor complex that travels to the cell nucleus. The hormone–messenger complex binds to DNA elements or specific DNA sequences called *hormone response elements* (HREs) that then activate or suppress intracellular mechanisms such as gene activity, with subsequent production or inhibition of messenger RNA and protein synthesis.

CONTROL OF HORMONE LEVELS

Hormone secretion varies widely during a 24-hour period. Some hormones, such as growth hormone (GH) and adrenocorticotropic hormone (ACTH), have diurnal fluctuations that vary with the sleep-wake cycle. Others, such as the female sex hormones, are secreted in a complicated cyclic manner. The levels of hormones such as insulin and antidiuretic hormone (ADH) are regulated by feedback mechanisms that monitor substances such as glucose (insulin) and water (ADH) in the body. The levels of many of the hormones are regulated by feedback mechanisms that involve the hypothalamic-pituitary–target cell system.

Hypothalamic-Pituitary Regulation

The hypothalamus and pituitary (*i.e.*, hypophysis) form a unit that exerts control over many functions of several endocrine glands as well as a wide range of other physiologic functions. These two structures are connected by blood flow in the hypophyseal portal system, which begins in the hypothalamus and drains into the anterior pituitary gland, and by the nerve axons that connect the supraoptic and paraventricular nuclei of the hypothalamus with the posterior pituitary gland (Fig. 30-3). The pituitary is enclosed in the bony sella turcica ("Turkish saddle") and is bridged by the diaphragma sellae. Embryo-

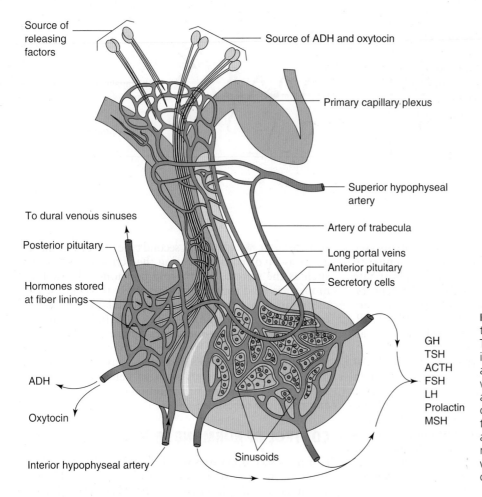

FIGURE 30-3 The hypothalamus and the anterior and posterior pituitary. The hypothalamic releasing or inhibiting hormones are transported to the anterior pituitary by way of the portal vessels. Antidiuretic hormone (ADH) and oxytocin are produced by nerve cells in the supraoptic and paraventricular nuclei of the hypothalamus and then transported through the nerve axon to the posterior pituitary, where they are released into the circulation.

logically, the anterior pituitary gland developed from glandular tissue and the posterior pituitary developed from neural tissue.

Hypothalamic Hormones. The synthesis and release of anterior pituitary hormones are largely regulated by the action of releasing or inhibiting hormones from the hypothalamus, which is the coordinating center of the brain for endocrine, behavioral, and autonomic nervous system function. It is at the level of the hypothalamus that emotion, pain, body temperature, and other neural inputs are communicated to the endocrine system (Fig. 30-4). The posterior pituitary hormones, ADH and oxytocin, are synthesized in the cell bodies of neurons in the hypothalamus that have axons that travel to the posterior pituitary. The release and function of ADH are discussed in Chapter 6.

The hypothalamic hormones that regulate the secretion of anterior pituitary hormones include GH-releasing hormone (GHRH), somatostatin, dopamine, thyrotropin-releasing hormone (TRH), corticotropin-releasing hormone (CRH), and gonadotropin-releasing hormone (GnRH). With the exception of GH and prolactin, most of the pituitary hormones are regulated by hypothalamic stimulatory hormones. GH secretion is stimulated by GHRH; thyroid-stimulating hormone (TSH) by TRH; ACTH by CRH; and luteinizing hormone (LH) and FSH by GnRH. Somatostatin functions as an inhibitory hormone for GH and TSH. Prolactin secretion is inhibited by dopamine; thus, persons receiving antipsychotic drugs that block dopamine often have increased prolactin levels.

The activity of the hypothalamus is regulated by both hormonally mediated signals (*e.g.*, negative feedback signals) and by neuronal input from a number of sources. Neuronal signals are mediated by neurotransmitters such as acetylcholine, dopamine, norepinephrine, serotonin, γ-aminobutyric acid, and opioids. Cytokines that are involved in immune and inflammatory responses, such as the interleukins, also are involved in the regulation of hypothalamic function. This is particularly true of the hormones involved in the hypothalamic-pituitary-adrenal axis. Thus, the hypothalamus can be viewed as a bridge by which signals from multiple systems are relayed to the pituitary gland.

Pituitary Hormones. The pituitary gland has been called the *master gland* because its hormones control the functions of many target glands and cells. The anterior pituitary gland contains five cell types: (1) somatotrophs, which produce growth hormone (GH); (2) thyrotrophs, which produce thyrotropin, also called thyroid-stimulating hormone (TSH); (3) corticotrophs, which produce corticotrophin, also called adrenocorticotropic hormone (ACTH); (4) gonadotrophs, which produce the gonadotropins, luteinizing hormone (LH), and follicle-stimulating hormone (FSH); and (5) lactotrophs, which produce prolactin. Hormones produced by the anterior pituitary control body growth and metabolism (GH), thyroid gland function (TSH), glucocorticoid hormone levels

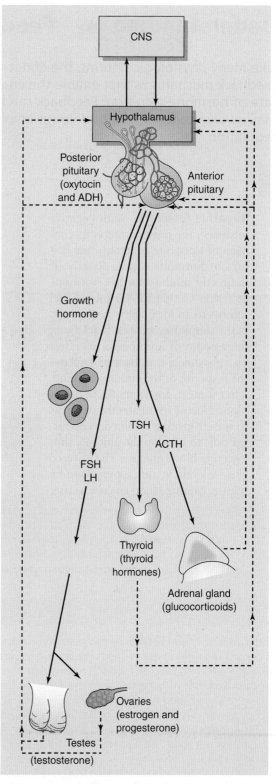

FIGURE 30-4 Control of hormone production by hypothalamic-pituitary–target cell feedback mechanism. Hormone levels from the target glands regulate the release of hormones from the anterior pituitary by means of a negative feedback system. The *dashed line* represents feedback control.

Understanding ➤ Feedback Regulation of Hormone Levels

Like many physiologic systems, the endocrine system is regulated by feedback mechanisms that enable the endocrine cells to change their rate of hormone secretion. Feedback can be negative or positive and may involve complex feedback loops involving hypothalamic-pituitary regulation.

1

Negative feedback. With negative feedback, the most common mechanism of hormone control, some feature of hormone action directly or indirectly inhibits further hormone secretion so that the hormone level returns to an ideal level or set point. In the simple negative feedback loop, the amount of hormone or its effect on a physiologic mechanism regulates the response of the endocrine gland. After a meal, for example, a rise in blood glucose stimulates the pancreas to secrete insulin; insulin acts on target cells to take up the glucose, thus lowering blood glucose. The lowered glucose levels, in turn, suppress insulin release, causing blood glucose to rise.

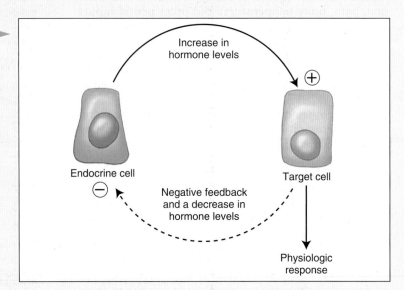

2

Hypothalamic-pituitary–target cell feedback. Hormones of the thyroid, adrenal cortex, and the gonads are regulated by more complex loops involving the hypothalamus and anterior pituitary gland. The hypothalamus produces a releasing hormone that stimulates the production of a tropic hormone by the anterior pituitary. The tropic hormone then stimulates the peripheral target gland to secrete its hormone, which acts on target cells to produce a physiologic response. A rise in blood levels of the target gland hormone also feeds back to the hypothalamus and anterior pituitary gland, resulting in a decrease in tropic hormone secretion and a subsequent reduction in hormone secretion by the target gland. As a result, blood levels of the hormone vary only within a narrow range.

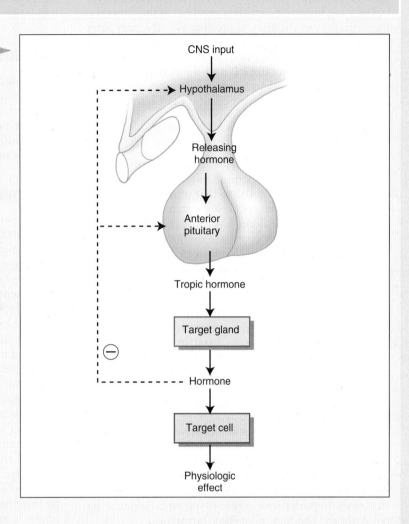

3

Positive feedback. A small number of hormones are regulated by positive feedback. In this type of regulation, a hormone stimulates continued secretion until appropriate levels are reached. An example of positive feedback is the preovulatory surge in luteinizing hormone (LH) levels that trigger ovulation. At that time, an increase in estrogen levels exerts a positive feedback effect on the anterior pituitary secretion of LH.

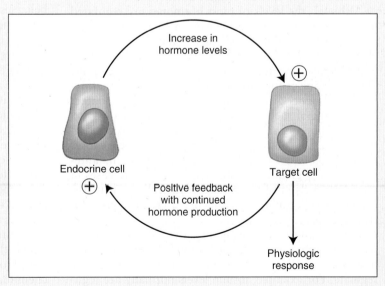

(ACTH), gonadal function (FSH) and LH), and breast growth and milk production (prolactin). Melanocyte-stimulating hormone, which is involved in the control of pigmentation of the skin, is produced by the pars intermedia of the pituitary gland. The functions of many of these hormones are discussed in other parts of this book (*e.g.*, thyroid hormone, GH, and the corticosteroids in Chapter 31, the sex hormones in Chapters 38 and 39, and ADH from the posterior pituitary in Chapter 6).

Feedback Regulation

The level of many of the hormones in the body is regulated by negative feedback mechanisms. The function of this type of system is similar to that of the thermostat in a heating system. In the endocrine system, sensors detect a change in the hormone level and adjust hormone secretion so that body levels are maintained within an appropriate range. When the sensors detect a decrease in hormone levels, they initiate changes that cause an increase in hormone production; when hormone levels rise above the set point of the system, the sensors cause hormone production and release to decrease. For example, an increase in thyroid hormone is detected by sensors in the hypothalamus or anterior pituitary gland, and this causes a reduction in the secretion of TSH, with a subsequent decrease in the output of thyroid hormone from the thyroid gland. The feedback loops for the hypothalamic-pituitary feedback mechanisms are illustrated in Figure 30-4.

Exogenous forms of hormones (given as drug preparations) can influence the normal feedback control of hormone production and release. One of the most common examples of this influence occurs with the administration of the corticosteroid hormones, which causes suppression of the hypothalamic-pituitary–target cell system that regulates the production of these hormones.

Although the levels of most hormones are regulated by negative feedback mechanisms, a small number are under positive feedback control, in which increasing levels of a hormone cause another gland to release a hormone that is stimulating to the first. However, there must be a mechanism for shutting off the release of the first hormone, or its production would continue unabated. An example of such a system is that of the female ovarian hormone estradiol. Increased estradiol production during the follicular stage of the menstrual cycle causes increased gonadotropin (FSH) production by the anterior pituitary gland. This stimulates further increases in estradiol levels until the demise of the follicle, which is the source of estradiol, resulting in a decrease in gonadotropin levels.

In addition to positive and negative feedback mechanisms that monitor changes in hormone levels, some hormones are regulated by the level of the substance they regulate. For example, insulin levels normally are regulated in response to blood glucose levels and those of aldosterone in response to body levels of sodium and potassium. Other factors such as stress, environmental temperature, and nutritional status can alter feedback regulation of hormone levels.

DIAGNOSTIC TESTS

Several techniques are available for assessing endocrine function and hormone levels. One technique measures the effect of a hormone on body function. For example, measurement of blood glucose reflects insulin levels and is an indirect method of assessing insulin availability. Another method is to measure hormone levels.

Blood Tests

Hormones circulating in the plasma were first detected by bioassays using the intact animal or a portion of tissue from the animal. At one time, female rats or male frogs were used to test women's urine for the presence of human chorionic gonadotropin, which is produced by the placenta during pregnancy. Unfortunately, most bioassays lack the precision, sensitivity, and specificity to measure low concentrations of hormones in plasma, and they are inconvenient to perform.

Blood hormone levels provide information about hormone levels at a specific time. For example, blood insulin levels can be measured along with blood glucose after administration of a challenge dose of glucose to measure the time course of change in blood insulin levels. Real progress in measuring plasma hormone levels came more than 40 years ago with the use of competitive binding and the development of radioimmunoassay (RIA) methods. This method uses a radiolabeled form of the hormone and a hormone antibody that has been prepared by injecting an appropriate animal with a purified form of the hormone. The unlabeled hormone in the sample being tested competes with the radiolabeled hormone for attachment to the binding sites of the antibody. Measurement of the radiolabeled hormone–antibody complex then provides a means of arriving at a measure of the hormone level in the sample. Because hormone binding is competitive, the amount of radiolabeled hormone–antibody complex that is formed decreases as the amount of unlabeled hormone in the sample is increased. Newer techniques of RIA have been introduced, including the immunoradiometric assay (IRMA). IRMA uses two antibodies instead of one. These two antibodies are directed against two different parts of the molecule, so IRMA assays are more specific. RIA has several disadvantages, including limited shelf-life of the radiolabeled hormone and the cost for the disposal of radioactive waste.

Nonradiolabeled methods have been developed in which the antigen of the hormone being measured is linked to an enzyme-activated label (*e.g.*, fluorescent label, chemiluminescent label) or latex particles that can be agglutinated with an antigen and measured. The enzyme-linked immunosorbent assays (ELISA) use antibody-coated plates and an enzyme-labeled reporter antibody. Binding of the hormone to the enzyme-labeled reporter antibody produces a colored reaction that can be measured using a spectrophotometer.

Urine Tests

Measurements of urinary hormone or hormone metabolite excretion often are done on a 24-hour urine sample and provide a better measure of hormone levels during that period than hormones measured in an isolated blood sample. The advantages of a urine test include the relative ease of obtaining urine samples and the fact that blood sampling is not required. The disadvantage is that reliably timed urine collections often are difficult to obtain. For example, a person may be unable to urinate at specific timed intervals, and urine samples may be accidentally discarded or inaccurately preserved. Because many urine tests involve the measure of a hormone metabolite, rather than the hormone itself, drugs or disease states that alter hormone metabolism may interfere with the test result. Some urinary hormone metabolite measurements include hormones from more than one source and are of little value in measuring hormone secretion from a specific source. For example, urinary 17-ketosteroids are a measure of both adrenal and gonadal androgens.

Stimulation and Suppression Tests

Stimulation tests are used when hypofunction of an endocrine organ is suspected. A tropic or stimulating hormone can be administered to test the capacity of an endocrine organ to increase hormone production. The capacity of the target gland to respond is measured by an increase in the appropriate hormone. For example, the function of the hypothalamic-pituitary-thyroid system can be evaluated through stimulation tests using TRH and measuring TSH response. Failure to effect an increase in TSH after a TRH stimulation test suggests inadequate production of TSH by the pituitary.

Suppression tests are used to determine if negative feedback control mechanisms are intact. For example, a glucocorticoid hormone can be administered to persons suspected of having hypercortisolism to assess the capacity to inhibit CRH.

Genetic Tests

The diagnosis of genetic diseases, using deoxyribonucleic acid (DNA) analysis, is rapidly becoming a routine part of endocrine practice. Identification of a gene for a given disorder (*e.g.,* the RET protooncogene in certain multiple endocrine neoplasia syndromes) using DNA analysis means not only a faster diagnosis and more appropriate treatment for the affected individual, but that the timely screening of family members for the mutation can be undertaken.

Imaging

Imaging studies are important in the diagnosis and follow-up of endocrine disorders. Imaging modalities related to endocrinology can be divided into those that use isotopes and those that do not. Isotopic imaging includes radioactive scanning of the thyroid (*e.g.,* using radioiodine), parathyroids (*e.g.,* using sestamibi), and adrenals (*e.g.,* using MIBG to detect pheochromocytoma). Nonisotopic imaging includes magnetic resonance imaging (MRI); computed tomography (CT) scanning; ultrasound scanning (especially for anatomic images for thyroid, parathyroid, and neighboring structures); selective venography (venous sampling to determine hormonal output from a gland or organ); positron emission tomography (PET) scanning (for evaluation of endocrine tumors); and dual electron x-ray absorptiometry (DEXA) for the diagnosis and monitoring of osteoporosis and metabolic bone diseases.

In summary, the endocrine system acts as a communication system that uses chemical messengers, or hormones, for the transmission of information from cell to cell and from organ to organ. Hormones act by binding to receptors that are specific for the different types of hormones. Many of the endocrine glands are under the regulatory control of other parts of the endocrine system. The hypothalamus and the pituitary gland form a complex integrative network that joins the nervous system and the endocrine system; this central network controls the output from many of the other glands in the body.

Endocrine function can be assessed directly by measuring hormone levels or indirectly by assessing the effects that a hormone has on the body (*e.g.,* assessment of insulin function through blood glucose). Imaging techniques are increasingly used to visualize endocrine structures, and genetic techniques are used to determine the presence of genes that contribute to the development of endocrine disorders.

Review Exercises

Thyroid hormones are transported in the serum bound to transport proteins such as thyroid-binding globulin and albumin.

A. Explain why free thyroxine (T_4) levels are usually used to assess thyroid function rather than total T_4 levels.

People who are being treated with exogenous forms of corticosteroid hormones often expe-

rience diminished levels of ACTH and exoge-
nously produced cortisol.

A. Explain, using information regarding the
hypothalamic-pituitary feedback control of
cortisol production by the adrenal cortex.

**Visit the Porth: Essentials of Pathophysiology:
Concepts of Altered Health States web site**
(http://thePoint.LWW.com/PorthEssentials) for links to
chapter-related resources on the Internet, all-new
exclusive animations, chapter review questions, and more!

BIBLIOGRAPHY

Belchetz P., Hammond P. (2003). *Mosby's color atlas and text of
diabetes and endocrinology.* New York: Mosby.

Greenspan F. S., Gardner D. G. (Eds.). (2004). *Basic and clinical
endocrinology* (7th ed.). New York: Lange Medical
Books/McGraw-Hill.

Griffin J. E., Sergio R. O. (Eds.). (2000). *Textbook of endocrine
physiology* (4th ed.). New York: Oxford University Press.

Larsen P. R., Kronenberg H. M., Melmed S., et al. (Eds.). (2003).
Williams textbook of endocrinology (10th ed.). Philadelphia:
Saunders.

Lavin N. (Ed.). (2002). *Manual of endocrinology and metabolism*
(3rd ed.). New York: Lippincott Williams & Wilkins.

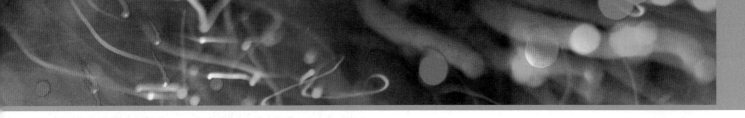

Chapter *31*

Disorders of Endocrine Function

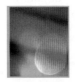
The endocrine system affects all aspects of body function, including growth and development, energy metabolism, muscle and adipose tissue distribution, sexual development, fluid and electrolyte balance, and inflammation and immune responses. This chapter focuses on disorders of pituitary function, growth and growth hormone, thyroid function, and adrenocortical function.

General Aspects of Altered Endocrine Function

HYPOFUNCTION AND HYPERFUNCTION

Disturbances of endocrine function usually can be divided into two categories: hypofunction and hyperfunction. Hypofunction of an endocrine gland can occur for a variety of reasons. Congenital defects can result in the absence or impaired development of the gland or the absence of an enzyme needed for hormone synthesis. The gland may be destroyed by a disruption in blood flow, infection, inflammation, autoimmune responses, or neoplastic growth. There may be a decline in function with aging, or the gland may atrophy as the result of drug therapy or for unknown reasons. Some endocrine-deficient states are associated with receptor defects: hormone receptors may be absent, the receptor binding of hormones may be defective, or the cellular responsiveness to the hormone may be impaired. It is suspected that in some cases a gland may produce a biologically inactive hormone or that an active hormone may be destroyed by circulating antibodies before it can exert its action.

Hyperfunction usually is associated with excessive hormone production. This can result from excessive stimulation and hyperplasia of the endocrine gland or from a hormone-producing tumor of the gland. An ectopic tumor can produce hormones; for example, certain bronchogenic tumors produce hormones such as antidiuretic hormone (ADH) and adrenocorticotropic hormone (ACTH).

PRIMARY, SECONDARY, AND TERTIARY DISORDERS

Endocrine disorders in general can be divided into primary, secondary, and tertiary groups. *Primary defects* in endocrine function originate in the target gland responsible for producing the hormone. In *secondary disorders* of endocrine function, the target gland is essentially normal, but its function is altered by defective levels of stimulating hormones or releasing factors from the pituitary system. For example, adrenalectomy produces a primary deficiency of adrenal corticosteroid hormones. Removal or destruction of the pituitary gland eliminates ACTH stimulation of the adrenal cortex and brings about a secondary deficiency. A *tertiary disorder* results from hypothalamic dysfunction (as may occur with craniopharyngiomas or cerebral irradiation); thus, both the pituitary and target organ are understimulated.

In summary, endocrine disorders are the result of hypofunction or hyperfunction of an endocrine gland. They can occur as a primary defect in hormone production by a target gland or as a secondary or tertiary disorder resulting from a defect in the hypothalamic-pituitary system that controls a target gland's function.

Pituitary and Growth Disorders

The pituitary gland is located in a saddlelike bony formation on the upper surface of the sphenoid bone, called the *sella turcica*. Usually said to be the size and shape of a pea, the pituitary gland is more accurately described as a pea on a stalk (see Chapter 30, Fig. 30-3). Its stalk, called the *infundibulum*, connects the pituitary gland to the hypothalamus. The pituitary gland has two lobes, an anterior and a posterior lobe. The posterior lobe is composed largely of neural tissue and releases the antidiuretic hormone (see Chapter 6). The anterior lobe is composed of glandular tissue. It synthesizes and releases ACTH, thyroid-stimulating hormone (TSH), growth hormone (GH), the gonadotrophic hormones (follicle-stimulating hormone [FSH] and luteinizing hormone [LH]), and prolactin.[1] Four of these, ACTH, TSH, LH, and FSH, control the secretion of hormones from other endocrine glands. ACTH controls the release of cortisol from the adrenal gland, TSH controls the secretion of thyroid hormone from the thyroid gland, LH regulates sex hormones, and FSH regulates fertility. Releasing and inhibiting hormones from the hypothalamus, which reach the anterior pituitary through blood vessels that travel in the infundibulum, control the synthesis and release of these hormones.

PITUITARY TUMORS

Pituitary tumors can be divided into primary or secondary tumors (*i.e.*, metastatic lesions). Tumors of the pituitary can be further divided into functional tumors that secrete pituitary hormones (*e.g.*, thyrotrope that secretes TSH) and nonfunctional tumors that do not secrete hormones. They can range in size from small lesions that do not enlarge the gland (microadenomas, <10 mm) to large, expansive tumors (macroadenomas, >10 mm) that erode the sella turcica and impinge on surrounding cranial structures.[1] Small, nonfunctioning tumors are found in approximately 25% of adult autopsies. Benign adenomas account for most of the functioning anterior pituitary tumors. Carcinomas of the pituitary are less common tumors.

HYPOPITUITARISM

Hypopituitarism, which is characterized by a decreased secretion of pituitary hormones, is a condition that affects many of the other endocrine systems.[1] Typically, 70% to 90% of the anterior pituitary must be destroyed before hypopituitarism becomes clinically evident. The cause may be congenital or result from a variety of acquired abnormalities (Chart 31-1). The manifestations of hypopituitarism usually occur gradually, but it can present as an acute and life-threatening condition. Affected persons usually complain of being chronically unfit, with weakness, fatigue, loss of appetite, impairment of sexual function, and cold intolerance. However, ACTH deficiency (secondary adrenal failure) is the most serious endocrine deficiency, leading to weakness, nausea, anorexia, fever, and postural hypotension. Hypopituitarism is associated with increased morbidity and mortality.

Anterior pituitary hormone loss tends to follow a typical sequence, especially with progressive loss of pituitary

---

CHART 31-1

Causes of Hypopituitarism

- Tumors and mass lesions—pituitary adenomas, cysts, metastatic cancer, and other lesions
- Pituitary surgery or radiation
- Infiltrative lesions and infections—hemochromatosis, lymphocytic hypophysitis
- Pituitary infarction—infarction of the pituitary gland after substantial blood loss during childbirth (Sheehan syndrome)
- Pituitary apoplexy—sudden hemorrhage into the pituitary gland
- Genetic diseases—rare congenital defects of one or more pituitary hormones
- Empty sella syndrome—an enlarged sella turcica that is not entirely filled with pituitary tissue
- Hypothalamic disorders—tumors and mass lesions (*e.g.*, craniopharyngiomas and metastatic malignancies), hypothalamic radiation, infiltrative lesions (*e.g.*, sarcoidosis), trauma, infections

reserve due to tumors or previous pituitary radiation therapy (which may take 10 to 20 years to produce hypopituitarism). Usually GH secretion is lost first, then LH and FSH, followed by TSH deficiency. ACTH is usually the last hormone to become deficient.

Treatment of hypopituitarism includes treating any identified underlying cause. Hormone deficiencies should be treated as dictated by baseline hormone levels, and more sophisticated pituitary testing where appropriate (and safe). Cortisol replacement is started when ACTH deficiency is present; thyroid replacement when TSH deficiency is detected; and sex hormone replacement when LH and FSH are deficient. GH replacement is being used increasingly to treat GH deficiency.[1-3]

ASSESSMENT OF HYPOTHALAMIC-PITUITARY FUNCTION

The assessment of hypothalamic-pituitary function has been made possible by many newly developed imaging and radioimmunoassay methods. Assessment of the baseline status of the hypothalamic-pituitary–target cell hormones involves measuring the following (ideally performed at 8:00 AM): (1) serum cortisol, (2) serum prolactin, (3) serum thyroxine and TSH, (4) serum testosterone (male)/serum estrogen (female) and serum LH/FSH, (5) serum GH/insulin-like growth factor-1, and (6) plasma osmolality and urine osmolality. Imaging studies (*e.g.*, magnetic resonance imaging [MRI] of the hypothalamus/pituitary) are also performed as required. When further information regarding pituitary function is required, combined hypothalamic-pituitary function tests are undertaken (although these are performed less often today).[1] These tests consist mainly of hormone stimulation tests (*e.g.*, rapid ACTH stimulation test) or suppression tests (*e.g.*, GH suppression test).

GROWTH AND GROWTH HORMONE DISORDERS

Several hormones are essential for normal body growth and maturation, including GH, insulin, thyroid hormone, and androgens.[3] In addition to its actions on carbohydrate and fat metabolism, insulin plays an essential role in growth processes. Children with diabetes, particularly those with poor control, often fail to grow normally even though GH levels are normal. When levels of thyroid hormone are lower than normal, bone growth and epiphyseal closure are delayed. Androgens such as testosterone and dihydrotestosterone exert anabolic growth effects through their actions on protein synthesis. Glucocorticoids at excessive levels inhibit growth, apparently because of their antagonistic effect on GH secretion.

Growth Hormone

Growth hormone, also called *somatotropin*, is a 191–amino-acid polypeptide hormone synthesized and secreted by special cells in the anterior pituitary called *somatotropes*. For many years, it was thought that GH was produced primarily during periods of growth. However,

KEY CONCEPTS

Growth Hormone

➤ Growth hormone (GH), which is produced by somatotropes in the anterior pituitary, is necessary for linear bone growth in children. It also stimulates cells to increase in size and divide more rapidly; it enhances amino acid transport across cell membranes and increases protein synthesis; and it increases the rate at which cells use fatty acids and decreases the rate at which they use carbohydrates.

➤ The effects of GH on cartilage growth require insulin-like growth factors (IGFs), also called somatomedins, which are produced mainly by the liver.

➤ In children, GH deficiency interferes with linear bone growth, resulting in short stature or dwarfism. In a rare condition called *Laron-type dwarfism*, GH levels are normal or elevated, but there is a hereditary defect in IGF production.

➤ GH excess in children results in increased linear bone growth, or gigantism. In adults, GH excess results in overgrowth of the cartilaginous parts of the skeleton, enlargement of the heart and other organs of the body, and metabolic disturbances resulting in altered fat metabolism and impaired glucose tolerance.

this has proved to be incorrect because the rate of GH production in adults is almost as great as in children. GH is necessary for growth and contributes to the regulation of metabolic functions (Fig. 31-1). All aspects of cartilage growth are stimulated by GH; one of the most striking effects of GH is on linear bone growth, resulting from its action on the epiphyseal growth plates of long bones. The width of bone increases because of enhanced periosteal growth; visceral and endocrine organs, skeletal and cardiac muscle, skin, and connective tissue all undergo increased growth in response to GH. In many instances, the increased growth of visceral and endocrine organs is accompanied by enhanced functional capacity. For example, increased growth of cardiac muscle is accompanied by an increase in cardiac output.

In addition to its effects on growth, GH facilitates the rate of protein synthesis by all of the cells of the body; it enhances fatty acid mobilization and increases the use of fatty acids for fuel; and it maintains or increases blood glucose levels by decreasing the use of glucose for fuel. GH has an initial effect of increasing insulin levels. However, the predominant effect of prolonged GH excess is to increase glucose levels despite an insulin increase. This is because GH induces a resistance to insulin in the peripheral tissues, inhibiting the uptake of glucose by muscle and adipose tissues.[1]

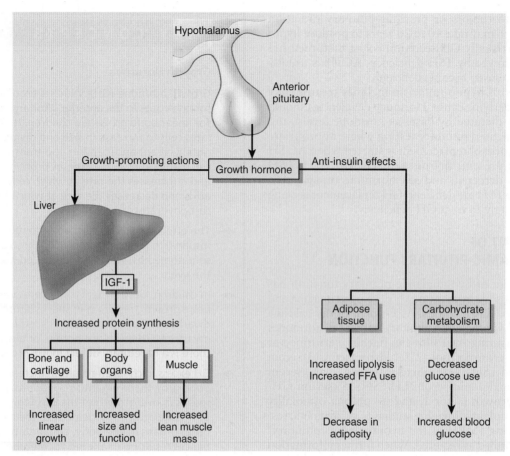

FIGURE 31-1 Growth-promoting and anti-insulin effects of growth hormone. FFA, free fatty acids; IGF-1, insulin-like growth factor-1.

Many of the effects of GH depend on a family of peptides called *insulin-like growth factors* (IGFs), also called *somatomedins,* which are produced mainly by the liver.[3] GH cannot directly produce bone growth; instead, it acts indirectly by causing the liver to produce IGFs. These peptides act on cartilage and bone to promote their growth. At least four IGFs have been identified; of these, IGF-1 (somatomedin C) appears to be the more important in terms of growth, and it is the one that usually is measured in laboratory tests. The IGFs have been sequenced and have structures that are similar to that of proinsulin. This undoubtedly explains the insulin-like activity of the IGFs and the weak action of insulin on growth. IGF levels are themselves influenced by a family of at least six binding factors called *IGF-binding proteins* (IGFBPs).

Growth hormone is carried unbound in the plasma and has a half-life of approximately 20 to 50 minutes. The secretion of GH is regulated by two hypothalamic hormones: GH-releasing hormone (GHRH), which increases GH release, and somatostatin, which inhibits GH release. These hypothalamic influences (*i.e.,* GHRH and somatostatin) are tightly regulated by neural, metabolic, and hormonal factors. The secretion of GH fluctuates over a 24-hour period, with peak levels occurring 1 to 4 hours after onset of sleep. The nocturnal sleep bursts, which

account for 70% of daily GH secretion, are greater in children than in adults. A third hormone, the recently identified ghrelin, also may be important in influencing GH secretion. Its location in the stomach suggests a new mechanism for regulation of GH (see Chapter 27).

Growth hormone secretion is stimulated by hypoglycemia, fasting, starvation, increased blood levels of amino acids (particularly arginine), and stress conditions such as trauma, excitement, emotional stress, and heavy exercise. GH is inhibited by increased glucose levels, free fatty acid release, cortisol, and obesity. Impairment of secretion, leading to growth retardation, is not uncommon in children with severe emotional deprivation.

Short Stature and Growth Hormone Deficiency in Children

Short stature is a condition in which the attained height is well below the fifth percentile or linear growth is below normal for age and sex. Short stature, or growth retardation, has a variety of causes, including chromosomal abnormalities such as Turner syndrome (see Chapter 4), GH deficiency, hypothyroidism, and panhypopituitarism.[3] Other conditions known to cause short stature include protein-calorie malnutrition, chronic diseases such as renal failure and poorly controlled diabetes mellitus, malabsorption syndromes, and certain therapies such as corticosteroid administration. Emotional disturbances can lead to functional endocrine disorders, causing psychosocial dwarfism. The causes of short stature are summarized in Chart 31-2.

Accurate measurement of height is an extremely important part of the physical examination of children. Completion of the developmental history and growth charts is essential. Growth curves and growth velocity studies also are needed. Diagnosis of short stature is not made on a single measurement, but is based on actual height and on velocity of growth and parental height.[3]

The diagnostic procedures for short stature include tests to exclude nonendocrine causes. If the cause is hormonal, extensive hormonal testing procedures are initiated. Usually, GH and IGF-1 levels are determined (IGFBP-3 levels also are useful). Tests can be performed using insulin (to induce hypoglycemia), levodopa, arginine, or clonidine, all of which stimulate GH secretion so that GH reserve can be evaluated.[2,3] Because administration of pharmacologic agents can result in false-negative responses, two or more tests usually are performed. If a prompt rise in GH is realized, the child is considered normal. Physiologic tests of GH reserve (e.g., GH response to exercise) also can be performed. Levels of IGF-1 usually reflect those of GH and may be used to indicate GH deficiency. Radiologic films are used to assess bone age, which most often is delayed. Lateral skull x-rays may be used to evaluate the size and shape of the sella turcica (i.e., depression in the sphenoid bone that contains the pituitary gland) and determine if a pituitary tumor exists. However, MRI or computed tomography (CT) scans of the hypothalamic-pituitary area are recommended if a lesion is clinically suspected. After the cause of short stature has been determined, treatment can be initiated.

Genetic and Constitutional Short Stature. Two forms of short stature, genetic short stature and constitutional short stature, are not disease states but variations from population norms. Genetically short children tend to be well proportioned and to have a height close to mid-parental height. The mid-parental height for boys can be calculated by adding 13 cm (5 inches) to the height of the mother, adding the father's height, and dividing the total by two. For girls, 13 cm (5 inches) is subtracted from the father's height, the result is added to the mother's height, and the total is divided by two. Ninety-five percent of normal children are within 8.5 cm of the mid-parental height.

Constitutional short stature is a term used to describe children (particularly boys) who have moderately short stature, thin build, delayed skeletal and sexual maturation, and absence of other causes of decreased growth. *Catch-up growth* is a term used to describe an abnormally high growth rate that occurs as a child approaches normal height for age. It occurs after the initiation of therapy for GH deficiency and hypothyroidism and the correction of chronic diseases.[3]

Psychosocial Dwarfism. Psychosocial dwarfism involves a functional hypopituitarism and is seen in some emotionally deprived children. These children usually present with poor growth, potbelly, and poor eating and drinking habits. Typically, there is a history of disturbed family relationships in which the child has been severely neglected or disciplined. Often, the neglect is confined to one child in the family. GH function usually returns to normal after the child is removed from the constraining environment. The prognosis depends on improvement in behavior and catch-up growth. Family therapy usually is indicated, and foster care may be necessary.

Growth Hormone Deficiency in Children. There are several forms of GH deficiency that present in childhood. Children with idiopathic GH deficiency lack the hypothalamic GHRH but have adequate somatotropes, whereas

---

CHART 31-2

Causes of Short Stature

Variants of Normal

Genetic or "familial" short stature
Constitutional short stature

Low Birth Weight (*e.g.,* **intrauterine growth retardation)**

Endocrine Disorders

Growth hormone (GH) deficiency
  Primary GH deficiency
    Idiopathic GH deficiency
    Pituitary agenesis
Secondary GH deficiency (panhypopituitarism)
Biologically inactive GH production
Deficient IGF-1 production in response to normal or
    elevated GH (Laron-type dwarfism)
Hypothyroidism
Diabetes mellitus in poor control
Glucocorticoid excess
  Endogenous (Cushing disease)
  Exogenous (glucocorticoid drug treatment)
Abnormal mineral metabolism (*e.g.,* pseudohypopara-
    thyroidism)

Chronic Illness and Malnutrition

Chronic organic or systemic disease (*e.g.,* asthma,
    especially when treated with glucocorticoids; heart
    or renal disease)
Nutritional deprivation
Malabsorption syndrome (*e.g.,* celiac sprue)

**Functional Endocrine Disorders
(Psychosocial Dwarfism)**

Chromosomal Disorders (*e.g.,* **Turner syndrome)**

Skeletal Abnormalities (*e.g.,* **achondroplasia)**

children with pituitary tumors or agenesis of the pituitary lack somatotropes. The term *panhypopituitarism* refers to conditions that cause a deficiency of all of the anterior pituitary hormones. In a rare condition called *Laron-type dwarfism,* GH levels are normal or elevated, but there is a hereditary defect in IGF production that can be treated directly with IGF-1 replacement.[4]

Congenital GH deficiency is associated with normal birth length, followed by a decrease in growth rate that can be identified by careful measurement during the first year and that becomes obvious by 1 to 2 years of age. Persons with classic GH deficiency have normal intelligence, short stature, obesity with immature facial features, and some delay in skeletal maturation (Fig. 31-2). Puberty often is delayed, and boys with the disorder have microphallus (abnormally small penis), especially if the condition is accompanied by gonadotropin-releasing hormone (GnRH) deficiency. In the neonate, GH deficiency can lead to hypoglycemia and seizures; if ACTH deficiency also is present, the hypoglycemia often is more severe. Acquired GH deficiency develops in later childhood; it may be caused by a hypothalamic-pituitary tumor, particularly if it is accompanied by other pituitary hormone deficiencies.

When short stature is caused by a GH deficiency, GH replacement therapy is the treatment of choice. GH is species specific, and only human GH is effective in humans.

GH previously was obtained from human cadaver pituitaries, but now is produced by recombinant DNA technology and is available in adequate supply. GH is administered subcutaneously in multiple weekly doses during the period of active growth, and can be continued into adulthood.[2,3]

Children with short stature due to Turner syndrome and chronic renal insufficiency also are treated with GH. GH therapy may be considered for children with short stature but without GH deficiency. Several studies suggest that short-term treatment with GH increases the rate of growth in these children. Although the effect of GH on adult height is not great, it can result in improved psychological well-being. There are concerns about misuse of the drug to produce additional growth in children with normal GH function who are of near-normal height. Guidelines for use of the hormone continue to be established.[2,3]

Growth Hormone Deficiency in Adults

There are two categories of GH deficiency in adults: (1) GH deficiency that was present in childhood; and (2) GH deficiency that developed during adulthood, mainly as the result of hypopituitarism resulting from a pituitary tumor or its treatment. GH levels also can decline with aging, and there has been interest in the effects of declining GH levels in the elderly (described as the *somatopause*). GH replacement obviously is important in the growing child; however, the role in adults (especially for the somatopause) is being assessed. Some of the differences between childhood and adult-onset GH deficiency are described in Table 31-1.

Several studies have shown that cardiovascular mortality is increased in GH-deficient adults. Increased arterial intima-media thickness and a higher prevalence of atherosclerotic plaques and endothelial dysfunction have been reported in both childhood and adult GH deficiency. The GH deficiency syndrome is associated with a cluster of cardiovascular risk factors, including central adiposity (increased waist-hip ratio), increased visceral fat, insulin resistance, and dyslipidemia. These

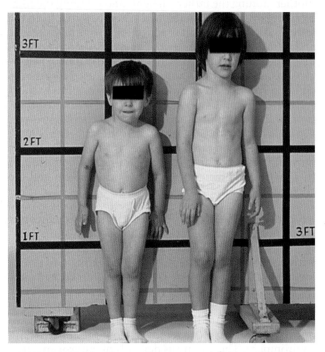

FIGURE 31-2 Child with growth hormone deficiency. A 5.5-year-old boy (**left**) with growth hormone deficiency was significantly shorter than his fraternal twin sister (**right**), with discrepancy beginning early in childhood. Notice his chubby, immature appearance compared with his sister. (From Shulman D., Bercu B. [2000]. *Atlas of clinical endocrinology, neuroendocrinology, and pituitary diseases* [edited by S. Korenman]. Philadelphia: Current Medicine.)

TABLE 31-1	Differences Between Childhood and Adult-Onset Growth Hormone Deficiency	
Characteristic	**Childhood Onset**	**Adult Onset**
Adult height	↓	NL
Body fat	↑	↑
Lean body mass	↓↓	↓
Bone mineral density	↓	NL,↓
Insulin-like growth factor (IGF)-1	↓↓	NL,↓
IGF binding protein-3	↓	NL
Low-density lipoprotein cholesterol	↑	↑
High-density lipoprotein cholesterol	NL,↓	↓

NL, normal

features also are associated with the *metabolic syndrome* (see Chapter 32). In addition to these so-called traditional cardiovascular risk factors, nontraditional cardiovascular risk factors (*e.g.*, C-reactive protein and interleukin-6, which are markers of the inflammatory pathway) also are elevated. GH therapy can improve many of these factors.[2,3,5]

The diagnosis of GH deficiency in adults is made by finding subnormal serum GH responses to provocative (*e.g.*, insulin, arginine, levodopa, clonidine) stimulation tests. Measurements of the serum IGF-1 or basal GH do not distinguish reliably between normal and subnormal GH secretion in adults. Insulin-induced hypoglycemia is the gold standard test for GH reserve. The levodopa test probably is the next best test. Other stimulation tests involve the use of arginine or arginine plus GHRH, clonidine (an α-adrenergic agonist), glucagon, or GHRH.

The approval of several recombinant human GH preparations for treating adults with GH deficiency allows physicians in the United States and elsewhere to prescribe this treatment. In the United States, persons with GH deficiency acquired as an adult must meet at least two criteria for therapy: a poor GH response to at least two standard stimuli, and hypopituitarism due to pituitary or hypothalamic damage. Difficulties can occur with the diagnosis of adult-onset GH deficiency, determining the GH dosage to be given, and monitoring the GH therapy.[1,2]

GH replacement therapy may lead to increased lean body mass and decreased fat mass, increased bone mineral density, increased glomerular filtration rate, decreased lipid levels, increased exercise capacity, and improved sense of well-being in GH-deficient adults. The most common side effects of GH treatment in adults with hypopituitarism are peripheral edema, arthralgias and myalgias, carpal tunnel syndrome, paresthesias, and decreased glucose tolerance. Side effects appear to be more common in people who are older and heavier and are overtreated, as judged by a high serum IGF-1 concentration during therapy. Women seem to tolerate higher doses better then men.

Tall Stature and Growth Hormone Excess in Children

Just as there are children who are short for their age and sex, there also are children who are tall for their age and sex.[6] Normal variants of tall stature include genetic tall stature and constitutional tall stature. Children with exceptionally tall parents tend to be taller than children with shorter parents. The term *constitutional tall stature* is used to describe a child who is taller than his or her peers and is growing at a velocity that is within the normal range for bone age. Other causes of tall stature are genetic or chromosomal disorders such as Marfan syndrome or XYY syndrome (see Chapter 4). Endocrine causes of tall stature include sexual precocity because of early onset of estrogen and androgen secretion and excessive GH.

Exceptionally tall children (*i.e.*, genetic tall stature and constitutional tall stature) can be treated with sex hormones—estrogens in girls and testosterone in boys—

to effect early epiphyseal closure. Such treatment is undertaken only after full consideration of the risks involved. To be effective, such treatment must be instituted 3 to 4 years before expected epiphyseal fusion.[3,6]

Growth Hormone Excess in Children. Growth hormone excess occurring before puberty and the fusion of the epiphyses of the long bones results in *gigantism* (Fig. 31-3). Excessive secretion of GH by somatotrope adenomas causes gigantism in the prepubertal child. It occurs when the epiphyses are not fused and high levels of IGF stimulate excessive skeletal growth. Fortunately, the condition is rare because of early recognition and treatment of the adenoma.

Growth Hormone Excess in Adults

When GH excess occurs in adulthood or after the epiphyses of the long bones have fused, the condition is referred to as *acromegaly*. Acromegaly results from excess levels

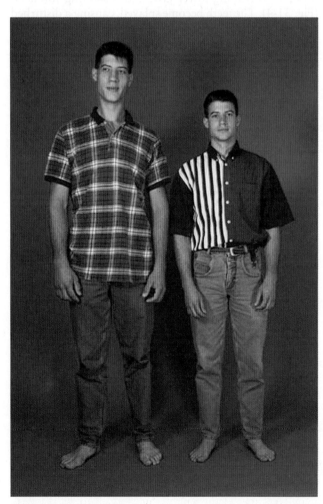

FIGURE 31-3 Primary gigantism. A 22-year-old man with gigantism due to excess growth hormone is shown to the left of his identical twin. (From Gagel R. F., McCutcheon I. E. [1999]. Images in clinical medicine. *New England Journal of Medicine* 340, 524. Copyright © 2003. Massachusetts Medical Society.)

of GH that stimulate the hepatic secretion of IGF-1, which causes most of the clinical manifestations of acromegaly. The annual incidence of acromegaly is 3 to 4 cases per 1 million people, with a mean age at the time of diagnosis of 40 to 45 years.[1,7,8]

The most common cause (95%) of acromegaly is a somatotropic adenoma. The other causes of acromegaly (<5%) are excess secretion of GHRH by hypothalamic tumors, ectopic GHRH secretion by nonendocrine tumors such as carcinoid tumors or small cell lung cancers, and ectopic secretion of GH by nonendocrine tumors.[1,7,8]

The disorder usually has an insidious onset, and symptoms often are present for a considerable period before a diagnosis is made. When the production of excessive GH occurs after the epiphyses of the long bones have closed, as in the adult, the person cannot grow taller, but the soft tissues continue to grow. Enlargement of the small bones of the hands and feet and of the membranous bones of the face and skull results in a pronounced enlargement of the hands and feet, a broad and bulbous nose, a protruding lower jaw, and a slanting forehead (Fig. 31-4). The teeth become splayed, causing a disturbed bite and difficulty in chewing. The cartilaginous structures in the larynx and respiratory tract also become enlarged, resulting in a deepening of the voice and tendency to develop bronchitis. Vertebral changes often lead to kyphosis, or hunchback. Bone overgrowth often leads to arthralgias and degenerative arthritis of the spine, hips, and knees. The skin may also manifest thickening and hypertrophy of the sebaceous and sweat glands. Virtually every organ of the body is increased in size. Enlargement of the heart and accelerated atherosclerosis may lead to an early death.

The metabolic effects of excess levels of GH include alterations in fat and carbohydrate metabolism. GH causes increased release of free fatty acids from adipose tissue, leading to increased concentration of free fatty acids in body fluids. In addition, GH enhances the formation of ketones and the use of free fatty acids for energy in preference to use of carbohydrates and proteins. GH exerts multiple effects on carbohydrate metabolism, including decreased glucose uptake by tissues such as skeletal muscle and adipose tissue, increased glucose production by the liver, and increased insulin secretion. Each of these changes results in GH-induced insulin resistance (see Chapter 32). This leads to glucose intolerance, which stimulates the beta cells of the pancreas to produce additional insulin. Long-term elevation of GH results in overstimulation of the beta cells, causing them literally to "burn out." Impaired glucose tolerance occurs in as many as 50% to 70% of persons with acromegaly; overt diabetes mellitus subsequently can result.

The pituitary gland is located in the pituitary fossa (i.e., sella turcica) of the sphenoid bone, which lies directly below the optic nerve. Almost all persons with acromegaly have a recognizable adenohypophysial tumor. Enlargement of the pituitary gland eventually causes erosion of the surrounding bone, and because of its location, this can lead to headaches, visual field defects resulting from

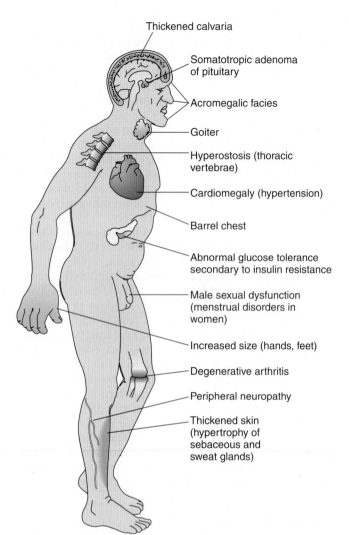

FIGURE 31-4 Clinical manifestations of acromegaly. (From Rubin E., Rubin R. [2005]. The endocrine system. In Rubin E., Gorstein F., Rubin R., et al. [Eds.], *Rubin's pathology: Clinico-pathologic foundations of medicine* [4th ed., p. 1132]. Philadelphia: Lippincott Williams & Wilkins.)

compression of the optic nerve (classically, bitemporal hemianopia), and palsies of cranial nerves III, IV, and VI. Compression of other pituitary structures can cause secondary hypothyroidism, hypogonadism, and adrenal insufficiency. GH-secreting pituitary tumors usually cause some degree of hypogonadism, either from direct damage to the hypothalamic or pituitary system, or indirectly from the hyperprolactinemia that can occur because the prolactin inhibitory factor (i.e., dopamine) is prevented from reaching the pituitary gland. In women, consistently elevated levels of prolactin inhibit the surge in pituitary LH necessary for ovulation. Men tend to suffer from decreased libido and erectile dysfunction.

Other manifestations of acromegaly include excessive sweating with an unpleasant odor, oily skin, heat intolerance, moderate weight gain, muscle weakness and fatigue, menstrual irregularities, and decreased libido.

Hypertension is relatively common. Sleep apnea syndrome is present in up to 90% of patients. The pathogenesis of the sleep apnea syndrome is obstructive in the majority of patients, due to increased pharyngeal soft tissue accumulation. Paresthesias may develop because of nerve entrapment and compression caused by excess soft tissue and accumulation of subcutaneous fluid (especially carpal tunnel syndrome). Acromegaly also is associated with an increased risk of colonic polyps and colorectal cancer. The mortality rate of patients with acromegaly is two to three times the expected rate, mostly from cardiovascular diseases and cancer. The cardiovascular disease results from the combination of cardiomyopathy, hypertension, insulin resistance and hyperinsulinemia, and hyperlipidemia.

Acromegaly often develops insidiously, and only a small number of persons seek medical care because of changes in appearance. The diagnosis of acromegaly is facilitated by the typical features of the disorder—enlargement of the hands and feet and coarsening of facial features. Laboratory tests to detect elevated levels of GH not suppressed by a glucose load are used to confirm the diagnosis. MRI and CT scans can detect and localize the pituitary lesions. Because most of the effects of GH are mediated by IGF-1, IGF-1 levels may provide information about disease activity.

The treatment goals for acromegaly focus on the correction of metabolic abnormalities, and include normalization of the GH response to an oral glucose load; normalization of IGF-1 levels to age- and sex-matched control levels; removal or reduction of the tumor mass; relieving the central pressure effects; improvement of adverse clinical features; and normalization of the mortality rate.[7-9] Pituitary tumors can be removed surgically using the transsphenoidal approach or, if that is not possible, a transfrontal craniotomy. Radiation therapy may be used, but remission (reduction in GH levels) may not occur for several years after therapy. Radiation therapy also significantly increases the risk of hypopituitarism, hypothyroidism, hypoadrenalism, and hypogonadism.

Medical therapy is usually given in an adjunctive role.[1,7,8] Octreotide acetate, an analog of somatostatin that produces feedback inhibition of GH, has been effective in the medical management of acromegaly. However, the medication must be given subcutaneously three times per week for effective dosing. Newer, longer-acting analogs of somatostatin are now available. Bromocriptine, a long-acting dopamine agonist, reduces GH levels and has been used with some success in the medical management of acromegaly. However, high doses often are required, and side effects may be troublesome. Several newly available dopamine agonists (*e.g.*, cabergoline, quinagolide) also can be considered as an alternative or adjunctive therapy.[7,8,10] The growth hormone receptor antagonists are structurally altered analogs of human GH that bind to GH receptors on cell surfaces, blocking the actions of endogenous GH and thus decreasing serum IGF-1 levels.[7,8,11]

ISOSEXUAL PRECOCIOUS PUBERTY

Isosexual precocious puberty is defined as early activation of the hypothalamic-pituitary-gonadal axis, resulting in the development of appropriate sexual characteristics and fertility.[12,13] Classically, sexual development was considered precocious and warranting investigation when it occurred before 8 years of age for girls and before 9 years of age for boys. However, these criteria were revised recently based on an office pediatric study of more than 17,000 American girls.[14] Precocious puberty is now defined as the appearance of secondary sexual development before the age of 7 years in white girls and 6 years in African-American girls.[13] In boys of either race, the lower age limit remains 9 years, although it is recognized that puberty can develop earlier in boys with obesity (an increasingly common problem).[13] Precocious sexual development may be idiopathic or may be caused by gonadal, adrenal, or hypothalamic disease.[12,13] Benign and malignant tumors of the central nervous system (CNS) can cause precocious puberty. These tumors are thought to remove the inhibitory influences normally exerted on the hypothalamus during childhood. CNS tumors are found more often in boys with precocious puberty than in girls. In girls, most cases are idiopathic.

Diagnosis of precocious puberty is based on physical findings of early thelarche (*i.e.*, beginning of breast development), adrenarche (*i.e.*, beginning of augmented adrenal androgen production), and menarche (*i.e.*, beginning of menstrual function) in girls. The most common sign in boys is early genital enlargement. Radiologic findings may indicate advanced bone age. Persons with precocious puberty usually are tall for their age as children but short as adults because of the early closure of the epiphyses. MRI or CT should be used to exclude intracranial lesions.

Depending on the cause of precocious puberty, the treatment may involve surgery, medication, or no treatment. The treatment of choice is administration of a long-acting GnRH agonist. Constant levels of the hormone cause a decrease in pituitary responsiveness to GnRH, leading to decreased secretion of gonadotropic hormones and sex steroids. Parents often need education, support, and anticipatory guidance in dealing with their feelings and the child's physical needs and in relating to a child who appears older than his or her years.[12,13]

In summary, pituitary tumors can result in deficiencies or excesses of pituitary hormones. Hypopituitarism, which is characterized by a decreased secretion of pituitary hormones, is a condition that affects many of the other endocrine systems. Depending on the extent of the disorder, it can result in decreased levels of GH, thyroid hormones, adrenal corticosteroid hormones, and testosterone in the male and of estrogens and progesterone in the female.

A number of hormones are essential for normal body growth and maturation, including GH, insulin, thyroid hormone, and androgens. GH exerts its growth effects through a group of IGFs. GH also exerts an effect on metabolism and is produced in the adult and in the child. Its metabolic effects include a decrease in peripheral use of carbohydrates and an increased mobilization and use of fatty acids.

In children, alterations in growth include short stature, isosexual precocious puberty, and tall stature. Short stature is a condition in which the attained height is well below the fifth percentile or the linear growth velocity is below normal for a child's age or sex. Short stature can occur as a variant of normal growth (*i.e.*, genetic short stature or constitutional short stature) or as the result of endocrine disorders, chronic illness, malnutrition, emotional disturbances, or chromosomal disorders. Short stature resulting from GH deficiency can be treated with human GH preparations. In adults, GH deficiency represents a deficiency carried over from childhood or one that develops during adulthood as the result of a pituitary tumor or its treatment. GH levels also can decline with aging, and there has been interest in the effects of declining GH levels in the elderly (described as the *somatopause*).

Tall stature refers to the condition in which children are tall for their age and sex. It can occur as a variant of normal growth (*i.e.*, genetic tall stature or constitutional tall stature) or as the result of a chromosomal abnormality or GH excess. GH excess in adults results in acromegaly, which involves proliferation of bone, cartilage, and soft tissue along with the metabolic effects of excessive hormone levels. Isosexual precocious puberty defines a condition of early activation of the hypothalamic-pituitary-gonadal axis (*i.e.*, before 6 years of age in African-American girls and 7 years in white girls; and before 9 years of age in boys of either race), resulting in the development of appropriate sexual characteristics and fertility. It causes tall stature during childhood but results in short stature in adulthood because of early closure of the epiphyses.

Thyroid Disorders

CONTROL OF THYROID FUNCTION

The thyroid gland is a shield-shaped structure located immediately below the larynx in the anterior middle portion of the neck. It is composed of a large number of tiny, saclike structures called *follicles* (Fig. 31-5). These are the functional units of the thyroid. Each follicle is formed by a single layer of epithelial (follicular) cells and is filled with a secretory substance called *colloid*, which consists largely of a glycoprotein-iodine complex called *thyroglobulin*. The thyroglobulin that fills the thyroid follicles is a large glycoprotein molecule that contains 140 tyrosine amino acids. In the process of thyroid synthesis, iodine is attached to these tyrosines. Both thyroglobulin and iodide are secreted into the colloid of the follicle by the follicular cells.

The thyroid is remarkably efficient in its use of iodide. A daily absorption of 150 to 200 µg of dietary iodide is sufficient to form normal quantities of thyroid hormone. In the process of removing it from the blood and storing it for future use, iodide is pumped into the follicular cells against a concentration gradient. Iodide (I^-) is transported across the basement membrane of the thyroid cells by an intrinsic membrane protein called the Na^+/I^- symporter (NIS).[15] At the apical border, a second I^- transport protein called *pendrin* moves iodine into the colloid, where it is involved in hormonogenesis. The NIS derives its energy from Na^+/K^+ adenosine triphosphatase (ATPase), which drives the process. As a result, the concentration of iodide in the normal thyroid gland is approximately 40 times that in the blood. The NIS is stimulated by both TSH and by the TSH receptor–stimulating antibody found in Graves disease. Pendrin, encoded by the Pendred syndrome gene (PDS), is a transporter of chloride and iodide. Mutations in the PDS gene have been found in persons with goiter and congenital deafness (Pendred syndrome).

Once inside the follicle, most of the iodide is oxidized by the enzyme thyroperoxidase (TPO) in a reaction that facilitates combination with a tyrosine molecule to form monoiodotyrosine and then diiodotyrosine. Two diiodotyrosine residues are coupled to form thyroxine (T_4), or a monoiodotyrosine and a diiodotyrosine are coupled to form triiodothyronine (T_3). Only T_4 (90%) and T_3 (10%) are released into the circulation. There is evidence that T_3 is the active form of the hormone and that T_4 is converted to T_3 before it can act physiologically.

Thyroid hormones are bound to thyroid-binding globulin and other plasma proteins for transport in the blood. Only the free hormone enters cells and regulates the pituitary feedback mechanism. Protein-bound thyroid hormone forms a large reservoir that is slowly drawn on as free thyroid hormone is needed. There are three major thyroid-binding proteins: thyroid hormone–binding globulin (TBG), thyroxine-binding prealbumin (TBPA), and albumin. More than 99% of T_4 and T_3 are carried in the bound form. TBG carries approximately 70% of T_4 and T_3; TBPA binds approximately 10% of circulating T_4 and lesser amounts of T_3; and albumin binds approximately 15% of circulating T_4 and T_3.

A number of disease conditions and pharmacologic agents can decrease the amount of binding protein in the plasma or influence the binding of hormone. Congenital TBG deficiency is an X-linked trait that occurs in 1 of every 2500 live births. Corticosteroid medications and systemic disease conditions such as protein malnutrition, nephrotic syndrome, and cirrhosis decrease TBG concentrations. Medications such as phenytoin, salicylates, and diazepam can affect the binding of thyroid hormone to normal concentrations of binding proteins.

The secretion of thyroid hormone is regulated by the hypothalamic-pituitary-thyroid feedback system (Fig. 31-6). In this system, thyrotropin-releasing hormone (TRH), which is produced by the hypothalamus, controls the release of TSH from the anterior pituitary gland. TSH increases the overall activity of the thyroid gland by

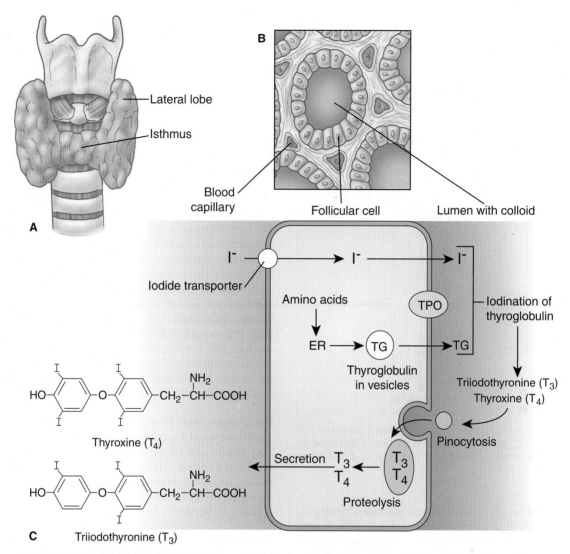

FIGURE 31-5 (**A**) Location, (**B**) microscopic structure of the thyroid gland, and (**C**) cellular mechanisms for transport of iodide (I^-), oxidation of I^- by thyroperoxidase (TPO), coupling of oxidized I^- with thyroglobin to form thyroid hormones, and pinocytotic movement of T_3 and T_4 into the follicular cell and release into the blood.

increasing thyroglobulin breakdown and the release of thyroid hormone from follicles into the bloodstream, activating the iodide pump (by increasing NIS activity), increasing the oxidation of iodide and the coupling of iodide to tyrosine, and increasing the number and the size of the follicle cells. The effect of TSH on the release of thyroid hormones occurs within approximately 30 minutes, but the other effects require days or weeks.

Increased levels of thyroid hormone act in the feedback inhibition of TRH or TSH. High levels of iodide (*e.g.*, from iodide-containing cough syrup or kelp tablets) can also cause a temporary decrease in thyroid activity, probably the result of a transient increase in hormone levels, followed by feedback inhibition of hormone production.[15] Cold exposure is one of the strongest stimuli

for increased thyroid hormone production and probably is mediated through TRH from the hypothalamus. Various emotional reactions also can affect the output of TRH and TSH and therefore indirectly affect secretion of thyroid hormones.

Actions of Thyroid Hormone

Thyroid hormone has two major functions: it increases metabolism and protein synthesis, and it is necessary for growth and development in children, including mental development and attainment of sexual maturity. Circulating T_4 is converted to T_3 in the periphery. In the cell, T_3 binds to a nuclear receptor, resulting in transcription of specific thyroid hormone–responsive genes.[15]

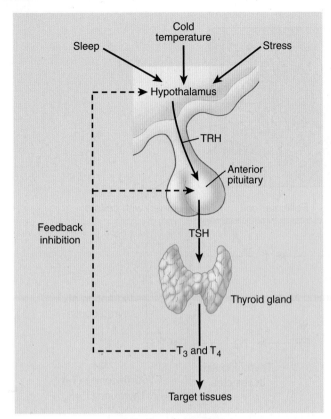

FIGURE 31-6 The hypothalamic-pituitary-thyroid feedback system, which regulates the body levels of thyroid hormone. TRH, thyrotropin-releasing hormone; TSH, thyroid-stimulating hormone.

Metabolic Rate. Thyroid hormone increases metabolic rate in all body tissues except the retina, spleen, testes, and lungs. The basal metabolic rate can increase by 60% to 100% above normal when large amounts of T_4 are present. As a result of this higher metabolism, the rate of

---

KEY CONCEPTS

Thyroid Hormone

➤ Thyroid hormone increases the metabolism and protein synthesis in nearly all of the tissues of the body.

➤ Hypothyroidism produces a decrease in metabolic rate, an accumulation of a hydrophilic mucopolysaccharide substance (myxedema) in the connective tissues throughout the body, and an elevation in serum cholesterol.

➤ Hyperthyroidism has an effect opposite that of hypothyroidism. It produces an increase in metabolic rate and oxygen consumption, increased use of metabolic fuels, and increased sympathetic nervous system responsiveness.

---

glucose, fat, and protein use increases. Lipids are mobilized from adipose tissue, and the catabolism of cholesterol by the liver is increased. Blood levels of cholesterol are decreased in hyperthyroidism and increased in hypothyroidism. Muscle proteins are broken down and used as fuel, probably accounting for some of the muscle fatigue that occurs with hyperthyroidism. The absorption of glucose from the gastrointestinal tract is increased. Because vitamins are essential parts of metabolic enzymes and coenzymes, an increase in metabolic rate "speeds up" the use of vitamins and tends to cause vitamin deficiency.

Cardiovascular Function. Cardiovascular and respiratory functions are strongly affected by thyroid function. With an increase in metabolism, there is a rise in oxygen consumption and production of metabolic end products, with an accompaning increase in vasodilatation. Blood flow to the skin, in particular, is augmented as a means of dissipating the body heat that results from the higher metabolism. Blood volume, cardiac output, and ventilation all are increased as a means of maintaining blood flow and oxygen delivery to body tissues. Heart rate and cardiac contractility are enhanced to maintain the needed cardiac output. On the other hand, blood pressure is likely to change little because the increase in vasodilatation tends to offset the increase in cardiac output.

Gastrointestinal Function. Thyroid hormone enhances gastrointestinal function, causing an increase in motility and production of gastrointestinal secretions that often results in diarrhea. An increase in appetite and food intake accompanies the higher metabolic rate that occurs with increased thyroid hormone levels. At the same time, weight loss occurs because of the increased use of calories.

Neuromuscular Effects. Thyroid hormone has marked effects on neural control of muscle function and tone. Slight elevations in hormone levels cause skeletal muscles to react more vigorously, and a drop in hormone levels causes muscles to react more sluggishly. In the hyperthyroid state, a fine muscle tremor is present. The cause of this tremor is unknown, but it may represent an increased sensitivity of the neural synapses in the spinal cord that control muscle tone.

In the infant, thyroid hormone is necessary for normal brain development. The hormone enhances cerebration; in the hyperthyroid state, it causes extreme nervousness, anxiety, and difficulty in sleeping.

Evidence suggests a strong interaction between thyroid hormone and the sympathetic nervous system. Many of the signs and symptoms of hyperthyroidism suggest overactivity of the sympathetic division of the autonomic nervous system, such as tachycardia, palpitations, and sweating. Tremor, restlessness, anxiety, and diarrhea also may reflect autonomic nervous system imbalances. Drugs that block sympathetic activity have proved to be valuable adjuncts in the treatment of hyperthyroidism because of their ability to relieve some of these undesirable symptoms.

Tests of Thyroid Function

Various tests aid in the diagnosis of thyroid disorders.[15,16] Measures of T_3, T_4, and TSH have been made available through immunoassay methods. The free T_4 test measures the unbound portion of T_4 that is free to enter cells to produce its effects. The resin uptake test is an inverse test of TBG. A high resin test result indicates that the serum sample contains low amounts of TBG or high T_4 levels. TSH levels are used to differentiate between primary and secondary thyroid disorders. T_3, T_4, and free T_4 levels are low in primary hypothyroidism, and the TSH level is elevated.

The assessment of thyroid autoantibodies (*e.g.*, antithyroid peroxidase [anti-TPO] antibodies in Hashimoto thyroiditis) is important in the diagnostic work-up and consequent follow-up of persons with thyroid disease. The radioiodine (^{123}I) uptake test measures the ability of the thyroid gland to remove and concentrate iodine from the blood. Thyroid scans (*i.e.*, ^{123}I, ^{99m}Tc-pertechnetate) can be used to detect thyroid nodules and determine the functional activity of the thyroid gland.

Ultrasonography can be used to differentiate cystic from solid thyroid lesions, and CT and MRI scans are used to demonstrate tracheal compression or impingement on other neighboring structures. Fine-needle aspiration biopsy of a thyroid nodule is used to differentiate benign from malignant thyroid disease.

Alterations in Thyroid Function

An alteration in thyroid function can represent a hypofunctional or a hyperfunctional state. The manifestations of these two altered states are summarized in Table 31-2. Disorders of the thyroid may be due to a congenital defect in thyroid development, or they may develop later in life, with a gradual or sudden onset.

Goiter is an increase in the size of the thyroid gland. It can occur in hypothyroid, euthyroid, and hyperthyroid states. Goiters may be diffuse, involving the entire gland without evidence of nodularity, or they may contain nodules. Diffuse goiters usually become nodular. Goiters may be toxic, producing signs of extreme hyperthyroidism, or thyrotoxicosis, or they may be nontoxic. Diffuse nontoxic and multinodular goiters are the result of compensatory hypertrophy and hyperplasia of follicular epithelium from some derangement that impairs thyroid hormone output.

The degree of thyroid enlargement usually is proportional to the extent and duration of thyroid deficiency. Multinodular goiters produce the largest thyroid enlargements and often are associated with thyrotoxicosis. When sufficiently enlarged, they may compress the esophagus and trachea, causing difficulty in swallowing, a choking sensation, and inspiratory stridor. Such lesions also may compress the superior vena cava, producing distention of the veins of the neck and upper extremities, edema of the eyelids and conjunctiva, and syncope with coughing.

HYPOTHYROIDISM

Hypothyroidism can occur as a congenital or an acquired defect. Congenital hypothyroidism develops prenatally and is present at birth. Acquired hypothyroidism develops later in life because of primary disease of the thyroid gland or secondary to disorders of hypothalamic or pituitary origin.

Congenital Hypothyroidism

Congenital hypothyroidism is a common cause of preventable mental retardation. It affects approximately 1 of

Level of Organization	Hypothyroidism	Hyperthyroidism
Basal metabolic rate	Decreased	Increased
Sensitivity to catecholamines	Decreased	Increased
General features	Myxedematous features	Exophthalmos (in Graves disease)
	Deep voice	Lid lag
	Impaired growth (child)	Decreased blinking
Blood cholesterol levels	Increased	Decreased
General behavior	Mental retardation (infant)	Restlessness, irritability, anxiety
	Mental and physical sluggishness	Hyperkinesis
	Somnolence	Wakefulness
Cardiovascular function	Decreased cardiac output	Increased cardiac output
	Bradycardia	Tachycardia and palpitations
Gastrointestinal function	Constipation	Diarrhea
	Decreased appetite	Increased appetite
Respiratory function	Hypoventilation	Dyspnea
Muscle tone and reflexes	Decreased	Increased, with tremor and fibrillatory twitching
Temperature tolerance	Cold intolerance	Heat intolerance
Skin and hair	Decreased sweating	Increased sweating
	Coarse and dry skin and hair	Thin and silky skin and hair
Weight	Gain	Loss

TABLE 31-2 **Manifestations of Hypothyroid and Hyperthyroid States**

5000 infants. Hypothyroidism in the infant may result from a congenital lack of the thyroid gland or from abnormal biosynthesis of thyroid hormone or deficient TSH secretion. With congenital lack of the thyroid gland, the infant usually appears normal and functions normally at birth because of thyroid hormones that have been supplied in utero by the mother. The manifestations of untreated congenital hypothyroidism are referred to as *cretinism*. However, the term does not apply to the normally developing infant in whom replacement thyroid hormone therapy was instituted shortly after birth.

Thyroid hormone is essential for normal brain development and growth, almost half of which occurs during the first 6 months of life. If untreated, congenital hypothyroidism causes mental retardation and impairs growth. Long-term studies show that closely monitored T_4 supplementation begun in the first 6 weeks of life results in normal intelligence. Fortunately, neonatal screening tests have been instituted to detect congenital hypothyroidism during early infancy. Screening usually is done in the hospital nursery. In this test, a drop of blood is taken from the infant's heel and analyzed for T_4 and TSH.

Transient congenital hypothyroidism has been recognized more frequently since the introduction of neonatal screening. It is characterized by high TSH levels and low thyroid hormone levels. The fetal and infant thyroids are sensitive to iodine excess. Iodine crosses the placenta and mammary glands and is readily absorbed by infant skin. Transient hypothyroidism may be caused by maternal or infant exposure to substances such as povidone-iodine used as a disinfectant (*i.e.*, vaginal douche or skin disinfectant, in the nursery). Antithyroid drugs, such as propylthiouracil and methimazole, can cross the placenta and block fetal thyroid function.

Congenital hypothyroidism is treated by hormone replacement. Evidence indicates that it is important to normalize T_4 levels as rapidly as possible because a delay is accompanied by poorer psychomotor and mental development. Dosage levels are adjusted as the child grows. Infants with transient hypothyroidism usually can have the replacement therapy withdrawn at 6 to 12 months. When early and adequate treatment regimens are followed, the risk of mental retardation in infants detected by screening programs essentially is nonexistent.

Acquired Hypothyroidism and Myxedema

Hypothyroidism in older children and adults causes a general slowing down of metabolic processes and myxedema (a nonpitting mucous type of edema). The hypothyroid state may be mild, with only a few signs and symptoms, or it may progress to a life-threatening condition called *myxedematous coma*. It can result from destruction or dysfunction of the thyroid gland (*i.e.*, primary hypothyroidism), or it can be a secondary disorder caused by impaired pituitary function or a tertiary disorder caused by a hypothalamic dysfunction.

Primary hypothyroidism is much more common than secondary (and tertiary) hypothyroidism. It may result

from thyroidectomy (*i.e.*, surgical removal) or ablation of the gland with radiation. Certain goitrogenic agents, such as lithium carbonate (*i.e.*, used in the treatment of bipolar disorders), and the antithyroid drugs propylthiouracil and methimazole in continuous dosage can block hormone synthesis and produce hypothyroidism with goiter. Large amounts of iodine (*i.e.*, ingestion of kelp tablets or iodide-containing cough syrups, or administration of iodide-containing radiographic contrast media or the cardiac drug amiodarone [which contains 75 mg of iodine per 200-mg tablet]) also can block thyroid hormone production and cause goiter, particularly in persons with autoimmune thyroid disease. Iodine deficiency, which can cause goiter and hypothyroidism, is rare in the United States because of the widespread use of iodized salt and other iodide sources.

The most common cause of hypothyroidism is Hashimoto thyroiditis, an autoimmune disorder in which the thyroid gland may be totally destroyed by an immunologic process.[17] It is the major cause of goiter and hypothyroidism in children and adults. Hashimoto thyroiditis is predominantly a disease of women, with a female-to-male ratio of 5:1. The course of the disease varies. At the onset, only a goiter may be present. In time, hypothyroidism usually becomes evident. Although the disorder usually causes hypothyroidism, a hyperthyroid state may develop midcourse in the disease. The transient hyperthyroid state is caused by leakage of preformed thyroid hormone from damaged cells of the gland. Subacute thyroiditis, which can occur in up to 10% of pregnancies postpartum (postpartum thyroiditis), also can result in hypothyroidism.

Hypothyroidism affects almost all of the organ systems in the body (see Table 31-2). The manifestations of the disorder are related largely to two factors: the hypometabolic state resulting from thyroid hormone deficiency and myxedematous involvement of body tissues. The hypometabolic state associated with hypothyroidism is characterized by a gradual onset of weakness and fatigue, a tendency to gain weight despite a loss of appetite, and cold intolerance (Fig. 31-7). As the condition progresses, the skin becomes dry and rough and acquires a pale yellowish cast, which primarily results from carotene deposition, and the hair becomes coarse and brittle. There can be loss of the lateral one third of the eyebrows. Gastrointestinal motility is decreased, producing constipation, flatulence, and abdominal distention. Nervous system involvement is manifested in mental dullness, lethargy, and impaired memory.

Myxedema is a hard nonpitting type of edema caused by increased quantities of mucins that trap water in the interstitial space. Although the myxedema is most obvious in the face and other superficial parts, it also affects many of the body organs and is responsible for many of the manifestations of the hypothyroid state. As a result of myxedematous fluid accumulation, the face takes on a characteristic puffy look, especially around the eyes. The tongue is enlarged, and the voice is hoarse and husky. Myxedematous fluid can collect in the interstitial spaces

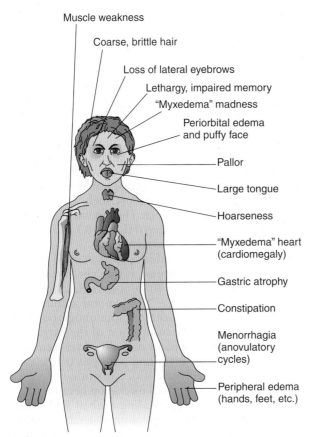

Muscle weakness
Coarse, brittle hair
Loss of lateral eyebrows
Lethargy, impaired memory
"Myxedema" madness
Periorbital edema and puffy face
Pallor
Large tongue
Hoarseness
"Myxedema" heart (cardiomegaly)
Gastric atrophy
Constipation
Menorrhagia (anovulatory cycles)
Peripheral edema (hands, feet, etc.)

FIGURE 31-7 Dominant clinical features of hypothyroidism. (From Rubin E., Rubin R. [2005]. The endocrine system. In Rubin E., Gorstein F., Rubin R., et al. [Eds.], *Rubin's pathology: Clinicopathologic foundations of medicine* [4th ed., p. 1137]. Philadelphia: Lippincott Williams & Wilkins.)

of almost any organ system. Pericardial or pleural effusion may develop. Mucopolysaccharide deposits in the heart cause generalized cardiac dilatation, bradycardia, and other signs of altered cardiac function.

Diagnosis of hypothyroidism is based on history, physical examination, and laboratory tests. A low serum T_4 and elevated TSH levels are characteristic of primary hypothyroidism. The tests for antithyroid antibodies should be done when Hashimoto thyroiditis is suspected (anti-TPO antibody titers are the preferred test). A TRH stimulation test may be helpful in differentiating pituitary (secondary hypothyroidism) from hypothalamic (tertiary hypothyroidism) disease.

Hypothyroidism is treated by replacement therapy with synthetic preparations of T_3 or T_4. Most people are treated with T_4. Serum TSH levels are used to estimate the adequacy of T_4 replacement therapy. When the TSH level is normalized, the T_4 dosage is considered satisfactory (for primary hypothyroidism only). A "go-low and go-slow" approach should be considered in the treatment of elderly with hypothyroidism because of the risk of inducing acute coronary syndromes in the susceptible individual.

Myxedematous Coma. Myxedematous coma is a life-threatening, end-stage expression of hypothyroidism. It is characterized by coma, hypothermia, cardiovascular collapse, hypoventilation, and severe metabolic disorders that include hyponatremia, hypoglycemia, and lactic acidosis. The pathophysiology of myxedema coma involves three major aspects: (1) carbon dioxide retention and hypoxia, (2) fluid and electrolyte imbalance, and (3) hypothermia.[15] It occurs most often in elderly women who have chronic hypothyroidism from a spectrum of causes. The fact that it occurs more frequently in winter months suggests that cold exposure may be a precipitating factor. The severely hypothyroid person is unable to metabolize sedatives, analgesics, and anesthetic drugs, and buildup of these agents may precipitate coma.

Treatment includes aggressive management of precipitating factors; supportive therapy such as management of cardiorespiratory status, hyponatremia, and hypoglycemia; and thyroid replacement therapy. If hypothermia is present (a low-reading thermometer should be used), active rewarming of the body is contraindicated because it may induce vasodilatation and vascular collapse. Prevention is preferable to treatment and entails special attention to high-risk populations, such as women with a history of Hashimoto thyroiditis. These persons should be informed about the signs and symptoms of severe hypothyroidism and the need for early medical treatment.

HYPERTHYROIDISM

Thyrotoxicosis is the clinical syndrome that results when tissues are exposed to high levels of circulating thyroid hormone.[15,18,19] In most instances, thyrotoxicosis is due to hyperactivity of the thyroid gland, or hyperthyroidism. The most common cause of hyperthyroidism is Graves disease (to be discussed). Other causes of hyperthyroidism are multinodular goiter, adenoma of the thyroid, and, occasionally, ingestion of excessive thyroid hormone. Iodine-containing agents can induce hyperthyroidism as well as hypothyroidism. Thyroid crisis, or storm, is an acutely exaggerated manifestation of the thyrotoxic state.

Many of the manifestations of hyperthyroidism are related to the increase in oxygen consumption and use of metabolic fuels associated with the hypermetabolic state, as well as to the increase in sympathetic nervous system activity that occurs[18] (see Table 31-2). The fact that many of the signs and symptoms of hyperthyroidism resemble those of excessive sympathetic nervous system activity suggests that thyroid hormone may heighten the sensitivity of the body to the catecholamines or that it may act as a pseudocatecholamine. With the hypermetabolic state, there are frequent complaints of nervousness, irritability, and fatigability (Fig. 31-8). Weight loss is common despite a large appetite. Other manifestations include tachycardia, palpitations, shortness of breath, excessive sweating, muscle cramps, and heat intolerance. The person appears restless and has a fine muscle tremor. Even

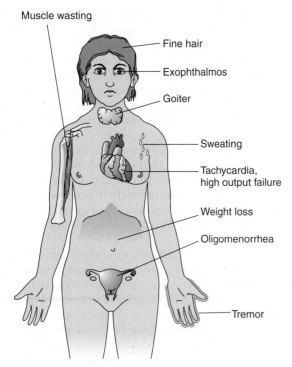

Muscle wasting

Fine hair

Exophthalmos

Goiter

Sweating

Tachycardia,
high output failure

Weight loss

Oligomenorrhea

Tremor

FIGURE 31-8 Dominant clinical features of Graves disease. (From Rubin E., Rubin R. [2005]. The endocrine system. In Rubin E., Gorstein F., Rubin R., et al. [Eds.], *Rubin's pathology: Clinico-pathologic foundations of medicine* [4th ed., p. 1140]. Philadelphia: Lippincott Williams & Wilkins.)

in persons without exophthalmos (i.e., bulging of the eyeballs seen in ophthalmopathy), there is an abnormal retraction of the eyelids and infrequent blinking such that they appear to be staring. The hair and skin usually are thin and have a silky appearance. About 15% of elderly individuals with new-onset atrial fibrillation have thyrotoxicosis.[18]

The treatment of hyperthyroidism is directed toward reducing the level of thyroid hormone. This can be accomplished with eradication of the thyroid gland with radioactive iodine, through surgical removal of part or all of the gland, or the use of drugs that decrease thyroid function and thereby the effect of thyroid hormone on the peripheral tissues. Eradication of the thyroid with radioactive iodine is used more frequently than surgery. The β-adrenergic–blocking drugs (propranolol, metoprolol, atenolol, and nadolol are preferred) are administered to block the effects of the hyperthyroid state on sympathetic nervous system function. They are given in conjunction with antithyroid drugs such as propylthiouracil and methimazole. These drugs prevent the thyroid gland from converting iodine to its organic (hormonal) form and block the conversion of T_4 to T_3 in the tissues. Iodinated contrast agents (iopanoic acid and ipodate sodium) may be given orally to block thyroid hormone synthesis and release as well as the peripheral conversion of T_4 to T_3. These agents may be used in treatment of thyroid storm or in persons who are intolerant of propylthiouracil or methimazole.

Graves Disease

Graves disease is a state of hyperthyroidism that is often accompanied by goiter, ophthalmopathy (exophthalmos or bulging of eyeballs), or less commonly dermopathy (marked thickening of the skin over the pretibial area).[15,18,19] The onset usually is between the ages of 20 and 40 years, and women are five times more likely to develop the disease than men. Graves disease is an autoimmune disorder characterized by abnormal stimulation of the thyroid gland by thyroid-stimulating antibodies (thyroid-stimulating immunoglobulins [TSI]) that act through the normal TSH receptors. It may be associated with other autoimmune disorders such as myasthenia gravis and pernicious anemia. The disease is associated with human leukocyte antigen (HLA)-DR3 and HLA-B8, and a familial tendency is evident.

The ophthalmopathy, which occurs in up to one third of persons with Graves disease, is thought to result from a cytokine-mediated activation of fibroblasts in orbital tissue behind the eyeball.[15,18–20] Humoral autoimmunity also is important; an ophthalmic immunoglobulin may exacerbate lymphocytic infiltration of the extraocular muscles. The ophthalmopathy of Graves disease can cause severe eye problems, including paralysis of the extraocular muscles; involvement of the optic nerve, with some visual loss; and corneal ulceration because the lids do not close over the protruding eyeball with exophthalmos. The ophthalmopathy usually tends to stabilize after treatment of the hyperthyroidism. Because ophthalmopathy can worsen acutely after radioiodine treatment, some physicians prescribe glucocorticoids for several weeks surrounding the treatment if the person had signs of ophthalmopathy; others do not to use radioiodine therapy under these circumstances, but prefer antithyroid therapy with drugs. Unfortunately, not all of the ocular changes are reversible with treatment. Ophthalmopathy also can be aggravated by smoking, which should be strongly discouraged. Figure 31-9 shows a woman with Graves disease.

Thyroid Storm

Thyroid storm, or crisis, is an extreme and life-threatening form of thyrotoxicosis, rarely seen today because of improved diagnosis and treatment methods.[15,18] When it does occur, it is seen most often in undiagnosed cases or in persons with hyperthyroidism who have not been adequately treated. It often is precipitated by stress such as an infection (usually respiratory), by diabetic ketoacidosis, by physical or emotional trauma, or by manipulation of a hyperactive thyroid gland during thyroidectomy. Thyroid storm is manifested by a very high fever, extreme cardiovascular effects (*i.e.*, tachycardia, congestive failure, and angina), and severe CNS effects (*i.e.*, agitation, restlessness, and delirium). The mortality rate is high.

Thyroid storm requires rapid diagnosis and implementation of treatment. Peripheral cooling is initiated with cold packs and a cooling mattress. For cooling to be effective, the shivering response must be prevented. General supportive measures to replace fluids, glucose, and electrolytes are essential during the hypermetabolic state. A

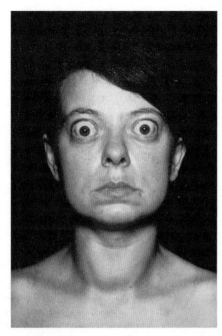

FIGURE 31-9 Graves disease. A young woman with hyperthyroidism presented with a mass in the neck and exophthalmos. (From Rubin E., Rubin R. [2005]. The endocrine system. In Rubin E., Gorstein F., Rubin R., et al. [Eds.], *Rubin's pathology: Clinicopathologic foundations of medicine* [4th ed., p. 1138]. Philadelphia: Lippincott Williams & Wilkins.)

β-adrenergic–blocking drug, such as propranolol, is given to block the undesirable effects of T_4 on cardiovascular function. Glucocorticoids are used to correct the relative adrenal insufficiency resulting from the stress imposed by the hyperthyroid state and to inhibit the peripheral conversion of T_4 to T_3. Propylthiouracil or methimazole may be given to block thyroid synthesis. Aspirin increases the level of free thyroid hormones by displacing the hormones from their protein carriers, and should not be used during thyroid storm. The iodide-containing radiographic contrast medium sodium ipodate also can be useful for blocking thyroid hormone production.

In summary, thyroid hormones play a role in the metabolic process of almost all body cells and are necessary for normal physical and mental growth in the infant and young child. Alterations in thyroid function can manifest as a hypothyroid or a hyperthyroid state. Hypothyroidism can occur as a congenital or an acquired defect. Congenital hypothyroidism leads to mental retardation and impaired physical growth unless treatment is initiated during the first months of life. Acquired hypothyroidism leads to a decrease in metabolic rate and an accumulation of a mucopolysaccharide substance in the intercellular spaces; this substance attracts water and causes a mucous type of edema called *myxedema*. Hyperthyroidism causes an increase in metabolic rate and alter-

ations in body function similar to those produced by enhanced sympathetic nervous system activity. Graves disease is characterized by the triad of hyperthyroidism, goiter, and ophthalmopathy (or dermopathy).

Disorders of Adrenal Cortical Function

CONTROL OF ADRENAL CORTICAL FUNCTION

The adrenal glands are small, bilateral structures (Fig. 31-10A) that weigh approximately 5 g each and lie retroperitoneally at the apex of each kidney. The medulla or inner portion of the gland secretes epinephrine and norepinephrine and is part of the sympathetic nervous system. The cortex forms the bulk of the adrenal gland and is responsible for secreting three types of hormones: the glucocorticoids, the mineralocorticoids, and the adrenal sex hormones.[21] Because the sympathetic nervous system also secretes epinephrine and norepinephrine, adrenal medullary function is not essential for life, but adrenal cortical function is. The total loss of adrenal cortical function is fatal in 4 to 14 days if untreated.

Biosynthesis, Transport, and Metabolism

More than 30 hormones are produced by the adrenal cortex. Of these hormones, aldosterone is the principal mineralocorticoid, cortisol (hydrocortisone) is the major glucocorticoid, and androgens are the chief sex hormones. All of the adrenal cortical hormones have a similar structure in that all are steroids and are synthesized from acetate and cholesterol (Fig. 31-10B). Each of the steps involved in the synthesis of the various hormones requires a specific enzyme. The secretion of the glucocorticoids and the adrenal androgens is controlled by the ACTH secreted by the anterior pituitary gland.

Cortisol and the adrenal androgens are secreted in an unbound state and bind to plasma proteins for transport in the circulatory system. Cortisol binds largely to corticosteroid-binding globulin and to a lesser extent to albumin. Aldosterone circulates mostly bound to albumin. It has been suggested that the pool of protein-bound hormones may extend the duration of their action by delaying metabolic clearance.

The main site for metabolism of the adrenal cortical hormones is the liver, where they undergo a number of metabolic conversions before being conjugated and made water soluble. They are then eliminated in either the urine or the bile.

Adrenal Sex Hormones

The adrenal sex hormones are synthesized primarily by the zona reticularis and the zona fasciculata of the cortex (see Fig. 31-10A). These sex hormones probably exert little effect on normal sexual function. There is evidence, however, that the adrenal sex hormones (the most important

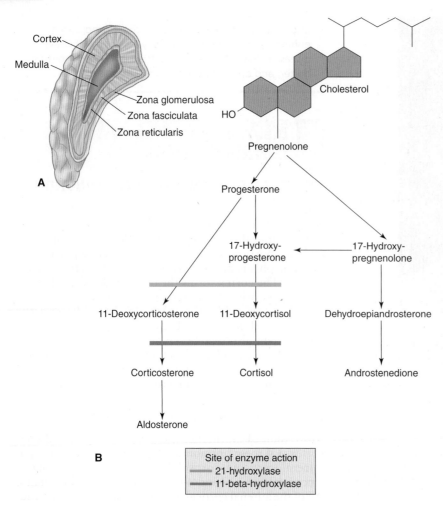

Site of enzyme action
- 21-hydroxylase
- 11-beta-hydroxylase

FIGURE 31-10 (**A**) The adrenal gland, showing the medulla and the three layers of the cortex. The outer layer of the cortex (zona glomerulosa) is primarily responsible for mineralocorticoid production, and the middle layer (zona fasciculata) and inner layer (zona reticularis) produce the glucocorticoids and adrenal sex hormones. (**B**) Predominant biosynthetic pathways of the adrenal cortex. Critical enzymes in the biosynthetic process include 11-β-hydroxylase and 21-hydroxylase. A deficiency in one of these enzymes blocks the synthesis of hormones dependent on that enzyme and routes the precursors into alternative pathways.

of which is dehydroepiandrosterone [DHEA]) contribute to the pubertal growth of body hair, particularly pubic and axillary hair in women. They also may play a role in the steroid hormone economy of the pregnant woman and the fetal-placental unit. Dehydroepiandrosterone sulfate (DHEAS) is increasingly being used in the treatment of both adrenal insufficiency (*i.e.,* Addison disease) and adults who have decreased levels of DHEAS. Adrenal androgens are physiologically important in women with Addison disease, and replacement therapy with DHEAS should be considered.[22] Because the testes produce these hormones, there is no rationale for using it in men. The levels of DHEAS decline to approximately one sixth the levels of a 20-year-old by 60 years of age (the *adrenopause*). The significance if this is unknown, but replacement may improve general well-being and sexuality, and have other important effects in women. The value of routine replacement of DHEAS in the adrenopause is largely unproven.

Mineralocorticoids

The mineralocorticoids play an essential role in regulating potassium and sodium levels and water balance. They are produced in the zona glomerulosa, the outer layer of cells of the adrenal cortex (see Fig. 31-10A). Aldosterone secretion is regulated by the renin-angiotensin mechanism and by blood levels of potassium. Increased levels of aldosterone promote sodium retention by the distal tubules of the kidney while increasing urinary losses of potassium. The influence of aldosterone on fluid and electrolyte balance is discussed in Chapter 6.

Glucocorticoids

The glucocorticoid hormones, mainly cortisol, are synthesized in the zona fasciculata and the zona reticularis of the adrenal gland (see Fig. 31-10A). The blood levels of these hormones are regulated by negative feedback mechanisms of the hypothalamic-pituitary-adrenal (HPA) system (Fig. 31-11). Just as other pituitary hormones are controlled by releasing factors from the hypothalamus, corticotropin-releasing hormone (CRH) is important in controlling the release of ACTH. Cortisol levels increase as ACTH levels rise and decrease as ACTH levels fall. There is considerable diurnal variation in ACTH levels, which reach their peak in the early morning (around 6 to

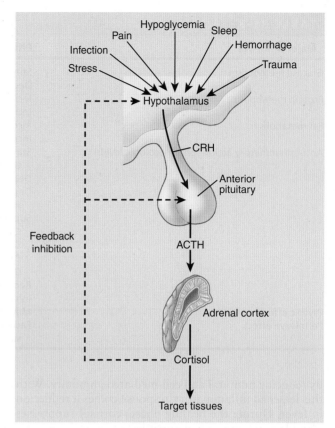

FIGURE 31-11 The hypothalamic-pituitary-adrenal (HPA) feedback system that regulates glucocorticoid (cortisol) levels. Cortisol release is regulated by adrenocorticotropic hormone (ACTH). Stress exerts its effects on cortisol release through the HPA system and corticotropin-releasing hormone (CRH), which controls the release of ACTH from the anterior pituitary gland. Increased cortisol levels incite a negative feedback inhibition of ACTH release.

8 AM) and decline as the day progresses. This appears to be due to rhythmic activity in the CNS, which causes bursts of CRH secretion and, in turn, ACTH secretion. This diurnal pattern is reversed in people who work during the night and sleep during the day. The rhythm also may be changed by physical and psychological stresses, endogenous depression, bipolar disorder, and liver disease or other conditions that affect cortisol metabolism. One of the earliest signs of Cushing syndrome, a disorder of cortisol excess, is the loss of diurnal variation in CRH and ACTH secretion. This is why late-night (between 11 PM and midnight) serum or salivary cortisol levels can be inappropriately elevated, aiding in the diagnosis of Cushing syndrome (to be discussed).[21]

The glucocorticoids perform a necessary function in response to stress and are essential for survival. When produced as part of the stress response, these hormones aid in regulating the metabolic functions of the body and in controlling the inflammatory response. The actions of cortisol are summarized in Table 31-3. Many of the anti-inflammatory actions attributed to cortisol result from the administration of pharmacologic levels of the hormone.

Metabolic Effects. Cortisol stimulates glucose production by the liver, promotes protein breakdown, and causes mobilization of fatty acids. As body proteins are broken down, amino acids are mobilized and transported to the liver, where they are used in the production of glucose (*i.e.,* gluconeogenesis). Mobilization of fatty acids converts cell metabolism from the use of glucose for energy to the use of fatty acids instead. As glucose pro-

duction by the liver rises and peripheral glucose use falls, a moderate resistance to insulin develops. In persons with diabetes and those who are diabetes prone, this has the effect of raising the blood glucose level.

Psychological Effects. The glucocorticoid hormones appear to be involved directly or indirectly in emotional behavior. Receptors for these hormones have been identified in brain tissue, which suggests that they play a role in the regulation of behavior. Persons treated with adrenal cortical hormones have been known to display behavior ranging from mildly aberrant to psychotic.

Immunologic and Inflammatory Effects. Cortisol influences multiple aspects of immunologic function and inflammatory responsiveness. Large quantities of cortisol are required for an effective anti-inflammatory action. This is achieved by the administration of pharmacologic rather than physiologic doses of synthetic cortisol. The increased cortisol blocks inflammation at an early stage by decreasing capillary permeability and stabilizing the lysosomal membranes so that inflammatory mediators are not released. Cortisol suppresses the immune response

TABLE 31-3	Actions of Cortisol
Major Influence	**Effect on Body**
Glucose metabolism	Stimulates gluconeogenesis
	Decreases glucose use by the tissues
Protein metabolism	Increases breakdown of proteins
	Increases plasma protein levels
Fat metabolism	Increases mobilization of fatty acids
	Increases use of fatty acids
Anti-inflammatory action (pharmacologic levels)	Stabilizes lysosomal membranes of the inflammatory cells, preventing the release of inflammatory mediators
	Decreases capillary permeability to prevent inflammatory edema
	Depresses phagocytosis by white blood cells to reduce the release of inflammatory mediators
	Suppresses the immune response
	Causes atrophy of lymphoid tissue
	Decreases eosinophils
	Decreases antibody formation
	Decreases the development of cell-mediated immunity
	Reduces fever
	Inhibits fibroblast activity
Psychic effect	May contribute to emotional instability
Permissive effect	Facilitates the response of the tissues to humoral and neural influences, such as that of the catecholamines, during trauma and extreme stress

by reducing humoral and cell-mediated immunity. With this lessened inflammatory response comes a reduction in fever. During the healing phase, cortisol suppresses fibroblast activity and thereby lessens scar formation. Cortisol also inhibits prostaglandin synthesis, which may account in large part for its anti-inflammatory actions.

Pharmacologic Suppression of Adrenal Function

A highly significant aspect of long-term therapy with pharmacologic preparations of the adrenal cortical hormones is adrenal insufficiency on withdrawal of the drugs. The deficiency results from suppression of the HPA system. Chronic suppression causes atrophy of the adrenal gland, and the abrupt withdrawal of drugs can cause acute adrenal insufficiency. Recovery to a state of normal adrenal function may be prolonged, requiring up to 12 months or more.

Tests of Adrenal Function

Several diagnostic tests can be used to evaluate adrenal cortical function and the HPA system.[21] Blood levels of cortisol, aldosterone, and ACTH can be measured using immunoassay methods. A 24-hour urine specimen measuring the excretion of various metabolic end products of the adrenal hormones and the male androgens provides information about alterations in the biosynthesis of the adrenal cortical hormones. The 24-hour urinary free cortisol, late-night (between 11 PM and midnight) serum or salivary cortisol levels, and the overnight 1-mg dexamethasone suppression test (see later) are excellent screening tests for Cushing syndrome.[21,23,24]

Suppression and stimulation tests afford a means of assessing the state of the HPA feedback system. For exam-

ple, a test dose of ACTH can be given to assess the response of the adrenal cortex to stimulation. Similarly, administration of dexamethasone, a synthetic glucocorticoid drug, provides a means of measuring negative feedback suppression of ACTH. Adrenal tumors and ectopic ACTH-producing tumors usually are unresponsive to ACTH suppression by dexamethasone. CRH tests can be used to diagnose a pituitary ACTH-secreting tumor (*i.e.*, Cushing disease), especially when combined with inferior petrosal venous sampling (this allows the blood drainage of the pituitary to be sampled directly). Metyrapone blocks the final step in cortisol synthesis, resulting in the production of 11-dehydroxycortisol, which does not inhibit ACTH. This test measures the ability of the pituitary to release ACTH. The gold standard test for assessing the HPA axis is the insulin hypoglycemic stress test.

 ## CONGENITAL ADRENAL HYPERPLASIA

Congenital adrenal hyperplasia (CAH), or the adrenogenital syndrome, describes a congenital disorder caused by an autosomal recessive trait in which a deficiency exists in any of the enzymes necessary for the synthesis of cortisol[25] (Fig. 31-10B). A common characteristic of all types of CAH is a defect in the synthesis of cortisol that results in increased levels of ACTH and adrenal hyperplasia. The increased levels of ACTH overstimulate the pathways for production of adrenal androgens. Mineralocorticoids may be produced in excessive or insufficient amounts, depending on the precise enzyme deficiency. Infants of both sexes are affected. Boys seldom are diagnosed at birth unless they have enlarged genitalia or lose salt and manifest adrenal crisis. In female infants, an increase in andro-

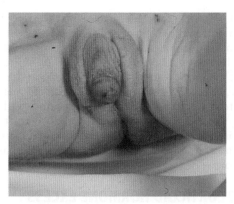

FIGURE 31-12 A female infant with congenital adrenal hyperplasia demonstrating virilization of the genitalia with hypertrophy of the clitoris and partial fusion of labioscrotal folds. (From Rubin E., Rubin R. [2005]. The endocrine system. In Rubin E., Gorstein F., Rubin R., et al. [Eds.], *Rubin's pathology: Clinicopathologic foundations of medicine* [4th ed., p. 1156]. Philadelphia: Lippincott Williams & Wilkins.)

gens is responsible for creating the virilization syndrome of ambiguous genitalia with an enlarged clitoris, fused labia, and urogenital sinus (see Fig. 31-12). In male and female children, other secondary sex characteristics are normal, and fertility is unaffected if appropriate therapy is instituted.

The two most common enzyme deficiencies are 21-hydroxylase (accounting for >90% of cases) and 11-β-hydroxylase deficiency (see Fig. 31-10B). The clinical manifestations of both deficiencies are largely determined by the functional properties of the steroid intermediates and the completeness of the block in the cortisol pathway.

A spectrum of 21-hydroxylase deficiency states exists, ranging from simple virilizing CAH to a complete salt-losing enzyme deficiency.[25,26] Simple virilizing CAH impairs the synthesis of cortisol, and steroid synthesis is shunted to androgen production. Persons with these deficiencies usually produce sufficient aldosterone or aldosterone intermediates to prevent signs and symptoms of mineralocorticoid deficiency. The salt-losing form is accompanied by deficient production of aldosterone and its intermediates. This results in fluid and electrolyte disorders after the fifth day of life (including hyponatremia, hyperkalemia, vomiting, dehydration, and shock).

The 11-β-hydroxylase deficiency is rare and manifests a spectrum of severity. Affected persons have excessive androgen production and impaired conversion of 11-deoxycorticosterone to corticosterone. The overproduction of 11-deoxycorticosterone, which has mineralocorticoid activity, is responsible for the hypertension that accompanies this deficiency. Diagnosis of the adrenogenital syndrome depends on the precise biochemical evaluation of metabolites in the cortisol pathway and on clinical signs and symptoms. Genetic testing is also invaluable, however, because the correlation between the phenotype and genotype is not always straightforward.[25,26]

Medical treatment of adrenogenital syndrome includes oral or parenteral cortisol replacement. Fludrocortisone

acetate, a mineralocorticoid, also may be given to children who are salt losers. Depending on the degree of virilization, reconstructive surgery during the first 2 years of life is indicated to reduce the size of the clitoris, separate the labia, and exteriorize the vagina. Advances in surgical techniques have led to earlier use of single-stage surgery—between 2 and 6 months of life in girls with 21-hydroxylase deficiency, a time when the tissues are maximally pliable and psychological trauma to the child is minimized.[25] Surgery has provided excellent results and does not usually impair sexual function.

ADRENAL CORTICAL INSUFFICIENCY

There are two forms of adrenal insufficiency: primary and secondary.[27] Primary adrenal insufficiency, or Addison disease, is caused by destruction of the adrenal gland. Secondary adrenal insufficiency results from a disorder of the HPA system.

Primary Adrenal Cortical Insufficiency

In 1855, Thomas Addison, an English physician, provided the first detailed clinical description of primary adrenal insufficiency, now called *Addison disease*. The use of this term is reserved for primary adrenal insufficiency in which adrenal cortical hormones are deficient and ACTH levels are elevated because of lack of feedback inhibition.

Addison disease is a relatively rare disorder in which all the layers of the adrenal cortex are destroyed. Autoimmune destruction is the most common cause of Addison disease in the United States. Before 1950, tuberculosis was the major cause of Addison disease in the United States, and it continues to be a major cause of the disease in countries where it is more prevalent. Rare causes include metastatic carcinoma, fungal infection (particularly histoplasmosis), cytomegalovirus infection, amyloid disease, and hemochromatosis. Bilateral adrenal hemorrhage may occur in persons taking anticoagulants, during open heart surgery, and during birth or major trauma. Adrenal insufficiency can be caused by acquired immunodeficiency syndrome, in which the adrenal gland is destroyed by a variety of opportunistic infectious agents.

Addison disease, like type 1 diabetes mellitus, is a chronic metabolic disorder that requires lifetime hormone replacement therapy. The adrenal cortex has a large reserve capacity, and the manifestations of adrenal insufficiency usually do not become apparent until approximately 90% of the gland has been destroyed. These manifestations are related primarily to mineralocorticoid deficiency, glucocorticoid deficiency, and hyperpigmentation resulting from elevated ACTH levels. Although lack of the adrenal androgens (*i.e.,* DHEAS) exerts few effects in men because the testes produce these hormones, women have sparse axillary and pubic hair. Mineralocorticoid deficiency causes increased urinary losses of sodium, chloride, and water, along with decreased excretion of potassium. The result is hyponatremia, loss of extracellular fluid, decreased cardiac output, and hyperkalemia. There may be an abnormal appetite for salt. Orthostatic hypotension is common. Dehydration, weakness, and fatigue are common early symptoms. If loss of sodium and water is extreme, cardiovascular collapse and shock ensue. Because of a lack of glucocorticoids, the person with Addison disease has poor tolerance to stress. This deficiency causes hypoglycemia, lethargy, weakness, fever, and gastrointestinal symptoms such as anorexia, nausea, vomiting, and weight loss.

Hyperpigmentation results from elevated levels of ACTH. The skin looks bronzed or suntanned in exposed and unexposed areas, and the normal creases and pressure points tend to become especially dark. The gums and oral mucous membranes may become bluish-black. The amino acid sequence of ACTH is strikingly similar to that of melanocyte-stimulating hormone; hyperpigmentation occurs in greater than 90% of persons with Addison disease and is helpful in distinguishing the primary and secondary forms of adrenal insufficiency.

The daily regulation of the chronic phase of Addison disease usually is accomplished with oral replacement therapy, with higher doses being given during periods of stress. The pharmacologic agent that is used should have both glucocorticoid and mineralocorticoid activity. Mineralocorticoids are needed only in primary adrenal insufficiency. Hydrocortisone usually is the drug of choice. In mild cases, hydrocortisone alone may be adequate. Fludrocortisone (a mineralocorticoid) is used for persons who do not obtain a sufficient salt-retaining effect from hydrocortisone. DHEAS replacement also may be helpful in the female patient.[22,27]

Because persons with the disorder are likely to have episodes of hyponatremia and hypoglycemia, they need to have a regular schedule for meals and exercise. Persons with Addison disease also have limited ability to respond to infections, trauma, and other stresses. Such situations require immediate medical attention and treatment. All persons with Addison disease should be advised to wear a medical alert bracelet or medal.

Secondary Adrenal Cortical Insufficiency

Secondary adrenal insufficiency can occur as the result of hypopituitarism or because the pituitary gland has been surgically removed. Tertiary adrenal insufficiency results from a hypothalamic defect. However, a far more common cause than either of these is the rapid withdrawal of glucocorticoids that have been administered therapeutically. These drugs suppress the HPA system, with resulting adrenal cortical atrophy and loss of cortisol production. This suppression continues long after drug therapy has been discontinued and can be critical during periods of stress or when surgery is performed.

Acute Adrenal Crisis

Acute adrenal crisis is a life-threatening situation.[27] If Addison disease is the underlying problem, exposure to even a minor illness or stress can precipitate nausea, vomiting, muscular weakness, hypotension, dehydration, and vascular collapse. The onset of adrenal crisis may be sudden, or it may progress over a period of several days. The symptoms may occur suddenly in children with salt-losing forms of the adrenogenital syndrome. Massive bilateral adrenal hemorrhage causes an acute fulminating form of adrenal insufficiency. Hemorrhage can be caused by meningococcal septicemia (*i.e.,* Waterhouse-Friderichsen syndrome), adrenal trauma, anticoagulant therapy, adrenal vein thrombosis, or adrenal metastases.

Acute adrenal insufficiency is treated with intravenous fluids and corticosteroid replacement therapy. Corticosteroid replacement is accomplished through the intravenous administration of either dexamethasone or hydrocortisone.

GLUCOCORTICOID HORMONE EXCESS (CUSHING SYNDROME)

The term *Cushing syndrome* refers to the manifestations of hypercortisolism from any cause.[21,23,24] Three important forms of Cushing syndrome result from excess glucocorticoid production by the body. One is a pituitary form, which results from excessive production of ACTH by a tumor of the pituitary gland. This form of the disease was the one originally described by Cushing; therefore; it is called *Cushing disease*. The second form is the adrenal form, caused by a benign or malignant adrenal tumor. The third form is ectopic Cushing syndrome, caused by a nonpituitary ACTH-secreting tumor. Certain extrapituitary malignant tumors such as small cell carcinoma of the lung may secrete ACTH or, rarely, CRH, and produce Cushing syndrome. Cushing syndrome also can result from long-term therapy with one of the potent pharmacologic preparations of glucocorticoids; this form is called *iatrogenic Cushing syndrome*.

The major manifestations of Cushing syndrome represent an exaggeration of the many actions of cortisol (Fig. 31-13). Altered fat metabolism causes a peculiar deposition of fat characterized by a protruding abdomen; subclavicular fat pads or "buffalo hump" on the back; and a round, plethoric "moon face" (Fig. 31-14). There is muscle weakness, and the extremities are thin because of protein breakdown and muscle wasting. In advanced cases, the skin over the forearms and legs becomes thin, having the appearance of parchment. Purple striae, or stretch marks, from stretching of the catabolically weakened skin and subcutaneous tissues are distributed over the breast, thighs, and abdomen. Osteoporosis may develop because of destruction of bone proteins and alterations in calcium metabolism, resulting in back pain, compression fractures of the vertebrae, and rib fractures. As calcium is mobilized from bone, renal calculi may develop.

Derangements in glucose metabolism are found in approximately 75% of persons with Cushing syndrome, with clinically overt diabetes mellitus occurring in approximately 20%. The glucocorticoids possess mineralocorticoid properties; this causes hypokalemia as a result of excessive potassium excretion and hypertension resulting from sodium retention. Inflammatory and immune responses are inhibited, resulting in increased susceptibility to infection. Cortisol increases gastric acid secretion, which may provoke gastric ulceration and bleeding. An accompanying increase in androgen levels causes hirsutism, mild acne, and menstrual irregularities in women.

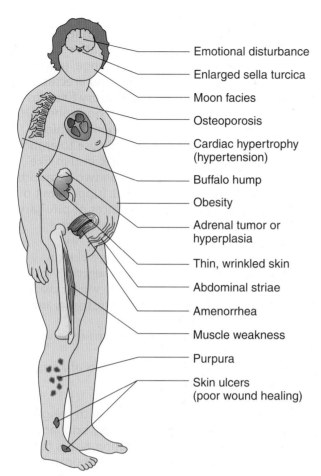

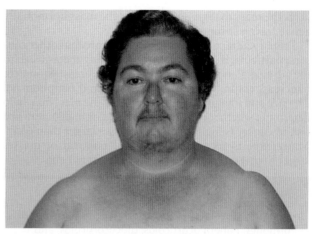

FIGURE 31-14 Cushing syndrome. A woman who suffered from a pituitary adenoma that produced adrenocorticotropic hormone exhibits a moon face, buffalo hump, increased facial hair, and thinning of the scalp hair. (From Rubin E., Rubin R. [2005]. The endocrine system. In Rubin E., Gorstein F., Rubin R., et al. [Eds.], *Rubin's pathology: Clinicopathologic foundations of medicine* [4th ed., p. 1162]. Philadelphia: Lippincott Williams & Wilkins.)

Emotional disturbance

Enlarged sella turcica

Moon facies

Osteoporosis

Cardiac hypertrophy (hypertension)

Buffalo hump

Obesity

Adrenal tumor or hyperplasia

Thin, wrinkled skin

Abdominal striae

Amenorrhea

Muscle weakness

Purpura

Skin ulcers (poor wound healing)

FIGURE 31-13 Major clinical manifestations of Cushing syndrome. (From Rubin E., Rubin R. [2005]. The endocrine system. In Rubin E., Gorstein F., Rubin R., et al. [Eds.], *Rubin's pathology: Clinicopathologic foundations of medicine* [4th ed., p. 1162]. Philadelphia: Lippincott Williams & Wilkins.)

Excess levels of the glucocorticoids may give rise to extreme emotional lability, ranging from mild euphoria and absence of normal fatigue to grossly psychotic behavior.

Diagnosis of Cushing syndrome depends on the finding of cortisol hypersecretion. The determination of 24-hour excretion of cortisol in urine provides a reliable and practical index of cortisol secretions. One of the prominent features of Cushing syndrome is loss of the diurnal pattern of cortisol secretion. This is why late-night (between 11 PM and midnight) serum or salivary cortisol levels can be inappropriately elevated, aiding in the diagnosis of Cushing syndrome.[21,23,24] The overnight 1-mg dexamethasone suppression test is also used as a screening tool for Cushing syndrome.

Other tests include measurement of the plasma levels of ACTH.[21,23,24] ACTH levels should be normal or elevated in ACTH-dependent Cushing syndrome (Cushing disease and ectopic ACTH), and low in non–ACTH-dependent Cushing syndrome (adrenal tumors). Various suppression or stimulation tests of the HPA system are performed to further delineate the cause. MRI or CT scans are used to locate adrenal or pituitary tumors.

Untreated, Cushing syndrome produces serious morbidity and even death. The choice of surgery, irradiation, or pharmacologic treatment is determined largely by the cause of the hypercortisolism. The goal of treatment for Cushing syndrome is to remove or correct the source of hypercortisolism without causing any permanent pituitary or adrenal damage. Transsphenoidal removal of a pituitary adenoma or a hemihypophysectomy is the preferred method of treatment for Cushing disease. This allows removal of only the tumor rather than the entire pituitary gland. After successful removal, the person must receive cortisol replacement therapy for 6 to 12 months or until adrenal function returns. Patients also may receive pituitary radiation therapy, but the full effects of treatment may not be realized for 3 to 12 months. Unilateral or bilateral adrenalectomy may be done in the case of a cortisol-producing adrenal adenoma. When possible, ectopic ACTH-producing tumors are removed. Pharmacologic agents that block steroid synthesis may be used to treat persons with ectopic tumors or adrenal carcinomas that cannot be resected.[21,23] Many of these patients also require *Pneumocystis carinii* pneumonia prophylaxis because of the profound immunosuppression caused by the excessive glucocorticoid levels.

INCIDENTAL ADRENAL MASS

An incidentaloma is a mass lesion found unexpectedly in an adrenal gland by an imaging procedure (done for other reasons), most commonly CT (but also MRI and ultrasonography). They have been increasingly recognized since the early 1980s. The prevalence of adrenal incidentalomas at autopsy is approximately 10 to 100 per 1000. In CT series, 0.4% to 0.6% are the usual figures published. Incidentalomas also can occur in other organs (*e.g.*, pituitary, thyroid).[28] The two most important questions are

(1) is the mass malignant, and (2) is the mass hormonally active (*i.e.*, is it functioning)?

Primary adrenal carcinoma is quite rare, but other cancers, particularly lung cancers, commonly metastasize to the adrenal gland (other cancers include breast, stomach, pancreas, colon, kidney, melanomas, and lymphomas). The size and imaging characteristics of the mass may help determine whether the tumor is benign or malignant. The risk of cancer is high in adrenal masses larger than 6 cm. Many experts recommend surgical removal of masses larger than 4 cm, particularly in younger patients.[29]

In summary, the adrenal cortex produces three types of hormones: mineralocorticoids, glucocorticoids, and adrenal sex hormones. The mineralocorticoids along with the renin-angiotensin mechanism aid in controlling body levels of sodium and potassium. The glucocorticoids have anti-inflammatory actions and aid in regulating glucose, protein, and fat metabolism during periods of stress. These hormones are under the control of the HPA system. The adrenal sex hormones exert little effect on daily control of body function, but they probably contribute to the development of body hair in women. The adrenogenital syndrome describes a genetic defect in the cortisol pathway resulting from a deficiency of one of the enzymes needed for its synthesis. Depending on the enzyme involved, the disorder causes virilization of female infants and, in some instances, fluid and electrolyte disturbances because of impaired mineralocorticoid synthesis.

Chronic adrenal insufficiency can be caused by destruction of the adrenal gland (Addison disease) or by dysfunction of the HPA system. Adrenal insufficiency requires replacement therapy with cortical hormones. Acute adrenal insufficiency is a life-threatening situation. Cushing syndrome refers to the manifestations of excessive cortisol levels. This syndrome may be a result of pharmacologic doses of cortisol, a pituitary or adrenal tumor, or an ectopic tumor that produces ACTH. The clinical manifestations of Cushing syndrome reflect the very high level of cortisol that is present. An incidentaloma is a mass lesion found unexpectedly in an adrenal gland (and other glands) by an imaging procedure done for other reasons. They are being recognized with increasing frequency, emphasizing the need for correct diagnosis and treatment.

Review Exercises

A 59-year-old man was referred to a neurologist for evaluation of headaches. Subsequent MRI studies revealed a large suprasellar mass (2.5 × 2.4 cm), consistent with a pituitary tumor. His history was positive for hypertension, and on direct inquiry, he thought his hands were slightly larger than previously, with increased sweating. Family history was negative, as were questions about weight change, polyuria/polydipsia, visual disturbance, and erectile dysfunction. Subsequent laboratory findings reveal a baseline serum growth hormone (GH) of 8.7 ng/mL (normal, 0 to 5 ng/mL), which was unsuppressed after oral glucose tolerance testing, and glucose intolerance; insulin-like growth factor-1 (IGF-1) levels on two occasions were high (1044 and 1145 μg/L [upper limit of normal is 480 μg/L]). Other indices of pituitary function were within the normal range.

A. What diagnosis would this man's clinical, MRI, and laboratory findings suggest?
B. Why was an inquiry made into weight change, polyuria/polydipsia, visual disturbance, and erectile dysfunction?
C. How would you explain his impaired glucose tolerance?
D. What are the possible local effects of a large pituitary tumor?

A 76-year-old woman presents with weight gain, subjective memory loss, dry skin, and cold intolerance. On examination, she is found to have a multinodular goiter. Laboratory findings reveal a low serum T_4 and elevated TSH.

A. What diagnosis would this woman's history, physical examination, and laboratory test results suggest?
B. Explain the possible relationship between the diagnosis and her weight gain, dry skin, cold intolerance, and subjective memory loss.
C. What type of treatment would be indicated?

A 45-year-old woman presents with a history of progressive weakness, fatigue, weight loss, nausea, and increased skin pigmentation (especially of creases, pressure areas, and nipples). Her blood pressure is 120/78 when supine and 105/52 when standing. Laboratory findings revealed a serum sodium of 120 mEq/L (normal, 135 to 145 mEq/L); potassium 5.9 mEq/L (normal, 3.5 to 5.0 mEq/L); low plasma cortisol levels; and high ACTH levels.

A. What diagnosis would this woman's clinical features and laboratory findings suggest?
B. Would her diagnosis be classified as a primary or secondary endocrine disorder?
C. What is the significance of her darkened skin?
D. What type of treatment would be indicated?

REFERENCES

1. Aron D. C., Findling J. W., Tyrrell J. B. (2004). Hypothalamus and pituitary gland. In Greenspan F. S., Gardner D. G. (Eds.), *Basic and clinical endocrinology* (7th ed., pp. 106–175). New York: Lange Medical Books/McGraw-Hill.

2. AACE Growth Hormone Task Force. (2003). AACE medical guidelines for clinical practice for growth hormone use in adults and children—2003 update. *Endocrine Practice* 9, 64–76.

3. Styne D. (2004). Growth. In Greenspan F. S., Gardner D. G. (Eds.), *Basic and clinical endocrinology* (7th ed., pp. 176–214). New York: Lange Medical Books/McGraw-Hill.

4. Laron Z. (1995). Laron syndrome (primary GH resistance) from patient to laboratory to patient. *Journal of Clinical Endocrinology and Metabolism* 80, 1526–1531.

5. Sesmilo G., Biller B. M., Levadot J., et al. (2000). Effects of GH administration on inflammatory and other cardiovascular risk markers in men with GH deficiency. *Annals of Internal Medicine* 133, 111–122.

6. Root A. (2001). The tall, rapidly growing infant, child, and adolescent. *Current Opinion in Endocrinology and Diabetes* 8, 6–16.

7. Katznelson L. (2002). Acromegaly: Current concepts. *Endocrinology Rounds* 10, 1–6. [On-line]. Available: www.endocrinologyrounds.org.

8. Merza Z. (2003). Modern treatment of acromegaly. *Postgraduate Medical Journal* 79, 189–194.

9. Giustina A., Barkan A., Casanaeva F. F., et al. (2000). Criteria for cure of acromegaly: A consensus statement. *Journal of Clinical Endocrinology and Metabolism* 85, 526–529.

10. Abs R., Verhelst J., Maitero D., et al. (1998). Cabergoline in the treatment of acromegaly: A study in 64 patients. *Journal of Clinical Endocrinology and Metabolism* 83, 374–378.

11. Utiger R. D. (2000). Treatment of acromegaly. *New England Journal of Medicine* 342, 1210–1211.

12. Lebrethon M. C., Bourguignon J. P. (2001). Central and peripheral isosexual precocious puberty. *Current Opinion in Endocrinology and Diabetes* 8, 17–22.

13. Styne D. (2004). Puberty. In Greenspan F. S., Gardner D. G. (Eds.), *Basic and clinical endocrinology* (7th ed., pp. 608–636). New York: Lange Medical Books/McGraw-Hill.

14. Kaplowitz P. B., Oberfield S. E. (1999). Reexamination of the age limit for defining when puberty is precocious in girls in the United States: Implications for evaluation and treatment. *Pediatrics* 104, 936–941.

15. Greenspan F. S. (2004). The thyroid gland. In Greenspan F. S., Gardner D. G. (Eds.), *Basic and clinical endocrinology* (7th ed., pp. 215–294). New York: Lange Medical Books/McGraw-Hill.

16. Dayan C. M. (2001). Interpretation of thyroid function tests. *Lancet* 357, 619–624.

17. Pearce E. N., Farwell A. P., Braverman L. E. (2003). Thyroiditis. *New England Journal of Medicine* 348, 2646–2655.

18. Cooper D. S. (2003). Hyperthyroidism. *Lancet* 362, 459–468.

19. McKenna T. J. (2001). Graves' disease. *Lancet* 357, 1793–1796.

20. Bahn R. (2003). Pathophysiology of Graves' ophthalmopathy: The cycle of disease. *Journal of Clinical Endocrinology and Metabolism* 88, 1939–1946.

21. Aron D. C., Findling J. W., Tyrrell J. B. (2004). Glucocorticoids and adrenal androgens. In Greenspan F. S., Gardner D. G. (Eds.), *Basic and clinical endocrinology* (7th ed., pp. 362–413). New York: Lange Medical Books/McGraw-Hill.

22. Ackermann J. C., Silverman B. L. (2001). Dehydroepiandrosterone replacement for patients with adrenal insufficiency. *Lancet* 357, 1381–1382.

23. Boscaro M. (2001). Cushing's syndrome. *Lancet* 357, 783–791.

24. Raff H., Findling J. W. (2003). A physiological approach to the diagnosis of Cushing's syndrome. *Annals of Internal Medicine* 138, 980–991.

25. Speiser P. W., White P. C. (2003). Congenital adrenal hyperplasia. *New England Journal of Medicine* 349, 776–788.

26. Boos C. J., Rumsby G., Matfin G. (2002). Multiple tumors associated with late onset congenital hyperplasia due to aberrant splicing of adrenal 21-hydroxylase gene. *Endocrine Practice* 8, 470–473.

27. Arlt W., Allolio B. (2003). Adrenal insufficiency. *Lancet* 361, 1881–1893.

28. Aron D. C. (Ed.). (2000). Endocrine incidentalomas. *Endocrinology and Metabolism Clinics of North America* 29, 1–230.

29. Grumbach M. M., Biller B. M. K., Braunstein G. D., et al. (2003). Management of the clinically inapparent adrenal mass ("incidentaloma"). *Annals of Internal Medicine* 138, 424–429.

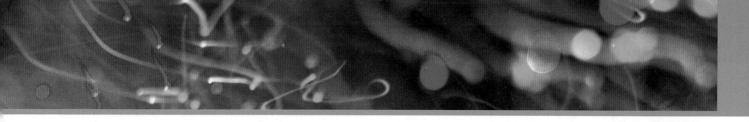

Chapter 32

Diabetes Mellitus and the Metabolic Syndrome

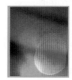 Diabetes mellitus is a chronic health problem affecting more than 18 million people in the United States.[1] Approximately 13 million of these people have been diagnosed, leaving about 5 million undiagnosed. There are 800,000 new cases of diabetes per year; almost all of these are type 2 diabetes. The disease affects people in all age groups and from all walks of life. It is more prevalent among African Americans (11.4%) and Hispanic Americans (8.2%) compared with whites (8.4%).[1]

The acute complications of diabetes are the most common causes of medical emergencies resulting from metabolic disease. Diabetes is a significant risk factor in coronary heart disease and stroke, and it is the leading cause of blindness and end-stage renal disease, as well as a major contributor to lower extremity amputations.

Hormonal Control of Glucose, Fat, and Protein Metabolism

The body uses glucose, fatty acids, and other substrates as fuel to satisfy its energy needs. Although the respiratory and circulatory systems combine efforts to furnish the body with the oxygen needed for metabolic purposes, it is the liver, in concert with the endocrine pancreas, that controls the body's fuel supply (Fig. 32-1).

GLUCOSE, FAT, AND PROTEIN METABOLISM

Glucose Metabolism

Glucose is a six-carbon molecule; it is an efficient fuel that, when metabolized in the presence of oxygen, breaks down to form carbon dioxide and water. Although many tissues and organ systems are able to use other forms of fuel, such as fatty acids and ketones, the brain and nervous system rely almost exclusively on glucose as a fuel

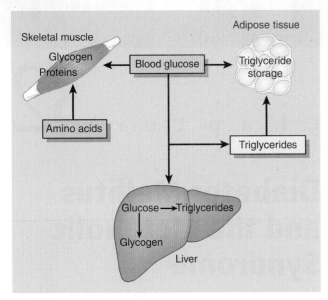

FIGURE 32-1 Effect of insulin on glucose, fat, and protein metabolism.

source. Because the brain can neither synthesize nor store more than a few minutes' supply of glucose, normal cerebral function requires a continuous supply from the circulation. Severe and prolonged hypoglycemia can cause brain death, and even moderate hypoglycemia can result in substantial brain dysfunction.

Body tissues obtain glucose from the blood. Blood glucose levels usually reflect the difference between the amount of glucose released into the circulation by the liver and the amount of glucose removed from the blood by body cells. Glucose is ingested in the diet and transported from the gastrointestinal tract, through the portal vein, to the liver before it gains access to the circulatory system. The liver regulates blood glucose through three processes: (1) glycogen synthesis (glycogenesis), (2) glycogen breakdown (glycogenolysis), and (3) synthesis of glucose from noncarbohydrate sources (gluconeogenesis). When blood glucose levels rise, it is removed from the blood and converted to glycogen, the main short-term storage form of glucose. When blood glucose levels fall, the liver glycogen stores are broken down and released into the circulation. Although skeletal muscle also participates in glycogen storage, it lacks the enzyme glucose-6-phosphatase that allows glucose to be broken down sufficiently to pass through the cell membrane and enter the circulation, limiting its usefulness to the muscle cell.

In addition to mobilizing its glycogen stores, the liver synthesizes glucose from noncarbohydrate sources such as amino acids, lactic acid, and the glycerol part of triglycerides. This glucose may be stored as glycogen or it may be released directly into the circulation.

Fat Metabolism

Fat is the most efficient form of fuel storage. It provides 9 kcal/g of stored energy, compared with the 4 kcal/g provided by carbohydrates and proteins. About 40% of the

calories in the normal American diet are obtained from fats, which is about equal to the amount obtained from carbohydrates.[2] Therefore, the use of fats by the body for energy is as important as the use of carbohydrates. In addition, many of the carbohydrates consumed in the diet are converted to triglycerides for storage in adipose tissue.

A triglyceride contains three fatty acids linked by a glycerol molecule. The mobilization of fatty acids for use as an energy source is facilitated by the action of enzymes (lipases) that break triglycerides into a glycerol molecule and three fatty acids. The glycerol molecule can enter the glycolytic pathway and be used along with glucose to produce energy, or it can be used to produce glucose. The fatty acids are transported to tissues where they are used for energy. Almost all cells, with the exception of brain tissue and red blood cells, can use fatty acids interchangeably with glucose for energy. Although many cells use fatty acids as a fuel source, fatty acids cannot be converted to glucose that can be used by the brain for energy.

A large share of the initial degradation of fatty acids occurs in the liver, especially when excessive amounts of fatty acids are being used for energy. The liver uses only a small amount of the fatty acids for its own energy needs; it converts the rest into ketones and releases them into the blood. In situations that favor fat breakdown, such as diabetes mellitus and fasting, large amounts of ketones are released into the bloodstream. Because ketones are organic acids, they cause ketoacidosis when they are present in excessive amounts.

Protein Metabolism

Approximately three fourths of body solids are proteins.[2] Proteins are essential for the formation of all body structures, including genes, enzymes, contractile structures in muscle, matrix of bone, and hemoglobin of red blood cells.

Amino acids are the building blocks of proteins. Significant quantities of amino acids are present in body proteins. Unlike glucose and fatty acids, there is only a limited facility for the storage of excess amino acids in the body. Most of the stored amino acids are contained in body proteins. Amino acids in excess of those needed for protein synthesis are converted to fatty acids, ketones, or glucose and are stored or used as metabolic fuel. Because fatty acids cannot be converted to glucose, the body must break down proteins and use the amino acids as a major substrate for gluconeogenesis during periods when metabolic needs exceed food intake.

GLUCOSE-REGULATING HORMONES

The hormonal control of blood glucose resides largely with the endocrine pancreas. The pancreas is made up of two major tissue types: the acini and the islets of Langerhans (Fig. 32-2). The acini secrete digestive juices into the duodenum, and the islets of Langerhans secrete glucose-regulating hormones into the blood. Each islet is composed of beta cells that secrete insulin and amylin, alpha cells that secrete glucagon, and delta cells that secrete somatostatin. In addition, at least one other type of the

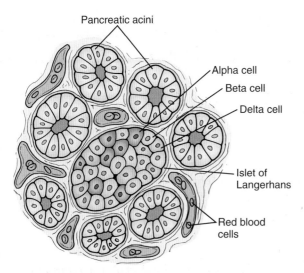

Pancreatic acini

Alpha cell

Beta cell

Delta cell

Islet of Langerhans

Red blood cells

FIGURE 32-2 Islet of Langerhans in the pancreas.

cell, the PP cell, is present in small numbers in the islets and secretes a hormone of uncertain function called *pancreatic polypeptide.*

Insulin lowers the blood glucose concentration by facilitating the movement of glucose into body tissues. Glucagon maintains blood glucose by increasing the release of glucose from the liver into the blood. Amylin is a 37–amino-acid peptide that is cosecreted with insulin from the beta cells in response to glucose and other beta cell stimulators.[2] Studies indicate that amylin acts as a neuroendocrine hormone, with several effects that complement the actions of insulin in regulating postprandial (postmeal) glucose levels. These include a suppression of glucagon secretion and a slowing of the rate at which glucose is delivered to the small intestine for absorption. A synthetic version of human amylin hormone has recently been approved for use in the treatment of type 1 diabetes as an adjunct therapy to insulin.

Somatostatin is a polypeptide hormone containing only 14 amino acids that has an extremely short half life.[2] Somatostatin acts locally in the islets of Langerhans to inhibit the release of insulin and glucagon. It also decreases gastrointestinal activity after ingestion of food. Almost all factors related to ingestion of food stimulate somatostatin secretion. By decreasing gastrointestinal activity, somatostatin is thought to extend the time during which food is absorbed into the blood, and by inhibiting insulin and glucagon, it is thought to extend the use of absorbed nutrients by the tissues.[2]

Several gut-derived hormones have been identified as having what is termed an *incretin* effect, meaning that they increase insulin release after an oral nutrient load (see Chapter 27). This suggests that gut-derived factors can stimulate insulin secretion after a predominantly carbohydrate meal. The two hormones that account for about 90% of the incretin effect are glucagon-like peptide-1 (GLP-1), which is released from L cells in the distal small bowel, and glucose-dependent insulinotropic polypeptide (GIP, previously known as *gastric inhibitory polypeptide*),

which is released by K cells in the upper gut (mainly the jejunum). An injectable GLP-1 analog (an "incretin mimetic") has recently been approved for use in type 2 diabetes.

Insulin

Although several hormones are known to increase blood glucose levels, insulin is the only hormone known to have a direct effect in lowering blood glucose levels. The actions of insulin are threefold: it (1) promotes glucose uptake by target cells and provides for glucose storage as glycogen, (2) prevents fat and glycogen breakdown and inhibits gluconeogenesis, and (3) increases protein synthesis (Table 32-1). Insulin acts to promote fat storage by increasing the transport of glucose into fat cells. It also facilitates triglyceride synthesis from glucose in fat cells and inhibits the intracellular breakdown of stored triglycerides. Insulin also inhibits protein breakdown and increases protein synthesis by increasing the active transport of amino acids into body cells. Insulin inhibits gluconeogenesis, or the building of glucose from new sources, mainly amino acids. When sufficient glucose and insulin are present, protein breakdown is minimal because the body is able to use glucose and fatty acids as a fuel source. In children and adolescents, insulin is needed for normal growth and development.

Insulin is produced by the pancreatic beta cells in the islets of Langerhans. The active form of the hormone is composed of two polypeptide chains, an A chain and a B chain (Fig. 32-3). Active insulin is formed in the beta cells from a larger molecule called *proinsulin.* In converting proinsulin to insulin, enzymes in the beta cell cleave proinsulin at specific sites to form two separate substances: active insulin and a biologically inactive connecting peptide (C-peptide) chain that joined the A and B chains before they were separated. Active insulin and the inactive C-peptide chain are packaged into secretory granules and released simultaneously from the beta cell. The C-peptide chains can be measured clinically, and this measurement can be used to study beta cell activity. The release of insulin from the pancreatic beta cells is regulated by blood glucose levels, increasing as blood glucose levels rise and decreasing when blood glucose levels decline.[3] Secretion of insulin occurs in an oscillatory or pulsatile fashion. After exposure to glucose, a first-phase release of stored preformed insulin occurs, followed by a second-phase release of newly synthesized insulin (Fig. 32-4). Serum insulin levels begin to rise within minutes after a meal, reach a peak in approximately 3 to 5 minutes, and then return to baseline levels within 2 to 3 hours.

Insulin secreted by the beta cells enters the portal circulation and travels directly to the liver, where approximately 50% is used or degraded. Insulin, which is rapidly bound to peripheral tissues or destroyed by the liver or kidneys, has a half-life of approximately 15 minutes once it is released into the general circulation.

To initiate its effects on target tissues, insulin binds to and activates a membrane receptor. It is the activated receptor that is responsible for the cellular effects of

TABLE 32-1   Actions of Insulin and Glucagon on Glucose, Fat, and Protein Metabolism

	Insulin	Glucagon
Glucose		
Glucose transport	Increases glucose transport into skeletal muscle and adipose tissue	
Glycogen synthesis	Increases glycogen synthesis	Promotes glycogen breakdown
Gluconeogenesis	Decreases gluconeogenesis	Increases gluconeogenesis
Fats		
Triglyceride synthesis	Increases triglyceride synthesis	
Triglyceride transport into adipose tissue	Increases fatty acid transport into adipose cells	Enhances lipolysis in adipose tissue, liberating fatty acids and glycerol for use in gluconeogenesis
Activation of adipose cell lipase	Inhibits adipose cell lipase and release of free fatty acids from adipose tissue	Activates adipose cell lipase
Proteins		
Amino acid transport	Increases active transport of amino acids into cells	Increases transport of amino acids into hepatic cells
Protein synthesis	Increases protein synthesis by increasing transcription of messenger RNA and accelerating protein synthesis by ribosomal RNA	Increases breakdown of proteins into amino acids for use in gluconeogenesis
Protein breakdown	Decreases protein breakdown by enhancing the use of glucose and fatty acids as fuel	Increases conversion of amino acids into glucose precursors

insulin.[2] The insulin receptor is a combination of four subunits—two large α subunits that extends outside the cell membrane and are involved in insulin binding and two smaller β subunits that are predominantly inside the cell membrane and contain a kinase enzyme that becomes activated during insulin binding (Fig. 32-5). Activation of the kinase enzyme results in phosphorylation of the β subunit, which in turn activates a number of signaling proteins that mediate the intracellular effect of insulin on glucose, fat, and protein metabolism.

Because cell membranes are impermeable to glucose, they require a special carrier, called a *glucose transporter*, to move glucose from the blood into the cell. Within seconds after insulin binds to its membrane receptor, the membranes of about 80% of body tissues increase their uptake of glucose by means of special glucose transporters.

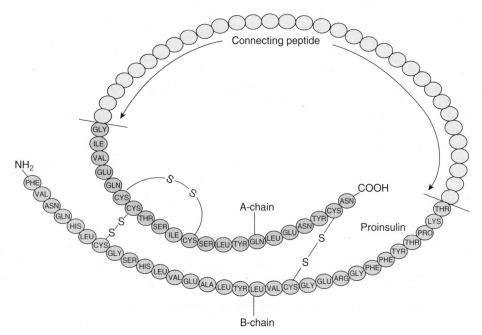

FIGURE 32-3 Structure of proinsulin. With removal of the connecting peptide (C-peptide), proinsulin is converted to insulin.

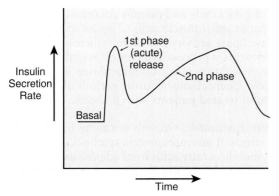

FIGURE 32-4 Biphasic insulin response to a constant glucose stimulus. The peak of the first phase in humans is 3 to 5 minutes; the second phase begins at 2 minutes and continues to increase slowly for at least 60 minutes or until the stimulus stops. (From Ward W. K., Beard J. C., Halter J. B., et al. [1984]. Pathology of insulin secretion in non-insulin-dependent diabetes mellitus. *Diabetes Care* 7, 491–502. Reprinted with permission from The American Diabetes Association. Copyright © 1984 American Diabetes Association.)

This is particularly true of skeletal muscle and adipose tissues. Considerable research has revealed a family of glucose transporters termed *GLUT-1*, *GLUT-2*, and so forth.[4] GLUT-4 is the insulin-dependent glucose transporter for skeletal muscle and adipose tissue (Fig. 32-6). It is sequestered inside the membrane of these cells and thus is unable to function as a glucose transporter until a signal from insulin causes it to move from its inactive site into the cell membrane, where it facilitates glucose entry. GLUT-2 is the major transporter of glucose into beta cells and liver cells. It has a low affinity for glucose and acts as a transporter only when plasma glucose levels are relatively high, such as after a meal. GLUT-1 is present in all tissues. It does not require the actions of insulin and is important in transport of glucose into the nervous system.

Glucagon

Glucagon, a polypeptide molecule produced by the alpha cells of the islets of Langerhans, maintains blood glucose between meals and during periods of fasting. Like insulin, glucagon travels through the portal vein to the liver, where it exerts its main action. Unlike insulin, glucagon produces an increase in blood glucose (see Table 32-1). The most dramatic effect of glucagon is its ability to initiate *glycogenolysis* or the breakdown of liver glycogen as a means of raising blood glucose, usually within a matter of minutes. Because liver glycogen stores are limited, gluconeogenesis is important in maintaining blood glucose levels over time. Glucagon also increases the transport of amino acids into the liver and stimulates their conversion into glucose.

As with insulin, glucagon synthesis and secretion is regulated by blood glucose. A decrease in blood glucose concentration to a hypoglycemic level produces an immediate

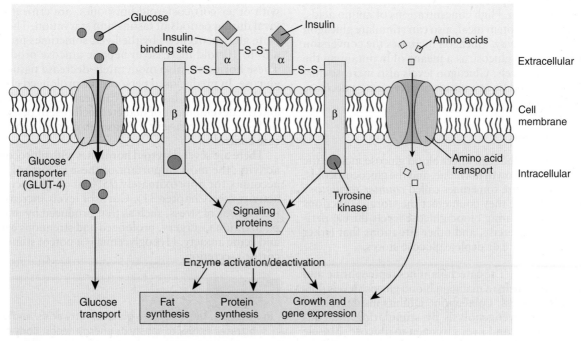

FIGURE 32-5 Insulin receptor. Insulin binds to the α subunits of the insulin receptor, which increases glucose and amino acid transport and causes autophosphorylation of the β subunit of the receptor, which induces tyrosine kinase activity. Tyrosine phosphorylation, in turn, activates a cascade of intracellular signaling proteins that mediate the effects of insulin on glucose, fat, and protein metabolism.

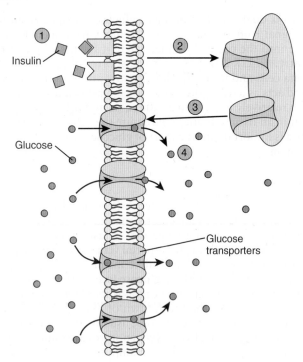

FIGURE 32-6 Insulin-dependent glucose transporter (GLUT-4). (1) Binding of insulin to insulin receptor on the surface of the cell membrane, (2) generation of intracellular signal, (3) insertion of GLUT-4 receptor from its inactive site into the cell membrane, and (4) transport of glucose across the cell membrane.

increase in glucagon secretion, and an increase in blood glucose to hyperglycemic levels produces a decrease in glucagon secretion. High concentrations of amino acids, as occur after a protein meal, also can stimulate glucagon secretion. In this way, glucagon increases the conversion of amino acids to glucose as a means of maintaining the body's glucose levels. Glucagon levels also increase during strenuous exercise as a means of preventing a decrease in blood glucose.

Other Hormones

Other hormones that can affect blood glucose include the catecholamines, growth hormone, and the glucocorticoids. These hormones are sometimes called *counter-regulatory hormones* because they counteract the storage functions of insulin in regulating blood glucose levels during periods of fasting, exercise, and other situations that either limit glucose intake or deplete glucose stores.

Catecholamines. The catecholamines (epinephrine and norepinephrine) help to maintain blood glucose levels during periods of stress. Epinephrine inhibits insulin release and promotes glycogenolysis by stimulating the conversion of muscle and liver glycogen to glucose. Muscle glycogen cannot be released into the blood; nevertheless, the mobilization of these stores for muscle use conserves blood glucose for use by other tissues such as the brain and the nervous system. During periods of exercise and other types of stress, epinephrine inhibits insulin release

from the beta cells and thereby decreases the movement of glucose into muscle cells. The catecholamines also increase lipase activity and thereby increase mobilization of fatty acids, a process that conserves glucose. The blood glucose–elevating effect of epinephrine is an important homeostatic mechanism during periods of hypoglycemia in insulin-treated patients with diabetes.

Growth Hormone. Growth hormone has many metabolic effects. It increases protein synthesis in all cells of the body, mobilizes fatty acids from adipose tissue, and antagonizes the effects of insulin. Growth hormone decreases cellular uptake and use of glucose, thereby increasing the level of blood glucose. The increased blood glucose level stimulates further insulin secretion by the beta cells. The secretion of growth hormone normally is inhibited by insulin and increased levels of blood glucose. During periods of fasting, when both blood glucose levels and insulin secretion fall, growth hormone levels increase. Exercise, such as running and cycling, and various stresses, including anesthesia, fever, and trauma, produce an increase in growth hormone levels.

Chronic hypersecretion of growth hormone, as occurs in a condition called *acromegaly* (see Chapter 31), can lead to glucose intolerance and the development of diabetes mellitus. In children who already have diabetes, moderate elevations in growth hormone levels that occur during periods of growth can produce the entire spectrum of metabolic abnormalities associated with poor regulation, despite optimized insulin treatment.

Glucocorticoid Hormones. The glucocorticoid hormones, which are synthesized in the adrenal cortex along with other corticosteroid hormones, are critical to survival during periods of fasting and starvation. They stimulate gluconeogenesis by the liver, sometimes producing a 6- to 10-fold increase in hepatic glucose production. These hormones also moderately decrease tissue use of glucose. In predisposed persons, the prolonged elevation of glucocorticoid hormones can lead to hyperglycemia and the development of diabetes mellitus. In people with diabetes, even transient increases in cortisol can complicate control.

There are several steroid hormones with glucocorticoid activity; the most important of these is cortisol, which accounts for approximately 95% of all glucocorticoid activity (see Chapter 31). Cortisol levels increase during periods of stress, such as that produced by infection, pain, trauma, surgery, prolonged and strenuous exercise, and acute anxiety. Hypoglycemia is a potent stimulus for cortisol secretion.

In summary, the body uses glucose, fatty acids, and other substrates as fuel to satisfy its energy needs. Body tissues, including the brain, which depends exclusively on glucose for its energy, obtain glucose from the blood. The liver stores excess glucose as glycogen and uses gluconeogenesis to convert amino acids, lactate, and glycerol into glucose during fasting or when glucose intake does not keep pace with demand. Blood glucose levels reflect the difference between the amount of glucose released into the circulation by the liver and the amount of glucose removed from the blood by body tissues. Fats, which serve as an efficient source of fuel for the body, are stored in adipose tissue as triglycerides, which consist of three fatty acids linked to a glycerol molecule. In situations that favor fat breakdown, such as fasting or diabetes mellitus, the triglycerides in adipose tissue are broken down and the fatty acids are used as fuel or transported to the liver, where they are converted to ketones. Proteins, which are made up of amino acids, are essential for the formation of all body structures. Unlike glucose and fatty acids, there is only a limited facility for storage of excess amino acids in the body. Because fatty acids cannot be converted to glucose, the body must break down proteins and use the amino acids for gluconeogenesis.

Energy metabolism is controlled by insulin and glucagon. Of these hormones, only insulin has the effect of lowering the blood glucose level. Insulin's blood glucose–lowering action results from its ability to increase the transport of glucose into body cells and to decrease the production and release of glucose into the bloodstream by the liver. Other hormones—glucagon, epinephrine, growth hormone, and the glucocorticoids—maintain or increase blood glucose concentrations and are referred to as *counter-regulatory hormones*. Glucagon and epinephrine promote glycogenolysis. Glucagon and the glucocorticoids increase gluconeogenesis. Growth hormone decreases the peripheral use of glucose. Insulin has the effect of decreasing lipolysis and the use of fats as a fuel source; glucagon and epinephrine increase fat use.

Diabetes Mellitus

The term *diabetes* is derived from a Greek word meaning "going through" and *mellitus* from the Latin word for "honey" or "sweet." Reports of the disorder can be traced to the first century AD, when Aretaeus the Cappadocian described the disorder as a chronic affliction characterized by intense thirst and voluminous, honey-sweet urine: "the melting down of flesh into urine." It was the discovery of insulin by Banting and Best in 1922 that transformed the once-fatal disease into a manageable chronic health problem.[5]

Diabetes is a disorder of carbohydrate, protein, and fat metabolism resulting from an imbalance between insulin availability and insulin need. It can represent an absolute insulin deficiency, impaired release of insulin by the pancreatic beta cells, inadequate or defective insulin receptors, or the production of inactive insulin or insulin that is destroyed before it can carry out its action. A person with uncontrolled diabetes is unable to transport glucose into fat and muscle cells; as a result, the body cells

are starved, and the breakdown of fat and protein is increased.

CLASSIFICATION AND ETIOLOGY

Although diabetes mellitus clearly is a disorder of insulin availability, it probably is not a single disease. A revised system for the classification of diabetes was developed in 1997 by the Expert Committee on the Diagnosis and Classification of Diabetes Mellitus.[6] The intent of the revised system, which replaces the 1979 classification system, was to move away from a system that focused on the type of pharmacologic treatment used in management of diabetes to one based on disease etiology. The revised system continues to include type 1 and type 2 diabetes, but uses Arabic, rather than Roman, numerals and eliminates the use of "insulin-dependent" and "non–insulin-dependent" diabetes mellitus (Table 32-2). Type 1 diabetes is due to pancreatic beta cell destruction predominantly by an autoimmune process. Type 2 diabetes is the more prevalent type and results from a combination of beta cell dysfunction and insulin resistance. Included in the classification system are the categories of gestational diabetes mellitus (GDM; *i.e.*, diabetes that develops during pregnancy) and other specific types of diabetes, many of which occur secondary to other conditions (*e.g.*, Cushing syndrome, pancreatitis, acromegaly).

The revised classification system also includes a system for diagnosing diabetes according to stages of glucose intolerance[5] (Table 32-3). The revised criteria have retained the former category of *impaired glucose tolerance* (IGT) and have added a new category of *impaired fasting plasma glucose* (IFG). The categories of IFG and IGT refer to metabolic stages intermediate between normal glucose homeostasis and diabetes, and are labeled together as *prediabetes*. A fasting plasma glucose (FPG) of less than 100 mg/dL or a 2-hour oral glucose tolerance test (OGTT) result of less than 140 mg/dL is considered normal. IFG is defined as an FPG of 100 to 125 mg/dL. IGT reflects abnormal plasma glucose measurements (≥140 mg/dL but <200 mg/dL) 2 hours after an oral glucose load.[6,7] IFG and IGT (*i.e.*, prediabetes) are associated with an increased risk of atherosclerotic heart disease and for progression to type 2 diabetes. Persons with an FPG of 126 mg/dL or more or an OGTT of 200 mg/L or more are considered to have *provisional diabetes*.[6,7] The criteria in Chart 32-1 are used to confirm the diagnosis of diabetes in persons with provisional diabetes.

Type 1 Diabetes Mellitus

Type 1 diabetes mellitus is characterized by destruction of the pancreatic beta cells.[8] Type 1 diabetes is subdivided into two types: type 1A, immune-mediated diabetes, and type 1B, idiopathic diabetes. In the United States and Europe, approximately 5% to 10% of people with diabetes mellitus have type 1 diabetes, with 95% of them having type 1A, immune-mediated diabetes.

Type 1A diabetes is characterized by autoimmune destruction of beta cells. This type of diabetes, formerly

TABLE 32-2	Etiologic Classification of Diabetes Mellitus	
Type	**Subtypes**	**Etiology of Glucose Intolerance**
I. Type 1*	*(Beta cell destruction usually leading to absolute insulin deficiency)*	
	A. Immune-mediated	Autoimmune destruction of beta cells
	B. Idiopathic	Unknown
II. Type 2*	May range from predominantly insulin resistance with relative insulin deficiency to a predominantly secretory defect with insulin resistance	
III. Other Specific Types	A. Genetic defects of beta cell function, *e.g.,* chromosome 7, glucokinase	Regulates insulin secretion due to defect in glucokinase generation
	B. Genetic defects in insulin action, *e.g.,* leprechaunism, Rabson-Mendenhall syndrome	Pediatric syndromes that have mutations in insulin receptors
	C. Diseases of the exocrine pancreas, *e.g.,* pancreatitis, neoplasms, cystic fibrosis	Loss or destruction of insulin-producing beta cells
	D. Endocrine disorders, *e.g.,* acromegaly, Cushing syndrome	Diabetogenic effects of excess hormone levels
	E. Drug or chemical-induced, *e.g.,* Vacor, glucocorticoids, thiazide diuretics, α-Interferon	Toxic destruction of beta cells Insulin resistance Impaired insulin secretion Production of islet cell antibodies
	F. Infections, *e.g.,* congenital rubella, cytomegalovirus	Beta cell injury followed by autoimmune response
	G. Uncommon forms of immune-mediated diabetes, *e.g.,* "stiff man syndrome"	Autoimmune disorder of central nervous system with immune-mediated beta cell destruction
	H. Other genetic syndromes sometimes associated with diabetes, *e.g.,* Down syndrome, Klinefelter syndrome, Turner syndrome	Disorders of glucose tolerance related to defects associated with chromosomal abnormalities
IV. Gestational diabetes mellitus (GDM)	*(Any degree of glucose intolerance with onset or first recognition during pregnancy)*	Combination of insulin resistance and impaired insulin secretion

*Patients with any form of diabetes may require insulin treatment at some stage of their disease. Such use of insulin does not, of itself, classify the patient.
(Adapted from The Expert Committee on the Diagnosis and Classification of Diabetes Mellitus. [1997]. Report of the Expert Committee on the Diagnosis and Classification of Diabetes Mellitus. *Diabetes Care 20,* 1183–1197. Reprinted with permission from The American Diabetes Association. Copyright © 1997 American Diabetes Association.)

called *juvenile diabetes,* occurs more commonly in young persons but can occur at any age. The rate of beta cell destruction is quite variable, being rapid in some individuals and slow in others. The rapidly progressive form commonly is observed in children, but also may occur in adults. The slowly progressive form usually occurs in adults and is sometimes referred to as *latent autoimmune diabetes in adults* (LADA). LADA may account for up to 10% of adults who are currently classified as having type 2 diabetes.

Type 1 diabetes is a catabolic disorder characterized by an absolute lack of insulin, an elevation in blood glucose,

TABLE 32-3	Expert Committee on the Diagnosis and Classification of Diabetes Mellitus Using Fasting Plasma Glucose (FPG) and Oral Glucose Tolerance Test (OGTT)			
Test	**Normoglycemic**	**Impaired FPG (IFG)***	**Impaired GT (IGT)***	**Diabetes Mellitus†**
FPG‡	<100 mg/dL (5.6 mmol/L)	100–125 mg/dL (5.6–6.9 mmol/L)		≥126 mg/dL (7.0 mmol/L)
2-h OGTT§	<140 mg/dL (7.8 mmol/L)		140–199 mg/dL (7.8–11.1 mmol/L)	≥200 mg/dL (11.1 mmol/L)
Other				Symptoms of diabetes mellitus and casual plasma glucose ≥200 mg/dL

*IFG and IGT are prediabetic states and can occur in isolation or together in a given subject.
†In the absence of unequivocal hyperglycemia with acute metabolic decompensation, these criteria should be confirmed by repeat testing on a separate day.
‡Fasting is defined as no caloric intake for at least 8 hours.
§OGTT with 2-h measurement of venous plasma or serum glucose following a 75-g carbohydrate load.
(Developed from data in American Diabetes Association. [2004]. Diagnosis and classification of diabetes mellitus. *Diabetes Care 27*[Suppl. 1], S5–10.)

CHART 32-1

Criteria for Diagnosis of Diabetes Mellitus

1. Symptoms of diabetes plus casual plasma glucose concentration >200 mg/dL (11.1 mmol/L). *Casual* is defined as any time of the day without regard to time since last meal. The classic symptoms of diabetes include polydipsia, and unexplained weight loss.

   or

2. Fasting plasma glucose ≥126 mg/dL (7.0 mmol/L). *Fasting* is defined as no caloric intake for at least 8 h.

   or

3. 2-h postload glucose ≥200 mg/dL (11.1 mmol/L) during oral glucose tolerance test (OGTT). The test should be performed as described by the World Health Organization, using a glucose load containing the equivalent of 75 g anhydrous glucose dissolved in water.

In the absence of unequivocal hyperglycemia, these criteria should be confirmed by repeat testing on a different day. The third measure (OGTT) is not recommended for routine use. (Developed from data in American Diabetes Association. [2004]. Diagnosis and classification of diabetes mellitus. *Diabetes Care 27*[Suppl. 1], S5–10.)

and a breakdown of body fats and proteins. The absolute lack of insulin in people with type 1 diabetes mellitus means that they are particularly prone to the development of ketoacidosis. One of the actions of insulin is the inhibition of *lipolysis* (*i.e.*, fat breakdown) and release of free fatty acids (FFA) from fat cells. In the absence of insulin, ketosis develops when these fatty acids are released from fat cells and converted to ketones in the liver. Because of the loss of the first-phase insulin (preformed insulin) response, all people with type 1A diabetes require exogenous insulin replacement to reverse the catabolic state, control blood glucose levels, and prevent ketosis.

Type 1A diabetes is thought to be an autoimmune disorder resulting from a genetic predisposition (*i.e.*, diabeto-

KEY CONCEPTS

Diabetes Mellitus

➤ Diabetes mellitus is a disorder of carbohydrate, fat, and protein metabolism brought about by impaired beta cell synthesis or release of insulin, or the inability of tissues to use glucose.

➤ Type 1 diabetes results from loss of beta cell function and an absolute insulin deficiency.

➤ Type 2 diabetes results from impaired ability of the tissues to use insulin accompanied by a relative lack of insulin or impaired release of insulin in relation to blood glucose levels.

genic genes); an environmental triggering event, such as an infection; and a T-lymphocyte–mediated hypersensitivity reaction against some beta cell antigen (see Chapter 15). Much evidence has focused on the inherited major histocompatibility complex (MHC) genes on chromosome 6 that encode human leukocyte antigens HLA-DQ and HLA-DR, especially DR-3 and DR-4.[3] In addition to the MHC susceptibility genes for type 1 diabetes on chromosome 6, an insulin gene regulating beta cell replication and function has been identified on chromosome 11.

Type 1 diabetes–associated autoantibodies may exist for years before the onset of hyperglycemia. There are two major types of autoantibodies: insulin autoantibodies (IAAs), and islet cell autoantibodies and antibodies directed at other islet autoantigens, including glutamic acid decarboxylase (GAD) and the protein tyrosine phosphatase IA-2.[9] Testing for antibodies to GAD or IA-2 and for IAAs using sensitive radiobinding assays can identify more than 85% of cases of new or future type 1 diabetes with 98% specificity.[10]

The fact that type 1 diabetes is thought to result from an interaction between genetic and environmental factors has led to research into methods directed at prevention and early control of the disease. These methods include the identification of genetically susceptible persons and early intervention in newly diagnosed persons with type 1 diabetes. After the diagnosis of type 1 diabetes, there often is a short period of beta cell regeneration, during which symptoms of diabetes disappear and insulin injections are not needed. This is sometimes called the *honeymoon period*. Immune interventions (immunomodulation) designed to interrupt the destruction of beta cells before development of type 1 diabetes are being investigated in various trials, including the Diabetes Prevention Trial-1 (DPT-1). Unfortunately, none of the interventions studied to date has shown any clinical utility.

The term *idiopathic type 1B diabetes* is used to describe those cases of beta cell destruction in which no evidence of autoimmunity is present. Only a small number of people with type 1 diabetes fall into this category; most are of African or Asian descent. Type 1B diabetes is strongly inherited. People with the disorder have episodic ketoacidosis due to varying degrees of insulin deficiency with periods of absolute insulin deficiency that may come and go.

Type 2 Diabetes Mellitus and the Metabolic Syndrome

Type 2 diabetes mellitus describes a condition of hyperglycemia that occurs despite the availability of insulin (*i.e.*, relative insulin deficiency). It accounts for 90% to 95% of persons with diabetes. Most people with type 2 diabetes are adults older than 40 years of age with some degree of obesity. Recently, however, type 2 diabetes is becoming more common in obese adolescents and children.[11] Although type 1 diabetes remains the main form of diabetes in children worldwide, it seems likely that type 2 diabetes will become the predominant form within 10 years in some ethnic groups.[11]

The pathophysiology of type 2 diabetes involves both genetic and acquired (environmental) factors.[12,13] Although lifestyle and overeating seem to be the triggering event in the pathogenesis of type 2 diabetes, genetic elements are also involved. A positive family history confers a two- to fourfold increased risk for type 2 diabetes, and 15% to 25% of first-degree relatives of persons with type 2 diabetes develop impaired glucose tolerance or diabetes.[13]

Among the acquired factors, obesity and physical activity are of paramount importance. Obese people have increased resistance to the action of insulin and impaired suppression of glucose production by the liver, resulting in both hyperglycemia and hyperinsulinemia.[14] The risk of diabetes increases as the body mass index (a measure of body fat content) increases. It is not only the absolute amount of fat, but its distribution that has an effect on insulin resistance. Central obesity (abdominal fat) is more closely linked with insulin resistance than is peripheral (gluteal/subcutaneous) obesity[15] (see Chapter 8). Waist circumference, which is a measure of central obesity, has been shown to correlate well with insulin resistance. The new terminology that is emerging for persons with obesity and type 2 diabetes is *diabesity*. Over time, insulin resistance may improve with weight loss, to the extent that many people with type 2 diabetes can manage their condition with a weight-reduction program and exercise.

The metabolic abnormalities that lead to type 2 diabetes include (1) peripheral insulin resistance, (2) deranged secretion of insulin by the pancreatic beta cells, and (3) increased glucose production by the liver[12,13] (Fig. 32-7). Before the onset of postprandial and fasting hyperglycemia, individuals who are genetically predisposed to type 2 diabetes are known to be resistant to the action of insulin. Insulin resistance initially stimulates an increase in insulin secretion, often to a level of modest hyperinsulinemia, as the beta cells attempt to maintain a normal blood glucose level. In time, the increased demand for insulin secretion leads to beta cell exhaustion and failure. This results in elevated postprandial blood glucose levels and an eventual increase in glucose production by the liver. Because people with type 2 diabetes do not have an absolute insulin deficiency, they are less prone to ketoacidosis than are people with type 1 diabetes.

Although many details of the relationship between adipose tissue and insulin resistance remain to be elucidated, several pathways have been proposed, including the role of FFAs, adipose tissue cytokines (adipokines), and the peroxisome proliferator–activated nuclear receptor.[12–14] A large number of circulating hormones, cytokines, and metabolic fuels such as FFAs originate in fat cells and modify insulin action. It has been theorized that the insulin resistance and increased glucose production in obese people with type 2 diabetes may stem from an increased concentration of FFAs.[12–14] Visceral obesity is especially important because it is accompanied by increases in fasting and postprandial FFA concentrations. The increased storage of triglycerides (the source of FFAs) leads to large adipose cells that are resistant to the action of insulin in suppressing lipolysis. The resulting increase in release and circulating levels of FFAs can contribute to increased insulin resistance, beta cell dysfunction/failure, and increased glucose production by liver. First, FFAs act at the level of the beta cell to stimulate insulin secretion, which, with excessive and chronic stimulation causes beta cell failure. Second, they act at the level of the peripheral tissues to cause insulin resistance by inhibiting

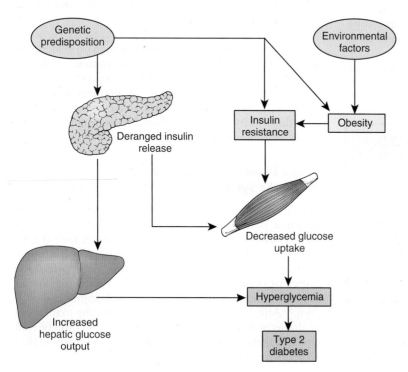

FIGURE 32-7 Pathogenesis of type 2 diabetes mellitus.

glucose uptake and glycogen storage. Third, an accumulation of FFAs reduces hepatic insulin sensitivity, leading to increased hepatic glucose production and hyperglycemia, especially fasting blood glucose levels. The uptake of FFAs from the portal blood can lead to hepatic triglyceride accumulation and nonalcoholic fatty liver disease (NAFLD; see Chapter 29).

Another proposed link to the insulin resistance associated with obesity is an adipokine or substance that causes mobilization of stored fat called *adiponectin*.[12,16] Adiponectin is secreted by adipose tissue and circulates in the blood. It has been shown that decreased levels of adiponectin coincide with insulin resistance in animal models and persons with obesity and type 2 diabetes. Moreover, there is evidence that the secretion of adiponectin might be partially regulated by peroxisome proliferator–activated receptor-γ (PPAR-γ), a nuclear receptor that leads to the regulation of genes controlling FFA levels and glucose metabolism (discussed with thiazolidinediones in the section on Oral Antidiabetic Agents). In skeletal muscle, adiponectin has been shown to decrease tissue triglyceride content by increasing the utilization of fatty acids as a fuel source.

Insulin Resistance and the Metabolic Syndrome. There is increasing evidence to suggest that when people with type 2 diabetes present predominantly with insulin resistance, the diabetes may represent only one aspect of a syndrome of metabolic abnormalities. Hyperglycemia in these people is frequently associated with obesity, high levels of plasma triglycerides and low levels of high-density lipoproteins (HDL), hypertension, systemic inflammation (as detected by C-reactive protein [CRP] and other mediators), abnormal fibrinolysis, abnormal function of the vascular endothelium, and macrovascular disease (coronary artery, cerebrovascular, and peripheral arterial disease). This constellation of abnormalities often is referred to as the *insulin resistance syndrome, syndrome X*, or, the preferred term, *metabolic syndrome*.[17] In clinical practice, the National Cholesterol Education Program (Adult Treatment Panel III) definition of "metabolic syndrome" is widely used[18] (Chart 32-2). Insulin resistance and an increased risk of developing type 2 diabetes are also seen in women with polycystic ovary syndrome[19] (see Chapter 39).

Other Specific Types

The category of other specific types of diabetes, formerly known as *secondary diabetes*, describes diabetes that is associated with certain other conditions and syndromes. Such diabetes can occur with pancreatic disease or the removal of pancreatic tissue and with endocrine diseases, such as acromegaly or Cushing syndrome. Endocrine disorders that produce hyperglycemia do so by increasing the hepatic production of glucose or decreasing the cellular use of glucose. Several specific types of diabetes are associated with monogenetic defects in beta cell function. These specific types of diabetes, which resemble type 2 diabetes but occur at an earlier age (usually before 25 years of age), were formerly referred to as *maturity-onset diabetes of the young* (MODY).[20]

CHART 32-2

NCEP ATP III Criteria for a Diagnosis of Metabolic Syndrome*

Three or more of the following:
- Abdominal obesity: waist circumference >35 inches in women or >40 inches in men
- Triglycerides ≥150 mg/dL
- High-density lipoproteins (HDL) <50 mg/dL in women or <40 mg/dL in men
- Blood pressure >130/85 mm Hg
- Fasting plasma glucose >110 mg/dL†

---

*Developed from: Grundy S. M., Panel Chair. (2001). Third Report of the National Cholesterol Education Program (NCEP) Expert Panel on Detection, Evaluation, and Treatment Panel III). (NIH publication no. 01-3670.) Bethesda, MD: National Institutes of Health.
†In view of the recent changes in the definition of abnormal glucose levels (American Diabetes Association. [2004]. Diagnosis and classification of diabetes mellitus. *Diabetes Care* 27[Suppl. 1], S5–10), an FPG value >100 mg/dL should now be used in the diagnosis of the metabolic syndrome.

Environmental agents that have been associated with altered pancreatic beta cell function include viruses (*e.g.*, mumps, congenital rubella, coxsackievirus) and chemical toxins. Among the suspected chemical toxins are the nitrosamines, which sometimes are found in smoked and cured meats. The nitrosamines are related to streptozocin, which is used to induce diabetes in experimental animals, and to the rat poison Vacor, which can produce diabetes when ingested by humans.

Several diuretics—thiazides and loop diuretics—elevate blood glucose. These diuretics increase potassium loss, which is thought to impair insulin release. Other drugs known to cause hyperglycemia are diazoxide, glucocorticoids, levodopa, oral contraceptives, sympathomimetics, phenothiazines, phenytoin, and total parenteral nutrition (*i.e.*, hyperalimentation). Drug-related increases in blood glucose usually are reversed after use of the drug has been discontinued.

Gestational Diabetes

Gestational diabetes mellitus refers to glucose intolerance that is detected first during pregnancy. It occurs to various degrees in 2% to 14% of pregnancies.[21] It most frequently affects women with a family history of diabetes; with glycosuria; and with a history of stillbirth or spontaneous abortion, fetal anomalies in a previous pregnancy, or a previous large- or heavy-for-date infant; and those who are obese, of advanced maternal age, or have had five or more pregnancies.

All pregnant women should undergo risk assessment for diabetes during their first prenatal visit. Those with significant risk should undergo plasma glucose testing as soon as feasible. If they are not found to have GDM at the initial screening, they should be retested between 24 and 28 weeks. Women with average risk should be tested at 24 to 28 weeks' gestation. Women with an FPG greater than 126 mg/dL or casual glucose greater than 200 mg/dL meet the threshold for diabetes, if confirmed on a subsequent day, and do not need to undergo OGTT.[21] Women with high or average GDM risk who do not demonstrate this degree of hyperglycemia on FPG testing should undergo further screening using the OGTT. This screening test consists of 50 g of glucose given without regard to the last meal and followed in 1 hour by a venous blood sample for glucose concentration. If the plasma glucose level is greater than 140 mg/dL, then a 100-g 3-hour glucose tolerance test is indicated to establish the diagnosis of GDM[21] (Table 32-4). On the other hand, women who are younger than 25 years of age, were of normal body weight before pregnancy, have no family history of diabetes or poor obstetric outcome, and are not members of a high-risk ethnic/racial group (*e.g.*, Hispanic, Native American, Asian, African American) may not need to be screened.

Diagnosis and careful medical management are essential because women with GDM are at higher risk for complications of pregnancy, mortality, and fetal abnormalities.[3] Fetal abnormalities include macrosomia (*i.e.*, large body size), hypoglycemia, hypocalcemia, polycythemia, and hyperbilirubinemia.

Treatment of GDM includes close observation of mother and fetus because even mild hyperglycemia has been shown to be detrimental to the fetus. Maternal fasting and postprandial blood glucose levels should be measured regularly. Fetal surveillance depends on the degree of risk for the fetus. The frequency of growth measurements and determinations of fetal distress depends on available technology and gestational age. All women with GDM require nutritional guidance because nutrition is the cornerstone of therapy. The nutrition plan should provide the necessary nutrients for maternal and fetal health, result in normoglycemia and proper weight gain, and prevent ketosis.[21] If dietary management alone

TABLE 32-4	Diagnosis of Gestational Diabetes Mellitus With a 100-g Glucose Load
100-g Glucose Load	**mg/dL (mmol/L)**
Fasting	95 (5.3)
1 hour	180 (10.0)
2 hour	155 (8.6)
3 hour	140 (7.8)

Two or more of the venous plasma concentrations must be met or exceeded for a positive diagnosis. The test should be done in the morning after an overnight fast of between 8 and 14 hours and after at least 3 days of unrestricted diet (>150 g carbohydrate/day) and unlimited physical activity. The subject should remain seated and should not smoke throughout the test. (Developed from data in American Diabetes Association. [2004]. Diagnosis and classification of diabetes mellitus. *Diabetes Care 27*[Suppl 1], S5–10.)

does not achieve a fasting blood glucose level no greater than 105 mg/dL or a 2-hour postprandial blood glucose no greater than 120 mg/dL, the Third International Workshop on GDM recommends therapy with human insulin. Oral antidiabetic agents may be teratogenic and are not recommended in pregnancy. Self-monitoring of blood glucose levels is essential.

Women with GDM are at increased risk for the development of diabetes 5 to 10 years after delivery. Women in whom GDM is diagnosed should be followed up after delivery to detect diabetes early in its course. These women should be evaluated during their first postpartum visit with a 2-hour OGTT with a 75-g glucose load.

CLINICAL MANIFESTATIONS

Diabetes mellitus may have a rapid or an insidious onset. In type 1 diabetes, signs and symptoms often arise suddenly. Type 2 diabetes usually develops more insidiously. Its presence may be detected during a routine medical examination or when a patient seeks medical care for other reasons.

The most commonly identified signs and symptoms of diabetes are referred to as the *three polys*—polyuria (*i.e.*, excessive urination), polydipsia (*i.e.*, excessive thirst), and polyphagia (*i.e.*, excessive hunger). These three symptoms are closely related to the hyperglycemia and glycosuria of diabetes. Glucose is a small, osmotically active molecule. When blood glucose levels are sufficiently elevated, the amount of glucose filtered by the glomeruli of the kidney exceeds the amount that can be reabsorbed by the renal tubules. This results in glycosuria accompanied by large losses of water in the urine. Thirst results from the intracellular dehydration that occurs as blood glucose levels rise and water is pulled out of body cells, including those in the thirst center. Cellular dehydration also causes dryness of the mouth. This early symptom may be easily overlooked in people with type 2 diabetes, particularly in those who have had a gradual increase in blood glucose levels. Polyphagia usually is not present in people with type 2 diabetes. In type 1 diabetes, it probably results from cellular starvation and the depletion of cellular stores of carbohydrates, fats, and proteins.

Weight loss despite normal or increased appetite is a common occurrence in people with uncontrolled type 1 diabetes. The cause of weight loss is twofold. First, loss of body fluids results from osmotic diuresis. Vomiting may exaggerate the fluid loss in ketoacidosis. Second, body tissue is lost because the lack of insulin forces the body to use its fat stores and cellular proteins as sources of energy. In terms of weight loss, there often is a marked difference between type 2 diabetes and type 1 diabetes. Weight loss is a common phenomenon in people with uncontrolled type 1 diabetes, whereas many people with uncomplicated type 2 diabetes have problems with obesity.

Other signs and symptoms of hyperglycemia include recurrent blurred vision, fatigue, paresthesias, and skin infections. In type 2 diabetes, these often are the symptoms that prompt a person to seek medical treatment. Blurred vision develops as the lens and retina are exposed to hyperosmotic effects of elevated blood glucose levels. Lowered plasma volume produces weakness and fatigue. Paresthesias reflect a temporary dysfunction of the peripheral sensory nerves. Chronic skin infections are common in people with type 2 diabetes. Hyperglycemia and glycosuria favor the growth of yeast organisms. Pruritus and vulvovaginitis resulting from candidal infections are common initial complaints in women with diabetes.

DIAGNOSTIC METHODS

The diagnosis of diabetes mellitus in nonpregnant adults is based on fasting blood glucose levels, random blood glucose tests, or the results of a glucose challenge test (see Table 32-4). Testing for diabetes should be considered in all individuals 45 years of age and older. Testing should be considered at a younger age in people who are obese, have a first-degree relative with diabetes, are members of a high-risk group, are women who have delivered an infant weighing more than 9 pounds or have received a diagnosis of GDM, have hypertension or hyperlipidemia, or have met the criteria for IGT or IFG (*i.e.*, prediabetes) on previous testing.[22]

Blood Tests

Blood glucose measurements are used in both the diagnosis and management of diabetes. Diagnostic tests include the fasting plasma glucose, casual plasma glucose, and the glucose tolerance test. Laboratory and capillary or "finger stick" glucose tests are used for glucose management in people with diagnosed diabetes. Glycated hemoglobin (A1C, previously termed HbA_{1c}) provides a measure of glucose control over time. Table 32-5 shows the correlation of mean plasma glucose levels with A1C values for people with diabetes.[23]

Fasting Blood Glucose Test. The fasting plasma glucose has been suggested as the preferred diagnostic test because of ease of administration, convenience, patient acceptability, and cost.[22] Glucose levels are measured after food has been withheld for at least 8 hours. An FPG level below 100 mg/dL is considered normal. A level between 100 and 126 mg/dL is significant and is defined as impaired fasting glucose. If the FPG level is 126 mg/dL or more on two occasions, diabetes is diagnosed.

Casual Blood Glucose Test. A casual plasma glucose is one that is done without regard to the time or the last meal. A casual plasma glucose concentration that is unequivocally elevated (≥200 mg/dL) in the presence of classic symptoms of diabetes such as polydipsia, polyphagia, polyuria, and blurred vision is diagnostic of diabetes mellitus at any age.

Oral Glucose Tolerance Test. The OGTT is an important screening test for diabetes. The test measures the body's ability to store glucose by removing it from the blood. In men and women, the test measures the plasma glucose response to 75 g of concentrated glucose solution at selected intervals, usually 1 hour and 2 hours. In pregnant women, a glucose load of 100 g is given (see the Gestational Diabetes section) with an additional 3-hour plasma glucose determination. In people with normal glucose tolerance, blood glucose levels return to normal within 2 to 3 hours after ingestion of a glucose load, in which case it can be assumed that sufficient insulin is present to allow glucose to leave the blood and enter body cells. Because a person with diabetes lacks the ability to respond to an increase in blood glucose by releasing adequate insulin to facilitate storage, blood glucose levels rise above those observed in normal people and remain elevated for longer periods.

Capillary Blood Glucose Monitoring. Technological advances have provided the means for monitoring of blood glucose levels by using a drop of capillary blood. This procedure has provided health professionals with a rapid and economical means for monitoring blood glucose and has given people with diabetes a way of maintaining near-normal blood glucose levels through self-monitoring of blood glucose. These methods use a drop of capillary blood obtained by pricking the finger or forearm with a special needle or small lancet. Small trigger devices make use of the lancet virtually painless. The drop of capillary blood is placed on or absorbed by a reagent strip, and glucose levels are determined electronically using a glucose meter.

Laboratory tests that use plasma for measurement of blood glucose give results that are 10% to 15% higher than the finger stick method, which uses whole blood.[23] Many blood glucose monitors approved for home use and some test strips now calibrate blood glucose readings to plasma values. It is important that people with diabetes know whether their monitors or glucose strips provide whole blood or plasma test results.

Glycated Hemoglobin Testing. Glycated hemoglobin, also referred to as glycohemoglobin, glycosylated hemoglobin, HbA_{1c}, or A1C (the preferred term), is a term used to describe hemoglobin into which glucose has been incorporated. Hemoglobin normally does not contain glucose when it is released from the bone marrow. During its 120-day life span in the red blood cell, hemoglobin normally becomes glycated to form hemoglobins A_{1a} and A_{1b}

TABLE 32-5	Correlation Between Hemoglobin A1C Level and Mean Plasma Glucose Levels	
Hemoglobin A1C (%)	**Mean Plasma Glucose mg/dL (mmol/L)**	
6	135 (7.5)	
7	170 (9.5)	
8	205 (11.5)	
9	240 (13.5)	
10	275 (13.5)	
11	310 (17.5)	
12	345 (19.5)	

(2% to 4%) and A_{1c} (termed A1C, 4% to 6%). Because glucose entry into the red blood cell is not insulin dependent, the rate at which glucose becomes attached to the hemoglobin molecule depends on blood glucose levels. Glycosylation is essentially irreversible, and the level of A1C present in the blood provides an index of blood glucose levels over the previous 6 to 12 weeks. In uncontrolled diabetes or diabetes with hyperglycemia, there is an increase in the level of A1C. The American Diabetes Association (ADA) recommends that the goal of therapy for people with diabetes should be an A1C result of less than 7.0%.[23]

Urine Tests

The ease, accuracy, and convenience of self-administered blood glucose monitoring techniques have made urine testing for glucose obsolete for most people with diabetes. Unlike glucose tests, urine ketone determinations remain an important part of monitoring diabetic control, particularly in people with type 1 diabetes who are at risk for developing ketoacidosis, and in pregnant diabetic women to check the adequacy of nutrition and glucose control.[21]

DIABETES MANAGEMENT

The desired outcomes for management of both type 1 and type 2 diabetes is normalization of blood glucose as a means of preventing short- and long-term complications. Treatment plans usually involve nutrition therapy, exercise, and antidiabetic agents. People with type 1 diabetes require insulin from the time of diagnosis. Weight loss and dietary management may be sufficient to control blood glucose levels in people with type 2 diabetes. However, they require follow-up care because insulin secretion from the beta cells may decrease or insulin resistance may persist, in which case oral antidiabetic agents are prescribed.

Among the methods used to achieve these goals are education in self-management and problem solving. Individual treatment goals should take into account the person's age and other disease conditions, the person's capacity to understand and carry out the treatment regimen, and socioeconomic factors that might influence compliance with the treatment plan. Optimal control of type 2 diabetes is associated with prevention or delay of chronic diabetes complications.[24]

Dietary Management

Dietary management usually is prescribed to meet the specific needs of each person with diabetes. Goals and principles of diet therapy differ between type 1 and type 2 diabetes, as well as for lean and obese people. Integral to diabetes management is a prescribed plan for nutrition therapy.[25] Therapy goals include maintenance of near-normal blood glucose levels, achievement of optimal lipid levels, adequate calories to maintain and attain reasonable weights, prevention and treatment of chronic diabetes complications, and improvement of overall health through optimal nutrition.

For a person with type 1 diabetes, the usual food intake is assessed and used as a basis for adjusting insulin therapy to fit with the person's lifestyle. Eating consistent amounts and types of food at specific and routine times is encouraged. Home blood glucose monitoring is used to fine-tune the plan. Newer forms of therapy, such as multiple daily insulin injections and the use of an insulin pump, provide many options. Most people with type 2 diabetes are overweight. Nutrition therapy goals focus on achieving glucose, lipid, and blood pressure goals, and weight loss if indicated. Mild to moderate weight loss (5% to 10% of total body weight) has been shown to improve diabetes control, even if desirable weight is not achieved.

A coordinated team effort, including the person with diabetes, is needed to individualize the nutrition plan. The diabetic diet has undergone marked changes over the years, particularly in the recommendations for distribution of calories among carbohydrates, proteins, and fats. There no longer is a specific diabetic or ADA diet but rather a dietary prescription based on nutrition assessment and treatment goals. Information is assessed regarding metabolic parameters and medical history of factors such as renal impairment and gastrointestinal autonomic neuropathy. Evaluating the effectiveness of the meal plan requires monitoring metabolic parameters such as blood glucose, A1C, lipids, blood pressure, body weight, and quality of life. Self-management education is essential to facilitate understanding of the associations among food, exercise, medication, and blood glucose.

Exercise

The benefits of exercise include cardiovascular fitness and psychological well-being. For many people with type 2 diabetes, the benefits of exercise include a decrease in body fat, better weight control, and improvement in insulin sensitivity.[26] In general, sporadic exercise has only transient benefits; a regular exercise or training program is the most beneficial. It is better for cardiovascular conditioning and can maintain a muscle–fat ratio that enhances peripheral insulin receptivity.

In people with insulin-dependent diabetes, the beneficial effects of exercise are accompanied by an increased risk of hypoglycemia. Although muscle uptake of glucose increases significantly, the ability to maintain blood glucose levels is hampered by failure to suppress the absorption of injected insulin and activate the counter-regulatory mechanisms that maintain blood glucose. Even after exercise ceases, insulin's lowering effect on blood glucose levels continues. In some people with type 1 diabetes, the symptoms of hypoglycemia occur many hours after cessation of exercise. People with diabetes should be aware that delayed hypoglycemia can occur after exercise and that they may need to alter their diabetes medication dose, their carbohydrate intake, or both.

Although of benefit to people with diabetes, exercise must be weighed on the risk-benefit scale. Before beginning an exercise program, persons with diabetes should undergo an appropriate evaluation for macrovascular and microvascular disease.[26] The goal of exercise is safe participation in activities consistent with an individual's lifestyle. Considerations include the potential for hypoglycemia, hyperglycemia, ketosis, cardiovascular ischemia and arrhythmias (particularly silent ischemic heart disease), exacerbation of proliferative retinopathy, and lower extremity injury. For those with chronic diabetes, the complications of vigorous exercise can be harmful and cause eye hemorrhage and other problems. For people with type 1 diabetes who exercise during periods of poor control (*i.e.*, when blood glucose is elevated, exogenous insulin levels are low, and ketonemia exists), blood glucose and ketone levels rise even higher because the stress of exercise is superimposed on preexisting insulin deficiency and increased counter-regulatory hormone activity.

Oral Antidiabetic Agents

Historically, two categories of antidiabetic agents existed: insulin and oral medications. However, this classification has now become somewhat blurred because of the introduction of new injectable antidiabetic agents for use as adjunctive therapy in type 1 diabetes (amylin analogs) and type 2 diabetes (amylin and GLP-1 analogs). Because people with type 1 diabetes are deficient in insulin, they are in need of exogenous insulin replacement therapy from the start. People with type 2 diabetes have increased hepatic glucose production; decreased peripheral utilization of glucose; decreased utilization of ingested carbohydrates; and, over time, impaired insulin secretion from the pancreas (Fig. 32-8). The oral antidiabetic agents used in the treatment of type 2 diabetes exert their action in one or sometimes all of these areas.[27–29] If good glycemic

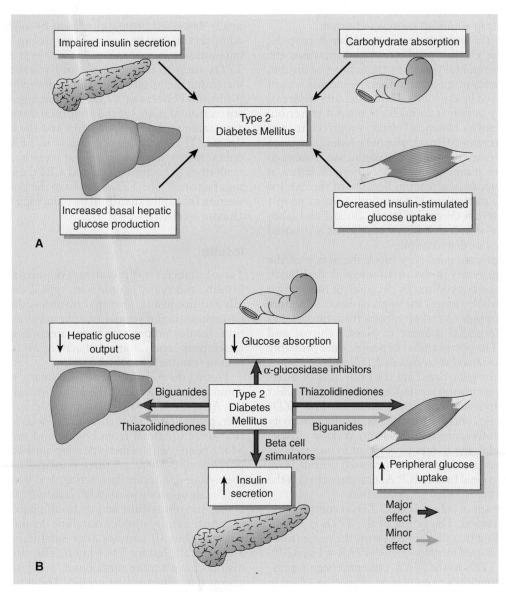

FIGURE 32-8 (**A**) Mechanisms of elevated blood glucose in type 2 diabetes. (**B**) Action sites of oral hypoglycemic agents and mechanisms of lowering blood glucose in type 2 diabetes mellitus.

control cannot be achieved with a combination of oral agents, insulin can be used with the oral agents or by itself. The oral antidiabetic agents that are used in the treatment of type 2 diabetes fall into four categories: beta cell stimulators (sulfonylureas, repaglinide, and nateglinide), biguanides (Metformin), α-glucosidase inhibitors, and thiazolidinediones (TZDs).

The *beta cell stimulators* act at the level of the pancreatic beta cells to stimulate insulin release. They require the presence of functioning beta cells, are used only in the treatment of type 2 diabetes, and have the potential for producing hypoglycemia. The *sulfonylureas* reduce blood glucose by stimulating the release of insulin from beta cells in the pancreas and increasing the sensitivity of peripheral tissues to insulin. *Repaglinide* and *nateglinide* are non-sulfonylurea beta cell stimulators. These agents, which are rapidly absorbed from the gastrointestinal tract, are taken shortly before meals. Both repaglinide and nateglinide can produce hypoglycemia; thus, proper timing of meals in relation to drug administration is important.

Metformin, the only currently available biguanide, inhibits hepatic glucose production and increases the sensitivity of peripheral tissues to the actions of insulin. Secondary benefits of metformin therapy include weight loss and improved lipid profiles. Unlike the sulfonylureas, whose primary action is to increase insulin secretion, metformin exerts its beneficial effects on glycemic control through decreased hepatic glucose production (main effect) and increased peripheral use of glucose. This medication does not stimulate insulin secretion; therefore, it does not produce hypoglycemia. Because of the risk for lactic acidosis, metformin is contraindicated in people with elevated serum creatinine levels, clinical and laboratory evidence of liver disease, or conditions associated with hypoxemia or dehydration.

The *α-glucosidase inhibitors* block the action of the brush border enzymes in the small intestine that break down complex carbohydrates. By delaying the breakdown of complex carbohydrates, the α-glucosidase inhibitors delay the absorption of carbohydrates from the gut and blunt the postprandial increase in plasma glucose and insulin levels. The postprandial hyperglycemia probably accounts for sustained increases in A1C levels.

The *TZDs* (or glitazones) are the only class of drugs that directly target insulin resistance, a fundamental defect in the pathophysiology of type 2 diabetes. The TZDs improve glycemic control by increasing insulin sensitivity in the insulin-responsive tissues—liver, skeletal muscle, and fat—allowing the tissues to respond to endogenous insulin more efficiently without increased output from already dysfunctional beta cells.[29] A secondary effect is the suppression of hepatic glucose production.

The mechanism of action of the TZDs is complex and not fully understood. The action of the TZDs is associated with binding to a nuclear receptor, the *peroxisome proliferator–activated receptor-γ*[12,13,29] (PPAR-γ; Fig. 32-9). Binding of the TZDs to the PPAR-γ receptor begins a cascade of events that leads to regulation of genes involved in lipid and glucose metabolism. They result in an increase in the number of GLUT-4 transporters and increased insulin-

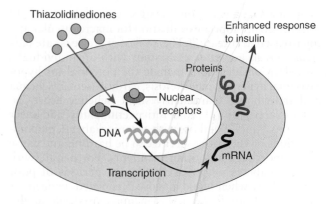

FIGURE 32-9 Action of the thiazolidinediones on activation of the PPAR-γ receptor, which regulates gene transcription of proteins that regulate glucose uptake and reduce fatty acid release.

mediated uptake of glucose in the peripheral tissues. A newly described protein produced by adipocytes, called *adiponectin*, may be a part of the missing link in explaining insulin resistance in persons with type 2 diabetes. The TZDs seem to decrease insulin resistance, in part, by increasing the production of adiponectin by adipocytes.[30] Additional effects of TZDs are numerous, and include correction of many of the abnormal metabolic features associated with type 2 diabetes and the metabolic syndrome. This includes a decrease in FFAs and triglycerides, microalbuminuria, blood pressure, inflammatory mediators (*e.g.*, fibrinogen and CRP), and procoagulation factors.[29] The TZDs also have the potential for preventing beta cell exhaustion by reducing FFAs and blood glucose levels.

Insulin

Type 1 diabetes mellitus always requires treatment with insulin, and many people with type 2 diabetes eventually require insulin therapy. Insulin is destroyed in the gastrointestinal tract and must be administered by injection. Insulin preparations are categorized according to onset, peak, and duration of action. An inhaled form of insulin is in the clinical trial stage.

During the past several decades, many pharmaceutical companies have entered the insulin-manufacturing market. After much research, human insulin has become available, providing an alternative to previous forms of insulin that were obtained from bovine and porcine sources. Many people with diabetes develop antibodies to beef and pork insulin. There are three principal types of insulin: short-acting, intermediate-acting, and long-acting.

The short-acting insulins fall into two categories: short-acting and ultra–short-acting. Insulin injection (Regular) is a short-acting soluble crystalline insulin whose effects begin within 30 minutes after subcutaneous injection and generally last for 5 to 8 hours. The ultra–short-acting insulins have a more rapid onset, peak, and duration of action than short-acting insulin. The ultra–short-acting insulins, which are used in combination with intermediate- or long-acting insulins, are usually administered immediately before a meal. Intermediate-acting insulins (NPH and Lente) have a slower onset and duration of action. Because the intermediate-acting insulins require several hours to reach therapeutic levels, their use in type 1 diabetes requires supplementation with an ultra–short- or short-acting insulin. The long-acting Ultralente insulin has an even longer onset and duration of action than the intermediate-acting insulins. As with intermediate-acting insulins, it is used in combination with the shorter-acting insulins. Glargine is a new long-acting human insulin analog. It has a slower, more prolonged absorption than NPH insulin and provides a relatively constant concentration over 24 hours. It is usually taken as a single bedtime dose and is used in combination with preprandial injections of short-acting insulin. All forms of insulin have the potential of producing hypoglycemia or "insulin reaction" as a side effect (to be discussed).

Two intensive treatment regimens—multiple daily injections (MDI) and continuous subcutaneous infusion of insulin (CSII)—closely simulate the normal pattern of insulin secretion by the body.[31] With each regimen, a basal insulin level is maintained, and bolus doses of short-acting insulin are delivered before meals. The choice of management is determined by the person with diabetes in collaboration with the health care team.

Pancreas or Islet Cell Transplantation

Pancreas or islet cell transplantation is not a lifesaving procedure.[32,33] However, it does afford the potential for significantly improving the quality of life. The most serious problems are the requirement for immunosuppression and the need for diagnosis and treatment of rejection. Investigators are looking for methods of transplanting islet cells and protecting the cells from destruction without the use of immunosuppressive drugs.

ACUTE COMPLICATIONS

The three major acute complications of diabetes are diabetic ketoacidosis, the hyperglycemic hyperosmolar state, and hypoglycemia. The Somogyi effect and dawn phenomenon, which result from the mobilization of counter-regulatory hormones, contribute to difficulties with diabetic control.

Diabetic Ketoacidosis

Diabetic ketoacidosis (DKA) occurs when ketone production by the liver exceeds cellular use and renal excretion.[34] DKA most commonly occurs in a person with type 1 diabetes, in whom the lack of insulin leads to mobilization of fatty acids from adipose tissue because of the unsuppressed adipose cell lipase activity that breaks down triglycerides into fatty acids and glycerol. The increase in fatty acid levels leads to ketone production by the liver (Fig. 32-10). It can occur at the onset of the disease, often before the disease has been diagnosed. For example, a mother may bring a child into the clinic or emergency department with reports of lethargy, vom-

iting, and abdominal pain, unaware that the child has diabetes. Stress increases the release of cortisol and other gluconeogenic hormones and predisposes the person to the development of ketoacidosis. DKA often is preceded by physical or emotional stress, such as infection, pregnancy, or extreme anxiety. In clinical practice, ketoacidosis also occurs with the omission or inadequate use of insulin.

The three major metabolic derangements in DKA are hyperglycemia, ketosis, and metabolic acidosis. The definitive diagnosis of DKA consists of hyperglycemia (blood glucose levels >250 mg/dL), low bicarbonate (<15 mEq/L), and low pH (<7.3), with ketonemia (positive at 1:2 dilution) and moderate ketonuria.[34] Hyperglycemia leads to osmotic diuresis, dehydration, and a critical loss of electrolytes. Hyperosmolality of extracellular fluids from hyperglycemia leads to a shift of water and potassium from the intracellular to the extracellular compartment. Extracellular sodium concentration frequently is low or normal despite enteric water losses because of the intracellular-extracellular fluid shift. This dilutional effect is referred to as *pseudohyponatremia*. Serum potassium levels may be normal or elevated, despite total potassium depletion resulting from protracted polyuria and vomiting. Metabolic acidosis is caused by the excess ketoacids that require buffering by bicarbonate ions; this leads to a marked decrease in serum bicarbonate levels.

Compared with an insulin reaction, DKA usually is slower in onset, and recovery is more prolonged. The person typically has a history of 1 or 2 days of polyuria, polydipsia, nausea, vomiting, and marked fatigue, with eventual stupor that can progress to coma. Abdominal pain and tenderness may be experienced without abdominal disease. The breath has a characteristic fruity smell because of the presence of the volatile ketoacids. Hypotension and tachycardia may be present because of a decrease in blood volume. A number of the signs and symptoms that occur in DKA are related to compensatory mechanisms. The heart rate increases as the body compensates for a decrease in blood volume, and the rate and depth of respiration increase (*i.e.,* Kussmaul's respiration) as the body attempts to prevent further decreases in pH. Metabolic acidosis is discussed further in Chapter 6.

The goals in treating DKA are to improve circulatory volume and tissue perfusion, decrease serum glucose, correct the acidosis, and correct electrolyte imbalances. These objectives usually are accomplished through the administration of insulin and intravenous fluid and electrolyte replacement solutions. Because insulin resistance accompanies severe acidosis, low-dose insulin therapy is used. Frequent laboratory tests are used to monitor blood glucose and serum electrolyte levels and to guide fluid and electrolyte replacement. Identification and treatment of the underlying cause, such as infection, also are important.

Hyperglycemic Hyperosmolar State

The hyperglycemic hyperosmolar state (HHS) is characterized by hyperglycemia (blood glucose >600 mg/dL), hyperosmolarity (plasma osmolarity >310 mOsm/L),

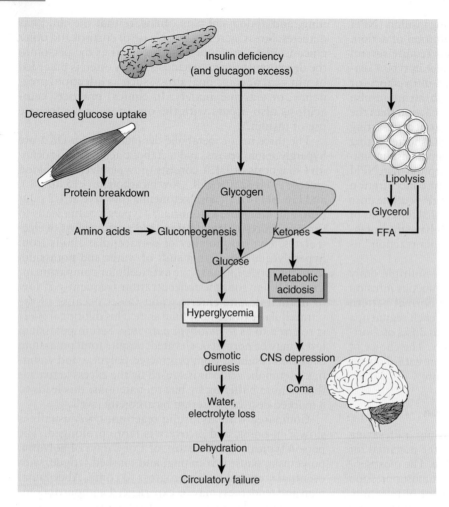

Insulin deficiency
(and glucagon excess)

Decreased glucose uptake

Protein breakdown

Amino acids → Gluconeogenesis

Glycogen

Gluconeogenesis   Ketones ← FFA

Glucose

Lipolysis

Glycerol

Metabolic
acidosis

Hyperglycemia

Osmotic
diuresis   CNS depression

Water,
electrolyte loss Coma

Dehydration

Circulatory failure

FIGURE 32-10 Mechanisms of diabetic ketoacidosis. CNS, central nervous system; FFA, free fatty acids.

and dehydration, the absence of ketoacidosis, and depression of the sensorium.[34] HHS may occur in various conditions, including type 2 diabetes, acute pancreatitis, severe infection, myocardial infarction, and treatment with oral or parenteral nutrition solutions. It is seen most frequently in people with type 2 diabetes. Two factors appear to contribute to the hyperglycemia that precipitates the condition: an increased resistance to the effects of insulin and an excessive carbohydrate intake.

In hyperosmolar states, the increased serum osmolarity has the effect of pulling water out of body cells, including brain cells. The condition may be complicated by thromboembolic events arising because of the high serum osmolality. The most prominent manifestations are dehydration, neurologic signs and symptoms, and excessive thirst. The neurologic signs include grand mal seizures, hemiparesis, aphasia, muscle fasciculations, hyperthermia, visual field loss, nystagmus, and visual hallucinations. The onset of HHS often is insidious, and because it occurs most frequently in older people, it may be mistaken for a stroke.

The treatment of HHS requires judicious medical observation and care because water moves back into brain cells during treatment, posing a threat of cerebral edema. Extensive potassium losses that also have occurred during the diuretic phase of the disorder require correction.

Because of the problems encountered in the treatment of HHS and the serious nature of the disease conditions that cause it, the prognosis for this disorder is less favorable than that for ketoacidosis.

Hypoglycemia

Hypoglycemia, sometimes referred to as an *insulin reaction*, occurs from a relative excess of insulin in the blood and is characterized by below-normal blood glucose levels.[35] It occurs most commonly in people treated with insulin injections, but prolonged hypoglycemia also can result from some oral hypoglycemic agents (*i.e.*, beta cell stimulators).

Hypoglycemia usually has a rapid onset and progression of symptoms. Because the brain relies on blood glucose as its main energy source, hypoglycemia produces behaviors related to altered cerebral function. Headache, difficulty in problem solving, disturbed or altered behavior, coma, and seizures may occur. At the onset of the hypoglycemic episode, activation of the parasympathetic nervous system often causes hunger. The initial parasympathetic response is followed by activation of the sympathetic nervous system; this causes anxiety, tachycardia, sweating, and constriction of the skin vessels (*i.e.*, the skin is cool and clammy).

There is wide variation in the manifestation of signs and symptoms; not every person with diabetes manifests all or even most of the symptoms. The signs and symptoms of hypoglycemia are more variable in children and in elderly people. Elderly people may not display the typical autonomic responses associated with hypoglycemia but frequently have signs of impaired function of the central nervous system, including mental confusion. Some people experience hypoglycemic unawareness. Unawareness of hypoglycemia should be suspected in people who do not experience symptoms when their blood glucose concentrations are less than 50 to 60 mg/dL. This occurs most commonly in people who have a longer duration of diabetes and A1C levels within the normal range.[35] Some medications, such as β-adrenergic–blocking drugs, interfere with the sympathetic response normally seen in hypoglycemia.

Many factors precipitate an insulin reaction in a person with type 1 diabetes, including error in insulin dose, failure to eat, increased exercise, decreased insulin need after removal of a stress situation, medication changes, and a change in insulin site. Alcohol decreases liver gluconeogenesis, and people with diabetes need to be cautioned about its potential for causing hypoglycemia, especially if it is consumed in large amounts or on an empty stomach.

The most effective treatment of an insulin reaction is the immediate ingestion of a concentrated carbohydrate source, such as glucose, honey, candy, or orange juice. Alternative methods for increasing blood glucose may be required when the person having the reaction is unconscious or unable to swallow. Glucagon may be given intramuscularly or subcutaneously. Glucagon acts by hepatic glycogenolysis to raise blood sugar. Because the liver contains only a limited amount of glycogen (approximately 75 g), glucagon is ineffective in people whose glycogen stores have been depleted. In situations of severe or life-threatening hypoglycemia, it may be necessary to administer glucose intravenously.

THE SOMOGYI EFFECT AND DAWN PHENOMENON

The Somogyi effect describes a cycle of insulin-induced posthypoglycemic episodes. In 1924, Joslin and associates noticed that hypoglycemia was associated with alternate episodes of hyperglycemia.[36] It was not until 1959 that Somogyi presented the results of his 20 years of studies, which confirmed the observation that "hypoglycemia begets hyperglycemia." In people with diabetes, insulin-induced hypoglycemia produces a compensatory increase in blood levels of catecholamines, glucagon, cortisol, and growth hormone. These counter-regulatory hormones cause blood glucose to become elevated and produce some degree of insulin resistance. The cycle begins when the increase in blood glucose and insulin resistance is treated with larger insulin doses. The hypoglycemic episode often occurs during the night or at a time when it is not recognized, rendering the diagnosis of the phenomenon more difficult.

Research suggests that even rather mild insulin-associated hypoglycemia, which may be asymptomatic, can cause hyperglycemia in those with type 1 diabetes through the recruitment of counter-regulatory mechanisms. A concomitant waning of the effect of insulin (i.e., end of the duration of action) on blood glucose, when it occurs, exacerbates the posthypoglycemic hyperglycemia and accelerates its development. These findings may explain the labile nature of the disease in some people with diabetes. Measures to prevent hypoglycemia and the subsequent activation of counter-regulatory mechanisms include a redistribution of dietary carbohydrates and an alteration in insulin dose or time of administration.[37]

The dawn phenomenon is characterized by increased levels of fasting blood glucose or insulin requirements, or both, between 5 and 9 AM without preceding hypoglycemia. It occurs in people with type 1 or type 2 diabetes. It has been suggested that the normal circadian rhythm for glucose tolerance, which usually is higher during the later part of the morning, is altered in people with diabetes.[38] Growth hormone has been suggested as a possible factor. When the dawn phenomenon occurs alone, it may produce only mild hyperglycemia, but when it is combined with the Somogyi effect, it may produce profound hyperglycemia.

CHRONIC COMPLICATIONS

The chronic complications of diabetes include disorders of the microcirculation (microvascular disease, i.e., neuropathies, nephropathies, and retinopathies), macrovascular complications, and foot ulcers. The microvascular disorders occur in the insulin-independent tissues of the body—tissues that do not require insulin for glucose entry into the cell.[39] This probably means that intracellular glucose concentrations in many of these tissues approach or equal those in the blood. The level of chronic glycemia is the most clearly established factor associated with diabetic microvascular complications. The Diabetes Control and Complications Trial (DCCT), which was conducted with 1441 people with type 1 diabetes, has demonstrated that the incidence of retinopathy, nephropathy, and neuropathy can be reduced by intensive diabetic treatment.[40] Similar results have been demonstrated by the United Kingdom Prospective Diabetes Study (UKPDS) in people with type 2 diabetes.[41]

Peripheral Neuropathies

Although the incidence of peripheral neuropathies is high among people with diabetes, it is difficult to document exactly how many people are affected by these disorders because of the diversity in clinical manifestations and because the condition often is far advanced before it is recognized. Results of the DCCT study showed that intensive therapy can reduce the incidence of clinical neuropathy by 60% compared with conventional therapy.[40]

Two types of pathologic changes have been observed in connection with diabetic peripheral neuropathies. The first is a thickening of the walls of the nutrient vessels that supply the nerve, leading to the assumption that vessel ischemia plays a major role in the development of

KEY CONCEPTS

Chronic Complications of Diabetes

➤ The chronic complications of diabetes result from elevated blood glucose levels and associated impairment of lipid and other metabolic pathways.

➤ Diabetic peripheral neuropathies, which affect both the somatic and autonomic nervous systems, result from the demyelinating effect of long-term uncontrolled diabetes.

➤ Diabetic nephropathy, which is a leading cause of end-stage renal disease, is associated with the increased work demands and microalbuminemia imposed by poorly controlled blood glucose levels.

➤ Diabetic retinopathy, which is a leading cause of blindness, is closely linked to elevations in blood glucose and hyperlipidemia seen in persons with uncontrolled diabetes.

➤ Macrovascular disorders such as coronary heart disease, stroke, and peripheral vascular disease reflect the combined effects of unregulated blood glucose levels, elevated blood pressure, and hyperlipidemia.

➤ The chronic complications of diabetes are best prevented by measures aimed at tight control of blood glucose levels, maintenance of normal lipid levels, and control of hypertension.

CHART 32-3

Classification of Diabetic Peripheral Neuropathies

Somatic

Polyneuropathies (bilateral sensory)
  Paresthesias, including numbness and tingling
  Impaired pain, temperature, light touch, two-point discrimination, and vibratory sensation
  Decreased ankle and knee-jerk reflexes
Mononeuropathies
  Involvement of a mixed nerve trunk that includes loss of sensation, pain, and motor weakness
Amyotrophy (muscle atrophy)
  Associated with muscle weakness, wasting, and severe pain of muscles in the pelvic girdle and thigh

Autonomic

Impaired vasomotor function
  Postural hypotension
Impaired gastrointestinal function
  Gastric atony
  Diarrhea, often postprandial and nocturnal
Impaired genitourinary function
  Paralytic bladder
  Incomplete voiding
  Impotence
  Retrograde ejaculation
Cranial nerve involvement
  Extraocular nerve paralysis
  Impaired pupillary responses
  Impaired special senses

these neural changes. The second finding is a segmental demyelinization process that affects the Schwann cell. This demyelinization process is accompanied by a slowing of nerve conduction.

The clinical manifestations of the diabetic peripheral neuropathies vary with the location of the lesion. Although there are several methods for classifying the diabetic peripheral neuropathies, a simplified system divides them into the somatic and autonomic nervous system neuropathies (Chart 32-3).

Somatic Neuropathy. The somatic neuropathies involve sensory and motor nerves of the somatic nervous system. A distal symmetric polyneuropathy, in which loss of function occurs in a stocking–glove pattern, is the most common form of somatic peripheral neuropathy. Somatic sensory involvement usually occurs first and usually is bilateral, symmetric, and associated with diminished perception of vibration, pain, and temperature, particularly in the lower extremities. In addition to the discomforts associated with the loss of sensory or motor function, lesions in the peripheral nervous system predispose a person with diabetes to other complications. The loss of feeling, touch, and position sense increases the risk of falling. Impairment of temperature and pain sensation increases the risk of serious burns and injuries to the feet.

Painful diabetic neuropathy involves the somatosensory neurons that carry pain impulses. This disorder, which causes hypersensitivity to light touch and occasionally severe "burning pain," particularly at night, can become physically and emotionally disabling.[42]

Autonomic Neuropathy. With autonomic nervous system neuropathies, there are defects in vasomotor responses, decreased cardiac responses, impaired motility of the gastrointestinal tract, inability to empty the bladder, and sexual dysfunction. Defects in vasomotor reflexes can lead to dizziness and syncope when the person moves from the supine to the standing position (see Chapter 17). Incomplete emptying of the bladder predisposes to urinary stasis and bladder infection and increases the risk of renal complications.

Gastrointestinal motility disorders are common in persons with long-standing diabetes. Although the pathogenesis of these disorders is poorly understood, neuropathy and metabolic abnormalities secondary to hyperglycemia are thought to play an important role.[43] The symptoms vary in severity and include constipation, diarrhea and fecal incontinence, nausea and vomiting, and upper abdominal discomfort referred as *dyspepsia*. Gastroparesis (delayed emptying of stomach) is commonly seen in persons with diabetes. The disorder is characterized by complaints of epigastric discomfort, nausea, postprandial vomiting, bloating, and early satiety. Abnormal gastric emptying also jeopardizes the regulation of the blood glucose level. Diarrhea is another common symptom seen mostly in persons with poorly controlled type 1 diabetes and autonomic neuropathy.[44] The pathogenesis is thought to be multifactorial. Diabetic diarrhea is typically intermittent, watery, painless, and nocturnal, and may be associated with fecal incontinence.

In the man, disruption of sensory and autonomic nervous system function may cause sexual dysfunction (see Chapter 38). Diabetes is the leading physiologic cause of erectile dysfunction, and it occurs in both type 1 and type 2 diabetes. Of the 7.8 million men with diabetes in the United States, 30% to 60% have erectile dysfunction.[45]

Nephropathies

Diabetic nephropathy is the leading cause of end-stage renal disease (ESRD), accounting for 43% of new cases.[1] In the United States, 40% of all people who seek renal replacement therapy (see Chapter 25) have diabetes.[46] The complication affects people with both type 1 and type 2 diabetes. According to the reports of the U.S. Renal Data System, the increase in ESRD since the early 1980s has been predominantly among people with type 2 diabetes.[47]

The term *diabetic nephropathy* is used to describe the combination of lesions that often occur concurrently in the diabetic kidney. The most common kidney lesions in people with diabetes are those that affect the glomeruli. Various glomerular changes may occur, including capillary basement membrane thickening, diffuse glomerular sclerosis, and nodular glomerulosclerosis (see Chapter 24).

Because not all people with diabetes experience clinically significant nephropathy, attention is focusing on risk factors for the development of this complication. Among the suggested risk factors are genetic and familial predisposition, elevated blood pressure, poor glycemic control, smoking, hyperlipidemia, and microalbuminemia.[46–48] The risk for development of ESRD also is greater among Native Americans, people of Hispanic descent (especially Mexican Americans), and African Americans.

One of the first manifestations of diabetic nephropathy is an increase in urinary albumin excretion (*i.e.*, microalbuminuria), which is easily assessed by laboratory methods. Microalbuminuria is defined as a urine protein loss of between 30 and 300 mg/day.[46] The risk of microalbuminuria increases abruptly with hemoglobin A1C levels greater than 8.1%.[49] Both systolic and diastolic hypertension accelerate the progression of diabetic nephropathy. Even moderate lowering of blood pressure can decrease the risk of ESRD. Smoking increases the risk of ESRD in both people with diabetes and those without the disease. People with type 2 diabetes who smoke have a greater risk of microalbuminuria, and their rate of progression to ESRD is approximately twice as rapid as in those who do not smoke.[48]

Measures to prevent diabetic nephropathy or its progression in persons with diabetes include achievement of glycemic control, maintenance of blood pressure in the mid-normal range (125 to 130/75 to 85 mm Hg), prevention or reduction in the level of proteinuria, treatment of hyperlipidemia, and smoking cessation in people who smoke.[46,47]

Retinopathies

Diabetes is the leading cause of acquired blindness in the United States. Although people with diabetes are at increased risk for the development of cataracts and glaucoma, retinopathy is the most common pattern of eye disease. Diabetic retinopathy is estimated to be the most common cause of newly diagnosed blindness among Americans between the ages of 20 and 74 years.[50] Diabetic retinopathy is characterized by abnormal retinal vascular permeability, microaneurysm formation, neovascularization and associated hemorrhage, scarring, and retinal detachment[50,51] (see Chapter 37). Twenty years after the onset of diabetes, nearly all people with type 1 diabetes and more than 60% of people with type 2 diabetes have some degree of retinopathy. Pregnancy, puberty, and cataract surgery can accelerate these changes.[50,51]

Although there has been no extensive research on risk factors associated with diabetic retinopathy, they appear to be similar to those for other complications. Among the suggested risk factors associated with diabetic retinopathy are poor glycemic control, elevated blood pressure, and hyperlipidemia. Because of the risk of retinopathy, it is important that people with diabetes have regular dilated eye examinations. They should have an initial examination for retinopathy shortly after the diagnosis of diabetes is made, with appropriate follow-up examinations.[50]

People with macular edema, moderate to severe nonproliferative retinopathy, or any proliferative retinopathy should receive the care of an ophthalmologist. Methods used in the treatment of diabetic retinopathy include the destruction and scarring of the proliferative lesions with laser photocoagulation. The Diabetic Retinopathy Study provides evidence that photocoagulation may delay or prevent visual loss in more than 50% of eyes with proliferative retinopathy.[51]

Macrovascular Complications

Diabetes mellitus is a major risk factor for coronary artery disease, cerebrovascular disease, and peripheral vascular disease. The prevalence of these vascular complications is increased two- to fourfold in people with diabetes.

Multiple risk factors for vascular disease, including obesity, hypertension, hyperglycemia, hyperinsulinemia, hyperlipidemia, altered platelet function, and elevated fibrinogen levels, frequently are found in people with diabetes and the metabolic syndrome. The prevalence of coronary artery disease, stroke, and peripheral vascular disease is substantially increased in people with diabetes, even in the absence of these risk factors. There appear to be differences between type 1 and type 2 diabetes in terms of duration of disease and the development of macrovascular disease. In people with type 2 diabetes, macrovascular disease may be present at the time of diagnosis. In type 1 diabetes, the attained age and the duration of diabetes appear to correlate with the degree of macrovascular disease. These discrepancies have been attributed to the associated cardiovascular risk factors that exist as part of the metabolic syndrome before the actual diagnosis of type 2 diabetes.[52]

Aggressive management of cardiovascular risk factors should include smoking cessation, control of hypertension, lipid lowering, diabetes control, and antiplatelet agents (aspirin or clopidogrel) if not contraindicated (see Chapter 17). If treatment is warranted for peripheral vascular disease, the peroneal arteries between the knees and ankles commonly are involved in persons with diabetes, making revascularization difficult.

Diabetic Foot Ulcers

Foot problems are common among people with diabetes and may become severe enough to cause ulceration and infection, eventually resulting in amputation. Foot problems have been reported as the most common complication leading to hospitalization among people with diabetes. In a controlled study of 854 outpatients with diabetes followed up in a general medical clinic, foot problems accounted for 16% of hospital admissions during a 2-year period and 23% of total hospital days.[53] In people with diabetes, lesions of the feet represent the effects of neuropathy and vascular insufficiency. Approximately 60% to 70% of people with diabetic foot ulcers have neuropathy without vascular disease, 15% to 20% have vascular disease, and 15% to 20% have neuropathy and vascular disease.[53]

Distal symmetric neuropathy is a major risk factor for foot ulcers. People with sensory neuropathies have impaired pain sensation and often are unaware of the constant trauma to the feet caused by poorly fitting shoes, improper weight bearing, hard objects or pebbles in the shoes, or infections such as athlete's foot. Neuropathy prevents people from detecting pain; they are unable to adjust their gait to avoid walking on an area of the foot where pressure is causing trauma and necrosis. Motor neuropathy with weakness of the intrinsic muscles of the foot may result in foot deformities, which lead to focal areas of high pressure. When the abnormal focus of pressure is coupled with loss of sensation, a foot ulcer can occur. Common sites of trauma are the back of the heel, the plantar metatarsal area, or the great toe, where weight is borne during walking (Fig. 32-11).

All persons with diabetes should receive a full foot examination at least once a year.[53] This examination should include assessment of protective sensation, foot structure and biomechanics, vascular status, and skin integrity. Evaluation of neurologic function should include a somatosensory test using either the Semmes-Weinstein monofilament or vibratory sensation. The

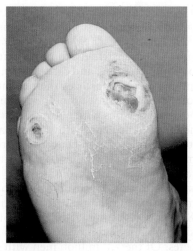

FIGURE 32-11 Neuropathic ulcers occur on pressure points in areas with diminished sensation in diabetic polyneuropathy. Pain is absent (and therefore the ulcer may go unnoticed). (From Bates B. B. [1995]. *A guide to physical examination and history taking* [6th ed.]. Philadelphia: J. B. Lippincott.)

Semmes-Weinstein monofilament is a simple, inexpensive device for testing sensory status (Fig. 32-12).

Because of the constant risk of foot problems, it is important that people with diabetes wear shoes that have been fitted correctly and inspect their feet daily, looking for blisters, open sores, and fungal infection (*e.g.*, athlete's foot) between the toes. If their eyesight is poor, a family member should do this for them. In the event a lesion is detected, prompt medical attention is needed to prevent serious complications. Specially designed shoes have been demonstrated to be effective in preventing relapses in people with previous ulcerations. Smoking should be avoided because it causes vasoconstriction and contributes

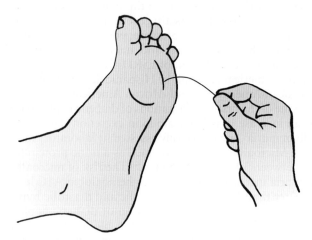

FIGURE 32-12 Use of a monofilament in testing for impaired sensation in the foot of a person with diabetes. When the unsupported end of the monofilament is pressed against the skin until it buckles or bends slightly, it delivers 10 g of pressure at the point of contact. Usually between 4 and 10 sites are tested for impaired sensation.

to vascular disease. Because cold produces vasoconstriction, appropriate foot coverings should be used to keep the feet warm and dry. Toenails should be cut straight across to prevent ingrown toenails. The toenails often are thickened and deformed, requiring the services of a podiatrist.

INFECTIONS

Although not specifically an acute or a chronic complication, infections are a common concern of people with diabetes. Certain types of infections occur with increased frequency in people with diabetes: soft tissue infections of the extremities, osteomyelitis, urinary tract infections and pyelonephritis, candidal infections of the skin and mucous surfaces, dental caries and infections, and tuberculosis.[54] Controversy exists about whether infections are more common in people with diabetes or whether infections seem more prevalent because they often are more serious in people with diabetes.

Suboptimal response to infection in a person with diabetes is caused by the presence of chronic complications, such as vascular disease and neuropathies, and by the presence of hyperglycemia and altered neutrophil function. Sensory deficits may cause a person with diabetes to ignore minor trauma and infection, and vascular disease may impair circulation and delivery of blood cells and other substances needed to produce an adequate inflammatory response and effect healing. Pyelonephritis and urinary tract infections are relatively common in persons with diabetes, and it has been suggested that these infections may bear some relation to the presence of a neurogenic bladder or nephrosclerotic changes in the kidneys. Hyperglycemia and glycosuria may influence the growth of microorganisms and increase the severity of the infection. Diabetes and elevated blood glucose levels also may impair host defenses such as the function of neutrophils and immune cells. Polymorphonuclear leukocyte function, particularly adherence, chemotaxis, and phagocytosis, are depressed in persons with diabetes, particularly those with poor glycemic control.

In summary, diabetes mellitus is a disorder of carbohydrate, protein, and fat metabolism resulting from an imbalance between insulin availability and insulin need. The disease can be classified as type 1 diabetes, in which there is destruction of beta cells and an absolute insulin deficiency, or type 2 diabetes, in which there is a lack of insulin availability or effectiveness. Type 1 diabetes can be further subdivided into type 1A immune-mediated diabetes, which is thought to be caused by autoimmune mechanisms, and type 1B idiopathic diabetes, for which the cause is unknown. Other specific types of diabetes include secondary forms of carbohydrate intolerance, which occur secondary to some other condition that destroys beta cells (e.g., pancreatic disorders) or endocrine diseases that cause increased production of glucose by the liver and decreased use of glucose by the tissues (e.g., Cushing syndrome). GDM develops during pregnancy, and although glucose tolerance often returns to normal after childbirth, it indicates an increased risk for the development of diabetes.

The diagnosis of diabetes mellitus is based on clinical signs of the disease, fasting plasma glucose levels, random plasma glucose measurements, and results of the glucose tolerance test. Self-monitoring provides a means of maintaining near-normal blood glucose levels through frequent testing of blood glucose and adjustment of insulin dosage. Glycosylation involves the irreversible attachment of glucose to the hemoglobin molecule; the measurement of A1C provides an index of blood glucose levels during a period of several months.

The treatment of diabetes includes diet, exercise, and, in many cases, the use of an antidiabetic agent. Dietary management focuses on maintaining a well-balanced diet, controlling calories to achieve and maintain an optimum weight, and regulating the distribution of carbohydrates, proteins, and fats. Two types of antidiabetic agents are used in the management of diabetes: injectable insulin (and newer injectable agents including amylin and GLP-1 analogs) and oral antidiabetic drugs. Type 1 diabetes, and sometimes type 2, requires treatment with injectable insulin. Oral antidiabetic drugs include the beta cell–stimulating agents, biguanides, α-glucosidase inhibitors, and TZDs. These drugs require a functioning pancreas and may be used in the treatment of type 2 diabetes.

The metabolic disturbances associated with diabetes affect almost every body system. The acute complications of diabetes include hypoglycemia in insulin-treated patients with diabetes, diabetic ketoacidosis, and hyperglycemic hyperosmolar state. The chronic complications of diabetes include the microvascular disorders that affect the non–insulin-dependent tissues, including the retina, kidneys, and peripheral nervous system, and the macrovascular disorders. Diabetic foot problems usually combine both microvascular and macrovascular disease.

Review Exercises

A 6-year-old boy is admitted to the emergency department with nausea, vomiting, and abdominal pain. He is very lethargic; his skin is warm, dry, and flushed; his pulse is rapid; and he has a sweet smell to his breath. His parents relate that he has been very thirsty during the past several weeks, his appetite has been poor, and he has been urinating frequently. His initial plasma glucose is 420 mg/dL and a urine test for ketones is strongly positive.

A. What is the most likely cause of this boy's elevated blood glucose and ketonuria? Explain his presenting signs and symptoms in terms of the elevated blood glucose and metabolic acidosis.

B. What type of treatment will this boy require?

A 53-year-old accountant presents for his routine yearly examination and was found to have a fasting glucose of 120 mg/dL on two occasions. Currently, he is asymptomatic. He has no other medical problems and does not use any medications. He neither smokes nor drinks alcohol. His father had type 2 diabetes at age 60 years. His physical examination reveals a blood pressure of 125/80, a BMI (body mass index) of 32 kg/m², and waist circumference of 45 inches. Laboratory study results are as follows: complete blood count (CBC), thyroid-stimulating hormone (TSH), alanine aminotransferase (ALT) are within normal limits; lipid panel: high-density lipoprotein (HDL) 30 mg/dL, low-density lipoprotein (LDL) 136 mg/dL, and triglycerides 290 mg/dL (normal <165 mg/dL).

A. What is this man's probable diagnosis?

B. Based on this man's blood glucose level and the ADA diabetes classification system, what diabetic status would you place this man in? Does he need a 75-g oral glucose tolerance test (OGTT) for further assessment of his impaired fasting plasma glucose (IFG)?

C. His OGTT results revealed 2-hour glucose value of 175 mg/dL. What is the diagnosis? What type of treatment would be appropriate for this man?

Visit the Porth: Essentials of Pathophysiology: Concepts of Altered Health States web site (http://thePoint.LWW.com/PorthEssentials) for links to chapter-related resources on the Internet, all-new exclusive animations, chapter review questions, and more!

REFERENCES

1. American Diabetes Association. (2005). Diabetes facts and figures. [On-line]. Available: www.diabetes.org.
2. Guyton A., Hall J. E. (2006). *Medical physiology* (11th ed., pp. 852, 865, 961–977). Philadelphia: W. B. Saunders.
3. Masharani U., Karam J. H., German M. S. (2004). Pancreatic hormones and diabetes. In Greenspan F. S., Gardner D. G. (Eds.), *Basic and clinical endocrinology* (7th ed., pp. 658–746), New York: Lange Medical Books/McGraw-Hill.
4. Shepard P. R., Kahn B. (1999). Glucose transporters and insulin action. *New England Journal of Medicine* 341, 248–256.
5. Goldfine I. R., Youngren J. F. (1998). Contributions of the *American Journal of Physiology* to the discovery of insulin. *American Journal of Physiology* 274, E207–E209.
6. Expert Committee on the Diagnosis and Classification of Diabetes Mellitus. (1997). Report of the Expert Committee on the Diagnosis and Classification of Diabetes Mellitus. *Diabetes Care* 20, 1183–1199.
7. Expert Committee on Diagnosis and Classification of Diabetes Mellitus (2003). Report of the Expert Committee on the Diagnosis and Classification of Diabetes Mellitus. *Diabetes Care* 26, 3160–3167.
8. Atkinson M. A., Eisenbarth G. S. (2001). Type 1 diabetes: New perspectives on disease pathogenesis and treatment. *Lancet* 358, 221–229.
9. Atkinson M. A. (2000). The $64,000 question in diabetes continues. *Lancet* 356, 4–5.
10. Bingley P. J., Bonifacio E., Ziegler A. G., et al. (2001). Proposed guidelines for screening for risk of type 1 diabetes. *Diabetes Care* 24, 398.
11. The International Diabetes Federation Consensus Workshop. (2004). Type 2 diabetes in the young: The evolving epidemic. *Diabetes Care* 27, 1798–1811.
12. Bays H., Mandarino L., DeFronzo R. A. (2004). Role of adipocyte, free fatty acid, and ectopic fat in pathogenesis of type 2 diabetes: Peroxisomal proliferator-activated receptor agonists provide a rational therapeutic approach. *Journal of Clinical Endocrinology and Metabolism* 89, 463–478.
13. Barry M. S. (2005). Type 2 diabetes: Principles of pathogenesis and therapy. *Lancet* 365, 1333–1346.
14. Gerich J. E. (2003). Contributions of insulin-resistance and insulin-secretory defects to the pathogenesis of type 2 diabetes. *Mayo Clinic Proceedings* 78, 447–456.
15. Guven S., El-Bershawi A., Sonnenberg G. E., et al. (1999). Persistent elevation in plasma leptin level in ex-obese with normal body mass index: Relation to body composition and insulin sensitivity. *Diabetes* 48, 347–352.
16. Yamauchi T., Kamon J., Waki H., et al. (2001). The fat-derived hormone adiponectin reverses insulin resistance associated with both lipoatrophy and obesity. *Nature Medicine* 7, 941–946.
17. Eckel R. H., Grundy S. M., Zimmet P. Z. (2005). The metabolic syndrome. *Lancet* 365, 1415–1428.
18. Grundy S. M., Panel Chair. (2001). *Third report of the National Cholesterol Education Program (NCEP) Expert Panel on Detection, Evaluation, and Treatment of High Blood Cholesterol in Adults (Adult Treatment Panel III).* NIH publication no. 01-3670. Bethesda, MD: National Institutes of Health.
19. Ehrmann D. A. (2005). Medical progress: Polycystic ovary syndrome. *New England Journal of Medicine* 352, 1223–1236.
20. Winter W. E., Kamura M., House D. W. (1999). Monogenic diabetes mellitus in youth: The MODY syndrome. *Metabolic Clinics of North America* 28, 765–785.
21. American Diabetes Association. (2004). Gestational diabetes mellitus. *Diabetes Care* 27(Suppl. 1), S88–S90.
22. American Diabetes Association. (2005). Standards of medical care for patients with diabetes mellitus. *Diabetes Care* 28 (Suppl. 1), S14–S36.
23. American Diabetes Association. (2004). Tests of glycemia in diabetes. *Diabetes Care* 27(Suppl. 1), S91–S93.
24. Shichiri M., Kishikquq H., Ohkubo Y., et al. (2000). Long-term results of Kumamoto Study on optimal diabetes control in type 2 diabetes patients. *Diabetes Care* 23(Suppl. 2), B21–B29.
25. American Diabetes Association. (2004). Evidence-based nutrition principles and recommendations for the treatment and prevention of diabetes and related complications (position statement). *Diabetes Care* 27(Suppl. 1), S36–S46.

26. American Diabetes Association. (2004). Physical activity/ exercise and diabetes mellitus. *Diabetes Care* 27(Suppl. 1), S55–S59.

27. Nathan D. M. (2002). Initial management of glycemia in type 2 diabetic mellitus. *New England Journal of Medicine* 347, 1342–1349.

28. Chan J. L., Abrahamson M. J. (2003). Pharmacological management of type 2 diabetes. *Mayo Clinic Proceedings* 78, 459–467.

29. Zangeneh F., Kudva Y. C., Basu A. (2003). Insulin sensitizers. *Mayo Clinic Proceedings* 78, 471–479.

30. Kadowaki T., Yamauchi T. (2005). Adiponectin and adiponectin receptors. *Endocrine Reviews* 26, 439–451.

31. American Diabetes Association. (2004). Continuous subcutaneous insulin infusion. *Diabetes Care* 27(Suppl. 1), S110.

32. American Diabetes Association. (2004). Pancreas transplantation for patients with type 1 diabetes. *Diabetes Care* 27 (Suppl. 1), S105.

33. Shapiro J., Lakey J., Ryan E., et al. (2000). Islet transplantation with type 1 diabetes mellitus using glucocorticoid-free immunosuppressive regimen. *New England Journal of Medicine* 343, 230–238.

34. American Diabetes Association. (2004). Hyperglycemic crises in patients with diabetes mellitus. *Diabetes Care* 27(Suppl. 1), S94–S102.

35. Karam J. H., Masharani U. (2004). Hypoglycemic disorders. In Greenspan F. S., Gardner D. G. (Eds.), *Basic and clinical endocrinology* (7th ed., pp. 747–765). New York: Lange Medical Books/McGraw-Hill.

36. Somogyi M. (1957). Exacerbation of diabetes in excess insulin action. *American Journal of Medicine* 26, 169–191.

37. Bolli G. B., Gotterman I. S., Campbell P. J. (1984). Glucose counterregulation and waning of insulin in the Somogyi phenomenon (posthypoglycemic hyperglycemia). *New England Journal of Medicine* 311, 1214–1219.

38. Bolli G. B., Gerich J. E. (1984). The dawn phenomenon: A common occurrence in both non-insulin and insulin dependent diabetes mellitus. *New England Journal of Medicine* 310, 746–750.

39. Sheetz M. J., King G. L. (2002). Molecular understanding of hyperglycemia's adverse effects for diabetic complications. *Journal of the American Medical Association* 288, 2579–2588.

40. The Diabetes Control and Complications Trial Research Group. (1993). The effect of intensified treatment of diabetes on the development and progression of long-term complications in insulin-dependent diabetes mellitus. *New England Journal of Medicine* 329, 955–977.

41. Stratton I. M., Adler A. I., Neil H. A., et al. (2000). Association of glycaemia with macrovascular and microvascular complications in type 2 diabetes (UKPDS 35): Prospective observational study. *British Medical Journal* 321, 405–412.

42. Vinik A. I. (1999). Diabetic neuropathy: Pathogenesis and therapy. *American Journal of Medicine* 107(Suppl. 2B), 17S–26S.

43. Camilleri M., Prather C. M. (1998). Gastric motor physiology and motor disorders. In Feldman M., Sleisenger M. H., Scharschmidt B. F., et al. (Eds.), *Sleisenger and Fordtran's gastrointestinal and liver disease* (6th ed., pp. 572–586). Philadelphia: W. B. Saunders.

44. Lysy J., Israeli E., Goldin E. (1999). The prevalence of chronic diarrhea among diabetic patients. *American Journal of Gastroenterology* 94, 2165–2170.

45. AACE Male Sexual Dysfunction Taskforce. (2003). AACE medical guidelines for clinical practice for the evaluation and treatment of male sexual dysfunction: a couple's problem— 2003 update. *Endocrine Practice* 9, 77–95.

46. American Diabetes Association. (2004). Diabetic nephropathy. *Diabetes Care* 27(Suppl. 1), S79–S83.

47. Renal Data System. (1998, April). *USRDS 1998 annual data report.* NIH publication no. 98:3176. Bethesda, MD: National Institute of Diabetes and Digestive and Kidney Diseases.

48. Ritz E., Orth S. R. (1999). Nephropathy in patients with type 2 diabetes mellitus. *New England Journal of Medicine* 341, 1127–1133.

49. Krolewski A. S., Laffel L. M. B., Krolewski M., et al. (1995). Glycosylated hemoglobin and the risk of microalbuminemia in patients with insulin-dependent diabetes mellitus. *New England Journal of Medicine* 332, 1251–1255.

50. American Diabetes Association. (2004). Diabetic retinopathy. *Diabetes Care* 27(Suppl. 1), S84–S87.

51. Aiello L. P., Gardner T. W., King G. L., et al. (1998). Diabetic retinopathy [technical review]. *Diabetes Care* 21, 143–156.

52. American College of Endocrinology. (2003). ACE position statement on the insulin resistance syndrome. *Endocrine Practice* 9, 237–252.

53. American Diabetes Association. (2004). Preventative foot care in people with diabetes. *Diabetes Care* 27(Suppl. 1), S63–S64.

54. Joshi N., Caputo G. M., Weitekamp M. R., et al. (1999). Infections in patients with diabetes mellitus. *New England Journal of Medicine* 341, 1906–1912.

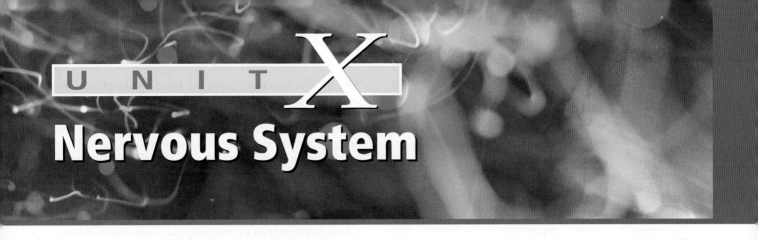

UNIT X
Nervous System

Chapter *33*

Organization and Control of Neural Function

 The nervous system, in coordination with the endocrine system, provides the means by which cell and tissue functions are integrated into a solitary, surviving organism. It controls skeletal muscle movement and helps to regulate cardiac and visceral smooth muscle activity. The nervous system enables the reception, integration, and perception of sensory information; it provides the substratum necessary for intelligence, anticipation, and judgment; and it facilitates adjustment to an ever-changing external environment.

Nervous Tissue Cells

The nervous system can be divided into two basic components: the central nervous system (CNS) and the peripheral nervous system (PNS). The CNS consists of the brain and spinal cord, which is protected by the skull and vertebral column, whereas the PNS is found outside these structures. Inherent in the basic design of the nervous system is the provision for the concentration of computational and control functions in the CNS, with the PNS relaying somatic and visceral sensory (afferent) input to the CNS for processing and transmitting efferent or motor output from the CNS to effector organs throughout the body (Fig. 33-1). Functionally, the nervous system is divided into the somatic and visceral or autonomic nervous systems. The somatic (Greek *soma,* "body") nervous system provides sensory and motor innervation for all parts of the CNS and PNS except viscera, smooth muscle, and glands. The autonomic nervous system (ANS) provides efferent

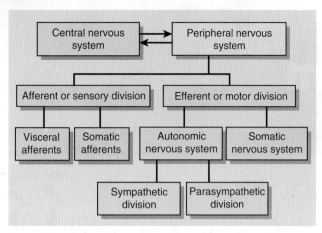

FIGURE 33-1 Organization of the central nervous system and the afferent input and efferent output of the peripheral nervous system.

motor innervation to smooth muscle, the conducting system of the heart, and glands. The ANS is further divided into a sympathetic division and a parasympathetic division.

Nervous tissue consists of two principal types of cells, neurons and supporting cells. The neurons are the functional cells of the nervous system. They exhibit membrane excitability and conductivity and secrete neurotransmitters and hormones, such as epinephrine and antidiuretic hormone. The supporting cells, such as the Schwann cells in the PNS and the glial cells in the CNS, protect the nervous system and provide metabolic support for the neurons.

NEURONS

Neurons, which are the functioning cells of the nervous system, have three distinct parts: the cell body and its cytoplasm-filled processes, the dendrites and axons (Fig.

KEY CONCEPTS

The Structural Organization of the Nervous System

➤ The nervous system is divided into two parts: the CNS, which consists of the brain and spinal cord, and the PNS, which contains the input and output neurons that lie outside the CNS.

➤ The neurons, which are functioning cells of the nervous system, consist of a cell body with cytoplasm-filled processes, the dendrites, and the axons, which form the functional connections with other nerve or effector cells.

➤ There are two types of neurons: afferent neurons or sensory neurons, which carry information to the CNS, and efferent neurons or motoneurons, which carry information from the CNS to the effector organs.

33-2B). The processes form the functional connections, or synapses, with other nerve cells, receptor cells, or effector cells. Axonal processes are particularly designed for rapid communication with other neurons and the many body structures innervated by the nervous system. Afferent, or sensory, neurons of the PNS transmit information to the CNS (see Fig. 33-2A), whereas efferent, or motor neurons, carry information away from the CNS (see Fig. 33-2B). Interspersed between the afferent and efferent neurons is a network of interconnecting neurons (also called *interneurons* or *internuncial* neurons) that modulate and control the body's response to changes in the internal and external environments.

The *cell body* of a neuron, also known as the *soma*, contains a large vesicular nucleus with one or more distinct nucleoli and a well-developed rough endoplasmic reticulum. A neuron's nucleus has the same deoxyribonucleic acid (DNA) and genetic code content that is present in other cells of the body, and its nucleolus, which is composed of portions of several chromosomes, produces ribonucleic acid (RNA) associated with protein synthesis. The cytoplasm contains large masses of ribosomes that are prominent in most neurons. These acidic RNA masses, which are involved in protein synthesis, stain as dark Nissl bodies with basic histologic stains (see Fig. 33-2B). The Nissl bodies and free ribosomes extend into the dendrites, but not into the axon. This area of the cell body, called the *axon hillock*, is free of large cytoplasmic organelles and serves as a landmark to distinguish between axons and dendrites in microscopic preparations.

The *dendrites* (*i.e.,* "treelike") are multiple, branched extensions of the nerve cell body; they conduct information toward the cell body and are the main source of information for the neuron. The dendrites and cell body are studded with synaptic terminals that communicate with axons and dendrites of other neurons.

Axons are long efferent processes that project from the cell body and carry impulses away from the cell. Most neurons have only one axon; however, axons may exhibit multiple branching that results in many axonal terminals. The cytoplasm of the cell body extends to fill the dendrites and the axon. The proteins and other materials used by the axon are synthesized in the cell body and then flow down the axon through its cytoplasm.

The cell body of the neuron is equipped for a high level of metabolic activity. This is necessary because the cell body must synthesize the cytoplasmic and membrane constituents required to maintain the function of the axon and its terminals. Some of these axons extend for a distance of 1 to 1.5 m and have a volume that is 200 to 500 times greater than the cell body itself. Two axonal transport systems, one slow and one rapid, move molecules from the cell body through the cytoplasm of the axon to its terminals. Replacement proteins and nutrients slowly diffuse from the cell body, where they are transported, down the axon, moving at the rate of approximately 1 mm/day. Other molecules, such as some neurosecretory granules (*e.g.,* neurotransmitters, neuromodulators, and neurohormones) or their precursors, are conveyed by a rapid,

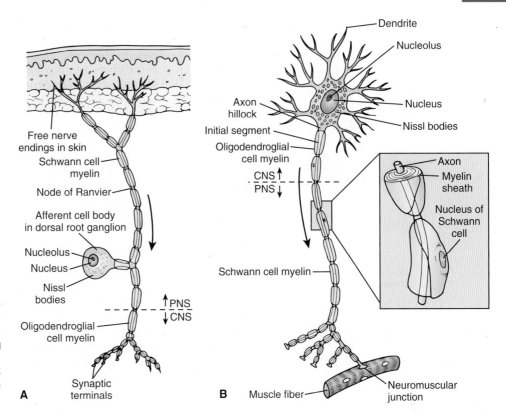

FIGURE 33-2 (**A**) Afferent and (**B**) efferent neurons, showing the soma or cell body, dendrites, and axon. Long arrows indicate the direction for conduction of action potentials.

energy-dependent active transport system, moving at the rate of approximately 400 mm/day. For example, antidiuretic hormone and oxytocin, which are synthesized by neurons in the hypothalamus, are carried by rapid axonal transport to the posterior pituitary, where the hormones are released into the blood. A reverse rapid (*i.e.,* retrograde) axonal transport system moves materials, including target cell messenger molecules, from axonal terminals back to the cell body.

SUPPORTING CELLS

Supporting cells of the nervous system, the Schwann and satellite cells of the PNS and the several types of glial cells of the CNS, give the neurons protection and metabolic support. The supporting cells segregate the neurons into isolated metabolic compartments, which are required for normal neural function. Astrocytes, together with the tightly joined endothelial cells of the capillaries in the CNS, contribute to what is called the *blood-brain barrier*. This term is used to emphasize the impermeability of the nervous system to large or potentially harmful molecules.

The many-layered myelin wrappings of Schwann cells of the PNS and the oligodendroglia of the CNS produce the myelin sheaths that serve to increase the velocity of nerve impulse conduction in axons. Myelin has a high lipid content, which gives it a whitish color, and hence the name *white matter* is given to the masses of myelinated fibers of the spinal cord and brain. Besides its role in increasing conduction velocity, the myelin sheath is essential for the survival of larger neuronal processes, perhaps by the secretion of neurotrophic compounds.

In some pathologic conditions, such as multiple sclerosis in the CNS and Guillain-Barré syndrome in the PNS, the myelin may degenerate or be destroyed, leaving a section of the axonal process without myelin while leaving the nearby Schwann or oligodendroglial cells intact. Unless remyelination takes place, the axon eventually dies.

Supporting Cells of the Peripheral Nervous System

Schwann cells and satellite cells are the two types of supporting cells in the PNS. Normally, the nerve cell bodies in the PNS are collected into ganglia, such as the dorsal root and autonomic ganglia. The cell bodies and processes of the peripheral nerves are separated from the connective tissue framework of the ganglion by a single layer of flattened capsular cells called *satellite cells*. Satellite cells secrete a basement membrane that protects the cell body from the diffusion of large molecules.

The processes of larger afferent and efferent neurons are surrounded by the cell membrane and cytoplasm of Schwann cells, which are close relatives of the satellite cells. During myelination, the Schwann cell wraps around the nerve process many times in a "jelly roll" fashion (Fig. 33-3). Schwann cells line up along the neuronal process, and each of these cells forms its own discrete myelin segment. Successive Schwann cells are separated by short extracellular fluid gaps called the *nodes of Ranvier*, where the myelin is missing and voltage-gated sodium channels are concentrated. The nodes of Ranvier increase nerve conduction by allowing the impulse to jump from node to node through the extracellular fluid in a process called

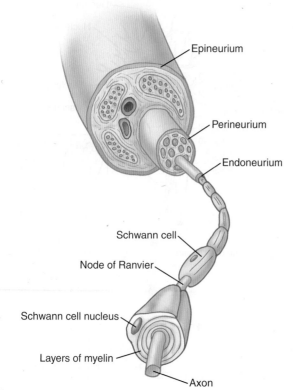

Epineurium

Perineurium

Endoneurium

Schwann cell

Node of Ranvier

Schwann cell nucleus

Layers of myelin

Axon

FIGURE 33-3 Section of a peripheral nerve. Schwann cells form a myelin sheath around the nerve fiber. Successive Schwann cells are separated by short extracellular fluid gaps called the *nodes of Ranvier,* where the myelin is missing and the voltage-gated sodium channels are concentrated. Each of the Schwann cells along a peripheral nerve is encased in an endoneurial sheath, with small bundles of nerves or fascicles being surrounded by another protective covering called the *perineurium* and several fascicles being surrounded by the epineurium.

saltatory conduction (from the Latin *saltare,* "to jump"). In this way, the impulse can travel more rapidly than it could if it were required to move systematically along the entire nerve process. This increased conduction velocity greatly reduces reaction time, or time between the application of a stimulus and the subsequent motor response. The short reaction time is of particular importance in peripheral nerves with long distances (sometimes 1 to 1.5 m) for conduction between the CNS and distal effector organs.

Each of the Schwann cells along a peripheral nerve is encased in a continuous tube of basement membrane, which in turn is surrounded by a multilayered sheath of loose connective tissue known as the *endoneurium* (see Fig. 33-3). The endoneurial sheath, which is essential to the regeneration of injured peripheral nerves, provides a collagenous tube through which a regenerating axon can again reach its former target. The endoneurial sheath does not penetrate the CNS. The absence of the endoneurial sheath is thought to be a major factor in the limited axonal regeneration of CNS nerves compared with those of the PNS.

The endoneurial sheaths are bundled with blood vessels into small bundles or clusters of nerves called *fascicles.* In the nerve, the fascicles consisting of bundles of nerve fibers are surrounded by another protective covering called the *perineurium.* Usually, several fascicles are further surrounded by the heavy, protective *epineurial sheath* of the peripheral nerve. The protective layers that surround the peripheral nerve processes are continuous with the connective tissue capsule of the sensory nerve endings and the connective tissue that surrounds the effector structures, such as the skeletal muscle cell. Centrally, the connective tissue layers continue along the dorsal and ventral roots of the nerve and fuse with the meninges that surround the spinal cord and brain.

Supporting Cells of the Central Nervous System

Supporting cells of the CNS consist of the oligodendrocytes, astrocytes, microglial cells, and ependymal cells (Fig. 33-4). The *oligodendrocytes* form the myelin in the CNS. Instead of forming a myelin covering for a single axon, these cells reach out with several processes, each wrapping around and forming a multilayered myelin segment around several different axons. The coverings of axons in the CNS function in increasing the velocity of nerve conduction, similar to the peripheral myelinated fibers.

A second type of glial cell, the *astrocyte,* is particularly prominent in the gray matter of the CNS. These large cells have many processes, some reaching to the surface of the capillaries, others reaching to the surface of the nerve cells, and still others filling most of the intercellular space of the CNS. The astrocytic linkage between the blood vessels and the neurons may provide a transport mechanism for the exchange of oxygen, carbon dioxide, and metabolites. The astrocytes also have an important role in sequestering cations such as calcium and potassium from the intercellular fluid. Astrocytes can fill their cytoplasm with microfibrils (*i.e.,* fibrous astrocytes), and masses of these cells form the special type of scar tissue called *gliosis* that develops in the CNS when tissue is destroyed.

A third type of glial cell, the *microglial cell,* is a small phagocytic cell that is available for cleaning up debris after cellular damage, infection, or cell death. The fourth type of cell, the *ependymal cell,* forms the lining of the neural tube cavity, the ventricular system. In some areas, these cells combine with a rich vascular network to form the *choroid plexus,* where production of the cerebrospinal fluid (CSF) takes place.

METABOLIC REQUIREMENTS OF NERVOUS TISSUE

Nervous tissue has a high rate of metabolism. Although the brain comprises only 2% of the body's weight, it receives approximately 15% of the resting cardiac output and consumes 20% of its oxygen. Despite its substantial energy requirements, the brain can neither store oxygen nor engage in anaerobic metabolism. An interruption in the blood or oxygen supply to the brain rapidly leads to

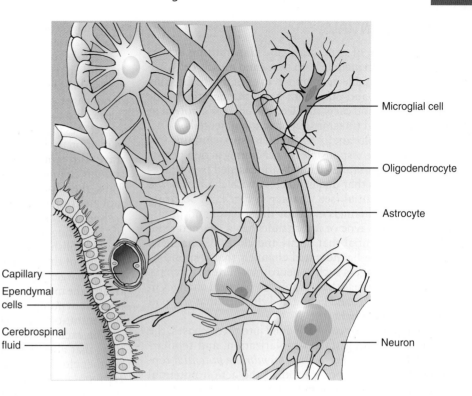

FIGURE 33-4 Supporting cells of the central nervous system (CNS). Diagrammatic view of the relationships among the glial elements (astrocyte, oligodendrocyte, microglial cell, and ependymal cells), capillaries, cerebrospinal fluid, and cell bodies of neurons in the CNS.

clinically observable signs and symptoms. Without oxygen, brain cells continue to function for approximately 10 seconds. Unconsciousness occurs almost simultaneously with cardiac arrest, and the death of brain cells begins within 4 to 6 minutes. Interruption of blood flow also leads to the accumulation of metabolic byproducts that are toxic to neural tissue.

Glucose is the major fuel source for the nervous system. Unlike muscle cells, however, neurons have no glycogen stores and must rely on glucose from the blood or the glycogen stores of supporting glial cells to meet their energy needs. Persons receiving insulin for diabetes may experience signs of neural dysfunction and unconsciousness (*i.e.,* insulin reaction or shock) when blood glucose drops because of insulin excess (see Chapter 32).

In summary, the nervous system can be divided into two basic components: the CNS or brain and spinal cord, which are located within the skull and vertebral column, and PNS, which is located outside these structures. Inherent in the basic design of the nervous system is the provision for the concentration of computational and control functions in the CNS, with the PNS relaying input to the CNS for processing and transmitting output from the CNS to effector organs throughout the body.

Nervous tissue consists of two types of cells: neurons and supporting cells. Neurons, which are the functional components of the nervous system, are composed of three parts: a cell body, which controls cell activity; the dendrites, which conduct information toward the cell body; and the axon, which carries impulses from the cell body. The supporting cells consist of Schwann and satellite cells of the PNS and the oligodendrocytes, astrocytes, microglial cells, and ependymal cells of the CNS. The supporting cells protect and provide metabolic support for the neurons and aid in segregating them into isolated compartments, which is necessary for normal neuronal function. The Schwann cells of the PNS and the oligodendroglial cells of the CNS form the myelin sheath that allows for rapid conduction of impulses.

The nervous system has a high level of metabolic activity, requiring a continuous supply of oxygen and glucose. Although the brain comprises only 2% of the body's weight, it receives approximately 15% of the resting cardiac output and consumes 20% of its oxygen.

 Nerve Cell Communication

Neurons are characterized by the ability to communicate with other neurons and body cells through pulsed electrical impulses or action potentials, which are abrupt, pulsatile changes in the membrane potential that last a few ten thousandths to a few thousandths of a second. The frequency and pattern of action potentials constitute the code used by neurons to transfer information from one location to another.

ACTION POTENTIALS

Tissues capable of generating and transmitting action potentials, which include both nerve and muscle cells, are said to have excitable membranes. In excitable tissue, ions such as sodium and potassium move through the membrane channels and carry the electrical charges involved in the initiation and transmission of action potentials.

The cell membrane of excitable tissues contains ion channels that are responsible for generating action potentials. These membrane channels are guarded by voltage-dependent gates that open and close with changes in the membrane potential (see Chapter 1, Fig. 1-9). Separate voltage-gated channels exist for the sodium and potassium ions. Each type of ion channel has a characteristic membrane potential that opens and closes its channels. Also present are ligand-gated channels that respond to chemical messengers such as neurotransmitters, mechanically gated channels that respond to physical changes in the cell membrane, and light-gated channels that respond to fluctuations in light levels.

Action potentials can be divided into three phases: the polarized or resting state, depolarization, and repolarization (Fig. 33-5). The *resting membrane potential* represents the undisturbed period of the action potential during which the nerve is not transmitting impulses (discussed in Chapter 1). During this time the inside of the membrane is negatively charged with respect to the outside, and the membrane is said to be *polarized*. The resting phase of the membrane potential continues until some event causes the membrane to increase its permeability to sodium. The *threshold potential* represents the membrane potential at which neurons or other excitable tissues are stimulated to fire. When the threshold potential is reached, the gatelike structures in the ion channels open. The gates are either fully open or fully closed (all-or-none). Under ordinary circumstances, the threshold stimulus is sufficient to open large numbers of ion channels, triggering massive depolarization of the membrane (the action potential).

Depolarization is characterized by the flow of electrically charged ions across the membrane, causing a reversal in the resting membrane potential. During the depolarization phase, the membrane suddenly becomes permeable to sodium ions. The rapid inflow of sodium ions causes the inside of the membrane to become positive in relation to the outside and produces local currents that travel through the adjacent cell membrane, causing the sodium channels in this part of the membrane to open. Thus, the impulse travels longitudinally along the nerve, moving from one part of the axon to another.

Repolarization is the phase during which the polarity of the resting membrane potential is reestablished. This is accomplished with closure of the sodium channels and opening of the potassium channels. The outflow of positively charged potassium ions across the cell membrane returns the membrane potential to negativity. The sodium-potassium pump gradually reestablishes the resting ionic concentrations on each side of the membrane.

The excitability of neurons can be affected by conditions that alter the resting membrane potential, moving it either closer to or further from the threshold potential. *Hypopolarization* increases the excitability of the postsynaptic neuron by bringing the membrane potential closer to the threshold potential so that a smaller subsequent stimulus is needed to cause the neuron to fire. *Hyperpolarization* brings the membrane potential further from threshold and has the opposite effect. It has an inhibitory effect and decreases the likelihood that an action potential will be generated.

SYNAPTIC TRANSMISSION

Neurons communicate with each other through structures known as *synapses*. Two types of synapses are found in the nervous system: electrical and chemical. *Electrical synapses* permit the passage of current-carrying ions through small openings called *gap junctions* that penetrate the cell junction of adjoining cells and allow current to travel in either direction. The gap junctions allow an action potential to pass directly and quickly from one neuron to another and often serve to link neurons having close functional relationships into circuits.

The most common type of synapse is the *chemical synapse*. Chemical synapses involve special presynaptic and postsynaptic membrane structures, separated by a synaptic cleft. The presynaptic terminal secretes one and often several chemical transmitter molecules (*i.e.*, neurotransmitters or neuromodulators). The secreted neurotransmitters diffuse into the synaptic cleft and unite with receptors on the postsynaptic membrane. In contrast to an electrical synapse, a chemical synapse serves as a rectifier, permitting only one-way communication. Chemical synapses are divided into two types: excitatory and inhibitory. In excitatory synapses, binding of the neurotransmitter to the receptor produces depolarization of the postsynaptic membrane. Binding of the neurotransmitter to the receptor in an inhibitory synapse reduces the post-

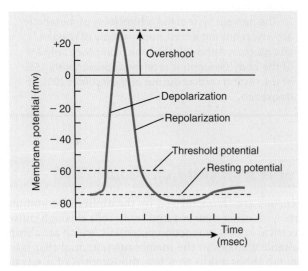

FIGURE 33-5 Time course of the action potential recorded at one point of an axon with one electrode inside and one on the outside of the plasma membrane.

synaptic neuron's ability to generate an action potential. Most inhibitory neurotransmitters induce hyperpolarization of the postsynaptic membrane by making the membrane more permeable to potassium or chloride, or both (see Chapter 6).

Chemical synapses are the slowest component in progressive communication through a sequence of neurons, such as in a spinal reflex. In contrast to the conduction of electrical synapses, each successive event at the chemical synapse—transmitter secretion, diffusion across the synaptic cleft, interaction with postsynaptic receptors, and generation of a subsequent action potential in the postsynaptic neuron—consumes time.

A neuron's cell body and dendrites are covered by thousands of synapses, any or many of which can be active at any moment. Because of the interaction of this rich synaptic input, each neuron resembles a little integrator, in which circuits of many neurons interact with one another. It is the complexity of these interactions and the subtle integrations involved in producing behavioral responses that give rise to the nervous system's intelligence.

MESSENGER MOLECULES

The function of the nervous system relies on chemical messengers. These messengers include the neurotransmitters, neuromodulators, and neurotrophic or nerve growth factors.

Neurotransmitters

Neurotransmitters are small molecules that incorporate a positively charged nitrogen atom; they include several amino acids, peptides, and monoamines. *Amino acids* are the building blocks of proteins and are present in body fluids. The amino acids glutamine, glycine, and γ-aminobutyric acid (GABA) serve as neurotransmitters at most CNS synapses. GABA mediates most synaptic inhibition in the CNS. Drugs such as the benzodiazepines (*e.g.*, the tranquilizer diazepam [Valium]) and the barbiturates exert their action by binding to their own distinct receptor on a GABA-operated ion channel. The drugs by themselves do not open the channel, but they change the effect that GABA has when it binds to the channel at the same time as the drug. *Peptides* are low–molecular-weight molecules that are made up of two or more amino acids. They include substance P and the endorphins and enkephalins, which are involved in pain sensation and perception (see Chapter 34). A *monoamine* is an amine molecule containing one amino group (NH_2). Serotonin, dopamine, norepinephrine, and epinephrine are monoamines synthesized from amino acids. Fortunately, the blood-brain barrier protects the nervous system from circulating amino acids and other molecules with potential neurotransmitter activity.

The process of neurotransmission involves the synthesis, storage, and release of a neurotransmitter; the reaction of the neurotransmitter with a receptor; and termination of the receptor action. Neurotransmitters are synthesized in the cytoplasm of the axon terminal. The synthesis of

transmitters may require one or more enzyme-catalyzed steps (*e.g.*, one for acetylcholine and three for norepinephrine). Neurons are limited as to the type of transmitter they can synthesize by their enzyme systems. After synthesis, the neurotransmitter molecules are stored in the axon terminal in tiny, membrane-bound sacs called *synaptic vesicles*. These vesicles protect the neurotransmitters from enzyme destruction in the nerve terminal. There may be thousands of vesicles in a single terminal, each containing 10,000 to 100,000 transmitter molecules. The arrival of an impulse at a nerve terminal causes the vesicles to move to the cell membrane and release their transmitter molecules into the synaptic space.

Neurotransmitters exert their actions through specific proteins, called *receptors,* embedded in the postsynaptic membrane. These receptors are tailored precisely to match the size and shape of the transmitter. In each case, the interaction between a transmitter and receptor results in a specific physiologic response. The action of a transmitter is determined by the type of receptor (excitatory or inhibitory) to which it binds. For example, acetylcholine is excitatory when it is released at a myoneural junction, and it is inhibitory when it is released at the sinoatrial node in the heart. Receptors are named according to the type of neurotransmitter with which they interact. For example, a *cholinergic receptor* is a receptor that binds acetylcholine.

Rapid removal of a transmitter, once it has exerted its effects on the postsynaptic membrane, is necessary to maintain precise control of neural transmission. A released transmitter can undergo one of three fates: (1) it can be broken down into inactive substances by enzymes; (2) it can be taken back up into the presynaptic neuron in a process called *reuptake;* or (3) it can diffuse away into the intercellular fluid until its concentration is too low to influence postsynaptic excitability. For example, acetylcholine is rapidly broken down by acetylcholinesterase into acetic acid and choline, with the choline being taken back into the presynaptic neuron for reuse in acetylcholine synthesis. The catecholamines are largely taken back into the neuron in an unchanged form for reuse. Catecholamines also can be degraded by enzymes in the synaptic space or in the nerve terminals.

Humoral neurotransmitters reach their target cells through the bloodstream. Both the nervous system and the endocrine system use chemical molecules as messengers. As more information is obtained about the chemical messengers of these systems, the distinction between them becomes less evident. Many neurons, such as those in the adrenal medulla, secrete transmitters into the bloodstream, and it has been found that other neurons possess receptor sites for hormones. Many hormones have turned out to be neurotransmitters. Vasopressin (also known as *antidiuretic hormone*), a peptide hormone released from the posterior pituitary gland, acts as a hormone in the kidney and as a neurotransmitter for nerve cells in the hypothalamus. More than a dozen of these cell-to-cell and blood-borne messengers can relay signals in the nervous system or the endocrine system.

Understanding ➤ Synaptic Transmission

Neurons communicate with each other through chemical synapses and the use of neurotransmitters. Chemical synapses consist of a presynaptic neuron, a synaptic cleft, and a postsynaptic neuron. The communication process relies on (1) synthesis and release of the neurotransmitter from a presynaptic neuron, (2) binding of the neurotransmitter to receptors in the postsynaptic neuron, and (3) removal of the neurotransmitter from the receptor site.

1

Neurotransmitter synthesis and release. Neurotransmitter synthesis takes place in the presynaptic neuron, where it is stored in synaptic vesicles. Communication between the two neurons begins with a nerve impulse that stimulates the presynaptic neuron, followed by movement of the synaptic vesicles to the cell membrane and release of neurotransmitter into the synaptic cleft.

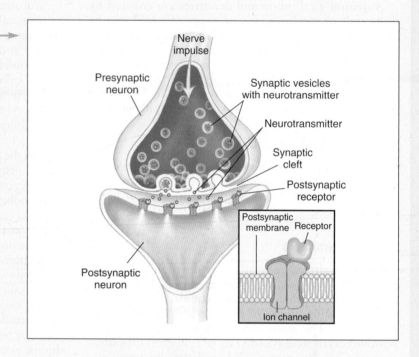

2

Receptor binding. Once released from the presynaptic neuron, the neurotransmitter moves across the synaptic cleft and binds to receptors on the postsynaptic neuron. The action of a neurotransmitter is determined by the type of receptor (excitatory or inhibitory) to which it binds. Binding of a neurotransmitter to a receptor with an excitatory function often results in the opening of an ion channel, such as the sodium channel. Many presynaptic neurons also have receptors to which a neurotransmitter binds. The presynaptic receptors function in a negative feedback manner to inhibit further release of the neurotransmitter.

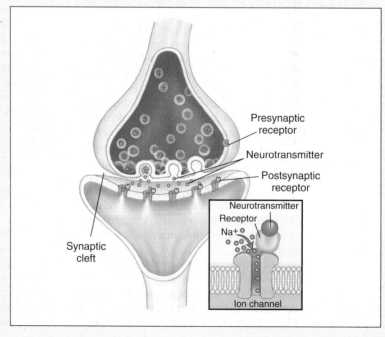

3

Neurotransmitter removal. Precise control of synaptic function relies on the rapid removal of the neurotransmitter from the receptor site. A released neurotransmitter can (1) be taken back up into the neuron in a process called *reuptake*, (2) diffuse out of the synaptic cleft, or (3) be broken down by enzymes into inactive substances or metabolites. The action of norepinephrine is largely terminated by the reuptake process, in which the neurotransmitter is taken back into the neuron in an unchanged form and reused. It can also be broken down by enzymes in the synaptic cleft or in the nerve terminals. The neurotransmitter acetylcholine is rapidly broken down by the enzyme acetylcholinesterase.

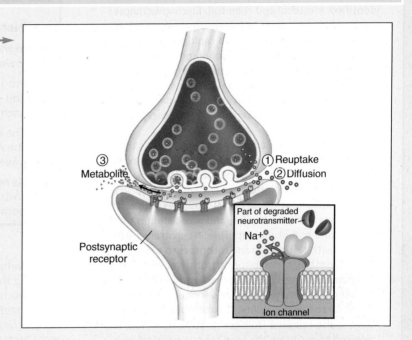

Neuromodulators

Other classes of messenger molecules, known as *neuro-modulators*, also may be released from axon terminals. Neuromodulator molecules react with presynaptic or postsynaptic receptors to alter the release of or response to neurotransmitters. Neuromodulators may act on postsynaptic receptors to produce slower and longer-lasting changes in membrane excitability. This alters the action of the faster-acting neurotransmitter molecules by enhancing or decreasing their effectiveness. By combining with autoreceptors on its own presynaptic membrane, a transmitter can act as a neuromodulator to augment or inhibit further nerve activity. In some nerves, such as the peripheral sympathetic nerves, a messenger molecule can have both transmitter and modulator functions. For example, norepinephrine can activate an α_1-adrenergic postsynaptic receptor to produce vasoconstriction or stimulate an α_2-adrenergic presynaptic receptor to inhibit further norepinephrine release.

Neurotrophic Factors

Neurotrophic or nerve growth factors are required to maintain the long-term survival of the postsynaptic cell and are secreted by axon terminals independent of action potentials. Examples include neuron-to-neuron trophic factors in the sequential synapses of CNS sensory neurons. Trophic factors from target cells that enter the axon and are necessary for the long-term survival of presynaptic neurons also have been demonstrated. Target cell–to-neuron trophic factors probably have great significance in establishing specific neural connections during normal embryonic development.

In summary, neurons communicate with other neurons and body cells through pulsed electrical signals called *action potentials*. The cell membranes of neurons contain ion channels that are responsible for generating action potentials. Action potentials are divided into three parts: the resting membrane potential, during which the membrane is polarized but no electrical activity occurs; the depolarization phase, during which sodium channels open, allowing rapid inflow of the sodium ions that generate the electrical impulse; and the repolarization phase, during which the membrane is permeable to the potassium ion, allowing for the efflux of potassium ions and return to the resting membrane potential.

Synapses are structures that permit communication between neurons. Two types of synapses have been identified: electrical and chemical. Electrical synapses consist of gap junctions between adjacent cells that allow action potentials to move rapidly from one cell to another. Chemical synapses involve special presynaptic and postsynaptic structures, separated by a synaptic cleft. They rely on chemical messengers, released from the presynaptic neuron, that cross the synaptic cleft and then interact with receptors on the postsynaptic neuron.

Neurotransmitters are chemical messengers that control neural function; they selectively cause excitation or inhibition of action potentials. Three major types of neurotransmitters are known: amino acids such as glutamic acid and GABA, peptides such as the endorphins and enkephalins, and monoamines such as epinephrine and norepinephrine. Neurotransmitters interact with cell membrane receptors to produce either excitatory or inhibitory actions. Neuromodulators are chemical messengers that react with membrane receptors to produce slower and longer-acting changes in membrane permeability. Neurotrophic or growth factors, also released from presynaptic terminals, are required to maintain the long-term survival of postsynaptic neurons.

Developmental Organization of the Nervous System

The organization of the nervous system can be described in terms of its development in which newer functions and greater complexity resulted from the modification and enlargement of more primitive structures. Thus, the rostral or front end of the CNS became specialized, with the more ancient organization being retained in the brain stem and spinal cord. The dominance of the front end of the CNS is reflected in what has been termed a *hierarchy of control*, with the forebrain having control over the brain stem and the brain stem having control over the spinal cord. In the developmental process, newer functions were added to the surface of functionally older systems. As newer functions became concentrated at the rostral end of the nervous system, they also became more vulnerable to injury. Nothing exemplifies this principle better than the persistent vegetative state (discussed in Chapter 36) that occurs when severe brain injury causes irreversible damage to higher cortical centers, while lower stem centers such as those that control breathing remain functional.

EMBRYONIC DEVELOPMENT

Throughout life, the organization of the nervous system retains many patterns that were established during embryonic life. It is this early pattern of segmental development

KEY CONCEPTS

Hierarchy of Nervous System Control

➤ In the nervous system, higher centers control lower centers.

➤ Progressively greater complexity in the responses and greater precision in their control occur at each higher level of the nervous system.

➤ The more rostral, recently developed parts of the neural tube gain dominance or control over lower levels.

➤ As newer functions became concentrated at the rostral end of the nervous system, they also became more vulnerable to injury.

in the embryo that is presented as a framework for understanding the nervous system.

All body tissues and organs, including those of the nervous system, have developed from the three embryonic layers (*i.e.*, endoderm, ectoderm, and mesoderm) that were present during the third week of embryonic life (Fig. 33-6). The mesoderm, which extends along the entire midline of the embryo, forms a specialized rod of embryonic tissue called the *notochord*. The notochord and adjacent mesoderm provide the necessary induction signal for the overlying ectoderm to differentiate and form a thickened

KEY CONCEPTS

The Developmental Organization of the Nervous System

➤ On cross section, the embryonic neural tube develops into a central canal surrounded by gray matter, or cellular portion (cell columns), and white matter, or tract system of the central nervous system (CNS).

➤ As the nervous system develops, it becomes segmented, with a repeating pattern of afferent neuron axons forming the dorsal roots of each succeeding segmental nerve and the exiting efferent neurons forming the ventral roots of each succeeding segmental nerve.

➤ The nerve cells in the gray matter are arranged longitudinally in cell columns, with afferent sensory neurons located in the dorsal columns and efferent motor neurons located in the ventral columns.

➤ The axons of the cell column neurons project out into the white matter of the CNS, forming the longitudinal tract systems.

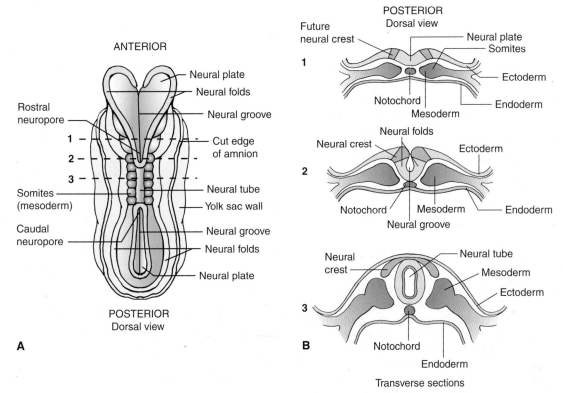

FIGURE 33-6 Folding of the neural tube. (**A**) Dorsal view of a six-somite embryo (22–23 days) showing the neural folds, neural groove, and the fused neural tube. The anterior neuropore closes at about day 25 and the posterior neuropore at about day 27. (**B**) Three cross-sections showing the ectoderm, mesoderm, endoderm, notochord, and neural crest cells taken at the levels indicated in (**A**). The sections indicate where the neural tube is just beginning to form. During development, the neural tube develops into the CNS and the notochord becomes the foundation on which the vertebral column develops. The neural crest cells become the progenitors of the neurons and supporting cells of the peripheral nervous system.

structure called the *neural plate*, the primordium of the nervous system. Within the neural plate an axial groove (*i.e.*, neural groove) develops that sinks into the underlying mesoderm; its walls fuse across the top, forming an ectodermal tube called the *neural tube*. This process, called *closure*, occurs during the later third and fourth weeks of gestation and is vital to the survival of the embryo. During development, the neural tube develops into the CNS, while the notochord becomes the foundation around which the vertebral column ultimately develops. The surface ectoderm separates from the neural tube and fuses over the top to become the outer layer of skin. Initial closure of the neural tube begins at the cervical and high thoracic levels and zippers rostrally toward the cephalic end of the embryo and caudally toward the sacrum. Complete closure occurs at the rostral-most end of the brain (*i.e.*, anterior neuropore) around day 25, and about day 27 in the lumbosacral region (*i.e.*, posterior neuropore). Most congenital abnormalities of the spinal cord result from defective closure of the neural tube during the fourth week of development. These neural tube defects affect the tissues overlying the spinal cord: meninges (*e.g.*, meningocele, meningomyelocele), vertebral arches (*e.g.*, spina bifida), muscles, and skin. Incomplete closure

of the vertebral arches is referred to as *spina bifida;* when it involves protrusion of a sac containing the meninges and CSF, it is referred to as *spina bifida with meningocele. Myelo* refers to the spinal cord; if the spinal cord is included in the sac, the defect is referred to as *spina bifida with meningomyelocele.*

As the neural tube closes, ectodermal cells called *neural crest cells* migrate away from the dorsal surface of the neural tube to become the progenitors of the neurons and supporting cells of the PNS (see Fig. 33-6). The more rostral portions of the embryonic neural tube—approximately 10 segments—undergo extensive modification and enlargement to form the brain. In the early embryo, 3 swellings, or primary vesicles, develop, subdividing these 10 segments into the prosencephalon, or forebrain, containing the first 2 segments; the mesencephalon, or midbrain, which develops from segment 3; and the rhombencephalon, or hindbrain, which develops from segments 4 to 10. All brain segments, except segment 2, retain some portion of the basic segmental organization of the nervous system. The evolutionary development of the brain is reflected in the cranial and upper cervical paired segmental nerves. This reflects the original pattern of a segmented neural tube, each segment of which has multiple paired branches containing a grouping of component axons. One segment would have paired branches to body muscles and another set to visceral structures, and so on. The classic pattern of spinal nerve organization, which consists of a pair of dorsal and a pair of ventral roots, is a later evolutionary development that has not occurred in the cranial nerves. Consequently, the cranial nerves, which are arbitrarily numbered 1 through 12, retain the ancient pattern, with more than one cranial nerve branching from a single segment. The truly segmental nerve pattern of the cranial nerves is altered because all branches from segment 2 and most of the branches from segment 1 are missing. Cranial nerve 2, also called the *optic nerve,* is not a segmental nerve. It is a brain tract connecting the retina (modified brain) with the first forebrain segment from which it developed.

Soma and Viscera

The body is organized into the soma and viscera. The *soma,* or body wall, includes all of the structures derived from the embryonic ectoderm, such as the epidermis of the skin and the CNS. Mesodermal connective tissues of the soma include the dermis of the skin, skeletal muscle, bone, and the outer lining of the body cavity (*i.e.,* parietal pleura and peritoneum). These structures are innervated by the somatic nervous system. The *viscera* include the great vessels derived from the intermediate mesoderm, the urinary system, and the gonadal structures; they also include the inner lining of the body cavities, such as the visceral pleura and peritoneum, and the mesodermal tissues that surround the endoderm-lined gut and its derivative organs (*e.g.,* lungs, liver, and pancreas). The visceral nerves supply the visceral organs of the body, with the ANS transmitting efferent or motor information to the smooth muscles, cardiac muscle, and glandular structures of the body.

SEGMENTAL ORGANIZATION

Developmentally, the basic organizational pattern of the body is that of a longitudinal series of segments, each repeating the same fundamental pattern. Although the early muscular, skeletal, vascular, and excretory systems and the nerves that supply the somatic and visceral structures have the same segmental pattern, it is the nervous system that most clearly retains this organization in postnatal life. The CNS and its associated peripheral nerves consist of approximately 43 segments, 33 of which form the spinal cord and spinal nerves, and 10 of which form the brain and its cranial nerves.

The basic pattern of the CNS is that seen in the spinal cord—a central cavity surrounded by inner core of gray matter and a superficial layer of white matter (Fig. 33-7). The brain retains this organization, but it also contains additional regions of gray matter that are not evident in the spinal cord. The gray matter is functionally divided into longitudinal columns of nerve cell bodies called the *cell columns.* The superficial white matter region contains the longitudinal tract systems of the CNS. The dorsal half

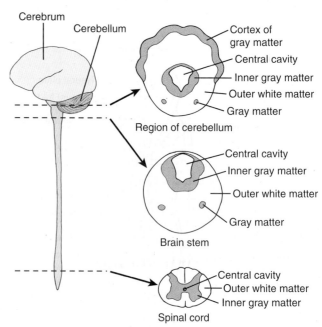

FIGURE 33-7 Segmental organization of gray and white matter in the CNS (highly simplified). From top to bottom, the diagrams represent cross-sections at the levels of cerebellum, brain stem, and spinal cord. In each section, the dorsal aspect is on top. In general, white matter lies external to gray matter; however, collections of gray matter migrate externally into the white matter in the developing brain (*arrows*). The cerebrum resembles the cerebellum in its external cortex of gray matter. (From Marieb E. N. [1995]. *Human anatomy and physiology* [3rd ed., p. 383]. Redwood City, CA: Benjamin/Cummings.)

or dorsal horn of the gray matter contains afferent neurons. The ventral portion, or *ventral horn,* contains efferent neurons that communicate by way of the ventral roots with effector cells of the body segment. Many CNS neurons develop axons that grow longitudinally as tract systems that communicate between neighboring and distal segments of the neural tube.

Each segment of the CNS is accompanied by bilateral pairs of bundled nerve fibers, or roots, a ventral pair and a dorsal pair (Fig. 33-8). The paired dorsal roots connect a pair of dorsal root ganglia and their corresponding CNS segment. The dorsal root ganglia contain many afferent nerve cell bodies, each having two axon-like processes—one that ends in a peripheral receptor and the other that enters the dorsal horn of its respective CNS segment. The axon-like process that enters the dorsal horn communicates with a neuron called an *input association (IA) neuron.* The paired ventral roots of each segment are bundles of axons that provide efferent output to effector sites such as the muscles and glandular cells of the body segment.

Cell Columns

The organizational structure of the nervous system can be best explained and simplified as a pattern in which functionally specific PNS and CNS neurons are repeated as parallel cell columns running lengthwise along the ner-

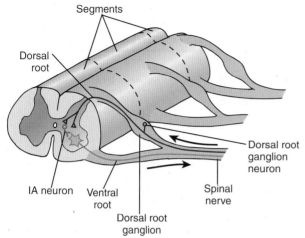

FIGURE 33-8 Three segments of the spinal cord depicting the left side of its bilateral pair of dorsal and ventral nerve roots. The dorsal root ganglia contain many afferent nerve cell bodies, each having two axon-like processes: one ends in a peripheral receptor and the other enters the dorsal horn of the spinal cord, where it communicates with an input association (IA) neuron. The ventral roots contain nerves that supply efferent output to effector sites such as muscles and glandular cells of the body.

vous system. In this organizational pattern, afferent neurons, dorsal horn cells, and ventral horn cells are organized as a bilateral series of 11 cell columns.

The cell columns on each side can be further grouped according to their location in the PNS: four in the dorsal root ganglia that contain sensory neurons; four in the dorsal horn containing sensory IA neurons; and three in the ventral horn that contain motor neurons (Fig. 33-9). Each column of dorsal root ganglia projects to its particular column of IA neurons in the dorsal horn. The IA neurons distribute afferent information to local reflex cir-

cuitry and to more rostral segments of the CNS. The ventral horns contain output association (OA) neurons and lower motor neurons, which project to the effector muscles. The afferent and efferent cell columns of the PNS and CNS, their projections, and the type of information they transmit are summarized in Table 33-1.

Between the IA neurons and the OA neurons are networks of small internuncial neurons arranged in complex circuits. Internuncial neurons provide the discreteness, appropriateness, and intelligence of responses to stimuli. Most of the billions of CNS cells in the spinal cord and brain gray matter are internuncial neurons.

Dorsal Horn Cell Columns. Four columns of afferent (sensory) neurons in the dorsal root ganglia directly innervate four corresponding columns of IA neurons in the dorsal horn. These columns are categorized as special and general afferents: special somatic afferent (SSA), general somatic afferent (GSA), special visceral afferent (SVA), and general visceral afferent (GVA).

The SSA fibers are concerned with internal sensory information such as joint and tendon sensation (*i.e.*, proprioception). Neurons in the special sensory IA cell columns relay their information to local reflexes concerned with posture and movement. These neurons also relay information to the cerebellum, contributing to coordination of movement, and to the forebrain, contributing to experience. Afferents innervating the vestibular system of the inner ear also belong to the special somatic afferent category.

The GSA neurons innervate the skin and other somatic structures, responding to stimuli such as those that produce pressure or pain. General sensory IA column neurons relay information to protective and other local reflex circuits and project the information to the forebrain, where it is perceived as painful, warm, cold, and the like.

FIGURE 33-9 Cell columns of the central nervous system. The cell columns in the dorsal horn contain input association (IA) neurons for the general visceral afferent (GVA), special visceral afferent (SVA), special sensory afferent (SSA), and general somatic afferent (GSA) neurons with cell bodies in the dorsal root ganglion. The cell columns in the ventral horn contain the general visceral efferent (GVE), pharyngeal efferent (PE), and general somite efferent (GSE) neurons and their output association (OA) neurons.

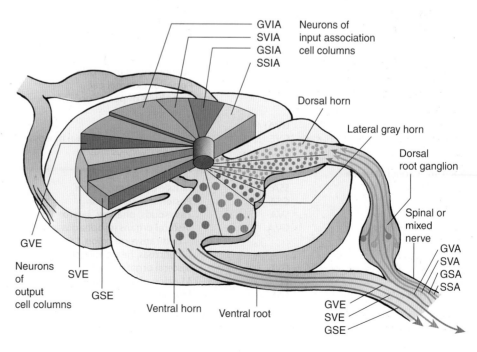

TABLE 33-1   The Segmental Nerves and Their Components

Segment and Nerve	Component	Innervation	Function
1. Forebrain			
I. Olfactory	SVA	Receptors in olfactory mucosa	Reflexes, olfaction (smell)
2. II. Optic nerve		Optic nerve and retina (part of brain system, not a peripheral nerve)	
3. Midbrain			
V. Trigeminal (V₁) ophthalmic division	SSA	Muscles: upper face: forehead, upper lid	Facial expression, proprioception
III. Oculomotor	GSA	Skin, subcutaneous tissue; conjunctiva; frontal/ethmoid sinuses	Somesthesia
	GVE	Iris sphincter and ciliary muscle of the eye	Reflexes (blink) Pupillary constriction Accommodation
	GSE	Extrinsic eye muscles	Eye movement, lid movement
4. Pons			
V. Trigeminal (V₂) maxillary division	SSA	Muscles: facial expression	Proprioception Reflexes (sneeze), somesthesia
	GSA	Skin, oral mucosa, upper teeth, hard palate, maxillary sinus	
V. Trigeminal (V₃) mandibular division	SSA	Lower jaw, muscles: mastication	Proprioception, jaw jerk
	GSA	Skin, mucosa, teeth, anterior ⅔ of tongue	Reflexes, somesthesia
	PE	Muscles: mastication tensor tympani tensor veli palatini	Mastication: speech Protects ear from loud sound Tenses soft palate
IV. Trochlear	GSE	Extrinsic eye muscle	Moves eye down and in
5. Caudal Pons			
VIII. Vestibular, cochlear (vestibulocochlear)	SSA	Vestibular end organs Organ of Corti	Reflexes, sense of head position Reflexes, hearing
VII. Facial nerve, intermedius portion	GSA	External auditory meatus	Somesthesia
	GVA	Nasopharynx	Gag reflex: sensation
	SVA	Taste buds of anterior ⅔ of tongue	Reflexes: gustation (taste)
	GVE	Nasopharynx Lacrimal, sublingual, submandibular glands	Mucous secretion, reflexes Lacrimation, salivation
Facial nerve	PE	Muscles: facial expression, stapedius	Facial expression Protects ear from loud sounds
VI. Abducens	GSE	Extrinsic eye muscle	Lateral eye deviation
6. Middle Medulla			
IX. Glossopharyngeal	SSA	Stylopharyngeus muscle	Proprioception
	GSA	Posterior external ear	Somesthesia
	SVA	Taste buds of posterior ⅓ of tongue	Gustation (taste)
	GVA	Oral pharynx	Gag reflex: sensation
	GVE	Parotid gland; pharyngeal mucosa	Salivary reflex: mucous secretion
	PE	Stylopharyngeus muscle	Assists swallowing
7,8,9,10. Caudal Medulla			
X. Vagus	SSA	Muscles: pharynx, larynx	Proprioception
	GSA	Posterior external ear	Somesthesia
	SVA	Taste buds, pharynx, larynx	Reflexes, gustation
	GVA	Visceral organs (esophagus to midtransverse colon, liver, pancreas, heart, lungs)	Reflexes, sensation
	GVE	Visceral organs as above	Parasympathetic efferent
	PE	Muscles: pharynx, larynx	Swallowing, phonation, emesis
XIII. Hypoglossal	GSE	Muscles of tongue	Tongue movement, reflexes

(continued)

TABLE 33-1	The Segmental Nerves and Their Components *(Continued)*		
Segment and Nerve	**Component**	**Innervation**	**Function**
Spinal Segments			
C1–C4 Upper Cervical	PE	Muscles: sternocleidomastoid, trapezius	Head, shoulder movement
XI. Spinal accessory nerve			
Spinal nerves	SSA	Muscles of neck	Proprioception, DTRs
	GSA	Neck, back of head	Somesthesia
	GSE	Neck muscles	Head, shoulder movement
C5–C8 Lower Cervical	SSA	Upper limb muscles	Proprioception, DTRs
	GSA	Upper limbs	Reflexes, somesthesia
	GSE	Upper limb muscles	Movement, posture
T1–L2 Thoracic, Upper Lumbar	SSA	Muscles: trunk, abdominal wall	Proprioception
	GSA	Trunk, abdominal wall	Reflexes, somesthesia
	GVA	All of viscera	Reflexes and sensation
	GVE	All of viscera	Sympathetic reflexes, vasomotor control, sweating, piloerection
	GSE	Muscles: trunk, abdominal wall, back	Movement, posture, respiration
L2–S1 Lower Lumbar, Upper Sacral	SSA	Lower limb muscles	Proprioception, DTRs
	GSA	Lower trunk, limbs, back	Reflexes, somesthesia
	GSE	Muscles: trunk, lower limbs, back	Movement, posture
S2–S4 Lower Sacral	SSA	Muscles: pelvis, perineum	Proprioception
	GSA	Pelvis, genitalia	Reflexes, somesthesia
	GVA	Hindgut, bladder, uterus	Reflexes, sensation
	GVE	Hindgut, visceral organs	Visceral reflexes, defecation, urination, erection
S5–Co2 Lower Sacral, Coccygeal	SSA	Perineal muscles	Proprioception
	GSA	Lower sacrum, anus	Reflexes, somesthesia
	GSE	Perineal muscles	Reflexes, posture

Afferent (sensory) components: SSA, special somatic afferent; GSA, general somatic afferent; SVA, special visceral afferent; GVA, general visceral afferent.
Efferent (motor) components: GVE, general visceral efferent (autonomic nervous system); PE, pharyngeal efferent; GSE, general somatic efferent; DTRs, deep tendon reflexes.

The SVAs innervate specialized gut-related receptors, such as the taste buds and receptors of the olfactory mucosa. Their central processes communicate with special visceral IA column neurons that project to reflex circuits producing salivation, chewing, swallowing, and other responses. Forebrain projection fibers from these association cells provide sensations of taste (*i.e.,* gustation) and smell (*i.e.,* olfaction).

GVA neurons innervate visceral structures such as the gastrointestinal tract, urinary bladder, and heart and great vessels; they project to the general visceral IA column, which relays information to vital reflex circuits and sends information to the forebrain regarding visceral sensations such as stomach fullness and bladder pressure.

Ventral Horn Cell Columns. The ventral horn contains three longitudinal cell columns: the general visceral efferent (GVE), pharyngeal efferent (PE), and general somatic efferent (GSE; see Fig. 33-9). The efferent neurons for the OA in the ventral horn originate in brain centers (motor cortex and ANS centers) that control skeletal muscle and visceral function. Each of these cell columns contains OA and efferent neurons. The OA neurons coordinate and integrate the function of the efferent motor neurons of its column.

The GVE neurons transmit the efferent output of the ANS and are called *preganglionic neurons.* These neurons are structurally and functionally divided between either the sympathetic or the parasympathetic nervous systems (discussed later in this chapter). Their axons project through the segmental ventral roots to innervate smooth and cardiac muscle and glandular cells of the body, most of which are in the viscera. In the viscera, three additional cell columns are present on each side of the body. These become the postganglionic neurons of the ANS. In the sympathetic nervous system, the columns are represented by the paravertebral or sympathetic chain ganglia and the prevertebral series of ganglia (*e.g.,* celiac ganglia) associated with the dorsal aorta. For the parasympathetic nervous system, these become the enteric plexus in the wall of the gut-derived organs and a series of ganglia in the head.

The PE neurons innervate the muscles of mastication and facial expression, as well as the muscles of the pharynx and larynx. PE neurons also innervate the muscles responsible for moving the head.

The GSE neurons supply skeletal muscles of the body and head, including those of the trunk, limbs, and tongue and the extrinsic eye muscles. These efferent neurons of the PNS transmit the commands of the CNS to peripheral effectors, the skeletal muscles. They are the "final common pathway neurons" in the sequence leading to motor activity. They often are called *lower motor neurons (LMNs)* because they are under the control of *upper motor neurons (UMNs)* that have their origin in the CNS.

Longitudinal Tracts

The gray matter of the cell columns in the CNS is surrounded by bundles of myelinated axons (*i.e.,* white matter) and unmyelinated axons that travel longitudinally along the length of the neural axis. This white matter can be divided into three layers: an inner, a middle, and an outer layer (Fig. 33-10). The inner layer contains short fibers that project for a maximum of approximately five segments before reentering the gray matter. The middle layer projects to six or more segments. The inner and middle layer fibers have many branches, or collaterals, that enter the gray matter of intervening segments. The outer layer contains large-diameter axons that can travel the entire length of the nervous system (Table 33-2). *Suprasegmental* is a term that refers to higher levels of the CNS, such as the brain stem and cerebrum and structures above a given CNS segment. The middle and outer layer fibers have suprasegmental projections.

The longitudinal layers are arranged in bundles, or fiber tracts, that contain axons that have either the same destination, origin, or function (Fig. 33-11). These longitudinal tracts are named systematically to reflect their origin and destination; the origin is named first, and the destination is named second. For example, the spinothalamic tract originates in the spinal cord and terminates in the thalamus. The corticospinal tract originates in the cerebral cortex and ends in the spinal cord.

The Inner Layer. The inner layer of white matter contains the axons of neurons that connect neighboring segments of the nervous system. Axons of this layer permit the pool of motor neurons of several segments to work together as a functional unit. They also allow the afferent neurons of one segment to trigger reflexes that activate motor units in neighboring and in the same segments. In terms of evolution, this is the oldest of the three layers, and it is sometimes called the *archilayer*. It is the first of the longitudinal layers to become functional, and its circuitry may be limited to reflex types of movements, including reflex movements of the fetus (*i.e.,* quickening) that begin during the fifth month of intrauterine life.

The archilayer of the white matter differs from the other two layers in one important aspect. Many neurons in the embryonic gray matter migrate out into this layer, resulting in a rich mixture of neurons and local fibers called the *reticular formation*. The circuitry of most reflexes is contained in the reticular formation. In the brain stem, the reticular formation becomes quite large and contains major portions of vital reflexes, such as those controlling respiration, cardiovascular function, swallowing, and vomiting. A functional system called the *reticular activating system* operates in the lateral portions of the reticular formation of the medulla, pons, and especially the midbrain. Information converging from all sensory modalities, including those of the somesthetic, auditory, visual, and visceral afferent nerves, bombards the neurons of this system.

The reticular activating system has descending and ascending portions. The descending portion communicates with all spinal segmental levels through middle-layer reticulospinal tracts and serves to facilitate many cord-level reflexes. For example, it speeds reaction time and stabilizes postural reflexes. The ascending portion accelerates brain activity, particularly thalamic and cortical activity. This is reflected by the appearance of awake brain-wave patterns. Sudden stimuli result in protective and attentive postures and cause increased awareness.

The Middle Layer. The middle layer of the white matter contains most of the major fiber tract systems required for sensation and movement. It contains the ascending spinoreticular and spinothalamic tracts. This layer consists of larger-diameter and longer suprasegmental fibers, which ascend to the brain stem and are largely functional at birth. In terms of evolutionary development, these tracts are quite old, and this layer is sometimes called the *paleolayer*. It facilitates many primitive functions, such as the auditory startle reflex, which occurs in response to loud noises. This reflex consists of turning the head and body toward the sound, dilating the pupils of the eyes, catching of the breath, and quickening of the pulse.

The Outer Layer. The outer layer of the tract systems is the newest of the three layers with respect to evolutionary development, and it is sometimes called the *neolayer*. This pathway, which becomes functional at about 2 years of age, contains the pathways needed for bladder training. Myelination of these suprasegmental tracts, which include many pathways required for delicate and highly coordinated skills, is not complete until approximately the fifth year of life. This includes the development of tracts needed

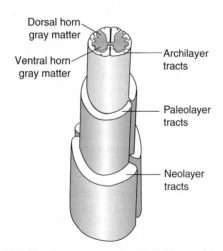

FIGURE 33-10 The three concentric subdivisions of the tract systems of the white matter. Migration of neurons into the archilayer converts it into the reticular formation of the white matter.

Labels on figure:
Dorsal horn gray matter
Ventral horn gray matter
Archilayer tracts
Paleolayer tracts
Neolayer tracts

TABLE 33-2	Characteristics of the Concentric Subdivisions of the Longitudinal Tracts in the White Matter of the Central Nervous System		
Characteristics	**Archilayer Tracts**	**Paleolayer Tracts**	**Neolayer Tracts**
Segmental span	Intersegmental (<5 segments)	Suprasegmental (≥5 segments)	Suprasegmental
Number of synapses	Multisynaptic	Multisynaptic but fewer than archilayer tracts	Monosynaptic with target structures
Conduction velocity	Very slow	Fast	Fastest
Examples of functional systems	Flexor withdrawal reflex circuitry	Spinothalamic tracts	Corticospinal tracts

for fine manipulative skills, such as the finger-thumb coordination required for using tools and the toe movements needed for acrobatics. Being the most recently evolved and more superficial, the neolayer tracts are the most vulnerable to injury.

Collateral Communication Pathways. Axons in the archilayer and paleolayer characteristically possess many collateral branches that move into the gray cell columns or synapse with fibers of the reticular formation as the axon passes each succeeding CNS segment. Should a major axon be destroyed at some point along its course, these collaterals provide multisynaptic alternative pathways that bypass the local damage. Damage usually is followed by slow return of function, presumably through the collateral connections.

Neolayer tracts do not possess these collaterals but instead project mainly to the target neurons with which they communicate. When neolayer tracts are damaged, the paleolayer and archilayer tracts often remain functional, and rehabilitation methods can result in effective use of the older systems. Delicacy and refinement may be lost, but basic function remains. For example, when the corticospinal system, an important neolayer system that

permits the fine manipulative control required for writing, is damaged, the remaining paleolayer systems, if intact, permit the grasping and holding of objects. The hand can still be used to perform its basic function, but the individual manipulation of the fingers is permanently lost.

In summary, the organization of the nervous system retains many early patterns of segmental development that were established during early embryonic life. Developmentally, the basic organizational pattern of the body is that of a longitudinal series of segments, each repeating the same fundamental pattern—a central cavity surrounded by an inner core of gray matter made up of nerve cells and a superficial layer of white matter containing axons of the longitudinal tract systems.

The 43 or more body segments are connected to their corresponding CNS or neural tube segments by segmental afferent and efferent PNS neurons. Afferent neuronal processes that carry sensory information enter the CNS through the dorsal root ganglia and are of four

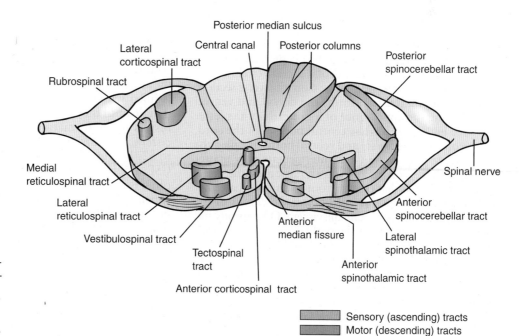

FIGURE 33-11 Transverse section of the spinal cord showing selected sensory and motor tracts. The tracts are bilateral but are indicated only on one half of the cord.

types: GSA, SSA, GVA, and SVA. Each of these afferent neurons synapses with its appropriate IA neurons in the cell columns of the dorsal horn. There are three cells columns of OA neurons in the ventral horn that synapse with LMNs that exit the CNS in the ventral roots: GSE neurons that innervate skeletal muscles; PE neurons that innervate pharyngeal muscles; and GVE neurons that innervate visceral structures.

Longitudinal communication between CNS segments is provided by tracts that are arranged in three layers: an inner, middle, and outer layer. The inner layer of white matter contains the axons of neurons that connect neighboring segments of the nervous system. It contains a mix of nerve cells and axons called the *reticular formation* and is the site of many important spinal cord and brain stem reflex circuits. The middle layer tracts provide the longitudinal communication between more distant segments of the nervous system; it contains most of the major fiber tract systems required for sensation and movement. The recently evolved outer or neolayer systems, which become functional during infancy and childhood, provide the means for very delicate and discriminative function.

Spinal Cord and Brain

THE SPINAL CORD

In the adult, the spinal cord is found in the upper two thirds of the spinal canal of the vertebral column (Fig. 33-12A). It extends from the foramen magnum at the base of the skull to a cone-shaped termination, the conus medullaris, usually at the level of the first or second lumbar vertebra (L1 or L2) in the adult. The dorsal and ventral roots of the more caudal portions of the cord elongate during development and angle downward from the cord, forming what is called the *cauda equina* (from the Latin for "horse's tail"). The filum terminale, which is composed of non-neural tissues and the pia mater, continues caudally and attaches to the second sacral vertebra (S2).

The spinal cord is somewhat oval on transverse section, with the gray matter that forms the dorsal and ventral horns having the appearance of a butterfly or the letter "H" (see Fig. 33-12B). The central portion of the cord, which connects the dorsal and ventral horns, is called the *intermediate gray matter*. The intermediate gray matter surrounds the central canal. In the thoracic area, the small, slender projections that emerge from the intermediate gray matter are called the *intermediolateral columns* of the horns. These columns contain the visceral OA neurons and the efferent neurons of the sympathetic nervous system.

The gray matter is proportional to the amount of tissue innervated by a given segment of the cord (see Fig. 33-12B). Larger amounts of gray matter are present in the lower lumbar and upper sacral segments, which supply the lower extremities, and in the fifth cervical segment to the first thoracic segment, which supply the upper limbs.

The white matter in the spinal cord also increases progressively toward the brain because ever more ascending fibers are added and the number of descending axons is greater.

The spinal cord and the dorsal and ventral roots are covered by a connective tissue sheath, the pia mater, which also contains the blood vessels that supply the white and gray matter of the cord (Fig. 33-13). On the lateral sides of the spinal cord, extensions of the pia mater, the denticulate ligaments, attach the sides of the spinal cord to the bony walls of the spinal canal. Thus, the cord is suspended by both the denticulate ligaments and the segmental nerves. A fat- and vessel-filled epidural space intervenes between the spinal dura mater and the inner wall of the spinal canal.

The spinal cord, spinal nerves, and their supporting structures are protected by the vertebral column. The vertebral body is the anterior, more massive part of the bone that gives strength to the vertebral column and supports body weight. Each vertebral body has two pedicles that extend posteriorly and support the laterally oriented transverse processes of the laminae, which arch medially and fuse to continue as the spinal processes. The vertebral arch and posterior surface of the vertebral body form the wall of the vertebral foramen. The succession of vertebral foramina in the articulated spinal column forms the vertebral canal (spinal canal), which contains the spinal cord, meninges, fat, and spinal nerve roots. The spaces between the vertebral bodies are filled with fibrocartilaginous discs and stabilized with tough ligaments. A gap, the intervertebral foramen, occurs between each two succeeding pedicles, allowing for the exit of the segmental nerves and passage of blood vessels. Supporting structures of the spinal cord are discussed further in Chapter 35.

Early in fetal life, the spinal cord extends the entire length of the vertebral column and the spinal nerves exit through the intervertebral foramina (openings) near their level of origin. Because the vertebral column and spinal dura grow faster than the spinal cord, a disparity develops between each succeeding cord segment and the exit of its dorsal and ventral nerve roots through the corresponding intervertebral foramina. In the newborn, the cord terminates at the level of L2 or L3. In the adult, the cord usually terminates in the inferior border of L1, and the arachnoid and its enclosed subarachnoid space, which is filled with CSF, do not close down on the filum terminale until they reach the level of S2 (Fig. 33-14). This results in the formation of a pocket of CSF, the *dural cisterna spinalis*, which extends from approximately L2 to S2. Because this area contains an abundant supply of CSF and the spinal cord does not extend this far, the area often is used for sampling the CSF. A procedure called a *spinal tap*, or puncture, can be done by inserting a special needle into the dural sac at L3 or L4. The spinal roots, which are covered with pia mater, are in little danger of trauma from the needle used for this purpose.

Spinal Nerves

The peripheral nerves that carry information to and from the spinal cord are called *spinal nerves*. There are 32 or

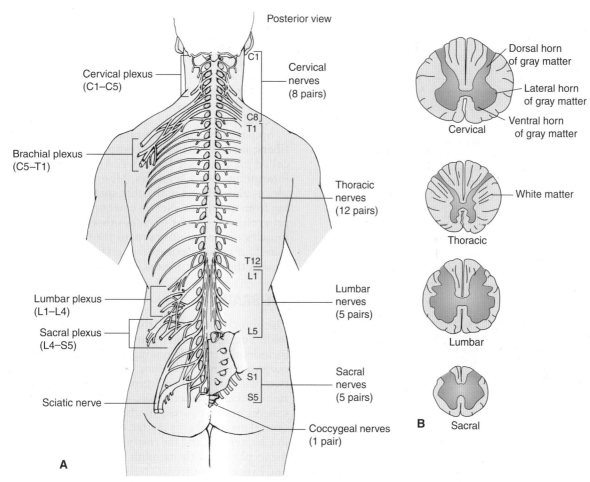

FIGURE 33-12 (**A**) Dorsal view of the spinal cord, including portions of the major spinal nerves and some of the components of the major nerve plexuses. (**B**) Cross-sectional views of the spinal cord, showing regional variations in gray matter and increasing white matter as the cord ascends.

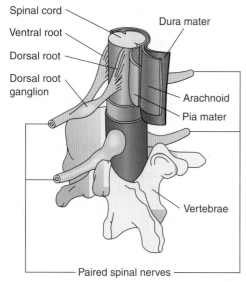

FIGURE 33-13 Spinal cord and meninges.

more pairs of spinal nerves (*i.e.*, 8 cervical, 12 thoracic, 5 lumbar, 5 sacral, and 2 or more coccygeal); each pair is named for the segment of the spinal cord from which it exits. Because the first cervical spinal nerve exits the spinal cord just above the first cervical vertebra (C1), the nerve is given the number of the bony vertebra just below it (see Fig. 33-12A). However, the numbering is changed for all lower levels. An extra cervical nerve, the C8 nerve, exits above the T1 vertebra, and each subsequent nerve is numbered for the vertebra just above its point of exit.

Each spinal cord segment communicates with its corresponding body segment through the paired segmental spinal nerves. Each spinal nerve, accompanied by the blood vessels supplying the spinal cord, enters the spinal canal through an intervertebral foramen, where it divides into two branches, or roots. One branch enters the dorsolateral surface of the cord (*i.e.*, dorsal root), carrying the axons of afferent neurons into the CNS. The other branch leaves the ventrolateral surface of the cord (*i.e.*, ventral root), carrying the axons of efferent neurons into the

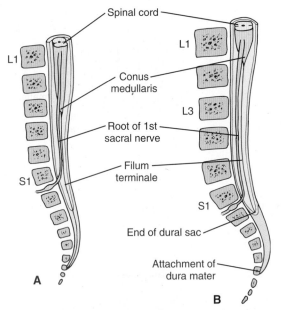

FIGURE 33-14 Position of the caudal end of the spinal cord in relation to the vertebral column in newborn (**A**) and adult (**B**). The increasing inclination of the root of the first sacral nerve is also illustrated. (Adapted from Moore K. L., Persaud T. V. N. [1998]. *The developing human* [6th ed., p. 459]. Philadelphia: W. B. Saunders, with permission from Elsevier Science.)

periphery. These two branches or roots fuse at the intervertebral foramen, forming the mixed spinal nerve—"mixed" because it has both afferent and efferent axons.

After emerging from the vertebral column, the spinal nerve divides into two branches or *rami* (singular, *ramus*): a small dorsal primary ramus and a larger ventral primary ramus (Fig. 33-15). The thoracic and upper lumbar spinal

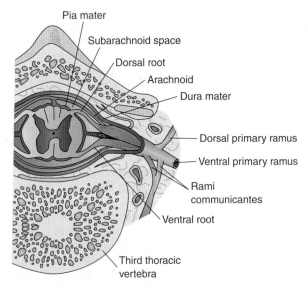

FIGURE 33-15 Cross section of vertebral column at the level of the third thoracic vertebra, showing the meninges, the spinal cord, and the origin of a spinal nerve and its branches or rami.

nerves also lead to a third branch, the ramus communicans, which contains sympathetic axons supplying the blood vessels, the genitourinary system, and the gastrointestinal system. The dorsal ramus contains sensory fibers from the skin and motor fibers to muscles of the back. The ventral primary ramus contains motor fibers that innervate the skeletal muscles of the anterior body wall and the legs and arms.

Spinal nerves do not go directly to skin and muscle fibers; instead, they form complicated nerve networks called *plexuses* (see Fig. 33-12A). A plexus is a site of intermixing nerve branches. Many spinal nerves enter a plexus and connect with other spinal nerves before exiting from the plexus. Nerves emerging from a plexus form progressively smaller branches that supply the skin and muscles of the various parts of the body. The PNS contains four major plexuses: the cervical plexus, the brachial plexus, the lumbar plexus, and the sacral plexus.

THE BRAIN

The brain is divided into three regions, the hindbrain, the midbrain, and the forebrain (Fig. 33-16A). The hindbrain includes the medulla oblongata, the pons, and its dorsal outgrowth, the cerebellum. Midbrain structures include two pairs of dorsal enlargements, the superior and inferior colliculi. The forebrain, which consists of two hemispheres and is covered by the cerebral cortex, contains central masses of gray matter, the basal ganglia (discussed in Chapter 35), and the rostral end of the neural tube, the diencephalon with its adult derivatives—the thalamus and hypothalamus.

An important concept is that the more rostral, recently developed parts of the neural tube gain dominance or control over regions and functions at lower levels. They do not replace the more ancient circuitry but merely dominate it. After damage to the more vulnerable parts of the forebrain, as occurs with brain death, a brain stem–controlled organism remains that is capable of breathing and may survive if the environmental temperature is regulated and nutrition and other aspects of care are provided. However, all aspects of intellectual function, experience, perception, and memory usually are permanently lost. The organization of content in this section moves from the more ancient circuitry of the hindbrain to the more dominant and recently developed structures of the forebrain.

Hindbrain

The term *brain stem* often is used to include the medulla, pons, and the midbrain (see Fig. 33-16B). These regions of the neural tube have the organization of spinal cord segments, except that more of the longitudinal cell columns are present, reflecting the increased complexity of the cranial segmental nerves. In the brain stem, the structure and function of the reticular formation have been greatly expanded. In the pons and medulla, the reticular formation contains neural networks controlling basic breathing, eating, and locomotion functions. Higher-level

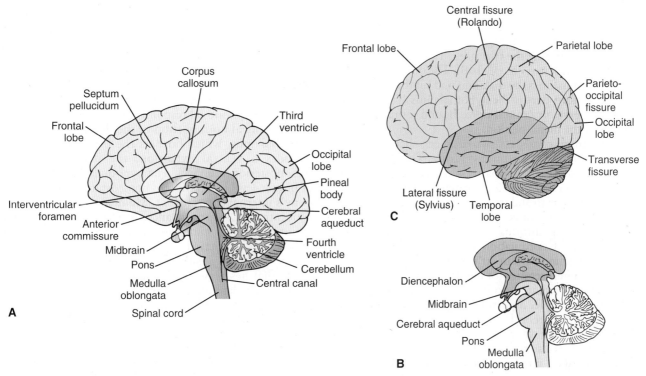

FIGURE 33-16 (**A**) Midsagittal section of the brain showing the structures of the forebrain, midbrain, and hindbrain. (**B**) Diencephalon, brain stem, and the cerebral aqueduct connecting the third and fourth ventricles. (**C**) Lateral view of the cerebral hemispheres.

integration of these functions occurs in the midbrain. The reticular formation is surrounded on the outside by the long tract systems that connect the forebrain with lower parts of the CNS.

Medulla. The *medulla oblongata* represents the caudal five segments of the brain part of the neural tube; the cranial nerve branches entering and leaving it have functions similar to the spinal segmental nerves. Although the ventral horn areas in the medulla are quite small, the dorsal horn areas are enlarged, processing the large amount of the information pouring through the cranial nerves. Cranial nerves XII (hypoglossal), X (vagus), and IX (glossopharyngeal) have their origin in the medulla (see Table 33-1).

Pons. The pons, which develops from the fifth neural tube segment, is located between the medulla oblongata and the midbrain. Dorsally, it forms part of the anterior wall of the fourth ventricle (see Fig. 33-16A).

As the name implies (*pons*, Latin for "bridge"), the pons is composed chiefly of conduction fibers. The enlarged area on the ventral surface of the pons contains the pontine nuclei, which receive information from all parts of the cerebral cortex. The axons of these neurons form a massive bundle that swings around the lateral side of the fourth ventricle to enter the cerebellum. In the pons, the reticular formation is large and contains the circuitry for masticating food and manipulating the jaws during speech. Cranial nerves VIII, VII, and VI have their origin in the pons (see Table 33-1).

Midbrain

The midbrain develops from the fourth segment of the neural tube, and its organization is similar to that of a spinal segment. The central canal is reestablished as the cerebral aqueduct, connecting the fourth ventricle with the third ventricle (see Fig. 33-16A).

Two prominent bundles of nerve fibers, the *cerebral peduncles*, pass along the ventral surface of the midbrain. These fibers include the corticospinal tracts and are the main motor pathways between the forebrain and the pons. On the dorsal surface, four "little hills," the *superior* and *inferior colliculi*, are areas of cortical formation. The inferior colliculus is involved in directional turning and, to some extent, in experiencing the direction of sound sources. The superior colliculi are essential to the reflex mechanisms that control conjugate eye movements when the visual environment is surveyed. Two general somatic efferent cranial nerves, the oculomotor nerve, or cranial nerve III, and the trochlear nerve, or cranial nerve IV, exit the midbrain (see Table 33-1).

Forebrain

The most rostral part of the brain, the forebrain consists of the telencephalon, or "end brain," and the diencephalon, or "between brain." The diencephalon forms the core of the forebrain, and the telencephalon forms the cerebral hemispheres.

Diencephalon. Three of the most forward brain segments form an enlarged dorsal horn and ventral horn with a narrow, deep, enlarged central canal—the third ventricle—separating the two sides. This region is called the *diencephalon* (see Fig. 33-16B). The dorsal horn part of the diencephalon is the thalamus and subthalamus, and the ventral horn part is the hypothalamus (Fig. 33-17). The optic nerve, or cranial nerve II, and retina are outgrowths of the diencephalon.

The thalamus consists of two large, egg-shaped masses, one on either side of the third ventricle. The thalamus is divided into several major parts, and each part is divided into distinct nuclei, which are the major relay stations for information going to and from the cerebral cortex. All sensory pathways have direct projections to thalamic nuclei, which convey the information to restricted areas of the sensory cortex. Coordination and integration of peripheral sensory stimuli occur in the thalamus, along with some crude interpretation of highly emotion-laden auditory experiences that not only occur but can be remembered. For example, a person can recover from a deep coma in which cerebral cortex activity is minimal and remember some of what was said at the bedside.

The thalamus also plays a role in relaying critical information regarding motor activities to and from selected areas of the motor cortex. Two neuronal circuits are significant in this regard. One is the pathway from the cerebral cortex to the pons and cerebellum and then, by way of the thalamus, back to the motor cortex. The second is the feedback circuit that travels from the cortex to the basal ganglia, then to the thalamus, and from the thalamus back to the cortex. The subthalamus also contains movement control systems related to the basal ganglia.

Through its connections with the ascending reticular activating system, the thalamus processes neural influences that are basic to cortical excitatory rhythms (*i.e.*, those recorded on the electroencephalogram), to essential sleep-wakefulness cycles, and to the process of attending to stimuli. Besides their cortical connections, the thalamic nuclei have connections with each other and with neighboring nonthalamic brain structures such as the limbic system. Through their connections with the limbic system, some thalamic nuclei are involved in relating stimuli with the emotional responses they evoke.

The ventral horn portion of the diencephalon is the hypothalamus, which borders the third ventricle and includes a ventral extension, the neurohypophysis (*i.e.*, posterior pituitary). The hypothalamus is the area of master-level integration of homeostatic control of the body's internal environment. Maintenance of blood gas concentration, water balance, food consumption, and major aspects of endocrine and ANS control require hypothalamic function.

The internal capsule is a broad band of projection fibers that lies between the thalamus medially and the basal ganglia laterally (see Fig. 33-17). It contains all of the fibers that connect the cerebral cortex with deeper structures, including the basal ganglia, thalamus, midbrain, pons, medulla, and spinal cord.

Cerebral Hemispheres. The two cerebral hemispheres are lateral outgrowths of the diencephalon. The cerebral hemispheres contain the lateral ventricles (*i.e.*, ventricles I and II), which are connected with the third ventricle of the diencephalon by a small opening called the *interventricular foramen* (see Fig. 33-16A). Axons of the olfactory nerve, or cranial nerve I, terminate in the most ancient portion of the cerebrum—the olfactory bulb, where initial processing of olfactory information occurs. Projection axons from the olfactory bulb relay information through the olfactory tracts to the thalamus and to other parts of the cerebral cortex (*i.e.*, orbital cor-

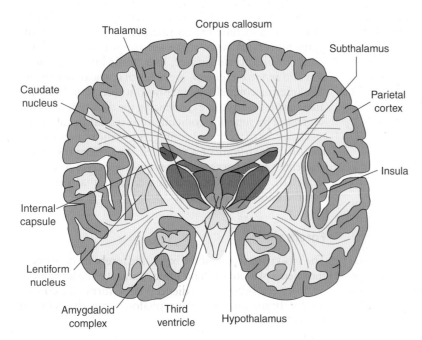

FIGURE 33-17 Frontal section of the brain passing through the third ventricle, showing the thalamus, subthalamus, hypothalamus, internal capsule, corpus callosum, basal ganglia (caudate nucleus, lenticular nucleus), amygdaloid complex, insula, and parietal cortex.

tex), where olfactory-related reflexes and olfactory experience occur.

The *corpus callosum* is a massive commissure, or bridge, of myelinated axons that connects the cerebral cortex of the two sides of the brain. Two smaller commissures, the anterior and posterior commissures, connect the two sides of the more specialized regions of the cerebrum and diencephalon.

The surface of the hemispheres, which contains the recently evolved six-layered neocortex, can be described as lateral (side), medial (area between the two sides of the brain), and basal (ventral). The surface of the hemispheres contains many ridges and grooves. A *gyrus* is the ridge between two grooves, and the groove is called a *sulcus* or *fissure*. The cerebral cortex is arbitrarily divided into lobes named after the bones that cover them: the frontal, parietal, temporal, and occipital lobes (see Fig. 33-16C).

Frontal Lobe. The frontal lobe extends from the frontal pole to the central sulcus (*i.e.,* fissure) and is separated from the temporal lobe by the lateral sulcus. The frontal lobe can be subdivided rostrally into the frontal pole and laterally into the superior, middle, and inferior gyri, which continue on the undersurface over the eyes as the orbital cortex. These areas are associated with the medial thalamic nuclei, which also are related to the limbic system. In terms of function, the prefrontal cortex is thought to be involved in anticipation and prediction of consequences of behavior.

The precentral gyrus (area 4), next to the central sulcus, is the *primary motor cortex* (Fig. 33-18). This area of the cortex provides precise movement control for distal flexor muscles of the hands and feet and of the phonation apparatus required for speech. Just rostral to the precentral gyrus is a region of the frontal cortex called the *premotor* or *motor association cortex*. This region (area 8 and rostral area 6) is involved in the planning of complex learned movement patterns. The primary motor cortex and the association motor cortex are connected with lateral thalamic nuclei, through which they receive feedback information from the basal ganglia and cerebellum. On the medial surface of the hemisphere, the premotor area includes a *supplementary motor cortex* involved in the control of bilateral movement patterns requiring great dexterity.

Parietal Lobe. The parietal lobe of the cerebrum lies behind the central sulcus (*i.e.,* postcentral gyrus) and above the lateral sulcus. The strip of cortex bordering the central sulcus is called the *primary somatosensory cortex* (areas 3, 1, and 2) because it receives very discrete sensory information from the lateral nuclei of the thalamus. Just behind the primary sensory cortex is the *somatosensory association cortex* (areas 5 and 7), which is connected with the thalamic nuclei and with the primary sensory cortex. This region is necessary for perceiving the meaningfulness of integrated sensory information from various sensory systems, especially the perception of "where" the stimulus is in space and in relation to body parts. Localized lesions of this region can result in the inability to recognize the meaningfulness of an object (*i.e.,* agnosia). With the person's eyes closed, a screwdriver can be felt and described as to shape and texture. Nevertheless, the person cannot integrate the sensory information required to identify it as a screwdriver.

Temporal Lobe. The temporal lobe lies below the lateral sulcus and merges with the parietal and occipital lobes. It includes the temporal pole and three primary gyri: the superior, middle, and inferior gyri. The primary auditory cortex (area 41) involves the part of the superior temporal gyrus that extends into the lateral sulcus (see Fig. 33-18). This area is particularly important in discrimination of sounds entering opposite ears. It receives

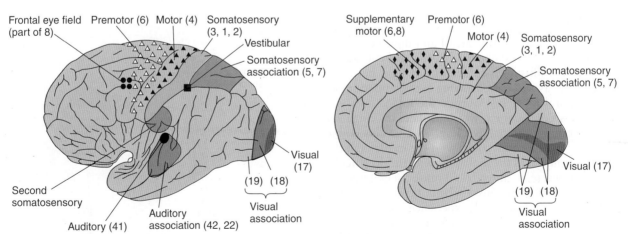

FIGURE 33-18 Motor and sensory areas of the cerebral cortex. (**Left**) The lateral view of the left (dominant) side is drawn as though the lateral sulcus had been pried open, exposing the insula. (**Right**) The diagram represents the areas in a brain that has been sectioned in the median plane. (From Nolte J. [1981]. *The human brain*. St. Louis: C. V. Mosby, with permission from Elsevier Science.)

auditory input projections by way of the inferior colliculus of the midbrain and a ventrolateral thalamic nucleus. The more exposed part of the superior temporal gyrus involves the auditory association area (area 22). The recognition of certain sound patterns and their meaning requires the function of this area. The remaining portion of the temporal cortex is less defined functionally but apparently is important in long-term memory recall. This is particularly true with respect to perception and memory of complex sensory patterns, such as geometric figures and faces (*i.e.*, recognition of "what" or "who" the stimulus is). Irritation or stimulation can result in vivid hallucinations of long-past events.

Occipital Lobe. The occipital lobe lies posterior to the temporal and parietal lobes and is only arbitrarily separated from them. The medial surface of the occipital lobe contains a deep sulcus extending from the limbic lobe to the occipital pole, the *calcarine sulcus*, which is surrounded by the primary visual cortex (area 17). Stimulation of this cortex causes the experience of bright lights (phosphenes) in the visual field. Just superior and inferior and extending onto the lateral side of the occipital pole is the *visual association cortex* (areas 18 and 19). This area is closely connected with the primary visual cortex and with complex nuclei of the thalamus. Integrity of the association cortex is required for gnostic visual function, by which the meaningfulness of visual experience, including experiences of color, motion, depth perception, pattern, form, and location in space, occurs.

The neocortical areas of the parietal lobe, between the somatosensory and the visual cortices, have a function in relating the texture, or "feel," and location of an object with its visual image. Between the auditory and visual association areas, the *parieto-occipital region* is necessary for relating the meaningfulness of a sound and image to an object or person.

Limbic System. The medial aspect of the cerebrum is organized into concentric bands of cortex, the *limbic system* (from the Latin *limbus*, "border"), which surrounds the connection between the lateral and third ventricles. The innermost band just above and below the cut surface of the corpus callosum is folded out of sight but is an ancient, three-layered cortex ending as the hippocampus in the temporal lobe. Just outside the folded area is a band of transitional cortex, which includes the cingulate and the parahippocampal gyri (Fig. 33-19). This limbic lobe has reciprocal connections with the medial and the intralaminar nuclei of the thalamus, with the deep nuclei of the cerebrum (*e.g.*, amygdaloid nuclei, septal nuclei), and with the hypothalamus. Overall, this region of the brain is involved in emotional experience and in the control of emotion-related behavior. Stimulation of specific areas in this system can lead to feelings of dread, high anxiety, or exquisite pleasure. It also can result in violent behaviors, including attack, defense, or explosive and emotional speech.

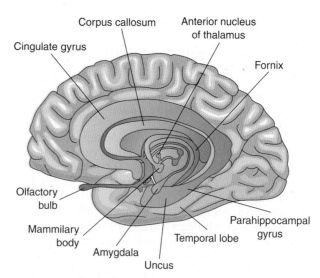

FIGURE 33-19 The limbic system includes the limbic cortex (cingulate gyrus, parahippocampal gyrus, uncus) and associated subcortical structures (thalamus, hypothalamus, amygdala).

Meninges

Inside the skull and vertebral column, the brain and spinal cord are loosely suspended and protected by several connective tissue sheaths called the *meninges* (Fig. 33-20). The surfaces of the spinal cord, brain, and segmental nerves are covered with a delicate connective tissue layer called the *pia mater* (Latin for "delicate mother"). The surface blood vessels and those that penetrate the brain and spinal cord are encased in this protective tissue layer. A second, very delicate, nonvascular, and waterproof layer, called the *arachnoid*, encloses the entire CNS. The arachnoid layer is named for its spider-web appearance.

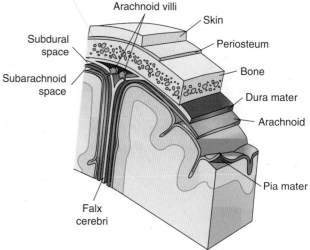

FIGURE 33-20 The cranial meninges. Arachnoid villi, shown within the superior sagittal sinus, are one site of cerebrospinal fluid absorption into the blood.

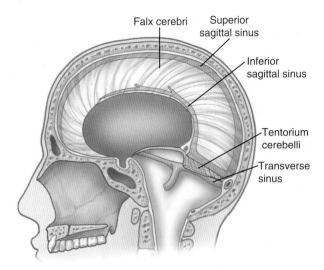

FIGURE 33-21 Cranial dura mater. The skull is open to show the falx cerebri and the tentorium cerebelli, as well as some of the cranial venous sinuses.

The CSF is contained in the subarachnoid space. Immediately outside the arachnoid is a continuous sheath of strong connective tissue, the *dura mater* (*i.e.,* "tough mother"), which provides the major protection for the brain and spinal cord. The cranial dura often splits into two layers, with the outer layer serving as the periosteum of the inner surface of the skull.

The inner layer of the dura forms two major folds. The first, a longitudinal fold called the *falx cerebri*, separates the cerebral hemispheres and fuses with a second transverse fold, called the *tentorium cerebelli* (Fig. 33-21). The tentorium cerebelli separates the anterior and middle depression in the skull (cranial fossae), which contains the cerebral hemispheres, from the posterior fossa, found interiorly and containing the brain stem and cere-

bellum. A semicircular gap, or incisura, is formed at the midline to permit the midbrain to pass forward from the posterior fossa.

Ventricular System and Cerebrospinal Fluid

The ventricular system is a series of CSF-filled cavities in the brain (Fig. 33-22). The CSF is a supporting and protective fluid in which the brain and spinal cord float. CSF helps maintain a constant ionic environment that serves as a medium for diffusion of nutrients, electrolytes, and metabolic end products into the extracellular fluid surrounding CNS neurons and glia. Filling the ventricles, the CSF supports the mass of the brain. Because it fills the subarachnoid space surrounding the CNS, a physical force delivered to either the skull or spine is to some extent diffused and cushioned.

The lining of the ventricles and central canal of the spinal cord is called the *ependyma*. There is a tremendous expansion of the ependyma in the roof of the lateral, third, and fourth ventricles. The CSF is produced by tiny reddish masses of specialized capillaries from the pia mater, called the *choroid plexus,* that project into the ventricles. CSF is an ultrafiltrate of blood plasma, composed of 99% water with other constituents, making it close to the composition of the brain extracellular fluid. Humans secrete approximately 500 mL of CSF each day. However, only approximately 150 mL is in the ventricular system at any one time, meaning that the CSF is continuously being absorbed.

Once produced, the CSF flows freely through the ventricles. Three openings, or foramina, allow the CSF to pass into the subarachnoid space. Two of these, the foramina of Luschka, are located at the lateral corners of the fourth ventricle. The third, the median foramen of Magendie, is in the midline at the caudal end of the fourth ventricle (see Fig. 33-22). Approximately 30% of the CSF passes down

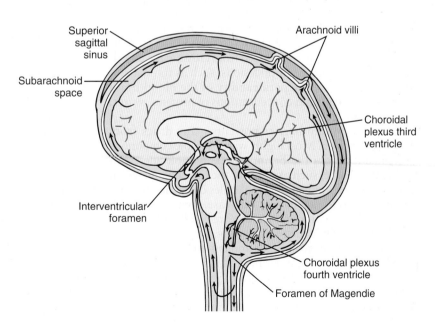

FIGURE 33-22 The flow of cerebrospinal fluid from the time of its formation from blood in the choroid plexuses until its return to the blood in the superior sagittal sinus. Plexuses in the lateral ventricles are not illustrated.

into the subarachnoid space that surrounds the spinal cord, mainly on its dorsal surface, and moves back up to the cranial cavity along its ventral surface.

Reabsorption of CSF into the vascular system occurs along the sides of the superior sagittal sinus in the anterior and middle fossa. Here, the waterproof arachnoid has protuberances, the *arachnoid villi* that penetrate the inner dura and venous walls of the superior sagittal sinus. The arachnoid villi function as one-way valves, permitting CSF outflow into the blood but not allowing blood to pass into the arachnoid spaces.

Blood-Brain and Cerebrospinal Fluid–Brain Barriers

Maintenance of a chemically stable environment is essential to the function of the brain. In most regions of the body, extracellular fluid undergoes small fluctuations in pH and concentrations of hormones, amino acids, and potassium ions during routine daily activities such as eating and exercising. If the brain were to undergo such fluctuations, the result would be uncontrolled neural activity because some substances such as amino acids act as neurotransmitters, and ions such as potassium influence the threshold for neural firing. Two barriers, the blood-brain barrier and the CSF-brain barrier, provide the means for maintaining the stable chemical environment of the brain. Only water, carbon dioxide, and oxygen enter the brain with relative ease; the transport of other substances between the brain and the blood is slower and more controlled.

Blood-Brain Barrier. The blood-brain barrier depends on the unique characteristics of the brain capillaries. The endothelial cells of brain capillaries are joined by continuous tight junctions. In addition, most brain capillaries are completely surrounded by a basement membrane and by the processes of previously described supporting astrocyte cells of the brain (Fig. 33-23). The blood-brain barrier permits passage of essential substances while excluding unwanted materials. Reverse transport systems remove materials from the brain. Large molecules such as proteins and peptides are largely excluded from crossing the blood-brain barrier. Acute cerebral lesions, such as trauma and infection, increase the permeability of the blood-brain barrier and alter brain concentrations of proteins, water, and electrolytes.

The blood-brain barrier prevents many drugs from entering the brain. Most highly water-soluble compounds are excluded from the brain, especially molecules with high ionic charge, such as many of the catecholamines. In contrast, many lipid-soluble molecules cross the lipid layers of the blood-brain barrier with ease. Some drugs, such as the antibiotic chloramphenicol, are highly lipid soluble and therefore enter the brain readily. Other medications have a low solubility in lipids and enter the brain slowly or not at all. Alcohol, nicotine, and heroin are very lipid soluble and rapidly enter the brain. Some substances that enter the capillary endothelium are converted by metabolic processes to a chemical form incapable of moving into the brain.

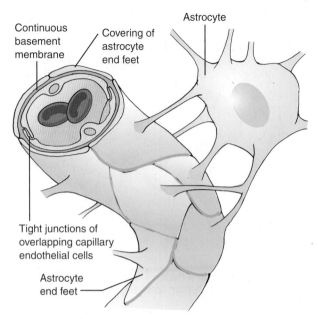

FIGURE 33-23 The three components of the blood-brain barrier: the astrocyte and astrocytic feet that encircle the capillary, the capillary basement membrane, and the tight junctions that join the overlapping capillary endothelial cells.

The cerebral capillaries are much more permeable at birth than in adulthood, and the blood-brain barrier develops during the early years of life. In severely jaundiced infants, bilirubin can cross the immature blood-brain barrier; producing kernicterus and brain damage (see Chapter 11). In adults, the mature blood-brain barrier prevents bilirubin from entering the brain, and the nervous system is not affected.

Cerebrospinal Fluid–Brain Barrier. The ependymal cells covering the choroid plexus are linked together by tight junctions, forming a blood-CSF barrier to diffusion of many molecules from the blood plasma of choroid plexus capillaries to the CSF. Water is transported through the choroid epithelial cells by osmosis. Oxygen and carbon dioxide move into the CSF by diffusion, resulting in partial pressures roughly equal to those of plasma. The high sodium and low potassium contents of the CSF are actively regulated and kept relatively constant. Lipids and nonpeptide hormones diffuse through the barrier rather easily, but most large molecules, such as proteins, peptides, many antibiotics, and other medications, do not normally get through. Many substances such as proteins, sodium ions, and a number of micronutrients such as vitamins C, B_6 (pyridoxine), and folate are actively secreted into the CSF by the choroid epithelium. Because the resultant CSF has relatively high sodium content, the negatively charged chloride and bicarbonate diffuse into the CSF along an ionic gradient. The choroid cells also generate bicarbonate from carbon dioxide in the blood. The generation of bicarbonate is important to the regulation of the pH of the CSF.

Mechanisms exist that facilitate the transport of other molecules such as glucose without energy expenditure.

Ammonia, a toxic metabolite of neuronal activity, is converted to glutamine by astrocytes. Glutamine moves by facilitated diffusion through the choroid epithelium into the plasma. This exemplifies a major function of the CSF, that of providing a means of removal of toxic waste products from the CNS. Because the brain and spinal cord have no lymphatic channels, the CSF serves this function.

There are several specific areas of the brain where the blood-CSF barrier does not exist. One area is at the caudal end of the fourth ventricle, where specialized receptors for the carbon dioxide level of the CSF influence respiratory function. Another area consists of the walls of the third ventricle, which permit hypothalamic neurons to monitor blood glucose levels. This mechanism permits hypothalamic centers to respond to these blood glucose levels, contributing to hunger and eating behaviors.

In summary, in the adult, the spinal cord is in the upper two thirds of the spinal canal of the vertebral column. On transverse section, the spinal cord has an oval shape, and the internal gray matter has the appearance of a butterfly or letter "H." The dorsal horns contain the IA neurons and receive afferent information from dorsal root and other connecting neurons. The ventral horns contain the OA neurons and efferent LMNs that leave the cord by the ventral roots. Thirty-two pairs of spinal nerves (i.e., 8 cervical, 12 thoracic, 5 lumbar, 5 sacral, and 2 or more coccygeal) are present. Each pair communicates with its corresponding body segments. The spinal nerves and the blood vessels that supply the spinal cord enter the spinal canal through an intervertebral foramen. After entering the foramen, they divide into two branches, or roots, one of which enters the dorsolateral surface of the cord (i.e., dorsal root), carrying the axons of afferent neurons into the CNS. The other root leaves the ventrolateral surface of the cord (i.e., ventral root), carrying the axons of efferent neurons into the periphery. These two roots fuse at the intervertebral foramen, forming the mixed spinal nerve.

The brain can be divided into three regions: the hindbrain, the midbrain, and the forebrain. The hindbrain, consisting of the medulla oblongata, pons, and cerebellum, contains the neuronal circuits for the eating, breathing, and locomotive functions required for survival. Cranial nerves XII, XI, X, IX, VIII, VII, VI, and V are located in the hindbrain. The midbrain contains cranial nerves IV and III.

The forebrain is the most rostral part of the brain; it consists of the diencephalon and the telencephalon. The diencephalon forms the core of the forebrain, and the telencephalon forms the cerebral hemispheres. The dorsal horn part of the diencephalon contains the thalamus and subthalamus, and the ventral horn contains the hypothalamus. All sensory pathways have direct projections to the thalamic nuclei, which convey the information to restricted parts of the sensory cortex.

The hypothalamus functions in the homeostatic control of the internal environment. The cerebral hemispheres are the lateral outgrowths of the diencephalon and are arbitrarily divided into lobes—the frontal, parietal, temporal, and occipital lobes. The premotor area and primary motor cortex are located in the frontal lobe; the primary sensory cortex and somatosensory association area are in the parietal cortex; the primary auditory cortex and the auditory association area are in the temporal lobe; and the primary visual cortex and association visual cortex are in the occipital lobe. The limbic system, which is involved in emotional experience and release of emotional behaviors, is located in the medial aspect of the cerebrum.

The brain is enclosed and protected by connective tissue sheaths (i.e., the pia mater, arachnoid, and dura mater) called the *meninges.* The protective CSF in which the brain and spinal cord float isolates them from minor and moderate trauma. The CSF is secreted into the ventricles, circulates through the ventricular system, passes outside to surround the brain, and is reabsorbed into the venous system through the arachnoid villi. The blood-brain barrier and CSF-brain barrier protect the brain from substances in the blood that would disrupt brain function.

The Autonomic Nervous System

The ability to maintain homeostasis and perform the activities of daily living in an ever-changing physical environment is largely vested in the autonomic nervous system (ANS). The ANS functions at the subconscious level and is involved in regulating, adjusting, and coordinating vital visceral functions such as blood pressure and blood flow, body temperature, respiration, digestion, metabolism, and elimination. The ANS is strongly affected by emotional influences and is involved in many of the expressive aspects of behavior. Blushing, pallor, palpitations of the heart, clammy hands, and dry mouth are several emotional expressions that are mediated through the ANS.

As with the somatic nervous system, the ANS is represented in both the CNS and the PNS. Traditionally, the ANS has been defined as a general efferent system innervating visceral organs. The efferent outflow from the ANS has two divisions: the sympathetic nervous system and the parasympathetic nervous system. The afferent input to the ANS is provided by visceral afferent neurons, usually not considered to be part of the ANS.

The functions of the sympathetic nervous system include maintaining body temperature and adjusting blood flow and blood pressure to meet the changing needs of the body that occur with activities of daily living, such as moving from the supine to the standing position. The sympathoadrenal system also can discharge as a unit when there is a critical threat to the integrity of the individual—

the so-called fight-or-flight response. During a stress situation, the heart rate accelerates; the blood pressure rises; blood flow shifts from the skin and gastrointestinal tract to the skeletal muscles and brain; blood sugar increases; the bronchioles and pupils dilate; the sphincters of the stomach and intestine and the internal sphincter of the urethra constrict; and the rate of secretion of exocrine glands that are involved in digestion diminishes. Emergency situations often require vasoconstriction and shunting of blood away from the skin and into the muscles and brain, a mechanism that, should a wound occur, provides for a reduction in blood flow and preservation of vital functions needed for survival. Sympathetic function often is summarized as catabolic in that its actions predominate during periods of pronounced energy expenditure, such as when survival is threatened.

In contrast to the sympathetic nervous system, the functions of the parasympathetic nervous system are concerned with conservation of energy, resource replenishment and storage (*i.e.*, anabolism), and maintenance of organ function during periods of minimal activity. The parasympathetic nervous system slows heart rate, stimulates gastrointestinal function and related glandular secretion, promotes bowel and bladder elimination, and contracts the pupil, protecting the retina from excessive light during periods when visual function is not vital to survival. The two divisions of the ANS usually are viewed as having opposite and antagonistic actions (*i.e.*, if one activates, the other inhibits a function). Exceptions are functions, such as sweating and regulation of arteriolar blood vessel diameter, that are controlled by a single division of the ANS, in this case the sympathetic nervous system.

The sympathetic and parasympathetic nervous systems are continually active. The effect of this continual or basal (baseline) activity is referred to as *tone*. The tone of an effector organ or system can be increased or decreased and usually is regulated by a single division of the ANS. For example, vascular smooth muscle tone is controlled by the sympathetic nervous system. Increased sympathetic activity produces local vasoconstriction from increased vascular smooth muscle tone, and decreased activity results in vasodilatation caused by decreased tone. In structures such as the sinoatrial node and atrioventricular node of the heart, which are innervated by both divisions of the ANS, one division predominates in controlling tone. In this case, the tonically active parasympathetic nervous system exerts a constraining or braking effect on heart rate, and when parasympathetic outflow is withdrawn, similar to releasing a brake, the heart rate increases. The increase in heart rate that occurs with vagal withdrawal can be further augmented by sympathetic stimulation.

AUTONOMIC EFFERENT PATHWAYS

The outflow of both divisions of the ANS follows a two-neuron pathway. The first motor neuron, called the *preganglionic neuron,* lies in the intermediolateral cell column in the ventral horn of the spinal cord or its equivalent location in the brain stem. The second motor neuron, called the *postganglionic neuron,* synapses with a preganglionic neuron in an autonomic ganglion located in the PNS. The two divisions of the ANS differ in terms of location of preganglionic cell bodies, relative length of preganglionic fibers, general function, nature of peripheral responses, and preganglionic and postganglionic neuromediators (Table 33-3). This two-neuron outflow pathway and the interneurons in the autonomic ganglia that add further modulation to ANS function are features distinctly different from the arrangement in somatic motor innervation.

Most visceral organs are innervated by both sympathetic and parasympathetic fibers. Exceptions include structures such as blood vessels and sweat glands that have input from only one division of the ANS. The fibers of the sympathetic nervous system are distributed to effectors throughout the body, and as a result, sympathetic actions tend to be more diffuse than those of the parasympathetic nervous system, in which there is a more localized distribution of fibers. The preganglionic fibers of the sympathetic nervous system may traverse a considerable distance and pass through several ganglia before synapsing with postganglionic neurons, and their terminals make contact with a large number of postganglionic fibers. In some ganglia, the ratio of preganglionic to postganglionic cells may be 1:20; because of this, the effects of sympathetic stimulation are diffuse. There is considerable overlap, and one ganglion cell may be supplied by several preganglionic fibers. In contrast to the sympathetic nervous system, the parasympathetic nervous system has its postganglionic neurons located very near or in the organ of innervation. Because the ratio of pregan-

TABLE 33-3 Characteristics of the Sympathetic and Parasympathetic Nervous Systems

Characteristic	Sympathetic Outflow	Parasympathetic Outflow
Location of preganglionic cell bodies	T1–T12, L1 and L2	Cranial nerves III, VII (intermedius), IX, X; sacral segments 2, 3, and 4
Relative length of preganglionic fibers	Short—to paravertebral chain of ganglia or to aortic prevertebral of ganglia	Long—to ganglion cells near or in the innervated organ
General function	Catabolic—mobilizes resources in anticipation of challenge for survival (preparation for "fight-or-flight" response)	Anabolic—concerned with conservation, renewal, and storage of resources
Nature of peripheral response	Generalized	Localized
Transmitter between preganglionic terminals and postganglionic neurons	ACh	ACh
Transmitter of postganglionic neuron	ACh (sweat glands and skeletal muscle vasodilator fibers); norepinephrine (most synapses); norepinephrine and epinephrine (secreted by adrenal gland)	ACh

ACh, acetylcholine.

glionic to postganglionic communication often is 1:1, the effects of the parasympathetic nervous system are much more circumscribed.

Sympathetic Nervous System

The preganglionic neurons of the sympathetic nervous system are located primarily in the thoracic and upper lumbar segments (T1 to L2) of the spinal cord; thus, the sympathetic nervous system often is referred to as the *thoracolumbar division* of the ANS. These preganglionic neurons, which are located primarily in the ventral horn intermediolateral cell column, have axons that are largely myelinated and relatively short. The postganglionic neurons of the sympathetic nervous system are located in the paravertebral ganglia of the sympathetic chain that lie on either side of the vertebral column, or in prevertebral sympathetic ganglia such as the celiac ganglia (Fig. 33-24). Besides postganglionic efferent neurons, the sympathetic ganglia contain neurons of the internuncial, short-axon type, similar to those associated with complex circuitry in the brain and spinal cord. Many of these inhibit and others modulate preganglionic-to-postganglionic transmission.

The axons of the preganglionic neurons leave the spinal cord through the ventral root of the spinal nerves (T1 to L2), enter the ventral primary rami, and leave the spinal nerve through white rami of the rami communicantes to reach the paravertebral ganglionic chain (Fig. 33-25). In the sympathetic chain of ganglia, preganglionic fibers may synapse with neurons of the ganglion they enter, pass up or down the chain and synapse with one or more ganglia, or pass through the chain and move outward through a splanchnic nerve to terminate in one of the prevertebral ganglia (*i.e.*, celiac, superior mesenteric, or inferior mesenteric) that are scattered along the dorsal aorta and its branches. The adrenal medulla, which is part of the sympathetic nervous system, contains postganglionic sympathetic neurons that secrete sympathetic neurotransmitters directly into the bloodstream.

Parasympathetic Nervous System

The preganglionic fibers of the parasympathetic nervous system, also referred to as the *craniosacral division* of the ANS, originate in some segments of the brain stem and sacral segments of the spinal cord (see Fig. 33-24). The central regions of origin are the midbrain, pons, medulla oblongata, and the sacral part of the spinal cord. The outflow from the midbrain passes through the oculomotor nerve (cranial nerve III) to supply the pupillary sphincter muscle of each eye and the ciliary muscles that control lens thickness for accommodation. Caudal pontine outflow comes from branches of the facial nerve (cranial nerve VII) that supply the lacrimal and nasal glands. The medullary outflow develops from cranial nerves VII, IX, and X. Fibers in the glossopharyngeal nerve (cranial nerve IX) supply the parotid salivary glands. Approximately 75% of parasympathetic efferent fibers are carried in the vagus nerve (cranial nerve X). The vagus nerve provides parasympathetic innervation for the heart, trachea, lungs, esophagus, stomach, small intestine, proximal half of the colon, liver, gallbladder, pancreas, kidneys, and upper portions of the ureters.

Sacral preganglionic axons leave the S2 to S4 segmental nerves by gathering into the pelvic nerves. The pelvic nerves leave the sacral plexus on each side of the cord and distribute their peripheral fibers to the bladder, uterus, urethra, prostate, distal portion of the transverse colon, descending colon, and rectum. The sacral parasympathetic fibers also supply the venous outflow from the external genitalia to facilitate erectile function.

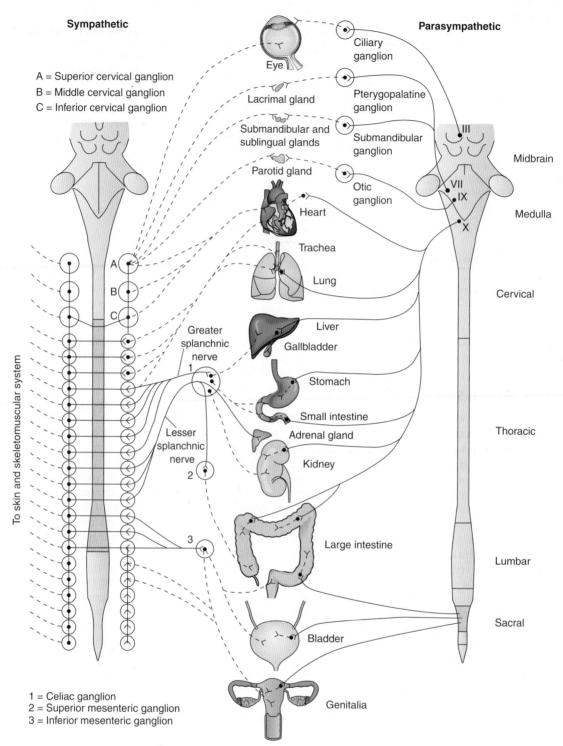

Sympathetic

A = Superior cervical ganglion
B = Middle cervical ganglion
C = Inferior cervical ganglion

To skin and skeletomuscular system

A
B
C

Greater
splanchnic
nerve

1

Lesser
splanchnic
nerve

2

3

1 = Celiac ganglion
2 = Superior mesenteric ganglion
3 = Inferior mesenteric ganglion

Parasympathetic

Eye

Ciliary
ganglion

Lacrimal gland

Pterygopalatine
ganglion

Submandibular and
sublingual glands

Submandibular
ganglion

Parotid gland

Otic
ganglion

Heart

Trachea

Lung

Liver

Gallbladder

Stomach

Small intestine

Adrenal gland

Kidney

Large intestine

Bladder

Genitalia

III

VII
IX
X

Midbrain

Medulla

Cervical

Thoracic

Lumbar

Sacral

FIGURE 33-24 The autonomic nervous system. The involuntary organs are depicted with their parasympathetic innervation (craniosacral) indicated on the right and sympathetic innervation (thoracolumbar) on the left. Preganglionic fibers are *solid lines;* postganglionic fibers are *dashed lines.* For purposes of illustration, the sympathetic outflow to the skin and skeletomuscular system is shown separately (to the far left); effectors include sweat glands, pilomotor muscles and blood vessels of the skin, and blood vessels of the skeletal muscles and bones. (Modified from Heimer L. [1983]. *The human brain and spinal cord: Functional neuroanatomy and dissection guide.* New York: Springer-Verlag.)

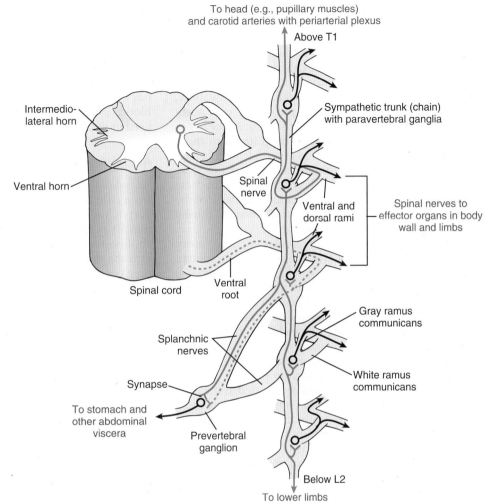

FIGURE 33-25 Sympathetic pathways. Preganglionic fibers (shown in blue) leave the spinal cord by way of the ventral root of the spinal nerves, enter the ventral primary rami, and pass through the white rami to the prevertebral or paravertebral ganglia of the sympathetic chain, where they synapse with postganglionic neurons. Some postganglionic fibers (shown in black) from the paravertebral ganglia reenter the segmental nerves through the gray rami and are then distributed in the spinal nerve branches that innervate the effector organs (*e.g.,* sweat glands and arrector pili muscles of skin and vascular smooth muscle of blood vessels). Other preganglionic neurons (*dotted lines*) travel directly to their destination in the various effector organs.

Labels in figure:
To head (e.g., pupillary muscles) and carotid arteries with periarterial plexus
Above T1
Intermedio-lateral horn
Ventral horn
Spinal cord
Ventral root
Splanchnic nerves
Synapse
To stomach and other abdominal viscera
Prevertebral ganglion
Spinal nerve
Ventral and dorsal rami
Sympathetic trunk (chain) with paravertebral ganglia
Spinal nerves to effector organs in body wall and limbs
Gray ramus communicans
White ramus communicans
Below L2
To lower limbs

With the exception of cranial nerves III, VII, and IX, which synapse in discrete ganglia, the long parasympathetic preganglionic fibers pass uninterrupted to short postganglionic fibers located in the organ wall. In the walls of these organs, postganglionic neurons send axons to smooth muscle and glandular cells that modulate their functions.

The gastrointestinal tract has its own intrinsic network of ganglionic cells located between the smooth muscle layers, called the *enteric* (or *intramural*) *plexus,* which controls local peristaltic movements and secretory functions. This network of parasympathetic postganglionic neurons and interneurons runs from the upper portion of the esophagus to the internal anal sphincter. Local afferent sensory neurons respond to mechanical and chemical stimuli and communicate these influences to motor fibers in the enteric plexus. The number of neurons in the enteric neural network (10^8) is so large that it approximates that of the spinal cord. It is thought that this enteric nervous system is capable of independent function without control from CNS fibers. The CNS has a modulating role, by way of preganglionic innervation of the plexus, converting local peristalsis to longer-distance movements, thereby speeding the transit of intestinal contents.

CENTRAL INTEGRATIVE PATHWAYS

General visceral afferent fibers accompany the sympathetic and parasympathetic outflow into the spinal and cranial nerves, bringing chemoreceptor, pressure, and nociceptive information from organs of the viscera to the brain stem, thoracolumbar cord, and sacral cord. Local reflex circuits relating visceral afferent and autonomic efferent activity are integrated into a hierarchic control system in the spinal cord and brain stem. Progressively greater complexity in the responses and greater precision in their control occur at each higher level of the nervous system. Most visceral reflexes contain contributions from the LMNs that innervate skeletal muscles as part of their response patterns.

For most autonomic-mediated functions, the hypothalamus serves as the major control center. The hypothalamus, which has connections with the cerebral cortex, the limbic system, and the pituitary gland, is in a prime position to receive, integrate, and transmit information to other areas of the nervous system. The neurons concerned with thermoregulation, thirst, and feeding behaviors are found in the hypothalamus. The hypothalamus also is the site for integrating neuroendocrine function. Hypothalamic releasing and inhibiting hormones control the secretion of anterior pituitary hormones (see Chapter 31).

The organization of many life-support reflexes occurs in the reticular formation of the medulla and pons. These areas of reflex circuitry, often called *centers*, produce complex combinations of autonomic and somatic efferent functions required for the cough, sneeze, swallow, and vomit reflexes, as well as for the more purely autonomic control of the cardiovascular system. At the hypothalamic level, these reflexes are integrated into more general response patterns, such as rage, defensive behavior, eating and drinking, voiding, and sexual function. Forebrain and especially limbic system control of these behaviors involves inhibiting or facilitating release of the response patterns according to social pressures during learned emotion-provoking situations.

Reflex adjustments of cardiovascular and respiratory function occur at the level of the brain stem. A prominent example is the carotid sinus baroreflex (see Chapter 17). One of the striking features of ANS function is the rapidity and intensity with which it can change visceral function. Within 3 to 5 seconds, it can increase heart rate to approximately twice its resting level. Bronchial smooth muscle tone is largely controlled by parasympathetic fibers carried in the vagus nerve. These nerves produce mild to moderate constriction of the bronchioles.

Other important ANS reflexes are located at the level of the spinal cord. As with other spinal reflexes, these reflexes are modulated by input from higher centers. When there is loss of communication between the higher centers and the spinal reflexes, as occurs in spinal cord injury, these reflexes function in an unregulated manner (see Chapter 35).

AUTONOMIC NEUROTRANSMISSION

The generation and transmission of impulses in the ANS occur in the same manner as in the CNS. There are self-propagating action potentials with transmission of impulses across synapses and other tissue junctions by way of neurohumoral transmitters. The postganglionic fibers of the ANS form a diffuse neural plexus at the site of innervation. The membranes of the cells of many smooth muscle fibers are connected by conductive protoplasmic bridges, called *gap junctions*, that permit rapid conduction of impulses through whole sheets of smooth muscle, often in repeating waves of contraction. Autonomic neurotransmitters released near a limited portion of these fibers provide a modulating function extending to a large number of effector cells. The muscle layers of the gut and of the bladder wall are examples.

The main neurotransmitters of the ANS are acetylcholine and the catecholamines, epinephrine and norepinephrine. Acetylcholine is released at all of the sites of preganglionic transmission in the autonomic ganglia of sympathetic and parasympathetic nerve fibers and at the sites of postganglionic transmission in parasympathetic nerve endings. It also is released at sympathetic nerve endings that innervate the sweat glands and cholinergic vasodilator fibers found in skeletal muscle. Norepinephrine is released at most sympathetic nerve endings. The

adrenal medulla, which is a modified neural crest tissue, produces epinephrine along with small amounts of norepinephrine. Dopamine, which is an intermediate compound in the synthesis of norepinephrine, also acts as a neurotransmitter. It is the principal inhibitory transmitter of internuncial neurons in the sympathetic ganglia. It also has vasodilator effects on renal, splanchnic, and coronary blood vessels when given intravenously and is sometimes used in the treatment of shock (see Chapter 19).

Acetylcholine and Cholinergic Receptors

Acetylcholine is synthesized in the cholinergic neurons from choline and acetyl coenzyme A (acetyl CoA). After acetylcholine is secreted by the cholinergic nerve endings, it is rapidly broken down by the enzyme acetylcholinesterase. The choline molecule is transported back into the nerve ending, where it is used again in the synthesis of acetylcholine.

Receptors that respond to acetylcholine are called *cholinergic receptors*. There are two types of cholinergic receptors: muscarinic and nicotinic. Muscarinic receptors are present on the innervational targets of postganglionic fibers of the parasympathetic nervous system and the sweat glands, which are innervated by the sympathetic nervous system. Nicotinic receptors are found in autonomic ganglia and the end plates of skeletal muscle. Acetylcholine has an excitatory effect on muscarinic and nicotinic receptors, except for those in the heart and lower esophagus, where it has an inhibitory effect. The drug atropine is an antimuscarinic or muscarinic cholinergic-blocking drug that prevents the action of acetylcholine at excitatory and inhibitory muscarinic receptor sites. Because it is a muscarinic-blocking drug, it exerts little effect at nicotinic receptor sites.

Catecholamines and Adrenergic Receptors

The catecholamines, which include norepinephrine, epinephrine, and dopamine, are synthesized in the sympathetic nervous system. Synthesis of dopamine and norepinephrine begins in the axoplasm of sympathetic nerve terminals with the conversion of the amino acid tyrosine to dopa; dopa to dopamine; and dopamine to norepinephrine. In the adrenal gland an additional step takes place during which approximately 80% of the norepinephrine is transformed into epinephrine.

Each of the steps in sympathetic neurotransmitter synthesis requires a different enzyme, and the type of neurotransmitter that is produced depends on the types of enzymes that are available in a nerve terminal. For example, the postganglionic sympathetic neurons that supply blood vessels have the needed enzymes for the synthesis of norepinephrine, whereas those in the adrenal medulla have the enzymes needed to convert norepinephrine into epinephrine. As the catecholamines are synthesized, they are stored in vesicles. The final step of norepinephrine synthesis occurs in these vesicles. When an action potential reaches an axon terminal, the neurotransmitter molecules are released from the storage vesicles. The storage vesicles provide a means for concentrated storage of the catecholamines and protect them from the cytoplasmic enzymes that degrade the neurotransmitters.

In addition to neuronal synthesis, there is a second major mechanism for replenishment of norepinephrine in sympathetic nerve terminals. This mechanism consists of the active reuptake of the released neurotransmitter into the nerve terminal. Between 50% and 80% of the norepinephrine that is released during an action potential is removed from the synaptic area by an active reuptake process. This process terminates the action of the neurotransmitter and allows it to be reused by the neuron. The remainder of the released catecholamines diffuses into the surrounding tissue fluids or is degraded by two special enzymes: catechol-O-methyltransferase, which is diffusely present in all tissues, and monoamine oxidase (MAO), which is found in the nerve endings themselves.

Catecholamines can cause excitation or inhibition of smooth muscle contraction, depending on the site, dose, and type of receptor present. The excitatory or inhibitory responses of organs to sympathetic neurotransmitters are mediated by interaction with special structures in the cell membrane called *receptors*. There are two types of sympathetic receptors: α and β receptors. In vascular smooth muscle, excitation of α-adrenergic receptors causes vasoconstriction, and excitation of β-adrenergic receptors causes vasodilatation. Constriction of blood vessels in the skin, kidneys, and splanchnic circulation is mediated by α-adrenergic receptors. The β-adrenergic receptors are most prevalent in the heart, the blood vessels of skeletal muscle, and the bronchioles.

α-Adrenergic receptors have been further subdivided into α_1 and α_2 receptors, and β-adrenergic receptors into β_1 and β_2 receptors. β_1-Adrenergic receptors are found primarily in the heart and can be selectively blocked by β_1-receptor–blocking drugs. β_2-Adrenergic receptors are found in the bronchioles and in other sites that have β-mediated functions. The α_1 receptors are found primarily in postsynaptic effector sites; they mediate responses in vascular smooth muscle. The α_2 receptors are mainly located presynaptically and can inhibit the release of norepinephrine from sympathetic nerve terminals. The α_2 receptors are abundant in the CNS and are thought to influence the central control of blood pressure.

In summary, the ANS regulates, adjusts, and coordinates the visceral functions of the body. The ANS, which is divided into the sympathetic and parasympathetic systems, is an efferent system. It receives its afferent input from visceral afferent neurons. The ANS has CNS and PNS components. The outflow of the sympathetic and parasympathetic nervous system follows a two-neuron pathway, which consists of a preganglionic neuron located in the CNS and a postganglionic neuron located outside the CNS. Sympathetic fibers leave the CNS at the thoracolumbar level, and the parasympathetic fibers leave at the craniosacral level.

In general, the sympathetic and parasympathetic nervous systems have opposing effects on visceral function—if one excites, the other inhibits. The hypothalamus serves as the major control center for most ANS functions; local reflex circuits relating visceral afferent and autonomic efferent activity are integrated in a hierarchic control system in the spinal cord and brain stem.

The main neurotransmitters for the ANS are acetylcholine, the catecholamines, epinephrine, and norepinephrine. Acetylcholine is the transmitter for all preganglionic neurons, for postganglionic parasympathetic neurons, and for selected postganglionic sympathetic neurons. The catecholamines are the neurotransmitters for most postganglionic sympathetic neurons. The ANS neurotransmitters exert their action through specialized cell surface receptors—cholinergic receptors that bind acetylcholine and adrenergic receptors that bind the catecholamines. The cholinergic receptors are divided into nicotinic and muscarinic receptors, and adrenergic receptors are divided into α and β receptors.

Review Exercises

An event such as cardiac arrest, which produces global ischemia of the brain, can produce a selective loss of memory and cognitive skills while preserving more vegetative and life-sustaining functions such as breathing.

A. Use principles related to the development of the nervous system and hierarchy of control to explain why this occurs.

Usually spinal cord injury or disease produces both sensory and motor deficits. An exception is infection by the poliomyelitis virus, which produces weakness and paralysis without loss of sensation in the affected extremities.

A. Explain this phenomenon using information on the organization of the nervous system into cell columns.

The functions of the sympathetic nervous system are often described in relation to the "fight-or-flight" response. Using this description, explain the physiologic advantage for the following distribution of sympathetic nervous system receptors:

A. The distribution of β_2 receptors to the blood vessels that provide blood flow to the skeletal muscles during "flight" and α_1 receptors to the resistance vessels that control blood pressure.

B. The presence of acetylcholine receptors on the sweat glands that allow for evaporative loss of body heat during "flight" and the presence of α_1 receptors that constrict the skin vessels that control blood flow to the skin.

C. The presence of β_2 receptors that produce relaxation in the detrusor muscle of the bladder during "fight or flight" and the α_1 receptors that produce contraction of the smooth muscle in the internal sphincter of the bladder.

Visit the Porth: Essentials of Pathophysiology: Concepts of Altered Health States web site

(http://thePoint.LWW.com/PorthEssentials) for links to chapter-related resources on the Internet, all-new exclusive animations, chapter review questions, and more!

BIBLIOGRAPHY

Araque A., Parpura V., Sanzgiri R. P., et al. (1999). Tri-partite synapses: Glia, the unacknowledged partner. *Trends in Neuroscience* 22, 208–215.

Bear M. F., Connors B. W., Paradiso M. A. (2001). *Neuroscience: Exploring the brain* (2nd ed.). Philadelphia: Lippincott Williams & Wilkins.

Dambska M., Wisniewski K. E. (1999). *Normal and pathologic development of the human brain and spinal cord.* London: John Libbey.

Gartner L. P., Hiatt J. L. (2001). *Color textbook of histology* (2nd ed., pp. 183–217). Philadelphia: W. B. Saunders.

Guyton A. C., Hall J. E. (2000). *Textbook of medical physiology* (10th ed.). Philadelphia: W. B. Saunders.

Kandel E. R., Schwartz J. H., Jessell T. M. (2000). *Principles of neural science* (4th ed.). New York: McGraw-Hill.

Kierszenbaum A. L. (2002). *Histology and cell biology: An introduction to pathology* (pp. 199–225). St. Louis: Mosby.

Matthews G. G. (1998). *Neurobiology: Molecules, cells, and systems.* Malden, MA: Blackwell Science.

Moore K. L., Persaud T. V. N. (2003). *The developing human: Clinically oriented embryology* (7th ed., pp. 59–76, 427–463). Philadelphia: Elsevier Saunders.

Parent A. (1996). *Carpenter's human neuroanatomy* (9th ed., pp. 186–192, 268–292, 748–756). Baltimore: Williams & Wilkins.

Ross M. H., Kaye G. I., Pawlina W. (2003). *Histology: A text and atlas* (4th ed., pp. 282–324). Philadelphia: Lippincott Williams & Wilkins.

Zigmond M. J., Bloom E. F., Landis S. C., et al. (1999). *Fundamental neuroscience.* San Diego: Academic Press.

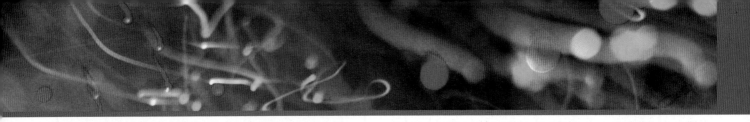

Chapter 34

Disorders of Somatosensory Function and Pain

Sensory mechanisms provide individuals with a continuous stream of information about their bodies, the outside world, and the interactions between the two. The somatosensory component of the nervous system provides an awareness of body sensations such as touch, temperature, limb position, and pain. Other sensory components of the nervous system include the special senses of vision and hearing, which are discussed in Chapter 37. This chapter provides an introduction to the somatosensory functions of the nervous system and discusses pain as a somatosensory modality, focusing on pain and its management; alterations in pain sensitivity and special types of pain; headache; and pain in children and older adults.

Organization and Control of Somatosensory Function

The somatosensory system is designed to provide the central nervous system (CNS) with information about the body. Sensory neurons can be divided into three types that vary in distribution and the type of sensation detected: general somatic, special somatic, and general visceral afferent neurons (see Chapter 33). *General somatic afferent neurons* have branches with widespread distribution throughout the body and with many distinct types of receptors that result in sensations such as pain, touch, and temperature. *Special somatic afferent neurons* have receptors located primarily in muscles, tendons, and joints. These receptors sense position and movement of the body. *General visceral afferent neurons* have receptors on various visceral structures and sense fullness and discomfort.

SENSORY SYSTEMS

Sensory systems can be conceptualized as a serial succession of neurons consisting of first-order, second-order, and third-order neurons. The *first-order neurons* contain the sensory receptors and transmit sensory information from the periphery to the CNS. The *second-order neurons* communicate with various reflex networks and sensory pathways in the spinal cord and contain the ascending pathways that travel to the thalamus. *Third-order neurons* relay information from the thalamus to the cerebral cortex (Fig. 34-1). Many interneurons process and modify the sensory information at the level of the second- and third-order neurons, and many more participate before coordinated and appropriate learned-movement responses occur.

The Sensory Unit

The somatosensory experience arises from information provided by a variety of receptors distributed throughout the body. There are four major modalities of somatosensory experience: discriminative touch (required to identify the size and shape of objects and their movement across the skin); proprioception (sense of movement of the limbs and joints of the body); temperature sense (perception of warmth and cold); and nociception (process whereby pain or itch is perceived).[1]

Each of the somatosensory modalities is mediated by a distinct system of receptors and pathways to the brain. However, all somatosensory information from the limbs and trunk shares a common class of sensory neurons called *dorsal root ganglion neurons*, whereas somatosensory information from the face and cranial structures is transmitted by *trigeminal sensory neurons*, which function in the same manner as the dorsal root ganglion neurons. The cell body of a dorsal root ganglion neuron,

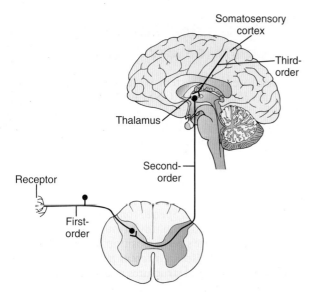

FIGURE 34-1 Arrangement of first-order, second-order, and third-order neurons of the somatosensory system.

KEY CONCEPTS

The Somatosensory System

➤ The somatosensory system relays information to the CNS about four major body sensations: touch, temperature, pain, and body position. Stimulation of receptors on regions of the body wall is required to initiate the sensory response.

➤ The somatosensory system is organized into dermatomes, with each segment supplied by a single dorsal root ganglion that sequentially relays the sensory information to the spinal cord, the thalamus, and the sensory cortex.

➤ Two pathways carry somatosensory information through the CNS. The dorsal column-medial lemniscal pathway crosses in the medulla and relays touch and body position. The anterolateral pathway crosses in the spinal cord and relays temperature and pain sensation from the opposite side of the body.

its receptors (which innervate a small area of periphery), and its central axon (which projects to the CNS) form a *sensory unit*. Individual dorsal root ganglion neurons respond selectively to specific types of stimuli because of their specialized peripheral terminals, or receptors.

Dermatomal Pattern of Dorsal Root Innervation

The somatosensory innervation of the body, including the head, retains a basic segmental organizational pattern that was established during embryonic development. The region of the body wall that is supplied by a single pair of dorsal root ganglia is called a *dermatome*.[1–3] These dorsal root ganglion–innervated strips occur in a regular sequence moving upward from the second coccygeal segment through the cervical segments, reflecting the basic segmental organization of the body and the nervous system (Fig. 34-2). The cranial nerves that innervate the head send their axons to equivalent nuclei in the brain stem. Neighboring dermatomes overlap one another sufficiently so that a loss of one dorsal root or root ganglion results in reduced but not a total loss of sensory innervation of a dermatome (Fig. 34-3). Dermatome maps are helpful in interpreting the level and extent of sensory deficits that result from segmental nerve and spinal cord damage.

Spinal Circuitry and Ascending Neural Pathways

On entry into the spinal cord, the central axons of the somatosensory neurons branch extensively and project to nuclei in the spinal gray matter. Some branches become involved in local spinal cord reflexes and directly initiate motor reflexes (*e.g.*, flexor-withdrawal reflex). Two parallel pathways, the rapid-conducting *dorsal column-medial*

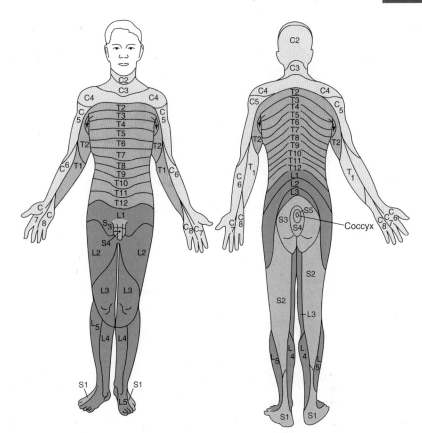

FIGURE 34-2 Cutaneous distribution of spinal nerves (dermatomes). (From Barr M. [1993]. *The human nervous system.* New York: Harper & Row.)

lemniscal pathway and the slower-conducting *anterolateral pathway*, transmit information from the spinal cord to the thalamic level of sensation, each taking a different route through the CNS.[1]

The Dorsal Column-Medial Lemniscal Pathway. The dorsal column-medial lemniscal pathway, which crosses at the base of the medulla, is used for the rapid transmission of discriminative touch sensation and proprioception[1-3] (Fig. 34-4A). It contains branches of primary

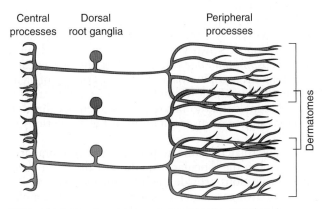

FIGURE 34-3 The dermatomes formed by the peripheral processes of adjacent spinal nerves overlap on the body surface. The central processes of these fibers also overlap in their spinal distribution.

afferent axons that travel up the ipsilateral (*i.e.,* same side) dorsal columns of the spinal cord white matter and synapse with highly evolved somatosensory input association neurons in the medulla. The dorsal column-medial lemniscal pathway uses only three neurons to transmit information from a sensory receptor to the somatosensory strip of parietal cerebral cortex of the opposite side of the brain: (1) the primary dorsal root ganglion neuron, which projects its central axon to the dorsal column nuclei; (2) the dorsal column neuron, which sends its axon through a rapid conducting tract, called the *medial lemniscus,* that crosses at the base of the medulla and travels to the thalamus on the opposite side of the brain, where basic sensation begins; and (3) the thalamic neuron, which projects its axons through the somatosensory radiation to the primary sensory cortex. The medial lemniscus is joined by fibers from the sensory nucleus of the trigeminal nerve (cranial nerve V) that supplies the face. Sensory information arriving at the sensory cortex by this route can be discretely localized and discriminated in terms of intensity.

One of the distinct features of the dorsal column-medial lemniscal pathway is that it relays precise information regarding spatial orientation. This is the only pathway taken by the sensations of muscle and joint movement, vibration, and delicate discriminative touch that are required to differentiate the location of touch on the skin at two neighboring points (*i.e.,* two-point discrimination). One of the important functions of this pathway is to integrate the input from multiple receptors. The

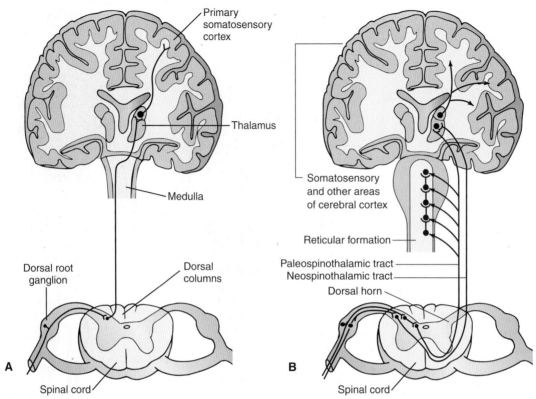

FIGURE 34-4 (**A**) Rapid-transmitting dorsal column-medial lemniscal pathway carrying axons mediating tactile sensation and proprioception. (**B**) Neospinothalamic and paleospinothalamic subdivisions of the anterolateral sensory pathway. The neurons of anterolateral pathways cross within the same segment as the cell body and ascend in the contralateral side of the spinal cord. The neospinothalamic tract travels mainly to thalamic nuclei that have third-order fibers projecting to the somatosensory cortex. The paleospinothalamic tract sends collaterals to the reticular formation and other structures, from which further fibers project to the thalamus.

sense of shape and size of an object in the absence of visualization, called *stereognosis*, is based on precise afferent information from muscle, tendon, and joint receptors. For example, a screwdriver is perceived as being different from a knife in terms of its texture (tactile sensibility) and shape based on the relative position of the fingers as they move over the object. This complex interpretive perception requires that the dorsal column-medial lemniscal pathway must be functioning optimally and that higher-order parietal association cortex processing and prior learning must have occurred. If the dorsal column-medial lemniscal pathway is functional but the parietal association cortex has become discretely damaged, the person can correctly describe the object but does not recognize that it is a screwdriver. This deficit is called *astereognosis*.

The Anterolateral Pathway. The anterolateral pathway is a multisynaptic slow-conducting pathway that uses the anterior and lateral spinothalamic tracts (see Chapter 33, Fig. 33-11), which cross within the first few segments of entering the spinal cord, to transmit sensory information to the brain (see Fig. 34-4B). In contrast to the dorsal column-medial lemniscal pathway, it transmits sensory sig-

nals such as pain, thermal sensations, crude touch, and pressure that do not require highly discrete localization of the signal source or fine discrimination of intensity.

There are two subdivisions in the anterolateral pathway: the outer neospinothalamic tract and the inner paleospinothalamic tract. The *neospinothalamic tract*, which carries bright pain, consists of a sequence of at least three neurons with long axons. It provides for relatively rapid transmission of sensory information to the thalamus. The *paleospinothalamic tract*, which is phylogenetically older than the neospinothalamic system, consists of bilateral, multisynaptic slow-conducting tracts that transmit sensory signals that do not require discrete localization of signal source or discrimination of fine gradations in intensity.

The anterolateral pathway gives off numerous branches that travel to the reticular formation of the brain stem. These projections provide the basis for increased wakefulness or awareness after strong somatosensory stimulation and for the generalized startle reaction that occurs with sudden and intense stimuli. They also stimulate autonomic nervous system responses, such as an increase in blood pressure and heart rate, dilation of the pupils, and the pale, moist skin that results from constriction of the cutaneous blood vessels and activation of the sweat glands. This slower-conducting pathway also projects into the intralaminar nuclei of the thalamus, which have close connections with the limbic cortical systems. This circuitry provides touch with its affective or emotional aspects.

Central Processing of Somatosensory Information

Perception, or the final processing of somatosensory information, involves awareness of the stimuli, localization and discrimination of their characteristics, and interpretation of their meaning. As sensory information reaches the thalamus, it begins to enter the level of consciousness. In the thalamus, the sensory information is roughly localized and perceived as a crude sense. The full localization, discrimination of the intensity, and interpretation of the meaning of the stimuli require processing by the somatosensory cortex.

The somatosensory cortex is located in the parietal lobe, which lies behind the central sulcus and above the lateral sulcus (Fig. 34-5). The strip of parietal cortex that borders the central sulcus is called the *primary somatosensory cortex* because it receives primary sensory information by way of direct projections from the thalamus. A distorted map of the body and head surface, called the *sensory homunculus*, reflects the density of cortical neurons devoted to sensory input from afferents in corresponding peripheral areas. As depicted in Figure 34-6, most of the cortical surface is devoted to areas of the body such as the thumb, forefinger, lips, and tongue where fine touch and pressure discrimination are essential for normal function.

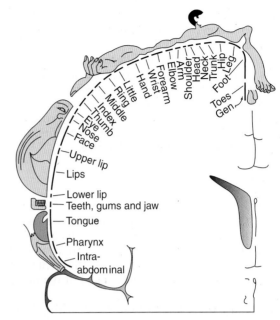

FIGURE 34-6 Homunculus, as determined by stimulation studies on the human cortex during surgery. (From Penfield E., Rasmussen T. [1955]. *The cerebral cortex of man.* New York: Macmillan. Copyright © by Macmillan Publishing Co., Inc., renewed 1978 by Theodore Rasmussen.)

The somatosensory association cortex, which lies parallel to and just behind the primary somatosensory cortex, is required to transform the raw material of sensation into a meaningful experience. It is here that the stimulus pattern from the present sensory experience is integrated with past learning. For instance, a person's past learning plus present tactile sensation provide the perception of sitting on a soft chair, rather than on a hard bicycle seat.

SENSORY MODALITIES

Somatosensory experience can be divided into *modalities,* a term used for qualitative subjective distinctions between sensations such as touch, heat, and pain. Such experiences require the function of sensory receptors and forebrain structures in the thalamus and cerebral cortex. Sensory experience also involves quantitative sensory discrimination or the ability to distinguish between different levels of sensory stimulation.

The receptive endings of different afferent neurons are particularly sensitive to specific forms of physical and chemical energy. For instance, a receptive ending may be particularly sensitive to a small increase in local skin temperature. Other afferent sensory terminals may be particularly sensitive to slight indentations of the skin, and their signals subjectively interpreted as touch. Cool versus warm, delicate touch versus deep pressure, and sharp versus dull pain are all based on different populations of afferent neurons or on central integration of simultaneous input from several differently tuned afferents. For example, the sensation of itch results from a combination

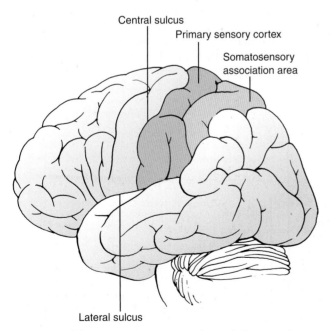

FIGURE 34-5 Primary somatosensory and association somatosensory cortex.

of high activity in pain- and touch-sensitive afferents, and the sensation of tickle requires a gently moving tactile stimulus over cool skin.

When information from different primary afferents reaches the forebrain, where subjective experience occurs, the qualitative differences between warmth and touch are called *sensory modalities*. Although the receptor-detected information is relayed to the thalamus and cortex over separate pathways, the experience of a modality, such as cold versus warm, is uniquely subjective.

Tactile Sensation

The tactile system, which relays sensory information regarding touch, pressure, and vibration, is considered the basic somatosensory system. Loss of temperature or pain sensitivity leaves the person with no awareness of deficiency. However, when input from the tactile system is lost, total anesthesia (*i.e.*, numbness) of the involved body part results.

Touch sensation results from stimulation of tactile receptors in the skin and in tissues immediately beneath the skin, pressure from deformation of deeper tissues, and vibration from rapidly repetitive sensory signals. There are at least six types of specialized tactile receptors in the skin and deeper structures: free nerve endings, Meissner corpuscles, Merkel disks, pacinian corpuscles, hair follicle end-organs, and Ruffini end-organs[1-3] (Fig. 34-7).

Free nerve endings are found in skin and many other tissues, including the cornea. They detect touch and pressure. *Meissner corpuscles* are present in nonhairy parts of the skin. They are particularly abundant in the fingertips, lips, and other areas where the sense of touch is highly developed. *Meissner corpuscles* are particularly sensitive to movement of very light objects over the surface of the skin and to low-frequency vibration. *Merkel disks* are found in nonhairy areas and in hairy parts of the skin. They are responsible for giving steady-state signals that allow for continuous determination of touch against the skin.

The *pacinian corpuscle* is located immediately beneath the skin and deep in the fascial tissues of the body and is important in detecting tissue vibration. The *hair follicle end-organs* detect movement on the surface of the body. *Ruffini end-organs* are found in the skin and deeper structures, including the joint capsules. These receptors are important for signaling continuous states of deformation, such as heavy and continuous touch and pressure.

The sensory information for tactile sensation enters the spinal cord through the dorsal roots of the spinal nerves. All tactile sensation that requires rapid transmission is transmitted through the dorsal column-medial lemniscal pathway to the thalamus by way of the medial lemniscus. This includes touch sensation requiring a high degree of localization or fine gradations of intensity, vibratory sensation, and sensation that signals movement against the skin. In addition to the ascending dorsal column-medial lemniscal pathway, tactile sensation also uses the more primitive and crude anterolateral pathway. The second-order dorsal horn neurons of this pathway have many branches or collaterals. After several synapses, axons are projected up both sides of the anterolateral aspect of the spinal cord to the thalamus. Few fibers travel all the way to the thalamus. Most synapse on reticular formation neurons that then send their axons on toward the thalamus, where a crude, poorly localized sensation from the opposite side of the body is received. From the thalamus, some projections travel to the somatosensory cortex.

Because of these multiple routes, total destruction of the pathways for tactile sensation seldom occurs. The only time the crude alternative system becomes essential is when the dorsal column-medial lemniscal pathway is damaged. Then, despite projection of the anterolateral system information to the somatosensory cortex, only a poorly localized, high-threshold sense of touch remains. Such persons lose all sense of joint and muscle movement, body position, and two-point discrimination.

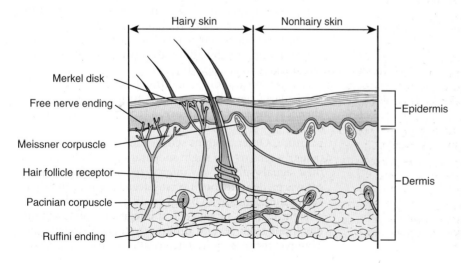

FIGURE 34-7 Somatic sensory receptors in the skin. There are a variety of sensory receptors within hairy and non-hairy skin. (Adapted from Bear M. F., Connors B. W., Paradiso M. A. [1996]. *Neuroscience: Exploring the brain* [p. 311]. Baltimore: Williams & Wilkins.)

Thermal Sensation

Thermal sensation is discriminated by three types of receptors: cold receptors, warmth receptors, and pain receptors. The cold and warmth receptors are located immediately under the skin at discrete but separate points. In some areas, there are more cold receptors than warmth receptors. For example, the lips have 15 to 25 cold receptors per square centimeter, compared with 3 to 5 in the same-sized area of the finger.[4] There are also correspondingly fewer warmth receptors in these areas. The gradations of heat and cold sensation result from selective stimulation of the different types of thermal receptors. The thermal receptors are very sensitive to differences between the temperature of skin and the temperature of objects that are touched. Warmth receptors respond proportionately to increases in skin temperature above resting values of 34°C and cool receptors to temperatures below 34°C.

The thermal pain receptors are stimulated only by extremes of temperature such as "freezing cold" (temperatures below 5°C) and "burning hot" (temperatures above 45°C) sensations.[4] With the exception of pain receptors, thermal receptors tend to adapt rapidly during the first few minutes and then more slowly during the next 30 minutes or so. However, these receptors do not appear to adapt completely, as evidenced by the experience of an intense sense of heat on entering a tub of hot water or the extreme degree of cold initially sensed when going outside on a cold day. On entering the dorsal horn, thermal signals are transmitted by neurons whose axons then cross to the opposite side of the cord and ascend in the multisynaptic, slow-conducting anterolateral system to the opposite side of the brain.

Conduction of thermal information through peripheral nerves is quite slow compared with the rapid tactile afferents that travel through the dorsal column-medial lemniscal pathway. If a person places a foot in a tub of hot water, the tactile sensation occurs well in advance of the burning sensation. The foot has been removed from the hot water by the local withdrawal reflex well before the excessive heat is perceived by the forebrain. Local anesthetic agents block the small-diameter afferents that carry thermal sensory information before they block the large-diameter axons that carry touch information.

Proprioception

Proprioception, or position sense, refers to the sense of joint and limb movement and position without using vision. It is mediated by input from proprioceptive receptors (muscle spindle receptors and Golgi tendon organs) found primarily in muscles, tendons, and joint capsules (see Chapter 35). There are two submodalities of proprioception: the stationary or static component (limb position sense) and the dynamic aspect of position sense (kinesthesia). Both of these depend on constant transmission of information to the CNS regarding the rate of change and degree of angulation of all joints. In addition, stretch-sensitive receptors in the skin (*i.e.,* Ruffini endings, pacinian corpuscles, and Merkel cells) also signal postural information.

In summary, the somatosensory component of the nervous system provides an awareness of body sensations such as touch, temperature, position sense, and pain. Somatosensory systems consist of first-order neurons, which contain the sensory receptors and transmit information from the periphery to the CNS; second-order neurons, which communicate with various reflex and sensory pathways in the spinal cord and contain ascending pathways that travel to the thalamus; and third-order neurons, which relay information from the thalamus to the cerebral cortex. A sensory unit consists of a single dorsal root ganglion neuron, its receptors, and its central axon that terminates in the dorsal horn of the spinal cord or medulla. The part of the body innervated by the somatosensory afferent neurons of one set of dorsal root ganglia is called a *dermatome.* Ascending pathways include the dorsal column-medial lemniscal pathway, which crosses at the base of the medulla, and the anterolateral pathway, which crosses within the first few segments of entering the spinal cord. Perception, or the final processing of somatosensory information, involves centers in the thalamus and the somatosensory cortex. In the thalamus, the sensory information is crudely localized and perceived. The full localization, discrimination of the intensity, and interpretation of the meaning of the stimuli require processing by the somatosensory cortex. A distorted map of the body and head surface, called the *sensory homunculus,* reflects the density of cortical neurons devoted to sensory input from afferents in corresponding peripheral areas.

The tactile system relays the sensations of touch, pressure, and vibration. It uses two anatomically separate pathways to relay touch information to the opposite side of the forebrain: the dorsal column-medial lemniscal pathway and the anterolateral pathway. Delicate touch, vibration, position, and movement sensations use the dorsal column-medial lemniscal pathway to reach the thalamus, where third-order neurons relay the tactile sensation to the primary somatosensory strip of parietal cortex. Crude tactile sensation is carried by the bilateral slow-conducting anterolateral pathway. Temperature sensations of warm-hot and cool-cold are the result of stimulation to thermal receptors of sensory units projecting to the thalamus and cortex through the anterolateral system on the opposite side of the body. Proprioception is the sense of limb and body movement and position without using vision. It is mediated by input from muscle spindle receptors and Golgi tendon organs found in muscles, tendons, and joint capsules and from mechanoreceptors (*e.g.,* Ruffini end-organs, pacinian corpuscles, and Merkel cells) in the joint capsules and ligaments.

 Pain

Pain, which like touch and position sense is a submodality of somatic sensation, is an unpleasant sensory and emotional experience associated with actual and potential tissue damage. Unlike other somatic modalities, pain has an urgent and primitive quality, a quality responsible for the psychological, social, cultural, and cognitive aspects of the pain experience. Despite its unpleasantness, pain can serve a useful purpose because it warns of impending tissue injury, motivating the person to seek relief. For example, an inflamed appendix could progress in severity, rupture, and even cause death were it not for the warning afforded by the pain.

PAIN THEORIES

Traditionally, two theories have been offered to explain the physiologic basis for the pain experience. The first, *specificity theory*, regards pain as a separate sensory modality evoked by the activity of specific receptors that transmit information to pain centers or regions in the forebrain where pain is experienced.[5] The second theory includes a group of theories collectively referred to as the *pattern theory*. It proposes that pain receptors share endings or pathways with other sensory modalities but that

different patterns of activity (*i.e.*, spatial or temporal) of the same neurons can be used to signal painful and non-painful stimuli.[5] For example, light touch applied to the skin would produce the sensation of touch through low-frequency firing of the receptor; intense pressure would produce pain through high-frequency firing of the same receptor. Both theories focus on the neurophysiologic basis of pain, and both probably apply. Specific nociceptive afferents have been identified; however, almost all afferent stimuli, if driven at a very high frequency, can be experienced as painful.

Gate control theory, a modification of specificity theory, was proposed by Melzack and Wall in 1965 to meet the challenges presented by the pattern theories.[6] This theory postulated the presence of neural gating mechanisms at the segmental spinal cord level to account for interactions between pain and other sensory modalities. According to the gate control theory, the internuncial neurons involved in the gating mechanism are activated by large-diameter, faster-propagating fibers that carry tactile information. The simultaneous firing of the large-diameter touch fibers has the potential for blocking the transmission of impulses from the small-diameter myelinated and unmyelinated pain fibers.

More recently, Melzack has developed the *neuromatrix theory* to address further the brain's role in pain as well as the multiple dimensions and determinants of pain.[7] This theory is particularly useful in understanding chronic pain and phantom limb pain, in which there is not a simple one-to-one relationship between tissue injury and pain experience. The neuromatrix theory proposes that the brain contains a widely distributed neural network, called the *body-self neuromatrix*, that contains somatosensory, limbic, and thalamocortical components. Genetic and sensory influences determine the synaptic architecture of an individual's neuromatrix that integrates multiple sources of input and evokes the sensory, affective, and cognitive dimensions of pain experience and behavior. These multiple input sources include somatosensory; other sensory impulses affecting interpretation of the situation; inputs from the brain addressing such things as attention, expectation, culture, and personality; intrinsic neural inhibitory modulatory circuits; and various components of stress regulation systems.

PAIN MECHANISMS AND PATHWAYS

Pain usually is viewed in the context of tissue injury. The term *nociception*, which means "pain sense," comes from the Latin word *nocere* ("to injure"). Nociceptive stimuli are objectively defined as stimuli of such intensity that they cause or are close to causing tissue damage. Researchers often use the withdrawal reflex (*e.g.*, the reflexive withdrawal of a body part from a tissue-damaging stimulus) to determine when a stimulus is nociceptive. Stimuli used include pressure from a sharp object, strong electric current to the skin, or application of heat or cold of approximately 10°C above or below normal skin temperature. At low levels of intensity, these stimuli may activate nociceptors, but are typically not perceived as

---

 KEY CONCEPTS

Pain Sensation

➤ Pain is both a protective and an unpleasant physical and emotionally disturbing sensation originating in pain receptors that respond to a number of stimuli that threaten tissue integrity.

➤ There are two pathways for pain transmission:

  ➤ The fast pathway for sharply discriminated pain that moves directly from the receptor to the spinal cord using myelinated Aδ fibers and from the spinal cord to the thalamus using the neospinothalamic tract

  ➤ The slow pathway for continuously conducted pain that is transmitted to the spinal cord using unmyelinated C fibers and from the spinal cord to the thalamus using the more circuitous and slower-conducting paleospinothalamic tract

➤ The central processing of pain information includes transmission to the somatosensory cortex, where pain information is perceived and interpreted; to the limbic system, where the emotional components of pain are experienced; and to brain stem centers, where autonomic nervous system responses are recruited.

➤ Modulation of the pain experience occurs by way of the endogenous analgesic center in the midbrain, the pontine noradrenergic neurons, and the nucleus raphe magnus in the medulla, which sends inhibitory signals to dorsal horn neurons in the spinal cord.

painful until the intensity reaches a level where tissue damage occurs or is imminent.

The mechanisms of pain are many and complex (Fig. 34-8). As with other forms of somatic sensation, the pathways are composed of first-, second-, and third-order neurons. The first-order neurons and their receptive endings detect stimuli that threaten the integrity of innervated tissues. Second-order neurons in the spinal cord process nociceptive information and transmit it to the brain stem reticular formation and the thalamus. Third-order neurons project pain information from the thalamus to the somatosensory cortex where the perception and subjective meaning of pain take place.

Pain Receptors, Primary Afferents, and Neuromediators

Nociceptors, or pain receptors, are sensory receptors that are activated by noxious insults to peripheral tissues. Structurally, the receptive endings of the peripheral pain

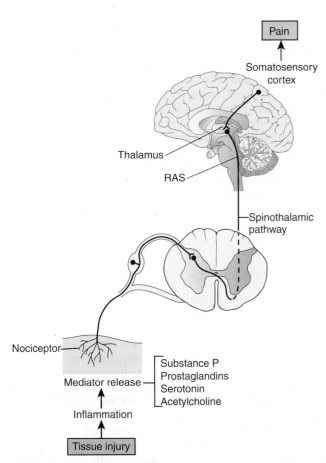

FIGURE 34-8 Mechanisms of acute pain. Tissue injury leads to release of inflammatory mediators with subsequent nociceptor stimulation. Pain impulses are then transmitted to the dorsal horn of the spinal cord, where they make contact with second-order neurons that cross to the opposite side of the cord and ascend through the spinothalamic tract to the reticular activating system (RAS) and thalamus. The localization and meaning of pain occur at the level of the somatosensory cortex.

fibers are free nerve endings. These receptive endings, which are widely distributed in the skin, dental pulp, periosteum, meninges, and some internal organs, translate the noxious stimuli into action potentials that are transmitted by a dorsal root ganglion to the dorsal horn of the spinal cord.

Nociceptive action potentials are transmitted through two types of afferent nerve fibers: myelinated Aδ fibers and unmyelinated C fibers.[1–4] The larger *Aδ fibers* have considerably greater conduction velocities, transmitting impulses at a rate of 6 to 30 m/second. The *C fibers* are the smallest of all peripheral nerve fibers; they transmit impulses at the rate of 0.5 to 2.5 m/second.[4] Pain conducted by Aδ fibers traditionally is called *fast pain* and typically is elicited by mechanical or thermal stimuli. C-fiber pain often is described as *slow-wave pain* because it is slower in onset and longer in duration. It typically is incited by chemical stimuli or by persistent mechanical or thermal stimuli. The slow-wave potentials generated in C fibers are now believed to be responsible for central sensitization to chronic pain.

Stimulation of Nociceptors. Unlike other sensory receptors, nociceptors respond to several forms of stimulation, including mechanical, thermal, and chemical. Some receptors respond to a single type of stimulus (mechanical or thermal), and others, called *polymodal receptors*, respond to all three types of stimuli (mechanical, thermal, and chemical).[1] Mechanical stimuli can arise from intense pressure applied to the skin or from the violent contraction or extreme stretch of a muscle. Both extremes of heat and cold can stimulate nociceptors. Chemical stimuli arise from a number of sources, including tissue trauma, ischemia, and inflammation. A wide range of chemical mediators are released from injured and inflamed tissues, including hydrogen and potassium ions, prostaglandins, leukotrienes, histamine, bradykinin, acetylcholine, and serotonin.[4] These chemical mediators produce their effects by directly stimulating nociceptors or sensitizing them to the effects of nociceptive stimuli; perpetuating the inflammatory responses that lead to the release of chemical agents that act as nociceptive stimuli; or inciting neurogenic reflexes that increase the response to nociceptive stimuli. For example, bradykinin, histamine, serotonin, and potassium activate and also sensitize nociceptors.[8–10] Prostaglandins, which are released from inflamed tissues, enhance the sensitivity of pain endings but do not directly stimulate them. Aspirin and other nonsteroidal analgesic drugs are effective in controlling pain because they block the enzyme needed for prostaglandin synthesis.

Nociceptive stimulation that activates C fibers can cause a response known as *neurogenic inflammation* that produces vasodilatation and an increased release of chemical mediators to which nociceptors respond.[9] This mechanism is thought to be mediated by a dorsal root neuron reflex that produces retrograde transport and release of chemical mediators, which in turn causes increasing inflammation of peripheral tissues. This reflex can set up a vicious cycle, which has implications for persistent pain and hyperalgesia.[8]

Mediators in the Spinal Cord. In the spinal cord, the transmission of impulses is mediated by neurotransmitters released from endings of the nociceptive neurons.[8–10] Some of these neurotransmitters are amino acids (*e.g.,* glutamate), others are amino acid derivatives (*e.g.,* norepinephrine), and still others are low–molecular-weight peptides composed of two or more amino acids. It is thought that glutamate is the excitatory neurotransmitter released in the spinal cord from the Aδ pain nerve fiber endings. It is one of the most widely used excitatory transmitters in the central nervous system, with a duration of action of usually only a few milliseconds.[4] C pain fibers entering the spinal cord release both glutamate and substance P in response to nociceptive stimulation. The glutamate transmitter acts instantaneously and lasts only a few milliseconds, whereas substance P is released more slowly, building up in concentration over seconds or even minutes.[4] In fact, it has been suggested that the "double pain" that is felt after a pinprick reflects the fast pain that results from the rapid action of glutamate and the lagging pain that results from the slower action of substance P.[4] Unlike glutamate, which confines its action to the immediate area of the synaptic terminal, substance P and perhaps other neuropeptides released in the dorsal horn can diffuse an additional distance before they are inactivated. This may help to explain the excitability and diffuse nature of many persistent painful conditions. Neuropeptides such as substance P also appear to prolong and enhance the action of glutamate. Understanding how chemical mediators function in nociception is an active area of research that has implications for the development of new treatments for pain.

Spinal Circuitry and Ascending Pathways

On entering the spinal cord through the dorsal roots, the pain fibers bifurcate and ascend or descend one or two segments before synapsing with second-order association neurons in the dorsal horn. From the dorsal horn, the axons of association projection neurons cross through the anterior commissure to the opposite side and then ascend upward in the previously described neospinothalamic and paleospinothalamic tracts of the anterolateral pathway (Fig. 34-9).

The faster-conducting fibers in the neospinothalamic tract are associated mainly with the transmission of sharp-fast pain information to the thalamus.[4] In the thalamus, synapses are made and the pathway continues to the somatosensory cortex to provide the precise location of the pain. Typically, the pain is experienced as bright, sharp, or stabbing in nature. There is also a local cord-level withdrawal reflex that is designed to remove endangered tissue from a damaging stimulus.

The paleospinothalamic tracts are slower-conducting, multisynaptic pathways concerned with the diffuse, dull, aching, and unpleasant sensations that commonly are associated with chronic and visceral pain.[4] Fibers of this pathway terminate widely in the brain stem. Only one tenth to one fourth pass directly to the thalamus. Instead, they terminate principally in the reticular formation in the medulla, pons, and midbrain; in the midbrain they project deep to the superior and inferior colliculi and to the periaqueductal gray region (to be discussed).[4] These lower regions of the brain appear to be important in the suffering aspects of pain. From the brain stem areas, multiple short-fiber neurons project to nuclei in the thalamus and into the hypothalamus and basal regions of the brain. These projections facilitate avoidance reflexes at all levels. This component of the paleospinothalamic system also contributes to an increase in the electroencephalographic activity associated with alertness and indirectly influences hypothalamic functions associated with other responses, such as increased heart rate and blood pressure.

Brain Centers and Pain Perception

The basic sensation of hurtfulness, or pain, occurs at the level of the thalamus. In the neospinothalamic system, interconnections between the lateral thalamus and the somatosensory cortex are necessary to add precision and discrimination to the pain sensation. In addition, association areas of the parietal cortex are essential to the learned meaningfulness of the pain experience (see Fig. 34-9). For example, if a person is stung on the index finger by a bee and only the thalamus is functional, the person reports pain somewhere on the hand. With the primary sensory cortex functional, the person can localize the pain to the precise area on the index finger. With the association cortex functional, the person can interpret the buzzing and sight of the bee that preceded the pain as being related to the bee sting. The paleospinothalamic system projects diffusely from the intralaminar nuclei of the thalamus to large areas of the limbic cortex. These connections probably are associated with the hurtfulness and the mood-altering and attention-narrowing effect of pain.

Central Pathways for Pain Modulation

A major advance in understanding pain was the discovery of neuroanatomic pathways that arise in the midbrain and brain stem, descend to the spinal cord, and modulate ascending pain impulses. One such pathway begins in an area of the midbrain called the *periaqueductal gray* (PAG) region.[1,4] Through research it was found that electrical stimulation of the midbrain PAG regions produced a state of analgesia that lasted for many hours. This stimulation-induced analgesia was found to be remarkably specific and was not associated with changes in either the levels of consciousness or the reactions to auditory and visual stimuli.[1] Subsequently, opioid receptors were found to be highly concentrated in this and other regions of the CNS where electrical stimulation produced analgesia. Because of these findings, the PAG area of the midbrain often is referred to as the *endogenous analgesia center.*

The PAG area receives input from widespread areas of the CNS, including the cerebral cortex, hypothala-

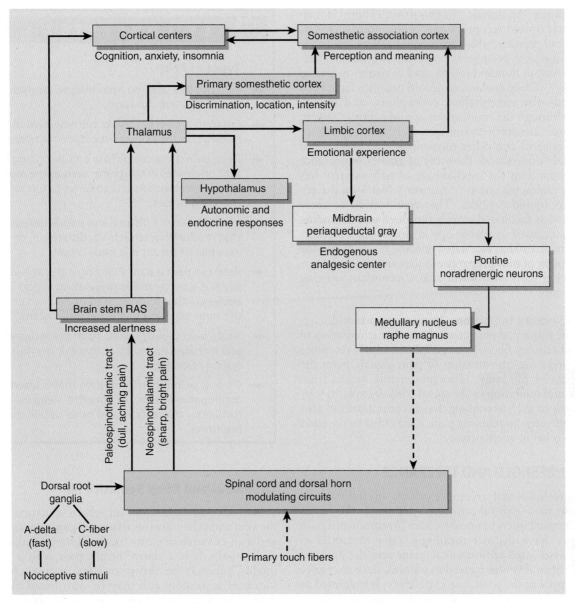

FIGURE 34-9 Primary pain pathways. The transmission of incoming nociceptive impulses is modulated by dorsal horn circuitry that receives input from primary touch receptors and from descending pathways that involve the limbic cortical systems, hypothalamus, periaqueductal endogenous analgesic center in the midbrain, pontine noradrenergic neurons, and the nucleus raphe magnus in the medulla. *Dashed lines* indicate inhibition or modulation. RAS, reticular activating system.

mus, brain stem reticular formation, and spinal cord by way of the paleospinothalamic and neospinothalamic tracts. This region is intimately connected to the limbic system, which is associated with emotional experience. The neurons of the PAG have axons that descend into an area of the rostral medulla called the *nucleus raphe magnus* (NRM).[2] Axons of the NRM neurons project to the dorsal horn of the spinal cord, where they terminate in the same layers as the entering primary pain fibers (see Fig. 34-9). In the spinal cord, these descending pathways inhibit pain transmission by dorsal horn projection neurons.[1] Serotonin has been identified as a

neurotransmitter in the NRM medullary nuclei. Tricyclic antidepressant drugs (*e.g.,* amitriptyline, nortriptyline, desipramine), which enhance the effects of serotonin by blocking its presynaptic uptake, have been found to be effective in the management of certain types of chronic pain.[11,12] Additional inhibitory spinal projections arise from noradrenergic neurons in the pons and medulla, which also receive input from the PAG region.[1] The discovery that norepinephrine can block pain transmission led to studies directed at the combined administration of opioids and clonidine, a central-acting α-adrenergic agonist, for pain relief.[13]

Endogenous Analgesic Mechanisms. There is evidence that opioid receptors and endogenously synthesized opioid peptides, which are morphine-like substances, are found on the peripheral processes of primary afferent neurons, in human synovia, and in many regions of the CNS. [14] Three families of opioid peptides have been identified—the enkephalins, endorphins, and dynorphins. Although the endogenous opioid peptides appear to function as neurotransmitters, their full significance in pain control and other physiologic functions is not completely understood. Probably of greater importance in understanding the mechanisms of pain control has been the characterization of receptors that bind the endogenous opioid peptides. The identification of these receptors has facilitated a more thorough understanding of the actions of available opioid drugs, such as morphine, and it also has facilitated ongoing research into the development of new preparations that are more effective in relieving pain with fewer side effects than existing preparations.[14]

Tactile Sensory Inhibition. Another important discovery in the history of pain control was that stimulation of large Aδ sensory fibers from peripheral tactile receptors can depress the transmission of pain signals from the same area of the body.[4] This presumably results from local lateral inhibition in the spinal cord. It explains why interventions such as rubbing the skin near a painful area is often effective in relieving pain; it may also be the basis for pain relief in acupuncture.

PAIN THRESHOLD AND TOLERANCE

Pain threshold and tolerance affect an individual's response to a painful stimulus. Although the terms often are used interchangeably, *pain threshold* and *pain tolerance* have distinct meanings. *Pain threshold* is closely associated with tissue damage and the point at which a stimulus is perceived as painful. *Pain tolerance* relates more to the total pain experience; it is defined as the maximum intensity or duration of pain that a person is willing to endure before the person wants something done about the pain. Psychological, familial, cultural, and environmental factors significantly influence the amount of pain a person is willing to tolerate. The threshold to pain is fairly uniform from one person to another, whereas pain tolerance is extremely variable.[8] Separation and identification of the role of each of these two aspects of pain continue to pose fundamental problems for the pain management team and for pain researchers.

TYPES OF PAIN

The most widely accepted classifications of pain are according to source or location, referral, and duration (acute or chronic). Classification based on associated medical diagnosis (*e.g.*, surgery, trauma, cancer, sickle cell disease, fibromyalgia) is useful in planning appropriate interventions.

KEY CONCEPTS

Types of Pain

➤ Pain can be classified according to location, site of referral, and duration.

➤ Cutaneous pain is a sharp, burning pain that has its origin in the skin or subcutaneous tissues.

➤ Deep pain is a more diffuse and throbbing pain that originates in structures such as the muscles, bones, and tendons and radiates to the surrounding tissues.

➤ Visceral pain is a diffuse and poorly defined pain that results from stretching, distention, or ischemia of tissues in a body organ.

➤ Referred pain is pain that originates at a visceral site but is perceived as originating in part of the body wall that is innervated by neurons entering the same segment of the nervous system.

➤ Acute pain usually results from tissue damage and is characterized by autonomic nervous system responses.

➤ Chronic pain is persistent pain that is often accompanied by loss of appetite, sleep disturbances, depression, and other debilitating responses.

Cutaneous and Deep Somatic Pain

Cutaneous pain arises from superficial structures, such as the skin and subcutaneous tissues. A paper cut on the finger is an example of easily localized superficial, or cutaneous, pain. It is a sharp, bright pain with a burning quality and may be abrupt or slow in onset. It can be localized accurately and may be distributed along the dermatomes. Because there is an overlap of nerve fiber distribution between the dermatomes, the boundaries of pain frequently are not as clear-cut as the dermatomal diagrams indicate.

Deep somatic pain originates in deep body structures, such as the periosteum, muscles, tendons, joints, and blood vessels. This pain is more diffuse than cutaneous pain. Various stimuli, such as strong pressure exerted on bone, ischemia to a muscle, and tissue damage, can produce deep somatic pain. This is the type of pain a person experiences from a sprained ankle. Radiation of pain from the original site of injury can occur. For example, damage to a nerve root can cause a person to experience pain radiating along its fiber distribution.

Visceral Pain

Visceral, or splanchnic, pain has its origin in the visceral organs and is one of the most common pains produced by disease. Although similar to somatic pain in many ways, both the neurologic mechanisms and the perception of visceral pain differ from somatic pain. One of the most important differences between surface pain and visceral pain is in the type of damage causing the pain. For example, "a surgeon can cut the bowel entirely in two in a patient who is awake without causing significant pain."[4] In contrast, strong contractions, distention, or ischemia affecting the walls of the viscera can induce severe pain. Also, visceral pain is not evoked from all viscera (*e.g.*, the liver, lung parenchyma).[15] Another difference is the diffuse and poorly localized nature of visceral pain—its tendency to be referred to other locations and to be accompanied by symptoms associated with autonomic reflexes (*e.g.*, nausea).[16] There are several explanations for this. There is a low density of nociceptors in the viscera compared with the skin. There is functional divergence of visceral input within the CNS, which occurs when many second-order neurons respond to stimulus from a single visceral afferent. There is also convergence between somatic and visceral afferents in the spinal cord and in the supraspinal centers, and possibly also between visceral afferents (*e.g.*, bladder, uterus, cervix and vagina).[16]

Visceral afferents are predominantly small, unmyelinated pain fibers that terminate in the dorsal horn of the spinal cord and express peptide neurotransmitters such as substance P.[14] There are thought to be two classes of nociceptive receptors that innervate the viscera: high-threshold and intensity-coding receptors.[15,16] High-threshold receptors have a high threshold for stimulation and respond only to stimuli within the noxious range. Intensity-coding receptors have a lower threshold for stimulation and an encoding function that incorporates the intensity of the stimulus into the magnitude of their discharge. Acute visceral pain, such as pain produced by intense contraction of a hollow organ, is thought to be triggered initially by high-threshold receptors. More extended forms of visceral stimulation, such as those caused by hypoxia and inflammation, often result in sensitization of the high-threshold receptors along with that of the intensity-coding receptors. Once sensitized, these receptors begin to respond to otherwise innocuous stimuli (*e.g.*, motility and secretory activity) that normally occur in the viscera. This sensitization may resolve more slowly than the initial injury, and thus visceral pain may persist longer than expected based on the initial injury.[16]

Referred Pain

Referred pain is pain that is perceived at a site different from its point of origin but innervated by the same spinal segment. It is hypothesized that visceral and somatic afferent neurons converge on the same dorsal horn projection neurons[1–4] (Fig. 34-10). For this reason, it can be difficult for the brain to correctly identify the original source of pain. Pain that originates in the abdominal or thoracic viscera is diffuse and poorly localized and often perceived at a site far removed from the affected area. For example, the pain associated with myocardial infarction commonly is referred to the left arm, neck, and chest.

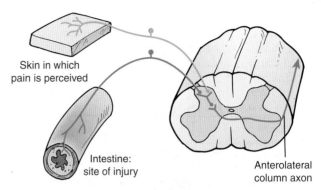

FIGURE 34-10 Convergence of cutaneous and visceral inputs onto the same second-order projection neuron in the dorsal horn of the spinal cord. Although virtually all visceral inputs converge with cutaneous inputs, most cutaneous inputs do not converge with other sensory inputs.

Referred pain may arise alone or concurrent with pain located at the origin of the noxious stimuli. This lack of correspondence between the location of the pain and the location of the painful stimuli can make diagnosis difficult. Although the term *referred* usually is applied to pain that originates in the viscera and is experienced as if originating from the body wall, it also may be applied to pain that arises from somatic structures. For example, pain referred to the chest wall could be caused by nociceptive stimulation of the peripheral portion of the diaphragm, which receives somatosensory innervation from the intercostal nerves. An understanding of pain referral is of great value in diagnosing illness. The typical pattern of pain referral can be derived from our understanding that the afferent neurons from visceral or deep somatic tissue enter the spinal cord at the same level as the afferent neurons from the cutaneous areas to which the pain is referred (Fig. 34-11).

The sites of referred pain are determined embryologically with the development of visceral and somatic structures that share the same site for entry of sensory information into the CNS and then move to more distant locations. For example, a person with peritonitis may report pain in the shoulder. Internally, there is inflammation of the peritoneum that lines the central part of the diaphragm. In the embryo, the diaphragm originates in the neck, and its central portion is innervated by the phrenic nerve, which enters the cord at the level of the third to fifth cervical segments (C3 to C5). As the fetus develops, the diaphragm descends to its adult position between the thoracic and abdominal cavities, while maintaining its embryonic pattern of innervation. Thus, fibers that enter the spinal cord at the C3 to C5 level carry information from both the neck area and the diaphragm, and the diaphragmatic pain is interpreted by the forebrain as originating in the shoulder or neck area.

Muscle spasm, or *guarding*, often occurs when somatic structures are involved. Guarding is a protective reflex rigidity; its purpose is to protect the affected body parts (*e.g.*, an abscessed appendix or a sprained muscle). This protective guarding may cause blood vessel compression

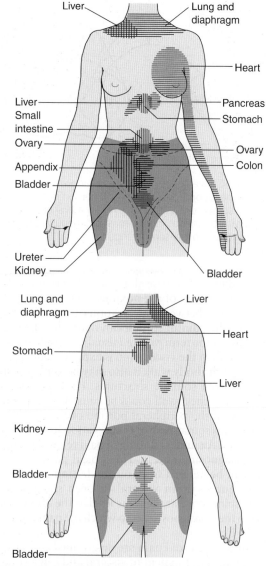

FIGURE 34-11 Areas of referred pain. (**Top**) Anterior view. (**Bottom**) Posterior view.

and give rise to the pain of muscle ischemia, causing local and referred pain.

Acute and Chronic Pain

It is common to classify pain according to its duration. Pain research of the past three decades has emphasized the importance of differentiating acute pain from chronic pain.[17] The diagnosis and therapy for each are distinctive because they differ in cause, function, mechanisms, and psychological sequelae.

Traditionally, the distinction between acute and chronic pain has relied on a time interval since the time of pain onset, such as 6 months, to designate the transition from acute to chronic pain.[18] A more recent conceptualization includes both the time and the physical dimensions of a disease process.[18,19] For example, some conditions such as osteoarthritis exhibit dimensions of both acute and chronic pain.

Acute Pain. Acute pain is elicited by injury to body tissues and activation of nociceptive stimuli at the site of local tissue damage. It is generally of short duration and remits when the underlying pathologic process has resolved.[18] The purpose of acute pain is to serve as a warning system. Besides alerting the person to the existence of actual or impending tissue damage, it prompts a search for professional help. The pain's location, radiation, intensity, and duration, as well as those factors that aggravate or relieve it, provide essential diagnostic clues.

Acute pain can lead to anxiety and secondary reflex musculoskeletal spasms, which in turn tend to worsen the pain.[17] Interventions that alleviate the pain usually alleviate the anxiety and musculoskeletal spasms as well. Inadequately treated pain can provoke physiologic responses that alter circulation and tissue metabolism and produce physical manifestations, such as tachycardia, reflective of increased sympathetic activity. Inadequately treated acute pain tends to decrease mobility and respiratory movements such as deep breathing and coughing to the extent that it may complicate or delay recovery.

Chronic Pain. Chronic pain is usually elicited by an injury but may be perpetuated by factors that are both pathologically and physically remote from the originating cause. Chronic pain extends for long periods of time and generally represents low levels of an underlying pathologic process that does not explain the presence or extent of the pain.[18] Chronic pain can be quite variable. It may be unrelenting and extremely severe, as in metastatic bone pain. It can be relatively continuous with or without periods of escalation, as with some forms of back pain. Some conditions with recurring episodes of acute pain are particularly problematic because they have characteristics of both acute and chronic pain. These include the pain associated with sickle cell crisis or migraine headaches.

Chronic pain is a leading cause of disability in the United States. Unlike acute pain, persistent chronic pain usually serves no useful function. On the contrary, it imposes physiologic, psychological, familial, and economic stresses and may exhaust a person's resources. In contrast to acute pain, psychological and environmental influences may play an important role in the development of behaviors associated with chronic pain.

The biologic factors that contribute to chronic pain include peripheral mechanisms, peripheral-central mechanisms, and central mechanisms.[19] Peripheral mechanisms result from persistent stimulation of nociceptors. They contribute to the pain associated with chronic musculoskeletal, visceral, and vascular disorders. Peripheral-central mechanisms involve abnormal function of the peripheral and central portions of the somatosensory system. These disorders include conditions such as those resulting from partial or complete loss of descending inhibitory pathways or spontaneous firing of regenerated nerve fibers. They include conditions such as causalgia, phantom limb pain, and postherpetic neuralgia. Central pain mechanisms are associated with disease or injury of the CNS. Central pain is characterized by burning, aching, hyperalgesia, dysesthesia, and other abnormal sensations. Central pain is associated with conditions such as thalamic lesions (thalamic pain), spinal cord injury, surgical interruption of pain pathways, and multiple sclerosis.

Persons with chronic pain may not exhibit the somatic, autonomic, or affective behaviors often associated with acute pain. As painful conditions become prolonged and continuous, autonomic nervous system responses tend to decrease. In addition, chronic pain often is associated with loss of appetite, sleep disturbances, and depression.[17] Amazingly, depression commonly is relieved once the pain is removed. The link between depression and decreased pain tolerance may be explained by the similar manner in which both respond to changes in the biologic pathways of serotonergic and noradrenergic systems. Tricyclic antidepressants and other medications with serotonergic and noradrenergic effects have been shown to relieve a variety of chronic pain syndromes, lending credence to the theory that chronic pain and depression share a common biologic pathway.[20]

PAIN MANAGEMENT

Assessment

Careful assessment of pain assists clinicians in diagnosing, managing, and relieving the patient's pain. Assessment includes such things as the nature, severity, location, and radiation of the pain. As is true of other disease states, it is preferable to eliminate the cause of the pain, rather than simply to treat the symptoms. A careful history often provides information about the triggering factors (*i.e.,* injury, infection, or disease) and the site of nociceptive stimuli (*i.e.,* peripheral receptor or visceral organ). Although the observation of facial expression and posture may provide additional information, the Agency for Health Care Policy and Research (AHCPR) practice guidelines emphasize that "the single most reliable indicator of the existence and intensity of acute pain—and any resultant affective discomfort or distress—is the patient's self report."[21] A comprehensive pain history should include pain onset; description, localization, radiation, intensity, quality, and pattern of the pain; anything that relieves or exacerbates it; and the individual's personal reaction to the pain.

Unlike many other bodily responses, such as temperature and blood pressure, the nature, severity, and distress of pain cannot be measured objectively. To overcome this problem, various methods have been developed for quantifying a person's pain. Most of these are based on the patient's report. They include numeric pain intensity, visual analog, and verbal descriptor scales.

Treatment

The approaches to treatment of acute and chronic pain differ markedly. In acute pain, therapy is directed at providing pain relief by interrupting the nociceptive stimulus. Because the pain is self-limited, in that it resolves as the injured tissues heal, long-term therapy usually is not needed. Chronic pain management is much more complex and is based on multiple considerations, including life expectancy. Persons with conditions such as musculoskeletal disorders who experience both acute and chronic pain require special considerations.

Acute Pain. Acute pain should be aggressively managed and pain medication provided before the pain becomes severe. This allows the person to be more comfortable and active and to assume a greater role in directing his or her own care. One reason for the reluctance of health care workers to provide adequate relief for acute pain has been fear of addiction. However, addiction to opioid medications is thought to be virtually nonexistent when these drugs are prescribed for acute pain. Usually, less medication is needed when the drug is given before the pain becomes severe and the pain pathways become sensitized.

The AHCPR guidelines, which address pain from surgery, medical procedures, and trauma, emphasize the need for (1) a collaborative, interdisciplinary approach to pain control, which includes members of the health care team and input from the patient and the patient's family when appropriate; (2) an individualized, proactive pain control plan developed before surgery (if possible) by patients and providers; (3) the assessment and frequent reassessment of the patient's pain, facilitated by a pain management log or flow sheet; (4) the use of drug and nondrug therapies to control or prevent pain; and (5) a formal, institutional approach to management of acute pain with clear lines of responsibility.[21]

Chronic Pain. Management of chronic pain requires early attempts to prevent pain and adequate therapy for acute bouts of pain. Specific treatment depends on the cause of the pain, the natural history of the underlying health problem, as well as the life expectancy of the individual. If the organic illness causing the pain cannot be cured, then noncurative methods of pain control become the cornerstone of treatment. Treatment methods for chronic pain can include neural blockade, electrical modalities (*e.g.,* transcutaneous electrical nerve stimulation), physical therapy, cognitive behavioral interventions, and nonnarcotic and narcotic medications. Non-narcotic medications such as tricyclic antidepressants, anticonvulsant medications, and nonsteroidal anti-inflammatory drugs (NSAIDs) serve as useful adjuncts to opioids for the treatment of different types of chronic pain. Chronic pain is best handled by a multidisciplinary team that includes specialists in areas such as anesthesiology, nursing, physical therapy, and social services.

Cancer is a common cause of chronic pain. The goal of chronic cancer pain management should be pain alleviation and prevention.[22] Preemptive therapy tends to reduce sensitization of pain pathways and provides for more effective pain control. Pharmacologic and nonpharmacologic interventions are the same as those used for other types of chronic pain. Depending on the form and stage of the cancer, other treatments such as palliative radiation, antineoplastic therapies, and palliative surgery may help to control the pain. The World Health Organization (WHO) has created an analgesic ladder for cancer pain that assists clinicians in choosing the appropriate analgesic medications.[23]

Nonpharmacologic Treatment.

A number of nonpharmacologic methods of pain control often are used in pain management. These include cognitive-behavioral interventions (*e.g.*, relaxation, distraction, imagery, and biofeedback), physical agents (*e.g.*, heat and cold), electroanalgesia (*e.g.*, transcutaneous electrical stimulation [TENS]), and acupuncture. Often these methods are used in addition to analgesics rather than as the only form of pain management.

Pharmacologic Treatment.

Pharmacologic treatment involves the use of drugs in the management of pain. They include non-narcotic and narcotic analgesics, as well adjuvant medications such as antidepressants, anticonvulsants, and muscle relaxants. Topical medications are a new aspect of pain management whose ultimate utility has yet to be determined.[19]

An analgesic drug is a medication that acts on the nervous system to decrease or eliminate pain without inducing loss of consciousness. Analgesic drugs do not cure the underlying cause of the pain, but their appropriate use may prevent acute pain from progressing to chronic pain.

Non-narcotic Analgesics.

Common non-narcotic oral analgesic medications include aspirin, other NSAIDs, and acetaminophen. Aspirin, or acetylsalicylic acid, acts centrally and peripherally to block the transmission of pain impulses. It also has antipyretic and anti-inflammatory properties. Aspirin and the other NSAIDs inhibit several forms of prostaglandins through the inhibition of cyclooxygenase, an enzyme needed for their synthesis. Prostaglandins affect the sensation of pain by sensitizing nociceptors to chemical mediators such as bradykinin and histamine. Independent of prostaglandins, NSAIDs also decrease the sensitivity of blood vessels to bradykinin and histamine, affect lymphokine production by T lymphocytes, reverse vasodilatation, and decrease the release of inflammatory mediators from granulocytes, mast cells, and basophils. Acetaminophen is an alternative to the NSAIDs. Although usually considered equivalent to aspirin as an analgesic and antipyretic agent, it lacks anti-inflammatory properties.

Opioid Analgesics.

The term *opioid* or *narcotic* is used to refer to a group of medications, natural or synthetic, with morphine-like actions. The opioids (*e.g.*, morphine, codeine, and many other semisynthetic congeners of morphine) exert their action through opioid receptors. There are three major categories of opioid receptors in the CNS, designated as mu (μ, for "morphine"), delta (δ), and kappa (κ).[24] Analgesia, as well as respiratory depression, miosis, reduced gastrointestinal motility (causing constipation), feelings of well-being or euphoria, and physical dependence result principally from morphine and morphine-like opioid analgesics that act at the mu receptors. Part of the pain-relieving properties of exogenous opioids such as morphine involve the release of endogenous opioids.[24]

Opioids are used in the management of acute and chronic pain. When given for temporary relief of severe pain, such as that occurring after surgery, there is much evidence that opioids given routinely before the pain starts or becomes extreme are far more effective than those administered in a sporadic manner. Persons who are treated in this manner usually require fewer doses and are able to resume regular activities sooner. Opioids also are used for persons with chronic pain such as that caused by cancer. Too often, because of undue concern about the possibility of addiction, many individuals with chronic pain receive inadequate pain relief. Addiction is not considered a problem in patients with cancer. Most pain experts agree that it is appropriate to provide the level of opioid necessary to relieve the severe, intractable pain of persons whose life expectancy is limited. Morphine remains the most useful strong opioid, and the WHO has recommended that oral morphine be part of the essential medication list and be made available throughout the world as the medication of choice for cancer pain.[23]

Adjuvant Pain Medications.

Adjuvant pain medications include drugs such as tricyclic antidepressants and anticonvulsant medications.[12,13] The fact that the pain suppression system has nonendorphin synapses raises the possibility that potent, centrally acting, nonopioid medications may be useful in relieving pain. Serotonin has been shown to play an important role in producing analgesia. The tricyclic antidepressant medications block the removal of serotonin from the synaptic cleft to produce pain relief in some persons. These medications are particularly useful in some chronic painful conditions, such as postherpetic neuralgia. Certain anticonvulsant medications, such as carbamazepine and phenytoin, have analgesic effects in some pain conditions. These medications, which suppress spontaneous neuronal firing, are particularly useful in the management of pain that occurs after nerve injury. Other agents, such as the corticosteroids, may be used to decrease inflammation and nociceptive stimuli responsible for pain.

Surgical Intervention.

The effects of surgical interventions may be curative or palliative. Surgical interventions that remove the source of the pain (*e.g.*, inflamed appendix) are curative. In other instances, surgery is used for symptom management, rather than for cure. Surgery for severe, intractable pain of peripheral or central origin has met with some success. It can be used to remove the cause or block the transmission of intractable pain from phantom limb pain, severe neuralgia, and inoperable cancer of certain types.

In summary, pain is an elusive and complex phenomenon; it is a symptom common to many illnesses. It is a highly individualized experience that is shaped by a person's culture and previous life experiences, and it is difficult to measure. Traditionally, there have been two principal theories of pain: the specificity theory and the pattern theory. Scientifically, pain is viewed within the context of nociception or tissue injury. The neural pathways for pain include the nociceptors or pain receptors, the afferent neurons that carry pain information to the dorsal horn of spinal cord, and the transmission of pain information from the spinal cord to the brain through the neospinothalamic and the paleospinothalamic pathways. The perception and meaningfulness of pain occur at the level of the somatosensory cortex. Nociceptors respond to several types of stimuli, including mechanical (*e.g.*, pressure applied to the skin), thermal (heat and cold), and chemical stimuli (*e.g.*, hydrogen and potassium ions, prostaglandins, histamine, bradykinin) resulting from tissue trauma and inflammation. Chemical neurotransmitters, such as glutamate and substance P, function in the transmission of pain impulses in the CNS. Several neuroanatomic pathways, as well as endogenous opioid peptides, modulate the transmission of pain impulses in the CNS.

Pain can arise from cutaneous, deep somatic, or visceral locations. Referred pain is pain perceived at a site different from its origin. Acute pain is self-limiting pain that ends when the injured tissue heals, whereas chronic pain is pain that lasts much longer than the anticipated healing time for the underlying cause of the pain. Pain threshold, pain tolerance, age, gender, and other factors affect an individual's reaction to pain.

Treatment modalities for pain include the use of nonpharmacologic and pharmacologic agents either singly or in combination. In acute pain, therapy is directed at providing pain relief by interrupting the nociceptive stimulus. Chronic pain management is much more complex and is based on multiple considerations, including life expectancy. It is becoming apparent that with both acute and chronic pain, the most effective approach is early interventions.

 ## Alterations in Pain Sensitivity and Special Types of Pain

ALTERATIONS IN PAIN SENSITIVITY

Sensitivity to and perception of pain vary among persons and in the same person under different conditions and in different parts of the body. Irritation, mild hypoxia, and mild compression of a peripheral nerve often result in hyperexcitability of the sensory nerve fibers or cell bodies. This is experienced as unpleasant hypersensitivity (*i.e.*, *hyperesthesia*) or increased painfulness (*i.e.*, *hyperalgesia*). Possible causes of increased sensitivity to noxious stimuli include a decrease in the threshold of nociceptors or an increase in pain produced by suprathreshold stimuli.

Primary hyperalgesia occurs at the site of injury. Secondary hyperalgesia occurs in nearby uninjured tissue.

Hyperpathia is a syndrome in which the sensory threshold is raised, but when it is reached, continued stimulation, especially if repetitive, results in a prolonged and unpleasant experience. This pain can be explosive and radiates through a peripheral nerve distribution. It is associated with pathologic changes in peripheral nerves, such as localized ischemia. Spontaneous, unpleasant sensations called *paresthesias* occur with more severe irritation (*e.g.*, the pins-and-needles sensation that follows temporary compression of a peripheral nerve). The general term *dysesthesia* is given to distortions (usually unpleasant) of somesthetic sensation that typically accompany partial loss of sensory innervation.

More severe pathologic processes can result in reduced or lost tactile (*e.g.*, *hypoesthesia*, *anesthesia*), temperature (*e.g.*, *hypothermia*, *athermia*), and pain sensation (*i.e.*, *hypalgesia*). *Analgesia* is the absence of pain on noxious stimulation or the relief of pain without loss of consciousness. The inability to sense pain may result in trauma, infection, and even loss of a body part or parts. Inherited insensitivity to pain may take the form of congenital indifference or congenital insensitivity to pain. In the former, transmission of nerve impulses appears normal, but the appreciation of painful stimuli at higher levels appears to be absent. In the latter, a peripheral nerve defect apparently exists such that transmission of painful nerve impulses does not result in perception of pain. Whatever the cause, persons who lack the ability to perceive pain are at constant risk of tissue damage because pain is not serving its protective function.

Allodynia (Greek *allo*, "other," and *odynia*, "painful") is the term used for the puzzling phenomenon of pain that follows a non-noxious stimulus to apparently normal skin. This term is intended to refer to instances in which otherwise normal tissues may be abnormally innervated or may be referral sites for other loci that give rise to pain with non-noxious stimuli. It may be that an area is hypersensitive because of inflammation, injury, or another cause, and a normally subthreshold stimulus is sufficient to trigger the sensation of pain. This response is thought to be chemically mediated, possibly the result of tissue damage in the surrounding area. *Trigger points* are highly localized points on the skin or mucous membrane that can produce immediate intense pain at that site or elsewhere when stimulated by light tactile stimulation. Myofascial trigger points are foci of exquisite tenderness found in many muscles and can be responsible for pain projected to sites remote from the points of tenderness. Trigger points, which are widely distributed in the back of the head and neck and in the lumbar and thoracic regions, cause reproducible myofascial pain syndromes in specific muscles.

NEUROPATHIC TYPES OF PAIN

Neuropathic pain represents unusual and sometimes intractable sensory disturbances associated with disease or injury of the peripheral or central nervous system.[25]

These include numbness, paresthesias, and pain. Depending on the cause, few or many axons could be damaged, and the condition could be unilateral or bilateral. Causes of neuropathic pain can be categorized according to the extent of peripheral nerve involvement. Conditions that can lead to pain by causing damage to peripheral nerves in a single area include nerve entrapment, nerve compression from a tumor mass, and various neuralgias (e.g., trigeminal, postherpetic, and post-traumatic). Conditions that can lead to pain by causing damage to peripheral nerves in a wide area include diabetes mellitus, long-term alcohol use, hypothyroidism, renal insufficiency, and drug treatment with neurotoxic agents.[26] Other causes of neuropathic pain include the complex regional pain syndrome, a multisystem syndrome, and phantom limb pain, which follows nerve damage associated with amputation.

Neuropathic pain can vary with the extent and location of disease or injury. There may be allodynia or pain that is stabbing, jabbing, burning, or shooting. The pain may be persistent or intermittent. The diagnosis depends on the mode of onset, the distribution of abnormal sensations, the quality of the pain, and other relevant medical conditions (e.g., diabetes, hypothyroidism, alcohol use, rash, or trauma). Injury to peripheral nerves sometimes results in pain that persists beyond the time required for the tissues to heal. Peripheral pathologic processes (e.g., neural degeneration, neuroma formation, and generation of abnormal spontaneous neural discharges from the injured sensory neuron) and neural plasticity (i.e., changes in CNS function) are the primary working hypotheses to explain persistent neuropathic pain.

Treatment methods include measures aimed at restoring or preventing further nerve damage (e.g., surgery to resect a tumor causing nerve compression, improving glycemic control for diabetic patients with painful neuropathies) and interventions for the palliation of pain. Although many adjuvant analgesics are used for neuropathic pain, pain control often is difficult. If there has been a poor response to the adjuvant analgesics, opioids also can be used. The initial approach in seeking adequate pain control is to try these drugs in sequence and then in combination. Nonpharmacologic therapies such as electrical stimulation of the peripheral nerve or spinal cord can be used for radiculopathies and neuralgias. As a last resort, neurolysis or neurosurgical blockade sometimes is used.

Neuralgia

Neuralgia is characterized by severe, brief, often repetitive attacks of lightning-like or throbbing pain. It occurs along the distribution of a spinal or cranial nerve and usually is precipitated by stimulation of the cutaneous region supplied by that nerve.

Trigeminal Neuralgia. Trigeminal neuralgia, or *tic douloureux,* is one of the most common and severe neuralgias. It is manifested by facial tics or grimaces and characterized by stabbing, paroxysmal attacks of pain that usually are limited to the unilateral sensory distribution of one or more branches of the trigeminal nerve, most often the maxillary or mandibular divisions. Although intermittent, the pain often is excruciating and may be triggered by such factors as light touch, movement, drafts, and eating. Spontaneous remissions for several months or longer may occur. As the disorders progresses, however, the episodes become more frequent, remissions become shorter, and a dull ache may persist between episodes of stabbing pain.

Diagnosis is usually based on presenting symptoms. Neurologic examination findings are usually normal in persons with classic trigeminal neuralgia, as are computed tomography (CT) scans and radiologic contrast studies. In young persons presenting with trigeminal neuralgia, multiple sclerosis should be suspected even if other neurologic signs are normal.[27]

The drug that is most helpful in the treatment of trigeminal neuralgia is carbamazepine, an anticonvulsant medication. Other anticonvulsant drugs (e.g., phenytoin, gabapentin) may be tried if carbamazepine is ineffective. Surgical release of vessels, dural structures, or scar tissue surrounding the semilunar ganglion or root in the middle cranial fossa often eliminates the symptoms. If not, destruction or blocking of peripheral branches or the central root of cranial nerve V (CN V) produces loss of all sensation, including pain. A more satisfactory treatment is sectioning of the descending spinal tract of CN V in the brain stem. This may be effective because it removes background inflow of impulses on which spontaneous attacks depend. Dissociation of facial sensation occurs, in that the ability to detect pain and temperature disappears, but there is only a slight decrease in ability to detect touch. Other interventions include avoidance of precipitating factors (e.g., stimulation of trigger spots) and eye injury due to irritation; provision for adequate nutrition; and avoidance of social isolation.

Postherpetic Neuralgia. Herpes zoster (also called *shingles*) is caused by the same herpesvirus that causes varicella (i.e., chickenpox) and is thought to represent a localized recurrent infection by the varicella virus that has remained latent in the dorsal root ganglia since the initial attack of chickenpox.[28,29] Reactivation of viral replication is associated with a decline in immunity, such as that which occurs with aging or certain diseases. Postherpetic neuralgia develops in 10% to 70% of patients with shingles.[28] Both the incidence and the duration of postherpetic neuralgia are directly correlated with the person's age.[29]

The pain associated with postherpetic neuralgia occurs in the areas of innervation of the infected ganglia. During the acute attack of herpes zoster, the reactivated virus travels from the ganglia to the skin of the corresponding dermatomes, causing localized vesicular eruption and hyperpathia (i.e., abnormally exaggerated subjective response to pain). In the acute infection, proportionately more of the large nerve fibers are destroyed. Regenerated fibers appear to have smaller diameters. Because there is a shift in the proportion of large- to small-diameter fibers that occurs with aging due to a loss of large nerve fibers, elderly persons tend to have greater pain, dysesthesia, and hyperesthesia after the acute phase. Normally, the pain of acute herpes zoster tends to resolve spontaneously. Postherpetic neuralgia describes the presence of pain more than 1 month after the onset of herpes zoster.

Early treatment of herpes zoster with an oral antiviral drug such as acyclovir or valacyclovir, medications that inhibit herpesvirus deoxyribonucleic acid (DNA) replication, may reduce the incidence of postherpetic neuralgia. Initially, postherpetic neuralgia can be treated with a topical anesthetic agent (*e.g.,* lidocaine-prilocaine cream or 5% lidocaine gel). A tricyclic antidepressant medication, such as amitriptyline or desipramine, may be used for pain relief. Regional nerve blockade (*i.e.,* stellate ganglion, epidural, local infiltration, or peripheral nerve block) has been used with limited success. Topical capsaicin cream is approved for treatment of postherpetic neuralgia and acts presumably by causing temporary degeneration of C pain fiber terminals in the skin of the treated area. However, many persons are intolerant of the burning sensation that precedes anesthesia after application.[28]

Complex Regional Pain Syndrome

Complex regional pain syndrome, formerly known as *reflex sympathetic dystrophy,* is a regional post-traumatic pain problem usually affecting one or more limbs.[30,31] Most persons with the disorder have had an identifiable inciting or irritating injury, which may be trivial, such as a minor joint sprain, or severe, such as trauma involving a major nerve or nerves. The hallmark is pain and mobility problems more severe than the injury warrants. Characteristically, the pain is severe and burning with or without deep aching. Usually, the pain can be elicited with the slightest movement or touch to the affected area, it increases with repetitive stimulation, and it lasts even after the stimulation has stopped. The pain can be exacerbated by emotional upsets or any increased peripheral sympathetic nerve stimulation. Symptoms of sympathetic nervous system dysfunction may be present and may manifest as vascular and trophic (*e.g.,* dystrophic or atrophic) changes to the skin, soft tissue, and bone. They may include rubor or pallor, sweating or dryness, edema (often sharply demarcated), skin atrophy, and, with time, patchy osteoporosis.

The pathophysiology of the complex regional pain syndromes remains obscure. Although abnormalities in sympathetic activity are observed, local sensitivity due to an increase in the number or sensitivity of peripheral receptors, rather than increased outflow of catecholamines, appears to be the cause. Increased vascular sensitivity to the catecholamines may lead to the decreased cutaneous blood flow observed in the later stages of the disease. Other likely mechanisms include neurogenic inflammation caused by the activation of neuromediators, such as substance P and histamine, that also mediate inflammation and vasodilatation of microvessels.[31]

According to the clinical practice guideline proposed by the Reflex Sympathetic Dystrophy Syndrome Associ-ation of America, the cornerstone of treatment is promoting normal use of the affected part to the extent possible.[32] Initially, oral analgesics (including the adjuvant analgesics), TENS, and physical activity are used. If this does not lead to improvement, treatment by sympathetic blockade may provide relief from pain; it also determines the extent to which the pain is sympathetically maintained. If the block successfully treats the pain, then sympathectomy may be an effective treatment. If not, electrical stimulation of the spinal cord or narcotics may be considered.

Phantom Limb Pain

Phantom limb pain, a type of neurologic pain, follows amputation of a limb or part of a limb. As many as 70% of those who undergo amputation experience phantom pain.[33] The pain often begins as sensations of tingling, heat and cold, or heaviness, followed by burning, cramping, or shooting pain. It may disappear spontaneously or persist for many years. One of the more troublesome aspects of phantom pain is that the person may experience painful sensations that were present before the amputation, such as that of a painful ulcer or bunion.

Several theories have been proposed as to the causes of phantom pain.[33] One theory is that the end of a regenerating nerve becomes trapped in the scar tissue of the amputation site. It is known that when a peripheral nerve is cut, the scar tissue that forms becomes a barrier to regenerating outgrowth of the axon. The growing axon often becomes trapped in the scar tissue, forming a tangled growth (*i.e.,* neuroma) of small-diameter axons, including primary nociceptive afferents and sympathetic efferents. It has been proposed that these afferents show increased sensitivity to innocuous mechanical stimuli and to sympathetic activity and circulating catecholamines. A related theory moves the source of phantom limb pain to the spinal cord, suggesting that the pain is caused by the spontaneous firing of spinal cord neurons that have lost their normal sensory input from the body. In this case, a closed, self-exciting neuronal loop in the posterior horn of the spinal cord is postulated to send impulses to the brain, resulting in pain. Even the slightest irritation to the amputated limb area can initiate this cycle. Other theories propose that the phantom limb pain may arise in the brain. In one hypothesis, the pain is caused by changes in the flow of signals through somatosensory areas of the brain. Phantom limb pain has been treated using sympathetic blocks, TENS of the large myelinated afferents innervating the area, hypnosis, and relaxation training.

In summary, pain may occur with or without an adequate stimulus, or it may be absent in the presence of an adequate stimulus—either of which describes a pain disorder. There may be analgesia (absence of pain), hyperalgesia (increased sensitivity to pain), hypalgesia (a decreased sensitivity to painful stimuli), hyperpathia (an unpleasant and prolonged response to pain), hyperesthesia (an abnormal increase in sensitivity to sensation), hypoesthesia (an abnormal decrease in sensitivity to sensations), paresthesia (abnormal touch sensation such as tingling or "pins and needles" in the absence of external stimuli), or allodynia (pain produced by stimuli that do not normally cause pain).

Neuropathic pain may be caused by trauma or disease of neurons in a focal area or in a more global distribution (*e.g.*, from endocrine disease or neurotoxic medications). Neuralgia is characterized by severe, brief, often repetitiously occurring attacks of lightning-like or throbbing pain that occurs along the distribution of a spinal or cranial nerve and usually is precipitated by stimulation of the cutaneous region supplied by that nerve. Trigeminal neuralgia, or tic douloureux, is one of the most common and severe neuralgias. It is manifested by facial tics or grimaces. Postherpetic neuralgia is a chronic pain that can occur after shingles, an infection by the herpes zoster virus of the dorsal root ganglia and corresponding areas of innervation. The complex regional pain syndrome is an extremely painful condition that may follow sudden and traumatic deformation of peripheral nerves. Phantom limb pain, a neurologic pain, can occur after amputation of a limb or part of a limb.

Headache

Headache is a very common health problem, with over 90% of adults reporting having a headache at least once. Seventy-six percent of women and 57% of men report at least one headache a month.[34] Twenty-five percent of adults report having recurrent severe headaches and 4% report having daily or nearly daily headaches.[35] Although head and facial pain have characteristics that distinguish them from other pain disorders, they also share many of the same features.

Headache is caused by a number of conditions. Some headaches represent primary disorders and others occur secondary to other disease conditions in which head pain is a symptom. The most common types of primary chronic headaches are migraine headache, cluster headache, and tension-type headache. Although most causes of secondary headache are benign, some are indications of serious disorders such as meningitis, brain tumor, or cerebral aneurysm. The sudden onset of a severe, intractable headache in an otherwise healthy person is more likely related to a serious intracranial disorder, such as subarachnoid hemorrhage or meningitis, than to a chronic headache disorder. Headaches that disturb sleep, exertional headaches (*e.g.*, triggered by physical or sexual activity or a Valsalva maneuver), and headaches accompanied by neurologic symptoms such as drowsiness, visual or limb disturbances, or altered mental status also are suggestive of underlying intracranial lesions or other pathologic processes. Other red flags for secondary headache disorder include fundamental change or progression in

headache pattern or a new headache in individuals younger than 5 or older than 50 years of age or in individuals with cancer, immunosuppression, or pregnancy.[35]

The diagnosis and classification of headaches often is difficult. It requires a comprehensive history and physical examination to exclude secondary causes. The history should include factors that precipitate headache, such as foods and food additives, missed meals, and association with the menstrual period. A careful medication history is essential because many medications can provoke or aggravate headaches. Alcohol also can cause or aggravate headache. A headache diary in which the person records his or her headaches and concurrent or antecedent events may be helpful in identifying factors that contribute to headache onset. Appropriate laboratory and imaging studies of the brain may be done to rule out secondary headaches.

In 2004, the International Headache Society (IHS) published the second edition of its classification of headache disorders. The classification system is divided into three sections: (1) primary headaches, (2) headaches secondary to other medical conditions, and (3) cranial neuralgias and facial pain[36] (see Chart 34-1 for a summary of the components of the system).

MIGRAINE HEADACHE

Migraine headaches affect approximately 20 million persons in the United States. They occur in about 18% of women and 6% of men and result in considerable time lost from work and other activities.[37] Migraine headaches tend to run in families and are thought to be inherited as an autosomal dominant trait with incomplete penetrance.[34] It is noteworthy that the genetic influence is stronger for migraine with aura than in migraine without aura.[37]

There are two categories of migraine headache—migraine without aura, which accounts for approximately 85% of migraines, and migraine with aura, which accounts for most of the remaining migraines. Migraine without aura is a pulsatile, throbbing, unilateral headache that typically lasts 1 to 2 days and is aggravated by routine physical activity. The headache is accompanied by nausea and vomiting, which often is disabling, and sensitivity to light and sound. Visual disturbances occur quite commonly and consist of visual hallucinations such as stars, sparks, and flashes of light. Migraine with aura has similar symptoms, but with the addition of visual or neurologic symptoms that precede the headache. The aura usually develops over a period of 5 to 20 minutes and lasts less than an hour. Although only a small percentage of persons with migraine experience an aura before an attack, many persons without aura have prodromal symptoms, such as fatigue and irritability, that precede the attack by hours or even days.

Subtypes of migraine include ophthalmoplegic migraine, hemiplegic migraine, aphasic migraine, and retinal migraine, in which transient visual and motor deficits occur. Ophthalmoplegic migraine is characterized by diplopia, due to a transient paralysis of the muscles that

CHART 34-1

Classification of Headache Disorders

1. Migraine
   1.1. Migraine without aura
   1.2. Migraine with aura
   1.3. Childhood periodic syndromes that are common precursors of migraine
   1.4. Retinal migraine
   1.5. Complications of migraine
   1.6. Probable migraine
2. Tension-type headache
   2.1. Infrequent episodic tension-type headache
   2.2. Frequent episodic tension-type headache
   2.3. Chronic tension-type headache
   2.4. Probable tension-type headache
3. Cluster headache and other trigeminal autonomic cephalalgias
4. Other primary headaches
5. Headache attributed to head and/or neck trauma
6. Headache attributed to cranial or cervical vascular disorder
7. Headache attributed to nonvascular intracranial disorder
8. Headache attributed to a substance or its withdrawal
9. Headache attributed to infection
10. Headache attributed to disorder of homeostasis
11. Headache or facial pain attributed to disorder of cranium, neck, eyes, ears, nose, sinuses, teeth, mouth, or other facial or cranial structures
12. Headache attributed to psychiatric disorder
13. Cranial neuralgias and central causes of facial pain
14. Other headache, cranial neuralgia, central or primary facial pain

(Adapted from Headache Classification Subcommittee of the International Headache Society. [2004]. The international classification of headache disorders, ed. 2. *Cephalalgia 24*[Suppl. 1], 1–152.)

control eye movement, and localized pain around the eye. Migraine headache also can present as a mixed headache, including symptoms typically associated with tension-type headache, sinus headache, or chronic daily headache. These are called *transformed migraine* and are difficult to classify. Although nasal symptoms are not one of the diagnostic criteria for migraine, they frequently accompany migraine and are probably due to cranial parasympathetic activation. Sinus pain may indicate either a headache due to sinus inflammation or migraine. In a recent study, 96% of those self-diagnosed with sinus headache in fact met the IHS criteria for migraine or migrainous headache.[36]

Migraine headaches occur in children as well as adults.[38,39] Before puberty, migraine headaches are equally distributed between sexes. The essential diagnostic crite-

rion for migraine in children is the presence of recurrent headaches separated by pain-free periods. Diagnosis is based on at least three of the following symptoms or associated findings: abdominal pain, nausea or vomiting, throbbing headache, unilateral location, associated aura (visual, sensory, motor), relief during sleep, and a positive family history.[39] Symptoms vary widely among children, from those that interrupt activities and cause the child to seek relief in a dark environment to those detectable only by direct questioning. A common feature of migraine in children is intense nausea and vomiting. The vomiting may be associated with abdominal pain and fever; thus, migraine may be confused with other conditions such as appendicitis. More than half of children with migraine undergo spontaneous prolonged remission after their 10th birthday. Because headaches in children can be a symptom of other, more serious disorders, including intracranial lesions, it is important that other causes of headache that require immediate treatment be ruled out.

The pathophysiologic mechanisms of the pain associated with migraines remain poorly understood. Although many different theories exist, it is well established that during a migraine the trigeminal nerve becomes activated.[40,41] Activation of the trigeminal sensory fibers may lead to the release of neuropeptides, causing painful neurogenic inflammation of the meningeal vasculature characterized by plasma protein extravasation, vasodilatation, and mast cell degranulation.[41] Another possible mechanism implicates neurogenic vasodilatation of meningeal blood vessels as a key component of the inflammatory processes that occur during migraine. Activation of trigeminal sensory fibers evokes a neurogenic dural vasodilatation mediated by calcitonin gene–related peptide. It also has been observed that the calcitonin gene–related peptide level is elevated during migraine and is normalized after successful treatment with sumatriptan.[41] Supporting the neurogenic basis for migraine is the frequent presence of premonitory symptoms before the headache begins; the presence of focal neurologic disturbances, which cannot be explained in terms of cerebral blood flow; and the numerous accompanying symptoms, including autonomic and constitutional dysfunction.[34]

Hormonal variations, particularly in estrogen levels, are thought to play a role in the pattern of migraine attacks. For many women, migraine headaches coincide with their menstrual periods. The greater predominance of migraine headaches in women is thought to be related to the aggravating effect of estrogen on the migraine mechanism.[37] Dietary substances, such as monosodium glutamate, aged cheese, and chocolate, also may precipitate migraine headaches. The actual triggers for migraine are the chemicals in the food, not allergens.[42]

The treatment of migraine headaches includes preventative and abortive nonpharmacologic and pharmacologic treatment. In 2002, the American College of Physicians–American Society of Internal Medicine and the American Academy of Family Physicians produced a set of evidence-based guidelines for the nonpharmacologic and pharmacologic management and prevention of migraine headaches in primary care settings.[43]

Nonpharmacologic treatment includes the avoidance of migraine triggers, such as foods, that precipitate an attack. Many persons with migraines benefit from maintaining regular eating and sleeping habits. Measures to control stress, which also can precipitate an attack, also are important. During an attack, many persons find it helpful to retire to a quiet, darkened room until symptoms subside.

Pharmacologic treatment involves both abortive therapy for acute attacks and preventive therapy. A wide range of medications is used to treat the acute symptoms of migraine headache. Based on clinical trials, first-line agents include acetylsalicylic acid; combinations of acetaminophen, acetylsalicylic acid, and caffeine and NSAIDs analgesics (*e.g.*, naproxen sodium, ibuprofen); serotonin (5-HT$_1$) receptor agonists (*e.g.*, sumatriptan, naratriptan, rizatriptan, zolmitriptan); ergotamine derivatives (*e.g.*, dihydroergotamine); and antiemetic medications (*e.g.*, prochlorperazine, metoclopramide). Nonoral routes of administration may be preferred in individuals who develop severe pain rapidly or upon awakening or in those with severe nausea and vomiting. Both sumatriptan and dihydroergotamine have been approved for intranasal administration. For intractable migraine headache, dihydroergotamine may be administered parenterally with an antiemetic (metoclopramide or prochlorperazine) or opioid analgesic (transnasal butorphanol).[44] Frequent use of abortive headache medications may cause rebound headache.

Preventative pharmacologic treatment may be necessary if migrainous headaches are disabling, if they occur more than two or three times a month, if abortive treatment is being used more than two times a week, or if the individual has hemiplegic migraine, migraine with prolonged aura, or migrainous infarction.[43] In most cases, preventative treatment must be taken daily for months to years. First-line agents include β-adrenergic blocking medications (*e.g.*, propranolol, timolol, atenolol), antidepressants (*e.g.*, amitriptyline), and antiseizure medications (divalproex sodium, sodium valproate).[43] When a decision to discontinue preventive therapy is made, the medications should be withdrawn gradually.

Other effective medications are available, but they can have serious side effects in some individuals. Because of the risk of coronary vasospasm, the 5-HT$_1$ receptor agonists should not be given to persons with coronary artery disease. Ergotamine preparations can cause uterine contractions and should not be given to pregnant women. They also can cause vasospasm, and should be used with caution in persons with peripheral vascular disease.

CLUSTER HEADACHE

Cluster headaches are relatively uncommon headaches that occur in about 1 in 1000 individuals, affecting men (80% to 85%) more frequently than women. These headaches tend to be episodic, characterized by periods (clusters or bouts) of headaches and periods of remission. During a bout, the person may experience one to eight headaches per day, and bouts may last from 7 days to 12 months.[45]

Cluster headache is a type of primary neurovascular headache that typically includes severe, unrelenting, unilateral pain located, in order of decreasing frequency, in the orbital, retro-orbital, temporal, supraorbital, and infraorbital region. The pain is of rapid onset and builds to a peak in approximately 10 to 15 minutes, lasting for 15 to 180 minutes. The pain behind the eye radiates to the ipsilateral trigeminal nerve (*e.g.*, temple, cheek, gum). The headache frequently is associated with one or more symptoms such as restlessness or agitation, conjunctival redness, lacrimation, nasal congestion, rhinorrhea, forehead and facial sweating, miosis, ptosis, and eyelid edema. Because of their location and associated symptoms, cluster headaches are often mistaken for sinus infections or dental problems.[42]

To fulfill the IHS criteria for diagnosis, the person must have at least five attacks occurring from one every other day to eight per day, that are not attributable to any other disorder.[36] In addition, headaches must cause severe or very severe unilateral, supraorbital, or temporal pain lasting 15 to 180 minutes and be accompanied by ipsilateral conjunctival injection or lacrimation (*i.e.*, redness or tearing of the eyes), ipsilateral nasal congestion or rhinorrhea, ipsilateral eyelid edema, ipsilateral forehead or facial sweating, ipsilateral miosis or ptosis, or a sense of restlessness or agitation. Episodic cluster headache is defined as at least two cluster periods lasting from 7 to 365 days and separated by pain-free remission periods of 1 month or longer.

Although the underlying pathophysiologic mechanisms of cluster headache are not completely known, the hypothalamus is believed to play a key role. In some families, an autosomal dominant gene may be involved. The possible role of the regulating centers in the anterior hypothalamus is implicated from observations of circadian rhythm changes (attacks often begin during sleep) and neuroendocrine disturbances (*e.g.*, changes in cortisol, prolactin, and testosterone) that occur during attacks and in remission. Activation of the trigeminal vascular system and cranial parasympathetic reflexes is thought to explain the pain and autonomic symptoms. Positron emission tomography (PET) has demonstrated increased blood flow as well as structural changes in the hypothalamic gray area on the painful side during an attack. Magnetic resonance imaging (MRI) has demonstrated dilated intracranial arteries on the painful side. Loss of vascular tone is believed to result from abnormalities in autonomic function with increased parasympathetic drive and decreased sympathetic function.[45]

Because of the relatively short duration and self-limited nature of cluster headache, oral preparations typically take too long to reach therapeutic levels. The most effective treatments are those that act quickly (*e.g.*, oxygen inhalation and subcutaneous sumatriptan). Intranasal lidocaine also may be effective.[33] Oxygen inhalation may be indicated for home use. Prophylactic medications for cluster headaches include ergotamine, verapamil, methysergide, lithium carbonate, corticosteroids, sodium valproate, and indomethacin.

TENSION-TYPE HEADACHE

The most common type of headache is tension-type headache. Unlike migraine and cluster headaches, tension-type headache usually is not sufficiently severe that it interferes with daily activities. Tension-type headaches frequently are described as dull, aching, diffuse, nondescript headaches, occurring in a hatband distribution around the head, and not associated with nausea or vomiting or worsened by activity. They can be infrequent, episodic, or chronic.

The exact mechanisms of tension-type headache are not known, and the hypotheses of causation are contradictory. One popular theory is that tension-type headache results from sustained tension of the muscles of the scalp and neck; however, some research has found no correlation between muscle contraction and tension-type headache. Many authorities now believe that tension-type headaches are forms of migraine headache.[34] It is thought that migraine headache may be transformed gradually into chronic tension-type headache. Tension-type headaches also may be caused by oromandibular dysfunction, psychogenic stress, anxiety, depression, and muscular stress. They also may result from overuse of analgesics or caffeine. Daily use of caffeine, whether in beverages or medications, can produce addiction, and a headache can develop in such persons who go without caffeine for several hours.[46]

Tension-type headaches often are more responsive to nonpharmacologic techniques, such as biofeedback, massage, acupuncture, relaxation, imagery, and physical therapy, than are other types of headache. For persons with poor posture, a combination of range-of-motion exercises, relaxation, and posture improvement may be helpful.[46]

The medications of choice for acute treatment of tension-type headaches are analgesics, including acetylsalicylic acid, acetaminophen, and NSAIDs. Persons with infrequently occurring tension-type headaches usually self-medicate using over-the-counter analgesics to treat the acute pain and do not require prophylactic medication. These agents should be used cautiously because rebound headaches can develop when the medications are taken regularly.

Because the "dividing lines" between tension-type headache, migraine, and chronic daily headache often are vague, addition of medications as well as the entire range of migraine medications may be tried in refractory cases. Other medications used concomitantly with analgesics include sedatives, anxiolytics, and skeletal muscle relaxants. Prophylactic treatment can include antidepressants.

TEMPOROMANDIBULAR JOINT PAIN

Another cause of head pain is temporomandibular joint (TMJ) syndrome. It usually is caused by an imbalance in joint movement because of poor bite, bruxism (*i.e.*, teeth grinding), or joint problems such as inflammation, trauma, and degenerative changes.[47] The pain almost always is referred and commonly presents as facial muscle pain, headache, neck ache, or earache. Referred pain is aggravated by jaw function. Headache associated with this syndrome is common in adults and children and can cause chronic pain problems.

Treatment of TMJ pain is aimed at correcting the problem, and in some cases this may be difficult. The initial therapy for TMJ should be directed toward relief of pain and improvement in function. Pain relief often can be achieved with use of the NSAIDs. Muscle relaxants may be used when muscle spasm is a problem. In some cases, the selected application of heat or cold, or both, may provide relief. Referral to a dentist who is associated with a team of therapists, such as a psychologist, physical therapist, or pain specialist, may be indicated.[47]

In summary, head pain is a common disorder that is caused by a number of conditions. Some headaches represent primary disorders and others occur secondary to another disease state in which head pain is a symptom. Primary headache disorders include migraine headache, tension-type headache, and cluster headache. Although most causes of secondary headache are benign, some are indications of serious disorders, such as meningitis, brain tumor, or cerebral aneurysm. TMJ syndrome is one of the major causes of headaches. It usually is caused by an imbalance in joint movement because of poor bite, teeth grinding, or joint problems such as inflammation, trauma, and degenerative changes.

Pain in Children and Older Adults

Pain frequently is underrecognized and undertreated in both children and the elderly. In addition to the common obstacles to adequate pain management, such as concern about the effects of analgesia on respiratory status and the potential for addiction to opioids, there are additional deterrents to adequate pain management in children and the elderly. With regard to both children and the elderly, there are stereotypic beliefs that they feel less pain than other patients.[48–51] These beliefs may affect a clinician's opinion about the need for pain control. In very young children and confused elderly, there are several additional factors. These include the extreme difficulty of assessing the location and intensity of pain in individuals who are cognitively immature or cognitively impaired, and the argument that even if they feel pain, they do not remember it. Research during the past few decades has added a great deal to the body of knowledge about pain in children and the elderly.

PAIN IN CHILDREN

Human responsiveness to painful stimuli begins in the neonatal period and continues through the life span. Although the specific and localized behavioral reactions are less marked in the younger neonate or the more cognitively impaired individual, protective or withdrawal reflexes in response to nociceptive stimuli are clearly demonstrated. Pain pathways, cortical and subcortical centers, and neurochemical responses associated with pain transmission are developed and functional by the last trimester of pregnancy. As infants and children grow, their responses to pain become more complex and reflective of their maturing cognitive and developmental processes.[49] Children do feel pain and have been shown to report pain reliably and accurately at as young as 3 years of age. They also remember pain, as evidenced in studies of children with cancer, whose distress during painful procedures increases over time without intervention, and in neonates in intensive care units, who demonstrate protective withdrawal responses to a heel stick after repeated episodes.

To treat pain adequately, ongoing assessment of the presence of pain and response to treatment is essential.[49,50] Self-report is usually regarded as the most reliable estimate of pain. With children 8 years of age or older, numeric scales (*i.e.*, 1 to 10) and word graphic scales (*i.e.*, "none," "a little," "most I have ever experienced") can be used. With children 3 to 8 years of age, scales with faces of actual children or cartoon faces can be used to obtain a report of pain. Another supplementary strategy for assessing a child's pain is to use a body outline and ask the child to indicate where the hurt is located. Particular care must be taken in assessing children's reports of pain because their reports may be influenced by a variety of factors, including age, anxiety and fear levels, and parental presence. In very young children, infants, and neonates as well as in children with disabilities that impair cognition or communication, clinicians must reply on physiologic parameters or age/development-appropriate behavioral pain scales.[49] Some physiologic measures, such as heart rate, are convenient to measure and respond rapidly to brief nociceptive stimuli, but they are nonspecific. Relying on indicators of sympathetic nervous system activity and behaviors can also be problematic because they can be caused by conditions other than pain (*e.g.*, anxiety and activity) and they do not always accompany pain, particularly chronic pain.

The management of children's pain basically falls into two categories: pharmacologic and nonpharmacologic. In terms of pharmacologic interventions, many of the analgesics used in adults can be used safely and effectively in children and adolescents. However, it is critical when using specific medications to determine that the medication has been approved for use with children and that it is dosed appropriately according to the child's weight and level of physiologic development. Age-related differences in physiologic functioning, notably in neonates, will affect drug action. Neonates have decreased fat and muscle and increased water, which increases the duration of action for some water-soluble drugs; neonates also have decreased concentration of plasma proteins (albumin and α_1-glycoprotein), which increases the unbound concentration of protein-binding drugs. Neonates and infants have decreased metabolic clearances of drugs metabolized in the liver. In addition, they have decreased glomerular filtration rates, leading to delayed clearance of renally excreted drugs and active metabolites.[52] Children 2 to 6 years of age have an increased hepatic mass compared with adults, leading to increased metabolic clearance of similar drugs.[52]

As with any person in pain, the type of analgesic used should be matched to the type and intensity of pain; and whether the patient is a child or adult, the management of chronic pain may require a multidisciplinary team. The overriding principle in all pediatric pain management is to treat each child's pain on an individual basis and to match the analgesic agent with the cause and the level of pain. A second principle involves maintaining the balance between the level of side effects and pain relief such that pain relief is obtained with as little opioid and sedation as possible. One strategy toward this end is to time the administration of analgesia so that a steady blood level is achieved and, as much as possible, pain is prevented. This requires that the child receive analgesia on a regular dosing schedule, rather than on an "as-needed" basis.

Nonpharmacologic strategies can be very effective in reducing the overall amount of pain and amount of analgesia used. In addition, some nonpharmacologic strategies can reduce anxiety and increase the child's level of self-control during pain. For infants and younger children, comfort measures such as cuddling, swaddling, auditory and tactile stimulation, and sucking may reduce behavioral and physiologic responses to acute pain.[49] Children as young as 4 years of age can be taught to use simple distraction and relaxation and other techniques such as application of heat and cold.[53] Other nonpharmacologic techniques can be taught to the child to provide psychological preparation for a painful procedure or surgery. These include positive self-talk, imagery, play therapy, modeling, and rehearsal. The nonpharmacologic interventions must be developmentally appropriate and, if possible, the child and parent should be taught these techniques when the child is not in pain (*e.g.*, before surgery or a painful procedure) so that it is easier to practice the technique.

PAIN IN OLDER ADULTS

Among adults, the prevalence of pain in the general population increases with age: 32% of those between 18 and 34 years of age report daily pain, whereas 55% of Americans aged 65 years and older report daily pain. Among the elderly, the most common self-attributed causes of pain are getting older (88%) and arthritis (69%).[54] In long-term care facilities, it has been estimated that 45% to 80% of residents experience pain on a regular basis.[51] Research is inconsistent about whether there are age-related changes in pain perception. Some apparent age-related differences in pain may be due to differences in willingness to report the pain rather than actual differences in pain. The elderly may be reluctant to report pain so as not to be a burden or out of fear of the diagnoses, tests, medications, or costs that may result from an attempt to diagnose or treat their pain.

The assessment of pain in the elderly can range from relatively simple in a well-informed, alert, cognitively intact individual to extraordinarily difficult in a frail individual with severe dementia and many concurrent health problems. When possible, a person's report of pain is the gold standard, but outward signs of pain should be considered as well. Accurately diagnosing pain when the individual has many health problems or some decline in cognitive function can be particularly challenging. In recent years, there has been increased awareness of the need to address issues of pain in individuals with dementia. The Assessment for Discomfort in Dementia Protocol is one example of the efforts to improve assessment and pain management in these individuals. It includes behavioral criteria for assessing pain and recommended interventions for pain. Its use has been shown to improve pain management.[55]

When prescribing pharmacologic and nonpharmacologic methods of pain management for the older population, care must be taken to consider the cause of the pain, the patient's health status, the concurrent therapies, and the patient's mental status. In the older population, where the risk of adverse events is higher, the nonpharmacologic options are usually less costly and cause fewer side effects.

Common nonpharmacologic interventions include application of cold (which suppresses the release of products from tissue damage) and heat (which promotes the release of endogenous endorphins).[51] The role of mental focus and anxiety is important, and relaxation techniques, massage, and biofeedback may be useful. Physical therapy and occupational therapy bring a variety of modalities, including the use of braces or splints, changes in biomechanics, and exercise, all of which have been shown to promote pain relief.

Although efficacy is important when considering the use of pharmacologic agents for pain relief in the elderly population, cost and safety must also be considered. Safety issues that must be considered among older adults include changes in drug metabolism, other disease comorbidity, and polypharmacy. The elderly may have physiologic changes that affect the pharmacokinetics of medications prescribed for pain management. These changes include decreased blood flow to organs, delayed gastric motility, reduced kidney function, and decreased albumin related to poor nutrition. Also, the elderly often have many coexisting health problems, leading to polypharmacy. On average, a 70-year-old takes seven different medications.[51] The addition of analgesics to a complex medication regimen is even more likely to cause drug interactions and complicate compliance in the elderly. However, these considerations should not preclude the appropriate use of analgesic drugs to achieve pain relief. Nonopioids are generally the first line of therapy for mild to moderate pain, and acetaminophen is usually the first choice because it is relatively safe for older adults.[51] Opioids are used for more severe pain and for palliative care. As with younger persons, adjuvant analgesics are effectively used for treatment of pain in older adults. The use of some assessment tool to evaluate the level of pain and effectiveness of treatment is essential. Monitoring for side effects is also critical.

In summary, pain frequently is underrecognized and undertreated in both children and the elderly. As well as the common obstacles to adequate pain management, such as concern about the effects of analgesia on respiratory status and the potential for addiction to opioids, there are additional deterrents to adequate pain management in children and the elderly.

Children experience and remember pain, and even fairly young children are able to report their pain accurately and reliably. Recognition of this has changed the clinical practice of health professionals involved in the assessment of children's pain. Pain management in children is improving as exaggerated fears and misconceptions concerning the risks of addiction and respiratory depression in children treated with opioids also are dispelled. Pharmacologic (including opioids) and nonpharmacologic pain management interventions have been shown to be effective in children. Nonpharmacologic techniques must be based on the developmental level of the child and should be taught to both children and parents.

Pain is a common symptom in the elderly. Assessment, diagnosis, and treatment of pain in the elderly can be challenging. The elderly may be reluctant or cognitively unable to report their pain. Diagnosis and treatment can be complicated by comorbidities and age-related changes in cognitive and physiologic function.

Review Exercises

A 25-year-old man is admitted to the emergency department with acute abdominal pain that began in the epigastric area and has now shifted to the lower right quadrant of the abdomen. There is localized tenderness and guarding or spasm of the muscle over the area. His heart rate and blood pressure are elevated and his skin is moist and cool from perspiring. He is given a tentative diagnosis of appendicitis and referred for surgical consultation.

A. Describe the origin of the pain stimuli and the neural pathways involved in the pain this man is experiencing.

B. Explain the neural mechanisms involved in the spasm of the overlying abdominal muscles.

C. What is the significance of his cool, moist skin and increased heart rate and blood pressure?

A 65-year-old woman with breast cancer is receiving hospice care in her home. She is currently receiving a long-acting opioid analgesic supplemented with a short-acting combination opioid and non-narcotic medication for breakthrough pain.

A. Explain the difference between the mechanisms and treatment of acute and chronic pain.

B. Describe the action of opioid drugs in the treatment of pain.

A 42-year-old woman presents with sudden, stabbing-type facial pain that arises near the right side of her mouth and then shoots toward the right ear, eye, and nostril. She is holding her hand to protect her face because the pain is "triggered by touch, movement, and drafts." Her initial diagnosis is trigeminal neuritis.

A. Explain the distribution and mechanisms of the pain, particularly the triggering of the pain by stimuli applied to the skin.

B. What are possible treatment methods for this woman?

A 21-year-old woman presents in the student health center with complaints of a throbbing pain on the left side of her head, nausea and vomiting, and extreme sensitivity to light, noise, and head movement. She also tells you she had a similar headache 3 months ago that lasted for 2 days and states that she thinks she is developing migraine headaches like her mother. She is concerned because she has been unable to attend classes and has exams next week.

A. Are this woman's history and symptoms consistent with migraine headaches?

B. Use the distribution of the trigeminal nerve and the concept of neurogenic inflammation to explain this woman's symptoms.

Visit the Porth: Essentials of Pathophysiology: Concepts of Altered Health States web site (http://thePoint.LWW.com/PorthEssentials) for links to chapter-related resources on the Internet, all-new exclusive animations, chapter review questions, and more!

REFERENCES

1. Kandel E. R., Schwartz J. H., Jessell T. M. (2000). *Principles of neural science* (4th ed., pp. 430–450). New York: McGraw-Hill.
2. Bear M. F., Connors B. W., Paradiso M. A. (2001). *Neuroscience: Exploring the brain* (2nd ed., pp. 397–435). Philadelphia: Lippincott Williams & Wilkins.
3. Berne R. M., Levy M. N. (2000). *Principles of physiology* (3rd ed., pp. 78–94). St. Louis: Mosby.
4. Guyton A., Hall J. E. (2005). *Textbook of medical physiology* (11th ed., pp. 598–604). Philadelphia: Elsevier Saunders.
5. Bonica J. J. (1991). History of pain concepts and pain theory. *Mount Sinai Journal of Medicine* 58, 191–202.
6. Melzack R., Wall P. D. (1965). Pain mechanisms: A new theory. *Science* 150, 971–979.
7. Melzack R. (1999). From the gate to the neuromatrix. *Pain* 6(Suppl.), S121–S126.
8. Cross S. A. (1994). Pathophysiology of pain. *Mayo Clinic Proceedings* 69, 375–383.
9. Julius D., Basbaum A. I. (2001). Molecular mechanisms of nociception. *Nature* 413, 203–210.
10. McHugh J. M., McHugh W. B. (2000). Pain: Neuroanatomy, chemical mediators, and clinical implications. *AACN Clinical Issues* 11(2), 168–179.
11. Fields H. L., Heinricher M. M., Mason P. (1991). Neurotransmitters in nociceptive modulatory circuits. *Review of Neuroscience* 14, 219–245.
12. Maizels M., McCorberg B. (2005). Antidepressant and antiepileptic drugs for chronic non-cancer pain. *American Family Physician* 71, 483–490.
13. Goldstein F. J. (2002). Adjuncts to opioid therapy. *Journal of the American Osteopathic Association* 102(9), S15–S20.
14. Stein C. (2003). Opioid receptors on peripheral sensory neurons. In Machelska H., Stein C. (Eds.), *Immune mechanisms of pain and analgesia* (pp. 69–76). New York: Kluwer Academic/Plenum.
15. Cervero F., Laird J. M. (1999). Visceral pain. *Lancet* 353, 2145–2148.
16. Al-Chaer E. D., Traub R. J. (2002). Biological basis of visceral pain: Recent developments. *Pain* 96, 221–225.
17. Grichnick K., Ferrante F. M. (1991). The difference between acute and chronic pain. *Mount Sinai Journal of Medicine* 58, 217–220.
18. Turk D. C., Okifuji A. (2001). Pain terms and taxonomies of pain. In Loser J. D. (Ed.), *Bonica's management of pain* (3rd ed., pp. 17–25). Philadelphia: Lippincott Williams & Wilkins.
19. Jacobson L., Mariano A. J. (2001). General considerations in chronic pain. In Loser J. D. (Ed.), *Bonica's management of pain* (3rd ed., pp. 241–254). Philadelphia: Lippincott Williams & Wilkins.
20. Ruoff G. E. (1996). Depression in the patient with chronic pain. *Journal of Family Practice* 43(6 Suppl.), S25–S33.
21. Acute Pain Management Guideline Panel. (1992). *Clinical practice guideline no. 1. Acute pain management: Operative or medical procedures and trauma*. AHCPR publication no. 92-0032. Rockville, MD: Agency for Health Care Policy and Research, Public Health Service, U.S. Department of Health and Human Services.
22. Jacox A., Carr D. B., Payne R., et al. (1994). *Clinical practice guideline no. 9. Management of cancer pain*. AHCPR publication no. 94-0592. Rockville, MD: Agency for Health Care Policy and Research, Public Health Service, U.S. Department of Health and Human Services.
23. World Health Organization. (1990). *Cancer pain relief and palliative care: Report of the WHO Expert Committee*. Technical Report Series 804. Geneva, Switzerland: Author.

24. Inturrisi C. E. (2002). Clinical pharmacology of opioids for pain. *Clinical Journal of Pain* 18(Suppl. 4), S3–S13.

25. Jensen T. S., Gottup H., Sindrup S. H., et al. (2001). The clinical picture of neuropathic pain. *European Journal of Pharmacology* 429, 1–11.

26. Vaillancourt P. D., Langevin H. M. (1999). Painful peripheral neuropathies. *Medical Clinics of North America* 83, 627–643.

27. Aminoff M. J. (2006). Nervous system. In Tierney L. M., McPhee S. J., Papadakis M. A. (eds.), *Current medical diagnosis and treatment* (43rd ed., pp. 978–979). New York: Lange Medical Books/McGraw-Hill.

28. Kost R. G., Straus S. E. (1996). Postherpetic neuralgia: Pathogenesis, treatment and prevention. *New England Journal of Medicine* 335, 32–42.

29. Gnann J. W., Whitley R. J. (2002). Herpes zoster. *New England Journal of Medicine* 347, 340–346.

30. Rho R. H., Brewer R. P., Lamer T. J., et al. (2002). Complex regional pain syndrome. *Mayo Clinic Proceedings* 77, 174–180.

31. Pham T., Lafforgue P. (2003). Reflex sympathetic dystrophy syndrome and neuromediators. *Joint, Bone, Spine* 70, 12–17.

32. Reflex Sympathetic Dystrophy Syndrome Association of America. (2000). Clinical practice guideline for treatment of reflex sympathetic dystrophy syndrome. [On-line]. Available: www.rsds.org/cpgeng.htm.

33. Melzack R. (1992). Phantom limb. *Scientific American* 226, 120–126.

34. Saper J. R. (1999). Headache disorders. *Medical Clinics of North America* 83, 663–670.

35. Kaniecki R. (2003). Headache assessment and management. *Journal of the American Medical Association* 289, 1430–1433.

36. Headache Classification Subcommittee of the International Headache Society. (2004). The international classification of headache disorders, ed. 2. *Cephalalgia* 24(Suppl. 1), 1–152.

37. Mathew N. T. (2001). Pathophysiology, epidemiology, and impact of migraine. *Clinical Cornerstone* 4, 1–17.

38. Annequin D., Tourniare B., Massoui H. (2000). Migraine and headache in childhood and adolescence. *Pediatric Clinics of North America* 47, 617–631.

39. Haslam R. H. A. (2004). Headaches. In Behrman R. E., Kliegman R. M., Jenson H. B. (Eds.), *Nelson textbook of pediatrics* (17th ed., pp. 2012–2015). Philadelphia: Elsevier Saunders.

40. Tepper S. J., Rapoport A., Sheftell F. (2001). The pathophysiology of migraine. *Neurologist* 7, 279–786.

41. Williamson D. H., Hargreaves R. J. (2001). Neurogenic inflammation in the context on migraine. *Microscopy Research and Technique* 53, 167–178.

42. Kunkel R. S. (2000). Managing primary headache syndromes. *Patient Care* January 30. [On-line]. Available: www.patient-careonline.com.

43. Snow V., Weiss K., Wall E. M., et al. (2002). Pharmacologic management of acute attacks of migraine and prevention of migraine headache. *Annals of Internal Medicine* 137, 840–849.

44. Silberstein S. D. (2000). Practice parameter: Evidence-based guidelines for migraine headache. *Neurology* 55, 754–763.

45. May A. (2005). Cluster headache: Pathogenesis, diagnosis, and management. *Lancet* 366, 843–855.

46. Millea, P. J., Brodie, J. J. (2002). Tension-type headache. *American Family Physician* 66, 797–804.

47. Okeson J. P. (1996). Temporomandibular disorders in the medical practice. *Journal of Family Practice* 43, 347–356.

48. Broome M., Richtsmeier A., Maikler V., et al. (1996). Pediatric pain practices: A survey of health professionals. *Journal of Pain and Symptom Management* 4, 315–319.

49. Howard R. F. (2003). Current status of pain management in children. *Journal of the American Medical Association* 29, 2464–2469.

50. Committee on Psychological Aspects of Child and Family Health. (2001). The assessment and management of acute pain in infants, children, and adolescents. *Pediatrics* 108, 793–797.

51. Gloth M. F. (2001). Pain management in older adults: Prevention and treatment. *Journal of the American Geriatrics Society* 49, 188–199.

52. Berde C. B., Sethna N. F. (2002). Analgesics for the treatment of pain in children. *New England Journal of Medicine* 347, 1094–1103.

53. Vessey J., Carlson K., McGill J. (1995). Use of distraction with children during an acute pain experience. *Nursing Research* 43, 369–372.

54. Gallup Survey. (1999). Conducted by the Gallup Organization from May 21 to June 9, 1999. Supported by the Arthritis Foundation and Merck & Company, Inc. [On-line]. Available: http://www.asaging.org/at/at-213/gallupsurvey.html. Accessed December 7, 2005.

55. Kovach C. R., Weissman, D. E., Griffie J., et al. (1999). Assessment and treatment of discomfort for people with late-stage dementia. *Journal of Pain and Symptom Management* 18, 412–419.

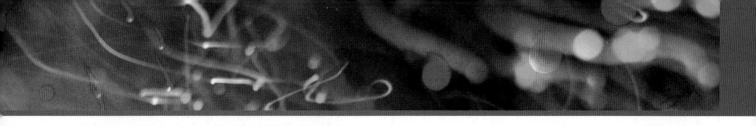

C h a p t e r *35*

Disorders of Neuromuscular Function

 Effective motor function requires that muscles move and that the mechanics of their movement be programmed in a manner that provides for smooth and coordinated movement. In some cases, purposeless and disruptive movements can be almost as disabling as relative or complete absence of movement. This chapter provides an introduction to the organization and control of motor function and discusses disorders of skeletal muscles, the neuromuscular junction, and peripheral nerves; the basal ganglia and cerebellum; and upper and lower motor neurons.

Organization and Control of Motor Function

Motor function, whether it involves walking, running, or precise finger movements, requires movement and maintenance of posture. Posture can be described as the relative position of various parts of the body with respect to one another (limb extension, flexion) or to the environment (standing, supine).[1] Posture also can be described as the active muscular resistance to the displacement of the body by gravity or acceleration. The structures that control posture and movement are located throughout the neuromuscular system. The system consists of the neuromuscular unit, which includes the motor neurons, the neuromuscular junction, and the muscle fibers; the spinal cord, which contains the basic reflex circuitry for posture and movement; and the descending pathways from the brain stem circuits, the cerebellum, the basal ganglia, and the motor cortex.

As with other parts of the nervous system, the motor systems are organized in a functional hierarchy, each concerned with increased levels of motor function (Fig. 35-1). The highest level of function, which occurs at the level of the frontal cortex, is concerned with the purpose and planning of the motor movement.[1] The lowest level

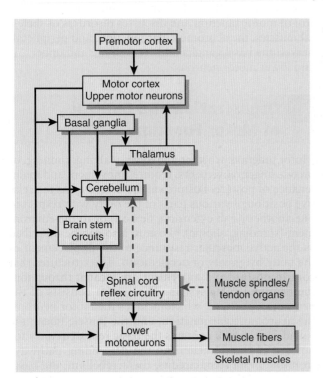

FIGURE 35-1 The motor control system. The final common pathway transmits all central nervous system commands to the skeletal muscles. This path is influenced by sensory input from the muscle spindles and tendon organs (*dashed lines*) and descending signals from the cerebral cortex and brain stem. The cerebellum and basal ganglia influence the motor function indirectly, using brain stem and cortical pathways.

of the hierarchy occurs at the spinal cord, which contains the basic reflex circuitry needed to coordinate the function of the motor units involved in the planned movement. Above the spinal cord is the brain stem, and above the brain stem are the cerebellum and basal ganglia, structures that modulate the actions of the brain stem systems. Overseeing these supraspinal structures are the motor centers in the cerebral cortex.

THE MOTOR UNIT

The neurons that control motor function are referred to as *motor neurons* or sometimes as *alpha motor neurons*. The motor neuron and the group of muscle fibers it innervates in a muscle is called a *motor unit*. When the motor neuron develops an action potential, all of the muscle fibers in the motor unit that it innervates develop action potentials, causing them to contract simultaneously. Thus, a motor neuron and the muscle fibers it innervates function as a single unit—the basic unit of motor control.

Each motor neuron undergoes multiple branching, making it possible for a single motor neuron to innervate a few to thousands of muscle fibers. In general, large muscles—those containing hundreds or thousands of muscle fibers and providing gross motor movement—have large motor units. This sharply contrasts with those that control the hand, tongue, and eye movements, for which the motor units are small and permit very precise control.

The motor neurons supplying a motor unit are located in the ventral horn of the spinal cord and are called *lower motor neurons* (LMNs). *Upper motor neurons* (UMNs), which exert control over LMNs, project from the motor strip in the cerebral cortex to the ventral horn and are fully contained within the central nervous system (CNS; Fig. 35-2).

THE MOTOR CORTEX

Precise, skillful, and intentional movements of the distal and especially flexor muscles of the limbs and speech apparatus are initiated and controlled by the motor cortex located in the posterior part of the frontal lobe. It consists of the primary, premotor, and supplementary motor cortex[1–3] (Fig. 35-3). These motor areas receive information from the thalamus and somatosensory (sensory) cortex and, indirectly, from the cerebellum and basal ganglia.

The primary motor cortex (area 4), also called the *motor strip,* is located on the rostral surface and adjacent to portions of the central sulcus. The primary motor cortex controls specific muscle movement sequences and is the first level of descending control for precise motor movements. The neurons in the primary motor cortex are arranged in a somatotopic array or distorted map of the body called the *motor homunculus* (Fig. 35-4). The body parts that require the greatest dexterity have the largest cortical areas devoted to them. More than one half of the primary motor cortex is concerned with controlling the muscles of the hands, of facial expression, and of speech.

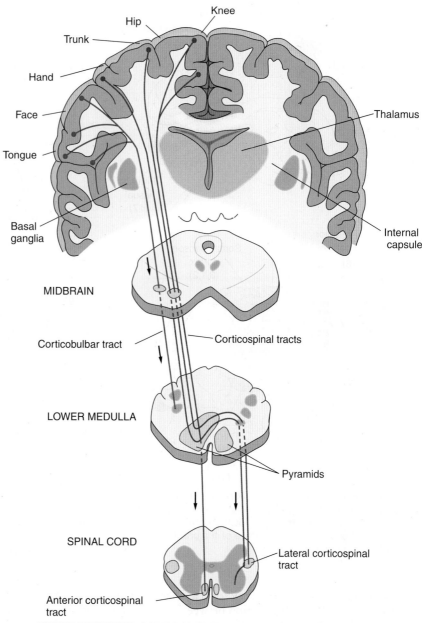

FIGURE 35-2 Motor pathways: corticospinal and corticobulbar tracts. (Modified from Bickley L. S. [2003]. *Bates guide to physical examination and history taking* [8th ed., p. 543]. Philadelphia: Lippincott Williams & Wilkins.)

MOTOR PATHWAYS: CORTICOSPINAL AND CORTICOBULBAR TRACTS

The premotor cortex (areas 6 and 8), which is located just anterior to the primary motor cortex, sends some fibers into the corticospinal tract but mainly innervates the primary motor strip. Nerve signals generated by the premotor cortex produce much more complex "patterns" of movement than the discrete patterns generated by the primary motor cortex. For example, the movement pattern to accomplish a particular objective, such as throwing a ball or picking up a fork, is programmed by the prefrontal association cortex and associated thalamic nuclei.

The supplementary motor cortex, which contains representations of all parts of the body, is located on the medial surface of the hemisphere (areas 6 and 8) in the premotor region. It is intimately involved in the performance of complex, skillful movements that involve both sides of the body.

The primary motor cortex contains many layers of pyramid-shaped output neurons that project to the premotor and somatosensory areas on the same side of the cortex (*i.e.*, premotor and somesthetic cortex), project to the opposite side of the cortex, or descend to subcortical structures such as the basal ganglia and thalamus. The large pyramidal cells located in the fifth layer project to the brain stem and spinal cord. The axons of these UMNs project through the subcortical white matter and internal capsule to the deep surface of the brain stem, through the ventral bulge of the pons, and to the ventral

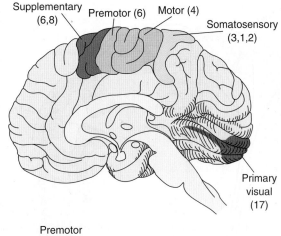

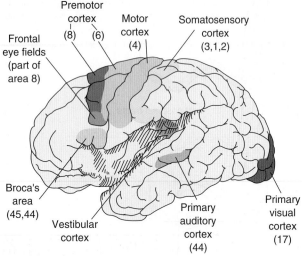

FIGURE 35-3 Primary motor cortex. (**Top**) The location of the primary, premotor, and supplementary cortex on the medial surface of the brain. (**Bottom**) The location of the primary and premotor cortex on the lateral surface of the brain. (Courtesy of Carole Russell Hilmer, C. M. I.)

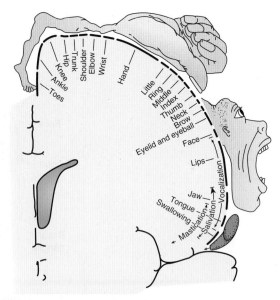

FIGURE 35-4 Representation of the relative extent of motor cortical area 4 devoted to muscles of the various body regions. Medial surface is at the left, lateral fissure is at the right, with pharyngeal and laryngeal muscle representation extending toward the insula. (From Penfield E., Rasmussen T. [1968]. *The cerebral cortex in man: A clinical study of localization of function.* New York: Macmillan.)

surface of the medulla, where they form a ridge or pyramid (see Fig. 35-2). At the junction between the medulla and cervical spinal cord, 80% or more of the UMN axons cross the midline to form the lateral corticospinal tract in the lateral white matter of the spinal cord. This tract extends throughout the spinal cord, with roughly 50% of the fibers terminating in the cervical segments, 20% in the thoracic segments, and 30% in the lumbosacral segments. Most of the remaining uncrossed fibers travel down the anterior corticospinal tract in the spinal cord, mainly to cervical levels, where they cross and innervate contralateral LMNs.

By convention, motor tracts have been classified as belonging to one of two motor systems: the pyramidal and extrapyramidal systems. According to this classification system, the pyramidal system consists of the corticobulbar and corticospinal tracts containing fibers that originate from the giant pyramidal cells, called *Betz cells*, that are found in the primary motor cortex. The fibers of the lateral corticospinal tract pass downward through the internal capsule and traverse the ventral surface of the medulla in a bundle called the *pyramid* before decussating or crossing to the opposite side of the brain at the medulla–spinal cord junction. Other fibers from the cortex and basal ganglia project to the brain stem reticular formation and reticulospinal systems, following a more ancient pathway to LMNs of proximal and extensor muscles. These fibers do not decussate in the pyramids, hence the name *extrapyramidal system*. Disorders of the pyramidal tracts (*e.g.*, stroke) are characterized by spasticity and paralysis, and those affecting the extrapyramidal tracts (*e.g.*, Parkinson disease) by involuntary movements, muscle rigidity, and immobility without paralysis. As increased knowledge regarding motor pathways has emerged, it has become evident that the extrapyramidal and pyramidal systems are extensively interconnected and cooperate in the control of movement.[1]

SPINAL REFLEXES

Reflexes are coordinated, involuntary motor responses initiated by a stimulus applied to peripheral receptors.[1,2] Some reflexes, such as the flexor-withdrawal reflex, initiate movements to avoid hazardous situations, whereas others, such as the stretch reflex or crossed-extensor reflex, serve to integrate motor movements so they function in a coordinated manner. The anatomic basis of a reflex consists of an afferent neuron, which synapses either directly with an effector neuron that innervates a muscle or with an interneuron that synapses with an effector neuron. Reflexes are essentially "wired into" the CNS so that they are always ready to function; with training, most reflexes can be modulated to become parts of more complicated movements. A reflex may involve neurons in a single cord segment (*i.e.,* segmental reflexes), several or many segments (*i.e.,* intersegmental reflexes), or structures in the brain (*i.e.,* suprasegmental reflexes).

The Stretch Reflex

The stretch reflex, a contraction of muscle fibers that occurs when a muscle is stretched, is essential to the control of muscle tone and maintenance of posture. Stretch reflexes can be evoked in many muscles throughout the body and are routinely tested (*e.g.,* knee-jerk reflex) during the clinical examination for the diagnosis of neurologic conditions. Disorders of muscle tone caused by dysregulated function of the stretch reflex are seen in persons with conditions such as spinal cord injury and stroke.

The stretch reflex uses specialized afferent sensory endings in skeletal muscles and tendons to relay information regarding the sense of body position, movement, and muscle tone to the CNS. Information from these sensory afferents is relayed to the cerebellum and cerebral cortex and is experienced as the sense of body movement and position (*proprioception*). To provide this information, the muscles and their tendons are supplied with two types of stretch receptors: muscle spindle receptors and Golgi tendon organs. The muscle spindles, which are distributed throughout the belly of a muscle, relay information about muscle length and rate of stretch. The *Golgi tendon organs* are found in muscle tendons and transmit information about muscle tension or force of contraction at the junction of the muscle and the tendon that attaches to bone. A likely role of the tendon organs is to equalize the contractile forces of the separate muscle groups, spreading the load over all the fibers to prevent the local muscle damage that might occur when small numbers of fibers are overloaded.

The muscle spindles consist of a group of specialized miniature skeletal muscle fibers called *intrafusal fibers* that are encased in a connective tissue capsule and attached to the extrafusal fibers of a skeletal muscle. In the center of the receptor area, a large sensory neuron spirals around the intrafusal fiber, forming the so-called *primary* or *annulospiral* ending. This nerve fiber is a type Ia fiber that transmits sensory signals to the spinal cord at the rate of 70 to 120 m/second, as rapidly as any nerve in the body. The extrafusal fibers and the intrafusal fibers are innervated by motor neurons that reside in the ventral horns of the spinal cord. Extrafusal fibers are innervated by large alpha motor neurons that produce contraction of the muscle. The intrafusal fibers are innervated by gamma motor neurons that control the sensitivity of the stretch reflex by adjusting intrafusal fiber length so it matches that of the extrafusal fibers.

The intrafusal muscle fibers function as stretch receptors. When a skeletal muscle is stretched, the spindle and its intrafusal fibers are stretched, resulting in increased firing of their afferent fibers. Increased firing of the afferent neurons, which synapse with alpha motor neurons in

the spinal cord, causes the extrafusal muscle fibers to contract, thereby shortening the muscle. The knee-jerk reflex that occurs when the knee is tapped with a reflex hammer tests for the intactness of the stretch reflex arc in the quadriceps muscle.

Axons of the Ia afferent neurons of the stretch reflex enter the spinal cord through several branches of the dorsal root. Some branches end in the segment of entry; others ascend to adjacent segments, influencing intersegmental reflex function; and still others ascend in the dorsal column of the cord to the medulla of the brain stem. Segmental branches make connections, along with other branches, that pass directly to the anterior gray matter of the spinal cord and establish monosynaptic contact with each of the LMNs that have motor units in the muscle containing the spindle receptor. This produces an opposing muscle contraction. Another segmental branch of the same Ia afferent neuron innervates an internuncial neuron that is inhibitory to motor units of antagonistic muscle groups. This disynaptic inhibitory pathway is the basis for reciprocal innervation; when a muscle is stretched, the antagonists relax.

Reciprocal innervation is useful not only for the stretch reflex, but for voluntary movements. Relaxation of the antagonist muscle during movements enhances the speed and efficiency because the muscles that act as prime movers are not working against the contraction of opposing muscle.[1] The Ia inhibitory interneurons involved in the stretch reflex also receive input from descending neurons that make direct connections with spinal motor neurons. This organizational feature simplifies the control of motor movements because higher centers do not have to send separate commands to the opposing muscles.

The role of afferent spindle fibers is also to inform the CNS of the status of muscle length. Ascending fibers from the stretch reflex ultimately provide information about muscle length to higher centers in the cerebellum and cerebral cortex. When a skeletal muscle lengthens or shortens against tension, a feedback mechanism needs to be available for readjustment such that the spindle apparatus remains sensitive to moment-to-moment changes in muscle stretch, even while changes in muscle length are occurring. This is accomplished by the gamma motor neurons that adjust spindle fiber length to match the length of the extrafusal muscle fiber. Descending fibers of motor pathways synapse with and simultaneously activate both alpha and gamma motor neurons so that the sensitivity of the spindle fibers is coordinated with muscle movement.

Central control over the gamma motor neurons also permits increases or decreases in muscle tone in anticipation of changes in the muscle force. The CNS, through its coordinated control of the muscle's alpha and the spindle's gamma motor neurons, can suppress the stretch reflex. This occurs during centrally programmed movements, such as pitching a baseball, that require a muscle to produce a full range of unopposed motion. Without this programmed adjustability of the stretch reflex, any movement is immediately opposed and prevented.

Understanding ➤ Stretch Reflex and Muscle Tone

Muscle tone is controlled by the stretch reflex, which monitors changes in muscle length. The activity of the stretch reflex can be divided into three steps: (1) activation of the stretch receptors, (2) integration of the reflex in the spinal cord, and (3) regulation of reflex sensitivity by higher centers in the brain. Testing the (4) knee-jerk reflex provides a means of assessing that reflex.

1

Stretch reflex receptors. Skeletal muscle is composed of two types of muscle fibers: a large number of extrafusal fibers, which control muscle movement, and a smaller number of intrafusal fibers, which control muscle tone. The intrafusal fibers are encapsulated in sheaths, forming a muscle spindle that runs parallel to the extrafusal fibers. Each intrafusal fiber is innervated by a large Ia sensory nerve fiber, which encircles the central noncontractile portion of the fiber to form the so-called *annulospiral ending*. Because the spindles are oriented parallel to the extrafusal muscle fibers, stretching of the extrafusal fibers also stretches the spindle fibers and stimulates the receptive endings of the Ia afferent neuron.

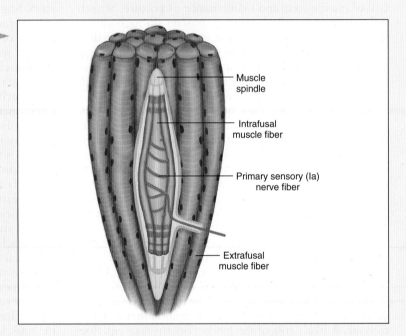

Muscle spindle

Intrafusal muscle fiber

Primary sensory (Ia) nerve fiber

Extrafusal muscle fiber

2

Spinal reflex centers. Afferent impulses from the Ia sensory fiber of the muscle spindle are transmitted to the spinal cord, where they synapse with alpha motor neurons of the stretched muscle to form a monosynaptic reflex arc—"monosynaptic" because only one synapse separates the primary sensory input from the motor neuron output. The reflex muscle contraction that follows resists further stretching of the muscle. As this spinal reflex activity is occurring, impulses providing information on muscle length are transmitted to higher centers in the brain. It is the coordinated activity of all the monosynaptic reflexes supplying the extrafusal fibers in a skeletal muscle that provides the muscle tone needed for organized movement.

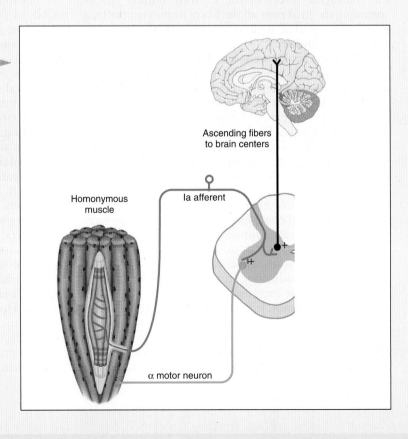

Ascending fibers to brain centers

Homonymous muscle

Ia afferent

α motor neuron

3

Brain center connections. Although a spinal reflex can function independently, its sensitivity is adjusted by higher centers in the brain. Both types of muscle fibers are supplied with motor neurons—the extrafusal fibers with large alpha motor neurons, which produce muscle contraction; and the intrafusal fibers with smaller gamma motor neurons, which control the sensitivity of the stretch reflex. Descending fibers of motor pathways synapse with both alpha and gamma motor neurons, and the impulses are sent simultaneously to the large extrafusal fibers and to the intrafusal fibers to maintain muscle spindle tension (and sensitivity) during muscle contraction.

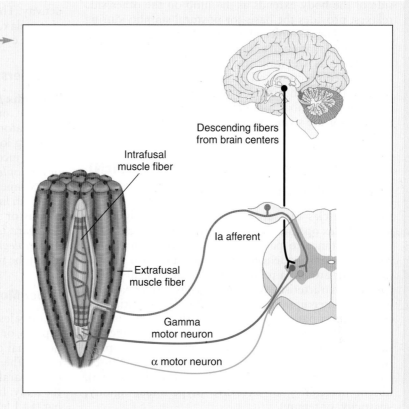

4

The knee-jerk reflex. The knee-jerk reflex that occurs when the knee is tapped with a reflex hammer tests for the intactness of the stretch reflex arc in the quadriceps muscle. Stretching of the extrafusal fibers by tapping with a reflex hammer leads to lengthening of the intrafusal fibers and increased firing of the type Ia afferent neuron. Impulses from the Ia fiber enter the dorsal horn of the spinal cord and make monosynaptic contact with the ventral horn alpha motor neuron supplying the extrafusal fibers in the quadriceps muscle. The resultant reflex contraction (shortening) of the quadriceps muscle is responsible for the knee jerk. These muscle reflexes are called *deep tendon reflexes* (DTRs). They can be checked at the wrists, elbows, knees, and ankles as a means of assessing the components of the stretch reflex at different spinal cord segments.

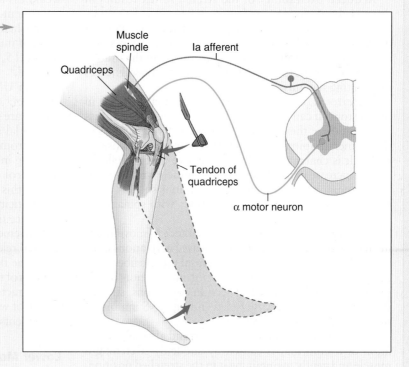

Crossed-Extensor Reflex

The crossed-extensor reflex, in which the limb on one side of the body extends as the limb on the other side relaxes, provides the basis for postural stability during walking.[2] For example, when the crossed-extensor reflex produces relaxation of antigravity muscles (with flexion) of one leg as we walk, the contralateral component produces contraction and extension of the opposite leg. Intersegmental connections of the crossed-extensor reflex between the lumbar and cervical spinal segments also account for the swinging of the arms that accompanies walking.

DISORDERS OF MUSCLE TONE AND MOVEMENT

Disorders of Muscle Tone

In the muscles that are supporting body weight, the stretch reflex operates continuously, producing a continuous resistance to passive stretch called *muscle tone*. Muscle tone is evidenced by the resistance to passive movement around a joint. Disorders of skeletal muscle tone are characteristic of many nervous system pathologies. Any interruption of the stretch reflex by peripheral nerve injury, pathologic process of the neuromuscular junction and of skeletal muscle fibers, damage to the corticospinal system, or injury to the spinal cord or spinal nerve root results in disturbance of muscle tone. Muscle tone may be described as less than normal (hypotonia), absent (flaccidity), or excessive (hypertonia, rigidity, spasticity, or tetany).

Reduced excitability of the stretch reflex results in decreased muscle tone, or *hypotonia*, ranging from postural weakness to total flaccid paralysis. It can result from decreased function of the descending facilitatory systems controlling the gamma LMNs that innervate the muscle spindle or damage to the stretch reflex or peripheral nerves innervating the muscle.

Hypertonia, or spasticity, is an abnormal increase in muscle tone. It can result from increased excitation or loss of inhibition of the spindle's gamma LMNs or changes in the segmental spinal cord circuitry controlling the stretch reflex. It is characterized by hyperactive tendon reflexes and an increase in resistance to rapid muscle stretch. Spasticity commonly occurs with UMN lesions such as those that exist after spinal shock in persons with spinal cord injury.

Rigidity is a greatly increased resistance to movements in all directions. It is caused by increased activation of the alpha LMNs innervating the extrafusal muscle fibers and does not depend on the dorsal root innervation of the intrafusal spindle fibers. It is seen in conditions, such as Parkinson disease, in which descending CNS inhibition of alpha LMNs is impaired.

Clonus is the rhythmic contraction and alternate relaxation of a limb that is caused by suddenly stretching a muscle and gently maintaining it in the stretched position. It is seen in the hypertonia of spasticity associated with UMN lesions, such as spinal cord injury. It is caused by an oscillating stimulation of the muscle spindles that occurs when the spindle fibers are activated by an initial muscle stretch. This results in reflex contraction of the muscle and unloading of the spindle fibers with decreased afferent activity. The reduced spindle fiber activity causes the muscle to relax, which causes the spindle fiber to stretch again, and the cycle starts over again.

Disorders of Muscle Movement

The suffix *plegia* comes from the Greek word for a blow, a stroke, or paralysis. Terms used to describe the extent and anatomic location of motor damage are *paralysis*, meaning loss of movement, and *paresis*, implying weakness or incomplete loss of muscle function. *Monoparesis* or *monoplegia* results from the destruction of pyramidal UMN innervation of one limb; *hemiparesis* or *hemiplegia*, both limbs on one side; *diparesis* or *diplegia* or *paraparesis* or *paraplegia*, both upper or lower limbs; and *tetraparesis* or *tetraplegia*, also called *quadriparesis* or *quadriplegia*, all four limbs (Fig. 35-5). Paresis or paralysis can be further designated as of UMN or LMN origin.

Upper Motor Neuron Lesions

A UMN lesion can involve the motor cortex, the internal capsule, or other brain structures through which the corticospinal or corticobulbar tracts descend, or the spinal cord. When the lesion is at or above the level of the pyramids, paralysis affects structures on the opposite side of the body. In UMN disorders involving injury to the lumbar (L) 1 level or above, there is an immediate, profound weakness and loss of fine, skilled voluntary lower limb movement, reduced bowel and bladder control, and diminished sexual functioning, followed by an exaggeration of muscle tone. With UMN damage above cervical (C) level 5, all function below the upper shoulders also is affected.[4]

With UMN lesions, the LMN spinal reflexes remain intact, but communication and control from higher brain centers are lost. Descending excitatory influences from the pyramidal system and some descending inhibitory influences from other cortical regions are lost after injury, resulting in immediate weakness accompanied by the loss of control of delicate, skilled movements. After several weeks, this weakness becomes converted to hypertonicity or spasticity, which is manifested by an initial increased resistance (stiffness) to the passive movement of a joint at the extremes of range of motion followed by a sudden or gradual release of resistance. The spasticity often is greatest in the flexor muscles of the upper limbs and extensor muscles of the lower limbs. Sometimes, a lesion of the pyramidal tract is less severe and results in a relatively minor degree of weakness. In this case, the finer and more skilled movements are most severely impaired.

Lower Motor Neuron Lesions

In contrast to UMN lesions, in which the spinal reflexes remain intact, LMN disorders disrupt communication between the muscle and all neural input and output from

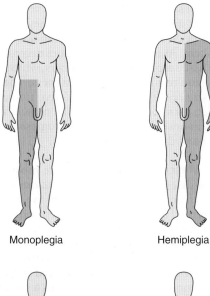

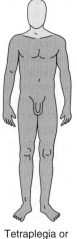

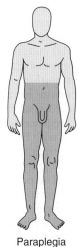

Monoplegia   Hemiplegia

Tetraplegia or   Paraplegia
quadriplegia

FIGURE 35-5 Areas of the body affected by monoplegia, hemiplegia, tetraplegia or quadriplegia, and paraplegia. The *shaded area* shows the extent of motor and sensory loss. (From Hickey J. V. [1997]. *The clinical practice of neurological and neurosurgical nursing* [3rd ed.]. Philadelphia: J. B. Lippincott.)

KEY CONCEPTS

Spastic Versus Flaccid Paralysis

➡ Afferent input from stretch receptors located in muscles and joints is incorporated into spinal cord reflexes that control muscle tone. The activity of the spinal cord reflexes that control muscle tone is constantly monitored and regulated by input from higher brain centers.

➡ Upper motor neuron lesions that interrupt communication between the spinal cord reflexes and higher brain centers result in unregulated reflex activity, increased muscle tone, and spastic paralysis.

➡ Lower motor neuron lesions that interrupt communication between the muscle and the spinal cord reflex result in a loss of reflex activity, decreased or absent muscle tone, and flaccid paralysis.

total weakness and total loss of reflexes, called *flaccid paralysis*, occurs.

With complete LMN lesions, the muscles of the affected limbs, bowel, bladder, and genital areas become atonic, and it is impossible to elicit contraction by stretching the tendons. One of the outstanding features of LMN lesions is the profound development of muscle atrophy. Damage to an LMN with or without spinal cord damage, often called *peripheral nerve injury*, may occur at any level of the spinal cord. For example, a C7 peripheral nerve injury leads to LMN hand weakness only. Usually, injury to the spinal cord at the lumbar (L) 1 level or below results in a LMN injury and flaccid paralysis to all areas below the level of injury. This occurs because the spinal cord ends at the L1 to L2 level, and from this level, the spinal roots of the LMNs continue caudally in the vertebral canal as part of the cauda equina.

spinal cord reflexes, including the stretch reflex, which maintains muscle tone.

Infection or irritation of the cell body of the LMN or its axon can lead to hyperexcitability, which causes spontaneous contractions of the muscle units. These can be observed as twitching and squirming movements on the muscle surface, a condition called *fasciculations*.[4] Toxic agents, such as the tetanus toxin, produce extreme hyperexcitability of the LMN, which results in continuous firing at maximum rate. The resultant sustained contraction of the muscles is called *tetany*. Tetany of muscles on both sides of a joint produces immobility or tetanic paralysis. When a virus, such as the poliomyelitis virus, attacks an LMN, it first irritates the LMN, causing fasciculations to occur. These fasciculations often are followed by the death of LMNs. Weakness and severe muscle wasting or denervation atrophy result. If muscles are totally denervated,

In summary, motor function, whether it involves walking, running, or precise finger movements, requires movement and maintenance of posture. It involves the LMNs, which are located in the ventral horn of the spinal cord, and the groups of muscle fibers they innervate in the muscle; spinal cord circuitry and reflexes; and the descending UMNs that project from the motor cortex to the opposite side of the medulla, where they form a pyramid before crossing the midline to form the lateral corticospinal tract in the spinal cord. Voluntary control of motor function is directed by the motor cortex, which consists of the primary, premotor, and supplementary motor cortex. The primary motor cortex is responsible for execution of a movement, the premotor cortex for generating a plan of movement, and the supplemental motor cortex for rehearsing the motor sequences of a movement, including those involving both sides of the body.

Proper control of muscle function requires not only excitation of the muscle by the LMNs located in the spinal cord but the function of reflex circuitry that monitors the functional status of the muscle fibers on a moment-by-moment basis. The muscle spindles of the stretch reflex function to monitor and correct for changes in muscle length when extrafusal fibers are either shortened (by contraction) or lengthened (by stretch).

Alterations in musculoskeletal function include weakness resulting from lesions of voluntary UMN pathways of the corticobulbar and corticospinal tracts and the LMNs of the peripheral nerves. Muscle tone is maintained through the combined function of the stretch reflex and the extrapyramidal system that monitors and buffers UMN innervation of the LMNs. Hypotonia is a condition of less-than-normal muscle tone, and hypertonia or spasticity is a condition of excessive tone. Paresis refers to weakness in muscle function, and paralysis refers to a loss of muscle movement. UMN lesions produce spastic paralysis and LMN lesions flaccid paralysis.

Skeletal Muscle, Neuromuscular Junction, and Peripheral Nerve Disorders

SKELETAL MUSCLE DISORDERS

Disorders of skeletal muscle groups involve atrophy and dystrophy. Atrophy describes a decrease in muscle mass and muscular dystrophy a primary defect in the muscle fibers.

Muscle Atrophy

Maintenance of muscle strength requires relatively frequent movements against resistance. Reduced use results in muscle atrophy, which is characterized by a reduction in the diameter of the muscle fibers because of a loss of protein filaments.[5] When a normally innervated muscle is not used for long periods, the muscle cells shrink in diameter, and although the muscle cells do not die, they lose much of their contractile protein and become weakened. This is called *disuse atrophy*, and it occurs with conditions such as immobilization and chronic illness. The most extreme examples of muscle atrophy are found in persons with disorders that deprive muscles of their innervation. This form is called *denervation atrophy*.

 ### Muscular Dystrophy

Muscular dystrophy is a term applied to a number of genetic disorders that produce progressive degeneration and necrosis of skeletal muscle fibers and eventual replacement with fat and connective tissue. They are primary diseases of muscle tissue and probably do not involve the nervous system. As the muscle undergoes necrosis, fat and connective tissue replace the muscle fibers, which increases muscle size and results in muscle weakness. The increase in muscle size resulting from connective tissue infiltration is called *pseudohypertrophy*. The muscle weakness is insidious in onset but continually progressive, varying with the type of disorder.

Duchenne Muscular Dystrophy. The most common form of the disease is *Duchenne muscular dystrophy* (DMD), which occurs once in every 3500 live male births.[5] DMD is inherited as a recessive single-gene on the X chromosome and is transmitted from the mother to her male offspring (see Chapter 4). A spontaneous (mutation) form may occur in girls. Another form of dystrophy, *Becker muscular dystrophy*, is similarly X-linked but manifests later in childhood or adolescence and has a slower course of progression.

The DMD mutation results in a defective form of a very large protein associated with the muscle cell membrane, called *dystrophin*, which fails to provide the normal attachment site for the contractile proteins. As a result there is necrosis of muscle fibers, a continuous effort at repair and regeneration, and progressive necrosis.

Children with DMD are usually asymptomatic at birth and during infancy.[6] Early gross movements such as rolling, sitting, and standing are usually achieved at the proper age. The postural muscles of hip and shoulder are usually the first to be affected (Fig 35-6). Pseudohypertrophy (enlargement of the muscle due to excessive replacement of muscle fibers with fibroadipose tissue) of the calf muscle eventually develops. Signs of muscle weakness usually become evident beginning at 2 to 3 years, when frequent falling begins to occur. Imbalances between agonist and antagonist muscles lead to abnormal postures and the development of contractures and joint immobility. Scoliosis is common. Wheelchairs usually are needed at

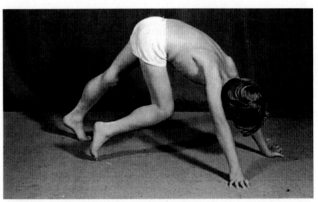

FIGURE 35-6 A boy with Duchenne muscular dystrophy demonstrating pseudohypertrophy of his calves and climbing from a sitting position because of proximal muscle weakness. (From Bird T., Sumi S. [2002]. *Atlas of clinical neurology.* Edited by Roger N. Rosenberg. © Current Medicine, Inc.)

approximately 7 to 12 years of age.[6] The function of the distal muscles usually is preserved well enough that the child can continue to use eating utensils and a computer keyboard. The function of the extraocular muscles also is well preserved, as is the function of the muscles controlling urination and defecation. Incontinence is an uncommon and late event. Respiratory muscle involvement results in weak and ineffective cough, frequent respiratory infections, and decreasing respiratory reserve. Cardiomyopathy is a common feature of the disease. The severity of cardiac involvement, however, does not necessarily correlate with skeletal muscle weakness. Some patients die early as the result of severe cardiomyopathy, whereas others maintain adequate cardiac function until the terminal stages of the disease. Death from respiratory and cardiac muscle involvement usually occurs in young adulthood.

Observation of the child's voluntary movement and a complete family history provide important diagnostic data for the disease. Serum levels of the enzyme creatine kinase, which leaks out of damaged muscle fibers, can be used to confirm the diagnosis. Muscle biopsy, which shows a mixture of muscle cell degeneration and regeneration and reveals fat and scar tissue replacement, is diagnostic of the disorder. Echocardiography, electrocardiography, and chest radiography are used to assess cardiac function. A specific molecular genetic diagnosis is possible by demonstrating defective dystrophin through the use of immunohistochemical staining of sections of muscle biopsy tissue or by deoxyribonucleic acid (DNA) analysis from the peripheral blood. The same methods of DNA analysis may be used on blood samples to establish carrier status in female relatives at risk, such as sisters and cousins. Prenatal diagnosis is possible as early as 12 weeks' gestation by sampling chorionic villi for DNA analysis[6] (see Chapter 4).

Management of the disease is directed toward maintaining ambulation and preventing deformities. Passive stretching, correct or counter posturing, and splints help to prevent deformities. Precautions should be taken to avoid respiratory infections. Although there have been exciting advances in identifying the gene and gene product involved in DMD, there is no known cure. Recent research has focused on interventions that target downstream events involved in the pathogenesis of the disorder. Many of these investigations have explored interventions that would slow the progression of DMD by increasing the regenerative capacity of the dystrophic muscle, slowing the catabolic processes that are important in the dystrophic process, or preventing exacerbation of dystrophic muscle cell death by the immune system.[7]

DISORDERS OF THE NEUROMUSCULAR JUNCTION

The neuromuscular junction serves as a synapse between a motor neuron and a skeletal muscle fiber.[2] It consists of the axon terminals of a motor neuron and a specialized region of the muscle membrane called the *endplate*. The transmission of impulses at the neuromuscular junction is mediated by the release of the neurotransmitter acetylcholine from the axon terminals. Acetylcholine binds to specific receptors in the endplate region of the muscle fiber surface to cause muscle contraction (Fig. 35-7). Acetylcholine is active in the neuromuscular junction only for a brief period, during which an action potential is generated in the innervated muscle cell. Some of the transmitter diffuses out of the synapse, and the remaining transmitter is rapidly inactivated by an enzyme called *acetylcholinesterase*. The rapid inactivation of acetylcholine allows repeated muscle contractions and gradations of contractile force.

Effects of Drugs and Chemicals

A number of drugs and agents can alter neuromuscular function by changing the release, inactivation, or receptor binding of acetylcholine. Curare acts on the postjunctional membrane of the motor endplate to prevent the depolarizing effect of the neurotransmitter. Neuromuscular transmission is blocked by curare-type drugs during many types of surgical procedures to facilitate relaxation

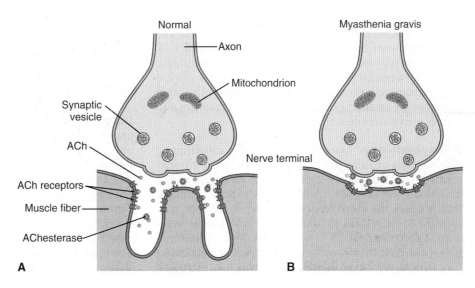

FIGURE 35-7 Neuromuscular junction. (**A**) Acetylcholine (ACh) released from the motor neurons in the myoneural junction crosses the synaptic space to reach receptors that are concentrated in the folds of the endplate of the muscle fiber. Once released, ACh is rapidly broken down by the enzyme acetylcholinesterase (AChesterase). (**B**) Decrease in ACh receptors in myasthenia gravis.

of involved musculature. Drugs such as physostigmine and neostigmine inhibit the action of acetylcholinesterase and allow acetylcholine released from the motor neuron to accumulate. These drugs are used in the treatment of myasthenia gravis.

Toxins from the botulism organism (*Clostridium botulinum*) produce paralysis by blocking acetylcholine release.[8] Spores from the botulism organism may be found in soil-grown foods that are not cooked at temperatures of at least 100°C in home canning procedures. A pharmacologic preparation of the botulism toxin (botulism toxin type A [Botox]) has become available for use in treating eyelid and eye movement disorders such as blepharospasm and strabismus. It also is used for treatment of spasmodic torticollis, spasmodic dysphonias (laryngeal dystonia), and other dystonias. The drug is injected into the target muscle using the electrical activity recorded from the tip of a special electromyographic injection needle to guide the injection. The treatment is not permanent and usually needs to be repeated approximately every 3 months.

The organophosphates (*e.g.*, malathion, parathion) that are used in some insecticides bind acetylcholinesterase to prevent the breakdown of acetylcholine. They produce excessive and prolonged acetylcholine action with a depolarization block of cholinergic receptors, including those of the neuromuscular junction.[8] The organophosphates are well absorbed from the skin, lungs, gut, and conjunctiva of the eye, making them particularly effective as insecticides but also potentially dangerous to humans. Malathion and certain other organophosphates are rapidly metabolized to inactive products in humans and are considered safe for sale to the general public. The sale of other insecticides, such as parathion, which is not effectively metabolized to inactive products, has been banned. Other organophosphate compounds (*e.g.*, soman) were developed as "nerve gases"; if absorbed in high enough concentrations, they produce lethal effects through depolarization block and loss of respiratory muscle function.

Myasthenia Gravis

Myasthenia gravis is a disorder of transmission at the neuromuscular junction that affects communication between the motor neuron and the innervated muscle cell. The disease may occur at any age, but the peak incidence occurs between 20 and 30 years of age, and the disease is approximately three times more common in women than men. A smaller second peak occurs in later life and affects men more often than women.[9]

Pathophysiology. Now recognized as an autoimmune disease, myasthenia gravis is caused by an antibody-mediated destruction of acetylcholine receptors in the neuromuscular junction.[5] Although the exact mechanism that triggers the autoimmune response is unclear, it is thought to be related to abnormal T-lymphocyte function. Approximately 75% of persons with myasthenia gravis also have thymic abnormalities, such as a thymoma (*i.e.*, thymus tumor) or thymic hyperplasia (*i.e.*, increased

thymus weight from an increased number of thymus cells).[9] Neonatal myasthenia gravis, caused by placental transfer of the acetylcholine receptor antibody, occurs in about 10% of infants born to mothers with the disease. Spontaneous resolution of symptoms usually occurs within a few months of birth.

The Lambert-Eaton myasthenic syndrome is a special type of myasthenic syndrome that develops in association with neoplasms, particularly small cell carcinoma of the lung[5] (see Chapter 5). Like myasthenia gravis, the disorder appears to have an autoimmune basis, but results from a decrease in release of acetylcholine from nerve terminals, rather than destruction of acetylcholine receptors.

Clinical Manifestations. In persons with myasthenia gravis who have fewer acetylcholine receptors in the postsynaptic membrane, each release of acetylcholine from the presynaptic membrane results in a lower-amplitude endplate potential. This results in muscle weakness and fatigability with sustained effort. Most commonly affected are the eye and periorbital muscles. Either ptosis due to eyelid weakness or diplopia due to weakness of the extraocular muscles is an initial symptom in approximately 50% of persons with the disease.[10] The disease may progress from ocular muscle weakness to generalized weakness, including respiratory muscle weakness. Chewing and swallowing may be difficult, and persons with the disease often choose to eat soft foods and cereals rather than meats and hard foods. Weakness in limb movement usually is more pronounced in proximal than in distal parts of the extremity, so that climbing stairs and lifting objects are difficult. As the disease progresses, the muscles of the lower face are affected, causing speech impairment. When this happens, the person often supports the chin with one hand to assist in speaking. In most persons, symptoms are least evident when arising in the morning, but they grow worse with effort and as the day proceeds.

Persons with myasthenia gravis may experience a sudden exacerbation of symptoms and weakness known as *myasthenia crisis*. Myasthenia crisis occurs when muscle weakness becomes severe enough to compromise ventilation to the extent that ventilatory support and airway protection are needed. This usually occurs during a period of stress, such as infection, emotional upset, pregnancy, alcohol ingestion, cold, or after surgery. It also can result from inadequate or excessive doses of the anticholinesterase drugs used in treatment of the disorder.

Diagnosis and Treatment. The diagnosis of myasthenia gravis is based on history and physical examination, the anticholinesterase test, nerve stimulation studies, and immunoassay tests for acetylcholine receptor antibodies. The anticholinesterase test uses a drug that inhibits acetylcholinesterase, the enzyme that breaks down acetylcholine. Edrophonium (Tensilon), a short-acting acetylcholinesterase inhibitor, commonly is used for the test. The drug, which is administered intravenously, decreases the breakdown of acetylcholine in the neuromuscular junction. When weakness is caused by myasthenia gravis, a dramatic transitory improvement in muscle function occurs. Electrophysiologic studies can be done to demonstrate a decremental muscle response to repetitive 2- or 3-Hz stimulation of motor nerves. An advance in diagnostic methods for myasthenia gravis is single-fiber electromyography, which is available in many medical centers. Single-fiber electromyography detects delayed or failed neuromuscular transmission in muscle fibers supplied by a single nerve fiber.[9,10] An immunoassay test can be used to detect the presence of acetylcholine receptor antibodies circulating in the blood.

Treatment methods include the use of pharmacologic agents; immunosuppressive therapy, including corticosteroid drugs; management of myasthenic crisis; thymectomy; and plasmapheresis or intravenous immunoglobulin.[9] Medications that may exacerbate myasthenia gravis, such as the aminoglycoside antibiotics, should be avoided.[11] Pharmacologic treatment with anticholinesterase drugs (*e.g.*, pyridostigmine and neostigmine) inhibits the breakdown of acetylcholine at the neuromuscular junction by acetylcholinesterase. Corticosteroid drugs, which suppress the immune response, are used in cases of a poor response to anticholinesterase drugs and thymectomy. Immunosuppressant drugs (*e.g.*, azathioprine, cyclosporine) also may be used, often in combination with plasmapheresis.

Plasmapheresis removes antibodies from the circulation and provides short-term clinical improvement. It is used primarily to stabilize the condition of persons in myasthenic crisis or for short-term treatment in persons undergoing thymectomy. Intravenous immunoglobulin also produces improvement in persons with myasthenia gravis. Although the effect is temporary, it may last for weeks to months. The indications for its use are similar to those for plasmapheresis. The mechanism of action of intravenous immunoglobulin is largely unknown. Intravenous immunoglobulin therapy is very expensive, which limits its use.

Thymectomy, or surgical removal of the thymus, may be used as a treatment for myasthenia gravis. Because the mechanism whereby surgery exerts its effect is unknown, the treatment is controversial.

PERIPHERAL NERVE DISORDERS

Peripheral nervous system (PNS) disorders involve neurons that are located outside the CNS. They include disorders of the motor and sensory branches of the somatic and visceral nervous systems and the peripheral branches of the autonomic nervous system (see Chapter 33). The result usually is muscle weakness, with or without atrophy and sensory changes. The disorder can involve a single nerve (mononeuropathy) or multiple nerves (polyneuropathy).

Unlike the nerves of the CNS, peripheral nerves are fairly strong and resilient. They contain a series of connective tissue sheaths that enclose their nerve fibers. An outer fibrous sheath called the *epineurium* surrounds the medium-sized to large nerves; inside, a sheath called the *perineurium* invests each bundle of nerve fibers; and

within each bundle, a delicate sheath of connective tissue known as the *endoneurium* surrounds each nerve fiber (see Chapter 33, Fig. 33-3). Inside the endoneurial sheath are the Schwann cells that produce the myelin sheath that surrounds the peripheral nerves. Each Schwann cell can myelinate only one segment of a single axon—the one that it covers—so that myelination of an entire axon requires the participation of a long line of these cells.

Peripheral Nerve Injury and Repair

There are two main types of peripheral nerve injury based on the target of the insult: segmental demyelination involving the Schwann cell and axonal degeneration involving the neuronal cell body or its axon.[5,12] The peripheral nerve disorders can affect a spinal nerve, plexus, or peripheral nerve trunk (mononeuropathies) or multiple peripheral nerves (polyneuropathies).

Segmental Demyelination. Segmental demyelination occurs when there is a disorder of the Schwann cell (as in Guillain-Barré syndrome) or damage to the myelin sheath (*e.g.*, sensory neuropathies) without a primary abnormality of the axon. It typically affects some Schwann cells while sparing others. The denuded axon provides a stimulus for remyelination and the population of cells within the endoneurium has the capacity to replace the injured Schwann cells. These cells proliferate and encircle the axon, and in time remyelinate the denuded portion. However, the new myelin sheath is thin in proportion to the axon, and in time, many chronic demyelinating neuropathies give way to axonal injury.

Axonal Degeneration. Axonal degeneration is caused by primary injury to a neuronal cell body or its axon. Damage to the axon may be due either to a focal event occurring at some point along the length of the nerve (*e.g.*, trauma or ischemia) or to a more generalized abnormality affecting the neuronal cell body (neuropathy).

Injury to a peripheral nerve axon, whether due to injury or neuropathy, results in degenerative changes, followed by breakdown of the myelin sheath and Schwann cells. In distal axonal degeneration, the proximal axon and neuronal cell body, which synthesizes the material required for nourishing and maintaining the axon, remain intact. In neuropathies and crushing injuries, in which the endoneurial tube remains intact, the outgrowing fiber grows down this tube to the structure that was originally innervated by the neuron (Fig. 35-8). However, it can take weeks or months for the regrowing fiber to reach its target organ and for communicative function to be reestablished. More time is required for the Schwann cells to form new myelin segments and for the axon to recover its original diameter and conduction velocity.

The successful regeneration of a nerve fiber in the PNS depends on many factors. If a nerve fiber is destroyed relatively close to the neuronal cell body, the chances are that the nerve cell will die, and if it does, it will not be replaced. If a crushing type of injury has occurred, partial or often

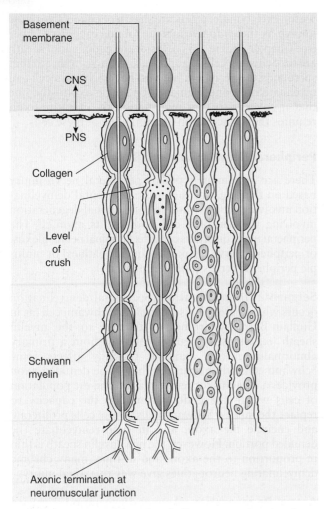

Basement membrane

CNS

PNS

Collagen

Level
of
crush

Schwann
myelin

Axonic termination at
neuromuscular junction

FIGURE 35-8 Sequential stages of efferent axon degeneration and regeneration within its endoneurial tube, after peripheral nerve crush injury.

full recovery of function occurs. Cutting-type trauma to a nerve is an entirely different matter. Connective scar tissue forms rapidly at the wound site, and when it does, only the most rapidly regenerating axonal branches are able to get through to the intact distal endoneurial tubes. A number of scar-inhibiting agents have been used in an effort to reduce this hazard, but have met with only moderate success. In another attempt to improve nerve regeneration, various types of tubular implants have been placed to fill longer gaps in the endoneurial tube.

Neuropathies involving the neuronal cell body are much less common than those affecting the axons. In these cases, there is little potential for recovery of function because death of the neuronal cells precludes axonal regeneration.

Mononeuropathies

Mononeuropathies usually are caused by localized conditions such as trauma, compression, or infections that affect a single spinal nerve, plexus, or peripheral nerve trunk. Fractured bones may lacerate or compress nerves; excessively tight tourniquets may injure nerves directly or produce ischemic injury; and infections such as herpes zoster may affect a single segmental afferent nerve. Recovery of nerve function usually is complete after compression lesions and incomplete or faulty after nerve transection.

Carpal Tunnel Syndrome. Carpal tunnel syndrome is an example of a compression-type mononeuropathy that is relatively common. The syndrome affects an estimated 3% of adult Americans and is approximately three times more common in women than men.[13] It is caused by compression of the median nerve as it travels with the flexor tendons through a canal made by the carpal bones and transverse carpal ligament (Fig. 35-9). The condition can be caused by a variety of conditions that produce a reduction in the capacity of the carpal tunnel (*i.e.*, bony or ligament changes) or an increase in the volume of the tunnel contents (*i.e.*, inflammation of the tendons, synovial swelling, or tumors).[14] Carpal tunnel syndrome can be a feature of many systemic diseases such as rheumatoid arthritis, hyperthyroidism, acromegaly, and diabetes mellitus.[13,14] The condition can result from wrist injury; it can occur during pregnancy and use of birth control drugs; and it is seen in persons with repetitive use of the wrist (*i.e.*, flexion-extension movements and stress associated with pinching and gripping motions).

Carpal tunnel syndrome is characterized by pain, paresthesia, and numbness of the thumb and first two

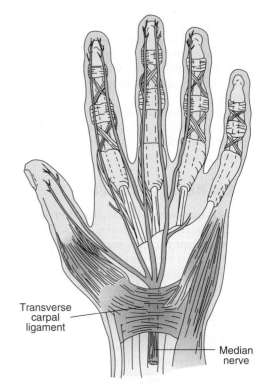

Transverse
carpal
ligament

Median
nerve

FIGURE 35-9 Carpal tunnel syndrome: compression of the median nerve by the transverse carpal ligament. (Courtesy of Carole Russell Hilmer, C. M. I.)

and one-half digits of the hand; pain in the wrist and hand, which worsens at night; atrophy of the abductor pollicis muscle; and weakness in precision grip. All of these abnormalities may contribute to clumsiness of fine motor activity.

Diagnosis usually is based on sensory disturbances confined to median nerve distribution. Electromyography and nerve conduction studies often are done to confirm the diagnosis and exclude other causes of the disorder.

Treatment includes avoidance of movements that cause nerve compression, splinting, and anti-inflammatory medications. Measures to decrease the causative repetitive movements should be initiated. Splints may be confined to nighttime use. When splinting is ineffective, corticosteroids may be injected into the carpal tunnel to reduce inflammation and swelling. Surgical intervention consists of operative division of the volar carpal ligaments as a means of relieving pressure on the medial nerve.

Polyneuropathies

Polyneuropathies involve demyelination or axonal degeneration of multiple peripheral nerves that leads to symmetric sensory, motor, or mixed sensorimotor deficits. Typically, the longest axons are involved first, with symptoms beginning in the distal part of the extremities. If the autonomic nervous system is involved, there may be postural hypotension, constipation, and impotence. Polyneuropathies can result from immune mechanisms (e.g., Guillain-Barré syndrome), toxic agents (e.g., arsenic polyneuropathy, lead polyneuropathy, alcoholic polyneuropathy), and metabolic diseases (e.g., diabetes mellitus, uremia). Different causes tend to affect axons of different diameters and to affect sensory, motor, or autonomic neurons to different degrees.

Guillain-Barré Syndrome. Guillain-Barré syndrome is an acute immune-mediated polyneuropathy.[15–17] The disorder defines a clinical entity that is characterized by rapidly progressive limb weakness and loss of tendon reflexes. It has been described as the most common cause of acute, flaccid paralysis in developed countries, now that poliomyelitis has been eliminated. As a syndrome, there are several subtypes of the disorder, including pure motor axonal degeneration, axonal degeneration of both motor and sensory nerves, and a variant characterized by ophthalmoplegia, ataxia, and areflexia.[15,16]

The cause of Guillain-Barré syndrome probably has an immune component. Controlled epidemiologic studies have linked it to infection with *Campylobacter jejuni*, cytomegalovirus, Epstein-Barr virus, and *Mycoplasma pneumoniae*.[15–17] Approximately two thirds of patients report having had an acute, influenza-like illness before the onset of symptoms. About one third have antibodies against nerve gangliosides, which in some cases also react with constituents of the lipopolysaccharide of *C. jejuni*.[17]

The disorder is characterized by progressive ascending muscle weakness of the limbs, producing a symmetric flaccid paralysis. Symptoms of paresthesia and numbness often accompany the loss of motor function. The rate of disease progression varies, and there may be disproportionate involvement of the upper or lower extremities. Paralysis may progress to involve the respiratory muscles; approximately 30% of persons with the disorder require ventilatory assistance. Autonomic nervous system involvement that causes postural hypotension, cardiac arrhythmias, facial flushing, abnormalities of sweating, and urinary retention is common. Pain is another common feature of Guillain-Barré syndrome. It is most common in the shoulder girdle, back, and posterior thighs and occurs with even the slightest of movements.[16]

Guillain-Barré syndrome usually is a medical emergency. There may be a rapid development of ventilatory failure and autonomic disturbances that threaten circulatory function. Treatment includes support of vital functions and prevention of complications such as skin breakdown and thrombophlebitis. Clinical trials have shown the effectiveness of plasmapheresis in decreasing morbidity and shortening the course of the disease. Treatment is most effective if initiated early in the course of the disease. High-dose intravenous immunoglobulin therapy also has proved effective.[15–17] Approximately 80% to 90% of persons with the disease achieve a full and spontaneous recovery within 6 to 12 months.

Back Pain and Herniated Intervertebral Disk

Back Pain. Back pain can result from a number of interrelated problems involving the structures of the vertebral column, the spinal nerve roots, or the muscles and ligamentous structures of the back. Perhaps the most common are musculoligamentous injuries and age-related degenerative changes in the intervertebral disks and facet joints.[18] Low back pain affects men and women equally, with onset most often between the ages of 30 and 50 years. It is the most common cause of work-related disability. Risk factors include heavy lifting, twisting, bodily vibration, obesity, and poor conditioning, although low back pain is common even in persons without these risk factors.

Although back problems commonly are attributed to a herniated disk, most acute back problems are caused by other, less serious conditions. It has been reported that 90% of persons with acute lower back problems of less than 3 months' duration recover spontaneously.[19,20] The diagnostic challenge is to identify those persons who require further evaluation for more serious problems such as tumors, compression fractures, or disk herniation. Diagnostic measures include history and physical examination, including a thorough neurologic examination. Other diagnostic methods include radiographs of the back and magnetic resonance imaging (MRI). These methods are usually used to rule out the possibility of impending neurologic infections and tumors.[20]

Treatment of back pain usually is conservative and consists of analgesic medications, muscle relaxants, and instruction in the correct mechanics for lifting and methods of protecting the back.[20,21] Pain relief is usually provided using nonsteroidal anti-inflammatory drugs. Muscle relaxants may be used on a short-term basis. Bed rest, once the mainstay of conservative therapy, is now understood to be ineffective for acute back pain. Conditioning exercises of the trunk muscles, particularly the back extensors, are often recommended.

Herniated Intervertebral Disk.

The intervertebral disk is considered the most critical component of the load-bearing structures of the spinal column. The intervertebral disk consists of a soft, gelatinous center called the *nucleus pulposus,* which is encircled by a strong, ringlike collar of fibrocartilage called the *annulus fibrosus.* The structural components of the disk make it capable of absorbing shock and changing shape while allowing movement. With dysfunction, the nucleus pulposus can be squeezed out of place and herniate through the annulus fibrosus, a condition referred to as a *herniated* or *slipped disk* (Fig. 35-10A and B).

The intervertebral disk can become dysfunctional because of trauma, the effects of aging, or degenerative disorders of the spine. Trauma accounts for 50% of disk herniations. It results from activities such as lifting while in the flexed position, slipping, falling on the buttocks or back, or suppressing a sneeze. With aging, the gelatinous center of the disk dries out and loses much of its elasticity, causing it to fray and tear. Degenerative processes such as osteoarthritis or ankylosing spondylitis predispose to malalignment of the vertebral column.

The cervical and lumbar regions are the most flexible areas of the spine and those most often involved in disk herniations. Usually, herniation occurs at the lower levels of the lumbar spine, where the mass being supported and the bending of the vertebral column are greatest. Approximately 90% to 95% of lumbar herniations occur in the L4 or L5 to S1 regions. With herniations of the cervical spine, the most frequently involved levels are C6 to C7 and C5 to C6. Protrusion of the nucleus pulposus usually occurs posteriorly and toward the intervertebral foramen and its contained spinal nerve root, where the annulus fibrosus is relatively thin and poorly supported by either the posterior or anterior ligaments[22] (see Fig. 35-10A).

The level at which a herniated disk occurs is important (see Fig. 35-10C). When the injury occurs in the lumbar area, only the cauda equina is involved. Because these elongated dorsal and ventral roots contain endoneurial tubes of connective tissue, regeneration of the nerve fibers is likely. However, several weeks or months are required for full recovery to occur because of the distance to the innervated muscle or skin of the lower limbs.

The signs and symptoms of a herniated disk are localized to the area of the body innervated by the nerve roots and include both motor and sensory manifestations (Fig. 35-11). Pain is the first and most common symptom of a herniated disk. The nerve roots of L4, L5, S1, S2, and S3

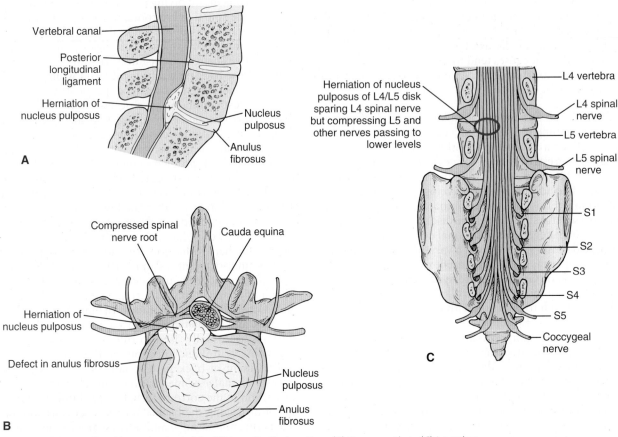

FIGURE 35-10 Herniated intervertebral disk. (**A**) Longitudinal section. (**B**) Cross-section. (**C**) Location of L4 to L5 and S1 to S5 spinal nerves, with site of L4/L5 herniation of nucleus pulposus indicated.

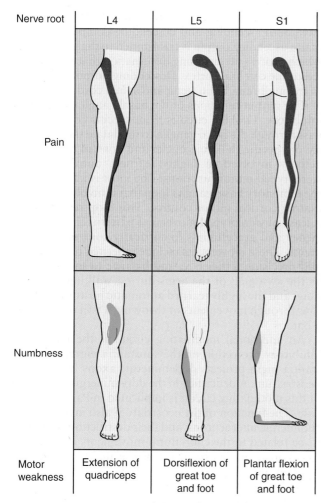

Nerve root	L4	L5	S1
Pain			
Numbness			
Motor weakness	Extension of quadriceps	Dorsiflexion of great toe and foot	Plantar flexion of great toe and foot

FIGURE 35-11 Dermatomes of the leg (L1 through S5) where pain and numbness would be experienced with spinal root irritation.

give rise to a syndrome of back pain that spreads down the back of the leg and over the sole of the foot. The pain is usually intensified with coughing, sneezing, straining, stooping, standing, and the jarring motions that occur during walking or riding. Slight motor weakness may occur, although major weakness is rare. The most common sensory deficits from spinal nerve root compression are paresthesias and numbness, particularly of the leg and foot. Knee and ankle reflexes also may be diminished or absent.

A herniated disk must be differentiated from other causes such as traumatic injury or fracture of the vertebral column, tumor, infection, cauda equina syndrome (see spinal cord injury), or other conditions that cause back pain. Diagnostic measures include history and physical examination. Neurologic assessment includes testing of muscle strength and reflexes. The straight leg test is done in the supine position and is performed by passively raising the person's leg. Normally, it is possible to raise the leg approximately 90 degrees without causing discomfort of the hamstring muscles. The test result is positive if pain is produced when the leg is raised to

60 degrees or less. Other diagnostic methods include radiographs of the back, MRI, myelography, and computed tomography (CT).[23]

Treatment usually is similar to that for back pain. Surgical treatment may be indicated when there is documentation of herniation by an imaging procedure, consistent pain, or consistent neurologic deficit that has failed to respond to conservative therapy.

In summary, the motor unit consists of the LMN, the neuromuscular junction, and the skeletal muscle that the nerve innervates. Disorders of the neuromuscular unit include muscular dystrophy, myasthenia gravis, and peripheral nerve disorders. *Muscular dystrophy* is a term used to describe a number of disorders that produce progressive deterioration of skeletal muscle. Muscle necrosis is followed by fat and connective tissue replacement. One form, Duchenne muscular dystrophy, is inherited as a X-linked trait and transmitted by the mother to her male offspring. Myasthenia gravis is a disorder of the neuromuscular junction resulting from a deficiency of functional acetylcholine receptors, which causes weakness of the skeletal muscles. Because the disease affects the neuromuscular junction, there is no loss of sensory function. The most common manifestations are weakness of the eye muscles, with ptosis and diplopia.

Peripheral nerve disorders involve motor and sensory neurons outside the CNS. There are two main types of peripheral nerve injury based on target of the insult: segmental demyelination involving the Schwann cell and axonal degeneration involving the nerve axon or its cell body. Peripheral nerve disorders include mononeuropathies, involving a single spinal nerve, plexus, or peripheral nerve, and polyneuropathies that involve demyelination or axonal degeneration of multiple peripheral nerves that leads to symmetric sensory, motor, or mixed sensorimotor deficits. Carpal tunnel syndrome, a mononeuropathy, is caused by compression of the medial nerve as it passes through the carpal tunnel in the wrist. Guillain-Barré syndrome is a subacute polyneuropathy, probably due to immune mechanisms, that causes progressive ascending motor, sensory, and autonomic nervous system manifestations. Respiratory involvement may occur and necessitate mechanical ventilation.

Acute back pain is most commonly the result of conditions such as musculoligamentous strain, with treatment that focuses on measures to improve activity tolerance. A herniated intervertebral disk is characterized by protrusion of the nucleus pulposus into the spinal canal with irritation or compression of the nerve root. Usually, herniation occurs at the lower levels of the lumbar and sacral (L4 or L5 to S1) and cervical (C6 to C7 and C5 to C6) regions of the spine. The signs and symptoms of a herniated disk are localized to the area of the body innervated by the affected nerve roots and include pain and both motor and sensory manifestations.

Basal Ganglia and Cerebellum Disorders

DISORDERS OF THE BASAL GANGLIA

Structure and Function of the Basal Ganglia

The basal ganglia are a group of deep, interrelated sub-cortical nuclei that constitute an accessory motor system that functions in close association with the motor cortex. The structural components of the basal ganglia include the caudate nucleus, putamen, and the globus pallidus in the forebrain.[1] The caudate and putamen are collectively referred to as the *neostriatum*, and the putamen and the globus pallidus form a wedge-shaped region called the *lentiform nucleus*. Two other structures, the *subthalamic nucleus* of the diencephalon and the *substantia nigra* of the midbrain, are considered part of the basal ganglia (Fig. 35-12). The dorsal part of the substantia nigra contains cells that synthesize the neurotransmitter dopamine and are rich in a black pigment called *melanin*. The high concentration of melanin gives the structure a black color, hence the name *substantia nigra*. The axons of the substantia nigra form the *nigrostriatal pathway*, which supplies dopamine to the striatum. The dopamine released from the substantia nigra regulates the overall excitability of the striatum and release of other neurotransmitters.

The basal ganglia have input structures that receive afferent information from the cerebral cortex and thalamus, internal circuits that connect the various structures of the basal ganglia, and output structures that deliver information to other brain centers. The neostriatum represents the major input structure for the basal ganglia. Virtually all areas of the cortex and afferents from the thalamus project to the neostriatum. The output areas of

the basal ganglia, including the lateral globus pallidus, have both ascending and descending components. The major ascending output is transmitted to thalamic nuclei, which process all incoming information that is transmitted to the cerebral cortex. Descending output is directed to the midbrain, brain stem, and spinal cord.

The output functions of the basal ganglia are mainly inhibitory. Looping circuits from specific cortical areas pass through the basal ganglia to modulate the excitability of specific thalamic nuclei and control the cortical activity involved in highly learned, automatic, and stereotyped motor functions. The most is known about the inhibitory basal ganglia loop that is involved in modulating cortical motor control. This loop regulates the release of stereotyped movement patterns that add efficiency and gracefulness to cortically controlled movements. These movements include inherited patterns that add precision, efficiency, and balance to motion, such as the swinging of the arms during walking and running, and the highly learned automatic postural and follow-through movements of throwing a ball or swinging a bat.

An additional modulating circuit is the neostriatal inhibitory projection on the substantia nigra. The substantia nigra projects dopaminergic axons back on the neostriatum. A deficiency in the dopaminergic projection of this modulating circuit is implicated in Parkinson disease. The function of the neostriatum also involves local cholinergic interneurons, and their destruction is thought to be related to the choreiform movements of Huntington chorea, another basal ganglia–related syndrome (see Chapter 36).

Movement Disorders

Disorders of the basal ganglia comprise a complex group of motor disturbances characterized by tremor and other involuntary movements, changes in posture and muscle tone, and poverty and slowness of movement. They include tremors and tics, hypokinetic disorders, and hyperkinetic disorders[1] (Table 35-1). Unlike disorders of the motor cortex and corticospinal (pyramidal) tract, lesions of the basal ganglia disrupt movement but do not cause paralysis.

Tremors and Tics. *Tremor* is caused by involuntary, oscillating contractions of opposing muscle groups around a joint. It usually is fairly uniform in frequency and amplitude. Certain tremors are considered physiologic in that they are transitory and normally occur under conditions of increased muscle tone, as in highly emotional situations, or they may be related to muscle fatigue or reduced body temperature (*i.e.*, shivering). Toxic tremors are produced by hyperexcitability related to conditions such as thyrotoxicosis. The tremor of Parkinson disease is caused by degenerative changes in the basal ganglia. *Tics* involve sudden and irregularly occurring contractions of whole muscles or major portions of a muscle. These are particularly evident in the muscles of the face, but can occur elsewhere.

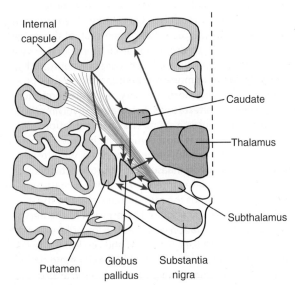

FIGURE 35-12 Basal ganglia. *Arrows* indicate the direction of communication between the motor cortex, thalamus, and structures of the basal ganglia.

Labels on figure: Internal capsule, Caudate, Thalamus, Subthalamus, Putamen, Globus pallidus, Substantia nigra

TABLE 35-1	Involuntary Movement Disorders Associated With Extrapyramidal Disorders
Movement Disorder	**Characteristics**
Tremor	Rhythmic oscillating contractions or movements of whole muscles or major portions of a muscle. They can occur as resting tremors, which are prominent at rest and decrease or disappear with movement; intention tremors, which increase with activity and become worse when the target is reached; and postural tremors, which appear when the affected part is maintained in a stabilized position.
Tics	Irregularly occurring, brief, repetitive, stereotyped, coordinated movements such as winking, grimacing, or shoulder shrugging
Chorea	Brief, rapid, jerky, and irregular movements that are coordinated and graceful. The face, head, and distal limbs are most commonly involved. They often interfere with normal movement patterns.
Athetosis	Continuous, slow, wormlike, twisting and turning motions of a limb or body that most commonly involve the face and distal extremities and are often associated with spasticity
Ballismus	Involve violent, sweeping, flinging-type limb movements, especially on one side of the body (hemiballismus)
Dystonia	Abnormal maintenance of posture results from a twisting, turning motion of the limbs, neck, or trunk. Motions are similar to athetosis but involve larger portions of the body. They can result in grotesque and twisted postures.
Dyskinesias	Rhythmic, repetitive, bizarre movements that chiefly involve the face, mouth, jaw, or tongue, causing grimacing, pursing of the lips, protrusion of the tongue, opening and closing of the mouth, and deviations of the jaw. The limbs are affected less often.

(From Bates B. [1991]. *A guide to physical examination and history taking* [5th ed., pp. 554–556]. Philadelphia: J.B. Lippincott.)

Hypokinetic Disorders. Hypokinetic disorders are characterized by bradykinesia or hypokinesia. They are caused by hyperfunction of the basal ganglia inhibitory loop, which produces excessive inhibition of cortical function. The results are slowness in a beginning movement, a reduced range and force of the movement ("poverty of movement"), reduced or absent emotional responses, including emotion-related facial expressions, and a loss of the balance and grace-producing movements and postures associated with skilled motion. An example of hypokinesia is seen in severely affected persons with the parkinsonian syndrome. These disorders are usually accompanied by muscular rigidity and tremor.

Basal ganglia–derived rigidity involves a strong resistance to movement that decreases to stiffness after the movement gets underway. In some instances, forcing a rigid joint to turn is met with a series of sudden releases followed by renewed resistance, a phenomenon called *cog-wheel rigidity.*

Hyperkinetic Disorders. Hyperkinetic disorders are characterized by excessive motor activity. They are caused by reduced function of the basal ganglia inhibitory loop, which results in *hyperkinesia*, or release of movement patterns at inappropriate times or sometimes continuously. Descending pathways to the LMNs involved in basal ganglia–related movement disorders involve the corticospinal systems and other descending systems. Because these movement patterns are not under cortical control, they often are referred to as *involuntary movements.* The involuntary movements may take several forms, including choreiform movements, athetoid movements, ballismus movements, dystonias, and dyskinesias. Various types of involuntary movements often occur in combination and some appear to have the same underlying cause. For example, chorea and ballismus may be simply distal (chorea) and proximal (ballismus) forms of the same underlying disorder.[1] The movements are manifested on the side of the body opposite to basal ganglia damage and are usually lost during sleep, although they may make falling asleep difficult.

Choreiform movements are sudden, jerky, and irregular but are coordinated and graceful. They can involve the distal limb, face, tongue, or swallowing muscles. Choreiform movements are accentuated by movement and by environmental stimulation; they often interfere with normal movement patterns. The word *chorea* originated from the Greek word meaning "to dance." There may be grimacing movements of the face, raising of the eyebrows, rolling of the eyes, and curling, protrusion and withdrawal of the tongue. In the limbs, the movements largely are distal; there may be piano-playing–type movements with alternating extension and flexion of the fingers. The shoulders may be elevated and depressed or rotated. Movements of the face or limbs may occur alone or, more commonly, in combination.

Athetoid movements are relatively continuous, wormlike twisting and turning motions of the joints of a limb or body. These result from continuous and prolonged contraction of agonist and antagonistic muscle groups. Normally, these are smooth and useful movements, but in extrapyramidal diseases, they occur continuously in a nonrhythmic, often irregular sequence.

The term *ballismus* originates from a Greek word meaning "to jump around." Ballistic movements are violent, sweeping, flinging motions, especially of the limbs on one side of the body (hemiballismus). They may occur as the result of a small vascular accident involving the subthalamic nucleus on the opposite side of the brain.

Dystonia refers to the abnormal maintenance of a posture resulting from a twisting, turning movement of the limbs, neck, or trunk. These postures often result from simultaneous contraction of agonist and antagonist muscles. Long-sustained simultaneous hypertonia across a joint can result in degenerative changes and permanent fixation in unusual postures. These effects can occur as a side effect of some antipsychotic medications. *Spasmodic torticollis*, the most common type of dystonia, affects the muscles of the neck and shoulder. The condition, which is characterized by bilateral and simultaneous contraction of the neck and shoulder muscles, results in unilateral head turning or head extension, sometimes limiting rotation. Elevations of the shoulder commonly accompany the spasmodic movements of the head and neck. Immobility of the cervical vertebrae eventually can lead to degenerative fixation in the twisted posture. Torsional spasm involving the trunk also can occur.

Dyskinesias are rhythmic, repetitive, bizarre movements. They frequently involve the face, mouth, jaw, and tongue, causing grimacing, pursing of the lips, or protrusion of the tongue. The limbs are affected less often. Tardive dyskinesia is an untoward reaction that can develop with long-term use of some of the antipsychotic medications.

Parkinson Disease

Parkinson disease (PD) is a degenerative disorder of the basal ganglia that results in variable combinations of tremor, rigidity, and bradykinesia. The disorder is characterized by progressive destruction of the nigrostriatal pathway with a subsequent reduction in striatal concentrations of dopamine. More than 1 million people in the United States are affected by the disease.[24,25] It usually begins after 50 years of age; most cases are diagnosed in the sixth and seventh decades of life.

The clinical syndrome arising from the degenerative changes in basal ganglia function often is referred to as *parkinsonism*. PD, the most common form of parkinsonism, is named after James Parkinson, a British physician who first described the disease in a paper he published in 1817 on the "shaking palsy."[26] In PD, also known as *idiopathic parkinsonism,* dopamine depletion results from degeneration of the dopamine-producing neurons of the nigrostriatal system. Parkinsonism can also develop as a postencephalitic syndrome, as a side effect of therapy with antipsychotic drugs that block dopamine receptors, as a toxic reaction to a chemical agent, or as an outcome of severe carbon monoxide poisoning. Symptoms of parkinsonism also may accompany conditions such as cerebral vascular disease, brain tumors, repeated head trauma, or degenerative neurologic diseases that structurally damage the nigrostriatal pathway.

Drug-induced parkinsonism can follow the administration of antipsychotic drugs in high doses (*e.g.,* phenothiazines, butyrophenones). These drugs block dopamine receptors and dopamine output by the cells of the substantia nigra. Of interest in terms of research was the development of PD in several persons who had attempted to make a narcotic drug and instead synthesized a compound called MPTP (1-methyl-phenyl-2,3,6-tetrahydropyridine).[5] This compound selectively destroys the dopaminergic neurons of the substantia nigra. This incident prompted investigations into the role of toxins that are produced by the body as a part of normal metabolic processes and those that enter the body from outside sources in the pathogenesis of PD. One theory is that the auto-oxidation of catecholamines such as dopamine during melanin synthesis injures neurons in the substantia nigra. There is increasing evidence that the development of PD may be related to oxidative metabolites of this process and the inability of neurons to render these products harmless.

Recent discovery of inherited forms of PD suggests that genetic factors may play a role in the pathogenesis of early-onset PD. Among the genes that have been found to be associated with inherited PD are the α-synuclein and parkin genes. α-Synuclein, a member of a small family of proteins that are expressed preferentially in the substantia nigra, was identified as the basis for an autosomally inherited form of PD. Although mutations in this gene appear to be a rare cause of PD, α-synuclein has received much attention because it is one of the major components of the Lewy bodies that are found in brain tissue of persons with PD.[5,25] A second gene, encoding the protein parkin, was linked to an autosomal recessive form of PD.[5,25] Alterations, including deletions and nonsense and missense mutations, resulting in loss of parkin functions have been found in various families. These mutations are most prevalent in people with early-onset PD.

Clinical Features. The cardinal symptoms of PD are tremor, rigidity, and bradykinesia or slowness of movement.[24,27] Other advanced-stage parkinsonian manifestations are falls, fluctuations in motor function, neuropsychiatric disorders, and sleep problems.

Tremor is the most visible manifestation of the disorder. The tremor affects the distal segments of the limbs, mainly the hands and feet; head, neck, face, lips, and tongue; or jaw. It is characterized by rhythmic, alternating flexion and contraction movements (four to six beats per minute) that resemble the motion of rolling a pill between the thumb and forefinger. Although the tremor usually is unilateral initially, occurs when the limb is supported and at rest, and disappears with movement and sleep, it eventually progresses to involve both sides of the body. While the most noticeable sign of PD, tremor usually is the least disabling manifestation of the disorder.

Rigidity is defined as resistance to movement of both flexors and extensors throughout the full range of motion. It is most evident during passive joint movement, and involves jerky, cog-wheel–type or ratchet-like movements that require considerable energy to perform. Flexion contractions may develop as a result of the rigidity. As with tremor, rigidity usually begins unilaterally but progresses to involve both sides of the body.

Bradykinesia is characterized by slowness in initiating and performing movements and difficulty in sudden, unexpected stopping of voluntary movements. Unconscious associative movements occur in a series of disconnected steps rather than in a smooth, coordinated manner. This is the most disabling of the symptoms of PD. Persons with PD have difficulty initiating walking and difficulty turning. While walking, they may freeze in place and feel as if their feet are glued to the floor, especially when moving through a doorway or preparing to turn. When they walk, they lean forward to maintain their center of gravity and take small, shuffling steps without swinging their arms, and they have difficulty in changing their stride (Fig. 35-13). Loss of postural reflexes predisposes them to falling, often backward. Emotional and voluntary facial movements become limited and slow as the disease progresses, and facial expression becomes stiff and mask-like. There is loss of the blinking reflex and a failure to express emotion. The tongue, palate, and throat muscles become rigid; the person may drool because of difficulty in moving the saliva to the back of the mouth and swallowing it. The speech becomes slow and monotonous, without modulation and poorly articulated.

Because the basal ganglia also influence the autonomic nervous system, persons with PD often have excessive and uncontrolled sweating, sebaceous gland secretion, and salivation. Autonomic symptoms such as lacrimation, dysphagia, orthostatic hypotension, impaired thermal regu-

lation, constipation, impotence, and urinary incontinence may be present, especially late in the disease.

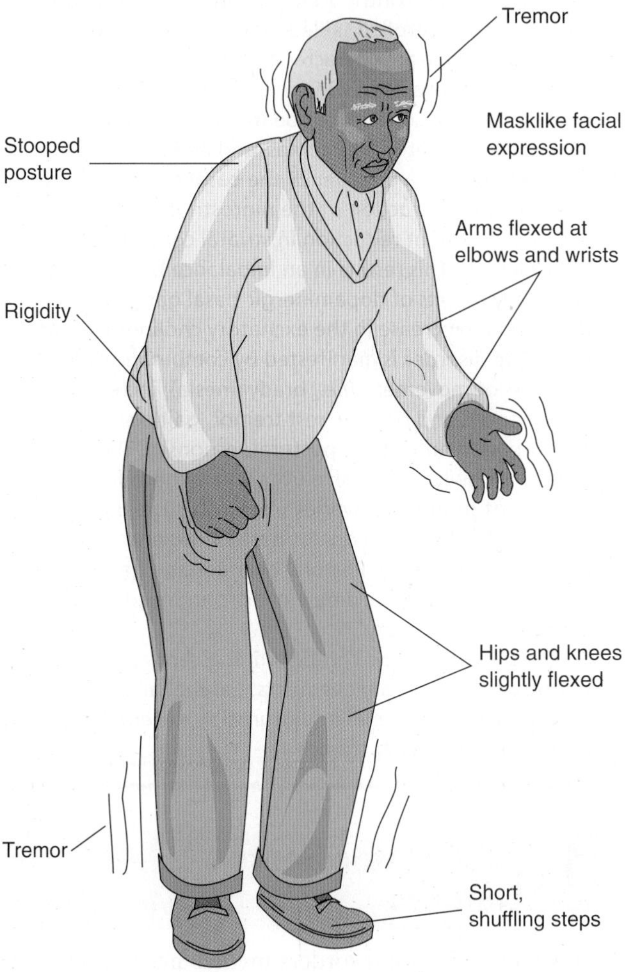

Dementia is an important feature associated with PD. It occurs in approximately 20% of persons with the disease and develops late in the course of the disease.[27] The mental state of some persons with PD may be indistinguishable from that seen in Alzheimer disease. It has been suggested that many of the brain changes in both diseases may result from degeneration of acetylcholine-containing neurons in a region of the brain called the *nucleus basalis of Meynert*, which is the main source of cholinergic innervation for the cerebral cortex. Persons with PD also have other neurochemical disturbances that can account for some of the features of dementia.

Treatment. The approach to treatment of PD must be highly individualized. It includes nonpharmacologic, pharmacologic, and, when indicated, surgical methods. Nonpharmacologic interventions include group support, education, daily exercise, and adequate nutrition.

Pharmacologic treatment usually is determined by the severity of symptoms. Antiparkinson drugs act by increasing the functional ability of the underactive dopaminergic system, or they reduce the excessive influence of excitatory cholinergic neurons.[24,28] They include drugs that increase dopamine levels (e.g., L-dopa, carbidopa L-dopa preparations), augment the release of dopamine (e.g., amantadine), or function as dopamine agonists or directly stimulate dopamine receptors (e.g., bromocriptine, pergolide, pramipexole, ropinirole). Selegiline is a monoamine oxidase type B inhibitor that inhibits the metabolic breakdown of dopamine. It has been proposed that in inhibiting dopamine metabolism and the generation of destructive metabolites, selegiline also may delay the progression of the disease.

Because dopamine transmission is disrupted in PD, there is a preponderance of cholinergic activity, which may be treated with anticholinergic drugs. Anticholinergic drugs (e.g., trihexyphenidyl, benztropine) are thought to restore a "balance" between reduced dopamine and uninhibited cholinergic neurons in the striatum. They are more useful in alleviating tremor and rigidity than bradykinesia.

Surgical treatment includes thalamotomy or pallidectomy performed using stereotactic surgery. With these procedures part of the thalamus or globus pallidum in the basal ganglia is destroyed using an electrical stimulator or the supercooled tip of a metal probe (cryothalamotomy). Brain mapping is done during the surgery to identify and prevent injury to sensory and motor tracts. Surgery is generally confined to one side of the brain and is usually restricted to persons who have failed to respond satisfactorily to drug therapy. Another surgical procedure involves the implantation of electrodes for deep brain stimulation into areas of the brain that are thought to account for rest tremors (thalamus) or motor dysfunction (subthalamic nuclei or the pars interna of the globus pallidus) in PD.[29] Electrical stimulation has the advantage of being reversible and of causing minimal or no damage to the brain. Surgical transplantation of

Tremor

Masklike facial expression

Arms flexed at elbows and wrists

Stooped posture

Rigidity

Hips and knees slightly flexed

Tremor

Short, shuffling steps

FIGURE 35-13 The clinical features of Parkinson disease. (From Timby B. K., Smith N. E. [2003]. *Introductory medical–surgical nursing* [8th ed., p. 626]. Philadelphia: Lippincott Williams & Wilkins.)

adrenal medullary tissue or fetal substantia nigra tissue is still experimental.

DISORDERS OF THE CEREBELLUM

The functions of the cerebellum, or "little brain," are essential for smooth, coordinated, skillful movement. The cerebellum does not initiate activity, but it is responsible for smoothing the temporal and spatial aspects of rapid movement anywhere in the body. It influences the motor systems by evaluating disparities between intention and action and by adjusting the operation of motor centers in the brain while a movement is in progress as well as during repetition of the movement.[1]

The signs of cerebellar dysfunction can be grouped into three classes: vestibulocerebellar disorders, cerebellar ataxia or decomposition of movement, and cerebellar tremor. These disorders occur on the side of cerebellar damage, whether because of congenital defect, vascular accident, or growing tumor. The abnormality of movement occurs whether the eyes are open or closed: visual monitoring of movement cannot compensate for cerebellar defects.

Damage to the part of the cerebellum associated with the vestibular system leads to difficulty or inability to maintain a steady posture of the trunk, which normally requires constant readjusting movements. This is seen as an unsteadiness of the trunk, called *truncal ataxia*, and it can be so severe that standing is not possible. The ability to fix the eyes on a target also can be affected. Constant conjugate readjustment of eye position, called *nystagmus*, results and makes reading extremely difficult, especially when the eyes are deviated toward the side of cerebellar damage.

Cerebellar ataxia and tremor are different aspects of defects in the smooth, continuously correcting functions. Cerebellar dystaxia or, if severe, ataxia includes a decomposition of movement; each succeeding component of a complex movement occurs separately instead of being blended into a smoothly proceeding action. Because ethanol specifically affects cerebellar function, persons who are inebriated often walk with a staggering and unsteady gait. Rapid alternating movements such as supination-pronation-supination of the hands are jerky and performed slowly (dysdiadochokinesia). Reaching to touch a target breaks down into small sequential components, each going too far, followed by overcorrection. The finger moves jerkily toward the target, misses, corrects in the other direction, and misses again, until the target is finally reached. This is called *over- and underreaching*, and the general term is *dysmetria*.

Cerebellar tremor is a rhythmic back-and-forth movement of a finger or toe that worsens as the target is approached. The tremor results from the inability of the damaged cerebellar system to maintain ongoing fixation of a body part and to make smooth, continuous corrections in the trajectory of the movement; overcorrection occurs, first in one direction and then the other. Often, the tremor of an arm or leg can be detected during the beginning of an intended movement. The common term for cerebellar tremor is *intention tremor*. Cerebellar func-

tion as it relates to tremor can be assessed by asking a person to touch one heel to the opposite knee, to move the toes gently along the back of the opposite shin, or to move the hand so as to touch the nose with a finger.

Cerebellar function also can affect the motor skills of chewing and swallowing (dysphagia) and of speech (dysarthria). Normal speech requires smooth control of respiratory muscles and highly coordinated control of the laryngeal, lip, and tongue muscles. Cerebellar dysarthria is characterized by slow, slurred speech of continuously varying loudness. Rehabilitative efforts directed by speech therapists include learning to slow the rate of speech and to compensate as much as possible through the use of less-affected muscles.

In summary, alterations in coordination of muscle movements and abnormal muscle movements result from disorders of the cerebellum and basal ganglia. The basal ganglia organize basic movement patterns into more complex patterns and release them when commanded by the motor cortex, contributing gracefulness to cortically initiated and controlled skilled movements. Disorders of the basal ganglia are characterized by involuntary movements, alterations in muscle tone, and disturbances in posture. These disorders include tremor, tics, hemiballismus, chorea, athetosis, dystonias, and dyskinesias.

Parkinsonism, a disorder of the basal ganglia, is characterized by destruction of the nigrostriatal pathway, with a subsequent reduction in striatal concentrations of dopamine. This results in an imbalance between the inhibitory effects of dopaminergic basal ganglia functions and an increase in the excitatory cholinergic functions. The disorder is manifested by combinations of slowness of movement (*i.e.*, bradykinesia), increased muscle tonus and rigidity, rest tremor, gait disturbances, and impaired autonomic postural responses. The disease usually is slowly progressive over several decades, but the rate of progression varies from 2 to 30 years. The tremor often begins in one or both hands and then becomes generalized. Postural changes and gait disturbances continue to become more pronounced, resulting in significant disability.

The function of the cerebellum is essential for smooth, coordinated movements. Cerebellar disorders include vestibulocerebellar dysfunction, cerebellar ataxia, and cerebellar tremor.

Upper Motor Neuron Disorders

Upper motor neuron disorders involve neurons that are fully contained within the CNS. They include the motor neurons arising in the motor areas of the cortex and their fibers as they project through the brain and descend in the spinal cord. Disorders that affect UMNs include multiple sclerosis and spinal cord injury (discussed later). Stroke, which is a common cause of UMN damage, is discussed in Chapter 36. Amyotrophic lateral sclerosis is a mixed UMN and LMN disorder.

AMYOTROPHIC LATERAL SCLEROSIS

Amyotrophic lateral sclerosis (ALS), also known as *Lou Gehrig disease* after the famous New York Yankees baseball player, is a devastating neurologic disorder that selectively affects motor function. ALS is primarily a disorder of middle to late adulthood, affecting persons between 55 and 60 years of age, with men developing the disease nearly twice as often as women.[30] The disease typically follows a progressive course, with a mean survival period of 2 to 5 years from the onset of symptoms.

Amyotrophic lateral sclerosis affects motor neurons in three locations: the anterior horn cells (LMNs) of the spinal cord; the motor nuclei of the brain stem, particularly the hypoglossal nuclei; and the UMNs of the cerebral cortex. The death of LMNs leads to denervation, with subsequent shrinkage of musculature and muscle fiber atrophy. It is this fiber atrophy, called *amyotrophy,* which appears in the name of the disease. The loss of nerve fibers in lateral columns of the white matter of the spinal cord along with fibrillary gliosis imparts a firmness or sclerosis to this CNS tissue; the term *lateral sclerosis* designates these changes. The fact that the disease is more extensive in the distal parts of the affected tracts in the lower spinal cord rather than the proximal parts suggests that affected neurons first undergo degeneration at their distal terminals and that the disease proceeds in a centripetal direction until ultimately the parent nerve cell dies. A remarkable feature of the disease is that the entire sensory system, the regulatory mechanisms of control and coordination of movement, and the intellect remain intact. The neurons for ocular motility and the parasympathetic neurons in the sacral spinal cord also are spared.

The cause of LMN and UMN destruction in ALS is uncertain. Five to 10% of cases are familial; the others are believed to be sporadic, with no family history of the disease. Recently, mutations to a gene encoding superoxide dismutase 1 (SOD1) were mapped to chromosome 21. This enzyme functions in the prevention of free radical formation (see Chapter 2). The mutation accounts for 20% of cases of familial ALS, with the remaining 80% being caused by mutations in other genes.[31] Five percent of persons with sporadic ALS also have SOD1 mutations. Possible targets of SOD1-induced toxicity include the neurofilament proteins, which function in the axonal transport of molecules necessary for the maintenance of axons.[31] Another suggested mechanism of pathogenesis in ALS is exotoxic injury through activation of glutamate-gated ion channels, which are distinguished by their sensitivity to N-methyl-D-aspartic acid (see Chapter 36). The possibility of glutamate excitotoxicity in the pathogenesis of ALS was suggested by the finding of increased glutamine levels in the cerebrospinal fluid of patients with sporadic ALS.[31] Although autoimmunity has been suggested as a cause of ALS, the disease does not respond to the immunosuppressant agents that normally are used in treatment of autoimmune disorders.

The symptoms of ALS may be referable to UMN or LMN involvement. Manifestations of UMN lesions include weakness, spasticity or stiffness, and impaired fine motor control.[30,32] Dysphagia (difficulty swallowing), dysarthria (impaired articulation of speech), and dysphonia (difficulty making the sounds of speech) may result from brain stem LMN involvement or from dysfunction of UMNs descending to the brain stem. Manifestations of LMN destruction include fasciculations, weakness, muscle atrophy, and hyporeflexia. Muscle cramps involving the distal legs often are an early symptom. The most common clinical presentation is slowly progressive weakness and atrophy in distal muscles of one upper extremity. This is followed by regional spread of clinical weakness, reflecting involvement of neighboring areas of the spinal cord. Eventually, UMNs and LMNs involving multiple limbs and the head are affected. In the more advanced stages, muscles of the palate, pharynx, tongue, neck, and shoulders become involved, causing impairment of chewing, swallowing, and speech. Dysphagia with recurrent aspiration and weakness of the respiratory muscles produces the most significant acute complications of the disease. Death usually results from involvement of cranial nerves and respiratory musculature.

Currently, there is no cure for ALS. Rehabilitation measures assist persons with the disorder to manage their disability, and respiratory and nutritional support allows persons with the disorder to survive longer than would otherwise have been the case. An antiglutamate drug, riluzole, is the only drug approved by the U.S. Food and Drug Administration (FDA) for treatment of ALS. The drug is designed to decrease glutamate accumulation and slow the progression of the disease. In two therapeutic trials, the drug prolonged survival by 3 to 6 months.[31]

DEMYELINATING DISORDERS

Multiple Sclerosis

Multiple sclerosis (MS), a demyelinating disease of the CNS, is the most common nontraumatic cause of neurologic disability among young and middle-aged adults. In approximately 80% of the cases, the disease is characterized by exacerbations and remissions over many years in several different sites in the CNS.[33] Initially, there is normal or near-normal neurologic function between exacerbations. As the disease progresses, there is less improvement between exacerbations and increasing neurologic dysfunction.

Multiple sclerosis is typically a disease of young adults, 20 to 45 years of age.[34] The incidence among women is almost double that among men, and persons of northern European descent appear to be at highest risk for the disease. Although MS is not directly inherited, a genetic predisposition is suggested by familial aggregation of the disease, an increased risk in second- and third-degree relatives of persons with MS, and a 25% concordance in monozygotic twins.[12] There also is a strong association between MS and certain human leukocyte antigens (HLA; see Chapter 13), with the presence of the HLA-DR2 allele substantially increasing the risk for development of the disease.[12,33]

Pathophysiology. The pathophysiology of MS involves the demyelination and subsequent degeneration of nerve fibers in the CNS. In the CNS, myelin is formed by the oligodendrocytes, whose function is equivalent to that of the Schwann cells in the PNS (see Chapter 33). The properties of the myelin sheath—high electrical resistance and low capacitance—permit it to function as an electrical insulator. Demyelinated nerve fibers display a variety of conduction abnormalities, ranging from decreased conduction velocity to conduction blocks, resulting in a variety of symptoms that depend on the location and duration of the lesion.

Pathogenesis. Multiple sclerosis generally is believed to be an immune-mediated disorder that occurs in genetically susceptible individuals. However, the sequence of events that initiates the process is largely unknown. The demyelination process in MS is marked by prominent lymphocytic invasion in the lesion. The infiltrate in plaques contains both CD8+ and CD4+ T cells as well as macrophages. Both macrophages and cytotoxic CD8+ T cells are thought to induce oligodendrocyte injury. There also is evidence of antibody-mediated damage involving myelin oligodendroglial protein.[5]

The lesions of MS consist of hard, sharp-edged demyelinated or sclerotic patches that are macroscopically visible throughout the white matter of the CNS [5,12] (Fig. 35-14). These lesions, which represent the end result of acute myelin breakdown, are called *plaques*. The lesions have a predilection for the optic nerves, periventricular white matter, brain stem, cerebellum, and spinal cord white matter.[33] In an active plaque, there is evidence of ongoing myelin breakdown. The sequence of myelin breakdown is not well understood, although it is known that the lesions contain small amounts of myelin basic proteins and increased amounts of proteolytic enzymes, macrophages, lymphocytes, and plasma cells. Oligodendrocytes are decreased in number and may be absent, especially in older lesions. Acute, subacute, and chronic lesions often are seen at multiple sites throughout the CNS.

Magnetic resonance imaging has shown that the lesions of MS may occur in two stages: a first stage that involves the sequential development of small inflammatory lesions, and a second stage during which the lesions extend and consolidate and when demyelination and gliosis (scar formation) occur. It is not known whether the inflammatory process, present during the first stage, is directed against the myelin or against the oligodendrocytes that produce myelin. Remyelination of the nervous system was considered to be impossible until the late 1990s. Evidence now suggests that remyelination can occur in the CNS if the process that initiated the demyelination is halted before the oligodendrocyte dies.[35]

Clinical Features. The interruption of neural conduction in the demyelinated nerves is manifested by a variety of symptoms, depending on the location and extent of the lesion. Areas commonly affected by MS are the optic nerve (visual field), corticobulbar tracts (speech and swallowing), corticospinal tracts (muscle strength), cerebellar tracts (gait and coordination), spinocerebellar tracts (balance), medial longitudinal fasciculus (conjugate gaze function of the extraocular eye muscles), and posterior cell columns of the spinal cord (position and vibratory sensation). Typically, an otherwise healthy person presents with an acute or subacute episode of paresthesias, optic neuritis (*i.e.*, visual clouding or loss of vision in part of the visual field with pain on movement of the globe), diplopia, or specific types of gaze paralysis.

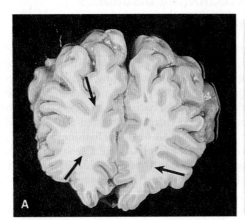 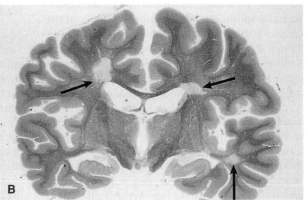

FIGURE 35-14 Multiple sclerosis. (**A**) In this unfixed brain, the plaques of multiple sclerosis in the white matter (*arrows*) assume the darker color of the cerebral cortex. (**B**) A coronal section of the brain from a patient with long-standing multiple sclerosis, which has been stained for myelin, shows discrete areas of demyelination (*arrows*) with characteristic involvement of the superior angles of the lateral ventricles. (From Trojanowski J. Q. [2005]. The central nervous system. In Rubin E., Gorstein F., Rubin R., et al. [Eds.], *Rubin's pathology: Clinicopathologic foundations of medicine* [4th ed., p. 1464]. Philadelphia: Lippincott Williams & Wilkins.)

Paresthesias are evidenced as numbness, tingling, a burning sensation, or pressure on the face or involved extremities; symptoms can range from annoying to severe. *Lhermitte symptom* is an electric shock–like tingling down the back and onto the legs that is produced by flexion of the neck. Pain from spasticity also may be a factor that can be ameliorated by appropriate stretching exercises. Although pain may not be a prominent symptom, approximately 80% of persons with MS experience some pain in the course of the disease. Other common symptoms are abnormal gait, bladder and sexual dysfunction, vertigo, nystagmus, fatigue, and speech disturbance. These symptoms usually last for several days to weeks, and then completely or partially resolve. After a period of normal or relatively normal function, new symptoms appear. Psychological manifestations, such as mood swings, may represent an emotional reaction to the nature of the disease or, more likely, involvement of the white matter of the cerebral cortex. Depression, euphoria, inattentiveness, apathy, forgetfulness, and loss of memory may occur.

Fatigue is one of the most common problems for persons with MS. Fatigue often is described as a generalized low-energy feeling not related to depression and different from weakness. Fatigue has a harmful impact on activities of daily living and sustained physical activity. Interventions such as spacing activities and setting priorities often are helpful.

The course of the disease may fall into one of several categories: relapsing-remitting, secondary progressive, or primary progressive.[35,36] The *relapsing-remitting* form of the disease is characterized by episodes of acute worsening with recovery and a stable course between relapses. *Secondary progressive disease* involves a gradual neurologic deterioration with or without superimposed acute relapses in a person with previous relapsing-remitting disease. *Primary progressive disease* is characterized by nearly continuous neurologic deterioration from onset of symptoms.

Diagnosis. The diagnosis of MS is based on established clinical and, when necessary, laboratory criteria. Advances in cerebrospinal fluid analysis and MRI have greatly simplified the procedure. A definite diagnosis of MS requires evidence of CNS lesions that are disseminated in time and space (*i.e.*, occur in different parts of the CNS at least 3 months apart), with no better explanation for the disease process.[34] MRI, which can detect the multiplicity of lesions even when CT scans appear normal, is used as an adjunct to clinical diagnosis. A computer-assisted MRI method can measure lesion size. Many new areas of myelin abnormality are asymptomatic. Serial MRI studies can be done to detect asymptomatic lesions, monitor the progress of existing lesions, and evaluate the effectiveness of treatment. Electrophysiologic evaluations (*e.g.*, evoked potential studies) and CT scans may assist in the identification and documentation of lesions.[34]

Although no laboratory test can be used to diagnose MS, examination of the cerebrospinal fluid is helpful. A large percentage of patients with MS have elevated immunoglobulin G (IgG) levels, and some have oligoclonal patterns (*i.e.*, discrete electrophoretic bands) even with normal IgG levels. Total protein or lymphocyte levels may be mildly elevated in the cerebrospinal fluid. These test results can be altered in a variety of inflammatory neurologic disorders and are not specific for MS.

Treatment. Most treatment measures for MS are directed at modifying the course and managing the primary symptoms of the disease. The variety of symptoms, unpredictable course, and lack of specific diagnostic methods has made the evaluation and treatment of MS difficult. Persons who are minimally affected by the disorder require no specific treatment. The person should be encouraged to maintain as healthy a lifestyle as possible, including good nutrition and adequate rest and relaxation. Physical therapy may help maintain muscle tone. Every effort should be made to avoid excessive fatigue, physical deterioration, emotional stress, viral infections, and extremes of environmental temperature, which may precipitate an exacerbation of the disease.

The pharmacologic agents used in the treatment of MS fall into four categories: those used to (1) treat acute relapses of the disease, (2) modify the course of the disease, (3) interrupt progression of the disease, and (4) treat symptoms of the disorder. Corticosteroids are the mainstay of treatment for acute relapses of MS.[34] These agents are thought to reduce the inflammation, improve nerve conduction, and have important immunologic effects. Long-term administration does not, however, appear to alter the course of the disease and can have harmful side effects.

Disease-modifying agents include interferon β, glatiramer acetate, and mitoxantone.[34,37] These agents have shown some benefit in reducing exacerbations in persons with relapsing-remitting MS. Interferon β is a cytokine that acts as an immune enhancer. Two forms of recombinant interferon have been approved by the FDA for treatment of MS—interferon β1-1a and interferon β1-1b. Both types of interferon are administered by injection and both are usually well tolerated. The most common side effects are flulike symptoms for 24 to 48 hours after each injection, and these usually subside after 2 to 3 months of treatment. Glatiramer acetate is a synthetic polypeptide that simulates parts of the myelin basic protein. Although the exact mechanism of action is unknown, the drug seems to block myelin-damaging T cells by acting as a myelin decoy. The drug is given daily by subcutaneous injection. Mitoxantrone, an anticancer drug, is recommended for persons with worsening forms of the disease. Because it is an anticancer drug, it is recommended that it be administered only by experienced health care professionals. Natalizumab, a monoclonal antibody directed against an adhesion molecule called VLA-4, is in the final stages of phase III clinical trials. It is administered intravenously once a month.

Progressive MS may be treated with immunosuppressive drugs such as methotrexate, cyclophosphamide, mitoxantrone, and cyclosporine.[37] Among the medications used to relieve symptoms associated with MS are dantrolene (Dantrium), baclofen (Lioresal), or diazepam (Valium) for spasticity; cholinergic drugs for bladder problems; and antidepressant drugs for depression.

SPINAL CORD INJURY

Spinal cord injury (SCI) represents damage to the neural elements of the spinal cord. SCI is primarily a disorder of young adults, with about 53% of cases occurring among persons in the 16- to 30-year age group. The most common cause of SCI is motor vehicle crashes, followed by falls, violence (primarily gunshot wounds), and recreational sporting activities.[38]

Most SCIs involve damage to the vertebral column or supporting ligaments as well as the spinal cord. Because of extensive tract systems that connect sensory afferent neurons and LMNs with higher brain centers, spinal cord injuries commonly involve both sensory and motor function.

Injury to the Vertebral Column

Injuries to the vertebral column include fractures, dislocations, and subluxations. A fracture can occur at any part of the bony vertebrae, causing fragmentation of the bone. It most often involves the pedicle, lamina, or processes (*e.g.*, facets). Dislocation or subluxation (partial dislocation) injury causes the vertebral bodies to become displaced, with one overriding another and preventing correct alignment of the vertebral column. Damage to the ligaments or bony vertebrae may make the spine unstable. In an unstable spine, further unguarded movement of the spinal column can impinge on the spinal canal, causing compression or overstretching of neural tissue.

Most injuries result from some combination of compressive force or bending movement.[39] Flexion injuries occur when forward bending of the spinal column exceeds the limits of normal movement. Typical flexion injuries result, for example, when the head is struck from behind, as in a fall with the back of the head as the point of impact. Extension injuries occur with excessive forced bending (*i.e.*, hyperextension) of the spine backward. A typical extension injury involves a fall in which the chin or face is the point of impact, causing hyperextension of the neck. Injuries of flexion and extension occur more commonly in the cervical spine (C4 to C6) than in any other area. Limitations imposed by the ribs, spinous processes, and joint capsules in the thoracic and lumbar spine make this area less flexible and less susceptible to flexion and extension injuries than the cervical spine.

A compression injury, causing the vertebral bones to shatter, squash, or even burst, occurs when there is spinal loading from a high-velocity blow to the top of the head or a forceful landing on the feet[39] (Fig. 35-15A). This typically occurs at the cervical level (*e.g.*, diving injuries) or in the thoracolumbar area (*e.g.*, falling from a distance and landing on the feet). Compression injuries may occur when the vertebrae are weakened by conditions such as osteoporosis and cancer with bone metastasis. Axial rotation injuries can produce highly unstable injuries. Maximal axial rotation occurs in the cervical region, especially between C1 and C2, and at the lumbosacral joint[39] (see Fig. 35-15B). Coupling of vertebral motions is common in injury when two or more individual motions occur (*e.g.*, lateral bending and axial rotation).

Acute Spinal Cord Injury

Spinal cord injury involves damage to the neural elements of the spinal cord. The damage may result from direct trauma to the cord such as occurs with penetrating wounds or from indirect injury resulting from vertebral fractures, fracture-dislocations, or subluxations of the spine. The spinal cord may be contused, not only at the site of injury

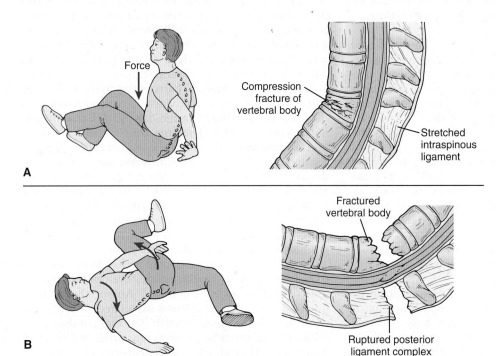

A

B

FIGURE 35-15 (A) Compression vertebral fracture secondary to axial loading as occurs when a person falls from a height and lands on the buttocks. **(B)** Rotational injury, in which there is concurrent fracture and tearing of the posterior ligamentous complex, is caused by extreme lateral flexion or twisting of the head or neck. (Modified from Hickey J. V. [2003]. *The clinical practice of neurological and neurosurgical nursing* [5th ed., pp. 411–412]. Philadelphia: Lippincott Williams & Wilkins.)

but above and below the trauma site[39] (Fig. 35-16). Traumatic injury may be complicated by loss of blood flow to the cord, with resulting infarction.

Sudden complete transection of the spinal cord results in complete loss of motor, sensory, reflex, and autonomic function below the level of injury. This immediate response to spinal cord injury is often referred to as *spinal cord shock*. It is characterized by flaccid paralysis with loss of tendon reflexes below the level of injury, absence of somatic and visceral sensations below the level of injury, and loss of bowel and bladder function. Loss of systemic sympathetic vasomotor tone may result in vasodilatation, increased venous capacity, and hypotension. These manifestations occur regardless of whether the level of the lesion eventually will produce spastic (UWM) or flaccid (LMN) paralysis. The basic mechanisms accounting for transient spinal shock are unknown. Spinal shock may last for hours, days, or weeks. Usually, if reflex function returns by the time the person reaches the health care facility, the neuromuscular changes are reversible. This type of reversible spinal shock may occur in football-type injuries, in which jarring of the spinal cord produces a concussion-like syndrome with loss of movement and reflexes, followed by full recovery within days. In persons in whom the loss of reflexes persists,

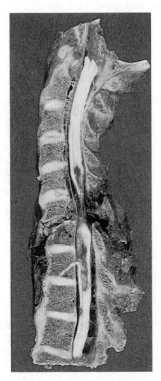

FIGURE 35-16 Cervical contusion. Hyperflexion injury caused forward angulation of the cervical cord, with fracture of the anterior lip of the underlying vertebral body. The cord is angulated over the superior-posterior ridge of the fixed underlying cervical body. (From Trojanowski J. Q. [2005]. The central nervous system. In Rubin E., Gorstein F., Rubin R., et al. [Eds.], *Rubin's pathology: Clinicopathologic foundations of medicine* [4th ed., p. 1434]. Philadelphia: Lippincott Williams & Wilkins.)

hypotension and bradycardia may become critical but manageable problems. In general, the higher the level of injury, the greater is the effect.

Pathophysiology. The pathophysiologic process of acute SCI can be divided into two types: primary and secondary.[40–42] The *primary neurologic injury* occurs at the time of mechanical injury and is irreversible. It is characterized by small hemorrhages in the gray matter of the cord, followed by edematous changes in the white matter that lead to necrosis of neural tissue. This type of lesion results from the forces of compression, stretch, and shear associated with fracture or compression of the spinal vertebrae, dislocation of vertebrae (*e.g.,* flexion, extension, subluxation), and contusions due to jarring of the cord in the spinal canal. Penetrating injuries produce lacerations and direct trauma to the cord and may occur with or without spinal column damage. Lacerations occur when there is cutting or tearing of the spinal cord, which injures nerve tissue and causes bleeding and edema.

Secondary injuries follow the primary injury and promote the spread of injury. Although there is considerable debate about the pathogenesis of secondary injuries, the tissue destruction that occurs ends in progressive neurologic damage. After SCI, several pathologic mechanisms come into play, including vascular damage, neuronal injury that leads to loss of reflexes below the level of injury, and release of vasoactive agents and cellular enzymes. Vascular lesions (*i.e.,* vessel trauma and hemorrhage) can lead to ischemia, increased vascular permeability, and edema. Blood flow to the spinal cord may be further compromised by spinal shock that results from a loss of vasomotor tone and neural reflexes below the level of injury. The release of vasoactive substances (*i.e.,* norepinephrine, serotonin, dopamine, and histamine) from the wound tissue causes vasospasm and impedes blood flow in the microcirculation, producing further necrosis of blood vessels and neurons. The release of proteolytic and lipolytic enzymes from injured cells causes delayed swelling, demyelination, and necrosis in the neural tissue in the spinal cord.

Management. The goal of management of acute SCI is to reduce the neurologic deficit and prevent any additional loss of neurologic function. The specific steps in resuscitation and initial evaluation can be carried out at the trauma site or in the emergency department, depending on the urgency of the situation.[39] Most traumatic injuries to the spinal column render it unstable, mandating measures such as immobilization with collars and backboards and limiting the movement of persons at risk for or with known SCI. Every person with multiple trauma or head injury, including victims of traffic and sporting accidents, should be suspected of having sustained an acute SCI.[39]

The nature of the injury determines further methods of stabilization and treatment. In unstable injuries of the cervical spine, cervical traction improves or restores spinal alignment, decompresses neural structures, and facilitates recovery. Fractures and dislocations of the thoracic and lumbar vertebrae may be initially stabilized by restricting the person to bed rest and turning him or her in a log-rolling manner to keep the spine rigid. Gunshot or stab wounds of the spinal column may not produce structural instability and may not require immobilization. The goal of early surgical intervention for an unstable spine is to provide internal skeletal stabilization so that early mobilization and rehabilitation can occur.

One of the more important aspects of early SCI care is the prevention and treatment of spinal or systemic shock and the hypoxia associated with compromised respiration. Correcting hypotension or hypoxia is essential to maintaining circulation to the injured cord.[39–43] The use of high-dose methylprednisolone has been shown to improve the outcome from SCI when given shortly after injury. Methylprednisolone is a short-acting corticosteroid that has been used extensively in the treatment of inflammatory and allergic disorders.[44] In acute SCI, it is thought to stabilize cell membranes, enhance impulse generation, improve blood flow, and inhibit free radical formation.

Types and Classification of Spinal Cord Injury

Alterations in body function that result from SCI depend on the level of injury and the amount of cord involvement. *Tetraplegia,* sometimes referred to as *quadriplegia,* is the impairment or loss of motor or sensory function (or both) after damage to neural structures in the cervical segments of the spinal cord.[45] It results in impairment of function in the arms, trunk, legs, and pelvic organs (see Fig. 35-5). *Paraplegia* refers to impairment or loss of motor or sensory function (or both) in the thoracic, lumbar, or sacral segments of the spinal cord from damage of neural elements in the spinal canal. With paraplegia, arm functioning is spared, but depending on the level of injury, functioning of the trunk, legs, and pelvic organs may be impaired. Paraplegia includes conus medullaris and cauda equina injuries (to be discussed).

Further definitions of SCI describe the extent of neurologic damage as *complete* or *incomplete.* Complete SCI implies there is an absence of motor and sensory function below the level of injury. Complete cord injuries can result from severance of the cord, disruption of nerve fibers although they remain intact, or interruption of blood supply to that segment, resulting in complete destruction of neural tissue and UMN or LMN paralysis.

Incomplete SCI implies there is some residual motor or sensory function below the level of injury.[41] The prognosis for return of function is better in an incomplete injury because of preservation of axonal function. Incomplete injuries may manifest in a variety of patterns but can be organized into certain patterns or "syndromes" that occur more frequently and reflect the predominant area of the cord that is involved. Types of incomplete lesions include the central cord syndrome, anterior cord syndrome, Brown-Séquard syndrome, and the conus medullaris syndrome.

Central Cord Syndrome. A condition called *central cord syndrome* occurs when injury is predominantly in the central gray or white matter of the cord.[39] Because the corticospinal tract fibers are organized with those controlling the arms located more centrally and those controlling the legs located more laterally, some external axonal transmission may remain intact. Motor function of the upper extremities is affected, but the lower extremities may not be affected or may be affected to a lesser degree, with some sparing of sacral sensation. Bowel, bladder, and sexual functions usually are affected to various degrees and may parallel the degree of lower extremity involvement. This syndrome occurs almost exclusively in the cervical cord, rendering the lesion a UMN lesion with spastic paralysis. Central cord damage is more frequent in elderly persons with narrowing or stenotic changes in the spinal canal that are related to arthritis. Damage also may occur in persons with congenital stenosis.

Anterior Cord Syndrome. Anterior cord syndrome usually is caused by damage from infarction of the anterior spinal artery, resulting in damage to the anterior two thirds of the cord[39] (Fig. 35-17). The deficits result in loss of motor function provided by the corticospinal tracts and loss of pain and temperature sensation from damage to the lateral spinothalamic tracts. The posterior one third of the cord is relatively unaffected, preserving the dorsal column axons that convey position, vibration, and touch sensation.

Brown-Séquard Syndrome. A condition called *Brown-Séquard syndrome* results from damage to a hemisection of the anterior and posterior cord[39] (Fig. 35-18). The effect is a loss of voluntary motor function from the

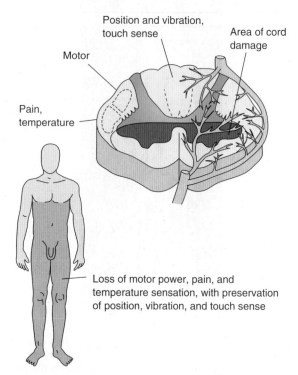

FIGURE 35-17 Anterior cord syndrome. Cord damage and associated motor and sensory loss are illustrated. (From Hickey J. V. [2003]. *The clinical practice of neurological and neurosurgical nursing* [5th ed., p. 420]. Philadelphia: Lippincott Williams & Wilkins.)

Right   Left

Area of cord damage

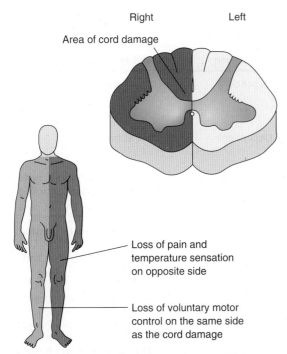

Loss of pain and
temperature sensation
on opposite side

Loss of voluntary motor
control on the same side
as the cord damage

FIGURE 35-18 Brown-Séquard syndrome. Cord damage and associated motor and sensory losses are illustrated. (From Hickey J. V. [2003]. *The clinical practice of neurological and neurosurgical nursing* [5th ed., p. 421]. Philadelphia: Lippincott Williams & Wilkins.)

corticospinal tract, proprioception loss from the ipsilateral side of the body, and contralateral loss of pain and temperature sensation from the lateral spinothalamic tracts for all levels below the lesion.

Conus Medullaris Syndrome. The conus medullaris syndrome involves damage to the conus medullaris or the sacral cord (*i.e.,* conus) and lumbar nerve roots in the neural canal. Functional deficits resulting from this type of injury usually result in flaccid bowel and bladder function, as well as altered sexual function. Sacral segments occasionally show preserved reflexes if only the conus is affected. Motor function in the legs and feet may be impaired without significant sensory impairment. Damage to the lumbosacral nerve roots in the spinal canal usually results in LMN and sensory neuron damage known as *cauda equina syndrome.* Functional deficits present as various patterns of asymmetric flaccid paralysis, sensory impairment, and pain.

Disruption of Functional Abilities

Functional abilities after SCI depend on degree of somatosensory and skeletal muscle function loss and altered reflex activity based on the level of cord injury and extent of cord damage (Table 35-2).

Motor and Somatosensory Function. Motor function in cervical injuries ranges from complete dependence to independence with or without assistive devices in activities

of mobility and self-care. The functional levels of cervical injury are related to C5, C6, C7, or C8 innervation. At the C5 level, deltoid and biceps function is spared, allowing full head, neck, and diaphragm control with good shoulder strength and full elbow flexion. At the C6 level, wrist dorsiflexion by way of wrist extensors is functional, allowing tenodesis, which is the natural bending inward and flexion of the fingers when the wrist is extended and bent backward. Tenodesis is a key movement because it can be used to pick up objects when finger movement is absent. A functional C7 injury allows full elbow flexion and extension, wrist plantar flexion, and some finger control. At the C8 level, finger flexion is added.

Thoracic cord injuries (T1 to T12) allow full upper extremity control with limited to full control of intercostal and trunk muscles and balance. Injury at the T1 level allows full fine motor control of the fingers. Because of the lack of specific functional indicators at the thoracic levels, the level of injury usually is determined by sensory level testing.

Functional capacity in the L1 through L5 nerve innervations allows hip flexors, hip abductors (L1 to L3), movement of the knees (L2 to L5), and ankle dorsiflexion (L4 to L5). Sacral (S1 to S5) innervation allows for full leg, foot, and ankle control and innervation of perineal musculature for bowel, bladder, and sexual function.

Reflex Activity. Spinal cord reflexes are fully integrated in the spinal cord and can function independent of input from higher centers. Altered spinal reflex activity after SCI is essentially determined by the level of injury and whether UMNs or LMNs are affected. With UMN injuries at T12 and above, the cord reflexes remain intact although communication pathways with higher centers have been interrupted. This results in spasticity of involved skeletal muscle groups and of smooth and skeletal muscles that control bowel, bladder, and sexual function. In LMN injuries at T12 or below, the reflex circuitry itself has been damaged at the level of the spinal cord or spinal nerve, resulting in decreased or absent reflex function. LMN injuries cause flaccid paralysis of involved skeletal muscle groups and the smooth and skeletal muscles that control bowel, bladder, and sexual function. However, injuries near the T12 level may result in mixed UMN and LMN deficits (*e.g.,* spastic paralysis of the bowel and bladder with flaccid skeletal muscle tone).

After the period of spinal shock in a UMN injury, isolated spinal reflex activity and muscle tone that is not under the control of higher centers returns. This may result in hypertonia and spasticity of skeletal muscles below the level of injury.[39] These spastic movements are involuntary instead of voluntary, a distinction that needs to be explained to persons with SCI and their families. The antigravity muscles, the flexors of the arms and extensors of the legs, are predominantly affected. Spastic movements are usually heightened initially after injury, reaching a peak and then becoming stable in approximately 1.5 to 2 years.[39]

The stimuli for reflex muscle spasm arise from somatic and visceral afferent pathways that enter the

TABLE 35-2   Functional Abilities by Level of Cord Injury

Injury Level	Segmental Sensorimotor Function	Dressing, Eating	Elimination	Mobility*
C1	Little or no sensation or control of head and neck; no diaphragm control; requires continuous ventilation	Dependent	Dependent	Limited. Voice or sip-n-puff controlled electric wheelchair
C2 to C3	Head and neck sensation; some neck control, independent of mechanical ventilation for short periods	Dependent	Dependent	Same as for C1
C4	Good head and neck sensation and motor control; some shoulder elevation; diaphragm movement	Dependent; may be able to eat with adaptive sling	Dependent	Limited to voice, mouth, head, chin, or shoulder-controlled electric wheelchair
C5	Full head and neck control; shoulder strength; elbow flexion	Independent with assistance	Maximal assistance	Electric or modified manual wheel-chair, needs transfer assistance
C6	Fully innervated shoulder; wrist extension or dorsiflexion	Independent or with minimal assistance	Independent or with minimal assistance	Independent in transfers and wheelchair
C7 to C8	Full elbow extension; wrist plantar flexion; some finger control	Independent	Independent	Independent; manual wheelchair
T1 to T5	Full hand and finger control; use of intercostal and thoracic muscles	Independent	Independent	Independent; manual wheelchair
T6 to T10	Abdominal muscle control, partial to good balance with trunk muscles	Independent	Independent	Independent; manual wheelchair
T11 to L5	Hip flexors, hip abductors (L1–L3); knee extension (L2–L4); knee flexion and ankle dorsiflexion (L4–L5)	Independent	Independent	Short distance to full ambulation with assistance
S1 to S5	Full leg, foot, and ankle control; innervation of perineal muscles for bowel, bladder, and sexual function (S2–S4)	Independent	Normal to impaired bowel and bladder function	Ambulate independently with or without assistance

*Assistance refers to adaptive equipment, setup, or physical assistance.

cord below the level of injury. The most common of these stimuli are muscle stretching, bladder infections or urinary tract stones, fistulas, bowel distention or impaction, pressure areas or irritation of the skin, and infections. Because the stimuli that precipitate spasms vary from person to person, careful assessment is required to identify the factors that precipitate spasm in each person. Passive range-of-motion exercises to stretch the spastic muscles help to prevent spasm induced by muscle stretching such as occurs with a change in body position.

Spasticity in and of itself is not detrimental and may even facilitate maintenance of muscle tone to prevent muscle wasting, improve venous return, and aid in mobility. Spasms become detrimental when they impair safety or reduce the ability to make functional gains in mobility and activities of daily living. Spasms also may cause trauma to bones and tissues, leading to joint contractures and skin breakdown.

Respiratory Muscle Function. Ventilation requires movement of the expiratory and inspiratory muscles, all of which receive innervation from the spinal cord. The main muscle of ventilation, the diaphragm, is innervated by segments C3 to C5 through the phrenic nerves.

The intercostal muscles, which function in elevating the rib cage and are needed for coughing and deep breathing, are innervated by spinal segments T1 through T7. The major muscles of expiration are the abdominal muscles, which receive their innervation from levels T6 to T12.

Although the ability to inhale and exhale may be preserved at various levels of SCI, functional deficits in ventilation are most apparent in the quality of the breathing cycle and the ability to oxygenate tissues, eliminate carbon dioxide, and mobilize secretions. Cord injuries involving C1 to C3 result in a lack of respiratory effort, and affected patients require assisted ventilation. Although a C3 to C5 injury allows partial or full diaphragmatic function, ventilation is diminished because of the loss of intercostal muscle function, resulting in shallow breaths and a weak cough. Below the C5 level, as less intercostal and abdominal musculature is affected, the ability to take a deep breath and cough is less impaired. Maintenance therapy consists of muscle training to strengthen existing muscles for endurance and mobilization of secretions. The ability to speak is compromised with assisted ventilation, whether continuous or intermittent. Thus, ensuring adequate communication of needs is also essential.

Disruption of Autonomic Nervous System Function

In addition to its effects on skeletal muscle function, SCI interrupts autonomic nervous system (ANS) function below the site of injury. This includes sympathetic outflow from the thoracic and lumbar cord and parasympathetic outflow from the sacral cord. Because of their sites of exit from the CNS, the cranial nerves, such as the vagus, are unaffected. Depending on the level of injury, the spinal reflexes that control ANS function are largely isolated from the rest of the CNS. Afferent sensory input that enters the spinal cord is unaffected, as is the efferent motor output from the cord. Lacking is the regulation and integration of reflex function by centers in the brain and brain stem. This results in a situation where the autonomic reflexes below the level of injury are uncontrolled, whereas those above the level of injury function in a relatively controlled manner.

The sympathetic nervous system regulation of circulatory function and thermoregulation presents some of the most severe problems in SCI. The higher the level of injury and the greater the surface area affected, the more profound are the effects on circulation and thermoregulation. Persons with injury at the T6 level or above experience problems in regulating vasomotor tone; those with injuries below the T6 level usually have sufficient sympathetic function to maintain adequate vasomotor function. The level of injury and its corresponding problems may vary among persons, and some dysfunctional effects may be seen at levels below T6. With lower lumbar and sacral injuries, sympathetic function remains essentially unaltered.

Vasovagal Response. The vagus nerve (cranial nerve X) normally exerts a continuous inhibitory effect on heart rate. Vagal stimulation that causes a marked bradycardia through the vagus nerve is called the *vasovagal response*. Visceral afferent input to the vagal centers in the brain stem of persons with tetraplegia or high-level paraplegia can produce marked bradycardia when unchecked by a dysfunctional sympathetic nervous system. Severe bradycardia and even asystole can result when the vasovagal response is elicited by deep endotracheal suctioning or rapid position change. Preventive measures, such as hyperoxygenation before, during, and after suctioning, are advised. Rapid position changes should be avoided or anticipated, and anticholinergic drugs should be immediately available to counteract severe episodes of bradycardia.

Autonomic Dysreflexia. Autonomic dysreflexia, also known as *autonomic hyperreflexia*, represents an acute episode of exaggerated sympathetic reflex responses that occur in persons with injuries at T6 and above, in which CNS control of spinal reflexes is lost (Fig. 35-19). It does not occur until spinal shock has resolved and autonomic reflexes return, most often within the first 6 months after injury. It is most unpredictable during the first year after injury but can occur throughout the person's lifetime.

Autonomic dysreflexia is characterized by vasospasm, hypertension ranging from mild (20 mm Hg above baseline) to severe (as high as 240/120 mm Hg or higher), skin pallor, and gooseflesh associated with the piloerector response.[46] Because baroreceptor function and parasympathetic control of heart rate travel by way of the cranial nerves, these responses remain intact. Continued hypertension produces a baroreflex-mediated vagal slowing of the heart rate to bradycardic levels. There is an accompanying baroreflex-mediated vasodilatation with flushed skin and profuse sweating above the level of injury, headache ranging from dull to severe and pounding, nasal stuffiness, and feelings of anxiety. A person may experience one, several, or all of the symptoms with each episode.

The stimuli initiating the dysreflexic response include visceral distention, such as a full bladder or rectum; stimulation of pain receptors, as occurs with pressure ulcers, ingrown toenails, dressing changes, and diagnostic or operative procedures; and visceral contractions, such as ejaculation, bladder spasms, or uterine contractions. In many cases, the dysreflexic response results from a full bladder.

Autonomic dysreflexia is a clinical emergency, and without prompt and adequate treatment, convulsions, loss of consciousness, and even death can occur. The major components of treatment include monitoring blood pressure while removing or correcting the initiating cause or stimulus. The person should be placed in an upright position, and all support hose or binders should be removed to promote venous pooling of blood and reduce venous return, thereby decreasing blood pressure. If the stimuli have been removed or the stimuli cannot be identified and the upright position is established, but the blood pressure remains elevated, drugs that block autonomic function are administered. Prevention of the type of stimuli that trigger the dysreflexic event is advocated.

Postural Hypotension. Postural, or orthostatic, hypotension usually occurs in persons with injuries at T4 to T6 and above and is related to the interruption of descending control of sympathetic outflow to blood vessels in the extremities and abdomen. Pooling of blood, along with gravitational forces, impairs venous return to the heart, and there is a subsequent decrease in cardiac output when the person is placed in an upright position. The signs of orthostatic hypotension include dizziness, pallor, excessive sweating above the level of the lesion, complaints of blurred vision, and possibly fainting. Postural hypotension usually is prevented by slow changes in position and measures to promote venous return.

Disruption of Other Functions

Temperature Regulation. The central mechanisms for thermoregulation are located in the hypothalamus. After SCI, the communication between the thermoregulatory centers in the hypothalamus and the sympathetic effector responses below the level of injury is disrupted; the ability to control blood vessel responses that conserve or dissipate heat is lost, as are the abilities to sweat and shiver. Higher levels of injury tend to produce greater

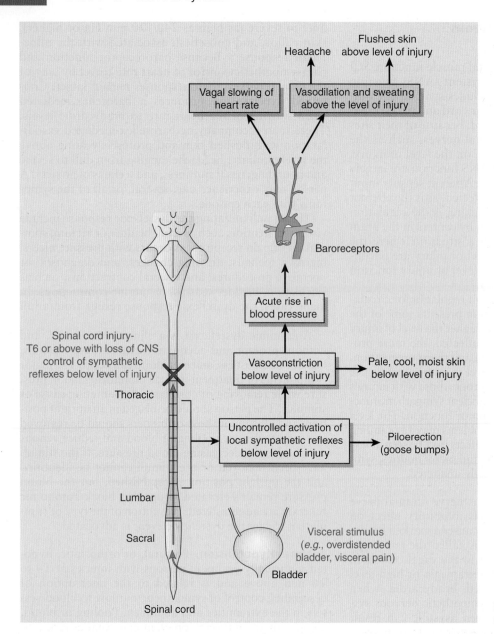

Headache Flushed skin above level of injury

Vagal slowing of heart rate

Vasodilation and sweating above the level of injury

Baroreceptors

Acute rise in blood pressure

Spinal cord injury- T6 or above with loss of CNS control of sympathetic reflexes below level of injury

Thoracic

Vasoconstriction below level of injury

Pale, cool, moist skin below level of injury

Uncontrolled activation of local sympathetic reflexes below level of injury

Piloerection (goose bumps)

Lumbar

Sacral

Visceral stimulus (*e.g.*, overdistended bladder, visceral pain)

Bladder

Spinal cord

FIGURE 35-19 Mechanisms of autonomic hyperreflexia.

disturbances in thermoregulation. In tetraplegia and high paraplegia, there are few defenses against changes in the environmental temperature, and body temperature tends to assume the temperature of the external environment, a condition known as *poikilothermy*. Persons with lower-level injuries have various degrees of thermoregulation. Disturbances in thermoregulation are chronic and may cause continual loss of body heat. Management consists of education in the adjustment of clothing and awareness of how environmental temperatures affect the person's ability to accommodate these changes.

Deep Vein Thrombosis and Edema. Persons with SCI are at high risk for development of deep vein thrombosis (DVT) and pulmonary emboli, particularly during the 2 to 3 weeks after injury.[47] The high risk of DVT in acute SCI is due to immobility, decreased vasomotor tone below the level of injury, and hypercoagulability and stasis of blood flow. Prevention strategies include the use of low–molecular-weight heparin, thigh-high graduated compression stockings, sequential compression boots, and early mobilization.[39,47] Electrical stimulation applied to the lower limbs has been reported to provide some benefit by achieving muscular contraction and improving venous flow. Local pain, a common symptom of DVT, is often absent because of sensory deficits. Thus, a regular schedule for visual inspection for local signs of DVT (*e.g.*, swelling) is important. Testing of persons at high risk of DVT include plethysmography and duplex ultrasonography.

Edema is also a common problem in persons with SCI. The development of edema is related to decreased peripheral vascular resistance, decreased muscle tone in the paralyzed limbs, and immobility that causes increased venous pressure and abnormal pooling of blood in the abdomen, lower limbs, and upper extremities. Edema in the dependent body parts usually is relieved by positioning to minimize gravitational forces or by using compression devices (*e.g.*, support stockings, binders) that encourage venous return.

Bladder, Bowel, and Sexual Function. Among the most devastating consequences of SCI is the loss of bowel, bladder, and sexual function.[48] Loss of bladder function results from disruption of neural pathways between the bladder and the reflex voiding center at the S2 to S4 level (*i.e.*, an LMN lesion) or between the reflex voiding center and higher brain centers for communication and coordinated sphincter control (*i.e.*, a UMN lesion). Persons with UMN lesions or spastic bladders lack awareness of bladder filling (*i.e.*, storage) and voluntary control of voiding (*i.e.*, evacuation). In LMN lesions or flaccid bladder dysfunction, lack of awareness of bladder filling and lack of bladder tone render the person unable to void voluntarily or involuntarily.

Bowel elimination is a coordinated function involving the enteric nervous system, the ANS, and the CNS. Persons with SCI above S2 to S4 develop spastic functioning of the defecation reflex and loss of voluntary control of the external anal sphincter. Damage to the cord at the S2 to S4 level causes flaccid functioning of the defecation reflex and loss of anal sphincter tone. Even though the enteric nervous system innervation of the bowel remains intact, without the defecation reflex, peristaltic movements are ineffective in evacuating stool.

Sexual function, as in bladder and bowel control, is mediated by the S2 to S4 segments of the spinal cord. The genital sexual response in SCI, which is manifested by an erection in men and vaginal lubrication in women, may be initiated by mental or touch stimuli, depending on the level of injury. The T11 to L2 cord segments have been identified as the mental-stimuli, or psychogenic, sexual response area, where autonomic nerve pathways in communication with the forebrain leave the cord and innervate the genitalia. The S2 to S4 cord segments have been identified as the sexual-touch reflex center. In T10 or higher injuries (UMN lesion), reflex sexual response to genital touch may occur freely. However, a sexual response to mental stimuli (T11 to L2) does not occur because of the spinal lesion blocking the communication pathway. In an injury at T12 or below (LMN lesion), the sexual reflex center may be damaged, and there may be no response to touch.

In men, the lack of normal erectile function or ability to experience penile sensations or orgasm is not a reliable indicator of fertility, which should be evaluated by an expert. In women, fertility is linked to resumption of menses, which usually is delayed 3 to 5 months after injury. There are hazards to pregnancy, labor, and use of birth control devices relative to SCI that require intervention from knowledgeable health care providers.

Skin Integrity. The entire surface of the skin is innervated by cranial or spinal nerves organized into dermatomes that show cutaneous distribution. The CNS and ANS also play a vital role in skin function. The sympathetic nervous system, through control of vasomotor and sweat gland activity, influences the health of the skin by ensuring adequate circulation, excretion of body fluids, and temperature regulation. The lack of sensory warning mechanisms and voluntary motor ability below the level of injury, coupled with circulatory changes, place the spinal cord–injured person at major risk for disruption of skin integrity. Significant factors associated with disruption of skin integrity are pressure, shearing forces, and localized trauma and irritation. Relieving pressure, allowing adequate circulation to the skin, and skin inspection are primary ways of maintaining skin integrity. Of all the complications after SCI, skin breakdown is the most preventable.

> **In summary,** UMN lesions are those involving neurons completely contained in the CNS. Amyotrophic lateral sclerosis is a progressive and devastating neurologic disorder that affects motor function. It affects both UMNs in the brain stem and cerebral cortex and LMNs in the spinal cord. Multiple sclerosis is a slowly progressive demyelinating disease of the CNS. The most frequent symptoms are paresthesia, optic neuritis, and motor weakness. The disease is usually characterized by exacerbations and remission. Initially, near-normal function returns between exacerbations.
>
> Spinal cord injury is a disabling neurologic condition most commonly caused by motor vehicle accidents, falls, and sports injuries. Dysfunctions of the nervous system after SCI comprise various degrees of sensorimotor loss and altered reflex activity based on the level of injury and extent of cord damage. Depending on the level of injury, the physical problems of SCI include spinal shock; ventilation and communication problems; ANS dysfunction that predisposes to the vasovagal response, autonomic hyperreflexia, impaired body temperature regulation, and postural hypotension; impaired muscle pump and venous innervation leading to edema of dependent areas of the body and risk of DVT; altered sensorimotor integrity that contributes to uncontrolled muscle spasms, altered pain responses, and threat to skin integrity; alterations in bowel and bladder elimination; and impaired sexual function.

Review Exercises

A 32-year-old woman presents with complaints of "drooping eyelids," difficulty chewing and swallowing, and weakness of her arms and legs that is less severe in the morning but becomes worse as the day progresses. She complains that climbing stairs and lifting objects is becoming increasingly difficult. Clinical examination confirms weakness of the eyelid and jaw muscles. She is told that she may have myasthenia gravis and is scheduled for testing using the short-acting acetylcholinesterase inhibitor edrophonium (Tensilon).

A. Explain the pathogenesis of this woman's symptoms as it relates to myasthenia gravis.

B. Explain how information from the administration of the acetylcholinesterase inhibitor edrophonium can be used to assist in the diagnosis of the disorder.

A 20-year-old man suffered spinal cord injury at the C2 to C3 level as the result of a motorcycle accident.

A. Explain the effects of this man's injury on ventilation and communication, sensorimotor function, autonomic nervous system function, bowel, bladder, and sexual function, and temperature regulation.

B. Autonomic dysreflexia, which is a threat to persons with spinal cord injuries at T6 or above, is manifested by hypertension, often to extreme levels, and bradycardia; constriction of skin vessels below the level of injury; and severe headache and nasal stuffiness. Explain the origin of the elevated blood pressure and bradycardia. The condition does not occur until spinal shock has resolved, and usually occurs only in persons with injuries at T6 and above. Explain.

Visit the Porth: Essentials of Pathophysiology: Concepts of Altered Health States web site (http://thePoint.LWW.com/PorthEssentials) for links to chapter-related resources on the Internet, all-new exclusive animations, chapter review questions, and more!

REFERENCES

1. Kandel E. R., Schwartz J. H., Jessell T. M. (Eds.). (2000). *Principles of neural science* (4th ed., pp. 816–831, 713–736, 853–867, 832–852). New York: McGraw-Hill.
2. Guyton A., Hall J. E. (2006). *Textbook of medical physiology* (11th ed., pp. 85–91, 673–613). Philadelphia: Elsevier Saunders.
3. Bear M. F., Connors B. W., Paradiso M. A. (2001). *Neuroscience: Exploring the brain* (2nd ed., pp. 473–477). Philadelphia: Lippincott Williams & Wilkins.
4. Hickey J. V. (2003). *Neurological and neurosurgical nursing* (5th ed., pp. 419–465, 469–480). Philadelphia: Lippincott Williams & Wilkins.
5. Kumar V., Abbas A. K., Fausto N. (Eds.). (2005). *Robbins and Cotran pathologic basis of disease* (7th ed., pp. 1325–1346). Philadelphia: Elsevier Saunders.
6. Sarnat H. B. (2004). Muscular dystrophies. In Behrman R. E., Kliegman R. M., Jenson H. B. (Eds.), *Nelson textbook of pediatrics* (17th ed., pp. 1873–1877). Philadelphia: Elsevier Saunders.
7. Tidball J. G., Wehling-Henricks, M. (2004). Evolving therapeutic strategies for Duchenne muscular dystrophy: Targeting downstream events. *Pediatric Research* 56, 831–841.
8. Katzung B. G. (2001). *Basic and clinical pharmacology* (8th ed., pp. 92–102). New York: Lange Medical Books/McGraw-Hill.
9. Vincent A., Palace J., Hilton-Jones D. (2001). Myasthenia gravis. *Lancet* 357, 2122–2128.
10. Drachman D. B. (1994). Myasthenia gravis. *New England Journal of Medicine* 330, 1797–1810.
11. Wittbrodt E. T. (1997). Drugs and myasthenia gravis. *Archives of Internal Medicine* 157, 399–408.
12. Bouldin T. W. (2005). The peripheral nervous system. In Rubin E., Gorstein F., Rubin R., et al. (Eds.), *Rubin's pathology: Clinicopathologic foundations of medicine* (4th ed., pp. 1491–1500). Philadelphia: Lippincott Williams & Wilkins.
13. Viera A. J. (2003). Management of carpal tunnel syndrome. *American Family Physician* 68, 265–272.
14. Katz J. N., Simmons B. P. (2002). Carpal tunnel syndrome. *New England Journal of Medicine* 346, 1807–1812.
15. Kuwabara S. (2004). Guillain-Barré syndrome. *Drugs* 64, 597–610.
16. Newswanger D. L., Warren C. R. (2004). Guillain-Barré syndrome. *American Family Physician* 69, 2405–2410.
17. Winer J. B. (2001). Guillain-Barré syndrome. *Molecular Pathology* 51, 381–385.
18. Deyo R. A. (1998). Low-back pain. *Scientific American* 283, 49–53.
19. Deyo R. A., Weinstein J. N. (2001). Low back pain. *New England Journal of Medicine* 344, 363–370.
20. Patel A. T., Ogle A. A. (2000). Diagnosis and management of acute low back pain. *American Family Physician* 61, 1779–1790.
21. Carragee E. J. (2005). Persistent low back pain. *New England Journal of Medicine* 352, 1891–1989.
22. Moore K. L., Dalley A. F. (2006). *Clinically oriented anatomy* (5th ed., pp. 497–519). Philadelphia: Lippincott Williams & Wilkins.
23. Bratton R. L. (1999). Assessment and management of acute low back pain. *American Family Physician* 60, 2299–2308.
24. Lang A. E., Lozano A. M. (1998). Parkinson's disease (Part 1 and Part 2). *New England Journal of Medicine* 339, 1044–1052, 1130–1143.
25. Steece-Collier K., Maries E., Kordower J. H. (2002). Etiology of Parkinson's disease: Genetics and environment revisited. *Proceedings of the National Academy of Science* 99, 1772–1374.
26. Parkinson J. (1817). *An essay on the shaking palsy.* London: Sherwood, Nelley & Jones.
27. Colcher A., Simuni T. (1999). Clinical manifestations of Parkinson's disease. *Medical Clinics of North America* 83, 327–347.
28. Guttman M., Kish S. J., Furukawa Y. (2003). Current concepts in the diagnosis and management of Parkinson disease. *Canadian Medical Association Journal* 168, 293–301.
29. The Deep-Brain Stimulation for Parkinson's Disease Group. (2001). Deep-brain stimulation of the subthalamic nucleus and of the pars interna of the globus pallidus in Parkinson's disease. *New England Journal of Medicine* 345, 956–963.

30. Mackin G. A. (1999). Optimizing care of patients with ALS. *Postgraduate Medicine* 105(4), 143–146.

31. Rowland L. P., Shneider N. A. (2001). Amyotropic lateral sclerosis. *New England Journal of Medicine* 344, 1688–1700.

32. Walling A. D. (1999). Amyotropic lateral sclerosis: Lou Gehrig's disease. *American Family Practitioner* 59, 1489–1496.

33. Noseworthy J. H., Lucchinetti C., Rodriguez M., et al. (2000). Multiple sclerosis. *New England Journal of Medicine* 343, 938–952.

34. Calabresi P. A. (2004). Diagnosis and management of multiple sclerosis. *American Family Physician* 70, 1935–1944.

35. Lublin F. D., Reingold S. C. (1996). Defining the clinical course of multiple sclerosis: Results of an international survey. *Neurology* 46, 907–911.

36. Keegan B. M., Noseworthy J. H. (2002). Multiple sclerosis. *Annual Review of Medicine* 53, 285–302.

37. Goodin D. S., Frohman E. M., Garmany G. P., Jr., et al. (2002). Disease modifying therapies in multiple sclerosis: Report of the Therapeutics and Technology Assessment Subcommittee of the American Academy of Neurology and the MS Council for Clinical Practice Guidelines. *Neurology* 58, 169–178.

38. National Spinal Cord Injury Statistical Center. (2003). *Spinal cord injury: Facts and figures at a glance.* Birmingham, AL: University of Alabama. [On-line]. Available: www.spinalcord.uab.edu.

39. Hickey J. V. (2003). *The clinical practice of neurological and neurosurgical nursing* (5th ed., pp. 407–480). Philadelphia: Lippincott Williams & Wilkins.

40. McDonald J. W. (2002). Spinal cord injury. *Lancet* 359, 417–425.

41. Buckley D. A., Guanci M. K. (1999). Spinal cord trauma. *Nursing Clinics of North America* 34, 661–687.

42. Chiles B. W., Cooper P. R. (1996). Acute spinal cord injury. *New England Journal of Medicine* 334, 514–520.

43. Atkinson P. P., Atkinson J. L. D. (1996). Spinal shock. *Mayo Clinic Proceedings* 71, 384–389.

44. Tator C. H., Fehlings M. G. (1999). Review of clinical trials in neuroprotection in acute spinal cord injury. *Neurosurgical Focus* 6(1), 1–14.

45. American Spinal Injury Association. (1992). *Standards of neurological and functional classification of spinal cord injury.* Chicago: Author.

46. Blackner J. (2003). Rehabilitation medicine: Autonomic dysreflexia. *Canadian Medical Association Journal* 169, 931–935.

47. Aito S., Pieri A., Marcelli F., et al. (2002). Primary prevention of deep venous thrombosis and pulmonary embolism in acute spinal cord injured patients. *Spinal Cord* 40, 300–303.

48. Benevento B. T., Sipski M. L. (2002). Neurogenic bladder, neurogenic bowel, and sexual dysfunction in people with spinal cord injury. *Physical Therapy* 62, 601–612.

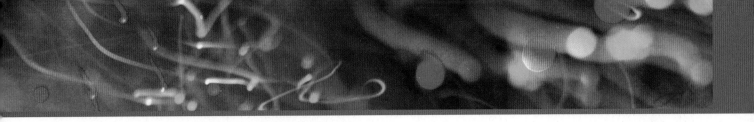

Chapter 36

Disorders of Brain Function

Anatomically and functionally, the brain is the most complex structure in the body. It controls our ability to think, our awareness of things around us, and our interactions with the outside world. Signals to and from various parts of the body are controlled by very specific areas in the brain. Therefore, the brain is much more vulnerable to focal lesions that in other organs might produce no significant effects. For example, an isolated renal infarct would not be expected to have a significant effect on kidney function, whereas an infarct of comparable size in a specific area of the brain could produce complete paralysis on one side of the body.[1]

Mechanisms and Manifestations of Brain Injury

The brain is protected from external forces by the rigid confines of the skull and the cushioning afforded by the cerebrospinal fluid (CSF). The metabolic stability required by its electrically active cells is maintained by a number of regulatory mechanisms, including the blood-brain barrier and autoregulatory mechanisms that ensure its blood supply.

MECHANISMS OF BRAIN INJURY

Injury to brain tissue can result from a number of conditions, including ischemia, trauma, tumors, degenerative processes, and metabolic derangements. Brain damage resulting from these disorders involves several common pathways, including the effects of hypoxia and ischemia; excitatory amino acid injury; cerebral edema; and increased intracranial pressure, herniation, and hydrocephalus. In many cases, the mechanisms of injury are interrelated.

Hypoxic and Ischemic Injury

The brain relies on the ability of the cerebral circulation to deliver sufficient oxygen for its energy needs. Although the brain makes up only 2% of the body weight, it receives one sixth of the resting cardiac output and accounts for 20% of the body's oxygen consumption.[1,2] By definition, *hypoxia* denotes a deprivation of oxygen with maintained blood flow, whereas *ischemia* represents a situation of greatly reduced or interrupted blood flow. The cellular effects of hypoxia and ischemia are quite different, and the brain tends to have different sensitivities to the two conditions. Hypoxia interferes with the delivery of oxygen, and ischemia interferes with the delivery of oxygen and glucose as well as the removal of metabolic wastes.

Hypoxia usually is seen in conditions such as exposure to reduced atmospheric pressure, carbon monoxide poisoning, severe anemia, and failure of the lungs to oxygenate the blood. Contrary to popular belief, hypoxia is fairly well tolerated, particularly in situations of chronic hypoxia. Neurons are capable of substantial anaerobic metabolism and are fairly tolerant of pure hypoxia; it commonly produces euphoria, listlessness, drowsiness, and impaired problem solving. Unconsciousness and convulsions may occur when hypoxia is sudden and severe. However, the effects of severe hypoxia (*i.e.*, anoxia) on brain function seldom are seen because the condition rapidly leads to cardiac arrest and ischemia.

Ischemia is seen in conditions of low blood flow. It can result from generalized low blood flow that leads to global ischemia, as in cardiac arrest, or from occlusion of a cerebral blood vessel, as in a stroke, that produces focal ischemia and often a localized infarct. If blood flow is not promptly restored, severe pathologic changes take place. Energy sources (*i.e.*, glucose and glycogen) are exhausted in 2 to 4 minutes, and cellular adenosine triphosphate (ATP) stores are depleted shortly thereafter. Much of the total energy requirement of neuronal tissue is spent on mechanisms for maintenance of ionic gradients across the cell membrane (*e.g.*, sodium-potassium pump), and breakdown of these mechanisms results in fluxes of sodium, potassium, and calcium ions. Excessive influx of sodium results in neuronal and interstitial edema. When ischemia is sufficiently severe or prolonged, infarction or death of all the cellular elements of the brain occurs.

Within the brain, certain regions and cell populations are more susceptible than others to hypoxic-ischemic injury.[1,3] For example, neurons are more susceptible than are the glial cells. Among the neurons, the pyramidal cells of the hippocampus, the Purkinje cells of the cerebellum, and the neurons of the globus pallidus of the basal ganglia are particularly sensitive to hypoxic-ischemic injury. Areas of the brain located at the border zones between the overlapping territories supplied by the major cerebral arteries, sometimes called the *watershed areas,* are also extremely vulnerable to ischemia. During events such as severe hypotension, these distal territories undergo a profound lowering of blood flow, predisposing to ischemia and infarction of brain tissues. As a consequence, areas of the cortex that are supplied by the major cerebral arteries usually regain function on recovery of adequate blood flow; however, infarctions may occur in the watershed boundary strips, resulting in focal neurologic deficits.

Although the threshold for ischemic neuronal injury is unknown, there is a period during which neurons can survive if blood flow is reestablished. Unfortunately, brain injury may not be reversible if the duration of ischemia is

such that the threshold of injury has been reached. Even after circulation has been reestablished, damage to blood vessels and changes in blood flow can prevent return of adequate tissue perfusion. This period of postischemic hypoperfusion is thought to be associated with mechanisms such as the level of desaturation of venous blood, capillary and venular clotting, or sludging of blood.[2] Because of sludging, blood viscosity increases and there is increased resistance to blood flow. There is also evidence of compromised flow resulting from an immediate vasomotor paralysis of the surface conducting blood vessels due to extracellular acidosis, followed by ischemic vasoconstriction.

Excitatory Amino Acid Injury

In many neurologic disorders, injury to neurons may be caused by overstimulation of receptors for specific amino acids such as glutamate and aspartate that act as excitatory neurotransmitters.[4,5] These neurologic conditions range from acute insults such as stroke, hypoglycemic injury, and trauma to chronic degenerative disorders such as Huntington disease and possibly Alzheimer dementia. The term *excitotoxicity* has been coined for the final common pathway for neuronal cell injury and death associated with excessive activity of the excitatory neurotransmitters and their receptor-mediated functions.

Glutamate is the principal excitatory neurotransmitter in the brain, and its interaction with specific receptors is responsible for many higher-order functions, including memory, cognition, movement, and sensation.[4,5] Many of the actions of glutamate are coupled with receptor-operated ion channels. One subtype in particular, called the *glutamate–N-methyl-D-*aspartate (NMDA) receptor, has been implicated in causing central nervous system (CNS) injury. This subtype of glutamate receptor opens a large-diameter calcium channel that permits calcium and sodium ions to enter the cell and allows potassium ions to exit, resulting in prolonged (seconds) action potentials. The uncontrolled opening of NMDA receptor–operated channels produces an increase in intracellular calcium and leads to a series of calcium-mediated processes called the *calcium cascade* (Fig. 36-1). Activation of the calcium cascade leads to the release of intracellular enzymes that cause protein breakdown, free radical formation, lipid peroxidation, fragmentation of deoxyribonucleic acid (DNA), and nuclear breakdown.

The effects of acute glutamate toxicity do not necessarily lead to cell death; they are reversible if excess glutamate can be removed or if its effects can be blocked. Drugs called *neuroprotectants* are being developed to interfere with the glutamate-NMDA pathway and thus reduce brain cell injury. These pharmacologic strategies may protect viable brain cells from irreversible damage in the setting of excitotoxicity. Pharmacologic strategies that are being explored include those that inhibit the synthesis or release of excitatory amino acid transmitters; block the NMDA receptors; stabilize the membrane potential to prevent initiation of the calcium cascade using lidocaine and certain barbiturates; and specifically block certain intracellular proteases, endonucleases, and lipases that are known to be cytotoxic.[5] The drug riluzole, which

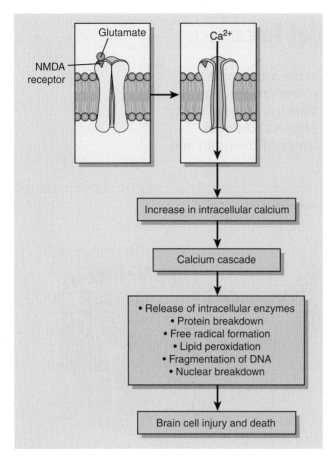

FIGURE 36-1 The role of the glutamate-NMDA receptor in brain cell injury.

acts presynaptically to inhibit glutamate release, currently is being used in the treatment of amyotrophic lateral sclerosis (see Chapter 35). Nimodipine, a calcium channel blocker that acts at the level of the NMDA receptor–operated channels, is being investigated for use in subarachnoid hemorrhage and acquired immunodeficiency syndrome dementia.[6] In the setting of ischemic stroke, multiple mechanisms of pharmacologic action, including NMDA receptor blockade, nitric oxide potentiation, and potassium channel opening, are being studied.[7]

Cerebral Edema

Cerebral edema, or brain swelling, is an increase in tissue volume secondary to abnormal fluid accumulation.[8] There are two types of brain edema: vasogenic and cytotoxic.[1]

Vasogenic edema occurs when integrity of the blood-brain barrier is disrupted, allowing fluid to escape into the extracellular fluid that surrounds brain cells. It occurs with conditions such as tumors, prolonged ischemia, hemorrhage, brain injury, and infectious processes (*e.g.,* meningitis) that impair the function of the blood-brain barrier and allow water and plasma proteins to leave the capillary and move into the interstitium. Vasogenic edema can be localized, as in the case of abscesses or neoplasms, or it may be more generalized. The functional manifestations of vasogenic edema include focal neurologic deficits,

disturbances in consciousness, and severe intracranial hypertension.

Cytotoxic edema involves the swelling of brain cells due to an increase in fluid in the intracellular space, chiefly the gray matter. Depending on the nature of the insult, cellular edema can also occur in the vascular endothelium, astrocytes, and the myelin-forming processes of oligodendrocytes. Cytotoxic edema can result from hypo-osmotic states, such as water intoxication or severe ischemia, that impair the function of the sodium-potassium membrane pump. This causes rapid accumulation of sodium in the cell, followed by movement of water along the osmotic gradient. Major changes in cerebral function, such as stupor and coma, occur with cytotoxic edema.

INCREASED INTRACRANIAL PRESSURE, HERNIATION, AND HYDROCEPHALUS

Increased intracranial pressure (ICP) is a common pathway for brain injury from different types of insults and agents. Excessive ICP can obstruct cerebral blood flow, destroy brain cells, displace brain tissue as in herniation, and otherwise damage delicate brain structures.

The cranial cavity contains blood, brain tissue, and CSF within the rigid confines of a nonexpandable skull.[9] Each of these three volumes contributes to the ICP, which normally is maintained within a range of 0 to 15 mm Hg when measured in the lateral ventricles. The volumes of each of these components can vary slightly without causing marked changes in ICP. This is because small increases in the volume of one component can be compensated for by a decrease in the volume of one or both of the other two components.[9] This association is called the *Monro-Kellie hypothesis.*

Abnormal variation in intracranial volume with subsequent change in ICP can occur because of a volume change in any of the three intracranial compartments. For example, an increase in tissue volume can result from a brain tumor, brain edema, or bleeding into brain tissue. An increase in blood volume develops when there is vasodilatation of cerebral vessels or obstruction of venous outflow. Excess production, decreased absorption, or obstructed circulation of CSF affords the potential for an increase in the CSF component.

According to the Monro-Kellie hypothesis, reciprocal compensation occurs among the three intracranial compartments.[9] Initial increases in ICP are largely buffered by a translocation of CSF to the spinal subarachnoid space and increased reabsorption of CSF. Of the three intracranial volumes, the tissue volume is relatively restricted in its ability to undergo change. The compensatory ability of the blood compartment is also limited by the small amount of blood that is in the cerebral circulation. The cerebral blood vessels contain less than 10% of the intracranial volume, most of which is contained in the low-pressure venous system. As the volume-buffering capacity of this compartment becomes exhausted, venous pressure increases and cerebral blood volume and ICP rise. In addition, cerebral blood flow is highly controlled by autoregulatory mechanisms (discussed later), which affect its compensatory capacity.

Understanding ➤ Intracranial Pressure

The intracranial pressure (ICP) is the pressure within the intracranial cavity. It is determined by (1) the pressure-volume relationships among the brain tissue, cerebrospinal fluid (CSF), and blood in the intracranial cavity; (2) the Monro-Kellie hypothesis, which relates to reciprocal changes among the intracranial volumes; and (3) the compliance of the brain and its ability to buffer changes in intracranial volume.

1

Intracranial volumes and pressure. The ICP represents the pressure exerted by the essentially incompressible tissue and fluid volumes of the three compartments contained within the rigid confines of the skull—the brain tissue and interstitial fluid (80%), the blood (10%), and the CSF (10%).

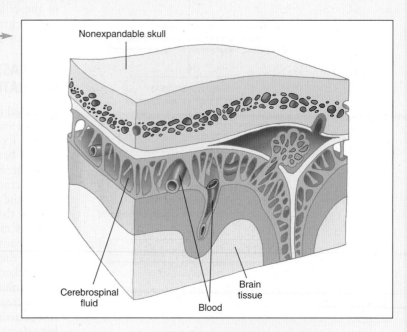

Nonexpandable skull

Cerebrospinal fluid

Blood

Brain tissue

2

Monro-Kellie hypothesis. Normally, a reciprocal relationship exists among the three intracranial volumes such that the ICP is maintained within normal limits. Because these volumes are practically incompressible, a change in one component must be balanced by an almost equal and opposite effect in one or both of the remaining components. This is known as the *Monro-Kellie hypothesis.*

Of the three intracranial volumes, the fluid in the CSF compartment is the most easily displaced. The CSF (**A**) can be displaced from the ventricles and cerebral subarachnoid space to the spinal subarachnoid space, and it can also undergo increased absorption or decreased production. Because most of the blood in the cranial cavity is contained in the low-pressure venous system, venous compression (**B**) serves as a means of displacing blood volume.

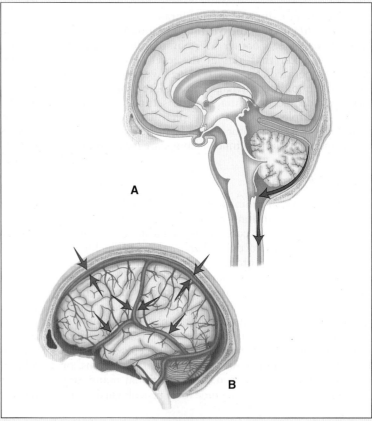

A

B

3

Compliance and the volume-pressure curve. Compliance, which refers to the ease with which a substance can be compressed or deformed, is a measure of the brain's ability to maintain its ICP during changes in intracranial volume. Compliance (C) represents the ratio of change (Δ) in volume (V) to change in pressure (P): $C = \Delta V/\Delta P$.

The dynamic effects of changes in intracranial volume and compliance on ICP can be illustrated on a graph with the volume represented on the horizontal axis and ICP on the vertical axis. The shape of the curve demonstrates the effect on ICP of adding volume to the intracranial cavity. From points A to B, the compensatory mechanisms are adequate, compliance is high, and the ICP remains relatively constant as volume is added to the intracranial cavity. At point B, the ICP is relatively normal, but the compensatory mechanisms have reached their limits, compliance is decreased, and ICP begins to rise with each change in volume. From points C to D, the compensatory mechanisms have been exceeded and ICP rises significantly with each increase in volume as compliance is lost.

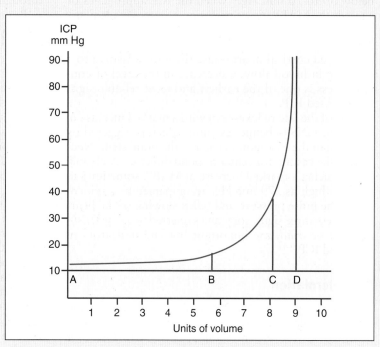

(From Hickey J. V. (2003). *Neurological and neurosurgical nursing* (5th ed., p. 286). Philadelphia: Lippincott Williams & Wilkins.)

The impact that increases in brain tissue, CSF, or blood volume have on ICP varies among individuals and depends on the extent of the increase, the effectiveness of the compensatory mechanisms, and the compliance of the brain tissue. Compliance is the measure of adaptive capacity or stiffness of the brain. It represents the ratio of change in volume to the resulting change in pressure.[9] In the case of intracranial volumes and pressure, an increase in intracranial volume will have little or no effect on ICP as long as compliance is high. Factors that influence compliance include the amount of volume increase, the time frame for accommodation, and the size of the intracranial compartments. For example, small volume increments over long periods of time can be accommodated more easily than a comparable amount introduced over a short period of time.

The cerebral perfusion pressure (CPP), which represents the difference between the mean arterial blood pressure (MABP) and the ICP, is the pressure perfusing the brain.[9,10] CPP is determined by the pressure gradient between the internal carotid artery and the subarachnoid veins. The MABP and ICP are often monitored frequently in persons with brain conditions that increase ICP and impair brain perfusion. Normal CPP ranges from 70 to 100 mm Hg. Brain ischemia develops at levels below 50 to 70 mm Hg.[9] When the ICP approaches or exceeds the MABP, tissue perfusion becomes inadequate, cellular hypoxia results, and, if the elevated pressure is maintained, neuronal death may occur. Because the highly specialized cortical neurons are the most sensitive to a decrease in blood flow, a decrease in the level of consciousness is one of the earliest and most reliable signs of increased ICP.

One of the late reflexes seen with a marked increase in ICP is the CNS ischemic response, which is triggered by ischemia of the vasomotor center in the brain stem. Neurons in the vasomotor center respond directly to ischemia by producing a marked increase in MABP, sometimes to levels as high as 270 mm Hg, accompanied by a widening of the pulse pressure and reflex slowing of the heart rate. These three signs, sometimes referred to as the *Cushing sign* or *triad,* are important but late indicators of increased ICP.[9–11]

Brain Herniation

The brain is protected by the nonexpandable skull and supporting septa, the falx cerebri and the tentorium cerebelli, that divide the intracranial cavity into *fossae* or compartments that normally protect against excessive movement. The falx cerebri is a sickle-shaped septum that separates the two hemispheres. The tentorium cerebelli is a tentlike structure, higher in the center than at the sides of the skull, which separates the occipital lobes of the brain from the cerebellum and much of the brain stem (Fig. 36-2A). It creates the area above the tentorium, called the *supratentorial space,* and the area below the tentorium, called the *infratentorial space.* Extending pos-

teriorly into the center of the tentorium is a large semicircular opening called the *incisura* or *tentorial notch.* The brain stem, blood vessels, and accompanying nerves pass through the incisura (see Fig. 36-2B).

Brain herniation is displacement of brain tissue under the falx cerebri or through the incisura of the tentorium cerebelli. It occurs when the pressure exerted by brain edema or a mass lesion is not evenly distributed, resulting in shifting or herniation of brain tissue from a compartment of higher pressure to one of lower pressure. The type of herniation syndrome that occurs is determined by the area of the brain that has herniated and the structure under which it has been pushed (see Fig. 36-2C). They are commonly divided into two broad categories, supratentorial and infratentorial, based on whether they are located above or below the tentorium.

Supratentorial Herniation. There are three major patterns of supratentorial herniation: cingulate or across the falx cerebri, uncal or lateral, and transtentorial or central.[1,9] *Cingulate herniation* (see Fig. 36-2C [1]) involves displacement of the cingulate gyrus and hemisphere beneath the sharp edges of the falx cerebri to the opposite side of the brain. *Uncal herniation* occurs when a lateral mass pushes the brain tissue centrally and forces the medial aspect of the temporal lobe, which contains the uncus and hippocampal gyrus, under the edge of the tentorial incisura, into the posterior fossa (see Fig. 36-2C [3]). *Transtentorial* or *central herniation* involves the downward displacement of the cerebral hemispheres, basal ganglia, diencephalon, and midbrain through the tentorial incisura.

Each supratentorial herniation syndrome has distinguishing features in the early phases, but as the forced downward displacement on the pons and medulla continues, clinical signs become similar (Table 36-1). Any

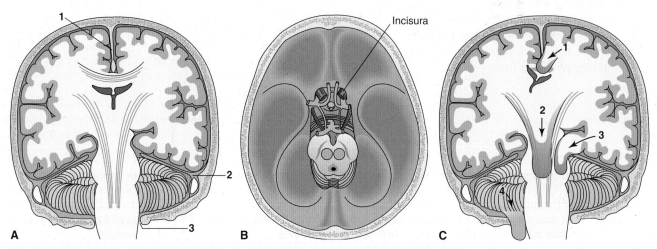

FIGURE 36-2 Supporting septa of the brain and patterns of herniation. (**A**) The falx cerebri [1], tentorium cerebelli [2], and foramen magnum [3]. (**B**) The location of the incisura or tentorial notch in relation to the cerebral arteries and oculomotor nerve. (**C**) Herniation of the cingulate gyrus under the falx cerebri [1], central or transtentorial herniation [2], uncal herniation of the temporal lobe into the tentorial notch [3], and infratentorial herniation of the cerebellar tonsils [4]. (Courtesy of Carole Russell Hilmer, C. M. I.)

TABLE 36-1	Key Structures and Clinical Signs of Cingulate, Transtentorial, and Uncal Herniation	
Herniation Syndrome	**Key Structures Involved**	**Key Clinical Signs**
Cingulate	Anterior cerebral artery	Leg weakness
Transtentorial	Reticular activating system	Altered level of consciousness
	Corticospinal tract	Decorticate posturing
		Rostral–caudal deterioration
Uncal	Cerebral peduncle	Hemiparesis
	Oculomotor nerve	Pupil dilatation
	Posterior cerebral artery	Visual field loss
	Cerebellar tonsils	
	Respiratory center	Respiratory arrest

of the supratentorial herniation syndromes can compress vascular and CSF flow, which can further complicate the neurologic manifestations of brain lesions. The progressive downward displacement from any of the supraventricular herniation syndromes can result in infratentorial or brain stem herniation, in which the medulla herniates into the foramen magnum. Death is immediate, caused by compression of cardiorespiratory centers in the medulla.

Infratentorial Herniation. Infratentorial herniation results from increased pressure in the infratentorial compartment. Herniation may occur superiorly (upward) through the tentorial incisura or inferiorly (downward) through the foramen magnum. Upward displacement of brain tissue can cause blockage of the aqueduct of Sylvius and lead to hydrocephalus and coma. Downward displacement of the midbrain through the tentorial notch or of the cerebellar tonsils through the foramen magnum can interfere with medullary functioning and cause cardiac or respiratory arrest. In cases of preexisting ICP, herniation may occur when the pressure is released from below, such as in a lumbar puncture.

Hydrocephalus

Enlargement of the CSF compartment occurs with hydrocephalus, which is defined as an abnormal increase in CSF volume in any part or all of the ventricular system (see Chapter 33, Fig. 33-22). There are two types of hydrocephalus: noncommunicating and communicating. *Hydrocephalus ex vacuo* refers to dilatation of the ventricular system and a compensatory increase in CSF volume secondary to a loss of brain tissue. It is commonly associated with other evidence of brain atrophy.[1,9]

Noncommunicating or obstructive hydrocephalus occurs when obstruction in the ventricular system prevents the CSF from reaching the arachnoid villi. CSF flow can be obstructed by congenital malformations, tumors encroaching on the ventricular system, inflammation, or hemorrhage.

Communicating hydrocephalus occurs as the result of impaired reabsorption of CSF from the arachnoid villi into the venous system. Decreased absorption can result from a block in the CSF pathway to the arachnoid villi or a failure of the villi to transfer the CSF to the venous system. It can occur if too few villi are formed, if postinfective (meningitis) scarring occludes them, or if the villi become obstructed with fragments of blood or infectious debris. Normal-pressure hydrocephalus is an important type of communicating hydrocephalus seen in older adults. It is accompanied by ventricular enlargement with compression of cerebral tissue but normal CSF pressure.

Similar pathologic patterns occur with both noncommunicating and communicating types of hydrocephalus. The cerebral hemispheres become enlarged, and the ventricular system is dilated behind the point of obstruction. The gyri on the surface of the brain tend to become less prominent as the sulci are compressed and the white matter is reduced in volume. The presence and extent of the increased ICP is determined by the amount of fluid accumulation and the type of hydrocephalus, the age at onset, and the rapidity and degree of pressure rise.

When hydrocephalus develops in utero or before the cranial sutures have fused in infancy, the ventricles expand beyond the point of obstruction, the cranial sutures separate, the head expands, and there is bulging of the fontanels[1,3] (Fig. 36-3). Because the skull is able to expand, signs of increased ICP usually are absent. Children with hydrocephalus are at risk for developmental disorders. Visual problems, including strabismus, visual field defects, and atrophy of the optic nerve, are common. Surgical placement of a shunt (*e.g.,* a ventriculoperitoneal shunt) that allows for diversion of excess CSF fluid is often used to prevent extreme enlargement of the head. The major complication of shunts is bacterial infection.

In contrast to hydrocephalus that develops in utero or during infancy, head enlargement does not occur in adults, and increases in ICP depend on whether the condition developed rapidly or slowly. Acute-onset hydrocephalus in adults usually is marked by symptoms of increased ICP, including headache, vomiting, and edema of the optic disk (papilledema).[9] If the obstruction is not relieved, mental deterioration eventually occurs. Slowly developing hydrocephalus is less likely to produce an increase in ICP, but it may produce deficits such as progressive dementia and gait changes.

Computed tomographic (CT) scans are used to diagnose all types of hydrocephalus. Treatment depends on the cause of the disorder. In noncommunicating hydrocephalus, shunting procedures are used to provide an

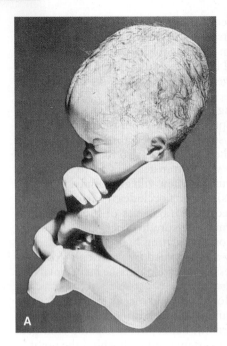

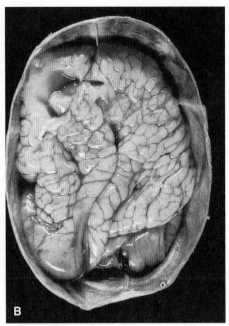

FIGURE 36-3 Congenital hydrocephalus. (**A**) Hydrocephalus occurring before the fusion of the cranial sutures causes pronounced enlargement of the head. (**B**) Removal of the calvarium demonstrates an atrophic and collapsed cerebral cortex. (From Trojanowski J. Q. [2005]. The central nervous system. In Rubin E., Gorstein F., Rubin R., et al. [Eds.], *Rubin's pathology: Clinicopathologic foundations of medicine* [4th ed., p. 1423]. Philadelphia: Lippincott Williams & Wilkins.)

alternative route for return of CSF to the circulation. In communicating hydrocephalus, attempts to clear the arachnoid villi of exudate may be made, and if this is unsuccessful, surgical shunting may be required.[9]

TRAUMATIC HEAD AND BRAIN INJURY

The term *head injury* is used to describe all structural damage to the skull and brain and has become synonymous with traumatic brain injury.[12–14] In the United States, traumatic brain injury is a leading cause of death among persons younger than 24 years of age. Of all the reasons for traumatic brain injury, lack of helmets for motorcyclists and bicycles, lack of restraint for auto passengers, and consumption of alcohol are the most common.[14]

Head injuries can involve both closed injuries and open wounds. Skull fractures can be divided into three groups: simple, depressed, and basilar. A *simple* or *linear* skull fracture is a break in the continuity of bone. A *comminuted* skull fracture refers to a splintered or multiple fracture line. When bone fragments are embedded into the brain tissue, the fracture is said to be *depressed.*

A fracture of the bones that form the base of the skull is called a *basilar* skull fracture. The ethmoid cribriform plate, through which the olfactory fibers enter the skull, represents the most fragile portion of the neurocranium and is shattered in basal skull fractures. A frequent complication of basilar skull fractures is leakage of CSF from the nose (rhinorrhea) or ear (otorrhea); this occurs because of the proximity of the base of the skull to the nose and ear. This break in protection of the brain becomes a possible source of infection of the meninges or of brain substance. There may be lacerations to the vessels of the dura, with resultant intracranial bleeding. Skull fractures may also damage

the cranial nerves (I, II, III, VII, VIII) as they exit the cranial vault.

Types of Injury

The effects of traumatic head injuries can be divided into two categories: primary and secondary injuries.[9,14] Primary injuries are those that occur at the time of injury. The cerebral injury may be focal (contusion or laceration) or diffuse (concussion or diffuse axonal injury). Secondary injuries result from complicating processes, such as hemorrhage, ischemia, and infection, that are initiated at the moment of injury, but which present later in the clinical course.

The major mechanisms of primary craniocerebral injury include direct-contact phenomena and head motions of acceleration and deceleration. When the mechanical forces inducing head injury cause bouncing of the brain in the closed confines of the rigid skull, a phenomenon called *coup-contrecoup injury* occurs.[3,9] Because the brain floats freely in the CSF, blunt force to the head can cause the brain to accelerate in the skull, and then abruptly decelerate on hitting the inner confines of the skull. The direct contusion of the brain at the site of external force is referred to as a *coup* injury, whereas the opposite side of the brain receives the *contrecoup* injury from rebound against the inner skull surfaces (Fig. 36-4). As the brain strikes the rough surface of the cranial vault, brain tissue, blood vessels, nerve tracts, and other structures are bruised and torn, resulting in contusions and hematomas.

Secondary injuries include the various processes that lead to cellular injury and death. They include biochemical changes, ischemic brain injury, intracranial hemorrhage, cerebral edema, and increased ICP. Ischemia is

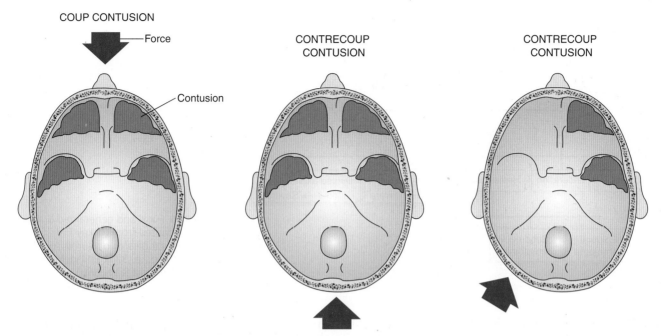

COUP CONTUSION

Force

Contusion

CONTRECOUP
CONTUSION

CONTRECOUP
CONTUSION

FIGURE 36-4 Mechanisms of cerebral contusion. The cerebral hemispheres float in the cerebrospinal fluid. Rapid deceleration or acceleration of the skull causes the cortex to impact forcefully on the anterior or middle fossa. The position of the contusion is determined by the direction of the force and the intracranial anatomy. (Courtesy of Dmitri Karetnikov, artist.) (From Trojanowski J. Q. [2005]. The central nervous system. In Rubin E., Gorstein F., Rubin R., et al. [Eds.], *Rubin's pathology: Clinicopathologic foundations of medicine* [4th ed., p. 1430]. Philadelphia: Lippincott Williams & Wilkins.)

considered to be the most common cause of secondary brain injury. It can result from the hypoxia and hypotension that occur during the resuscitation process or from the impairment of regulatory mechanisms by which cerebrovascular responses maintain an adequate blood flow and oxygen supply.[15] Insults that occur immediately after injury or in the course of resuscitation efforts are important determinants of the outcome from severe brain injury. The significance of secondary injuries depends on the extent of damage caused by the primary injury.

Even if there is no break in the skull a blow to the head can cause severe and diffuse brain damage. Such closed injuries can vary in severity and can be classified as focal or diffuse[1,9,14] (Fig. 36-5). Diffuse injuries include concussion and diffuse axonal injury and focal injuries, contusions, lacerations, and hemorrhage.

Concussion. The term *concussion* refers to a momentary interruption of brain function with or without loss of consciousness.[1,9,14] In mild head injury, there may be momentary loss of consciousness without demonstrable neurologic symptoms or residual damage, except for possible residual amnesia. Microscopic changes usually can be detected in the neurons and supporting tissues within hours of injury. Although recovery usually takes place within 24 hours, mild symptoms, such as headache, irritability, insomnia, and poor concentration and memory,

may persist for months. This is known as the *postconcussion syndrome*. Because these complaints are vague and subjective, they sometimes are regarded as being of psychological origin.

Diffuse Axonal Injury. Diffuse axonal injury is a primary injury with diffuse microscopic damage to axons in the cerebral hemisphere, corpus callosum, and brain stem[1,9] (Fig. 36-6). It is responsible for most cases of posttraumatic dementia and, in conjunction with hypoxic-ischemic injury, is the most common cause of persistent vegetative state. The lesions of diffuse axonal injury result from sudden deceleration or acceleration forces sufficient to stretch or, in extreme cases, tear nerve cell processes within the white matter of the brain.

Contusion. A *contusion* is a bruise to the cortical surface of the brain caused by blunt head trauma.[1,7] Contusions may be single or multiple and occur at any place where the brain comes in contact with the skull. The apices of the gyri are most susceptible, whereas the cerebral cortex along the sulci is less vulnerable. They are most common in the frontal lobes along the orbital gyri, and the temporal lobes.[1]

Contusions are usually the result of anteroposterior displacement, when the moving head strikes a fixed object. As the brain strikes the rough surface of the cranial vault, brain tissue, blood vessels, nerve tracts, and

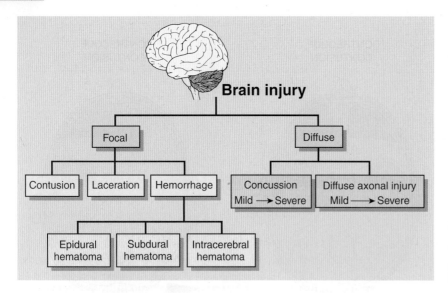

FIGURE 36-5 Focal and generalized brain injuries. (Adapted from Hickey J. V. [2005]. *Neurological and neurosurgical nursing* [5th ed., p. 374]. Philadelphia: Lippincott Williams & Wilkins.)

other structures are bruised and torn. The extent of brain damage that occurs depends on the force causing the injury. If the force is minimal, the contusion is limited to the apices of the gyri. Greater forces destroy larger expanses of the cortex, creating deeper lesions that extend into the white matter or lacerate the cortex and initiate cortical and subcortical hemorrhages. Cerebral contusions, particularly those accompanied by tearing of the superficial layers of the brain, are an important cause of traumatic subarachnoid hemorrhage.

Contusions cause permanent damage to brain tissue. The bruised, necrotic tissue is phagocytized by macrophages, and scar tissue formed by astrocyte proliferation persists as a crater.

Hematomas

Hematomas result from vascular injury and bleeding. Depending on the anatomic position of the ruptured vessel, bleeding may involve the development of an epidural hematoma, subdural hematoma, or an intracerebral hematoma[1,3,9] (Fig. 36-7).

Epidural Hematoma. An epidural hematoma is one that develops between the inner table of the bones of the skull and the dura. It usually results from a tear in an artery, most often the middle meningeal, which is located under the thin temporal bone. Because bleeding is arterial in origin, rapid compression of the brain occurs from the expanding hematoma. Epidural hematomas are more common in young persons because the dura is not as firmly attached to the skull surface as it is in older persons. Typically, a person with an epidural hematoma presents with a history of head injury and a brief period of unconsciousness, followed by a lucid period in which consciousness is regained, followed by rapid progression to unconsciousness. The lucid interval does not always occur, but when it does, it is of great diagnostic value. With rapidly developing unconsciousness, there are focal symptoms related to the area of the brain involved. These symptoms can include ipsilateral (same side) pupil dilation and contralateral (opposite side) hemiparesis. If the hematoma is not removed, the condition progresses, with increased ICP, tentorial herniation, and death. However, prognosis is excellent if the hematoma is removed before loss of consciousness occurs.

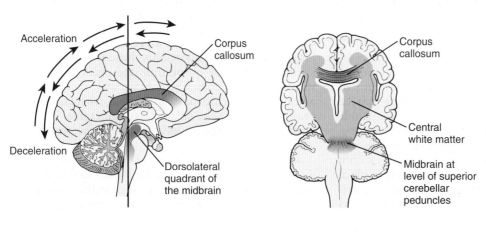

FIGURE 36-6 Diffuse axonal injury. Diffuse axonal injury results from acceleration-deceleration and shearing of the brain. Depending on the severity of the injury, the areas of brain most affected are the corpus callosum, the dorsolateral area of the midbrain, and the parasagittal white matter (Adapted from Hickey J. V. [2003]. *Neurological and neurosurgical nursing* [5th ed., p. 382]. Philadelphia: Lippincott Williams & Wilkins.)

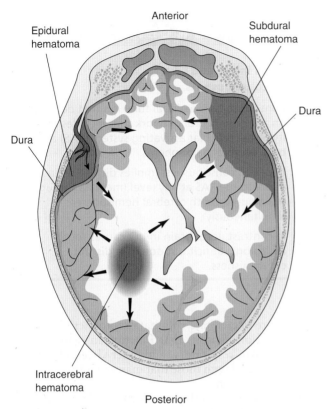

FIGURE 36-7 Location of epidural, subdural, and intracerebral hematomas.

Subdural Hematoma. A subdural hematoma develops in the area between the dura and the arachnoid (subdural space) and usually is the result of a tear in the small bridging veins that connect veins on the surface of the cortex to dural sinuses (Fig. 36-8). These veins are readily snapped in head injury when the brain moves suddenly in relation to the skull. A subdural hematoma develops more slowly than an epidural hematoma because the tear is in the venous, rather than the arterial, system.

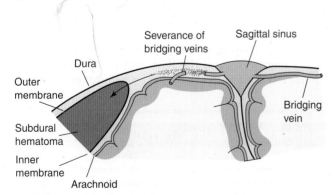

FIGURE 36-8 Mechanism of bleeding in subdural hematoma. (Courtesy of Dmitri Karetnikov, artist.) (From Trojanowski J. Q. [2005]. The central nervous system. In Rubin E., Gorstein F., Rubin R., et al. [Eds.], *Rubin's pathology: Clinicopathologic foundations of medicine* [4th ed., p. 1430]. Philadelphia: Lippincott Williams & Wilkins.)

Subdural hematomas are classified as acute, subacute, or chronic. Symptoms of an acute subdural hematoma are seen within 24 hours of the injury. Acute subdural hematomas progress rapidly and are associated with a high mortality rate because of the severe secondary injuries related to edema and uncontrolled rise in ICP. Subacute hematomas do not produce symptoms until 2 to 10 days after injury. There may be a period of improvement in the level of consciousness and neurologic symptoms, followed by deterioration if the hematoma is not removed.

The symptoms of chronic subdural hematomas may not arise until several weeks after the injury, so much later that the person may not remember having had a head injury. This is especially true of the older person with fragile vessels whose brain has shrunk away from the dura. Seepage of blood into the subdural space may occur slowly. Because the blood in the subdural space is not absorbed, fibroblastic activity begins, and the hematoma becomes encapsulated.[3] Within this encapsulated area, the blood cells are slowly lysed, and a fluid with a high osmotic pressure is formed. This creates an osmotic gradient, with fluid from the surrounding subarachnoid space being pulled into the hematoma, causing the mass to increase in size and exert pressure on the surrounding intracranial contents. In some instances, the clinical picture is less defined, with the most prominent symptom being a decreasing level of consciousness indicated by drowsiness, confusion, and apathy. The person also may have a headache.

Traumatic Intracerebral Hematomas. Traumatic intracerebral hematomas may be single or multiple. They can occur in any lobe of the brain but are most common in the frontal or temporal lobes. They may occur in association with the severe motion that the brain undergoes during head injury, or a contusion can coalesce into a hematoma. Intracerebral hematomas occur more frequently in older persons and alcoholics whose brain vessels are more friable.

The signs and symptoms produced by an intracerebral hematoma depend on its size and location in the brain. Signs of increased ICP can be manifested if the hematoma is large and encroaching on vital structures. A hematoma in the temporal lobe can be dangerous because of the potential for lateral herniation.

MANIFESTATIONS OF GLOBAL BRAIN INJURY

Global, or diffuse, brain injury, whether due to head trauma, stroke, or other pathologic processes, is manifested by alterations in sensory and motor function and by changes in the level of consciousness. Severe injury that seriously compromises brain function may result in brain death.

The cerebral hemispheres are the most susceptible to damage, and the most frequent sign of brain dysfunction is altered level of consciousness and change in behavior. As the brain structures in the diencephalon, midbrain, pons, and medulla are affected, additional respiratory signs, pupillary and eye movement reflexes, and motor signs become evident (Table 36-2). Hemodynamic and respiratory instability are the last signs to occur because their regulatory centers are located low in the medulla.

In progressive brain deterioration, the person's neurologic capabilities appear to deteriorate in stepwise fashion. Similarly, as neurologic function returns, there appears to be stepwise progress to higher levels of consciousness. Deterioration of brain function from supratentorial lesions tends to follow a rostral-to-caudal stepwise progression, which is observed as the brain initially compensates for injury and subsequently decompensates with loss of autoregulation and cerebral perfusion. Infratentorial (brain stem) lesions may lead to an early, sometimes abrupt disturbance in consciousness without any orderly rostrocaudal progression of neurologic signs.

Levels of Consciousness

Consciousness is the state of awareness of self and the environment and of being able to become oriented to new stimuli.[12,16] It has traditionally been divided into two components: (1) arousal and wakefulness and (2) content and cognition. The content and cognition aspects of consciousness are determined by a functioning cerebral cortex. Arousal and wakefulness require the concurrent functioning of both cerebral hemispheres and an intact reticular activating system (RAS) in the brain stem.

The reticular formation is a diffuse, primitive system of interlacing nerve cells and fibers in the brain stem that receives input from multiple sensory pathways (Fig. 36-9). Anatomically, the reticular formation constitutes the central core of the brain stem, extending from the medulla through the pons to the midbrain, which is continuous caudally with the spinal cord and rostrally with the subthalamus, the hypothalamus, and the thalamus.[9,16] Fibers from the RAS also project to the autonomic nervous system and motor systems. The hypothalamus plays a predominant role in maintaining homeostasis through integration of somatic, visceral, and endocrine functions. Inputs from the reticular formation, vestibulospinal projections, and other motor systems are integrated to provide a continuously adapting background of muscle tone

---

KEY CONCEPTS

Brain Injury and Levels of Consciousness

➤ Consciousness is a global function that depends on a diffuse neural network that includes activity of the reticular activating system (RAS) and both cerebral hemispheres.

➤ Impaired consciousness implies diffuse brain injury to the RAS at any level (medulla through thalamus) or both cerebral hemispheres simultaneously.

➤ In contrast, local brain injury causes focal neurologic deficit but does not disrupt consciousness.

---

and posture to facilitate voluntary motor actions. Reticular formation neurons that function in regulation of cardiovascular, respiratory, and other visceral functions are intermingled with those that maintain other reticular formation functions.

Ascending fibers of the reticular formation, known as the *ascending RAS*, transmit activating information to all parts of the cerebral cortex. The flow of information in the ascending RAS activates the hypothalamic and limbic structures that regulate emotional and behavioral responses such as those that occur in response to pain and loud noises, and they exert facilitatory effects on cortical neurons. Without cortical activation, a person is less able to detect specific stimuli, and the level of consciousness is reduced. The pathways for the ascending RAS travel through the midbrain, and lesions of the midbrain can interrupt RAS activity, leading to altered levels of consciousness and coma.

Any deficit in level of consciousness, from mild confusion to stupor or coma, indicates injury to either the RAS or to both cerebral hemispheres concurrently. For example, consciousness may decline owing to severe systemic metabolic derangements that affect both hemispheres, or from head trauma causing shear injuries to white matter of both the RAS and the cerebral hemispheres. Brain injuries that affect a hemisphere unilater-

---

TABLE 36-2	Key Signs in Rostral-to-Caudal Progression of Brain Lesions
Level of Brain Injury	**Key Clinical Signs**
Diencephalon	Impaired consciousness (see Table 36-3); small, reactive pupils; intact oculocephalic reflex; decorticate posturing; Cheyne-Stokes respirations
Midbrain	Coma, fixed, midsize pupils; impaired oculocephalic reflex; neurogenic hyperventilation; decerebrate posturing
Pons	Coma, fixed, irregular pupils; dysconjugate gaze; impaired cold caloric stimulation; loss of corneal reflex; hemiparesis/quadriparesis; decerebrate posturing; apneustic respirations
Medulla	Coma, fixed pupils, flaccidity, loss of gag and cough reflexes, ataxic/apneic respirations

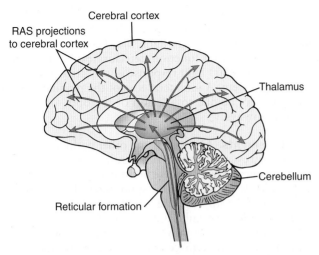

FIGURE 36-9 The ascending reticular activating system. Ascending sensory tracts send axon collateral fibers to the reticular formation. These give rise to fibers synapsing in the nonspecific nuclei of the thalamus. From there, the nonspecific thalamic projections influence widespread areas of the cerebral cortex and limbic system.

ally and also spare the RAS, such as cerebral infarction, usually do not impair consciousness.

Altered Levels of Consciousness. Consciousness is evaluated clinically as the ability of a person to respond appropriately to environmental stimuli. A fully conscious person is totally aware of her or his surroundings. Two aspects of consciousness must be assessed: arousability and content of consciousness in terms of the appropriateness of a person's responses.[9,16]

Arousability exists on a continuum that includes consciousness, confusion, delirium, obtundation, stupor, and coma (Table 36-3). The earliest signs of diminution in level of consciousness are inattention, mild confusion, disorientation, and blunted responsiveness. With further deterioration, the delirious person becomes markedly inattentive and variably lethargic or agitated. Persons who cannot be fully aroused are obtunded, and those who remain in a sleeplike state are stuporous. A person who cannot make a purposeful response to stimulation is comatose.

Because of its simplicity of application, the Glasgow Coma Scale has gained almost universal acceptance as a method for assessing the level of consciousness in persons with brain injury[9,17,18] (Table 36-4). Numbered scores are given to responses of eye opening, verbal utterances, and motor responses. The total score is the sum of the best response in each category.

The content of consciousness may be assessed in terms of the appropriateness of the person's responses. Impairment of specific cognitive processes may leave the person unable to appreciate or respond to entire classes of stimuli. Delirium occurs when a person with diffuse cortical impairment misinterprets sensory information, causing inappropriate excitement or arousal.

Other Manifestations of Deteriorating Brain Function

Additional elements in the initial neurologic evaluation of a person with brain injury provide important clues to the cause of coma. These elements include respiratory patterns, level of arousal and motor responses, the pupillary light response, and eye movements.[16]

Respiratory Responses. The first systems to be evaluated in a comatose person are the cardiovascular and respiratory systems. Diffuse forebrain impairment without brain stem injury induces a pattern yawning and sighing, with progression to Cheyne-Stokes breathing (*i.e.*, waxing and waning of respirations with periods of apnea). With progression continuing to the mid-brain, respirations change to neurogenic hyperventilation, in which the frequency of respirations may exceed 40 breaths per minute because of uninhibited stimulation of inspiratory and expiratory centers. With medullary involvement, respirations become ataxic (*i.e.*, totally uncoordinated and irregular). Only a bilateral lesion at the level of the ventrolateral medulla or more caudally will cause complete apnea. Complete ventilatory assistance is often required at this point.

Level of Arousability and Motor Responses. Depressed responsiveness to painful stimuli indicates the depth of coma. With the early onset of unconsciousness there is some combative movement and purposeful

TABLE 36-3	Descending Levels of Consciousness and Their Characteristics
Level of Consciousness	**Characteristics**
Confusion	Disturbance of consciousness characterized by impaired ability to think clearly, and to perceive, respond to, and remember current stimuli; also disorientation
Delirium	State of disturbed consciousness with motor restlessness, transient hallucinations, disorientation, and sometimes delusions
Obtundation	Disorder of decreased alertness with associated psychomotor retardation
Stupor	A state in which the person is not unconscious but exhibits little or no spontaneous activity
Coma	A state of being unarousable and unresponsive to external stimuli or internal needs; often determined by the Glasgow Coma Scale

(Data from Bates D. [1993]. The management of medical coma. *Journal of Neurology, Neurosurgery, and Psychiatry* 56, 59.)

TABLE 36-4	The Glasgow Coma Scale	
Test		**Score***
Eye Opening (E)		
Spontaneous		4
To call		3
To pain		2
None		1
Motor Response (M)		
Obeys commands		6
Localizes pain		5
Normal flexion (withdrawal)		4
Abnormal flexion (decorticate)		3
Extension (decerebrate)		2
None (flaccid)		1
Verbal Response (V)		
Oriented		5
Confused conversation		4
Inappropriate words		3
Incomprehensible sounds		2
None		1

*GCS Score = E + M + V. Best possible score = 15; worst possible score = 3.

movement in response to pain. As coma progress, noxious stimuli can initiate rigidity and abnormal postures if the motor tracts are interrupted at specific levels.[16] *Decorticate* (flexion) *posturing* is characterized by flexion of the arms, wrists and fingers, with abduction of the upper extremities, internal rotation, and plantar flexion of the lower extremities (Fig. 36-10A). It results from lesions of the cerebral hemisphere or internal capsule. *Decerebrate* (extensor) *posturing* results from increased muscle excitability (see Fig. 36-10B). It is characterized by rigidity of the arms with palms of the hands turned away from the body and stiffly extended legs with plantar flexion of the feet. This response occurs when lesions of the diencephalon extend to involve the midbrain and upper brain stem. Both decerebrate and decorticate posturing are poor prognostic signs.

Pupillary Reflexes. The pupillary reflex is elicited by shining a bright light in one eye. Although the pupils may initially respond briskly to light, they become unreactive and dilated as brain function deteriorates.[16] A bilateral loss of the pupillary light response is indicative of lesions of the brain stem. A unilateral loss of the pupillary light response may be due to a lesion of the optic or oculomotor pathways.

Eye Movements. More than any other pathways, those that control eye movements run parallel to the ascending RAS.[16] In persons with diffuse brain injury, the eyes often rove aimlessly or do not move spontaneously. However, there should be appropriate conjugate eye movements when a vestibular stimulus is provided. The oculocephalic reflex (doll's-head eye movement) can be used to determine if the brain stem centers for eye movement are intact (Fig. 36-11). If the oculocephalic reflex is inconclusive, and if there are no contraindications, the oculovestibular (*i.e.*, cold caloric test, in which cold water is instilled into the ear canal) may be used to elicit nystagmus (see Chapter 37).

Brain Death

Brain death is defined as the irreversible loss of function of the brain, including the brain stem.[19-21] Irreversibility implies that brain death cannot be reversed. Some conditions such as drug and metabolic intoxication can cause cessation of brain functions that is completely reversible, even when they produce clinical cessation of brain functions and electroencephalographic silence. This needs to be excluded before declaring that a person is brain dead.

With advances in scientific knowledge and technology that have provided the means for artificially maintaining ventilatory and circulatory function, the definition of death has had to be continually reexamined. In 1995, the Quality of Standards Subcommittee of the American Academy of Neurology published the clinical parameters for determining brain death and procedures for testing

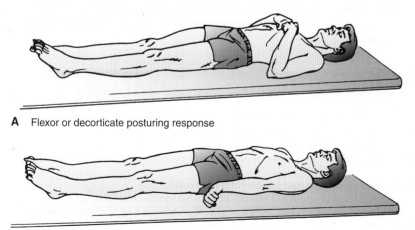

A   Flexor or decorticate posturing response

B   Extensor or decerebrate posturing

FIGURE 36-10 Abnormal posturing. (**A**) Decorticate rigidity. In decorticate rigidity, the upper arms are held at the sides, with elbows, wrists, and fingers flexed. The legs are extended and internally rotated. The feet are plantar flexed. (**B**) Decerebrate rigidity. In decerebrate rigidity, the jaws are clenched and neck extended. The arms are adducted and stiffly extended at the elbows with the forearms pronated, wrists and fingers flexed. (From Fuller J., Schaller-Ayers J. [1994]. *Health assessment: A nursing approach* [2nd ed.]. Philadelphia: J. B. Lippincott.)

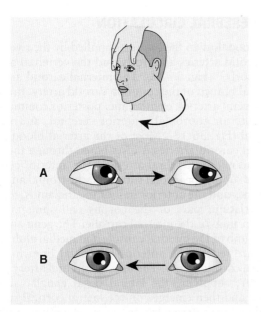

FIGURE 36-11 The *doll's-head eye response* demonstrates the always-present vestibular static reflexes without forebrain interference or suppression. Severe damage to the forebrain or to the brain stem rostral to the pons often results in loss of rostral control of these static vestibular reflexes. If the person's head is moved from side to side or up and down, the eyes will move in conjugate gaze to the opposite side (**A**), much like those of a doll with counterweighted eyes. If the doll's-head phenomenon is observed, brain stem function at the level of the pons is considered intact (in a comatose person). In the unconscious person without intact brain stem function and vestibular static reflexes, the eyes stay in midposition (fixed) or turn in the same direction (**B**) as the head is turned.

persons older than 18 years of age.[21] According to these parameters, "brain death is the absence of clinical brain function when the proximate cause is known and demonstrably irreversible."[21] Clinical examination must disclose at least the absence of responsiveness, brain stem reflexes, and respiratory effort. Brain death is a clinical diagnosis, and a repeat evaluation at least 6 hours later is recommended. Longer periods of observation of absent brain activity are required in cases of children, drug overdose (*e.g.*, barbiturates, other CNS depressants), drug toxicity (*e.g.*, neuromuscular blocking drugs, aminoglycoside antibiotics), neuromuscular diseases such as myasthenia gravis, hypothermia, and shock. Medical circumstances may require use of confirmatory tests.

Medical documentation should include cause and irreversibility of the condition, absence of brain stem reflexes and motor responses to pain, absence of respiration with a PCO_2 of 60 mm Hg or more, and the justification for use of confirmatory tests and their results. Apnea is confirmed after ventilation with pure oxygen 10 minutes before withdrawal from the ventilator, followed by passive flow of oxygen. This method allows blood levels of carbon dioxide to rise to a PCO_2 of 60 mm Hg after a 10-minute period of apnea, without hazardously lowering the oxygen content of the blood. If respiratory reflexes are intact, the hypercarbia that devel-

ops should stimulate ventilatory effort within 30 seconds. Spontaneous breathing efforts indicate that the brain stem is functioning. Confirmatory tests of brain death include conventional angiography (*i.e.*, no intracerebral filling at the level of the carotid bifurcation or circle of Willis), transcranial Doppler ultrasonography, technetium-99m hexamethylpropyleneamineoxime brain scan (*i.e.*, no uptake of isotope in brain parenchyma), somatosensory evoked potentials, and electroencephalography (EEG). In the United States, EEG testing is often used to establish brain death. EEG testing should reveal no electrical activity during at least 30 minutes of recording that adheres to the minimal technical criteria for EEG recording in suspected brain death as adopted by the American Electroencephalographic Society, including use of 16-channel EEG instruments.

Persistent Vegetative State

Advances in the care of brain-injured persons during the past several decades have resulted in survival of many persons who previously would have died. Unfortunately, most persons in prolonged coma who survive evolve to what often is called the *persistent vegetative state*. The vegetative state is characterized by loss of all cognitive functions and the unawareness of self and surroundings. Reflex and vegetative functions remain, including sleepwake cycles.[22] Persons in the vegetative state must be fed and require full nursing care.

The criteria for diagnosis of vegetative state include the absence of awareness of self and environment and an inability to interact with others; the absence of sustained or reproducible voluntary behavioral responses; lack of language comprehension; sufficiently preserved hypothalamic and brain stem function to maintain life; bowel and bladder incontinence; and variably preserved cranial nerve (*e.g.*, pupillary, gag) and spinal cord reflexes.[22] The diagnosis of persistent vegetative state requires that the condition has continued for at least 1 month.

In summary, many of the agents that cause brain damage do so through common pathways, including hypoxia or ischemia, accumulation of excitatory neurotransmitters, cerebral edema, and increased ICP. Deprivation of oxygen (*i.e.*, hypoxia) or blood flow (*i.e.*, ischemia) can have deleterious effects on the brain structures. Ischemia can be focal, as in stroke, or global. Global ischemia occurs when blood flow is inadequate to meet the metabolic needs of the entire brain, as in cardiac arrest. The term *excitotoxicity* has been coined for the final common pathway for neuronal cell injury and death associated with excessive activity of excitatory neurotransmitters, particularly glutamine.

Cerebral edema represents an increase in tissue volume secondary to abnormal fluid accumulation. Vasogenic edema occurs when integrity of the blood-brain barrier is disrupted, allowing fluid to escape into the extracellular fluid that surrounds brain cells, whereas cytotoxic edema involves the swelling of brain cells. ICP is the pressure normally exerted by the CSF as it circulates around the brain. It reflects the volumes of the brain tissue, blood, and CSF in the intracranial cavity. Excessive ICP can obstruct cerebral blood flow, destroy brain cells, displace brain tissue as in herniation, and otherwise damage delicate brain structures. Hydrocephalus represents enlargement of the CSF compartment owing to an abnormal CSF volume. It can result from impaired reabsorption from the arachnoid villi into the venous system (communicating hydrocephalus) or from obstruction of the ventricular system (noncommunicating hydrocephalus), which prevents the CSF from reaching the arachnoid villi.

Head injury is the term used to describe all structural damage to the skull and brain and has become synonymous with *brain injury*. The effects of traumatic head injuries can be divided into two categories: primary or secondary injuries. Secondary injuries result from complicating processes that are initiated at the time of injury. Primary injuries come from direct contact of the head and brain as an immediate result of the initial insult. The injuries may be focal (contusion or laceration) or diffuse (concussion and diffuse axonal injury). Hematomas result from vascular injury and bleeding. Depending on its location, the bleeding may result in an epidural hematoma, subdural hematoma, or intracerebral hematoma.

Deterioration of brain function is manifested by alterations in sensory and motor function and by changes in the level of consciousness. Consciousness is a state of awareness of self and environment. It exists on a normal continuum of wakefulness and sleep and a pathologic continuum of wakefulness and coma. Any deficit in level of consciousness, from mild confusion to stupor or coma, indicates injury to either the RAS or to both cerebral hemispheres concurrently. In progressive brain injury, coma may follow a rostral-to-caudal progression with characteristic changes in levels of consciousness, respiratory patterns, level of arousal and motor responses, the pupillary light response, and eye movements.

Brain death is defined as the irreversible loss of function of the brain, including that of the brain stem. Clinical examination must disclose at least the absence of responsiveness, brain stem reflexes, and respiratory effort. The vegetative state is characterized by loss of all cognitive functions and the unawareness of self and surroundings, while reflex and vegetative functions remain intact.

Cerebrovascular Disease

Cerebrovascular disease encompasses a number of disorders involving vessels in the cerebral circulation. These disorders include ischemic and hemorrhage stroke, aneurysmal subarachnoid hemorrhage, and arteriovenous malformations.

THE CEREBRAL CIRCULATION

The blood flow to the brain is supplied by the two internal carotid arteries anteriorly and the vertebral arteries posteriorly[23] (Fig. 36-12). The internal carotid artery, a terminal branch of the common carotid artery, branches into several arteries: ophthalmic, posterior communicating, anterior choroidal, anterior cerebral, and middle cerebral (Fig. 36-13). Most of the arterial blood in the internal carotid arteries is distributed through the anterior and middle cerebral arteries. The anterior cerebral arteries supply the medial surface of the frontal and parietal lobes and the anterior half of the thalamus, the corpus striatum, part of the corpus callosum, and the anterior limb of the internal capsule. The genu and posterior limb of the internal capsule and medial globus pallidus are fed by the anterior choroidal branch of the internal carotid artery. The middle cerebral artery passes laterally, supplying the lateral basal ganglia and the insula, and then emerges on the lateral cortical surface, supplying the inferior frontal gyrus, the motor and premotor frontal cortex concerned with delicate face and hand control. It is the major vascular source for the language cortices (frontal and superior temporal), the primary and association auditory cortex (superior temporal gyrus), and primary and association somesthetic cortex for the face and hand (postcentral gyrus, parietal). The middle cerebral artery is functionally a continuation of the internal carotid; emboli of the internal carotid most frequently become lodged in branches of the middle cerebral artery. The consequences of ischemia of these areas may be most devastating, resulting in damage to the fine manipulative skills of the face or upper limb and to receptive and expressive communication functions (*e.g.*, aphasia).

The two vertebral arteries arise from the subclavian artery and enter the foramina in the transverse spinal processes at the level of the sixth cervical vertebra and continue upward through the foramina of the upper six vertebrae; they wind behind the atlas and enter the skull through the foramen magnum and unite to form the basilar artery, which then diverges to terminate in the posterior cerebral arteries. Branches of the basilar and vertebral arteries supply the medulla, pons, cerebellum, midbrain, and caudal part of the diencephalon. The posterior cerebral arteries supply the remaining occipital and inferior regions of the temporal lobes, and the thalamus.

The distal branches of the internal carotid and vertebral arteries communicate at the base of the brain through the circle of Willis; this anastomosis of arteries can provide continued circulation if blood flow through one of the main vessels is disrupted.[23] Without collateral input, cessation of blood flow in cerebral arteries may result in neural damage as metabolic needs of electrically active cells exceed nutrient supply. Because the vertebral arteries supply the structures in the brain stem that maintain basic life support reflexes, interruption of blood flow in the carotid arteries with preserved vertebral supply may result in severe coma, although not necessarily death.

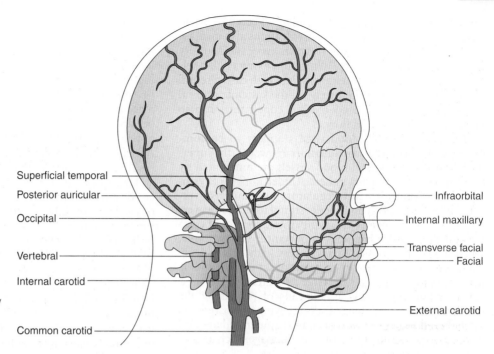

FIGURE 36-12 Branches of the right external carotid artery. The internal carotid artery ascends to the base of the brain. The right vertebral artery is also shown as it ascends through the transverse foramina of the cervical vertebrae.

The cerebral blood is drained by two sets of veins that empty into the dural venous sinuses: the deep (great) cerebral venous system and the superficial venous system.[23] In contrast to the superficial cerebral veins that travel through the pia mater on the surface of the cerebral cortex, the deep system is well protected. These vessels connect directly to the sagittal sinuses in the falx cerebri by way of bridging veins. They travel through the CSF-filled subarachnoid space and penetrate the arachnoid and then the dura to reach the dural venous sinuses. This system of sinuses returns blood to the heart primarily by way of the internal jugular veins. Alternate routes for venous flow also exist; for example, venous blood may exit through the emissary veins that pass through the skull and through veins that traverse various foramina to empty into extracranial veins.

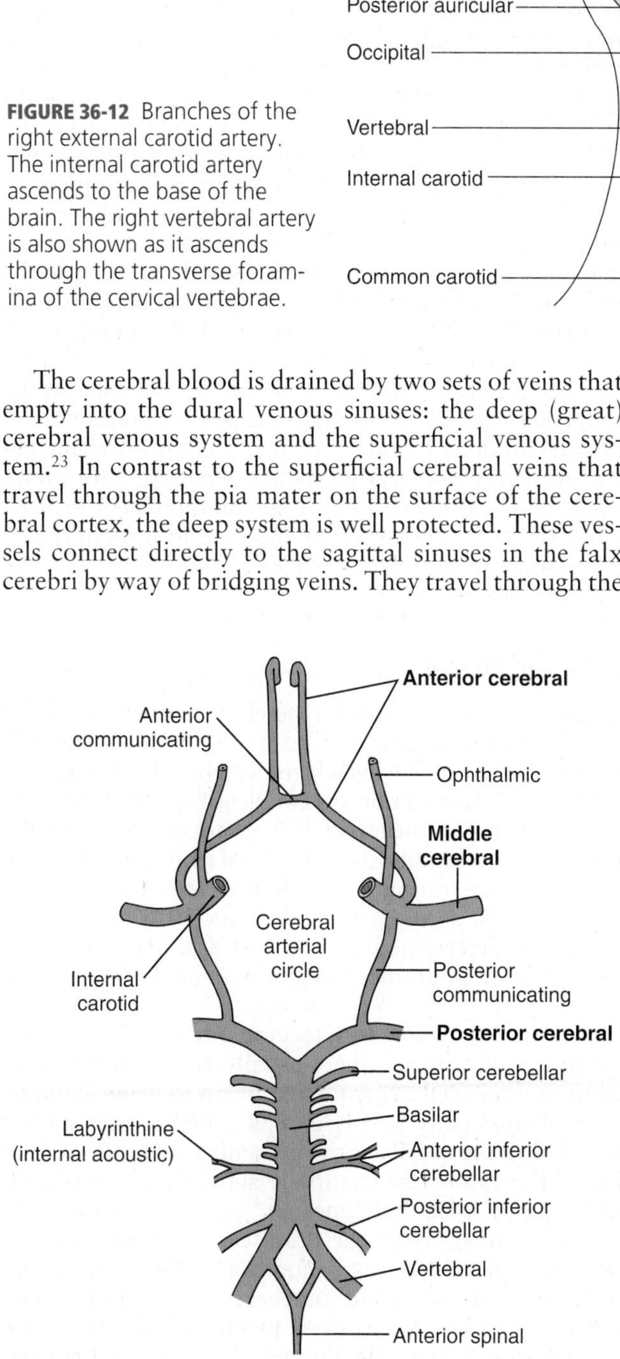

Regulation of Cerebral Blood Flow

The blood flow to the brain is maintained at approximately 750 to 900 mL/minute or 15% of the resting cardiac output.[11] The regulation of blood flow to the brain is controlled largely by autoregulatory or local mechanisms that respond to the metabolic needs of the brain. Cerebral autoregulation has been classically defined as the ability of the brain to maintain constant cerebral blood flow despite changes in systemic arterial pressure. This allows the cerebral cortex to adjust cerebral blood flow locally to satisfy its metabolic needs. The autoregulation of cerebral blood flow is efficient within a MABP range of approximately 60 to 140 mm Hg.[11] Although total cerebral blood flow remains relatively stable throughout marked changes in cardiac output and arterial blood pressure, regional blood flow may vary markedly in response to local changes in metabolism. If blood pressure falls below 60 mm Hg, cerebral blood flow becomes severely compromised, and if it rises above the upper limit of autoregulation, blood flow increases rapidly and overstretches the cerebral vessels. In persons with hypertension, this autoregulatory range shifts to a higher level.

At least three metabolic factors affect cerebral blood flow: carbon dioxide, hydrogen ion, and oxygen concentration. Increased carbon dioxide provides a potent stimulus for vasodilatation—a 70% increase in the PCO_2 in

FIGURE 36-13 The cerebral arterial circle (circle of Willis).

the arterial blood results in a doubling of cerebral blood flow. Increased hydrogen ion concentrations also increase cerebral blood flow, serving to wash away the neurally depressive acidic materials.[11] Profound extracellular acidosis induces vasomotor paralysis, in which case cerebral blood flow may depend entirely on the systemic arterial blood pressure. Decreased oxygen concentration also increases cerebral blood flow.

The deep cerebral blood vessels appear to be completely controlled by autoregulation. However, the superficial and major cerebral blood vessels are innervated by the sympathetic nervous system. Under normal physiologic conditions, local autoregulatory mechanisms override the effects of sympathetic stimulation. However, when local mechanisms fail, sympathetic control of cerebral blood pressure becomes important.[11] For example, when the arterial pressure rises to very high levels during strenuous exercise or in other conditions, the sympathetic nervous system constricts the large and intermediate-sized superficial blood vessels as a means of protecting the smaller, more easily damaged vessels. Sympathetic reflexes are believed to cause vasospasm in the intermediate and large arteries in some types of brain damage, such as that caused by rupture of a cerebral aneurysm.

STROKE (BRAIN ATTACK)

Stroke is an acute focal neurologic deficit caused by a vascular disorder that injures brain tissue. Stroke remains one of the leading causes of mortality and morbidity in the United States. Each year, 700,000 Americans are afflicted with stroke.[24] The term *brain attack* has been promoted to highlight that time-dependent tissue damage occurs and to raise awareness of the need for rapid emergency treatment, similar to that with heart attack.

 K E Y   C O N C E P T S

Stroke/Brain Attack

➤ Stroke is an acute focal neurologic deficit from an interruption of blood flow in a cerebral vessel (ischemic stroke, the most common type) due to thrombi or emboli or to bleeding into the brain tissue (hemorrhagic stroke).

➤ During the evolution of an ischemic stroke, there usually is a central core of dead or dying cells surrounded by an ischemic band of minimally perfused cells called a penumbra. Whether the cells of the penumbra continue to survive depends on the successful timely return of adequate circulation.

➤ The realization that there is a window of opportunity during which ischemic but viable brain tissue can be salvaged has led to the use of thrombolytic agents in the early treatment of ischemic stroke.

Among the major risk factors for stroke are age, gender, race, heart disease, hypertension, high cholesterol levels, cigarette smoking, prior stroke, and diabetes mellitus.[25] Other risk factors include sickle cell disease (during sickle cell crisis), polycythemia, blood dyscrasias, obesity, and sedentary lifestyle. The incidence of stroke increases with age, with a 1% per year increased risk for persons 65 to 74 years of age; the incidence of stroke is approximately 19% greater in men than women; and African Americans have a 60% greater risk of death and disability from stroke than do whites.[26]

Heart disease, particularly atrial fibrillation and other conditions that predispose to clot formation on the wall of the heart or valve leaflets or to paradoxical embolism through right-to-left shunting, predisposes to cardioembolic stroke. Alcohol abuse can contribute to stroke in several ways: induction of cardiac arrhythmias and defects in ventricular wall motion that lead to cerebral embolism, induction of hypertension, enhancement of blood coagulation disorders, and reduction of cerebral blood flow.[27] Another cause of stroke is cocaine. Cocaine use causes both ischemic and hemorrhagic strokes by inducing vasospasm, enhanced platelet activity, and increased blood pressure, heart rate, body temperature, and metabolic rate.[28]

There are two main types of strokes: ischemic stroke and hemorrhagic stroke. Ischemic strokes are caused by an interruption of blood flow in a cerebral vessel and are the most common type of stroke, accounting for about 88% of all strokes.[24] The less common hemorrhagic strokes, which are caused by bleeding into brain tissue, are associated with a much higher fatality rate than are ischemic strokes.

Ischemic Stroke

Ischemic strokes are caused by cerebrovascular obstruction by thrombosis or emboli (Fig. 36-14). Various methods have been used to classify ischemic cerebrovascular disease. A common classification system identifies five stroke subtypes and their frequency; 20% large artery atherosclerotic disease (both thrombosis and arterial emboli); 25% small vessel or penetrating artery disease (so-called *lacunar stroke*); 20% cardiogenic embolism; 30% cryptogenic stroke (undetermined cause); and 5% other, unusual causes[29] (*i.e.*, migraine, dissection, coagulopathy).

Ischemic Penumbra in Evolving Stroke. During the evolution of a stroke, there usually is a central core of dead or dying cells, surrounded by an ischemic band or area of minimally perfused cells called the *penumbra* (*i.e.*, halo). Brain cells of the penumbra receive marginal blood flow and their metabolic activities are impaired; although the area undergoes an "electrical failure," the structural integrity of the brain cells is maintained.[3,30] Whether the cells of the penumbra continue to survive depends on the successful timely return of adequate circulation, the volume of toxic products released by the neighboring dying cells, the degree of cerebral edema, and alterations in local blood flow. If the toxic products

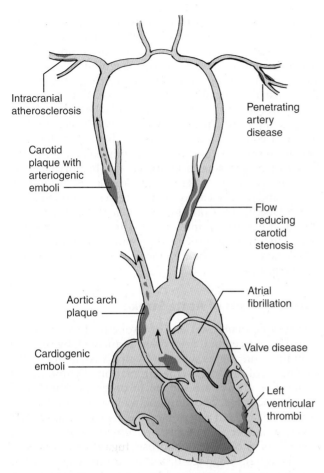

FIGURE 36-14 The most frequent sites of arterial and cardiac abnormalities causing ischemic stroke. (From Albers G. W., Easton D., Sacco R. L., et al. [1999]. Antithrombotic and thrombotic therapy for ischemic stroke. *Chest* 114[5], 684S.)

result in additional death of cells in the penumbra, the core of dead or dying tissue enlarges, and the volume of surrounding ischemic tissue increases.

Transient Ischemic Attacks. Transient ischemic attacks (TIAs) are characterized by focal ischemic cerebral neurologic deficits that last for less than 24 hours (usually less than 1 to 2 hours).[31] TIA or "ministroke" is equivalent to "brain angina" and reflects a temporary disturbance in focal cerebral blood flow, which reverses before infarction occurs, analogous to angina in relation to heart attack. The term *TIA* and the qualification of a deficit resolving within 24 hours were defined before the mechanisms of ischemic cell damage and the penumbra were known. A more accurate definition now is a deficit lasting less than 1 hour, and it may best be described as a zone of penumbra without central infarction. The causes of TIAs are the same as those of ischemic stroke, and include atherosclerotic disease of cerebral vessels and emboli. TIAs are important because they may provide warning of impending stroke. In fact, the risk of stroke after a TIA is similar to the risk after a first stroke, and is maximal immediately after the event: 4% to 8%

risk of stroke within 1 month, 12% to 13% risk during the first year, and 24% to 29% risk over 5 years.[32] Diagnosis of TIA before a stroke may permit surgical or medical intervention that prevents an eventual stroke and the associated neurologic deficits.[32]

Large Vessel (Thrombotic) Stroke. Thrombi are the most common cause of ischemic strokes, usually occurring in atherosclerotic blood vessels. In the cerebral circulation, atherosclerotic plaques are found most commonly at arterial bifurcations. Common sites of plaque formation include larger vessels of the brain, notably the origins of the internal carotid and vertebral arteries, and junctions of the basilar and vertebral arteries (see Fig. 36-14). Cerebral infarction can result from an acute local thrombosis and occlusion at the site of chronic atherosclerosis, with or without embolization of the plaque material distally, or from critical perfusion failure distal to a stenosis (watershed). These infarcts often affect the cortex, causing aphasia or neglect, visual field defects, or transient monocular blindness (amaurosis fugax). In most cases of stroke, a single cerebral artery and its territories are affected. Usually, thrombotic strokes are seen in older persons and frequently are accompanied by evidence of atherosclerotic heart or peripheral arterial disease. The thrombotic stroke is not usually associated with activity and may occur in a person at rest.

Small Vessel Stroke (Lacunar Infarct). Lacunar infarcts are small (1.5 to 2.0 cm) to very small (3 to 4 mm) infarcts located in the deeper, noncortical parts of the brain or in the brain stem.[1] They are found in the territory of single deep penetrating arteries supplying the internal capsule, basal ganglia, or brain stem. They result from occlusion of the smaller penetrating branches of large cerebral arteries, commonly the middle cerebral and posterior cerebral arteries. In the process of healing, lacunar infarcts leave behind small cavities, or lacunae (lakes). They are thought to result from arteriolar lipohyalinosis or microatheroma, commonly in the settings of chronic hypertension or diabetes. Six basic causes of lacunar infarcts have been proposed: embolism, hypertension, small vessel occlusive disease, hematologic abnormalities, small intracerebral hemorrhages, and vasospasm. Because of their size and location, lacunar infarcts usually do not cause cortical deficits like aphasia or apraxia. Instead, they produce classic recognizable "lacunar syndromes" such as pure motor hemiplegia, pure sensory hemiplegia, and dysarthria with the clumsy hand syndrome. Because CT scans are not sensitive enough to detect these tiny infarcts, diagnosis is usually determined by clinical features alone. The use of magnetic resonance imaging (MRI) has allowed frequent visualization of small vessel infarcts and is obligatory to confirm such a lesion.

Cardiogenic Embolic Stroke. An embolic stroke is caused by a moving blood clot that travels from its origin to the brain. It usually affects the larger proximal cerebral vessels, often lodging at bifurcations. The most frequent site of embolic strokes is the middle cerebral artery, reflecting the large territory of this vessel and its position as the terminus of the carotid artery. Although most cerebral emboli originate from a thrombus in the left heart, they also may originate in an atherosclerotic plaque in the carotid arteries. The embolus travels quickly to the brain and becomes lodged in a smaller artery through which it cannot pass. Embolic stroke usually has a sudden onset with immediate maximum deficit.

Various cardiac conditions predispose to formation of emboli that produce embolic stroke, including rheumatic heart disease, atrial fibrillation, recent myocardial infarction, ventricular aneurysm, mobile aortic arch atheroma and bacterial endocarditis. More recently, the use of transesophageal echocardiography, which better images the interatrial septum, has implicated a patent foramen ovale as a source for paradoxical venous emboli to the arterial system. Advances in the diagnosis and treatment of heart disease can be expected to alter favorably the incidence of embolic stroke.

Hemorrhagic Stroke

The most frequently fatal stroke is a spontaneous hemorrhage into the brain substance.[33-35] With rupture of a blood vessel, hemorrhage into the brain tissue occurs, resulting in edema, compression of the brain contents, or spasm of the adjacent blood vessels (Fig. 36-15). The

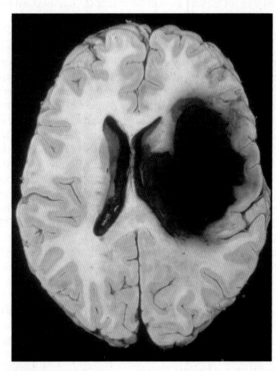

FIGURE 36-15 Cerebral hemorrhage. A spontaneous cerebral hemorrhage began near the external capsule and produced a hematoma that threatened rupture of a lateral ventricle. (From Trojanowski J. Q. [2005]. The central nervous system. In Rubin E., Gorstein F., Rubin R., et al. [Eds.], *Rubin's pathology: Clinicopathologic foundations of medicine* [4th ed., p. 1437]. Philadelphia: Lippincott Williams & Wilkins.)

most common predisposing factors are advancing age and hypertension. Other causes of hemorrhage are aneurysm, trauma, erosion of the vessels by tumors, arteriovenous malformations, blood coagulation disorders, vasculitis, and drugs. A cerebral hemorrhage occurs suddenly, usually when the person is active. Vomiting commonly occurs at the onset, and headache often occurs. Focal symptoms depend on which vessel is involved. In the most common situation, hemorrhage into the basal ganglia results in contralateral hemiplegia, with initial flaccidity progressing to spasticity. The hemorrhage and resultant edema exert great pressure on the brain substance, and the clinical course progresses rapidly to coma and frequently to death. Recent research has focused on the ultra-early (within 4 hours after onset of hemorrhage) use of hemostatic therapy with recombinant activated factor VII in the treatment of acute intracerebral hemorrhage.[36]

Manifestations of Acute Stroke

The specific manifestations of stroke or TIA are determined by the cerebral artery that is affected, by the area of brain tissue that is supplied by that vessel, and by the adequacy of the collateral circulation. Symptoms of stroke/TIA always are sudden in onset and focal, and usually one-sided. The most common symptom is weakness of the face and arm, sometimes also of the leg. Other frequent stroke symptoms are unilateral numbness, vision loss in one eye (amaurosis fugax) or to one side (hemianopia), language disturbance (aphasia), slurred speech (dysarthria), and sudden, unexplained imbalance or ataxia. In the event of TIA, symptoms rapidly resolve spontaneously, although the underlying mechanisms are the same as for stroke. The specific stroke signs depend on the specific vascular territory compromised (Table 36-5). Discrete subsets of these vascular syndromes occur, depending on which branches of the involved artery are blocked.

Diagnosis and Treatment

Diagnosis. Accurate diagnosis of acute stroke is based on a complete history and thorough physical and neurologic examination. A careful history, including documentation of previous TIAs, the time of onset and pattern and rapidity of system progression, the specific focal symptoms (to determine the likely vascular territory), and the existence of any coexisting diseases, can help to determine the type of stroke that is involved. The diagnostic evaluation should aim to determine the presence of hemorrhage or ischemia, identify the stroke or TIA mechanism (large vessel or small vessel atherothrombotic, cardioembolic, hemorrhagic), characterize the severity of clinical deficits, and unmask the presence of risk factors.

Imaging studies document the brain infarction and the anatomy and pathology of the related blood vessels. CT scans and MRI have become essential tools in diagnosing stroke, differentiating cerebral hemorrhage from ischemia, and excluding intracranial lesions that mimic

TABLE 36-5	Signs and Symptoms of Stroke by Involved Cerebral Artery	
Cerebral Artery	**Brain Area Involved**	**Signs and Symptoms***
Anterior cerebral	Infarction of the medial aspect of one frontal lobe if lesion is distal to communicating artery; bilateral frontal infarction if flow in other anterior cerebral artery is inadequate	Paralysis of contralateral foot or leg; impaired gait; paresis of contralateral arm; contralateral sensory loss over toes, foot, and leg; problems making decisions or performing acts voluntarily; lack of spontaneity, easily distracted; slowness of thought; aphasia depends on the hemisphere involved; urinary incontinence; cognitive and affective disorders
Middle cerebral	Massive infarction of most of lateral hemisphere and deeper structures of the frontal, parietal, and temporal lobes; internal capsule; basal ganglia	Contralateral hemiplegia (face and arm); contralateral sensory impairment; aphasia; homonymous hemianopia; altered consciousness (confusion to coma); inability to turn eyes toward paralyzed side; denial of paralyzed side or limb (hemiattention); possible acalculia, alexia, finger agnosia, and left–right confusion; vasomotor paresis and instability
Posterior cerebral	Occipital lobe; anterior and medial portion of temporal lobe	Homonymous hemianopia and other visual defects such as color blindness, loss of central vision, and visual hallucinations; memory deficits, perseveration (repeated performance of same verbal or motor response)
	Thalamus involvement	Loss of all sensory modalities; spontaneous pain; intentional tremor; mild hemiparesis; aphasia
	Cerebral peduncle involvement	Oculomotor nerve palsy with contralateral hemiplegia
Basilar and vertebral	Cerebellum and brain stem	Visual disturbance such as diplopia, dystaxia, vertigo, dysphagia, dysphonia

*Depend on hemisphere involved and adequacy of collaterals.

stroke clinically. CT scans are a necessary screening tool in the acute setting for rapid identification of hemorrhage, but are insensitive to ischemia within 24 hours, and to any brain stem or small infarcts. MRI is superior for imaging ischemic lesions in all territories. Arteriography can demonstrate the site of the vascular abnormality and afford visualization of most intracranial vascular areas. Although angiography still is required for invasive treatments and for maximal sensitivity, magnetic resonance angiography (MRA) has largely replaced angiography as a screening tool for vascular lesions.

Two other types of imaging, positron emission tomography (PET) and single-photon emission computed tomography (SPECT), are nuclear studies used to assess the distribution of blood flow and metabolic activity of the brain. These tests rarely are used in routine stroke management because of limited availability, and are applied more often in clinical research of cerebral ischemia. The introduction of several Doppler ultrasonographic techniques has facilitated the noninvasive evaluation of the cerebral circulation, especially for detection of carotid stenosis.

Treatment. The treatment of acute ischemic stroke has changed markedly since the early 1990s, with an emphasis on salvaging brain tissue and minimizing long-term disability. The realization that there is a window of opportunity during which ischemic but viable brain tissue can be salvaged has led to the use of reperfusion techniques and neuroprotective strategies in the early treatment of ischemic stroke.[37] Although the results of emergent treatment of hemorrhagic stroke have been less

dramatic, continued efforts to reduce disability have been promising.

Intravenous thrombolytic therapy is effective in reducing the neurologic deficits in selected patients without CT evidence of intracranial pressure when administered within 3 hours of the onset of symptoms.[37–39] The first and only agent approved by the U.S. Food and Drug Administration (FDA) for treatment of acute ischemic stroke is recombinant tissue plasminogen activator (tPA), which was approved in 1996.[39] A subcommittee of the Stroke Council of the American Heart Association has developed guidelines for the use of tPA for acute stroke.[38] The major risk of treatment with thrombolytic agents is intracranial hemorrhage of the infarcted brain. A number of conditions, including therapeutic levels of oral anticoagulant medications, a history of gastrointestinal bleeding, previous stroke or head injury within 3 months, surgery within the past 14 days, and a blood pressure greater than 200/120 mm Hg, are considered contraindications to thrombolytic therapy.[38]

The successful treatment of stroke depends on education of the public, paramedics, and health care professionals about the need for early diagnosis and treatment. As with heart attack, the message should be "do not wait to decide if the symptoms subside but seek immediate treatment." Effective medical and surgical procedures may preserve brain function and prevent disability.

Post-stroke treatment is aimed at preventing complications and recurrent stroke and promoting the fullest possible recovery of function. During the acute phase, proper positioning and range-of-motion exercises are essential. Early rehabilitation efforts include all members of the rehabilitation team—physician, nurse, speech therapist, physical therapist, and occupational therapist—and the family. Much research is ongoing into the determinants and mechanisms of stroke recovery.

Stroke-Related Deficits

Deficits from stroke include motor and sensory deficits, language and speech problems, and higher cognitive deficits. Motor deficits are most common, followed by deficits of language, sensation, and cognition.

Motor Deficits. After a stroke affecting the corticospinal tract such as the motor cortex, posterior limb of the internal capsule, basis pontis, or medullary pyramids, there is profound weakness on the contralateral side (hemiparesis; see Chapter 35, Fig. 35-2). Involvement at the level of the motor cortex is most often in the territory of the middle cerebral artery, usually with a sparing of the leg, which is supplied by the anterior cerebral artery. Subcortical lesions of the corticospinal tracts cause equal weakness of the face, arm, and leg. Within 6 to 8 weeks, the initial weakness and flaccidity is replaced by hyperreflexia and spasticity. Spasticity involves an increase in the tone of affected muscles and usually an element of weakness. The flexor muscles usually are more strongly affected in the upper extremities and the extensor muscles more strongly affected in the lower extremities. There is a tendency toward foot drop; outward rotation and circumduction of the leg with gait; flexion at the wrist, elbow, and fingers; lower facial paresis; slurred speech; upward movement of the big toe to plantar stimulation (*Babinski sign*); and dependent edema in the affected extremities. A slight corticospinal lesion may be indicated only by clumsiness in carrying out fine coordinated movements rather than obvious weakness. Passive range-of-motion exercises help to maintain joint function; prevent edema, shoulder subluxation (*i.e.*, incomplete dislocation), and muscle atrophy; and may help to reestablish motor patterns. If no voluntary movement or movement on command appears within a few months, significant function usually will not return to that extremity.

Dysarthria and Aphasia. Two key aspects of verbal communication are speech and language. Speech involves the mechanical act of articulating language, the "motor act" of verbal expression, whereas language involves the written or spoken use of symbolic formulations, such as words or numbers.[40] *Dysarthria* is a disorder of speech, manifest as the imperfect articulation of speech sounds or changes in voice pitch or quality. It results from a stroke affecting the muscles of the pharynx, palate, tongue, lips, or mouth, and does not relate to the content of speech. A person with dysarthria may demonstrate slurred speech while still retaining language ability, or may have a concurrent language problem as well. *Aphasia* is a general term that encompasses varying degrees of inability to comprehend, integrate, and express language. Aphasia may be localized to the dominant cerebral cortex or thalamus, usually the left side in 95% of people who are right handed and 70% of people who are left handed. In children, language dominance can readily shift to the unaffected hemisphere, resulting in more transient language deficits after stroke. A stroke in the territory of the middle cerebral artery is the most common aphasia-producing stroke.

Aphasia can be categorized as fluent (many words) or nonfluent (few words). Expressive or *nonfluent aphasia* is characterized by an inability to spontaneously communicate or translate thoughts or ideas into meaningful speech or writing. Speech production is limited, effortful, and halting and often may be poorly articulated because of a concurrent dysarthria. The person may be able, with difficulty, to utter or write two or three words, especially those with an emotional overlay. Comprehension is normal, and the person seems to be aware of his or her deficits but is unable to correct them. This often leads to frustration, anger, and depression. Expressive, nonfluent aphasia is associated with lesions of Broca area of the dominant frontal lobe (areas 44 and 45).

Fluent speech requires little or no effort, is articulate, and is of increased quantity. The term *fluent* refers only to the ease and rate of verbal output, and does not relate to the content of speech or the ability of the person to comprehend what is being said. There are three categories of fluent aphasia: Wernicke, anomic, and conductive aphasia. *Wernicke aphasia* is characterized by an inability to comprehend the speech of others or to comprehend written material. Lesions of the posterior temporal or lower parietal lobe (areas 22 and 39) are associated with receptive, fluent aphasia. *Anomic aphasia* is speech that is nearly normal except for a difficulty with finding singular words. *Conduction aphasia* is manifest as impaired repetition and speech riddled with letter substitutions, despite good comprehension and fluency. Conduction aphasia (*i.e.*, disconnection syndrome) results from destruction of the fiber system under the insula that connects the Wernicke and Broca areas.

Cognitive and Other Deficits. Stroke can also cause cognitive, sensory, visual, and behavioral deficits. One distinct cognitive syndrome is that of hemineglect or hemi-inattention, usually from strokes affecting the nondominant (right) hemisphere. Hemineglect is the inability to attend to and react to stimuli coming from the contralateral (left) side of space. Patients may not visually track, orient, or reach to the neglected side. They may neglect to use the limbs on that side, despite normal motor function, and may not shave, wash, or comb that side. Such persons are unaware of this deficit, which is another form of their neglect. Other cognitive deficits include apraxia (impaired ability to carry out previously learned motor activities despite normal sensory and motor function), agnosia (impaired recognition with normal sensory function), memory loss, behavioral syndromes, and depression.

Sensory deficits affect the body contralateral to the lesion, and can manifest as numbness, tingling paresthesias, or distorted sensations such as dysesthesia and neuropathic pain. Visual disturbances from stroke are diverse, but most common are hemianopia from a lesion of the optic radiations between the lateral geniculate body and the temporal or occipital lobes, or monocular blindness from occlusion of the ipsilateral central retinal artery, a branch of the internal carotid.

ANEURYSMAL SUBARACHNOID HEMORRHAGE

Aneurysmal subarachnoid hemorrhage represents bleeding into the subarachnoid space caused by a ruptured cerebral aneurysm. Bleeding into the subarachnoid space can extend well beyond the site of origin, flooding the basal cistern, ventricles, and spinal subarachnoid space.[1,3,41] An aneurysm is a bulge at the site of a localized weakness in the muscular wall of an arterial vessel. Most cerebral aneurysms are small saccular aneurysms called *berry aneurysms* (Fig. 36-16). They usually occur at bifurcations and other junctions of vessels such as those in the circle of Willis (Fig. 36-17). They are thought to arise from a congenital defect in the media of the involved vessels. Their incidence is higher in persons with certain disorders, including polycystic kidney disease, Marfan syndrome, fibromuscular dysplasia, coarctation of aorta, and arteriovenous malformations of the brain.[1]

Rupture of a cerebral aneurysm results in subarachnoid hemorrhage.[41,42] The probability of rupture increases with the size of the aneurysm; aneurysms larger than 10 mm in diameter have a 50% chance of bleeding per year. Rupture often occurs with acute increases in ICP. Of the various environmental factors that may predispose to aneurysmal subarachnoid hemorrhage, cigarette smoking and hypertension appear to constitute the greatest threat. Intracranial aneurysms are rare in children, and the mean age for subarachnoid hemorrhage is approximately 50 years. The mortality and morbidity rates with aneurysmal subarachnoid hemorrhage are high,

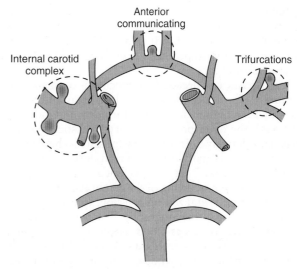

FIGURE 36-17 Common sites of berry aneurysms.

with only a third of persons recovering without major disability.[9]

The signs and symptoms of cerebral aneurysms can be divided into two phases: those presenting before rupture and bleeding and those presenting after rupture and bleeding. Most small aneurysms are asymptomatic; intact aneurysms frequently are found at autopsy as an incidental finding.[1] Large aneurysms may cause chronic headache, neurologic deficits, or both. Approximately 50% of persons with subarachnoid hemorrhage have a history of atypical headaches occurring days to weeks before the onset of hemorrhage, suggesting the presence of a small leak.[41,42] These headaches are characterized by sudden onset and often are accompanied by nausea, vomiting, and dizziness. Persons with these symptoms may be mistakenly diagnosed as having tension or migraine headaches.

The onset of subarachnoid aneurysmal rupture often is heralded by a sudden and severe headache, described as "the worst headache of my life." If the bleeding is severe, the headache may be accompanied by collapse and loss of consciousness. Vomiting may accompany the presenting symptoms. Other manifestations include signs of meningeal irritation such as nuchal rigidity (neck stiffness) and photophobia (light intolerance); cranial nerve deficits, especially cranial nerve II, and sometimes III and IV (diplopia and blurred vision); stroke syndrome (focal motor and sensory deficits); cerebral edema and increased ICP; and pituitary dysfunction (diabetes insipidus and hyponatremia). Hypertension, a frequent finding, and cardiac dysrhythmias result from massive release of catecholamines triggered by the subarachnoid hemorrhage.

The complications of aneurysmal rupture include rebleeding, vasospasm with cerebral ischemia, hydrocephalus, hypothalamic dysfunction, and seizure activity. Rebleeding and vasospasm are the most serious and most difficult to treat. Rebleeding, which has its highest incidence on the first day after the initial rupture, results

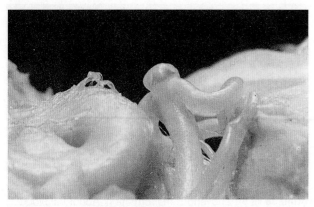

FIGURE 36-16 Berry aneurysm. A thin-walled aneurysm protrudes from the arterial bifurcation in the circle of Willis. (From Trojanowski J. Q. [2005]. The central nervous system. In Rubin E., Gorstein F., Rubin R., et al. [Eds.], *Rubin's pathology: Clinicopathologic foundations of medicine* [4th ed., p. 1435]. Philadelphia: Lippincott Williams & Wilkins.)

in further and usually catastrophic neurologic deficits. Another complication of aneurysm rupture is the development of hydrocephalus. It is caused by plugging of the arachnoid villi with products from lysis of blood in the subarachnoid space.

Vasospasm is a dreaded complication of aneurysmal rupture.[43] The condition is difficult to treat and is associated with a high incidence of morbidity and mortality. Although the description of aneurysm-associated vasospasm is relatively uniform, its proposed mechanisms are controversial. Usually, the condition develops within 3 to 10 days (peak, 7 days) after aneurysm rupture and involves a focal narrowing of the cerebral artery or arteries that can be visualized on arteriography or by transcranial Doppler ultrasonography. The neurologic status gradually deteriorates as blood supply to the brain in the region of the spasm is decreased; this usually can be differentiated from the rapid deterioration seen in rebleeding. Vasospasm is treated by attempting to maintain adequate CPP through the use of vasoactive drugs or administration of large amounts of intravenous fluids to increase intravascular volume and produce hemodilution. There is a risk of rebleeding from this therapy. Early surgery may provide some protection from vasospasm. Endovascular techniques, including balloon dilatation, have been developed to treat spasmed arterial segments mechanically. Nimodipine, a drug that blocks calcium channels and selectively acts on cerebral blood vessels, may be used to prevent or treat vasospasm.

The diagnosis of subarachnoid hemorrhage and intracranial aneurysms is made by clinical presentation, CT scan, lumbar puncture, and angiography. Lumbar puncture may reveal the presence of blood in the CSF, whereas CT may demonstrate the location and extent of subarachnoid blood. To identify the aneurysm at the source of bleeding, conventional angiography, MRA, and helical (spiral) CT angiography are used. Conventional catheter angiography is the definitive diagnostic tool for detecting the aneurysm. MRA is noninvasive and does not require the intravascular administration of contrast, but is less sensitive. Helical CT angiography does require intravenous contrast, but can be used in persons after aneurysmal clipping when the use of MRI may be contraindicated.

The course of treatment after aneurysm rupture depends on the extent of neurologic deficit. Persons with mild to no neurologic deficits may undergo cerebral arteriography and early surgery, usually within 24 to 72 hours. Surgery involves craniotomy and inserting a specially designed silver clip that is tightened around the neck of the aneurysm. This procedure offers protection from rebleeding and may permit removal of the hematoma. Some persons with subarachnoid hemorrhage are managed medically for 10 days or more in an attempt to improve their clinical status before surgery. The use of endovascular techniques such as balloon embolization and platinum coil electrothrombosis is emerging as an alternative to surgery, particularly in surgically inaccessible aneurysms or poor surgical candidates.

ARTERIOVENOUS MALFORMATIONS

Arteriovenous malformations are complex tangles of abnormal arteries and veins linked by one or more fistulas[44,45] (Fig. 36-18). These vascular networks lack a capillary bed and the small arteries have a deficient muscularis layer. Arteriovenous malformations are thought to arise from failure in development of the capillary network in the embryonic brain. As the child's brain grows, the malformation acquires additional arterial contributions that enlarge to form a tangled collection of thin-walled vessels that shunt blood directly from the arterial to the venous circulation. Arteriovenous malformations typically present before 40 years of age and affect men and women equally. Rupture of vessels in the malformation causing hemorrhagic stroke accounts for approximately 2% of all strokes.[44]

The hemodynamic effects of arteriovenous malformations are twofold. First, blood is shunted from the high-pressure arterial system to the low-pressure venous system without the buffering advantage of the capillary network. The draining venous channels are exposed to high levels of pressure, predisposing them to rupture and hemorrhage. Second, the elevated arterial and venous pressures divert blood away from the surrounding tissue, impairing tissue perfusion. Clinically, this is evidenced by slowly progressive neurologic deficits. The major clinical manifestations of arteriovenous malformations are intracerebral and subarachnoid hemorrhage, seizures, headache, and progressive neurologic deficits. Headaches often are severe, and persons with the disorder may describe them as being throbbing and synchronous with their heartbeat. Other, focal symptoms depend on the location of the lesion and include visual symptoms (*i.e.,* diplopia and hemianopia), hemiparesis, mental deterioration, and speech deficits. Learning disorders have been documented in 66% of adults with arteriovenous malformations.[44]

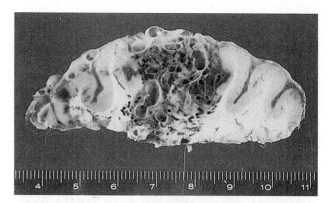

FIGURE 36-18 Arteriovenous malformation. Abnormal blood vessels replace the cortical gray matter and extend deeply into the underlying white matter. (From Trojanowski J. Q. [2005]. The central nervous system. In Rubin E., Gorstein F., Rubin R., et al. [Eds.], *Rubin's pathology: Clinicopathologic foundations of medicine* [4th ed., p. 1435]. Philadelphia: Lippincott Williams & Wilkins.)

Definitive diagnosis often is obtained through cerebral angiography. Treatment methods include surgical excision, endovascular occlusion, and radiation therapy. Because of the nature of the malformation, each of these methods is accompanied by some risk of complications. If the arteriovenous malformation is accessible, surgical excision usually is the treatment of choice.[44,45] Radiation therapy (also known as *radiosurgery*) may involve the use of a gamma knife, proton beam, or linear accelerator.

In summary, a stroke, or brain attack, is an acute focal neurologic deficit caused by a vascular disorder that injures brain tissue. It is a leading cause of death in the United States and a major cause of disability. There are two main types of stroke: ischemic and hemorrhagic. Ischemic stroke, which is the most common type, is caused by cerebrovascular obstruction by a thrombus or emboli. Hemorrhagic stroke, which is associated with greater morbidity and mortality, is caused by the rupture of a blood vessel and bleeding into the brain. The acute manifestations of stroke depend on the location of the blood vessel that is involved and can include motor, sensory, language, speech, and cognitive disorders. Early diagnosis and treatment with thrombolytic agents have improved the outlook for many persons with ischemic stroke.

A subarachnoid hemorrhage involves bleeding into the subarachnoid space. Most subarachnoid hemorrhages are the result of a ruptured cerebral aneurysm. Presenting symptoms include headache, nuchal rigidity, photophobia, and nausea. Complications include rebleeding, vasospasm, and hydrocephalus. Arteriovenous malformations are congenital abnormal communications between arterial and venous channels that result from failure in the development of the capillary network in the embryonic brain. The vessels in the arteriovenous malformations may enlarge to form a space-occupying lesion, become weak and predispose to bleeding, and divert blood away from other parts of the brain; they can cause brain hemorrhage, seizures, headache, and other neurologic deficits.

Infections and Brain Tumors

INFECTIONS

Infections of the CNS may be classified according to the structure involved: the meninges (meningitis); the brain parenchyma (encephalitis); the spinal cord (myelitis); and the brain and spinal cord (encephalomyelitis). They also may be classified by the type of invading organism: bacterial, viral, or other. In general, the pathogens enter the CNS through the bloodstream by crossing the blood-brain barrier or by direct invasion through a skull fracture or bullet hole or, rarely, by contamination during surgery or lumbar puncture.

Meningitis

Meningitis is an inflammation of the pia mater, the arachnoid, and the CSF-filled subarachnoid space. Inflammation spreads rapidly because of CSF circulation around the brain and spinal cord. The inflammation usually is caused by an infection, but chemical meningitis can occur. There are two types of acute infectious meningitis: acute pyogenic meningitis (usually bacterial) and acute lymphocytic (usually viral) meningitis.[1]

Bacterial Meningitis. Most cases of bacterial meningitis are caused by *Streptococcus pneumoniae* (pneumococcus), *Haemophilus influenzae*, or *Neisseria meningitidis* (the meningococcus), except in neonates (infected most often by *Escherichia coli* and group B streptococci). The incidence of *H. influenzae* infection in children younger than 5 years of age has declined dramatically during recent years because of vaccination against *H. influenzae*. Epidemics of meningococcal meningitis occur in settings such as the military, where the recruits must reside in close contact. The very young and the very old are at highest risk for pneumococcal meningitis. Other pathogens in adults are gram-negative bacilli and staphylococci. Risk factors associated with contracting meningitis include head trauma with basilar skull fractures, otitis media, sinusitis or mastoiditis, neurosurgery, dermal sinus tracts, systemic sepsis, or immunocompromise.

In the pathophysiologic process of bacterial meningitis, the bacterial organisms replicate and undergo lysis in the CSF, releasing endotoxins or cell wall fragments. These substances initiate the release of inflammatory mediators, which set off a complex sequence of events permitting pathogens, neutrophils, and albumin to move across the capillary wall into the CSF. As the pathogens enter the subarachnoid space, they cause inflammation, characterized by a cloudy, purulent exudate. Thrombophlebitis of the bridging veins and dural sinuses may develop, followed by congestion and infarction in the surrounding tissues. Ultimately, the meninges thicken, and adhesions form. These adhesions may impinge on the cranial nerves, giving rise to cranial nerve palsies, or may impair the outflow of CSF, causing hydrocephalus.

The most common manifestations of acute bacterial meningitis are fever and chills; headache; stiff neck (nuchal rigidity) and back; abdominal and extremity pains; and nausea and vomiting. Other signs include seizures, cranial nerve damage (especially the eighth nerve, with resulting deafness), and focal cerebral signs.[46] Meningococcal meningitis causes a petechial rash with palpable purpura in most people. These petechiae vary from pinhead size to large ecchymoses or even areas of skin gangrene that slough if the person survives. Other types of meningitis also may produce a petechial rash. Persons infected with *H. influenzae* or *S. pneumoniae* may present with difficulty in arousal and seizures, whereas those with *N. meningitidis* infection may present with delirium or coma.[47] The development of brain edema, hydrocephalus, or increased cerebral blood flow can result in increased ICP.

Diagnosis of bacterial meningitis is based on the history and physical examination, along with laboratory data. Lumbar puncture (*i.e.,* spinal tap), which is necessary for accurate diagnosis, reveals the presence of a cloudy and purulent CSF under increased pressure. The CSF typically contains large numbers of polymorphonuclear neutrophils (up to 90,000/mm^3), increased protein content, and reduced sugar content. Bacteria can be seen on smears and can usually be cultured with appropriate media.

Treatment includes antibiotics and corticosteroids. Optimal antibiotic treatment requires that the drug have a bactericidal effect in the CSF. Because bactericidal therapy often results in rapid lysis of the pathogen, treatment can promote the release of biologically active cell wall products into the CSF. The release of these cell wall products can increase the production of inflammatory mediators that have the potential for exacerbating the abnormalities of the blood-brain barrier and the inflammatory process. Because of evidence linking the inflammatory mediators to the pathogenesis of bacterial meningitis, adjunctive corticosteroid therapy usually is administered with or just before the first dose of antibiotics in infants and children. Growing evidence also supports the adjunctive use of corticosteroid therapy in adults.[48]

Persons who have been exposed to someone with meningococcal meningitis should be treated prophylactically with antibiotics.[49] Effective polysaccharide vaccines are available to protect against meningococcal groups A, C, Y, and W-135. These vaccines are recommended for military recruits and college students, who are at increased risk of invasive meningococcal disease.

Viral Meningitis. Viral meningitis manifests in much the same way as bacterial meningitis, but the course is less severe, and the CSF findings are markedly different. There are lymphocytes in the CSF fluid rather than polymorphonuclear cells, the protein content is only moderately elevated, and the sugar content usually is normal. Viral meningitis can be caused by many different viruses, most often enteroviruses (coxsackie B and echovirus).[3] Other causes include the Epstein-Barr, mumps, herpes simplex (HSV), and West Nile viruses. In many cases, the virus cannot be identified. The acute viral meningitides are self-limited and require only symptomatic treatment.

Encephalitis

Encephalitis represents a generalized infection of the parenchyma of the brain or spinal cord. It is usually caused by a virus, but it also may be caused by bacteria, fungi, and other organisms. The nervous system is subjected to invasion by many viruses, such as arbovirus, poliovirus, and rabies virus. The mode of transmission may be the bite of a mosquito (arbovirus), a rabid animal (rabies virus), or ingestion (poliovirus). A common cause of encephalitis in the United States is HSV. Less frequent causes of encephalitis are toxic substances such as ingested lead and vaccines for measles and mumps. Encephalitis

caused by human immunodeficiency virus (HIV) infection is discussed in Chapter 15.

The pathologic picture of encephalitis includes local necrotizing hemorrhage, which ultimately becomes generalized, with prominent edema. There is progressive degeneration of nerve cell bodies. Like meningitis, encephalitis is characterized by fever, headache, and nuchal rigidity, but more often patients also experience neurologic disturbances, such as lethargy, disorientation, seizures, focal paralysis, delirium, and coma. Diagnosis of encephalitis is made by clinical history and presenting symptoms, in addition to traditional CSF studies.

BRAIN TUMORS

Brain tumors account for 2% of all aggressive neoplasms, and mostly affect older persons.[3] Metastases to the brain from other sites are more common. One estimate suggests that more than 100,000 people per year die with symptomatic intracranial metastasis.[50] In children, primary brain tumors are second only to leukemia as a cause of death from cancer, with 2,200 primary brain tumors being diagnosed each year. The mortality rate among this age group approaches 45%.[51]

Types of Tumors

The term *brain tumor* refers to a collection of intracranial neoplasms, each with its own histology, site of origin, prognosis, and treatment.[50–53] For most neoplasms, the term *malignant* is used to describe the tumor's lack of cell differentiation, its invasive nature, and its ability to metastasize. However, the terms *benign* and *malignant* do not apply to brain tumors in the same sense as to tumors in other parts of the body. In the brain, even a well-differentiated and histologically benign tumor may grow and cause death because of its location. Also, tumors in the brain are rarely benign because surgery rarely cures.[51] Most histologically benign tumors infiltrate the normal brain tissue, preventing total resection and allowing for tumor recurrence. Furthermore, brain tumors seldom metastasize, except within the CNS itself.[51] Because of difficulty with pathologic discrimination and absence of metastasis, the clinical staging systems used for other cancers are not used for describing brain tumors. Instead, the terms *low-grade tumors* and *high-grade tumors* are often used.[51]

Brain tumors can be divided into three basic types: primary intracranial tumors of neuroepithelial tissue (*e.g.,* neurons, neuroglia), primary intracranial tumors that originate in the skull cavity but are not derived from the brain tissue itself (*e.g.,* meninges, pituitary gland, pineal gland, primary CNS lymphoma), and metastatic tumors. Collectively, neoplasms of astrocytic origin are the most common type of primary brain tumor in the adult, followed by primary CNS lymphoma. Tumors of neuronal origin (*e.g.,* medulloblastoma) usually occur during infancy and early childhood. This is in accord with the principle that a cell must be capable of replication to undergo neoplastic transformation. In fact, many neuronal tumors probably have their origin during embryonic development.[3]

Glial Tumors. Glial tumors are divided into two main categories: astrocytic and oligodendroglial. For purposes of classification astrocytic tumors can be subdivided into fibrillary (infiltrating) astrocytic tumors and pilocytic astrocytomas.

Fibrillary or *diffuse astrocytomas* account for 80% of adult primary brain tumors.[50] They are most common in middle age, with the anaplastic astrocytomas having a peak incidence in the sixth decade. Although they usually are found in the cerebral hemispheres, they also can occur in the cerebellum, brain stem, or spinal cord. Astrocytomas of the cerebral hemispheres commonly are divided into three grades of increasingly pathologic anaplasia and rapidity of progression: well-differentiated lesions, designated *astrocytomas;* intermediate-grade tumors, termed *anaplastic astrocytomas;* and the least differentiated and most aggressive, designated *glioblastoma multiforme*. Clinically, infiltrating astrocytic tumors present with symptoms of increased ICP (*e.g.,* headache) or focal abnormalities related to their position (*e.g.,* seizures).

Pilocytic astrocytomas are distinguished from other astrocytomas by their cellular appearance and their benign behavior. Typically, they occur in children and young adults and usually are located in the cerebellum, but they also can be found in the floor and walls of the third ventricle, the optic chiasm and nerves, and occasionally in the cerebral hemispheres. The prognosis of persons with pilocytic astrocytomas is influenced primarily by their location. The prognosis is usually better for persons with surgically resectable tumors, such as those located in the cerebellar cortex, than for persons with less accessible tumors such as those involving the hypothalamus or brain stem.

Oligodendrogliomas are tumors of the oligodendrocytes or their precursors, or they have histologic features characteristic of both oligodendrocytes and astrocytes. They represent approximately 5% of glial tumors and are most common in middle life.[52] The prognosis of persons with oligodendrogliomas is less predictable than for persons with infiltrating astrocytomas, and depends on the histologic grade and location of the tumor. Oligodendroglial tumors are prone to spontaneous hemorrhage because of their delicate vasculature.[50]

Ependymomas. Ependymomas are tumors derived from the single layer of epithelium that lines the ventricles and spinal canal. Although they can occur at any age, they are most likely to occur in the first two decades of life and most frequently affect the fourth ventricle; they constitute 5% to 10% of brain tumors in this age group.[1] The spinal cord is the most common site for ependymomas occurring in middle age. The clinical features depend on the location of the neoplasm. Intracranial tumors are often associated with hydrocephalus and evidence of increased ICP.

Meningiomas. Meningiomas develop from the meningothelial cells of the arachnoid and are outside the brain. They usually have their onset in the middle or later years of life and constitute approximately 20% of primary brain tumors in this age group.[3] Meningiomas are slow-growing, well-circumscribed, and often highly vascular tumors. They usually are benign, and complete removal is possible if the tumor does not involve vital structures.

Primary Central Nervous System Lymphomas. Primary CNS lymphoma has increased in incidence by a factor of 10 in the past two decades. These deep, periventricular, and diffuse tumors are especially common in immunocompromised patients and are associated with the Epstein-Barr virus and derived from large B cells. Most are malignant and recurrence is common despite treatment. Behavioral and cognitive changes, which are the most common presenting symptoms, occur in about 65% of patients; hemiparesis, aphasia, and visual field deficits in about 50%; and seizures in 15% to 20%.[50]

Clinical Features

Tumors may be located intra-axially (*i.e.,* within brain tissue) or extra-axially (*i.e.,* outside brain tissue, within the cranium). Disturbances in brain function usually are greatest with fast-growing, infiltrative, intra-axial tumors because of compression, infiltration, and necrosis of brain tissue. Extra-axial tumors, such as meningiomas, may reach a large size without producing signs and symptoms. Cysts may form in tumors and contribute to brain compression. Cerebral edema usually is of the vasogenic type, which develops around brain tumors and is characterized by increased brain water and expanded extracellular fluid. The edema is thought to result from increased permeability of tumor capillary endothelial cells.

Because the volume of the intracranial cavity is fixed, brain tumors cause a generalized increase in ICP when they reach sufficient size. Tumors can obstruct the flow of CSF in the ventricular cavities and produce hydrocephalic dilatation of the proximal ventricles and atrophy of the cerebral hemispheres. Complete compensation of ventricular volumes can occur with very slow-growing tumors, but with rapidly growing tumors, increased ICP is an early sign. Depending on the location of the tumor, brain displacement and herniation of the uncus or cerebellum may occur.

Clinical Manifestations. The clinical manifestations of brain tumors depend on the size and location of the tumor. General signs and symptoms include headache, nausea, vomiting, mental changes, papilledema, visual disturbances (*e.g.,* diplopia), alterations in sensory and motor function, and seizures.

The brain itself is insensitive to pain. The headache that accompanies brain tumors results from compression or distortion of pain-sensitive dural or vascular structures. It may be felt on the same side of the head as the tumor but more commonly is diffuse. In the early stages, the headache is mild and occurs in the morning upon awakening, and improves with head elevation. The headache becomes more constant as the tumor enlarges and often is worsened by coughing, bending, or sudden movements of the head.

Vomiting occurs with or without nausea, may be projectile, and is a common symptom of increased ICP and brain stem compression. Direct stimulation of the vomiting center, which is located in the medulla, may contribute to the vomiting that occurs with brain tumors. The vomiting is often associated with headache. Papilledema (edema of the optic disk) results from increased ICP and obstruction of the CSF pathways. It is associated with decreased visual acuity, diplopia, and deficits in the visual fields. Visual defects associated with papilledema often are the reason persons with brain tumor seek medical care.

Personality and mental changes are common with brain tumors. Persons with brain tumors often are irritable initially and later become quiet and apathetic. They may become forgetful, seem preoccupied, and appear to be psychologically depressed. Because of the mental changes, a psychiatric consultation may be sought before a diagnosis of brain tumor is made.

Focal signs and symptoms are determined by the location of the tumor. Tumors arising in the frontal lobe may grow to large size, increase the ICP, and cause signs of generalized brain dysfunction before focal signs are recognized. Tumors that impinge on the visual system cause visual loss or visual field defects long before generalized signs develop. Certain areas of the brain have a relatively low threshold for seizure activity. Temporal lobe tumors often produce seizures as their first symptom. Hallucinations of smell or hearing and *déjà vu* phenomena are common focal manifestations of temporal lobe tumors. Brain stem tumors commonly produce upper and lower motor neuron signs, such as weakness of facial muscles and ocular palsies, that occur with or without involvement of sensory or long motor tracts. Cerebellar tumors often cause ataxia of gait.

Diagnosis. Diagnostic procedures for brain tumor include physical and neurologic examinations, visual field and funduscopic examination, CT scans and MRI, skull x-ray films, technetium pertechnetate brain scans, EEG, and cerebral angiography.[50,52] Physical examination is used to assess motor and sensory function. Because the visual pathways travel through many areas of the cerebral lobes, detection of visual field defects can provide information about the location of tumors. A funduscopic examination is done to detect papilledema. Although CT scanning is used as a screening test, MRI scans are more sensitive than CT for detecting mass lesions. Skull x-ray films are used to detect calcified areas in a neoplasm or erosion of skull structures due to tumors. Approximately 75% of persons with a brain tumor have an abnormal EEG; in some cases, the results of the test can be used to localize the tumor. Cerebral angiography can be used to locate a tumor and visualize its vascular supply, infor-

mation that is important when planning surgery. MRI can be used to distinguish vascular masses from tumors.

Treatment. The three general methods for treatment of brain tumors are surgery, irradiation, and chemotherapy. Surgery is part of the initial management of virtually all brain tumors; it establishes the diagnosis and achieves tumor removal in many cases. The development of microsurgical neuroanatomy, the operating microscope, and advanced stereotactic and ultrasonographic technology; the fusion of imaging systems with resection techniques; and the intraoperative monitoring of evoked potentials or EEG have improved the effectiveness of surgical resection. However, removal may be limited by the location of the tumor and its invasiveness.

Most malignant brain tumors respond to external irradiation. Irradiation can increase longevity and sometimes can allay symptoms when tumors recur. The treatment dose depends on the tumor's histologic type, radioresponsiveness, and anatomic site and on the level of tolerance of the surrounding tissue. A newer technique called *gamma knife* combines stereotactic localization of tumor with radiosurgery, allowing delivery of high-dose radiation to deep tumors, sparing surrounding brain. Radiation therapy is avoided in treating children younger than 2 years of age because of the long-term effects, which include developmental delay, panhypopituitarism, and secondary tumors.

The use of chemotherapy for brain tumors is somewhat limited by the blood-brain barrier. Chemotherapeutic agents can be administered intravenously, intraarterially, intrathecally (*i.e.*, into the spinal canal), or intraventricularly. A promising area of improved delivery of chemotherapeutic agents is the use of biodegradable anhydrous wafers impregnated with a drug and implanted into the tumor at the time of surgery. These wafers are constructed so they release the drug over a period of many months.

In summary, infections of the CNS may be classified according to the structures involved—the meninges (meningitis) or brain parenchyma (encephalitis)—and the type of organism causing the infection (bacteria or virus). The damage caused by infection may predispose to hydrocephalus, seizures, or other neurologic defects.

Brain tumors account for 2% of all aggressive neoplasms and are the second most common type of cancer in children. Brain tumors can arise primarily from intracranial structures, and tumors from other parts of the body often metastasize to the brain. Primary brain tumors can arise from any structure in the cranial cavity. The clinical manifestations of brain tumor depend on the size and location of the tumor. Focal disturbances result from brain compression, tumor infiltration, disturbances in blood flow, and cerebral edema. General signs and symptoms include headache, nausea, vomiting, mental changes, papilledema, visual disturbances, alterations in motor and sensory function, and seizures. Diagnostic tests include physical examination, visual field testing and funduscopic examination, CT scans, MRI studies, skull x-ray films, brain scans, EEG, and cerebral angiography. Treatment includes surgery, irradiation, and chemotherapy.

Seizure Disorders

A seizure represents the clinical manifestations of an abnormal, uncontrolled electrical discharge from a group of neurons in the cerebral cortex. It is a discrete clinical event with associated signs and symptoms that vary according to the site of neuronal discharge in the brain. Manifestations of seizure generally include sensory, motor, autonomic, or psychic phenomena. A convulsion refers to the specific type of motor seizure involving the entire body.

A seizure is not a disease but a symptom of underlying CNS dysfunction. Seizures may occur during almost all serious illnesses or injuries affecting the brain, including infections, tumors, drug abuse, vascular lesions, congenital deformities, and brain injury. Seizure activity is the most common disorder encountered in pediatric neurology, and among adults, its incidence is exceeded only by cerebrovascular disorders.

PROVOKED AND UNPROVOKED SEIZURES

Many theories have been proposed to explain the cause of the abnormal brain electrical activity that occurs with seizures. Seizures may be caused by alterations in cell membrane permeability or distribution of ions across the neuronal cell membranes. Another cause may be decreased inhibition of cortical or thalamic neuronal activity or structural changes that alter the excitability of neurons. Neurotransmitter imbalances such as an acetylcholine excess or γ-aminobutyric acid (GABA, an inhibitory neurotransmitter) deficiency have been proposed as causes.

Clinically, seizures may be categorized as unprovoked (primary or idiopathic) or provoked (secondary or acute symptomatic).[54–56] Unprovoked or idiopathic seizures are those for which no identifiable cause can be determined, and are thought to be genetic. Most unprovoked seizures occur in the setting of an epileptic syndrome. These patients usually require chronic administration of antiepileptic medications to limit seizure recurrences.

Provoked or symptomatic seizures include febrile seizures, seizures precipitated by systemic metabolic conditions, and those that follow a primary insult to the CNS. Most provoked seizures are best prevented by treatment of the underlying cause. For example, the most common subgroup is that of febrile seizures in children.[57] In susceptible children, a high fever, usually over 104°F, will provoke a generalized seizure. Treatment includes aggressive use of antipyretics to prevent seizures during a febrile illness. Transient systemic metabolic disturbances

KEY CONCEPTS

Seizures

➤ Seizures are paroxysmal motor, sensory, or cognitive manifestations of spontaneous, abnormally synchronous electrical discharges from collections of neurons in the cerebral cortex that are thought to result directly or indirectly from changes in excitability of single neurons or groups of neurons.

➤ Partial seizures originate in a small group of neurons in one hemisphere with secondary spread of seizure activity to other parts of the brain. Simple partial seizures usually are confined to one hemisphere and do not involve loss of consciousness. Complex partial seizures begin in a localized area, spread to both hemispheres, and involve impairment of consciousness.

➤ Generalized seizures show simultaneous disruption of normal brain activity in both hemispheres from the onset. They include unconsciousness and varying bilateral degrees of symmetric motor responses with evidence of localization to one hemisphere. Absence seizures are generalized nonconvulsive seizure events that are expressed mainly by brief periods of unconsciousness. Tonic-clonic seizures involve unconsciousness along with both tonic and clonic muscle contractions.

may precipitate seizures. Examples include electrolyte imbalances, hypoglycemia, hypoxia, hypocalcemia, uremia, alkalosis, and rapid withdrawal of sedative drugs. Specific CNS injuries such as toxemia of pregnancy, water intoxication, meningoencephalitis, trauma, cerebral hemorrhage and stroke, and brain tumors may precipitate a seizure. In all cases of provoked seizures, treatment of the immediate underlying cause often results in their resolution.

EPILEPTIC SYNDROMES

Recurrent seizures are one feature of epileptic syndromes. In most persons, the first seizure episode occurs before 20 years of age. After 20 years of age, a seizure is caused most often by a structural change, trauma, tumor, or stroke. Approximately 2 million persons in the United States are subject to recurrent seizures.[54]

Patients with an epileptic syndrome may have several seizure types. The current classification system endorsed by the International League Against Epilepsy identifies seizure type by clinical symptoms and EEG activity. It divides seizures into two broad categories: partial seizures, in which the seizure begins in a specific or focal area of one cerebral hemisphere, and generalized seizures, which begin simultaneously in both cerebral hemispheres[58,59] (Chart 36-1). Further classification of epileptic *syndromes* characterizes the underlying diseases that cause the seizures, and divides them into idiopathic (suspected to be genetic), symptomatic (resulting from some CNS injury), and cryptogenic (presumed to be symptomatic of some unidentified cause).[59] The system also has categories for seizures of undetermined origin such as neonatal seizures and a category of special syndromes such as febrile seizures.

Partial Seizures

Partial or focal seizures are the most common type of seizure among newly diagnosed cases in all persons older than 10 years of age. Partial seizures can be subdivided into three major groups: simple partial (consciousness is not impaired), complex partial (impairment of consciousness), and secondarily generalized partial seizures.

Simple Partial Seizures. Simple partial seizures usually involve only one hemisphere and are not accompanied by loss of consciousness or responsiveness. These seizures

---

CHART 36-1

Classification of Epileptic Seizures

Partial Seizures

Simple partial seizures (no impairment of consciousness)
  With motor symptoms
  With sensory symptoms
  With autonomic signs
  With psychic symptoms
Complex partial seizures (impairment of consciousness)
  Simple partial onset followed by impaired consciousness
  Impairment of consciousness at onset
Partial seizures evolving to secondarily generalized seizures
  Simple partial leading to generalized seizures
  Complex partial leading to generalized seizures

Unclassified Seizures

Classification not possible because of inadequate or incomplete data

Generalized Seizures

Absence seizures (typical or atypical)
Atonic seizures
Myoclonic seizures
Clonic seizures
Tonic
Tonic-clonic seizures

(Adapted from Commission on Classification and Terminology of the International League Against Epilepsy. [1981]. Proposal for revised clinical and electroencephalographic classification of epileptic seizures. *Epilepsia* 22, 489.)

---

also have been referred to as *elementary partial seizures, partial seizures with elementary symptoms,* or *focal seizures.* Simple partial seizures are classified according to motor signs, sensory symptoms, autonomic manifestations, and psychic symptoms.

The observed clinical signs and symptoms depend on the area of the brain where the abnormal neuronal discharge is taking place. If the motor area of the brain is involved, the earliest symptom is motor movement corresponding to the location of onset on the contralateral side of the brain. The motor movement may remain localized or may spread to other cortical areas, with sequential involvement of body parts in an epileptic-type "march," known as a *Jacksonian seizure.* If the sensory portion of the brain is involved, there may be no observable clinical manifestations. Sensory symptoms correlating with the location of seizure activity on the contralateral side of the brain may involve somatic sensory disturbance (*e.g.,* tingling and crawling sensations) or special sensory disturbance (*i.e.,* visual, auditory, gustatory, or olfactory phenomena). When abnormal cortical discharge stimulates the autonomic nervous system, flushing, tachycardia, diaphoresis, hypotension or hypertension, or pupillary changes may be evident.

The term *prodrome* or *aura* traditionally has meant a sensory warning sign of impending seizure activity or the onset of seizure that affected persons could describe because they were conscious. The aura itself now is considered part of the seizure. Because only a small area of the brain is involved and consciousness is maintained, an aura is considered a simple partial seizure. Simple partial seizures may progress to complex partial seizures or generalized tonic-clonic seizures that result in unconsciousness. Therefore, the aura, a simple partial seizure, may be considered a warning sign of impending complex partial seizures.

Complex Partial Seizures. Complex partial seizures involve impairment of consciousness and often arise from the temporal lobe. The seizure begins in a localized area of the brain but may progress rapidly to involve both hemispheres. These seizures also may be referred to as *temporal lobe seizures* or *psychomotor seizures.*

Complex partial seizures often are accompanied by automatisms. Automatisms are repetitive, nonpurposeful activity such as lip smacking, grimacing, patting, or rubbing clothing. Confusion during the postictal state (after a seizure) is common. Hallucinations and illusional experiences such as *déjà vu* (familiarity with unfamiliar events or environments) or *jamais vu* (unfamiliarity with a known environment) have been reported. There may be overwhelming fear, uncontrolled forced thinking or a flood of ideas, and feelings of detachment and depersonalization. A person with a complex partial seizure disorder sometimes is misunderstood and believed to require hospitalization for a psychiatric disorder.

Secondarily Generalized Partial Seizures. These seizures are focal at onset but then become generalized as the seizure activity spreads, involving deeper structures of the brain, such as the thalamus or the reticular formation. Discharges spread to both hemispheres, resulting in progression to tonic-clonic seizure activity. These seizures may start as simple or complex partial seizures and may be preceded by an aura. The aura, often a stereotyped peculiar sensation that precedes the seizure, is the result of partial seizure activity. A history of an aura is clinically useful to identify the seizure as partial and not generalized in onset. However, absence of an aura does not reliably exclude a focal onset because many partial seizures generalize too rapidly to generate an aura.

Generalized Seizures

Generalized seizures begin with initial involvement of both hemispheres. Generalized-onset seizures are the most common type in young children. These seizures are classified as primary or generalized when clinical signs, symptoms, and supporting EEG changes indicate involvement of both hemispheres at onset. The clinical symptoms include unconsciousness and involve varying degrees of symmetric bilateral motor responses without evidence of localization to one hemisphere.

These seizures are divided into four broad categories: absence seizures (typical and atypical), atonic seizures, myoclonic seizures, and major motor (tonic-clonic) seizures.[54,55]

Absence Seizures. Absence seizures, formerly referred to as *petit mal seizures,* are generalized, nonconvulsive epileptic events and are expressed mainly as disturbances in consciousness. Absence seizures typically occur only in children and cease in adulthood or evolve to generalized motor seizures. Children may present with a history of school failure that predates the first evidence of seizure episodes. Although *typical absence seizures* have been characterized as manifesting with a blank stare, motionlessness, and unresponsiveness, motion occurs in many cases of typical absence seizures. This motion may take the form of automatisms such as lip smacking, mild clonic motion (usually in the eyelids), increased or decreased postural tone, and autonomic phenomena. There often is a brief loss of contact with the environment. The seizure usually lasts only a few seconds, and then the child is able to resume normal activity immediately. The manifestations often are so subtle that they may pass unnoticed.

Atypical absence seizures are similar to typical absence seizures except for greater alterations in muscle tone and less abrupt onset and cessation. In practice, it is difficult to distinguish typical from atypical absence seizures without benefit of supporting EEG findings. Because automatisms and unresponsiveness are common to complex partial seizures, the latter may be mistakenly labeled as absence seizures. However, it is important to distinguish between the two types of seizures because the drug treatment is different. Medications that are effective for partial seizures may increase the frequency of absence seizures.

Atonic Seizures. In atonic or akinetic seizures, there is a sudden, split-second loss of muscle tone leading to slackening of the jaw, drooping of the limbs, or falling to the ground. These seizures also are known as *drop attacks.*

Myoclonic Seizures. Myoclonic seizures involve brief involuntary muscle contractions induced by stimuli of cerebral origin. A myoclonic seizure involves bilateral jerking of muscles, generalized or confined to the face, trunk, or one or more extremities. Tonic seizures are characterized by a rigid, violent contraction of the muscles, fixing the limbs in a strained position. Clonic seizures consist of repeated contractions and relaxations of the major muscle groups.

Tonic-Clonic Seizures. Tonic-clonic seizures, formerly called *grand mal seizures,* are the most common major motor seizure. Frequently, a person has a vague warning (probably a simple partial seizure) and experiences a sharp tonic contraction of the muscles with extension of the extremities and immediate loss of consciousness. Incontinence of bladder and bowel is common. Cyanosis may occur from contraction of airway and respiratory muscles. The tonic phase is followed by the clonic phase, which involves rhythmic bilateral contraction and relaxation of the extremities. At the end of the clonic phase, the person remains unconscious until the RAS begins to function again. This is called the *postictal phase.* The tonic-clonic phases last approximately 60 to 90 seconds.

Unclassified Seizures

Unclassified seizures are those that cannot be placed in one of the previous categories. These seizures are observed in the neonatal and infancy periods. Determination of whether the seizure is focal or generalized is not possible. Unclassified seizures are difficult to control with medication.

DIAGNOSIS AND TREATMENT

The diagnosis of seizure disorders is based on a thorough history and neurologic examination, including a full description of the seizure. The physical examination and laboratory studies help exclude any metabolic disease (*e.g.,* hyponatremia) that could precipitate seizures. Skull radiographs and CT or MRI scans are used to identify structural defects. One of the most useful diagnostic tests is the EEG, which is used to record changes in the brain's electrical activity. It is used to support the clinical diagnosis of epilepsy, to provide a guide for prognosis, and to assist in classifying the seizure disorder.

The first rule of treatment is to protect the person from injury during a seizure, preserve brain function by aborting or preventing seizure activity, and treat any underlying disease. Persons with epilepsy should be advised to avoid situations that could be dangerous or life threatening if seizures occur.

Pharmacologic Treatment

More than 20 drugs are available in the United States for the treatment of epilepsy. This group includes six anti-epileptic drugs that have been approved for use in the United States since 1996.[60]

Antiepileptic drugs act mainly by suppressing repetitive firing of isolated neurons that act as epileptogenic foci for seizure activity or by inhibiting the transmission of electrical impulses involved in seizure activity.[61] Because of their selective mechanisms of action, different drugs are used to treat the different types of seizures. For example, ethosuximide, which suppresses the brain wave activity associated with lapses of consciousness, is used in the treatment of absence seizures, but is not effective for tonic-clonic seizures that progress from partial seizures.

The goal of pharmacologic treatment is to bring the seizures under control with the least possible disruption in lifestyle and minimum side effects from medication. When possible, a single drug should be used. Monotherapy eliminates drug interactions and additive side effects. Determining the proper dose of the anticonvulsant drug is often a long and tedious process, which can be very frustrating for the person with epilepsy. Often blood tests are used to determine that the blood concentration is within the therapeutic range. Consistency in taking the medication is essential. Antiepileptic drug use never should be discontinued abruptly. Special consideration is needed when a person taking an antiepileptic medication becomes ill and must take additional medications. Some drugs act synergistically, and others interfere with the actions of other antiepileptic medications. This situation needs to be carefully monitored to avoid overmedication or interference with successful seizure control.

Women of childbearing age require special consideration concerning fertility, contraception, and pregnancy. Many of the drugs interact with oral contraceptives; some affect hormone function or decrease fertility. All such women should be advised to take folic acid supplementation. For women with epilepsy who become pregnant, antiepileptic drugs increase the risk of congenital abnormalities and other perinatal complications.

Surgical Therapy

Surgical treatment may be an option for persons with epilepsy that is refractory to drug treatment.[62] With the use of modern neuroimaging and surgical techniques, a single epileptogenic lesion can be identified and removed without leaving a neurologic deficit.

GENERALIZED CONVULSIVE STATUS EPILEPTICUS

Seizures that do not stop spontaneously or occur in succession without recovery are called *status epilepticus*. There are as many types of status epilepticus as there are types of seizures. Tonic-clonic status epilepticus is a medical emergency and, if not promptly treated, may lead to respiratory failure and death.

The disorder occurs most frequently in the young and old. Morbidity and mortality rates are highest in elderly persons and persons with acute symptomatic seizures, such as those related to anoxia or cerebral infarction.[63] Approximately one third of patients have no history of a seizure disorder, and in another one third, status epilepticus occurs as an initial manifestation of epilepsy.[63]

Treatment consists of appropriate life-support measures. If status epilepticus is caused by neurologic or systemic disease, the cause needs to be identified and treated immediately. Medications are given to control seizure activity.

In summary, seizures are caused by spontaneous, uncontrolled, paroxysmal, transitory discharges from cortical centers in the brain. Seizures may occur as a reversible symptom of another disease condition or as a recurrent condition called *epilepsy*. Epileptic seizures are classified as partial or generalized seizures. Partial seizures have evidence of local onset, beginning in one hemisphere. They include simple partial seizures, in which consciousness is not lost, and complex partial seizures, which begin in one hemisphere but progress to involve both. Generalized seizures involve both hemispheres and include unconsciousness and rapidly occurring, widespread, bilateral symmetric motor responses. They include absence, atonic, myotonic, and tonic-clonic seizures. Control of seizures is the primary goal of treatment and is accomplished with anticonvulsant medications. Anticonvulsant medications interact with each other and need to be monitored closely when more than one drug is used.

Dementias

Dementia is a syndrome of intellectual deterioration severe enough to interfere with occupational and social performance. It may involve disturbances in memory, language use, perception, and motor skills and may interrupt the ability to learn necessary skills, solve problems, think abstractly, and make judgments. The dementias include Alzheimer disease, multi-infarct dementia, Pick disease, Creutzfeldt-Jakob disease, Wernicke-Korsakoff syndrome, and Huntington chorea.

Depression is the most common treatable illness that may masquerade as dementia, and must be excluded when a diagnosis of dementia is considered. This is important because cognitive functioning usually returns to baseline levels after depression is treated.

ALZHEIMER DISEASE

Dementia of the Alzheimer type occurs in middle or late life and accounts for 50% to 70% of all cases of dementia. The disorder affects approximately 4.5 million Americans.[64] The risk of developing Alzheimer disease increases with age, and the prevalence doubles for every 5 years beyond age 65 years. As the elderly population in the United States continues to increase, the number of persons with Alzheimer-type dementia also is expected to increase.

Pathophysiology

Alzheimer disease is characterized by cortical atrophy and loss of neurons, particularly in the parietal and temporal lobes (Fig. 36-19). With significant atrophy, there is ventricular enlargement (*i.e.*, hydrocephalus) from the loss of brain tissue.

The major microscopic features of Alzheimer disease are the presence of amyloid-containing neuritic plaques and neurofibrillary tangles.[1,3,65] The neurofibrillary tangles, found in the cytoplasm of abnormal neurons, consist of fibrous proteins that are wound around each other in a helical fashion. These tangles are resistant to chemical or enzymatic breakdown, and they persist in brain tissue long after the neuron in which they arose has died and disappeared. The senile plaques are patches or flat areas composed of clusters of degenerating nerve terminals arranged around a central core of amyloid β-protein (Aβ).[3] These plaques are found in areas of the cerebral cortex that are linked to intellectual function. Aβ is a fragment of a much larger membrane-spanning amyloid precursor protein (APP). The function of APP is unclear, but it appears to be associated with the cytoskeleton of nerve fibers. Normally, the degradation of APP involves cleavage in the middle of the Aβ portion of the molecule, with both fragments being lost in the extracellular fluid. These fragments are not amyloidogenic. In Alzheimer disease, the APP molecule is cut at both ends of the Aβ segment, thereby releasing an intact Aβ molecule that accumulates in neuritic plaques as amyloid fibrils.[3]

Some plaques and tangles can be found in the brains of older persons who do not show cognitive impairment. The number and distribution of the plaques and tangles appear to contribute to the intellectual deterioration that occurs with Alzheimer disease. In persons with the disease, the plaques and tangles are found throughout the neocortex and in the hippocampus and amygdala, with relative sparing of the primary sensory cortex.[1] Hippocampal function in particular may be compromised by the pathologic changes that occur in Alzheimer disease. The hippocampus is crucial to information processing, acquisition of new memories, and retrieval of old memories. The development of neurofibrillary tangles in the entorhinal cortex and superior portion of the hippocampal gyrus interferes with cortical input and output, thereby isolating the hippocampus from the remainder of the cortex and rendering it functionless.

Neurochemically, Alzheimer disease has been associated with a decrease in the level of choline acetyltransferase activity in the cortex and hippocampus. This enzyme is required for the synthesis of acetylcholine, a neurotransmitter that is associated with memory. The reduction in choline acetyltransferase is quantitatively related to the numbers of neuritic plaques and severity of dementia.

Several drugs have been shown to be effective in slowing the progression of the disease by potentiating the available acetylcholine. The drugs—tacrine, donepezil, rivastigmine, and galantamine—inhibit acetylcholinesterase, preventing the metabolism of endogenous acetylcholine. Thus far, such therapy has not halted disease progression, but it can establish a meaningful plateau in decline.

It is likely that Alzheimer disease is caused by several factors that interact differently in different persons. Progress on the genetics of inherited early-onset Alzheimer disease shows that mutations in at least three genes—the APP gene on chromosome 21; presenilin-1 (PS1), a gene on chromosome 14; and presenilin-2 (PS2), a gene on

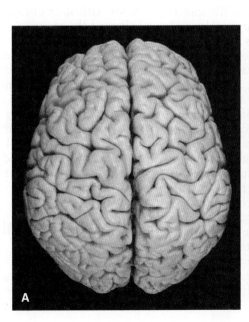
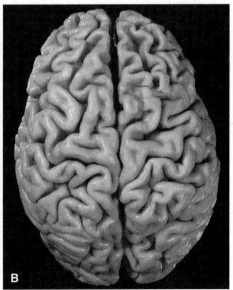

FIGURE 36-19 Alzheimer disease. (**A**) Normal brain. (**B**) The brain of a patient with Alzheimer disease shows cortical atrophy, characterized by slender gyri and prominent sulci. (From Trojanowski J. Q. [2005]. The central nervous system. In Rubin E., Gorstein F., Rubin R., et al. [Eds.], *Rubin's pathology: Clinicopathologic foundations of medicine* [4th ed., p. 1476]. Philadelphia: Lippincott Williams & Wilkins.)

chromosome 1—can cause Alzheimer disease in certain families.[1,3] The APP gene is associated with an autosomal dominant form of early-onset Alzheimer disease, and can be tested clinically. Persons with Down syndrome (trisomy 21) develop the pathologic changes of Alzheimer disease and a comparable decline in cognitive functioning at a relatively young age. Virtually all persons with Down syndrome who survive past 50 years of age develop the full-blown pathologic features of dementia. Because the APP gene is located on chromosome 21, it is thought that the additional dosage of the gene product in trisomy 21 predisposes to accumulation of $A\beta$.[3] There is some indication that PS1 and PS2 mutant proteins alter the processing of APP.[3] A fourth gene, an allele of the apolipoprotein E gene, APOE e4, has been identified as a risk factor for late-onset Alzheimer disease.[1]

Clinical Features

Alzheimer-type dementia follows an insidious and progressive course. The hallmark symptoms are loss of short-term memory and a denial of such memory loss, with eventual disorientation, impaired abstract thinking, apraxias, and changes in personality and affect.[66] Three stages of Alzheimer dementia have been identified, each of which is characterized by progressive degenerative changes. The *first stage,* which may last for 2 to 4 years, is characterized by short-term memory loss that often is difficult to differentiate from the normal forgetfulness that occurs in the elderly, and usually is reported by caregivers and denied by the patient. Although most elderly have trouble retrieving from memory incidental information and proper names, persons with Alzheimer disease randomly forget important and unimportant details. They forget where things are placed, get lost easily, and have trouble remembering appointments and performing novel tasks. Mild changes in personality, such as lack of spontaneity, social withdrawal, and loss of a previous sense of humor, occur during this stage.

As the disease progresses, the person with Alzheimer disease enters the *second* or *confusional stage* of dementia. This stage may last several years and is marked by a more global impairment of cognitive functioning. During this stage, there are changes in higher cortical functioning needed for language, spatial relationships, and problem solving. Depression may occur in persons who are aware of their deficits. There is extreme confusion, disorientation, lack of insight, and inability to carry out the activities of daily living. Personal hygiene is neglected, and language becomes impaired because of difficulty in remembering and retrieving words. Wandering, especially in the late afternoon or early evening, becomes a problem. The *sundown syndrome,* which is characterized by confusion, restlessness, agitation, and wandering, may become a daily occurrence late in the afternoon. Some persons may become hostile and abusive toward family members. Persons who enter this stage become unable to live alone and should be assisted in making decisions about supervised placement with family members or friends or in a community-based facility.

Stage 3 is the terminal stage. It usually is relatively short (1 to 2 years) compared with the other stages, but it has been known to last for as long as 10 years.[67] The person becomes incontinent, apathetic, and unable to recognize family or friends. It usually is during this stage that the person is institutionalized.

Diagnosis and Treatment. Alzheimer disease is essentially a diagnosis of exclusion. There are no peripheral biochemical markers or tests for the disease. The diagnosis can be confirmed only by microscopic examination of tissue obtained from a cerebral biopsy or at autopsy. The diagnosis is based on clinical findings. Guidelines for the early recognition and assessment of Alzheimer disease have been published by the Agency for Health Care Policy and Research (AHCPR).[67] A diagnosis of Alzheimer disease requires the presence of dementia established by clinical examination and documented by results of a Mini-Mental State Examination, Blessed Dementia Test, or similar mental status test; no disturbance in consciousness; onset between ages 40 and 90 years, most often after age 65 years; and absence of systemic or brain disorders that could account for the memory or cognitive deficits.[68] Brain imaging, CT scan, or MRI is done to exclude other brain disease. Metabolic screening should be done for known reversible causes of dementia such as vitamin B_{12} deficiency, thyroid dysfunction, and electrolyte imbalance.

There is no curative treatment for Alzheimer dementia. Drugs are used primarily to slow the progression and to control depression, agitation, or sleep disorders. Two major goals of care are maintaining the person's socialization and providing support for the family. Self-help groups that provide support for family and friends have become available, with support from the Alzheimer Disease and Related Disorders Association. Day care and respite centers are available in many areas to provide relief for caregivers and appropriate stimulation for the patient.

Although there is no current drug therapy that is curative for Alzheimer disease, some show promise in terms of slowing the progress of the disease. The use of pharmacologic agents such as tacrine, donepezil, rivastigmine, and galantamine has been approved for symptomatic therapy in Alzheimer disease.[64,65,68] Memantine, an NMDA receptor antagonist recently approved by the FDA for treatment of moderate to severe Alzheimer disease, may interfere with glutamatergic excitotoxicity and may provide symptomatic relief through effects on functioning hippocampal neurons.[64] There also is interest in the use of agents such as antioxidants (*e.g.,* vitamin E, ginkgo) and anti-inflammatory agents to prevent or delay the onset of the disease.

OTHER TYPES OF DEMENTIA

Vascular Dementia

Vascular dementia is the second most common cause of dementia, after Alzheimer disease. It results from a variety of cerebrovascular disorders and produces a pattern of cognitive impairments that vary with the location and extent of the underlying pathologic process.[69] The most common causes are single, strategically placed infarcts; multiple cortical infarcts; and subcortical small vessel disease. The two most potent risk factors are hypertension and stroke. Other contributing factors include cardiac arrhythmias, peripheral vascular disease, diabetes, and smoking.

The symptoms of vascular dementia are often different from those of Alzheimer disease. The memory deficits that occur early in Alzheimer disease are not always observed in vascular dementia. Instead, there tends to be greater impairment of executive function such as organizing thoughts, time, materials, and belongings; and difficulty in initiating tasks, switching between tasks, or sustaining focus on the relevant aspects of a stimulus or task.[69] The disease also differs from Alzheimer dementia in its presentation and tissue abnormalities. The onset may be gradual or abrupt, the course usually is a stepwise progression, and there may be focal neurologic symptoms related to local areas of infarction.

Pick Disease

Pick disease is a rare form of dementia characterized by atrophy of the frontal and temporal areas of the brain. The neurons in the affected areas contain cytoplasmic inclusions called *Pick bodies*.[3] The average age at onset of Pick disease is 38 years. The disease is more common in women than men. Behavioral manifestations may be noticed earlier than memory deficits, taking the form of a striking absence of concern and care, a loss of initiative, echolalia (*i.e.,* automatic repetition of anything said to the person), hypotonia, and incontinence. The course of the disease is relentless, with death ensuing within 3 to 10 years.[3] The immediate cause of death usually is infection.

Creutzfeldt-Jakob Disease

Creutzfeldt-Jakob disease is a rare transmissible form of dementia thought to be caused by an infective protein agent called a *prion*[70] (see Chapter 12). Similar diseases occur in animals, including scrapie in sheep and goats and bovine spongiform encephalitis (BSE; mad cow disease) in cattle. The pathogen is resistant to chemical and physical methods commonly used for sterilizing medical and surgical equipment. The disease reportedly has been transmitted through corneal transplants and human growth hormone obtained from cadavers. The National Hormone and Pituitary Program halted the distribution of human pituitary hormone in 1985 after reports that three young persons who had received the hormone had died of Creutzfeldt-Jakob disease.[71]

Creutzfeldt-Jakob disease causes degeneration of the pyramidal and extrapyramidal systems and is distinguished most readily by its rapid course.[1] Affected persons usually are demented within 6 months of onset. The disease is uniformly fatal, with death often occurring within months, although a few persons may survive for several years. The early symptoms consist of abnormalities in personality and visual-spatial coordination. Extreme dementia, insomnia, and ataxia follow as the disease progresses.

Wernicke-Korsakoff Syndrome

Wernicke-Korsakoff syndrome most commonly results from chronic alcoholism. Wernicke syndrome is characterized by acute weakness and paralysis of the extraocular muscles, nystagmus, ataxia, and confusion.[1] The affected person also may have signs of peripheral neuropathy. The person has an unsteady gait and complains of diplopia. There may be signs attributable to alcohol withdrawal such as delirium, confusion, and hallucinations. This disorder is caused by a deficiency of thiamine (vitamin B$_1$), and many of the symptoms are reversed when nutrition is improved with supplemental thiamine.

The Korsakoff component of the syndrome involves the chronic phase with severe impairment of recent memory. There often is difficulty in dealing with abstractions, and the person's capacity to learn is defective. Confabulation (*i.e.,* recitation of imaginary experiences to fill in gaps in memory) probably is the most distinctive feature of the disease. Polyneuritis also is common. Unlike Wernicke disease, Korsakoff psychosis does not improve significantly with treatment.

Huntington Disease

Huntington disease is a hereditary disorder characterized by chronic progressive chorea, psychological changes, and dementia. Although the disease is inherited as an autosomal dominant disorder, the age of onset most commonly is in the fourth and fifth decades.[1] By the time the disease has been diagnosed, the person often has passed the gene on to his or her children. Approximately 10% of Huntington cases involve juvenile onset.[72] Children with the disease rarely live to adulthood.

The pathologic process in Huntington disease involves a localized loss of brain cells. The frontal cortex is moderately and symmetrically atrophic and there is symmetric atrophy of the caudate nuclei and, to a lesser extent, of the putamen of the basal ganglia. There is loss of most of the cell bodies of the GABA-secreting neurons in the caudate and the putamen and of the acetylcholine-secreting neurons in other parts of the brain.[11] The GABA-secreting neurons normally inhibit portions of the globus pallidus and substantia nigra and the loss of inhibition is thought to result in spontaneous outbursts from the globus pallidus and substantia nigra that cause the choreiform movements. The dementia probably results from loss of acetylcholine-secreting neurons in the cortex.

Depression and personality changes are the most common early psychological manifestations; memory loss often is accompanied by impulsive behavior, moodiness, antisocial behavior, and a tendency toward emotional outbursts.[73] Other early signs of the disease are lack of initiative, loss of spontaneity, and inability to concentrate. Fidgeting or restlessness may represent early signs of dyskinesia, followed by choreiform and some dystonic posturing. Eventually, progressive rigidity and akinesia (rather than chorea) develop in association with dementia. Symptoms of juvenile onset include dystonias and seizures.

There is no cure for Huntington disease. The treatment is largely symptomatic. Drugs may be used to treat the dyskinesias and behavioral disturbances. Study of the genetics of Huntington disease led to the discovery that the gene for the disease is located on chromosome 4.[3] The discovery of a marker probe for the gene locus has enabled testing that can predict whether a person will develop the disease.

In summary, dementia is a syndrome of intellectual deterioration severe enough to interfere with occupational or social performance. It may involve disturbances in memory, language use, perception, and motor skills and may interrupt the ability to learn necessary skills, solve problems, think abstractly, and make judgments. Dementia can be caused by any disorder that permanently damages large association areas of the cerebral hemispheres or subcortical areas subserving memory and learning. The dementias include Alzheimer disease, vascular dementia, Pick disease, Creutzfeldt-Jakob disease, Wernicke-Korsakoff syndrome, and Huntington chorea. By far the most common cause of dementia (50% to 70%) is Alzheimer disease. The condition is a major health problem among the elderly. It is characterized by cortical atrophy and loss of neurons, the presence of neuritic plaques, granulovacuolar degeneration, and cerebrovascular deposits of amyloid. The disease follows an insidious and progressive course that begins with memory impairment and terminates in an inability to recognize family or friends and the loss of control over bodily functions.

Review Exercises

A 20-year-old man who was an unbelted driver involved in a motor vehicle accident presents in coma.

A. What are the clinical signs of coma?

B. Where does the source of coma localize in the brain?

C. Which complications of traumatic head injury might lead to coma?

D. What are the key treatment options to manage elevated intracranial pressure?

A 65-year-old woman presents with a 1-hour history of right-sided weakness and aphasia. An immediate CT scan of the brain is negative.

A. Where in the brain is the pathology?

B. What are the indications to administer intravenous tissue plasminogen activator?

C. What are the possible causes of this stroke, and what diagnostic tests would reveal the cause?

A child is taken to the emergency department with lethargy, fever, and a stiff neck on examination.

A. What findings on initial lumbar puncture indicate bacterial versus viral meningitis?

B. In the case of bacterial meningitis, what are the most likely organisms, and which antibiotics should be started?

A 60-year-old man develops involuntary shaking of his right arm that spreads to the face, after which he collapses with wholebody shaking and loss of consciousness. After 1 minute, the shaking stops and he is confused and disoriented.

A. What type of seizure is suggested by the clinical manifestations?

B. Assuming this is his first seizure, what diagnostic tests should be performed to identify a cause for the seizure?

C. If he has a long history of similar recurrent seizures, what treatments should be instituted? What treatments should be considered if he has failed multiple adequate trials of anticonvulsant medications?

Visit the Porth: Essentials of Pathophysiology: Concepts of Altered Health States web site (http://thePoint.LWW.com/PorthEssentials) for links to chapter-related resources on the Internet, all-new exclusive animations, chapter review questions, and more!

REFERENCES

1. Frosch M. P., Anthony D. C., DeGirolani U. (2005). The central nervous system. In Kumar V., Abbas A. K., Fausto N. (Eds.), *Robbins and Cotran pathologic basis of disease* (7th ed., pp. 1347–1419). Philadelphia: Elsevier Saunders.
2. Meyer F. B. (1992). Brain metabolism, blood flow, and ischemic thresholds. In Awad I. A. (Ed.), *Neurosurgical topics: Cerebrovascular occlusive disease and brain ischemia* (pp. 1–24). Cleveland: American Association of Neurological Surgeons.
3. Trojanowski J. Q. (2005). The central nervous system. In Rubin E., Gorstein F., Rubin E., et al. (Eds.), *Rubin's pathology: Clinicopathologic foundations of medicine* (4th ed., pp. 1413–1491). Philadelphia: Lippincott Williams & Wilkins.
4. Lipton S. A., Rosenberg P. A. (1994). Excitatory amino acids as a final common pathway in neurologic disorders. *New England Journal of Medicine* 330, 613–622.

5. Arundine M., Tymianski M. (2004). Molecular-mechanisms of glutamine-dependent neurodegeneration in ischemia and traumatic brain injury. *Cellular and Molecular Life Sciences* 61, 634–668.

6. Feurerstein G., Hunter J., Barone F. C. (1992). Calcium blockers and neuroprotection. In Marangos P. J., Lal H. (Eds.), *Advances in neuroprotection: Emerging strategies in neuroprotection* (p. 129). Boston: Birkhauser.

7. Albers G. W., Clark W. M., DeGraba T. J. (1998). *The evolving paradigm of neuronal protection following stroke*. Englewood, CO: Postgraduate Institute for Medicine.

8. Xiao F. (2002). Bench to bedside: Brain edema and cerebral resuscitation: The present and the future. *Academic Emergency Medicine* 9, 933–946.

9. Hickey J. V. (2003). *The clinical practice of neurological and neurosurgical nursing* (5th ed., pp. 159–184, 295–327, 378–385). Philadelphia: Lippincott Williams & Wilkins.

10. Lang E. W., Chestnut R. M. (1995). Intracranial pressure and cerebral perfusion pressure in severe head injury. *New Horizons* 3, 400–409.

11. Guyton A. C., Hall J. E. (2006). *Textbook of medical physiology* (11th ed., pp. 213, 711–712, 761–767). Philadelphia: Elsevier Saunders.

12. Ghajar J. (2000). Traumatic brain injury. *Lancet* 356, 923–929.

13. White R. J., Likavec M. J. (1992). The diagnosis and initial management of head injury. *New England Journal of Medicine* 327, 1507–1511.

14. Nolan S. (2005). Traumatic brain injury. *Critical Nursing Care Quarterly* 28, 188–194.

15. Teasdale G. M. (1995). Head injury. *Journal of Neurology, Neurosurgery, and Psychiatry* 58, 526–539.

16. Saper C. B. (2000). Brain stem modulation of sensation, movement, and consciousness. In Kandell E. R., Schwartz J. H., Jessel T. M. (Eds.), *Principles of neural science* (4th ed., pp. 896–909). New York: McGraw-Hill.

17. Ingersoll G. L., Leyden D. B. (1987). The Glasgow Coma Scale for patients with head injuries. *Critical Care Nurse* 7(5), 26–32.

18. Teasdale G. M. (2000). Revisiting the Glasgow Coma Scale and Coma Score. *Intensive Care Medicine* 26, 153–154.

19. Wijdicks E. F. M. (2001). The diagnosis of brain death. *New England Journal of Medicine* 344, 1215–1221.

20. Henneman E. A., Karras G. E. (2004). Determining brain death in adults: A guideline for use in critical care. *Critical Care Nurse* 24(5), 50–56.

21. Quality Standards Subcommittee of the American Academy of Neurology. (1995). Practice parameters for determining brain death in adults. *Neurology* 45, 1012–1014.

22. Quality Standards Subcommittee of the American Academy of Neurology. (1995). Practice parameters: Assessment and management of patients with persistent vegetative state. *Neurology* 45, 1015–1018.

23. Moore K. L., Dalley A. F. (2006). *Clinically oriented anatomy* (5th ed., pp. 927–933). Philadelphia: Lippincott Williams & Wilkins.

24. American Heart Association. (2005). *Heart disease and stroke statistics—2005 update*. Dallas: Author.

25. Goldstein L. B. (Chairperson, Stroke Council of American Heart Association). (2001). Primary prevention of ischemic stroke: A statement for health care professionals. *Circulation* 103, 163–182.

26. Stroke Council of the American Heart Association. (1999). *The latest news about stroke*. Dallas: American Heart Association.

27. Gorelick P. B. (1987). Alcohol and stroke. *Current Concepts in Cerebrovascular Disease* 21(5), 21.

28. Blank-Reid C. (1996). How to have a stroke at an early age: The effects of crack, cocaine and other illicit drugs. *Journal of Neuroscience Nursing* 28(1), 19–27.

29. Albers W. A. (Chair). (1998). Antithrombotic and thrombolytic therapy for ischemic stroke. *Chest* 114, 683S–698S.

30. Zambramski J. M., Anson J. A. (1992). Diagnostic evaluation of ischemic cerebrovascular disease. In Awad I. A. (Ed.), *Neurosurgical topics: Cerebrovascular occlusive disease and brain ischemia* (pp. 73–101). Cleveland: American Association of Neurological Surgeons.

31. Johnston S. C. (2002). Transient ischemic attack. *New England Journal of Medicine* 347, 1687–1692.

32. Gregory W. (Chair, Ad Hoc Committee on Guidelines for Management of Transient Ischemic Attacks, Stroke Council, American Heart Association). (1999). Supplement to the guidelines for transient ischemic attacks. *Stroke* 30, 2502–2511.

33. Qureshi A. I., Tuhrim S., Broderick J. P., et al. (2001). Spontaneous intracerebral hemorrhage. *New England Journal of Medicine* 344, 1450–1460.

34. Fewel M. E., Thompson M. G., Hoff J. T. (2003). Spontaneous intracerebral hemorrhage: A review. *Neurosurgical Focus* 15, 1–17.

35. Broderick J. P., Adams H. P., Barson W., et al. (1999). American Heart Association scientific statement: Guidelines to the management of spontaneous intracerebral hemorrhage. *Stroke* 30, 905–915.

36. Mayer S. A., Brun N. C., Begtrup K., et al. (2005). Recombinant activated factor VII for acute intracerebral hemorrhage. *New England Journal of Medicine* 352, 777–785.

37. Brott T., Bogousslavsy J. (2000). Treatment of acute ischemic stroke. *New England Journal of Medicine* 343, 709–721.

38. Adams H., Adams R., Del Zoppo G., et al. (Committee). (2005). Guidelines for early management of patients with ischemic stroke: A scientific statement from the Stroke Council at the American Heart Association/American Stroke Association. *Stroke* 36, 916–921.

39. Broderick J. P., Hacke W. (2002). Recanalization strategies. *Circulation* 106, 1563–1569.

40. Bronstein K. S., Popovich J. M., Stewart-Amidei C. (1991). *Promoting stroke recovery: A research based approach for nurses* (p. 200). St. Louis: C. V. Mosby.

41. Schievink W. I. (1997). Intracranial aneurysms. *New England Journal of Medicine* 336, 28–39.

42. Mayberg M. R. (Chair). (1994). Guidelines for the management of aneurysmal subarachnoid hemorrhage: A statement for healthcare professionals from a Special Writing Group of the Stroke Council, American Heart Association. *Stroke* 25, 2315–2327.

43. Oyama K., Criddle L. (2004). Vasospasm after aneurysmal subarachnoid hemorrhage. *Critical Care Nurse* 24(5), 58–67.

44. Arteriovenous Malformations Study Group. (1999). Arteriovenous malformations of the brain in adults. *New England Journal of Medicine* 340, 1812–1818.

45. Ogilvy C. S. (Chair, Special Writing Group of the Stroke Council, American Heart Association). (2001). Recommendations for management of intracranial arteriovenous malformations. *Stroke* 32, 1458–1471.

46. Tunkel A. R., Scheld W. M. (1997). Issues in management of bacterial meningitis. *American Family Physician* 56, 1355–1365.

47. Quagliarello V. J., Scheld W. M. (1997). Treatment of bacterial meningitis. *New England Journal of Medicine* 336, 708–716.

48. De Gans J., Van De Beek D. (2002). Dexamethasone in adults with bacterial meningitis. *New England Journal of Medicine* 349, 1549–1556.

49. Mehta N., Levin M. (2000). Management and prevention of meningococcal disease. *Hospital Practice* 35(8), 75–86.

50. DeAngelo L. M. (2001). Brain tumors. *New England Journal of Medicine* 344, 114–123.

51. Kuttesch J. F., Jr., Ater J. L. (2004). Brain tumors in childhood. In Behrman R. E., Kliegman R. M., Jenson H. B. (Eds.), *Nelson textbook of pediatrics* (17th ed., pp. 1702–1711). Philadelphia: Elsevier Saunders.

52. DeAngelis L. M., Posner J. B. (2001). Cancer of the central nervous system and pituitary gland. In Lenhard R. E., Osteen R. T., Gansler T. (Eds.), *The American Cancer Society's clinical oncology* (pp. 655–703). Atlanta: American Cancer Society.

53. Behin A., Hoang-Xuan K., Carpenter A. F., et al. (2003). Primary brain tumors in adults. *Lancet* 361, 323–331.

54. Browne T. R., Holmes G. L. (2001). Epilepsy. *New England Journal of Medicine* 344, 1145–1151.

55. Chang B. S., Lowenstein D. H. (2003). Mechanisms of disease: Epilepsy. *New England Journal of Medicine* 349, 1257–1266.

56. Benbadis S. (2001). Epileptic seizures and syndromes. *Neurologic Clinics* 19, 251–270.

57. Johnston M. V. (2004). Seizures in childhood. In Behrman R. E., Kliegman R. M., Jenson H. B. (Eds.), *Nelson textbook of pediatrics* (17th ed., pp. 1993–2009). Philadelphia: Elsevier Saunders.

58. Commission on Classification and Terminology of the International League Against Epilepsy. (1981). Proposal for revised clinical and electroencephalographic classification of epileptic seizures. *Epilepsia* 22, 489–501.

59. Commission on Classification and Terminology of the International League Against Epilepsy. (1989). Proposal for revised classification of epilepsies and epileptic syndromes. *Epilepsia* 30, 389–399.

60. Subcommittee and Quality Standards Subcommittee of the American Academy of Neurology and American Epilepsy Society. (2004). Efficacy and tolerability of new antiepileptic drugs: I. Treatment of new onset epilepsy; II. Treatment of refractory epilepsy. *Neurology* 62, 1252–1260, 1261–1273.

61. Nguyen D. K., Spencer S. S. (2003). Recent advances in the treatment of epilepsy. *Archives of Neurology* 60, 929–935.

62. Engel J. (1996). Surgery for seizures. *New England Journal of Medicine* 334, 647–652.

63. Cascino G. D. (1996). Generalized convulsive status epilepticus. *New England Journal of Medicine* 71, 787–792.

64. Cummings J. L. (2004). Alzheimer's disease. *New England Journal of Medicine* 351, 56–67.

65. Clark C. M., Karawish J. H. T. (2003). Alzheimer disease: Current concepts and emerging diagnostic and therapeutic strategies. *Annals of Internal Medicine* 138, 400–410.

66. Morris J. C. (1997). Alzheimer's disease: A review of clinical assessment and management issues. *Geriatrics* 52(Suppl. 2), S22–S25.

67. U.S. Department of Health and Human Services. (1996). Recognition and initial assessment of Alzheimer's disease and related disorders. AHCPR publication no. 97-0702. Washington, DC: Public Health Service, Agency for Health Care Policy and Research.

68. Kawas C. H. (2003). Early Alzheimer disease. *New England Journal of Medicine* 349, 1056–1063.

69. Black S. E. (2005). Vascular dementia. *Postgraduate Medicine* 117, 19–25.

70. Prusiner S. B. (2001). Shattuck lecture: Neurodegenerative diseases and prions. *New England Journal of Medicine* 344, 1516–1526.

71. Rappaport E. B. (1987). Iatrogenic Creutzfeldt-Jakob disease. *Neurology* 37, 1520–1522.

72. Huntington's Disease Society of America. (2000). Juvenile Huntington's disease. [On-line]. Available: www.geocities.com/hdsarmc/juvenile_hd.htm. Accessed September 6, 2005.

73. Martin J., Gusella J. (1987). Huntington's disease: Pathogenesis and management. *New England Journal of Medicine* 315, 1267–1276.

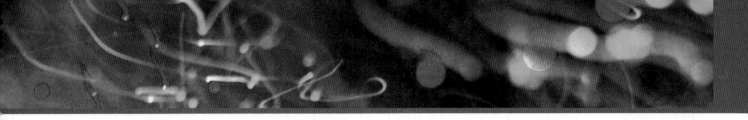

Chapter *37*

Disorders of Special Sensory Function: Vision, Hearing, and Vestibular Function

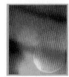 The special senses allow us to view and hear what is going on around us, to maintain our balance, and to communicate effectively with others. This chapter focuses on the eye and disorders of vision; the ear and disorders of hearing; and the vestibular system and disorders of equilibrium and balance.

The Eye and Disorders of Vision

An estimated 12 million people in the United States have some degree of visual impairment that cannot be corrected with glasses; of these, 1.3 million are legally blind.[1] The prevalence of vision impairment increases with age. An estimated 26% of persons 75 years of age and older report visual impairment severe enough to interfere with recognizing a friend across the room or reading newspaper print even when wearing glasses.[1] At the other end of the age spectrum, an estimated 2,600 children younger than 5 years of age and approximately 51,000 aged 5 to 19 years are legally blind.[1]

The optic globe, or eyeball, is a remarkable, mobile, nearly spherical structure contained in a pyramid-shaped cavity of the skull called the *orbit* (Fig. 37-1). The eyeball consists of three layers: an outer supporting fibrous layer, the sclera; a vascular layer, the uveal tract; and a neural layer, the retina. Its interior is filled with transparent media, the aqueous and vitreous humors, which allow the penetration and transmission of light to photoreceptors in the retina. Exposed surfaces of the eyes are protected by the eyelids, which are mucous membrane–lined skin flaps that provide a means for shutting out most light. Tears bathe the anterior surface of the eye; they prevent friction between it and the lid, maintain hydration of

KEY CONCEPTS

Vision

➤ Vision is a special sensory function that incorporates the visual receptor functions of the eyeball, the optic nerve, and visual pathways that carry and distribute sensory information from the optic globe to the central nervous system, and the primary and visual association cortices that translate the sensory signals into visual images.

➤ The eyeball is a fluid-filled spherical structure that functions in the reception of the light rays that provide the stimuli for vision. The refractive surface of the cornea and accommodative properties of the lens serve to focus the light signals from near and far objects on the photoreceptors in the retina.

➤ Visual information is carried to the brain by axons of the retinal cells that form the optic nerve. The two optic nerves fuse in the optic chiasm, where axons of the nasal retina of each eye cross to the contralateral side and travel with axons of the ipsilateral temporal retina to form the fibers of the optic radiations that travel to the visual cortex.

➤ Binocular vision depends on the coordination of three pairs of extraocular nerves that provide for the conjugate eye movements, with optical axes of the two eyes maintained parallel to one another.

the cornea, and protect the eye from irritation by foreign objects. The two eyes, with their associated extraocular muscles that permit directional rotation of the eyeball, provide different images of the same object. This results in binocular vision with depth perception.

THE CONJUNCTIVA

The conjunctiva is a thin layer of mucous membrane that lines the anterior surface of both eyelids as the *palpebral conjunctiva* and folds back over the anterior surface of the optic globe as the *ocular* or *bulbar conjunctiva* (see Fig. 37-1). The ocular conjunctiva covers only the sclera or white portion of the optic globe, not the cornea. When both eyes are closed, the conjunctiva lines the closed conjunctival sac. Although the conjunctiva protects the eye by preventing foreign objects from entering beyond the conjunctival sac, its main function is the production of a lubricating mucus that bathes the eye and keeps it moist.

Conjunctivitis

Conjunctivitis, or inflammation of the conjunctiva (*i.e.,* red eye or pink eye), is one of the most common forms of eye disease.[2–5] It may result from bacterial or viral infection, allergens, chemical agents, physical irritants, or radiant energy. Infections may extend from areas adjacent to the conjunctiva or may be blood-borne, such as in measles or chickenpox. Newborns can contract conjunctivitis during the birth process.[6] Infectious forms of conjunctivitis are often bilateral and may involve other family members and close associates.

Depending on the cause, conjunctivitis can vary in severity from a mild hyperemia (redness) with tearing to

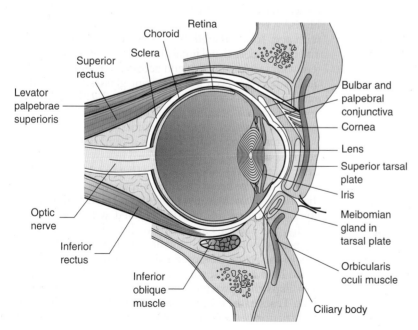

FIGURE 37-1 The eye and its appendages, lateral view.

severe conjunctivitis with purulent drainage. Unilateral symptoms suggest sources of irritation such as foreign bodies or chemical irritation. The conjunctiva is extremely sensitive to irritation and inflammation. Important symptoms of conjunctivitis are a foreign body sensation, a scratching or burning sensation, itching, and photophobia. Severe pain suggests corneal rather than conjunctival disease. Itching is common in allergic conditions. A discharge, or exudate, may be present with all types of conjunctivitis and may cause transient blurring of vision. It is usually watery when the conjunctivitis is caused by allergy, a foreign body, or viral infection and mucopurulent in the presence of bacterial or fungal infection.

The diagnosis of conjunctivitis is based on history, physical examination, and microscopic and culture studies to identify the cause. Because a red eye may be the sign of several eye conditions, it is important to differentiate between redness due to conjunctivitis that is caused by more serious eye disorders, such as corneal lesions and acute glaucoma. In contrast to corneal lesions and acute glaucoma, conjunctivitis produces injection (*i.e.*, enlargement and redness) of the peripheral conjunctival blood vessels rather than those radiating around the corneal limbus (Fig. 37-2). Conjunctivitis also produces only mild discomfort compared with the moderate to severe discomfort associated with corneal lesions or the severe and deep pain associated with acute glaucoma.

Bacterial Conjunctivitis. Bacterial conjunctivitis may present as a hyperacute, acute, or chronic infection. Common agents of acute bacterial conjunctivitis are *Streptococcus pneumoniae, Staphylococcus aureus,* and *Haemophilus influenzae.* The infection usually has an abrupt onset and is characterized by large amounts of yellow-green drainage. The eyelids are sticky, and there may be excoriation of the lid margins. Treatment may include local application of antibiotics. The disorder usually is self-limited, lasting approximately 10 to 14 days if untreated and 1 to 3 days if properly treated.[2]

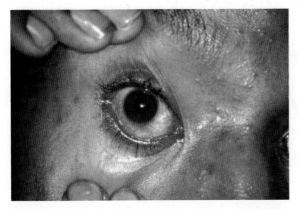

FIGURE 37-2 Gonococcal conjunctivitis of right eye. Note injection of the peripheral conjunctival blood vessels. (From Centers for Disease Control and Prevention, Public Health Images Library. [On-line]. Available: http://phil.cdc.gov/phil/details/asp.)

Hyperacute conjunctivitis is a severe, sight-threatening ocular infection. The most common causes of hyperacute purulent conjunctivitis are *Neisseria gonorrhoeae* and *Neisseria meningitidis,* with *N. gonorrhoeae* being the most common.[3] The symptoms, which typically are progressive, include conjunctival redness and edema (chemosis); lid swelling and tenderness; and swollen preauricular lymph nodes. Gonococcal ocular infections that are left untreated result in corneal ulceration with ultimate perforation and sometimes permanent loss of vision.[3] Treatment includes systemic antibiotics supplemented with ocular antibiotics. Because of the increasing prevalence of penicillin-resistant *N. gonorrhoeae,* antibiotic choice should be determined by current information regarding antibiotic sensitivity.

Chronic bacterial conjunctivitis most commonly occurs in people with obstruction of the nasolacrimal duct or chronic infection of the lacrimal sac (dacryocystitis) and is usually unilateral.[2] The symptoms of chronic bacterial conjunctivitis vary and can include itching, burning, foreign body sensation, and morning eyelash crusting. There may be flaky debris and erythema along the lid margins, as well as eyelash loss and eye redness. Treatment includes good eyelid hygiene and application of topical antibiotics.

Chlamydial Conjunctivitis. Inclusion conjunctivitis usually is a benign suppurative conjunctivitis transmitted by the type of *Chlamydia trachomatis* (serotypes D through K) that causes venereal infections. It is spread by contaminated genital secretions and occurs in newborns of mothers with *C. trachomatis* infections of the birth canal. It also can be contracted through swimming in unchlorinated pools. The incubation period varies from 5 to 12 days, and the disease may last for several months if untreated. The infection usually is treated with appropriate oral antibiotics.

A more serious form of infection is caused by a different strain of *C. trachomatis* (serotypes A through C). This form of chlamydial infection affects the conjunctiva and causes ulceration and scarring of the cornea. It is the leading cause of preventable blindness in the world. Although the agent is widespread, it is seen mostly in developing countries, particularly those of Asia, the Middle East, and parts of Africa.[5] It is transmitted by direct human contact, contaminated objects (fomites), and flies.

Viral Conjunctivitis. One of the most common causes of viral conjunctivitis is adenovirus type 3. Conjunctivitis caused by this agent usually is associated with pharyngitis, fever, and malaise.[3,4] It causes generalized hyperemia, excessive tearing, and minimal exudate. Children are affected more often than adults. Swimming pools contaminated because of inadequate chlorination are common sources of infection. Infections caused by adenoviruses types 4 and 7 often are associated with acute respiratory disease. These viruses are rapidly disseminated when large groups mingle with infected individuals (*e.g.*, military recruits). There is no specific treatment for this type of viral conjunctivitis; it usually lasts 7 to 14 days. Preventive measures include hygienic measures and avoiding shared use of eyedroppers, eye makeup, goggles, and towels.

Herpes simplex virus (HSV) conjunctivitis is characterized by unilateral infection, irritation, mucoid discharge, pain, and mild photophobia. Herpetic vesicles may develop on the eyelids and lid margins. The infection usually is caused by the HSV type 1, but can be caused by the HSV type 2. It often is associated with HSV keratitis, in which the cornea shows discrete epithelial lesions. Treatment involves the use of systemic or local antiviral agents. Local corticosteroid preparations increase the activity of the herpes virus, apparently by enhancing the destructive effect of collagenase on the collagen of the cornea. The use of these medications should be avoided in those suspected of having herpes simplex conjunctivitis or keratitis.

Allergic Conjunctivitis. Allergic conjunctivitis encompasses a spectrum of conjunctival conditions usually characterized by itching. The most common of these is seasonal allergic rhinoconjunctivitis, or hay fever. Seasonal allergic conjunctivitis is an immunoglobulin E (IgE)–mediated hypersensitivity reaction precipitated by small airborne allergens such as pollens.[7] It typically causes bilateral tearing, itching, and redness of the eyes.

The treatment of seasonal allergic rhinoconjunctivitis includes allergen avoidance and the use of cold compresses, oral antihistamines, and vasoconstrictor eye drops. Allergic conjunctivitis also has been successfully treated with oral antihistamines, topical mast cell stabilizers, and topical nonsteroidal anti-inflammatory drugs.[2] All three types of agents are well tolerated and have a rapid onset of action. In severe cases, a short course of topical corticosteroids may be required to afford symptomatic relief.

Ophthalmia Neonatorum. Ophthalmia neonatorum is a form of conjunctivitis that occurs in newborns younger than 1 month of age and is usually contracted during or soon after vaginal delivery. Many causes are known, including N. gonorrhoeae, Pseudomonas, and C. trachomatis.[6] Epidemiologically, these infections reflect those sexually transmitted diseases most common in a particular area. Once the most common form of conjunctivitis in the newborn, gonococcal ophthalmia neonatorum has an incidence of 0.3% of live births in the United States; C. trachomatis has an incidence of 8.2% of live births.[6] Drops of 0.5% erythromycin or 1% silver nitrate are applied immediately after birth to prevent gonococcal ophthalmia. Silver nitrate instillation may cause mild, self-limited conjunctivitis.

THE CORNEA

The cornea functions as a transparent membrane through which light passes as it moves toward the retina (Fig. 37-3). The cornea also contributes to the refraction (i.e., bending) of light rays and focusing of vision. Three

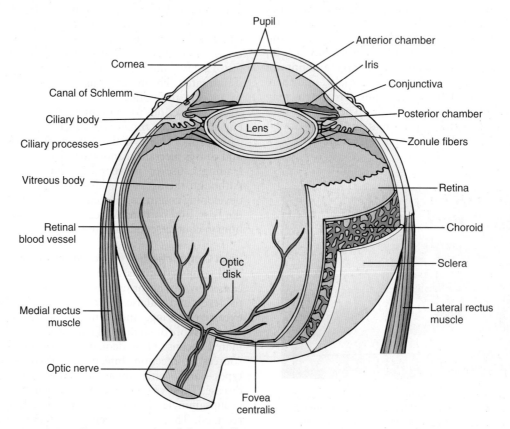

FIGURE 37-3 Transverse section of the eyeball.

layers of tissue form the cornea: an extremely thin outer epithelial layer, which is continuous with the ocular or bulbar conjunctiva; a middle stromal layer called the *substantia propria stroma;* and an inner endothelial layer, which lies next to the aqueous humor of the anterior chamber. A thin membrane (Bowman membrane) lies between the epithelial layer and the underlying stromal layer. The Bowman membrane acts as a barrier to the spread of infection. The substantia propria is composed of regularly arranged collagen bundles embedded in a mucopolysaccharide matrix. This organization of the collagen fibers makes the substantia propria transparent and is necessary for light transmission. Hydration within a limited range is necessary to maintain the spacing of the collagen fibers and transparency.

The cornea is avascular and obtains its nutrient and oxygen supply by diffusion from blood vessels of the adjacent sclera, from the aqueous humor at its deep surface, and from tears. The corneal epithelium is heavily innervated by sensory neurons. Epithelial injury causes discomfort that ranges from a foreign body sensation and burning of the eyes to severe pain. Photophobia may occur as the result of painful contraction of the inflamed iris. Reflex tearing is common.

Corneal Trauma

The integrity of the epithelium and the endothelium is necessary to maintain hydration of the cornea within a limited range. Damage to either layer leads to edema and loss of transparency. Among the causes of corneal edema is the prolonged and uninterrupted wearing of hard contact lenses, which can deprive the epithelium of oxygen. With corneal edema, the cornea appears dull, uneven, and hazy; visual acuity decreases; and iridescent vision (*i.e.,* rainbows around lights) occurs.

Trauma that causes abrasions of the cornea can be extremely painful, but if minor, the abrasions usually heal in a few days. The epithelium is an effective barrier to entrance of microorganisms into the cornea. It is capable of regeneration, and small defects heal without scarring. If the stroma is damaged, healing occurs more slowly, and the danger of infection is increased. Injuries to the Bowman membrane and the stromal layer heal with scar formation and permanent opacification. Opacities of the cornea impair the transmission of light. Even a minor scar can severely distort vision because it disturbs the refractive surface of the eye.

Keratitis

Keratitis refers to inflammation of the cornea. It can be caused by infections, hypersensitivity reactions, ischemia, defective tear production, and interruption in sensory innervation, as occurs with local anesthesia.[8] Scar tissue formation caused by keratitis is the leading cause of blindness and impaired vision throughout the world. Most of this vision loss is preventable if the condition is diagnosed early and appropriate treatment is instituted.

Keratitis can be divided into two types: nonulcerative and ulcerative. In *nonulcerative* or *interstitial* keratitis, all the layers of the epithelium are affected, but the epithelium remains intact. It is associated with a number of diseases, including syphilis, tuberculosis, and lupus erythematosus. It also may result from a viral infection entering through a small defect in the cornea. Treatment usually is symptomatic.

Ulcerative keratitis is an inflammatory process in which parts of the epithelium, stroma, or both are destroyed. Causes of ulcerative keratitis include infectious agents such as those causing conjunctivitis (*e.g., Staphylococcus, S. pneumoniae, Chlamydia*), exposure trauma, and use of extended-wear contact lens. Bacterial keratitis tends to be aggressive and demands immediate care. Exposure trauma may result from deformities of the lid, paralysis of the lid muscles, or severe exophthalmos (protrusion of the eyeball). *Mooren ulcer* is a chronic, painful, indolent ulcer that occurs in the absence of infection. It usually is seen in older persons and may affect both eyes. Although the cause is unknown, an autoimmune origin is suspected.

Herpes Simplex Keratitis. Herpes simplex keratitis is the most common cause of corneal ulceration and most common corneal cause of blindness in the Western world.[8] Most cases are caused by HSV type 1 infections. An exception is neonatal keratitis, which is caused by HSV type 2 acquired during the birth process.[8] HSV keratitis occurs as an initial primary or recurrent infection. Primary HSV type 1 ocular disease usually occurs in young children. It is manifested by vesicular blepharoconjunctivitis, occasionally with corneal involvement. It usually is self-limited, without causing corneal damage. After the initial primary infection, the virus may persist in a quiescent or latent state, remaining in the trigeminal ganglion and possibly in the cornea without causing signs of infection.

Recurrent infection may be precipitated by various poorly understood, stress-related factors that reactivate the virus. Involvement is usually unilateral. The first symptoms are irritation, photophobia, and tearing. Some reduction in vision may occur when the lesion affects the central part of the cornea. Because corneal anesthesia occurs early in the disease, the symptoms may be minimal, and the person may delay seeking medical care. A history of fever blisters or other herpetic infection is often noted, but corneal lesions may be the only sign of recurrent herpes infection. Most typically, the corneal lesion involves the epithelium and has a typical branching pattern. These epithelial lesions heal without scarring. Herpetic lesions that involve the stromal layer of the cornea produce increasingly severe corneal opacities. They are thought to have an immune rather than an infectious cause.

The treatment of HSV keratitis focuses on eliminating viral replication within the cornea while minimizing the damaging effects of the inflammatory process. It involves the use of epithelial debridement and drug therapy. Debridement is used to remove the virus from the corneal epithelium. Topical antiviral agents are used to promote healing. Corticosteroid drugs increase viral replication. With a few exceptions, their use is usually contraindicated.

Herpes Zoster Ophthalmicus. Herpes zoster or shingles is a relatively common infection caused by the varicella-zoster virus, the same virus that causes varicella (chickenpox).[9] It occurs when the varicella-zoster virus, which has remained dormant in the neurosensory ganglia since the primary infection, is reactivated. Herpes zoster ophthalmicus, which represents 10% to 25% of all cases of herpes zoster, occurs when reactivation of the latent virus occurs in the ganglia of the ophthalmic division of the trigeminal nerve.[9] Immunocompromised persons, particularly those with human immunodeficiency virus (HIV) infection, are at higher risk for developing herpes zoster ophthalmicus than those with a normally functioning immune system.

Herpes zoster ophthalmicus usually presents with malaise, fever, headache, and burning and itching of the periorbital area. These symptoms commonly precede the eruption by 1 or 2 days. The rash, which is initially vesicular, becomes pustular and then crusting (see Chapter 45). Involvement of the tip of the nose and lid margins indicates a high likelihood of ocular involvement. Ocular signs include conjunctivitis, keratitis, and anterior uveitis, often with elevated intraocular pressure. Persons with corneal disease present with varying degrees of decreased vision, pain, and light insensitivity.

Treatment includes the use of high-dose oral antiviral drugs (acyclovir, valacyclovir). Initiation of treatment within the first 72 hours after the appearance of the rash reduces the incidence of ocular complications but not the postherpetic neuralgia (see Chapter 34).

Corneal Transplantation

Advances in ophthalmologic surgery permit corneal transplantation using a cadaver cornea. Unlike kidney or heart transplantation procedures, which are associated with considerable risk of rejection of the transplanted organ, the use of cadaver corneas entails minimal danger of rejection because this tissue is not exposed to the vascular and therefore the immunologic defense system. Instead, the success of this type of transplantation operation depends on the prevention of scar tissue formation, which would limit the transparency of the transplanted cornea.

INTRAOCULAR PRESSURE AND GLAUCOMA

Glaucoma includes a group of conditions that feature an optic neuropathy accompanied by optic disk cupping and visual field loss. It is usually associated with an increase in intraocular pressure, although some people with normal intraocular pressure may develop characteristic optic nerve and visual field changes.[10] An estimated 60 million people worldwide currently have glaucoma. About 6 million people worldwide are blind from glaucoma, including 100,000 Americans, making it the leading cause of blindness in the United States.[10] African Americans are three to four times more likely to have open angle-glaucoma as whites, and even greater racial disparities exist in terms of blindness from the disease.

The intraocular pressure largely reflects that of the aqueous humor, which fills the anterior and posterior chambers of the eye. The aqueous humor is produced by the ciliary body and passes from the posterior chamber through the pupil into the anterior chamber (Fig. 37-4A). Aqueous humor leaves through the iridocorneal angle between the anterior surface of the iris and the sclera. Here it filters through the trabecular meshwork and enters the canal of Schlemm for return to the venous circulation. The canal of Schlemm is actually a thin-walled vein that extends circumferentially around the iris of the eye. Its endothelial membrane is so porous that even large protein molecules up to the size of a red blood cell can pass from the anterior chamber into the canal of Schlemm.

The pressure of the aqueous humor results from a balance of several factors, including the rate of secretion, the resistance to flow between the iris and the ciliary body, and the resistance to resorption at the trabeculated region of the sclera at the iridocorneal angle. Normally, the rate of aqueous production is equal to the rate of aqueous outflow, and the intraocular pressure is maintained within a normal range of 9 to 21 mm Hg.[11]

Glaucoma usually results from congenital or acquired lesions of the anterior segment of the eye that mechanically obstruct aqueous outflow.[10,12] Glaucoma is commonly classified as angle-closure (*i.e.*, narrow-angle) or open-angle (*i.e.*, wide-angle) glaucoma, depending on the location of the compromised outflow, and may occur as a primary or secondary disorder. Primary glaucoma occurs without evidence of preexisting ocular or systemic disease. Secondary glaucoma can result from inflammatory processes that affect the eye, from tumors, or from blood cells of trauma-produced hemorrhage that obstruct the outflow of aqueous humor.

In persons with glaucoma, temporary or permanent impairment of vision results from degenerative changes in the retina and optic nerve and from corneal edema and opacification. Damage to optic nerve axons in the region of the optic nerve can be recognized on ophthalmoscopic examination. The normal optic disk has a central depression called the *optic cup*. With progressive atrophy of axons caused by increased intraocular pressure, pallor of the optic disk develops, and the size and depth of the optic cup increase. Because changes in the optic cup precede visual field loss, regular ophthalmoscopic examinations are important for detecting eye changes that occur with increased intraocular pressure. Many attempts have been made to quantify the optic disk changes in people with glaucoma using various photographic techniques and, more recently, scanning laser imaging systems.

Open-Angle Glaucoma

Primary open-angle glaucoma is the most common form of glaucoma. It tends to manifest after 35 years of age, with an incidence of 0.5% to 2% among persons 40 years of age and older. The condition is characterized

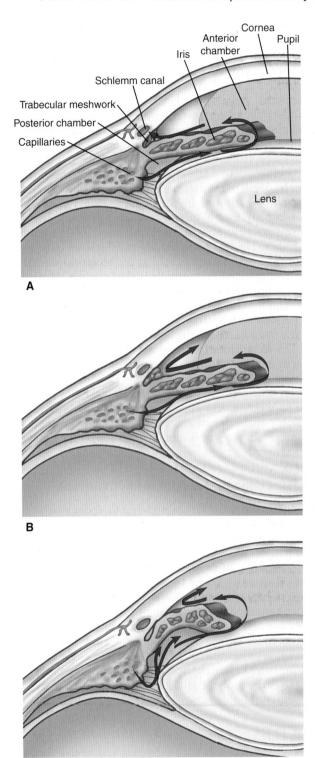

FIGURE 37-4 (A) Normally, aqueous humor, which is secreted in the posterior chamber, gains access to the anterior chamber by flowing through the pupil. In the angle of the anterior chamber, it passes through the canal of Schlemm into the venous system. **(B)** In open-angle glaucoma, the outflow of aqueous humor is obstructed at the trabecular meshwork. **(C)** In angle-closure glaucoma, the aqueous humor encounters resistance to flow through the pupil. Increased pressure in the posterior chamber produces a forward bowing of the peripheral iris, so that the iris blocks the trabecular meshwork.

by an abnormal increase in intraocular pressure that occurs without obstruction at the iridocorneal angle, hence the name *open-angle glaucoma*. Instead, it usually occurs because of an abnormality of the trabecular meshwork that controls the flow of aqueous humor into the canal of Schlemm[12] (see Fig. 37-4B).

Primary open-angle glaucoma is usually asymptomatic and chronic, causing progressive damage to the optic nerve and visual field loss unless it is appropriately treated. Elevated intraocular pressure is the major risk factor for open-angle glaucoma, but it is not the only diagnostic factor. Some people maintain a higher intraocular pressure without evidence of optic nerve or visual field loss. It is suggested that these people be described as "glaucoma suspects" or "ocular hypertensives."[13]

The etiology of primary open-angle glaucoma remains unclear. The only known causative risk factors are elevated intraocular pressure and insults to the eye, including trauma, uveitis, and corticosteroid therapy. Risk factors for this disorder include an age of 40 years and older, black race, a positive first-degree family history, diabetes mellitus, and myopia.[13] In some persons, the use of moderate amounts of topical or inhaled corticosteroid medications can cause an increase in intraocular pressure. Sensitive persons also may sustain an increase in intraocular pressure with the use of systemic corticosteroid drugs.

Diagnostic methods include applanation tonometry (measurement of intraocular pressure), ophthalmoscopic visualization of the optic nerve, and central visual field testing. Measurement of intraocular pressures provides a means of assessing glaucoma risk. Because the condition is usually asymptomatic, persons at risk for open-angle glaucoma should have regular direct ophthalmoscopic examinations, on both eyes, concentrating on the optic disk. Optic disk changes frequently are noted before visual field defects become apparent.

The elevation in intraocular pressure in persons with open-angle glaucoma is usually treated pharmacologically or, in cases where pharmacologic treatment fails, by increasing aqueous outflow through a surgically created pathway. Drugs used in the long-term management of glaucoma fall into five classes: β-adrenergic antagonists, prostaglandin analogs, adrenergic agonists, carbonic anhydrase inhibitors, and cholinergic agonists.[14] Most glaucoma drugs are applied topically. However, systemic side effects may occur.

Topical β-adrenergic antagonists are usually the drugs of first choice for lowering intraocular pressure. The β-adrenergic antagonists are thought to lower intraocular pressure by decreasing aqueous humor production in the ciliary body.[14] Prostaglandins are locally acting substances found in most tissues. At low concentrations, prostaglandin $F_{2\alpha}$ increases the outflow of aqueous humor through the iris root and ciliary body, either by decreasing the extracellular matrix or by relaxing the ciliary musculature. Adrenergic agonists cause an early decrease in production of aqueous humor by constricting the vessels supplying the ciliary body. Carbonic anhydrase inhibitors reduce the secretion of aqueous humor by the ciliary epithelium. Until recently, these drugs had to be taken orally, and systemic side effects were common. A topical carbonic anhydrase inhibitor, which acts locally, is now available. Cholinergic drugs exert their effects by increasing the effects of acetylcholine. Acetylcholine is the postganglionic neurotransmitter for the parasympathetic nervous system; it increases aqueous outflow through contraction of the ciliary muscle and pupillary constriction (miosis).

When a reduction in intraocular pressure cannot be maintained through pharmacologic methods, surgical treatment may become necessary. Until recently, the main surgical treatment for open-angle glaucoma was a filtering procedure in which an opening was created between the anterior chamber and the subconjunctival space. An argon or neodymium–yttrium–aluminum garnet (Nd:YAG) laser technique, in which multiple spots are applied 360 degrees around the trabecular meshwork, has been developed.[10] The microburns resulting from the laser treatment scar rather than penetrate the trabecular meshwork, a process thought to enlarge the outflow channels by increasing the tension exerted on the trabecular meshwork. Cryotherapy, diathermy, and high-frequency ultrasound may be used in some cases to destroy the ciliary epithelium and reduce aqueous humor production.

Angle-Closure Glaucoma

Angle-closure glaucoma, which accounts for 5% to 10% of cases of glaucoma, results from occlusion of the anterior chamber angle by the iris (see Fig. 37-4C). It is most likely to develop in eyes with preexisting narrow anterior chambers. An acute attack is often precipitated by pupillary dilation, which causes the iris to thicken with blockage of the anterior chamber angle by the peripheral iris.[10] Angle-closure glaucoma usually occurs as the result of an inherited anatomic defect that causes a shallow anterior chamber. It is seen more commonly in people of East Asian, Asian, or Inuit (Eskimo) descent and in people with hypermetropic eyes that cause nearsightedness.[10,12] This defect is exaggerated by the anterior displacement of the peripheral iris that occurs in older persons because of the increase in lens size that occurs with aging.

Symptoms of acute angle-closure glaucoma are related to sudden, intermittent increases in intraocular pressure. These often occur after prolonged periods in the dark, emotional upset, and other conditions that cause extensive and prolonged dilation of the pupil. Administration of pharmacologic agents such as atropine that cause pupillary dilation (mydriasis) also can precipitate an acute episode of increased intraocular pressure in persons with the potential for angle-closure glaucoma. Attacks of increased intraocular pressure are manifested by ocular pain and blurred or iridescent vision caused by corneal edema.[10] The pupil may be enlarged and fixed. Symptoms are often spontaneously relieved by sleep and conditions that promote pupillary constriction. With repeated or prolonged attacks, the eye becomes reddened, and edema of the cornea may develop, giving the eye a hazy appearance. A unilateral, often excruciating, headache is common. Nausea and vomiting may occur, causing the headache to be confused with a migraine headache.

Some persons with congenitally narrow anterior chambers never develop symptoms, and others develop symptoms only when they are elderly. Because of the dangers of vision loss, people with narrow anterior chambers should be warned about the significance of blurred vision, halos, and ocular pain. Sometimes, decreased visual acuity and an unreactive pupil may be the only clues to angle-closure glaucoma in the elderly.

The depth of the anterior chamber can be evaluated by transillumination or by a technique called *gonioscopy*. Gonioscopy uses a special contact lens and mirrors or prisms to view and measure the angle of the anterior chamber. The transillumination method uses only a penlight. The light source is held at the temporal side of the eye and directed horizontally across the iris. In persons with a normal-sized anterior chamber, the light passes through the chamber to illuminate both halves of the iris. In persons with a narrow anterior chamber, only the half of the iris adjacent to the light source is illuminated.

The treatment of acute angle-closure glaucoma is primarily surgical. It involves creating an opening between the anterior and posterior chambers with laser or incisional iridectomy to allow the aqueous humor to bypass the pupillary block. The anatomic abnormalities responsible for angle-closure glaucoma are usually bilateral, and prophylactic surgery is often performed on the other eye.

Congenital and Infantile Glaucoma

Congenital glaucoma is caused by a disorder in which the anterior chamber retains its fetal configuration, with aberrant trabecular meshwork extending to the root of the iris, or is covered by a membrane. It is bilateral in 65% to 80% of cases, and occurs more commonly in boys than girls. About 10% of cases have a familial origin.[15] The earliest symptoms are excessive lacrimation and photophobia. Affected infants tend to be fussy, have poor eating habits, and rub their eyes frequently. Diffuse edema of the cornea usually occurs, giving the eye a grayish-white appearance. Chronic elevation of the intraocular pressure before the age of 3 years causes enlargement of the entire globe. Early surgical treatment is necessary to prevent blindness.

THE LENS

The lens is a remarkable structure that functions to bring images into focus on the retina. The lens is an avascular, transparent, biconvex body, the posterior side of which is more convex than the anterior side. A thin, highly elastic lens capsule is attached to the surrounding ciliary body by delicate suspensory radial ligaments called *zonules*, which hold the lens in place (see Fig. 37-3). The suspensory ligaments and lens capsule are normally under tension, causing the lens to have a flattened shape for distant vision. Contraction of the muscle fibers of the ciliary body narrows the diameter of the ciliary body, relaxes the fibers of the suspensory ligaments, and allows the lens to relax to a more spherical or convex shape for near vision.

Disorders of Refraction

Refraction can be defined as the bending of light rays as they pass from one transparent medium (such as air) to a second transparent medium with a different density (such as a glass lens). When light rays pass through the center of a lens, their direction is not changed; however, other rays passing peripherally through the lens are bent. The refractive power of a lens is usually described as the distance (in meters) from its surface to the point at which the rays come into focus (*i.e.,* focal length). Usually, this is reported as the reciprocal of this distance (*i.e.,* diopters).[16] For example, a lens that brings an object into focus at 0.5 m has a refractive power of 2 diopters (1.0/0.5 = 2.0). With a fixed-power lens, the closer an object is to the lens, the further behind the lens is its focus point. The closer the object, the stronger and more precise the focusing system must be.

In the eye, the major refraction of light begins at the convex corneal surface. Further refraction occurs as light moves from the posterior corneal surface to the aqueous humor, from the aqueous humor to the anterior lens surface, from the anterior lens surface to the posterior lens surface, and from the posterior lens surface to the vitreous humor. A perfectly shaped optic globe and cornea result in optimal visual acuity, producing a sharp image in focus at all points on the retinal surface in the posterior part, or fundus, of the eye (Fig. 37-5A). Unfortunately, individual differences in formation and growth of the eyeball and cornea frequently can result in inappropriate focal image formation. If the anterior-posterior dimension of the eyeball is too short, the image is focused posterior to (behind) the retina (see Fig. 37-5B). This is called *hyperopia* or *farsightedness.* In such cases, the accommodative changes of the lens can bring distant images into focus, but near images become blurred. Hyperopia is corrected by appropriate biconvex lenses. If the anterior-posterior dimension of the eyeball is too long, the focus point for an infinitely distant target is anterior to the retina. This condition is called *myopia* or *nearsightedness* (see Fig. 37-5C). Persons with myopia can see close objects without problems because accommodative changes in their lens bring near objects into focus, but distant objects are blurred. Myopia can be corrected with an appropriate biconcave lens. Radial keratotomy, a form of refractive corneal surgery, can be performed to correct the defect. This surgical procedure involves the use of radial incisions to alter the corneal curvature.

Nonuniform curvature of the refractive medium (*e.g.,* horizontal versus vertical plane) is called *astigmatism.* Astigmatism is usually the result of a defect in the cornea, but it can result from defects in the lens or the retina. Spherical aberration, another refractive error, involves a cornea with nonspherical surfaces. Lens correction is available for both refractive errors.

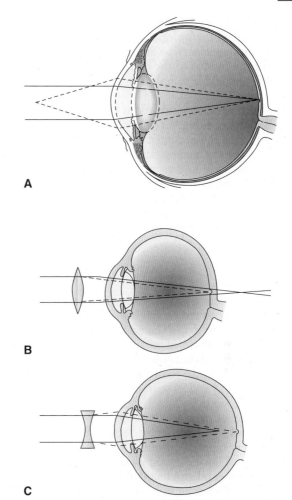

FIGURE 37-5 (**A**) Accommodation. The *solid lines* represent rays of light from a distant object, and the *dotted lines* represent rays from a near object. The lens is flatter for the former and more convex for the latter. In each case, the rays of light are brought to a focus on the retina. (**B**) Hyperopia corrected by a biconvex lens, shown by the *dotted lines.* (**C**) Myopia corrected by a biconcave lens, shown by the *dotted lines.*

Disorders of Accommodation

Accommodation is the process whereby a clear image is maintained as gaze is shifted from far to near objects. Accommodation requires convergence of the eyes, pupillary constriction, and thickening of the lens through contraction of the ciliary muscle. Contraction of the ciliary muscles is controlled mainly by the parasympathetic fibers of the oculomotor cranial nerve (CN III).

In near vision, pupillary constriction (*i.e., miosis*) improves the clarity of the retinal image. This must be balanced against the resultant decrease in light intensity reaching the retina. During changes from near to far vision, pupillary dilation partially compensates for the reduced size of the retinal image by increasing the light entering the pupil. A third component of accommodation involves the reflex narrowing of the palpebral opening during near vision and widening during far vision.

Paralysis of the ciliary muscle, with loss of accommodation, is called *cycloplegia.* Pharmacologic cycloplegia is sometimes necessary to aid ophthalmoscopic examination of the fundus of the eye, especially in small children who are unable to hold a steady fixation during the examination.

The term *presbyopia* refers to changes in vision that occur because of aging.[17] The lens consists of transparent fibers arranged in concentric layers, of which the external layers are the newest and softest. No loss of lens fibers occurs with aging; instead, additional fibers are added to the outermost portion of the lens. As the lens ages, it thickens, and its fibers become less elastic, so that the range of focus or accommodation is diminished to the point where reading glasses become necessary for near vision.

Cataracts

A cataract is a lens opacity that interferes with the transmission of light to the retina. It has been estimated that 13 million persons in the United States 40 years of age or older are visually disabled because of cataracts.[1] Cataracts are the most common cause of age-related visual loss in the world[18]; they are found in approximately 50% of those between 65 and 74 years of age, and in 70% of those older than 75 years.[1]

The cause of cataract development is thought to be multifactorial, with different factors being associated with different types of opacities. Several risk factors have been proposed, including the effects of aging, genetic factors, environmental and metabolic influences, drugs, and injury.[17] Metabolically induced cataracts are caused by disorders of carbohydrate metabolism (diabetes) or inborn errors of metabolism. Long-term exposure to sunlight (ultraviolet B radiation) and heavy smoking have been associated with increased risk of cataract formation.[17] Occasionally, cataracts occur as a developmental defect (*i.e.,* congenital cataracts) or secondary to trauma or diseases. Corticosteroids drugs have been implicated as causative agents in cataract formation. Both systemic and inhaled corticosteroids have been cited as risk factors.[19] Traumatic cataracts most often are caused by foreign body injury to the lens or blunt trauma to the eye. Foreign body injury that interrupts the lens capsule allows aqueous and vitreous humor to enter the lens and initiate cataract formation. Other causes of traumatic cataract are overexposure to heat (*e.g.,* glassblower's cataract) or to ionizing radiation. The radiation dose necessary to cause a cataract varies with the amount and type of energy; younger lenses are most vulnerable.

With normal aging, the nucleus and the cortex of the lens enlarge as new fibers are formed in the cortical zones of the lens.[18] In the nucleus, the old fibers become more compressed and dehydrated. Metabolic changes also occur. Lens proteins become more insoluble, and concentrations of calcium, sodium, potassium, and phosphate increase. During the early stages of cataract formation, a yellow pigment and vacuoles accumulate in the lens fibers.

Manifestations. The manifestations of cataracts depend on the extent of opacity and whether the defect is bilateral or unilateral. With the exception of traumatic or congenital cataract, most cataracts are bilateral. Age-related cataracts, which are the most common type, are characterized by increasingly blurred vision and visual distortion. Vision for far and near objects decreases. Dilation of the pupil in dim light improves vision. With nuclear cataracts (those involving the lens nucleus), the refractive power of the anterior segment often increases to produce an acquired myopia. Persons with hyperopia may experience a "second sight" or improved reading acuity until increasing opacity reduces acuity. Central lens opacities may divide the visual axis and cause an optical defect in which two or more blurred images are seen. Posterior subcapsular cataracts are located in the posterior cortical layer and usually involve the central visual axis. In addition to decreased visual acuity, cataracts tend to scatter the light entering the eye, thereby producing glare or the abnormal presence of light in the visual field.

Diagnosis and Treatment. Diagnosis of cataract is based on ophthalmoscopic examination and the degree of visual impairment on the Snellen vision test. On ophthalmoscopic examination, cataracts may appear as a gross opacity filling the pupillary aperture or as an opacity silhouetted against the red background of the fundus. A Snellen test acuity of 20/50 is a common requirement for drivers of motor vehicles. Other tests that determine the ability to see well after surgery, such as electrophysiologic testing in which the response to visual stimuli is measured electronically, may be done.

There is no effective medical treatment for cataract. Strong bifocals, magnification, appropriate lighting, and visual aids may be used as the cataract progresses. Surgery is the only treatment for correcting cataract-related vision loss. Surgery usually involves lens extraction and intraocular lens implantation. It is commonly performed on an outpatient basis with the use of local anesthesia. The use of extracapsular surgery, which leaves the posterior capsule of the lens intact, has significantly improved the outcomes of cataract surgery. The cataract lens is usually removed using phacoemulsification, a process that involves the ultrasonic fragmentation of the lens into fine pieces, which then are aspirated from the eye.[17,18]

One of the greatest advances in cataract surgery has been the development of reliable intraocular implants. Until recently, only monofocal intraocular lenses that correct for distance vision were available, and eyeglasses were needed for near vision. This has been remedied by the recent introduction of multifocal lenses.

Congenital Cataract. A congenital cataract is one that is present at birth. Among the causes of congenital cataracts are genetic defects, toxic environmental agents, and viruses such as rubella.[6] A maternal rubella infection during the first trimester can cause congenital cataract. Cataracts and other developmental defects of the ocular apparatus depend on the total dose and the embryonic stage at the time of exposure.

Most congenital cataracts are not progressive and are not dense enough to cause significant visual impairment. However, if the cataracts are bilateral and the opacity is significant, lens extraction should be done on one eye by the age of 2 months to permit the development of vision and prevent amblyopia (discussed later). If the surgery is successful, the contralateral lens should be removed soon after.

THE RETINA

The function of the retina is to receive visual images, partially analyze them, and transmit this modified information to the brain. Disorders of the retina and its function include ischemic conditions caused by disorders of the retinal blood supply; disorders of the retinal vessels such as retinopathies that cause hemorrhage and the development of opacities; separation of the pigment and sensory layers of the retina (*i.e.*, retinal detachment); and macular degeneration. Because the retina has no pain fibers, most diseases of the retina are painless and do not cause redness of the eye.

The retina is composed of two layers: an outer pigment (melanin-containing) epithelium and an inner neural layer[20] (Fig. 37-6). The outer surface of the pigmented layer, a single-cell–thick lining called the *Bruch membrane*, abuts the choroid, and extends anteriorly to cover the ciliary body and the posterior side of the iris. Its pigmented epithelial cells, like those of the choroid, absorb light and prevent it from scattering. The pigment layer stores large quantities of vitamin A, which is an important precursor of the photosensitive visual pigments.

The importance of melanin in the pigment layer is well illustrated by its absence in people with a condition called *albinism*. Albinism is a genetic deficiency of tyrosinase, the enzyme needed for the synthesis of melanin by the melanocytes. Affected persons have white hair, pink skin, and light blue eyes. In these persons, excessive light penetrates the unpigmented iris and choroid and is reflected in all directions, so that their photoreceptors are flooded with excess light, and visual acuity is markedly reduced. Excess stimulation of the photoreceptors at normal or high illumination levels is experienced as painful photophobia.

The inner light-sensitive neural retina covers the inner aspect of the eyeball.[20] The neural retina is composed of three layers of neurons: a posterior layer of photoreceptors (rods and cones), a middle layer of bipolar cells, and an inner layer of ganglion cells that communicate with the photoreceptors (see Fig. 37-5). Light must pass through the transparent inner layers of the sensory retina before it reaches the photoreceptors. Local currents produced in response to light spread from the photoreceptors to the bipolar neurons and other interneurons and then to the ganglionic cells, where action potentials are generated. The interneurons, which are composed of horizontal and amacrine cells, have cell bodies in the bipolar layer, and they play an important role in modulating retinal function. A superficial marginal layer contains the axons of the ganglion cells as they collect and leave the eye by way of the optic nerve. The optic disk, where the optic nerve exits the eye, is the weak part of the eye because it is not reinforced by the sclera. It also forms the blind spot because it is not backed by photoreceptors, and light focused on it cannot be seen. People do not notice the blind spot because of a sophisticated visual function called "filling in," which the brain uses to deal with missing visual input. Local retinal damage caused by small vascular lesions (*i.e.*, retinal stroke) and other localized pathologic processes can produce additional blind spots.

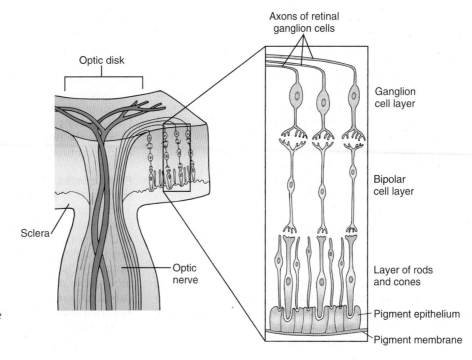

FIGURE 37-6 Organization of the human retina. The visual pathway begins with photoreceptors (rods and cones) in the retina. The responses of the photoreceptors are transmitted by the bipolar cells to the ganglion cell layer of the retina.

Two types of photoreceptors are present in the retina: rods, capable of black-white discrimination, and cones, capable of color discrimination. Rod-based vision is particularly sensitive to detecting light, especially moving light stimuli, at the expense of clear pattern discrimination. Rod vision is particularly adapted for night and low-level illumination. Dark adaptation is the process by which rod sensitivity increases to the optimum level. This requires approximately 4 hours in total or near-total darkness and involves only rods. Cone receptors, which are selectively sensitive to different wavelengths of light, provide the basis for color vision. Three types of cones, or cone-color systems, respond to the blue, green, and red portions of the visible electromagnetic spectrum. Cones do not have the dark adaptation capacity of rods. Consequently, the dark-adapted eye is a rod receptor eye with only black-gray-white experience (*scotopic* or *night vision*). The light-adapted eye (*photopic vision*) adds the capacity for color discrimination.

Both rods and cones contain chemicals that change configuration on exposure to light and, in the process, generate the currents that lead to the action potentials generated by the ganglionic cells. The light-sensitive chemical in the rods is called *rhodopsin*, and the light-sensitive chemicals in the cones are called *cone* or *color pigments*. Both types of photoreceptors are thin, elongated, mito-chondria-filled cells with a single, highly modified cilium (Fig. 37-7). The cilium has a short base, or inner segment, and a highly modified outer segment. The plasma membrane of the outer segment is tightly folded to form membranous disks (rods) or conical shapes (cones) containing visual pigment. Both rhodopsin and color pigment are incorporated into membranes of these disks in the form of transmembrane proteins. These disks are continuously synthesized at the base of the outer segment and shed at the distal end. The discarded membranes are phagocytized by the retinal pigment cells. If this phagocytosis is disrupted, as in *retinitis pigmentosa*, the sensory retina degenerates.

An area approximately 1.5 mm in diameter near the center of the retina, called the *macula lutea* (*i.e.,* "yellow spot"), is especially adapted for acute and detailed vision. This area is composed entirely of cones. In the central portion of the macula, the *fovea centralis*, the blood vessels and innermost layers are displaced to one side instead of resting on top of the cones (see Fig. 37-3). This allows light to pass unimpeded to the cones without passing through several layers of the retina. Many of these cones are connected one-to-one with ganglion cells, an arrangement that favors high acuity.

Retinal Blood Supply and Vascular Lesions

The blood supply for the retina is derived from two sources: the choriocapillaris of the choroid and the branches of the central retinal artery. The cones and rods of the outer neural layer receive nutrients from the choriocapillaris, a fine layer of capillaries on the inner surface of the choroid against which the retina is pressed (see Fig. 37-3). Because the choriocapillary layer

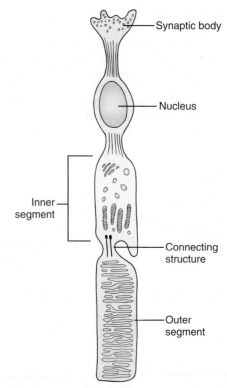

FIGURE 37-7 Retinal rod, showing its component parts and the distribution of its organelles. Its outer segment contains the disks (rods). The connecting structure joins the outer and inner segments. The inner segment contains the mitochondria, the ribosomal endoplasmic reticulum, the free ribosomes, and the Golgi saccules. The synaptic body forms the site where the photoreceptors synapse with subsequent nerve cells.

provides the only blood supply for the fovea centralis, detachment of this part of the sensory retina from the pigment epithelium causes irreparable visual loss. The central retinal artery, which is a branch of the ophthalmic, supplies the rest of the retina. A corresponding system of retinal veins unites to form the central vein of the retina.

Funduscopic examination of the eye with an ophthalmoscope provides an opportunity to examine the retinal blood vessels and other aspects of the retina (Fig. 37-8). Dilating the pupil pharmacologically enables more thorough examination of the retina.

Papilledema. The central retinal artery enters the eye through the *optic papilla* in the center of the optic nerve. The central vein of the retina exits the eye along the same path. The entrance and exit of the central artery and vein of the retina through the tough scleral tissue at the optic papilla can be compromised by any condition causing persistent increased intracranial pressure. The most common of these conditions are cerebral tumors, subdural hematomas, hydrocephalus, and malignant hypertension.

The thin-walled, low-pressure veins are the first to collapse, with the consequent backup and slowing of arterial

KEY CONCEPTS

Disorders of the Retinal Blood Supply

➤ The blood supply for the retina is derived from the central retinal artery, which supplies blood flow for the entire inside of the retina, and from vessels in the choroid, which supply the rods and cones.

➤ Central retinal occlusion interrupts blood flow to the inner retina and results in unilateral blindness.

➤ The retinopathies, which are disorders of the retinal vessels, interrupt blood flow to the visual receptors, leading to visual impairment.

➤ Retinal detachment separates the visual receptors from the choroid, which provides their major blood supply.

blood flow. Under these conditions, capillary permeability increases, and leakage of fluid results in edema of the optic papilla, called *papilledema*. The interior surface of the papilla normally is cup-shaped and can be evaluated through an ophthalmoscope. With papilledema, sometimes called *choked disk*, the optic cup is distorted by protrusion into the interior of the eye (Fig. 37-9). Because this sign does not occur until the intracranial pressure is significantly elevated, compression damage to the optic nerve fibers may have begun. As a warning sign, papilledema occurs quite late. Unresolved papilledema results in destruction of the optic nerve axons and blindness.

Retinopathies

The retinopathies involve the small blood vessels of the retina, with changes in blood vessel structure and the development of microaneurysms, neovascularization, and hemorrhage. *Microaneurysms* are outpouchings of the retinal vasculature. The microaneurysms may bleed, but areas of hemorrhage and edema tend to clear spontaneously. However, they reduce visual acuity if they encroach on the macula and cause degeneration before they are absorbed.

Neovascularization involves the formation of new blood vessels. They can develop from the choriocapillaris, extending between the pigment layer and the sensory layer, or from the retinal veins, extending between the sensory retina and the vitreous cavity and sometimes into the vitreous. These new blood vessels are fragile, leak protein, and are likely to bleed. Neovascularization occurs in many conditions that impair retinal circulation, including stasis because of hyperviscosity of blood or decreased flow, vascular occlusion, sickle cell disease, sarcoidosis, diabetes mellitus, and retinopathy of prematurity.[21] Although the cause of neovascularization is uncertain, research links the process with a vascular endothelial growth factor (VEGF) produced by the endothelial cells of blood vessels.[22,23] It is likely that other growth factors and signaling systems are also involved.

Retinal hemorrhages can be preretinal, intraretinal, or subretinal. Preretinal hemorrhages occur between the retina and the vitreous. These hemorrhages are usually large because the blood vessels are only loosely restricted; they may be associated with a subarachnoid or subdural hemorrhage and are usually regarded as a serious manifestation of the disorder. They usually reabsorb without complications unless they penetrate into the vitreous.

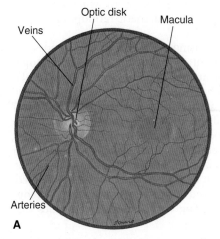
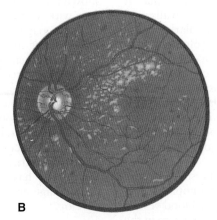
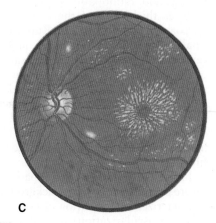

FIGURE 37-8 Fundus of the eye as seen in retinal examination with an ophthalmoscope: (**A**) normal fundus; (**B**) diabetic retinopathy—combination of microaneurysms, deep hemorrhages, and hard exudates of background retinopathy; (**C**) hypertensive retinopathy with purulent exudates. Some exudates are scattered, whereas others radiate from the fovea to form a macular star. (From Bates B. [1995]. *A guide to physical examination and history taking* (pp. 208, 210). Philadelphia: J. B. Lippincott.)

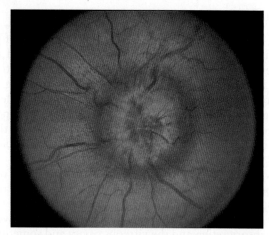

FIGURE 37-9 Chronic papilledema. The optic nerve head is congested and protrudes anteriorly toward the interior of the eye. It has blurred margins, and vessels within it are poorly seen. (From Klintworth G. K. [2005]. The eye. In Rubin E., Gorstein F., Rubin R., et al. [Eds.], *Rubin's pathology: Clinicopathologic foundations of medicine* [4th ed., p. 1521]. Philadelphia: Lippincott Williams & Wilkins.)

Intraretinal hemorrhages occur because of abnormalities of the retinal vessels, diseases of the blood, increased pressure in the retinal vessels, or vitreous traction on the vessels. Systemic causes include diabetes mellitus, hypertension, and blood dyscrasias. Subretinal hemorrhages are those that develop between the choroid and pigment layer of the retina. A common cause of subretinal hemorrhage is neovascularization.

Diabetic Retinopathy. Diabetic retinopathy is the third leading cause of blindness for all ages in the United States. It ranks first as the cause of newly reported cases of blindness in persons between the ages of 20 and 74 years.[22]

Diabetic retinopathy can be divided into two types: *nonproliferative* and *proliferative*.[22] Nonproliferative or background retinopathy is confined to the retina. It involves thickening of the retinal capillary walls and microaneurysm formation. Ruptured capillaries cause small intraretinal hemorrhages, and microinfarcts may cause cotton-wool exudates. A sensation of glare (because of the scattering of light) is a common complaint. The most common cause of decreased vision in persons with background retinopathy is macular edema.[22–24] It involves the breakdown of the blood-retinal barrier with leakage of plasma from the small blood vessels in the macula, which is responsible for the major part of visual function.

Proliferative diabetic retinopathy represents a more severe retinal change than background retinopathy. It is characterized by formation of new, fragile blood vessels (*i.e.*, neovascularization) at the disk and elsewhere in the retina. These vessels grow in front of the retina along the posterior surface of the vitreous or into the vitreous. They threaten vision in two ways. First, because they are abnormal, they often bleed easily, leaking blood into the vitreous cavity and decreasing visual acuity. Second, the blood vessels attach firmly to the retinal surface and posterior surface of the vitreous, such that normal movement of the vitreous may exert a pull on the retina, causing retinal detachment and progressive blindness.

Because early proliferative diabetic retinopathy is likely to be asymptomatic, it must be identified early, before bleeding occurs and obscures the view of the fundus or leads to fibrosis and retinal detachment. The American Diabetes Association, American College of Physicians, and American Academy of Ophthalmology have developed screening guidelines for diabetic retinopathy.[25] These guidelines recommend that persons with type 1 diabetes should have an initial dilated and comprehensive eye examination by an ophthalmologist or optometrist within 3 to 5 years after the onset of diabetes. Usually, screening is not indicated before the start of puberty. Persons with type 2 diabetes should have an initial comprehensive examination shortly after diagnosis. Subsequent examinations for persons with either type 1 or type 2 diabetes should be repeated annually. When planning pregnancy, women with preexisting diabetes should be counseled about the risk of developing retinopathy or progression of existing retinopathy. Women who become pregnant should have a comprehensive eye examination just before or soon after conception and at least every 3 months throughout pregnancy.

Preventing diabetic retinopathy from developing or progressing is considered the best approach to preserving vision. Growing evidence suggests that careful control of blood glucose levels in persons with diabetes mellitus may retard the onset and progression of retinopathy. The Diabetes Control and Complications Trial Research Group demonstrated that intensive management of persons with type 1 diabetes to maintain blood glucose levels at near-normal levels reduced the risk of retinopathy by 76% in persons with no retinopathy and slowed the progress by 54% in persons with early disease.[26] There also is a need for intensive management of hypertension and hyperlipidemia, both which have been shown to increase the risk of diabetic retinopathy in persons with diabetes.

Photocoagulation using an argon laser provides the major direct treatment modality for diabetic retinopathy.[27] Treatment strategies include laser photocoagulation applied directly to leaking microaneurysms and grid photocoagulation with a checkerboard pattern of laser burns applied to diffuse areas of leakage and thickening. Because laser photocoagulation destroys the proliferating vessels and the ischemic retina, it reduces the stimulus for further neovascularization. However, photocoagulation of neovascularization near the disk is not recommended. Vitrectomy has proved effective in removing vitreous hemorrhage and severing vitreoretinal membranes that develop.

Hypertensive Retinopathy. Long-standing systemic hypertension results in the compensatory thickening of arteriolar walls, which effectively reduces capillary perfusion pressure.[21] Ordinarily, a retinal blood vessel is transparent and seen as a red line; in venules, the red cells resemble a string of boxcars. On ophthalmoscopy, arteries in persons with long-standing hypertension appear paler than veins because they have thicker walls. The thickened arterioles in chronic hypertension become opaque and have a copper-wiring appearance. Edema, microaneurysms, intraretinal hemorrhages, exudates, and cotton-wool spots all are observed (see Fig. 37-7). Malignant hypertension involves swelling of the optic disk because of the local edema produced by escaped fluid. If the condition is permitted to progress long enough, serious visual deficits result.

Protective thickening of arteriolar walls cannot occur with sudden increases in blood pressure. Therefore, hemorrhage is likely to occur. Trauma to the optic globe or the head, sudden high blood pressure in eclampsia, and some types of renal disease characteristically are accompanied by edema of the retina and optic disk and by an increased likelihood of hemorrhage.

Retinal Detachment

Retinal detachment involves the separation of the sensory retina from the pigment epithelium (Fig. 37-10). It occurs when traction on the inner sensory layer or a tear in this layer allows fluid, usually vitreous, to accumulate between the two layers.[28] Retinal detachment that results from breaks in the sensory layer of the retina is called *rhegmatogenous detachment* (from the Greek *rhegma*, meaning "rent" or "hole"). The vitreous normally adheres to the retina at the optic disk, macula, and periphery of the retina. When the vitreous shrinks, it separates from the retina at the posterior pole of the eye (posterior vitreous detachment). However, at the periphery, the vitreous pulls on the attached retina, which can lead to tearing of the retina. Vitreous fluid can enter the tear and contribute to further separation of the retina from its overlying pigment layer.

Factors that predispose to retinal detachment include myopia, cataract extraction, and conditions that lead to preretinal fibrosis or formation of an exudate between the two layers of the retina. Persons with high grades of myopia may have abnormalities in the peripheral retina that predispose to sudden detachment. Intraocular surgery such as cataract extraction may produce traction on the peripheral retina that causes eventual detachment months or even years after surgery. Detachment may result from exudates that separate the two retinal layers. Exudative retinal detachment may be caused by intraocular inflammation, intraocular tumors, or certain systemic diseases. Inflammatory processes include posterior scleritis, uveitis, or parasitic invasion. Retinal detachment also can follow trauma immediately or at some later time.

Detachment of the neural retina from the retinal pigment layer separates the receptors from their major blood supply, the choroid. If retinal detachment continues for some time, permanent destruction and blindness of that part of the retina occur. The bipolar and ganglion cells survive because their blood supply, by way of the retinal arteries, remains intact. Without receptors, however, there is no visual function. The primary symptom of retinal detachment is loss of vision. Sometimes, flashing lights or sparks, followed by small floaters or spots in the field of vision, occur as the retina pulls away from the posterior pole of the eye. No pain is associated with this retinal detachment. As detachment progresses, the person perceives a dark curtain progressing across the visual field. Because the process begins in the periphery and spreads circumferentially and posteriorly, initial visual disturbances may involve only one quadrant of the visual field. Large peripheral detachments may occur without involvement of the macula, so that visual acuity remains unaffected. The tendency, however, is for detachments to enlarge until the entire retina is detached.

Diagnosis is based on the ophthalmoscopic appearance of the retina. Treatment is aimed at closing retinal tears and reattaching the retina. Rhegmatogenous detachment usually requires surgical treatment. Scleral buckling or pneumatic retinopexy is the most commonly used surgical technique.[28] Scleral buckling is the primary surgical procedure performed to reattach the retina. The procedure requires careful location of the retinal break and treatment with diathermy, cryotherapy, or laser to produce chorioretinal adhesions that seal the retinal tears so that the vitreous can no longer leak into the subretinal space. With scleral buckling, a piece of silicone (*i.e.*, the buckle) is sutured and infolded into the sclera, physically indenting the sclera so it contacts the separated pigment and retinal layers. Pneumatic retinopexy involves the intraocular injection of an expandable gas instead of a piece of silicone to form the indentation.

Macular Degeneration

Macular degeneration is characterized by the loss of central vision due to destructive changes of the macular or yellow-pigmented area surrounding the central fovea. Age-related macular degeneration is the most common cause of reduced vision in the United States. It is the leading cause of blindness among persons older than 75 years

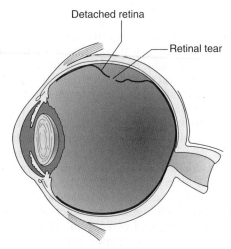

Detached retina

Retinal tear

FIGURE 37-10 Detached retina.

and of newly reported cases of blindness among those older than 65 years of age.[1] The cause of age-related macular degeneration is poorly understood. In addition to older age, identifiable risk factors include female sex, white race, cigarette smoking, and low dietary intake of carotenoids (precursors of vitamin A). Increasing evidence suggests that genetic factors may also play a role.[29]

There are two types of age-related macular degeneration: an atrophic nonexudative or "dry" form and an exudative or "wet" form. While both types are progressive, they differ in manifestations, prognosis, and management. Although most people with age-related macular degeneration manifest nonproliferative changes only, the majority of people who experience severe vision loss do so from the development of the exudative form of the disease.[28]

Nonexudative age-related macular degeneration is characterized by various degrees of atrophy and degeneration of the outer retina, Bruch membrane, and the choriocapillaris. It does not involve leakage of blood or serum; hence it is called *dry age-related macular degeneration*. On ophthalmoscopic examination, there are visible changes in the retinal pigmentary epithelium and pale yellow spots, called *drusen*, that may occur individually or in groups throughout the macula. Histopathologically, most drusen contain remnants of materials representative of focal detachment of the pigment epithelium. With time, the drusen enlarge, coalesce, and increase in number. The level of associated visual impairment is variable and may be minimal. Most people with macular drusen do not experience significant loss of central vision, and the atrophic changes may stabilize or progress slowly. However, people with the nonexudative form of age-related macular degeneration need to be followed closely because the exudative stage may develop suddenly at any time.

The exudative form of macular degeneration is characterized by the formation of a choroidal neovascular membrane that separates the pigmented epithelium from the neural retina. These new blood vessels have weaker walls than normal and are prone to leakage; therefore, the condition is called *wet age-related macular degeneration*. The leakage of serous or hemorrhagic fluid into the subretinal space causes separation of the pigmented epithelium from the neurosensory retina. Over time, the subretinal hemorrhages organize to form scar tissue. When this happens, retinal tissue death and loss of all visual function in the corresponding macular area occurs. The early stages of subretinal neovascularization may be difficult to detect ophthalmoscopically. Therefore, there is a need to be alert for recent or sudden changes in central vision, blurred vision, or scotoma in persons with evidence of age-related macular degeneration.

Although some subretinal neovascular membranes may regress spontaneously, the natural course of exudative macular degeneration is toward irreversible loss of central vision. Persons with late-stage disease often find it difficult to see at long distances (*e.g.*, in driving), do close work (*e.g.*, reading), see faces clearly, or distinguish colors. However, they may not be severely incapacitated because the peripheral retinal function usually remains intact. With the help of low-vision aids, many of them are able continue many of their normal activities.

Although there is no treatment for the nonexudative form of macular degeneration, argon laser photocoagulation may be useful in treating the neovascularization that occurs with the exudative form.[30,31] Another method used to halt neovascularization is photodynamic therapy, a nonthermal process leading to localized production of reactive oxygen species that mediate cellular, vascular, and immunologic injury and destruction of new blood vessels.

NEURAL PATHWAYS AND CORTICAL CENTERS

Full visual function requires the normally developed brain-related functions of photoreception and the pupillary reflex. These functions depend on the integrity of all visual pathways, including retinal circuitry and the pathway from the optic nerve to the visual cortex and other visual regions of the brain and brain stem.

Visual information is carried to the brain by axons of the retinal ganglion cells, which form the optic nerve. The two optic nerves meet and fuse in the optic chiasm, beyond which they are continued as the optic tracts (Fig. 37-11). In the optic chiasm, axons from the nasal retina of each eye cross to the opposite side and join with the axons of the temporal retina of the contralateral eye to form the optic tracts. One optic tract contains fibers from both eyes that transmit information from the same visual field.

Fibers of the optic tracts synapse in the lateral geniculate nucleus (LGN) of the thalamus. Axons from these neurons in the LGN form the optic radiations to the primary visual cortex in the occipital lobe. The pattern of information transmission established in the optic tract is retained in the optic radiations. For example, the axons from the right visual field, represented by the nasal retina of the right eye and the temporal retina of the left eye, are united at the chiasm. They continue through the left optic tract and left optic radiation to the left visual cortex, where visual experience is first perceived. The left primary visual cortex receives two representations of the right visual field. Physical separation of information from the left and right visual fields is maintained in the visual cortex. Interaction between these disparate representations occurs and provides the basis for the sensation of depth in the near visual field.

The primary visual cortex (area 17) surrounds the calcarine fissure, which lies in the occipital lobe. It is at this level that visual sensation is first experienced (Fig. 37-12). Immediately surrounding area 17 are the visual association cortices (areas 18 and 19) and several other association cortices. These association cortices, with their thalamic nuclei, must be functional for added meaningfulness of visual perception. This higher-order aspect of the visual experience depends on previous learning.

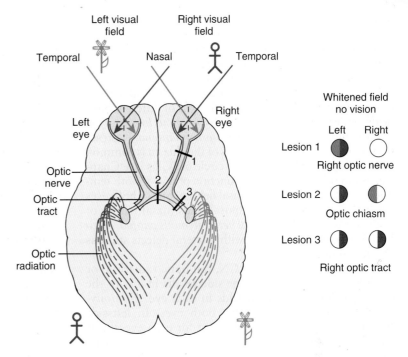

FIGURE 37-11 Diagram of optic pathways. The red lines indicate the right visual field and the blue lines the left visual field. Note the crossing of fibers from the medial half of each retina at the optic chiasm. Lesion 1 (right optic nerve) produces unilateral blindness. Lesion 2 (optic chiasm) may involve only those fibers that originate in the nasal half of each retina and cross to the opposite side in the optic chiasm; visual loss involves the temporal half of each field (bitemporal hemianopia). Lesion 3 (right optic tract) interrupts fibers (and vision) originating on the same side of both eyes (homonymous), with loss of vision from half of each field (hemianopia).

Disorders of the Optic Pathways

Among the disorders that can interrupt the visual pathway are trauma, tumors, and vascular lesions. Trauma and tumors can produce direct injury or impinge on the optic pathways. Vascular insufficiency in any one of the arterial systems of the retina or visual pathways can seriously affect vision. For example, normal visual function depends on adequacy of blood flow in the ophthalmic artery and its branches; the central artery of the retina; the anterior and middle cerebral arteries, which supply the intracranial optic nerve, chiasm, and optic tracts; and the posterior cerebral artery, which supplies the LGN,

optic radiation, and visual cortex. The adequacy of posterior cerebral artery function depends on that of the vertebral and basilar arteries that supply the brain stem.

Visual Field Defects

The *visual field* refers to the area that is visible during fixation of vision in one direction (see Fig. 37-11). As with a camera, the simple lens system of the eye inverts the image of the external world on each retina. In addition, the right and left sides of the visual field also are reversed. The right binocular visual field (the nasal half of the right eye and the temporal half of the left eye) is seen by the left retinal halves of each eye. Likewise, the left binocular field is seen by the right retinal halves of each eye.

Most of the visual field is *binocular*, or seen by both eyes. This binocular field is subdivided into *central* and *peripheral* portions. Central portions of the retina provide high visual acuity and correspond to the field focused on the central fovea. The peripheral and surrounding portion provides the capacity to detect objects, particularly moving objects. Beyond the visual field shared by both eyes, the left lateral periphery of the visual field is seen exclusively by the left nasal retina, and the right peripheral field by the right nasal retina.

Visual field defects result from damage to the visual pathways or the visual cortex (see Fig. 37-11). The testing of visual fields of each eye and of the two eyes together is useful in localizing lesions affecting the system. Perimetry or visual field testing, in which the visual field of each eye is measured and plotted in an arc, is used to identify defects and determine the location of lesions.

Blindness in one eye is called *anopia*. If half of the visual field for one eye is lost, the defect is called *hemianopia*; loss

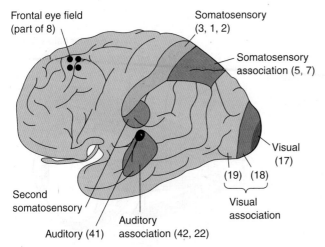

FIGURE 37-12 Lateral view of the cortex illustrating the location of the visual, visual association, auditory, and auditory association areas.

of a quarter-field is called *quadrantanopia.* Enlarging pituitary tumors can produce longitudinal damage through the optic chiasm with loss of the medial fibers of the optic nerve representing both nasal retinas and both temporal visual half-fields. Loss of the temporal or peripheral visual fields on both sides results in a narrow binocular field, commonly called *tunnel vision.* The loss of different half-fields in the two eyes is called a *heteronymous loss,* and the abnormality is called *heteronymous hemianopia.* Destruction of one or both lateral halves of the chiasm is common with multiple aneurysms of the circle of Willis (see Chapter 36). In this condition, the function of one or both temporal retinas is lost, and the nasal fields of one or both eyes are lost. The loss of the temporal fields (nasal retina) of both eyes is called *bitemporal heteronymous anopia.* With both eyes open, the person with bilateral defects still has the full binocular visual field.

Loss of the optic tract, LGN, full optic radiation, or complete visual cortex on one side results in loss of the corresponding visual half-fields in each eye. *Homonymous* means "the same" for both eyes. In left-side lesions, the right visual field is lost for each eye and is called *complete right homonymous hemianopia.* Partial injury to the left optic tract, LGN, or optic radiation can result in the loss of a quarter of the visual field in both eyes. This is called *homonymous quadrantanopia,* and depending on the lesion, it can involve the upper (superior) or lower (inferior) fields. The LGN, optic radiation, and visual cortex all receive their major blood supply from the posterior cerebral artery; unilateral occlusion of this artery results in complete loss of the opposite field (*i.e.,* homonymous hemianopia). Bilateral occlusion of these arteries results in total cortical blindness.

THE EXTRAOCULAR EYE MUSCLES AND DISORDERS OF EYE MOVEMENTS

For complete function of the eyes, it is necessary that the two eyes point toward the same fixation point and that the retinal and central nervous system (CNS) visual acuity mechanisms function. Despite slight variations in the view of the external world for each eye, it is important that these two images become fused, which is a forebrain function. Binocular fusion is controlled by ocular reflex mechanisms that adjust the orientation of each eye to produce a single image. If these reflexes fail, diplopia or double vision occurs.

Binocular vision depends on three pairs of extraocular muscles—the medial and lateral recti, the superior and inferior recti, and the superior and inferior obliques (Fig. 37-13). Each of the three sets of muscles in each eye is reciprocally innervated so that one muscle relaxes when the other contracts. Reciprocal contraction of the medial and lateral recti moves the eye from side to side (adduction and abduction); the superior and inferior recti move the eye up and down (elevation and depression). The oblique muscles rotate (intorsion and extorsion) the eye around its optic axis. A seventh muscle, the levator palpebrae superioris, elevates the upper lid.

The extraocular muscles are innervated by three cranial nerves. The trochlear nerve (CN IV) innervates the superior oblique, the abducens nerve (CN VI) innervates the lateral rectus, and the oculomotor nerve (CN III) innervates the remaining four muscles. Table 37-1 describes the function and innervation of the extraocular muscles.

Normal vision depends on the coordinated action of the entire visual system and a number of central control systems. It is through these mechanisms that an object is simultaneously imaged on the fovea of both eyes and perceived as a single image. Strabismus and amblyopia are two disorders that affect this highly integrated system. Although strabismus may develop in later life, it is seen most commonly in children.

 Strabismus

Strabismus, or squint, refers to any abnormality of eye coordination or alignment that results in loss of binocular vision (Fig. 37-14). When images from the same spots

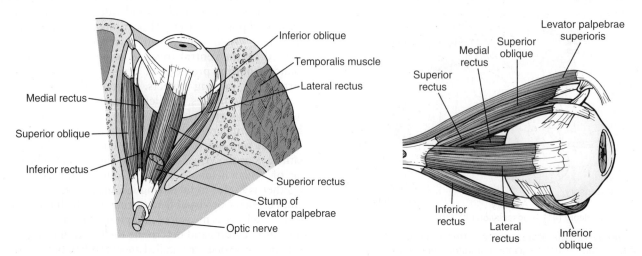

FIGURE 37-13 Extraocular muscles of the right eye.

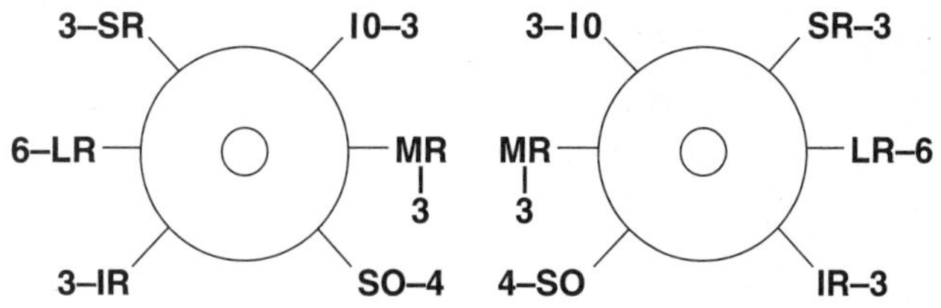

TABLE 37-1 Eye in Primary Position: Extrinsic Ocular Muscle Actions

Muscle*	Innervation	Primary	Secondary	Tertiary
MR: medial rectus	III	Adduction		
LR: lateral rectus	VI	Abduction		
SR: superior rectus	III	Elevation	Intorsion	Adduction
IR: inferior rectus	III	Depression	Extorsion	Adduction
SO: superior oblique	IV	Intorsion	Depression	Abduction
IO: inferior oblique	III	Extorsion	Elevation	Abduction

*In the schema of the functional roles of the six extraocular muscles, the major directional force applied by each muscle is indicated on the top. These muscles are arranged in functionally opposing pairs per eye and in parallel opposing pairs for conjugate movements of the two eyes. The numbers associated with each muscle indicate the cranial nerve innervation: 3, oculomotor (III) cranial nerve; 4, trochlear (IV) cranial nerve; 6, abducens (VI) cranial nerve.

in visual space do not fall on corresponding points of the two retinas, diplopia, or double vision, occurs.

In standard terminology, the disorders of eye movement are described according to the direction of movement. Esotropia refers to medial deviation, exotropia refers to lateral deviation, hypertropia refers to upward deviation, hypotropia refers to downward deviation, and cyclotropia refers to torsional deviation. The term *concomitance* refers to equal deviation in all directions of gaze. A nonconcomitant strabismus is one that varies with the direction of gaze. Strabismus may be divided into paralytic (nonconcomitant) forms, in which there is weakness or paralysis of one or more of the extraocular muscles, and nonparalytic (concomitant) forms, in which there is no primary muscle impairment. Strabismus is called *intermittent,* or *periodic,* when there are periods in which the eyes are parallel. It is monocular when the same eye always deviates and the fellow eye fixates. Figure 37-15 illustrates abnormalities in eye movement associated with esotropia, hypertropia, and exotropia.

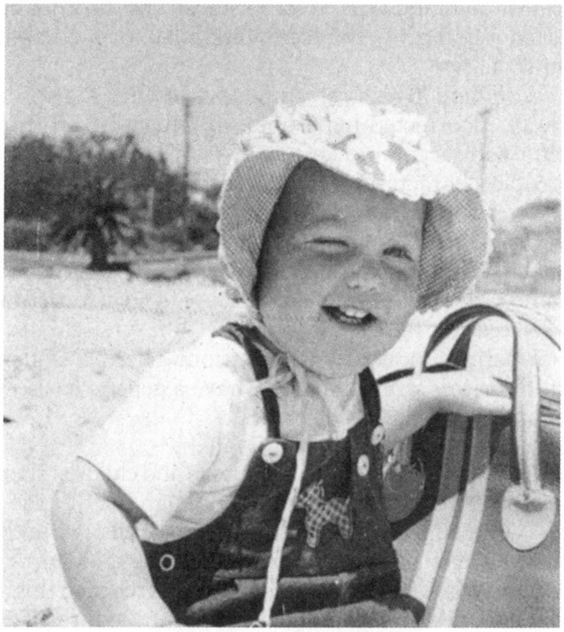

FIGURE 37-14 A child with intermittent exotropia squinting in the sunlight. (From Vaughan D. G., Asbury T., Riordan-Eva P. [Eds.]. [1995]. *General ophthalmology* [14th ed., p. 239]. Stamford, CT: Appleton & Lange.)

Strabismus affects approximately 4% of children younger than 6 years of age.[32] Because 30% to 50% of these children sustain permanent secondary loss of vision, or amblyopia, if the condition is left untreated, early diagnosis and treatment are essential.[33]

Paralytic Strabismus. Paralytic strabismus results from paresis (*i.e.,* weakness) or plegia (*i.e.,* paralysis) of one or more of the extraocular muscles. When the normal eye fixates, the affected eye is in the position of primary deviation. In the case of esotropia, there is weakness of one of the lateral rectus muscles, usually the result of weakness of the abducens nerve (CN VI). When the affected eye fixates, the unaffected eye is in a position of secondary deviation. The secondary deviation of the unaffected eye is greater than the primary deviation of the affected eye. This is because the affected eye requires an excess of innervational impulse to maintain fixation; the excess impulses also are distributed to the unaffected eye, causing overaction of its muscles.

Paralytic strabismus is uncommon in children but accounts for nearly all cases of adult strabismus; it can be caused by a number of conditions. Paralytic strabis-

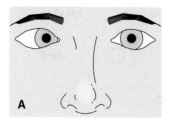

Primary position: right esotropia

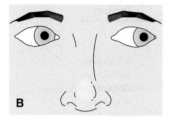

Left gaze: no deviation

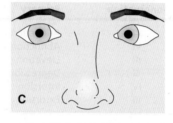

Right gaze: left esotropia

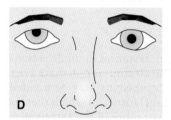

Right hypertropia

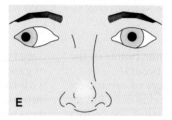

Right exotropia

FIGURE 37-15 Paralytic strabismus associated with paralysis of the right lateral rectus muscle: (**A**) primary position (looking straight ahead) of the eyes; (**B**) left gaze with no deviation; and (**C**) right gaze with left esotropia. Primary position of the eyes with weakness of the right inferior rectus and (**D**) right hypertropia. Primary position of the eyes with weakness of the right medial rectus and (**E**) right exotropia.

mus is seen most commonly in adults who have had cerebral vascular accidents and also may occur as the first sign of a tumor or inflammatory condition involving the CNS. One type of muscular dystrophy exerts its effects on the extraocular muscles. Initially, eye movements in all directions are weak, with later progression to bilateral optic immobility. Weakness of eye movement and lid elevation often is the first evidence of myasthenia gravis. The pathway of the oculomotor (CN III), trochlear (CN IV), and abducens (CN VI) nerves through the cavernous sinus and the back of the orbit make them vulnerable to basal skull fracture and tumors of the cavernous sinus (*e.g.,* cavernous sinus syndrome) or orbit (*e.g.,* orbital syndrome).[33] In infants, paralytic strabismus can be caused by birth injuries affecting the extraocular muscles or the cranial nerves supplying these muscles. It also can result from congenital anomalies of the muscles. In general, paralytic strabismus in an adult with previously normal binocular vision causes diplopia. This does not occur in persons who have never developed binocular vision.

Nonparalytic Strabismus. In nonparalytic strabismus, there is no extraocular muscle weakness or paralysis, and the angle of deviation is always the same in all fields of gaze. With persistent deviation, secondary abnormalities may develop because of over- or under-action of the muscles in some fields of gaze. Nonparalytic esotropia is the most common type of strabismus. The disorder may be accommodative, nonaccommodative, or a combination of the two.

Accommodative strabismus is caused by disorders such as uncorrected hyperopia, in which the esotropia occurs with accommodation. The onset of this type of esotropia characteristically occurs between 18 months and 4 years of age because accommodation is not well developed until that time. The disorder most often is monocular but may be alternating. The causes of nonaccommodative strabismus are obscure. The disorder may be related to faulty muscle insertion, muscle fascia abnormalities, or faulty innervation. There is evidence that idiopathic strabismus may have a genetic basis; siblings may have similar disorders.

Diagnosis and Treatment. All infants and children should be examined for visual alignment. Alignment of the visual axis occurs in the first 3 months of life. All infants should have consistent, synchronized eye movement by 5 to 6 months of age.[34] Infants who have reached this age and whose eyes are not aligned at all times during waking hours should be examined by a qualified health care practitioner.

Treatment of strabismus is directed toward the development of normal visual acuity, correction of the deviation, and superimposition of the retinal images to provide binocular vision. Nonsurgical and surgical methods can be used. In children, early treatment is important; the ideal age to begin is 6 months. Nonsurgical treatment includes occlusive patching, pleoptics (*i.e.*, eye exercises), and prism glasses. Because prolonged occlusive patching leads to loss of useful vision in the covered eye, patching is alternated between the affected and unaffected eye. This improves the vision in the affected eye without sacrificing vision in the unaffected eye. Prism glasses compensate for an abnormal alignment of an optic globe. Occasionally, long-acting miotics in low doses are used to cause pharmacologic accommodation in place of or in combination with corrective lenses.[32] Surgical procedures may be used to strengthen or weaken a muscle by altering its length or attachment site. A relatively new form of treatment involves the injection of botulinum toxin type A (Botox) into the extraocular muscle to produce a dose-dependent paralysis of that extraocular muscle. Paralysis of the muscle shifts the eye into the field of action of the antagonist muscle. During the time the eye is deviated the paralyzed muscle is stretched, whereas the antagonistic muscle is contracted. Usually two or more injections of the drug are necessary to obtain a lasting effect.

Amblyopia

Amblyopia describes a condition of diminished vision (uncorrectable by lenses) in which no detectable organic lesion of the eye is present.[34–36] This condition is sometimes called *lazy eye.* Types of amblyopia include deprivation occlusion, strabismus, refractive, and organic amblyopia. It is caused by visual deprivation (*e.g.*, cataracts, severe ptosis) or abnormal binocular interactions (*e.g.*, strabismus, anisometropia) during visual immaturity. In infants with unilateral cataracts that are dense, central, and larger than 2 mm in diameter, this time is before 2 months of age.[32] Normal development of the thalamic and cortical circuitry necessary for binocular visual perception requires simultaneous binocular use of each fovea during a critical period early in life (0 to 5 years).

In conditions causing abnormal binocular interactions, one image is suppressed to provide clearer vision. In esotropia, vision of the deviated eye is suppressed to prevent diplopia. A similar situation exists in anisometropia, in which the refractive indexes of the two eyes are different. Although the eyes are correctly aligned, they are unable to focus together, and the image of one eye is suppressed. The reversibility of amblyopia depends on the maturity of the visual system at the time of onset and the duration of the abnormal experience. If esotropia is involved, some persons alternate eyes and do not experience diplopia. With late adolescent or adult onset, this habit pattern must be unlearned after correction.

Peripheral vision is less affected than central foveal vision in amblyopia. Suppression becomes more evident with high illumination and high contrast. It is as if the affected eye did not possess central vision and the person

learns to fixate with the nonfoveal retina. If bilateral congenital blindness or near blindness (*e.g.*, from cataracts) occurs and remains uncorrected during infancy and early childhood, the person remains without pattern vision and has only overall field brightness and color discrimination. This is essentially bilateral amblyopia.

The treatment of children with the potential for development of amblyopia must be instituted well before the age of 6 years to avoid the suppression phenomenon. Surgery for congenital cataracts and ptosis should be done early. Severe refractive errors should be corrected. In strabismus, the alternate blocking of vision in one eye and then the other forces the child to use both eyes for form discrimination. The duration of occlusion of vision in the good eye must be short (2 to 5 hours per day) and closely monitored, or deprivation amblyopia can develop in the good eye as well.

In summary, the optic globe, or eyeball, is a nearly spherical structure protected posteriorly by the bony structures of the orbit and anteriorly by the eyelids. A conjunctiva lines the inner surface of the eyelids and covers the optic globe to the junction of the cornea and sclera. Conjunctivitis, also called *red eye* or *pink eye,* may result from bacterial or viral infection, allergic reactions, or the injurious effects of chemical agents, physical agents, or radiant energy. Keratitis, or inflammation of the cornea, can be caused by infections, hypersensitivity reactions, ischemia, defects in tearing, or trauma. Trauma or disease that involves the stromal layer of the cornea heals with scar formation and permanent opacification. These opacities interfere with the transmission of light and may impair vision.

Interiorly, the eye is divided into a smaller, fluid-filled anterior cavity and a larger, vitreous-filled posterior segment. The anterior segment of the eye is divided into an anterior and posterior chamber, separated by the pupil and closely adjacent lens. Glaucoma, which is one of the leading causes of blindness in the United States, is characterized by an increase in intraocular pressure resulting from the overproduction or impeded outflow of aqueous humor from the anterior chamber of the eye. Angle-closure glaucoma is caused by a narrow anterior chamber and blockage of the outflow channels at the angle formed by the iris and the cornea. Open-angle glaucoma is caused by an imbalance between aqueous humor production and outflow.

Refraction refers to the ability to focus an object on the retina. In hyperopia, or farsightedness, the image falls behind the retina. In myopia, or nearsightedness, the image falls in front of the retina. Accommodation is the process by which a clear image is maintained as the gaze is shifted from afar to a near object. Presbyopia is a change in the lens that occurs because of aging such that the lens becomes thicker and less able to change shape and accommodate for near vision. A cataract is characterized by increased lens opacity. It can occur as the result of congenital influences, metabolic disturbances, infection, injury, and aging.

The retina covers the inner aspect of the posterior two thirds of the eyeball and is continuous with the optic nerve. It contains the photoreceptors for vision: the rods, for black and white discrimination, and the cones, for color vision. Disorders of retinal vessels can result from a number of local and systemic disorders, including diabetes mellitus and hypertension. They cause vision loss through changes that result in hemorrhage, the production of opacities, and the separation of the pigment epithelium and sensory retina. Retinal detachment involves separation of the sensory receptors from their blood supply; it causes blindness unless reattachment is accomplished promptly. Macular degeneration, which is a leading cause of blindness in the elderly, is characterized by loss of central vision resulting from destructive changes in the central fovea.

Visual information is carried to the brain by axons of the retinal ganglion cells that form the optic nerve. The two optic nerves meet and cross at the optic chiasm, with the axons from each nasal retina joining the uncrossed fibers of the temporal retina of the opposite eye in the optic tract. The fibers in the optic tract pass to the LGN in the thalamus and then to the primary visual cortex, which is located in the occipital lobe. Damage to the visual pathways causes visual field defects that can be identified through visual field testing or perimetry.

Eye movement, which is controlled by the extraocular muscles, provides for alignment of the eyes and binocular vision. Strabismus refers to abnormalities in the coordination of eye movements with loss of binocular eye alignment. This inability to focus a visual image on corresponding parts of the two retinas results in diplopia. Paralytic strabismus is caused by weakness or paralysis of the extraocular muscles. Nonparalytic strabismus results from the inappropriate length or insertion of the extraocular muscles or from accommodation disorders. The neural pathways for vision develop during infancy. Amblyopia (*i.e.,* lazy eye) is a condition of diminished vision that cannot be corrected by lenses and in which no detectable organic lesion in the eye can be observed. It results from inadequately developed CNS circuitry because of visual deprivation (*e.g.,* cataracts) or abnormal binocular interactions (*e.g.,* strabismus, anisometropia) during the period of visual immaturity.

The Ear and Disorders of Auditory Function

The ears are paired organs consisting of an external and middle ear, which function in capturing, transmitting, and amplifying sound, and an inner ear that contains the receptive organs that are stimulated by sound waves (*i.e.,* hearing) or head position and movement (*i.e.,* vestibular function). Otitis media, or inflammation of the middle ear, is a common disorder of childhood. Hearing loss is one of the most common disabilities experienced by persons in the United States, particularly among the elderly.

THE EXTERNAL EAR

The external ear is a funnel-shaped structure that conducts sound waves to the tympanic membrane. It consists of the auricle, the external acoustic meatus, and the lateral surface of the tympanic membrane (Fig. 37-16). A thin layer of skin containing fine hairs, sebaceous glands, and ceruminous glands lines the ear canal. Ceruminous glands secrete cerumen, or earwax, which has certain antimicrobial properties and is thought to serve a protective function.

Disorders of the External Ear

The function of the external ear is disturbed when sound transmission is obstructed by impacted cerumen, inflammation (*i.e.,* otitis externa), or drainage from the external ear (otorrhea).

Impacted Cerumen. Although the ear normally is self-cleaning, the cerumen can accumulate and narrow the canal. Impacted cerumen is a common cause of reversible hearing loss.[37] It usually produces no symptoms until the canal becomes completely occluded, at which point the person experiences a feeling of fullness, loss of hearing, tinnitus (*i.e.,* ringing in the ears), or coughing because of vagal stimulation.

In most cases, cerumen can be removed by gentle irrigation using a bulb syringe and warm tap water. Warm water is used to avoid inducing a feeling of disequilibrium caused by the vestibular caloric response. Alternatively, health care professionals may remove cerumen using an otoscope and a wire loop or blunt cerumen curette.

Otitis Externa. Otitis externa is an inflammation of the external ear that can vary in severity from mild eczematoid dermatitis to severe cellulitis. It can be caused by infectious agents, irritation (*e.g.,* wearing earphones), or allergic reactions. Predisposing factors include moisture in the ear canal after swimming (*i.e.,* swimmer's ear) or bathing and trauma resulting from scratching or attempts to clean the ear. Most infections are caused by gram-negative bacteria (*e.g., Pseudomonas, Proteus*) or fungi (*e.g., Aspergillus*) that grow in the presence of excess moisture.[38] Otitis externa commonly occurs in the summer and is manifested by itching, redness, tenderness, and narrowing of the ear canal because of swelling. Inflammation of the auricle and external acoustic meatus makes movement of the ear painful. There may be watery or purulent drainage and intermittent hearing loss. Treatment usually includes the use of ear drops containing an appropriate antimicrobial or antifungal agent in combination with a corticosteroid to reduce inflammation.

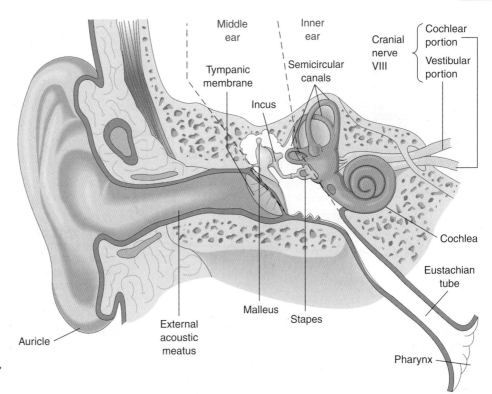

FIGURE 37-16 External, middle, and internal subdivisions of the ear.

THE MIDDLE EAR AND EUSTACHIAN TUBE

The middle ear is a small air-filled cavity located within the petrous (stony) portion of the middle ear. Its lateral wall is formed by the tympanic membrane and its medial wall by the bone dividing the middle and inner ear (see Fig. 37-16). Posteriorly, the middle ear is connected with small air pockets in the temporal bone called *mastoid air spaces* or *cells*.

Three tiny bones, the auditory ossicles, are suspended from the roof of the middle ear cavity and connect the tympanic membrane with the oval window.[39] They are connected by synovial joints and are covered with the epithelial lining of the cavity. The malleus ("hammer") has its handle firmly fixed to the upper portion of the tympanic membrane. The head of the malleus articulates with the *incus* ("anvil"), which articulates with the *stapes* ("stirrup"), which is inserted and sealed into the oval window by an annular ligament. Arrangement of the ear ossicles is such that their lever movements transmit vibrations from the tympanic membrane to the oval window and from there to the fluid in the inner ear. Two tissue-covered openings in the medial wall of the middle ear, the oval and the round windows, provide for the transmission of sound waves between the air-filled middle ear and the fluid-filled inner ear. It is the piston-like action of the stapes footplate that sets up compression waves in the inner ear fluid.

The middle ear is connected to the nasopharynx by the eustachian or auditory tube, which is located in a gap

---

KEY CONCEPTS

Disorders of the Middle Ear

➤ The middle ear is a small air-filled compartment in the temporal bone. It is separated from the outer ear by the tympanic membrane, contains tiny bony ossicles that aid in the amplification and transmission of sound to the inner ear, and is ventilated by the eustachian tube, which is connected to the nasopharynx.

➤ The eustachian tube, which is lined with a mucous membrane that is continuous with the nasopharynx, provides a passageway for pathogens to enter the middle ear.

➤ Otitis media (OM) refers to inflammation of the middle ear, usually associated with an acute infection (acute OM) or an accumulation of fluid (OME). It commonly is associated with disorders of eustachian tube function.

➤ Impaired conduction of sound waves and hearing loss occur when the tympanic membrane has been perforated; air in the middle ear has been replaced with fluid (OME); or the function of the bony ossicles has been impaired (otosclerosis).

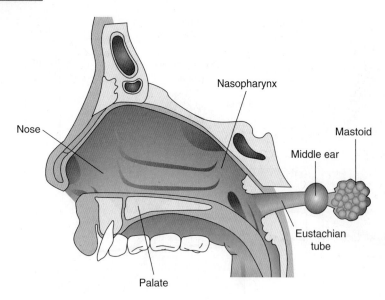

FIGURE 37-17 Nasopharynx–eustachian tube–mastoid air cell system. (From Bluestone C. D. [1981]. Recent advances in pathogenesis, diagnosis, and management of otitis media. *Pediatric Clinics of North America* 28, 736, with permission from Elsevier Science.)

in the bone between the anterior and medial walls of the middle ear (Fig. 37-17). The eustachian tube is lined with a mucous membrane that is continuous with the pharynx and the mastoid air cells.[40] The nasopharyngeal entrance to the eustachian tube, which usually is closed, is opened by the action of the *tensor veli palatini muscles* (Fig. 37-18). Opening of the eustachian tube, which normally occurs with swallowing and yawning reflexes, provides the mechanism for equalizing the pressure of the middle ear with that of the atmosphere. This equalization ensures that the pressures on both sides of the tympanic membrane are the same, so that sound transmission is not reduced and rupture does not result from sudden changes in external pressure, as occurs during plane travel.

Disorders of the Eustachian Tube

Abnormalities in eustachian tube function are important factors in the pathogenesis of middle ear infections. There are two important types of eustachian tube dysfunction: abnormal patency and obstruction. The *abnormally patent tube* does not close or does not close completely. In infants and children with an abnormally patent tube, air and secretions often are pumped into the eustachian tube during crying and nose blowing.

Obstruction can be functional or mechanical (see Fig. 37-18). *Functional obstruction* results from the persistent collapse of the eustachian tube due to a lack of tubal stiffness or poor function of the tensor veli palatini muscle that controls the opening of the eustachian tube. It is common in infants and young children because the amount and stiffness of the cartilage supporting the eustachian tube are less than in older children and adults. Changes in the craniofacial base also render the tensor muscle less efficient for opening the eustachian tube in this age group. In infants and children with craniofacial disorders, such as a cleft palate, abnormalities in attachment of the tensor muscles may produce functional obstruction of the eustachian tube.

Mechanical obstruction results from internal obstruction or external compression of the eustachian tube. The most common cause of internal obstruction is swelling and secretions resulting from allergy and viral respiratory infections. With obstruction, air in the middle ear is absorbed, causing a negative pressure and the transudation of serous capillary fluid into the middle ear.

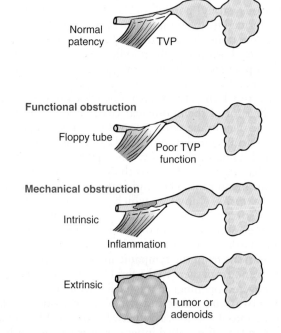

FIGURE 37-18 Pathophysiology of the eustachian tube. TVP, tensor veli palatini. (From Bluestone C. D. [1981]. Recent advances in the pathogenesis, diagnosis, and management of otitis media. *Pediatric Clinics of North America* 28, 737, with permission from Elsevier Science.)

Otitis Media

Otitis media (OM) is an infection of the middle ear that is associated with a collection of fluid. Although OM may occur in any age group, it is the most common diagnosis made by health care providers who care for children.[41–44] Infants and young children are at highest risk for OM, with the peak occurrence between 6 and 20 months of age. The occurrence of the disease tends to decrease as a function of age, with a marked decline after 6 years of age. The incidence is higher in boys, non–breast-fed infants, those who use pacifiers beyond infancy, children in large day care settings, children exposed to tobacco smoke, those with siblings or parents with a significant history of OM, those with allergic rhinitis, and children with congenital or acquired immune deficiencies (e.g., acquired immunodeficiency syndrome). The incidence of OM also is higher among children with craniofacial anomalies (e.g., cleft palate, Down syndrome) and among Canadian and Alaskan Inuit, and Native Americans. It is more common during the winter months, reflecting the seasonal patterns of upper respiratory tract infections.

There are two reasons for the increased risk of OM in infants and young children: the eustachian tube is shorter, more horizontal, and wider in this age group than in older children and adults; and infection can spread more easily through the eustachian canal of infants who spend most of their day lying supine. Bottle-fed infants have a higher incidence of OM than breast-fed infants, probably because they are held in a more horizontal position during feeding, and swallowing while in the horizontal position facilitates the reflux of milk into the middle ear. Breast-feeding also provides for the transfer of protective maternal antibodies to the infant.

Otitis media may present as acute OM (AOM), recurrent OM, or OM with effusion (OME) or fluid in the middle ear. This effusion may be thin and watery (serous), thick and mucus-like (mucoid), or purulent (containing pus). The characteristics of the fluid vary depending on the type of OM.

Acute Otitis Media.

Acute OM is characterized by the presence of fluid in the middle ear in combination with signs and symptoms of an acute or systemic infection. AOM can fail to resolve despite antibiotic treatment (persistent OM), or it may resolve and then recur (recurrent OM).

Most cases of AOM follow an upper respiratory tract infection that has been present for several days. The mucosal lining of the middle ear is continuous with the eustachian tube and nasopharynx, and most middle ear infections enter through the eustachian tube (see Fig. 33-17). AOM may be of either bacterial or viral origin. S. pneumoniae, H. influenzae, and Moraxella catarrhalis are the three major bacterial pathogens isolated from the middle ear in children with AOM.[41–44] There may be more than one type of bacteria present in some children. S. pneumoniae causes the largest proportion (40% to 50%) of cases generated by a single organism, and it is the least likely to resolve without treatment.[44] Emergence of

a multiple–drug-resistant strain of S. pneumoniae (DRSP) has led to increased numbers of treatment failures.[45]

Acute OM is characterized by otalgia (earache), fever, and hearing loss. Children older than 3 years of age may have rhinorrhea or running nose, vomiting, and diarrhea. In contrast, younger children often have nonspecific signs and symptoms that manifest as ear tugging, irritability, nighttime awakening, and poor feeding. Ear pain usually increases as the effusion accumulates behind the tympanic membrane. Perforation of the tympanic membrane may occur acutely, allowing purulent material from the eustachian tube to drain into the external auditory canal. This may prevent spread of the infection into the temporal bone or intracranial cavity.

Diagnosis of AOM is made by associated signs and symptoms and otoscopic examination. Although diagnosis of AOM often can be made by otoscopic examination alone, pneumatic otoscopy usually is performed to document middle ear effusion and immobility of the tympanic membrane. The use of the pneumatic otoscope permits the introduction of air into the ear canal for the purpose of determining tympanic membrane flexibility.

The treatment of AOM includes the judicious use of antibiotic therapy in high-risk children, especially those younger than 2 years of age who are at increased risk of intracranial complications and speech and language impairment.[44] Older children who have no fever or a low-grade fever usually do not require antibiotic treatment provided follow-up evaluation of symptoms occurs within 1 to 3 days. Regardless of whether antibiotic therapy is indicated, supportive therapy that includes analgesics, antipyretics, and local heat often is helpful. If the tympanic membrane is bulging and painful because of the accumulation of purulent drainage, a tympanotomy (incision in the tympanic membrane) may be done to relieve the pressure, thus reducing pain and hearing loss. In addition, this procedure prevents the ragged opening that can follow spontaneous rupture of the tympanic membrane.

Residual middle ear effusions are part of the continuum of AOM and persist regardless of whether antibiotics have been used. The effusion usually clears spontaneously within 1 to 3 months and does not require further treatment unless it persists beyond this period.

Recurrent Otitis Media.

Recurrent OM is defined as three new AOM episodes within 6 months or four episodes in 1 year that occur with almost every upper respiratory tract infection. Reinforcement of environmental controls, such as avoidance of passive tobacco smoke, is important. Children with recurrent OM should be evaluated to rule out any anatomic variations (e.g., enlarged adenoids) and immunologic disorders.

Recurrent OM may be managed with prophylactic antibiotic therapy. However, the emergence of bacterial resistance has raised concerns about the injudicious use of prophylactic antibiotics. Another approach to prevent recurrent OM is immunization with pneumococcal and influenza vaccines. Placement of tympanostomy tubes is another alternative, particularly for children who have experienced five or more OM episodes within a 12-month period.

Otitis Media with Effusion. Otitis media with effusion is a condition in which the tympanic membrane is intact and there is an accumulation of fluid in the middle ear without signs or symptoms of infection. The type of effusion often is described as serous, nonsuppurative, or secretory, but these terms may not be correct in all cases. Compared with children with AOM, those with OME do not have a fever or other signs and symptoms of infection, although some may report a feeling of ear fullness.

Most cases of persistent middle ear effusion resolve spontaneously within 3 months. The management options for this period include observation only, antibiotic therapy, or combination antibiotic and corticosteroid therapy. Because there is concern about hearing loss and its effect on learning and speech, a hearing evaluation may be indicated and usually is done after 6 weeks. If the effusion persists for 3 months or longer and is accompanied by hearing loss of 20 decibels (dB) or greater in children of normal development, tympanostomy tube placement may be indicated.[44]

Complications of Otitis Media. The complications of OM include hearing loss and extratemporal complications, including those affecting the middle ear, mastoid, adjacent structures of the temporal bone, and intracranial structures.

Hearing loss, which is a common complication of OM, usually is conductive and temporary based on the duration of the effusion. Hearing loss that is associated with fluid collection usually resolves when the effusion clears. Permanent hearing loss may occur as the result of damage to the tympanic membrane or other middle ear structures. Cases of sensorineural hearing loss are rare. Persistent and episodic conductive hearing loss in children may impair their cognitive, linguistic, and emotional development. However, the degree and duration of hearing loss required to produce such effects are unknown.

Adhesive OM involves an abnormal healing reaction in an inflamed middle ear. It produces irreversible thickening of the mucous membranes and may cause impaired movement of the ossicles and possibly conductive hearing loss. Tympanosclerosis involves the formation of whitish plaques and nodular deposits on the submucosal surface of the tympanic membrane, with possible adherence of the ossicles and conductive hearing loss.

A *cholesteatoma* is a saclike mass containing silvery-white keratin debris, which is shed by the squamous epithelial lining of the tympanic membrane.[46] As the lining of the epithelium sheds and desquamates, the lesion expands and erodes the surrounding tissues. The lesion, which is associated with chronic middle ear infection, is insidiously progressive, and erosion may involve the temporal bone, causing intracranial complications. Treatment involves microsurgical techniques to remove the cholesteatomatous material.

The mastoid antrum and air cells constitute a portion of the temporal bone and may become inflamed as an extension of acute or chronic OM. The disorder causes necrosis of the mastoid process and destruction of the bony intercellular matrix, which are visible by radiologic examination. Mastoid tenderness and drainage of exudate through a perforated tympanic membrane can occur. Chronic mastoiditis can develop as the result of chronic middle ear infection. Mastoid or middle ear surgery, along with other medical treatment, may be indicated.

Intracranial complications are uncommon since the advent of antimicrobial therapy. Although rare, these complications can develop if the infection spreads through vascular channels, by direct extension, or through preformed pathways such as the round window. These complications are seen more often with chronic suppurative OM and mastoiditis. They include meningitis, focal encephalitis, brain abscess, lateral sinus thrombophlebitis or thrombosis, labyrinthitis, and facial nerve paralysis.

Otosclerosis

Otosclerosis refers to the formation of new spongy bone around the stapes and oval window, which results in progressive deafness.[47] In most cases, the condition is familial and follows an autosomal dominant pattern with variable penetrance. Otosclerosis may begin at any time in life but usually does not appear until after puberty, most frequently between the ages of 20 and 30 years. The disease process accelerates during pregnancy.

Otosclerosis begins with resorption of bone in one or more foci. During active bone resorption, the bone structure appears spongy and softer than normal (*i.e.,* osteospongiosis). The resorbed bone is replaced by an overgrowth of new, hard, sclerotic bone. The process is slowly progressive, involving more areas of the temporal bone, especially in front of and posterior to the stapes footplate. As it invades the footplate, the pathologic bone increasingly immobilizes the stapes, reducing the transmission of sound. The pressure of otosclerotic bone on inner ear structures or the vestibulocochlear nerve (CN VIII) may contribute to the development of tinnitus, sensorineural hearing loss, and vertigo (discussed later in this chapter).

The symptoms of otosclerosis involve an insidious hearing loss. Initially, the affected person is unable to hear a whisper or someone speaking at a distance. In the earliest stages, the bone conduction by which the person's own voice is heard remains relatively unaffected. At this point, the person's own voice sounds unusually loud, and the sound of chewing becomes intensified. Because of bone conduction, most of these persons can hear fairly well on the telephone, which provides an amplified signal. Many are able to hear better in a noisy environment, probably because the masking effect of background noise causes other persons to speak more loudly.

The treatment of otosclerosis can be medical or surgical. A carefully selected, well-fitting hearing aid may allow a person with conductive deafness to lead a normal life. Sodium fluoride has been used with some success in the medical treatment of osteospongiosis. Because much of the conductive hearing loss associated with otosclerosis is caused by stapedial fixation, surgical treatment involves stapedectomy with reconstruction using the patient's own stapes or a prosthetic device.

THE INNER EAR AND AUDITORY PATHWAYS

The inner ear contains a labyrinth, or system of intercommunicating channels, and the receptors for hearing and position sense. An outer bony wall, or bony labyrinth, encloses a thin-walled, membranous labyrinth, which floats in the bony labyrinth.[39] Two separate fluids are found in the inner ear. The *periotic fluid* or *perilymph* separates the bony labyrinth from the membranous labyrinth, and the *otic fluid* or *endolymph* fills the membranous labyrinth. Periotic fluid composition is similar to that of the cerebrospinal fluid (CSF), and a tubular perilymphatic duct connects the periotic fluid with the CSF in the arachnoid space of the posterior fossa. Otic fluid has a potassium content that is similar to that of intracellular fluid.

Localized dilatations of the membranous labyrinth develop into three specialized sensory regions: the ampulla of each semicircular canal, the maculae of the utricle and sacculus, and the cochlea (Fig. 37-19). The cochlea is enclosed in a bony tube shaped like a snail shell that winds around a central bone column called the *modiolus*. Running through its center is the triangular membranous cochlear duct, which houses the spiral organ of Corti, the receptor organ for hearing. The cochlear duct and the spiral lamina, a thin, shelflike extension that spirals up the modiolus, divides the cavity of the cochlea into three chambers: the scala vestibuli, the scala tympani, and the scala media (Fig. 37-20A). The organ of Corti, which rests atop the basilar membrane in the scala media, is composed of supporting cells and several long rows of cochlear hair cells: one row of inner hair cells and three rows of outer hair cells (see Fig. 37-20B). Afferent fibers from the cochlear nerve are coiled around the bases of the hair cells. Sound waves, delivered to the oval window by the stapes footplate, are transmitted to the periotic fluid in the scala vestibuli and scala tympani. Transduction of sound stimuli occurs when the trapped cilia of the hair cells in the organ of Corti are bent by the sound-induced movement of the basilar membrane.

Afferent fibers from the organ of Corti have their cell bodies in the spiral ganglion in the central portion of the cochlea. Nerve fibers from the spiral ganglion (*i.e.,* vestibulocochlear or auditory nerve [CN VIII]) travel to the cochlear nuclei in the caudal pons. Many secondary nerve fibers from the cochlear nuclei pass to the nuclei on the opposite side of the pons or rostrally toward the inferior colliculus of the midbrain. From the inferior colliculus, the auditory pathway passes to the primary auditory cortex (area 41) in the temporal lobe through relays in the medial geniculate nucleus of the thalamus (see Fig. 37-12). The auditory association cortex (areas 42 and 22), which is necessary for the meaningfulness of sound, borders the primary cortex. Because some of the fibers from each ear cross, each auditory cortex receives impulses from both ears.

Disorders of the Inner Ear and Central Auditory Pathways

Disorders of the cochlear component of the inner ear and auditory pathways can lead to the presence of tinnitus or sensorineural hearing loss.

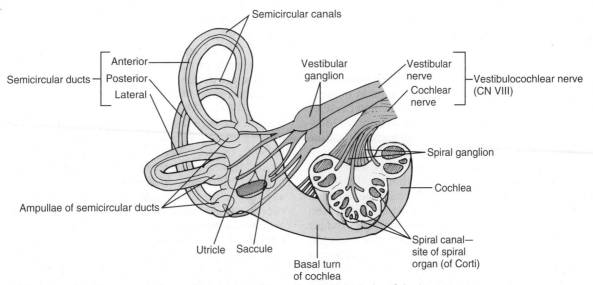

FIGURE 37-19 Schematic lateral view of the bony and membranous labyrinths of the inner ear showing the ducts and chambers filled with endolymph and bathed in perilymph within the bony labyrinth. Observe the cochlea, parts of the membranous labyrinth (the saccule and utricle within the vestibule, and the semicircular ducts within the semicircular canals), and the vestibular and cochlear branches of the vestibulocochlear nerve (cranial nerve [CN] VIII).

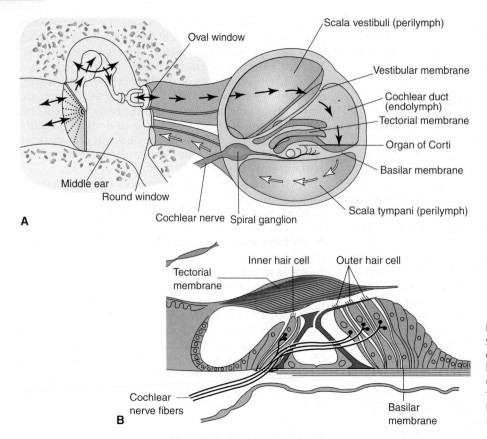

A

B

FIGURE 37-20 (**A**) Path taken by sound waves reaching the inner ear. (**B**) Spiral organ of Corti has been removed from the cochlear duct and greatly enlarged to show the inner and outer hair cells, the basilar membrane, and cochlear nerve fibers.

Tinnitus. Tinnitus (from the Latin *tinniere*, "to ring") is the perception of abnormal ear or head noises not produced by an external stimulus.[48,49] Although it often is described as "ringing of the ears," it may also assume a hissing, roaring, buzzing, or humming sound. It has been estimated that 35 million people in the United States have the disorder. The condition affects men and women equally, is most prevalent between 40 and 70 years of age, and occasionally affects children.[48]

Tinnitus may be constant, intermittent, and unilateral or bilateral. Intermittent periods of mild, high-pitched tinnitus lasting for several minutes are common in normal-hearing persons. Impacted cerumen is a benign cause of tinnitus, which resolves after the earwax is removed. Medications such as aspirin and stimulants such as nicotine and caffeine can cause transient tinnitus. Although tinnitus is a subjective experience, for clinical purposes it is subdivided into objective and subjective tinnitus. *Objective tinnitus* refers to those rare cases in which the sound is detected or potentially detectable by another observer. Typical causes of objective tinnitus include vascular abnormalities or neuromuscular disorders. For example, in some vascular disorders, sounds generated by turbulent blood flow (*e.g.*, arterial bruits or venous hums) are conducted to the auditory system. Vascular disorders typically produce a pulsatile form of tinnitus. *Subjective tinnitus* refers to noise perception when there is no noise stimulation of the cochlea. The physiologic mechanism underlying subjective tinnitus is largely unknown. It seems likely that there are several mechanisms, including abnormal firing of auditory receptors, dysfunction of cochlear neurotransmitter function or ionic balance, and alterations in central processing of the signal.

Treatment measures for tinnitus are designed to treat the symptoms, rather than effect a cure. They include elimination of drugs or other substances such as caffeine, some cheeses, red wine, and foods containing monosodium glutamate that are suspected of causing tinnitus. The use of an externally produced sound (noise generators or tinnitus-masking devices) may be used in severe cases to mask or inhibit the tinnitus.

Disorders of the Central Auditory Pathways. The auditory pathways in the brain involve communication between the two sides of the brain at many levels. As a result, strokes, tumors, abscesses, and other focal abnormalities seldom produce more than a mild reduction in auditory acuity on the side opposite the lesion. For auditory language to have meaning, lateral dominance becomes important. On the dominant side, usually the left side, the more medial and dorsal portion of the auditory association cortex is of crucial importance. This area is called *Wernicke's area*, and damage to it is associated with auditory receptive aphasia (and agnosia of speech). Persons with damage to this area of the brain can speak intelligibly and read normally but are unable to understand the meaning of major aspects of audible speech.

Irritative foci that affect the auditory radiation or the primary auditory cortex can produce roaring or clicking sounds, which appear to come from the auditory environment of the opposite side (*i.e.*, auditory hallucinations). Focal seizures that originate in or near the auditory cortex often are immediately preceded by the perception of ringing or other sounds preceded by a prodrome (*i.e.*, aura). Damage to the auditory association cortex, especially if bilateral, results in deficiencies of sound recognition and memory (*i.e.*, auditory agnosia). If the damage is in the dominant hemisphere, speech recognition can be affected (*i.e.*, sensory or receptive aphasia).

HEARING LOSS

Nearly 30 million Americans have hearing loss.[50–52] It affects persons of all age groups. One of every 1000 infants born in the United States is completely deaf, and more than 3 million children have hearing loss. Between 25% and 40% of people older than 65 years have hearing loss.[53]

The level of hearing is measured in decibels, where 0 dB is the threshold for perception of sound at a given frequency in persons with normal hearing. A 10-fold increase in sound pressure level from 0 dB is measured as 20 dB. Hearing loss is classified as mild, moderate, severe, or profound. "Hard of hearing" is defined as hearing loss greater than 20 to 25 dB in adults and greater than 15 dB in children. Profound deafness is defined as hearing loss greater than 100 dB in adults[54] or 70 dB in children.[55]

There are many causes of hearing loss or deafness. Most fit into the categories of conductive, sensorineural, or mixed deficiencies that involve a combination of conductive and sensorineural function deficiencies of the same

ear. Chart 37-1 summarizes common causes of hearing loss. Hearing loss may be genetic or acquired, sudden or progressive, unilateral or bilateral, partial or complete, reversible or irreversible. Age and suddenness of onset provide important clues as to the cause of hearing loss.

Conductive Hearing Loss

Conductive hearing loss occurs when auditory stimuli are not adequately transmitted through the auditory canal, tympanic membrane, middle ear, or ossicle chain to the inner ear. Temporary hearing loss can occur as the result of impacted cerumen in the outer ear or fluid in the middle ear. Foreign bodies, including pieces of cotton and insects, may impair hearing. More permanent causes of hearing loss are thickening or damage of the tympanic

---

KEY CONCEPTS

Hearing Loss

→ Hearing is a special sensory function that incorporates the sound-transmitting properties of the external ear canal, the eardrum that separates the external and middle ear, the bony ossicles of the middle ear, the sensory receptors of the cochlea in the inner ear, the neural pathways of the vestibulocochlear or auditory nerve, and the primary auditory and auditory association cortices.

→ Hearing loss represents impairment of the ability to detect and perceive sound.

→ Conductive hearing loss is caused by disorders in which auditory stimuli are not transmitted through the structures of the outer and middle ears to the sensory receptors in the inner ear.

→ Sensorineural hearing loss is caused by disorders that affect the inner ear, auditory nerve, or auditory pathways.

CHART 37-1

Common Causes of Conductive and Sensorineural Hearing Loss

Conductive Hearing Loss

- External ear conditions
  - Impacted earwax or foreign body
  - Otitis externa
- Middle ear conditions
  - Trauma
  - Otitis media (acute and with effusion)
  - Otosclerosis
  - Tumors

Sensorineural Hearing Loss

- Trauma
  - Head injury
  - Noise
- Central nervous system infections (*e.g.*, meningitis)
- Degenerative conditions
  - Presbycusis
- Vascular
  - Atherosclerosis
- Ototoxic drugs (*e.g.*, aminoglycosides, salicylates, loop diuretics)
- Tumors
  - Vestibular schwannoma (acoustic neuroma)
  - Meningioma
  - Metastatic tumors
- Idiopathic
  - Ménière disease

Mixed Conductive and Sensorineural Hearing Loss

- Middle ear conditions
  - Barotrauma
  - Cholesteatoma
  - Otosclerosis
- Temporal bone fractures

membrane or involvement of the bony structures (ossicles and oval window) of the middle ear caused by otosclerosis or Paget disease.

Sensorineural Hearing Loss

Sensorineural, or perceptive, hearing loss occurs with disorders that affect the inner ear, auditory nerve, or auditory pathways of the brain. With this type of deafness, sound waves are conducted to the inner ear, but abnormalities of the cochlear apparatus or auditory nerve decrease or distort the transfer of information to the brain. Tinnitus often accompanies cochlear nerve irritation. Abnormal function resulting from damage or malformation of the central auditory pathways and circuitry is included in this category.

Sensorineural hearing loss may have a genetic cause or may result from intrauterine infections, such as maternal rubella, or developmental malformations of the inner ear. Genetic hearing loss may result from mutation in a single gene (monogenetic) or from a combination of mutations in different genes and environmental factors (multifactorial). It has been estimated that 50% of profound deafness in children has a monogenetic basis.[53,54] The inheritance pattern for monogenetic hearing loss is autosomal recessive in approximately 75% of cases.[55] Hearing loss may begin before development of speech (prelingual) or after speech development (postlingual). Most prelingual forms are present at birth. Genetic forms of hearing loss also can be classified as being part of a syndrome in which other abnormalities are present, or as nonsyndromic, in which deafness is the only abnormality.

Sensorineural hearing loss also can result from trauma to the inner ear, tumors that encroach on the inner ear or sensory neurons, vascular disorders with hemorrhage, or thrombosis of vessels that supply the inner ear. Other causes of sensorineural deafness are infections and drugs. Sudden sensorineural hearing loss represents an abrupt loss of hearing that occurs instantaneously or on awakening. It most commonly is caused by viral infections or circulatory disorders. Hypothyroidism is a potential cause of sensorineural hearing loss in older persons.

Environmentally induced deafness can occur through direct exposure to excessively intense sound, as in the workplace or at a concert. This is a particular problem in older adults who were working in noisy environments before the mid-1960s, when there were no laws mandating use of devices for hearing protection. Sustained or repeated exposure to noise pollution at sound intensities greater than 100 to 120 dB can cause corresponding mechanical damage to the organ of Corti. Severe damage can result in permanent sensorineural deafness to the affected sound frequencies. Wearing earplugs or ear protection is important under many industrial conditions and for musicians and music listeners exposed to high sound amplification.

A number of infections can cause sensorineural hearing loss. Deafness or some degree of hearing impairment is the most common serious complication of bacterial meningitis in infants and children, reportedly resulting in sensorineural hearing loss in 5% to 35% of persons who survive the infection.[53] The mechanism causing hearing impairment seems to be a suppurative labyrinthitis or neuritis resulting in the loss of hair cells and damage to the auditory nerve. Untreated suppurative OM also can extend into the inner ear and cause sensorineural hearing loss through the same mechanisms.

Among the neoplasms that impair hearing are *acoustic neuromas*. Acoustic neuromas are benign Schwann cell tumors affecting CN VIII. These tumors usually are unilateral and cause hearing loss by compressing the cochlear nerve or interfering with blood supply to the nerve and cochlea. Other neoplasms that can affect hearing include meningiomas and metastatic brain tumors. The temporal bone is a common site of metastases.

Drugs that damage inner ear structures are labeled *ototoxic*. Vestibular symptoms of ototoxicity include lightheadedness, giddiness, and dizziness; if toxicity is severe, cochlear symptoms consisting of tinnitus or hearing loss occur. Hearing loss is sensorineural and may be bilateral or unilateral, transient or permanent. Several classes of drugs have been identified as having ototoxic potential, including the aminoglycoside antibiotics and some other basic antibiotics, antimalarial drugs, some chemotherapeutic drugs, loop diuretics, and salicylates. The symptoms of drug-induced hearing loss may be transient, as often is the case with salicylates and diuretics, or they may be permanent. The risk of ototoxicity depends on the total dose of the drug and its concentration in the bloodstream. It is increased in persons with impaired kidney functioning and in those previously or currently treated with another potentially ototoxic drug.

Diagnosis and Treatment of Hearing Loss

Diagnosis of hearing loss is aided by careful history of associated otologic factors such as otalgia, otorrhea, tinnitus, and self-described hearing difficulties; physical examination to detect the presence of conditions such as otorrhea, impacted cerumen, or injury to the tympanic membrane; and hearing tests. Testing for hearing loss includes a number of methods, including a person's reported ability to hear an observer's voice, use of a tuning fork to test air and bone conduction, audioscopes, and auditory brain stem evoked responses (ABRs).

Tuning forks are used to differentiate conductive and sensorineural hearing loss. Audioscopes can be used to assess a person's ability to hear pure tones at 1000 to 2000 Hz (usual speech frequencies). The ABR uses electroencephalographic (EEG) electrodes and high-gain amplifiers to produce a record of brain wave activity elicited during repeated acoustic stimulations of either or both ears. It involves subjecting the ear to loud clicks and using a computer to analyze nerve impulses as they are processed in the midbrain. Imaging studies such as computed tomography (CT) scans and magnetic resonance imaging (MRI) can be done to determine the site of a lesion and the extent of damage.[50]

Treatment. Untreated hearing loss can have many consequences. Social isolation and depressive disorders are common in hearing-impaired elderly. Hearing-impaired people may avoid social situations where background noise makes conversation difficult to hear. Safety issues, both in and out of the home, may become significant. Treatment measures for hearing loss range from simple removal of impacted cerumen in the external auditory canal to surgical procedures such as those used to reconstruct the tympanic membrane. For other people, particularly the frail elderly, hearing aids remain an option. Cochlear implants also are an option for some people.

Hearing aids remain the mainstay of treatment for many persons with conductive and sensorineural hearing loss. With the advent of microcircuitry, hearing aids are now being designed with computer chips that allow multiple programs to be placed in a single hearing aid. The various programs allow the user to select a specific setting for different listening situations. The development of microcircuitry has also made it possible for hearing aids to be miniaturized to the point that, in many cases, they can be placed deep in the ear where they take advantage of the normal shape of the external ear and ear canal. Although modern hearing aids have improved greatly, they cannot replicate the hearing person's ability to hear both soft and loud noises. They also fail consistently to filter out distorted or background noise. Other aids for the hearing impaired include alert and signal devices, assisted-listening devices from telephone companies, and dogs trained to respond to various sounds.

Surgically implantable cochlear prostheses for the profoundly deaf have been developed and are available for use in adults and children 2 years of age or older. These prostheses are inserted into the scala tympani of the cochlea and work by providing direct stimulation to the auditory nerve, bypassing the stimulation that typically is provided by transducer cells but that is absent or nonfunctional in a deaf cochlea. For the implant to work, the auditory nerve must be functional. Although early implants used a single electrode, current implants use multielectrode placement, enhancing speech perception. Much of the progress in implant performance has been achieved through improvements in the speech processors that convert sound into electrical stimuli. Advances in the development of the multichannel implant have improved performance such that cochlear implants have been established as an effective option for adults and children with profound hearing impairment.[56] Most persons who are deafened after learning speech derive substantial benefit when cochlear implants are used in conjunction with lip reading; some are able to understand some speech without lip reading; and some are able to communicate by telephone.

 Hearing Loss in Infants and Children

Even mild or unilateral hearing loss can have a detrimental effect on the language development and hearing-associated learning of the young child. Although estimates vary depending on the group surveyed and testing methods used, from 1 to 2 per 1000 newborns have moderate (30 to 50 dB), severe (50 to 70 db), or profound (≥70 dB) sensorineural hearing loss.[44] An additional 1 to 2 per 1000 may have milder or unilateral impairments. For the less severe or transient conductive hearing loss that is commonly associated with middle ear disease in young children, the numbers are even greater.

The cause of hearing impairment in children depends on whether the hearing loss is conductive or sensorineural. Conductive hearing loss is usually the result of middle ear infections. Causes of sensorineural hearing impairment include genetic, infectious, traumatic, and ototoxic factors. The most common infectious cause of congenital sensorineural hearing loss is cytomegalovirus (CMV), which infects 1 in 100 newborns in the United States each year; of these, about 4500 to 6000 per year have sensorineural hearing loss.[44] Of particular concern is the fact that congenital CMV can cause both symptomatic and asymptomatic hearing loss in the newborn. Some children with congenital CMV infection, who were asymptomatic as newborns, have suddenly lost residual hearing at 4 to 5 years of age.[44] Postnatal causes of sensorineural hearing loss include beta-streptococcal sepsis in the newborn and bacterial meningitis. *S. pneumoniae* is the most common cause of bacterial meningitis that results in sensorineural hearing loss after the neonatal period; this cause may become less frequent with the availability of the conjugate pneumococcal vaccine. Other causes of sensorineural hearing loss are toxins and trauma. Early in pregnancy, the embryo is particularly sensitive to toxic substances including ototoxic drugs such as the aminoglycosides and loop diuretics. Trauma, particularly head trauma, may cause sensorineural hearing loss.

Hearing impairment can have a major impact on the development of a child; therefore, early identification through screening programs is strongly advocated. The American Academy of Pediatrics (AAP) and the Joint Commission on Infant Hearing (JCIH) recently published a position paper calling for universal screening of all infants by physiologic measurements before 3 months of age, with proper intervention no later than 6 months of age.[57,58] Many states have now enacted legislation supporting the position paper; as a result, newborn hearing screening programs have been implemented in newborn nurseries throughout the United States. The currently recommended screening techniques are either the evoked otoacoustic emissions (EOAE) or the ABR. Both methodologies are noninvasive, relatively quick (<5 minutes), and easy to perform.[59] The EOAE measures sound waves generated in the inner ear (cochlea) in response to clicks or tone bursts emitted and recorded by a minute microphone placed in the external ear canals of the infant. The ABR uses three electrodes pasted to the infant's scalp to measure the EEG waves generated by clicks. Because many children become hearing impaired after the neonatal period and are not identified by neonatal screening programs, the AAP and JCIH recommend that all infants with risk factors for delayed onset of progressive hearing loss receive ongoing audiologic monitoring for 3 years and at appropriate intervals thereafter.

Once hearing loss has been identified, a full developmental and speech and language evaluation is needed. Parental involvement and counseling are essential. Children with sensorineural hearing loss should be evaluated for possible hearing aid use by a pediatric audiologist.[60] Hearing aids may be fitted for infants as young as 2 months of age. The use of surgically implanted cochlear implants in children with profound hearing loss has been approved for children 2 years of age and older.[56,61]

Hearing Loss in the Elderly

The term *presbycusis* is used to describe the degenerative hearing loss that occurs with advancing age. Approximately 23% of persons between 65 and 75 years of age and 40% of the population older than 75 years of age are affected.[62] Men are affected earlier and experience a greater loss than women.

The degenerative changes that impair hearing may begin in the fifth decade of life and may not be clinically apparent until later.[63] Onset may be associated with chronic noise exposure or vascular disorders.[63] The disorder involves loss of neuroepithelial (hair) cells, neurons, and the stria vascularis. High-frequency sounds are affected more than low-frequency sounds because high and low frequencies distort the base of the basilar membrane, but only low frequencies affect the distal (apical) region. Through the years, permanent mechanical damage to the organ of Corti is more likely to occur near the base of the cochlea, where the high sonic frequencies are discriminated.

Although hearing loss is a common problem in the elderly, many older persons are not appropriately assessed for hearing loss. When assessing an older person's ability to hear, it is important to ask both the person and the family about awareness of hearing loss. The ability to hear high-frequency sounds usually is lost first. Loss of high-frequency discrimination is characterized by difficulty in understanding words in noisy environments, in hearing a speaker in an adjacent room, or hearing a speaker whose back is turned. Hearing loss may be estimated by having the person report hearing of softly whispered, normally spoken, or shouted words. In the English language, vowels are low-frequency sounds, whereas consonants are of higher frequency. A ticking watch also may be used to test for the higher frequencies.

In summary, disorders of the auditory system include infections of the external and middle ear, otosclerosis, and conduction and sensorineural deafness. Otitis externa is an inflammatory process of the external ear. Otitis media is an infection of the middle ear. It may present as AOM, recurrent OM, or OME. AOM usually follows an upper respiratory tract infection and is char-

acterized by otalgia, fever, and hearing loss. The effusion that accompanies OM can persist for weeks or months, interfering with hearing and impairing speech development. Otosclerosis is a familial disorder of the otic capsule that results in hearing loss due to immobilization of the stapes and conduction deafness.

Deafness, or hearing loss, can develop as the result of a number of auditory disorders. It can be conductive, sensorineural, or mixed. Conduction deafness occurs when transmission of sound waves from the external to the inner ear is impaired. Sensorineural deafness can involve cochlear structures of the inner ear or the neural pathways that transmit auditory stimuli. Sensorineural hearing loss can result from genetic or congenital disorders, trauma, infections, vascular disorders, tumors, or ototoxic drugs. Hearing loss that occurs in young children and the elderly can have special implications. Even mild or unilateral hearing loss can affect the development and hearing-associated learning of the young child. The age-related degenerative changes that impair hearing may begin in the fifth decade and not be clinically apparent until later. Treatment of hearing loss includes the use of hearing aids and, in some cases of profound deafness, implantation of a cochlear prosthesis.

Disorders of Vestibular Function

The vestibular receptive organs, which are located in the inner ear, and their CNS connections provide for the sense of equilibrium and orientation in space. Because the vestibular apparatus is part of the inner ear and located in the head, it is head position and acceleration that is sensed. The equilibrium sense, which is also dependent on vision and input from stretch receptors in muscles and tendons, serves to maintain and assist recovery of a stable body and head position through control of postural reflexes and it serves to maintain a stable visual field despite marked changes in head position.

THE VESTIBULAR SYSTEM AND MAINTENANCE OF EQUILIBRIUM

The Vestibular Apparatus

The peripheral apparatus of the vestibular system is contained in the bony labyrinth of the inner ear next to and continuous with the cochlea of the auditory system.[16,39] It is divided into five prominent structures: three semicircular ducts, which occupy the semicircular canals, and two large chambers, the utricle and saccule, which occupy the vestibule (Fig. 37-21A). Receptors in these structures are differentiated into those of the semicircular ducts that monitor rotational movement of the head and those of the utricle and saccule that monitor straight line changes in speed and direction.

KEY CONCEPTS

Disorders of the Vestibular System

➤ The vestibular system, which is located in the inner ear and senses head motion and acceleration, contributes to the reflex activity needed for effective posture and movement, and it serves to maintain a stable visual field despite changes in head position.

➤ The vestibular system has extensive interconnections with neural pathways controlling vision, hearing, chemotactic receptor trigger zone, the cerebellum, and the autonomic nervous system. Its disorders are characterized by vertigo, nystagmus, tinnitus, nausea and vomiting, and autonomic nervous system manifestations.

➤ Disorders of vestibular function can result from repeated stimulation of the vestibular system, such as during car, air, and boat travel (motion sickness); distention of the endolymphatic compartment of the inner ear (Ménière disease); or dislodgment of otoliths that participate in the receptor function of the vestibular system (benign paroxysmal positional vertigo).

The receptors of the vestibular system consist of small patches of hair cells located in the membranous ampullae of the three semicircular ducts and the maculae of the utricle and saccule. Each patch of hair cells has a number of small cilia called *stereocilia*, plus one large cilium, the *kinocilium*. The kinocilium is always located at one end, and the stereocilia become progressively shorter toward the other side of the cell (Fig. 37-22). Minute filamentous attachments connect the tip of each stereocilium to the next longer stereocilium, and finally to the kinocilium. Movement of the adjoined stereocilia and kinocilium in one direction causes depolarization or activation of the receptor, and movement in the other direction causes hyperpolarization or inactivation of the receptor.

The three semicircular ducts, which monitor head rotation, are arranged at right angles to one another. These are the receptors that help you maintain your balance when you turn suddenly or twirl on a dance floor. The horizontal ducts in the inner ears on the two sides of the head are in the same plane, whereas the superior (anterior) duct of one side is parallel with the inferior (posterior) duct on the other side, and the two function as a pair. Each duct is filled with endolymph and has a swelling at the base called the *ampulla*. Each ampulla contains a hair cell sensory surface raised into a crest, or crista, at right angles to the duct. The hair bundles extend into a flexible gelatinous mass, called the *cupula*, which essentially closes off fluid flow through the semicircular ducts (see Fig. 37-21B).

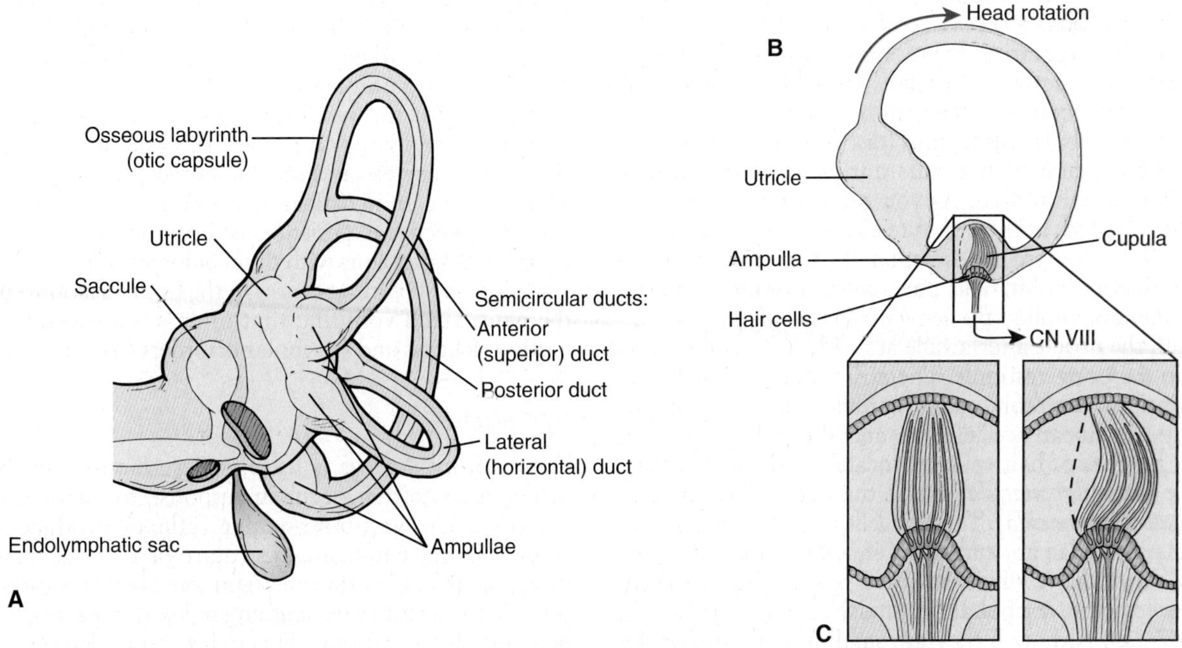

FIGURE 37-21 (A) The osseous and membranous labyrinth of the left ear. (B) Location of the ampulla. (C) The cupula and movement of hair bundles with head movement.

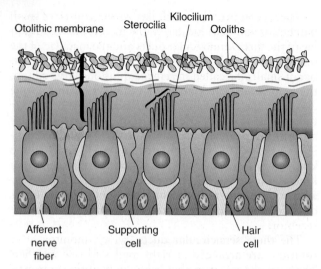

Otolithic membrane   Sterocilia   Kilocilium   Otoliths

Afferent nerve fiber   Supporting cell   Hair cell

FIGURE 37-22 The relation of the otoliths to the sensory cells in the macula of the utricle and saccule. (Adapted from Selkurt F. D. [Ed.]. [1982]. *Basic physiology for the health sciences* [2nd ed.]. Boston: Little, Brown.)

When the head begins to rotate around the axis of a semicircular canal (*i.e.,* undergoes angular acceleration), the momentum of the endolymph causes an increase in pressure on one side of the cupula (see Fig. 37-21C). This is similar to the lagging behind of the water in a glass that is suddenly rotated, except that the endolymph cannot flow past the cupula. Instead, the endolymph applies a differential pressure to the two sides of the cupula, bending the hair bundles. Because all the hair bundles in each semicircular canal share a common orientation, angular acceleration in one direction depolarizes hair cells and excites afferent neurons, whereas acceleration in the opposite direction hyperpolarizes the receptor cells and diminishes afferent nerve activity. Impulses from the semicircular ducts are particularly important to reflex movements of the eyes. Vestibular nystagmus (discussed later) is a complex phenomenon that occurs during and immediately after rotational motion. As you rotate your head, your eyes slowly drift in the opposite direction and then jump rapidly back toward the direction of rotation to establish a new fixation point. This phenomenon results from the flow of endolymph in the semicircular canals.

Both the utricle and saccule are widened membranous sacs in the bony vestibule. The utricle and saccule house equilibrium receptors called *maculae* that respond to changes in linear acceleration and the pull of gravity. Small patches of hair cells are located in the floor of the utricle (*utricular macula*) and in the side wall of the saccule (*saccular macula*). The hair cells in both utricular and saccular maculae are embedded in a flattened gelatinous mass, the *otolithic membrane,* which is studded with tiny stones (calcium carbonate crystals) called *otoliths* (see Fig. 37-22). Although they are small, the density of the otoliths increases the membrane's weight and its resistance to change in motion. When the head is tilted, the gelatinous mass shifts its position because of the pull of

the gravitational field, bending the stereocilia of the macular hair cells. Although each hair cell becomes more or less excitable depending on the direction in which the cilia are bending, the hair cells are oriented in all directions, making these sense organs sensitive to static or changing head position in relation to the gravitational field. In a condition called *benign positional vertigo,* the otoliths become dislodged from their gelatinous base, causing positional vertigo (to be discussed).

Neural Pathways

Our response to body imbalance, such as stumbling, must be fast and reflexive. Hence, information from the vestibular system goes directly to reflex centers in the brain stem, rather than to the cerebral cortex. Ganglionic cells, homologous with the dorsal root ganglion cells, form afferent ganglia: the superior and inferior vestibular ganglia that innervate the hair cells in the peripheral vestibular apparatus. The central axons of these ganglionic cells become the superior and inferior vestibular nerves, which become part of the vestibulocochlear nerve (CN VIII).

Impulses from the vestibular nerves initially pass to one of two destinations: the vestibular nuclear complex in the brain stem or the cerebellum. The vestibular nuclei, which form the main integrative center for balance, also receive input from visual and somatic receptors, particularly from stretch receptors in the neck muscles that report the angle or inclination of the head. The vestibular nuclei integrate this information and then send impulses to the brain stem centers that control the extraocular eye movements (CN III, IV, and VI) and reflex movements of the neck, limb, and trunk muscles (through the vestibulospinal tracts). These reflex movements include the vestibulo-ocular reflexes that keep the eyes still as the head moves and vestibulospinal reflexes that enable the skeletomotor system to make the quick adjustments needed to maintain or regain balance.

Neurons of the vestibular nuclei also project to the thalamus, the temporal cortex, the somesthetic area of the parietal cortex, and the chemoreceptor trigger zone. The thalamic and cortical projections provide the basis for the subjective experiences of position in space and of rotation. Connections with the chemoreceptor trigger zone stimulate the vomiting center in the brain, accounting for the nausea and vomiting that often are associated with motion sickness and vestibular disorders (see Chapter 27).

Nystagmus

The term *nystagmus* is used to describe the vestibulo-ocular reflexes that occur in response to ongoing head rotation. The vestibulo-ocular reflexes produce slow compensatory conjugate eye rotations that occur in the direction precisely opposite to ongoing head rotation and provide for continuous, ongoing reflex stabilization of the binocular fixation point. This reflex can be demonstrated by holding a pencil vertically in front of the eyes and moving it from side to side through a 10-degree arc at a rate of approximately five times per second. At this rate of motion, the pencil appears blurred, because a different and more complex reflex, smooth pursuit, cannot compensate quickly enough. However, if the pencil is maintained in a stable position and the head is moved back and forth at the same rate, the image of the pencil is clearly defined. The eye movements are the same in both cases. The reason that the pencil image remains clear in the second situation is because the vestibulo-ocular reflexes keep the image of the pencil on the retinal fovea. When compensatory vestibulo-ocular reflexes carry the conjugate eye rotations to their physical limit, a very rapid conjugate movement (*i.e.*, saccade) moves the eyes in the direction of head rotation to a new fixation point, followed by a slow vestibulo-ocular reflex as the head continues to rotate past the new fixation point.

Spontaneous nystagmus that occurs without head movement or visual stimuli is always pathologic. It seems to appear more readily and more severely with fatigue and to some extent can be influenced by psychological factors. Nystagmus caused by CNS disease, in contrast to vestibular end-organ or vestibulocochlear nerve sources, seldom is accompanied by vertigo. If present, the vertigo is of mild intensity. Nystagmus can be tested by electronystagmography (discussed later)

Vertigo

Disorders of vestibular function are characterized by a condition called *vertigo*, in which an illusion of motion occurs. Persons with vertigo frequently describe a sensation of spinning or tumbling, a "to-and-fro" motion, or falling forward or backward. Vertigo should be differentiated from lightheadedness, faintness, unsteadiness, or syncope (loss of consciousness).[64-66] Vertigo or dizziness can result from peripheral or central vestibular disorders. Approximately 85% of persons with vertigo have a peripheral vestibular disorder, whereas only 15% have a central disorder. Vertigo caused by peripheral disorders tends to be severe in intensity and episodic or brief in duration. In contrast, vertigo attributable to central causes tends to be mild and constant and chronic in duration.

Diagnostic methods include the Romberg test (discussed later in this section), an evaluation of gait, and observations for the presence of nystagmus.[65] Laboratory investigations include audiologic evaluation, electronystagmography, CT scan or MRI, and ABRs. These tests help to distinguish between central and peripheral causes of vertigo and to identify causes requiring specific treatment.

Motion Sickness

Motion sickness is a form of normal physiologic vertigo. It is caused by repeated rhythmic stimulation of the vestibular system, such as is encountered in car, air, or boat travel. Vertigo, malaise, nausea, and vomiting are the principal symptoms. Autonomic signs, including lowered blood pressure, tachycardia, and excessive sweating, may occur. Some persons experience a variant of motion sickness, reporting sensing the rocking motion of the boat after returning to ground. This usually resolves after the vestibular system becomes accustomed to the stationary influence of being back on land. Among the drugs used to suppress, reduce, or ameliorate the symptoms of motion sickness are the antihistamines (*e.g.*, meclizine, dimenhydrinate, and promethazine).

DISORDERS OF PERIPHERAL VESTIBULAR FUNCTION

Disorders of peripheral vestibular function occur when signals from the vestibular organs in the inner ear are distorted, such as in benign paroxysmal positional vertigo, or unbalanced by unilateral involvement of one of the vestibular organs, such as in Ménière disease. The inner ear is vulnerable to injury caused by fracture of the petrous portion of the temporal bones; by infection of nearby structures, including the middle ear and meninges; and by blood-borne toxins and infections. Alcohol can cause transient episodes of vertigo.

Ménière Disease

Ménière disease is a disorder of the inner ear caused by distention of the endolymphatic compartment of the inner ear, causing a triad of hearing loss, vertigo, and tinnitus.[67,68] The primary lesion appears to be in the endolymphatic sac, which is thought to be responsible for endolymph filtration and excretion. A number of pathogenic mechanisms have been postulated, including an increased production of endolymph, decreased production of perilymph accompanied by a compensatory increase in volume of the endolymphatic sac, and decreased absorption of endolymph caused by malfunction of the endolymphatic sac or blockage of endolymphatic pathways.

The cause of Ménière disease is unknown. A number of conditions, such as trauma, infection (*e.g.*, syphilis), and immunologic, endocrine (adrenal-pituitary insufficiency and hypothyroidism), and vascular disorders have been proposed as possible causes of Ménière disease.[68] The most common form of the disease is an idiopathic form thought to be caused by a viral injury to the fluid transport system of the inner ear.

Ménière disease is characterized by fluctuating episodes of tinnitus, feelings of ear fullness, and violent rotary vertigo that often renders the person unable to sit or walk. There is a need to lie quietly with the head fixed in a comfortable position, avoiding all head movements that aggravate the vertigo. Symptoms referable to the autonomic nervous system, including pallor, sweating, nausea, and vomiting, usually are present. The more severe the attack, the more prominent are the autonomic manifestations. A fluctuating hearing loss occurs, with a return to normal after the episode subsides. Initially the symptoms tend to be unilateral, resulting in rotary nystagmus caused by an imbalance in vestibular control of eye movements. Because initial involvement usually is unilateral and because the sense of hearing is bilateral, many persons with the disorder are not aware of the full extent of their hearing loss. However, as the disease progresses, the hearing loss stops fluctuating and progressively worsens, with both ears tending to be affected so that the prime disability becomes one of deafness. The episodes of vertigo diminish and then disappear, although the person may be unsteady, especially in the dark.

Methods used in the diagnosis of Ménière disease include audiograms, vestibular testing by electronystagmography, and petrous pyramid radiographs. The administration of hyperosmolar substances, such as glycerin and urea, often produces acute temporary hearing improvement in persons with Ménière disease and sometimes is used as a diagnostic measure of endolymphatic distention.

The management of Ménière disease focuses on attempts to reduce the distention of the endolymphatic space and can be medical or surgical. Pharmacologic management consists of suppressant drugs (e.g., prochlorperazine, promethazine, diazepam), which act centrally to decrease the activity of the vestibular system. Diuretics are used to reduce endolymph fluid volume. A low-sodium diet is recommended in addition to these medications. Corticosteroid medications (e.g., prednisone) may be used to maintain satisfactory hearing and resolve dizziness. Gentamicin therapy has been used for ablation of the vestibular system.[69] This treatment is mainly effective in controlling vertigo and does not alter the underlying pathologic process.

Surgical methods include the creation of an endolymphatic shunt, in which excess endolymph from the inner ear is diverted into the subarachnoid space or the mastoid (endolymphatic sac surgery), and vestibular nerve section.

Benign Paroxysmal Positional Vertigo

Benign paroxysmal positional vertigo (BPPV) is the most common cause of pathologic vertigo and usually develops after the fourth decade. It is characterized by brief periods of vertigo, usually lasting less than 1 minute, that are precipitated by a change in head position.[70,71] The most prominent symptom of BPPV is vertigo that occurs in bed when the person rolls into a lateral position. It also commonly occurs when the person is getting in and out of bed, bending over and straightening up, or extending the head to look up. It also can be triggered by amusement park rides that feature turns and twists.

Benign paroxysmal positional vertigo is thought to result from damage to the delicate sensory organs of the inner ear, the semicircular ducts and otoliths. In persons with BPPV, the calcium carbonate particles (otoliths) from the utricle become dislodged and become free-floating debris in the endolymph (otic fluid) of the posterior semicircular duct, which is the most dependent part of the inner ear.[70] Movement of the free-floating debris causes this portion of the vestibular system to become more sensitive, such that any movement of the head in the plane parallel to the posterior duct may cause vertigo and nystagmus. There usually is a several-second delay between head movement and onset of vertigo, representing the time it takes to generate the exaggerated endolymph activity. Symptoms usually subside with continued movement, probably because the movement causes the debris

to be redistributed throughout the endolymph system and away from the posterior duct.

Diagnosis is based on tests that involve the use of a change in head position to elicit vertigo and nystagmus. BPPV often is successfully treated with drug therapy to control vertigo-induced nausea. Nondrug therapies using habituation exercises and otolith repositioning are successful in many people (to be discussed).[70,71] Otolith repositioning involves a series of maneuvers in which the head is moved to different positions in an effort to reposition the free-floating debris in the endolymph of the semicircular canals.

DISORDERS OF CENTRAL VESTIBULAR FUNCTION

Abnormal nystagmus and vertigo can occur as a result of CNS lesions involving the cerebellum and lower brain stem. Central causes of vertigo include brain stem ischemia, tumors, and the demyelinating effects of multiple sclerosis.[72] When brain stem ischemia is the cause of vertigo, it usually is associated with other brain stem signs, such as diplopia, ataxia, dysarthria, or facial weakness. Compression of the vestibular nuclei by cerebellar tumors invading the fourth ventricle results in progressively severe signs and symptoms. In addition to abnormal nystagmus and vertigo, vomiting and a broad-based and dystaxic gait become progressively more evident.

In contrast to peripherally generated nystagmus, CNS-derived nystagmus is relatively constant, rather than episodic; can occur in any direction, rather than being primarily in the horizontal or torsional (rotatory) dimensions; often changes direction through time; and cannot be suppressed by visual fixation. Repeated induction of nystagmus results in rapid diminution or "fatigue" of the reflex with peripheral abnormalities, but fatigue is not characteristic of central lesions.

DIAGNOSIS AND TREATMENT

Tests of Vestibular Function

Diagnosis of vestibular disorders is based on a description of the symptoms, a history of trauma or exposure to agents that are destructive to vestibular structures, and physical examination. Tests of eye movements (i.e., nystagmus) and muscle control of balance and equilibrium often are used.

Electronystagmography (ENG) is a precise and objective diagnostic method of evaluating nystagmic eye movements. Electrodes are placed lateral to the outer canthus of each eye and above and below each eye, and a ground electrode is placed on the forehead. With ENG, the velocity, frequency, and amplitude of spontaneous or induced nystagmus and the changes in these measurements brought by a loss of fixation, with the eyes open or closed, can be quantified. The advantages of ENG are that it is easily administered, is noninvasive, does not interfere with vision, and does not require head restraint.

Caloric testing involves elevating the head 30 degrees and irrigating each external auditory canal separately with 30 to 50 mL of ice water. The resulting changes in temperature, which are conducted through the petrous portion of the temporal bone, set up convection currents in the otic fluid that mimic the effects of angular acceleration. In an unconscious person with a functional brain stem and intact vestibulo-ocular reflexes, the eyes exhibit a jerk nystagmus lasting 2 to 3 minutes, with the slow component toward the irrigated ear followed by rapid movement away from the ear. With impairment of brain stem function, the response becomes perverted and eventually disappears. An advantage of the caloric stimulation method is the ability to test the vestibular apparatus on one side at a time. The test is never done on a person who does not have an intact eardrum or those who have blood or fluid collected behind the eardrum.

Rotational testing involves the use of a motor-driven revolving chair or platform. Unlike caloric testing, rotational testing depends only on the inner ear and is unrelated to conditions of the external ear or temporal bone. A major disadvantage of the method is that both ears are tested simultaneously. Motor-driven chairs or platforms can be precisely controlled, and multiple graded stimuli can be delivered in a relatively short period. Testing usually is performed in the dark without visual influence and with selected light stimuli. Eye movements are usually monitored using ENG.

The *Romberg test* is used to demonstrate disorders of static vestibular function. The person being tested is requested to stand with feet together and arms extended forward so that the degree of sway and arm stability can be observed. The person then is asked to close his or her eyes. When visual clues are removed, postural stability is based on proprioceptive sensation from the joints, muscles, and tendons and from static vestibular reception. Deficiency in vestibular static input is indicated by greatly increased sway and a tendency for the arms to drift toward the side of deficiency. If vestibular input is severely deficient, the subject falls toward the deficient side.

Treatment of Vestibular Disorders

Pharmacologic Treatment. Depending on the cause, vertigo may be treated pharmacologically. There are two types of drugs used in the treatment of vertigo. First are the drugs used to suppress the illusion of motion. These include drugs such as antihistamines (*e.g.,* meclizine, cyclizine, dimenhydrinate, and promethazine) and anticholinergic drugs (*e.g.,* scopolamine, atropine) that suppress the vestibular system. Although the antihistamines have long been used in treating vertigo, little is known about their mechanism of action. The second type includes drugs used to relieve the nausea and vomiting that commonly accompany the condition. Antidopaminergic drugs (*e.g.,* phenothiazines) and benzodiazepines commonly are used for this purpose.

Vestibular Rehabilitation. Vestibular rehabilitation, a relatively new treatment modality for peripheral vestibular disorders, has met with considerable success.[73,74] It commonly is done by physical therapists and uses a home exercise program that incorporates habituation exercises, balance retraining exercises, and a general conditioning program. The habituation exercises take advantage of physiologic fatigue of the neurovegetative response to repetitive movement or positional stimulation and are done to decrease motion-provoked vertigo, lightheadedness, and unsteadiness. The exercises are selected to provoke the vestibular symptoms. The person moves quickly into the position that causes symptoms, holds the position until the symptoms subside (*i.e.,* fatigue of the neurovegetative response), relaxes, and then repeats the exercise for a prescribed number of times. The exercises usually are repeated twice daily. The habituation effect is characterized by decreased sensitivity and duration of symptoms. It may occur in as little as 2 weeks or take as long as 6 months.

Balance retraining exercises consist of activities directed toward improving individual components of balance that may be abnormal. General conditioning exercises, a vital part of the rehabilitation process, are individualized to the person's preferences and lifestyle. They should consist of motion-oriented activity that the person is interested in and should be done on a regular basis, usually four to five times per week.

In summary, the vestibular system plays an essential role in the equilibrium sense, which is closely integrated with the visual and proprioceptive (position) senses. Receptors for the vestibular system, in the semicircular ducts of the inner ear, respond to changes in linear and angular acceleration of the head. The vestibular nerve fibers travel in CN VIII to the vestibular nuclei at the junction of the medulla and pons; some fibers pass through the nuclei to the cerebellum.

Disorders of peripheral vestibular function, which involve the inner ear sensory organs, include Ménière disease and BPPV. Ménière disease, which is caused by an overaccumulation of endolymph, is characterized by severe, disabling episodes of tinnitus, feelings of ear fullness, and violent rotary vertigo. BPPV is thought to be caused by free-floating particles in the posterior semicircular canal. It presents as a sudden onset of dizziness or vertigo that is provoked by certain changes in head position. Among the methods used in treatment of the vertigo that accompanies vestibular disorders are habituation exercises (for BPPV) and antivertigo drugs.

Review Exercises

The mother of a 3-year-old boy notices that his left eye is red and watering when she picks him up from day care. He keeps rubbing his eye as though it itches. The next morning, however, she notices that both eyes are red, swollen, and watering. Being concerned, she takes him to the pediatrician in the morning and is told that he has "pink eye." She is told that the infection should go away by itself.

A. What part of the eye is involved?
B. What type of conjunctivitis do you think this child has (bacterial, viral, or allergic)?
C. Why didn't the pediatrician order an antibiotic?
D. Is the condition contagious? What measures should she take to prevent its spread?

During a routine eye examination to get new glasses because she had been having difficulty with her distant vision, a 75-year-old woman is told that she is developing cataracts.

A. What types of visual changes occur as the result of a cataract?
B. What can the woman do to prevent the cataracts from getting worse?
C. What treatment may she eventually need?

A 50-year-old woman is told by her eye doctor that her intraocular pressure is slightly elevated and that although there is no evidence of damage to her eyes at this time, she is at risk for developing glaucoma and should have regular eye examinations.

A. Describe the physiologic mechanisms involved in the regulation of intraocular pressure.
B. What are the risk factors for development of glaucoma?
C. Explain how an increase in intraocular pressure produces its damaging effects.

The parents of a newborn infant have been told that their son has congenital cataracts in both eyes and will require cataract surgery to prevent losing his sight.

A. Explain why the infant is at risk for losing his sight if the cataracts are not removed.
B. When should this procedure be done to prevent loss of vision?

A mother notices that her 13-month-old child is fussy and tugging at his ear and refuses to eat his breakfast. When she takes his temperature, it is 100°F. Although the child attends day care, his mother has kept him home and made an appointment with the child's pedia-

trician. In the physician's office, his temperature is 100.2°F, he is somewhat irritable, and he has a clear nasal drainage. His left tympanic membrane shows normal landmarks and motility on pneumatic otoscopy. His right tympanic membrane is erythematous and there is decreased motility on pneumatic otoscopy.

A. What risk factors are present that predispose this child to the development of acute otitis media?
B. Are his signs and symptoms typical of otitis media in a child of this age?
C. What are the most likely pathogens? What treatment would be indicated?
D. Later in the week, the mother notices that the child does not seem to hear as well as he did before developing the infection. Is this a common occurrence, and should the mother be concerned about transient hearing loss in a child of this age?

A granddaughter is worried that her grandfather is "losing his hearing." Lately, he has been staying away from social gatherings that he always enjoyed, saying everybody mumbles. He is defiant in maintaining that there is nothing wrong with his hearing. However, he does complain that his ears have been ringing a lot lately.

A. What are common manifestations of hearing loss in the elderly?
B. What type of evaluation would be appropriate for determining if this man has a hearing loss, and the extent of his hearing loss?
C. What are some things the granddaughter might do so that her grandfather could hear her better when she is talking to him?

A 70-year-old man complains that he gets this terrible feeling "like the room is moving around" and becomes nauseated when he rolls over in bed or bends over suddenly. It usually goes away once he has been up for a while. He has been told that his symptoms are consistent with benign paroxysmal positional vertigo.

A. What is the pathophysiology associated with this man's vertigo?
B. Why do the symptoms subside once he has been up for a while?
C. What methods are available for treatment of the disorder?

REFERENCES

1. Leonard R. (2002). Statistics on visual impairment: A resource manual. Lighthouse International. [On-line]. Available: www.lighthouse.org. Accessed July 15, 2005.

2. Garcia-Ferrier F. J., Schwab I. R., Shetlar D. J. (2004). Conjunctiva. In Riordan-Eva P., Asbury T., Whitcher J. P. (Eds.), *Vaughan & Asbury's general ophthalmology* (16th ed., pp. 100–128). New York: Lange Medical Books/McGraw-Hill.

3. Morrow G. L., Abbott R. L. (1998). Conjunctivitis. *American Family Physician* 57, 735–746.

4. Riordan-Eva P. (2006). Eye. In Tierney L. M., McPhee S. J., Papadakis M. A. (Eds.), *Current medical diagnosis and treatment* (45th ed., pp. 150–179). New York: Lange Medical Books/McGraw-Hill.

5. Klintworth G. K. (2005). The eye. In Rubin E., Gorstein F., Rubin R., et al. (Eds.), *Rubin's pathology: Clinicopathologic foundations of medicine* (4th ed., pp. 1502–1526). Philadelphia: Lippincott Williams & Wilkins.

6. Olitsky S. E., Nelson L. (2004). Disorders of the eye. In Behrman R. E., Kliegman R. M., Jenson H. B. (Eds.), *Nelson textbook of pediatrics* (17th ed., pp. 2099–2102, 2105–2110). Philadelphia: Elsevier Saunders.

7. Collum L. M. T., Kilmartin D. J. (2001). Acute allergic conjunctivitis. In Abelson M. B. (Ed.), *Allergic diseases of the eye* (pp. 112–131). Philadelphia: W. B. Saunders.

8. Biswell R. (2004). Cornea. In Riordan-Eva P., Asbury T., Whitcher J. P. (Eds.), *Vaughan & Asbury's general ophthalmology* (16th ed., pp. 129–153). New York: Lange Medical Books/McGraw-Hill.

9. Shaikh S., Ta C. (2002). Evaluation and management of herpes zoster ophthalmicus. *American Family Physician* 66, 1723–1732.

10. Riordan-Eva P. (2004). Glaucoma. In Riordan-Eva P., Asbury T., Whitcher J. P. (Eds.), *Vaughan & Asbury's general ophthalmology* (16th ed., pp. 212–229). New York: Lange Medical Books/McGraw-Hill.

11. Martin X. D. (1992). Normal intraocular pressure in man. *Ophthalmologica* 205, 57–63.

12. Coleman A. L. (1999). Glaucoma. *Lancet* 354, 1803–1810.

13. Distellhorst J. S., Hughes G. M. (2003). Open-angle glaucoma. *American Family Physician* 67, 1937–1950.

14. Lee D. A., Higginbotham E. J. (2005). Glaucoma and its treatment: A review. *American Journal of Health-System Pharmacists* 62, 691–699.

15. Kipp M. A. (2003). Childhood glaucoma. *Pediatric Clinics of North America* 50, 89–104.

16. Guyton A. C., Hall J. E. (2006). *Textbook of medical physiology* (11th ed., pp. 613–650, 651–661). Philadelphia: Elsevier Saunders.

17. Harper R. A., Shock J. P. (2004). Lens. In Riordan-Eva P., Asbury T., Whitcher J. P. (Eds.), *Vaughan & Asbury's general ophthalmology* (16th ed., pp. 173–188). New York: Lange Medical Books/McGraw-Hill.

18. Solomon B., Donnenfeld E. D. (2003). Recent advances and future frontiers in treating age-related cataracts. *Journal of the American Medical Association* 290, 248–251.

19. Jobling A. J., Augusteyn R. C. (2002). What causes steroid cataracts? A review of steroid-induced posterior subcapsular cataracts. *Clinical and Experimental Optometry* 852, 61–75.

20. Kandel E. R., Schwartz J. H., Jessell T. M. (2000). *Principles of neural science* (4th ed., pp. 523–547). New York: McGraw-Hill.

21. Poole T. R. G., Graham E. M. (2004). Ocular disorders associated with systemic disease. In Riordan-Eva P., Asbury T., Whitcher J. P. (Eds.), *Vaughan & Asbury's general ophthalmology* (16th ed., pp. 307–342). New York: Lange Medical Books/McGraw-Hill.

22. Fong D. S., Aiello L., Gardner T. W., et al. (2003). Diabetic retinopathy. *Diabetes Care* 26, 226–229.

23. Cuilla T. A., Amador A. G., Zinman B. (2003). Diabetic retinopathy and diabetic macular edema. *Diabetes Care* 26, 2653–2664.

24. Frank R. N. (2004). Diabetic retinopathy. *New England Journal of Medicine* 350, 48–58.

25. Donaldson M., Dockson P. (2003). Medical treatment of diabetic neuropathy. *Eye* 17, 550–562.

26. Diabetes Control and Complications Trial Research Group. (1993). The effect of intensive treatment of diabetes on the development and progression of long-term complications in insulin-dependent diabetes mellitus. *New England Journal of Medicine* 329, 977–986.

27. Ferris F. L., Davis M. D., Aiello L. M. (1999). Treatment of diabetic retinopathy. *New England Journal of Medicine* 341, 667–678.

28. Hardy R. A., Shetlar D. J. (2004). Retina. In Riordan-Eva P., Asbury T., Whitcher J. P. (Eds.), *Vaughan & Asbury's general ophthalmology* (16th ed., pp. 189–211). New York: Lange Medical Books/McGraw-Hill.

29. Fine S. L., Berger J. W., MacGuire M., et al. (2000). Age-related macular degeneration. *New England Journal of Medicine* 342, 483–492.

30. Chopdar A., Chakravarthy U., Verma D. (2003). Age-related macular degeneration. *British Medical Journal* 326, 484–488.

31. Gottlieb J. L. (2002). Age-related macular degeneration. *Journal of the American Medical Association* 288, 2233–2236.

32. Fredrick D. P., Asbury T. (2004). Strabismus. In Riordan-Eva P., Asbury T., Whitcher J. P. (Eds.), *Vaughan & Asbury's general ophthalmology* (16th ed., pp. 230–249). New York: Lange Medical Books/McGraw-Hill.

33. Ticho B. H. (2003). Strabismus. *Pediatric Clinics of North America* 50, 173–188.

34. Mills M. D. (1999). The eye in childhood. *American Family Physician* 60, 907–918.

35. Mittelman D. (2003). Amblyopia. *Pediatric Clinics of North America* 50, 189–196.

36. Simon J. W., Kaw P. (2001). Commonly missed diagnoses in childhood eye exams. *American Family Physician* 64, 623–628.

37. Grossan M. (2000). Safe, effective techniques for cerumen removal. *Geriatrics* 55, 83–86.

38. Jackler R. K., Kaplan M. J. (2006). Ear, nose, and throat. In Tierney L. M., McPhee S. J., Papadakis M. A. (Eds.), *Current medical diagnosis and treatment* (45th ed., pp. 180–181). New York: Lange Medical Books/McGraw-Hill.

39. Moore K. L., Dallen A. F. (2006). *Clinically oriented anatomy* (5th ed., pp. 1021–1037). Philadelphia: Lippincott Williams & Wilkins.

40. Licameli G. R. (2002). The eustachian tube: Update on anatomy, development and function. *Otolaryngology Clinics of North America* 35, 803–809.

41. Hendley J. O. (2002). Otitis media. *New England Journal of Medicine* 347, 1169–1174.

42. Weber S. M., Grundfast K. M. (2003). Modern management of otitis media. *Pediatric Clinics of North America* 50, 399–411.

43. Perkins J. A. (2002). Medical and surgical management of otitis media in children. *Otolaryngology Clinics of North America* 35, 811–825.

44. Haddad J., Jr. (2004). The ear. In Behrman R. E., Kliegman R. M., Jenson H. B. (Eds.), *Nelson textbook of pediatrics* (17th ed., pp. 2127–2152). Philadelphia: Elsevier Saunders.

45. Pichichero, M. E. (2000). Acute otitis media: Part II. Treatment in an era of increasing antibiotic resistance. *American Family Physician* 61, 2410–2415.

46. Shohet J. A., deJong A. L. (2002). The management of pediatric cholesteatoma. *Otolaryngology Clinics of North America* 35, 841–851.

47. Wenig B. M., Cunnane M., Bálogh K. (2005). The head and neck. In Rubin E., Gorstein F., Rubin R., et al. (Eds.), *Rubin's pathology: Clinicopathologic foundations of medicine* (4th ed., pp. 1296–1302). Philadelphia: Lippincott Williams & Wilkins.

48. Fortune D. S. (1999). Tinnitus: Current evaluation and management. *Medical Clinics of North America* 83, 153–162.

49. Lockwood A. H., Salvi R. J., Burckard R. F. (2002). Tinnitus. *New England Journal of Medicine* 347, 904–910.

50. Weissman J. L. (1996). Hearing loss. *Radiology* 199, 593–611.

51. Isaacson J. E., Vora N. M. (2003). Differential diagnosis and treatment of hearing loss. *American Family Physician* 68, 1125–1132.

52. Yueh B., Shapiro N., MacLean C. H., et al. (2003). Screening and management of hearing loss in primary care: Scientific review. *Journal of the American Medical Association* 289, 1976–1985.

53. Nadol J. G. (1993). Hearing loss. *New England Journal of Medicine* 329, 1092–1101.

54. Shohet J. A., Bent T. (1998). Hearing loss: The invisible disability. *Postgraduate Medicine* 104(3), 81–83, 87–90.

55. Willems P. J. (2000). Genetic causes of hearing loss. *New England Journal of Medicine* 342, 1101–1109.

56. Francis H. W., Niparko J. K. (2003). Cochlear implantation update. *Pediatric Clinics of North America* 50, 341–361.

57. Task Force on Newborn and Infant Hearing of the American Academy of Pediatrics. (1999). Newborn and infant hearing loss: Detection and intervention. *Pediatrics* 103, 527–530.

58. Joint Commission on Infant Hearing. (2000). Year 2000 position statement: Principles and guidelines for early hearing detection and intervention programs. *Pediatrics* 106, 798–817.

59. Kenna M. A. (2003). Neonatal hearing screening. *Pediatric Clinics of North America* 50, 301–313.

60. Johnson K. C. (2002). Audiologic assessment of children with suspected hearing loss. *Otolaryngology Clinics of North America* 35, 711–732.

61. Rubinstein J. T. (2002). Paediatric cochlear implantation: Prosthetic hearing and language development. *Lancet* 360, 483–485.

62. Saeed S., Ramsden R. (1994). Hearing loss. *Practitioner* 238, 454–460.

63. Gates G. A. (Chairperson). (1989). Invitational Geriatric Otorhinolaryngology Workshop: Presbycusis. *Otolaryngology–Head and Neck Surgery* 100, 266–271.

64. Baloh, R. W. (1999). The dizzy patient: Presence of vertigo points to vestibular cause. *Postgraduate Medicine* 105(5), 161–172.

65. Derebery J. M. (1999). The diagnosis and treatment of dizziness. *Medical Clinics of North America* 83, 163–176.

66. Ruckenstein M. J. (2001). The dizzy patient: How you can help. *Consultant* 41(1), 29–33.

67. Paparella M. M., Djalilian H. R. (2002). Etiology, pathophysiology of symptoms and pathogenesis of Ménière's disease. *Otolaryngology Clinics of North America* 35, 529–545.

68. Dickins J. R. E., Graham S. S. (1990). Ménière's disease: 1983–1989. *American Journal of Otology* 11, 51–65.

69. Brooks C. B. (1996). The pharmacological treatment of Ménière's disease. *Clinical Otolaryngology* 21, 3–11.

70. Furman J. M., Cass S. P. (1999). Benign paroxysmal positional vertigo. *New England Journal of Medicine* 341, 1590–1596.

71. Parnes L. S., Agrawal S. K., Atlas J. (2003). Diagnosis and management of benign paroxysmal positional vertigo (BPPV). *Canadian Medical Association Journal* 169, 681–693.

72. Derebery M. J. (1999). The diagnosis and treatment of dizziness. *Medical Clinics of North America* 83, 163–176.

73. Horak F. B., Jones-Rycewicz C., Black F. W., et al. (1992). Effects of vestibular rehabilitation on dizziness and imbalance. *Otolaryngology–Head and Neck Surgery* 106, 175–180.

74. Brandt T. (2000). Management of vestibular disorders. *Journal of Neurology* 247, 491–499.

UNIT XI
Genitourinary and Reproductive Function

Chapter 38

Disorders of the Male Genitourinary System

The male genitourinary system is subject to structural defects, inflammation, and neoplasms, all of which can affect urine elimination, sexual function, and fertility. This chapter focuses on spermatogenesis and hormonal control of male reproductive function; neural control of sexual function and erectile dysfunction; disorders of the penis, scrotum, testes, and prostate; disorders of the male reproductive system in children; and changes in function as a result of the aging process.

Physiologic Basis of Male Reproductive Function

The male genitourinary system is composed of the paired gonads, or testes, genital ducts, accessory organs, and penis (Fig. 38-1). The dual function of the testes is to produce male sex androgens (*i.e.*, male sex hormones), mainly testosterone, and spermatozoa (*i.e.*, male germ cells). The internal accessory organs produce the fluid constituents of semen, and the ductile system aids in the storage and transport of spermatozoa. The penis functions in urine elimination and sexual function.

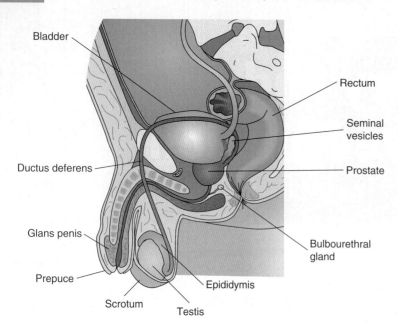

FIGURE 38-1 The structures of the male reproductive system, including the testes, the scrotum, and the excretory ducts.

SPERMATOGENESIS

Spermatogenesis refers to the generation of spermatozoa or sperm. It begins at an average age of 13 years and continues throughout the reproductive years of a man's life. Spermatogenesis occurs in the seminiferous tubules of the testes (Fig. 38-2). Internally, the testes are composed of several hundred compartments or lobules. Each lobule contains one or more coiled seminiferous tubules. The

outer layer of the seminiferous tubules is made up of connective tissue and smooth muscle; the inner lining is composed of Sertoli cells, which are embedded with sperm in various stages of development (Fig. 38-3). Sertoli cells secrete a special fluid that contains nutrients to bathe and nourish the immature germ cells; they provide digestive enzymes that play a role in spermiation (*i.e.*, converting the spermatocytes to sperm); and they are thought to play a role in shaping the head and tail of the sperm. Sertoli cells also secrete several hormones, including the principal feminizing sex hormone, estradiol, which seems to be required in the man for spermatogenesis, and inhibin, which controls the function of Sertoli cells through feedback inhibition of follicle-stimulating hormone (FSH) from the anterior pituitary gland.

KEY CONCEPTS

Male Reproductive System

➤ The male genitourinary system functions in both urine elimination and reproduction.

➤ The testes function in both production of male germ cells (spermatogenesis) and secretion of the male sex hormone, testosterone.

➤ The ductile system (epididymides, vas deferens, and ejaculatory ducts) transports and stores sperm and assists in their maturation, and the accessory glands (seminal vesicles, prostate gland, and bulbourethral glands) prepare the sperm for ejaculation.

➤ Sperm production requires temperatures that are 2°C to 3°C below body temperature. The position of the testes in the scrotum and the unique blood flow-cooling mechanisms provide this environment.

➤ The urethra, which is enclosed in the penis, is the terminal portion of the male genitourinary system. Because it conveys both urine and semen, it serves both urinary and reproductive functions.

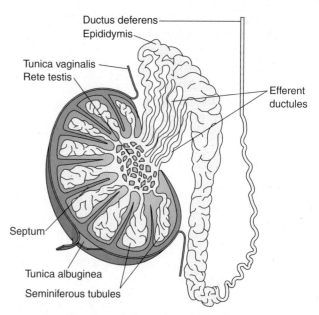

FIGURE 38-2 The parts of the testis and epididymis.

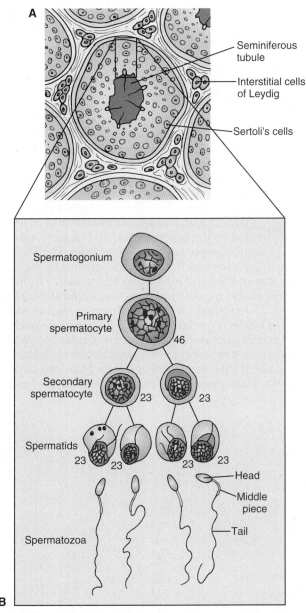

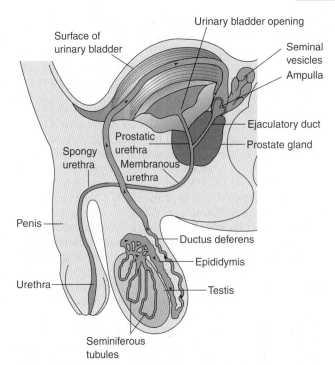

FIGURE 38-4 The excretory ducts of the male reproductive system and the path that sperm follows as it leaves the testis and travels to the urethra.

FIGURE 38-3 (**A**) Cross section of seminiferous tubule and (**B**) stages of development of spermatozoa. (46, 23 = number of chromosomes.)

After the spermatozoa are formed in the seminiferous tubules, they travel through the efferent ductules to the epididymis, which is the final site for sperm maturation. Because the spermatozoa are not motile at this stage of development, peristaltic movements of the ductal walls of the epididymis aid in their movement.[1] The spermatozoa continue their migration through the ductus deferens, also called the *vas deferens*. The ampulla of the vas deferens serves as a storage reservoir for sperm. Sperm are stored in the ampulla until they are released through the penis during ejaculation (Fig. 38-4). Spermatozoa can be stored in the genital ducts for as long as 42 days and still maintain their fertility. Surgical disconnection of the vas deferens in the scrotal area (*i.e.*, vasectomy) serves as an effective method of male contraception. Because sperm are stored in the ampulla, men can remain fertile for 4 to 5 weeks after performance of a vasectomy.

The seminal vesicles, the prostate gland, and the bulbourethral glands form the accessory reproductive structures of the male genitourinary system. The spermatozoa plus the secretions from the genital ducts and accessory organs make up the semen (from the Latin word meaning *seed*). The seminal vesicles consist of two highly tortuous tubes that secrete fluid for the semen. Each of the paired seminal vesicles is lined with secretory epithelium containing an abundance of fructose, prostaglandins, and several other proteins. The fructose secreted by the seminal vesicles provides the energy for sperm motility. The prostaglandins are thought to assist in fertilization by making the cervical mucus more receptive to sperm and by causing reverse peristaltic contractions in the uterus and fallopian tubes to move the sperm toward the ovaries. Each seminal vesicle joins its corresponding vas deferens to form the ejaculatory duct, which enters the posterior part of the prostate and continues through until it ends in the prostatic portion of the urethra. During the emission phase of coitus, each vesicle empties fluid into the ejaculatory duct, adding bulk to the semen. Approximately 70% of the ejaculate originates in the seminal vesicles.

HORMONAL CONTROL OF MALE REPRODUCTIVE FUNCTION

The male sex hormones are called *androgens*. The testes secrete several male sex hormones, including *testosterone*, *dihydrotestosterone*, and *androstenedione*.[2] Testosterone, which is the most abundant of these hormones, is considered the main testicular hormone. The adrenal cortex also produces androgens, although in much smaller quantities (<5% of the total male androgens) than those produced in the testes. The testes also secrete small quantities of estradiol and estrone.

Testosterone is produced and secreted by the interstitial Leydig cells in the testes. It is metabolized in the liver and excreted by the kidneys. In the bloodstream, testosterone exists in a free (unbound) or a bound form. The bound form is attached to plasma proteins, including albumin and the sex hormone–binding protein produced by the liver. Only approximately 2% of circulating testosterone is unbound and therefore able to enter the cell and exert its metabolic effects. Much of the testosterone that becomes fixed to the tissues is converted to dihydrotestosterone, especially in certain target tissues such as the prostate gland. Some of the actions of testosterone depend on this conversion, whereas others do not. Testosterone also can be aromatized or converted to estradiol in the peripheral tissues.

Testosterone exerts a variety of biologic effects in the male (Chart 38-1). In the male embryo, testosterone is essential for the appropriate differentiation of the internal and external genitalia, and it is necessary for descent of the testes in the fetus. Testosterone is essential to the development of primary and secondary male sex characteristics during puberty and for the maintenance of these characteristics during adult life. It causes growth of pubic, chest, and facial hair; it produces changes in the larynx that result in the male bass voice; and it increases the thickness of the skin and the activity of the sebaceous glands, predisposing to acne.

All or almost all of the actions of testosterone and other androgens result from increased protein synthesis in target tissues. Androgens function as anabolic agents in males and females to promote metabolism and musculoskeletal growth. Testosterone and the androgens have a great effect on the development of increasing musculature during puberty, with boys averaging approximately 50% more of an increase in muscle mass than girls.

Action of the Hypothalamic and Anterior Pituitary Hormones

The hypothalamus and the anterior pituitary gland play an essential role in promoting spermatogenic activity in the testes and maintaining the endocrine function of the testes by means of the gonadotropic hormones (*i.e.*, anterior pituitary hormones that promote the function and growth of the testes in the male). The synthesis and release of the gonadotropic hormones from the pituitary gland are regulated by gonadotropin-releasing hormone (GnRH), which is synthesized by the hypothalamus and secreted into the hypothalamohypophysial portal circulation (Fig. 38-5).

Two gonadotropic hormones are secreted by the pituitary gland: FSH and luteinizing hormone (LH). In the male, LH also is called *interstitial cell–stimulating hormone*. The production of testosterone by the interstitial cells of Leydig is regulated by LH. FSH binds selectively to Sertoli cells surrounding the seminiferous tubules, where it functions in the initiation of spermatogenesis. Under the influence of FSH, Sertoli cells produce androgen-binding protein, plasminogen activator, and inhibin. Androgen-

---

CHART 38-1

Main Actions of Testosterone

Induces the development of male genitalia in the embryo and descent of testes in the fetus
Induces the development and maintenance of primary and secondary male sexual characteristics
  Gonadal function
  External genitalia and accessory organs
  Male voice timbre
  Male skin characteristics
  Male hair distribution
Anabolic effects
  Promotes protein metabolism
  Promotes musculoskeletal growth
  Influences subcutaneous fat distribution
Promotes spermatogenesis (in FSH-primed tubules) and maturation of sperm

---

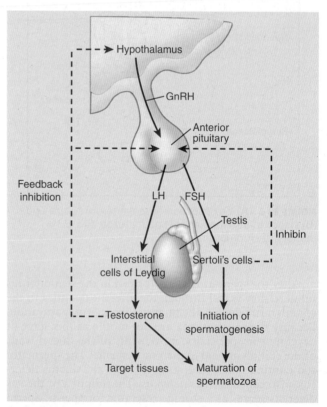

FIGURE 38-5 Hypothalamic-pituitary feedback control of spermatogenesis and testosterone levels in the male. The *dashed line* represents negative feedback. FSH, follicle-stimulating hormone; GnRH, gonadotropin-releasing hormone; LH, luteinizing hormone.

binding protein binds testosterone and serves as a carrier of testosterone in Sertoli cells and as a storage site for testosterone. Although FSH is necessary for the initiation of spermatogenesis, full maturation of the spermatozoa requires testosterone. Androgen-binding protein also serves as a carrier of testosterone from the testes to the epididymis. Plasminogen activator, which converts plasminogen to plasmin, functions in the final detachment of mature spermatozoa from Sertoli cells.

Circulating levels of the gonadotropic hormones are regulated in a negative feedback manner by testosterone. High levels of testosterone suppress LH secretion through a direct action on the pituitary and an inhibitory effect on the hypothalamus. FSH is thought to be inhibited by a substance called *inhibin,* produced by Sertoli cells. Inhibin suppresses FSH release from the pituitary gland. The pituitary gonadotropic hormones and Sertoli cells in the testes form a classic negative feedback loop in which FSH stimulates inhibin and inhibin suppresses FSH. Unlike the cyclic hormonal pattern in the woman, in the man, FSH, LH, and testosterone secretion and spermatogenesis occur at relatively unchanging rates during adulthood.

NEURAL CONTROL OF SEXUAL FUNCTION

The penis is the male external genital organ through which the urethra passes. It functions both as a sexual organ and as an organ of urine elimination. Anatomically, the external penis consists of a shaft that ends in a tip called the *glans* (see Fig. 38-1). The loose skin of the penis shaft folds to cover the glans, forming the prepuce, or foreskin. The glans of the penis contains many sensory nerves, making this the most sensitive portion of the penile shaft. The cylindrical body or shaft of the penis is composed of three masses of erectile tissue held together by fibrous strands and covered with a thin layer of skin (Fig. 38-6). The two lateral masses of tissue are called the *corpora cavernosa.* The third, ventral mass is called the *corpus spongiosum* (see Fig. 38-7A). The corpora cavernosa and corpus spongiosum are cavernous sinuses that normally are relatively empty but become engorged with blood during penile erection.

The physiology of the male sex act involves a complex interaction between autonomic-mediated spinal cord reflexes, higher neural centers, and the vascular system. It involves erection, emission, ejaculation, and detumescence. Erection involves increased inflow of blood into the corpora cavernosa and penile rigidity. Emission involves the contraction of the vas deferens and ampulla with expulsion of sperm into the internal urethra, and ejaculation, the expulsion of semen from the urethra. Detumescence, or penile relaxation, results from outflow of blood from the corpora cavernosa.

Erection is a neurovascular process involving the autonomic nervous system, neurotransmitters and endothelial relaxing factors, the vascular smooth muscle of the arteries and veins supplying the penile tissue, and the trabecular smooth muscle of the sinusoids of the corpora cavernosa (see Fig. 38-6). The penis is innervated by both

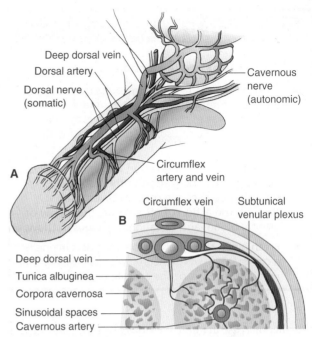

FIGURE 38-6 Anatomy and mechanism of penile erection. (**A**) Innervation and arterial and venous blood supply to penis. (**B**) Cross-section of the sinusoidal system of the corpora cavernosa.

the autonomic and somatic nervous systems. In the pelvis, the sympathetic and parasympathetic components of the autonomic nervous system merge to form what are called the *cavernous nerves.*[3] Erection is under the control of the parasympathetic nervous system, and ejaculation and detumescence (penile relaxation) are under the control of the sympathetic nervous system. Somatic innervation, which occurs through the pudendal nerve, is responsible for penile sensation and contraction and relaxation of the extracorporeal striated muscles (bulbocavernous and ischiocavernous).[3]

Penile erection is the first effect of male sexual stimulation, whether psychological or physical. It involves increased inflow of blood into the corpora cavernosa due to relaxation of the trabecular smooth muscle that surrounds the sinusoidal spaces and compression of the veins controlling outflow of blood from the venous plexus. Erection is mediated by parasympathetic impulses that pass from the sacral segments of the spinal cord through the pelvic nerves to the penis. Parasympathetic stimulation results in release of nitric oxide, a nonadrenergic-noncholinergic neurotransmitter, which causes relaxation of the trabecular smooth muscle of the corpora cavernosa. This relaxation permits inflow of blood into the sinuses of the cavernosa at pressures approaching those of the arterial system. Because the erectile tissues of the cavernosa are surrounded by a nonelastic fibrous covering, high pressure in the sinusoids causes ballooning of the erectile tissue to such an extent that the penis becomes hard and elongated. At the same time, contraction of the somatic-innervated ischiocavernous muscles forcefully compresses the blood-filled corpora cavernosa, producing a further increase in intercavernous pressures. During this phase of erection, inflow and outflow of blood cease.

Parasympathetic innervation must be intact and nitric oxide synthesis must be active for erection to occur. Nitric oxide activates guanyl cyclase, an enzyme that increases the concentration of cyclic guanosine monophosphate (cGMP), which in turn causes smooth muscle relaxation. Other smooth muscle relaxants (*e.g.*, prostaglandin E_1 analogs and α-adrenergic antagonists), if present in high enough concentrations, can independently cause sufficient cavernosal relaxation to result in erection.[3] Many of the drugs that have been developed to treat erectile dysfunction act at the levels of these mediators.

Detumescence or penile relaxation is largely a sympathetic nervous system response. It can result from a cessation of neurotransmitter release, the breakdown of second messengers such as cGMP, or sympathetic discharge during ejaculation. Contraction of the trabecular smooth muscle opens the venous channels so that the trapped blood can be expelled and penile flaccidity return.

ERECTILE DYSFUNCTION

"Erectile dysfunction is defined as the inability to achieve and maintain an erection sufficient to permit satisfactory sexual intercourse."[4] It has been estimated that the disorder affects up to 30 million men in the United States.[5] Erectile dysfunction is commonly classified as psychogenic, organic, or mixed psychogenic or organic.[5,6] Organic etiologies are the most common. Psychogenic causes of erectile dysfunction include performance anxiety, a strained relationship with a sexual partner, depression, and overt psychotic disorders such as schizophrenia. Depression is a common cause of erectile dysfunction.[5]

Organic causes span a wide range of pathologic processes. They include neurogenic, hormonal, vascular, drug-induced, and penile-related etiologies. Neurogenic disorders such as Parkinson disease, stroke, and cerebral trauma often contribute to erectile dysfunction by decreas-

ing libido or preventing the initiation of erection. In spinal cord injury, the extent of neural impairment depends on the level, location, and extent of the lesion. Somatosensory innervation of the genitalia is essential to the reflex mechanisms involved in erection; this becomes important with aging and conditions such as diabetes that impair peripheral nerve function.

Hormonal causes of erectile dysfunction include a decrease in androgen levels. Androgen levels may be decreased because of aging. Hyperprolactinemia from any cause interferes with both reproduction and erectile function. This is because prolactin acts centrally to inhibit release of the hypothalamic GnRH that controls the release of pituitary gonadotropic hormones.

Common risk factors for generalized penile arterial insufficiency include hypertension, hyperlipidemia, cigarette smoking, diabetes mellitus, and pelvic irradiation.[5] In hypertension, erectile function is impaired not so much by the increased blood pressure as by the associated stenotic arterial lesions. Focal stenosis of the common penile artery most often occurs in men who sustained blunt pelvic or perineal trauma. Failure of the veins to close completely during an erection (veno-occlusive dysfunction) may occur in men with large venous channels that drain the corpora cavernosa. Other disorders that impair venous occlusion are degenerative changes involving the tunica albuginea, as in Peyronie disease. Poor relaxation of the trabecular smooth muscle may accompany anxiety with excessive adrenergic tone.

Many drugs are reported to cause erectile dysfunction, including antidepressant, antipsychotic, antiandrogen, and antihypertensive medications. Cigarette smoking can induce vasoconstriction and penile venous leakage because of its effects on cavernous smooth muscle.[5] Alcohol in small amounts may increase libido and improve erection; however, in large amounts it can cause central sedation, decreased libido, and transient erectile dysfunction.

Aging is known to increase the risk of erectile dysfunction.[7] Many of the pathologic processes that contribute to erectile dysfunction are more common in older men, including diabetes, hyperlipidemia, hypertension, vascular disease, and the long-term effects of cigarette smoking. Many of these factors (*i.e.*, diabetes, hyperlipidemia, and hypertension) are also components of the metabolic syndrome (see Chapter 32), which is a constellation of various cardiovascular risk factors. Indeed, erectile dysfunction can be viewed as a risk marker of cardiovascular disease, and hence all patients with erectile dysfunction should be screened for cardiovascular disease.[7] Age-related declines in testosterone also may play a role. Psychosocial problems such as depression, esteem issues, partner relationships, history of substance abuse, and anxiety and fear of performance failure also may contribute to erectile dysfunction in older men.

A diagnosis of erectile dysfunction requires careful history (medical, sexual, and psychosocial), physical examination, and laboratory tests aimed at determining what other tests are needed to rule out organic causes of the disorder.[6] Because many medications, including prescribed, over-the-counter, and illicit drugs, can cause erectile dysfunction, a careful drug history is indicated.

Treatment methods include psychosexual counseling, androgen replacement therapy (when androgen deficiency is confirmed), oral and intracavernous drug therapy, vacuum constriction devices, and surgical treatment (prosthesis and vascular surgery).[6] Among the commonly prescribed drugs are sildenafil, vardenafil, tadalafil, yohimbine, alprostadil, and phentolamine. Sildenafil (Viagra), vardenafil (Levitra), and tadalafil (Cialis) are all selective inhibitors of phosphodiesterase type 5 (PDE5 inhibitors), the enzyme that inactivates cGMP. Yohimbine, an α_2-adrenergic receptor antagonist, acts at the adrenergic receptors in brain centers associated with libido and penile erection. Both the PDE5 inhibitors and yohimbine are taken orally. Alprostadil, a prostaglandin E analog, acts by producing relaxation of cavernous smooth muscle. It is either injected directly into the cavernosa or placed in the urethra as a minisuppository. Phentolamine, an α_2-adrenergic receptor antagonist, also is administered by intracavernous injection.

In summary, the male genitourinary system consists of the testes, genital ducts, accessory organs, and penis. Spermatogenesis occurs in Sertoli cells of the seminiferous tubules of the testes. After formation in seminiferous tubules, the spermatozoa travel through the efferent tubules to the epididymis, then to the ductus deferens, and on to the ampulla, where they are stored until released through the penis during ejaculation. The male accessory organs consist of the seminal vesicles, prostate gland, and bulbourethral glands.

The function of the male reproductive system is under the negative feedback control of the hypothalamus and the anterior pituitary gonadotropic hormones FSH and LH. Spermatogenesis is initiated by FSH, and the production of testosterone is regulated by LH. Testosterone, the major male sex hormone, is produced by interstitial Leydig cells in the testes. In addition to its role in the differentiation of the internal and external genitalia in the male embryo, testosterone is essential for the development of secondary male characteristics during puberty, the maintenance of these characteristics during adult life, and spermatozoa maturation.

The male sex act involves erection, emission, ejaculation, and detumescence. The physiology of these functions involves a complex interaction between autonomic-mediated spinal cord reflexes, higher neural centers, and the vascular system. Erection is mediated by the parasympathetic nervous system and emission and ejaculation by the sympathetic nervous system. Erectile dysfunction is defined as the inability to achieve and maintain an erection sufficient to permit satisfactory sexual intercourse. It can be due to psychogenic factors, organic disorders, or mixed psychogenic and organic conditions.

Disorders of the Penis, the Scrotum and Testes, and the Prostate

DISORDERS OF THE PENIS

Disorders of the penis include congenital defects (discussed in the section on Disorders of Childhood), acute and chronic inflammatory conditions, Peyronie disease, priapism, and neoplasms.

Inflammation and Infection

Balanitis and Balanoposthitis. *Balanitis* is an acute or chronic inflammation of the glans penis. *Balanoposthitis* refers to inflammation of the glans and prepuce. It usually is encountered in males with phimosis (a tight foreskin) or a large, redundant prepuce that interferes with cleanliness and predisposes to bacterial growth in the accumulated secretions and smegma (*i.e.*, debris from the desquamated epithelia). If left untreated, the condition may cause ulcerations of the mucosal surface of the glans; these ulcerations may lead to inflammatory scarring of the phimosis and further aggravate the condition.

Acute superficial balanoposthitis is characterized by erythema of the glans and prepuce. An exudate in the form of malodorous discharge may be present. Extension of the erythema and edema may result in phimosis. The condition may result from infection, trauma, or irritation. Infective balanoposthitis may be caused by a wide variety of organisms. Chlamydiae and mycoplasmas have been identified as causative organisms in this disease. The inflammatory reaction is nonspecific and correct identification of the specific agent requires microscopic examination or culture of the exudate.

Balanitis due to candidal infection may be a presenting feature or result from poorly controlled diabetes mellitus. Noninfectious types of balanitis also occur. These include circinate balanitis, which is seen in reactive arthritis (see Chapter 43). Lesions are superficial, painless ulcers that heal without scarring.

Balanitis xerotica obliterans is a chronic white, patchy lesion that originates on the glans and usually progresses to involve the meatus. It is clinically and histologically similar to the lichen sclerosus seen in women. It commonly is observed in middle-aged diabetic men. Treatment measures include topical or intralesional injections of corticosteroids.[8]

Peyronie Disease

Peyronie disease involves a localized and progressive fibrosis of unknown origin that affects the tunica albuginea (*i.e.*, the tough, fibrous sheath that surrounds the corpora cavernosa) of the penis. It is named after François de la Peyronie, who in 1743 described a patient who had "rosary beads of scar tissue to cause upward curvature of the penis during erection."[9] The disorder is characterized initially by an inflammatory process that results in dense fibrous plaque formation. The plaque usually is on the dorsal midline of the shaft, causing upward bowing of the shaft during erection (Fig. 38-7). Some men may develop scarring on both the dorsal and ventral aspects of the shaft, causing the penis to be straight but shortened or have a lateral bend.[9] The fibrous tissue prevents lengthening of the involved area during erection, making intercourse difficult and painful. The disease usually occurs in middle-aged or elderly men. Although the cause of the disorder is unknown, the dense microscopic plaques are consistent with findings of severe vasculitis. As much as 47% of men with Peyronie disease have another condition associated with fascial tissue fibrosis, such as Dupuytren contracture (fibrosis of the palmar fascia).[9]

The manifestations of Peyronie disease include painful erection, bent erection, and the presence of a hard mass at the site of fibrosis. Approximately two thirds of men report pain as a symptom. The pain is thought to be generated by inflammation of the adjacent fascial tissue and usually disappears as the inflammation resolves.[10] During the first year or so after formation of the plaque, while the scar tissue is undergoing the process of remodeling, penile distortion may increase, remain static, or resolve and disappear completely.[9] In some cases, the scar tissue may progress to calcification and formation of bonelike tissue.

Diagnosis is based on history and physical examination. Doppler ultrasonography may be used to assess the cause of the disorder. Although surgical intervention can be used to correct the disorder, it often is delayed because in many cases the disorder is self-limiting.[10] Less invasive treatments include the administration of oral agents with antioxidant properties (*e.g.*, vitamin E, colchicine), and intralesional treatments, including corticosteroids.

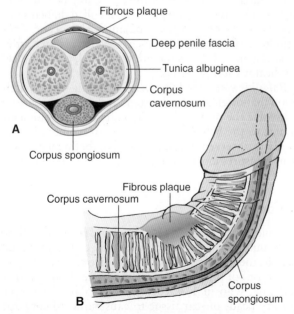

A

B

FIGURE 38-7 Peyronie disease. (**A**) Penile cross-section showing plaque between the corpora. (**B**) Penile curvature.

Labels in figure: Fibrous plaque; Deep penile fascia; Tunica albuginea; Corpus cavernosum; Corpus spongiosum; Fibrous plaque; Corpus cavernosum; Corpus spongiosum

Priapism

Priapism is an involuntary, prolonged (lasting more than 4 to 6 hours), abnormal, and painful erection that is not associated with sexual excitement. Priapism is a true urologic emergency because the prolonged erection can result in ischemia and fibrosis of the erectile tissue with significant risk of subsequent impotence. Priapism can occur at any age, in the newborn as well as other age groups. Sickle cell disease and neoplasms are the most common causes in boys between 5 and 10 years of age.

Priapism is due to impaired blood flow in the corpora cavernosa of the penis. Two mechanisms for priapism have been proposed: low-flow (ischemic) priapism, in which there is stasis of blood flow in the corpora cavernosa with a resultant failure of detumescence, and high-flow (nonischemic) priapism, which involves persistent arterial flow into the corpora cavernosa.[11] In high-flow priapism, there is no hypoxia of local tissue, the penis is less rigid, the pain is less than in stasis priapism, and permanent corporal fibrosis and cellular damage are rare.[11]

Priapism is classified as primary (idiopathic) or secondary to a disease or drug effect. Primary priapism is the result of conditions such as trauma, infection, and neoplasms. Secondary causes include hematologic conditions such as leukemia, sickle cell disease, and thrombocytopenia; neurologic conditions such as stroke, spinal cord injury, and other central nervous system lesions; and renal failure. Between 6% and 42% of males with sickle cell disorders are affected at some stage by priapism.[11] The relative deoxygenation and stasis of cavernosal blood during erection is thought to increase sickling. Various medications, such as antihypertensive drugs, anticoagulant drugs, antidepressant drugs, alcohol, and marijuana, can contribute to the development of priapism. Androstenedione, sold as an over-the-counter drug to enhance muscle building and athletic performance, has been implicated in the disorder.[12] Currently, intracavernous injection therapy for erectile dysfunction is one of the more common causes of priapism.

The diagnosis of priapism usually is based on clinical findings. Doppler studies of penile blood flow, penile ultrasonography, and computed tomography (CT) scans may be used to determine intrapelvic pathology.

Initial treatment measures include analgesics, sedation, and hydration. Urinary retention may necessitate catheterization. Local measures include application of ice packs and irrigation of the corpus cavernosum with plain or heparinized saline, or instillation of α-adrenergic drugs. If less aggressive treatment does not produce detumescence, a temporary surgical shunt may be established between the corpus cavernosum and the corpus spongiosum.

The prognosis for whether fibrosis or erectile failure will occur is determined by the severity and duration of blood stasis. In high-flow priapism, the damaging effects of decreased oxygen tension and intracavernosal blood pressure are less pronounced than in stasis priapism. Normal erectile potency can be restored even after a long duration of high-flow priapism. In contrast, persistent stasis priapism is known to result in impaired erectile function and tissue fibrosis unless resolved within 24 to 48 hours of onset.[11]

Cancer of the Penis

While a relatively uncommon form of cancer in the United States, accounting for less than 1% of all male genital tumors, cancer of the penis is much more common in less-developed countries, accounting for up to 10% of male cancers in some parts of Asia and Africa. The average age of onset is 60 years of age.[13,14] When it is diagnosed early, penile cancer is highly curable. The greatest hindrance to early diagnosis is a delay in seeking medical attention.

The cause of penile cancer is unknown. Several risk factors have been suggested, including poor hygiene, human papillomavirus (HPV) infections, ultraviolet radiation exposure, and immunodeficiency states. There is an association between penile cancer and poor genital hygiene and phimosis. One theory postulates that smegma accumulation under the phimotic foreskin may produce chronic inflammation, leading to carcinoma. The HPVs have been implicated in the genesis of several genital cancers, including cancer of the penis.[13] Ultraviolet radiation also is thought to have a carcinogenic effect on the penis. Men who were treated for psoriasis with ultraviolet A or B therapies (*i.e.,* PUVA or PUVB) have had a reported increased incidence of genital squamous cell carcinomas.[13] Because of this observation, it is suggested that men should shield their genital area when using tanning salons. Immunodeficiency states also may play a role in the pathogenesis of penile cancer. Approximately 18% of men with acquired immunodeficiency syndrome (AIDS)–related Kaposi sarcoma have lesions of the penis or genitalia.[13]

Dermatologic lesions with precancerous potential include balanitis xerotica obliterans (discussed earlier) and giant condylomata acuminata.[14] Giant condylomata acuminata are cauliflower-like lesions arising from the prepuce or glans that result from HPV infection.

Approximately 95% of penile cancers are squamous cell carcinoma.[13] It is thought to progress from an in situ lesion to an invasive carcinoma. Bowen disease and erythroplasia of Queyrat are penile lesions with histologic features of carcinoma in situ.[14] Bowen disease appears as a solitary, thickened, dull red, opaque plaque with shallow ulceration and crusting. It commonly involves the skin of the shaft of the penis and the scrotum. Erythroplasia of Queyrat involves the mucosal surface of the glans or prepuce. It is characterized by single or multiple shiny red, sometimes velvety, plaques.[14] These lesions require careful follow-up because of their potential to progress to invasive carcinoma.

Invasive carcinoma of the penis begins as a small lump or ulcer. If phimosis is present, there may be painful swelling, purulent drainage, or difficulty urinating. Palpable lymph nodes may be present in the inguinal region. Diagnosis usually is based on physical examination and biopsy results. CT scans, penile ultrasonographic studies, and magnetic resonance imaging (MRI) may be used in the diagnostic workup.

Treatment options vary according to stage, size, location, and invasiveness of the tumor. Carcinoma in situ may be treated conservatively with fluorouracil cream application or laser treatment.[14] Surgery remains the mainstay of treatment for invasive carcinoma. Partial or total penectomy is indicated for invasive lesions.

DISORDERS OF THE SCROTUM AND TESTES

The testes, or male gonads, are two egg-shaped structures located outside the abdominal cavity in the scrotum. Embryologically, the testes develop in the abdominal cavity and then descend through the inguinal canal into a pouch of peritoneum (which becomes the tunica vaginalis) in the scrotum during the seventh to ninth months of fetal life. As they descend, the testes pull their arteries, veins, lymphatics, nerves, and conducting excretory ducts with them. These structures are encased by the cremaster muscle and layers of fascia that constitute the spermatic cord (Fig. 38-8A). The descent of the testes is thought to

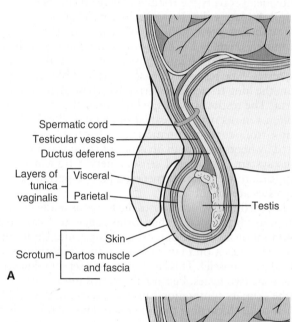

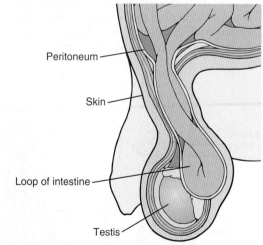

FIGURE 38-8 (**A**) Anterior view of the spermatic cord and inguinal canal and coverings of the spermatic cord and testes. (**B**) Indirect inguinal hernia. (Adapted from Moore K. L., Agur A. M. [2002]. *Essentials of clinical anatomy* [2nd ed., pp. 130, 138]. Philadelphia: Lippincott Williams & Wilkins.)

be mediated by testosterone, which is active during this stage of development.

After descent of the testes, the inguinal canal closes almost completely. Failure of this canal to close predisposes to the development of an inguinal hernia later in life (see Fig. 38-8B). An inguinal hernia or "rupture" is a protrusion of the parietal peritoneum and part of the intestine through an abnormal opening from the abdominal cavity. A loop of small bowel may become incarcerated in an inguinal hernia (strangulated hernia), in which case the lumen may become obstructed and the vascular supply compromised (see Chapter 28).

The testes and epididymis are completely surrounded by the tunica vaginalis, a serous pouch derived from the peritoneum during fetal descent of the testes into the scrotum. The tunica vaginalis has an outer parietal layer and a deeper visceral layer that adheres to the dense fibrous covering of the testes, the tunica albuginea. The tunica albuginea protects the testes and gives them their ovoid shape. A space exists between these two layers that typically contains a few milliliters of clear fluid. The cremaster muscles, which are bands of skeletal muscle arising from the internal oblique muscles of the trunk, elevate the testes. The testes receive their arterial blood supply from the long testicular arteries, which branch from the aorta. The testicular veins, which drain the testes, arise from a venous network called the *pampiniform plexus* that surrounds the spermatic artery. The testes are innervated by fibers from both divisions of the autonomic nervous system. Associated sensory nerves transmit pain impulses, resulting in excruciating pain, especially when the testes are hit forcibly.

The scrotum, which houses the testes, is made up of a thin outer layer of skin that forms rugae, or folds, and is continuous with the outer skin of the groin. Under the outer skin lies a thin layer of fascia and smooth muscle (*i.e.,* dartos muscle). This layer contains a septum that separates the two testes. Because the dartos muscle attaches to the skin, its contraction causes the scrotum to wrinkle when cold, thickening the outer skin layer while reducing scrotal surface area and assisting the cremaster muscles in holding the testes close to the body. When it is

warmer, the muscle relaxes, allowing the scrotum to fall away from the body.

The location of the testes in the scrotum is important for sperm production, which is optimal at 2°C to 3°C below body temperature. Two systems maintain the temperature of the testes at a level consistent with sperm production. One is the pampiniform plexus of testicular veins that surround the testicular artery. This plexus absorbs heat from the arterial blood, cooling it as it enters the testes. The other is the dartos and cremaster muscles, which respond to decreases in testicular temperature by moving the testes closer to the body. Prolonged exposure to elevated temperatures, as a result of prolonged fever or the dysfunction of thermoregulatory mechanisms, can impair spermatogenesis. Some tight-fitting undergarments hold the testes against the body and are thought to contribute to a decrease in sperm counts and infertility by interfering with the thermoregulatory function of the scrotum. Cryptorchidism, the failure of the testes to descend into the scrotum, also exposes the testes to the higher temperature of the body.

Disorders of the Testicular Tunica

Hydrocele. A hydrocele forms when excess fluid collects between the layers of the tunica vaginalis (Fig. 38-9C). It may be unilateral or bilateral and can develop as a primary congenital defect or as a secondary condition. Acute hydrocele may develop after local injury, epididymitis or orchitis, gonorrhea, lymph obstruction, or germ cell testicular tumor, or as a side effect of radiation therapy. Chronic hydrocele is more common. Fluid collects about the testis, and the mass grows gradually. Its cause is unknown, and it usually develops in men older than 40 years.

Most cases of hydrocele in male infants and children are due to a patent processus vaginalis, which is continuous with the peritoneal cavity. In many cases they are associated with an indirect inguinal hernia.[15] Most hydroceles of infancy close spontaneously; therefore, they are not usually repaired before the age of 1 year. Hydroceles that persist beyond 2 years of age may require surgical treatment.

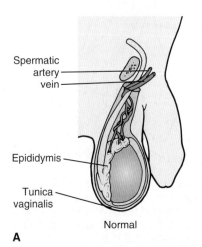

Spermatic
artery
vein

Epididymis

Tunica
vaginalis

A   Normal

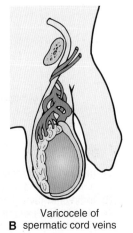

B Varicocele of
spermatic cord veins

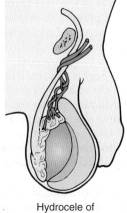

C Hydrocele of
tunica vaginalis

FIGURE 38-9 (**A**) Normal testis and appendages, (**B**) varicocele, and (**C**) hydrocele.

Hydroceles are palpated as cystic masses that may attain massive proportions. If there is enough fluid, the mass may be mistaken for a solid tumor. Transillumination of the scrotum (*i.e.,* shining a light through the scrotum for the purposes of visualizing its internal structures) or ultrasonography can help to determine whether the mass is solid or cystic and whether the testicle is normal.[16] A dense hydrocele that does not illuminate should be differentiated from a testicular tumor. If a hydrocele develops in a young man without apparent cause, careful evaluation is needed to exclude cancer or infection.

In an adult man, a hydrocele is a relatively benign condition. The condition often is asymptomatic, and no treatment is necessary. When symptoms do occur, the feeling may be that of heaviness in the scrotum or pain in the lower back. In cases of secondary hydrocele, the primary condition is treated. If the hydrocele is painful or cosmetically undesirable, surgical correction is indicated. Surgical repair may be done inguinally or transcrotally.

Hematocele. A hematocele is an accumulation of blood in the tunica vaginalis, which causes the scrotal skin to become dark red or purple. It may develop as a result of an abdominal surgical procedure, scrotal trauma, a bleeding disorder, or a testicular tumor.

Spermatocele. A spermatocele is a painless, sperm-containing cyst that forms at the end of the epididymis. It is located above and posterior to the testis, is attached to the epididymis, and is separate from the testes. Spermatoceles may be solitary or multiple and usually are less than 1 cm in diameter. They are freely movable and should transilluminate. Spermatoceles rarely cause problems, but a large one may become painful and require excision.

Varicocele. A varicocele is characterized by varicosities of the pampiniform plexus, a network of veins supplying the testes (see Fig. 38-9B). The left side is more commonly affected because the left internal spermatic vein inserts into the left renal vein at a right angle, whereas the right spermatic vein usually enters the inferior vena cava. Incompetent valves are more common in the left internal spermatic veins, causing a reflux of blood back into the veins of the pampiniform plexus. The force of gravity resulting from the upright position also contributes to venous dilatation. If the condition persists, there may be damage to the elastic fibers and hypertrophy of the vein walls, as occurs in formation of varicose veins in the leg. Sperm concentration and motility are decreased in 65% to 75% of men with varicocele because of changes in testicular temperature resulting from altered blood flow.[16]

Varicoceles rarely are found before puberty, and the incidence is highest in men between 15 and 35 years of age. Symptoms of varicocele include an abnormal feeling of heaviness in the left scrotum, although many varicoceles are asymptomatic. Usually, the varicocele is readily diagnosed on physical examination with the patient in the standing and recumbent positions. Typically, the varicocele disappears in the lying position because of a decrease in venous pressure. Scrotal palpation of a varicocele has been compared to feeling a "bag of worms."

Treatment options include surgical ligation or sclerosis using a percutaneous transvenous catheter under fluoroscopic guidance. It has been suggested that men with abnormalities in their semen and a varicocele show some degree of improvement in fertility after obliteration of the dilated veins. However, the effectiveness of varicocele treatment in men from subfertile couples is still debated, especially when other assisted reproductive techniques (intracytoplasmic sperm injection [ICSI]) may be effective with as few as 20 sperm.[16] Aside from improving fertility, other reasons for surgery include the relief of the sensation of "heaviness" and cosmetic improvement.

Testicular Torsion

Testicular torsion is a twisting of the spermatic cord that suspends the testis (Fig. 38-10). It is the most common acute scrotal disorder in the pediatric and young adult population. Testicular torsion can be divided into two distinct clinical entities, depending on the level of spermatic cord involvement: extravaginal and intravaginal torsion.[17]

Extravaginal torsion, which occurs almost exclusively in neonates, is the less common form of testicular torsion. It occurs when the testicle and the fascial tunicae that surround it rotate around the spermatic cord at a level well above the tunica vaginalis. *Intravaginal torsion* is considerably more common than extravaginal torsion. It occurs when the testis rotates on the long axis in the tunica vaginalis. In most cases, congenital abnormalities of the tunica vaginalis or spermatic cord exist.[17] The tunica vaginalis normally surrounds the testes and epididymis, allowing the testicle to rotate freely in the tunica. Although anomalies of suspension vary, the epididymal attachment may be loose enough to permit torsion between the testis and the epididymis. More commonly, the testis rotates about the distal spermatic cord. Because this abnormality is developmental, bilateral anomalies are common.

Intravaginal torsion occurs most frequently between the ages of 8 and 18 years and rarely is seen after 30 years

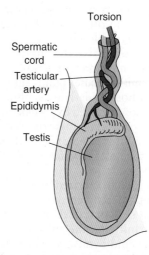

FIGURE 38-10 Testicular torsion with twisting of the spermatic cord that suspends the testis and the spermatic vessels that supply the testis with blood.

of age. Males usually present in severe distress within hours of onset and often have nausea, vomiting, and tachycardia. The affected testis is large and tender, with pain radiating to the inguinal area. Extensive cremaster muscle contraction causes a thickening of the spermatic cord.

Testicular torsion must be differentiated from epididymitis, orchitis, and trauma to the testis. On physical examination, the testicle often is high in the scrotum and in an abnormal orientation. These changes are due to the twisting and shortening of the spermatic cord. The degree of scrotal swelling and redness depends on the duration of symptoms. The testes are firm and tender. The cremasteric reflex, normally elicited by stroking the medial aspect of the thigh and observing testicular retraction, frequently is absent.[17] Color Doppler ultrasonography is increasingly used in the evaluation of suspected testicular torsion.[17]

Intravaginal testicular torsion is a true surgical emergency, and early recognition and treatment are necessary if the testicle is to be saved. Treatment includes surgical detorsion (repositioning and fixation) and orchiectomy. Orchiectomy is carried out when the testis is deemed nonviable after surgical detorsion. Testicular salvage rates are directly related to the duration of torsion. Because the opposite testicle usually is affected by the same abnormal attachments, prophylactic fixation of that testis often is performed.

Inflammation and Infection

Epididymitis. Epididymitis is an inflammation of the epididymis. There are two major types of epididymitis: sexually transmitted infections associated with urethritis and primary nonsexually transmitted infections associated with urinary tract infections and prostatitis. Most cases of epididymitis are caused by bacterial pathogens.

In primary nonsexual infections, the pressure associated with voiding or physical strain may force pathogen-containing urine from the urethra or prostate up the ejaculatory duct and through the vas deferens and into the epididymis. Infections also may reach the epididymis through the lymphatics of the spermatic cord. In rare cases, organisms from other foci of infection reach the epididymis through the bloodstream. In children, the disorder usually is associated with congenital urinary tract abnormalities and infection with gram-negative rods.

Sexually transmitted acute epididymitis occurs mainly in young men without underlying genitourinary disease and is most commonly caused by *Chlamydia trachomatis* and *Neisseria gonorrhoeae* (singly or in combination). In men older than 35 years, epididymitis often is associated with pathogens such as *Escherichia coli*, *Pseudomonas*, and gram-positive cocci.

Epididymitis is characterized by unilateral pain and swelling, accompanied by erythema and edema of the overlying scrotal skin that develops during a period of 24 to 48 hours. Initially, the swelling and induration are limited to the epididymis. However, the distinction between the testis and epididymis becomes less evident as the inflammation progresses, and the testis and epididymis become one mass. There may be tenderness over

the groin (spermatic cord) or in the lower abdomen. Fever and reports of dysuria occur in approximately one half of cases. Whether urethral discharge is present depends on the organism causing the infection; it usually accompanies gonorrheal infections, is common in chlamydial infections, and is less common in infections caused by gram-negative organisms.

Laboratory findings usually reveal an elevated white blood cell count. Urinalysis and urine culture are important in the diagnosis of epididymitis, with bacteriuria and pyuria suggestive of the disorder. Treatment during the acute phase (which usually lasts for 3 to 4 days) includes bed rest, scrotal elevation and support, and antibiotics.[18] Bed rest with scrotal support improves lymphatic drainage. The choice of antibiotics is determined by age, physical findings, urinalysis, Gram stain results, cultures, and sexual history. Oral analgesics and antipyretics usually are indicated. Sexual partners should be screened and treated in cases of sexually transmitted infections.

Orchitis. Orchitis is an infection of the testes. It can be precipitated by a primary infection in the genitourinary tract, or the infection can be spread to the testes through the bloodstream or lymphatics. Epididymitis with subsequent infection of the testis is commonly related to genitourinary tract infections (cystitis, urethritis, genitoprostatitis) that travel to the epididymis and testis through the vas deferens or the lymphatics of the spermatic cord.

Orchitis can develop as a complication of a systemic infection, such as parotitis (*i.e.,* mumps), scarlet fever, or pneumonia. Probably the best known of these complications is orchitis caused by the mumps virus. Mumps orchitis does not occur in prepubertal boys. However, approximately 20% to 35% of adolescent boys and young men with mumps develop this form of orchitis.[18] The onset of mumps orchitis is sudden; it usually occurs approximately 3 to 4 days after the onset of the parotitis and is characterized by fever, painful enlargement of the testes, and small hemorrhages into the tunica albuginea. The residual effects seen after the acute phase include hyalinization of the seminiferous tubules and atrophy of the testes. Spermatogenesis is irreversibly impaired in approximately 30% of testes damaged by mumps orchitis.[18] If both testes are involved, permanent sterility results, but androgenic hormone function usually is maintained. Fortunately, the incidence of mumps has greatly declined since the introduction of the mumps vaccine.

Cancer of the Scrotum and Testes

Tumors can develop in the scrotum or the testes. Benign scrotal tumors are common and often do not require treatment. Carcinoma of the scrotum is rare and usually is associated with exposure to carcinogenic agents. Almost all solid tumors of the testes are malignant.

Scrotal Cancer. Cancer of the scrotum was the first cancer directly linked to a specific occupation when, in the 18th century, it was associated with chimney sweeps.[19] Studies have linked this cancer to exposure to tar, soot, and oils. Most squamous cell cancers of the scrotum are linked to poor hygiene and chronic inflammation. Exposure to ultraviolet A radiation (*e.g.,* PUVA) or HPV also has been associated with the disease. The mean age of presentation with the disease is 60 years, often preceded by 20 to 30 years of chronic irritation.

In the early stages, cancer of the scrotum may appear as a small tumor or wartlike growth that eventually ulcerates. The thin scrotal wall lacks the tissue reactivity needed to block the malignant process; more than one half of the cases seen involve metastasis to the lymph nodes. Because this tumor does not respond well to chemotherapy or irradiation, the treatment includes wide local excision of the tumor with inguinal and femoral node dissection.[20]

Testicular Cancer. Testicular cancer accounts for 1% of all male cancers and 3% of male urogenital cancers. Although relatively rare, it is the most common cause of cancer in the 15- to 35-year-old age group.[21] In the past, testicular cancer was a leading cause of death among men entering their most productive years. However, since the late 1970s, advances in therapy have transformed an almost invariably fatal disease into one that is highly curable. With appropriate treatment, the prognosis for men with testicular cancer is excellent. The 5-year survival rate for patients with early disease exceeds 95%. Even patients with more advanced disease have excellent chances for long-term survival.

Although the cause of testicular cancer is unknown, several predisposing influences may be important: cryptorchidism, genetic factors, and disorders of testicular development.[22] The strongest association has been with cryptorchid or undescended testes. The higher the location of the undescended testis, the greater the risk.[22] Genetic predisposition also appears to be important. Family clustering of the disorder has been described, although a well-defined pattern of inheritance has not been established. Men with disorders of testicular development, including those with Klinefelter syndrome and testicular feminization, have a higher risk of germ cell tumors.

Approximately 95% of malignant tumors arising in the testis are germ cell tumors.[21,23] Germ cell tumors can be classified as seminomas and nonseminomas based on their origin in primordial germ cells and their ability to differentiate in vivo. Because these tumors derive from germ cells in the testis, they are multipotential (able to differentiate into different tissue types) and often secrete polypeptide hormones or enzymes representing earlier stages of development (see Chapter 5). *Seminomas* and *nonseminoma tumors* equally account for approximately 50% of germ cell tumors. Seminomas occur most frequently during the fourth decade of life.[21] Seminomas are thought to arise from the seminiferous epithelium of the testes and are the type of germ cell tumor most likely to produce a uniform population of cells.

The *nonseminoma tumors* include embryonal carcinoma, teratoma, choriocarcinoma, and yolk cell carcinoma derivatives. Nonseminoma tumors usually contain more than one cell type and are less differentiated than seminomas. Embryonal carcinomas are the least differentiated of the tumors, with totipotential capacity to differentiate into other nonseminomatous cell types. They occur most commonly in the 20- to 30-year-old age group. Choriocarcinoma is a rare and highly malignant form of testicular cancer that is identical to tumors that arise in placental tissue. Yolk sac tumors mimic the embryonic yolk sac histologically. They are the most common type of testicular tumors in infants and children up to 3 years of age, and in this age group are associated with a very good prognosis.[22] Teratomas are composed of somatic cell types from two or more germ-line layers (ectoderm, mesoderm, or endoderm). They constitute less than 2% to 3% of germ cell tumors and can occur at any age from infancy to old age. They usually behave as benign tumors in children; in adults, they often contain minute foci of cancer cells.

Often the first sign of testicular cancer is a slight enlargement of the testicle that may be accompanied by some degree of discomfort. This may be an ache in the abdomen or groin or a sensation of dragging or heaviness in the scrotum. Frank pain may be experienced in the later stages, when the tumor is growing rapidly and hemorrhaging occurs. Testicular cancer can spread when the tumor may be barely palpable. Signs of metastatic spread include swelling of the lower extremities, back pain, cough, hemoptysis, or dizziness. Gynecomastia (breast enlargement) may result from human chorionic gonadotropin (hCG)–producing tumors.

Early diagnosis of testicular cancer is important because a delay in seeking medical attention often results in presentation with a later stage of the disease and decreased treatment effectiveness. The diagnosis of testicular cancer requires a thorough urologic history and physical examination. A painless testicular mass may be cancer. The examination for masses should include palpation of the testes and surrounding structures, transillumination of the scrotum, and abdominal palpation. Testicular ultrasonography can be used to differentiate testicular masses. CT scans and MRI are used in assessing metastatic spread.

Tumor markers, which measure protein antigens produced by malignant cells, provide information about the existence of a small or undetected tumor and the type of tumor present. Three tumor markers are useful in evaluating the tumor response: α-fetoprotein, a glycoprotein that normally is present in fetal serum in large amounts; β-hCG, a hormone that is produced by the placenta in pregnant women and not normally found in men; and lactate dehydrogenase (LDH), a cellular enzyme normally found in muscle, liver, kidney, and brain.

The basic treatment of all testicular cancers includes orchiectomy, which is done at the time of diagnostic exploration. Depending on the histologic characteristics of the tumor and the clinical stage of the disease, radiation or chemotherapy may be used after orchiectomy. Rigorous follow-up in all men with testicular cancer is necessary to detect recurrence, which most often occurs within the first year.[23]

DISORDERS OF THE PROSTATE

The prostate is a fibromuscular and glandular organ lying just inferior to the bladder. The prostate gland secretes a thin, milky, alkaline fluid containing citric acid, calcium, acid phosphate, a clotting enzyme, and a profibrinolysin. During ejaculation, the capsule of the prostate contracts, and the added fluid increases the bulk of the semen. Both vaginal secretions and the fluid from the vas deferens are strongly acidic. Because sperm mobilization occurs at a pH of 6.0 to 6.5, the alkaline nature of the prostatic secretions is essential for successful fertilization of the ovum. The bulbourethral glands (see Fig. 38-1) lie on either side of the membranous urethra and secrete an alkaline mucus, which further aids in neutralizing acids from the urine that remain in the urethra.

The prostate gland, which forms a fibrous capsule that surrounds the urethra where it joins the bladder, also functions in the elimination of urine. The segment of urethra that travels through the prostate gland is called the *prostatic urethra*. The prostatic urethra is lined by a thin layer of smooth muscle that is continuous with the bladder wall. This smooth muscle represents the true involuntary sphincter of the male posterior urethra. Because the prostate surrounds the urethra, enlargement of the gland can produce urinary obstruction.

The prostate gland is made up of many secretory glands arranged in three concentric areas surrounding the prostatic urethra, into which they open. The component glands of the prostate include the (1) small mucosal glands associated with the urethral mucosa, (2) the intermediate submucosal glands that lie peripheral to the mucosal glands, and (3) the large main prostatic glands that are situated toward the outside of the gland. It is the overgrowth of the mucosal glands that causes benign prostatic hyperplasia in older men.

Prostatitis

Prostatitis refers to a variety of inflammatory disorders of the prostate gland, some of which are bacterial and some not. It may occur spontaneously, as a result of catheterization or instrumentation, or secondary to other diseases of the male genitourinary system. As an outcome of 1995 and 1998 consensus conferences, the National Institutes of Health established a classification system with four categories of prostatitis syndromes: asymptomatic inflammatory prostatitis, acute bacterial prostatitis, chronic bacterial prostatitis, and chronic prostatitis/pelvic pain syndrome.[24] Men with asymptomatic inflammatory prostatitis have no subjective symptoms and are detected incidentally on biopsy or examination of prostatic fluid.

Acute Bacterial Prostatitis. Acute bacterial prostatitis often is considered a subtype of urinary tract infection. The most likely etiology of acute bacterial prostatitis is an ascending urethral infection or reflux of infected urine into the prostatic ducts. The most common organism is *E. coli*. Other frequently found species include *Pseudomonas*, *Klebsiella*, and *Proteus*. Less frequently, the infection is caused by *Staphylococcus aureus*, *Streptococcus faecalis*, *Chlamydia*, or anaerobes such as *Bacteroides* species.[25,26]

The manifestations of acute bacterial prostatitis include fever and chills, malaise, myalgia, arthralgia, frequent and urgent urination, dysuria, and urethral discharge. Dull, aching pain often is present in the perineum, rectum, or sacrococcygeal region. The urine may be cloudy and malodorous because of urinary tract infection. Rectal examination reveals a swollen, tender, warm prostate with scattered soft areas. Prostatic massage produces a thick discharge with white blood cells that grows large numbers of pathogens on culture.

Acute prostatitis usually responds to appropriate antimicrobial therapy chosen in accordance with the sensitivity of the causative agents in the urethral discharge. Depending on the urine culture results, antibiotic therapy usually is continued for at least 4 weeks. Because acute prostatitis often is associated with anatomic abnormalities, a thorough urologic examination usually is performed after treatment is completed.

A persistent fever indicates the need for further investigation for an additional site of infection or a prostatic abscess. CT scans and transrectal ultrasonography of the prostate are useful in the diagnosis of prostatic abscesses. Prostatic abscesses, which are relatively uncommon since the advent of effective antibiotic therapy, are found more commonly in men with diabetes mellitus. Because prostatic abscesses usually are associated with bacteremia, prompt drainage by transperitoneal or transurethral incision followed by appropriate antimicrobial therapy usually is indicated.[25]

Chronic Bacterial Prostatitis. In contrast to acute bacterial prostatitis, chronic bacterial prostatitis is a subtle disorder that is difficult to treat. Men with the disorder typically have recurrent urinary tract infections with persistence of the same strain of pathogenic bacteria in prostatic fluid and urine. Organisms responsible for chronic bacterial prostatitis usually are the gram-negative enterobacteria (*E. coli*, *Proteus*, or *Klebsiella*) or *Pseudomonas*. Occasionally, a gram-positive organism such as *S. faecalis* is the causative organism. Infected prostatic calculi may develop and contribute to the chronic infection.

The symptoms of chronic prostatitis are variable and include frequent and urgent urination, dysuria, perineal discomfort, and low back pain. Occasionally, myalgia and arthralgia accompany the other symptoms. Secondary epididymitis sometimes is associated with the disorder. Many men develop relapsing lower or upper urinary tract infections because of recurrent invasion of the bladder by the prostatic bacteria. Bacteria may exist in the prostate gland even when the prostatic fluid is sterile.

The most accurate method of establishing a diagnosis is by urine cultures. Even after an accurate diagnosis has been established, treatment of chronic prostatitis often is difficult and frustrating. Unlike their action in the acutely inflamed prostate, antibacterial drugs penetrate poorly into the chronically inflamed prostate. Long-term therapy (3 to 4 months) with an appropriate low-dose oral antimicrobial agent often is used to treat the infection. Transurethral prostatectomy may be indicated when the infection is not cured or adequately controlled by medical therapy, particularly when prostate stones are present.

Chronic Prostatitis/Chronic Pelvic Pain Syndrome.

Chronic prostatitis/pelvic pain syndrome is both the most common and least understood of the prostatitis syndromes.[27] The category is divided into two types, inflammatory and noninflammatory, based on the presence of leukocytes in the prostatic fluid. The inflammatory type was previously referred to as *nonbacterial prostatitis*, and the noninflammatory type as *prostatodynia*.

Men with nonbacterial prostatitis have inflammation of the prostate with an elevated leukocyte count, inflammatory cells in their prostatic secretions, but no evidence of bacteria. The cause of the disorder is unknown, and efforts to prove the presence of unusual pathogens (*e.g.*, mycoplasmas, chlamydiae, trichomonads, viruses) have been largely unsuccessful. It also is thought that nonbacterial prostatitis may be an autoimmune disorder. Manifestations of *inflammatory prostatitis* include pain along the penis, testicles, and scrotum; painful ejaculation; low back pain; rectal pain along the inner thighs; urinary symptoms; decreased libido; and erectile dysfunction.

Men with noninflammatory prostatitis have symptoms resembling those of nonbacterial prostatitis but have negative urine culture results and no evidence of prostatic inflammation (*i.e.*, normal leukocyte count). The cause of noninflammatory prostatitis is unknown, but because of the absence of inflammation, the search for the cause of symptoms has been directed toward extraprostatic sources. In some cases, there is an apparent functional obstruction of the bladder neck near the external urethral sphincter; during voiding, this results in higher than normal pressures in the prostatic urethra that cause intraprostatic urine reflux and chemical irritation of the prostate by urine. In other cases, there is an apparent myalgia (*i.e.*, muscle pain) associated with prolonged tension of the pelvic floor muscles. Emotional stress also may play a role.

Treatment methods for chronic prostatitis/pelvic pain syndrome are highly variable. Antibiotic therapy is used when an occult infection is suspected. Sitz baths and nonsteroidal anti-inflammatory drugs may provide some symptom relief. In men with irritative urination symptoms, anticholinergic agents or α-adrenergic–blocking agents may be beneficial.

Benign Prostatic Hyperplasia

Benign prostatic hyperplasia (BPH) is an age-related, nonmalignant enlargement of the prostate gland (Fig. 38-11). It is characterized by the formation of large, nodular lesions in the periurethral region of the prostate, rather than the peripheral zones, which commonly are affected by prostate cancer (Fig. 38-12). BPH is one of the most common diseases of aging men. It has been reported that more than 50% of men older than 60 years of age have BPH.[28]

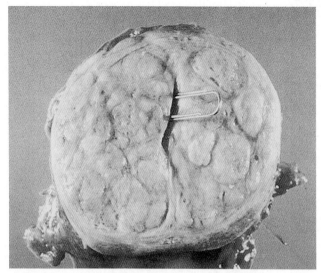

FIGURE 38-11 Nodular hyperplasia of the prostate. Cut surface of a prostate enlarged by nodular hyperplasia shows numerous, well-circumscribed nodules of prostatic tissue. The prostatic urethra (*paper clip*) has been compressed to a narrow slit. (From Damjanov I. [2005]. The lower urinary tract and male reproductive system. In Rubin E., Gorstein F., Rubin R., et al. [Eds.], *Rubin's pathology: Clinicopathologic foundations of medicine* [4th ed., p. 920]. Philadelphia: Lippincott Williams & Wilkins.)

The exact cause of BPH is unknown. Potential risk factors include age, family history, race, ethnicity, dietary fat and meat consumption, and hormonal factors. The incidence of BPH increases with advancing age, is highest in African Americans, and is lowest in native Japanese. Men with a family history of BPH are reported to have had larger prostates than those of control subjects, and higher rates of BPH were found in monozygotic twins than in dizygotic twins.[28]

Both androgens (testosterone and dihydrotestosterone) and estrogens appear to contribute to the development of BPH. Dihydrotestosterone (DHT), the biologically active metabolite of testosterone, is thought to be the ultimate mediator of prostatic hyperplasia, with estrogen serving to sensitize the prostatic tissue to the growth-producing effects of DHT. Free plasma testosterone enters prostatic cells, where at least 90% is converted into DHT by the action of 5α-reductase. The discovery that DHT is the active factor in BPH is the rationale for use of 5α-reductase inhibitors in the treatment of the disorder. Although the exact source of estrogen is uncertain, small amounts of estrogen are produced in the male. It has been postulated that a relative increase in estrogen levels that occurs with aging may facilitate the action of androgens in the prostate despite a decline in the testicular output of testosterone.

The anatomic location of the prostate at the bladder neck contributes to the pathophysiology and symptomatology of BPH. There are two prostatic components to the obstructive properties of BPH and the development of lower urinary tract symptoms: dynamic and static.[29] The static component of BPH is related to an increase in

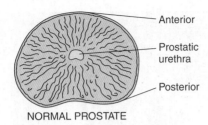

NORMAL PROSTATE

Anterior

Prostatic
urethra

Posterior

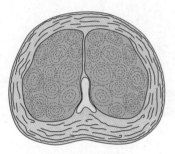

NODULAR PROSTATIC
HYPERPLASIA

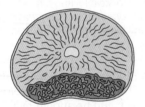

CARCINOMA
OF PROSTATE

FIGURE 38-12 Normal prostate, nodular benign prostatic hyperplasia, and cancer of the prostate. (From Damjanov I. [2005]. The lower urinary tract and male reproductive system. In Rubin E., Gorstein F., Rubin R., et al. [Eds.], *Rubin's pathology: Clinicopathologic foundations of medicine* [4th ed., p. 920]. Philadelphia: Lippincott Williams & Wilkins. Artist: Dimitri Karetnikov.)

prostatic size and gives rise to symptoms such as a weak urinary stream, postvoid dribbling, frequency of urination, and nocturia. The dynamic component of BPH is related to prostatic smooth muscle tone. The α_1-adrenergic receptors are the main receptors for the smooth muscle component of the prostate. The recognition of the role of α_1-adrenergic receptors in neuromuscular function in the prostate is the basis for use of α_1-adrenergic receptor blockers in treating BPH. A third component, detrusor instability and impaired bladder contractility, may contribute to the symptoms of BPH independent of the outlet obstruction created by an enlarged prostate[29,30] (see Chapter 26). It has been suggested that some of the symptoms of BPH might be related to a decompensating or aging bladder, rather than being primarily related to outflow obstruction. An example is the involuntary contraction that results in urgency and an attempt to void that occurs because of a decrease in bladder compliance.[29]

Clinical Course. The clinical significance of BPH resides in its tendency to compress the urethra and cause partial or complete obstruction of urinary outflow. As the obstruction increases, acute retention may occur with overdistention of the bladder. The residual urine in the bladder causes increased frequency of urination and a constant desire to empty the bladder, which becomes worse at night. With marked bladder distention, overflow incontinence may occur with the slightest increase in intra-abdominal pressure. The resulting obstruction to urinary flow can give rise to urinary tract infection, destructive changes of the bladder wall, hydroureter, and hydronephrosis. Hypertrophy and changes in bladder wall structure develop in stages. Initially, the hypertrophied fibers form trabeculations and then herniations, or sacculations; finally, diverticula develop as the herniations extend through the bladder wall (see Chapter 26, Fig. 26-4). Because urine seldom is completely emptied from them, these diverticula are readily infected. Back-pressure on the ureters and collecting system of the kidneys predisposes to hydroureter, hydronephrosis, and eventual renal failure.

It is now thought that the single most important factor in the evaluation and treatment of BPH is the man's own experiences related to the disorder. The American Urological Society Symptom Index consists of seven questions about symptoms regarding incomplete emptying, frequency, intermittency, urgency, weak stream, straining, and nocturia.[31] Each question is rated with a score of 0 (mild) to 7 (severe). A maximum score of 35 indicates severe symptoms. Total scores below 7 are considered mild; those between 8 and 20, moderate; and scores over 20, severe. A final question relates to quality of life related to urinary problems.

Diagnosis of BPH is based on history, physical examination, digital rectal examination, urinalysis, blood tests for serum creatinine and prostate-specific antigen (PSA), and urine flow rate.[32] Blood and urine analyses are used as adjuncts to determine BPH complications. Urinalysis is done to detect bacteria, white blood cells, or microscopic hematuria in the presence of infection and inflammation. The serum creatinine test is used as an estimate of the glomerular filtration rate and kidney function. The PSA test is used to screen for prostatic cancer. These evaluation measures, along with the symptom index, are used to describe the extent of obstruction, determine if other diagnostic tests are needed, and establish the need for treatment.

Transabdominal or transrectal diagnostic ultrasonography can be used to evaluate the kidneys, ureters, and bladder. Abdominal radiographs may be used to reveal the size of the gland. Urethrocystoscopy is indicated in men with a history of hematuria, stricture disease, urethral injury, or prior lower urinary tract surgery. It is used to evaluate the length and diameter of the urethra, the size and configuration of the prostate, and bladder capacity. It also detects the presence of trabeculations, bladder stones, and small bladder cancers. CT scans, MRI studies, and radionuclide scans are reserved for rare instances of tumor detection.

Treatment of BPH is determined by the degree of symptoms that the condition produces and complications due to obstruction. When a man develops mild symptoms related to BPH, a "watch and wait" stance often is taken. The condition does not always run a predictable course; it may remain stable or even improve. Until the 1980s, surgery was the mainstay of treatment to alleviate urinary obstruction due to BPH. Currently, there is an emphasis on less invasive methods of treatment, including use of pharmacologic agents. However, when more severe signs of obstruction develop, surgical treatment (e.g., transurethral resection of the prostate [TURP]) usually is indicated to provide comfort and avoid serious renal damage. For men who have heart or lung disease or a condition that precludes major surgery, a stent may be used to widen and maintain the patency of the urethra.

Pharmacologic management includes the use of 5α-reductase inhibitors and α_1-adrenergic–blocking drugs.[28,29] The 5α-reductase inhibitors such as finasteride reduce prostate size by blocking the effect of androgens on the prostate. The presence of α-adrenergic receptors in prostatic smooth muscle has prompted the use of α_1-adrenergic–blocking drugs to relieve prostatic obstruction and increase urine flow.

Cancer of the Prostate

Prostatic cancer is the most common male cancer in the United States and is second to lung cancer as a cause of cancer-related death in men. The American Cancer Society estimates that during 2005, approximately 232,090 men in the United States received a diagnosis of prostate cancer, and 30,350 men died of the disorder.[33] The increase in diagnosed cases is thought to reflect earlier diagnosis because of the widespread use of PSA testing since the early 1990s.[34] The incidence of prostate cancer varies markedly from country to country and among races in the same country.[33,34] African-American men have the highest reported incidence for prostate cancer at all ages, and Asian and Native American men have the lowest rate. Prostate cancer also is a disease of aging. The incidence increases rapidly after 50 years of age; more than 85% of all prostate cancers are diagnosed in men older than 65 years of age.[33]

Etiology. The precise cause of prostatic cancer is unclear. As with other cancers, it appears that the development of prostate cancer is a multistep process involving genes that control cell differentiation and growth (see Chapter 5). Several risk factors, such as age, race, heredity, and environmental influences (including dietary fat and meat consumption), are suspected of playing a role.[34,35] Male hormone levels also may play a role. There is insufficient evidence linking socioeconomic status, infectious agents, smoking, vasectomy, sexual behavior, or BPH to the pathogenesis of prostate cancer.

The incidence of prostate cancer appears to be higher in relatives of men with prostate cancer. Diet may also play a role. It has been suggested that a diet high in fats may alter the production of sex hormones and increase the risk of prostate cancer. Supporting the role of dietary fats as a risk factor for prostate cancer has been the observation that the diet of Japanese men, who have a low rate of prostate cancer, is much lower in fat content than that of U.S. men, who have a much higher incidence.

In terms of hormonal influence, androgens are believed to play a role in the pathogenesis of prostate cancer.[34,35] Evidence favoring a hormonal influence includes the presence of steroid receptors in the prostate, the requirement of sex hormones for normal growth and development of the prostate, and the fact that prostate cancer almost never develops in men who have been castrated. The response of prostatic cancer to estrogen administration or androgen deprivation further supports a correlation between the disease and testosterone levels.

Pathology. Prostatic adenocarcinomas, which account for 98% of all primary prostatic cancers, are commonly multicentric and located in the peripheral zones of the prostate (see Fig. 38-12). The high frequency of invasion of the prostatic capsule by adenocarcinoma relates to its subcapsular location. Invasion of the urinary bladder is less common and occurs later in the clinical course. Metastasis to the lung reflects lymphatic spread through the thoracic duct and dissemination from the prostatic venous plexus to the inferior vena cava. Bony metastases, particularly to the vertebral column, ribs, and pelvis, produce pain that often presents as a first sign of the disease.

Manifestations. Most men with early-stage prostate cancer are asymptomatic. The presence of symptoms often suggests locally advanced or metastatic disease. Depending on the size and location of prostatic cancer at the time of diagnosis, there may be changes associated with the voiding pattern similar to those found in BPH. These include urgency, frequency, nocturia, hesitancy, dysuria, hematuria, or blood in the ejaculate. On physical examination, the prostate is nodular and fixed. Bone metastasis often is characterized by low back pain. Pathologic fractures can occur at the site of metastasis. Men with metastatic disease may experience weight loss, anemia, or shortness of breath.

Screening. Because early cancers of the prostate usually are asymptomatic, screening tests are important. The screening tests currently available are digital rectal examination, PSA testing, and transrectal ultrasonography. PSA is a glycoprotein secreted into the cytoplasm of benign and malignant prostatic cells that is not found in other normal tissues or tumors.[36] However, a positive PSA test indicates only the possible presence of prostate cancer. It also can be positive in cases of BPH and prostatitis. The American Cancer Society and the American Urological Association recommend that men 50 years of age or older should undergo annual measurement of PSA and rectal examination for early detection of prostate cancer.[33] Men at high risk for prostate cancer, such as blacks and those with a strong family history, should undergo annual screening beginning at 45 years of age.[33]

Diagnosis. The diagnosis of prostate cancer is based on history and physical examination and confirmed through biopsy methods. Transrectal ultrasonography, a continuously improving method of imaging, is used to guide a biopsy needle and document the exact location of the sampled tissue. It also is used for providing staging information. Newly developed small probes for transrectal MRI have been shown to be effective in detecting the presence of cancer in the prostate. Radiologic examination of the bones of the skull, ribs, spine, and pelvis can be used to reveal metastases, although radionuclide bone scans are more sensitive. Excretory urograms are used to delineate changes due to urinary tract obstruction and renal involvement.

Cancer of the prostate, like other forms of cancer, is graded and staged (see Chapter 5). Prostatic adenocarcinoma commonly is classified using the Gleason grading system.[35] Well-differentiated tumors are assigned a grade of 1, and poorly differentiated tumors a grade of 5. Two tumor markers, PSA and serum acid phosphatase, are important in the staging and management of prostatic cancer. In untreated cases, the level of PSA correlates with the volume and stage of disease.[37] A rising PSA after treatment is consistent with progressive disease, whether it is locally recurring or metastatic. Measurement of PSA is used to detect recurrence after total prostatectomy. Because the prostate is the source of PSA, levels of the antigen should drop to zero after surgery; a rising PSA indicates recurring disease. Serum acid phosphatase is less sensitive than PSA and is used less frequently. However, it is more predictive of metastatic disease and may be used for that purpose.

Treatment. Cancer of the prostate is treated by surgery, radiation therapy, and hormonal manipulations.[35,37] Chemotherapy has shown limited effectiveness in the treatment of prostate cancer. Treatment decisions are based on tumor grade and stage and on the age and health of the man. Expectant therapy (watching and waiting) may be used if the tumor is not producing symptoms,

is expected to grow slowly, and is small and contained in one area of the prostate. This approach is particularly suited for men who are elderly or have other health problems. Most men with an anticipated survival greater than 10 years are considered for surgical or radiation therapy.[38] Radical prostatectomy involves complete removal of the seminal vesicles, prostate, and ampullae of the vas deferens. Radiation therapy can be delivered by a variety of techniques, including external-beam radiation therapy and transperineal implantation of radioisotopes.

Metastatic disease often is treated with androgen deprivation therapy.[39] Androgen deprivation may be induced by orchiectomy (surgical castration) or at several levels along the pituitary-gonadal axis using a variety of methods or agents (medical castration). Orchiectomy often is effective in reducing symptoms and extending survival. The GnRH analogs (e.g., leuprolide, buserelin, nafarelin) block LH release from the pituitary and reduce testosterone levels without orchiectomy. When given continuously and in therapeutic doses, these drugs desensitize GnRH receptors in the pituitary, thereby preventing the release of luteinizing hormone. The antiandrogens (e.g., flutamide) block the uptake and actions of androgens in the target tissues. Complete androgen blockade can be achieved by combining an antiandrogen with a GnRH agent or orchiectomy.

In summary, disorders of the penis include balanitis, an acute or chronic inflammation of the glans penis, and balanoposthitis, an inflammation of the glans and prepuce. Peyronie disease is characterized by the growth of a band of fibrous tissue on top of the penile shaft. Priapism is prolonged, painful, and nonsexual erection that can lead to thrombosis with ischemia and necrosis of penile tissue. Cancer of the penis accounts for less than 1% of male genital cancers in the United States. Although the tumor is slow growing and highly curable when diagnosed early, the greatest hindrance to successful treatment is a delay in seeking medical attention.

Disorders of the scrotum and testes include hydrocele, hematocele, spermatocele, varicocele, and testicular torsion. Inflammatory conditions can involve the scrotal sac, epididymis, or testes. Tumors can arise in the scrotum or the testes. Scrotal cancers usually are associated with exposure to petroleum products such as tar, pitch, and soot. Testicular cancers account for 1% of all male cancers and 3% of cancers of the male genitourinary system. With current treatment methods, a large percentage of men with these tumors can be cured. Testicular self-examination is recommended as a means of early detection of this form of cancer.

The prostate is a firm, glandular structure that surrounds the urethra. Inflammation of the prostate occurs as an acute or a chronic process. Chronic prostatitis probably is the most common cause of relapsing urinary tract infections in men. BPH is a common disorder in men older than 50 years. Because the prostate encircles the urethra, BPH exerts its effect through obstruction of urinary outflow from the bladder. Advances in the treatment of BPH include laser surgery, balloon dilatation, prostatic stents, and pharmacologic treatment.

Prostatic cancer is the most common male cancer in the United States and is second to lung cancer as a cause of cancer-related death in men. A recent increase in diagnosed cases is thought to reflect earlier diagnosis because of widespread use of PSA testing. Most prostate cancers are asymptomatic and are incidentally discovered on rectal examination. Cancer of the prostate, like other forms of cancer, is graded according to the histologic characteristics of the tumor and staged clinically using the TNM system. Treatment, which is based on the extent of the disease, includes surgery, radiation therapy, and hormonal manipulation.

Disorders in Childhood and Aging Changes

DISORDERS OF CHILDHOOD

Disorders of the male reproductive system that present in childhood include hypospadias, epispadias, phimosis and paraphimosis, and cryptorchidism.

Hypospadias and Epispadias

Hypospadias and epispadias are congenital disorders of the penis resulting from embryologic defects in the development of the urethral groove and penile urethra (Fig. 38-13). In hypospadias, which affects approximately 1 in 300 male infants, the termination of the urethra is on the

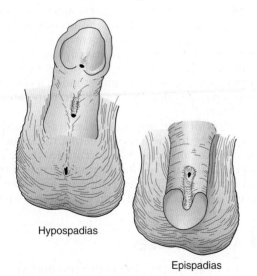

Hypospadias

Epispadias

FIGURE 38-13 Hypospadias and epispadias.

ventral surface of the penis.[40,41] The testes are undescended in 10% of boys born with hypospadias and chordee (*i.e.*, ventral bowing of the penis), and inguinal hernia also may accompany the disorder. In the newborn with severe hypospadias and cryptorchidism (undescended testes), the differential diagnosis should consider ambiguous genitalia and masculinization that is seen in female infants with congenital adrenal hyperplasia (see Chapter 31). Because many chromosomal aberrations result in ambiguity of the external genitalia, chromosomal studies often are recommended for male infants with hypospadias and cryptorchidism.[40]

Surgery is the treatment of choice for hypospadias.[40] Circumcision is avoided because the foreskin is used for surgical repair. Factors that influence the timing of surgical repair include anesthetic risk, penile size, and the psychological effects of the surgery on the child. In mild cases, the surgery is done for cosmetic reasons only. In more severe cases, surgical repair becomes essential for normal sexual functioning and to prevent the psychological effects of having malformed genitalia. When indicated, surgical repair is usually done between the ages of 6 to 12 months.

Epispadias, in which the opening of the urethra is on the dorsal surface of the penis, is a less common defect. Although epispadias may occur as a separate entity, it often is associated with exstrophy of the bladder, a condition in which the abdominal wall fails to cover the bladder. The treatment depends on the extent of the developmental defect.

Phimosis and Paraphimosis

Phimosis refers to a tightening of the prepuce or penile foreskin that prevents its retraction over the glans. Embryologically, the foreskin begins to develop during the eighth week of gestation as a fold of skin at the distal edge of the penis that eventually grows forward over the base of the glans.[42] By the 16th week of gestation, the prepuce and the glans are adherent. Only a small percentage of newborns have a fully retractable foreskin. With growth, a space develops between the glans and foreskin, and by 3 years of age, approximately 90% of male children have retractable foreskins.

Because the foreskin of many boys cannot be fully retracted in early childhood, it is important that the area be cleaned thoroughly. There is no need to retract the foreskin forcibly because this could lead to infection, scarring, or paraphimosis. As the child grows, the foreskin becomes retractable, and the glans and foreskin should be cleaned routinely. If symptomatic phimosis occurs after childhood, it can cause difficulty with voiding or sexual activity. Circumcision is then the treatment of choice.

In a related condition called *paraphimosis*, the foreskin is so tight and constricted that it cannot cover the glans. A tight foreskin can constrict the blood supply to the glans and lead to ischemia and necrosis. Many cases of paraphimosis result from the foreskin being retracted for an extended period, as in the case of catheterized uncircumcised males.

Cryptorchidism

Cryptorchidism, or undescended testes, occurs when one or both of the testicles fail to move down into the scrotal sac. The condition is bilateral in 10% to 20% of cases. The testes develop intra-abdominally in the fetus and usually descend into the scrotum through the inguinal canal during the seventh to ninth months of gestation.[41] The undescended testes may remain in the lower abdomen or at a point of descent in the inguinal canal (Fig. 38-14).

The incidence of cryptorchidism is directly related to birth weight and gestational age; infants who are born prematurely or are small for gestational age have the highest incidence of the disorder. Up to one third of premature infants and 3% to 5% of full-term infants are born with undescended testicles.[42,43] The cause of cryptorchidism in full-term infants is poorly understood. Most cases are idiopathic, but some may result from genetic or hormonal factors.[42]

The major manifestation of cryptorchidism is the absence of one or more of the testes in the scrotum. The testis either is not palpable or can be felt external to the inguinal ring. Spontaneous descent often occurs during the first 3 months of life, and by 6 months of age the incidence decreases to 0.8%.[40,43] Spontaneous descent rarely occurs after 6 months of age.

In children with cryptorchidism, histologic abnormalities of the testes reflect intrinsic defects in the testicle or adverse effects of the extrascrotal environment. The undescended testicle is normal at birth, but pathologic changes can be demonstrated at 6 to 12 months.[40] There is a delay in germ cell development, changes in the spermatic tubules, and reduced number of Leydig cells. These changes are progressive if the testes remain undescended. When the disorder is unilateral, it also may produce morphologic changes in the contralateral descended testis.

The consequences of cryptorchidism include infertility, malignancy, and the possible psychological effects of an empty scrotum. Indirect inguinal hernias usually accompany the undescended testes but rarely are symptomatic. Recognition of the condition and early treatment are important steps in preventing adverse consequences. The risk of malignancy in the undescended testis is four to six times higher than in the general population.[40,43]

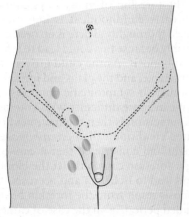

FIGURE 38-14 Possible locations of undescended testicles.

The increased risk of testicular cancer is not significantly affected by orchiopexy, hormonal therapy, or late spontaneous descent after the age of 2 years. However, orchiopexy does allow for earlier detection of a testicular malignancy by positioning the testis in a more easily palpable location.

As a group, men with unilateral or bilateral cryptorchidism usually have decreased sperm counts, poorer-quality sperm, and lower fertility rates than do men whose testicles descend normally. The likelihood of decreased fertility increases when the condition is bilateral. Unlike the risk of testicular cancer, there seems to be some advantage to early orchiopexy for protection of fertility.[40,43]

Diagnosis is based on careful examination of the genitalia in male infants. Undescended testes due to cryptorchidism should be differentiated from retractable testes that retract into the inguinal canal in response to an exaggerated cremaster muscle reflex. Retractable testes usually are palpable at birth but become nonpalpable later. They can be brought down with careful palpation in a warm room. Retractable testes usually assume a scrotal position during puberty. They have none of the complications associated with undescended testicles due to cryptorchidism.[40]

Improved techniques for testicular localization include ultrasonography (*i.e.*, visualization of the testes by recording the pulses of ultrasonic waves directed into the tissues), gonadal venography and arteriography (*i.e.*, radiography of the veins and arteries of the testes after the injection of a contrast medium), and laparoscopy (*i.e.*, examination of the interior of the abdomen using a visualization instrument).

The treatment goals for the child with cryptorchidism include measures to enhance future fertility potential, placement of the gonad in a favorable place for cancer detection, and improved cosmetic appearance. Regardless of the type of treatment used, it should be carried out between 6 months and 2 years of age.[40,43] Treatment modalities for children with unilateral or bilateral cryptorchidism include initial hormone therapy with hCG or GnRH agonists (a hypothalamic hormone that stimulates production of the gonadotropic hormones by the anterior pituitary gland). For children who do not respond to hormonal treatment, surgical placement and fixation of the testes in the scrotum (*i.e.*, orchiopexy) has proven to be effective. Approximately 95% of infants who have orchiopexy for a unilateral undescended testis will be fertile, compared with a 30% to 50% fertility rate in uncorrected men.[43]

Treatment of men with undescended testis should include lifelong follow-up, considering the sequelae of testicular cancer and infertility. Parents need to be aware of the potential issues of infertility and increased risk of testicular cancer. On reaching puberty, boys should be instructed in the necessity of testicular self-examination.

AGING CHANGES

Like other body systems, the male reproductive system undergoes degenerative changes as a result of the aging process; it becomes less efficient with age. The declining physiologic efficiency of male reproductive function occurs gradually and involves the endocrine, circulatory, and neuromuscular systems.[44] Compared with the marked physiologic change in aging women, the changes in the aging man are more gradual and less drastic. Gonadal and reproductive failures usually are not related directly to age because a man remains fertile into advanced age; 80- and 90-year-old men have been known to father children.

As the man ages, his reproductive system becomes measurably different in structure and function from that of the younger man. Male sex hormone levels, particularly of testosterone, decrease with age, with the decline starting later on average than in women. The term *andropause* has been used to describe an ill-defined collection of symptoms in aging men, typically those older than 50 years, who may have a low androgen level.[44,45]

The sex hormones play a part in the structure and function of the reproductive system and other body systems from conception to old age; they affect protein synthesis, salt and water balance, bone growth, and cardiovascular function. Decreasing levels of testosterone affect sexual energy, muscle strength, and the genital tissues. The testes become smaller and lose their firmness. The seminiferous tubules, which produce spermatozoa, thicken and begin a degenerative process that finally inhibits sperm production, resulting in a decrease of viable spermatozoa. The prostate gland enlarges, and its contractions become weaker. The force of ejaculation decreases because of a reduction in the volume and viscosity of the seminal fluid. The seminal vesicle changes little from childhood to puberty. The pubertal increases in the fluid capacity of the gland remain throughout adulthood and decline after the age of 60 years. After age 60 years, the walls of the seminal vesicles thin, the epithelium decreases, and the muscle layer is replaced by connective tissue. Age-related changes in the penis consist of fibrotic changes in the trabeculae in the corpus spongiosum, with progressive sclerotic changes in arteries and veins. Sclerotic changes also follow in the corpora cavernosa, with the condition becoming generalized in 55- to 60-year-old men.

Erectile dysfunction in the elderly man often is directly related to the general physical condition of the person. Diseases that accompany aging can have direct bearing on male reproductive function. Various cardiovascular, respiratory, hormonal, neurologic, and hematologic disorders can be responsible for secondary impotence. For example, vascular disease affects male potency because it may impair blood flow to the pudendal arteries or their tributaries, resulting in loss of blood volume with subsequent poor distention of the vascular spaces of erectile tissue. Other diseases affecting potency include hypertension, diabetes, cardiac disease, and malignancies of the reproductive organs. In addition, certain medications can have an effect on sexual function.

Testosterone and other synthetic androgens may be used in older men with low androgen levels to improve muscle strength and vigor. Preliminary studies of androgen replacement in aging men with low androgen levels show an increase in lean body mass and a decrease in bone turnover. Before testosterone replacement therapy is initiated, all men should be screened for prostate cancer and other androgen-related diseases. Testosterone is available in an injectable form that is administered every 2 to 4 weeks, as a buccal tablet, or as a transdermal patch or gel. Side effects of replacement therapy may include acne, gynecomastia, and reduced high-density lipoprotein levels. It also may contribute to a worsening of sleep apnea in men who are troubled by this problem.

In summary, childhood disorders of the male reproductive system include congenital disorders in which the urethral opening is located on the ventral surface of the penis (hypospadias) or on the dorsal surface (epispadias). Phimosis is the condition in which the opening of the foreskin is too tight to permit retraction over the glans. Disorders of the scrotum and testes include cryptorchidism or undescended testicles. Early diagnosis and treatment are important because of the risk of malignancy and infertility.

Like other body systems, the male reproductive system undergoes changes as a result of the aging process. The changes occur gradually and involve parallel changes in endocrine, circulatory, and neuromuscular function. Testosterone levels decrease, the size and firmness of the testes decrease, sperm production declines, and the prostate gland enlarges. There usually is a decrease in frequency of intercourse, intensity of sensation, speed of attaining erection, and force of ejaculation.

Review Exercises

A 64-year-old man presents to his family physician with erectile dysfunction. He is on multiple medications for "his heart disease." An initial physical examination is unremarkable.

A. What additional information should be obtained?
B. Given his medical history, what are possible factors contributing to his problem?

A 23-year-old man presents in the emergency department in severe distress. His left testicle is large and tender and he has pain radiating to the inguinal area.

A. What would be a tentative diagnosis for this man?
B. Why would this problem necessitate immediate diagnosis and surgical intervention?

A 72-year-old man had a radical prostatectomy for localized prostate cancer. After surgery his PSA level was undetectable. He presents 5 years later having been "lost to follow-up." He complains of pain in his hip and lower back. His PSA level is now markedly elevated.

A. What initial investigations are warranted?
B. What therapies are available for this complication?

Visit the Porth: Essentials of Pathophysiology:
Concepts of Altered Health States web site
(http://thePoint.LWW.com/PorthEssentials) for links to chapter-related resources on the Internet, all-new exclusive animations, chapter review questions, and more!

REFERENCES

1. Guyton A. C., Hall J. E. (2006). *Textbook of medical physiology* (11th ed., p. 999). Philadelphia: Elsevier Saunders.
2. Braunstein G. D. (2004). Testes. In Greenspan F. S., Gardner D. G. (Eds.), *Basic and clinical endocrinology* (7th ed., pp. 478–510). New York: Lange Medical Books/McGraw-Hill.
3. Anderson K. E., Wagner G. (1995). Physiology of penile erection. *Physiology Review* 75, 191–236.
4. NIH Consensus Development Panel on Impotence. (1993). NIH Consensus Conference: Impotence. *Journal of the American Medical Association* 270, 83–90.
5. Lue T. F. (2000). Erectile dysfunction. *New England Journal of Medicine* 342, 1802–1813.
6. AACE Male Sexual Dysfunction Taskforce. (2003). AACE medical guidelines for clinical practice for the evaluation and treatment of male sexual dysfunction: A couple's problem—2003 update. *Endocrine Practice* 9, 77–95.
7. Matfin G. (2005). Erectile dysfunction: Interrelationship with the metabolic syndrome. *Current Diabetes Reports* 5, 64–69.
8. Edwards S. (1996). Balanitis and balanoposthitis: A review. *Genitourinary Medicine* 72, 155–159.
9. Fitkin J., Ho G. T. (1999). Peyronie's disease: Current management. *American Family Physician* 60, 549–554.
10. McAninch J. W. (2004). Disorders of the penis and male urethra. In Tanagho E. A., McAninch J. W. (Eds.), *Smith's general urology* (16th ed., pp. 612–626). New York: Lange Medical Books/McGraw-Hill.
11. Harmon W. J., Nehra A. (1997). Priapism: Diagnosis and treatment. *Mayo Clinic Proceedings* 72, 350–355.
12. Kachhi P. N., Henderson S. O. (2000). Priapism after androstenedione intake for athletic performance enhancement. *Annals of Emergency Medicine* 35, 391–393.
13. Krieg R., Hoffman R. (1999). Current management of unusual genitourinary cancers: Part 1. Penile cancer. *Oncology* 13, 1347–1352.
14. Presti J. C. (2004). Genital tumors. In Tanagho E. A., McAninch J. W. (Eds.), *Smith's general urology* (16th ed., pp. 386–399). New York: Lange Medical Books/McGraw-Hill.
15. Kapur P., Caty M. G., Glick P. L. (1998). Pediatric hernias and hydroceles. *Pediatric Clinics of North America* 45, 773–789.
16. Templeton A. (2003). Varicocele and infertility. *Lancet* 361, 1838–1839.
17. Galejs L. E., Kass E. J. (1999). Diagnosis and treatment of acute scrotum. *American Family Physician* 59, 817–824.
18. Meares E. M. (2000). Nonspecific infections of the genitourinary tract. In Tanagho E. A., McAninch J. W. (Eds.), *Smith's general urology* (15th ed., pp. 237–238). Norwalk, CT: Appleton & Lange.
19. Melicow M. M. (1975). Percivall Pott (1713–1788): 200th anniversary of first report of occupation-induced cancer of the scrotum in chimney sweepers (1775). *Urology* 6, 745–749.
20. Lowe F. C. (1992). Squamous cell carcinoma of the scrotum. *Urologic Clinics of North America* 19, 297–305.
21. Bosl G. J. (1997). Testicular germ-cell cancer. *New England Journal of Medicine* 337, 242–252.
22. Pillai S. B., Besner G. E. (1998). Pediatric testicular problems. *Pediatric Clinics of North America* 45, 813–818.
23. Motzer R. J., Bosl G. J. (2004). Testicular cancer. In Kasper D. L., Braunwald E., Fauci A., et al. (Eds.), *Harrison's principles of internal medicine* (16th ed., pp. 550–552). New York: McGraw-Hill.
24. Krieger J. N., Nyberg L., Nickel J. C. (1999). NIH consensus definition and classification of prostatitis. *Journal of the American Medical Association* 282, 721–725.
25. Nguyen H. T. (2005). Bacterial infections of the genitourinary system. In Tanagho E. A., McAninch J. W. (Eds.), *Smith's general urology* (16th ed., pp. 203–227). New York: Lange Medical Books/McGraw-Hill.
26. Stevermer J. J., Easley S. K. (2000). Treatment of prostatitis. *American Family Physician* 61, 3015–3026.
27. Collins M. M., MacDonald R., Wilt T. J. (2000). Diagnosis and treatment of chronic abacterial prostatitis: A systemic review. *Annals of Internal Medicine* 133, 367–381.
28. Thorpe A., Neal D. (2003). Benign prostatic hyperplasia. *Lancet* 361, 1359–1367.
29. Zida A., Rosenblum M., Crawford E. D. (1999). Benign prostatic hyperplasia: An overview. *Urology* 53(Suppl. 3A), 1–6.
30. Elbadawi A. (1998). Voiding dysfunction in benign prostatic hyperplasia: Trends, controversies and recent revelations: Pathology and pathophysiology. *Urology* 51(Suppl. 5A), 73–82.
31. Barry M. J., Cherkin D. C., Chang Y., et al. (1992). The American Urological Association index of benign prostatic hypertrophy. *Journal of Urology* 148, 1549–1557.
32. Agency of Health Care Policy and Research. (1994). *Clinical practice guidelines for benign prostatic hyperplasia.* AHCPR publication no. 94-0582. Rockville, MD: U.S. Department of Health and Human Services.
33. American Cancer Society. (2005). Prostate cancer resource center. [On-line]. Available: www.cancer.org.
34. Gronberg H. (2003). Prostate cancer epidemiology. *Lancet* 361, 859–864.
35. Nelson W. G., De Manzo A. M., Isaacs W. B. (2003). Prostate cancer. *New England Journal of Medicine* 349, 366–381.
36. Balk S. P., Ko Y. J., Bubley G. J. (2003). Biology of prostate-specific antigen. *Journal of Clinical Oncology* 21, 383–391.
37. Stoller M. L., Presti J. C., Carroll P. R. (2005). Urology. In Tierney L. M., McPhee S. J., Papadakis M. A. (Eds.), *Current medical diagnosis and treatment* (44th ed., pp. 956–961). New York: Lange Medical Books/McGraw-Hill.
38. Scher H. I. (2004). Hyperplastic and malignant diseases of the prostate. In Kasper D. L., Braunwald E., Fauci A., et al. (Eds.), *Harrison's principles of internal medicine* (16th ed., pp. 543–551). New York: McGraw-Hill.
39. Sharifi N., Gulley J. L., Dahut W. L. (2005). Androgen deprivation therapy for prostate cancer. *Journal of the American Medical Association* 294, 238–244.

40. Behrman R., Kleigman R. M., Jenson H. B. (2004). *Nelson textbook of pediatrics* (16th ed., pp. 1812–1815, 1817–1818). Philadelphia: Elsevier Saunders.

41. Moore K. L., Persaud T. V. N. (2003). *The developing human: Clinically oriented embryology* (7th ed., pp. 304–327). Philadelphia: W. B. Saunders.

42. Epstein J. I. (2005). The lower urinary tract and male genital system. In Kumar V., Abbas A. K., Fausto N. (Eds.), *Robbins and Cotran pathologic basis of disease* (7th ed., pp. 1034–1058). Philadelphia: Elsevier Saunders.

43. Docimo S. G., Silver R. I., Cromie W. (2000). The undescended testicle: Diagnosis and management. *American Family Physician* 62, 2037–2048.

44. Muller M., Grobbee D. E., Thijssen J. H. H., et al. (2003). Sex hormones and male health: Effects on components of the frailty syndrome. *Trends in Endocrinology and Metabolism* 14, 289–296.

45. Yialamas M. A., Hayes F. J. (2003) Androgens and the aging male. *Endocrinology Rounds* 2, 1–6. [On-line]. Available: www.endocrinologyrounds.org.

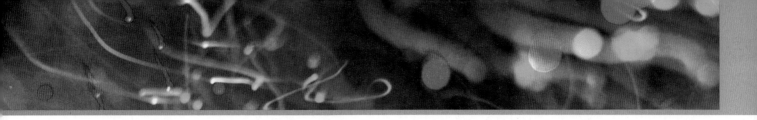

Chapter 39

Disorders of the Female Genitourinary System

The reproductive function of the woman is far more complex than the man's. Not only must the woman produce germ cells, she must nourish the developing embryo and prepare to nurse the infant once childbirth has occurred. This chapter includes a review of the structure and function of the female reproductive system and a discussion of disorders of the internal and external female reproductive organs.

Structure and Function of the Female Reproductive System

The female genitourinary system consists of the external and internal genital organs. The external female sex organs are referred to as the *genitalia* or *vulva*. The internal genital organs, which are largely located within the pelvic cavity, include the vagina, uterus, fallopian (or uterine) tubes, and ovaries (Fig. 39-1).

EXTERNAL GENITALIA

The external genitalia are located at the base of the pelvis in the perineal area. The external genitalia, also called the *vulva*, include the mons pubis, labia majora, labia minora, clitoris, and perineal body (Fig. 39-2). Because of their location, the urethra and anus usually are considered in a discussion of the external genitalia.

The *mons pubis* is a rounded, skin-covered fat pad located anterior to the symphysis pubis. Running posteriorly from the mons pubis are two elongated, hair-covered, fatty folds, the *labia majora*. The labia majora are analogous to the male scrotum. The labia majora enclose the *labia minora*, which are smaller than the labia majora and are composed of skin, fat, and some erectile tissue. The *clitoris* is located below the clitoral hood, which is formed

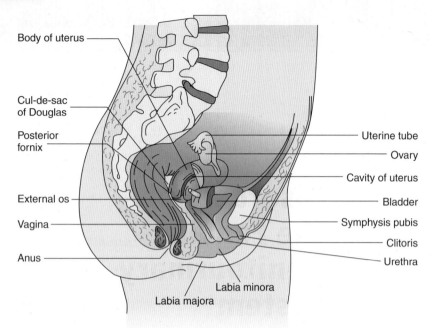

Body of uterus

Cul-de-sac
of Douglas

Posterior
fornix

External os

Vagina

Anus

Uterine tube
Ovary
Cavity of uterus
Bladder
Symphysis pubis
Clitoris
Urethra

Labia minora
Labia majora

FIGURE 39-1 Female reproductive system as
seen in sagittal section.

by the joining of the two labia minora. The female clitoris
is an erectile organ, rich in vascular and nervous supply.
Analogous to the male penis, it is a highly sensitive organ
that becomes distended during sexual stimulation.

The area between the labia minora is called the *vestibule*.
Located in the vestibule are the urethral and vaginal openings and Bartholin lubricating glands. The urethra is
located posterior to the clitoris and usually is closer to the
vaginal opening than to the clitoris. The urethral open-

ing is the site of *Skene glands*, which have a lubricating
function. The vaginal orifice, commonly known as the
introitus, is the opening between the external and internal
genitalia.

INTERNAL GENITALIA

Vagina

The vagina is a fibromuscular tube that connects the external and internal genitalia. The vagina, which is essentially
free of sensory nerve fibers, is located behind the urinary
bladder and urethra and anterior to the rectum (Fig. 39-3).

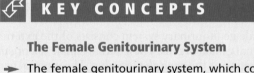

KEY CONCEPTS

The Female Genitourinary System

➤ The female genitourinary system, which consists
of the external and internal genitalia, has both
sexual and reproductive functions.

➤ The external genitalia (labia majora, labia minora,
clitoris, and vestibular glands) surround the
openings of the urethra and vagina. Although
the female urinary and genital structures are
anatomically separate, their close proximity
provides a means for cross-contamination and
shared symptomatology.

➤ The internal genitalia of the female reproductive system are specialized to participate in sexual intercourse (the vagina), to produce and
maintain the female egg cells (the ovaries), to
transport these cells to the site of fertilization
(the fallopian tubes), to provide a favorable
environment for development of the offspring
(the uterus), and to produce the female sex
hormones (the ovaries).

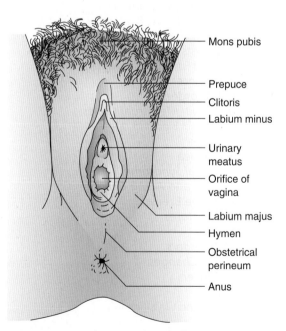

Mons pubis

Prepuce
Clitoris
Labium minus

Urinary
meatus
Orifice of
vagina

Labium majus
Hymen
Obstetrical
perineum

Anus

FIGURE 39-2 Female external genitalia.

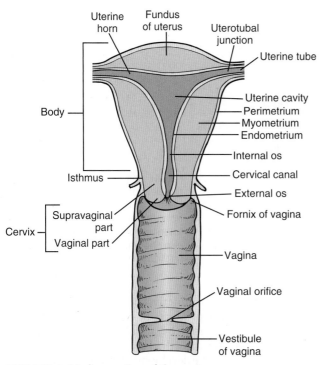

FIGURE 39-3 Median section of the vagina.

The uterine cervix projects into the vagina at its upper end, forming recesses called *fornices*. The vagina functions as a route for discharge of menses and other secretions. It also serves as an organ of sexual fulfillment and reproduction.

Uterus and Cervix

The uterus is a thick-walled muscular organ. This pear-shaped, hollow structure is located between the bladder and the rectum. The uterus can be divided into three parts: the upper portion above the insertion of the fallopian tubes, called the *fundus;* the central tapering portion, called the *body;* and the inferior constricted part, called the *cervix* (see Fig. 39-3).

The wall of the uterus is composed of three layers: the perimetrium, the myometrium, and the endometrium. The *perimetrium* is the outer serous covering that is derived from the abdominal peritoneum. This outer layer merges with the peritoneum that covers the broad ligaments. Anteriorly, the perimetrium is reflected over the bladder wall, forming the vesicouterine pouch; posteriorly, it extends to form the rectouterine pouch (see Fig. 39-1). Because of the proximity of the perimetrium to the urinary bladder, a bladder infection often causes uterine symptoms, particularly during pregnancy.

The middle muscle layer, the *myometrium,* forms the major portion of the uterine wall. It is continuous with the myometrium of the fallopian tubes and the vagina and extends into all the supporting ligaments with the exception of the broad ligaments. The inner fibers of the myometrium run in various directions, giving it an interwoven appearance. Contractions of these muscle fibers help to expel menstrual flow and the products of conception during miscarriage or childbirth.

The *endometrium,* or inner layer of the uterus, is continuous with the lining of the fallopian tubes and vagina. It consists of two distinct layers, or zones, that are responsive to hormonal stimulation: a basal layer and a functional layer.[1] The *basal layer* lies adjacent to the myometrium and is not sloughed during menstruation. The *functional layer,* which can be subdivided into a thin, compact superficial layer and a deeper spongiosa layer, arises from the basal layer and undergoes proliferative changes and menstrual sloughing. The endometrial cycle can be divided into three phases: proliferative, secretory, and menstrual. The proliferative, or preovulatory, phase is the period during which the glands and stroma of the superficial layer grow rapidly under the influence of estrogen. The secretory, or postovulatory, phase is the period during which progesterone produces glandular dilatation and active mucus secretion and the endometrium becomes highly vascular and edematous. The menstrual phase is the period during which the superficial layer degenerates and sloughs off.

The round cervix forms the neck of the uterus. The opening, or os, of the cervix forms a pathway between the uterus and the vagina. The vaginal opening is called the *external os* and the uterine opening, the *internal os.* The space between these two openings is called the *endocervical (cervical) canal.* Secretions from the columnar epithelium of the endocervix protect the uterus from infection, alter receptivity to sperm, and form a mucoid "plug" during pregnancy. The endocervical canal provides a route for menstrual discharge and entry of sperm.

Uterine Tubes

The *fallopian,* or uterine, tubes are slender cylindrical structures attached bilaterally to the uterus and supported by the upper folds of the broad ligament. The end of the fallopian tube nearest the ovary forms a funnel-like opening with fringed, finger-like projections, called *fimbriae,* that pick up the ovum after its release into the peritoneal cavity after ovulation (Fig. 39-4). The fallopian tubes are formed of smooth muscle and lined with a ciliated, mucus-producing epithelial layer. The beating of the cilia, along with contractile movements of the smooth muscle, propels the nonmobile ovum toward the uterus. Besides providing a passageway for ova and sperm, the fallopian tubes permit drainage of tubal secretions into the uterus.

OVARIES

In the adult, the ovaries are flat, almond-shaped structures that measure $4 \times 2.5 \times 1.5$ cm.[2] They are located on either side of the uterus below the ends of the two fallopian tubes. The ovaries are attached to the posterior surface of the broad ligament and to the uterus by the ovarian ligament (see Fig. 39-4). They are covered with a thin layer of surface epithelium that is continuous with the lining of the peritoneum. The integrity of this covering is periodically broken at the time of ovulation.

The tissues of the adult ovary can be conveniently divided into four compartments, or units: (1) the stroma, or supporting tissue; (2) the interstitial cells; (3) the follicles;

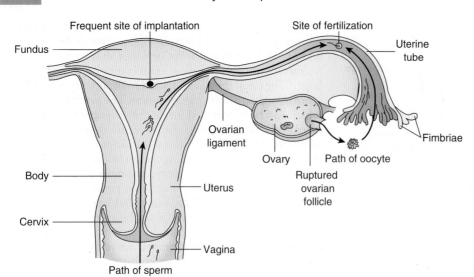

FIGURE 39-4 Schematic drawing of female reproductive organs, showing the path of the oocyte as it moves from the ovary into the fallopian (uterine) tube; the path of sperm is also shown, as is the usual site of fertilization.

and (4) the corpus luteum. The *stroma* is the connective tissue substance of the ovary in which the follicles are distributed. The *interstitial cells* are estrogen-secreting cells that resemble Leydig cells, the interstitial cells of the testes. The *follicles* contain the female germ cells or ova. The *corpus luteum* ("yellow body") develops after expulsion of the ovum from the follicle.

Ovarian Hormones

The ovaries produce estrogens, progesterone, and androgens.[1,3] Ovarian hormones are secreted in a cyclic pattern as a result of the interaction between the hypothalamic gonadotropin-releasing hormone (GnRH) and the pituitary gonadotropic hormones, follicle-stimulating hormone (FSH) and luteinizing hormone (LH). The secretion of LH and FSH is stimulated by GnRH from the hypothalamus (Fig. 39-5). In addition to LH and FSH, the anterior pituitary secretes a third hormone called *prolactin*. The primary function of prolactin is the stimulation of lactation in the postpartum period. During pregnancy, prolactin and other hormones such as estrogen, progesterone, insulin, and cortisol contribute to breast development in preparation for lactation.

Estrogens. Estrogens are a family of structurally related female sex hormones synthesized and secreted by cells in the ovaries and, in small amounts, by cells in the adrenal cortex. Androgens can be converted to estrogens peripherally, especially in fat tissue. Three estrogens occur naturally in humans: estrone, estradiol, and estriol. Of these, estradiol is the most biologically potent and the most abundantly secreted product of the ovary. Estrogens are secreted throughout the menstrual cycle. Two peaks occur: one before ovulation and the other in the middle of the luteal phase. Estrogens are transported in the blood bound to specific plasma globulins, inactivated and conjugated in the liver, and then excreted in the bile.

Estrogens are necessary for normal female physical maturation.[4] In concert with other hormones, estrogens

provide for the reproductive processes of ovulation, implantation of the products of conception, pregnancy, parturition, and lactation by stimulating the development and maintaining the growth of the accessory organs. The estrogens stimulate the development of the vagina, uterus, and uterine tubes in the embryo. They also stimulate the stromal development and ductal growth of the breasts

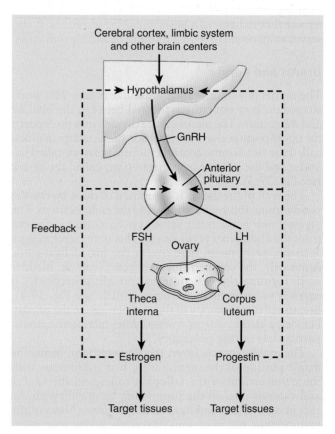

FIGURE 39-5 Hypothalamic-pituitary feedback control of estrogen and progesterone levels in the woman. The *dashed line* represents negative feedback.

at puberty, are responsible for the accelerated pubertal skeletal growth phase and for closure of the epiphyses of the long bones, contribute to the growth of axillary and pubic hair, and alter the distribution of body fat to produce the typical female body contours.

Estrogens have a number of important extragenital metabolic effects. They are responsible for maintaining the normal structure of skin and blood vessels in women. Estrogens decrease the rate of bone resorption by antagonizing the effects of calcitonin on bone; for this reason, osteoporosis is a common problem in estrogen-deficient post-menopausal women (see Chapter 43). In the liver, estrogens increase the synthesis of transport proteins for thyroxine, estrogen, testosterone, and other hormones. Estrogens also affect the composition of the plasma lipoproteins. They produce an increase in high-density lipoproteins (HDLs), a slight reduction in low-density lipoproteins (LDLs), and a reduction in cholesterol levels (see Chapter 17). Estrogens also increase plasma triglyceride levels, and they enhance the coagulability of blood by increasing the circulating levels of plasminogen and factors II, VII, IX, and X.

The estrogens cause moderate retention of sodium and water. Most women retain sodium and water and gain weight just before menstruation. This occurs because the estrogens facilitate the movement of intravascular fluids into the extracellular spaces, producing edema and increased sodium and water retention by the kidneys because of the decreased plasma volume. The actions of estrogens are summarized in Table 39-1.

Progesterone. Although the word *progesterone* refers to a substance that maintains pregnancy, progesterone is secreted as part of the normal menstrual cycle. The corpus luteum of the ovary secretes large amounts of progesterone after ovulation, and the adrenal cortex secretes small amounts. The hormone circulates in the blood attached to a specific plasma protein. It is metabolized in the liver and conjugated for excretion in the bile.

The local effects of progesterone on reproductive organs include the glandular development of the lobular and alveolar tissue of the breasts and the cyclic glandular development of the endometrium. Progesterone also can compete with aldosterone at the level of the renal tubule, causing a decrease in sodium reabsorption, with a resultant increase in secretion of aldosterone by the adrenal cortex (as occurs in pregnancy). Although the mechanism is uncertain, progesterone increases basal body temperature and is responsible for the increase in body temperature that occurs with ovulation. Smooth muscle relaxation under the influence of progesterone plays an important role in maintaining pregnancy by decreasing uterine contractions and is responsible for many of the common discomforts of pregnancy, such as edema, nausea, constipation, flatulence, and headaches. The increased progesterone present during pregnancy and the luteal phase of the menstrual cycle enhances the ventilatory response to carbon dioxide, leading to a measurable change in arterial and alveolar carbon dioxide (PCO_2) levels.

Androgens. The normal female also produces androgens. Approximately 25% of these androgens are secreted from the ovaries, 25% from the adrenal cortex, and 50% from ovarian or adrenal precursors. In the female, androgens contribute to normal hair growth at puberty and may have other important metabolic effects.

Ovarian Follicle Development and Ovulation

Unlike the male gonads, which produce sperm throughout a man's reproductive life, the female gonads contain a fixed number of ova at birth that diminishes throughout a woman's life. The process of oogenesis begins during the sixth week of fetal life and proceeds to the development of the primary oocytes, which become surrounded by a single layer of granulosa cells. The primary oocytes with their surrounding granulosa cells are referred to as

TABLE 39-1	Actions of Estrogens	
General Function	**Specific Actions**
Growth and Development	
Reproductive organs	Stimulate development of vagina, uterus, and fallopian tubes in utero and of secondary sex characteristics during puberty
Skeleton	Accelerate growth of long bones and closure of epiphyses at puberty
Reproductive Processes	
Ovulation	Promote growth of ovarian follicles
Fertilization	Alter the cervical secretions to favor survival and transport of sperm
	Promote motility of sperm within the fallopian tubes by decreasing mucus viscosity
Implantation	Promote development of endometrial lining in the event of pregnancy
Vagina	Promote proliferation and maturation of the vaginal mucosa
Cervix	Increase mucus consistency
Breasts	Stimulate stromal development and ductal growth
General Metabolic Effects	
Bone resorption	Decrease rate of bone resorption
Plasma proteins	Increase production of thyroid and other binding globulins
Lipoproteins	Increase high-density and slightly decrease low-density lipoproteins

primordial follicles. These primitive germ cells provide the 1 to 2 million oocytes that are present in the ovaries at birth. Throughout childhood, the granulosa cells provide nourishment for the ovum and secrete an inhibiting factor that keeps the ovum suspended in a primordial state.[3] After puberty, when FSH and LH from the anterior pituitary begin to be secreted in sufficient amounts, the ovaries, together with some of the follicles within them, begin to grow.

Ovarian Cycle. The monthly series of events associated with the maturation of the ovum is called the *ovarian cycle*. It consists of two phases, the follicular phase and the luteal phase. The follicular phase, typically days 1 to 14, is the period of follicle growth. The luteal phase, days 14 to 28, is the period of corpus luteum activity. The typical ovarian cycle repeats at intervals of 28 days, with ovulation occurring at mid-cycle. However, cycles as long as 40 days and as short as 21 days are not uncommon.

Follicles at all stages of development can be found in both ovaries, except in menopausal women (Fig. 39-6). Most follicles exist as primary follicles, each of which consists of a round oocyte surrounded by a single layer of flattened, epithelium-derived granulosa cells and a basement membrane. The primary follicles constitute an inactive pool of follicles from which all the ovulating follicles develop.

Under the influence of FSH and LH stimulation, 6 to 12 primary follicles develop into secondary (preantral) follicles once every ovulatory cycle. During the development of the secondary follicle, the primary oocyte increases in size, and the surrounding granulosa cells proliferate to form a multilayered wall around it. In addition, cells from the surrounding ovarian interstitium align themselves to form a cellular wall called the *theca*. The cells of the theca become differentiated into two layers:

an inner theca interna, which lies adjacent to the follicular cells, and an outer theca externa. The cells in the theca interna take on epithelioid characteristics similar to those of the granulosa cells and develop the ability to secrete additional sex hormones (estrogen and progesterone). The theca externa develops into a highly vascular connective tissue capsule that becomes the capsule for the developing preantral follicle.

As the follicle enlarges, a single large cavity, or *antrum*, is formed, and some of the granulosa cells and the oocytes are displaced to one side of the follicle by the fluid that accumulates. The secondary oocyte remains surrounded by a crown of granulosa cells, the *corona radiata*. As the granulosa cells continue to divide and the follicle grows, the thecal and granulosa cells cooperate to secrete a follicular fluid that contains a high concentration of estrogen. Selection of a dominant follicle occurs with the conversion to an estrogen microenvironment. The dominant (preovulatory) follicle accumulates a greater mass of granulosa cells, and the theca becomes richly vascular, giving the follicle a hyperemic appearance. The lesser follicles, although continuing to produce some estrogen, atrophy or become atretic.

High levels of estrogen also exert a negative feedback effect on FSH, inhibiting further follicular development and causing an increase in LH levels. This represents the follicular stage of the menstrual cycle. As estrogen suppresses FSH, the actions of LH predominate, and the mature follicle bursts; the oocyte, along with the corona radiata, is ejected from the follicle. The ovum normally is then picked up and transported through the fallopian tube toward the uterus. After ovulation, the follicle collapses, and the luteal stage of the menstrual cycle begins. The granulosa cells are invaded by blood vessels and yellow lipochrome-bearing cells from the theca layer. A rapid accumulation of blood and fluid forms a mass called the *corpus luteum*. Leakage of this blood onto the peritoneal surface that surrounds the ovary is thought to contribute to the *mittelschmerz* ("middle [or intermenstrual] pain") of ovulation. During the luteal stage, progesterone is secreted from the corpus luteum. If fertilization does not take place, the corpus luteum atrophies and is replaced by white scar tissue called the *corpus albicans;* the hormonal support of the endometrium is withdrawn, and menstruation occurs. In the event of fertilization, the corpus luteum remains functional for 3 months and provides hormonal support for pregnancy until the placenta is fully functional.

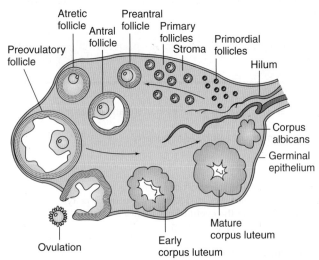

FIGURE 39-6 Schematic diagram of an ovary, showing the sequence of events in the origin, growth, and rupture of an ovarian follicle and the formation and retrogression of a corpus luteum. The atretic follicles are those that show signs of degeneration and death.

In summary, the genitourinary system as a whole serves sexual and reproductive functions throughout a woman's life. The female reproductive system consists of external and internal genitalia. The internal genitalia consist of the vagina, uterus, uterine tubes, and paired ovaries. The uterus is a thick-walled, muscular organ. The wall of the uterus is composed of three layers: the outer perimetrium; the myometrium or muscle layer, which is continuous with the myometrium of the fallopian tubes and the vagina; and the inner lining or endometrium, which is continuous with the lining of the fallopian tubes and vagina.

The gonads, or ovaries, which are internal in the female (unlike the testes in the male), have the dual function of storing the female germ cells, or ova, and producing the female sex hormones. Through the regulation and release of sex hormones, the ovaries influence the development of secondary sexual characteristics, regulation of menstrual cycles, maintenance of pregnancy, and advent of menopause.

Disorders of the Female Reproductive Organs

Disorders of the female genitourinary system have widespread effects on physical and psychological function, affecting sexuality and reproductive function. The reproductive organs are located close to other pelvic structures, particularly those of the urinary system, and disorders of the reproductive system may affect urinary function. This section of the chapter focuses on infections and benign and malignant disorders of the external and internal genitalia.

DISORDERS OF THE EXTERNAL GENITALIA

Bartholin's Gland Cyst and Abscess

A Bartholin's gland cyst is a fluid-filled sac that results from the occlusion of the duct system of the gland.[2] When the cyst becomes infected, the contents become purulent; if the infection goes untreated, an abscess can result. Most commonly cyst and abscess formation follows a bacterial, chlamydial, or gonococcal infection. Cysts can attain the size of an orange and frequently recur. Abscesses can be extremely tender and painful. Treatment of symptomatic cysts consists of the administration of appropriate antibiotics, local application of moist heat, and incision and drainage.

Non-neoplastic Epithelial Disorders

The term *non-neoplastic epithelial disorders* refers to nonmalignant atrophic and hyperplastic changes of the vulvar skin and mucosa.[2] The condition, commonly referred to as *leukoplakia*, presents as white lesions of the vulva. Itching is the most common symptom, and dyspareunia (painful intercourse) is common.

There are two forms of non-neoplastic epithelial lesions: lichen sclerosus and lichen simplex chronicus. *Lichen sclerosus* patches are hypopigmented, parchment-thin, and atrophic. Such lesions occur in all age groups but are most common in postmenopausal women. They may also occur on other areas of the skin. Although slowly progressive in its development, lichen sclerosus is not premalignant. *Lichen simplex chronicus* lesions are thick, gray-white plaques. The thickened epithelium displays a marked increase in superficial keratin, which imparts a white

appearance to the vulva. Because squamous carcinoma may also appear as white plaques, biopsy is required to distinguish benign from malignant lesions.

Vulvodynia

Vulvodynia is a syndrome of unexplained vulvar pain, also referred to as *vulvar pain syndrome* or *burning vulva syndrome*. It is a chronic disorder characterized by burning, stinging, irritation, and rawness. Several forms or subsets of vulvodynia have been identified, including cyclic vulvovaginitis, vulvar dermatoses, vulvar vestibular syndrome, and vulvar dysesthesia. Because vulvodynia is a multifaceted condition, certain subsets may coexist with others.

Cyclic vulvodynia demonstrates episodic flares that occur only before menses or after coitus. *Vulvar dermatoses* are manifested by pruritus, and in some cases pain develops progressively during the perimenopausal or postmenopausal period. Vulvar dermatoses include thick and scaly (*e.g.*, papulosquamous) lesions. Erosions may occur from excessive scratching.

Vulvar vestibulitis syndrome (VVS) is characterized by pain at onset of intercourse (*i.e.*, insertional dyspareunia), localized point tenderness near the vaginal opening, and sensitivity to tampon placement, tight-fitting pants, bicycling, or prolonged sitting. It is the leading cause of dyspareunia in women younger than 50 years of age. VVS can be primary (present from first contact) or secondary (developing after a period of comfortable sexual relations). Etiology is unknown, but VVS can evolve from chronic vulvar inflammation or trauma. Nerve fibers to the vestibular epithelium become highly sensitized, causing neurons in the dorsal horn to respond abnormally, which transforms the sensation of touch in the vestibule into pain (allodynia).[5]

Vulvar dysesthesia, also known as *idiopathic* or *essential vulvodynia*, involves severe, constant, widespread burning that interferes with daily activities. No abnormalities are found on examination, but there is diffuse and variable hypersensitivity and altered sensation to light touch. The quality of pain shares many of the features of neuropathic pain, particularly complex regional pain syndrome (see Chapter 34) or pudendal neuralgia. Although the cause of the neuropathic pain is unknown, it has been suggested that it may result from myofascial restrictions affecting sacral and pelvic floor nerves. Surface electromyography–assisted pelvic floor muscle rehabilitation has been shown to be an effective and long-term cure for dysesthetic vulvodynia.[6]

Possible causes for other forms of vulvodynia include candidal hypersensitivity related to chronic recurrent yeast infections; chemical irritation or drug effects, especially prolonged use of topical steroid creams; the irritating effects of elevated urinary levels of calcium oxalate; immunoglobulin A (IgA) deficiency; and dermatoses such as lichen sclerosus, lichen planus, or squamous cell hyperplasia. Herpes simplex virus may be related to episodic vulvodynia, and long-term viral suppressive therapy may be of benefit to women with known herpes simplex virus infection who experience multiple outbreaks each year.

Treatment for this chronic, often debilitating problem is aimed at symptom relief and elimination of suspected underlying problems. Careful history taking and physical assessment are essential for differential diagnosis and treatment. Regimens can include long-term vaginal or oral antifungal therapy, avoidance of potential irritants, cleaning with water only or a gentle soap, sitz baths with baking soda, emollients such as vitamin E or vegetable oil for lubrication, low-oxalate diet plus calcium citrate supplements (calcium binds oxalate in the bowel and citrate inhibits the formation of oxalate crystals), and topical anesthetic or steroid ointments. The tricyclic antidepressants are often used to treat the neuropathic pain associated with vulvar dysesthesia. Psychosocial support often is needed because this condition can cause strain in sexual, family, and work relationships. Vulvodynia often needs to be managed from a multidimensional, chronic pain perspective.[6]

Premalignant and Malignant Neoplasms

Carcinoma of the vulva accounts for approximately 3% of all cancers of the female genitourinary system, occurring most often in women 60 years of age or older.[2,7,8] Approximately 85% of vulvar malignancies are squamous cell carcinomas; the remainder are adenocarcinomas, melanomas, and basal cell carcinomas.

Vulvar intraepithelial neoplasia (VIN), which is a precursor lesion of squamous cell carcinoma, represents a spectrum of neoplastic changes that range from minimal cellular atypia to invasive cancer. VIN appears to be caused by the oncogenic (cancer-promoting) potential of certain strains of human papillomavirus (HPV) and is associated with the type of vulvar cancer found in younger women (see Chapter 40).[7] This virus is the known cause of sexually transmitted vulvar condyloma acuminatum (genital warts). VIN lesions may take many forms. The lesions may be singular or multicentric, macular, papular, or plaquelike. VIN frequently is multicentric, and 10% to 30% are associated with squamous neoplasms in the vagina and cervix.[2] Microscopically, VIN presents as a proliferative process characterized by cells with abnormal epithelial maturation, nuclear enlargement, and nuclear atypia. The same system that is used for grading cervical cancer is used for vulvar cancer.[2] Spontaneous regression of VIN lesions has been reported, usually in younger women. The risk of progression to invasive cancer increases in older women (>45 years) and in immunosuppressed women.

A second form of vulvar cancer, which is seen more often in older women, is usually preceded by vulvar non-neoplastic disorders (VNED) such as chronic vulvar irritation or lichen sclerosus. The pruritus associated with VNED causes an itch-scratch cycle that can lead to squamous cell hyperplasia. If left untreated, the hyperplasia progresses to atypia (differentiated VIN), and invasive cell carcinoma develops in many of these women after 6 to 7 years.[8] The etiology of this type of VIN is infrequently associated with HPV infection.

The initial lesion of squamous cell vulvar carcinoma may appear as an inconspicuous thickening of the skin, a small raised area or lump, or an ulceration that fails to heal. It may be single or multiple and vary in color from white to velvety red or black. The lesions may resemble eczema or dermatitis and may produce few symptoms other than pruritus, local discomfort, and exudation. A recurrent, persistent, pruritic vulvitis may be the only complaint. The symptoms frequently are treated with various home remedies before medical treatment is sought. The lesion may become secondarily infected, causing pain and discomfort. The malignant lesion gradually spreads superficially or as a deep furrow involving all of one labial side. Because there are many lymph channels around the vulva, the cancer metastasizes freely to the regional lymph nodes. The most common extension is to the superficial inguinal, deep femoral, and external iliac lymph nodes.

Early diagnosis is important in the treatment of vulvar carcinoma. Because malignant lesions can vary in appearance and commonly are mistaken for other conditions, biopsy and treatment often are delayed. Any vulvar lesion that is increasing in size or has an unusual warty appearance should be sampled for biopsy.[7] Treatment is primarily wide surgical excision of the lesion for noninvasive cancer and radical excision or vulvectomy with node resection for invasive cancer.[8]

DISORDERS OF THE VAGINA

The normal vaginal ecology depends on the delicate balance of hormones and bacterial flora. The vagina is lined with mucus-secreting stratified squamous epithelial cells. The epithelial cells of the vagina, like other tissues of the reproductive system, respond to changing levels of the ovarian sex hormones. Estrogen stimulates the proliferation and maturation of the vaginal mucosa; this results in a thickening of the vaginal mucosa and an increased glycogen content of the epithelial cells.

Vaginal tissue usually is moist, with a pH maintained within the bacteriostatic range of 3.8 to 4.2. Döderlein bacilli, part of the normal vaginal flora, metabolize glycogen, and in the process produce the lactic acid that normally maintains the vaginal pH below 4.5. The vaginal ecology can be disrupted at many levels, rendering the area susceptible to infection. Pregnancy and the use of oral contraceptive agents increase the amount of estrogen in the system. Diabetes or a prediabetic state may increase the glycogen content of the cells. The use of systemic antibiotics may decrease the number of lactobacilli in the vagina. Decreased estrogen stimulation after menopause causes the vaginal mucosa to become thin and dry, often resulting in dyspareunia (i.e., painful intercourse), atrophic vaginitis, and occasionally in vaginal bleeding.

Vaginitis

Vaginitis is an inflammatory condition of the vagina. It is characterized by vaginal discharge and burning, itching, redness, and swelling of vaginal tissues. Pain often occurs with urination and sexual intercourse. Vaginitis may be caused by chemical irritants, foreign bodies, and infectious agents. The causes of vaginitis differ in various age groups.

In premenarchal girls, most vaginal infections have non-specific causes, such as poor hygiene, intestinal parasites, or the presence of foreign bodies. *Candida albicans, Trichomonas vaginalis*, and bacterial vaginosis are the most common causes of vaginitis in the childbearing years, and some of these organisms can be transmitted sexually[9,10] (see Chapter 40). Atrophic vaginitis, which is caused by a decrease in estrogen levels, is the most common form in postmenopausal women or after removal of the ovaries. Estrogen deficiency results in a lack of regenerative growth of the vaginal epithelium, rendering these tissues more susceptible to infection and irritation. Döderlein's bacilli disappear, and the vaginal secretions become less acidic.

Every woman has a normal vaginal discharge during the menstrual cycle, but it should not cause burning or itching or have an unpleasant odor. These symptoms suggest inflammation or infection. Because these symptoms are common to the different types of vaginitis, precise identification of the organism is essential for proper treatment. A careful history should include information about systemic disease conditions, the use of drugs such as antibiotics that foster the growth of *C. albicans,* dietary habits, stress, and other factors that alter the resistance of vaginal tissue to infections. A physical examination usually is done to evaluate the nature of the discharge and its effects on the genital structures. Treatment is directed at the cause of the disorder.

Cancer of the Vagina

Primary cancers of the vagina are extremely rare. They account for approximately 1% of all cancers of the female reproductive system, and of these 95% are squamous cell carcinomas.[2] Adenocarcinoma of the vagina is a rare tumor that is seen almost exclusively in women exposed in utero to diethylstilbestrol (DES).[2,11] DES is a nonsteroidal synthetic estrogen that was commonly prescribed between 1940 and 1971 to prevent miscarriage. Fortunately, less than 0.14% of women exposed to DES actually develop adenocarcinoma. Vaginal cancers may also result from local extension of cervical cancer, from local irritation such as occurs with prolonged use of a pessary, or from exposure to sexually transmitted HPV infections.

Like vulvar carcinoma, carcinoma of the vagina is largely a disease of older women. Approximately half are women 60 years of age or older at the time of diagnosis. The most common symptom of vaginal carcinoma is abnormal bleeding. Twenty percent of women are asymptomatic, with the cancer being discovered during a routine pelvic examination. The anatomic proximity of the vagina to other pelvic structures (*e.g.,* urethra, bladder, rectum) permits early spread to these areas. Pelvic pain, dysuria, constipation, and vaginal discharge can be associated symptoms.

Vaginal cancer is often detected by vaginal cytology (Papanicolaou test [Pap smear]) or examination of the vagina during a pelvic examination. It is recommended that women who have been exposed to DES have an initial colposcopic examination to identify areas of abnormal vaginal epithelium, followed by yearly Pap smears. It is also important for women who have had a hysterectomy to continue to have vaginal Pap smears every 3 to 5 years for early detection of vaginal cancer. Diagnosis of vaginal cancer requires biopsy of suspect lesions or areas.

Treatment of vaginal cancer must take into consideration the type of cancer; the size, location, and spread of the lesion; and the woman's age. Local excision, laser vaporization, or a loop electrode excision procedure (LEEP) can be considered with stage 0 squamous cell cancer. Radical surgery (a total hysterectomy, pelvic lymph node dissection, partial vaginectomy) and radiation therapy are both curative with more advanced cancers.

DISORDERS OF THE UTERINE CERVIX

The cervix is composed of two distinct types of tissue. The exocervix, or visible portion, is covered with stratified squamous epithelium, which also lines the vagina. The endocervical canal is lined with columnar epithelium. The junction of these two tissue types (*i.e.,* squamocolumnar junction) appears at various locations on the cervix at different points in a woman's life (Fig. 39-7). During periods of high estrogen production, particularly fetal existence, menarche, and the first pregnancy, the cervix everts or turns outward, exposing the columnar epithelium to the vaginal environment. The combination of estrogen and low vaginal pH leads to a gradual transformation from columnar to squamous epithelium—a process called *metaplasia* (see Chapter 2). The dynamic area of change where metaplasia occurs is called the *transformation zone.*[12] The transformation zone is a critical area for the development of cervical cancer. During metaplasia, the newly developed squamous epithelial cells are vulnerable to the development of dysplastic changes.

The process of transformation is increased by trauma and infections occurring during the reproductive years.[12]

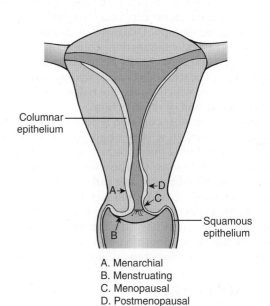

Columnar epithelium

Squamous epithelium

A. Menarchial
B. Menstruating
C. Menopausal
D. Postmenopausal

FIGURE 39-7 Location of squamocolumnar junction (transformation zone) in menarchial, menstruating, menopausal, and postmenopausal women.

As the squamous epithelium expands and obliterates the surface columnar papillae, it covers and obstructs crypt openings, with trapping of mucus in the deeper crypts (glands) to form retention cysts, called *nabothian cysts*.[2] These are benign cysts that require no treatment unless they become so numerous that they cause cervical enlargement. The nabothian cyst farthest away from the external cervical os indicates the outer aspect of the transformation zone.

Cervicitis and Cervical Polyps

Cervicitis is an acute or chronic inflammation of the cervix. Acute cervicitis may result from the direct infection of the cervix or may be secondary to a vaginal or uterine infection. It may be caused by a variety of infective agents, including *C. albicans, T. vaginalis, Neisseria gonorrhoeae, Chlamydia trachomatis, Ureaplasma urealyticum*, and herpes simplex virus. Chronic cervicitis represents a low-grade inflammatory process. It is common in parous women and may be a sequela to minute lacerations that occur during childbirth, instrumentation, or other trauma. The organisms usually are a nonspecific type, often staphylococcal, streptococcal, or coliform bacteria.

With acute cervicitis, the cervix becomes reddened and edematous. Irritation from the infection results in copious mucopurulent drainage and leukorrhea. The symptoms of chronic cervicitis are less well defined: the cervix may be ulcerated or normal in appearance; it may contain nabothian cysts; the cervical os may be distorted by old lacerations or everted to expose areas of columnar epithelium; and a mucopurulent drainage may be present.

Untreated cervicitis may extend to include the development of pelvic cellulitis, low back pain, painful intercourse, cervical stenosis, dysmenorrhea, and ascending infection of the uterus or fallopian tubes. Depending on the causative agent, acute cervicitis is treated with appropriate antibiotic therapy. Diagnosis of chronic cervicitis is based on vaginal examination, colposcopy, cytologic (Pap) smears, and occasionally biopsy to exclude malignant changes. The treatment usually involves cryosurgery or cauterization, which causes the tissues to slough and leads to eradication of the infection.

Polyps are the most common lesions of the cervix.[2,12] They can be found in women of all ages, but their incidence is higher during the reproductive years. Polyps are soft, velvety red lesions; they usually are pedunculated and often are found protruding through the cervical os. They usually develop as a result of inflammatory hyperplasia of the endocervical mucosa. Polyps typically are asymptomatic but may have associated postcoital bleeding. Most are benign, but they should be removed and examined by a pathologist to exclude malignant change.

Cancer of the Cervix

Cervical cancer is readily detected and, if detected early, is the most easily cured of all the cancers of the female reproductive system. Fifty years ago cervical cancer was the most common cause of cancer deaths in women in the United States. However, with early detection and treatment made possible by the introduction of the Pap smear, the death rate has declined by two thirds to its present rank of eighth leading cause of cancer mortality.[12] In sharp contrast to this reduced mortality rate, the detection rate of early cancer and precancerous conditions is high. However, worldwide the incidence of and mortality associated with cervical cancer are second only to breast cancer, and in parts of the developing world, cervical cancer is the major cause of death in women of reproductive age.[13]

Epidemiology and Pathogenesis. Carcinoma of the cervix is often considered a sexually transmitted disease. A preponderance of evidence suggests a causal link between HPV infection and cervical cancer. Certain strains of HPV (types 16 and 18) are associated with cervical cancer (high risk) versus condylomata (6, 11, 42, 44, 53, 54, 62, 66).[2,12] Because these viruses are spread by sexual contact, their association with cervical cancer provides a tempting hypothesis to explain the relation between sexual practices and cervical cancer. However, the evidence does not implicate HPV as the only factor. Other factors such as smoking, nutrition, and sexual partners may play a contributing role in determining whether a woman with HPV infection develops cervical cancer. The recent development of an HPV type 16 vaccine offers hope for the future prevention of cervical cancer.[14]

KEY CONCEPTS

Gynecologic Cancers

➤ Certain types of sexually transmitted human papillomaviruses are risk factors for cervical intraepithelial neoplasia, which can be a precursor lesion of invasive carcinoma.

➤ Endometrial cancers, which are seen most frequently in women 55 to 65 years of age, are strongly associated with conditions that produce excessive estrogen stimulation and endometrial hyperplasia.

➤ Ovarian cancer is the second most common female cancer and the most lethal because there are few early signs and no good screening tests. The most significant risk factors for ovarian cancers are the length of time that a woman's ovarian cycles are not suppressed by pregnancy, lactation, or oral contraceptive use, and family history.

➤ Breast cancer is the most common cancer in women and the second most common cause of cancer death in women. Risk factors include age, family history, and hormonal influences.

Precursor and Malignant Lesions. One of the most important advances in the early diagnosis and treatment of cancer of the cervix was made possible by the observation that this cancer arises from precursor lesions, which begin with the development of atypical cervical cells. These atypical cells gradually progress to carcinoma in situ and to invasive cancer of the cervix. Atypical cells differ from normal cervical squamous epithelium. There are changes in the nuclear and cytoplasmic parts of the cell and more variation in cell size and shape (*i.e.*, dysplasia). Carcinoma in situ is localized to the epithelial layer, whereas invasive cancer of the cervix spreads to deeper layers.[2,12]

A system of grading devised to describe the dysplastic changes of cancer precursors uses the term *cervical intraepithelial neoplasia* (CIN).[2,12] This histologic terminology system divides the precursors according to the extent of involvement of the epithelial thickness of the cervix. (Table 39-2). It was presumed that CIN represented a single, progressive disease process. Current understanding of the pathogenesis of cervical cancer precursors now suggests two distinct biologic entities: a productive viral infection (HPV) which can regress spontaneously (mild dysplasia or CIN1), and a true neoplastic process confined to the epithelium (CIN2 or CIN3). CIN histologic terminology has been largely replaced with cytopathology terms for these two biologic entities: *low-grade squamous intraepithelial lesion* (LSIL) and *high-grade squamous intraepithelial lesion* (HSIL).[12] The precursor lesions can exist in a reversible form, which may regress spontaneously, persist, or progress and undergo malignant change. Studies of the "natural history" of these precursor lesions have yielded variable rates of progression and regression. Generally, only a small percentage of lesions progress to invasive carcinoma. HSIL has a much greater potential for progressing than does LSIL. De novo development of HSIL has also been demonstrated, challenging the concept that LSIL is always a precursor to HSIL. Cancers of the cervix have a long latent period; untreated dysplasia gradually progresses to carcinoma in situ, which may remain static for 7 to 10 years before it becomes invasive. After the preinvasive period, growth may be rapid, and survival rates decline significantly depending on the extent of disease at the time of diagnosis.[2]

The atypical cellular changes that precede frank neoplastic changes consistent with cancer of the cervix can be recognized by a number of direct and microscopic techniques, including the Pap smear, colposcopy, and cervicography. Currently, Pap smears are used for cervical cancer screening. The purpose of the Pap smear is to detect the presence of abnormal cells on the surface of the cervix or in the endocervix (see Chapter 5). After an extensive review of the literature, the American Cancer Society (ACS) in late 2002 released revised guidelines for cervical cancer screening[15] (Chart 39-1). The U.S. Preventive Services Task Force (USPSTF) screening guidelines were also updated in 2002.[16] Although many clinicians and women themselves are reluctant to move away from yearly Pap smears, the evidence about the natural progression of cervical cancer supports the position that this is a more cost-effective approach to screening.

Clinical Course and Management. Cervical cancer in its early stages often manifests as a poorly defined lesion of the endocervix. Frequently, women with cervical cancer present with abnormal vaginal bleeding, spotting, and discharge.[11] Although bleeding may occur without a specific trigger, it is reported most frequently after intercourse. Women with more advanced disease may present with pelvic or back pain that may radiate down the leg, hematuria, fistulas (rectovaginal or vesicovaginal), or with evidence of metastatic disease to supraclavicular or inguinal lymph node areas.

Diagnosis of cervical cancer requires pathologic confirmation. Pap smear results demonstrating SIL often require further evaluation by colposcopy. This is a vaginal examination that is done using a colposcope, an instrument that affords a well-lit and magnified stereoscopic view of the cervix. During colposcopy, the cervical tissue may be stained with an iodine solution (*i.e.*, Schiller test) or acetic acid solution to accentuate topographic or vascular changes that can differentiate normal from abnormal tissue. A biopsy sample may be obtained from suspect areas and examined microscopically. An alternative diagnostic tool in areas where colposcopy is not readily available is

TABLE 39-2	**Classification Systems for Papanicolaou Smears**	
Dysplasia/Neoplasia	**CIN**	**Bethesda System**
Benign	Benign	Negative for intraepithelial lesion or malignancy
Benign with inflammation	Benign with inflammation	Negative for intraepithelial lesion or malignancy, ASC-US
Mild dysplasia	CIN 1	Low-grade SIL, ASC-H
Moderate dysplasia	CIN 2	High-grade SIL
Severe dysplasia and carcinoma in situ	CIN 3	
Invasive cancer	Invasive cancer	Invasive cancer

CIN, cervical intraepithelial neoplasia; SIL, squamous intraepithelial lesion; ASC-US, atypical squamous cell of undetermined significance; ASC-H, cannot rule out high-grade SIL.
Adapted from information in Rubin E., Gorstein F., Rubin R. et al. (Eds.). (2005). *Rubin's pathology: Clinicopathologic foundations of medicine* (4th ed., pp. 945–946). Philadelphia: Lippincott Williams & Wilkins; Solomon D., Davey D., Kurman R., et al., Forum Group Members and Bethesda 2001 Workshop. (2002). The 2001 Bethesda System. *Journal of the American Medical Association* 287(16), 2114–2119.

CHART 39-1

Guidelines for Cervical Cancer Screening Using Papanicolaou (Pap) Smear

- Screening should begin 3 years after first vaginal intercourse or after age 21, whichever comes first.*
- Women 30 years of age and older may be screened at longer intervals after three consecutive normal/negative cytology results.
- Screening may be discontinued in women aged 70 years and older if they had adequate screening with normal Pap smears and are not otherwise at increased risk for cervical cancer.
- Women who have had a total hysterectomy with removal of the cervix do not need screening unless the surgery was performed to treat cervical cancer or a precancerous condition.
- If a woman has risk factors, such as HPV infection, DES exposure in utero, or strong family history of cervical cancer, more frequent Pap smears may be recommended.

*Testing should be done every year with the regular Pap test or every 2 years using the newer liquid-based Pap test.
(Adapted from American Cancer Society. (2005). *Detailed guide: Cervical cancer.* Available: www.cancer.org.

cervicography, a noninvasive photographic technique that provides permanent objective documentation of normal and abnormal cervical patterns. Acetic acid (5%) is applied to the cervix, a cervicography camera is used to take photographs, and the projected cervicogram (*i.e.*, slide after film developing) can be sent for expert evaluation.[17]

Early treatment of cervical cancer involves removal of the lesion by one of various techniques. Biopsy or local cautery may itself be therapeutic. Electrocautery, cryosurgery, or carbon dioxide laser therapy may be used to treat moderate to severe dysplasia that is limited to the exocervix (*i.e.*, squamocolumnar junction clearly visible). Loop electrosurgical excision, which is performed on an outpatient basis, is often used. In certain situations, cervical conization (removal of tissue around the external os of the cervix), and (rarely) hysterectomy are performed.[11]

Depending on the stage of involvement of the cervix, invasive cancer is treated with radiation therapy, surgery, or both. External-beam radiation and intracavitary cesium irradiation (*i.e.*, insertion of a closed metal cylinder containing radioactive cesium) can be used in the treatment of cervical cancer.[11] Intracavitary radiation provides direct access to the central lesion and increases the tolerance of the cervix and surrounding tissues, permitting curative levels of radiation to be used. External-beam radiation eliminates metastatic disease in pelvic lymph nodes and other structures, as well as shrinking the cervical lesion to optimize the effects of intracavitary radiation. Surgery can include extended hysterectomy (*i.e.*, removal of the uterus, fallopian tubes, ovaries, and upper portion of the vagina) without pelvic lymph node dissection, radical hysterectomy with pelvic lymph node dissection, or pelvic exenteration (*i.e.*, removal of all pelvic organs, including the bladder, rectum, vulva, and vagina). The choice of treatment is influenced by the stage of the disease as well as the woman's age and health.

DISORDERS OF THE UTERUS

Infectious Disorders of the Uterus and Pelvic Structures

The uterus and pelvic structures are subject to infections by a number of agents, including *N. gonorrhoeae* and *C. trachomatis*, as well as endogenous microorganisms such as anaerobes, *Haemophilus influenzae*, enteric gram-negative rods, and streptococci. Tuberculosis salpingitis is rare in the United States but more common in developing countries.

Endometritis. The endometrium and myometrium are relatively resistant to infections, primarily because the endocervix normally forms a barrier to ascending infections. Acute endometritis is uncommon and usually occurs after the cervical barrier is compromised by abortion, delivery, or instrumentation.[2,12] Curettage is diagnostic and often curative because it removes the necrotic tissue that has served as a site of infection.

Chronic inflammation of the endometrium is associated with intrauterine devices (IUD), pelvic inflammatory disease, and retained products of conception after delivery or abortion. The presence of plasma cells (which are not present in the normal endometrium) is required for diagnosis. The clinical picture is variable, but often includes abnormal vaginal bleeding, mild to severe uterine tenderness, fever, malaise, and foul-smelling discharge. Treatment involves oral or intravenous antibiotic therapy, depending on the severity of the condition.

Pelvic Inflammatory Disease. Pelvic inflammatory disease (PID) is an inflammation of the upper reproductive tract that involves the uterus (endometritis), fallopian tubes (salpingitis), or ovaries (oophoritis). Most women with acute salpingitis have *N. gonorrhoeae* or *C. trachomatis* identified in the reproductive tract. PID is a polymicrobial infection, and the cause varies by geographic location and population.

The organisms that cause PID ascend through the endocervical canal to the endometrial cavity and then to the tubes and ovaries. The endocervical canal is slightly dilated during menstruation, allowing bacteria to gain entrance to the uterus and other pelvic structures. After entering the upper reproductive tract, the organisms multiply rapidly in the favorable environment of the sloughing endometrium and ascend to the fallopian tube. Factors that predispose women to the development of PID include an age of 16 to 24 years, unmarried status, nulliparity, history of multiple sexual partners, and previous history of PID.

The symptoms of PID include lower abdominal pain, which may start just after a menstrual period; purulent cervical discharge; pelvic tenderness; and an exquisitely painful cervix. Fever (>101°F), increased erythrocyte sedimentation rate, and an elevated white blood cell count (>10,000 cells/mL) commonly are seen, even though the woman may not appear acutely ill.[18]

Diagnosis is based on the presence of lower abdominal pain and pelvic or cervical tenderness. A newer test involves measurement of C-reactive protein in the blood. Elevated C-reactive protein levels equate with inflammation.[18] Endocervical cultures may be done to document the presence of *N. gonorrhoeae* or *C. trachomatis*. Transvaginal ultrasonography or imaging techniques may be used. Laparoscopy is often used to confirm a diagnosis of PID.

Treatment is aimed at preventing complications, which can include pelvic adhesions, infertility, ectopic pregnancy, chronic abdominal pain, and tubo-ovarian abscesses. It may involve hospitalization with intravenous administration of antibiotics. If the condition is diagnosed early, outpatient antibiotic therapy may be sufficient.

Endometriosis

Endometriosis is the condition in which functional endometrial tissue is found in ectopic sites outside the uterus. The site may be the ovaries, posterior broad ligaments, uterosacral ligaments, pouch of Douglas (cul-de-sac), pelvis, vagina, vulva, perineum, or intestines (Fig. 39-8). Rarely, endometrial implants have been found in the nostrils, umbilicus, lungs, and limbs.

The cause of endometriosis is unknown. There appears to have been an increase in its incidence in the developed Western countries during the past four to five decades. Approximately 10% to 15% of premenopausal women have some degree of endometriosis. The incidence may be higher in women with infertility (15% to 70%) or women younger than 20 years of age with chronic pelvic pain (47% to 73%).[19] It is more common in women who

have postponed childbearing. Risk factors for endometriosis may include early menarche; regular periods with shorter cycles (<27 days), longer duration (>7 days), or heavier flow; increased menstrual pain; and other first-degree relatives with the condition.

Several theories attempt to account for endometriosis.[2] One theory suggests that menstrual blood containing fragments of endometrium is forced upward through the fallopian tubes into the peritoneal cavity.[2,20] Retrograde menstruation is not an uncommon phenomenon, and it is unknown why endometrial cells implant and grow in some women but not in others. Another proposal is that dormant, immature cellular elements, spread over a wide area during embryonic development, persist into adult life and that the ensuing metaplasia accounts for the development of ectopic endometrial tissue.[2] Another theory suggests that the endometrial tissue may metastasize through the lymphatics or vascular system.[2] Genetics, immunity, and environmental factors also have been studied as contributing factors to the development of endometriosis.[20]

The gross pathologic changes that occur in endometriosis differ with location and duration. In the ovary, the endometrial tissue may form cysts (*i.e.*, endometriomas filled with old blood that resembles chocolate syrup [chocolate cysts]). Rupture of these cysts can cause peritonitis and adhesions. Elsewhere in the pelvis, the tissue may take the form of small hemorrhagic lesions that may be black, bluish, red, clear, or opaque. Some may be surrounded by scar tissue. These ectopic implants respond to hormonal stimulation in the same way normal endometrium does, becoming proliferative and then secretory, finally undergoing menstrual breakdown. Bleeding into the surrounding structures can cause pain and the development of significant pelvic adhesions. Extensive fibrotic tissue can develop and occasionally cause bowel obstruction.

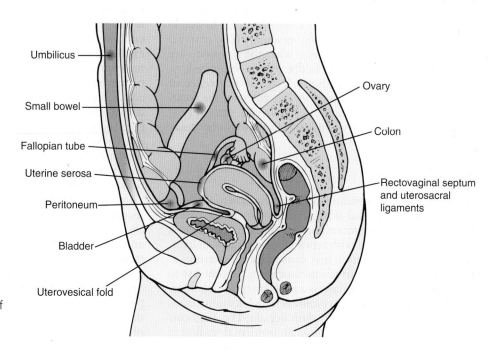

FIGURE 39-8 Common locations of endometriosis in the pelvis and abdomen.

Endometriosis may be difficult to diagnose because its symptoms mimic those of other pelvic disorders. The severity of the symptoms does not always reflect the extent of the disease. The classic triad of dysmenorrhea, dyspareunia, and infertility strongly suggests endometriosis. Accurate diagnosis can be accomplished only through laparoscopy. This minimally invasive surgery allows direct visualization of pelvic organs to determine the presence and extent of endometrial lesions. Imaging techniques including ultrasonography and magnetic resonance imaging (MRI) can be useful tools in evaluating endometriomas. CA-125 is a serum marker that may be elevated in the presence of endometriosis. It has limitations as a screening tool, but can be useful in monitoring response to therapy and recurrence.[19]

Treatment goals for endometriosis are pain management or restoration of fertility. Treatment modalities fall into three categories: pain relief, endometrial suppression, and surgery. In young, unmarried women, simple observation and antiprostaglandin analgesics (i.e., nonsteroidal anti-inflammatory drugs [NSAIDs]) may be sufficient treatment. The use of hormones to induce physiologic amenorrhea is based on the observation that pregnancy affords temporary relief by inducing atrophy of the endometrial tissue. This can be accomplished through administration of progesterone, oral contraceptive pills, danazol (a synthetic androgen), or long-acting GnRH analogs that inhibit the pituitary gonadotropins and suppress ovulation.[20–22]

Surgery is the definitive therapy for many women with endometriosis. In the past, laparoscopic cautery was limited to mild endometriosis without significant adhesions. More extensive treatment required laparotomy. With the advent of lasers, in-depth treatment of endometriosis or pelvic adhesions can be accomplished by means of laparoscopy. Advantages of laser surgery include better hemostasis, more precision in vaporizing lesions with less damage to surrounding tissue, and better access to areas that are not well visualized or would be difficult to reach with cautery. Radical treatment involves total hysterectomy and bilateral salpingo-oophorectomy (i.e., removal of the fallopian tubes and ovaries) when the symptoms are unbearable or the woman's childbearing is completed.

Treatment offers relief but not cure. Recurrence of endometriosis is not uncommon, regardless of the treatment (except for radical surgery). Recurrence rates appear to correlate with severity of disease. Pregnancy may delay but does not preclude recurrence.

Adenomyosis

Adenomyosis is the condition in which endometrial glands and stroma are found within the myometrium, interspersed between the smooth muscle fibers.[12] It is thought that events associated with repeated pregnancies, deliveries, and uterine involution may cause the endometrium to be displaced throughout the myometrium. In contrast to endometriosis, which usually is a problem of young, infertile women, adenomyosis typically is found in multiparous women in their late fourth or fifth decade. The diagnosis of adenomyosis often is made as an incidental finding in

a uterus removed for symptoms indicative of myoma or hyperplasia. Adenomyosis resolves with menopause. Conservative therapy using oral contraceptives or GnRH agonists is the first choice for treatment. Hysterectomy (with preservation of the ovaries in premenopausal women) is considered when this approach fails.

Endometrial Cancer

Endometrial cancer is the most common invasive cancer of the female reproductive tract. It accounts for 7% of all invasive cancers in women, excluding skin cancers.[2] Endometrial cancer occurs more frequently in postmenopausal women (peak age of 55 to 65 years) and is uncommon in women younger than 40 years of age.

A major risk factor for endometrial cancer is prolonged estrogenic stimulation with excessive growth (i.e., hyperplasia) of the endometrium.[11] Obesity, anovulatory cycles, conditions that alter estrogen metabolism, estrogen-secreting neoplasms, and unopposed estrogen therapy all increase the risk of endometrial cancer.[23] Estrogens are synthesized in body fats from adrenal and ovarian androgen precursors; endometrial hyperplasia and endometrial cancer appear to be related to obesity. The degree of risk correlates with body weight, with the risk increasing 10-fold for women who are more than 50 pounds overweight.[12] Ovulatory dysfunction that causes infertility at any age or occurs with declining ovarian function in perimenopausal women also can result in unopposed estrogen and increase the risk of endometrial cancer. Diabetes mellitus, hypertension, and polycystic ovary syndrome are conditions that alter estrogen metabolism and elevate estrogen levels.

Endometrial cancer risk also is increased in women with estrogen-secreting granulosa cell tumors and in women receiving unopposed estrogen therapy. It is the presence of progesterone in the second half of the normal menstrual cycle that matures the endometrium and the withdrawal of progesterone that ultimately results in endometrial sloughing. Long-term unopposed estrogen exposure without periodic addition of progesterone allows for continued endometrial growth and the development of hyperplasia, with or without the presence of atypical cells. A sharp increase in endometrial cancer was seen during the 1970s among middle-aged women who had received unopposed estrogen therapy (i.e., estrogen therapy without progesterone) for menopausal symptoms. It was later determined that it was not the estrogen exposure that increased the risk of cancer, but administration of estrogen without administration of progesterone. Tamoxifen (a selective inhibitor of estradiol at estrogen receptors), which is used in the treatment of breast cancer, exerts a weak estrogenic effect on the endometrium and represents another exogenous risk factor for endometrial cancer.[11]

A small subset of women in whom endometrial cancer develops do not exhibit increased estrogen levels or preexisting hyperplasia. These women usually acquire the disease at an older age. These tumors arise from clones of cancer-initiated mutant cells and are more poorly differentiated. This type of endometrial cancer usually is associated with a poorer prognosis than is the endometrial cancer associated with prolonged estrogen stimulation and endometrial hyperplasia.[23]

The major symptom of endometrial hyperplasia or overt endometrial cancer is abnormal, painless bleeding. In menstruating women, this takes the form of bleeding between periods or excessive, prolonged menstrual flow. In postmenopausal women, any bleeding is abnormal and warrants investigation. Abnormal bleeding is an early warning sign of the disease, and because endometrial cancer tends to be slow growing in its early stages, the chances of cure are good if prompt medical care is sought. Later signs of uterine cancer may include cramping, pelvic discomfort, postcoital bleeding, lower abdominal discomfort, and enlarged lymph nodes.

Although the Pap smear can identify a small percentage of endometrial cancers, it is not a good screening test for the tumor. Endometrial biopsy is far more accurate. Dilatation and curettage (D&C), which consists of dilating the cervix and scraping the uterine cavity, is the definitive procedure for diagnosis because it provides a more thorough evaluation. Transvaginal ultrasonography may be used to determine the endometrial thickness as an indicator of hypertrophy and possible neoplastic change.

The prognosis for endometrial cancer depends on the clinical stage of the disease when it is diagnosed and its histologic grade and type. Surgery and radiation therapy are the most successful methods of treatment for endometrial cancer. With early diagnosis and treatment, the 5-year survival rate is approximately 90%.[2]

Leiomyomas

Leiomyomas are benign neoplasms of smooth muscle origin. They also are known as *myomas* and sometimes are called *fibroids*. These are the most common form of pelvic tumor and are believed to occur in one of every four or five women older than 35 years of age. They are seen more often and their rate of growth is more rapid in black women than in white women. Leiomyomas usually develop in the corpus of the uterus; they may be submucosal, subserosal, or intramural (Fig. 39-9). Intramural fibroids are embedded in the myometrium. They are the most common type of fibroid and present as a symmetric enlargement of the nonpregnant uterus. Subserosal tumors are located beneath the perimetrium of the uterus. These tumors are recognized as irregular projections on the uterine surface; they may become pedunculated, displacing or impinging on other genitourinary structures and causing hydroureter or bladder problems. Submucosal fibroids displace endometrial tissue and are more likely to cause bleeding, necrosis, and infection than either of the other types.

Leiomyomas are asymptomatic approximately half of the time and may be discovered during routine pelvic examination, or they may cause menorrhagia (excessive menstrual bleeding), anemia, urinary frequency, rectal pressure/constipation, abdominal distention, and infrequently pain. Their rate of growth is variable, but they may

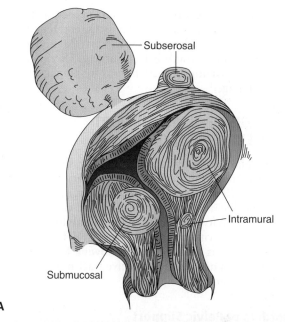

A

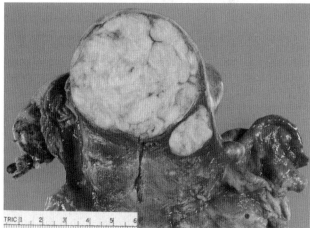

B

FIGURE 39-9 (**A**) Submucosal, intramural, and subserosal leiomyomas. (Redrawn from Green T. H. [1977]. *Gynecology: Essentials of clinical practice* [3rd ed.]. Boston: Little, Brown.) (**B**) A bisected uterus displays a prominent, sharply circumscribed, fleshy tumor. (From Robboy S., Kurman R. J., Merino M. J. [2005]. The female reproductive system. In Rubin E., Gorstein E., Rubin R., et al. [Eds.], *Rubin's pathology: Clinicopathologic foundations of medicine* [4th ed., p. 963]. Philadelphia: Lippincott Williams & Wilkins.)

increase in size during pregnancy or with exogenous estrogen stimulation (*i.e.*, oral contraceptives or menopausal estrogen replacement therapy). Interference with pregnancy is rare unless the tumor is submucosal and interferes with implantation or obstructs the cervical outlet. These tumors may outgrow their blood supply, become infarcted, and undergo degenerative changes.

Most leiomyomas regress with menopause, but if bleeding, pressure on the bladder, pain, or other problems persist, hysterectomy may be required. Myomectomy (removal of just the tumors) can be done to preserve the uterus for future childbearing. Cesarean section may be recommended if the uterine cavity is entered during myomectomy. Hypothalamic GnRH may be used to suppress leiomyoma growth before surgery. Uterine artery embolization is a nonsurgical therapy for management of heavy bleeding.[24]

DISORDERS OF PELVIC SUPPORT AND UTERINE POSITION

The muscular floor of the pelvis is a strong, slinglike structure that supports the uterus, vagina, urinary bladder, and rectum (Fig. 39-10). In the female anatomy, nature is faced with the problems of supporting the pelvic viscera against the force of gravity and increases in intra-abdominal pressure associated with coughing, sneezing, defecation, and laughing while at the same time allowing for urination, defecation, and normal reproductive tract function, especially the delivery of an infant.

Disorders of Pelvic Support

The uterus and the pelvic structures are maintained in proper position by the uterosacral ligaments, round ligaments, broad ligament, and cardinal ligaments. The two cardinal ligaments maintain the cervix in its normal position. The uterosacral ligaments normally hold the uterus in a forward position (Fig. 39-11A). The broad ligament suspends the uterus, fallopian tubes, and ovaries in the pelvis.

Three supporting structures are provided for the abdominal pelvic diaphragm. The bony pelvis provides support and protection for parts of the digestive tract and genitourinary structures, and the peritoneum holds the pelvic viscera in place. However, the main support for the viscera is the pelvic diaphragm, made up of muscles and connective tissue that stretch across the bones of the pelvic outlet. The openings that must exist for the urethra, rectum, and vagina cause an inherent weakness

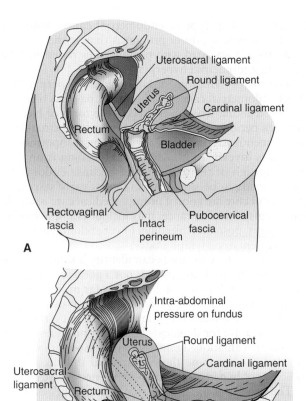

A

B

FIGURE 39-11 (**A**) Normal support of the uterus and vagina. (**B**) Relaxation of pelvic support structures with descent of the uterus as well as formation of cystocele and rectocele. (From Rock J. A., Thompson J. D. [1992]. *Te Linde's operative gynecology* [7th ed.]. Philadelphia: J. B. Lippincott.)

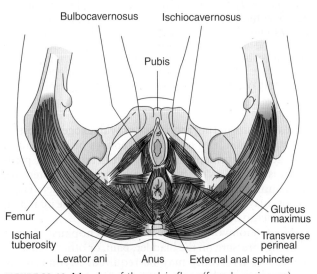

FIGURE 39-10 Muscles of the pelvic floor (female perineum).

in the pelvic diaphragm. Congenital or acquired weakness of the pelvic diaphragm results in widening of these openings, particularly that for the vagina, with the possible herniation of pelvic viscera through the pelvic floor (*i.e.*, prolapse).

Relaxation of the pelvic outlet usually comes about because of overstretching of the perineal supporting tissues during pregnancy and childbirth. Although the tissues are stretched only during these times, there may be no difficulty until later in life, such as the fifth or sixth decade, when further loss of elasticity and muscle tone occurs. Even in a woman who has not borne children, the combination of aging and postmenopausal changes may give rise to problems related to relaxation of the pelvic support structures. It also may result from pelvic tumors and neurologic conditions, such as spina bifida and diabetic neuropathy that interrupt the innervation of pelvic muscles. The three most common conditions associated with this relaxation are cystocele, rectocele, and uterine prolapse. These may occur separately or together.

Cystocele is a herniation of the bladder into the vagina (see Fig. 39-11B). It occurs when the normal muscle support for the bladder is weakened, and the bladder sags below the uterus. The vaginal wall stretches and bulges downward because of the force of gravity and the pressure from coughing, lifting, or straining at stool. The bladder herniates through the anterior vaginal wall, and a cystocele forms. The symptoms include an annoying bearing-down sensation, difficulty in emptying the bladder, frequency and urgency of urination, and cystitis. Stress incontinence may occur at times of increased abdominal pressure, such as during squatting, straining, coughing, sneezing, laughing, or lifting.

Rectocele is the herniation of the rectum into the vagina (see Fig. 39-11B). It occurs when the posterior vaginal wall and underlying rectum bulge forward, ultimately protruding through the introitus as the pelvic floor and perineal muscles are weakened. The symptoms include discomfort because of the protrusion of the rectum and difficulty in defecation. Digital pressure (*i.e.*, splinting) on the bulging posterior wall of the vagina may become necessary for defecation.

Uterine prolapse is the bulging of the uterus into the vagina that occurs when the primary supportive ligaments (*i.e.*, cardinal ligaments) are stretched. Prolapse is ranked as first, second, or third degree, depending on how far the uterus protrudes through the introitus. First-degree prolapse shows some descent, but the cervix has not reached the introitus. In second-degree prolapse, the cervix or part of the uterus has passed through the introitus. The entire uterus protrudes through the vaginal opening in third-degree prolapse (*i.e.*, procidentia). Prolapse often is accompanied by perineal relaxation, cystocele, or rectocele. The symptoms associated with uterine prolapse result from irritation of the exposed mucous membranes of the cervix and vagina and the discomfort of the protruding mass.

Most of the disorders of pelvic relaxation require surgical correction. These are elective surgeries and usually are deferred until after the childbearing years. The symptoms associated with the disorders often are not severe enough to warrant surgical correction. In other cases, the stress of surgery is contraindicated because of other physical disorders; this is particularly true of older women, in whom many of these disorders occur. Kegel exercises, which strengthen the pubococcygeus muscle, may be helpful in cases of mild cystocele or rectocele or after surgical repair to help maintain the improved function. In women with uterine prolapse, a pessary may be inserted to hold the uterus in place and may stave off surgical intervention in women who want to have children or in older women for whom the surgery may pose a significant health risk.

Variations in Uterine Position

Variations in the position of the uterus are common. Some variations are innocuous; others, which may be the result of weakness and relaxation of the perineum, give rise to various problems that compromise the structural integrity of the pelvic floor, particularly after childbirth. The uterus usually is flexed approximately 45 degrees anteriorly, with the cervix positioned posteriorly and downward in the anteverted position. When the woman is standing, the angle of the uterus is such that it lies practically horizontal, resting lightly on the bladder. Asymptomatic, normal variations in the axis of the uterus in relation to the cervix (*i.e.*, flexion) and physiologic displacements that arise after pregnancy or with pelvic pathology include anteflexion, retroflexion, and retroversion (Fig. 39-12). An anteflexed uterus is flexed forward on itself. Retroflexion is flexion backward at the isthmus. Retroversion describes the condition in which the uterus inclines posteriorly while the cervix remains tilted forward. Simple retroversion is the most common variation. It usually is a congenital condition caused by a short anterior vaginal wall and relaxed uterosacral ligaments. Retroversion also can follow certain diseases, such as endometriosis and PID, which produce fibrous tissue adherence with retraction of the fundus posteriorly. Large leiomyomas can also cause the uterus to move into a posterior position. Symptoms of retroversion include dyspareunia with deep penetration and low back pain with menses.

DISORDERS OF THE OVARIES

Disorders of the ovaries frequently cause menstrual and fertility problems. Benign conditions of the ovaries can present as primary lesions of the ovarian structures or as secondary disorders related to hypothalamic, pituitary, or adrenal dysfunction.

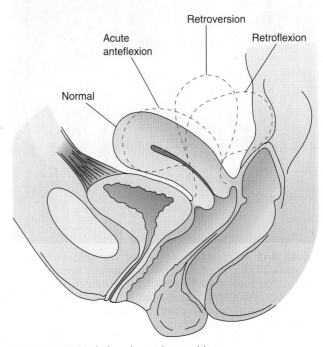

FIGURE 39-12 Variations in uterine position.

Ovarian Cysts

Cysts are the most common form of ovarian tumor.[12] Many are benign. A follicular cyst is one that results from occlusion of the duct of the follicle. Each month, several follicles begin to develop and are blighted at various stages of development. These follicles form cavities that fill with fluid, producing a cyst. The dominant follicle normally ruptures to release the egg (*i.e.*, ovulation) but occasionally persists and continues growing. Likewise, a luteal cyst is a persistent cystic enlargement of the corpus luteum that is formed after ovulation and does not regress in the absence of pregnancy. Functional cysts are asymptomatic unless there is substantial enlargement or bleeding into the cyst. This can cause considerable discomfort or a dull, aching sensation on the affected side. However, usually these regress spontaneously. The cyst may become twisted or may rupture into the intra-abdominal cavity (Fig. 39-13).

Polycystic Ovary Syndrome. Ovarian dysfunction associated with infrequent or absent menses in obese, infertile women was first reported in the 1930s by Stein and Leventhal, for whom the syndrome was originally named. Polycystic ovary syndrome (PCOS) is characterized by varying degrees of hirsutism, obesity, and infertility, and often is associated with hyperinsulinemia or insulin resistance (and is part of the insulin resistance or metabolic syndrome).[25–27]

Chronic anovulation, causing amenorrhea or irregular menses, is now thought to be the underlying cause of the bilaterally enlarged "polycystic" ovaries. Hence, the appearance of the ovary is a sign, not the disease itself. The precise etiology of this condition is still being debated. A possible genetic basis has been suggested with an autosomal dominant mode of inheritance and premature balding as the phenotype in men.[26]

Most women with PCOS have elevated LH levels with normal estrogen and FSH production. Elevated levels of testosterone, dehydroepiandrosterone sulfate (DHEAS), or androstenedione are not uncommon, and these women occasionally have hyperprolactinemia or hypothyroidism. Persistent anovulation results in an estrogen environment that alters the hypothalamic release of GnRH. Increased sensitivity of the pituitary to GnRH results in increased LH secretion and suppression of FSH. This altered LH:FSH ratio often is used as a diagnostic criterion for this condition, but it is not universally present. The presence of some FSH allows for new follicular development; however, full maturation is not attained, and ovulation does not occur. The elevated LH level also results in increased androgen production, which in turn prevents normal follicular development and contributes to the vicious cycle of anovulation.[26] The association between hyperandrogenism and insulin resistance is now well recognized. Evidence suggests that the hyperinsulinemia may lead to the excess androgen production, and several reports have shown that normal ovulation and sometimes pregnancy have occurred when women with hyperandrogenism were treated with insulin-sensitizing drugs.[28,29]

The diagnosis can be suspected from the clinical picture. Although there is no consensus over which laboratory tests should be used, laboratory evaluation to exclude hyperprolactinemia, late-onset adrenal hyperplasia, and adrenogenic-secreting tumors of the ovary and adrenal gland is commonly done. Because insulin resistance is common and may affect treatment, fasting blood glucose is often measured to evaluate for prediabetes or diabetes mellitus. Confirmation with ultrasonography or laparoscopic visualization of the ovaries is not required.

The overall goal of treatment of PCOS is to suppress insulin-facilitated, LH-driven androgen production. Although numerous medications and protocols are available, the choice depends on the manifestations that are bothersome to the woman and her stage in reproductive life. Weight loss also may be beneficial in restoring normal ovulation when obesity is present. If fertility is not desired, oral contraceptives or cyclic progesterone can induce regular menses and prevent the development of endometrial hyperplasia caused by unopposed estrogen. Chronic anovulation can increase a woman's risk of endometrial cancer, cardiovascular disease, and hyperinsulinemia leading to diabetes mellitus. Treatment is essential for anyone with this condition. When medication is ineffective, laser surgery to puncture the multiple follicles may restore normal ovulatory function, although adhesion formation is a potential problem.

When fertility is desired, the condition usually is treated by the administration of the hypothalamic-pituitary–stimulating drug clomiphene citrate or injectable gonadotropins to induce ovulation. These drugs must be used

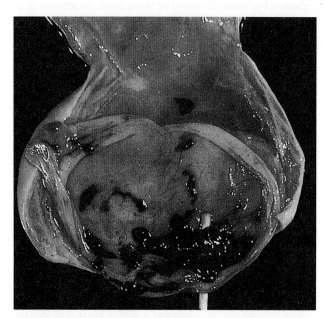

FIGURE 39-13 Follicular cyst of the ovary. The rupture of this thin-walled follicular cyst led to intra-abdominal hemorrhage. The cyst has been opened and rupture site indicated by the dowel stick. (From Robboy S., Kurman R. J., Merino M. J. [2005]. The female reproductive system. In Rubin E., Gorstein E., Rubin R., et al. [Eds.], *Rubin's pathology: Clinicopathologic foundations of medicine* [4th ed., p. 967]. Philadelphia: Lippincott Williams & Wilkins.)

carefully because they can induce extreme enlargement of the ovaries. Metformin, an insulin-sensitizing drug, has been used before or concurrent with ovulation-inducing medications.[29] Use of this drug has been associated with reductions in androgen and LH levels. Thiazolidinediones (TZDs) are also insulin sensitizers and have been used to treat PCOS-related ovulatory dysfunction (and the other features of the metabolic syndrome).

Benign and Functioning Ovarian Tumors

Benign ovarian tumors can be composed of epithelial tissue, endometriosis tissue, fibrocytes and collagen fibers, or primordial germ cells. Benign *epithelial tumors* are almost always serous or mucinous.[2,12] They generally occur in women between the ages of 20 and 60 years and are often large, growing 15 to 30 cm in diameter. They are often cystic, thus the term *cystadenomas.* However, some of the cystadenomas are considered to have low malignant potential. *Endometriomas* are the "chocolate cysts" that develop secondary to ovarian endometriosis (see the section on endometriosis earlier in this chapter). *Ovarian fibromas* are connective tissue tumors composed of fibrocytes and collagen. They range in size from 6 to 20 cm. *Cystic teratomas,* or *dermoid cysts,* are derived from primordial germ cells and are composed of various combinations of well-differentiated ectodermal, mesodermal, and endodermal elements. Not uncommonly, they contain sebaceous material, hair, or teeth.

Benign ovarian tumors are usually asymptomatic unless their size is sufficient to cause abdominal enlargement. Treatment for all ovarian tumors is surgical excision. Ovarian tissue that is not affected by the tumor can be left intact if frozen-section analysis does not reveal malignancy. When ovarian tumors are very large, as is frequently the case with serous or mucinous cystadenomas, the entire ovary must be removed.

The three types of functioning ovarian tumors are estrogen secreting, androgen secreting, and mixed estrogen-androgen secreting. These tumors may be benign or cancerous. One such tumor, the granulosa cell tumor, is associated with excess estrogen production. When it develops during the reproductive period, the persistent and uncontrolled production of estrogen interferes with the normal menstrual cycle, causing irregular and excessive bleeding, endometrial hyperplasia, or amenorrhea and fertility problems. When it develops after menopause, it causes postmenopausal bleeding, stimulation of the glandular tissues of the breast, and other signs of renewed estrogen production. Androgen-secreting tumors inhibit ovulation and estrogen production. They tend to cause hirsutism and development of masculine characteristics, such as baldness, acne, oily skin, breast atrophy, and deepening of the voice. The treatment of functioning ovarian tumors is surgical removal.

Ovarian Cancer

Ovarian cancer is the second most common female genitourinary cancer in the United States,[2] with an estimated 22,220 new cases and 16,210 deaths occurring in 2005.[2] The incidence of ovarian cancer increases with age, being greatest between 65 and 84 years of age. Ovarian cancer is difficult to diagnose, and as much as 75% of women have metastatic disease before the time of discovery.[12]

Cancer of the ovary is complex because of the diversity of tissue types that originate in the ovary. As a result of this diversity, there are several types of ovarian cancers. Malignant neoplasms of the ovary can be divided into three categories: epithelial tumors, germ cell tumors, and gonadal stromal tumors. About 90% of ovarian cancers derive from malignant transformation of the epithelium of the ovary, which is contiguous with the peritoneal mesothelium.[2,11,30] A strong family history of cancer, particularly breast and ovarian cancer, is the most important risk factor. Nulliparity is also associated with increased risk, whereas oral contraceptive use, pregnancy, and lactation are associated with decreased risk. These observations suggest that stimulation of the ovarian epithelium which occurs with nulliparity and uninterrupted ovulation may predispose to ovarian cancer. A strong family history of breast and ovarian cancer, sometimes at an early age, may be related to the presence of an inherited mutation in one of two genes, known as BRCA1 and BRCA2 (see Chapter 5).

Most cancers of the ovary produce no symptoms or the symptoms are so vague that the woman seldom seeks medical care until the disease is far advanced. These vague discomforts include abdominal distress, flatulence, and bloating, especially after ingesting food. These gastrointestinal manifestations may precede other symptoms by months. It is not fully understood why the initial symptoms of ovarian cancer are manifested as gastrointestinal disturbances. It is thought that biochemical changes in the peritoneal fluids may irritate the bowel or that pain originating in the ovary may be referred to the abdomen and be interpreted as a gastrointestinal disturbance. Clinically evident ascites (*i.e.,* fluid in the peritoneal cavity) is seen in approximately one fourth of women with malignant ovarian tumors and is associated with a worse prognosis.

At present, there are no good screening tests or other early methods of detection for ovarian cancer. The serum tumor marker CA-125 is a cell surface antigen that can be used in monitoring therapy and recurrences when preoperative levels have been elevated. Because it lacks sensitivity and specificity, CA-125 has limited value as a single screening test. Transvaginal ultrasonography (TVS) can be used to evaluate ovarian masses for malignant potential. However, cost has prohibited its use as a universal screening tool. The National Institutes of Health Consensus Panel convened in 1995 recommended against widespread screening of women for ovarian cancer.[30] CA-125 with TVS is suggested only for women who are part of a family with hereditary ovarian cancer syndrome (*i.e.,* two or more affected first-degree relatives).

When ovarian cancer is suspected, surgical evaluation is required for diagnosis, complete and accurate staging, and cytoreduction and debulking procedures to reduce the size of the tumor. Recommendations regarding treatment beyond surgery and prognosis depend on the stage of the disease. Most women with early-stage disease require postoperative adjuvant chemotherapy in an attempt to eradicate residual disease. In women with advanced disease, combination chemotherapy is used with the goal of effecting complete clinical remission.[30,31]

In summary, the external genitalia are affected by disorders that affect skin on other parts of the body. Bartholin cysts are the result of occluded ducts in Bartholin glands. They often are painful and can become infected. Vulvar dystrophies are characterized by thinning and hyperplastic thickening of vulvar tissues. Vulvodynia is a chronic vulvar pain syndrome with several classifications and variable treatment results. Cancer of the vulva, which accounts for 3% of all female genitourinary cancers, is associated with HPV infections.

The normal vaginal ecology depends on the delicate balance of hormones and bacterial flora. Vaginitis or inflammation of the vagina is characterized by vaginal discharge and burning, itching, redness, and swelling of vaginal tissues. It may be caused by chemical irritants, foreign bodies, and infectious agents. Primary cancers of the vagina are uncommon, accounting for 1% of all cancers of the female reproductive system. Daughters of women treated with DES to prevent miscarriage are at increased risk for the development of adenocarcinoma of the vagina.

Disorders of the cervix and uterus include inflammatory conditions (*i.e.*, cervicitis and endometritis), cancer (*i.e.*, cervical and endometrial cancer), endometriosis, and leiomyomas. Acute cervicitis, which may be caused by a number of agents, may result from the direct infection of the cervix or may be secondary to a vaginal or uterine infection. Chronic cervicitis represents a low-grade inflammatory process resulting from trauma or nonspecific infectious agents. Cervical cancer arises from precursor lesions that can be detected on a Pap smear, and if detected early, is the most easily cured of all the cancers of the female reproductive system.

Pelvic inflammatory disease is an inflammation of the upper reproductive tract that involves the uterus (endometritis), fallopian tubes (salpingitis), or ovaries (oophoritis). It is most commonly caused by *N. gonorrhoeae* or *C. trachomatis*. Endometriosis is the condition in which functional endometrial tissue is found in ectopic sites outside the uterus. It causes dysmenorrhea, dyspareunia, and infertility.

Adenomyosis is the condition in which endometrial glands and stroma are found in the myometrium interspersed between the smooth muscle fibers. Leiomyomas are benign uterine wall neoplasms of smooth muscle origin. They can develop in the corpus of the uterus and can be submucosal, subserosal, or intramural. Submucosal fibroids displace endometrial tissue and are more likely to cause bleeding, necrosis, and infection than either of the other types. Endometrial cancer is the most common cancer found in the female pelvis; it occurs twice as frequently as cervical cancer. Prolonged estrogen stimulation with hyperplasia of the endometrium has been identified as a major risk factor for endometrial cancer.

Alterations in pelvic support frequently occur because of weaknesses and relaxation of the pelvic floor and perineum. Cystocele and rectocele involve herniation of the bladder or rectum into the vagina. Uterine prolapse occurs when the uterus bulges into the vagina. Pelvic relaxation disorders typically result from overstretching of the perineal supporting muscles during pregnancy and childbirth. The loss of elasticity in these structures that is a normal accompaniment of aging contributes to these problems. Variations in uterine position are common; they include anteflexion, in which the uterus is flexed forward on itself; retroflexion, in which the uterus is flexed backward at the isthmus; and retroversion, in which the uterus inclines posteriorly while the cervix remains tilted forward.

Disorders of the ovaries include benign cysts, functioning ovarian tumors, and cancer of the ovary. Functional cysts usually are asymptomatic unless there is substantial enlargement or bleeding into the cyst or the cyst becomes twisted or ruptures. PCOS is characterized by numerous cystic follicles or follicular cysts; it causes various degrees of hirsutism, obesity, and infertility. Benign ovarian tumors consist of endometriomas, which are chocolate cysts that develop secondarily to ovarian endometriosis; ovarian fibromas, which are connective tissue tumors composed of fibrocytes and collagen; and cystic teratomas or dermoid cysts, which are derived from primordial germ cells and are composed of various combinations of well-differentiated ectodermal, mesodermal, and endodermal elements. Functioning ovarian tumors are of three types: estrogen secreting, androgen secreting, and mixed estrogen-androgen secreting, and may be benign or cancerous. Cancer of the ovary is the second most common female genitourinary cancer and the most lethal. A family history of cancer, particularly breast and ovarian cancer, and nulliparity increase the risk of developing ovarian cancer, whereas oral contraceptive use, pregnancy, and lactation decrease the risk. There are no effective screening methods for ovarian cancer, and often the disease is well advanced at the time of diagnosis.

Menstrual Disorders

Between menarche (*i.e.*, first menstrual bleeding) and menopause (*i.e.*, last menstrual bleeding), the female reproductive system undergoes cyclic changes called the *menstrual cycle*. This includes the maturation and release of oocytes from the ovary during ovulation and periodic vaginal bleeding resulting from the shedding of the endometrial lining. It is not necessary for a woman to ovulate to menstruate; anovulatory cycles do occur. The menstrual cycle produces changes in the breasts, uterus, skin, ovaries, and perhaps other unidentified tissues. The maintenance of the cycle affects biologic and sociologic aspects of a woman's life, including fertility, reproduction, sexuality, and femaleness.

The hormonal control of the menstrual cycle is complex. For example, the biosynthesis of estrogens that occurs in adipose tissue may be a significant source of the hormone. There is evidence that a certain minimum body weight (48 kg) and fat content (16% to 24%) are necessary for menarche to occur and for the menstrual cycle to be maintained. This is supported by the observation of amenorrhea in women with anorexia nervosa, chronic disease, and malnutrition and in those who are long-distance runners. In women with anorexia nervosa, gonadotropin and estradiol secretion, including LH release and responsiveness to the GnRH, can revert to prepubertal levels. With resumption of weight gain and attainment of sufficient body mass, the normal hormonal pattern usually is reinstated. Obesity or significant weight gain also is associated with oligomenorrhea or amenorrhea and infertility, although the mechanism is not well understood.

In addition to their effects on the growth of uterine muscle, estrogens play an important role in the development of the endometrial lining. During anovulatory cycles, continued exposure to estrogens for prolonged periods leads to abnormal hyperplasia of the endometrium and abnormal bleeding patterns. When estrogen production is poorly coordinated during the normal menstrual period, inappropriate bleeding and shedding of the endometrium also can occur.

DYSFUNCTIONAL MENSTRUAL CYCLES

Normal menstrual function results from interactions among the central nervous system, hypothalamus, anterior pituitary, ovaries, and associated target tissues. Although each part of the system is essential to normal function, the ovaries are primarily responsible for controlling the cyclic changes and the length of the menstrual cycle. In most women in the middle reproductive years, menstrual bleeding occurs every 25 to 35 days, with a median length of 28 days.

Dysfunctional Bleeding

Although unexplained uterine bleeding can occur for many reasons, such as pregnancy, abortion, bleeding dyscrasias, and neoplasms, the most frequent cause in the nonpregnant female is what is commonly called *dysfunctional menstrual cycles* or *bleeding*. Dysfunctional cycles may take the form of amenorrhea (absence of menstruation), hypomenorrhea (scanty menstruation), oligomenorrhea (infrequent menstruation, periods more than 35 days apart), menorrhagia (excessive menstruation), or metrorrhagia (bleeding between periods). Menometrorrhagia is heavy bleeding during and between menstrual periods.

Dysfunctional menstrual cycles are related to alterations in the hormones that support normal cyclic endometrial

KEY CONCEPTS

Dysfunctional Menstrual Cycles

→ The pattern of menstrual bleeding tends to be fairly consistent in most healthy women with regard to frequency, duration, and amount of flow.

→ Dysfunctional bleeding in postpubertal women can take the form of absent or scanty periods, infrequent periods, excessive and irregular periods, excessive bleeding during periods, and bleeding between periods.

→ When the basic pattern of bleeding is changed, it is most often due to a lack of ovulation and disturbances in the pattern of hormone secretion.

→ When the basic pattern is undisturbed and there are superimposed episodes of bleeding or spotting, the etiology is more likely to be related to organic lesions or hematologic disorders.

changes. Estrogen deprivation causes retrogression of a previously built-up endometrium and bleeding. Such bleeding often is irregular in amount and duration, with the flow varying with the time and degree of estrogen stimulation and with the degree of estrogen withdrawal. A lack of progesterone can cause abnormal menstrual bleeding; in its absence, estrogen induces development of a much thicker endometrial layer with a richer blood supply. The absence of progesterone results from the failure of any of the developing ovarian follicles to mature to the point of ovulation, with the subsequent formation of the corpus luteum and production and secretion of progesterone.

Periodic bleeding episodes alternating with amenorrhea are caused by variations in the number of functioning ovarian follicles present. If sufficient follicles are present and active and if new follicles assume functional capacity, high levels of estrogen develop, causing the endometrium to proliferate for weeks or even months. In time, estrogen withdrawal and bleeding develop. This can occur for two reasons: an absolute estrogen deficiency may develop when several follicles simultaneously degenerate, or a relative deficiency may develop as the needs of the enlarged endometrial tissue mass exceed the capabilities of the existing follicles, even though estrogen levels remain constant. Estrogen and progesterone deficiency are associated with the absence of ovulation, thus the term *anovulatory bleeding*. Because the vasoconstriction and myometrial contractions that normally accompany menstruation are caused by progesterone, anovulatory bleeding seldom is accompanied by cramps, and the flow frequently is heavy. Anovulatory cycles are common among adolescents during the first several years after menarche, when ovarian function is becoming established, and among perimenopausal women, whose ovarian function is beginning to decline.

Dysfunctional menstrual cycles can originate as a primary disorder of the ovaries or as a secondary defect in ovarian function related to hypothalamic-pituitary stimulation. The latter can be initiated by emotional stress, marked variation in weight (*i.e.*, sudden gain or loss), or nonspecific endocrine or metabolic disturbances. Organic causes of irregular menstrual bleeding include endometrial polyps, submucosal myoma (*i.e.*, fibroid), blood dyscrasia, infection, endometrial cancer, polycystic ovary syndrome, and pregnancy.

The treatment of dysfunctional bleeding depends on what is identified as the probable cause. The minimum evaluation should include a detailed history with emphasis on bleeding pattern and a physical examination. Endocrine studies (FSH:LH ratio, thyroid function tests, prolactin, testosterone, DHEAS), β-human chorionic gonadotropin (β-hCG) pregnancy test, endometrial biopsy, D&C with or without hysteroscopy, and progesterone withdrawal tests may be needed for diagnosis. If organic problems are excluded and alterations in hormone levels are the primary cause, treatment may include the use of oral contraceptives, cyclic progesterone therapy, or long-acting progesterone injections.

Amenorrhea

There are two types of amenorrhea: primary and secondary. Primary amenorrhea is the failure to menstruate by 16 years, or by 14 years of age if failure to menstruate is accompanied by absence of secondary sex characteristics. Secondary amenorrhea is the cessation of menses for at least 6 months in a woman who has established normal menstrual cycles. Primary amenorrhea usually is caused by gonadal dysgenesis, congenital müllerian agenesis, testicular feminization, or a hypothalamic-pituitary-ovarian axis disorder. Causes of secondary amenorrhea include ovarian, pituitary, or hypothalamic dysfunction and destruction of the endometrial cavity by chronic infections such as tuberculosis or destruction of the endometrium by curettage (surgical scraping). Another cause is anorexia nervosa or participation in athletic activities to the extent that there is an alteration in the critical body fat–muscle ratio needed for menses to occur.[32]

Diagnostic evaluation of amenorrhea resembles that for dysfunctional uterine bleeding, with the possible addition of a computed tomographic scan to exclude a pituitary tumor. Treatment is based on correcting the underlying cause and inducing menstruation with cyclic progesterone or combined estrogen-progesterone regimens.

DYSMENORRHEA

Dysmenorrhea is pain or discomfort with menstruation. Although not usually a serious medical problem, it causes some degree of monthly disability for a significant number of women. There are two forms of dysmenorrhea: primary and secondary. Primary dysmenorrhea is menstrual pain that is not associated with a physical abnormality or pathologic process.[33] It usually occurs with ovulatory menstruation beginning 6 months to 2 years after menarche. Symptoms may begin 1 to 2 days before menses, peak on the first day of flow, and subside within several hours to several days. Severe dysmenorrhea may be associated with systemic symptoms such as headache, nausea, vomiting, diarrhea, fatigue, irritability, dizziness, and syncope. The pain typically is described as dull, lower abdominal aching or cramping, spasmodic or colicky in nature, often radiating to the lower back, labia majora, or upper thighs.

Secondary dysmenorrhea is menstrual pain caused by specific organic conditions, such as endometriosis, uterine fibroids, adenomyosis, pelvic adhesions, or PID. Laparoscopy often is required for diagnosis of secondary dysmenorrhea if medication for primary dysmenorrhea is ineffective.

Treatment for primary dysmenorrhea is directed at symptom control. Although analgesic agents such as aspirin and acetaminophen may relieve minor uterine cramping or low back pain, prostaglandin synthetase inhibitors, such as ibuprofen, naproxen, mefenamic acid, and indomethacin, are more specific for dysmenorrhea. Ovulation suppression and symptomatic relief of dysmenorrhea can be instituted simultaneously with the use of oral contraceptives. Relief of secondary dysmenorrhea depends on identifying the cause of the problem. Medical or surgical intervention may be needed to eliminate the problem.

PREMENSTRUAL SYNDROME

The *premenstrual syndrome* (PMS) is a distinct clinical entity characterized by a cluster of physical and psychological symptoms limited to 3 to 14 days preceding menstruation and relieved by onset of the menses. The incidence of PMS seems to increase with age, with symptoms typically beginning between the ages of 25 to 35 years of age.[34]

Although the causes of PMS are poorly documented, they probably are multifactorial. Like dysmenorrhea, it is only recently that PMS has been recognized as a bona fide disorder, rather than merely a psychosomatic illness.

The physical symptoms of PMS include painful and swollen breasts, bloating, abdominal pain, headache, and backache. Psychologically, there may be depression, anxiety, irritability, and behavioral changes. In some cases, there are puzzling alterations in motor function, such as clumsiness and altered handwriting.[34,35] Women with PMS may report one or several symptoms, with symptoms varying from woman to woman and from month to month in the same patient. Signs and symptoms associated with this disorder are summarized in Table 39-3. PMS can significantly affect a woman's ability to perform at normal levels. She may lose time from or function ineffectively at work. Family responsibilities and relationships may suffer. More crimes are committed by women during the premenstrual phase of the cycle, and more lives are lost to suicide during this period. The term *premenstrual dysphoric disorder* is a psychiatric diagnosis that has been developed to distinguish women whose symptoms are severe enough to interfere signifi-

TABLE 39-3	Symptoms of Premenstrual Syndrome (PMS) by System
Body System	**Symptoms**
Cerebral	Irritability, anxiety, nervousness, fatigue, and exhaustion; increased physical and mental activity; lability; crying spells; depressions; inability to concentrate
Gastrointestinal	Craving for sweets or salts, lower abdominal pain, bloating, nausea, vomiting, diarrhea, constipation
Vascular	Headache, edema, weakness, or fainting
Reproductive	Swelling and tenderness of the breasts, pelvic congestion, ovarian pain, altered libido
Neuromuscular	Trembling of the extremities, changes in coordination, clumsiness, backache, leg aches
General	Weight gain, insomnia, dizziness, acne

cantly with activities of daily living or in whom the symptoms are not relieved with the onset of menstruation, as is usually the case with PMS.[36]

Diagnosis focuses on identification of the symptom clusters by means of prospective daily symptom diary for at least two cycles.[35] A complete history and physical examination are necessary to exclude other physical causes of the symptoms. Depending on the symptom pattern, blood studies, including thyroid hormones and glucose tests, may be done. Psychosocial evaluation is helpful to exclude emotional illness that is merely exacerbated premenstrually.

Treatment of PMS is directed toward an integrated program of regular exercise, avoidance of caffeine, and a diet emphasizing complex carbohydrates. Foods high in simple sugars and alcohol should be avoided. Drug therapy should be used cautiously until well-controlled studies establish criteria for use and effective treatment results.

 MENOPAUSE AND AGING CHANGES

Menopause is the cessation of menstrual cycles. Like menarche, it is more of a process than a single event. Most women stop menstruating between 48 and 55 years of age. *Perimenopause* (the years immediately surrounding menopause) precedes menopause by approximately 4 years and is characterized by menstrual irregularity and other menopausal symptoms. *Climacteric* is a more encompassing term that refers to the entire transition to the nonreproductive period of life. Premature ovarian failure describes the approximately 1% of women who experience menopause before the age of 40 years. A woman who has not menstruated for a full year or has an FSH level greater than 30 mIU/mL is considered menopausal.[37]

Menopause results from the gradual cessation of ovarian function and the resultant diminished levels of estrogen. Although estrogens derived from the adrenal cortex continue to circulate in a woman's body, they are insufficient to maintain the secondary sexual characteristics in the same manner as ovarian estrogens. As a result, breast tissue, body hair, skin elasticity, and subcutaneous fat decrease; the ovaries and uterus diminish in size; and the cervix and vagina become pale and friable. Problems that can arise as a result of this urogenital atrophy include vaginal dryness, urinary stress incontinence, urgency, nocturia, vaginitis, and urinary tract infection.[37,38] The woman may find intercourse painful and traumatic, although some type of vaginal lubrication may be helpful.

Systemically, a woman may experience significant vasomotor instability secondary to the decrease in estrogens and the relative increase in other hormones, including FSH, LH, GnRH, dehydroepiandrosterone, and androstenedione. This instability may give rise to "hot flashes," palpitations, dizziness, and headaches as the blood vessels dilate. Despite the association with these biochemical changes, the underlying cause of hot flashes is unknown. Tremendous variation exists in the onset, frequency, severity, and length of time that women experience hot flashes. When they occur at night and are accompanied by significant perspiration, they are referred to as *night sweats*. Insomnia as well as frequent awakening because of vasomotor symptoms can lead to sleep deprivation. A woman may experience irritability, anxiety, and depression as a result of these uncontrollable and unpredictable events.

Consequences of long-term estrogen deprivation include osteoporosis, due to an imbalance in bone remodeling (*i.e.*, bone resorption occurs at a faster rate than bone formation), and an increased risk for cardiovascular disease (atherosclerosis is accelerated), which is the leading cause of death for women after menopause.

Menopausal hormonal therapy has recently come under scrutiny. Vaginal estrogen preparations are available to treat symptoms related to vaginal atrophy. Selective estrogen receptor modulators (SERMs) may be used in place of estrogen to prevent osteoporosis. The National Institutes of Health State-of-the-Art Conference Panel on Menopause-Related Symptoms recommends that research is needed to define clearly the natural history of menopause, associated symptoms, and effectiveness of treatment for bothersome symptoms.[38]

 In summary, between the menarche and menopause, the female reproductive system undergoes cyclic changes called the *menstrual cycle*. Normal menstrual function results from complex interactions among the hypothalamus, which produces GnRH; the anterior pituitary gland, which synthesizes and releases FSH, LH, and prolactin; the ovaries, which synthesize and release estrogens, progesterone, and androgens; and associated target tissues, such as the endometrium and the vaginal mucosa. Although each component of the system is essential for normal functioning, the ovarian hormones are largely responsible for controlling the cyclic changes and length of the menstrual cycle.

Menstrual disorders include dysfunctional menstrual cycles, dysmenorrhea, and PMS. Dysfunctional menstrual cycles produce amenorrhea, oligomenorrhea, metrorrhagia, or menorrhagia. Dysmenorrhea is characterized by pain or discomfort during menses. It can occur as a primary or secondary disorder. Primary dysmenorrhea is not associated with other disorders and begins soon after menarche. Secondary dysmenorrhea is caused by a specific organic condition, such as endometriosis or pelvic adhesions. It occurs in women with previously painless menses. PMS represents a cluster of physical and psychological symptoms that precede menstruation by 1 to 2 weeks.

Menopause is the cessation of ovarian function and menstrual cycles. It is accompanied by a decline in secondary sexual characteristics, vasomotor instability, and long-term consequences, including osteoporosis and increased risk of heart disease.

Disorders of the Breast

Although anatomically separate, the breasts are functionally related to the female genitourinary system in that they respond to the cyclic changes in sex hormones and produce milk for infant nourishment. Most breast diseases may be described as benign or cancerous. Benign breast conditions are nonprogressive; however, some forms of benign disease increase the risk of malignant disease.

BREAST STRUCTURES

The breasts, or mammary tissues, are located between the third and seventh ribs of the anterior chest wall and are supported by the pectoral muscles and superficial fascia. They are specialized glandular structures that have an abundant shared nervous, vascular, and lymphatic supply (Fig. 39-14). Structurally the breast consists of fat, fibrous connective tissue, and glandular tissue. The superficial fibrous connective tissue is attached to the skin, a fact that is important in the visual observation of skin movement over the breast during breast self-examination. The breast mass is supported by the fascia of the pectoralis major and minor muscles and by the fibrous connective tissue of the breast. Fibrous tissue ligaments, called *Cooper ligaments*, extend from the outer boundaries of the breast to the nipple area in a radial manner, like the spokes on a wheel. These ligaments further support the breast and form septa that divide the breast into 15 to 25 lobes. Each lobe consists of grapelike clusters, alveoli or glands, which are interconnected by ducts. Estrogen stimulates the growth of the ductal system, whereas progesterone stimulates the growth and development of the ductile and alveolar secretory epithelium.

The alveoli are lined with secretory cells capable of producing milk or fluid under the proper hormonal conditions (Fig. 39-15). The route of descent of milk and other breast secretions is from alveoli to duct, to intralobar duct, to lactiferous duct and reservoir, to nipple. Breast milk is produced secondary to complex hormonal changes associated with pregnancy. The breasts respond to the cyclic changes in the menstrual cycle with fullness and discomfort.

The nipple is made up of epithelial, glandular, erectile, and nervous tissue. Areolar tissue surrounds the nipple and is recognized as the darker, smooth skin between the nipple and the breast. The small bumps or projections on the areolar surface known as *Montgomery tubercles* are sebaceous glands that keep the nipple area soft and

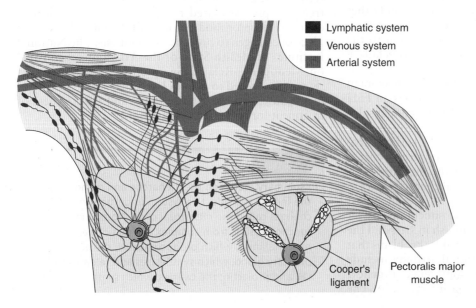

- ■ Lymphatic system
- ■ Venous system
- ■ Arterial system

Cooper's ligament

Pectoralis major muscle

FIGURE 39-14 The breasts, showing the shared vascular and lymphatic supply as well as the pectoral muscles.

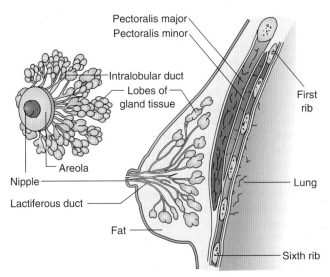

FIGURE 39-15 The breast, showing the glandular tissue and ducts of the mammary glands.

Pectoralis major
Pectoralis minor
Intralobular duct
Lobes of gland tissue
First rib
Areola
Nipple
Lung
Lactiferous duct
Fat
Sixth rib

elastic. At the time of puberty and during pregnancy, increased levels of estrogen and progesterone cause the areola and nipple to become darker and more prominent and Montgomery's glands to become more active. The erectile tissue of the nipple is responsive to psychological and tactile stimuli, which contributes to the sexual function of the breasts.

MASTITIS

Mastitis is inflammation of the breast. It most frequently occurs during lactation but may also result from other conditions. In the lactating woman, inflammation results from an ascending infection that travels from the nipple to the ductal structures. The most common organisms isolated are *Staphylococcus* and *Streptococcus*.[12] The offending organisms originate from the suckling infant's nasopharynx or the mother's hands. During the early weeks of nursing, the breast is particularly vulnerable to bacterial invasion because of minor cracks and fissures that occur with vigorous suckling. Infection and inflammation cause obstruction of the ductal system. The breast area becomes hard, inflamed, and tender if not treated early. Without treatment, the area becomes walled off and may abscess, requiring incision and drainage. It is advisable for the mother to continue breast-feeding during antibiotic therapy to prevent this.

Mastitis is not confined to the postpartum period; it can occur as a result of hormonal fluctuations, tumors, trauma, or skin infection. Cyclic inflammation of the breast occurs most frequently in adolescents, who commonly have fluctuating hormone levels. Tumors may cause mastitis secondary to skin involvement or lymphatic obstruction. Local trauma or infection may develop into mastitis because of ductal blockage of trapped blood, cellular debris, or the extension of superficial inflammation. The treatment for mastitis symptoms may include application of heat or cold, excision, aspiration, mild anal-

gesics, antibiotics, and a supportive brassiere or breast binder.

DUCTAL DISORDERS

Ductal ectasia manifests in older women as a spontaneous, intermittent, usually unilateral, grayish-green nipple discharge. Palpation of the breast increases the discharge. Ectasia occurs during or after menopause and is symptomatically associated with burning, itching, pain, and a pulling sensation of the nipple and areola. The disease results in inflammation of the ducts and subsequent thickening. Treatment requires removal of the involved ductal mass.

Intraductal papillomas are benign epithelial tissue tumors that range in size from 2 mm to 5 cm. Papillomas usually manifest with a bloody nipple discharge. The tumor may be palpated in the areolar area. The papilloma is probed through the nipple, and the involved duct is removed.

FIBROCYSTIC CHANGES

Fibrocystic changes, formerly called *fibrocystic breast disease*, is the most common lesion of the breast. It is most common in women 30 to 50 years of age and is rare in postmenopausal women not receiving hormone replacement.[39–41] The term implies women with lumpy breasts or breasts with nondiscrete nodules who do not have breast disease.

Fibrocystic changes encompass a wide variety of lesions and breast changes. Microscopically, fibrocystic changes refers to a constellation of morphologic changes manifested by (1) cystic dilatation of terminal ducts, (2) a relative increase in fibrous tissue, and (3) variable proliferation of terminal duct epithelial elements. Autopsy studies have demonstrated some degree of fibrocystic changes in 75% of adult women in the United States.[40] Symptomatic fibrocystic change, in which large, clinically detectable cysts are present, is much less common, occurring in approximately 10% of adult women between 35 and 55 years of age.[40] Although fibrocystic changes often has been thought to increase the risk of breast cancer, only certain variants in which proliferation of the epithelial components is demonstrated represent a true risk.

Diagnosis of fibrocystic changes is made by physical examination, mammography, ultrasonography, and biopsy (*i.e.*, aspiration or tissue sample). Ultrasonography is useful in differentiating a cystic from a solid mass. Because a mass caused by fibrocystic changes may be indistinguishable from carcinoma on the basis of clinical findings, suspect lesions should undergo biopsy. Fine-needle aspiration may be used, but if a suspect mass that was nonmalignant on cytologic examination does not resolve during the course of several months, it should be removed surgically.

Treatment for fibrocystic changes usually is symptomatic. Women should be encouraged to wear a good supporting brassiere and advised to avoid foods that contain xanthines (*e.g.*, coffee, cola, chocolate, and tea) in their daily diets, particularly premenstrually.[41] Mild analgesics (*e.g.,* aspirin, acetaminophen, and NSAIDs) may be used for pain relief. Tamoxifen or danazol, a synthetic androgen, may be used for treatment of severe pain.

BREAST CANCER

Cancer of the breast is the most common female cancer. One in eight women in the United States will have breast cancer in her lifetime. In 2005, breast cancer affected 211,240 American women and killed an estimated 40,410 women.[42] Although the breast cancer mortality rate has shown a slight decline, it is second only to lung cancer as a cause of cancer-related deaths in women. An additional 400 deaths occurred from breast cancer in men.[42] Incidence rates for carcinoma in situ have increased dramatically since the mid-1970s because of recommendations regarding mammography screening. The decline in the breast cancer mortality rate since 1989 is due to this earlier diagnosis as well as improvements in cancer treatments.[43]

Risk factors for breast cancer include sex, increasing age, personal or family history of breast cancer (*i.e.,* at highest risk are those with multiple affected first-order relatives), history of benign breast disease (*i.e.,* primary "atypical" hyperplasia), and hormonal influences that promote breast maturation and may increase the chance of cell mutation (*i.e.,* early menarche, late menopause, and no term pregnancies or first child after 30 years of age).[42] Most women with breast cancer have no identifiable risk factors.

Approximately 10% of all breast cancers are hereditary, with genetic mutations causing up to 80% of breast cancers in women younger than 50 years of age.[44] Two breast cancer susceptibility genes—BRCA1 on chromosome 17 and BRCA2 on chromosome 13—may account for most inherited forms of breast cancer[39,40] (see Chapter 5). BRCA1 is known to be involved in tumor suppression. A woman with known mutations in BRCA1 has a lifetime risk of 56% to 85% for breast cancer and an increased risk of ovarian cancer. BRCA2 is another susceptibility gene that carries an elevated cancer risk similar to that with BRCA1. A task force organized by the National Institutes of Health and the National Genome Research Institute has proposed a set of provisional consensus recommendations for monitoring known carriers of BRCA1 and BRCA2 mutations. The task force recommended that known carriers should begin monthly breast self-examination (BSE) at 18 years of age and begin having annual mammograms at 25 years of age.[44]

Detection

Cancer of the breast may manifest clinically as a mass, a puckering, nipple retraction, or unusual discharge. Many cancers are found by women themselves through BSE—sometimes when only a thickening or subtle change in breast contour is noticed. The variety of symptoms and potential for self-discovery underscore the need for regular, systematic self-examination. BSE should be done routinely by women older than 20 years of age. Premenopausal women should conduct the examination right after menses. This time is most appropriate in relation to cyclic breast changes that occur in response to fluctuations in hormone levels. Postmenopausal women and women who have had a hysterectomy should perform the examination on the same day of every month. Examination should be done in the shower or bath or at bedtime. The most important aspect of BSE is to devise a regular, systematic, convenient, and consistent method of examination. As an adjunct to BSE, women should have a clinical examination by a trained health professional at least every 3 years between 20 and 40 years of age, and annually after 40 years of age.

Mammography is the only effective screening technique for the early detection of clinically unapparent lesions. Although recent studies have brought into question the value of mammography,[45–47] in 2002 the USPSTF issued new guidelines concluding that there were sufficient data to justify recommending mammography every 1 to 2 years in women older than 40 years of age.[48] A generally slow-growing form of cancer, breast cancer may have been present for 2 to 9 years before it reaches 1 cm, the smallest mass normally detected by palpation. Mammography can disclose lesions as small as 1 mm and the clustering of calcifications that may warrant biopsy to exclude cancer. The American Cancer Society recommends annual evaluation for women after 40 years of age.[49] Approximately 40% of breast cancers can be detected only by palpation and another 40% only by mammography.[44] The most comprehensive approach to screening is a combination of BSE, clinical evaluation by a health professional, and mammography.

Diagnosis and Classification

Procedures used in the diagnosis of breast cancer include physical examination, mammography, ultrasonography, percutaneous needle aspiration, stereotactic needle biopsy (*i.e.,* core biopsy), and excisional biopsy. Figure 39-16 illustrates the appearance of breast cancer on mammography. Breast cancer often manifests as a solitary, painless, firm, fixed lesion with poorly defined borders. It can be found anywhere in the breast but is most common in the upper outer quadrant. Because of the variability in presentation, any suspect change in breast tissue warrants further investigation. The diagnostic use of mammography enables additional definition of the clinically suspect area (*e.g.,* appearance, character, calcification). Placement of a wire marker under radiographic guidance can ensure accurate surgical biopsy of nonpalpable suspect areas. Ultrasonography is useful as a diagnostic adjunct to differentiate cystic from solid tissue in women with nonspecific thickening.

Fine-needle aspiration is a simple in-office procedure that can be performed repeatedly in multiple sites and with minimal discomfort. It can be accomplished by stabilizing a palpable mass between two fingers or in conjunction with hand-held sonography to define cystic masses or fibrocystic changes and to provide speci-

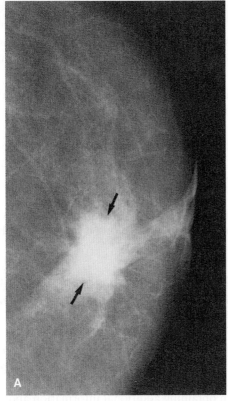
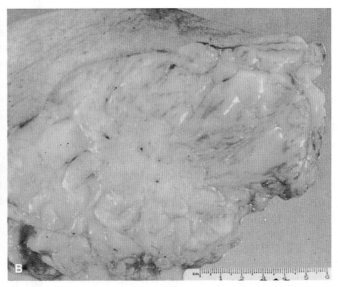

FIGURE 39-16 Carcinoma of the breast. (**A**) Mammogram. An irregularly shaped, dense mass (*arrows*) is seen in this otherwise fatty breast. (**B**) Mastectomy specimen. The irregular, white, firm mass in the center is surrounded by fatty tissue. (From Thor A. D., Wang J., Bartow S. A. [2005]. The breast. In Rubin E., Gorstein F., Rubin R., et al. [Eds.], *Rubin's pathology: Clinicopathologic foundations of medicine* [4th ed., p. 1088]. Philadelphia: Lippincott Williams & Wilkins.)

mens for cytologic examination. Fine-needle aspiration can identify the presence of malignant cells, but it cannot differentiate in situ from infiltrating cancers. Stereotactic needle biopsy is an outpatient procedure done with the guidance of a mammography machine. After the lesion is localized radiologically, a large-bore needle is mechanically thrust quickly into the area, removing a core of tissue. Discomfort is similar to that with ear piercing, and even when multiple cores are obtained, healing occurs quite rapidly. Cells are available for histologic evaluation with 96% accuracy in detecting cancer. This procedure is less costly than excisional biopsy. Excisional biopsy to remove the entire lump provides the only definitive diagnosis of breast cancer, and often is therapeutic without additional surgery. MRI techniques, positron emission tomography, and computer-based or digital mammography are being evaluated as additional diagnostic modalities for breast cancer, and may be recommended to supplement conventional mammography in women with a strong family history of cancer or who are known carriers of BRCA1 or BRCA2.

Tumors are classified histologically according to tissue characteristics and staged clinically according to tumor size, nodal involvement, and presence of metastasis. It is recommended that estrogen and progesterone receptor analysis be performed on surgical specimens.

Information about the presence or absence of estrogen and progesterone receptors can be used in predicting tumor responsiveness to hormonal manipulation. High levels of both receptors improve the prognosis and increase the likelihood of remission.

Treatment

The treatment methods for breast cancer are controversial. They may include surgery, chemotherapy, radiation therapy, and hormonal manipulation. Radical mastectomy (*i.e.*, removal of the entire breast, underlying muscles, and all axillary nodes) rarely is used today as a primary surgical therapy unless breast cancer is advanced at the time of diagnosis. Modified surgical techniques (*i.e.*, mastectomy plus axillary dissection or lumpectomy for breast conservation) accompanied by chemotherapy or radiation therapy have achieved outcomes comparable with those obtained with radical surgical methods and constitute the preferred treatment methods.

The prognosis is related more to the extent of nodal involvement than to the extent of breast involvement. Greater nodal involvement requires more aggressive postsurgical treatment, and many cancer specialists believe that a diagnosis of breast cancer is not complete until dissection and testing of the axillary lymph nodes has been accomplished. A newer technique for evaluating lymph node involvement is a sentinel lymph node (SLN) biopsy.[50] A radioactive substance or dye is injected into the region of the tumor. In theory, the dye is carried to the first (sentinel) node to receive lymph from the tumor. This would therefore be the node most likely to contain cancer cells if the cancer has spread. If the sentinel node biopsy is positive, more nodes are removed. If it is negative, further lymph node evaluation may not be needed.

Adjuvant systemic therapy refers to the administration of chemotherapy or hormonal therapy to women without detectable metastatic disease. Tamoxifen is a nonsteroidal antiestrogen that binds to estrogen receptors and blocks the effects of estrogens on the growth of malignant cells in the breast.[51] Studies have shown decreased cancer recurrence, decreased mortality rates, and increased 5-year survival rates in women with estrogen receptor–positive tissue samples who have been treated with the drug. Autologous bone marrow transplantation and peripheral stem cell transplantation are experimental therapies that may be used for treatment of advanced disease or in women at increased risk for recurrence. Immunotherapy, using a drug called trastuzumab (Herceptin), is used to stop the growth of breast tumors that express the HER2/neu receptor on their cell surface. The HER2/neu receptor binds an epidermal growth factor that contributes to cancer cell growth. Trastuzumab is a recombinant DNA–derived monoclonal antibody that binds to the HER2/neu receptor, thereby inhibiting proliferation of tumor cells that overexpress the receptor gene.

Paget Disease

Paget disease accounts for 1% of all breast cancers. The disease presents as an eczematoid lesion of the nipple and areola. Paget disease usually is associated with an infiltrating, intraductal carcinoma. When the lesion is limited to the nipple only, the rate of axillary metastasis is approximately 5%. Complete examination is required and includes a mammogram and biopsy. Treatment depends on the extent of spread.

In summary, the breasts are subject to benign and malignant disease. Mastitis is inflammation of the breast, occurring most frequently during lactation. Ductal ectasia and intraductal papilloma cause abnormal drainage from the nipple. Fibroadenoma and fibrocystic changes are characterized by abnormal masses in the breast that are benign. By far the most important disease of the breast is breast cancer, which is a significant cause of death for women. BSE and mammography afford a woman the best protection against breast cancer. They provide the means for early detection of breast cancer and, in many cases, allow early treatment and cure.

Review Exercises

Most oral contraceptive agents use low doses of estrogen and progestin to prevent conception.

A. Use Figure 39-4 to explain how these oral agents prevent ovulation and pregnancy.

Diabetes mellitus and treatment with broad-spectrum antibiotics increase the risk of vaginal infections.

A. Explain how these two conditions change the vaginal ecology, making it more susceptible to infection.

A 32-year-old woman has been told that the report of her annual Pap test revealed the presence of mild cervical dysplasia.

A. What questions should this woman ask to become informed about the significance of these findings?
B. In obtaining additional information about the results of her Pap test, the woman is informed that dysplastic changes are consistent with CIN1 classification.
   1. Does this mean that the woman has cervical cancer?
   2. Cervical cancer is often referred to as a sexually transmitted disease. Explain.
   3. What type of follow-up care would be indicated?

A 30-year-old woman consults her gynecologist because of amenorrhea and inability to become pregnant. Physical examination reveals an obese woman with hirsutism. The physician tells her that she might have a condition known as polycystic ovary syndrome and that further laboratory tests are indicated.

A. Among tests ordered were a fasting blood glucose and serum LH, FSH, and dehydroepiandrosterone levels. What information can these tests provide that would help in establishing a diagnosis of polycystic ovary syndrome?
B. What is the probable cause of this woman's amenorrhea, hirsutism, and failure to become pregnant?
C. What type of treatment might be used to help this woman become pregnant?

A 45-year-old woman makes an appointment to see her physician because of a painless lump in her breast that she discovered while doing her routine monthly breast examination.

A. What tests should be done to confirm the presence or absence of breast cancer?

B. During the removal of breast cancer, a sentinel node biopsy is often done to determine whether the cancer has spread to the lymph nodes. Explain how this procedure is done and its value in determining lymph node spread.

C. After surgical removal of breast cancer, tamoxifen may be used as an adjuvant systemic therapy for women without detectable metastatic disease. The presence or absence of estrogen receptors in the cytoplasm of tumor cells is important in determining the selection of an agent for use in adjuvant therapy. Explain.

Visit the Porth: Essentials of Pathophysiology: Concepts of Altered Health States web site

(http://thePoint.LWW.com/PorthEssentials) for links to chapter-related resources on the Internet, all-new exclusive animations, chapter review questions, and more!

REFERENCES

1. Rosen M., Cedars M. I. (2004). Female reproductive endocrinology and infertility. In Greenspan F. S., Gardner D. G. (Eds.), *Basic and clinical endocrinology* (7th ed., pp. 511–563). New York: Lange Medical Books/McGraw-Hill.

2. Crum C. P. (2005). The female genital tract. In Kumar V., Abbas A. K., Fausto N. (Eds.), *Robbins and Cotran pathologic basis of disease* (7th ed., pp. 1059–1117). Philadelphia: Elsevier Saunders.

3. Guyton A. C., Hall J. E. (2006). *Textbook of medical physiology* (11th ed., pp. 1011–1024). Philadelphia: Elsevier Saunders.

4. Gruber C. J., Tschugguel W., Huber J. (2002). Production and actions of estrogens. *New England Journal of Medicine* 346, 340–350.

5. Stewart E. G. (2003). Treatment options for vulvar vestibulitis. *Contemporary OB/GYN* 1, 47–61.

6. Edwards, L. (2003). New concepts in vulvodynia. *American Journal of Obstetrics and Gynecology* 189(3, Suppl. 1), S24–S30.

7. Canavan T. P., Cohen D. (2002). Vulvar cancer. *American Family Physician* 66, 1269–1274.

8. Tyring S. K. (2003). Vulvar squamous cell carcinoma: Guidelines for early diagnosis and treatment. *American Journal of Obstetrics and Gynecology* 189(3, Suppl. 1), S17–S23.

9. Sweet R. L., Gibbs R. S. (2002). *Infectious diseases of the female genital tract* (4th ed., pp. 337–340). Philadelphia: Lippincott Williams & Wilkins.

10. Sobel J. D. (1997). Vaginitis. *New England Journal of Medicine* 337, 1896–1903.

11. Fields A. L., Jones J. G., Thomas G. M., et al. (2001). Gynecological cancer. In Lenhard R. E., Jr., Osteen R. T., Gansler T. (Eds.), *The American Cancer Society's clinical oncology* (pp. 455–496). Atlanta: American Cancer Society.

12. Robboy S., Kurman R. J., Merino M. J. (2005). The female reproductive system. In Rubin E., Gorstein F., Rubin R., et al. (Eds.), *Rubin's pathology: Clinicopathologic foundations of medicine* (4th ed., pp. 927–1015): Philadelphia: Lippincott Williams & Wilkins.

13. Janicek M. F., Averette H. E. (2001). Cervical cancer: Prevention, diagnosis, and therapeutics. *CA: A Cancer Journal for Clinicians* 51, 92–114.

14. Crum C. P. (2002). The beginning of the end of cervical cancer. *New England Journal of Medicine* 347, 1703–1705.

15. Saslow D., Runowicz C. D., Solomon D., et al. (2002). American Cancer Society guideline for the early detection of cervical neoplasia and cancer. *CA: A Cancer Journal for Clinicians* 52, 342–362.

16. U.S. Preventive Services Task Force. (2003). Screening for cervical cancer: Recommendations and rationale. *American Journal of Nursing* 103(11), 101–109.

17. Eskridge C., Begneaud W. P., Landwehr C. (1998). Cervicography combined with repeat Papanicolaou test as triage for low grade cytologic abnormalities. *Obstetrics and Gynecology* 92, 351–355.

18. Mott A. M. (2000). Prevention and management of pelvic inflammatory disease by primary care providers. *American Journal of Nurse Practitioners* 8, 7–13.

19. Spaczynski R. Z., Duleba A. J. (2003). Diagnosis of endometriosis. *Seminars in Reproductive Medicine* 21, 193–207.

20. Giudice L. C., Kao L. C. (2004). Endometriosis. *Lancet* 365, 789–799.

21. Gambone J. C., Mittman B. S., Munro M. G., et al., and the Chronic Pelvic Pain/Endometriosis Working Group. (2002). Consensus statement for the management of chronic pelvic pain and endometriosis: Proceedings of an expert-panel consensus process. *Fertility and Sterility* 78, 961–972.

22. Olive D. L., Pritts E. A. (2001). Treatment of endometriosis. *New England Journal of Medicine* 345, 266–275.

23. Canavan T. P., Doshi N. R. (1999). Endometrial cancer. *American Family Practitioner* 59, 3069–3077.

24. Hutchins F. J. (1998). Fibroids in primary care. *The Clinical Advisor* 9, 29.

25. Ehrmann D. A. (2005). Polycystic ovary syndrome. *New England Journal of Medicine* 352, 1223–1236.

26. Mark T. L., Menta A. E. (2003). Polycystic ovary syndrome: Pathogenesis and treatment over the short and long term. *Cleveland Clinic Journal of Medicine* 70, 31–45.

27. Richardson M. B. (2003). Current perspectives in polycystic ovary syndrome. *American Family Physician* 68, 697–704.

28. Nestler J. E., Stovall D., Akhtar N., et al. (2002). Strategies for the use of insulin-sensitizing drugs to treat infertility in women with polycystic ovary syndrome. *Fertility and Sterility* 77, 209–215.

29. Costello M. F., Eden J. A. (2003). A systematic review of the reproductive system effects of metformin in patients with polycystic ovary syndrome. *Fertility and Sterility* 79, 1–13.

30. Cannistra S. A. (2004). Cancer of the ovary. *New England Journal of Medicine* 351, 2519–2529.

31. National Institutes of Health Consensus Development Panel on Ovarian Cancer. (1995). Ovarian cancer: Screening and follow-up. *Journal of the American Medical Association* 273, 491–497.

32. American College of Obstetricians and Gynecologists. (2000). Management of anovulatory bleeding. ACOG Practice Bulletin no. 14. In *2001 Compendium of selected publications* (pp. 961–968). Washington, DC: Author.

33. Coco A. S. (1999). Primary dysmenorrhea. *American Family Practitioner* 60, 489–496.

34. Dickerson L. M., Mazyck P. J., Hunter M. (2003). Premenstrual syndrome. *American Family Physician* 67, 1743–1745.

35. ACOG Practice Bulletin. (2000). Clinical management guidelines for obstetricians-gynecologists: Premenstrual syndrome. *Obstetrics and Gynecology* 95, 1–9.

36. Grady-Weliky T. A. (2003). Premenstrual dysphoric disorder. *New England Journal of Medicine* 348, 433–438.

37. Rebar R., Gass M. (2000). Menopause: Hormonal changes and symptomatic management. *Clinical Bulletins in Menopause* 1, 2.

38. National Institutes of Health State of the Art Panel. (2005). National Institutes of Health State-of-the-Science Conference Statement: Management of menopause-related symptoms. *Annals of Internal Medicine* 142, 1003–1010.

39. Lester S. C. (2005). The breast. In Kumar V., Abbas A. K., Fausto N. (Eds.), *Robbins and Cotran pathologic basis of disease* (7th ed., pp. 1119–1151). Philadelphia: Elsevier Saunders.

40. Thor A. D., Wang J., Bartow S. A. (2005). The breast. In Rubin E., Gorstein F., Rubin R., et al. (Eds.), *Rubin's pathology: Clinicopathologic foundations of medicine* (4th ed., pp. 997–1016). Philadelphia: Lippincott Williams & Wilkins.

41. Santen R. J., Mansel R. (2005). Benign breast tumors. *New England Journal of Medicine* 353, 275–285.

42. American Cancer Society. (2005). Cancer facts and figures. [On-line]. Available: www.cancer.org.

43. Osteen R. T. (2001). Breast cancer. In Lenhard R. E., Jr., Osteen R. T., Gansler T. (Eds.), *The American Cancer Society's clinical oncology* (pp. 251–268). Atlanta: American Cancer Society.

44. Zimmerman V. L. (2002). BRCA gene mutations and cancer. *American Journal of Nursing* 102(8), 28–36.

45. Gotzsche P. C., Olsen O. (2000). Is screening for breast cancer with mammography justifiable? *Lancet* 355, 129–134.

46. Olsen O., Gotzsche P. C. (2001). Cochrane Review on screening for breast cancer with mammography. *Lancet* 358, 1340–1342.

47. Miller A. B., To T., Baines C. J., et al. (2002). The Canadian National Breast Screening Study 1: Breast cancer mortality after 11 to 16 years of follow-up. *Annuals of Internal Medicine* 137, 305–312.

48. Humphrey L. L., Helfand M., Chan B. K. S., et al. (2002). Breast cancer screening: A summary of the evidence for the U.S. Preventive Service Task Force. *Annals of Internal Medicine* 137, 347–360.

49. Smith R. A., Saslow D., Sawyers K. A., et al. (2003). American Cancer Society guidelines for breast cancer screening updated 2003. *CA: A Cancer Journal for Clinicians* 53, 134–137.

50. Cox C. E., Salud C. J., Harrington M. A. (2000). The role of selective sentinel lymph node dissection in breast cancer. *Surgical Clinics of North America* 80, 1759–1775.

51. Hortobagyi G. N. (1998). Treatment of breast cancer. *New England Journal of Medicine* 339, 974–984.

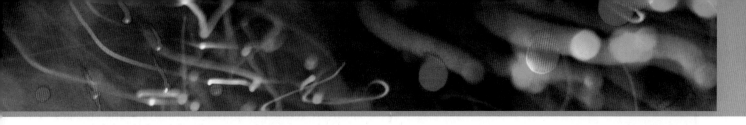

Chapter *40*

Sexually Transmitted Diseases

 The incidence and types of sexually transmitted diseases (STDs), as reported in the professional literature and public health statistics, are increasing. The incidence of disease is based on clinical reports, however, and many STDs are not reportable or not reported. The agents of transmission include bacteria, chlamydiae, viruses, fungi, protozoa, parasites, and unidentified microorganisms. Portals of entry include the mouth, genitalia, urinary meatus, rectum, and skin. All STDs are more common in persons who have more than one sexual partner, and it is not uncommon for a person to be concurrently infected with more than one type of STD. Many of the STDs, particularly those that produce ulcerative lesions, predispose to human immunodeficiency virus (HIV) transmission (see Chapter 15). This chapter discusses the manifestations of STDs in men and women in terms of infections of the external genitalia, vaginal infections, and infections that have both systemic effects and genitourinary manifestations.

Infections of the External Genitalia

Some STDs primarily affect the mucocutaneous tissues of the external genitalia. These include condylomata acuminata, genital herpes, chancroid, and granuloma inguinale.

CONDYLOMATA ACUMINATA (GENITAL WARTS)

Condylomata acuminata, or *genital warts,* are caused by the human papillomavirus (HPV). Although recognized for centuries, HPV-induced genital warts have become one of the fastest-growing STDs of the past decade. The Centers for Disease Control and Prevention (CDC) estimates that 20 million Americans carry the virus and that up to 5.5 million new cases are diagnosed each year.[1] The

vical intraepithelial neoplasia (CIN) and cancer (see Chapter 39). The first neoplastic changes noted on the Pap smear are termed *dysplasia*. These dysplastic changes regress in many women and only a subset of women infected with HPV go on to develop cervical cancer, suggesting that there may be variants of HPV-16 and HPV-18, each with differing oncogenic potential.[5] Cofactors that may increase the risk for development of cervical cancer include smoking, immunosuppression, and exposure to hormonal alteration (*e.g.*, pregnancy, oral contraceptives).[2–4]

Human papillomavirus infection begins with viral inoculation into stratified squamous epithelium, where infection stimulates the replication of the squamous epithelium, producing the various HPV-proliferative lesions. The incubation period for HPV-induced genital warts ranges from 6 weeks to 8 months. Genital warts typically present as soft, raised, fleshy lesions on the external genitalia, including the penis (Fig. 40-1), vulva, scrotum, perineum, and perianal skin. External warts appear as small bumps, or they may be flat, wartlike, or pedunculated. Less commonly, they can appear as reddish or brown, smooth, raised papules or as dome-shaped lesions on keratinized skin. Internal warts are cauliflower-shaped lesions that affect the mucous membranes of the vagina, urethra, anus, or mouth. They may cause discomfort, bleeding, or painful intercourse.[7]

Subclinical infection occurs more frequently than visible genital warts among men and women. Infection often is indirectly diagnosed on the cervix by Pap smear, col-

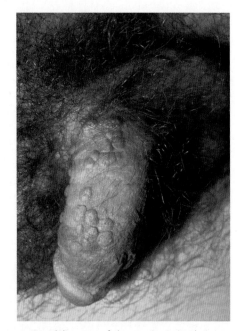

FIGURE 40-1 Condylomata of the penis. Raised circumscribed lesions are seen on the shaft of the penis. (From Damjanov I. [2005]. The lower urinary tract and male reproductive system. In Rubin E., Gorstein F., Rubin R., et al. [Eds.], *Rubin's pathology: Clinicopathologic foundations of medicine* [4th ed., p. 904]. Philadelphia: Lippincott Williams & Wilkins.)

true prevalence of HPV is difficult to determine because it is not a reportable disease in all states, it can be a transient infection, of short duration, with only a small number of people exposed remaining persistently infected, and most infections remain subclinical without development of overt lesions or abnormal cytologic changes.[2–4]

Human papillomaviruses cause proliferative lesions of the squamous epithelium, including verruca vulgaris (common warts) that occur anywhere but most frequently on the hands, verruca plana (flat warts) that are common the face or dorsal surfaces of the hands, verruca plantaris (plantar warts) that occur on the soles of the feet, and anogenital warts (condylomata acuminata).[4] Over 60 distinct types of HPV have been identified, and different types are associated with different diseases. HPV types 1, 2, and 4 produce common warts and plantar warts[5] (see Chapter 45); HPV types 6, 10, 11, and 40 through 45 cause anogenital warts[5]; and types 16 and 18 have been associated with squamous cell cancers of the genital tract.[5,6]

A relation between HPV and genital neoplasms has become increasingly apparent since the mid-1970s. Infection of the female genital tract by HPV-16 and HPV-18 and, rarely, by other types of HPV is associated with cer-

poscopy, or biopsy. Both spontaneous resolution and infection with new HPV types are common. Although reinfection from sexual partners was considered the main cause for the high prevalence of this disease, it is now thought that reinfection with the same HPV type is infrequent. Instead, it is thought that HPV may be a lifelong infection.

Genital warts should be considered in any woman who presents with the primary complaint of vulvar pruritus or who has had an abnormal Pap smear. Careful inspection of the vulva, with magnification as needed, usually reveals the characteristic lesions, and specimens for biopsy can be taken from questionable areas. Examination with a colposcope (instrument that magnifies cells of the cervix and vagina) may be advised as a follow-up measure when there is an abnormal Pap smear or when HPV lesions are identified on the vulva. Evaluation and treatment of sexual partners may be suggested, although this may be difficult considering that genital warts often do not become clinically apparent for several years after exposure.

The recent development and controlled trial of a vaccine to protect against HPV type 16 may eventually reduce the risk of cervical cancer associated with this strain of HPV.[8] Currently, however, there is no treatment to eradicate the virus once a person has become infected. Thus, treatment goals are aimed at elimination of symptomatic warts, surveillance for malignancy and premalignant changes, and education and counseling to decrease psychosocial distress.[9] Prevention of HPV transmission through condom use has not been adequately demonstrated.

The CDC identifies several pharmacologic treatments for symptomatic removal of visible genital warts, including patient-applied therapies (podofilox and imiquimod) and provider-administered therapies (podophyllin and trichloroacetic acid).[10] Podophyllin, a topical cytotoxic agent, has long been used for treatment of visible external growths. Multiple applications may be required for resolution of lesions. The amount of drug used and the surface area treated should be limited with each treatment session to avoid systematic absorption and toxicity. This treatment is contraindicated in pregnancy for the same reason. An alternative therapy is the topical application of a solution of trichloroacetic acid. This weak destructive agent produces an initial burning in the affected area, followed in several days by a sloughing of the superficial tissue. Several applications 1 to 2 weeks apart may be necessary to eradicate the lesion. Podofilox is a topical, patient-applied antimitotic agent that results in visible necrosis of wart tissue. It is a applied twice a day for 3 days, followed by 4 days of without treatment for a total of four cycles. The safety of podofilox during pregnancy has not been established. Imiquimod cream is a new type of therapeutic agent that stimulates the body's immune system (i.e., production of interferon-α and other cytokines). This cream is applied at home three times a week for up to 16 weeks. It must be washed off 6 to 10 hours after application to avoid excessive skin reaction. It is a category B drug and therefore potentially safe for use in pregnancy. Sexual abstinence is suggested during any type of treatment to enhance healing.

Genital warts also may be removed using cryotherapy, surgical excision, laser vaporization, or electrocautery. Because it can penetrate deeper than other forms of therapy, cryotherapy (i.e., freezing therapy) often is the treatment of choice for cervical HPV lesions. Laser surgery can be used to remove large or widespread lesions of the cervix, vagina, or vulva, or lesions that have failed to respond to other first-line methods of treatment. Electrosurgical treatment has become more widespread for these types of lesions because it is more readily available in outpatient settings and is much less expensive than laser.

GENITAL HERPES

Genital herpes is the most common cause of genital ulcers in the United States. Approximately 40 to 50 million Americans have genital herpes and approximately 1 million new cases occur each year.[11] Primary infection occurs mainly in adolescents and young adults. Women have a greater mucosal surface area exposed in the genital area and therefore are at greater risk of acquiring the infection. As with other ulcerative STDs, genital herpes increases the risk of HIV transmission and is believed to play an important role in the heterosexual spread of HIV.[11]

Herpesviruses are large, enveloped viruses that have a double-stranded genome.[12] There are nine types of herpesviruses, belonging to three groups, that cause infections in humans: neurotropic α-group viruses, including herpes simplex virus type 1 (HSV-1; usually associated with cold sores) and HSV-2 (usually associated with genital herpes); varicella-zoster virus (causes chickenpox and shingles); and lymphotropic β-group viruses, including cytomegalovirus (causes cytomegalic inclusion disease), Epstein-Barr virus (causes infectious mononucleosis and Burkitt lymphoma), and human herpesvirus type 8 (the apparent cause of Kaposi sarcoma).[5,12]

Herpes simplex virus type 1 and HSV-2 are genetically similar; both cause a similar set of primary and recurrent infections, and both can cause genital lesions. Both of these viruses replicate in the skin and mucous membranes at the site of infection (oropharynx or genitalia), where they cause vesicular lesions of the epidermis. HSV-1 and HSV-2 are neurotropic viruses, meaning that they grow in neurons and share the biologic property of latency. Latency refers to the ability to maintain disease potential in the absence of clinical signs and symptoms. In genital herpes, the virus ascends through the peripheral nerves to the sacral dorsal root ganglia (Fig. 40-2). The virus can remain dormant in the dorsal root ganglia, or it can reactivate, in which case the viral particles are transported back down the nerve root to the skin, where they multiply and cause a lesion to develop. During the dormant or latent period, the virus replicates in a different manner so that the immune system or available treatments have no effect on it. It is not known what reactivates the virus. It may be that the body's defense mechanisms are altered.

Herpes simplex virus is transmitted by contact with infectious lesions or secretions. HSV-1 is transmitted by oral secretions, and infections frequently occur in childhood.[5] It may be spread to the genital area by autoinoculation after poor hand washing or through oral intercourse.

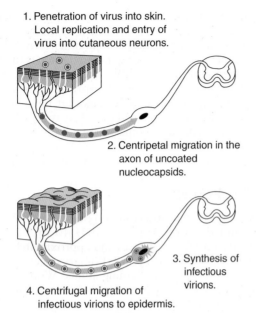

1. Penetration of virus into skin. Local replication and entry of virus into cutaneous neurons.

2. Centripetal migration in the axon of uncoated nucleocapsids.

3. Synthesis of infectious virions.

4. Centrifugal migration of infectious virions to epidermis.

FIGURE 40-2 Pathogenesis of primary mucocutaneous herpes simplex virus infection. (From Corey L., Spear P. G. [1986]. Infections with herpes simplex viruses. Part 1. *New England Journal of Medicine* 314, 686. Copyright © 2003. Massachusetts Medical Society.)

At least 15% of new cases of genital herpes are caused by HSV-1.[13] HSV-2 usually is transmitted by sexual contact but can be passed to an infant during childbirth if the virus is actively being shed from the genital tract. Most cases of HSV-2 infection are subclinical, manifesting as truly asymptomatic or symptomatic but unrecognized infections. These subclinical infections can occur in people who have never had a symptomatic outbreak or between recognized clinical recurrences. It has been estimated that 50% to 80% of genital herpes is spread through asymptomatic shedding by people who do not realize they have the infection.[13]

The incubation period for HSV is approximately 4 days (range, 2 to 12 days).[14] Genital HSV infection may manifest as a primary, nonprimary, or recurrent infection. *Primary infections* are infections that occur in a person who is seronegative for antibodies to HSV-1 or HSV-2. *Initial nonprimary infections* refer to the first clinical episode in a person who is seropositive for antibodies to the opposite HSV type (usually genital herpes in someone seropositive to HSV-1). *Recurrent infections* refer to the second or subsequent outbreak due to the same virus type. HSV-2 is responsible for greater than 90% of recurrent genital herpes infections.[9] Many "severe" presumed primary cases are actually first-recognized recurrences in persons with long-standing infection. Presence of antibodies to one type of HSV may decrease the symptomatic response to the initial infection with the other virus. Correct classification requires clinical correlation with viral isolation and type-specific serologic testing.[3]

The initial symptoms of primary genital herpes infections include tingling, itching, and pain in the genital area, followed by eruption of small pustules and vesicles. These lesions rupture on approximately the fifth day to form wet ulcers that are excruciatingly painful to touch and can be associated with dysuria, dyspareunia, and urine retention. Involvement of the cervix, vagina, urethra, and inguinal lymph nodes is common in women with primary infections. In men, the infection can cause urethritis and lesions of the penis and scrotum. Rectal and perianal infections are possible with anal contact. Systemic symptoms associated with primary infections include fever, headache, malaise, muscle ache, and lymphadenopathy.

Untreated primary infections typically are self-limited and last for approximately 2 to 4 weeks. The symptoms usually worsen for the first 10 to 12 days. This period is followed by a 10- to 12-day interval during which the lesions crust over and gradually heal. Recurrent episodes of genital herpes, which result from reactivation of the virus stored in the dorsal root ganglia of the infected dermatomes, manifest with less severe symptoms that usually are of shorter duration and have fewer systemic manifestations. Except for the greater tendency of HSV-2 to recur, the clinical manifestations of HSV-2 and genital HSV-1 are similar. Because the person has already developed immune lymphocytes from the primary infection, recurrent episodes have fewer lesions, fewer systemic symptoms, less pain, and a shorter duration (7 to 10 days). Frequency and severity of recurrences vary from person to person. Numerous factors, including emotional stress, lack of sleep, overexertion, other infections, vigorous or prolonged coitus, and premenstrual or menstrual distress have been identified as triggering mechanisms.

Diagnosis of genital herpes is based on the symptoms, appearance of the lesions, and identification of the virus from cultures taken from the lesions. Depending on the laboratory, a preliminary culture report takes from 2 to 5 days, and a final negative report takes from 10 to 12 days to establish. The likelihood of obtaining a positive culture decreases with each day that has elapsed after a lesion develops. The chance of obtaining a positive culture from a crusted lesion is slight, and persons suspected of having genital herpes should be instructed to have a culture within 48 hours of development of new lesions. Type-specific (HSV-1 and HSV-2) serologic tests are available for determining past infection. Because almost all HSV-2 infections are sexually acquired, the presence of type-specific HSV-2 antibodies usually indicates anogenital infection, whereas the presence of HSV-1 antibodies does not distinguish between anogenital and orolabial infections.

There is no known cure for genital herpes, and the methods of treatment are largely symptomatic. The antiviral drugs acyclovir, valacyclovir, and famciclovir have become the cornerstone for management of genital herpes. By interfering with viral deoxyribonucleic acid (DNA) replication, these drugs decrease the frequency of recurrences, shorten the duration of active lesions, reduce the number of new lesions formed, and decrease viral shedding with primary infections. Episodic intervention reduces the duration of viral shedding and the healing time for recurrent lesions. Continuous antiviral suppressive therapy may be advised when more than six outbreaks occur within 1 year.[10] These drugs are well tolerated, with few adverse effects. This long-term suppressive therapy does not limit latency, and reactivation of the disease frequently occurs after the drug is discontinued. In 2002 the U.S. Food and Drug Administration (FDA) approved long-term suppressive therapy with valacyclovir for the prevention of HSV-2 transmission to an uninfected sexual partner. Good hygiene is essential to prevent secondary HSV infection. Fastidious hand washing is recommended to avoid hand-to-eye spread of the infection. HSV infection of the eye is the most frequent cause of corneal blindness in the United States (see Chapter 37). To prevent spread of the disease, intimate contact should be avoided until lesions are completely healed.

Current information indicates the risk of neonatal infection is very low when the mother has developed type-specific antibodies, which are then protective to the neonate. Newborns at highest risk are those born to women who shed the virus and have not developed antibodies from previous infections. Disseminated neonatal infection is associated with high mortality and morbidity rates. Active infection during labor may necessitate cesarean delivery, ideally before membranes rupture. Recommendations from the American College of Obstetricians and Gynecologists direct care providers to obtain cultures when a woman has active lesions during pregnancy. Vaginal delivery is acceptable if visible lesions are not present at the onset of labor.[3]

CHANCROID

Chancroid is a disease of the external genitalia and lymph nodes caused by the gram-negative bacterium *Haemophilus ducreyi*. The disease is most common in tropical and subtropical regions. It is one of the most common causes of genital ulcers in less-developed countries, especially in Africa and parts of Asia, where it probably serves as an important cofactor in the transmission of HIV infection.[5,15] This STD, which has become uncommon in the United States (only 143 cases were reported in 1999), typically occurs in discrete outbreaks.[1] However, recent evidence suggests that chancroid may be underdiagnosed because many STD clinics do not have the facilities to test for *H. ducreyi*.[15]

Chancroid is highly infectious and is usually transmitted by sexual intercourse or through skin and mucous membrane abrasions. Autoinoculation may lead to multiple chancres. Lesions begin as macules, progress to pustules, and then rupture. This painful ulcer has a necrotic base and jagged edges. In contrast, the syphilitic chancre is nontender and indurated. Subsequent discharge can lead to further infection of self or others. On physical examination, lesions and regional lymphadenopathy (*i.e.*, buboes) may be found. Secondary infection may cause significant tissue destruction.

Diagnosis usually is made clinically but may be confirmed through culture. However, the culture method is expensive and requires special laboratory methods and experience.[15] Polymerase chain reaction (PCR) methods may soon be available commercially for definitive identification of *H. ducreyi*. The organism has shown resistance to treatment with sulfamethoxazole alone and to tetracycline. The CDC recommends treatment with azithromycin, erythromycin, ciprofloxacin, or ceftriaxone.[10]

GRANULOMA INGUINALE

Granuloma inguinale (*i.e.*, granuloma venereum) is caused by a gram-negative bacillus, *Calymmatobacterium donovani*, which is a tiny, encapsulated intracellular parasite. This disease is almost nonexistent in the United States. It is found most frequently in India, Brazil, the West Indies, and parts of China, Australia, and Africa.

Granuloma inguinale causes ulceration of the genitalia, beginning with an innocuous papule. The papule progresses through nodular or vesicular stages until it begins to break down as pink, granulomatous tissue. At this final stage, the tissue becomes thin and friable and bleeds easily. There are complaints of swelling, pain, and itching. Extensive inflammatory scarring may cause late sequelae, such as lymphatic obstruction with the development of enlarged and elephantoid external genitalia. The liver, bladder, bone, joint, lung, and bowel tissue may become involved. Genital complications include tubo-ovarian abscess, fistula, vaginal stenosis, and occlusion of vaginal or anal orifices. Lesions may become neoplastic.

Diagnosis is made through the identification of Donovan bodies (*i.e.*, large mononuclear cells filled with intracytoplasmic gram-negative rods) in tissue smears, biopsy samples, or culture. A 3-week period of treatment with doxycycline, tetracycline, erythromycin, or gentamicin is used in treating the disorder.[10]

In summary, STDs that primarily affect the external genitalia include condylomata acuminata, genital herpes (HSV-2), chancroid, and granuloma inguinale. Condylomata acuminata, or *genital warts,* are caused by HPV. Of concern is the relation between some subtypes of HPV and genital neoplasms, particularly cervical cancer. Genital herpes is caused by a neurotropic virus (HSV-2) that ascends through the peripheral nerves to reside in the sacral dorsal root ganglia. The herpesvirus can be reactivated, producing recurrent lesions in genital structures that are supplied by the peripheral nerves of the affected ganglia. There is no permanent cure for herpes infections. Chancroid, which is caused by the gram-negative bacterium *H. ducreyi,* is characterized by lymphadenopathy and painful ulcers of the genitalia. Granuloma inguinale produces external genital lesions with various degrees of inguinal lymph node involvement.

Vaginal Infections

Candidiasis, trichomoniasis, and bacterial vaginosis are vaginal infections that can be sexually transmitted. Although these infections can be transmitted sexually, the male partner usually is asymptomatic.

CANDIDIASIS

Candidiasis, also called *yeast infection, thrush,* and *moniliasis,* is the second leading cause of vulvovaginitis in the United States. Approximately 75% of reproductive-age women in the United States experience one episode in their lifetime; 40% to 45% experience two or more infections.[10]

Candida albicans is the most commonly identified organism in vaginal yeast infections, but other candidal species, such as *Candida glabrata* and *Candida tropicalis,* may also be present. These organisms are present in 10% to 20% of healthy women without causing symptoms, and alteration of the host vaginal environment usually is necessary before the organism can cause pathologic effects.[16] Although vulvovaginal candidiasis usually is not transmitted sexually, it is included in the CDC STD treatment guidelines because it often is diagnosed in women being evaluated for STDs.[10] The possibility of sexual transmission has been recognized for many years; however, candidiasis requires a favorable environment for growth. Despite studies that have documented the presence of *Candida* on the penis of male partners of women with vulvovaginal candidiasis, few men develop balanoposthitis that requires treatment. The gastrointestinal tract also serves as a reservoir for this organism, and candidiasis can develop through autoinoculation in women who are not sexually active.

Causes for the overgrowth of *C. albicans* include antibiotic therapy, which suppresses the normal protective bacterial flora; high hormone levels owing to pregnancy or the use of oral contraceptives, which cause an increase in vaginal glycogen stores; and diabetes mellitus or HIV infection, because they compromise the immune system.

Manifestations of vulvovaginal candidiasis include vulvovaginal irritation, pruritus, swelling, and erythema; dysuria; and dyspareunia. In obese persons, *Candida* may grow in skinfolds underneath breast tissue, the abdominal flap, and the inguinal folds. The characteristic vaginal discharge, when present, is usually odorless, thick, and cheesy. Accurate diagnosis is made by identification of budding yeast filaments (*i.e.,* hyphae) or spores on a wet-mount slide using a 10% to 20% potassium hydroxide preparation.[16,17] The pH of the discharge, which is checked with litmus paper, typically is less than 4.5. When the wet-mount technique is negative but the clinical manifestations are suggestive of candidiasis, a culture may be necessary.

Antifungal agents such as clotrimazole, miconazole, butoconazole, and terconazole, in various topical forms, are effective in treating candidiasis. These drugs, with the exception of terconazole, are available without prescription for use by women who have had a previously confirmed diagnosis of candidiasis. Oral fluconazole has been shown to be as safe and effective as the standard intravaginal regimens.[10] It is, however, a pregnancy class C drug. Tepid sodium bicarbonate baths, clothing that allows adequate ventilation, and the application of cornstarch to dry the area may increase comfort during treatment. Chronic vulvovaginal candidiasis, defined as four or more mycologically confirmed episodes within 1 year, affects approximately 5% of women and is difficult to manage. Subsequent prophylaxis (maintenance therapy) often is required for long-term management of this problem.[16]

TRICHOMONIASIS

Trichomonas vaginalis is credited with being a far more prevalent cause of STD than either *Chlamydia trachomatis* or *Neisseria gonorrhoeae.* In the United States, it has been estimated that 5 million new cases of trichomoniasis appear annually.[1,18] However, this number remains an estimate because trichomoniasis is not a reportable STD.

T. vaginalis is a large, anaerobic, pear-shaped, flagellated protozoan. Trichomonads can reside in the paraurethral glands of both sexes. Men harbor the organism in the urethra and prostate and are asymptomatic. Although 10% to 25% of women are asymptomatic, trichomoniasis is a common cause of vaginitis when some imbalance allows the protozoan to proliferate.[1] This extracellular parasite feeds on the vaginal mucosa and ingests bacteria and leukocytes. The infection causes a copious, frothy, malodorous, green or yellow discharge. There commonly is erythema and edema of the affected mucosa, with occasional itching and irritation. Sometimes, small hemorrhagic areas, called *strawberry spots,* appear on the cervix.

Trichomoniasis can cause a number of complications.[18] It is a risk factor for HIV transmission and infectivity in both men and women. In women, it increases the risk of tubal infertility and atypical pelvic inflammatory disease (see Chapter 39) and it is associated with adverse outcomes such as premature birth in pregnant women. Trichomonads attach easily to mucous membrane. They may serve as vectors for spread of other organisms, carrying pathogens attached to their surface into the fallopian tubes. In men, it a common cause of nongonococcal urethritis and is a risk factor for infertility by altering sperm motility and viability.[18] It has also been associated with chronic prostatitis.

Diagnosis is based on positive identification of the organism.[18] Wet-mount microscopic examination of vaginal secretions is the most common diagnostic method. Special culture media are available for diagnosis, but are costly and not necessary for diagnosis. Pap smear has been used for diagnosing trichomoniasis; however, this method has a low sensitivity compared with culture diagnosis. Diagnosis in men is more problematic because it is difficult to identify the organism in either urine or genital secretions in men.

The treatment of choice is oral metronidazole, a medication that is effective against anaerobic protozoans.[10] Metronidazole is chemically similar to disulfiram (Antabuse), a drug used in the treatment of alcohol addiction that causes nausea, vomiting, flushing of the skin, headache, palpitations, and lowering of the blood pressure when alcohol is ingested. Alcohol should be avoided during and for 24 to 48 hours after treatment. Metronidazole has not been proven safe for use during pregnancy and is used only after the first trimester for fear of potential teratogenic effects. Because trichomoniasis is an STD, sexual partners should be treated concurrently. When sexual partners are treated, the cure rates approach 100% and recurrence is rare.[18]

BACTERIAL VAGINOSIS

Bacterial vaginosis is a common condition with a poorly understood etiology. It is one of the most prevalent forms of vaginal infection seen by health care professionals. Its relation to sexual activity is not clear. Sexual activity is believed to be a catalyst rather than a primary mode of transmission, and endogenous factors play a role in the development of symptoms.

A number of terms have been used to describe the nonspecific vaginitis that cannot be attributed to one of the accepted pathogenic organisms, such as *T. vaginalis* or *C. albicans*. It appears to result from imbalance of the normal vaginal flora, overgrowth of anaerobic bacteria, and a reduction in the *Lactobacillus* species in the vagina.[19,20] The implicated microorganisms include *Gardnerella vaginalis*, *Mycoplasma hominis*, *Ureaplasma urealyticum*, *Mobiluncus* species, and other anaerobes.[20]

The predominant symptom of bacterial vaginosis is a thin, grayish-white discharge that has a foul, fishy odor. Burning, itching, and erythema usually are absent because the bacteria have only minimal inflammatory potential. The organisms responsible for bacterial vaginosis may be carried asymptomatically by men and women. Bacterial vaginosis has been shown to be a risk factor for premature labor and perinatal infection. It may also increase the risk of infectious complications of certain gynecologic procedures, such as hysterectomy.[17,20]

The diagnosis is made when at least three of the following characteristics are present: homogeneous discharge, production of a fishy, amine odor when a 10% potassium hydroxide solution is dropped onto the secretions, vaginal pH above 4.5 (usually 5.0 to 6.0), and the presence of characteristic "clue cells" in the vaginal fluid on light microscopy.[17,20] *Clue cells* are squamous epithelial cells covered with masses of coccobacilli, often with large clumps of organisms floating free from the cell. Because *G. vaginalis* can be part of the normal vaginal flora, cultures should not be done routinely.

The mere presence of *G. vaginalis* in an asymptomatic woman is not an indication for treatment. According to CDC guidelines, treatment for bacterial vaginosis is indicated to reduce symptoms and prevent infectious complications associated with pregnancy and hysterectomy. When indicated, treatment is aimed at eradicating the anaerobic component of bacterial vaginosis to reestablish the normal balance of the vaginal flora. The CDC recommends oral metronidazole.[10] Alternative therapies include metronidazole vaginal gel, clindamycin vaginal cream, or oral clindamycin. The CDC guidelines also support testing and treatment of pregnant women with a history of premature delivery. Women who are undergoing hysterectomy should also be tested and treated. Treatment of sexual partners is not recommended.[10]

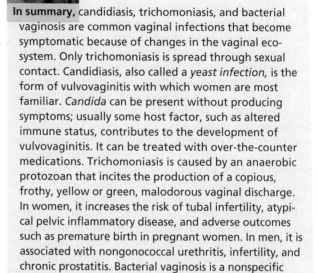

In summary, candidiasis, trichomoniasis, and bacterial vaginosis are common vaginal infections that become symptomatic because of changes in the vaginal ecosystem. Only trichomoniasis is spread through sexual contact. Candidiasis, also called a *yeast infection*, is the form of vulvovaginitis with which women are most familiar. *Candida* can be present without producing symptoms; usually some host factor, such as altered immune status, contributes to the development of vulvovaginitis. It can be treated with over-the-counter medications. Trichomoniasis is caused by an anaerobic protozoan that incites the production of a copious, frothy, yellow or green, malodorous vaginal discharge. In women, it increases the risk of tubal infertility, atypical pelvic inflammatory disease, and adverse outcomes such as premature birth in pregnant women. In men, it is associated with nongonococcal urethritis, infertility, and chronic prostatitis. Bacterial vaginosis is a nonspecific type of infection that produces a characteristic fishy-smelling discharge. It appears to result from imbalance of the normal vaginal flora, overgrowth of anaerobic bacteria, and a reduction in vaginal *Lactobacillus* species.

 Urogenital-Systemic Infections

Some STDs produce both urogenital lesions and systemic manifestations. Among the infections of this type are chlamydial infections, gonorrhea, and syphilis. Many of these infections also pose a risk to infants born to infected mothers. Some infections, such as syphilis, may be spread to the infant in utero; others, such as chlamydial and gonorrheal infections, can be spread to the infant during the birth process.

CHLAMYDIAL INFECTIONS

Infection with *C. trachomatis* is the most common reportable STD in the United States.[21] As of December 2000, chlamydial infections are reportable in all 50 states and the District of Columbia. According to the latest CDC estimates, chlamydial infections occur at a rate of almost 3 million new cases each year.[21] Rates for chlamydial infections have risen significantly over the past 15 years because of an increase in screening programs, improved sensitivity of diagnostic tests, and improved surveillance and reporting systems. Reported rates are higher in women largely because of screening efforts, although actual occurrence rates are thought to be the same for men and women. Significant declines in prevalence have been noted in areas where screening programs have been initiated.

Chlamydiae are intracellular parasites that are smaller than most bacteria.[12] They lack the enzymes necessary to generate adenosine triphosphate (ATP) and must parasitize the machinery of the host cell to reproduce. *C. trachomatis* causes a wide variety of genitourinary infections,

...luding nongonococcal urethritis in men and pelvic inflammatory disease in women. The closely related organisms *Chlamydia pneumoniae* and *Chlamydia psittaci* cause mild and severe pneumonia, respectively. *C. trachomatis* can be serologically subdivided into types A, B, and C, which are associated with trachoma and chronic keratoconjunctivitis; types D through K, which are associated with genital infections and their complications; and types L1, L2, and L3, which are associated with lymphogranuloma venereum. *C. trachomatis* can cause significant ocular disease in neonates; it is a leading cause of blindness in underdeveloped countries. In these countries, the organism is spread primarily by flies, fomites, and nonsexual personal contact. In industrial countries, the organism is spread almost exclusively by sexual contact and therefore affects primarily the genitourinary structures.

Chlamydiae exist in two forms: elementary bodies, which are the infectious particles capable of entering uninfected cells, and reticulate bodies, which multiply by binary fission to produce the inclusions identified in stained cells.[5] The growth cycle starts with attachment of the elementary body to the susceptible host cell, after which it is ingested by a process that resembles phagocytosis. Once inside the cell, the elementary body is organized into the reticulate body, the metabolically active form of the organism that is capable of reproduction. The reticulate body is not infectious and cannot survive outside the body. The reticulate bodies divide repeatedly, forming daughter elementary bodies and destroying the host cell. Necrotic debris elicits inflammation and immunologic responses that further damage infected tissue.

The signs and symptoms of *C. trachomatis* infection resemble those produced by gonorrhea. The most significant difference between chlamydial and gonococcal salpingitis is that chlamydial infections may be asymptomatic or subclinically nonspecific. As many as 85% to 95% of *C. trachomatis* infections in men and women are asymptomatic; therefore, most cases are undiagnosed, unreported, and untreated.[22]

Despite the frequent absence of symptoms, at least one third of women have local signs of infection (*e.g.*, mucopurulent drainage, hypertrophic cervical changes) on examination. Clinical manifestations of *T. trachomatis* infection in women depend on the site of infection.[22] Infection of the urethra and lower genital tract causes urinary frequency, dysuria, abnormal vaginal discharge, and postcoital bleeding. Infection of the upper genital tract (endometritis or salpingitis) may be manifested as irregular uterine bleeding and abdominal or pelvic discomfort. In women, untreated infection can lead to severe reproductive complications, including infertility, ectopic pregnancy, and chronic pelvic pain. Up to two thirds of cases of infertility due to tubal factors and one third of cases of ectopic pregnancy may be attributable to *C. trachomatis* infection.[22] Chlamydial infection during pregnancy is associated with a number of adverse effects, including preterm labor, premature rupture of the membranes, low-birth–weight infants, and postpartum endometritis. The infection may also be transmitted to the infant during delivery.[22] Approximately 30% to 50% of infants born to mothers with active infection will have conjunctivitis, and at least 50% of these will also have nasopharyngeal infection. Chlamydial pneumonia develops in about 30% of infants with nasopharyngeal infection.

In men, chlamydial infections cause urethritis, including meatal erythema and tenderness, urethral discharge, dysuria, and urethral itching. Prostatitis and epididymitis with subsequent infertility may develop. The most serious complication that can develop with nongonococcal urethritis is Reiter syndrome, a systemic condition characterized by urethritis, conjunctivitis, arthritis, and mucocutaneous lesions (see Chapter 43). Infection with *C. trachomatis* is believed to be a cofactor in transmission of HIV infection in both men and women.

Routine screening for sexually active adolescents and young adults has been suggested by the CDC and the U.S. Preventive Services Task Force (USPSTF) as a means of decreasing the incidence of the serious sequelae of untreated asymptomatic infections.[21] Because reinfection rates are high and occur within several months, it is recommended that sexual partners be treated and women be rescreened 4 to 6 months after initial infection.[23]

Until recently, culture was the accepted method of diagnosis, but it requires special handling and laboratory services. The direct fluorescent antibody test and the enzyme-linked immunosorbent assay that use antibodies against an antigen in the *Chlamydia* cell wall are rapid tests that are highly sensitive and specific. Nucleic acid amplification tests (NAATs) do not require viable organisms for detection, and can produce a positive signal from as little as a single copy of the target DNA or ribonucleic acid (RNA). Tests such as PCR, ligase chain reaction (LCR), or transcription-mediated amplification (TMA) have demonstrated specificities of near 100% (same as culture) and sensitivities of 90% to 95%. Because NAATs can be performed on urine and swab specimens from the distal vagina as well as the traditional endocervical and urethral specimens, this easy, convenient means of accurate detection has become the diagnostic method of choice.[10,21,24] Nucleic acid hybridization assays detect *C. trachomatis* and *N. gonorrhoeae* in a single test. This type of test does not differentiate between the two organisms, and a positive result requires follow-up testing to obtain organism-specific results.[24] Cost often is a factor in determining which type of testing to use.

The CDC recommends the use of doxycycline or azithromycin in the treatment of chlamydial infection; penicillin is ineffective. Erythromycin or amoxicillin is the preferred choice in pregnancy.[10] Antibiotic treatment of both sexual partners simultaneously is recommended. Abstinence from sexual activity is encouraged to facilitate cure. Retesting of all women with chlamydial infection 3 to 4 months after treatment has been recommended to rule out recurrence.[10]

GONORRHEA

Gonorrhea is a reportable disease caused by the bacterium *N. gonorrhoeae*. In 1999, there were 360,076 reported cases of gonorrhea in the United States.[1] Of these reported cases, more than 90% involved persons between 15 and 44 years of age, with the heaviest concentration among young adults (15 to 24 years of age). There are an estimated 600,000 new cases every year.[10] Although the incidence of gonorrhea has declined steadily from its peak in 1975, there was an increase in occurrence between 1997 and 1998. Improved screening efforts as well as greater use of more sensitive nonculture methods of testing may have contributed to this increase. Higher rates of occurrence among homosexual men were documented in several states, leading to a concern that a rise in unsafe sexual behavior may be occurring because of the availability of highly active antiretroviral agents for treatment of HIV infection.[25]

The gonococcus is a pyogenic (*i.e.*, pus-forming), gram-negative diplococcus that evokes inflammatory reactions characterized by purulent exudates.[12] Humans are the only natural host for *N. gonorrhoeae*. The organism grows best in warm, mucus-secreting epithelia. The portal of entry can be the genitourinary tract, eyes, oropharynx, anorectum, or skin.

Transmission usually is by heterosexual or homosexual intercourse. Autoinoculation of the organism to the conjunctiva is possible. Neonates born to infected mothers can acquire the infection during passage through the birth canal and are in danger of developing gonorrheal conjunctivitis, with resultant blindness, unless treated promptly. An amniotic infection syndrome characterized by premature rupture of the membranes, premature delivery, and increased risk of infant morbidity and mortality has been identified as an additional complication of gonococcal infections in pregnancy. Genital gonorrhea in young children should raise the possibility of sexual abuse.

The infection commonly manifests 2 to 5 days after exposure.[12] It typically begins in the anterior urethra, accessory urethral glands, Bartholin's or Skene's glands, and the cervix. If untreated, gonorrhea spreads from its initial sites upward into the genital tract. In men, it spreads to the prostate and epididymis; in women, it commonly moves to the fallopian tubes. Pharyngitis may follow oral-genital contact. The organism also can invade the bloodstream (*i.e.*, disseminated gonococcal infection), causing serious sequelae such as bacteremic involvement of joint spaces, heart valves, meninges, and other body organs and tissues.

Persons with gonorrhea may be asymptomatic and may unwittingly spread the disease to their sexual partners. Men are more likely to be symptomatic than women. In men, the initial symptoms include urethral pain and a creamy, yellow, sometimes bloody discharge (Fig. 40-3). The disorder may become chronic and affect the prostate, epididymis, and periurethral glands. Rectal infections are common in homosexual men. In women, recognizable symptoms include unusual genital or urinary discharge, dysuria, dyspareunia, pelvic pain or tenderness, unusual vaginal bleeding (including bleeding after intercourse), fever, and proctitis. Symptoms may occur or increase during or immediately after menses because the bacterium is an intracellular diplococcus that thrives in menstrual blood but cannot survive long outside the human body. There may be infections of the uterus and development

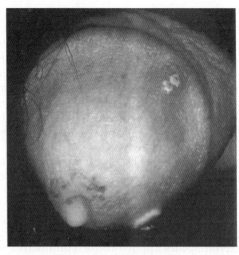

FIGURE 40-3 Purulent penile discharge due to gonorrhea with overlying pyodermal lesions. (From Centers for Disease Control and Prevention photographic images library. Available: http://phil.cdc.gov/phil/details.asp.)

of acute or chronic infection of the fallopian tubes with ultimate scarring and sterility (Fig. 40-4).

Diagnosis is based on the history of sexual exposure and symptoms. It is confirmed by identification of the organism on Gram stain or culture. A Gram stain usually is an effective means of diagnosis in symptomatic men (*i.e.*, those with discharge). In women and asymptomatic

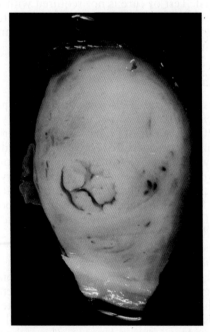

FIGURE 40-4 Gonorrhea of the fallopian tube. Cross-section of a "pus tube" shows thickening of the wall and lumen swollen with pus. (From Schwartz D., Genta R. M., Conner D. H. (2005). Infectious and parasitic diseases. In Rubin E., Gorstein F., Rubin R., et al. [Eds.], *Rubin's pathology: Clinicopathologic foundations of medicine* [4th ed., p. 386]. Philadelphia: Lippincott Williams & Wilkins.)

n, a culture usually is preferred because Gram stains often are unreliable. Culture detects more than 95% of male urethral gonorrhea and 80% to 90% of cervical, rectal, and pharyngeal infections.[10] An enzyme immunoassay for detecting gonococcal antigens (Gonozyme) is available but has several requirements that limit its usefulness. Detection by means of amplified DNA probes is possible using urine and urethral swab specimens. The sensitivity of these probes is similar to that of culture, and they may be cost-effective in high-risk populations.

Testing for other STDs, particularly syphilis and chlamydial infections, is suggested at the time of examination. Pregnant women are routinely screened at the time of their first prenatal visit; members of high-risk populations should have repeat cultures during the third trimester. Neonates are routinely treated with various antibacterial agents applied to the conjunctiva within 1 hour of birth to protect against undiagnosed gonorrhea and other diseases.

Penicillin-resistant strains of *N. gonorrhoeae* are prevalent worldwide and strains with other kinds of antibiotic resistance continue to evolve and spread. Currently, the CDC recommends the use of a single dose of ceftriaxone, cefixime, ciprofloxacin, or ofloxacin as initial therapy for uncomplicated cases of gonorrhea and that these agents be given in combination with doxycycline or azithromycin in the management of dual infection with chlamydiae. Fluoroquinolones are no longer recommended as first-line agents because of emerging resistance; the same is true of amoxicillin. All sex partners within 60 days before discovery of the infection should be contacted, tested, and treated. Test of cure is not required with observed single-dose therapy. Patients are instructed to refrain from intercourse until therapy is completed and symptoms are no longer present.[10]

SYPHILIS

Syphilis is a reportable disease caused by a spirochete, *Treponema pallidum*.[5,26] After declining every year from 1990 to 2000, the rate of primary and secondary syphilis in the United States increased between 2001 and 2002 by 12.4%. Syphilis continues to affect minority populations disproportionately. Although the rate of primary and secondary syphilis for blacks declined from 2001 to 2002, it was still 8.2 times higher than the rate reported for whites.[26] During the same time period, the rate for Hispanics and Asian/Pacific Islanders increased by 20%, primarily among men.

T. pallidum is a strict human pathogen that is spread by direct contact with an infectious, moist lesion, usually through sexual intercourse. Bacteria-laden secretions may transfer the organism during kissing or intimate contact. Skin abrasions provide another possible portal of entry. There is rapid transplacental transmission of the organism from the mother to the fetus after 16 weeks' gestation, so that active disease in the mother during pregnancy can produce congenital syphilis in the fetus. Untreated syphilis can cause prematurity, stillbirth, and congenital defects and active infection in the infant. Once treated for syphilis,

a pregnant woman usually is followed throughout pregnancy by repeat testing of serum titers.

The tissue destruction and lesions observed in syphilis are primarily the result of the person's immune response to the infection. The clinical disease is divided into three stages: primary, secondary, and tertiary. Primary syphilis is characterized by the appearance of a chancre at the site of exposure. Chancres typically appear within 3 weeks of exposure but may incubate for 1 week to 3 months. The primary chancre begins as a single, indurated, buttonlike papule up to several centimeters in diameter that erodes to create a clean-based ulcerated lesion on an elevated base.[5] These lesions usually are painless and located at the site of sexual contact. Primary syphilis is readily apparent in the man, where the lesion is on the penis or scrotum (Fig. 40-5). Although chancres can develop on the external genitalia in women, they are more common on the vagina or cervix, and primary syphilis therefore may go undetected and untreated. There usually is an accompanying regional lymphadenopathy. The disease is highly contagious at this stage, but because the symptoms are mild, it frequently goes unnoticed. The chancre usually heals within 3 to 12 weeks, with or without treatment.

Secondary syphilis features systemic dissemination and proliferation of *T. pallidum* and is characterized by lesions of the skin, mucous membranes, lymph nodes, meninges, stomach, and liver.[5] The most common presentation of secondary syphilis is an erythematous and maculopapular rash, involving the trunk and extremities, especially the

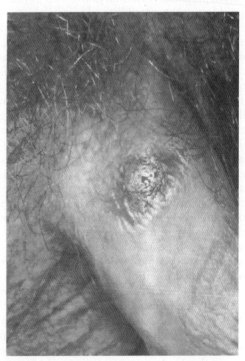

FIGURE 40-5 Syphilitic chancre of the penis shaft. (From Centers for Disease Control and Prevention photographic images library. Available: http://phil.cdc.gov/phil/details.asp.)

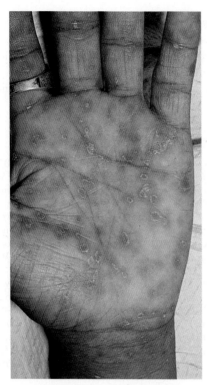

FIGURE 40-6 Secondary syphilis. A maculopapular rash is present on the palm. (From Schwartz D., Genta R. M., Conner D. H. (2005). Infectious and parasitic diseases. In Rubin E., Gorstein F., Rubin R., et al. [Eds.], *Rubin's pathology: Clinicopathologic foundations of medicine* [4th ed., p. 409]. Philadelphia: Lippincott Williams & Wilkins.)

palms of the hands (Fig. 40-6) and soles of the feet. The rash occurs 2 weeks to 3 months after the chancre of primary syphilis heals. Other skin manifestations may include alopecia and genital condylomata lata. Condylomata lata are elevated, red-brown lesions that may ulcerate and produce a foul discharge. They are 2 to 3 cm in diameter, contain many spirochetes, and are highly infectious. Lesions of the mucosal surfaces of the mouth and genital organs, called *mucous patches,* are rich in organisms and highly infectious. Although *T. pallidum* is commonly found in meninges, this involvement is frequently asymptomatic.

After the secondary stage, syphilis frequently enters a latent phase that may last for years to decades. Persons can be infective during the first 1 to 2 years of latency. During this time, the spirochetes continue to multiply and may cause progression to tertiary syphilis. Tertiary syphilis is a delayed response to the untreated disease. It can occur as long as 20 years after the initial infection. Approximately one third of people with untreated syphilis develop the tertiary stage of the disease.[5] When syphilis does progress to the symptomatic tertiary stage, it most frequently affects the cardiovascular system, central nervous system, and the liver, bones, and testes.[6] Cardiovascular manifestations usually result from scarring of the medial layer of the thoracic aorta with aneurysm formation. These aneurysms produce enlargement of the aortic valve ring with aortic valve insufficiency. Central nervous system lesions can produce dementia, blindness, or injury to the spinal cord, with ataxia and sensory loss (*i.e.,* tabes dorsalis). Syphilitic gummas are peculiar, rubbery, necrotic lesions caused by noninflammatory tissue necrosis. Gummas can occur singly or multiply and vary in size from microscopic to large, tumorous masses. They most commonly are found in the liver, testes, and bone.

T. pallidum cannot be cultured and it does not produce endotoxins or exotoxins, but evokes a humoral immune response that provides the basis for serologic tests. Two types of antibodies—nonspecific and specific—are produced. The nonspecific antibodies can be detected by flocculation tests such as the Venereal Disease Research Laboratory (VDRL) test or the rapid plasma reagin (RPR) test. Because these tests are nonspecific, positive results can occur with diseases other than syphilis. The tests are easy to perform, rapid, and inexpensive and frequently are used as screening tests for syphilis. Results become positive 4 to 6 weeks after infection or 1 to 3 weeks after the appearance of the primary lesion. Because these tests are quantitative, they can be used to measure the degree of disease activity or treatment effectiveness. The VDRL titer usually is high during the secondary stage of the disease and becomes less so during the tertiary stage. A falling titer during treatment suggests a favorable response. The fluorescent treponemal antibody absorption test or microhemagglutinin test is used to detect specific antibodies to *T. pallidum*. These qualitative tests are used to determine whether a positive result on a nonspecific test such as the VDRL is attributable to syphilis. The test results remain positive for life.

The treatment of choice for syphilis is penicillin. Because of the spirochetes' long generation time, effective tissue levels of penicillin must be maintained for several weeks. Long-acting injectable forms of penicillin are used. Tetracycline or doxycycline is used for treatment in persons who are sensitive to penicillin. Pregnant women should be desensitized and treated with penicillin because erythromycin does not treat fetal infection. Sexual partners should be evaluated and treated prophylactically even though they may show no sign of infection. All treated individuals should be reexamined clinically and serologically at 6 and 12 months after completing therapy; more frequent monitoring (3-month intervals) is suggested for individuals with HIV infection.[10]

In summary, the urogenital-systemic STDs—chlamydial infections, gonorrhea, and syphilis—can severely involve the urogenital structures and manifest as systemic infections. *C. trachomatis* infection is the most common reportable STD in the United States. In women, untreated infection can lead to severe reproductive complications, including infertility, ectopic pregnancy, and chronic pelvic pain, and in men it can cause urethritis, prostatitis, and epididymitis with subsequent infertility. Gonorrhea, which is caused by the gram-negative bacterium, *N. gonorrhoeae*, evokes an inflammatory reaction characterized by purulent exudates. The infection typically begins in the external genitalia and then moves upward in the genital tract, commonly to the fallopian tubes in women and to the prostate and epididymis in men. The organism also can invade the bloodstream (*i.e.*, disseminated gonococcal infection), causing serious sequelae such as bacteremic involvement of joint spaces, heart valves, meninges, and other body organs and tissues. Both gonorrhea and chlamydial infections can cause ocular disease and blindness in neonates born to infected mothers. Syphilis is caused by a spirochete, *T. pallidum*. It can produce widespread systemic effects and is transferred to the fetus of infected mothers through the placenta. Untreated, the disease progresses through a primary stage, which is characterized by the appearance of a chancre at the site of exposure; a secondary stage, which features systemic dissemination and proliferation of *T. pallidum;* and a latent stage, which lasts for years to decades and progresses to tertiary syphilis in about one third of untreated people.

Review Questions

A 25-year-old woman has been told that her Pap test indicates infection with HPV 16.

A. What are the possible implications of infection with HPV 16?
B. How might she have acquired this infection?
C. What treatments are currently available for treatment of this infection?

A 35-year-old woman presents with vulvar pruritus, dysuria, dyspareunia, and an odorless, thick, cheesy vaginal discharge. She has diabetes mellitus and has recently recovered from a respiratory tract infection, which required antibiotic treatment.

A. Given that these manifestations are consistent with a *Candida* infection, what tests might be used to confirm the diagnosis?
B. What risk factors does this woman have that predispose to this type of vaginitis?
C. How might this infection be treated?

Visit the Porth: Essentials of Pathophysiology: Concepts of Altered Health States web site (http://thePoint.LWW.com/PorthEssentials) for links to chapter-related resources on the Internet, all-new exclusive animations, chapter review questions, and more!

REFERENCES

1. Centers for Disease Control and Prevention. (2000). *Tracking the hidden epidemics: Trends in STDs in the United States.* [Online]. Available: www.cdc.gov/nchstp/dstd/dstdp.html. Accessed August 10, 2005.
2. Kurman R. J. (2002). *Blaustein's pathology of the female genital tract* (5th ed., pp. 258–276). New York: Springer.
3. Sweet R. L., Gibbs R. S. (2002). *Infectious diseases of the female genital tract* (5th ed., pp. 155–164). Baltimore: Williams & Wilkins.
4. Gunter J. (2003). Genital and perianal warts: New treatment opportunities for human papillomavirus infection. *American Journal of Obstetrics and Gynecology* 189(3), S3–S11.
5. Schwartz D., Genta R. M., Conner D. H. (2005). Infectious and parasitic diseases. In Rubin E., Gorstein F., Rubin R., et al. (Eds.), *Rubin's pathology: Clinicopathologic foundations of medicine* (4th ed., pp. 354–387, 408–411). Philadelphia: Lippincott Williams & Wilkins.
6. McAdam A. J., Sharpe A. H. (2005). Infectious diseases. In Kumar V., Abbas A. K., Fausto N. (Eds.), *Robbins and Cotran pathologic basis of disease* (7th ed., pp. 365–361). Philadelphia: Elsevier Saunders.
7. Kodner C. M., Nasraty S. (2004). Management of genital warts. *American Family Physician* 70, 2335–2342.
8. Koutsky L. A., Ault K. A., Wheeler C. M. (2002). A controlled trial of human papilloma virus type 16 vaccine. *New England Journal of Medicine* 347, 1645–1651.
9. Handsfield H. H. (2001). *Color atlas and synopsis of sexually transmitted diseases* (pp. 13, 23, 71, 87, 163). New York: McGraw-Hill.
10. Centers for Disease Control and Prevention. (2002). Sexually transmitted diseases: Treatment guidelines 2002. *MMWR Morbidity and Mortality Weekly Report* 51(RR-6), 1–118.
11. Miller K. E., Rutz D. E., Graves C. (2003). Update on prevention and treatment of sexually transmitted diseases. *American Family Physician* 67, 1915–1921.
12. Murray P. R., Rosenthal K. D., Kobayashi G. S., et al. (2002). *Medical microbiology* (4th ed., pp. 256, 475–498). St. Louis: Mosby.
13. Mark H. D., Hanahan A. P., Stender S. C. (2003). Herpes simplex virus type 2: An update. *Nurse Practitioner* 28(11), 34–41.
14. Kimberlin D. W., Rouse D. J. (2004). Genital herpes. *New England Journal of Medicine* 350, 1970–1977.
15. Lewis D. A. (2003). Chancroid: Clinical manifestations, diagnosis, and management. *Sexually Transmitted Infections* 79, 68–71.
16. Ringdahl E. N. (2000). Treatment of recurrent vulvovaginal candidiasis. *American Family Physician* 61, 3306–3317.
17. Owen M. K., Clenney T. L. (2004). Management of vaginitis. *American Family Physician* 70, 2125–2132.
18. Soper D. (2004). Trichomoniasis: Under control or undercontrolled? *American Journal of Obstetrics and Gynecology* 190, 281–290.
19. Weir E. (2004). Bacterial vaginosis: More questions than answers. *Journal of the Canadian Medical Association* 171, 448.

20. Sobel J. D. (2000). Bacterial vaginosis. *Annual Review of Medicine* 51, 349–356.

21. U.S. Preventive Services Task Force. (2001). Screening for chlamydial infection. *American Journal of Preventative Medicine* 20, 90–94.

22. Peipert J. F. (2003). Genital chlamydial infections. *New England Journal of Medicine* 349, 1414–2430.

23. Kohl K. S., Markowitz L. E., Koumans E. H. (2003). Development of screening for *Chlamydia trachomatis:* A review. *Obstetrics and Gynecology Clinics of North America* 30, 637–658.

24. U.S. Department of Health and Human Services. (2002). Screening tests to detect *Chlamydia trachomatis* and *Neisseria gonorrhoeae* infections. *MMWR Morbidity and Mortality Weekly Report* 51(RR15), 1–27.

25. Centers for Disease Control and Prevention. (2000). Gonorrhea—United States, 1998. *MMWR Morbidity and Mortality Weekly Report* 49, 538.

26. Centers for Disease Control and Prevention. (2003). Primary and secondary syphilis—United States, 2002. *MMWR Morbidity and Mortality Weekly Report* 52, 1117–1120.

UNIT XII
Musculoskeletal Function

Chapter

41

Structure and Function of the Skeletal System

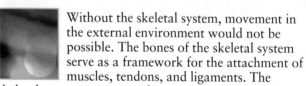

Without the skeletal system, movement in the external environment would not be possible. The bones of the skeletal system serve as a framework for the attachment of muscles, tendons, and ligaments. The skeletal system protects and maintains soft tissues in their proper position, provides stability for the body, and maintains the body's shape. The bones act as a storage reservoir for calcium, and the central cavity of some bones contains the hematopoietic connective tissue in which blood cells are formed.

The skeletal system consists of the axial and appendicular skeleton. The *axial skeleton*, which is composed of the bones of the skull, thorax, and vertebral column, forms the axis of the body. The *appendicular skeleton* consists of the bones of the upper and lower extremities, including the shoulder and hip. For our purposes, the skeletal system is considered to include the bones and cartilage of the axial and appendicular skeleton, as well as the connective tissue structures (*i.e.,* ligaments and tendons) that connect the bones and join muscles to bone.

Characteristics
of Skeletal Tissue

Two types of connective tissue are found in the skeletal system: cartilage and bone. Each of these connective tissue types consists of living cells, nonliving intercellular protein fibers, and an amorphous (shapeless) ground substance. The tissue cells are responsible for secreting and maintaining the intercellular substances in which they are housed. These substances provide the structural characteristics of the tissue. For example, the intercellular matrix of bone is impregnated with calcium salts, providing the hardness that is characteristic of this tissue.

Two main types of intercellular fibers are found in skeletal tissue: collagenous and elastic. Collagen is an inelastic and insoluble fibrous protein. Because of its molecular configuration, collagen has great tensile strength; the breaking point of collagenous fibers found in human tendons is reached with a force of several hundred kilograms per square centimeter. Fresh collagen is colorless, and tissues that contain large numbers of collagenous fibers generally appear white. The collagen fibers in tendons and ligaments give these structures their white color. Elastin is the major component of elastic fibers that allows them to stretch several times their length and rapidly return to their original shape when the tension

is released. Ligaments and structures that must undergo repeated stretching contain a high proportion of elastic fibers.

CARTILAGE

Cartilage is a firm but flexible type of connective tissue consisting of cells and intercellular fibers embedded in an amorphous, gel-like material. It has a smooth and resilient surface and a weight-bearing capacity exceeded only by that of bone.

Cartilage is essential for growth before and after birth. It is able to undergo rapid growth while maintaining a considerable degree of stiffness. In the embryo, most of the axial and appendicular skeleton is formed first as a cartilage model and is replaced by bone. In postnatal life, cartilage continues to play an essential role in the growth of long bones and persists as articular cartilage in the adult.

There are three types of cartilage: elastic cartilage, hyaline cartilage, and fibrocartilage. *Elastic cartilage* contains some elastin in its intercellular substance. It is found in areas, such as the ear, where some flexibility is important. Pure cartilage is called *hyaline cartilage* (from a Greek word meaning "glass") and is pearly white. It is the type of cartilage seen on the articulating ends of fresh soup bones found in the supermarket. *Fibrocartilage* has characteristics that are intermediate between dense connective tissue and hyaline cartilage. It is found in the intervertebral disks, in areas where tendons are connected to bone, and in the symphysis pubis.

Hyaline cartilage is the most abundant type of cartilage. It forms much of the cartilage of the fetal skeleton. In the adult, hyaline cartilage forms the costal cartilages that join the ribs to the sternum and vertebrae, many of the cartilages of the respiratory tract, the articular cartilages, and the epiphyseal plates. The free surfaces of most hyaline cartilage, with the exception of articular cartilage, are covered by a layer of fibrous connective tissue called the *perichondrium*.

Cartilage cells, which are called *chondrocytes*, are located in lacunae. These lacunae are surrounded by an uncalcified, gel-like intercellular matrix of collagen fibers and ground substance. Cartilage is devoid of blood vessels and nerves. It has been estimated that approximately 65% to 80% of the wet weight of cartilage is water held in its gel structure. Because cartilage has no blood vessels, this tissue fluid allows the diffusion of gases, nutrients, and wastes between the chondrocytes and blood vessels outside the cartilage. Diffusion cannot take place if the cartilage matrix becomes impregnated with calcium salts, and cartilage dies if it becomes calcified.

BONE

Bone is connective tissue in which the intercellular matrix has been impregnated with inorganic calcium salts so that it has great tensile and compressible strength but is light enough to be moved by coordinated muscle contractions. The intercellular matrix is composed of two

---

KEY CONCEPTS

The Skeletal System

➤ The skeletal system consists of the bones of the skull, thorax, and vertebral column, which form the axial skeleton, and the bones of the upper and lower extremities, which form the appendicular skeleton.

➤ Two types of connective tissue are found in the skeletal system: (1) cartilage, a semirigid and slightly flexible structure that plays an essential role in prenatal and childhood development of the skeleton and as a surface for the articulating ends of skeletal joints; and (2) bones, which provide for the firm structure of the skeleton and serve as a reservoir for calcium and phosphate storage.

➤ Both bone and cartilage are composed of living cells and a nonliving intercellular matrix that is secreted by the living cells.

➤ Bone matrix is maintained by three types of cells: osteoblasts, which synthesize and secrete the constituents of bone; osteoclasts, which resorb surplus bone and are required for bone remodeling; and the osteocytes, which make up the osteoid tissue of bone.

types of substances—organic matter and inorganic salts. The organic matter, including bone cells, blood vessels, and nerves, constitutes approximately one third of the dry weight of bone; the inorganic salts make up the other two thirds.

The organic matter consists primarily of collagen fibers embedded in an amorphous ground substance. The inorganic matter consists of hydroxyapatite, an insoluble macrocrystalline structure of calcium phosphate salts, and small amounts of calcium carbonate and calcium fluoride. Bone may also take up lead and other heavy metals, thereby removing these toxic substances from the circulation. This can be viewed as a protective mechanism. The antibiotic tetracycline is readily bound to calcium deposited in newly formed bones and teeth. When tetracycline is given during pregnancy, it can be deposited in the teeth of the fetus, causing discoloration and deformity. Similar changes can occur if the drug is given for long periods to children younger than 6 years of age.

Types of Bone

There are two types of mature bones, cancellous and compact bone (Fig. 41-1). Both types are formed in layers and thus are called *lamellar bone*. Cancellous (spongy) bone is found in the interior of bones and is composed of *trabeculae*, or *spicules*, of bone that form a lattice-like pattern. These lattice-like structures are lined with osteogenic cells and filled with red or yellow bone marrow. Cancellous bone is relatively light, but its structure is

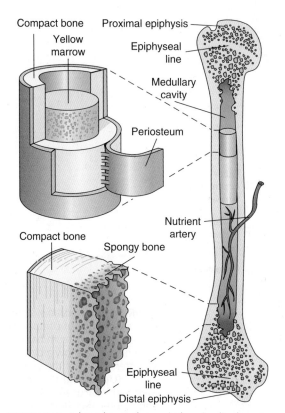

FIGURE 41-1 A long bone shown in longitudinal section.

such that it has considerable tensile strength and weight-bearing properties. Compact (cortical) bone, which forms the outer shell of a bone, has a densely packed calcified intercellular matrix that makes it more rigid than cancellous bone. The relative quantity of compact and cancellous bone varies in different types of bones throughout the body and in different parts of the same bone, depending on the need for strength and lightness. Compact bone is the major component of tubular bones. It is also found along the lines of stress on long bones and forms an outer protective shell on other bones.

Bone Cells

Four types of bone cells participate in the formation and maintenance of bone tissue: osteogenic cells, osteoblasts, osteocytes, and osteoclasts (Table 41-1).

Osteogenic Cells. The undifferentiated osteogenic cells are found in the periosteum, endosteum, and epiphyseal plate of growing bone. These cells differentiate into osteoblasts and are active during normal growth; they may also be activated in adult life during healing of fractures and other injuries. Osteogenic cells also participate in the continual replacement of worn-out bone tissue.

Osteoblasts. The osteoblasts, or bone-building cells, are responsible for the formation of the bone matrix. Bone formation occurs in two stages: ossification and calcification. Ossification involves the formation of osteoid, or prebone. Calcification of bone involves the deposition of calcium salts in the osteoid tissue. The osteoblasts synthesize collagen and other proteins that make up osteoid tissue. They also participate in the calcification process of the osteoid tissue, probably by controlling the availability of calcium and phosphate. Osteoblasts secrete the enzyme *alkaline phosphatase*, which is thought to act locally in bone tissue to raise calcium and phosphate

TABLE 41-1	Function of Bone Cells
Type of Bone Cell	**Function**
Osteogenic cells	Undifferentiated cells that differentiate into osteoblasts. They are found in the periosteum, endosteum, and epiphyseal growth plate of growing bones.
Osteoblasts	Bone-building cells that synthesize and secrete the organic matrix of bone. Osteoblasts also participate in the calcification of the organic matrix.
Osteocytes	Mature bone cells that function in the maintenance of bone matrix. Osteocytes also play an active role in releasing calcium into the blood.
Osteoclasts	Bone cells responsible for the resorption of bone matrix and the release of calcium and phosphate from bone.

levels to the point at which precipitation occurs. The activity of the osteoblasts undoubtedly contributes to the increase in serum levels of alkaline phosphatase that follows bone injury and fractures.

Osteocytes. The osteocytes are mature bone cells that are actively involved in maintaining the bony matrix. Death of the osteocytes results in the resorption of this matrix. The osteocytes lie in a small lake filled with extracellular fluid, called a *lacuna,* and are surrounded by a calcified intercellular matrix. Extracellular fluid-filled passageways permeate the calcified matrix and connect with the lacunae of adjacent osteocytes. These passageways are called *canaliculi.* Because diffusion does not occur through the calcified matrix of bone, the canaliculi serve as communicating channels for the exchange of nutrients and metabolites between the osteocytes and the blood vessels on the surface of the bone layer.

The osteocytes, together with their intercellular matrix, are arranged in layers, or lamellae. In compact bone, 4 to 20 lamellae are arranged concentrically around a central haversian canal, which runs essentially parallel to the long axis of the bone. Each of these units is called a *haversian system,* or *osteon.* The haversian canals contain blood vessels that carry nutrients and wastes to and from the canaliculi (Fig. 41-2). The blood vessels from the periosteum enter the bone through tiny openings called *Volkmann's canals* and connect with the haversian systems. Cancellous bone is also composed of lamellae, but its trabeculae usually are not penetrated by blood vessels. Instead, the bone cells of cancellous bone are nourished by diffusion from the endosteal surface through canaliculi, which interconnect their lacunae and extend to the bone surface.

Osteoclasts. Osteoclasts are "bone-chewing" cells that function in the resorption of bone, removing the mineral content and the organic matrix. They are large phagocytic cells of monocyte/macrophage lineage. Although the mechanism of osteoclast formation and activation remains elusive, it is known that parathyroid hormone (PTH) increases the number and resorptive function of the osteoclasts. Calcitonin is thought to reduce the number and resorptive function of the osteoclasts (to be discussed). Estrogen also reduces the number and function of the osteoclasts; thus, the decrease in estrogen levels that occurs at menopause results in increased reabsorption of bone. The mechanism whereby osteoclasts exert their

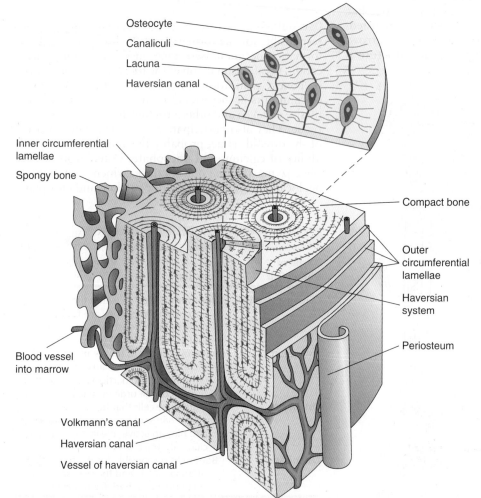

Osteocyte
Canaliculi
Lacuna
Haversian canal
Inner circumferential lamellae
Spongy bone
Compact bone
Outer circumferential lamellae
Haversian system
Periosteum
Blood vessel into marrow
Volkmann's canal
Haversian canal
Vessel of haversian canal

FIGURE 41-2 Haversian systems as seen in a wedge of compact bone tissue. The periosteum has been peeled back to show a blood vessel entering one of the Volkmann canals. (**Upper right**) Osteocytes lying within lacunae; canaliculi permit interstitial fluid to reach each lacuna.

resorptive effect on bone is unclear. These cells may secrete an acid that removes calcium from the bone matrix, releasing the collagenic fibers for digestion by osteoclasts or mononuclear cells. The osteoclastic cells, by virtue of their phagocytic lineage, also imbibe minute particles of bone matrix and crystals, eventually dissolving and releasing them into the blood.

Periosteum and Endosteum

Bones are covered, except at their articular ends, by a membrane called the *periosteum* (see Fig. 41-1). The periosteum has an outer fibrous layer and an inner layer that contains the osteogenic cells needed for bone growth and development. The periosteum contains blood vessels and acts as an anchorage point for vessels as they enter and leave the bone. The endosteum is the membrane that lines the spaces of spongy bone, the marrow cavities, and the haversian canals of compact bone. It is composed mainly of osteogenic cells. These osteogenic cells contribute to the growth and remodeling of bone and are necessary for bone repair.

BONE GROWTH AND REMODELING

The skeletal system develops from the mesoderm, the thin middle layer of embryonic tissue. Development of the vertebrae of the axial skeleton begins at approximately the fourth week in the embryo; during the ninth week, ossification begins with the appearance of ossification centers in the lower thoracic and upper lumbar vertebrae. The paddle-shaped limb buds of the lower extremities make their appearance late in the fourth week. The hand pads are developed by days 33 to 36, and the finger rays are evident on days 41 to 43 of embryonic development.

During the first two decades of life, the skeleton undergoes general overall growth. The long bones of the skeleton, which grow at a relatively rapid rate, are provided with a specialized structure called the *epiphyseal growth plate*. As long bones grow in length, the deeper layers of cartilage cells in the growth plate multiply and enlarge, pushing the articular cartilage farther away from the metaphysis and diaphysis of the bone. As this happens, the mature and enlarged cartilage cells at the metaphyseal end of the plate become metabolically inactive and are replaced by bone cells. This process allows bone growth to proceed without changing the shape of the bone or causing disruption of the articular cartilage. The cells in the growth plate stop dividing at puberty, at which time the epiphysis and metaphysis fuse.

Several factors can influence the growth of cells in the epiphyseal growth plate. Epiphyseal separation can occur in children as the result of trauma. The separation usually occurs in the zone of the mature enlarged cartilage cells, which is the weakest part of the growth plate. The blood vessels that nourish the epiphysis pass through the growth plate. These vessels are ruptured when the growth plate separates. This can cause cessation of growth and a shortened extremity.

The growth plate also is sensitive to nutritional and metabolic changes. Scurvy (*i.e.*, vitamin C deficiency) impairs the formation of the organic matrix of bone, causing slowing of growth at the epiphyseal plate and cessation of diaphyseal growth. In rickets (*i.e.*, vitamin D deficiency), calcification of the newly developed bone on the metaphyseal side of the growth plate is impaired. Thyroid and growth hormones are required for normal growth. Alterations in these and other hormones can affect growth (see Chapter 31).

Growth in the diameter of bones occurs as new bone is added to the outer surface of existing bone along with an accompanying resorption of bone on the endosteal or inner surface. Such oppositional growth allows for widening of the marrow cavity while preventing the cortex from becoming too thick and heavy. In this way, the shape of the bone is maintained. As a bone grows in diameter, concentric rings are added to the bone surface, much as rings are added to a tree trunk; these rings form the lamellar structure of mature bone. Osteocytes, which develop from osteoblasts, become buried in the rings. Haversian channels form as periosteal vessels running along the long axis become surrounded by bone.

HORMONAL CONTROL OF BONE FORMATION AND METABOLISM

The process of bone formation and mineral metabolism is complex. It involves the interplay among the actions of PTH, calcitonin, and vitamin D. Other hormones, such as cortisol, growth hormone, thyroid hormone, and the sex hormones, also influence bone formation directly or indirectly.

Parathyroid Hormone

Parathyroid hormone is one of the important regulators of calcium and phosphate levels in the blood. PTH prevents serum calcium levels from falling below and serum phosphate levels from rising above normal physiologic concentrations (see Chapter 6). The secretion of PTH is regulated by negative feedback levels of ionized calcium. PTH maintains serum calcium levels by initiation of calcium release from bone, by conservation of calcium by the kidney, by enhanced intestinal absorption of calcium through activation of vitamin D, and by reduction of serum phosphate levels (Fig. 41-3). PTH also increases the movement of calcium and phosphate from bone into the extracellular fluid. Calcium is immediately released from the canaliculi and bone cells; a more prolonged release of calcium and phosphate is mediated by increased osteoclast activity. In the kidney, PTH stimulates tubular reabsorption of calcium while reducing the reabsorption of phosphate. The latter effect ensures that increased release of phosphate from bone during mobilization of calcium does not produce an elevation in serum phosphate levels. This is important because an increase in calcium and phosphate levels could lead to crystallization in soft tissues. PTH increases intestinal absorption of calcium because of its ability to stimulate activation of vitamin D by the kidney.

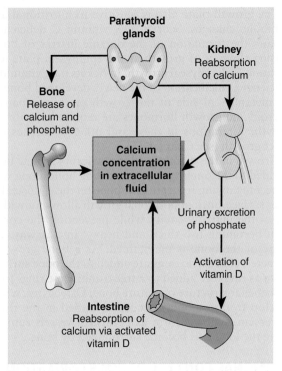

FIGURE 41-3 Regulation and actions of parathyroid hormone.

Calcitonin

Whereas PTH increases blood calcium levels, the hormone calcitonin lowers blood calcium levels. Calcitonin, sometimes called *thyrocalcitonin,* is secreted by the parafollicular, or C, cells of the thyroid gland. Calcitonin inhibits the release of calcium from bone into the extracellular fluid. It is thought to act by causing calcium to become sequestered in bone cells and by inhibiting osteoclast activity. Calcitonin also reduces the renal tubular reabsorption of calcium and phosphate; the decrease in serum calcium level that follows administration of pharmacologic doses of calcitonin may be related to this action.

The major stimulus for calcitonin synthesis and release is an increase in serum calcium. The role of calcitonin in overall mineral homeostasis is uncertain. There are no clearly definable syndromes of calcitonin deficiency or excess, which suggests that calcitonin does not directly alter calcium metabolism. It has been suggested that the physiologic actions of calcitonin are related to the postprandial handling and processing of dietary calcium. This theory proposes that after meals, calcitonin maintains parathyroid secretion at a time when it normally would be reduced by calcium entering the blood from the digestive tract. Although excess or deficiency states associated with alterations in physiologic levels of calcitonin have not been observed, it has been shown that pharmacologic doses of the hormone reduce osteoclastic activity. Because of this action, calcitonin has proved effective in the treatment of Paget disease (see Chapter 43). The hormone is also used to reduce serum calcium levels during hypercalcemic crises.

Vitamin D

Vitamin D and its metabolites are not vitamins but steroid hormones. There are two forms of vitamin D: vitamin D_2 (ergocalciferol) and vitamin D_3 (cholecalciferol). The two forms differ by the presence of a double bond, but they have identical biologic activity. The term *vitamin D* is used to indicate both forms.

Vitamin D has little or no activity until it has been metabolized to compounds that mediate its activity. Figure 41-4 depicts sources of vitamin D and pathways for activation. The first step of the activation process occurs in the liver, where vitamin D is hydroxylated to form the metabolite 25-hydroxyvitamin D_3 [25-$(OH)D_3$]. From the liver, 25-$(OH)D_3$ is transported to the kidneys, where it undergoes conversion to 1,25-dihydroxyvitamin D_3 [1,25-$(OH)_2D_3$] or 24,25-dihydroxyvitamin D_3 [24,25-$(OH)_2D_3$]. Other metabolites of vitamin D have been and still are being discovered.

There are two sources of vitamin D: intestinal absorption and skin production. Intestinal absorption occurs mainly in the jejunum and includes vitamin D_2 and vitamin D_3. The most important dietary sources of vitamin D are fish, liver, and irradiated milk. Because vitamin D is fat soluble, its absorption is mediated by bile salts and

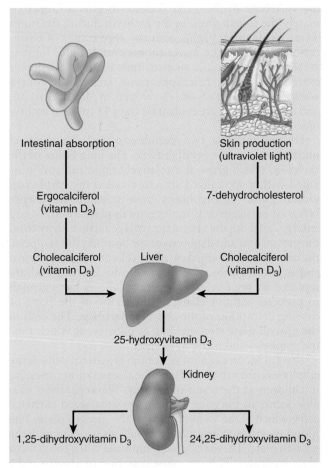

FIGURE 41-4 Sources and pathway for activation of vitamin D.

occurs by means of the lymphatic vessels. In the skin, ultraviolet radiation from sunlight spontaneously converts 7-dehydrocholesterol provitamin D_3 to vitamin D_3. A circulating vitamin D–binding protein provides a mechanism to remove vitamin D from the skin and make it available to the rest of the body.

With adequate exposure to sunlight, the amount of vitamin D that can be produced by the skin is usually sufficient to meet physiologic requirements. The importance of sunlight exposure is evidenced by population studies that report lower vitamin D levels in countries, such as England, that have less sunlight than the United States. Elderly persons who are housebound or institutionalized frequently have low vitamin D levels. The deficiency often goes undetected until there are problems such as pseudofractures or electrolyte imbalances. Seasonal variations in vitamin D levels probably reflect changes in sunlight exposure.

The most potent of the vitamin D metabolites is $1,25$-$(OH)_2D_3$. This metabolite increases intestinal absorption of calcium and promotes the actions of PTH on resorption of calcium and phosphate from bone. Bone resorption by the osteoclasts is increased, and bone formation by the osteoblasts is decreased; there is also an increase in acid phosphatase and a decrease in alkaline phosphatase. Intestinal absorption and bone resorption increase the amount of calcium and phosphorus available to the mineralizing surface of the bone. The role of $24,25$-$(OH)_2D_3$ is less clear. There is evidence that $24,25$-$(OH)_2D_3$, in conjunction with $1,25$-$(OH)_2D_3$, may be involved in normal bone mineralization.

The regulation of vitamin D activity is influenced by several hormones. PTH and prolactin stimulate $1,25$-$(OH)_2D_3$ production by the kidney. States of hyperparathyroidism are associated with increased levels of $1,25$-$(OH)_2D_3$, and hypoparathyroidism leads to lowered levels of this metabolite. Prolactin may have an ancillary role in regulating vitamin D metabolism during pregnancy and lactation. Calcitonin inhibits $1,25$-$(OH)_2D_3$ production by the kidney. In addition to hormonal influences, changes in the concentration of ions such as calcium, phosphate, hydrogen, and potassium exert an effect on $1,25$-$(OH)_2D_3$ and $24,25$-$(OH)_2D_3$ production. Under conditions of deprivation of phosphate and calcium, $1,25$-$(OH)_2D_3$ levels are increased, whereas hyperphosphatemia and hypercalcemia decrease the levels of this metabolite.

In summary, skeletal tissue is composed of two types of connective tissue: cartilage and bone. These skeletal structures are composed of similar tissue types; each has living cells and nonliving intercellular fibers and ground substance that is secreted by the cells. Cartilage is a firm, flexible type of skeletal tissue that is essential for growth before and after birth. There are three types of cartilage: elastic, hyaline, and fibrocartilage. Hyaline cartilage, which is the most abundant type, forms the costal cartilages that join the ribs to the sternum and vertebrae, many of the cartilages of the respiratory tract, and the articular cartilages.

The characteristics of the various skeletal tissue types are determined by the intercellular matrix. In bone, this matrix is impregnated with calcium salts to provide hardness and strength. There are four types of bone cells: osteocytes, or mature bone cells; osteoblasts, or bone-building cells; osteoclasts, which function in bone resorption; and osteogenic cells, which differentiate into osteoblasts. Densely packed compact bone forms the outer shell of a bone, and lattice-like cancellous bone forms the interior. The periosteum, the membrane that covers bones, contains blood vessels and acts as an anchorage point for vessels as they enter and leave the bone. The endosteum is the membrane that lines the spaces of spongy bone, the marrow cavities, and the haversian canals of compact bone.

The process of bone formation and mineral metabolism involves the interplay among the actions of PTH, calcitonin, and vitamin D. PTH acts to maintain serum levels of ionized calcium; it increases the release of calcium and phosphate from bone, the conservation of calcium and elimination of phosphate by the kidney, and the intestinal reabsorption of calcium through vitamin D. Calcitonin inhibits the release of calcium from bone and increases renal elimination of calcium and phosphate, thereby serving to lower serum calcium levels. Vitamin D functions as a hormone in regulating body calcium. It increases absorption of calcium from the intestine and promotes the actions of PTH on bone.

Skeletal Structures

CLASSIFICATION OF BONES

Bones are classified by shape as long, short, flat, and irregular. Long bones are found in the upper and lower extremities. Short bones are irregularly shaped bones located in the ankle and the wrist. Except for their surface, which is compact bone, these bones are spongy throughout. Flat bones are composed of a layer of spongy bone between two layers of compact bone. They are found in areas such as the skull and rib cage, where extensive protection of underlying structures is needed, or, as in the scapula, where a broad surface for muscle attachment must be provided. Irregular bones, because of their shapes, cannot be classified in any of the previous groups. This group includes bones such as the vertebrae and the bones of the jaw.

A typical long bone has a shaft, or *diaphysis*, and two ends, called *epiphyses* (Fig. 41-5). Long bones usually are narrow in the mid-portion and broad at the ends so that the weight they bear can be distributed over a wider surface. The shaft of a long bone is formed mainly of compact bone roughly hollowed out to form a marrow-filled medullary canal. The ends of long bones are covered with articular cartilage that rests on a bony plate, the subchondral bone.

In growing bones, the part of the bone shaft that funnels out as it approaches the epiphysis is called the *metaphysis* (see Fig. 41-5). It is composed of bony trabeculae that have cores of cartilage. In the child, the epiphysis is separated from the metaphysis by the cartilaginous growth plate. After puberty, the metaphysis and epiphysis merge, and the growth plate is obliterated.

Bone marrow occupies the medullary cavities of the long bones throughout the skeleton and the cavities of cancellous bone in the vertebrae, ribs, sternum, and flat bones of the pelvis. The cellular composition of the bone marrow varies with age and skeletal location. Red bone marrow contains developing red blood cells and is the site of blood cell formation. Yellow bone marrow is composed largely of adipose cells. At birth, nearly all of the marrow is red and hematopoietically active. As the need for red blood cell production decreases during postnatal growth, red marrow is gradually replaced with yellow bone marrow in most of the bones. In the adult, red marrow persists in the vertebrae, ribs, sternum, and ilia.

TENDONS AND LIGAMENTS

In the skeletal system, tendons and ligaments are dense connective tissue structures that connect muscles and bones. Tendons connect muscles to bone, and ligaments connect the movable bones of joints. Tendons can appear as cordlike structures or as flattened sheets, called *aponeuroses,* such as in the abdominal muscles.

The dense connective tissue found in tendons and ligaments has a limited blood supply and is composed largely of intercellular bundles of collagen fibers arranged in the same direction and plane. This type of connective tissue provides great tensile strength and can withstand tremendous pull in the direction of fiber alignment. At the sites where tendons or ligaments are inserted into cartilage or bone, a gradual transition from pure dense connective tissue to bone or cartilage occurs. In cartilage, this transitional tissue is called *fibrocartilage.*

Tendons that may rub against bone or other friction-generating surfaces are enclosed in double-layered sheaths. An outer connective tissue tube is attached to the structures surrounding the tendon, and an inner sheath encloses the tendon and is attached to it. The space between the inner and outer sheath is filled with a fluid similar to synovial fluid.

JOINTS AND ARTICULATIONS

Articulations, or joints, are areas where two or more bones meet. The term *arthro* is the prefix used to designate a joint. For example, *arthrology* is the study of joints, and *arthroplasty* is the repair of a joint. There are two classes of joints, based on movement and the presence of a joint cavity: synarthroses and diarthroses.

Synarthroses

Synarthroses are joints that lack a joint cavity and move little or not at all. There are three types of synarthroses: synostoses, synchondroses, and syndesmoses. *Synostoses* are nonmovable joints in which the surfaces of the bones are joined by dense connective tissue or bone. The bones of the skull are joined by synostoses; they are joined by dense connective tissue in children and young adults and by bone in older persons. *Synchondroses* are joints in

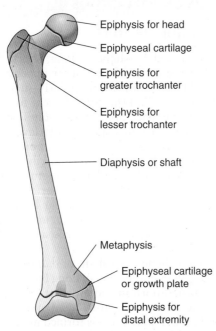

FIGURE 41-5 A femur, showing epiphyseal cartilages for the head, metaphysis, trochanters, and distal end of the bone.

- Epiphysis for head
- Epiphyseal cartilage
- Epiphysis for greater trochanter
- Epiphysis for lesser trochanter
- Diaphysis or shaft
- Metaphysis
- Epiphyseal cartilage or growth plate
- Epiphysis for distal extremity

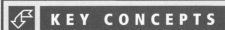

KEY CONCEPTS

Skeletal Joints

➤ Joints, or articulations, are sites where two or more bones meet to hold the skeleton together and give it mobility.

➤ There are two types of joints: synarthroses, which are immovable joints, and diarthroses, which are freely movable joints.

➤ All limb joints are synovial diarthrodial joints, which are enclosed in a joint cavity containing synovial fluid.

➤ The articulating surfaces of synovial joints are covered with a layer of avascular cartilage that relies on oxygen and nutrients contained in the synovial fluid.

➤ Regeneration of articular cartilage of synovial joints is slow, and the healing of injuries often is slow and unsatisfactory.

which bones are connected by hyaline cartilage and have limited motion. The ribs are attached to the sternum by this type of joint. *Syndesmoses* permit a certain amount of movement; they are separated by a fibrous disk and joined by interosseous ligaments. The symphysis pubis of the pelvis and the bodies of the vertebrae that are joined by intervertebral disks are examples of syndesmoses.

Diarthroses

Diarthrodial joints (*i.e.*, synovial joints) are freely movable joints. Most joints in the body are of this type. Although they are classified as freely movable, their movement ranges from almost none (*e.g.*, sacroiliac joint), to simple hinge movement (*e.g.*, interphalangeal joint), to movement in many planes (*e.g.*, shoulder or hip joint). The bony surfaces of these joints are covered with thin layers of articular cartilage, and the cartilaginous surfaces of these joints slide past each other during movement. As discussed in Chapter 43, diarthrodial joints are the joints most frequently affected by rheumatic disorders.

In a diarthrodial joint, the articulating ends of the bones are not connected directly but are indirectly linked by a strong fibrous capsule (*i.e.*, joint capsule) that surrounds the joint and is continuous with the periosteum (Fig. 41-6). This capsule supports the joint and helps to hold the bones in place. Additional support may be provided by ligaments that extend between the bones of the joint.

The joint capsule consists of two layers: an outer fibrous layer and an inner membrane, the synovium. The synovium surrounds the tendons that pass through the joints and the free margins of other intra-articular structures, such as ligaments and menisci. The synovium forms folds that surround the margins of articulations but do not cover the weight-bearing articular cartilage. These folds permit stretching of the synovium so that movement can occur without tissue damage.

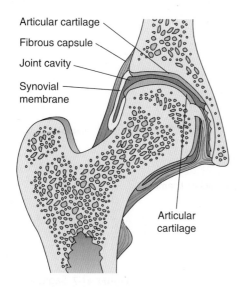

FIGURE 41-6 Diarthrodial joint, showing the articular cartilage, fibrous joint capsule, joint cavity, and synovial membrane.

Articular cartilage
Fibrous capsule
Joint cavity
Synovial membrane
Articular cartilage

The synovium secretes a slippery fluid with the consistency of egg white called *synovial fluid*. This fluid acts as a lubricant and facilitates the movement of the articulating surfaces of the joint. Normal synovial fluid is clear or pale yellow, does not clot, and contains fewer than 100 cells/mm³. The cells are predominantly mononuclear cells derived from the synovium. The composition of the synovial fluid is altered in many inflammatory and pathologic joint disorders. Aspiration and examination of the synovial fluid play an important role in the diagnosis of joint diseases.

The articular cartilage is an example of hyaline cartilage and is unique in that its free surface is not covered with perichondrium. It has only a peripheral rim of perichondrium, and calcification of the portion of cartilage abutting the bone may limit or preclude diffusion from blood vessels supplying the subchondral bone. Articular cartilage is apparently nourished by the diffusion of substances contained in the synovial fluid bathing the cartilage. Regeneration of most cartilage is slow; it is accomplished primarily by growth that requires the activity of perichondrium cells. In articular cartilage, which has no perichondrium, superficial injuries heal slowly.

Blood Supply and Innervation

The blood supply to a joint arises from blood vessels that enter the subchondral bone at or near the attachment of the joint capsule and form an arterial circle around the joint. The synovial membrane has a rich blood supply, and constituents of plasma diffuse rapidly between these vessels and the joint cavity. Because many of the capillaries are near the surface of the synovium, blood may escape into the synovial fluid after relatively minor injuries. Healing and repair of the synovial membrane usually are rapid and complete. This is important because synovial tissue is injured in many surgical procedures that involve the joint.

The nerve supply to joints is provided by the same nerve trunks that supply the muscles that move the joints. These nerve trunks also supply the skin over the joints. As a rule, each joint of an extremity is innervated by all the peripheral nerves that cross the articulation; this accounts for the referral of pain from one joint to another. For example, hip pain may be perceived as pain in the knee.

The tendons and ligaments of the joint capsule are sensitive to position and movement, particularly stretching and twisting. These structures are supplied by the large sensory nerve fibers that form proprioceptor endings. The proprioceptors function reflexively to adjust the tension of the muscles that support the joint and are particularly important in maintaining muscular support for the joint. For example, when a weight is lifted, there is a proprioceptor-mediated reflex contraction and relaxation of appropriate muscle groups to support the joint and protect the joint capsule and other joint structures. Loss of proprioception and reflex control of muscular support leads to destructive changes in the joint.

The synovial membrane is innervated only by autonomic fibers that control blood flow. It is relatively free of pain fibers, as evidenced by the fact that surgical procedures on the joint are often done under local anesthesia. The joint capsule and the ligaments have pain receptors; these receptors are more easily stimulated by stretching and twisting than are other joint structures. Pain arising from the capsule tends to be diffuse and poorly localized.

Bursae

In some diarthrotic joints, the synovial membrane forms closed sacs that are not part of the joint. These sacs, called *bursae*, contain synovial fluid. Their purpose is to prevent friction on a tendon. Bursae occur in areas where pressure is exerted because of close approximation of joint structures (Fig. 41-7). Such conditions occur when tendons are deflected over bone or where skin must move freely over bony tissue. Bursae may become injured or inflamed, causing discomfort, swelling, and limitation in movement of the involved area. A bunion is an inflamed bursa of the metatarsophalangeal joint of the great toe.

Intra-Articular Menisci

Intra-articular menisci are fibrocartilaginous structures that develop from portions of the articular disk that occupied the space between articular cartilage surfaces during fetal development. Menisci may extend part way through the joint and have a free inner border, as at the lateral and medial articular surfaces of the knee, or they may extend through the joint, separating it into two separate cavities, as in the sternoclavicular joint. The menisci of the knee joint may be torn as the result of an injury (see Chapter 42).

In summary, bones are classified on the basis of their shape as long, short, flat, or irregular. Long bones are found in the upper and lower extremities; short bones in the ankle and wrist; flat bones in the skull and rib cage; and irregular bones in the vertebrae and jaw. Tendons and ligaments are dense connective skeletal tissue that connect muscles and bones. Tendons connect muscles to bones, and ligaments connect the movable bones of joints.

Articulations, or joints, are areas where two or more bones meet. Synarthroses are joints in which bones are joined together by fibrous tissue, cartilage, or bone; they lack a joint cavity and have little or no movement. Diarthrodial, or synovial, joints are freely movable. The surfaces of the articulating ends of bones in diarthrodial joints are covered with a thin layer of articular cartilage, and they are enclosed in a fibrous joint capsule. The joint capsule consists of two layers: an outer fibrous layer and an inner membrane, the synovium. The synovial fluid, which is secreted by the synovium into the joint capsule, acts as a lubricant and facilitates movement of the joint's articulating surfaces. Bursae, which are closed sacs containing synovial fluid, prevent friction in areas where tendons are deflected over bone or where skin must move freely over bony tissue.

Menisci are fibrocartilaginous structures that develop from portions of the articular disk that occupied the space between the articular cartilage during fetal development. The menisci may have a free inner border, or they may extend through the joint, separating it into two cavities.

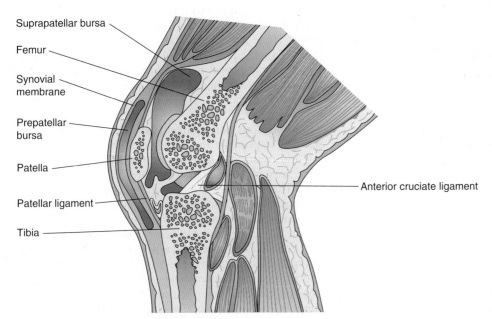

FIGURE 41-7 Sagittal section of knee joint, showing prepatellar and suprapatellar bursae.

Review Exercises

Pain from injury to the knee often is experienced as pain in the hip.

A. Explain why this might occur.

Persons with end-stage kidney disease have a deficiency of activated vitamin D.

A. Explain why this occurs and what effect it would have on their bones.

Recent studies have revealed that estrogen deficiency as well as normal aging may produce a decrease in osteoblast activity.

A. Explain how this could contribute to the development of osteoporosis.

Visit the Porth: Essentials of Pathophysiology: Concepts of Altered Health States web site (http://thePoint.LWW.com/PorthEssentials) for links to chapter-related resources on the Internet, all-new exclusive animations, chapter review questions, and more!

BIBLIOGRAPHY

DeLuca H. F. (1988). The vitamin D story: A collaborative effort of basic science and clinical medicine. *FASEB Journal 2*, 236–242.

Guyton A. C., Hall J. E. (2006). *Textbook of medical physiology* (11th ed., pp. 978–990). Philadelphia: Elsevier Saunders.

Moore K. L., Dalley A. F. (2006). *Clinically oriented anatomy* (5th ed., pp. 18–30). Philadelphia: Lippincott Williams & Wilkins.

Rhoades R. A., Tanner G. A. (2003). *Medical physiology* (2nd ed., pp. 634–648). Philadelphia: Lippincott Williams & Wilkins.

Rosenberg A. (2005). Bones, joints, and soft tissue tumors. In Kumar V., Abbas A. K., Fausto N. (Eds.), *Robbins and Cotran pathologic basis of disease* (7th ed., pp. 1273–1288). Philadelphia: Elsevier Saunders.

Ross M. H., Kay G. I., Pawlina W. (2003). *Histology* (4th ed., pp. 180–213). Philadelphia: Lippincott Williams & Wilkins.

Schiller A. L., Wang B. Y., Klein M. J. (2005). Bones and joints. In Rubin E., Gorstein F., Rubin R., et al. (Eds.), *Rubin's pathology: Clinicopathologic foundations of medicine* (4th ed., pp. 1307–1315). Philadelphia: Lippincott Williams & Wilkins.

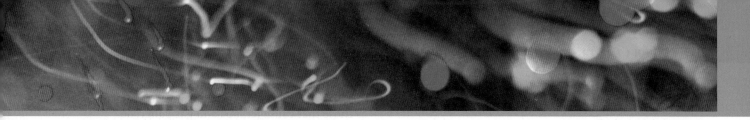

C h a p t e r *42*

Disorders of the Skeletal System: Trauma, Infection, and Childhood Disorders

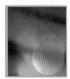 The musculoskeletal system includes the bones, joints, and muscles of the body together with associated structures such as ligaments and tendons. This system, which constitutes more than 70% of the body, is subject to a large number of disorders. These disorders affect persons in all age groups and walks of life and are a major cause of pain and disability. The discussion in this chapter focuses on injuries, infections, necrosis, and neoplasms of the musculoskeletal system. Disorders of skeletal growth and development in children are discussed at the end of the chapter.

Injury and Trauma of Musculoskeletal Structures

A broad spectrum of musculoskeletal injuries results from numerous physical forces, including blunt tissue trauma, disruption of tendons and ligaments, and fractures of bony structures. Many of the forces that cause injury to the musculoskeletal system are typical for a particular environmental setting, activity, or age group. Trauma resulting from high-speed motor accidents is a common cause of injury in adults younger than 45 years of age. In fact, the risk of motor vehicle accidents is higher among 16- to 19-year-olds than among any other age group.[1] The most common causes of childhood injuries are falls, bicycle-related injuries, and sports injuries. Falls are the most common cause of injury in people 65 years of age and older, with fractures of the hip and proximal humerus particularly common in this age group.

ATHLETIC INJURIES

Both acute and overuse injuries of the musculoskeletal system are particularly common among persons who engage in athletic activities. Acute injuries are caused by sudden trauma and include injuries to soft tissues (contusion, strains, and sprains) and to bone (fractures). Overuse injuries have been described as chronic injuries, including stress fractures that result from constant high levels of physiologic stress without sufficient recovery time.[2] They commonly occur in the elbow ("Little League elbow" or "tennis elbow") and in tissue where tendons attach to the bone, such as the heel, knee, and shoulder. Contact sports pose a greater threat for injury to the neck, spine, and growth plates in children and adolescents, who have not yet reached maturity. Injuries can often be prevented by proper training, use of safety equipment, and competition according to skill and size rather than chronologic age. Adequate warm-up time, hydration, and proper nutrition are also key factors in injury prevention.[3]

SOFT TISSUE INJURIES

Most skeletal injuries are accompanied by soft tissue (muscle, tendon, or ligament) injuries. These injuries include contusions, hematomas, and lacerations. They are discussed here because of their association with musculoskeletal injuries.

A contusion is an injury, or *bruise,* that results from direct trauma and is usually caused by striking a body part against a hard object.[4] Muscle bruises are common in all athletic events, even the so-called noncontact sports. The thigh and upper portion of the arm are the most commonly involved. In contusions, the skin overlying the injury remains intact while the injured tissue undergoes a well-defined sequence of events including microscopic rupture of blood vessels and damage to muscle cells, infiltrative bleeding, and inflammation. The area often becomes ecchymotic (*i.e.,* black and blue) because of local hemorrhage; later, the discoloration gradually changes to brown and then to yellow as the blood is reabsorbed.

A large area of local hemorrhage is called a *hematoma.* Hematomas cause pain as blood accumulates and exerts pressure on nerve endings. The pain increases with movement or when pressure is applied to the area. The pain and swelling of a hematoma take longer to subside than that accompanying a contusion.

The treatment for a contusion and a hematoma consists of elevating the affected part and applying cold for the first 24 hours to reduce the bleeding into the area. A compression wrapping is sometimes helpful in the early stages. Crutches may be necessary for lower extremity injuries. Reinjury is avoided by appropriately protecting the area and allowing for complete healing to occur before returning to activities.

A *laceration* is an injury in which the skin is torn or its continuity is disrupted. The seriousness of a laceration depends on the size and depth of the wound and on whether there is contamination from the object that caused the injury. Puncture wounds from nails or rusted material provide the setting for growth of anaerobic bacteria such as those that cause tetanus and gas gangrene.

Lacerations are usually treated by wound closure, which is done after the area is sufficiently cleaned; the closed wound is covered with a sterile dressing. It is important to minimize contamination of the wound and to control bleeding. Contaminated wounds and open fractures are copiously irrigated and debrided, and the skin usually is left open to heal to prevent the development of an anaerobic infection or a sinus tract. Antimicrobial agents are selectively used based on the suspected nature of the contaminants.

JOINT (MUSCULOTENDINOUS) INJURIES

Joints, or articulations, are sites where two or more bones meet. Joints (*i.e.,* diarthrodial) are supported by tough bundles of collagenous fibers called *ligaments* that attach to the joint capsule and bind the articular ends of bones together, and by *tendons* that join muscles to the periosteum of the articulating bones. Joint injuries involve mechanical overloading or forcible twisting or stretching.

Strains and Sprains

Sprains and strains are both musculoskeletal injuries, but they differ in terms of the tissue that is affected.[5] Strains involve muscles, or more precisely the muscle-tendon unit. Sprains involve the supporting ligaments of a joint. A complete tear in a muscle or tendon is described as a rupture.

A *strain* is a stretching or partial tear in a muscle or a muscle-tendon unit. Strains commonly result from sudden stretch of a muscle that is actively contracting. Strains can occur at any age, but are more common in middle-aged and older adults. With aging, the collagen in a muscle-

---

KEY CONCEPTS

Joint Injuries

➤ Joints are the weakest part of the skeletal system and common sites for injury due to mechanical overloading or forcible twisting or stretching.

➤ Injury can include damage to the tendons, which connect muscle to bone; ligaments, which hold bones together; or the cartilage that covers the articular surface.

➤ Healing of the dense connective tissue involved in joint injuries requires time to restore the structures so that they are strong enough to withstand the forces imposed on the joint. Ligamentous injuries may require surgical intervention with approximation of many fibrous strands to facilitate healing.

tendon unit changes; as result, muscles have decreased elasticity and are more susceptible to injury. Common sites of muscle strains are the lower back and the cervical region of the spine. The elbow and the shoulder are also supported by muscle-tendon units that are subject to strains. Foot strain is associated with the weight-bearing stresses of the feet; it may be caused by inadequate muscular and ligamentous support, overweight, or excessive exercise such as standing, walking, or running. Strains of muscle units around the hip, hamstring, and quadriceps are commonly associated with athletic activities.[5] Proper warm-up exercises increase the flexibility of muscle-tendon units and help prevent these types of injuries.[5]

Muscle strains are usually characterized by pain, stiffness, swelling, and local tenderness. Pain is increased with stretching of the muscle group. Although there usually is no external evidence of a specific injury, an inflammatory response develops at the injured site, followed by fibrous tissue replacement of the damaged muscle fibers.

A *sprain*, which involves the joint ligaments or capsule surrounding the joint, resembles a strain, but the pain and swelling subside more slowly. It usually is caused by abnormal or excessive movement of the joint. With a sprain, the ligaments may be incompletely torn or, as in a severe sprain, completely torn or ruptured (Fig. 42-1). The signs of sprain are pain, rapid swelling, heat, disability, discoloration, and limitation of function. Any joint may be sprained, but the ankle joint is most commonly involved, especially in high-risk sports such as basketball.[4] Most ankle sprains occur in the lateral ankle when the foot is turned inward under a person, forcing the ankle into inversion beyond its structural limits. Other common sites of sprain are the knee (the collateral ligament and anterior cruciate ligament) and elbow (the ulnar side). As with a strain, the soft tissue injury that occurs with a sprain is not evident on the radiograph. However, occasionally a chip of bone is evident when the entire ligament, including part of its bony attachment, has been ruptured or torn from the bone.

The treatment of muscle strains and ligamentous sprains involves rest, ice, compression, and elevation (RICE).[5] For an injured extremity, such as the ankle, elevation of the part followed by local application of cold may be sufficient. Compression, accomplished through the use of adhesive wraps or a removable splint, helps reduce swelling and provides support. A cast is applied for severe sprains, especially those severe enough to warrant surgical repair. Immobilization for a muscle strain is continued until the pain and swelling have subsided. In a sprain, the affected joint is immobilized for several weeks. Immobilization may be followed by graded active exercises. Early diagnosis, treatment, and rehabilitation are essential in preventing chronic ligamentous instability.

Healing of the dense connective tissues in tendons and ligaments is similar to that of other soft tissues.[6] If properly treated, injuries usually heal with the restoration of the original tensile strength. Repair is accomplished by fibroblasts from the inner tendon sheath or, if the tendon has no sheath, from the loose connective tissue that surrounds the tendon. Capillaries infiltrate the injured area during the initial healing process and supply the fibroblasts with the materials they need to produce large amounts of collagen. Formation of the long collagen bundles occurs within the first 2 weeks, and although tensile strength increases steadily thereafter, it is not sufficient to permit strong tendon pulls for 6 to 8 weeks.[7] During the healing process, there is a danger that muscle contraction will pull the injured ends apart, causing the tendon to heal in the lengthened position. There is also a danger that adhesions will develop in areas where tendons pass through fibrous channels, such as in the distal palm of the hands, rendering the tendon useless.

Dislocations

Dislocation of a joint is the loss of articulation of the bone ends in the joint capsule caused by displacement or separation of the bone ends from their position in the joint. It usually follows a severe trauma that disrupts the holding ligaments. Dislocations are seen most often in the shoulder and acromioclavicular joints. A *subluxation* is a partial dislocation in which the bone ends in the joint are still in partial contact with each other.

Dislocations can be congenital, traumatic, or pathologic. Congenital dislocations occur in the hip or knee. Traumatic dislocations occur after falls, blows, or rotational injuries. For example, auto accidents often cause dislocations of the hip and accompanying acetabular

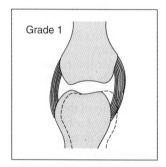
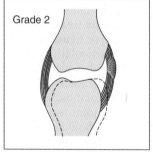
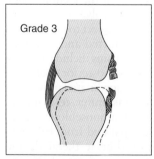
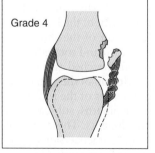

FIGURE 42-1 Degrees of sprain on the medial side of the right knee: grade 1, mild sprain of the medial collateral ligament; grade 2, moderate sprain with hematoma formation; grade 3, severe sprain with total disruption of the ligament; and grade 4, severe sprain with avulsion of the medial femoral condyle at the insertion of the medial collateral ligament. (Adapted from Spickler L. L. [1983]. Knee injuries of the athlete. *Orthopedic Nursing* 2[5], 12–13.)

fractures because of the direction of impact. In the shoulder and patella, dislocations may become recurrent, especially in athletes. They recur with the same motion but require less and less force each time. Less common sites of dislocation, seen mainly in young adults, are the wrist and mid-tarsal region. They usually are the result of direct force, such as a fall on an outstretched hand. Pathologic dislocation in the hip is a late complication of infection, rheumatoid arthritis, paralysis, and neuromuscular diseases.

Diagnosis of a dislocation is based on history, physical examination, and radiologic findings. The symptoms are pain, deformity, and limited movement. The treatment depends on the site, mechanism of injury, and associated injuries such as fractures. Dislocations that do not reduce spontaneously usually require manipulation or surgical repair. Various surgical procedures also can be used to prevent redislocation of the patella, shoulder, or acromioclavicular joints. Immobilization is necessary for several weeks after reduction of a dislocation to allow healing of the joint structures. In dislocations affecting the knee, alternatives to surgery are isometric quadriceps-strengthening exercises and a temporary brace. Surgical procedures, such as joint replacement, may be necessary in certain pathologic dislocations.

Loose Bodies

Loose bodies, commonly referred to as "joint mice," are small pieces of bone or cartilage within a joint space.[4] These can result from trauma to the joint or may occur when cartilage has worn away from the articular surface, causing a necrotic piece of bone to separate and become free floating. The symptoms are painful catching and locking of the joint. Loose bodies are commonly seen in the knee, elbow, hip, and ankle. The loose body repeatedly gets caught in the crevice of a joint, pinching the underlying healthy cartilage; unless the loose body is removed, it may cause osteoarthritis and restricted movement. The treatment consists of removal using operative arthroscopy.

Shoulder and Rotator Cuff Injuries

The shoulder is a complex series of joints that produce extraordinary range of motion. The extreme mobility is accomplished at the expense of instability. This instability, combined with its relatively exposed position, makes the shoulder extremely vulnerable to injuries such as sprains and dislocations and degenerative processes such as rotator cuff disorders.[8,9]

The shoulder includes the proximal humerus, the clavicle, and the scapula, and their connections with each other, to the sternum (clavicle), and to the ribs (scapula; Fig. 42-2). The scapula is a thin bone that articulates widely and closely with the chest wall.[4,8] It also articulates with the humerus by way of its small, shallow glenoid cavity and with the clavicle at the acromion process. The clavicle, which is held firmly in place by ligaments at the sternum and acromion, forms the only bony connec-

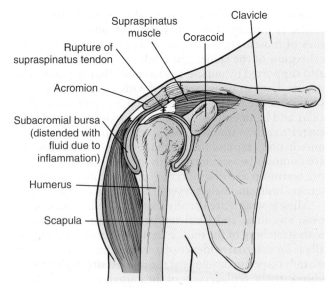

FIGURE 42-2 Structures of the shoulder showing the location of common rotator cuff injuries. The supraspinatus muscle is the most commonly injured part of the rotator cuff. (Adapted from Moore K. L., Dalley A. F. [1999]. *Clinically oriented anatomy* [4th ed., p. 698]. Philadelphia: Lippincott Williams & Wilkins.)

tion between the axial skeleton and the upper extremity. Clavicle fractures are among the most common fractures of childhood.[9] The typical mechanism of fracture is a fall on the lateral shoulder, or less commonly by a direct blow or by falling on an outstretched arm. Most clavicle fractures are treated nonoperatively, with either a simple arm sling or figure-of-eight clavicle strap.[5]

Four articulations form the shoulder joint: the acromioclavicular, glenohumeral, scapulothoracic, and sternoclavicular joints. The stability of these joints is provided by a series of muscles and tendons. Sprains of the acromioclavicular joint usually occur as a result of a blow to the top of the shoulder, but are known to occur with a fall to the lateral or posterior aspect of the shoulder.[9] The most common site of shoulder dislocation is the glenohumeral joint.[8-10] Most acute dislocations involve anterior displacement of the humeral head with respect to the glenoid, the result of the shoulder being abducted and forcefully extended and rotated. Other mechanisms include a fall on an outstretched arm or a blow to the posterior shoulder.

Motion of the arm involves the coordinated movement of muscles of the rotator cuff (supraspinous, teres minor, infraspinatus, subscapularis) and their musculotendinous attachments. These muscles are separated from the overlying "coracoacromial" arch by two bursae, the subdeltoid and subcoracoid. These two bursae, sometimes referred to as the *subacromial bursae*, often communicate and are affected by lesions of the rotator cuff.

Rotator cuff injuries and impingement disorders can result from a number of causes, including excessive use, a direct blow, or stretch injury, usually involving throwing or swinging, as with baseball pitchers or tennis players. Complete tears or rupture of the rotator cuff usually occur in young persons after severe trauma (see Fig. 42-2). Lesser degrees of injury can cause partial-thickness tears. Overuse injuries usually occur in athletes and increase with advancing age.[4] Degenerative disorders have a slower onset and are seen in older persons with minor or no trauma. The tendons of the rotator cuff are fused together near their insertions into the tuberositas of the humerus to form the musculotendinous cuff. Degeneration of these tendons can result from a number of factors, including repetitive microtrauma, impairment of vascularity as a result of age, or shoulder instability with secondary overload of the cuff. Degeneration is most severe near the tendon insertion, with the supraspinous being affected most often. Chronic irritation of the musculotendinous unit can lead to tendinitis with scarring and thickening of the tendon along with secondary inflammation of the overlying bursae.[5] Thickening of these tissues decreases the distance between the cuff and the overlying coracoacromial arch. Pain and impingement may be noted when motions of the arm squeeze and pinch these tissues between the humerus and the overlying arch. Severe tendinitis also can cause either a partial or complete rotator cuff tear.

Several physical examination maneuvers, including assessment of active and passive range of motion, are used to define shoulder pathology.[11] The history and mechanism of injury are important. In addition to standard radiographs, an arthrogram, computed tomography (CT) scan, or magnetic resonance imaging (MRI) scan may be obtained. Arthroscopic examination under anesthesia is done for diagnostic purposes, and operative arthroscopy is used to repair severe tears. Conservative treatment with anti-inflammatory agents, corticosteroid injections, and physical therapy often is used. A period of rest is followed by a customized exercise and rehabilitation program to improve strength, flexibility, and endurance. Surgical repair may be considered for persons with an acute traumatic cuff tear or those with significant symptoms and failed rehabilitation.[5]

Knee Injuries

The knee is a common site of injury, particularly sports-related injuries in which the knee is subjected to abnormal twisting and compression forces. These forces can result in injury to the menisci, patellar subluxation and dislocation, and chondromalacia. Knee injuries in young adulthood and both knee and hip injuries in middle age substantially increase the risk of osteoarthritis in the same joint later in life.

Meniscus Injuries. The menisci are C-shaped plates of fibrocartilage that are superimposed between the condyles of the femur and tibia. There are two menisci in each knee, a lateral and medial meniscus (Fig. 42-3). The menisci are thicker at their external margins and taper to thin, unattached edges at their interior margin. They are firmly attached at their ends to the intercondylar area of the tibia and they are supported by the coronary and transverse ligaments of the knee. The menisci play a major

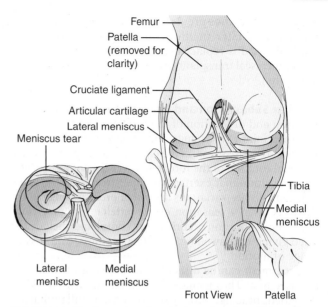

FIGURE 42-3 The knee showing the lateral and medial meniscus (with the patella removed for clarity). Insert (**lower left**) shows meniscus tear.

role in load bearing and shock absorption. They also help to stabilize the knee by deepening the tibial socket and maintaining the femur and tibia in proper position. In addition, the menisci assist in joint lubrication and serve as a source of nutrition for articular cartilage in the knee.

Any action of the knee that causes injury to the knee ligaments can also cause a meniscal tear.[12] Meniscus injury commonly occurs as the result of a rotational injury from a sudden or sharp pivot or a direct blow to the knee, as in hockey, basketball, or football. The type and location of the meniscal tear is determined by the magnitude and direction of the force that acts on the knee and the position of the knee at the time of injury. Meniscus tears can be described by their appearance (*e.g.,* parrot-beak, bucket handle) or their location (*e.g.,* posterior horn, anterior horn). The injured knee is edematous and painful, especially with hyperflexion and hyperextension. A loose fragment may cause knee instability and locking.

Diagnosis is made by examination and confirmed by methods such as arthroscopy, radiologic or CT scans, and radionuclide imaging. MRI has proven particularly useful in diagnosis of meniscal tears.[12] Initial treatment of meniscal injuries may be conservative. The knee may be placed in a removable knee immobilizer. Isometric quadriceps exercises may be prescribed. Activity usually is restricted until complete motion is recovered. Arthroscopic meniscectomy may be performed when there is recurrent or persistent locking, recurrent effusion, or disabling pain.

There is evidence that loss of meniscal function is associated with progressive deterioration of knee function.[13] Damaged articular cartilage has a limited capacity to heal because of its avascular nature and inadequate mobilization of regenerative cells. Meniscal reconstruction procedures have been developed to preserve these functions before development of significant degenerative changes occur, thus preventing the need for a total joint replacement later in life. Among the reconstruction methods used is replacement of the damaged meniscus with a meniscal transplant (fresh, frozen, or cryopreserved allografts).[13,14]

Patellar Subluxation and Dislocations.

Recurrent subluxation and dislocation of the patella (*i.e.*, knee cap) are common injuries in young adults. Sports such as skiing or tennis may cause stress on the patella. These sports involve external rotation of the foot and lower leg with knee flexion, a position that exerts rotational stresses on the knee. Congenital knee variations are also a predisposing factor. There is often a sensation of the patella "popping out" when the dislocation occurs. Other complaints include the knee giving out, swelling, crepitus, stiffness, and loss of range of motion.[4]

Treatment can be difficult, but nonsurgical methods are used first. They include immobilization with the knee extended, bracing, administration of anti-inflammatory agents, and isometric quadriceps-strengthening exercises. Surgical intervention often is necessary.

Chondromalacia.

Chondromalacia, or softening of the articular cartilage, is seen most commonly on the undersurface of the patella and occurs most frequently in young adults.[4] It can be the result of recurrent subluxation of the patella or overuse in strenuous athletic activities. Persons with this disorder typically complain of anterior knee pain, particularly when climbing stairs or sitting with the knees bent. Squatting and prolonged sitting with the knee flexed are also uncomfortable. Symptoms of the knee giving way or locking may be present. Occasionally, the person experiences weakness of the knee.

Treatment consists of rest, isometric exercises, and application of ice after exercise. Most cases recover spontaneously. Treatment is directed toward the underlying cause, if any is present. Surgery may rarely be indicated if symptoms persist. If needed, it usually consists of some procedure to realign the patella to prevent abnormal motion or relieve abnormal lateral pressure.

Hip Injuries

The hip is a ball-and-socket joint in which the femoral head articulates deeply in the acetabulum.[4] The proximal part of the femur consists of a head, neck, and greater trochanter. The vascular anatomy of the femoral head is of critical importance in any disorder of the hip. The main sources of blood supply are the retinacular and intramedullary vessels, both of which course from the intertrochanteric region proximally to nourish the femoral head (Fig. 42-4). Disease or injuries that compromise the circulation may damage the viability of the femoral head and lead to avascular necrosis or osteonecrosis (to be discussed). Disorders of the hip include dislocations and fractures of the hip. Congenital dysplasia of the hip, Legg-Calvé-Perthes disease, and slipped capital femoral epiphysis are discussed in the last part of the chapter.

Dislocations of the Hip.

Dislocations of the hip are the result of severe trauma and are usually posterior in direction.[4] They commonly result from the knee being struck while the hip and knee are in a flexed position. This force drives the femoral head out of the acetabulum posteriorly. Anterior dislocations are less common and usually result from a force on the knee with the thigh abducted.

Hip dislocation is an emergency.[4] In the dislocated position, great tension is placed on the blood supply to

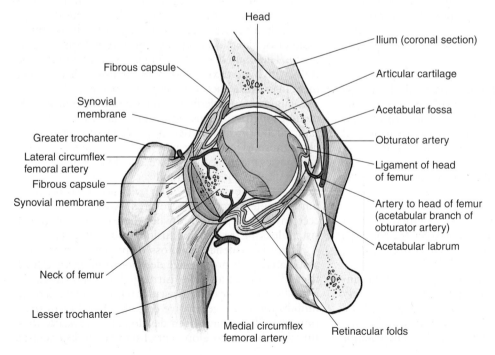

FIGURE 42-4 Blood supply of the head and neck of the femur, anterior view. A section of bone has been removed from the femoral neck. (Modified from Moore K., Agur A. M. R. [2002]. *Essential clinical anatomy* [2nd ed., p. 381]. Philadelphia: Lippincott Williams & Wilkins.)

the femoral head and avascular necrosis may result. To prevent this complication, early reduction is indicated. Weight bearing is usually limited after reduction to prevent dislocation from reoccurring and allow healing to occur.

Fractures of the Hip. Hip fracture is a major public health problem in the Western world, particularly among the elderly. It results in hospitalization, disability, and loss of independence. The incidence of hip fractures increases with age, doubling for each decade after 50 years of age, and is two to three times higher in women than men.[15,16] The incidence is also higher in white women compared with nonwhite women. Risk factors for hip fracture include excessive consumption of alcohol and caffeine, physical inactivity, low body weight, tall stature, use of certain psychotropic drugs, residence in an institution, visual impairment, and dementia.[16] Osteoporosis is an important contributing factor.

Most hip fractures result from falls. Occasionally, the person may actually fracture the hip before falling, the fracture representing the completion of an incomplete fracture. The characteristics of the fall (the direction, site of impact, and protective response) and environmental factors are recognized as important influences on the risk of hip fracture from a fall.

A hip fracture is usually a fracture of the proximal femur. Such fractures are commonly categorized according to the anatomic site in which they occur.[15,16] Femoral neck fractures are located in the area distal to the femoral head but proximal to the greater and lesser trochanters and are considered intracapsular because they are located within the capsule of the hip joint. Intertrochanteric fractures occur in the metaphyseal region between the greater and lesser trochanter. Subtrochanteric fractures are those that occur just below the greater trochanter. Femoral neck and intertrochanteric fractures account for over 90% of hip fractures, occurring in approximately equal proportions.[16]

The location of a hip fracture is important in terms of blood flow to the femoral head, which receives its blood supply from vessels that course proximally up the femoral neck (see Fig. 42-4). Subtrochanteric and intertrochanteric fractures that occur distal to these vessels do not usually disturb the blood supply to the femoral head, whereas femoral neck fractures, particularly those involving marked displacement, often disrupt the blood supply to the femoral head and are therefore associated with an increased incidence of complications (nonunion and avascular necrosis).

Most hip fractures are diagnosed based on clinical findings and standard radiographs. A bone scan or magnetic resonance imaging (MRI) may be done when the radiograph is negative but the clinical findings support the diagnosis of hip fracture.

The primary goal of treatment is a return to the preinjury level of function as soon as possible.[4] Undisplaced or impacted fractures have a better prognosis in terms of healing and are often treated nonoperatively or by simple internal fixation to provide stability. Displaced intra-capsular fractures in the elderly are usually best treated by surgical hip replacement and early mobilization. Young, healthy people are treated by reduction of the fracture (if needed) and internal fixation. This method allows for preservation of the femoral head, which in this age group is desirable because the long-term results are better than with prosthetic replacement.[16] Intertrochanteric fractures are usually treated with open reduction and internal fixation. This allows for early ambulation by eliminating pain at the fracture site.[16] Nonunion in this type of fracture is much less common than with intracapsular fractures. Weight bearing, however, is usually restricted for 3 months until union of the fracture has occurred.

FRACTURES

A fracture, or discontinuity of the bone, is the most common type of bone lesion. Normal bone can withstand considerable compression and shearing forces and, to a lesser extent, tension forces. A fracture occurs when more stress is placed on the bone than it is able to absorb. Grouped according to cause, fractures can be divided into three major categories: (1) fractures caused by sudden injury, (2) fatigue or stress fractures, and (3) pathologic fractures. The most common fractures are those resulting from sudden injury. The force causing the fracture may be direct, such as a fall or blow, or indirect, such as a massive muscle contraction or trauma transmitted along the bone. For example, the head of the radius or clavicle can be fractured by the indirect forces that result from falling on an outstretched hand.

A *fatigue fracture* results from repeated wear on a bone. Pain associated with overuse injuries of the lower extremities, especially posterior medial tibial pain, is one of the most common symptoms that physically active persons, such as runners, experience. *Stress fractures* in the tibia may be confused with "shin splints," a nonspecific term for pain in the lower leg from overuse in walking and running, because they frequently do not appear on x-ray films until 2 weeks after the onset of symptoms.

A *pathologic fracture* occurs in bones that already are weakened by disease or tumors. Fractures of this type may occur spontaneously with little or no stress. The underlying disease state can be local, as with infections, cysts, or tumors, or it can be generalized, as in osteoporosis, Paget disease, or disseminated tumors.

Classification

Fractures usually are classified according to location, type, and direction or pattern of the fracture line[4] (Fig. 42-5). A fracture of the long bone is described in relation to its position in the bone—proximal, midshaft, and distal. Other descriptions are used when the fracture affects the head or neck of a bone, involves a joint, or is near a prominence such as a condyle or malleolus.

The type of fracture is determined by its communication with the external environment, the degree of break in continuity of the bone, and the character of the fracture pieces. A fracture can be classified as open or closed.

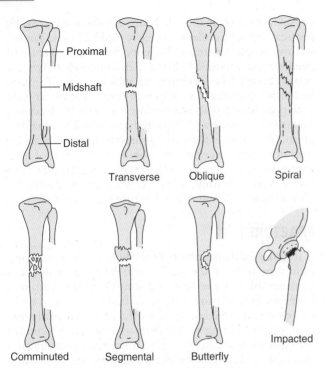

FIGURE 42-5 Classification of fractures. Fractures are classified according to location (proximal, midshaft, or distal), the direction of fracture line (transverse, oblique, or spiral), and type (comminuted, segmental, butterfly, or impacted).

When the bone fragments have broken through the skin, the fracture is called an *open* or *compound fracture*. In a closed fracture, there is no communication with the outside skin.

The degree of a fracture is described in terms of a complete or incomplete break in the continuity of bone.[4,17] A *greenstick fracture*, which is seen in children, is an example of a partial break in bone continuity and resembles that seen when a young sapling is broken. This kind of break occurs because children's bones, especially until approximately 10 years of age, are more resilient than the bones of adults.

The character of the fracture pieces may also be used to describe a fracture. A *comminuted fracture* has more than two pieces. A *compression fracture*, as occurs in the vertebral body, involves two bones that are crushed or squeezed together. A fracture is called *impacted* when the fracture fragments are wedged together. This type usually occurs in the humerus, often is less serious, and usually is treated without surgery.

The direction of the trauma or mechanism of injury produces a certain configuration or pattern of fracture. *Reduction* is the restoration of a fractured bone to its normal anatomic position. The pattern of a fracture indicates the nature of the trauma and provides information about the easiest method for reduction. *Transverse fractures* are caused by simple angulatory forces. A *spiral fracture* results from a twisting motion, or torque. A transverse fracture is not likely to become displaced or lose its position after it is reduced. On the other hand,

spiral, oblique, and comminuted fractures often are unstable and may change position after reduction.

Manifestations

The signs and symptoms of a fracture include pain, tenderness at the site of bone disruption, swelling, loss of function, deformity of the affected part, and abnormal mobility. The deformity varies according to the type of force applied, the area of the bone involved, the type of fracture produced, and the strength and balance of the surrounding muscles.

In long bones, three types of deformities—angulation, shortening, and rotation—are seen. Severely angulated fracture fragments may be felt at the fracture site and often push up against the soft tissue to cause a tenting effect on the skin. Bending forces and unequal muscle pulls cause angulation. Shortening of the extremity occurs as the bone fragments slide and override each other because of the pull of the muscles on the long axis of the extremity (Fig. 42-6). Rotational deformity occurs when the fracture fragments rotate out of their normal longitudinal axis; this can result from rotational strain produced by the fracture or unequal pull by the muscles that are attached to the fracture fragments. A crepitus or grating sound may be heard as the bone fragments rub against each other. In the case of an open fracture, there is bleeding from the wound where the bone protrudes. Blood loss from a pelvic fracture or multiple long bone fractures can cause hypovolemic shock in a trauma victim.

Shortly after the fracture has occurred, nerve function at the fracture site may be temporarily lost. The area may become numb, and the surrounding muscles may become flaccid. This condition has been called *local shock*. During this period, which may last for a few minutes to half an hour, fractured bones may be reduced with little or no pain. After this brief period, the pain sensation returns and, with it, muscle spasms and contractions of the surrounding muscles.

Diagnosis and Treatment

Diagnosis is the first step in the care of fractures and is based on history and physical manifestations. X-ray examination is used to confirm the diagnosis and direct the treatment. The ease of diagnosis varies with the location and severity of the fracture. In the trauma patient, the presence of other, more serious injuries may make diagnosis more difficult.

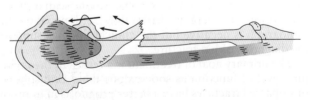

FIGURE 42-6 Displacement and overriding of fracture fragments of a long bone (femur) caused by severe muscle spasm.

Treatment depends on the general condition of the person, the presence of associated injuries, the location of the fracture and its displacement, and whether the fracture is open or closed. A *splint* is a device for immobilizing the movable fragments of a fracture. When a fracture is suspected, the injured part always should be splinted before it is moved. This is essential for preventing further injury.[4]

There are three objectives for treatment of fractures: (1) reduction of the fracture, (2) immobilization, and (3) preservation and restoration of the function of the injured part.[4] Reduction of a fracture is directed toward replacing the bone fragments to as near-normal an anatomic position as possible. This can be accomplished by closed manipulation or surgical (open) reduction. Closed manipulation uses methods such as manual pressure and traction. Fractures are held in reduction by external or internal fixation devices. Surgical reduction involves the use of various types of hardware to accomplish internal fixation of the fracture fragments. Immobilization prevents movement of the injured parts and is the single most important element in obtaining union of the fracture fragments. Immobilization can be accomplished through the use of external devices, such as splints, casts, external fixation devices, or traction, or by means of internal fixation devices inserted during surgical reduction of the fracture. Preservation and restoration of the function of muscles and joints is an ongoing process in the unaffected and affected extremities during the period of immobilization required for fracture healing. Exercises designed to preserve function, maintain muscle strength, and reduce joint stiffness should be started early.

Bone Healing

Bone healing occurs in a manner similar to soft tissue healing. However, it is a more complex process and takes longer. There are essentially four stages involved in bone healing: hematoma formation, fibrocartilaginous callus development, ossification, and remodeling.[17-19] The degree of response during each of these stages is in direct proportion to the extent of trauma.

Hematoma formation occurs during the first 1 to 2 days after fracture. It develops from torn blood vessels in the periosteum and adjacent muscles and soft tissue. Disruption of blood vessels also leads to death of bone cells at the fracture site. In 2 to 5 days, the hemorrhage forms a large blood clot. Neovascularization begins to occur peripheral to the blood clot. By the end of the first week, most of the clot is organized by invasion of blood vessels and early fibrosis. Hematoma formation is thought to be necessary for the initiation of the cellular events essential to bone healing.[18] As the result of hematoma formation, clotting factors remain in the injured area to initiate the formation of a fibrin meshwork, which serves as a framework for the ingrowth of fibroblasts and new capillary buds. At the same time, degranulated platelets and migrating inflammatory cells release growth factors, which stimulate osteoclast and osteoblast proliferation.[17,18]

The next event in fracture healing is formation of granulation tissue or soft tissue callus. During this stage of bone healing, fibroblasts and osteoblasts migrate into the fracture site from the nearby periosteal and endosteal membranes and begin reconstruction of bone. The fibroblasts produce collagen that spans the break and connects the broken bone ends, and some differentiate into chondrocytes that secrete collagen matrix. At about the same time, osteoblasts begin depositing bone into this matrix. After a few days, a fibrocartilage "collar" becomes evident around the fracture site. The collar edges on either side of the fracture eventually unite to form a bridge, which connects the bone fragments. The earliest bone, in the form of woven bone, begins its formation sometime after the first week. In an uncomplicated fracture, the repair tissue reaches its maximum girth at the end of the second to third week, which helps stabilize the fracture, but it is not yet strong enough for weight bearing.

Ossification represents the deposition of mineral salts into the callus. This stage usually begins during the third to fourth week of fracture healing. During this stage, mature bone gradually replaces the fibrocartilaginous callus, and the excess callus is gradually resorbed by the osteoclasts. The fracture site feels firm and immovable and appears united on the radiograph. At this point, it is usually safe to remove the cast.

Remodeling involves resorption of the excess bony callus that develops in the marrow space and encircles the external aspect of the fracture site. As the callus matures and transmits weight-bearing forces, the portions that are not stressed are resorbed. It is in this manner that the callus is reduced in size until the shape and outline of the bone have been reestablished. The medullary cavity of the bone is also restored. After this is completed, the bone usually appears as it did before the injury.

Healing Time. Healing time depends on the site of the fracture, the condition of the fracture fragments, hematoma formation, and other local and host factors. In children, fractures usually heal within 4 to 6 weeks; in adolescents, they heal within 6 to 8 weeks; and in adults, they heal within 10 to 18 weeks. The increased rate of healing among children compared with adults may be related to the increased cellularity and vascularity of the child's periosteum.[20] In general, fractures of long bones, displaced fractures, and fractures with less surface area heal more slowly. Function usually returns within 6 months after union is complete. However, return to complete function may take longer.

Impaired Bone Healing. Factors that influence bone healing are specific to the person, the type of injury sustained, and local factors that disrupt healing (Chart 42-1). Individual factors that may delay bone healing are the patient's age; current medications; debilitating diseases, such as diabetes and rheumatoid arthritis; local stress around the fracture site; circulatory problems and coagulation disorders; and poor nutrition.

Malunion is healing with deformity, angulation, or rotation that is visible on x-ray films.[20] Early and aggressive

Understanding ➤ Fracture Healing

A fracture, which is any break in a bone, undergoes a healing process to reestablish bone continuity and strength. The repair of simple fractures is commonly divided into four phases: (1) hematoma formation, (2) fibrocartilaginous callus formation, (3) bony callus formation, and (4) remodeling.

1

Hematoma formation. When a bone breaks, blood vessels in the bone and surrounding tissues are torn and bleed into and around the fragments of the fractured bone, forming a blood clot, or hematoma. The hematoma facilitates the formation of the fibrin meshwork that seals off the fracture site and serves as a framework for the influx of inflammatory cells, the ingrowth of fibroblasts, and the development of new capillary buds (vessels). It is also the source of signaling molecules that initiate the cellular events that are critical to the healing process.

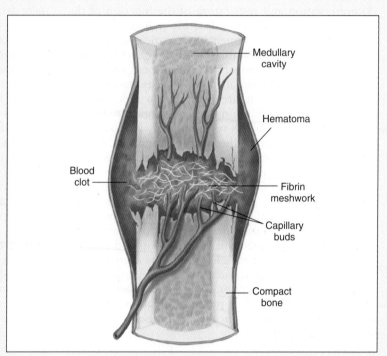

2

Fibrocartilaginous callus formation. As new capillaries infiltrate the hematoma at the fracture site, it becomes organized into a form of granulation tissue, called *procallus*. Fibroblasts from the periosteum, endosteum, and red bone marrow proliferate and invade the procallus. The fibroblasts produce a fibrocartilaginous soft callus bridge that connects the bone fragments. Although this repair tissue usually reaches its maximum girth at the end of the second or third week, it is not strong enough for weight bearing.

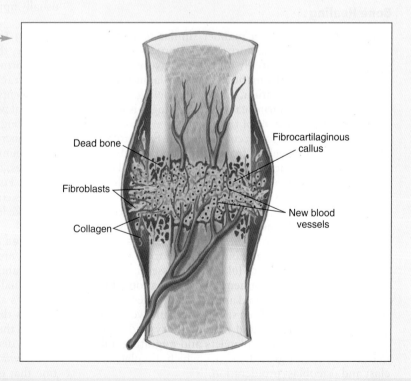

3

Bony callus formation. Ossification represents the conversion of the fibrocartilaginous cartilage to bony callus. In areas close to well-vascularized bone tissue, osteogenic cells develop into osteoblasts, or bone-building cells, which produce spongy bone trabeculae. The newly formed osteoblasts first deposit bone on the outer surface of the bone some distance from the fracture site. The formation of bone progresses toward the fracture site until a new bony sheath covers the fibrocartilaginous callus. In time, the fibrocartilage is converted to spongy bone, and the callus is then referred to as bony callus. Gradually, the bony callus calcifies and is replaced by mature bone. Bony callus formation begins 3 to 4 weeks after injury and continues until a firm bony union is formed months later.

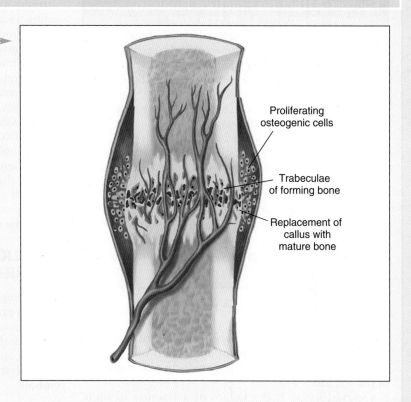

Proliferating osteogenic cells

Trabeculae of forming bone

Replacement of callus with mature bone

4

Remodeling. During remodeling of the bony callus, dead portions of the bone are gradually removed by osteoclasts. Compact bone replaces spongy bone around the periphery of the fracture, and there is reorganization of mineralized bone along the lines of mechanical stress. During this period, the excess material on the outside of the bone shaft and within the medullary cavity is removed and compact bone is laid down to reconstruct the shaft. The final structure of the remodeled area resembles that of the original unbroken bone; however, a thickened area on the surface of the bone may remain as evidence of a healed fracture.

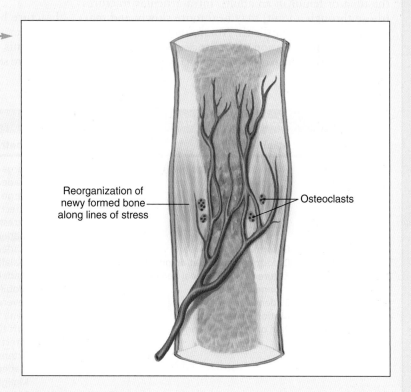

Reorganization of newy formed bone along lines of stress

Osteoclasts

CHART 42-1

Factors Affecting Fracture Healing

- Nature of the injury or the severity of the trauma, including fracture displacement, edema, and arterial occlusion with crushing injuries
- Degree of fibrocartilage bridge formation that develops during bone healing
- Amount of bone loss (e.g., it may be too great for the healing to bridge the gap)
- Type of bone that is injured (e.g., cancellous bone heals faster than cortical bone)
- Degree of immobilization that is achieved (e.g., movement disrupts the fibrin bridge and cartilage forms instead of bone)
- Local infection, which retards or prevents healing
- Local malignancy, which must be treated before healing can proceed
- Bone necrosis, which prevents blood flow into the fracture site

treatment, especially of the hand, can prevent malunion and result in earlier alignment and return of function. Malunion is caused by inadequate reduction or alignment of the fracture.

Delayed union is the failure of a fracture to unite within the normal period (e.g., 20 weeks for a fracture of the tibia or femur in an adult). Intra-articular fractures (those through a joint) may heal more slowly and may eventually produce arthritis. *Nonunion* is failure to produce union and cessation of the processes of bone repair. It is seen most often in the tibia, especially with open frac-

tures or crushing injuries. It is characterized by mobility of the fracture site and pain on weight bearing. Muscle atrophy and loss of range of motion may occur. Nonunion usually is established 6 to 12 months after the time of the fracture.[20] The complications of fracture healing are summarized in Table 42-1.

Treatment methods for impaired bone healing encompass surgical interventions, including bone grafts, bracing, external fixation, or electrical stimulation of the bone ends. Electrical stimulation is thought to stimulate the osteoblasts to lay down a network of bone. Three types of commercial bone growth stimulators are available: a noninvasive model, which is placed outside the cast; a semi-invasive model, in which pins are inserted around the fracture site; and a totally implantable type, in which a cathode coil is wound around the bone at the fracture site and operated by a battery pack implanted under the skin.[4]

COMPLICATIONS OF FRACTURES AND OTHER MUSCULOSKELETAL INJURIES

The complications of fractures and other orthopedic injuries are associated with loss of skeletal continuity, injury from bone fragments, pressure from swelling and hemorrhage (e.g., fracture blisters, compartment syndrome), involvement of nerve fibers (e.g., reflex sympathetic dystrophy and causalgia), or development of fat emboli.

Fracture Blisters

Fracture blisters are skin bullae and blisters representing areas of epidermal necrosis with separation of the epidermis from the underlying dermis by edema fluid. They are seen with more severe, twisting types of injuries

TABLE 42-1	Complications of Fracture Healing	
Complication	**Manifestations**	**Contributing Factors**
Delayed union	Failure of fracture to heal within predicted time as determined by x-ray	Large displaced fracture
		Inadequate immobilization
		Large hematoma
		Infection at fracture site
		Excessive loss of bone
		Inadequate circulation
Malunion	Deformity at fracture site	Inadequate reduction
	Deformity or angulation on x-ray	Malalignment of fracture at time of immobilization
Nonunion	Failure of bone to heal before the process of bone repair stops	Inadequate reduction
	Evidence on x-ray	Mobility at fracture site
	Motion at fracture site	Severe trauma
	Pain on weight bearing	Bone fragment separation
		Soft tissue between bone fragments
		Infection
		Extensive loss of bone
		Inadequate circulation
		Malignancy
		Bone necrosis
		Noncompliance with mobility restrictions

(*e.g.*, motor vehicle accidents and falls from heights) but can also occur after excessive joint manipulation, dependent positioning, and heat application, or from peripheral vascular disease. They can be solitary, multiple, or massive, depending on the extent of injury. Most fracture blisters occur in the ankle, elbow, foot, knee, or areas where there is little soft tissue between the bone and the skin. The development of fracture blisters reportedly is reduced by early surgical intervention in persons requiring operative repair.[21] This probably reflects the early operative release of the fracture hematoma, reapproximation of the disrupted soft tissues, ligation of bleeding vessels, and fixation of bleeding fracture surfaces. Prevention of fracture blisters is important because they pose an additional risk of infection.

Compartment Syndrome

The compartment syndrome has been described as a condition of increased pressure within a limited space (*e.g.*, abdominal and limb compartments) that compromises the circulation and function of the tissues within the space.[22] The abdominal compartment syndrome alters cardiovascular hemodynamics, respiratory mechanics, and renal function. The discussion in this chapter is limited to a discussion of the limb compartment syndromes.

The muscles and nerves of an extremity are enclosed in a tough, inelastic fascial envelope called a *muscle compartment*[5,22-24] (Fig. 42-7). If the pressure in the compartment is sufficiently high, tissue circulation is compromised, causing death of nerve and muscle cells. Permanent loss of function may occur. The amount of pressure required to produce a compartment syndrome depends on many factors, including the duration of the pressure elevation, the metabolic rate of the tissues, vascular tone, and local blood pressure. Less tissue pressure

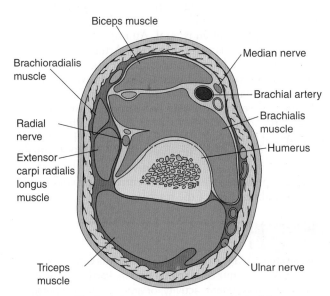

FIGURE 42-7 The proximal muscle compartment of the arm, showing the location of fascia, muscles, nerves, and blood vessels.

is required to stop circulation when hypotension or vasoconstriction is present. Intracompartmental pressures greater that 30 mm Hg (normal is approximately 6 mm Hg) are considered sufficient to impair capillary blood flow.[5]

Compartment syndrome can result from a decrease in compartment size, an increase in the volume of its contents, or a combination of the two factors. Among the causes of decreased compartment size are constrictive dressings and casts, closure of fascial defects, and burns. In persons with circumferential third-degree burns, the inelastic and constricting eschar decreases the size of the underlying compartments (see Chapter 45).

An increase in compartment volume can be caused by trauma, swelling, vascular injury and bleeding, and venous obstruction. One of the most important causes of compartment syndrome is bleeding and edema caused by fractures and bone surgery. Contusions and soft tissue injury also are common causes of compartment syndrome. Increased compartment volume may also follow ischemic events, such as arterial occlusion, that are of sufficient duration to produce capillary damage, causing increased capillary permeability and edema. Infiltration of intravenous fluids or bleeding from an arterial puncture can also cause compartment ischemia and postischemic swelling. During unattended coma caused by drug overdose or carbon monoxide poisoning, high compartment pressures are produced when an extremity is compressed by the weight of the overlying head or torso.

Compartment syndrome can be acute or chronic. Acute compartment syndrome can occur after a fracture or crushing injury, when excessive swelling around the site of injury results in increased pressure in a closed compartment. This increase in pressure occurs because fascia, which covers and separates muscles, is inelastic and unable to stretch and compensate for the extreme swelling. Chronic compartment syndrome may develop in long-distance runners and others involved in a major change in activity level. In this case, the symptoms are less severe and tend to improve with rest. Although the exact mechanism is unclear, exercise causes an increase in the compartment volume and intramuscular pressure that result in tissue ischemia and pain.[25]

The hallmark symptom of an acute compartment syndrome is severe pain that is out of proportion to the original injury or physical findings.[5] Nerve compression may cause changes in sensation (*e.g.*, paresthesias such as burning or tingling or loss of sensation), diminished reflexes, and eventually the loss of motor function. Symptoms usually begin within a few hours but can be delayed as long as 64 hours.[22]

Because muscle necrosis can occur in as little as 4 to 8 hours, it is important that persons at risk for compartment syndrome be identified and proper treatment methods instituted.[5] Assessment should include pain assessment, examination of sensory (*i.e.*, light touch and two-point discrimination) and motor function (*i.e.*, movement and muscle strength), tests of passive stretch, and palpation of the muscle compartments. Peripheral pulses frequently are normal in the presence of compartment syndrome because the major arteries are located outside the muscle compartments. Although edema may make it difficult to palpate the pulse, the increased compartment pressure seldom is sufficient to occlude flow in a major artery. Doppler methods usually confirm the existence of a pulse. Direct measurements of tissue pressure can be obtained using a needle or wick catheter inserted into the muscle compartment. This method is particularly useful in persons who are unresponsive and in those with nerve deficits.

Treatment consists of reducing compartmental pressures. This entails cast splitting or removal of restrictive dressings. These procedures often are sufficient to relieve most of the underlying pressure and symptoms. Elevating the extremity on pillows can help to reduce edema. However, excessive elevation should be avoided because the effects of gravity can lower the arterial pressure in the limb, thereby decreasing compartment perfusion.[5] When compartment syndrome cannot be relieved by conservative measures, a fasciotomy may become necessary. During this procedure, the fascia is incised longitudinally and separated so that the compartment volume can expand and blood flow can be reestablished. Because of potential problems with wound infection and closure, this procedure is performed as a last resort.

Complex Regional Pain Syndrome

The complex regional pain syndrome, also known as *reflex sympathetic dystrophy*, is a complication of orthopedic injuries that causes pain out of proportion to the injury and autonomic nervous system dysfunction manifested by hyperhidrosis (increased sweating) and vasomotor instability (either flushed and warm or cold and pale).[21,26] The disorder often produces long-term disability and chronic pain syndromes (see Chapter 34).

Pain, which is the prominent symptom of the disorder, is described as severe, aching, or burning. It usually increases in intensity with movement and with noxious and non-noxious stimuli. The cause of the pain is unclear, but it is thought to have a sympathetic nervous system component. Muscle wasting, thin and shiny skin, and abnormalities of the nails and bone can occur. Decreased muscle strength and disuse can lead to contractures and osteoporosis.

Treatment focuses on pain management and prevention of disability. Physical therapy interventions such as hot/cold baths and elevation of the limb are used to maximize range of motion and minimize pain. Medications include anti-inflammatory agents, vasodilators, and antidepressant medications. Sympathetic nerve blocks may be used.

Fat Embolism Syndrome

The fat embolism syndrome (FES) refers to a constellation of clinical manifestations resulting from the presence of fat droplets in the small blood vessels of the lung or other organs after a long bone fracture or other major trauma.[21,27–30] The fat emboli are thought to be released from the bone marrow or adipose tissue at the fracture site into the venous system through torn veins.

The pathophysiologic process of FES is unclear. It is important to point out that fat embolization and FES are not synonymous.[27] Fat embolization involves the presence of fat particles in the circulation. One suggestion is that when a bone is fractured, disruption of the venous sinusoids and fat cells allows fat globules to gain access to the venous circulation. The larger particles then become lodged in and block small pulmonary capillaries, whereas the smaller particles may pass through the lung capillaries and enter the systemic circulation. Although fat embolization occurs in many persons with fractures or operative fixation of fractures, FES occurs in only a small percentage of cases, supporting the hypothesis that factors other than fat embolization may be necessary in the development of FES.[27]

The main clinical features of FES are respiratory failure, cerebral dysfunction, and skin and mucosal petechiae.[21,27] Cerebral manifestations include encephalopathy, seizures, and focal neurologic deficits unrelated to head injury. Initial symptoms begin within a few hours to 3 to 4 days after injury and do not appear beyond 1 week after the injury. The first symptoms include a subtle change in behavior and signs of disorientation resulting from emboli in the cerebral circulation combined with respiratory depression. There may be complaints of substernal chest pain and dyspnea accompanied by tachycardia and a low-grade fever. Diaphoresis, pallor, and cyanosis become evident as respiratory function deteriorates. A petechial rash that does not blanch with pressure often occurs 2 to 3 days after the injury. This rash usually is found on the anterior chest, axillae, neck, and shoulders. It also may appear on the soft palate and conjunctiva. The rash is thought to be related to embolization of the skin capillaries or thrombocytopenia.

Three degrees of severity are seen: subclinical, overt clinical, and fulminating. Although the subclinical and overt clinical forms of FES respond well to treatment, the fulminating form often is fatal. An important part of the treatment of FES is early diagnosis. Arterial blood gases should be assayed immediately after recognition of clinical manifestations. Treatment is directed toward correcting hypoxemia and maintaining adequate fluid balance. Mechanical ventilation may be required. Corticosteroid drugs are administered to decrease the inflammatory response of lung tissues, decrease edema, stabilize the lipid membranes to reduce lipolysis, and combat bronchospasm. Corticosteroids are also given prophylactically to high-risk persons. The only preventive approach to FES is early stabilization of the fracture.

In summary, many external physical agents can cause trauma to the musculoskeletal system. Particular factors, such as environment, activity, or age, can place a person at greater risk for injury. Some soft tissue injuries such as contusions, hematomas, and lacerations are relatively minor and easily treated. Muscle strains and ligamentous sprains are caused by mechanical overload on the connective tissue. They heal more slowly than the minor soft tissue injuries and require some degree of immobilization. Healing of soft tissue begins within 4 to 5 days of the injury and is primarily the function of fibroblasts, which produce collagen. Joint dislocation is caused by trauma to the supporting structures. Repeated trauma to the joint can cause articular softening (*i.e.,* chondromalacia) or the separation of small pieces of bone or cartilage, called *loose bodies,* in the joint. The knee and shoulder are common sites for injuries in athletes. The rotator cuff is a common site for shoulder injuries. Knee injuries include injury to the menisci, anterior cruciate ligament tears, patellar subluxation and dislocation, and chondromalacia. Hip injuries include dislocations and fractures. The blood supply to the head of the femur travels through the femoral neck. Thus dislocations and hip fractures affecting the femoral neck often disrupt blood flow to the femoral head, predisposing to fracture malunion and avascular necrosis.

Fractures occur when more stress is placed on a bone than the bone can absorb. The nature of the stress determines the type of fracture and the character of the resulting bone fragments. Healing of fractures is a complex process that takes place in four stages: hematoma formation, fibrocartilaginous callus formation, bony callus formation, and remodeling. For satisfactory healing to take place, the affected bone has to be reduced and immobilized. This is accomplished with external fixation devices (*e.g.,* splints, casts, or traction) or surgically implanted internal fixation devices.

The complications of fractures are associated with loss of skeletal continuity (malunion or nonunion), pressure from swelling and hemorrhage (fracture blisters and compartment syndrome), involvement of nerve fibers (complex regional pain syndrome), or development of fat emboli. Compartment syndrome is a condition of increased pressure in a muscle compartment that compromises blood flow and potentially leads to death of nerve and muscle tissue. Complex regional pain syndrome is a complication of orthopedic injuries that cause excessive pain and autonomic nervous system dysfunction manifested by hyperhidrosis and vasomotor instability. FES refers to a constellation of symptoms including a petechial skin rash, respiratory failure, and cerebral dysfunction due to the presence of fat droplets in small blood vessels after a fracture.

Infections and Osteonecrosis

OSTEOMYELITIS

Osteomyelitis represents an acute or chronic infection of the bone.[30–32] The term *osteo* refers to bone and *myelo* to the marrow cavity, both of which are involved in this disease. Despite the common use of antibiotics, these infec-

tions remain difficult to treat and eradicate. All types of organisms, including parasites, viruses, bacteria, and fungi, can cause osteomyelitis, but certain pyogenic bacteria and mycobacteria are most common.

Acute Osteomyelitis

Acute osteomyelitis is usually caused by bacteria. The infection can be caused by direct extension or contamination of an open fracture or wound (contiguous invasion); by seeding through the bloodstream (hematogenous spread); or by spread from skin infections in persons with vascular insufficiency.

The specific agents isolated in bacterial osteomyelitis are often associated with the age of the person or the inciting condition (*e.g.,* trauma or surgery). *Staphylococcus aureus* is responsible for most cases of acute hematogenous osteomyelitis. *Staphylococcus epidermidis, S. aureus, Pseudomonas aeruginosa, Serratia marcescens,* and *Escherichia coli* are commonly isolated in persons with chronic osteomyelitis. *S. aureus* has several characteristics that favor its ability to produce osteomyelitis: it is able to produce collagen-binding adhesion molecules that allow it to adhere to the connective tissue elements of bone; and it has the ability to be internalized and survive in cells such as the osteoblast, which helps to explain the persistent nature of the infection. *S. aureus* and *S. epidermidis* can also form biofilms, making them more resistant to antimicrobial therapy.[32]

Osteomyelitis Due to Contiguous Spread. Osteomyelitis secondary to a contiguous focus of infection may occur as a result of direct inoculation from an exogenous source or from an adjacent extraskeletal site. The most common cause is the direct contamination of bone from an open wound. It may be the result of an open fracture, a gunshot wound, or a puncture wound.

Iatrogenic bone infections are those inadvertently brought about by surgery or other treatments. These

KEY CONCEPTS

Bone Infections

➤ Bone infections may be caused by a wide variety of microorganisms introduced during injury, during operative procedures, or from the bloodstream.

➤ Once localized in bone, the microorganisms proliferate, produce cell death, and spread within the bone shaft, inciting a chronic inflammatory response with further destruction of bone.

➤ Bone infections are difficult to treat and eradicate. Measures to prevent infection include careful cleaning and debridement of skeletal injuries and strict operating room protocols.

infections include complications of pin tract infection in skeletal traction, septic (infected) joints in joint replacement surgery, and wound infections after surgery. Measures to prevent these infections include preparation of the skin to reduce bacterial growth before surgery or insertion of traction devices or wires; strict operating room protocols; prophylactic use of antibiotics immediately before and for 24 hours after surgery and as a topical wound irrigation; and maintenance of sterile technique after surgery when working with drainage tubes and dressing changes.

Osteomyelitis after trauma or bone surgery usually is associated with persistent or recurrent fevers, increased pain at the operative or trauma site, and poor incisional healing, which often is accompanied by continued wound drainage and wound separation. Prosthetic joint infections present with joint pain, fever, and cutaneous drainage.

Treatment includes the use of antibiotics and selective use of surgical interventions. Antibiotics should be administered prophylactically to persons undergoing bone surgery. For persons with osteomyelitis, early antibiotic treatment, before there is extensive destruction of bone, produces the best results. The choice of antibiotics and method of administration depend on the microorganisms causing the infection. Antibiotic beads (*e.g.*, vancomycin, tobramycin, or other broad-spectrum antibiotics) can be embedded into the cement as part of the procedure for an infected hip arthroplasty. In acute osteomyelitis that does not respond to antibiotic therapy, surgical decompression is used to release intramedullary pressure and remove drainage from the periosteal area.

Hematogenous Osteomyelitis. Hematogenous osteomyelitis originates with infectious organisms that reach the bone through the bloodstream.[17,18,31-34] Acute hematogenous osteomyelitis occurs predominantly in children. In adults, it is seen most commonly in debilitated patients and in those with a history of chronic skin infections, chronic urinary tract infections, and intravenous drug use and in those who are immunologically suppressed. Intravenous drug users are at risk for infections with *Streptococcus* and *Pseudomonas*.

The pathogenesis of hematogenous osteomyelitis differs in children and adults. In children, the infection usually affects the long bones of the appendicular skeleton.[18,32] It starts in the metaphyseal region close to the growth plate, where termination of nutrient blood vessels and sluggish blood flow favor the attachment of blood-borne bacteria. With advancement of the infection, purulent exudate collects in the rigidly enclosed bony tissue. Because of the bone's rigid structure, there is little room for swelling, and the purulent exudate finds its way beneath the periosteum, shearing off the perforating arteries that supply the cortex with blood, thereby leading to necrosis of cortical bone. Eventually, the purulent drainage may penetrate the periosteum and skin to form a draining sinus. In children younger than 1 year of age, the adjacent joint is often involved because the periosteum is not firmly attached to the cortex.[32]

In adults, the long bone microvasculature no longer favors seeding and hematogenous infection rarely affects the appendicular skeleton. Instead, vertebrae, sternoclavicular and sacroiliac joints, and the symphysis pubis are involved. Infection typically first involves subchondral bone, and then spreads to the joint space. With vertebral infections, this causes sequential destruction of the endplate, adjoining disk, and contiguous vertebral body. Infection less commonly begins in the joint and spreads to the adjacent bone. There is a tendency for infectious organisms to seed sites of previous, often minor injury.

The manifestations of acute hematogenous osteomyelitis are those of bacteremia accompanied by symptoms referable to the site of the bone lesion. Bacteremia is characterized by chills, fever, and malaise. There often is pain on movement of the affected extremity, loss of movement, and local tenderness followed by redness and swelling. X-ray studies may appear negative initially, but they show evidence of periosteal elevation and increased osteoclastic activity after an abscess has formed. Changes are evident on a bone scan 10 to 14 days before any changes are seen on x-ray films.[32]

The diagnosis of skeletal infection requires both confirmation of the presence of infection and identification of the causative organism. Various imaging strategies, including conventional radiology, nuclear imaging studies, CT scans, and MRI, are used to confirm the presence of infection. Blood and bone aspiration cultures are used to identify the causative organism and direct the choice of antibiotics for use in treatment of the infection.[31-34] Antibiotics are given first parenterally and then orally. Debridement and surgical drainage also may be necessary.

Chronic Osteomyelitis

Chronic osteomyelitis usually occurs in adults. Generally, these infections occur secondary to an open wound, most often to the bone or surrounding tissue. Chronic osteomyelitis has long been recognized as a disease. However, the incidence has decreased in the past century because of improvements in surgical techniques and broad-spectrum antibiotic therapy. Chronic osteomyelitis may be the result of delayed or inadequate treatment of acute hematogenous osteomyelitis or osteomyelitis caused by direct contamination of bone. Acute osteomyelitis is considered to have become chronic when the infection persists beyond 6 to 8 weeks or when the acute process has been adequately treated and is expected to resolve but does not. Chronic osteomyelitis can persist for years; it may appear spontaneously, after a minor trauma, or when resistance is lowered.

The hallmark feature of chronic osteomyelitis is the presence of a *sequestrum* or piece of dead bone that has separated from the surrounding living bone. A sheath of new bone, called the *involucrum*, forms around the dead bone (Fig. 42-8). Radiologic techniques such as x-ray films, bone scans, and sinograms are used to identify the infected site. Chronic osteomyelitis or infection around a total joint prosthesis can be difficult to diagnose because the classic signs of infection are not apparent and the

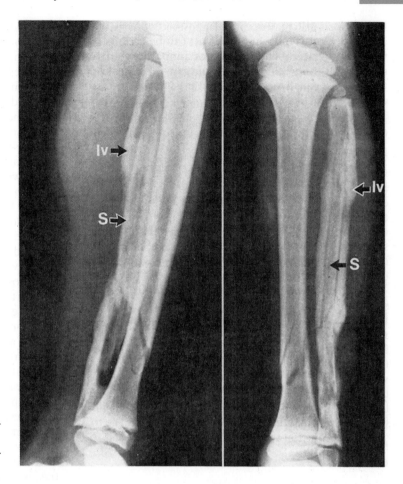

FIGURE 42-8 Hematogenous osteomyelitis of the fibula of 3 months' duration. The entire shaft has been deprived of its blood supply and has become a sequestrum (S) surrounded by new immature bone, involucrum (Iv). Pathologic fractures are present in the lower tibia and fibula. (From Wilson F. C. [1980]. *The musculoskeletal system* [2nd ed., p. 150]. Philadelphia: J. B. Lippincott.)

blood leukocyte count may not be elevated. A subclinical infection may exist for years. Bone scans are used in conjunction with bone biopsy for a definitive diagnosis.

The treatment of chronic bone infections begins with wound cultures to identify the microorganism and its sensitivity to antibiotic therapy. As a general rule, antibiotics are given for 4 to 6 weeks, usually by the intravenous route. Initial antibiotic therapy is followed by surgery to remove foreign bodies (*e.g.,* metal plates, screws) or sequestra and by long-term antibiotic therapy. Immobilization of the affected part usually is necessary, with restriction of weight bearing on a lower extremity. External fixation devices are sometimes used. With this method, full mechanical recovery can often be achieved and the fixation device removed after consolidation has occurred.

Osteomyelitis With Vascular Insufficiency

In persons with vascular insufficiency, osteomyelitis may develop from a skin lesion. It is most commonly associated with chronic or ischemic foot ulcers in persons with long-standing diabetes or other chronic vascular disorders. It is characterized by local cellulitis with inflammation and necrosis. Treatment depends on the oxygen tension of the involved tissues. Debridement and antibiotic therapy may benefit persons who have good oxygen

tension in the infected site. Amputation is indicated when oxygen tension is inadequate.

Tuberculosis of the Bone or Joint

Most tuberculosis infections of the bone and joint in the United States are caused by the human strain of *Mycobacterium tuberculosis*. A resurgence of tuberculosis osteomyelitis is occurring in industrialized nations, attributed to the influx of immigrants from developing countries and greater numbers of immunosuppressed people.[17]

Bone or joint infections are caused by hematogenic spread from a primary lesion in the respiratory tract. They may occur shortly after a primary infection or years later as disease reactivation. The spine (especially the thoracic and lumbar vertebrae) is the most common site of infection, followed by the hips and knees.[17,18] Tuberculosis osteomyelitis also can affect the joints and soft tissues. The disease is characterized by bone necrosis, and abscess formation tends be more destructive and resistant to control than in pyogenic osteomyelitis. In the spine (Pott disease), the infection spreads through the intervertebral disks to involve multiple vertebrae and extends into the soft tissues, forming abscesses.

Manifestations of the disease include pain, immobility, and muscle atrophy; joint swelling, mild fever, and leukocytosis also may occur. Diagnosis is confirmed by a positive culture. CT scans and MRI can be used as aids for early diagnosis. The most important part of the treatment is antituberculosis drug therapy. Conservative treatment is usually as effective as surgery, especially for earlier and milder cases.

OSTEONECROSIS

Osteonecrosis refers to necrosis or death of bone and marrow in the absence of infection[18] (Fig. 42-9). It is a relatively common disorder and can occur in the medullary cavity of the metaphysis and the subchondral region of the epiphysis, especially in the proximal femur, distal femur, and proximal humerus. All forms of bone necrosis result from ischemia. It is a common complicating disorder of Legg-Calvé-Perthes disease, sickle cell disease, corticosteroid therapy, and hip surgery.[35,36]

Bone has a rich blood supply that varies from site to site. The flow in the medullary portion of bone originates in nutrient vessels from an interconnecting plexus that supplies the marrow, trabecular bone, and endosteal half of the cortex. The outer cortex receives its blood supply from periosteal, muscular, metaphyseal, and epiphyseal vessels that surround the bone. Some bony sites, such as the head of the femur, have only limited collateral circulation so that interruption of the flow, such as with a hip fracture, can cause necrosis and irreversible damage to a substantial portion of medullary and cortical bone.

Although bone necrosis results from ischemia, the mechanisms producing the ischemia are varied and include mechanical vascular interruption such as occurs with a fracture; thrombosis and embolism (*e.g.*, sickle cell disease, nitrogen bubbles caused by inadequate decompression during deep sea diving); vessel injury (*e.g.*, vasculitis, radiation therapy); and increased intraosseous pressure with vascular compression. In many cases, the cause of the necrosis is uncertain. Other than fracture, the most common causes of bone necrosis are idiopathic (*i.e.*, those of unknown cause) and prior steroid therapy. Chart 42-2 lists disorders associated with osteonecrosis.

One of the most common causes of osteonecrosis is that associated with administration of corticosteroids.[35,36] Despite numerous studies, the mechanism of steroid-induced osteonecrosis remains unclear. The condition may develop after the administration of very high, short-term doses, during long-term treatment, or even from intra-articular injection. Although the risk increases with the dose and duration of treatment, it is difficult to predict who will be affected. The interval between corticosteroid administration and onset of symptoms rarely is less than 6 months and may be more than 3 years. There is no satisfactory method for preventing progression of the disease.

The pathologic features of bone necrosis are the same, regardless of cause. The site of the lesion is related to the vessels involved. There is necrosis of cancellous bone and marrow. The cortex usually is not involved because of collateral blood flow. In persons with subchondral infarcts (*i.e.*, ischemia below the cartilage), a triangular or wedge-shaped segment of tissue that has the subchondral bone plate as its base and the center of the epiphysis as its apex undergoes necrosis. In cases where medullary infarcts occur in fatty marrow, death of bone results in calcium release and necrosis of fat cells with the formation of free

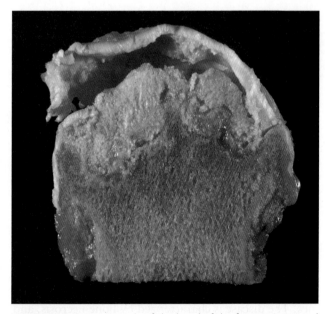

FIGURE 42-9 Osteonecrosis of the head of the femur. A coronal section shows a circumscribed area of subchondral infarction with partial detachment of the overlying articular cartilage and subarticular bone. (From Schiller A. L., Wang B. Y., Klein M. J. [2005]. Bones and joints. In Rubin E., Gorstein F., Rubin R., et al. [Eds.], *Rubin's pathology: Clinicopathologic foundations of medicine* [4th ed., p. 1326]. Philadelphia: Lippincott Williams & Wilkins.)

CHART 42-2

Causes of Osteonecrosis

Mechanical disruption of blood vessels
    Fractures
    Legg-Calvé-Perthes disease
    Blount disease
Thrombosis and embolism
    Sickle cell disease
    Nitrogen bubbles in decompression sickness
Vessel injury
    Vasculitis
    Connective tissue disease
        Systemic lupus erythematosus
        Rheumatoid arthritis
    Radiation therapy
Increased intraosseous pressure
Steroid-induced osteonecrosis

fatty acids. Released calcium forms an insoluble "soap" with free fatty acids. Because bone lacks mechanisms for resolving the infarct, the lesions remain for life.

The symptoms associated with osteonecrosis are varied and depend on the extent of infarction. Typically, subchondral infarcts cause chronic pain that is initially associated with activity but that gradually becomes more progressive until it is experienced at rest. Subchondral infarcts often collapse and predispose the patient to severe secondary osteoarthritis.

Diagnosis of osteonecrosis is based on history, physical findings, radiographic findings, and the results of special imaging studies, including CT scans and technetium-99m bone scans. MRI is particularly effective in the diagnosis of osteonecrosis. Plain radiographs are used to define and classify the course of the disease, particularly of the hip.

Treatment of osteonecrosis depends on the underlying pathologic process. In some cases, only short-term immobilization, nonsteroidal anti-inflammatory drugs, exercises, and limitation in weight bearing are used. Osteonecrosis of the hip is particularly difficult to treat. In persons with early disease, limitation of weight bearing through the use of crutches may allow the condition to stabilize. Although several surgical approaches have been used, the most definitive treatment of advanced osteonecrosis of the knee or hip is total joint replacement.

In summary, bone infections occur because of the direct or indirect invasion of the skeletal circulation by microorganisms, most commonly *S. aureus*. Osteomyelitis, or infection of the bone and marrow, can be an acute or chronic disease. Acute osteomyelitis is seen most often as a result of the direct contamination of bone by a foreign object. Chronic osteomyelitis is a long-term process that can recur spontaneously at any time throughout a person's life. Tuberculosis of the bone, which is characterized by bone destruction and abscess formation, is caused by spread of the infection from the lungs or lymph nodes.

Osteonecrosis, or death of a segment of bone, is a condition caused by the interruption of blood supply to the marrow, medullary bone, or cortex. Sites with poor collateral circulation, such as the femoral head, are most seriously affected. It is a common complicating disorder of Legg-Calvé-Perthes disease, sickle cell disease, corticosteroid therapy, and hip surgery. Symptoms include pain that varies in severity, depending on the extent of infarction. Total joint replacement is the most frequently used treatment for advanced osteonecrosis.

 Neoplasms

Neoplasms of the skeletal system, often referred to as bone tumors, can present as a primary or secondary lesion. Primary bone tumors may arise from any of the skeletal components, including osseous tissue, cartilage, and bone marrow. Primary malignant tumors are relatively rare, constituting approximately 1% of all adult cancers and 15% of pediatric malignancies.[37] Bone, however, is a common site for cancer metastasis.

Like other types of neoplasms, bone tumors may be benign or malignant. Benign tumors, such as osteochondromas, tend to grow rather slowly and usually do not destroy the supporting or surrounding tissue or spread to other parts of the body. Malignant tumors, such as osteosarcoma, grow rapidly and can spread to other parts of the body through the bloodstream or lymphatics.

There are three major symptoms of bone tumors: pain, presence of a mass, and impairment of function. Pain is a feature common to almost all malignant tumors but may or may not occur with benign tumors. For example, a benign tumor often is asymptomatic until a fracture occurs. Pain that persists at night and is not relieved by rest suggests malignancy. A mass or hard lump may be the first sign of a bone tumor. A malignant tumor is suspected when a painful mass exists that is enlarging or eroding the cortex of the bone. The ease of discovery of a mass depends on the location of the tumor; a small lump arising on the surface of the tibia is easy to detect, whereas a tumor that is deep in the medial portion of the femur may grow to a considerable size before it is noticed. Benign and malignant tumors may cause the bone to erode to the point where it cannot withstand the strain of ordinary use. In such cases, even a small amount of bone stress or trauma precipitates a pathologic fracture. A tumor may produce pressure on a peripheral nerve, causing decreased sensation, numbness, a limp, or limitation of movement.

BENIGN BONE TUMORS

Benign bone tumors usually are limited to the confines of the bone, have well-demarcated edges, and are surrounded by a thin rim of sclerotic bone. The most common types of benign bone tumors are osteoma, chondroma, osteochondroma, and giant cell tumor.

 KEY CONCEPTS

Bone Neoplasms

➤ Neoplasms of the skeletal system can affect bone tissue, cartilage, or bone marrow.

➤ Benign tumors tend to grow slowly, do not spread to other parts of the body, and exert their effects through the space-occupying nature of the tumor and their ability to weaken bone structures.

➤ Malignant bone tumors are rare before 10 years of age, have their peak incidence in the teenage years, tend to grow rapidly, and extend beyond the confines of the bone.

An *osteoma* is a small bony tumor found on the surface of a long bone, flat bone, or the skull. It usually is composed of hard, compact (ivory osteoma), or spongy (cancellous) bone. Pain, typically nocturnal, is proportional to the size of the lesion. It is usually relieved by aspirin, probably because of the high prostaglandin content of the tumor.[17] Surgical excision or electrocautery is usually curative.

A *chondroma* is a tumor composed of hyaline cartilage.[17] It may arise on the surface of the bone (*i.e.*, ecchondroma) or within the medullary cavity (*i.e.*, endochondroma). These tumors may become large and are especially common in the hands and feet. A chondroma may persist for many years and then take on the attributes of a malignant chondrosarcoma. A chondroma usually is not treated unless it becomes unsightly or uncomfortable.

An *osteochondroma*, also known as *exostosis*, is a benign cartilage-capped outgrowth that is attached to underlying bone by a bony stalk. It is the most common form of benign tumor in the skeletal system, representing 20% of all benign bone tumors, and is seen most frequently in adolescents 10 to 20 years of age.[17] It grows only during periods of skeletal growth, originating in the epiphyseal cartilage plate and growing out of the bone like a mushroom. An osteochondroma is composed of cartilage and bone and usually occurs singly, but may affect several bones in a condition called *multiple exostoses*. Malignant changes are rare, and excision of the tumor is done only when necessary.

A *giant cell tumor,* or *osteoclastoma,* is an aggressive tumor of multinucleated cells that often behaves like a malignant tumor, metastasizing through the bloodstream and recurring locally after excision. It occurs most often in young adults, predominantly women, and is found most commonly in the knee, wrist, or shoulder.[17] The tumor begins in the metaphyseal region, grows into the epiphysis, and may extend into the joint surface. Pathologic fractures are common because the tumor destroys the bone substance. Clinically, pain may occur at the tumor site, with gradually increasing swelling. X-ray films show destruction of the bone with expansion of the cortex. The treatment of giant cell tumors depends on their location. If the affected bone can be eliminated without loss of function, such as the clavicle or fibula, the entire bone or part of it may be removed. When the tumor is near a major joint, such as the knee or shoulder, a local excision is done. Irradiation may be used to prevent recurrence of the tumor.

MALIGNANT BONE TUMORS

Primary malignant tumors of the skeletal system include osteosarcoma, Ewing sarcoma, and chondrosarcoma. In contrast to benign tumors, primary malignant tumors tend to be ill defined, lack sharp borders, and extend beyond the confines of the bone. As a group, primary bone tumors occur in all age groups and may arise in any part of the body. However, certain types of tumors tend to target certain age groups and anatomic sites. For example, osteosarcoma and Ewing sarcoma are the two major forms of bone cancer in children and young adults,[38] whereas chondrosarcoma is most common in those between 20 and 50 years of age.[17]

Osteosarcoma

Osteosarcoma is an aggressive and highly malignant bone tumor. It is the most common primary malignant bone tumor, representing one fifth of all bone tumors. Osteosarcoma is the most common bone tumor in children and the third most common cancer in children and adolescents.[38,39] Although they can develop in any bone, osteosarcomas most commonly arise in the vicinity of the knee (*e.g.*, lower femur or upper tibia or fibula). The proximal humerus is the second most common site. Involvement of the hands, feet, skull, and jaw is less frequent and is usually seen in persons older than 25 years of age.[17]

The cause of osteosarcoma is unknown. The tumor has a bimodal distribution, with 75% occurring in persons younger than 20 years of age. A second peak occurs in the elderly with predisposing factors such as Paget disease, bone infarcts, or prior irradiation.[18] The correlation of age and location of most of the tumors with the period of maximum growth suggests some relation to increased osteoblastic activity. In younger persons, the primary tumor most often is located at the anatomic sites associated with maximum growth velocity—the distal femur, proximal tibia, and proximal humerus. Bone tumors in the elderly are more common in the humerus, pelvis, and proximal femur. Paget disease, which is linked to osteosarcoma in adults, also is associated with increased osteoblastic activity. Irradiation from an internal source, such as the radioactive pharmaceutical technetium used in bone scans, or an external source, such as radiography, also has been associated with osteosarcoma. Two genes are reported to increase the susceptibility to the development of osteosarcoma: the retinoblastoma gene (RB) and the p53 gene[38,40,41] (see Chapter 5).

Osteosarcomas are aggressive tumors that grow rapidly; they often are eccentrically placed in the bone and move from the metaphysis of the bone out into the periosteal surface, with subsequent spread to adjacent soft tissues (Fig. 42-10). The tumor infrequently metastasizes to the lymph nodes because the cells are unable to grow in the node. Nodal metastases usually occur only in the late course of disseminated disease. Most often, the tumor cells exit the primary tumor through the venous end of the capillary, and early metastasis to the lung is common. The prognosis for a person with osteosarcoma depends on the aggressiveness of the disease, radiologic features, presence or absence of pathologic fractures, size of the tumor, and rapidity of tumor growth.

The primary symptom of osteosarcoma is deep localized pain with nighttime awakening and swelling in the affected bone. Because the pain is often of sudden onset, patients and their families often associate the symptoms with recent trauma.[38,40] The skin overlying the tumor may be warm, shiny, and stretched, with prominent superficial veins. The range of motion of the adjacent joint may be restricted.

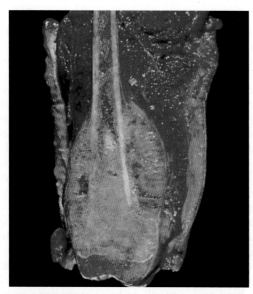

FIGURE 42-10 Osteosarcoma. The distal femur contains dense osteoblastic malignant tumor that extends through the cortex into the soft tissue and epiphysis. (From Schiller A. L., Wang B. Y., Klein M. J. [2005]. Bones and joints. In Rubin E., Gorstein F., Rubin R., et al. [Eds.], *Rubin's pathology: Clinicopathologic foundations of medicine* [4th ed., p. 1355]. Philadelphia: Lippincott Williams & Wilkins.)

History, physical examination, and radiographic studies are all part of the evaluation of a patient with osteosarcoma. Plain films of the primary site and of the chest are obtained first. An MRI, CT scan, and full-body scan are required to evaluate the extent of the local disease and to determine the extent of metastasis, if present. Radionuclide bone scans are done to evaluate for lung and bone metastasis.[38–40] An open biopsy is required to confirm the diagnosis and determine the histologic features and cell type of the tumor.

The treatment for osteosarcoma is surgery in combination with multiagent chemotherapy both before and after surgery.[38,39] In the past, treatment usually entailed amputation above the level of the tumor. Limb salvage surgical procedures, using a metal prosthesis or cadaver allograft, are becoming a standard alternative. In younger children who undergo arthroplasty, an expandable internal prosthesis is used to allow for bone growth. Chemotherapy using various drug combinations is the most effective treatment for metastatic osteosarcoma.

The primary objective of treatment of patients with osteosarcoma is to achieve long-term disease-free survival or cure. Preserving limb function is a secondary objective. In cases in which adequate limb salvage surgery cannot be achieved, limb amputation may be necessary.[38,39]

Ewing Sarcoma

Ewing sarcoma is a member of a group of small, round cell, undifferentiated tumors thought to be of neural crest origin[38] (see Chapter 33). The family of tumors includes Ewing sarcoma of the bone and soft tissue and peripheral primitive neuroectodermal tumor (PPNET).[17] Of the tumors in this family, Ewing sarcoma accounts for most cases. It is the second most common type of primary bone tumor in children and adolescents. It can occur at any age, but is seen most commonly in early teenage years. This tumor rarely presents in black or Asian children.[38]

The most frequent site for Ewing sarcoma is the femur, usually in the diaphysis. The pelvis represents the second most common site; other sites include the pubis, sacrum, humerus, vertebrae, ribs, skull, and other flat bones. The characteristic pathologic findings of Ewing sarcoma include densely packed, regularly shaped small cells with round or oval nuclei. The majority of cells have a characteristic reciprocal translocation of chromosomes 11 and 22.

Manifestations of Ewing sarcoma include pain, limitation of movement, and tenderness over the involved bone or soft tissue.[38] It often is accompanied by systemic manifestations such as fever or weight loss, which may serve to confuse the diagnosis. There may be a delay in diagnosis when the pain and swelling associated with the tumor are attributed to a sports injury. Pathologic fractures are common because of bone destruction. The most common sites of metastasis are the lungs, bone marrow, and other bones.

Because Ewing sarcoma is a difficult diagnosis to establish, the diagnostic biopsy is very important. Clinical evaluations include MRI and CT scans of the primary tumor, chest x-rays, CT of the chest, bone scan, bilateral bone marrow aspiration, and biopsy of the primary tumor site.[38] Treatment methods incorporate a combination of multiagent chemotherapy, surgery, and radiation therapy. Multiagent chemotherapy is important because it can shrink the tumor and is generally given before local control measures are initiated. Ewing sarcoma is considered to be a radiosensitive tumor and local control may be achieved through radiation or surgery. Persons with small, nonmetastatic, distally located tumors generally have the best prognosis, with up to a 75% cure rate.[38]

Chondrosarcoma

Chondrosarcoma, a malignant tumor of cartilage that can develop in the medullary cavity or peripherally, is the second most common form of malignant bone tumor. It occurs primarily in middle or later life and slightly more often in men. The tumor arises from points of muscle attachment to bone, particularly the knee, shoulder, hip, and pelvis. Chondrosarcomas can arise from underlying benign lesions such as osteochondroma, chondroblastoma, or fibrous dysplasia.[17,18]

Chondrosarcomas are slow growing, metastasize late, and often are painless. They can remain hidden in an area such as the pelvis for a long time. This type of tumor, like many primary malignancies, tends to destroy bone and extend into the soft tissues beyond the confines of the bone of origin. Chondrosarcomas mainly affect the bones of the trunk, pelvis, or proximal femur and rarely develop in the distal portion of a bone. Irregular flecks and ringlets of calcification often are prominent radiographic findings.

Early diagnosis is important because chondrosarcoma responds well to early radical surgical excision. It usually is resistant to radiation therapy and available chemotherapeutic agents. Not infrequently, these tumors transform into a highly malignant tumor, mesenchymal chondrosarcoma, which requires a more aggressive treatment, including combination chemotherapy.

METASTATIC BONE DISEASE

Skeletal metastases are the most common malignancy of osseous tissue.[17,42] Approximately half of all people with cancer have bone metastasis at some point in their disease.[43] Metastatic lesions are seen most often in the spine, femur, pelvis, ribs, sternum, proximal humerus, and skull, and are less common in anatomic sites that are further removed from the trunk of the body. Tumors that frequently spread to the skeletal system are those of the breast, lung, prostate, kidney, and thyroid, although any cancer can ultimately involve the skeleton. More than 85% of bone metastases result from primary lesions in the breast, lung, or prostate.[42] The incidence of metastatic bone disease is highest in persons older than 40 years of age.

The major symptom of bone metastasis is pain with evidence of an impending pathologic fracture. It usually develops gradually, over weeks, and is more severe at night. Pain is caused by stretching of the periosteum of the involved bone or by nerve entrapment, as in the nerve roots of the spinal cord by the vertebral body. Pathologic fractures occur in approximately 10% to 15% of persons with metastatic bone disease. The affected bone appears to be eaten away on x-ray images and, in severe cases, crumbles on impact, much like dried toast. Many pathologic fractures occur in the femur, humerus, and vertebrae.[39]

Radiographic examinations are used along with CT or bone scans to detect, diagnose, and localize metastatic bone lesions. Approximately one third of persons with skeletal metastases have positive bone scans without radiologic findings. This is because 50% of the trabecular bone must be destroyed before a lesion is visible on plain radiographs.[39] Arteriography using radiopaque contrast media may be helpful in outlining the tumor margins. A bone biopsy usually is done when there is a question regarding the diagnosis or treatment. A closed-needle biopsy with CT localization is particularly useful with spine lesions. Serum levels of alkaline phosphatase and calcium often are elevated in persons with metastatic bone disease.

The primary goals in treatment of metastatic bone disease are to prevent pathologic fractures and promote survival with maximum functioning, allowing the person to maintain as much mobility and pain control as possible. Standard treatment methods include chemotherapy, irradiation, and surgical stabilization. Radiation therapy is primarily used as a palliative treatment to alleviate pain and prevent pathologic fractures. After a pathologic fracture has occurred, bracing, intramedullary nailing of the femur, or spine stabilization may be done. Because adequate fixation often is difficult in diseased bone, cement (*i.e.*, methylmethacrylate) often is used with internal fixation devices to stabilize the bone.

Recent research has focused on the role of osteoclastic and osteoblastic activity in the pathogenesis of metastatic bone disease and on the use of the bisphosphonates (*e.g.*, pamidronate disodium, zoledronic acid) for its treatment.[43,44] Bone tissue contains a rich environment of growth factors and cells of various embryonic origins, including hematopoietic, stromal, endothelial, and other cell types. The osteoclasts and osteoblasts, in particular, appear to play a dominant role in the pathogenesis of bone metastasis. Osteoclasts are involved in osteolytic or destructive bone lesions and osteoblasts in the excessive production of new and poor-quality bone. The bisphosphonates, which are now well-established agents for the prevention and treatment of osteoporosis, have recently been shown to decrease symptoms associated with bone metastasis secondary to breast and prostate cancer. These agents bind preferentially to bone at sites of active bone metabolism, are released from the bone matrix during bone resorption, and potentially inhibit osteoclast activity and survival, thereby reducing osteoclast-mediated bone resorption. Recent studies suggest that besides their strong antiosteoclastic activity, these agents may have some direct antitumor effects.[44]

In summary, bone tumors, like any other type of neoplasm, may be benign or malignant. Benign bone tumors grow slowly and usually do not destroy the surrounding tissues. Malignant tumors can be primary or metastatic. Primary bone tumors are rare, grow rapidly, metastasize to the lungs and other parts of the body through the bloodstream, and are associated with a high mortality rate. Metastatic bone tumors usually are multiple, originating primarily from cancers of the breast, lung, and prostate. The incidence of metastatic bone disease is increasing, probably because improved treatment methods enable persons with cancer to live longer. Advances in chemotherapy, radiation therapy, and surgical procedures have substantially increased the survival and cure rates for many types of bone cancers. The bisphosphonate drugs, which directly target the osteolytic action of osteoclasts, are also used in the treatment of metastatic bone disease.

Skeletal Disorders in Children

During childhood, skeletal structures grow in length and diameter and sustain a large increase in bone mass. Alterations in musculoskeletal structure and function may develop as a result of normal growth and developmental processes or as a result of impairment of skeletal development caused by hereditary or congenital influences.

VARIATIONS OF NORMAL GROWTH AND DEVELOPMENT

Infants and children undergo changes in muscle tone and joint motion during growth and development. Intoeing, outtoeing, genu varum (bowlegs), and genu valgum (knock-knees) occur frequently in infancy and childhood.[45,46] These changes usually cause few problems and are corrected during normal growth processes. The normal folded position of the fetus in utero causes physiologic flexion contractures of the hips and a froglike appearance of the lower extremities (Fig. 42-11). The hips are externally rotated, and the patellae point outward, whereas the feet appear to point forward because of the internal pulling force of the tibiae. During the first year of life, the lower extremities begin to straighten out in preparation for walking. Internal and external rotations become equal, and the hips extend. Flexion contractures of the shoulders, elbows, and knees also are commonly seen in newborns, but they should disappear by 4 to 6 months of age.[47]

Musculoskeletal assessment of the newborn is important to identify abnormalities that require early intervention, facilitate treatment, establish baselines for future reference, and educate and counsel parents. There are many clinical deviations that are easily correctable in a newborn. Many others correct spontaneously as the child grows.

Torsional Deformities

All infants and toddlers have lax ligaments that become tighter with age and assumption of the weight-bearing posture. The hypermobility that accompanies joint laxity coupled with the torsional, or twisting, forces exerted

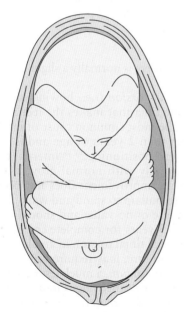

FIGURE 42-11 Position of fetus in utero, with tibial bowing and legs folded. (From Dunne K. B., Clarren S. K. [1986]. The origin of prenatal and postnatal deformities. *Pediatric Clinics of North America* 33[6], 1282, with permission from Elsevier Science.)

KEY CONCEPTS

Developmental Skeletal Disorders

➤ Many disorders of early infancy are caused by intrauterine positions and resolve as the child grows.

➤ Infants and toddlers have lax ligaments that predispose to skeletal disorders caused by twisting or torsional forces.

➤ Bone growth in infants and children occurs at the epiphysis. Injury to the epiphyseal growth plate ruptures the blood vessels that nourish the epiphysis, causing cessation of growth and shortened extremity length.

on the limbs during growth are responsible for a number of variants seen in young children. Torsional forces caused by intrauterine positions or sleeping and sitting patterns twist the growing bones and can produce deformities as a child grows and develops.

In infants, the femur normally is rotated to an anteverted position with the femoral head and neck rotated anteriorly with respect to the femoral condyles. Femoral anteversion (*i.e.*, medial rotation) decreases from an average 40 degrees at birth to approximately 15 degrees at maturity. The normal tibia is externally rotated approximately 5 degrees at birth and 15 degrees at maturity. Torsional abnormalities frequently demonstrate a familial tendency.

Intoeing and Outtoeing. The foot progression angle describes the angle between the axis of the foot and the line of progression.[5,45–47] It is determined by watching the child walking and running, although it is usually less noticeable when the child is running or barefoot. Figure 42-12 illustrates the position of the foot in intoeing and outtoeing.

Intoeing means that the foot turns in more than expected during walking or running activities. Intoeing may be

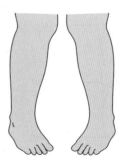
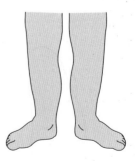

Intoeing   Outtoeing

FIGURE 42-12 The position of feet in intoeing and outtoeing.

secondary to foot deformities or may be due to inward rotation of the femur or tibia, or a combination of the two. Increased internal torsion of the femur (femoral anteversion) is the most common finding. In many cases intoeing is a variation of normal development.

Intoeing due to a condition called *metatarsus adductus* is a common congenital deformity characterized by adduction of the forefoot with a normal hindfoot, giving the foot a kidney-shaped appearance[45–47] (Fig. 42-13). It may occur in one foot or both feet. Diagnostic methods include examination of the plantar aspect of the foot, noting the overall shape of the foot and the presence or absence of an arch. The severity of the deformity can be determined by assessing the flexibility of the foot and using a heel bisection line.[5] Normally, a line bisecting the heel crosses the forefoot between the second and third toes. In mild metatarsus adductus, the foot is flexible and can be passively manipulated and the line crosses the third toe; in a moderate deformity, the foot is less flexible and the line falls between the third and fourth toes; and in a severe deformity, the foot is more rigid and the line crosses between the fourth and fifth toes. Most infants are not treated, although parents are advised to avoid positioning the infant in the prone position with the feet turned in, a position that accentuates metatarsus adductus. Because the condition often corrects itself spontaneously, treatment is usually not instituted until the infant is 6 months of age.[5] When needed, treatment consists of serial long leg casting or a brace that pushes the metatarsals (not the hindfoot) into abduction.

Outtoeing is a common problem in children and is caused by external femoral torsion. This occurs when the femur can be externally rotated to approximately 90 degrees but internally rotated only to a neutral position or slightly beyond. Because the femoral torsion persists when a child habitually sleeps in the prone position, an external tibial torsion also may develop. If external tibial torsion is present, the feet point lateral to the midline of the medial plane. External tibial torsion rarely causes outtoeing; it only intensifies the condition. Outtoeing usually corrects itself as the child becomes proficient in walking. Occasionally, a night splint is used.

Tibial Torsion. *Tibial torsion* refers to an abnormal internal or external angulation of the tibia. It is determined by measuring the thigh-foot angle. When the child is in the

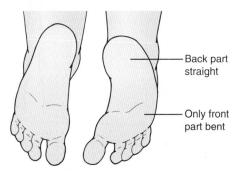

FIGURE 42-13 Shape of foot in metatarsus adductus. The left foot is normal, whereas the right foot has metatarsus adductus.

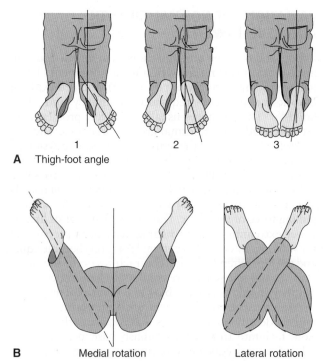

A Thigh-foot angle

B   Medial rotation   Lateral rotation

FIGURE 42-14 (**A**) Assessment for tibial torsion using thigh-foot angle. When the child is in the prone position with the knee flexed, with normal alignment there is slight external rotation (2); internal tibial torsion produces inward rotation (3), and external tibial torsion; outward rotation (1). (**B**) Hip rotation is measured with the child prone and knees flexed at a 90-degree angle. On outward rotation the leg produces internal (medial) hip and femoral rotation; on inward rotation the leg produces external (lateral) hip and femoral rotation. (Adapted from Staheli L. T. [1986]. Torsional deformity. *Pediatric Clinics of North America* 33[6], 1378, and Kliegman R. M., Neider M. I., Super D. M. [Eds.]. [1996]. *Practical strategies in pediatric diagnosis and therapy*. Philadelphia: W. B. Saunders.)

prone position, there is normally a slight external rotation (Fig. 42-14A).

Internal tibial torsion (*i.e.*, bowing of the tibia) is a rotation of the tibia that makes the feet appear to turn inward. It is the most common cause of intoeing in children younger than 2 years of age and is secondary to normal in utero positioning.[47,48] Internal tibial torsion improves naturally with normal growth and development, although improvement does not occur until the child begins to pull up to stand and walk independently. Night splints are of no value and should be avoided. It may take 1 to 3 years for complete correction to occur. Persistent internal tibial torsion in an older child or adolescent, although rare, may require surgical derotation.

External tibial torsion, a much less common disorder, is associated with calcaneovalgus foot and is caused by a normal variation of intrauterine positioning or a neuromuscular disorder. It is characterized by an abnormally positive thigh-foot angle of 30 to 50 degrees.[47] The condition corrects itself naturally, and treatment is observational. Significant improvement begins during the first year with the onset of ambulation and usually is complete by 2 to 3 years of age.

Femoral Torsion. *Femoral torsion* refers to abnormal angulation of the femur with abnormal hip rotation. Hip rotation is measured at the pelvic level with the child in the prone position and the knees flexed at a 90-degree angle. In this position, the hip is in a neutral position. Rotating the lower leg outward produces internal or medial femoral rotation; rotating it inward produces external or lateral rotation (see Fig. 42-14B). During measurement of hip rotation, the legs are allowed to fall to full internal rotation by gravity alone; lateral rotation is measured by allowing the legs to fall inward and cross. By 1 year of age, there is normally approximately 45 degrees of internal and 45 degrees of external rotation.[47] Hip rotation in flexion and extension also can be measured with CT scans.

Internal femoral torsion, also called *femoral anteversion*, is a normal variant commonly seen during the first 6 years of life, especially in 3- and 4-year-old girls.[47] The condition is thought to be related to increased laxity of the anterior capsule of the hip such that it does not provide the stable pressure needed to correct the anteversion that is present at birth. Children are most comfortable sitting in the "W" position with their hips between their knees (Fig. 42-15). It is believed that this position allows the lower leg to act as a lever, producing torsional changes in the femur. When the child stands, the knees turn in and the feet appear to point straight ahead, and when the child walks, the knees and toes point in. The treatment of internal femoral torsion is predominantly by observation. Children with this problem are encouraged to sit cross-legged or in the so-called *tailor position*. This sitting position usually allows the torsion to resolve with normal growth and development. Children 10 years of age or older may not have sufficient remaining musculoskeletal growth for correction to occur, and surgical intervention may be necessary.[47] The use of nighttime splints and daytime twister cables is not recommended and may produce external tibial torsion. The combination of internal tibial torsion and a compensatory external tibial torsion produces a pathologic genu valgum deformity, which can result in patellofemoral malalignment with patellar subluxation or dislocation and pain.[47]

External femoral torsion is an uncommon disorder unless associated with slipped capital femoral epiphysis (to be discussed). When idiopathic, it is usually bilateral. Because it produces no significant functional impairment, treatment is usually observational.

Genu Varum and Genu Valgum

Genu varum or bowlegs is an outward bowing of the knees greater than 1 inch when the medial malleoli of the ankles are touching (Fig. 42-16). Most infants and toddlers have some bowing of their legs up to age 18 months.[48] If there is a large separation between the knees (>15 degrees) after 2 years of age, the child may require bracing.

Genu valgum or *knock-knees* is a deformity in which there is decreased space between the knees (see Fig. 42-16). The medial malleoli in the ankles cannot be brought in

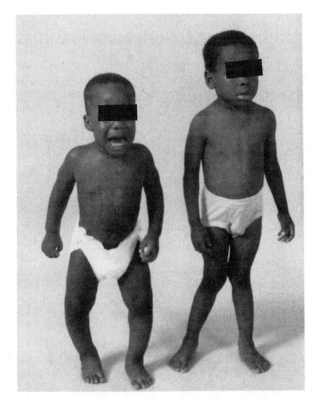

FIGURE 42-16 Normal genu varum (bowlegs) in a toddler (*left*) and genu valgum (knock-knees) in a toddler (*right*), which is often seen in children between 2 and 6 years of age. (From Weinstein S. L., Buckwalter J. A. [1994]. *Turek's orthopaedics* [5th ed.]. Philadelphia: J. B. Lippincott.)

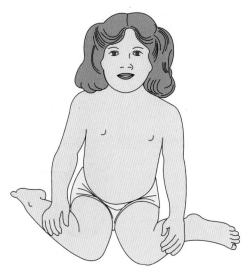

FIGURE 42-15 Typical sitting position of child with femoral anteversion. (Adapted from Staheli L. T. [1986]. Torsional deformities. *Pediatric Clinics of North America* 33[6], 1382, with permission from Elsevier Science.)

contact with each other when the knees are touching. It is seen most frequently in children between the ages of 3 and 5 years and should resolve by 5 to 8 years of age.[47] The condition usually is the result of lax medial collateral ligaments of the knee and may be exacerbated by sitting in the "M" position. Genu valgum can be ignored to age 7 years, unless it is more than 15 degrees, unilateral, or associated with short stature. It usually resolves spontaneously and rarely requires treatment.

If genu varum or genu valgum persists and is uncorrected, osteoarthritis may develop in adulthood as a result of abnormal intra-articular stress. Genu varum can cause gait awkwardness and increased risk of sprains and fractures. Uncorrected genu valgum may cause subluxation and recurrent dislocation of the patella, with a predisposition to chondromalacia and joint pain and fatigue.

Idiopathic tibia vara, or *Blount disease*, is a developmental deformity of the medial half of the proximal tibial epiphysis that results in a progressive varus angulation below the knee (Fig. 42-17). It is the most common cause of pathologic genu varum and seen most often in black children, girls, obese children, and early walkers.[49] Onset can occur early in infancy or later, during adolescence. Adolescent Blount disease occurs in the second decade of life, is seen in persons who are above the 95th percentile in height and weight, and is usually unilateral.[49] Long leg braces are used for treatment in early-onset disease. If progression occurs, or onset is late, surgery is done to correct the angulation and prevent further progression.

HEREDITARY AND CONGENITAL DEFORMITIES

Congenital deformities are abnormalities that are present at birth. Congenital deformities are caused by many factors, some unknown. These factors include genetic influences, external agents that injure the fetus (*e.g.*, radiation, alcohol, drugs, viruses), and intrauterine environmental factors. They range in severity from mild limb deformities, which are relatively common, to major limb malformations, which are relatively rare. There may be a simple webbing of the fingers or toes (syndactyly), the presence of an extra digit (*i.e.*, polydactyly), or the absence of a bone such as the phalanx, rib, or clavicle. Joint contractures and dislocations produce more severe deformity, as does the absence of entire bones, joints, or limbs.

Congenital Deformities of the Foot

Deformities of the foot are usually described according to the shape and position of the ankle and foot (Fig. 42-18). The term *talipes* refers to a deformity of the ankle and foot (Latin *talus*, "ankle," + *pes*, "foot"); additional terms include *equinus* (resembling a horse—i.e., a horse's hoof); *calcaneus* (pertaining to the heel); and *tarsus* (pertaining to the tarsal bones of the instep). Talipes varus refers to inversion or bending inward of the foot as it relates to the heel; talipes valgus, eversion or bending outward; talipes equinus, plantar flexion so the toes are lower than the heel; and talipes calcaneus, dorsiflexion, in which the toes are higher than the heel.

Talipes Equinovarus. Congenital clubfoot, or talipes equinovarus, is a congenital deformity of the foot that can affect one or both feet.[50,51] The condition has an incidence of 1 to 2 per 1000 live births and occurs twice

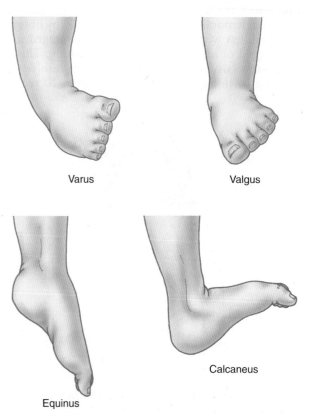

Varus   Valgus

Equinus   Calcaneus

FIGURE 42-18 Positions of the foot in varus, valgus, equinus, and calcaneus deformities.

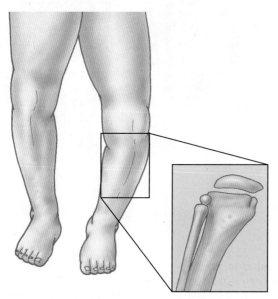

FIGURE 42-17 Rotational deformity of the proximal tibia, especially when unilateral, suggests tibia vera (Blount disease).

as often in boys as in girls.[51] Although there are many theories about the causes of clubfoot, none has been proven. It is most commonly idiopathic and found in healthy infants in whom no genetic or chromosomal abnormality or other extrinsic cause can be found. However, if a parent or sibling has clubfoot, the risk is increased. Neuromuscular clubfoot is secondary to disorders such as myelomeningocele. Maternal smoking is associated with occurrence of clubfoot, and the risk increases enormously when combined with a family history.[52]

The foot deformity in equinovarus consists of three major components: plantar flexion (equinus) of the ankle and forefoot, varus (twisted inward) of the heel, and adduction (turned toward the midline of the body) of the forefoot (see Fig. 42-18). The medial portion of the foot is concave and the lateral portion, convex. Infants with the disorder typically appear as if they could walk on the top or dorsolateral aspect of the foot.

Diagnosis is based on physical examination. Radiographs are usually necessary to confirm the diagnosis. A true idiopathic clubfoot cannot be corrected by manipulation; therefore, a foot that can be placed in normal position by manipulation is talipes equinovarus caused by intrauterine positioning rather than true clubfoot. Treatment is begun as soon as the diagnosis is made and usually is effective within a short period. Serial manipulations and casting are used to gently correct each component in the forefoot varus, the hindfoot varus, and the equinus. The casts initially are changed at semiweekly to weekly intervals and are continued until the deformity responds and is corrected fully. Surgery may be required for severe deformities or when nonoperative treatment methods are unsuccessful.

Talipes Calcaneovalgus. Talipes calcaneovalgus, in which the foot is dorsiflexed with the heel (calcaneus) down and the foot bent or twisted outward (valgus), is the most common neonatal foot disorder.[47] It is usually associated with external tibial torsion. It is often unilateral but occasionally may be bilateral. The condition occurs as the result of in utero positioning in which the plantar surface of the foot is against the wall of the uterus, forcing it into a hyperdorsiflexed position. The position also produces the external tibial torsion.

The typical calcaneovalgus foot usually requires no treatment and resolves during the first 6 months of life. However, the external tibial torsion persists. Spontaneous improvement does not occur until the child begins to pull up to stand and walk independently. It then takes about 6 to 12 months for complete correction to occur.

Developmental Dysplasia of the Hip

Developmental dysplasia of the hip, formerly known as *congenital dislocation of the hip*, is an abnormality in hip development that leads to a wide spectrum of hip problems in infants and children, including hips that are unstable, malformed, subluxated, or dislocated.[47,53–55] In less severe cases, the hip joint may be unstable, with excessive laxity of the joint capsule, or subluxated, so that the joint surfaces are separated and there is a partial dislocation (Fig. 42-19). With dislocated hips, the head of the femur is located outside of the acetabulum.

The results of newborn screening programs have shown that 1 of 100 infants have some evidence of hip instability; however, dislocation of the hip is seen in 1.5 of every 1000 live births.[53] The left hip is involved three times more frequently than the right hip because of the left occipital intrauterine positioning of most infants. In white infants, developmental dysplasia of the hips occurs most frequently in first-born children and is six times more common in female than in male infants. The cause of developmental dysplasia of the hip is multifactorial, with physiologic, mechanical, and postural factors playing a role. A positive family history and generalized laxity of the ligaments are related. The increased frequency in girls is thought to result from their susceptibility to maternal estrogens and other hormones associated with pelvic relaxation. Dislocation also may result from environmental factors such as fetal position, a tight uterus that prevents fetal movement, and breech delivery.

Early diagnosis of a developmental dysplasia of the hip is important because treatment is easiest and most effective if begun during the first 6 months of life. Repeated dislocation causes damage to the femoral head and the acetabulum. Clinical examinations to detect dislocation of the hip should be done at birth and every several months during the first year of life.[54,55] In infants, signs of dislocation include asymmetry of the hip or

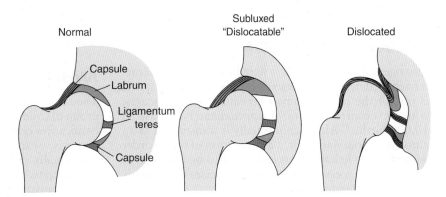

Normal   Subluxed "Dislocatable"   Dislocated

Capsule
Labrum
Ligamentum teres
Capsule

FIGURE 42-19 Normal and abnormal relationships of hip joint structure. (Adapted from Dunn P. M. [1969]. Congenital dislocation of the hip. *Proceedings of the Royal Society of Medicine* 62, 1035–1037.)

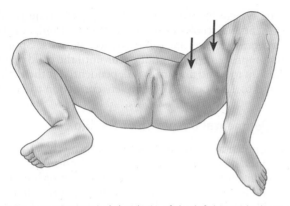

FIGURE 42-20 Congenital dysplasia of the left hip with shortening of the femur, as indicated by legs in abduction and asymmetric gluteal and thigh folds (indicated by *arrows*).

gluteal folds, shortening of the thigh so that one knee (on the affected side) is higher than the other knee, and limited abduction of the affected hip (Fig. 42-20). The asymmetry of gluteal folds is not definitive but indicates the need for further evaluation. In the older child, instability of the hip may produce a delay in walking or eventually cause a characteristic waddling gait. Diagnosis is confirmed by radiography. Ultrasonography may be used to diagnose the condition in newborns and infants from birth to 4 months of age.[47]

The treatment of a developmental dysplasia should be individualized and depends on whether the hip is subluxated or dislocated. Mild instability often resolves without treatment. The best results are obtained if the treatment is begun before changes in the hip structure (*e.g.*, 2 to 3 months) prevent it from being reduced by gentle manipulation or abduction devices. Infants with dislocated hips caused by anatomic changes and toddlers who may lack development of the acetabular socket require more aggressive treatment, such as open reduction and joint reconstruction. Treatment at any age includes reduction of the dislocation and immobilization of the legs in an abducted position. With children younger than 3 years, skin traction is used when reduction cannot be easily obtained. This treatment is followed by several months of immobilization in a hip spica cast, plaster splints, or an abduction splint. Older children or adults with an unreduced dislocatable hip may require hip surgery because of damage to the articulating surface of the joint.

OSTEOGENESIS IMPERFECTA

Osteogenesis imperfecta is a hereditary disease characterized by defective synthesis of type I collagen.[17,18,56,57] It is one of the most common hereditary bone diseases, with an occurrence rate of approximately 1 case in 10,000 births.[57] Although it usually is transmitted as an autosomal dominant trait, a distinct form of the disorder with multiple lethal defects is thought to be inherited as an autosomal recessive trait.[56] In some cases the defect is caused by a spontaneous mutation.

The clinical manifestations of osteogenesis imperfecta include a spectrum of disorders marked by increased bone fragility, low bone mass, and extraskeletal abnormalities associated with defective collagen synthesis. These problems include short stature, thin skin, blue or gray sclera, abnormal tooth development, hypotonic muscles, loose-jointedness, scoliosis, and a tendency toward hernia formation. Hearing loss caused by otosclerosis of the middle and inner ear is common in affected adults. There are at least four types of osteogenesis imperfecta (types I, II, III, and IV), each with a different genetic structural abnormality and clinical features.[17,18]

The pathogenesis of osteogenesis imperfecta involves mutations in the COL1A1 and COL1A2 genes, which encode the α_1 and α_2 chains of type I procollagen, the major structural protein of bone. These two genes are located on chromosomes 17 and 7, respectively.[17] Defects in COL1A1 are found in all types of osteogenesis imperfecta, whereas defects in COL1A2 are found in types II, III, and IV. Type I osteogenesis imperfecta, which is inherited as an autosomal dominant trait, is the mildest form of the disorder. It is characterized by multiple fractures after birth, blue sclera, and progressive hearing loss, which develops into total deafness in adulthood. The joint laxity associated with the condition eventually leads to kyphoscoliosis and flat feet. Type II is a lethal, perinatal form of the disease with a variable pattern of inheritance. It is most often inherited as an autosomal recessive trait, but some cases are inherited as an autosomal dominant trait, and still others are due to a new mutation.[18] Affected infants are either stillborn or die within a few days of birth. Type III is progressive and the most severely deforming type of osteogenesis imperfecta and is characterized by many fractures, growth retardation, and severe skeletal deformities. The inheritance pattern is autosomal dominant, although rare autosomal recessive forms have been reported. Type IV is inherited as an autosomal dominant trait and clinically is the most diverse type. The phenotype may vary from mild to severe, with the most severely affected persons presenting with fractures at birth, suffering moderate skeletal deformity, and attaining a relatively short stature.

There is no known medical treatment for correction of the defective collagen synthesis that is characteristic of osteogenesis imperfecta. Instead, current treatment modalities focus on preventing complications and improving functional outcomes.[56] Although there is no cure for osteogenesis imperfecta, research studies have shown that bisphosphonate (*e.g.*, pamidronate) treatment can improve bone mass in all types of the disorder.[56,57]

JUVENILE OSTEOCHONDROSES

The term *juvenile osteochondroses* is used to describe a group of children's diseases in which one or more growth ossification centers undergoes a period of degeneration, necrosis, or inactivity that is followed by regeneration and usually deformity. The osteochondroses are separated into two groups according to their causes. The first group consists of the true osteonecrotic osteochondroses, so called because the diseases are caused by localized osteonecrosis of an apophyseal or epiphyseal center (*e.g.*, Legg-Calvé-Perthes disease, Freiberg infarction, Panner disease, Kienböck disease). The second group of juvenile osteochondroses is caused by abnormalities in ossification of cartilaginous tissue resulting from a genetically determined normal variation or from trauma (*e.g.*, Osgood-Schlatter disease, Blount disease, Sever disease, Scheuermann disease). The discussion in this section focuses on Legg-Calvé-Perthes disease from the first group and Osgood-Schlatter disease from the second group.

Legg-Calvé-Perthes Disease

Legg-Calvé-Perthes disease, or coxa plana, is an osteonecrotic disease of the proximal femoral (capital) epiphysis, which is the growth center for the head of the femur. It occurs in 1 of 1200 children, affecting primarily those between 2 and 13 years of age, with a peak incidence between 4 and 9 years.[47,58] It occurs primarily in boys and is much more common in whites than African Americans. Although no definite genetic pattern has been established, it occasionally affects more than one family member.

The cause of Legg-Calvé-Perthes disease is unknown. The disorder usually is insidious in onset and occurs in otherwise healthy children. However, it may be associated with acute trauma. Affected children usually have a shorter stature. Undernutrition has been suggested as a causative factor. When girls are affected, they usually have a poorer prognosis than boys because they are skeletally more mature and have a shorter period for growth and remodeling than do boys of the same age. Although both legs can be affected, in 85% of cases only one leg is involved.[48]

The primary pathologic feature of Legg-Calvé-Perthes disease is an avascular necrosis of the bone and marrow involving the epiphyseal growth center in the femoral head. The disorder may be confined to part of the epiphysis, or it may involve the entire epiphysis. In severe cases, there is a disturbance in the growth pattern that leads to a broad, short femoral neck. The necrosis is followed by slow absorption of the dead bone over a period of 2 to 3 years. Although the necrotic bone is eventually replaced by healthy new bone, the epiphysis rarely regains its normal shape.

Legg-Calvé-Perthes disease has an insidious onset with a prolonged course. The main symptoms are pain in the groin, thigh, or knee and difficulty in walking. The child may have a painless limp with limited abduction and internal rotation and a flexion contracture of the affected hip. The age of onset is important because young children have a greater capability for remodeling of the femoral head and acetabulum, so less flattening of the femoral head occurs.

Early diagnosis is important and is based on correlating physical symptoms with radiographic findings that are related to the stage of the disease. The goal of treatment is to reduce deformity and preserve the integrity of the femoral head. Conservative and surgical interventions are used in the treatment of Legg-Calvé-Perthes disease. Children younger than 4 years of age with little or no involvement of the femoral head may require only periodic observation. In all other children, some intervention is needed to relieve the force of weight bearing, muscular tension, and subluxation of the femoral head. It is important to maintain the femur in a well-seated position in the concave acetabulum to prevent deformity. This is done by keeping the hip in abduction and mild internal rotation.

Treatment involves abduction casts or braces to keep the legs separated in abduction with mild internal rotation. The Atlanta Scottish Rite brace, which does not extend below the knee, is the most widely used orthosis because it provides containment while allowing free knee motion and ambulation without crutches or external support[47,48] (Fig. 42-21). Surgery may be done to contain the femoral head in the acetabulum. This treatment usually is reserved for children older than 6 years of age who at the time of diagnosis have more serious involvement of the femoral head. The best surgical results are obtained when surgery is done early, before the epiphysis becomes necrotic.

Osgood-Schlatter Disease

Osgood-Schlatter disease involves microfractures in the area where the patellar tendon inserts into the tibial tubercle, which is an extension of the proximal tibial epiphysis.[47] This area is particularly vulnerable to injury caused by sudden or continued strain from the patellar tendon during periods of growth, particularly in athletic individuals. It

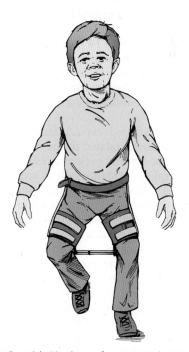

FIGURE 42-21 Scottish Rite brace for Legg-Calvé-Perthes disease produces containment for abduction and allows free knee motion. (From Crocetti M., Barone M. A. [2004]. *Oski's essential pediatrics* (2nd ed., p. 679). Philadelphia: Lippincott Williams & Wilkins.)

occurs most frequently in boys between the ages of 11 and 15 years and in girls between 8 and 13 years.

The disorder is characterized by pain in the front of the knee that is associated with inflammation and thickening of the patellar tendon. The pain usually is associated with specific activities, such as kneeling, running, bicycle riding, or stair climbing. There is swelling, tenderness, and increased prominence of the tibial tubercle. The symptoms usually are self-limiting. They may recur during growth periods but usually resolve after closure of the tibial growth plate. In some cases, limitations on activity, tibial bands or braces to immobilize the knee, anti-inflammatory agents, and application of cold are necessary to relieve the pain. The objective of treatment is to release tension on the quadriceps to permit revascularization and reossification of the tibial tubercle. Complete resolution of symptoms through physiologic healing (physeal closure) of the tibial tubercle usually requires 12 to 24 months.[47] Occasionally, minor symptoms or an increased prominence of the tibial tubercle may continue into adulthood. In some cases, a high-riding patella can cause dislocation with chondromalacia of the patella and result in degenerative arthritis.

SLIPPED CAPITAL FEMORAL EPIPHYSIS

Slipped capital femoral epiphysis, or coxa vara, is a disorder of the growth plate that occurs near the age of skeletal maturity. The condition occurs with an estimated frequency of 1 in 100,000 to 1 in 800,000 and is the most common disorder of the hip in adolescents.[48] Normally, the proximal capital femoral epiphysis unites with the neck of the femur between 14 and 16 years of age. Before this time (10 to 14 years of age in girls and 10 to 16 years in boys), slippage may occur with the capital femoral epiphysis remaining in the acetabulum and the femoral neck rotating anteriorly (although occasionally superiorly).[58] This results in a varus retroverted femoral head and neck.

The cause of slipped capital femoral epiphysis is obscure, but it may be related to the child's susceptibility to stress on the femoral neck as a result of genetic factors or structural abnormalities. Boys are affected twice as often as girls, and in approximately one half of cases, the condition is bilateral. Affected children often are overweight with poorly developed secondary sex characteristics or, in some instances, are extremely tall and thin. In many cases, there is a history of rapid skeletal growth preceding displacement of the epiphysis. The condition also may be affected by nutritional deficiencies or endocrine disorders such as hypothyroidism, hypopituitarism, and hypogonadism. Rapid growth after administration of growth hormone has been associated with displacement of the epiphysis.

Children with the condition often complain of referred knee pain accompanied by difficulty in walking, fatigue, and stiffness. The diagnosis is confirmed by radiographic studies in which the degree of slippage is determined and graded according to severity (mild, 0% to 33%; moderate, 34% to 50%; and severe, >50%). Early treatment is imperative to prevent lifelong crippling. Avoidance of weight bearing on the femur and bed rest are essential parts of the treatment. Traction or gentle manipulation under anesthesia is used to reduce the slippage. Surgical insertion of pins to keep the femoral neck and head aligned is a common method of treatment for children with moderate or severe slips. Crutches are used for several months after surgical correction to prevent full weight bearing until the growth plate closes.

Children with the disorder must be followed closely until the epiphyseal plate closes. Long-term prognosis depends on the amount of displacement that occurs. Complications include avascular necrosis, leg shortening, malunion, and problems with the internal fixation. Degenerative arthritis may develop, requiring joint replacement later in life.

SCOLIOSIS

Scoliosis is a lateral deviation of the spinal column that may or may not include rotation or deformity of the vertebrae. It has been estimated that more than 500,000 adults in the United States have scoliosis.[59] It is most commonly seen during adolescence and is eight times more common among girls than boys. Scoliosis can develop as the result of another disease condition, or it can occur without known cause. Idiopathic scoliosis accounts for 75% to 80% of cases of the disorder. The other 20% to 25% of cases result from more than 50 different causes, including poliomyelitis, congenital hemivertebrae, neurofibromatosis, and cerebral palsy. Although minor curves are relatively common (affecting approximately 2% of the population), it has been estimated that less than 0.1% of U.S. schoolchildren have severe idiopathic scoliosis.[60]

Types of Scoliosis

Scoliosis is classified as postural or structural. With postural scoliosis, there is a small curve that corrects with bending. It can be corrected with passive and active exercises. Structural scoliosis does not correct with bending. It is a fixed deformity classified according to the cause: congenital, neuromuscular, and idiopathic.

Congenital scoliosis is caused by disturbances in vertebral development during the sixth to eighth week of embryologic development. There are structural anomalies in the vertebrae that can cause a severe curvature. The child may have other anomalies and neurologic complications if the spine is involved. Early diagnosis and treatment of progressive curves are essential for children with congenital scoliosis.

Neuromuscular scoliosis develops from neuropathic or myopathic diseases. Neuropathic scoliosis is seen with cerebral palsy, myelodysplasia, and poliomyelitis. There is often a long, "C"-shaped curve from the cervical to the sacral region. In children with cerebral palsy, severe deformity may make treatment difficult. Myopathic neuromuscular scoliosis develops with Duchenne muscular dystrophy and usually is not severe.

Idiopathic scoliosis is a structural spinal curvature for which no cause has been established. The cause is most likely complex and multifactorial. Genetic factors, neurophysiologic predisposition, abnormal biomechanical forces, connective tissue abnormality, and collagen abnormalities have all been researched as possible causes of idiopathic scoliosis.[61] It seems likely that genetic influences are involved, and mother-daughter pairings are common.[61] Growth and mechanical factors also seem to play a role.

Idiopathic scoliosis can be divided into three groups on the basis of age at onset: infantile (birth to 3 years), juvenile (4 to 10 years), and adolescent (11 years and older).[62] Adolescent scoliosis is the most common type of idiopathic scoliosis. It accounts for approximately 80% of cases, and is seen most commonly in girls. An increase in joint laxity, which causes excessive joint motion and is found commonly in girls, has been associated with development of idiopathic scoliosis. Delayed puberty and menarche are other risk factors for the development of scoliosis.[63] Although the curve may be present in any area of the spine, the most common curve is a right thoracic curve, which produces a rib prominence on the convex side and hypokyphosis from rotation of the vertebral column around its long axis as the spine begins to curve.

Clinical Features

Manifestations. Scoliosis usually is first noticed because of the deformity it causes. A high shoulder, prominent hip, or projecting scapula may be noticed by a parent or in a school screening program. Idiopathic scoliosis usually is a painless process, although pain may be present in severe cases, usually in the lumbar region. The pain may be caused by pressure on the ribs or on the crest of the ilium. There may be shortness of breath as a result of diminished chest expansion and gastrointestinal disturbances from crowding of the abdominal organs. Adults with less severe deformity may experience mild backache. If scoliosis is left untreated, the curve may progress to an extent that compromises cardiopulmonary function and creates a risk for neurologic complications.

Diagnosis and Treatment. Early diagnosis of scoliosis can be important in the prevention of severe spinal deformity. The cardinal signs of scoliosis are uneven shoulders or iliac crests, prominent scapula on the convex side of the curve, malalignment of spinous processes, asymmetry of the flanks, asymmetry of the thoracic cage, and rib hump or paraspinal muscle prominence when bending forward (Fig. 42-22). A complete physical examination is necessary for children with scoliosis because the defect may be indicative of another, underlying pathologic process.

Diagnosis of scoliosis is made by physical examination and confirmed by radiographs. A scoliometer should be used at the apex of the curvature to quantify a prominence; a scoliometer reading of greater than 10 degrees requires referral to a physician. The curve is measured by determining the amount of lateral devia-

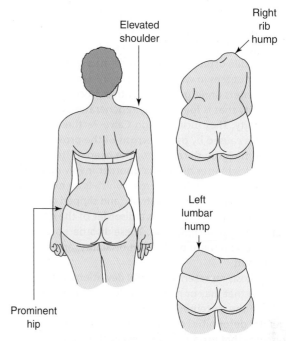

FIGURE 42-22 Scoliosis. Abnormalities to be determined at initial screening examination. (From Gore D. R., Passehl R., Sepic S., et al. [1981]. Scoliosis screening: Results of a community project. *Pediatrics* 67, 196–200. Copyright 1981 by the American Academy of Pediatrics.)

tion present on radiographs and is labeled "right" or "left" for the convex portion of the curve. Other radiographic procedures may be done, including CT, MRI, and myelography.

The treatment of scoliosis depends on the severity of the deformity and the likelihood of progression. A brace may be used to control the progression of the curvature and provide some correction. Surgical intervention with instrumentation and spinal fusion is done in severe cases. Unlike bracing, which is intended to halt progression of the curvature, surgical intervention is used to decrease the curve.

In summary, skeletal disorders in children result from congenital or hereditary influences or from factors that occur during normal periods of skeletal growth and development. Newborn infants undergo normal changes in muscle tone and joint motion, causing torsional and angulation deformities of the femur or tibia. Many of these conditions are corrected as skeletal growth and development take place.

Disorders such as congenital clubfoot and developmental dysplasia of the hip are present at birth. Developmental dysplasia of the hip includes a range of structural abnormalities. Dislocated hips are always treated to prevent changes in the anatomic structure. Osteogenesis imperfecta is a rare autosomal hereditary disorder characterized by defective synthesis of connective tissue, including bone matrix. It results in poorly developed bones that fracture easily.

Juvenile osteochondroses refer to a group of children's diseases in which one or more growth ossification centers undergo degeneration, necrosis, or inactivity that is followed by regeneration and usually deformity. They include Legg-Calvé-Perthes disease, which is caused by osteonecrosis of the proximal epiphysis, the growth center for the head of the femur; Osgood-Schlatter disease, a disorder involving microfractures in the tibial tubercle, which is an extension of the proximal tibial epiphysis; and slipped capital femoral epiphysis, which is a disorder of the proximal femoral (capital) epiphysis. These disorders are progressive, can cause permanent disability, and require treatment.

Scoliosis represents a lateral deviation of the spinal column that may or may not include rotation or deformity of the vertebrae. It can occur as the result of congenital deformities of the vertebrae, neuromuscular diseases that produce weakness of the muscles that support the spinal column, or curvature for which no cause has been established (idiopathic scoliosis). Idiopathic scoliosis, which is the most common form, occurs more frequently in girls than boys. Treatment depends on the severity of the deformity and the likelihood of progression.

Review Exercises

A 34-year-old football player dislocates his hip during one of the season's games.

A. Explain the need for immediate reduction of the dislocation based on the vascular anatomy of the hip.

A 39-year-old man is in intensive care after a motorcycle accident in which he skidded across the pavement on his right side. He has fractures of his right femur, pelvis, and several ribs on the right side. His right leg was crushed beneath the motorcycle, and he is beginning to lose movement in that leg.

A. What are the priorities in treating his orthopedic injuries? What are the options for stabilizing his leg?
B. What risk factors for complications of fractures are present?
C. What are the symptoms of compartment syndrome, and how is it treated?

A 73-year-old woman with a history of breast cancer sustained a comminuted fracture in the mid-diaphysis of her left humerus when her husband lifted her up in bed. She has multiple lucent lesions scattered throughout her proximal humerus, radius, and ulna. She was recently hospitalized for confusion and found to have diffuse bone metastases.

A. What would you consider to be the most likely cause of her fracture?
B. What are the most common sites for bone metastasis?
C. Explain the treatment goals for persons with pathologic fractures.

A 14-year-old boy complains of recent pain and swelling of the knee, with some restriction in movement. Although he thinks he may have injured his knee playing football, his mother insists that he be seen by an orthopedic specialist and raises the possibility that the boy may have an osteosarcoma.

A. Use the theory that osteosarcoma originates in sites of maximal growth velocity to explain the site of this boy's possible tumor.
B. What diagnostic tests could be used to establish a diagnosis of osteosarcoma?
C. The boy and his family are concerned that the boy will require radical surgery with amputation of the leg. How would you go about explaining possible treatment options to him?

A newborn girl was found to have developmental dysplasia of the hip during a routine screening examination.

A. Describe the anatomic abnormalities that are present in the disorder.
B. Explain the need for early treatment of developmental dysplasia of the hip.

A 12-year-old girl was noted to have asymmetry of the shoulders, scapular height, and pelvic height during routine physical examination. On x-ray examination she is found to have a 30-degree spinal curvature.

A. What possible treatments are available for this girl?
B. Describe the physical problems associated with progressive scoliosis.

REFERENCES

1. Centers for Disease Control and Prevention, National Center for Injury Prevention and Control. Web-based Injury Statistics Query and Reporting System (WISQARS). [On-line.] Available: www.cdc.gov/ncipc/wisqars/. Accessed September 12, 2005.

2. Hogan K. A., Gross R. H. (2003). Overuse injuries in pediatric athletes. *Orthopedic Clinics of North America* 34, 405–415.

3. American Academy of Orthopedic Surgeons. (2003). Pay attention to high school sports injuries. [On-line.] Available: http://orthoinfo.aaos.org.

4. Mercier L. R. (2000). *Practical orthopedics* (5th ed., pp. 6–18, 48–74, 159–175, 187–191). St. Louis: Mosby

5. Greene W. B. (Ed). (2001). *Essentials of musculoskeletal care* (2nd ed., pp. 17–19, 91–93, 136–156, 327–332). Rosemont, IL: American Academy of Orthopedic Surgeons.

6. Liu S. H., Yang R., Raad A., et al. (1995). Collagen in tendon, ligament, and bone healing. *Clinical Orthopedics and Related Research* 318, 265–278.

7. Wolfe M. W., Uhl T. L., McCluskey L. C. (2001). Management of ankle strains. *American Family Physician* 63, 93–104.

8. Quillen D. M., Wuchner M., Hatch R. L. (2004). Acute shoulder injuries. *American Family Physician* 70, 1949–1954.

9. Gómez J. E. (2002). Upper extremity injuries in youth sports. *Pediatric Clinics of North America* 49, 593–626.

10. Hegenroeder A., Chorley J. N. (2004). Sports injuries. In Behrman R. F., Kliegman R. M., Jenson H. B. (Eds.), *Nelson textbook of pediatrics* (17th ed., pp. 2302–2314). Philadelphia: Elsevier Saunders.

11. Fongeimie A. E., Buss D. B., Rolnick S. J. (1998). Management of shoulder impingement syndrome and rotator cuff tears. *American Family Physician* 57, 667–674.

12. Muellner T., Nikolic A., Vecsei V. (1999). Recommendations for the diagnosis of traumatic meniscal injuries in athletes. *Sports Medicine* 27, 337–345.

13. Maitra R. S., Miller M. D., Johnson D. L. (1999). Meniscal reconstruction: Part I. Indications, techniques, and graft considerations. *American Journal of Orthopedics* 28, 213–218.

14. Maitra R. S., Miller M. D., Johnson D. L. (1999). Meniscal reconstruction: Part II. Outcome, potential complications, and future directions. *American Journal of Orthopedics* 28, 280–286.

15. Brunner L., Eshilian-Oats L. (2003). Hip fractures in adults. *American Family Physician* 67, 537–542.

16. Zuckerman J. D. (1996). Hip fracture. *New England Journal of Medicine* 334, 1519–1525.

17. Rosenberg A. (2005). Bones, joints, and soft tissue tumors. In Kumar V., Abbas A., Fausto N. (Eds.), *Robbins and Cotran pathologic basis of disease* (7th ed., pp. 1273–1324). Philadelphia: Elsevier Saunders.

18. Schiller A. L., Wang B. Y., Klein M. J. (2005). Bones and joints. In Rubin E., Gorstein F., Rubin R., et al. (Eds.), *Rubin's pathology: Clinicopathologic foundations of medicine* (4th ed., pp. 1305–1384). Philadelphia: Lippincott Williams & Wilkins.

19. Einhorn T. A. (1998). The cell and molecular biology of fracture healing. *Clinical Orthopaedics and Related Research* 355(Suppl.), S7–S21.

20. Hayda R. A., Brighton C. T., Esterhai J. L. (1998). Pathophysiology of delayed healing. *Clinical Orthopaedics and Related Research* 355(Suppl.), S31–S36.

21. Hoover T. J., Siefert J. A. (2000). Soft tissue complications of orthopedic emergencies. *Emergency Medicine Clinics of North America* 18, 115–139.

22. Kostler W., Strohm P. C., Sudkamp N. P. (2004). Acute compartment syndrome of the limb. *Injury* 35, 1221–1227.

23. Harvey C. V. (2001). Compartment syndrome: When it is least expected. *Orthopedic Nursing* 20(3), 15–26.

24. Swain R., Ross D. (1999). Lower extremity compartment syndrome. *Postgraduate Medicine* 105, 159–168.

25. Mohler L. R., Styf J. R., Pedowitz R., et al. (1997). Intramuscular deoxygenation during exercise in patients who have chronic anterior compartment syndrome of the leg. *Journal of Bone and Joint Surgery* [American volume] 79, 844–849.

26. Schwartzman R. (2000). New treatments for reflex sympathetic dystrophy. *New England Journal of Medicine* 343, 654–656.

27. Parisi D. M., Koval K., Egot K. (2002). Fat embolism syndrome. *American Journal of Orthopedics* 31, 507–512.

28. Forteza A. M., Kock S., Romano J. O., et al. (1999). Transcranial detection of fat emboli. *Stroke* 30, 2687–2691.

29. Richards R. R. (1997). Fat emboli syndrome. *Canadian Journal of Surgery* 40, 334–339.

30. Mellor A., Soni M. (2001). Fat embolism. *Anesthesia* 56, 145–154.

31. Lew D. P., Waldvogel F. A. (1997). Osteomyelitis. *New England Journal of Medicine* 336, 999–1007.

32. Lew D. P., Waldvogel F. A. (2004). Osteomyelitis. *Lancet* 364 (9431), 369–379.

33. Carek P. J., Dickerson L. M., Sack J. L. (2001). Diagnosis and management of osteomyelitis. *American Family Physician* 63, 2413–2420.

34. Lampe R. (2004). Osteomyelitis and suppurative arthritis. In Behrman R. F., Kliegman R. M., Jenson H. B. (Eds.), *Nelson textbook of pediatrics* (17th ed., pp. 2297–2302). Philadelphia: Elsevier Saunders.

35. Assouline-Dayan Y., Chang C., Greenspan A., et al. (2002). Pathogenesis and natural history of osteonecrosis. *Seminars in Arthritis and Rheumatism* 32, 94–124.

36. Mont M. A., Jones J. C., Einhorn T. A., et al. (1998). Osteonecrosis of the femoral head. *Clinical Orthopaedics and Related Research* 355(Suppl.), S314–S335.

37. Rosen G., Forscher C. A., Mankin H. J., et al. (2000). Neoplasms of bone and soft tissue. In Bast R. C., Kufe D. W., Pollack R. E., et al. (Eds.), *Cancer medicine* (pp. 1870–1902). Hamilton, Ontario: B. C. Decker.

38. Arndt C. S. (2004). Neoplasms of bone. In Behrman R. E., Kliegman R. M., Jenson H. B. (Eds.), *Nelson textbook of pediatrics* (16th ed., pp. 1714–1723). Philadelphia: Elsevier Saunders.

39. Wittig J. D., Bickels J., Priebat D., et al. (2002). Osteosarcoma: A multidisciplinary approach to diagnosis and treatment. *American Family Physician* 65, 1123–1136.

40. Marina N., Gebhardt M., Teot L., et al. (2004). Biology and therapeutic advances for pediatric osteosarcoma. *Oncologist* 9, 422–421.

41. Marcus K. D. (2001). Pediatric solid tumors. In Lenhard R. E., Jr., Osteen R. T., Gansler T. (eds.), *The American Cancer Society's clinical oncology* (pp. 590–593). Atlanta: American Cancer Society.

42. O'Keefe R. J., Schwartz E. M., Boyce B. F. (2000). Bone metastasis: An update on bone resorption and therapeutic strategies. *Current Opinion in Orthopedics* 11, 353–359.

43. Juan J., Pollock C. B., Kelly K. (2005). Mechanisms of cancer metastasis to the bone. *Cell Research* 15, 57–62.

44. Hershey M. S. (2004). Toward new horizons: The future of bisphosphonate therapy. *Oncologist* 9(Suppl. 4), 38–47.

45. Sass P., Hassan G. (2003). Lower extremity abnormalities in children. *American Family Physician* 68, 461–468.

46. Bruce R. W. (1996). Torsional and angular deformities. *Pediatric Clinics of North America* 43, 867–881.

47. Thompson G. H. (2004). Bone and joint disorders. In Behrman R. E., Kliegman R. M., Jenson H. B. (Eds.), *Nelson textbook of pediatrics* (17th ed., pp. 2251–2290). Philadelphia: Elsevier Saunders.

48. Crocetti M., Barone M. A. (2004). *Oski's essential pediatrics* (2nd ed., pp. 160–166, 676–687). Philadelphia: Lippincott Williams & Wilkins.

49. Schoppee K. (1995). Blount disease. *Orthopedic Nursing* 14(5), 31–34.

50. Gore A. L., Spencer J. P. (2004). The newborn foot. *American Family Physician* 69, 865–872.

51. Weinstein S. L. (1994). The pediatric foot. In Weinstein S. L., Buckwalter J. A. (Eds.), *Turek's orthopaedics: Principles and their application* (5th ed., pp. 615–653). Philadelphia: J. B. Lippincott.

52. Honein M., Paulozzi L. J., Moore C. A. (2000). Family history, maternal smoking, and clubfoot: An indication of a gene–environment interaction. *American Journal of Epidemiology* 152, 658–665.

53. Novacheck T. F. (1996). Developmental dysplasia of the hip. *Pediatrics* 43, 829–848.

54. American Academy of Pediatrics. (2000). Clinical practice guideline: Early detection of developmental dysplasia of the hip. *Pediatrics* 105, 896–905.

55. Eastwood D. M. (2003). Neonatal hip screening. *Lancet* 361, 595–597.

56. Rauch F., Glorieux F. H. (2004). Osteogenesis imperfecta. *Lancet* 363, 1377–1385.

57. Roughley P. J., Rauch F., Glorieux F. H. (2003). Osteogenesis imperfecta: Clinical and molecular diversity. *European Cells & Materials Journal* 5, 41–47.

58. Koops S., Quanbeck D. (1996). Three common causes of childhood hip pain. *Pediatric Clinics of North America* 43, 1056–1065.

59. U.S. Preventive Services Task Force. (1993). Screening for adolescent idiopathic scoliosis. *Journal of the American Medical Association* 269, 2664–2672.

60. Reamy B. V., Slakey J. B. (2001). Adolescent scoliosis: Review and current comments. *American Family Physician* 64, 111–116.

61. Lowe T. G., Edgar M., Margulles F. Y., et al. (2000). Etiology of idiopathic scoliosis: Current trends in research. *Journal of Bone and Joint Surgery* [American volume] 82, 1157–1168.

62. Weinstein S. (1994). The thoracolumbar spine. In Weinstein S. L., Buckwalter J. A. (Eds.), *Turek's orthopaedics: Principles and their application* (5th ed., pp. 447–483). Philadelphia: J. B. Lippincott.

63. Omey M. L., Micheli L. J., Gerbino P. G. (2000). Idiopathic scoliosis and spondylolysis in the female athlete: Tips for treatment. *Clinical Orthopaedics and Related Research* 372, 74–84.

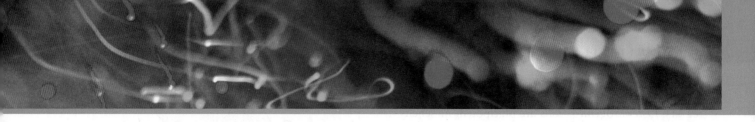

Chapter 43

Disorders of the Skeletal System: Metabolic and Rheumatic Disorders

 The skeletal system is as vital to body function as any other organ system because of its essential roles in mechanical support and mineral homeostasis. The bones of the skeletal system provide the basic framework that supports the body, protects its organs, and provides for movement. For example, the bones of the lower extremities act as a pillar when we stand, and the ribs provide a cage that supports and protects our heart and lungs. Joints hold the bones of our skeleton together, making movement possible. Bone is also one of the few tissues that normally undergoes mineralization. It is a storehouse for 99% of the body's calcium and 85% of its phosphorus. This chapter focuses on two types of skeletal disorders: metabolic bone disorders, which produce a decrease in bone mass and mineralization, and joint disorders, which disrupt mobility.

Metabolic Bone Disease

BONE REMODELING

Bone is made up of connective tissue, which is defined by its distinctive admixture of inorganic elements (65%) and it organic matrix (35%).[1] It is the inorganic elements (calcium hydroxyapatite) that give bone its strength. The organic component includes the bone cells and the proteins of its matrix. The formation of calcium hydroxyapatite and mineralization of bone requires the actions of the bone cells and the structural integrity of the organic matrix and is tightly regulated by a number of factors.

The cells of bone tissue include the osteoprogenitor cells, osteoblasts, osteocytes, and osteoclasts[1-3] (see Chapter 41). *Osteoprogenitor cells* are pluripotent mesenchymal cells that are found in the periosteum and all the stromal (supporting) structures in the marrow cavity. When appropriately stimulated by growth factors, they undergo cell division and differentiate into osteoblasts. The generation of osteoblasts from osteoprogenitor cells is essential to the growth, remodeling, and repair of bone throughout life.

Osteoblasts are specialized cells that synthesize and secrete the collagen and the ground substance that constitute the initial unmineralized bone, called *osteoid*. The osteoblasts are also responsible for mineralization of the bone matrix. Osteoblasts express cell surface receptors that bind many hormones, including parathyroid hormone (PTH), vitamin D, and estrogen. Metabolically active osteoblasts have a life span of about 3 months and then undergo apoptosis, become surrounded by osteoid or bone matrix and transform into osteocytes, or become quiescent, flattened bone surface–lining cells.

Osteocytes are mature bone cells that are housed in lacunae within the calcified bone matrix. Although encased in bone, the osteocyte has processes that extend through bony channels, called *canaliculi*, and communicate with other osteocytes. Recent evidence suggests that the osteocyte may be the cell that senses and responds to mechanical stress. It is also the cell that responds to changes in extracellular calcium and phosphate.

The *osteoclasts* are phagocytic cells, responsible for bone resorption. They are derived from hematopoietic bone marrow cells that also give rise to monocytes and macrophages. A number of cytokines and growth factors contribute to the differentiation and maturation of osteoclasts. These factors work by either stimulating osteoclast progenitor cells or participating in a signaling system in which osteoblasts and marrow stromal cells play a central role. Interleukin (IL)-6, which is produced in response to systemic hormones such as PTH and vitamin D, stimulates the early stages of osteoclast development.

The recent identification of a chemical messenger called the receptor activator for nuclear factor κB ligand (RANKL), its receptor RANK, and its decoy receptor osteoprotegerin (OPG), has provided new insights into osteoclast activation and bone remodeling[1,4] (Fig. 43-1). RANKL, a member of the tumor necrosis factor (TNF) superfamily, is produced by osteoblasts and their stromal precursor cells. RANKL binds to and activates the RANK receptor, which is produced by osteoclasts and their monocyte/macrophage precursors, thus promoting osteoclast proliferation and activation. The actions of RANKL can be blocked by OPG, a member of the TNF family of receptors, which is a soluble protein produced by a number of tissues, including bone, hematopoietic tissues, and immune cells. OPG inhibits osteoclast generation by acting as a decoy receptor that binds to RANKL, thus preventing it from binding to the RANK receptor. It is now believed that dysregulation of the RANKL/RANK

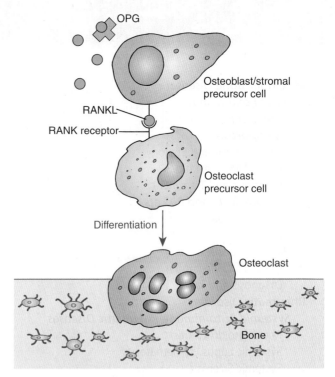

FIGURE 43-1 RANK ligand (RANKL), RANK receptor, and osteoprotegerin (OPG) interactions in the activation of osteoclasts and subsequent resorption of bone. RANKL, which is produced by osteoblasts and their stromal precursors, binds to the RANK receptor on osteoclast precursor cells, promoting osteoclast differentiation and proliferation. The soluble OPG molecule, which is produced by a number of tissues, acts as a decoy receptor, blocking the action of RANKL.

receptor pathway may play a prominent role in the pathogenesis of bone diseases such as osteoporosis.

Osteoblasts and osteoclasts act in coordination with each other and are considered to be the functional unit of bone. The processes of bone resorption by the osteoclasts and bone formation by the osteoblasts are tightly coupled, and their balance determines skeletal mass at any point in time. As the skeleton grows and enlarges in the fetus and growing child, bone formation predominates. This process is called *modeling*. Once the skeleton has reached its full adult size, the breakdown and replacement of bone that is responsible for its maintenance is called *remodeling*.

There are two different types of bone: the dense compact bone on the outside surface of a bone and the porous cancellous bone that lines the marrow cavity. Compact bone is composed of parallel or concentric layers, called *lamellae*. There are four lamellar systems in compact bone: an outer circumferential lamella that lies deep to the periosteum, an inner circumferential lamella that encircles the marrow cavity, osteons containing the haversian canal system, and the interstitial lamellae[1,4] (see Chapter 41, Fig. 41-2). Bone remodeling takes place in the osteons. It begins with osteoclastic resorption of existing bone, during which the organic (protein matrix) and the inorganic (mineral) components are removed. The sequence proceeds to the formation of new bone by osteoblasts. Remnants of osteons remain as irregular arcs of lamellar fragments known as interstitial lamellae, surrounded by osteons. In the adult, the length of one sequence (*i.e.*, bone resorption and formation) is approximately 4 months. Ideally, the replaced bone should equal the absorbed bone. If it does not, there is a net loss of bone. In the elderly, for example, bone resorption and formation no longer are perfectly coupled, and bone mass is lost.

The major influences on the equilibrium of bone tissue include mechanical stress; calcium and phosphate levels in the extracellular fluid; and cytokines, local growth factors, and hormones that influence bone resorption and formation. Mechanical stress stimulates osteoblastic activity and formation of the organic matrix. It is important in preventing bone atrophy and in healing fractures. Bone serves as a storage site for extracellular calcium and phosphate ions. Consequently, alterations in the extracellular levels of these ions affect their deposition in bone (see Chapter 6). Blood levels of calcium and phosphate are regulated by PTH and calcitonin. PTH promotes bone resorption and calcitonin inhibits bone resorption. Other hormones such as estrogens, testosterone, corticosteroids, and thyroid hormone also influence osteoclastic and osteoblastic activity.

Vitamins C, D, and K are also essential to proper bone formation.[4] Vitamin C is required for proper collagen formation. A deficiency of vitamin C can result in a disease called *scurvy*. In the absence of vitamin C, the epiphyseal plates and bony shaft of growing bone are so thin and fragile that they are predisposed to fractures. In the adult, vitamin C deficiency affects bone maintenance rather than growth. Vitamin D is needed for intestinal absorption of calcium and phosphate. Over the past several decades, several vitamin K–dependent proteins have been discovered. Recent studies have shown that in addition to their role in the synthesis of coagulation factors, the vitamin K–dependent proteins are also involved in bone metabolism and the inhibition of arterial calcification. One of these proteins, osteocalcin, which is synthesized mainly by osteoblasts, has molecular properties that allow it to bind hydroxyapatite tightly in bone, thereby prompting mineralization.[5]

OSTEOPENIA

Osteopenia is a condition that is common to all metabolic bone diseases. It is characterized by a reduction in bone mass greater than expected for age, race, or sex, and it occurs because of a decrease in bone formation, inadequate bone mineralization, or excessive bone deossification. *Osteopenia* is not a diagnosis but a term used to describe an apparent lack of bone mass seen on x-ray studies. The major causes of osteopenia are osteoporosis, osteomalacia, malignancies such as multiple myeloma, and endocrine disorders such as hyperparathyroidism and hyperthyroidism.

OSTEOPOROSIS

Osteoporosis is a skeletal disorder characterized by the loss of bone mass and deterioration of the architecture of cancellous bone with a subsequent increase in bone fragility and susceptibility to fractures. Although osteoporosis can occur as the result of an endocrine disorder or malignancy, it most often is associated with the aging process. An estimated 44 million U.S. women and men aged 50 years and older are affected by osteoporosis or low bone mass.[6] By the year 2010, it is estimated that this number will increase to over 52 million in this same age category, and if the current trend continues, the figure will climb to over 61 million by 2020.[6]

Pathogenesis and Etiology

The pathogenesis of osteoporosis is unclear, but most data suggest an imbalance between bone resorption and formation such that bone resorption exceeds bone formation.[7] Although both of these factors play a role in most cases of osteoporosis, their relative contribution to bone loss may vary depending on age, gender, nutritional status, and genetic predisposition.

Under normal conditions, bone mass increases steadily during childhood, reaching a peak in the young adult years. The peak bone mass is an important determinant of the subsequent risk of osteoporosis. It is determined in part by genetic factors, gonadal hormone

Understanding ➤ Bone Remodeling

Bone remodeling constitutes a process of skeletal maintenance once skeletal growth has reached maturity. It takes place in (1) the osteons of mature bone and consists of a cycle of (2) bone resorption by osteoclasts followed by (3) bone formation by osteoblasts.

1

Bone remodeling cycle. Mature bone is made up of osteons or units of concentric lamellae (bone layers) and the Haversian canals that they surround. Bone remodeling consists of a sequence of bone resorption within an osteon channel by osteoclasts followed by new bone formation by osteoblasts. In the adult, the length of one sequence (*i.e.,* bone resorption and formation) is approximately 4 months. Ideally, the replaced bone should equal the absorbed bone. If it does not, there is a net loss of bone. In the elderly, for example, bone resorption and formation no longer are perfectly coupled, and bone mass is lost.

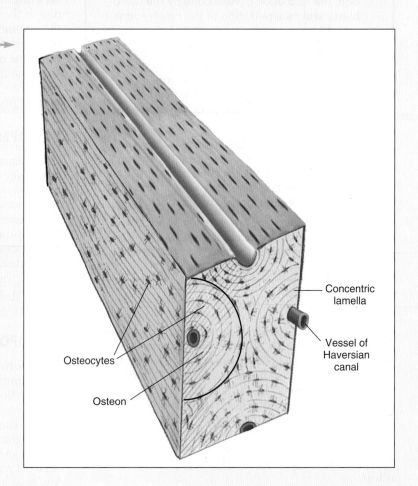

Concentric lamella

Vessel of Haversian canal

Osteocytes

Osteon

2

Bone resorption. The sequence of bone resorption and bone formation is activated by many stimuli, including the actions of parathyroid hormone (PTH) and calcitonin. It begins with osteoclastic resorption of existing bone, during which the organic (protein matrix) and the inorganic (mineral) components are removed, creating a tunnel-like space in the osteon.

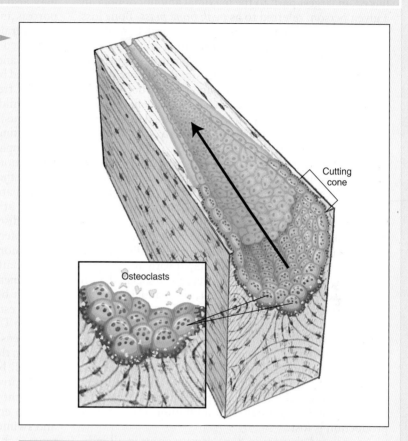

3

Bone formation. After the osteoclastic activity has ceased, osteoblasts begin to deposit the organic matrix (osteoid) on the wall of the osteon canal. As successive lamellae of bone are deposited, the canal ultimately attains the relative proportions of the original osteon. In the formation and maintenance of bone, osteoblasts provide much of the local control because they not only produce new bone matrix, but they also play an essential role in mediating osteoclast activity. Many of the primary stimulators of bone resorption, such as PTH, have minimal or no direct effect on osteoclasts. Once the osteoblast, which has receptors for these substances, receives the appropriate signal, it releases a soluble mediator that induces osteoclast activity.

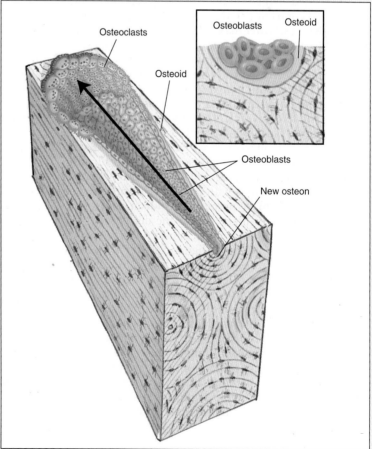

(estrogen) levels, exercise, calcium intake and absorption, and environmental factors. Genetic factors are linked, in largest part, to the maximal amount of bone in a given person, referred to as *peak bone mass*. Bone loss occurs in all races, but because of higher peak bone mass, blacks are less prone to osteoporosis than are Asians and whites.[4] Exercise may help to prevent osteoporosis by increasing peak bone mineral density during periods of growth. Poor nutrition or an age-related decrease in intestinal absorption of calcium because of deficient activation of vitamin D may contribute to the development of osteoporosis, particularly in the elderly.

Hormonal factors play a significant role in the development of osteoporosis, particularly in postmenopausal women. Postmenopausal osteoporosis, which is caused by an estrogen deficiency, is manifested by a loss of cancellous bone and a predisposition to fractures of the vertebrae and distal radius. The loss of bone mass is greatest during early menopause, when estrogen levels are withdrawing. Several factors appear to influence the increased loss of bone mass associated with an estrogen deficiency. Decreased estrogen levels are associated with an increase in cytokines (*e.g.,* IL-1, IL-6, and TNF) that stimulate the production of osteoclast precursors.[1] Recent studies indicate that estrogen deficiency also influences osteoclast differentiation through the RANK receptor pathway.[1] Estrogen stimulates the production of OPG and thus inhibits the formation of osteoclasts, and it also blunts the responsiveness of osteoclast precursors to RANKL. With menopause and its accompanying estrogen deficiency, this inhibition of osteoclast production is lost.

Age-related changes in bone density occur in all individuals and contribute to the development of osteoporosis in both sexes.[8] After maximal bone mass is attained at about 30 years of age, the rate of bone loss for both sexes is approximately 0.7% per year.[1] The age-related loss of bone reflects decreased osteoblast activity as well as an increase in osteoclastic activity. The greatest losses occur in areas containing abundant cancellous bone, such as the spine and femoral neck. Thus, these are common sites for fractures in older persons with osteoporosis.

Secondary osteoporosis is associated with many conditions, including endocrine disorders, malabsorption disorders, malignancies, alcoholism, and use of certain medications.[9,10] Persons with endocrine disorders such as hyperthyroidism, hyperparathyroidism, and Cushing syndrome are at high risk for the development of osteoporosis. Hyperthyroidism causes an acceleration of bone turnover. Some malignancies (*e.g.,* multiple myeloma) secrete osteoclast-activating factor, causing significant bone loss. Alcohol is a direct inhibitor of osteoblasts and may also inhibit calcium absorption. Corticosteroids are responsible for the most common form of drug-related osteoporosis, and their long-term use in treatment of disorders such as rheumatoid arthritis and chronic obstructive lung disease is associated with an increased rate of fractures. The prolonged use of medications that increase calcium excretion, such as aluminum-containing antacids, also is associated with bone loss.[10] Persons with human immunodeficiency virus (HIV) infection or acquired immunodeficiency syndrome (AIDS) who are being treated with antiretroviral therapy may also have a lower bone density and signs of osteoporosis and osteopenia.[11]

Several groups of children and adolescents are at increased risk of decreased bone mass, including premature and low–birth-weight infants who have lower than expected bone mass in the early weeks of life; children who require treatment with corticosteroid drugs (*e.g.,* those with childhood inflammatory diseases and transplant recipients); children with cystic fibrosis; and adolescents with eating disorders.[12] Children with cystic fibrosis often have impaired gastrointestinal function that reduces the absorption of calcium and other nutrients, and many also require the frequent use of corticosteroid drugs.

Premature osteoporosis is being seen increasingly in female athletes because of an increased prevalence of eating disorders and amenorrhea.[13,14] The *female athlete triad* refers to a pattern of disordered eating that leads to amenorrhea and eventually osteoporosis. Poor nutrition, combined with intense exercise training, can lead to an energy deficit that causes a lack of estrogen production by the ovary and secondary amenorrhea. The lack of estrogen combined with the lack of calcium and vitamin D from dietary deficiencies results in a loss of bone density and increased risk of fractures.[13] There is a concern that female athletes with low bone mineral density will be at increased risk for fractures during their competitive years. It is unclear if osteoporosis induced by amenorrhea is reversible. It most frequently affects women engaged in endurance sports, such as running and swimming; in activities where appearance is important, such as figure skating, diving, and gymnastics; or sports with weight categories, such as horse racing, martial arts, and rowing.[14]

Although commonly considered a women's health issue, men are also at risk for development of osteoporosis.[15] However, men usually develop osteoporosis at a later age than women and are at lower risk for osteoporotic fractures. This is largely because of their greater peak bone mass at skeletal maturity and because they do not undergo the period of accelerated bone loss that women do during menopause. At the same time, the risk factors that influence peak bone mass and bone loss, such as genetics, nutritional intake, exercise and lifestyle practices, and medications, are similar between men and women. Age-related osteoporosis tends to occur in men older than 70 years of age and is thought to result from a decreased absorption of calcium, reduced activation of vitamin D, a decline in osteoblast activity, and decreased concentration of sex hormones.

Clinical Manifestations

Osteoporotic changes occur largely in the diaphysis and metaphysis of bone. The diameter of the bone enlarges with age, causing the outer supporting cortex to become thinner. In severe osteoporosis, the bones begin to resemble the fragile structure of a fine porcelain vase. There is loss of trabeculae from cancellous bone and thinning of the cortex to such an extent that minimal stress causes fractures (Fig. 43-2). The changes that occur with osteoporosis have been explained by two distinct disease processes affecting women early and late in life.[1,4]

Type I is caused by early postmenopausal estrogen deficiency and is manifested by loss of trabecular bone, with a predisposition to fractures of the vertebrae and distal radius. Type II (*i.e.*, senile osteoporosis) is caused by a calcium deficiency and is a slower process in which cortical and trabecular bone are lost. Hip fractures, which are seen later in life, result from the second type.

Osteoporosis is usually a silent disorder. Often the first manifestations of the disorder are those that accompany a skeletal fracture—a vertebral compression fracture or fractures of the hip, pelvis, humerus, or any other bone.

Fractures often occur with a force less than typically would be needed. Wedging and collapse of vertebrae may cause a loss of height in the vertebral column and kyphosis, a condition commonly referred to as *dowager's hump*. Usually, there is no generalized bone tenderness. When pain occurs, it is related to fractures. Systemic symptoms such as weakness and weight loss suggest that the osteoporosis may be caused by another underlying disease.

Diagnosis and Treatment

An important advance in diagnostic methods for the identification of osteoporosis has been the use of bone mineral density (BMD) assessment. The clinical method of choice for bone density studies is dual-energy x-ray absorptiometry (DXA) of the spine and hip.[16] Whenever possible,

the first four vertebrae should be included. The site with the lowest score should be used to make a diagnosis. The National Institutes of Health consensus conference defined the diagnostic criterion for osteoporosis as 2.5 standard deviations (SD) below the young adult mean.[12] Measurement of BMD has become increasingly common for early detection and fracture prevention. Measurement of serial heights in older adults is another simple way to screen for osteoporosis. A further advance in the diagnosis of osteoporosis is the refinement of risk factors, permitting better analysis of risk pertaining to particular persons. Women older than 65 years of age who weigh less than 140 pounds at menopause or who have never used estrogens for more than 6 months should be screened for osteoporosis. The simple mnemonic ABONE (*A* = age, *B* = bulk, and *ONE* = never on estrogen) aids in remembering these criteria.[17]

Prevention and early detection of osteoporosis are essential to the prevention of the associated deformities and fractures. It is important to identify persons in high-risk groups so treatment can begin early. Postmenopausal women of small stature or lean body mass, those with sedentary lifestyles, those with poor calcium intake, and those with diseases that demineralize bone are at greatest risk.[18] Other risk factors found to be associated with osteoporosis are a diet high in protein, consumption of caffeine-containing beverages, cigarette smoking, and alcohol ingestion. Risk factors for osteoporosis are listed in Chart 43-1.

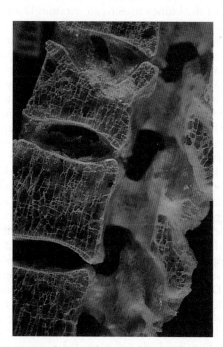

FIGURE 43-2 Osteoporosis. A section of the vertebral column, in which the bone marrow has been washed out, demonstrates a loss of bone tissue and a compression fracture of a vertebral body (*top*). (From Rubin E., Farber J. L. [Eds.]. [1999]. *Pathology* [3rd ed., p. 1367]. Philadelphia: Lippincott Williams & Wilkins.)

CHART 43-1

Risk Factors Associated With Osteoporosis

Primary

Advanced Age
Female
White (fair, thin skin)
Small bone structure
Postmenopausal
Family history
Contributing factors
    Sedentary lifestyle
    Calcium deficiency (long term)

Secondary

Cushing disease
Diabetes
Hyperparathyroidism
Hyperthyroidism
Malignancy
Malabsorption disorders
Chronic alcoholism
Medications
    Anticonvulsants
    Aluminum-containing antacids
    Corticosteroids
    Heparin

Regular exercise and adequate calcium intake are important factors in preventing osteoporosis. Weight-bearing exercises such as walking, jogging, rowing, and weight lifting are important in the maintenance of bone mass. Studies have indicated that premenopausal women need more than 1000 mg and postmenopausal women need 1500 mg of calcium daily.[18] Because most older women do not consume a sufficient quantity of dairy products to meet their calcium needs, calcium supplementation is recommended. Vitamin D is critical for intestinal absorption of calcium, and a daily intake of 400 to 800 IU of vitamin D is recommended.[18]

Active treatment of osteoporosis uses two main classes of drugs: antiresorptive agents (drugs that block bone resorption by osteoclasts) and anabolic agents (agents that stimulate bone formation by osteoblasts).[18] There are three main types of antiresorptive agent: estrogens and selective estrogen receptor modulators, bisphosphonates, and calcitonin. Although estrogen is one of the most effective interventions for reducing the incidence and progression of osteoporosis in postmenopausal women, the use of hormone therapy (estrogen plus progestin) has come under scrutiny after the recent release of data from the Women's Health Initiative.[18] Raloxifene, a selective estrogen receptor modulator (SERM) that acts only on specific estrogen receptors, was recently approved by the U.S. Food and Drug Administration (FDA) for prevention and treatment of osteoporosis in postmenopausal women. The use of phytoestrogens, naturally occurring plant compounds, has gained popularity as an alternative to estrogens; however, information regarding their effect on bone health is conflicting and incomplete.[19]

Bisphosphonates are effective inhibitors of bone resorption and the most effective agents for prevention and treatment of osteoporosis. The bisphosphonates (*e.g.,* alendronate, risedronate, ibandronate) are analogs of endogenous inorganic pyrophosphate that the body cannot break down. In bone, they bind to hydroxyapatite and prevent bone resorption through the inhibition of osteoclast activity. Bisphosphonates have been shown to reduce the risk of hip, vertebral, and nonvertebral fractures by up to 50%.[12,18] The most dramatic impact has been in the reduction of multiple spine fractures, showing that treatment can decrease progression of the disease.

Calcitonin is an endogenous peptide that partially inhibits osteoclastic activity. Nasal calcitonin and subcutaneous calcitonin have been approved for the treatment of postmenopausal osteoporosis.

Teriparatide is an analog of PTH that was recently approved by the FDA for the treatment of osteoporosis.[18] In addition to its effects on osteoclast activity and bone resorption, PTH increases bone formation through increased osteoblast production and activation of preexisting osteoblasts.

In men, testosterone appears to play an important role in bone homeostasis by stimulating osteoblasts and inhibiting osteoclasts. Testosterone can be administered by intramuscular injection, transdermal patch, or transscrotal patch.[15] The use of testosterone is contraindicated in men with prostate cancer. Men with osteoporosis may also benefit from bisphosphonate, calcitonin, or PTH

therapy. As with women, they have the same need for calcium and vitamin D supplementation.

OSTEOMALACIA AND RICKETS

In contrast to osteoporosis, which causes a loss of total bone mass, osteomalacia and rickets cause defective mineralization but not the loss of bone matrix. Defective mineralization of the growing skeleton in childhood causes permanent bone deformities and is referred to as *rickets;* in adults, it is known as *osteomalacia.*

Osteomalacia

Osteomalacia is a generalized bone condition in which inadequate mineralization of bone results from a calcium or phosphate deficiency, or both. There are two main causes of osteomalacia: (1) insufficient calcium absorption from the intestine because of a lack of dietary calcium or deficiency or resistance to the action of vitamin D, and (2) phosphate deficiency caused by altered elimination by the kidney or decreased intestinal absorption. Vitamin D deficiency is caused most commonly by reduced vitamin D absorption as a result of biliary tract or intestinal diseases that impair fat and fat-soluble vitamin absorption. Lack of vitamin D in the diet is rare in the United States because many foods are fortified with the vitamin. Anticonvulsant medications, such as phenobarbital and phenytoin, induce hepatic hydroxylases that accelerate breakdown of the active forms of vitamin D.

A form of osteomalacia called *renal rickets* occurs in persons with chronic renal failure. It is caused by the inability of the kidney to activate vitamin D and excrete phosphate and is accompanied by hyperparathyroidism, increased bone turnover, and increased bone resorption (see Chapter 25). Another form of osteomalacia results from renal tubular defects that cause excessive phosphate losses. This form of osteomalacia is commonly referred to as *vitamin D–resistant rickets* and often is a familial disorder.[4] It is inherited as an X-linked dominant gene passed by mothers to one half of their children and by fathers to their daughters only. This form of osteomalacia affects boys more severely than girls. Long-standing primary hyperparathyroidism causes increased calcium resorption from bone and hypophosphatemia, which can lead to rickets in children and osteomalacia in adults.

The incidence of osteomalacia is high among the elderly because of diets deficient in calcium and vitamin D, and often is compounded by the intestinal malabsorption problems that accompany aging. Osteomalacia often is seen in cultures in which the diet is deficient in vitamin D, such as in northern China, Japan, and northern India. Women in these areas have a higher incidence of the disorder than do men because of the combined effects of pregnancy, lactation, and more indoor confinement. Osteomalacia occasionally is seen in strict vegetarians, persons who have had a gastrectomy, and those on long-term anticonvulsant, tranquilizer, sedative, muscle relaxant, or diuretic drug therapy. There also is a greater incidence of osteomalacia in the colder regions of the world, particularly during the winter months, probably because of decreased exposure to sunlight.

The clinical manifestations of osteomalacia are bone pain, tenderness, and fractures as the disease progresses. In severe cases, muscle weakness often is an early sign. The cause of muscle weakness is unclear. The combined effects of gravity, muscle weakness, and bone softening contribute to the development of deformities. There may be a dorsal kyphosis in the spine, rib deformities, a heart-shaped pelvis, and marked bowing of the tibiae and femurs. Osteomalacia predisposes a person to pathologic fractures in the weakened areas, especially in the distal radius and proximal femur. In contrast to osteoporosis, it is not a significant cause of hip fractures. There may be delayed healing and poor retention of internal fixation devices. Osteomalacia usually is accompanied by a compensatory or secondary hyperparathyroidism stimulated by low serum calcium levels.

Diagnostic methods include x-ray studies and laboratory tests such as serum calcium, phosphate, PTH, and vitamin D levels. Bone density studies or bone biopsy may be done to confirm the diagnosis of osteomalacia.

The treatment of osteomalacia is directed at the underlying cause. If the problem is nutritional, restoring adequate amounts of calcium and vitamin D to the diet may be sufficient. Vitamin D is specific for adult osteomalacia and vitamin D–resistant rickets, but large doses usually are needed to overcome the resistance to its calcium absorption action and to prevent renal loss of phosphate. If osteomalacia is caused by malabsorption, the treatment is directed toward correcting the primary disease. For example, adequate replacement of pancreatic enzymes is of paramount importance in pancreatic insufficiency. In renal tubular disorders, the treatment is directed at the altered renal physiology.

Rickets

Rickets is a disorder of vitamin D deficiency, inadequate calcium absorption, and impaired mineralization of bone in children. Children with rickets manifest inadequate mineralization not only of bone, but of the cartilaginous matrix of the epiphyseal growth plate. Rickets occurs primarily in underdeveloped areas of the world and among immigrants to developed countries. The causes are inadequate exposure to sunlight (*e.g.,* children are often kept clothed and indoors) and prolonged breast-feeding without vitamin D supplementation.[20] Although the vitamin D content of human milk is low, the combination of breast milk and sunlight exposure usually provides sufficient vitamin D. Another cause of rickets is the use of commercial alternative milks (*e.g.,* soy or rice beverages) that are not fortified with vitamin D.[21] A dietary deficiency in calcium and phosphorus may also contribute to the development of rickets. A newly discovered genetic mutation also can cause vitamin D deficiency rickets, a condition that does not respond to simple vitamin supplementation. The mutation results in the absence of a critical enzyme in vitamin D metabolism.[22]

The pathologic process of rickets is the same as that of osteomalacia in adults. Because rickets affects children during periods of active growth, the structural changes seen in the bone are somewhat different. Bones become deformed; ossification at epiphyseal plates is delayed and disordered, resulting in widening of the epiphyseal cartilage plate. Any new bone that does grow is unmineralized.

The symptoms of rickets usually are noticed between 6 months and 3 years of age. The child usually has stunted growth, with a height sometimes far below the normal range. Weight often is not affected so that the children, many of whom present with a protruding abdomen (*i.e.,* rachitic potbelly), have been described as presenting a Buddha-like appearance when sitting. Early symptoms are lethargy and muscle weakness, which may be accompanied by convulsions or tetany related to hypocalcemia. Irritability is common. In severe cases, children lose their skin pigment, acquire flabby subcutaneous tissue, and have poorly developed musculature. The ends of long bones and ribs are enlarged. The thorax may be abnormally shaped, with prominent rib cartilage (*i.e.,* rachitic rosary). The legs exhibit bowlegged or knock-kneed deformities. The skull is enlarged and soft, and closure of the fontanels is delayed. Teeth are slow to develop, and the child may have difficulty standing.

Rickets is treated with a balanced diet sufficient in calcium, phosphorus, and vitamin D. Exposure to sunlight also is important, especially for premature infants and those receiving artificial milk feedings. Supplemental vitamin D in excess of normal requirements is given for several months. Maintenance of good posture, positioning, and bracing in older children are used to prevent deformities. After the disease is controlled, deformities may have to be surgically corrected as the child grows.

PAGET DISEASE

Paget disease (osteitis deformans) is the second most common bone disease after osteoporosis.[23,24] The disease is characterized by focal regions of excessive bone turnover and disorganized osteoid formation. The disease usually begins during mid-adulthood and becomes progressively more common thereafter.[1] Although the disease is often asymptomatic, 10% to 30% of persons experience pain, skeletal deformity, neurologic symptoms, pathologic fractures, and deafness.

Paget disease is characterized by a localized increase in osteoclast formation that leads to bone resorption. Subsequently, bone formation is also markedly increased, with increased numbers of osteoblasts rapidly depositing bone in a chaotic fashion such that the newly formed bone is of poor quality and is disorganized rather than lamellar. The poor quality of bone accounts for the bowing and even fractures of bones affected by Paget disease. The lesions of Paget disease may be solitary or may occur in multiple sites. They tend to localize to the bones of the axial skeleton, including the spine, skull, and pelvis. The proximal femur and tibia may be involved in more widespread forms of the disease. As rapid bone formation predominates in advanced stages of the disease, the lesions

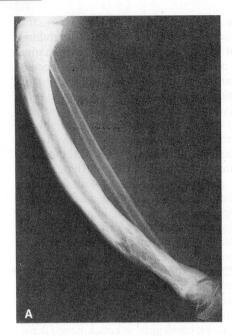
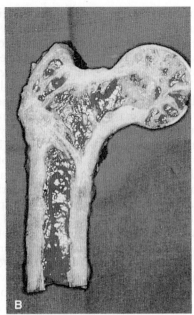

FIGURE 43-3 Paget disease. (**A**) Radiograph of the leg shows marked involvement of the tibia by Paget disease with thickening and disorganization of the cortex. Note the normal appearance of the fibula. (**B**) The proximal end of a femur affected by Paget disease shows replacement of the normal cancellous architecture by coarse, thick bundles of trabecular bone. The cortical bone is irregularly thickened and exhibits a coarse, granular appearance instead of normally smooth cortical bone. (From Rubin E., Farber J. L. [Eds.]. [1999]. *Pathology* [3rd ed., p. 1377]. Philadelphia: Lippincott Williams & Wilkins.)

become sclerotic and the bone marrow is replaced by vascular and fibrous tissue. The result is a thick layer of coarse bone with a rough and pitted outer surface that has the appearance of pumice (Fig. 43-3).

Although the cause of Paget disease remains unclear, there is evidence of both genetic and environmental influences. It has been reported that 15% to 40% of persons with the disease have a first-degree relative with Paget disease, and numerous studies have described extended family members with the disease.[23] It is likely that factors other than genetics are also involved in the pathogenesis of the disease. Current evidence suggests a probable association with a virus, possibly a paramyxovirus.[1,4,23] This has been supported by the observation of viral particles resembling the paramyxovirus nucleocapsid in the cytoplasm of osteoclasts in persons with Paget disease.

Clinical Manifestations

Clinical findings are extremely variable and depend on the extent and site of the disease. Many persons with Paget disease are totally asymptomatic, and the disease is discovered accidentally. When the disease is limited to a single bone, it may cause only mild pain and stiffness.

For those with symptomatic disease, pain is usually a first complaint. Involvement of the skull causes headaches, intermittent tinnitus, vertigo, and eventual hearing loss. In the spine, collapse of the anterior vertebrae causes kyphosis of the thoracic spine. The femur and tibia become bowed (see Fig. 43-3). Softening of the femoral neck can cause coxa vara (*i.e.*, reduced angle of the femoral neck). Coxa vara, in combination with softening of the sacral and iliac bones, causes a waddling gait. Pathologic fractures may occur, especially in the bones subjected to the greatest stress (*e.g.*, upper femur, lower spine, pelvic bones).

These fractures often heal poorly, with excessive and poorly distributed callus.

Other manifestations of Paget disease include nerve palsy syndromes from lesions in the upper extremities, mental deterioration, and cardiovascular disease. Cardiovascular disease is the most serious complication and is listed as the most common cause of death in those with advanced generalized Paget disease. It is caused by vasodilatation of the vessels in the skin and subcutaneous tissues overlying the affected bones. When one third to one half of the skeleton is affected, the increased blood flow may lead to high-output cardiac failure. Ventilatory capacity may be limited by rib and spine involvement.

Persons with Paget disease are also at risk for the development of a variety of tumors and tumor-like conditions. The most dreaded complication is the development of osteosarcoma, which occurs in up to 1% of all persons with Paget disease but has an increased incidence in those with more severe forms of the disease.[4]

Diagnosis and Treatment

Diagnosis of Paget disease is based on characteristic bone deformities and x-ray changes.[23,24] Technetium pyrophosphate bone scans are used to detect the rapid bone turnover indicative of active disease and to monitor the response to treatment. The scan cannot identify bone activity resulting from malignant lesions. Bone biopsy may be done to differentiate the lesion from osteomyelitis or a primary or metastatic bone tumor. Elevated serum alkaline phosphatase levels, which reflect osteoblast activity, can be used to support a diagnosis of Paget disease, and continued monitoring of these levels can be used to monitor the effectiveness of treatment.

The treatment of Paget disease is based on the degree of pain and the extent of the disease. Pain can be reduced with nonsteroidal or other anti-inflammatory agents. The bisphosphonates (*e.g.*, alendronate, pamidronate), which decrease bone resorption by inhibiting osteoclast activity, have become the treatment of choice for Paget disease.[23,25] Calcitonin, which is available in injectable and a nasal spray form, also inhibits bone resorption. However, many people develop antibodies to calcitonin and become resistant to its effects. Persons with Paget disease should receive adequate doses of calcium and vitamin D.[24]

In summary, the skeletal system is as vital to normal body function as any other body system because of its essential roles in mechanical support and mineral homeostasis. The bones of the skeletal system are composed of inorganic mineral elements (calcium and phosphorus) that give bone its strength; proteins and other organic elements that form its matrix; and bone cells that are responsible for its maintenance. Bone maintenance consists of a continuous process of remodeling of the bone matrix, which involves bone resorption by osteoclasts and bone formation by osteoblasts, and bone mineralization, which involves deposition of calcium and phosphate into the bone matrix.

Metabolic bone diseases such as osteoporosis, osteomalacia, rickets, and Paget disease are the result of a disruption in the equilibrium of bone formation and resorption. Osteoporosis, which is the most common metabolic bone disease, occurs when the rate of bone resorption is greater than that of bone formation. It is seen frequently in postmenopausal women and is the major cause of fractures in persons older than 45 years of age. Osteomalacia and rickets are caused by inadequate mineralization of bone matrix, primarily because of a deficiency of vitamin D. Paget disease, which is the second most common bone disease after osteoporosis, is characterized by focal regions of excessive bone turnover and disorganized osteoid formation. Although many people are asymptomatic, the disease can cause pain, skeletal deformities, neurologic symptoms, pathologic fractures, and deafness.

Rheumatic Disorders

Arthritis is a descriptive term applied to more than 100 rheumatic diseases, ranging from localized, self-limiting conditions to those that are systemic, autoimmune processes.[26,27] Arthritis affects persons in all age groups and is the leading cause of disability in the United States.

The common use of the term *arthritis* oversimplifies the nature of the varied disease processes, the difficulty in differentiating one form of arthritis from another, and the complexity of treatment of these usually chronic conditions. These diverse rheumatic conditions share inflammation of the joint as a prominent or accompanying symptom. In the systemic rheumatic diseases, such as rheumatoid arthritis, the inflammation is primary, resulting from an immune response, probably autoimmune in origin. In rheumatic conditions limited to a single or few diarthrodial joints, such as osteoarthritis, the inflammation is secondary, resulting from the degenerative process and joint irregularities.

SYSTEMIC AUTOIMMUNE RHEUMATIC DISEASES

Systemic autoimmune rheumatic diseases are a group of chronic disorders characterized by diffuse inflammatory vascular lesions and degenerative changes in connective tissue that share clinical features and may affect many of the same organs. They include rheumatoid arthritis, systemic lupus erythematosus, and systemic sclerosis, all of which share an autoimmune systemic pathogenesis.

Rheumatoid Arthritis

Rheumatoid arthritis (RA) is a systemic inflammatory disease that attacks joints by producing a proliferative synovitis that leads to the destruction of the articular cartilage and underlying bone. It affects 0.3% to 1.5% of the population, with women affected two to three times more frequently than men.[26] Although the disease occurs in all age groups, its prevalence increases with age. The peak incidence among women is between the ages of 40 and 60 years, with the onset at 30 to 50 years of age.

The cause of RA has not been established. However, evidence points to a genetic predisposition and the development of joint inflammation that is immunologically mediated. The importance of genetic factors in the pathogenesis of RA is supported by the increased frequency of the disease among first-degree relatives and monozygotic twins.[1,4] Multiple gene loci are believed to be responsible for susceptibility to the disease, but most have not yet been identified. An important genetic locus that is known to predispose to RA is present in human leukocyte antigen (HLA) class II genes, and a specific set of HLA-DR

KEY CONCEPTS

Arthritis

➤ Arthritis represents a diverse group of rheumatic conditions that share inflammation of the joint as a prominent or accompanying symptom.

➤ In the systemic rheumatic diseases, the inflammation is primary, resulting from an immune response, probably autoimmune in origin.

➤ In rheumatic conditions, such as osteoarthritis, which are limited to a single or few diarthrodial joints, the inflammation is secondary, resulting from the degenerative process and joint irregularities.

alleles (DR4, DR1, DR10, DR14).[4] These alleles share a common binding site, which forms the rheumatoid pocket on the HLA molecule.[1,4] It has been hypothesized that binding properties of this site may contribute to the pathogenesis of RA by binding and displaying the arthritogenic antigen to T cells[1,4] (see Chapter 13).

Pathogenesis. The pathogenesis of RA can be viewed as an aberrant immune response that leads to synovial inflammation and destruction of joint architecture. It has been suggested that the disease is initiated by the activation of CD4+ helper T cells, release of cytokines (e.g., TNF, IL-1), and antibody formation (Fig. 43-4). Approximately 70% to 80% of those with the disease have the *rheumatoid factor (RF)*, an autoantibody that reacts with a fragment of immunoglobulin G (IgG) to form immune complexes.[27] RF has been found in the blood, synovial fluid, and synovial membrane of affected individuals. Much of the RF produced by immune cells is present in the inflammatory infiltrate of the synovial tissue.[27]

The role of the autoimmune process in the joint destruction of RA remains obscure. At the cellular level, neutrophils, macrophages, and lymphocytes are attracted to the area. The neutrophils and macrophages phagocytize the immune complexes and, in the process, release lysosomal enzymes capable of causing destructive changes in the joint cartilage. The inflammatory response that follows attracts additional inflammatory cells, setting into motion a chain of events that perpetuates the condition. As the inflammatory process progresses, the synovial cells and subsynovial tissues undergo reactive hyperplasia. Vasodilatation and increased blood flow cause warmth and redness. The joint swelling that occurs is the result of the increased capillary permeability that accompanies the inflammatory process.

Characteristic of RA is the development of an extensive network of new blood vessels (angiogenesis) in the synovial membrane that contributes to the advancement of the disease. This destructive vascular granulation tissue, which is called *pannus*, extends from the synovium to involve the "bare area" of unprotected bone at the junction between cartilage and subchondral bone (Fig. 43-5). Pannus is a feature of RA that differentiates it from other forms of inflammatory arthritis.[28] The inflammatory cells found in the pannus have a destructive effect on the adjacent cartilage and bone. Eventually, pannus develops between the joint margins, leading to reduced joint motion and the possibility of eventual ankylosis. With progression of the disease, joint inflammation and the resulting structural changes can lead to joint instability, muscle atrophy from disuse, stretching of ligaments, and involvement of the tendons and muscles. The effect of the pathologic changes on joint structure and function is related to the degree of disease activity, which can change at any time. Unfortunately, the destructive changes are irreversible.

Clinical Manifestations. Rheumatoid arthritis often is associated with systemic as well as joint manifestations. The disease, which is characterized by exacerbations and remissions, may involve only a few joints for brief durations, or it may be relentlessly progressive and debilitating. Approximately one fourth of persons seem to recover completely; another fourth seem to remain for many years with only slight functional impairment; and the remaining half have serious progressive and disabling joint disease.[4]

Joint Manifestations. Joint involvement usually is symmetric and polyarticular. Any diarthrodial joint can be involved. The person may report joint pain and stiffness that lasts 30 minutes and frequently for several hours. The limitation of joint motion that occurs early in the disease usually is caused by pain; later, it is caused by fibrosis. The most frequently affected joints initially are the fingers, hands, wrists, knees, and feet. Later, other diarthrodial joints may become involved. Spinal involvement usually is limited to the cervical region.

In the hands, there usually is bilateral and symmetric involvement of the proximal interphalangeal (PIP) and metacarpophalangeal (MCP) joints in the early stages of RA; the distal interphalangeal (DIP) joints rarely

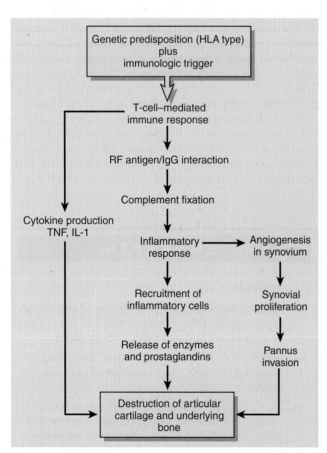

FIGURE 43-4 Disease process in rheumatoid arthritis.

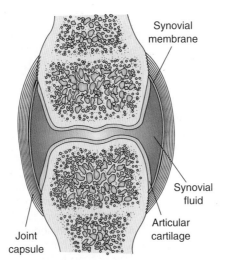
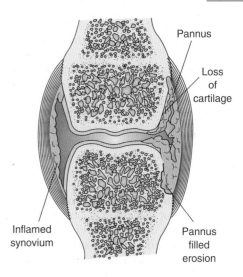

FIGURE 43-5 (Left) Normal joint structures. **(Right)** Joint changes in rheumatoid arthritis. The left side denotes early changes occurring within the synovium, and the right side shows progressive disease that leads to erosion and the formation of pannus.

are affected. The fingers often take on a spindle-shaped appearance because of inflammation of the PIP joints (Fig. 43-6).

Progressive joint destruction may lead to subluxation (*i.e.,* dislocation of the joint resulting in misalignment of the bone ends) and instability of the joint, resulting in limitation of movement. Swelling and thickening of the synovium can result in stretching of the joint capsule and ligaments. When this occurs, muscle and tendon imbalances develop, and mechanical forces applied to the joints through daily activities produce joint deformities. In the MCP joints, the extensor tendons can slip to the ulnar side of the metacarpal head, causing ulnar deviation of the finger (*Fig. 43-7*). Subluxation of the MCP joints may develop when this deformity is present. Hyperextension of the PIP joint and partial flexion of the DIP joint is called a *swan*

neck deformity. After this condition becomes fixed, severe loss of function occurs because the person can no longer make a fist. Flexion of the PIP joint with hyperextension of the DIP joint is called a *boutonnière deformity.*

The knee is one of the most commonly affected joints and is responsible for much of the disability associated with the disease.[26] Active synovitis may be apparent as visible swelling that obliterates the normal contour over the medial and lateral aspects of the patella. The *bulge sign,* which involves milking fluid from the lateral to the medial side of the patella, may be used to determine the presence of excess fluid when it is not visible. Joint contractures, instability, and genu valgum (knock-knee) deformity are other possible manifestations. Severe quadriceps atrophy can contribute to the disability. *Baker cyst* may occur in the popliteal area behind the knee. This is caused by enlargement of the bursa and

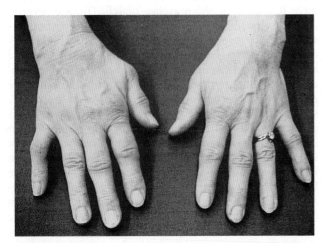

FIGURE 43-6 Inflammation of finger proximal interphalangeal joints in early stages of rheumatoid arthritis, giving the fingers a spindle-shaped appearance. (Reprinted from the ARHP Arthritis Teaching Slide Collection. Used with permission of the American College of Rheumatology.)

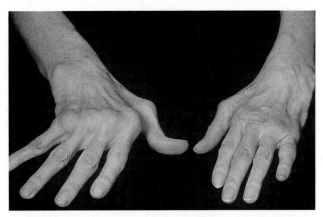

FIGURE 43-7 Subluxation of the metacarpophalangeal joints of the fingers in rheumatoid arthritis (swan neck deformity). (Reprinted from the ARHP Arthritis Teaching Slide Collection. Used with permission of the American College of Rheumatology.)

usually does not cause symptoms unless the cyst ruptures, in which case symptoms mimicking thrombophlebitis appear.

Ankle involvement can limit flexion and extension, which can create difficulty in walking. Involvement of the metatarsophalangeal joints can cause subluxation, hallux valgus, and hammer-toe deformities. Neck discomfort is common. In rare cases, long-standing disease can lead to neurologic complications such as occipital headaches, muscle weakness, and numbness and tingling in the upper extremities.

Extra-articular Manifestations. Although characteristically a joint disease, RA can affect a number of other tissues. Extra-articular manifestations probably are common but usually are mild enough to cause few problems. They are most likely to occur in persons with the RF.

Because RA is a systemic disease, it may be accompanied by complaints of fatigue, weakness, anorexia, weight loss, and low-grade fever when the disease is active. The erythrocyte sedimentation rate (ESR), which commonly is elevated during inflammatory processes, has been found to correlate with the amount of disease activity.[28] Anemia associated with a low serum iron level or low iron-binding capacity is common.[26] This anemia usually is resistant to iron therapy.

Rheumatoid nodules are granulomatous lesions that develop around small blood vessels. The nodules may be tender or nontender, movable or immovable, and small or large. Typically, they are found over pressure points such as the extensor surfaces of the ulna. The nodules may remain unless surgically removed, or they may resolve spontaneously.

Vasculitis, involving the small and medium-size arterioles, is an uncommon manifestation of RA in persons with a long history of active arthritis and high titers of RF (see Chapter 17). Manifestations include ischemic areas in the nail fold and digital pulp that appear as brown spots. Ulcerations may occur in the lower extremities, particularly around the malleolar areas. In some cases, neuropathy may be the only symptom of vasculitis. The visceral organs, such as the heart, lungs, and gastrointestinal tract, also may be affected.

Other extra-articular manifestations include eye lesions such as episcleritis and scleritis, hematologic abnormalities, pulmonary disease, cardiac complications, infection, and Felty syndrome (*i.e.,* leukopenia with or without splenomegaly).

Diagnosis and Treatment. The diagnosis of RA is based on findings of the history, physical examination, and laboratory tests. The criteria for RA developed by the American Rheumatism Association are useful in establishing the diagnosis[28] (Chart 43-2). The last four of the criteria must be present to make a diagnosis of RA. Although these criteria were developed for classification purposes and for use in epidemiologic studies, they can be used as guidelines for diagnosing the illness in individual patients.

Because changes in joint structure usually are not visible early in the disease, diagnosis is often difficult. On

---

CHART 43-2

Criteria for Classification of Rheumatoid Arthritis

Four or more of the following conditions must be present to establish a diagnosis of rheumatoid arthritis:

1. Morning stiffness for at least 1 hour and present for at least 6 weeks
2. Simultaneous swelling of three or more joints for at least 6 weeks
3. Swelling of wrist, metacarpophalangeal, or proximal interphalangeal joints for 6 or more weeks
4. Symmetric joint swelling for 6 or more weeks
5. Rheumatoid nodules
6. Serum rheumatoid factor identified by a method that is positive in less than 5% of normal subjects
7. Radiographic changes typical of rheumatoid arthritis on hand or wrist radiographs

(Adapted from Arnett F. C., Edworthy S. M., Block D. L., et al. [1988]. The American Rheumatism Association 1987 revised criteria for the clarification of rheumatoid arthritis. *Arthritis and Rheumatism,* 31, 315–324.)

---

physical examination, the affected joints show signs of inflammation, swelling, tenderness, and possibly warmth and reduced motion. The joints have a soft, spongy feeling because of the synovial thickening and inflammation. Body movements may be guarded to prevent pain.

Rheumatoid factor test results are not diagnostic for RA, but they can be of value in differentiating RA from other forms of arthritis. Between 1% and 5% of healthy persons have the factor, and its presence seems to be more common with advancing age.[26] Also, a person can have RA without the presence of RF. Disease severity and activity tend to correlate with RF levels; patients with high RF levels tend to have a significantly higher frequency of extra-articular involvement (*e.g.,* rheumatoid nodules, vasculitis, neuropathy).[4] The detection of anti-cyclic citrullinated peptide (CCP) antibodies may be more useful for diagnosing RA because of its higher specificity.[29] Citrulline is an unusual amino acid that is generated by the enzymatic digestion of arginine. Recent research suggests that citrulline-containing proteins may serve as specific targets for the IgG antibody response in RA.[29] The presence of anti-CCP antibodies, which have been detected very early in RA, appear to be a good prognostic marker for the disease and discriminate between erosive and nonerosive forms of the disease. Radiologic findings also are not diagnostic in RA because joint erosions often are not seen on radiographic images in the early stages of the disorder. Synovial fluid analysis can be helpful in the diagnostic process. The synovial fluid has a cloudy appearance, the white blood cell count is elevated as a result of inflammation, and the complement components are decreased.

The treatment goals for a person with RA are to reduce pain, minimize stiffness and swelling, maintain mobility, and become an informed health care consumer. The treatment plan includes education about the disease and its treatment, rest, therapeutic exercises, and medications. Because of the chronicity of the disease and the need for continuous, long-term adherence to the prescribed treatment modalities, it is important that the treatment be integrated with the person's lifestyle.[29]

Both physical rest and emotional rest are important aspects of care.[26] Physical rest reduces joint stress. Rest of specific joints is recommended to relieve pain. For example, sitting reduces the weight on an inflamed knee, and the use of lightweight splints reduces undue movement of the hand or wrist. Although rest is essential, therapeutic exercises also are important in maintaining joint motion and muscle strength. Range-of-motion exercises involve the active and passive movement of joints. Isometric (muscle-tensing) exercises may be used to strengthen muscles. Aerobic exercise and strengthening exercises can be an important component of the treatment regimen of selected patients.[30] Proper posture, positioning, body mechanics, and the use of supportive shoes can provide further comfort. There often is a need for information about the principles of joint protection and work simplification. Some persons need assistive devices to reduce pain and improve their ability to perform activities of daily living. Instruction in the safe use of heat and cold modalities to relieve discomfort and in the use of relaxation techniques also is important.

The goals of pharmacologic therapy for RA are to reduce pain, decrease inflammation, maintain or restore joint function, and prevent bone and cartilage destruction.[26] Medications used to achieve these goals are classified as those that provide relief of arthritis symptoms and those that have the potential for modifying the course of the disease. The trend in RA management is toward a more aggressive pharmacologic approach earlier in the disease. Ideally, disease-modifying antirheumatic drugs (DMARDs) should be used when the diagnosis of RA is established and before erosive changes appear on radiography.[26,31] Early treatment is based on the theory that T-cell–dependent pathways, which manifest early in the inflammatory process, are more responsive to treatment, and that later in the process, when disease progression may be dominated by activated fibroblasts and macrophages, the disease may be more resistant to treatment.

Nonsteroidal anti-inflammatory drugs (NSAIDs) usually are the first choice in the treatment of RA. The NSAIDs inhibit the production of prostaglandins, which have a damaging effect on joint structures. NSAIDs, including salicylates (e.g., aspirin), provide analgesic and anti-inflammatory effects. Effectiveness, side effects, cost, and dosing schedules are considered when selecting an NSAID. There is a wide range of responses to the various NSAIDs, and the particular NSAID that works best for any one individual is not always predictable. The incidence of adverse reactions to the NSAIDs (e.g., gastric irritation and bleeding, fluid retention, kidney damage) tends to increase with age and long-term use.

Second-line drug therapy requires rapid and sustained suppression of inflammation with DMARDs, which are defined as medications that retard or halt the progression of the disease.[31] The DMARDs include gold salts, hydroxychloroquine, sulfasalazine, methotrexate, and azathioprine. Methotrexate has become the drug of choice because of its potency, and it is relatively fast acting (i.e., improvement is seen in 1 month) compared with the slower-acting DMARDs, which can take 3 to 4 months to work. Methotrexate is thought to interfere with purine metabolism, leading to the release of adenosine, a potent anti-inflammatory compound. All of the DMARDs can be toxic and require close monitoring for adverse effects, especially those related to bone marrow suppression.[31]

Corticosteroid drugs may be used to reduce discomfort. These agents interrupt the inflammatory and immune cascade at several levels, such as interfering with inflammatory cell adhesion and migration, impairing prostaglandin synthesis, and inhibiting neutrophil superoxide production. To avoid long-term side effects, they are used only in specific situations for short-term therapy at a low dose level.[26] The corticosteroids do not modify the disease and are unable to prevent joint destruction. Intra-articular corticosteroid injections can provide rapid relief of acute or subacute inflammatory synovitis (after infection is excluded) in a few joints. They should not be repeated more than a few times each year.

Newer antirheumatic drugs include leflunomide, etanercept, infliximab, and adalimumab.[32] Leflunomide is a pyrimidine synthesis inhibitor that blocks the proliferation of T cells. Its efficacy is equal to that of methotrexate. Etanercept, infliximab, and adalimumab are biologic response–modifying agents that block TNF-α, one of the key proinflammatory cytokines in RA.[32] The anti–TNF-α blockers have shown significant efficacy and favorable safety profiles. These agents have also been shown to inhibit radiologic disease progression and improve functional outcomes.

Surgery also may be a part of the treatment of RA.[26] Synovectomy may be indicated to reduce pain and joint damage when synovitis does not respond to medical treatment. Total joint replacements (i.e., arthroplasty) may be performed to reduce pain and increase motion. Arthrodesis (i.e., joint fusion) is indicated only in extreme cases when there is so much soft tissue damage and scarring or infection that a replacement is impossible.

Systemic Lupus Erythematosus

Systemic lupus erythematosus (SLE) is a chronic inflammatory disease that can affect virtually any organ system, including the musculoskeletal system. It is a major rheumatic disease, with a prevalence of approximately 1 case per 2000 persons.[26] There is a female predominance of 10 to 1, and this ratio is closer to 30 to 1 during the childbearing years. SLE is more common in African Americans, Latin Americans, and Asians than whites, and the incidence in some families is higher than in others.[33]

Etiology and Pathogenesis. The cause of SLE is unknown. It is characterized by the formation of autoantibodies and immune complexes. Persons with SLE appear to have B-cell hyperreactivity and increased production of antibodies against self (*i.e.*, autoantibodies) and nonself antigens. These B cells are polyclonal, each producing a different type of antibody. The autoantibodies can directly damage tissues or combine with corresponding antigens to form tissue-damaging immune complexes. Antibodies have been identified against an array of cell components and cell types. Some autoantibodies that have been identified in SLE are anti-nuclear antibodies (ANA), including anti-deoxyribonucleic acid (anti-DNA). Other antibodies may be produced against cell surface antigens of blood cells, including red blood cells and platelets. Autoantibodies against red blood cells can lead to anemia, and those against platelets to thrombocytopenia.

The development of autoantibodies is thought to result from a combination of factors, including genetic, hormonal, immunologic, and environmental.[34] Genetic predisposition is evidenced by the occurrence of familial cases of SLE, especially among identical twins. As many as four genes may be involved in the expression of SLE in humans. Genes linked to the HLA-DR and HLA-DQ loci in the major histocompatibility complex (MHC) class II molecules show strong support for a genetic link in the development of SLE.[35] The genes involved in inherited complement deficiencies also seem to influence disease susceptibility.[26,36]

There are many indications that in addition to genetic factors, several environmental factors may be involved in the pathogenesis of SLE. Certain drugs may provoke a lupus-like disorder in susceptible persons, particularly in the elderly. The most common of these drugs are hydralazine and procainamide. Other drugs, such as quinidine, methyldopa, isoniazid, and phenytoin, also have been known to produce this syndrome.[26] The disease usually recedes when use of the drug is discontinued. Exposure to ultraviolet light is another environmental factor that exacerbates the disease in many individuals.[36] How ultraviolet light exerts is action is unclear, but it is suspected of modulating the immune response. For example, it is known to induce keratinocytes to produce IL-1, a factor known to influence the immune response.

Sex hormones also seem to exert an influence on the occurrence and manifestations of SLE. During the reproductive years, the frequency of SLE is 10 times greater in women than in men, and exacerbations have been noted during menses and pregnancy.[36]

Clinical Manifestations. Systemic lupus erythematosus can manifest in a variety of ways. The disease has been called the *great imitator* because it has the capacity for affecting many different body systems, including the musculoskeletal system, the skin, the cardiovascular system, the lungs, the kidneys, the central nervous system (CNS), and the red blood cells and platelets. The onset may be acute or insidious, and the course of the disease is characterized by exacerbations and remissions.

Arthralgia and arthritis are among the most commonly occurring early symptoms of SLE; approximately 90% of all persons with the disease report joint pain at some point during the course of their disease.[34] The polyarthritis of SLE initially can be confused with other forms of arthritis, especially RA, because of the symmetric arthropathy. Ligaments, tendons, and the joint capsule may be involved, causing varied deformities in approximately 30% of persons with the disease. Flexion contractures, hyperextension of the interphalangeal joint, and subluxation of the carpometacarpal joint contribute to deformity and subsequent loss of function in the hands. Other musculoskeletal manifestations include tenosynovitis, rupture of the intrapatellar and Achilles tendons, and avascular necrosis, frequently of the femoral head.

Skin manifestations can vary greatly and may be classified as acute, subacute, or chronic. The acute skin lesions include the classic malar or "butterfly" rash on the nose and cheeks (Fig. 43-8). This rash is seen in SLE but may be associated with other skin lesions, such as hives or livedo reticularis (*i.e.*, reticular cyanotic discoloration of the skin, often precipitated by cold). Fingertip lesions, such as periungual erythema, nail fold infarcts, and splinter hemorrhages, also are seen. Hair loss is common. Mucous membrane lesions tend to occur during periods of exacerbation. Sun sensitivity may occur in SLE even after mild sun exposure.

Renal involvement occurs in approximately one half to two thirds of persons with SLE.[26] Several forms of glomerulonephritis may occur, including mesangial, focal proliferative, diffuse proliferative, and membranous

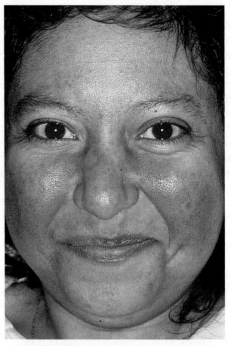

FIGURE 43-8 The butterfly (malar) rash of systemic lupus erythematosus. (Reprinted from the ARHP Arthritis Teaching Slide Collection. Used with permission of the American College of Rheumatology.)

(see Chapter 25). Interstitial nephritis also may occur. Nephrotic syndrome causes proteinuria with resultant edema in the legs, abdomen, and around the eyes. Renal failure may or may not be preceded by the nephrotic syndrome. Kidney biopsy is the best determinant of renal damage and the extent of treatment needed.

The heart and lungs frequently are sites of complications in people with SLE.[36] Pulmonary involvement in SLE occurs in more than 30% of persons and is manifested primarily by pleural effusions or pleuritis.[26] Less frequently occurring pulmonary problems include acute pneumonitis, pulmonary hemorrhage, chronic interstitial lung disease, and pulmonary embolism. Pericarditis is the most common of the cardiac manifestations, occurring in up to 30% to 40% of persons with SLE. Accelerated atherosclerosis has also received considerable attention and is an important cause of morbidity and mortality in SLE.[26] Hypertension may be associated with lupus nephritis and long-term corticosteroid use. Hematologic disorders may manifest as hemolytic anemia, leukopenia, lymphopenia, or thrombocytopenia.

The CNS is involved in approximately two thirds of persons with SLE.[26] The pathologic basis for CNS symptoms is not entirely clear. It has been ascribed to an acute vasculitis that impedes blood flow, causing strokes or hemorrhage; an immune response involving anti-neuronal antibodies that attack nerve cells; or production of anti-phospholipid antibodies that damage blood vessels and cause blood clots in the brain. Seizures can occur and are more common when renal failure is present. Psychotic symptoms, including depression and unnatural euphoria, as well as decreased cognitive functioning, confusion, and altered levels of consciousness, may develop.

There is also a localized cutaneous form of lupus erythematosus called *discoid lupus erythematosus*, with no associated systemic effects. The cutaneous form of lupus erythematosus involves plaquelike lesions of the head, scalp, and neck. These lesions first appear as red, swollen patches on the skin, and later there can be scarring, depigmentation, and plugging of hair follicles. The cutaneous lesions may develop or worsen with sun exposure. Although persons with discoid lupus erythematosus usually do not go on to develop systemic disease, about one third of persons with SLE may exhibit skin lesions that are indistinguishable from those of discoid type.[36]

Diagnosis and Treatment. The diagnosis of SLE is based on a complete history, physical examination, and analysis of blood work. No single test can diagnose SLE in all persons. The most common laboratory test performed is the immunofluorescence test for ANA. Ninety-five percent of persons with untreated SLE have high ANA levels. Although the ANA test is not specific for lupus, it establishes that the differential diagnosis includes autoimmunity. The anti-DNA antibody test is more specific for the diagnosis of SLE.[37] Other serum tests may reveal moderate to severe anemia, thrombocytopenia, and leukocytosis or leukopenia. Additional immunologic tests may be done to support the diagnosis or to differentiate SLE from other connective tissue diseases.

Treatment of SLE focuses on managing the acute and chronic symptoms of the disease. The goals of treatment include preventing progressive loss of organ function, reducing the possibility of exacerbations, minimizing disability from the disease process, and preventing complications from medication therapy.[38] Treatment with medications may be as simple as a drug to reduce inflammation, such as an NSAID. NSAIDs can control fever, arthritis, and mild pleuritis. An antimalarial drug (*e.g.*, hydroxychloroquine) may be the next medication considered to treat cutaneous and musculoskeletal manifestations of SLE. Corticosteroids are used to treat more significant symptoms of SLE, such as renal and CNS disorders. High-dose corticosteroid treatment is used for acute symptoms, and the drug is tapered to the lowest therapeutic dose as soon as possible to minimize adverse effects. Immunosuppressive drugs are used in cases of severe disease.

Systemic Sclerosis

Systemic sclerosis, sometimes called *scleroderma,* is an autoimmune disease of connective tissue characterized by excessive collagen deposition in the skin and internal organs, such as the lungs, gastrointestinal tract, heart, and kidneys. In this disorder, the skin is thickened through fibrosis, with an accompanying fixation of subdermal structures, including the sheaths or fascia covering tendons and muscles.[39] Systemic sclerosis affects women four times as frequently as men, with a peak incidence in the 35- to 50-year age group.[40] The cause of this rare disorder is poorly understood. There is evidence of both humoral and cellular immune system abnormalities.

Scleroderma presents as two distinct clinical entities: the diffuse or generalized form of the disease and the limited or CREST variant. In the CREST syndrome, hardening of the skin (scleroderma) is limited to the hands and face, whereas the skin changes in diffuse scleroderma also involve the trunk and proximal extremities. Almost all persons with scleroderma develop polyarthritis and Raynaud phenomenon, a vascular disorder characterized by reversible vasospasm of the arteries supplying the fingers (see Chapter 17).

Diffuse scleroderma is characterized by severe and progressive disease of the skin and the early onset of organ involvement. The typical person has a *stone facies* caused by tightening of the facial skin with restricted motion of the mouth. Involvement of the esophagus leads to hypomotility and difficulty swallowing. Malabsorption may develop if the submucosal and muscular atrophy affect the intestine. Pulmonary involvement leads to dyspnea and eventually respiratory failure. Vascular involvement of the kidneys is responsible for malignant hypertension and progressive renal insufficiency. Cardiac problems include pericarditis, heart block, and myocardial fibrosis.

The CREST syndrome is manifested by calcinosis (*i.e.*, calcium deposits in the subcutaneous tissue that erupt through the skin), Raynaud phenomenon, esophageal dysmotility, sclerodactyly (localized scleroderma of the fingers), and telangiectasia.

Treatment of systemic sclerosis is largely symptomatic and supportive. Studies have indicated that if heart, lung, or kidney involvement is to become severe, it tends to do so early in the disease and is a predictor of shortened survival. Advances in treatment, primarily the use of angiotensin-converting enzyme (ACE) inhibitors in renal involvement, have led to a substantial decrease in the mortality rate from hypertensive renal disease.[40] There is also some evidence that ACE inhibitors may be disease modifying.[41]

SERONEGATIVE SPONDYLOARTHROPATHIES

The *spondyloarthropathies* are an inter-related group of multisystem inflammatory disorders that primarily affect the axial skeleton, particularly the spine. Typically, the inflammation begins at sites where tendon and ligament insert into bone rather than in the synovium. Sacroiliitis is a pathologic hallmark of the disorders. Persons with the spondyloarthropathies may also have inflammation and involvement of the peripheral joints, in which case the signs and symptoms overlap with other inflammatory types of arthritis. Because the RF is absent, these disorders often are referred to as *seronegative spondyloarthropathies*.

The seronegative spondyloarthropathies include ankylosing spondylitis, juvenile ankylosing spondylitis, reactive arthritis (*e.g.,* Reiter syndrome), enteropathic arthritis (*i.e.,* inflammatory bowel disease), and psoriatic arthritis. Although they differ in terms of factors such as age and type of onset and extent of joint involvement, there is clinical evidence of overlap between the various seronegative spondyloarthropathies (Table 43-1). In none of these disorders is the cause or pathogenesis well understood. There is, however, a striking association with the HLA-B27 antigen, but the presence of the HLA-B27 antigen by itself is neither necessary nor sufficient for the development of any of the diseases.

Ankylosing Spondylitis

Ankylosing spondylitis is a chronic, systemic inflammatory disease of the joints of the axial skeleton manifested by pain and progressive stiffening of the spine. The disease is more common than once was believed, affecting approximately 2% to 8% of the HLA-B27–positive white population.[26] Clinical manifestations usually begin in late adolescence or early adulthood and are slightly more common in men than in women. The disease usually evolves more slowly and is less severe in women.

Ankylosing spondylitis produces an inflammatory erosion of the sites where tendons and ligaments attach to bone.[26] Typically, the disease process begins with bilateral involvement of the sacroiliac joints and then moves to the smaller joints of the posterior elements of the spine. The result is ultimate destruction of these joints with ankylosis or posterior fusion of the spine. The vertebrae take on a squared appearance and bone bridges fuse one vertebral body to the next across the intervertebral disks (Fig. 43-9). Progressive spinal changes usually follow an ascending pattern up the spine. Occasionally, large synovial joints (*i.e.,* hips, knees, and shoulders) may be involved. The small peripheral joints usually are not affected. The disease spectrum ranges from an asymptomatic sacroiliitis to a progressive disease that can affect many body systems.

Etiology and Pathogenesis. Although the pathogenesis of ankylosing spondylitis has not been established, the presence of mononuclear cells in acutely involved tissue suggests an immune response. Epidemiologic findings indicate that genetic and environmental factors play a role in the pathogenesis of the disease. The HLA-B27 antigen remains one of the best-known examples of an association between a disease and a hereditary marker.[26] Although approximately 90% of people with ankylosing spondylitis possess the HLA-B27 antigen, the HLA-B27 antigen also is present in approximately 8% of the normal population. Several theories have been advanced to explain the association between the HLA-B27 antigen and ankylosing spondylitis. One possibility is that the gene that determines the HLA-B27 antigen may be linked to other genes that predispose to the development of ankylosing spondylitis or lead to increased susceptibility to infections or environmental agents that are associated with the disorder. A second explanation focuses on molecular mimicry: an immune reaction to a foreign agent, usually an infectious organism, that expresses antigens that have the same amino acid sequence as self-antigens.[42]

TABLE 43-1	**Comparison of the Spondyloarthropathies**			
Characteristics	Ankylosing Spondylitis	Reiter Syndrome	Psoriatic Arthritis	Inflammatory Bowel Disease
Age at onset	Young adult	Young to middle age	Any age	Any age
Type of onset	Gradual	Sudden	Variable	Gradual
Sacroiliitis	>95%	20%	20%	10%
Peripheral joint involvement	25%	90%	All (about 5% to 7% of those patients with psoriasis)	Occasional
HLA-B27 (in whites)	>90%	75%	<50%	<50%
Eye involvement	25% to 30%	Common	Occasional	Occasional

(Developed from data in Arnett F. C., Khan M. A., Willikens R. F. [1989]. A new look at ankylosing spondylitis. *Patient Care* 23[19], 82–101.)

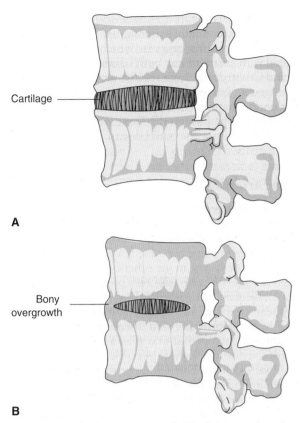

A

Cartilage

B

Bony overgrowth

FIGURE 43-9 The bony overgrowth (**B**) of the vertebra characteristic of ankylosing spondylitis is evident when compared with normal vertebra (**A**).

Clinical Manifestations. The person with ankylosing spondylitis typically reports low back pain, which may be persistent or intermittent. The pain, which becomes worse when resting, particularly when lying in bed, initially may be blamed on muscle strain or spasm from physical activity. Lumbosacral pain also may be present, with discomfort in the buttocks and hip areas. Sometimes, pain can radiate to the thigh in a manner similar to that of sciatic pain. Prolonged stiffness is present in the morning and after periods of rest. Mild physical activity or a hot shower helps reduce pain and stiffness. Sleep patterns frequently are interrupted because of these manifestations. Walking or exercise may be needed to provide the comfort necessary for a return to sleep.

Loss of motion in the spinal column is characteristic of the disease. The severity and duration of disease activity influence the degree of mobility. Loss of lumbar lordosis occurs as the disease progresses, and this is followed by kyphosis of the thoracic spine and extension of the neck. A spine fused in the flexed position is the end result in severe ankylosing spondylitis. A kyphotic spine makes it difficult for the patient to look ahead and to maintain balance while walking. The image is one of a person bent over looking at the floor and unable to straighten up. X-ray films show a rigid, bamboo-like spine. The heart and lungs are constricted in the chest cavity. Abnormal weight bearing can lead to degeneration and destruction of the hips, necessitating joint replacement procedures. Peripheral arthritis is more common in hips and shoulders. The incidence of hip joint involvement varies from 17% to 36% and potentially is more crippling than involvement in any other joint.[26]

The most common extraskeletal involvement is acute anterior uveitis, which occurs in 25% to 30% of patients at some time in the course of their disease.[26] Systemic features of weight loss, fever, and fatigue may be apparent. Sometimes, the fatigue is a greater problem than pain or stiffness. Osteoporosis can occur, especially in the spine, which contributes to the risk of spinal fracture. Fusion of the costovertebral joints can lead to reduced lung volume.

The disease process varies considerably among individuals. Exacerbations and remissions are common; their unpredictability can create uncertainty in planning daily activities and in setting goals. Fortunately, most of those affected are able to lead productive lives. The prognosis for ankylosing spondylitis in general is good. The progression of the disease during the first decade of disease predicts the remainder. Severe disease usually occurs early and is marked by peripheral arthritis, especially of the hip.

Diagnosis and Treatment. The diagnosis of ankylosing spondylitis is based on history, physical examination, and x-ray examination. Laboratory findings frequently include an elevated ESR. A mild normocytic normochromic anemia may be present. Because HLA-B27 is found in 8% of the normal population, it is not a specific diagnostic test for the disease. Radiologic evaluations help differentiate sacroiliitis from other diseases.

Treatment is directed at controlling pain and maintaining mobility by suppressing inflammation. Therapeutic exercises are important to assist in maintaining motion in peripheral joints and in the spine. Muscle-strengthening exercises for extensor muscle groups also are prescribed. Immobilizing joints is not recommended. Maintaining ideal weight reduces the stress on weight-bearing joints.

Pharmacologic treatment includes the use of NSAIDs to reduce inflammation, relieve pain, and reduce muscle spasm. Phenylbutazone is highly effective, but its use is usually limited to persons with severe disease in whom other agents have failed because of potential bone marrow suppression with long-term use. More recently, promising small-scale studies have suggested anti–TNF-α agents are efficacious in the treatment of active ankylosing spondylitis.[43]

Reactive Arthropathies

The reactive arthropathies may be defined as sterile inflammatory joint disorders that are distant in time and place from the initial inciting infective process. The infecting agents cannot be cultured, and are not viable once having reached the joints. The list of triggering agents is continuously increasing and may be divided into urogenic, enterogenic, and respiratory tract–associated, and the idiopathic arthritides. In some cases, the identity of the causative agent is unknown.[44]

Commonly recognized forms of reactive arthritis include those involving *Chlamydia pneumoniae* infection and *Pseudomonas*. Additional and frequently occurring pathogens include *Chlamydia trachomatis, Salmonella, Shigella, Yersinia, Campylobacter,* and *Streptococcus.*[44] Reactive arthritis also has been observed in persons with AIDS. Spondyloarthropathies such as Reiter syndrome and psoriatic arthritis are more severe and frequent in HIV-infected patients than in the general population. It is thought that the immune response to HIV infection is selective and largely spares the natural killer cells, which may be critical in the pathogenesis of these conditions.[45] This is in contrast to RA and SLE, which dramatically improve as immunodeficiency develops. Reactive arthritis may also result from the presence of a foreign substance in the joint tissue, such as silicone implants in the small joints of the hand or feet or after exposure to industrial gases and oils. However, there is no evidence for antigenicity of the causative substance.

In the strictest sense, the definition of reactive arthritis includes a possibility of immunologic sensitization before arthritic development.[45] Similarities exist between reactive arthritis and bacterial arthritis. Several bacteria cause both diseases. When cultured bacteria are isolated from the synovial fluid, the diagnosis is bacterial arthritis. When they cannot be isolated, even though there has been a preceding infection, the diagnosis of reactive arthritis is made.

Reactive arthritis may follow a self-limited course; it may involve recurrent episodes of arthritis; or, in a small number of cases, it may follow a continuous and unremitting course. The treatment is largely symptomatic. NSAIDs are used in treating the arthritic symptoms. Vigorous treatment of possible triggering infections is thought to prevent relapses of reactive arthritis, but in many cases, the triggering infection passes unnoticed or is mild, and the patient contacts a physician only with the onset of definite arthritis. Short antibiotic courses at this time are not effective.

Reiter Syndrome. Reiter syndrome is considered to be a clinical manifestation of reactive arthritis that may be accompanied by extra-articular symptoms such as uveitis, bowel inflammation, and carditis. The disease develops in a genetically susceptible host after a bacterial infection due to *C. trachomatis* in the genitourinary tract or *Salmonella, Shigella, Yersinia,* or *Campylobacter* in the gastrointestinal tract.

The term *Reiter syndrome* soon may be relegated to history as the pathogenesis becomes better understood. Alternative designations include SARA (sexually associated reactive arthritis) and the BASE syndrome (HLA-B27, arthritis, sacroiliitis, and extra-articular inflammation).[45] Reiter syndrome was the first rheumatic disease to be recognized in association with HIV infection. Symptoms of arthritis may precede any overt signs of HIV disease. Treatment with agents such as methotrexate and azathioprine may further suppress the immune response and provoke a full expression of AIDS.

Enteropathic Arthritis. Arthritis that is associated with an inflammatory bowel disease usually is considered an enteropathic arthritis because the intestinal disease is directly involved in the pathogenesis. Most cases of enteropathic arthritis are classified among the spondyloarthropathies. These include cases in which the arthritis is associated with inflammatory bowel disease (*i.e.,* ulcerative colitis and Crohn disease), the reactive arthritides triggered by enterogenic bacteria, some of the undifferentiated spondyloarthropathies, Whipple disease, and reactions after intestinal bypass surgery.[26] There is no direct relation between the activity of the bowel disease and the degree of arthritis activity.

Psoriatic Arthritis

Psoriatic arthritis is a seronegative inflammatory arthropathy that occurs in 5% to 7% of people with psoriasis. It is a heterogeneous disease with features of the spondyloarthropathies in some persons, RA in others, and features of both coexisting in yet others.

The etiology of psoriasis and psoriatic arthritis is unknown. Genetic, environmental, and immunologic factors appear to affect susceptibility and play a role in expression of the psoriatic skin disease and the arthritis. Environmental factors that may play a role in the pathogenesis of the disorder include infectious agents and physical trauma. T-cell–mediated immune responses also seem to play an important role in the skin and joint manifestations of the disease, as indicated by the observation that there is improvement in disease status after treatment with immunosuppressant agents such as cyclosporine.

Although the arthritis can antedate detectable skin rash, the definitive diagnosis of psoriatic arthritis cannot be made without evidence of skin or nail changes typical of psoriasis. Psoriatic arthritis falls into five subgroups: oligoarticular or asymmetric (48%); spondyloarthropathy (24%); polyarticular, or symmetric (18%); distal interphalangeal (8%); and mutilans, or disfiguring (2%).[46] This heterogeneous clinical presentation suggests more than one disease is associated with psoriasis, or that there are various clinical responses to a common cause. At least 20% of those with psoriatic arthritis have an elevated serum level of uric acid, which is caused by the rapid skin turnover of psoriasis and the subsequent breakdown of nucleic acids, followed by their metabolism to uric acid. This finding may lead to a misdiagnosis of gout. Psoriatic arthritis tends to be slowly progressive, but has a more favorable prognosis than RA.

Basic management is similar to the treatment of RA. Suppression of the skin disease may be important in helping to control the arthritis. Often, affected joints are surprisingly functional and only minimally symptomatic. The biologic response modifiers, specifically the TNF inhibitors (*e.g.,* etanercept and infliximab), have been found to be beneficial in controlling the arthritis as well as the psoriasis in patients with psoriatic arthritis.[46]

OSTEOARTHRITIS SYNDROME

Osteoarthritis (OA), formerly called *degenerative joint disease,* is the most prevalent form of arthritis and a leading cause of disability and pain in the elderly. Osteoarthritis is more of a disease process than a specific entity. The term encompasses a heterogeneous collection of syndromes, including osteoarthritis of the hand, knee, hip, foot, and spine.[47] It can occur as a primary idiopathic disorder or as a secondary disorder, although this distinction is not always clear. Idiopathic or primary variants of OA occur as localized or generalized (*i.e.*, involvement of more than three joints) syndromes.[26] Secondary OA has a known underlying cause such as congenital or acquired defects of joint structures, trauma, metabolic disorders, or inflammatory diseases (Chart 43-3).

The joint changes associated with OA, which include a progressive loss of articular cartilage and synovitis, result from the inflammation caused when cartilage attempts to repair itself, creating osteophytes or spurs. These changes are accompanied by joint pain, stiffness, limitation of motion, and in some cases by joint instability and deformity. Fortunately, changes in the traditional conservative management of this underemphasized condition are occurring. Attitudes regarding the inevitability of the limitations imposed by this condition are changing on the part of health care providers and persons with the disease.

Age and gender interact to influence the time of onset and, with race, the pattern of joint involvement in OA. Men are affected more commonly at a younger age than women, but the rate at which women are affected exceeds that of men by middle age.[26] Heredity influences the occurrence of hand OA in the DIP joint. Hand OA is more likely to affect white women, whereas knee OA is more common in black women. The incidence of hip OA is less among the Chinese than Europeans, perhaps representing the influence of other factors such as occupation, obesity, or heredity. Bone mass may also influence the risk of developing OA. In theory, thinner subchondral bone may provide a greater shock-absorbing function than denser bone, allowing less direct trauma to the cartilage.

Obesity is a particular risk factor for OA of the knee in women and a contributory biomechanical factor in the pathogenesis of the disease. Excess fat may have a direct metabolic effect on cartilage beyond the effects of excess joint stress. Weight loss reduces the risk of developing symptomatic arthritis of the knee.[48] Although the radiographic incidence of knee OA increases with advancing age, the incidence of symptomatic OA of the knee decreases.[48]

Pathogenesis

The pathogenesis of OA resides in the homeostatic mechanisms that maintain the articular cartilage. Articular cartilage plays two essential mechanical roles in joint physiology. First, it serves as a remarkably smooth weight-bearing surface. In combination with synovial fluid, the articular cartilage provides extremely low friction during movement of the joint. Second, the cartilage transmits the load down to the bone, dissipating the mechanical stress.[1] The subchondral bone protects the overlying articular cartilage, providing it with a pliable bed and absorbing the energy of the force (Fig. 43-10).

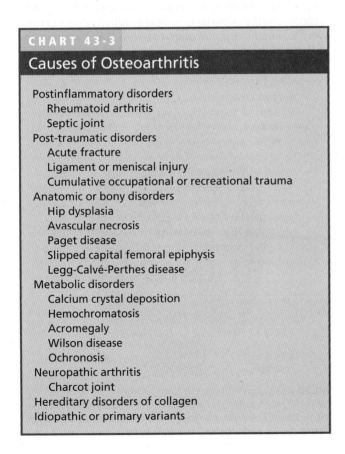

CHART 43-3

Causes of Osteoarthritis

Postinflammatory disorders
  Rheumatoid arthritis
  Septic joint
Post-traumatic disorders
  Acute fracture
  Ligament or meniscal injury
  Cumulative occupational or recreational trauma
Anatomic or bony disorders
  Hip dysplasia
  Avascular necrosis
  Paget disease
  Slipped capital femoral epiphysis
  Legg-Calvé-Perthes disease
Metabolic disorders
  Calcium crystal deposition
  Hemochromatosis
  Acromegaly
  Wilson disease
  Ochronosis
Neuropathic arthritis
  Charcot joint
Hereditary disorders of collagen
Idiopathic or primary variants

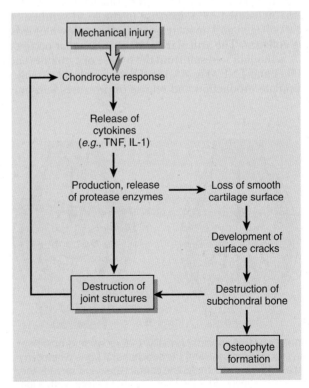

FIGURE 43-10 Disease process in osteoarthritis.

Cartilage is a specialized type of connective tissue. As with other types of tissue, it consists of cells (*i.e.,* chondrocytes) nested in an extracellular matrix. In articular cartilage, the extracellular matrix is composed of water, proteoglycans, collagen, and ground substance. The proteoglycans, which are large macromolecules made up of disaccharides and amino acids, afford elasticity and stiffness, permitting articular cartilage to resist compression. The ground substance constitutes a highly hydrated, semisolid gel. Collagen molecules consist of polypeptide chains that form long fibrous strands. They provide form and tensile strength. The primary function of the collagen fibers is to provide a rigid scaffold to support the chondrocytes and ground substance of cartilage. The hydrated proteoglycan molecules, because of their macromolecular size and charge, are trapped in the collagen meshwork of the extracellular matrix and prevented from expanding to their maximum size. This confers the high interstitial osmotic pressure and fluid volume that is needed for lubrication of the joint.[49] As in the case of adult bone, articular cartilage is not static; it undergoes turnover and its "worn out" matrix components are continually degraded and replaced. This turnover is maintained by the chondrocytes, which not only synthesize the matrix but secrete matrix-degrading enzymes. Thus, the health of the chondrocytes determines joint integrity.

Popularly known as *wear and tear* arthritis, OA is characterized by significant changes in both the composition and mechanical properties of cartilage. Early in the course of the disease, the cartilage contains increased water and decreased concentrations of proteoglycans compared with healthy cartilage. In addition, there appears to be a weakening of the collagen network, presumably caused by a decrease in the local synthesis of new collagen and an increase in the breakdown of existing collagen. The articular cartilage injury that occurs in OA is thought to result from the release of cytokines such as IL-1 and TNF[1] (Fig. 43-11). These chemical messengers stimulate production and release of proteases (enzymes)

that are destructive to joint structures.[1] The resulting damage predisposes the chondrocytes to more injury and impairs their ability to repair the damage by producing new collagen and proteoglycans. The combined effects of inadequate repair mechanisms and imbalances between the proteases and their inhibitors contribute further to disease progression.

The earliest structural changes in OA include enlargement and reorganization of the chondrocytes in the superficial part of the articular cartilage. This is accompanied by edematous changes in the cartilaginous matrix, principally the intermediate layer. The cartilage loses its smooth aspect and surface cracks or microfractures occur, allowing synovial fluid to enter and widen the crack. As the crack deepens, vertical clefts form and eventually extend through the full thickness of the articular surface and into the subchondral bone.[1] Portions of the articular cartilage eventually become completely eroded and the exposed surface of the subchondral bone becomes thickened and polished to an ivory-like consistency (eburnation). Fragments of cartilage and bone often become dislodged, creating free-floating osteocartilaginous bodies ("joint mice") that enter the joint cavity. Synovial fluid may leak though the defects in the residual cartilage to form cysts within the bone.[1] As the disease progresses, the underlying trabecular bone becomes sclerotic in response to increased pressure on the surface of the joint, rendering it less effective as a shock absorber. Sclerosis, or formation of new bone and cysts, usually occurs at the joint margins, forming abnormal bony outgrowths called *osteophytes,* or spurs (Fig. 43-12). As the joint begins to lose its integrity, there is trauma to the synovial membrane, which results in nonspecific inflammation. Compared with RA, however, the changes in the synovium that occur in OA are not as pronounced, nor do they occur as early.

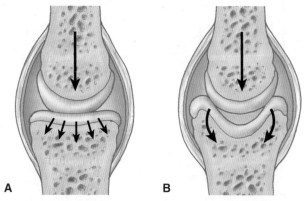

FIGURE 43-11 (**A**) A joint normally undergoes deformation of the articular cartilage and the subchondral bone when carrying a load. This maximizes the contact area and spreads the force of the load. (**B**) If the joint does not deform with a load, the stresses are concentrated and the joint breaks down.

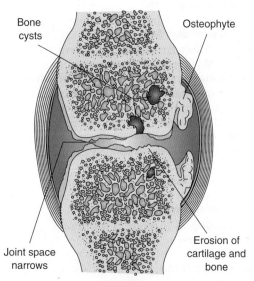

FIGURE 43-12 Joint changes in osteoarthritis. The left side shows early changes and joint space narrowing with cartilage breakdown. The right side shows more severe disease progression with lost cartilage and osteophyte formation.

In secondary forms of OA, repetitive impact loading contributes to joint failure, accounting for the high prevalence of OA specific to vocational or avocational sites, such as the shoulders and elbows of baseball pitchers, ankles of ballet dancers, and knees of basketball players. Immobilization also can produce degenerative changes in articular cartilage. Cartilage degeneration due to immobility may result from loss of the pumping action of lubrication that occurs with joint movement. These changes are more marked and appear earlier in areas of contact but occur also in areas not subject to mechanical compression. Although cartilage atrophy is rapidly reversible with activity after a period of immobilization, impact exercise during the period of remobilization can prevent reversal of the atrophy. Therefore, slow and gradual remobilization may be important in preventing cartilage injury. Clinically, it has implications for instructions concerning the recommended level of physical activity after removal of a cast.

Clinical Manifestations

The manifestations of OA may occur suddenly or insidiously. Initially, pain may be described as aching and may be somewhat difficult to localize. It worsens with use or activity and is usually relieved by rest. In later stages of disease activity, pain may be experienced during rest and for several hours after the use of the involved joints. Crepitus and grinding may be evident when the joint is moved. As the disease advances, even minimal activity may cause pain because of the limited range of motion resulting from intra-articular and periarticular structural damage.

The most frequently affected joints are the hips, knees, lumbar and cervical vertebrae, proximal and distal joints of the hand, the first carpometacarpal joint, and the first metatarsophalangeal joints of the feet. A single joint or several may be affected. Although a single weight-bearing joint may be involved initially, other joints often become affected because of the additional stress placed on them while trying to protect the original joint. It is not unusual for a person having a knee replacement to discover soon after the surgery is done that the second knee also needs to be replaced. Other clinical features are limitations of joint motion and joint instability. Joint enlargement usually results from new bone formation; the joint feels hard, in contrast to the soft, spongy feeling characteristic of the joint in RA. Sometimes, mild synovitis or increased synovial fluid can cause joint enlargement.

Diagnosis and Treatment

The diagnosis of OA usually is determined by history and physical examination, x-ray studies, and laboratory findings that exclude other diseases. Although OA often is contrasted with RA for diagnostic purposes, the differences are not always readily apparent. Other rheumatic diseases may be superimposed on OA.

Characteristic radiologic changes initially include medial joint space narrowing, followed by subchondral bony sclerosis, formation of spikes on the tibial eminence, and osteophytes. The results of laboratory studies usually are normal because the disorder is not a systemic disease. The ESR may be slightly elevated in generalized OA or erosive inflammatory variations of the disease. If inflammation is present, there may be a slight increase in the white blood cell count. The synovial fluid usually is normal.

Because there is no cure, the treatment of OA is symptomatic and includes physical rehabilitative, pharmacologic, and surgical measures. Physical measures are aimed at improving the supporting structures of the joint and strengthening opposing muscle groups involved in cushioning weight-bearing forces. These include a balance of rest and exercise, use of splints to protect and rest the joint, use of heat and cold to relieve pain and muscle spasm, and adjusting the activities of daily living. The involved joint should not be further abused, and steps should be taken to protect and rest it. This includes weight reduction (when weight-bearing surfaces are involved) and the use of a cane or walker if the hips and knees are involved. Muscle-strengthening exercises may help protect the joint and decrease pain.[47]

Pharmacologic treatment is aimed at reducing inflammation or providing analgesia. The most common medications used in the treatment of OA are the NSAIDs, many of which are available without a prescription. For many persons, acetaminophen in doses as high as 4000 mg/day may be as effective and less toxic than NSAIDs. The American College of Rheumatology (ACR) recommends the use of acetaminophen as the initial systemic treatment for OA.[50]

Intra-articular corticosteroid injections may be used for relieving symptoms, especially for those who have an effusion of the joint. Injections usually are limited to two to three times a year because their use is thought to accelerate joint destruction.[26] Vesicosupplementation, a newer concept in the treatment of OA, involves the injection of sodium hyaluronate into the joint with the goal of improving joint lubrication.[51]

Surgery is considered when the person is having severe pain and joint function is severely reduced. Procedures include arthroscopic lavage and debridement, bunion resections, osteotomies to change alignment of the knee and hip joints, and decompression of the spinal roots in osteoarthritic vertebral stenosis. Total hip replacements have provided effective relief of symptoms and improved range of motion for many persons, as have total knee replacements, although the latter procedure has produced less consistent results.

CRYSTAL-INDUCED ARTHROPATHIES

Crystal deposition in joints produces arthritis. In gout, monosodium urate or uric acid crystals are found in the joint cavity. Another condition in which calcium pyrophosphate dihydrate crystals are found in the joints sometimes is referred to as *pseudogout* (discussed in the section on rheumatic diseases in the elderly).

Gout

Gout is actually a group of diseases known as the *gout syndrome.*[52,53] It includes acute gouty arthritis with recurrent attacks of severe articular and periarticular inflammation; tophi or the accumulation of crystalline deposits in articular surfaces, bones, soft tissue, and cartilage; gouty nephropathy or renal impairment; and uric acid kidney stones.

The term *primary gout* is used to designate cases in which the cause of the disorder is unknown or an inborn error in metabolism and is characterized primarily by hyperuricemia and gout. Primary gout is predominantly a disease of men, with a peak incidence in the fourth or sixth decade. In secondary gout, the cause of the hyperuricemia is known but the accompanying arthritis is not the main disorder. Asymptomatic hyperuricemia is a laboratory finding and not a disease. Most persons with hyperuricemia do not develop gout.

Pathogenesis. The pathogenesis of gout resides in an elevation of the serum uric acid levels. Uric acid is the end product of purine (adenine and guanine from DNA and ribonucleic acid [RNA]) metabolism.[1] Two pathways are involved in purine synthesis: (1) a de novo pathway, in which purines are synthesized from nonpurine precursors, and (2) the salvage pathway, in which purine bases are recaptured from the breakdown of nucleic acids derived from exogenous (dietary) or endogenous sources. The elevation of uric acid and the subsequent development of gout can result from (1) overproduction of purines, (2) decreased salvage of free purine bases, (3) augmented breakdown of nucleic acids as a result of increased cell turnover, or (4) decreased urinary excretion of uric acid. Primary gout, which constitutes 90% of cases, is due to enzyme defects resulting from an overproduction of uric acid, inadequate elimination of uric acid by the kidney, or a combination of the two. In most

cases, the reason is unknown. In secondary gout, the hyperuricemia may be caused by increased breakdown of nucleic acids, as occurs with rapid tumor cell lysis during treatment for lymphoma or leukemia. Other cases of secondary gout result from chronic renal disease. Some of the diuretics, including the thiazides, can interfere with the excretion of uric acid.

An attack of gout occurs when monosodium urate crystals precipitate in the joint and initiate an inflammatory response. Synovial fluid is a poorer solvent for uric acid than plasma, and uric acid crystals are even less soluble at temperatures below 37°C.[1] Crystal deposition usually occurs in peripheral areas of the body, such as the great toe, where the temperatures are cooler than other parts of the body. With prolonged hyperuricemia, crystals and microtophi accumulate in the cells of the synovial lining and in the joint cartilage. The released crystals are chemotactic to leukocytes and also activate complement, leading to inflammation and destructive changes to the cartilage and subchondral bone. Repeated attacks of acute arthritis eventually lead to chronic arthritis and the formation of tophi. Tophi are large, hard nodules that have irregular surfaces and contain crystalline deposits of monosodium urate[4] (Fig. 43-13). They are found most commonly in the synovium, olecranon bursa, Achilles tendon, subchondral bone, and extensor surface of the forearm and may be mistaken for rheumatoid nodules. Tophi usually do not appear until 10 years or more after the first gout attack. This stage of gout, called *chronic tophaceous* gout, is characterized by more frequent and prolonged attacks, which often are polyarticular.

Clinical Manifestations. The typical acute attack of gout is monoarticular and usually affects the first metatarsophalangeal joint. The tarsal joints, insteps, ankles, heels, knees, wrists, fingers, and elbows also may be initial sites of involvement. Acute gouty arthritis often begins at night

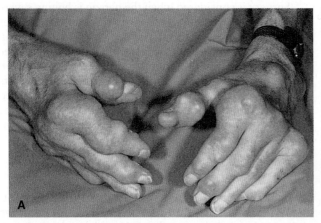
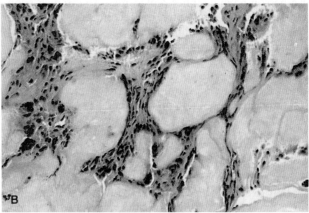

FIGURE 43-13 Gout. (**A**) Gouty tophi project from the fingers as rubbery nodules. (**B**) A section from a tophus shows extracellular masses of urate crystals with accompanying foreign-body giant cells. (From Rubin E., Farber J. L. [Eds.]. [1999]. *Pathology* [3rd ed., p. 1404]. Philadelphia: Lippincott Williams & Wilkins.)

and may be precipitated by excessive exercise, certain medications, foods, alcohol, or dieting. The onset of pain typically is abrupt, and redness and swelling are observed. The attack may last for days or weeks. Pain may be severe enough to be aggravated even by the weight of a bed sheet covering the affected area.

In the early stages of gout after the initial attack has subsided, the person is asymptomatic, and joint abnormalities are not evident. This is referred to as *intercritical gout*. After the first attack, it may be months or years before another attack. As attacks recur with increased frequency, joint changes occur and become permanent.

Diagnosis and Treatment. Although hyperuricemia is the biochemical hallmark of gout, the presence of hyperuricemia cannot be equated with gout because many persons with this condition never develop gout. A definitive diagnosis of gout can be made only when monosodium urate crystals are identified in the synovial fluid or in tissue sections of tophaceous deposits. Synovial fluid analysis is useful in excluding other conditions, such as septic arthritis, pseudogout, and RA. Diagnostic methods also include measures to determine if the disorder is related to overproduction or underexcretion of uric acid. This is done through measurement of serum uric acid levels and collection of a 24-hour urine sample for determination of urate excretion in the urine.[54]

The objectives for treatment of gout include the termination and prevention of the acute attacks of gouty arthritis and the correction of hyperuricemia, with consequent inhibition of further precipitation of sodium urate and absorption of urate crystal deposits already in the tissues. Some changes in lifestyle may be needed, such as maintenance of ideal weight, moderation in alcohol consumption, and avoiding purine-rich foods, such as liver, kidney, sardines, anchovies, and sweetbreads, particularly by persons with excessive tophaceous deposits.

Pharmacologic management of acute gout is directed toward reducing joint inflammation. Hyperuricemia and related problems of tophi, joint destruction, and renal problems are treated after the acute inflammatory process has subsided. NSAIDs, particularly indomethacin and ibuprofen, are used for treating acute gouty arthritis. Alternative therapies include colchicine and intra-articular deposition of corticosteroids. Treatment with colchicine is used early in the acute stage. Colchicine produces its antiinflammatory effects by inhibition of leukocyte migration and phagocytosis.

Treatment of hyperuricemia is aimed at maintaining normal uric acid levels and is lifelong. Two classes of drugs may be used. Allopurinol prevents the production of uric acid, and uricosuric drugs, such as probenecid or sulfinpyrazone, may be used to prevent the tubular reabsorption of urate and increase its excretion.[54] Prophylactic colchicine or NSAIDs may be used between gout attacks. If the uric acid level is normal and the person has not had recurrent attacks of gout, the use of these medications may be discontinued.

In summary, the systemic autoimmune rheumatic disorders are a group of chronic disorders with overlapping symptoms that are characterized by diffuse inflammatory lesions and progressive changes in connective tissue. RA is a chronic systemic inflammatory disorder affecting multiple joints. Joint involvement, which is symmetric, begins with inflammatory changes of the synovium and formation of a destructive granulation tissue called *pannus* that leads to joint instability and eventual deformity. Systemic lupus erythematosus is a chronic autoimmune disorder that affects multiple body systems, including the musculoskeletal system, skin, kidneys, cardiovascular system, hematologic system, and CNS. There is an exaggerated production of autoantibodies, which interact with antigens to produce an immune complex. These immune complexes produce an inflammatory response in affected tissues. Systemic sclerosis, often prefixed by the term *progressive,* is sometimes called *scleroderma.* In this disorder, the skin is thickened through fibrosis with an accompanying fixation to the subdermal structures, including the sheaths or fascia covering tendons and muscles.

The spondyloarthropathies affect the axial skeleton, particularly the spine. Inflammation develops at sites where ligaments insert into bone. Because they lack the RF, they are referred to as *seronegative spondyloarthropathies.* They include ankylosing spondylitis, reactive arthropathies, and psoriatic arthritis. Ankylosing spondylitis, which is characterized by bilateral ankylosing spondylitis and loss of motion in the spinal column, is considered a prototype of this classification category. The cause remains unknown; however, a strong association between the HLA-B27 antigen and ankylosing spondylitis has been identified.

Osteoarthritis, the most common form of arthritis, is a localized condition affecting primarily the weight-bearing joints. It can occur as a primary idiopathic disorder or as a secondary disorder due to congenital or acquired defects in joint structures. Risk factors for OA progression include older age, multiple joint involvement, neuropathy, and, for knees, obesity. The joint changes associated with OA, which include progressive loss of articular cartilage and subchondral bone, result from inflammatory changes that occur when cartilage tries to repair itself.

Gout is a crystal-induced arthropathy caused by the presence of monosodium urate crystals in the joint cavity. It includes acute gouty arthritis with recurrent attacks of auricular and periauricular inflammation, and tophi or the accumulation of crystalline deposits in articular surfaces, bones, and soft tissue surrounding joints. The disorder is accompanied by hyperuricemia, which results from overproduction of uric acid or from the reduced ability of the kidney to rid the body of excess uric acid.

Rheumatic Diseases in Children and the Elderly

RHEUMATIC DISEASES IN CHILDREN

Children can be affected with almost all of the rheumatic diseases that occur in adults. In addition to disease-specific differences, these conditions affect not only the child but the family. Growth and development require special attention. Rheumatic disorders of children include juvenile RA, SLE, and juvenile spondyloarthropathies.

Juvenile Rheumatoid Arthritis

Juvenile RA (JRA) is the most common form of childhood arthritis and one of the more common chronic childhood diseases.[26] The disease is characterized by synovitis of the peripheral joints, soft tissue swelling, and effusion. It can also influence epiphyseal growth, resulting in a discrepancy in leg length. Generalized stunted growth also may occur.

JRA can be subdivided into three types: systemic onset, pauciarticular, and polyarticular-onset. These subtypes demonstrate unique clinical presentations, immunologic characteristics, and clinical manifestations. Approximately 10% of children with JRA experience a systemic onset.[26] The symptoms of systemic JRA include a daily intermittent high fever, which usually is accompanied by a rash, generalized lymphadenopathy, hepatosplenomegaly, leukocytosis, and anemia. Most of these children also have joint involvement, which develops concurrently with fever and rash. Systemic symptoms usually subside in 6 to 12 months. This form of JRA also can make an initial appearance in adulthood.

The second subgroup of JRA, pauciarticular arthritis, affects no more than four joints. This disease affects approximately 50% of children with JRA.[26] Pauciarticular arthritis affects two distinct groups. The first group generally consists of girls younger than 6 years of age with chronic uveitis. The results of ANA testing in this group usually are positive. The second group, characterized by late-onset arthritis, is made up mostly of boys. The HLA-B27 test results are positive in more than half of this group. They are affected by sacroiliitis, and the arthritis usually occurs in the lower extremities.

The third subgroup of JRA, accounting for approximately 40% of the total, is polyarticular-onset disease.[26] It affects five or more joints during the first 6 months of the disease. This form of arthritis more closely resembles the adult form of the disease than the other two subgroups. RF sometimes is present and may indicate a more active disease process. Systemic features include a low-grade fever, weight loss, malaise, anemia, stunted growth, slight organomegaly (*e.g.,* hepatosplenomegaly), and adenopathy.[26]

The prognosis for most children with JRA is good. NSAIDs are the first-line drugs used in treating JRA. Salicylates have been replaced by agents such as naproxen, ibuprofen, and ketoprofen. Second-line agents are low-dose methotrexate and, less often, sulfasalazine. Gold salts, hydroxychloroquine, and D-penicillamine rarely are used.[55] Biologic response modifiers are also being used in JRA, with etanercept being the first to get FDA approval.[56] Other aspects of treatment of children with JRA require careful attention to growth and development and nutritional issues. Children are encouraged to lead as normal a life as possible.

Systemic Lupus Erythematosus

The features of SLE in children are similar to those in adults. The incidence in children is 10 times lower, with an estimated occurrence of 0.6 of 100,000 children. The occurrence in the sexes is almost equal until puberty, after which it approaches the sex ratio seen in adults. The clinical manifestations of SLE in children reflect the extent and severity of systemic involvement. The best prognostic indicator in children is the extent of renal involvement, which is more common and more severe in children than in adults with SLE. Infectious complications are the most common cause of death (40%) in children with SLE.

Children with SLE may present with constitutional symptoms, including fever, malaise, anorexia, and weight loss. Symptoms of the integumentary, musculoskeletal, central nervous, cardiac, pulmonary, and hematopoietic systems are similar to those of adults. Endocrine abnormalities include Cushing syndrome from long-term corticosteroid use and autoimmune thyroiditis. Adolescents often experience menstrual disturbances, which tend to resolve with disease remission.

Treatment of SLE in children is similar to that in adults. The use of NSAIDs, corticosteroids, antimalarials, and immunosuppressive agents depends on the symptoms. Corticosteroids may cause stunting of growth and necrosis of femoral heads and other joints. Immunization schedules should be maintained using attenuated rather than live vaccines. Rest periods should be balanced with exercise; children should be encouraged to maintain as normal a schedule as possible.[56] The diversity of the clinical manifestations of SLE in the young requires the establishment of a comprehensive treatment program.

Juvenile Dermatomyositis

Juvenile dermatomyositis (JDMS) is an inflammatory myopathy primarily involving skin and muscle and associated with a characteristic rash. JDMS can affect children of all ages, with a mean age at onset of 8 years. There is an increased incidence among girls. The cause is unknown. Symmetric proximal muscle weakness, elevated muscle enzymes, evidence of vasculitis, and electromyographic changes confirming an inflammatory myopathy are diagnostic for JDMS. Generalized vasculitis is not seen in the adult form of the disease. The rash may precede or follow the onset of proximal muscle weakness. Periorbital edema, erythema, and eyelid telangiectases are common.

Calcifications can occur in 30% to 50% of children with JDMS and are by far the most debilitating symptom. The calcifications appear at pressure points or sites of previous trauma. JDMS is treated primarily with corticosteroids to reduce inflammation. Occasionally, immunosuppressives are used in cases of refractory disease.[26] Adjunct therapies include using sun block (SPF >36), a calcium-sufficient diet, and vitamin D therapy.

Juvenile Spondyloarthropathies

Ankylosing spondylitis, reactive arthritis, psoriatic arthritis, and spondyloarthropathies associated with ulcerative colitis and regional enteritis can affect children as well as adults. In children, spondyloarthritis manifests in peripheral joints first, mimicking pauciarticular JRA, with no evidence of sacroiliac or spinal involvement for months to years after onset. The spondyloarthropathies are more common in boys and commonly occur in children who have a positive family history. HLA-B27 typing is helpful in diagnosing children because of the unusual presentation of the disease.

Management of the disease involves physical therapy, education, and attention to school and growth and development issues. Medication includes the use of salicylates or other NSAIDs such as tolmetin or indomethacin. More severe disease or symptoms may require systemic corticosteroids.[26] Etanercept and infliximab produce more dramatic improvement of disease activity, although their long-term effects and toxicity are not yet known.[57]

 ## RHEUMATIC DISEASES IN THE ELDERLY

Arthritis is the most common complaint of elderly persons. The pain, stiffness, and muscle weakness affect daily life, often threatening independence and quality of life. Symptoms of the rheumatic diseases also can have indirect effects and even threaten the duration of life for the elderly. The weakness and gait disturbance that often accompany the rheumatic diseases can contribute to the likelihood of falls and fracture, causing suffering, increased health care costs, further loss of independence, and the potential for a decreased life span.

The types of arthritis that affect the elderly are the same as those that affect younger persons, but there are often differences in the manifestations, diagnostic methods, and treatment modalities. The usual presentation of these conditions was discussed earlier in this chapter. One form of rheumatic disease that has a predilection for the elderly is polymyalgia rheumatica.

In general, the elderly tend to cope less well with mild to moderately severe disease that in younger persons is less likely to lead to serious disability for the same degree of impairment. Also, the elderly and their health care providers often assume that the problems associated with arthritis are an inevitable consequence of aging, thereby discounting the value of measures that can improve the quality of life. In addition, the elderly often have multiple health problems complicating diagnosis and management. The diagnosis must consider a wide variety of disorders that are usually outside the typical range of rheumatic diseases. Among these are metastatic bone disease, multiple myeloma, musculoskeletal disorders accompanying endocrine or metabolic disorders, other orthopedic conditions, and neurologic disease.

Systemic Autoimmune Rheumatic Disorders

Rheumatoid Arthritis. The prevalence of RA increases with advancing age, at least until 75 years of age.[58] Seropositive patients are more likely to have had an acute onset with systemic features and higher disease activity. Patients with seronegative, elderly-onset RA have a disease that usually follows a mild course. The close resemblance of the manifestations of seronegative RA in the elderly to those of polymyalgia rheumatica has led to speculation concerning the relation of these syndromes.[58] It may be that RA in the elderly is a broad disorder that includes a number of distinct subsets with characteristic manifestations, courses, and outcomes.

The goals for treatment for elderly persons with RA are similar to those for younger persons. The goals, however, take on more urgency because the potential for immobility places the elderly at high risk for complications and permanent loss of their independence. For this reason, corticosteroids may be used as an initial treatment.[59] Usually the dosages needed for suppression of the inflammatory process are low and long-term side effects are minimal. This contrasts with the use of NSAIDs, which must be given at high doses that are more likely to cause problems in the elderly. For those elderly who do not respond to low-dose corticosteroid therapy, or who have either erosive or destructive arthritis or systemic extra-articular disease, treatment with DMARDs may be used.

Systemic Lupus Erythematosus. Systemic lupus erythematosus is another condition with different manifestations in the elderly. The disease is accompanied less frequently by renal involvement. However, pleurisy, pericarditis, arthritis, and symptoms closely resembling polymyalgia rheumatica are more common than in younger patients. The characteristics of SLE in the elderly closely resemble those of drug-induced SLE, leading to speculation that the syndrome may result from one of the multiple drugs that are taken by many elderly patients.[60] As with RA, SLE in the elderly is often treated with corticosteroids.

Osteoarthritis

Osteoarthritis is by far the most common form of arthritis among the elderly. It is the greatest cause of disability and limitation of activity in older populations. It has been suggested that OA begins at a very young age, expressing itself in the elderly only after a long period of latency. Too often, it is accepted by the patient or expected by the physician. OA presents a major management problem, but there is much that can be done. Self-control by maintaining a positive attitude and sense of self-esteem is a frequent coping strategy.[61]

Treatment of OA in the elderly focuses on relief of pain and improvement of functional status. As with younger persons, treatment includes physical measures to reduce strain on the affected joints and providing a balance of rest with exercise. Acetaminophen may be used for pain relief.

Crystal-Induced Arthropathies

Gout. The incidence of clinical gout increases with advancing age, in part because of the increased involvement of joints after years of continued hyperuricemia. High serum urate levels rarely occur in women before menopause; initial attacks of clinical gout occur around the age of 70 years, or 20 years after menopause.[52] Gouty attacks in elderly women may be precipitated by the use of diuretics. The treatment of gout is often more difficult in the elderly. Although colchicine may be effective in controlling the symptoms of chronic gout, it may cause diarrhea in some patients, limiting its effectiveness in maintenance therapy.

Pseudogout. As part of the tissue aging process, OA develops with associated cartilage degeneration and the shedding of calcium pyrophosphate crystals into the joint cavity. These crystals may produce a low-grade chronic inflammation—the chronic pseudogout syndrome. The accumulation of calcium pyrophosphate and related crystalline deposits in articular cartilage is common in the elderly. There are no medications that can remove the crystals from the joints. Although it may be asymptomatic, presence of the crystals may also contribute to more rapid cartilage deterioration. This condition may coexist with severe OA.

Polymyalgia Rheumatica

Polymyalgia rheumatica is an inflammatory condition of unknown origin characterized by aching and morning stiffness in the cervical regions and shoulder and pelvic girdle areas.[62] Of the forms of arthritis affecting the elderly, it is one of the more difficult to diagnose and one of the most important to identify. Elderly women are especially at risk. Polymyalgia rheumatica is a common syndrome of older patients, rarely occurring before age 50 and usually after age 60 years. The onset can be abrupt, with the patient going to bed feeling well and awakening with pain and stiffness in the neck, shoulders, and hips.

Diagnosis is based on the pain and stiffness persisting for at least 1 month and an elevated ESR. The diagnosis is confirmed when the symptoms respond dramatically to a small dose of prednisone, a corticosteroid. Biopsies have shown that the muscles are normal, despite the name, but that a nonspecific inflammation affecting the synovial tissue is present. It is possible that a number of patients are erroneously diagnosed as having RA or OA. For patients with an elevated ESR, the diagnosis usually is based on a 3-day trial of prednisone treatment.[63] Patients with polymyalgia rheumatica typically exhibit striking clinical improvement on approximately the second day. Patients with RA also show improvement, although usually days later.

Treatment with NSAIDs provides relief for some patients, but most require continuing therapy with prednisone, with gradual reduction of the dose over the course of 1.5 to 2 years, using the person's symptoms as the primary guide. Persons with the disorder need close monitoring during the maintenance phase with prednisone therapy. Because their symptoms are relieved, they often quit taking the prednisone and their symptoms recur, or doses are missed and the decreased dosage leads to an increase in symptoms. Unless careful assessment reveals the frequency of missed doses, the health care provider may be misled into increasing the dosage when it is not needed. Because of the side effects of the corticosteroids, the goal is to use the lowest dose of the drug necessary to control the symptoms. Weaning patients off low-dose prednisone therapy after this length of time can be a difficult and extended process.

A certain percentage of patients with polymyalgia rheumatica also have giant cell arteritis (*i.e.,* temporal arteritis), frequently with involvement of the ophthalmic arteries. The two conditions are considered to represent different manifestations of the same disease. Giant cell arteritis, a form of systemic vasculitis, is a systemic inflammatory disease of large and medium-sized arteries (see Chapter 17).

The clinical symptoms suggesting a person has giant cell arteritis include a new type of headache; scalp tenderness (especially over the temporal area), visual symptoms (diplopia, loss of vision), and claudication of the jaw or arm. The temporal artery may be nodular, enlarged, tender, or pulseless. The symptoms often begin insidiously and may exist for some time before being recognized.[63] Some persons present with fever of unknown origin that is frequently accompanied by chills and sweating.

Diagnosis is usually based on physical findings, an elevated ESR, and temporal artery biopsy. Giant cell arteritis is potentially dangerous if missed or mistreated, especially if the temporal artery or other vessels supplying the eye are involved, in which case blindness can ensue quickly without treatment. Initial treatment, which consists of large doses of prednisone, is usually initiated immediately, and a temporal artery biopsy is obtained as soon as possible after instituting treatment. The prednisone is continued for 4 to 6 weeks and then decreased gradually.

Management of Rheumatic Diseases in the Elderly

In addition to diagnosis-specific treatment, the elderly require special considerations. Management techniques that rely on modalities other than drugs are particularly important for the elderly. These include splints, walking aids, muscle-building exercise, and local heat. Muscle-strengthening and stretching exercises are particularly effective in the elderly person with age-related losses in muscle function and should be instituted early. Rest, the cornerstone of conservative therapy, is hazardous in the elderly, who can rapidly lose muscle strength.

In terms of medications, the selection of drugs used in the treatment of arthritic disorders and their dosages may need to be considered when prescribing for the elderly. For example, the NSAIDs may be less well tolerated by the elderly, and their side effects are more likely to be serious. In addition to bleeding from the gastrointestinal tract and renal insufficiency, there may be cognitive dysfunction manifested by forgetfulness, inability to concentrate, sleeplessness, paranoid ideation, and depression.

Joint arthroplasty can also be used for pain relief and increased function. Chronologic age is not a contraindication to surgical treatment of arthritis. In appropriately selected elderly candidates, survival and functional outcome after surgery are equivalent to those in younger age groups. The more sedentary activity level of the elderly makes them even better candidates for joint replacement because they put less stress and demand on the new joint.

In summary, rheumatic diseases that affect children include RA, SLE, JDMS, and juvenile spondyloarthropathies. Although the childhood form of the disease may be similar to that seen in the adult, there are manifestations and treatment issues that are unique to the younger population. Managing rheumatic diseases in children requires a team approach to address issues related to the family, school, growth and development, and coping strategies, with development of a comprehensive disease management program.

Arthritis is the most common complaint of the elderly population. The pain, stiffness, and muscle weakness affect daily life, often threatening independence and quality of life. There is a difference in the manifestations, diagnosis, and treatment of some of the rheumatic diseases in the elderly compared with those in the younger population. OA is the most common form of arthritis among the elderly. The prevalence of RA and gout increases with advancing age. One form of rheumatic disease that has a predilection for the elderly is polymyalgia rheumatica. A certain percentage of patients with polymyalgia rheumatica also develop giant cell arteritis, a condition that can potentially cause blindness if not recognized and treated.

Review Exercises

A 60-year-old postmenopausal woman presents with a compression fracture of the vertebrae. She has also noticed increased backache and loss of height over the last few years.

A. Explain how the lack of estrogen and aging contribute to the development of osteoporosis.
B. What other factors should be considered when assessing the risk for developing osteoporosis?
C. What is the best way to measure bone density?
D. Name the two most important factors in preventing osteoporosis.
E. What medications might be used to treat this woman's condition?

A 30-year-old woman, recently diagnosed with rheumatoid arthritis (RA), complains of general fatigue and weight loss along with symmetric joint swelling, stiffness, and pain.

The stiffness is more prominent in the morning and subsides during the day. Laboratory measures reveal a rheumatoid factor (RF) of 120 IU/mL (nonreactive, 0 to 39 IU/mL; weakly reactive, 40 to 79 IU/mL; reactive, >80 IU/mL).

A. Describe the immunopathogenesis of the joint changes that occur with RA.
B. How do these changes relate to this woman's symptoms?
C. What is the significance of her RF test results?
D. How do her complaints of general fatigue and weight loss relate to the RA disease process?

A 65-year-old obese woman with a diagnosis of osteoarthritis (OA) has been having increased pain in her right knee that is made worse with movement and weight bearing and is relieved by rest. Physical examination reveals an enlarged joint with a varus deformity; coarse crepitus is felt over the joint on passive movement.

A. Compare the pathogenesis and articular structures involved in OA with those of RA.
B. What is the origin of the enlargement of the affected joint, the varus deformity, and the crepitus that is felt on movement of the affected knee?
C. Explain the predilection for involvement of the knee in persons such as this woman.
D. What types of treatment are available for this woman?

A 75-year-old woman is seen by a health care provider because of complaints of fever, malaise, and weight loss. She is having trouble combing her hair, putting on a coat, and getting out of a chair because of the stiffness and pain in her shoulders, hip, and lower back. Because of her age and symptoms, the health care provider suspects the woman has polymyalgia rheumatica.

A. What laboratory test can be used to substantiate the diagnosis?
B. What other diagnostic strategies are used to confirm the diagnosis?
C. How is the disease treated?

Visit the Porth: Essentials of Pathophysiology: Concepts of Altered Health States web site (http://thePoint.LWW.com/PorthEssentials) for links to chapter-related resources on the Internet, all-new exclusive animations, chapter review questions, and more!

REFERENCES

1. Rosenberg A. E. (2005). Bones, joints, and soft tissue tumors. In Kumar V., Abbas A. K., Fausto N. (Eds.), *Robbins and Cotran pathologic basis of disease* (7th ed., pp. 1273–1314). Philadelphia: Elsevier Saunders.

2. Manolagas S. C., Jilka R. L. (1995). Bone marrow, cytokines, and bone remodeling. *New England Journal of Medicine* 332, 305–310.

3. Hofbauer L. C., Schoppet M. (2004). Clinical implications of the osteoprotegerin/RANKL/RANK system for bone and vascular diseases. *Journal of the American Medical Association* 292, 490–495.

4. Schiller A. L., Wang B. Y., Klein M. J. (2005). Bones and joints. In Rubin E., Gorstein F., Rubin R., et al. (Eds.), *Rubin's pathology: Clinicopathologic foundations of medicine* (4th ed., pp. 1305–1335). Philadelphia: Lippincott Williams & Wilkins.

5. Adams J., Pepping J. (2005). Vitamin K in the treatment and prevention of osteoporosis and arterial calcification. *American Journal of Health-System Pharmacists* 62, 1574–1581.

6. National Osteoporosis Foundation. (2005). America's bone health: The state of osteoporosis and low bone mass. [On-line]. Available: www.nof.org/advocacy/prevalence.

7. Raisz L. G., Rodan G. A. (2003). Pathogenesis of osteoporosis. *Endocrinology Clinics of North America* 32, 15–24.

8. Seeman E. (2003). The structural and biomechanical basis of the gain and loss of bone strength in women and men. *Endocrinology Clinics of North America* 32, 25–38.

9. Stein E., Shane E. (2003). Secondary osteoporosis. *Endocrinology Clinics of North America* 32, 115–134.

10. Hansen L. B., Vondracek S. F. (2004). Prevention and treatment of nonpostmenopausal osteoporosis. *American Journal of Health-System Pharmacists* 61, 2637–2654.

11. Tebas P., Powerly W. G., Claxton S., et al. (2000). Accelerated bone mineral loss in HIV-infected patients receiving potent antiretroviral therapy. *AIDS* 14(4), F63–F67.

12. National Institutes of Health. (2000). National Institutes of Health Consensus Development Statement: Osteoporosis prevention, diagnosis, and therapy. [On-line]. Available: http://consensus.nih.gov/2000/2000Osteoporosis111html.htm. Accessed September 15, 2005.

13. Otis C. L., Drinkwater B., Johnson M., et al. (1997). American College of Sports Medicine position stand: The female athlete triad. *Medicine and Science in Sports and Exercise* 29(5), i–ix.

14. Hobart J. A., Smucker D. R. (2000). The female athlete triad. *American Family Physician* 61, 3357–3367.

15. Vondracek S. F., Hansen L. B. (2004). Current approaches to management of osteoporosis in men. *American Journal of Health-System Pharmacists* 61, 1801–1811.

16. Leid E. S., Lenchik L., Bilezikian J. P., et al. (2002). Position statements of the International Society of Clinical Densitometry: Methodology. *Journal of Clinical Densitometry* 5(Suppl.), S5–S10.

17. Weinstein L., Ullery B. (2000). Age, weight, and estrogen use determine need for osteoporosis screen. *American Journal of Obstetrics and Gynecology* 183, 547–549.

18. Rosen C. J. (2004). Postmenopausal osteoporosis. *New England Journal of Medicine* 353, 595–603.

19. National Institutes of Health, Osteoporosis and Related Bone Diseases—National Resource Center. (2003). Fact sheets: Phytoestrogens and bone health. [On-line]. Available: www.osteo.org.

20. Bishop M. (1999). Rickets today: Children still need milk and sunshine. *New England Journal of Medicine* 341, 602–604.

21. Centers for Disease Control and Prevention. (2001). Severe malnutrition among young children—Georgia, January 1997–June 1999. *MMWR Morbidity and Mortality Weekly Report* 50(12), 224–227.

22. Bouillon R. (1998). The many faces of rickets. *New England Journal of Medicine* 131, 935–942.

23. Schneider D., Hofmann M. T. (2002). Diagnosis and treatment of Paget's disease of bone. *American Family Physician* 65, 2069–2072.

24. Ankrom M. A., Shapiro J. R. (1998). Paget's disease of bone (osteitis deformans). *Journal of the American Geriatric Society* 46, 1025–1033.

25. Siris E. S. (1998). Paget's disease of bone. *Journal of Bone and Mineral Research* 13, 1061–1065.

26. Klippel J. R. (Ed.). (2001). *Primer on the rheumatic diseases* (12th ed., pp. 209–235, 239–258, 285–298, 307–324, 329–351, 534–540). Atlanta: Arthritis Foundation.

27. Zhang Z., Bridges S. L. (2001). Pathogenesis of rheumatoid arthritis: Role of B lymphocytes. *Annals of Rheumatic Disease* 27, 335–353.

28. American College of Rheumatology Subcommittee on Rheumatoid Arthritis Guidelines. (2002). Guidelines for the management of rheumatoid arthritis: 2002 update. *Arthritis and Rheumatism* 46, 328–346.

29. Lee D. M., Schur P. H. (2003). The detection of anti-cyclic citrullinated peptides (CCP). *Annals of Rheumatic Disease* 62, 870–874.

30. Stenstrom C. H., Minor M. A. (2003). Evidence for the benefit of aerobic and strengthening exercise in rheumatoid arthritis. *Arthritis Care and Research* 49, 428–434.

31. O'Dell J. R. (2004). Therapeutic strategies for rheumatoid arthritis. *New England Journal of Medicine* 350, 2591–2602.

32. Olson N. J., Stein M. (2004). New drugs for rheumatoid arthritis. *New England Journal of Medicine* 350, 2167–2179.

33. Mulvihill K. (2003). Systemic lupus erythematosus. *Advance for Nurse Practitioners* January, 32–37.

34. Edworthy S. M. (2001). Clinical manifestations of systemic lupus erythematosus. In Ruddy S., Harris E. D., Sledge C. B. (Eds.), *Kelley's textbook of rheumatology* (6th ed., pp. 1105–1123). Philadelphia: W. B. Saunders.

35. Criscione L. G. (2003). The pathogenesis of systemic lupus erythematosus. *Bulletin on the Rheumatic Diseases* 52(6), 1–7.

36. Abbas A. K. (2005). Diseases of immunity. In Kumar V., Abbas A. K., Fausto N. (Eds.), *Robbins and Cotran pathologic basis of disease* (7th ed., pp. 227–235). Philadelphia: Elsevier Saunders.

37. Tan E. M., Cohen A. S., Fries J. C., et al. (1982). The 1982 revised criteria for the classification of systemic lupus erythematosus. *Arthritis and Rheumatism* 25, 1271–1277.

38. Pigg J. S., Bancroft D. A. (2000). Management of patients with rheumatic diseases. In Smeltzer S. C., Bare B. C. (Eds.), *Brunner and Suddarth's textbook of medical-surgical nursing* (9th ed., pp. 1405–1433). Philadelphia: Lippincott Williams & Wilkins.

39. Steen V. D., Medsger T. A. (2000). Severe organ involvement in systemic sclerosis with diffuse scleroderma. *Arthritis and Rheumatism* 43, 2437–2444.

40. Mayes M. D. (2003). Scleroderma epidemiology. *Rheumatic Disease Clinics of North America* 29, 240–254.

41. Lin A. T. H., Clements P. J., Furst D. E. (2003). Update on disease modifying antirheumatic drugs in the treatment of systemic sclerosis. *Rheumatic Disease Clinics of North America* 29, 409–426.

42. Kuon W., Sieper J. (2003). Identification of HLA-B27 restricted peptides in reactive arthritis and other spondyloarthropathies. *Rheumatic Disease Clinics of North America* 29, 595–611.

43. Brandt J., Haibel H., Cornely D., et al. (2000). Successful treatment of active ankylosing spondylitis with the anti-tumor necrosis factor α monoclonal antibody infliximab. *Arthritis and Rheumatism* 43, 1346–1352.

44. Flores D., Marquez J., Garza M., et al. (2003). Reactive arthritis: Newer developments. *Rheumatic Disease Clinics of North America* 29, 37–59.

45. Sigal L. H. (2001). Update on reactive arthritis. *Bulletin on the Rheumatic Diseases* 50(4), 1–4.

46. Mease P. J. (2003). Current treatment of psoriatic arthritis. *Rheumatic Disease Clinics of North America* 29, 495–511.

47. Loeser R. F. (2003). A stepwise approach to the management of osteoarthritis. *Bulletin on the Rheumatic Diseases* 52(5).

48. Huang M., Chen C., Chen T., et al. (2000). The effects of weight reduction on the rehabilitation of patients with knee osteoarthritis and obesity. *Arthritis Care and Research* 13, 398–405.

49. Loeser R. F. (2000). Aging and the etiopathogenesis and treatment of osteoarthritis. *Rheumatic Disease Clinics of North America* 26, 547–567.

50. American College of Rheumatology Subcommittee on Osteoarthritis Guidelines. (2000). Recommendations for the medical management of osteoarthritis of the hip and knee: 2000 update. *Arthritis and Rheumatology* 43, 1905–1915.

51. Brandt K., Smith G. N., Simon L. S. (2000). Intraarticular injection of hyaluronan as treatment for knee osteoarthritis: What is the evidence? *Arthritis and Rheumatism* 43, 1192–1203.

52. Agudelo C. A., Wise K. M. (2000). Crystal-associated arthritis in the elderly. *Rheumatic Disease Clinics of North America* 26, 527–546.

53. Schlesinger N., Schumacher H. R. (2002). Update on gout. *Arthritis Care and Research* 47, 563–565.

54. Perez-Ruiz F., Calabozo M., Pijoan J. I., et al. (2002). Effect of urate lowering therapy on the velocity and size reduction of tophi in chronic gout. *Arthritis Care and Research* 47, 356–360.

55. Lomater C., Gerloni V., Gattinara M., et al. (2000). Systemic onset juvenile idiopathic arthritis: A retrospective study of 80 consecutive patients followed for 10 years. *Journal of Rheumatology* 27, 491–496.

56. Milojevic D. S., Ilowite N. T. (2002). Treatment of rheumatic diseases in children: Special considerations. *Rheumatic Disease Clinics of North America* 28, 461–482.

57. Burgos-Vargas R. (2002). The juvenile-onset spondyloarthritides. *Rheumatic Disease Clinics of North America* 28, 531–560.

58. Yaziu Y., Paget S. A. (2000). Elderly-onset rheumatoid arthritis. *Rheumatic Disease Clinics of North America* 26, 517–526.

59. Kerr L. D. (2003). Inflammatory arthritis in the elderly. *Mount Sinai Journal of Medicine* 70, 23–26.

60. Kammer G. M., Misha N. (2000). Systemic lupus erythematosus in the elderly. *Rheumatic Disease Clinics of North America* 26, 475–492.

61. Rapp S. R., Rejeski W. J., Miller M. E. (2000). Physical function among older adults with knee pain: The role of coping skills. *Arthritis Care and Research* 13, 270–279.

62. Salvarani C., Cantini F., Boiardi L., et al. (2002). Polymyalgia rheumatica and giant-cell arteritis. *New England Journal of Medicine* 347, 261–271.

63. Evans J. M., Hunder G. C. (2000). Polymyalgia rheumatica and giant cell arteritis. *Rheumatic Disease Clinics of North America* 26, 493–515.

UNIT XIII
Integumentary Function

Chapter 44

Structure and Function of the Skin

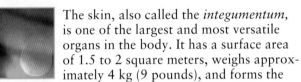 The skin, also called the *integumentum*, is one of the largest and most versatile organs in the body. It has a surface area of 1.5 to 2 square meters, weighs approximately 4 kg (9 pounds), and forms the major interface between the internal organs and the external environment. As the body's first line of defense, the skin is continuously subjected to potentially harmful environmental agents, including solid matter, liquids, gases, sunlight, and microorganisms. The skin also serves as an immunologic barrier. The Langerhans cells detect foreign antigens, playing an important part in allergic skin conditions and skin graft rejections.

Structure of the Skin

The skin is composed of three layers: the epidermis (outer layer), the dermis (inner layer), and the subcutaneous fat layer (Fig. 44-1). The basal lamina (basement membrane) divides the first two layers. The subcutaneous tissue, a layer of loose connective and fatty tissue, binds the dermis to the underlying tissues of the body and supports the blood vessels and nerves that pass from the underlying tissues to the dermis.

EPIDERMIS

The functions of the skin depend on the properties of its outermost layer, the epidermis. The epidermis covers the body, and it is specialized in areas to form the various skin appendages: hair, nails, and glandular structures. The

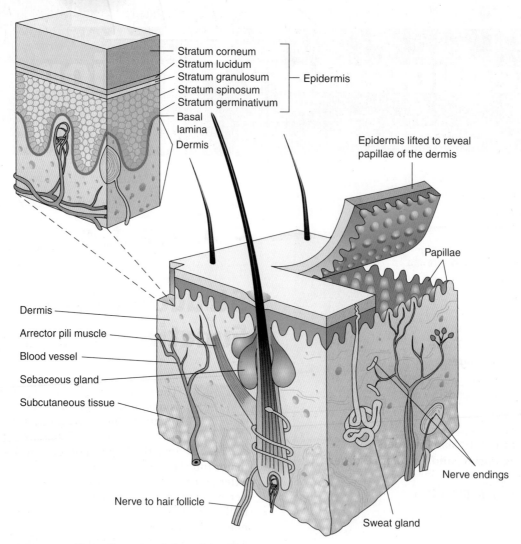

FIGURE 44-1 • Three-dimensional view of the skin.

keratinocytes of the epidermis produce a fibrous protein called *keratin,* which is essential to the protective function of skin. In addition to the keratinocytes, the epidermis has three other types of cells that arise from its basal layer: melanocytes that produce a pigment called *melanin,* which is responsible for skin color, tanning, and protecting against ultraviolet radiation; Merkel cells that provide sensory information (see Chapter 34); and Langerhans cells that link the epidermis to the immune system. The epidermis contains openings for two types of glands: sweat glands, which produce watery secretions, and sebaceous glands, which produce an oily secretion called *sebum.*

Keratinocytes

The keratinocytes, or keratin-forming cells, are the major cells of the epidermis. They develop into five distinct layers, or strata, as they divide and mature: the stratum germinativum, the stratum spinosum, the stra-

tum granulosum, the stratum lucidum, and the stratum corneum.

The deepest layer, the *stratum germinativum* or *stratum basale,* consists of a single layer of basal cells that are attached to the basal lamina. The basal cells are the only epidermal cells that are mitotically active. All cells of the epidermis arise from this layer. As new cells form in the basal layer, the older cells change shape and are pushed upward (Fig. 44-2). As these cells near the surface, they die and their cytoplasm is converted to keratin. It normally takes 3 to 4 weeks for the epidermis to replicate itself. This cell turnover is greatly accelerated in diseases such as psoriasis.

The second layer, the *stratum spinosum,* is formed as cells from the basal cell layer move upward toward the skin surface. The stratum spinosum is two to four layers thick. The cells of this layer are commonly referred to as *prickle cells* because they develop a spiny appearance as their cell borders interact. The third layer, the *stratum granulosum,* is only a few cells thick; it is com-

Organization of Skin Structures

➤ The skin has two layers, an outer epidermis and an inner dermis, separated by a basement membrane.

➤ The epidermis, which is avascular, is composed of four to five layers of stratified squamous keratinized epithelial cells that are formed in the deepest layer of the epidermis and migrate to the skin surface to replace cells that are lost during normal skin shedding.

➤ The basement membrane is a thin adhesive layer that cements the epidermis to the dermis. This is the layer involved in blister formation.

➤ The dermis is a connective tissue layer that separates the epidermis from the underlying subcutaneous tissue layer. It contains the blood vessels and nerve fibers that supply the epidermis.

posed of flatter cells containing protein granules called *keratohyalin granules*. The *stratum lucidum*, the fourth layer, which lies just superficial to the stratum granulosum, is a thin, transparent layer mostly confined to the palms of the hands and soles of the feet. It consists of transitional cells that retain some of the functions of living skin cells from the layers below but otherwise resemble the cells of the stratum corneum.

The top or surface layer of the epidermis is the *stratum corneum*. It is made up of stratified layers of dead keratinized cells that are constantly shedding. The stratum corneum contains the most cell layers and the largest cells of any zone of the epidermis. It ranges from 15 layers thick in areas such as the face to 25 layers or more on the arm. Specialized areas, such as the palms of the hands or soles of the feet, have 100 or more layers.

Melanocytes

The melanocytes are pigment-synthesizing cells that are located at or in the basal layer. They function to produce pigment granules called *melanosomes* that contain *melanin*, the black or brown substance that gives skin its color. The melanocytes have long, cytoplasm-filled extensions that extend between the keratinocytes. Although the melanocytes remain in the basal layer, melanin is transferred to the keratinocytes through these extensions (Fig. 44-3). Each melanocyte is capable of supplying several keratinocytes with melanin. The primary function of melanin is to protect the skin from harmful ultraviolet sun rays. Exposure to the sun's ultraviolet rays increases the production of melanin, causing tanning to occur. The amount of melanin in the keratinocytes determines a person's skin color. All people have relatively few or no melanocytes in the epidermis of the palms of the hands or the soles of the feet.

The ability to synthesize melanin depends on the ability of the melanocytes to produce an enzyme called *tyrosinase*, which converts the amino acid tyrosine to a precursor of melanin. A genetic lack of this enzyme results in a clinical condition called *albinism*. Persons with this disorder lack pigmentation in the skin, hair, and iris of the eye.

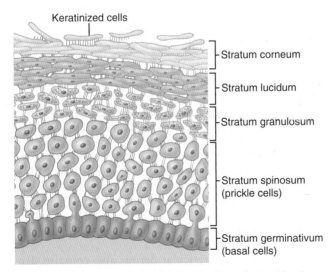

FIGURE 44-2 Epidermal cells. The basal cells undergo mitosis, producing keratinocytes that change their size and shape as they move upward, replacing cells that are lost during normal cell shedding.

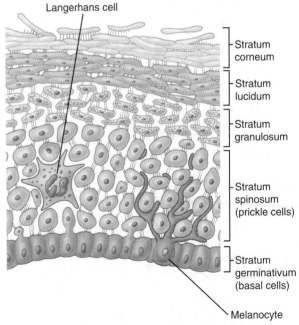

FIGURE 44-3 Melanocytes. The melanocytes, which are located in the basal layer of the skin, produce melanin pigment granules that give skin its color. The melanocytes have threadlike, cytoplasm-filled extensions that are used in passing the pigment granules to the keratinocytes.

Langerhans Cells

Langerhans cells, sometimes called dendritic cells, are star-shaped macrophages of the immune system. They arise from the bone marrow and migrate to the epidermis, where they help activate the immune system. Their slender dendritic, or threadlike, processes extend through the keratinocytes in the epidermis, forming a more or less continuous network recognizing foreign antigens (Fig. 44-4). The function of the Langerhans cell is to capture the foreign antigen, process it, and then, bearing the processed antigen, migrate from the epidermis into lymphatic vessels and then into the regional lymph nodes. During their migration from the epidermis to the lymph nodes, the Langerhans cells mature and develop into antigen-presenting cells. Mature Langerhans cells reside in the T cell zones of the lymph nodes and in this location they present antigens to the T cells. They are the only immune cells in the skin known to be capable of antigen-presentation

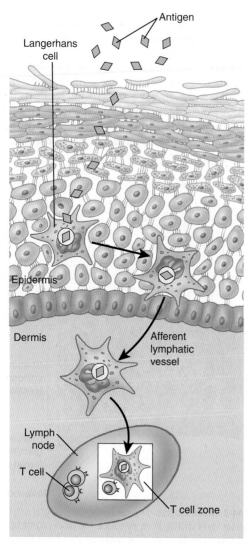

FIGURE 44-4 Langerhans cells.

and, therefore, may be responsible for many of the allergic reactions affecting the skin.

BASAL LAMINA

The basal lamina (basement membrane) is a layer of intercellular and extracellular matrices that serves as an interface between the dermis and the epidermis. It provides for adhesion of the dermis to the epidermis and serves as a selective filter for molecules moving between the two layers. It is also a major site of immunoglobulin and complement deposition in skin disease. The basal lamina is involved in skin disorders that cause bullae or blister formation.

DERMIS

The dermis is the connective tissue layer that separates the epidermis from the subcutaneous fat layer. It supports the epidermis and serves as its primary source of nutrition. The two layers of the dermis, the papillary dermis and the reticular dermis, are composed of cells, fibers, ground substances, nerves, and blood vessels. The hair and glandular structures are embedded in this layer and continue through the epidermis.

Papillary Dermis

The papillary dermis is a thin, superficial layer that lies adjacent to the epidermis. It consists of collagen fibers and ground substance. This layer is densely covered with conical projections called *dermal papillae* (see Fig. 44-1). The basal cells of the epidermis project into the papillary dermis, forming *rete ridges*. It is believed that the dense structure of the dermal papillae serves to minimize the separation of the dermis and the epidermis. Dermal papillae contain capillary venules that nourish the epidermal layers of the skin. Lymph vessels and nerve tissue also are found in this layer.

Reticular Dermis

The reticular dermis is the thicker area of the dermis and forms the bulk of the dermal layer. The reticular dermis is characterized by a complex meshwork of three-dimensional collagen bundles interconnected with large elastic fibers and ground substance, a viscid gel that is rich in mucopolysaccharides. The collagen fibers are oriented parallel to the body's surface in any given area. Collagen bundles may be organized lengthwise, as on the abdomen, or in round clusters, as in the heel. The direction of surgical incisions is often determined by this organizational pattern.

Immune Cells. The reticular dermis also contains dendritic cells with threadlike projections, called *dermal dendrocytes*. Dermal dendrocytes, which have phagocytic properties, are believed to possess an antigen-presenting capacity and play an important part in the immune function of the skin. Immune cells found in the dermis include macrophages, T cells, mast cells, and fibroblasts. The major type of T-cell–mediated immune response in the skin is delayed-type hypersensitivity (see Chapter 15). The mast cells play a prominent role in immunoglobulin E (IgE)–mediated hypersensitivity responses.

Innervation and Blood Supply. The innervation of the skin is complex. The skin, with its accessory structures, serves as an organ for receiving sensory information from the environment. The dermis is well supplied with sensory neurons as well as nerves that supply the blood vessels, sweat glands, and arrector pili muscles. The receptors for touch, pressure, heat, cold, and pain are widely distributed in the dermis. The papillary layer of the dermis is supplied with free nerve endings that serve as nociceptors (*i.e.*, pain receptors) and thermoreceptors. The dermis also contains encapsulated pressure-sensitive receptors that detect pressure and touch.

The arterial vessels that nourish the skin form two plexuses (*i.e.*, collections of blood vessels), one located between the papillary and reticular layers of the dermis and the other between the dermis and the subcutaneous tissue layer. Capillary flow that arises from vessels in this plexus extends up and nourishes the overlaying epidermis by diffusion. Blood leaves the skin by way of small veins that accompany the subcutaneous vessels. The lymphatic system of the skin, which aids in combating certain skin infections, also is limited to the dermis.

Most of the skin's blood vessels are under sympathetic nervous system control. The sweat glands are innervated by cholinergic fibers but controlled by the sympathetic nervous system.

SUBCUTANEOUS TISSUE

The subcutaneous tissue layer consists primarily of loose connective and fatty tissues that lend support to the vascular and neural structures supplying the outer layers of the skin. This layer serves as a major energy storage site and also provides insulation. Individual smooth muscle cells that originate in this layer form the arrector pili (pilomotor) muscles that connect the deep part of the hair follicles to the more superficial dermis. Contraction of these muscles tends to cause the skin to dimple, producing "goose bumps."

SKIN APPENDAGES

The skin houses a variety of appendages, including hair, nails, and sebaceous and sweat glands. The distribution and functions of the appendages vary.

Sweat Glands

There are two types of sweat glands: eccrine and apocrine. *Eccrine sweat glands* are simple tubular structures that originate in the dermis and open directly to the skin surface. They are numerous (several million), vary in density, and are located over the entire body surface. Their purpose is to transport sweat to the outer skin surface to regulate body temperature. *Apocrine sweat glands* are less numerous than eccrine sweat glands. They are larger and located deep in the dermal layer. They open through a hair follicle, even though a hair may not be present, and are found primarily in the axillae and groin. The major difference between these glands and the eccrine glands is that apocrine glands secrete an oily substance. In animals, apocrine secretions give rise to distinctive odors that enable animals to recognize the presence of others. In humans, apocrine secretions are sterile until mixed with bacteria on the skin surface; then they produce what is commonly known as body odor.

Sebaceous Glands

The sebaceous glands are located over the entire skin surface except for the palms, soles, and sides of the feet. They are part of the *pilosebaceous unit*. They secrete a mixture of lipids, including triglycerides, cholesterol, and wax. This mixture is called *sebum*; it lubricates hair and skin. Sebum is not the same as the surface lipid film. Sebum prevents undue evaporation of moisture from the stratum corneum during cold weather and helps to conserve body heat. Sebum production is under the control of genetic and hormonal influences. Sebaceous glands are relatively small and inactive until an individual approaches adolescence. The glands then enlarge, stimulated by the rise in sex hormones. Gland size directly influences the amount of sebum produced, and the level of androgens influences gland size. The sebaceous glands are the structures that become inflamed in acne (see Chapter 45).

Hair

Hair is a structure that originates from hair follicles in the dermis. Most hair follicles are associated with sebaceous glands, and these structures combine to form the pilosebaceous unit. The entire hair structure consists of the hair follicle, sebaceous gland, hair muscle (arrector pili), and, in some instances, the apocrine gland (Fig. 44-5). Hair is a keratinized structure that is pushed upward from the hair follicle. Growth of the hair is centered in the bulb (*i.e.*, base) of the hair follicle, and the hair undergoes changes as it is pushed outward. Hair has been found to go through cyclic phases identified as anagen (the growth phase), catagen (the atrophy phase), and telogen (the resting phase or no growth). Like most animals, human beings shed hair cyclically. However, human hair follicles work independently, and therefore, unlike most animals, human beings shed hair asynchronously.

A vascular network at the site of the follicular bulb nourishes and maintains the hair follicle. Melanocytes in the bulb transfer melanin-containing melanosomes to the cells of the bulb matrix in much the same way as in the skin and are therefore responsible for the color of

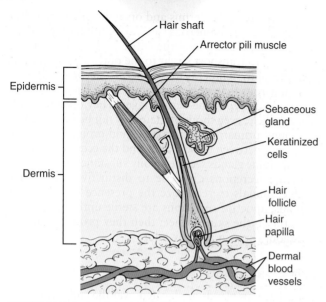

FIGURE 44-5 Parts of the hair follicle.

the hair. Similar to the skin, large melanosomes are found in the hair of darker-skinned persons; aggregated and encapsulated melanosomes are found in persons with light skin. Red hair has spherical melanosomes, whereas gray hair is the result of a decreased number of melanosome-producing melanocytes. The arrector pili muscle, located under the sebaceous gland, plays a role in thermoregulation by contracting to cause "goose bumps," thereby reducing the skin surface area that is available for the dissipation of body heat.

Nails

The nails are hardened keratinized plates, called *finger-nails* and *toenails*, that protect the fingers and toes and enhance dexterity. The nails grow out from a curved transverse groove called the *nail groove*. The floor of this groove, called the *nail matrix*, is the germinal region of the nail plate. The underlying epidermis, attached to the nail plate, is called the *nail bed*. Like hair, nails are the end product of dead matrix cells that are pushed outward from the nail matrix. Unlike hair, nails grow continuously rather than cyclically, unless permanently damaged or diseased. The epithelium of the fold of skin that surrounds the nail consists of the usual layers of skin. The stratum corneum forms the *eponychium* or cuticle. The nearly transparent nail plate provides a useful window for viewing the amount of oxygen in the blood, providing a view of the color of the blood in the dermal vessels. Changes or abnormalities of the nail can also serve to help diagnose skin or systemic diseases.

 In summary, the skin, which forms the major barrier between the internal organs and the external environ-

ment, is primarily an organ of protection. The skin is composed of two layers, the epidermis and dermis. The skin also houses a variety of appendages, including hair, nails, and sebaceous and sweat glands. The epidermis, the outermost layer of the skin, contains five layers, or strata. The major cells of the epidermis are the keratinocytes, melanocytes, Langerhans cells, and Merkel cells. The stratum germinativum, or basal layer, is the source of the cells in all five layers of the epidermis. The keratinocytes, which are the major cells of the epidermis, are transformed from viable keratinocytes to dead keratin as they move from the innermost layer of the epidermis (*i.e.*, stratum germinativum) to the outermost layer (*i.e.*, stratum corneum). The melanocytes are pigment-synthesizing cells that give skin its color.

The dermis provides the epidermis with support and nutrition and is the source of blood vessels, nerves, and skin appendages. Sensory receptors for touch, pressure, heat, cold, and pain are widely distributed in the dermis. Both the epidermis and dermis participate in the immune functions of the skin; the Langerhans cells of the epidermis capture and process foreign antigens for presentation to T cells of the immune system. The subcutaneous tissue layer consists primarily of fat and connective tissues that lend support to the vascular and neural structures supplying the outer layers of the skin.

 ## Manifestations of Skin Disorders

Skin disorders are manifested by a variety of primary lesions and rashes (Fig. 44-6). Commonly, secondary lesions result from overtreatment, scratching, and infection that accompany the primary skin disorders.

LESIONS, RASHES, AND VASCULAR DISORDERS

Rashes are temporary eruptions of the skin, such as those associated with childhood diseases, heat, diaper irritation, or drug-induced reactions. The term *lesion* refers to a traumatic or pathologic loss of normal tissue continuity, structure, or function. The components of a rash sometimes are referred to as *lesions*. Rashes and lesions may range in size from a fraction of a millimeter (*e.g.*, the pinpoint spots of petechiae) to many centimeters (*e.g.*, decubitus ulcer, or pressure sore). They may be blanched (white), erythematous (reddened), hemorrhagic or purpuric (containing blood), or pigmented. Repeated rubbing and scratching can lead to lichenification (thickened and roughened skin characterized by prominent skin markings caused by repeated scratching or rubbing) or excoriation (lesion caused by breakage of the epidermis, producing a raw linear area). Skin lesions may occur as

Circumscribed, flat, nonpalpable changes in skin color	Palpable elevated solid masses	Circumscribed superficial elevations of the skin formed by free fluid in a cavity within the skin layers
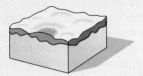	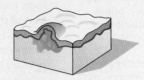	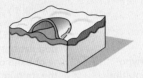
Macule—Small, up to 1 cm. Example: freckle, petechia *Patch*—Larger than 1 cm. Example: vitiligo	*Papule*—Up to 0.5 cm. Example: elevated nevus *Plaque*—A flat, elevated surface larger than 0.5 cm, often formed by the coalescence of papules *Nodule*—0.5 cm to 1–2 cm; often deeper and firmer than a papule *Tumor*—Larger than 1–2 cm *Wheal*—A somewhat irregular, relatively transient, superficial area of localized skin edema. Example: mosquito bite, hive	*Vesicle*—Up to 0.5 cm; filled with serous fluid. Example: herpes simplex *Bulla*—Greater than 0.5 cm; filled with serous fluid. Example: 2nd-degree burn *Pustule*—Filled with pus. Examples: acne, impetigo

FIGURE 44-6 Primary lesions may arise from previously normal skin. Authorities vary somewhat in their definitions of skin lesions by size. Dimensions given should be considered approximate. (From Bates B. B. [1995]. *A guide to physical examination and history taking* [6th ed.]. Philadelphia: J. B. Lippincott.)

primary lesions arising in previously normal skin, or they may develop as secondary lesions resulting from other disease conditions.

A *blister* is a vesicle or fluid-filled papule. Blisters of mechanical origin form from the friction caused by repeated rubbing on a single area of the skin. Friction blisters most commonly occur on the palmar and plantar surfaces of the hands and feet where the skin is thick enough to form a bleb. Blisters also develop from first-degree and second-degree partial-thickness burns. Histologically, there is degeneration of epidermal cells and a disruption of intercellular junctions that causes the layers of the skin to separate. As a result, fluid accumulates, and a noticeable bleb forms on the skin surface.

A *callus* is a hyperkeratotic plaque of skin caused by chronic pressure or friction. It represents a hyperplasia of the dead keratinized cells that make up the cornified or horny layer of the skin. Increased cohesion between cells results in hyperkeratosis and decreased skin shedding. *Corns* are small, well-circumscribed, conical keratinous thickenings of the skin. They usually appear on the toes from rubbing or ill-fitting shoes. The actual corn may be either hard with a central horny core or soft, as commonly seen between the toes. They may appear on the hands as an occupational hazard. Corns on the feet often are painful, whereas corns on the hands may be asymptomatic.

Telangiectases are dilated superficial blood vessels, capillaries, or terminal arteries that appear either red or bluish. They can appear by themselves or as a part of other skin disorders such as rosacea or basal cell carcinoma.

PRURITUS

Pruritus, or the sensation of itch, is a symptom common to many skin disorders. Generalized itching in the absence of a primary skin disease may be symptomatic of other organ disorders, such as chronic renal disease, diabetes, or biliary disease. Warmth, touch, and vibration also can act locally to trigger the itch phenomenon.

Itch sensation is mediated by cutaneous receptors. Substances such as histamine, bradykinin, substance P, and bile salts act locally to stimulate the itch receptors. Prostaglandins are modulators of the itch response, lowering the threshold for other mediators. One type of itch, sometimes referred to as *central itch*, is perceived as occurring on the skin, but originates in the central nervous system (CNS). For example, the pain reliever morphine promotes itch by acting on central opioid receptors in the CNS.

Scratching, the well-known response to itch, is a neurologic reflex that to varying degrees can be controlled by the individual. Although scratching may temporarily relieve itch, many types of itch are not easily localized and are not relieved by scratching. In many people, excoriations and thickened papular areas develop at the site of repeated scratching or rubbing.

VARIATIONS IN BLACK SKIN

Some skin disorders common to African Americans are not commonly found in European Americans. Similarly, some skin disorders, such as skin cancers, affect light-

TABLE 44-1	Common Normal Variations in Dark Skin
Variation	**Appearance**
Futcher (Voigt) line	Demarcation between darkly pigmented and lightly pigmented skin in upper arm; follows spinal nerve distribution; common in black and Japanese populations
Midline hypo-pigmentation	Line or band of hypopigmentation over the sternum, dark or faint, lessens with age; common in Latin American and black populations
Nail pigmentation	Linear dark bands down nails or diffuse nail pigmentation, brown, blue or blue-black
Oral pigmentation	Blue to blue-gray pigmentation of oral mucosa; gingivae also affected
Palmar changes	Hyperpigmented creases, small hyper-keratotic papules, and tiny pits increases
Plantar changes	Hyperpigmented macules, can be multiple with patchy distribution, irregular borders, and variance in color

Developed from information in Rosen T., Martin S. (1981). *Atlas of black dermatology*. Boston: Little, Brown.

skinned persons more commonly than dark-skinned persons. Because of these differences, serious skin disorders may be overlooked, and normal variations in darker skin may be mistaken for anomalies. Skin color is determined by the melanin produced by the melanocytes. Although the number of melanosomes in dark and white skin is the same, black skin produces more melanin and produces it faster than does white skin. Because of their skin color, blacks are better protected against skin cancer and the premature wrinkling and aging of the skin that occurs with sun exposure.

Some conditions common in people with black skin are too much or too little color. Areas of the skin may darken after injury, such as a cut or scrape, or after disease conditions, such as acne. These darkened areas may take many months or years to fade. Dry or "ashy" skin also can be a problem for people with black skin. It often is uncomfortable, and it also is easily noticed because it gives the skin an ashen, or grayish, appearance. Although using a moisturizer may help relieve the discomfort, it may cause a worsening of acne in predisposed persons.

Normal variations in skin structure and skin tones often make evaluation of dark skin difficult (Table 44-1). The darker pigmentation can make skin pallor, cyanosis, and erythema more difficult to observe. Therefore, verbal histories must be relied on to assess skin changes. The verbal history should include clients' descriptions of their normal skin tone. Changes in skin color, in particular hypopigmentation and hyperpigmentation, often accompany ethnic skin disorders and are very important signs to observe for when diagnosing skin conditions.

In summary, skin lesions and rashes are the most common manifestations of skin disorders. Rashes are temporary skin eruptions. Lesions result from traumatic or pathologic loss of the normal continuity, structure, or function of the skin. Lesions may be vascular in origin; they may occur as primary lesions in previously normal skin; or they may develop as secondary lesions resulting from primary lesions. Blisters, calluses, and corns result from rubbing, pressure, and frictional forces applied to the skin. Pruritus and dry skin are symptoms common to many skin disorders. Scratching because of pruritus can lead to excoriation, infection, and other complications.

Normal variations in black skin often make evaluation difficult and result in some disorders being overlooked. Changes in color, especially hypopigmentation or hyperpigmentation, often accompany the skin disorders of dark-skinned people.

Review Exercises

Psoriasis is a papulosquamous skin disorder that is characterized by well-demarcated, pink-to salmon-colored plaques covered by loosely adherent scales. The disease is thought to be caused by a T-cell–stimulated increase in keratocyte proliferation.

A. Hypothesize on the relationship between increased keratocyte proliferation and the lesions of psoriasis.

"Allergy tests" involve the application of an antigen to the skin, either through a small scratch or intradermal injection.

A. Explain how the body's immune system is able to detect and react to these antigens.

Visit the Porth: Essentials of Pathophysiology: Concepts of Altered Health States web site (http://thePoint.LWW.com/PorthEssentials) for links to chapter-related resources on the Internet, all-new exclusive animations, chapter review questions, and more!

BIBLIOGRAPHY

Choung C. M., Nickoloff B. J., Elias P. M., et al. (2002). What is the "true" function of the skin? *Experimental Dermatology* 11, 159–187.

Gartner L. P., Hiatt J. L. (2001). *Color textbook of histology* (2nd ed., pp. 325–342). Philadelphia: W. B. Saunders.

Hood A. F., Kwan T. H., Mihm M. C., et al. (2002). *Primer of dermatopathology* (3rd ed.). Philadelphia: Lippincott Williams & Wilkins.

Lotti T., Bianchi B., Ghersetich I., et al. (2002). Can the brain inhibit inflammation generated in the skin? The lesson of gamma-melanocyte-stimulating hormone. *International Journal of Dermatology* 41, 311–318.

Ross M. H. (2003). *Histology: A text and atlas* (4th ed., pp. 400–433). Philadelphia: Lippincott Williams & Wilkins.

Storm C. A., Elder D. E. (2005). The skin. In Rubin E., Gorstein F., Rubin R., et al. (Eds.), *Rubin's pathology: Clinicopathologic foundations of medicine* (4th ed., pp. 1203–1211). Philadelphia: Lippincott Williams & Wilkins.

Wysocki A. B. (2000). Skin anatomy, physiology, and pathophysiology. *Nursing Clinics of North America* 34, 777–798.

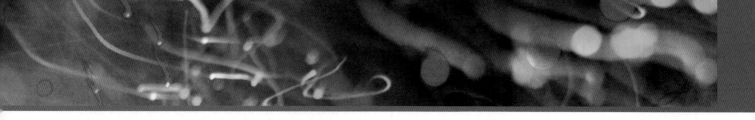

C h a p t e r 45

Disorders of the Skin

The skin is a unique organ in that numerous signs of disease or injury are immediately observable on the skin. The skin serves as the interface between the body's internal organs and the external environment. Therefore, skin disorders represent the culmination of environmental forces and the internal functioning of the body. Sunlight, infectious organisms, chemicals, and physical agents all play a role in the pathogenesis of skin diseases. Although most disorders are intrinsic to skin, many are external manifestations of systemic disease. Thus, the skin provides a valuable window for the recognition of many systemic disorders.

Primary Disorders of the Skin

Primary skin disorders are those originating in the skin. They include infectious processes, acne and rosacea, allergic and hypersensitivity disorders, and papulosquamous dermatoses. Although most of these disorders are not life threatening, they can cause intense discomfort and affect the quality of life.

INFECTIOUS PROCESSES

The skin is subject to invasion by a number of microorganisms, including fungi, bacteria, and viruses. Normally, the skin flora, sebum, immune responses, and other protective mechanisms guard the skin against infection. Depending on the virulence of the infecting agent and the competence of the host's resistance, infections may result.

Fungal Infections

Fungi are free-living, saprophytic, plantlike organisms, certain strains of which are considered part of the normal skin flora[1] (see Chapter 12). Fungal or mycotic infections of the skin are traditionally classified as superficial or deep infections. The superficial fungal infections are limited to the keratinized tissue of the skin, hair, and nails.[2,3] Deep fungal infections involve the epidermis, dermis, and subcutaneous tissue.

Superficial Fungal Infections. The fungi that cause superficial mycoses are called *dermatophytes* and require keratin for growth. Thus, these fungi do not infect deeper body tissues or mucosal surfaces. The dermatophytes emit an enzyme that enables them to digest keratin, which results in superficial skin scaling, nail disintegration, or hair breakage, depending on the location of the infection. Deeper reactions involving vesicles, erythema, and infiltration are caused by the inflammation that results from exotoxins liberated by the fungus. The dermatophytes also are capable of producing an allergic or immune response.[2]

The dermatophytes that cause skin disease have been classified into three genera: *Microsporum* (*M. audouinii, M. canis, M. fulvum*), *Epidermophyton* (*E. floccosum*), and *Trichophyton* (*T. gypseum, T. mentagrophytes, T. tonsurans, T. violaceum*). Only two of these invade the hair: *Microsporum* and *Trichophyton*. The dermatophytes can also be classified according to their ecologic origin—soil, animal, or human. Geophilic species are found in the soil. Zoophilic species (*M. canis, T. mentagrophytes*) cause parasitic infections in animals, some of which can be spread to humans. Anthropophilic species (*M. audouinii, M. tonsurans, T. violaceum*) are parasitic on humans and are spread by other infected humans. Transmission can also be indirect through fomites (*e.g.*, upholstery, hairbrushes, hats).

The clinical manifestations of dermatophyte infections are commonly referred to as *tinea* or *ringworm*.[2,3]

Tinea comes from the Latin meaning "worm" or "moth." It describes snakelike and annular (ringlike) lesions on the skin that resembles a worm burrowing at the margins. Tinea can affect the body (tinea corporis), face and neck (tinea faciei), scalp (tinea capitis), hands (tinea manus), feet (tinea pedis), or nails (tinea unguium). During an acute episode of any of the fungal infections, a dermatophytid or "id" eruption can develop. This is a manifestation of an allergic reaction to the fungus. The phenomenon is characterized by an erythematous, vesicular, or eczematous eruption that occurs in disseminated parts of the body. The most common id reaction occurs on the hands during an acute tinea infection of the feet. The id lesions do not contain fungi and disappear after adequate treatment of the acute focus.[1]

Tinea corporis (ringworm of the body) can be caused by any of the fungi, but is most frequently caused by *M. canis* and less commonly by *E. floccosum* and *T. mentagrophytes* from groin and foot lesions. Although tinea corporis affects all ages, children seem most prone to infection. Transmission is most commonly from kittens, puppies, and other children who have infections. The lesions vary, depending on the fungal agent. The most common types of lesions are oval or circular patches on exposed skin surfaces and the trunk, back, or buttocks (Fig. 45-1). Less common are foot and groin infections. The lesion begins as a red papule and enlarges, often with a central clearing. Patches have raised red borders consisting of vesicles, papules, or pustules. The borders are sharply defined, but lesions may coalesce. Pruritus, a mild burning sensation, and erythema frequently accompany the skin lesion. A secondary bacterial infection, particularly at the advancing border, is common in association with certain fungi, such as *M. canis* and *T. mentagrophytes*.

Tinea capitis (ringworm of the scalp), the most common type of dermatophytosis in children, is an infection

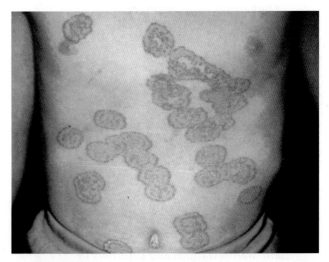

FIGURE 45-1 Tinea of the body caused by *Microsporum canis*. (From Sauer G. C., Hall J. C. [1996]. *Manual of skin diseases* [7th ed.]. Philadelphia: Lippincott-Raven.)

of the scalp and hair shaft. *Tinea capitis* can be divided into two clinical types: noninflammatory and inflammatory. The noninflammatory type is caused primarily by *T. tonsurans*. Children between 3 and 14 years of age are primarily affected, with a disproportionately higher incidence among African Americans.[1] Lower incidence rates among adults have been partially attributed to the fungistatic fatty acids in the sebum after puberty. The primary lesions can vary from grayish, round, hairless patches to balding spots, with or without black dots on the head. The lesions vary in size and are most commonly seen on the back of the head (Fig. 45-2). Mild erythema, crust, or scale may be present. The individual usually is asymptomatic, although pruritus may exist.

The inflammatory type of tinea capitis is most commonly caused by virulent strains of *T. tonsurans and M. canis*.[1] The onset is rapid, and inflamed lesions usually are localized to one area of the head. The inflammation is believed to be a delayed hypersensitivity reaction to the invading fungus. The initial lesion consists of a pustular, scaly, round patch with broken hairs. A secondary bacterial infection is common and may lead to a painful, circumscribed, boggy, and indurated lesion called a *kerion*. The highest incidence is among children and farmers who work with infected animals.

Tinea pedis (athlete's foot or ringworm of the feet) is a common dermatosis primarily affecting the spaces between the toes, the soles of the feet, or the sides of the feet (Fig. 45-3). The lesions vary from a mildly scaling lesion to a painful, exudative, erosive, inflamed lesion with fissuring. Lesions often are accompanied by pruritus, pain, and foul odor. Some persons are prone to chronic tinea pedis, whereas others have a milder form that is exacerbated during hot weather or when the feet are exposed to moisture or occlusive shoes. *Tinea manus* (ringworm of the hands) usually is a secondary infection with tinea pedis as the primary infection. In contrast to

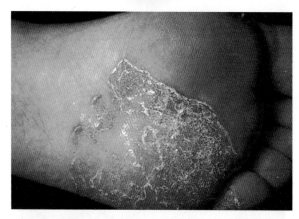

FIGURE 45-3 Chronic tinea of sole of the foot caused by *Trichophyton rubrum*. (Schering Corp.) (From Sauer G. C., Hall J. C. [1996]. *Manual of skin diseases* [7th ed.]. Philadelphia: Lippincott-Raven.)

other skin disorders such as contact dermatitis and psoriasis, which affect both hands, tinea manus usually occurs only on one hand. The characteristic lesion is a blister on the palm or finger surrounded by erythema. Chronic lesions are scaly and dry. Cracking and fissuring may occur. Usually there is a single patch as opposed to multiple patches. If chronic, tinea manus may lead to tinea of the fingernails.

Tinea unguium is a dermatophyte infection (onychomycosis) of the nails. Toenails are involved more commonly than fingernails. Toenail infection is common in persons prone to chronic infections of tinea pedis. Often, the infection in the toenails becomes a ready source for future infections of the foot. It may begin from a crushing injury to a toenail or from the spread of tinea pedis. The infection often begins at the tip of the nail, where the fungus digests the nail keratin. Initially, the nail appears opaque, white, or silvery (Fig. 45-4). The nail then turns yellow or brown. The condition often remains unchanged for years. During this time it may involve only one or two nails and may produce little or no discomfort. Gradually, the nail thickens and cracks as the infection spreads. Permanent discoloration and distortion result as the nail separates from the underlying epidermis.

Diagnosis of superficial fungal infections is primarily done by microscopic examination of skin scrapings for fungal spores, the reproducing bodies of fungi. Potassium hydroxide (KOH) preparations are used to prepare slides of skin scrapings.[1,3,4] KOH disintegrates human tissue and leaves behind the threadlike filaments, called *hyphae*, that grow from the fungal spores. Cultures also may be done.

Superficial fungal infections may be treated with topical or systemic antifungal agents. Topical agents, both prescription and over-the-counter preparations, are commonly used in the treatment of tinea infections. The two principal pharmacologic groups are the azoles and alkylamines.[3] The azoles (*e.g.*, clotrimazole, ketoconazole,

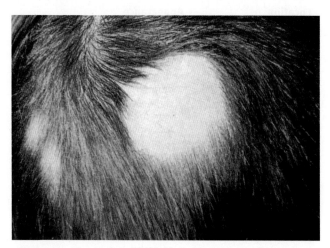

FIGURE 45-2 Tinea of the scalp caused by *Microsporum audouinii*. (From Sauer G. C., Hall J. C. [1996]. *Manual of skin diseases* [7th ed.]. Philadelphia: Lippincott-Raven.)

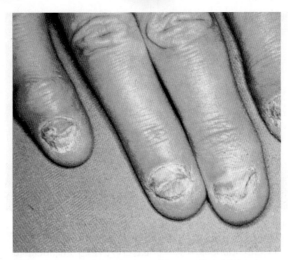

FIGURE 45-4 Tinea of the fingernail caused by *Trichophyton rubrum*. (Duke Laboratories, Inc.) (From Sauer G. C., Hall J. C. [1996]. *Manual of skin diseases* [7th ed.]. Philadelphia: Lippincott-Raven.)

miconazole, oxiconazole, econazole) are a group of synthetic antifungal drugs that act by inhibiting the fungal enzymes needed for the synthesis of ergosterol, which is an essential part of fungal cell membranes. The topical allylamines (*e.g.*, terbinafine, naftifine) act by interrupting ergosterol synthesis, causing the accumulation of a metabolite that is toxic to the fungus. Other agents that do not fit into these two main categories are tolnaftate (generic, Tinactin), haloprogin (Halotex), and butenafine (Lotrimin, Mentax). Because the topical agents do not penetrate hair or nails, they are usually ineffective in treating tinea capitis and tinea unguium. Ciclopirox, an antifungal agent that acts by inhibiting a fungal enzyme, is available as a nail lacquer for treatment of tinea unguium. It is reported to have a cure rate of 29% to 47% when applied daily for 48 weeks.[3]

The oral systemic antifungal agents include griseofulvin, the azoles (*e.g.*, ketoconazole, itraconazole), and an allylamine (terbinafine). Griseofulvin is a fungicidal agent derived from a species of *Penicillium* that is used only in the treatment of dermatophytoses.[2] It acts by binding to the keratin of newly forming skin, protecting the skin from new infection. Because its action is to prevent new infection, it must be administered for 2 to 6 weeks to allow for skin replacement. In contrast to griseofulvin, the azoles and terbinafine are fungicidal (*i.e.*, kill the fungus) and thus are more effective in shorter treatment periods. Some of the oral agents can produce serious side effects, such as hepatic toxicity, or interact adversely with other medications being taken.

Deep Fungal Infections. The deep fungal infections invade the skin more deeply and move into living tissue; they are also capable of involving other organs. They include candidiasis, sporotrichosis, and blastomycosis.

Candidiasis is a fungal infection caused by *Candida albicans*.[1] This yeastlike fungus is a normal inhabitant of the gastrointestinal tract, mouth, and vagina (see Chapter 40). The skin problems result from the release of irritating toxins on the skin surface. Some persons are predisposed to candidal infections by conditions such as diabetes mellitus, antibiotic therapy, pregnancy and use of birth control pills, poor nutrition, and immunosuppressive diseases. Oral candidiasis may be the first sign of infection with human immunodeficiency virus (HIV).

C. albicans thrives in warm, moist, intertriginous areas of the body. The rash is red with well-defined borders. Patches erode the epidermis, and there is scaling. Mild to severe itching and burning often accompany the infection. Severe forms of infection may involve pustules or vesiculopustules. In addition to microscopic analysis, a candidal infection often can be differentiated from a tinea infection by the presence of satellite lesions. These satellite lesions are maculopapular and are found outside the clearly demarcated borders of the candidal infection. Satellite lesions often are diagnostic of diaper rash complicated by *Candida*. The appearance of candidal infections varies according to the site (Table 45-1). Diagnosis of cutaneous candidiasis usually is based on microscopic examination of skin or mucous membrane scrapings placed in KOH solution. Depending on the site of infection and extent of involvement, topical and oral antifungal agents may be used in treatment.

Sporotrichosis is a granulomatous fungal infection of the skin and subcutaneous tissues that is caused by *Sporothrix schenckii*, a fungus that grows on wood and in soil.[1] It invades open wounds and is an occupational hazard of farmers, gardeners, laborers, and miners. Characteristically, a chancre-type lesion develops at the site of skin inoculation and precedes more extensive skin involvement. The chancre begins as a painless, moveable subcu-

TABLE 45-1	Candidal Infections: Locations and Appearance of Lesions
Location	**Appearance**
Breasts, groin, axillae, anus, umbilicus, toe or fingerwebs	Red lesions with well-defined borders and presence of satellite lesions; lesions may be dry or moist
Vagina	Red, oozing lesions with sharply defined borders and inflamed vagina; cervix may be covered with moist, white plaque; cheesy, foul-smelling discharge; presence of pruritus and burning
Glans penis (balanitis)	Red lesions with sharply defined borders; penis may be covered with white plaque; presence of pruritus and burning
Mouth (thrush)	Creamy white flakes on a red, inflamed mucous membrane; papillae on tongue may be enlarged
Nails	Red, painful swelling around nail bed; common in persons who often have their hands in water

taneous nodule that eventually softens and breaks down to form an ulcer. Within a few weeks subcutaneous nodules arise along the course of the draining lymphatics and form a chain of ulcers. The development of the skin lesions is slow and rarely affects general health.

Bacterial Infections

Bacteria are considered normal flora of the skin. Most bacteria are not pathogenic, but when pathogenic bacteria invade the skin, superficial or systemic infections may develop. Bacterial skin infections are commonly classified as primary or secondary infections. Primary infections are superficial skin infections such as impetigo or ecthyma. Secondary infections consist of deeper cutaneous infections, such as infected ulcers. Diagnosis usually is based on cultures taken from the infected site. Treatment measures include antibiotic therapy and measures to promote comfort and prevent the spread of infection.

Impetigo. Impetigo is a common superficial bacterial infection caused by staphylococci aureus or group A β-hemolytic streptococci, or both.[1,5,6] It is common among infants and young children, although older children and adults occasionally contract the disease. Impetigo initially appears as a small vesicle or pustule or as a large bulla on the face or elsewhere on the body. As the primary lesion ruptures, it leaves a denuded area that discharges a honey-colored serous liquid that hardens on the skin surface and dries as a honey-colored crust with a "stuck-on" appearance (Fig. 45-5). New vesicles erupt within hours. Pruritus often accompanies the lesions, and the skin excoriations that result from scratching multiply the infec-

tion sites. A possible complication of untreated group A β-hemolytic streptococcal impetigo is poststreptococcal glomerulonephritis (see Chapter 24). Topical mupirocin, which has few side effects, may be effective for limited disease. If the area is large or if there is concern about complications, systemic antibiotics are used. Impetigo is spread by direct person-to-person contact, so appropriate hygiene is important.

Ecthyma is another superficial bacterial infection that is seen less commonly and is deeper than impetigo. It is usually caused by group A β-hemolytic streptococci and occurs on the buttocks and thighs of children[1] (Fig. 45-6). The lesions are similar to those of impetigo. A vesicle or pustule ruptures, leaving a skin erosion or ulcer that weeps and dries to a crusted patch, often resulting in scar formation. With extensive ecthyma, there is a low-grade fever and extension of the infection to other organs. Treatment usually involves the use of systemic antibiotics.

Viral Infections

Viruses are intracellular pathogens that rely on living cells of the host for reproduction. They have no organized cell structure but consist of a deoxyribonucleic acid (DNA) or ribonucleic acid (RNA) core surrounded by a protein coat. The viruses seen in skin lesion disorders tend to be DNA-containing viruses. Viruses invade the keratinocyte, begin to reproduce, and cause cellular proliferation or cellular death. The rapid increase in viral skin diseases has been attributed to the use of corticosteroid drugs, which have immunosuppressive qualities, and the use of antibiotics, which alter the protective bacterial flora of the skin.

Verrucae. Verrucae, or *warts*, are common, benign papillomas caused by DNA-containing human papillomaviruses (HPV).[5–7] The lesions are circumscribed, symmetric epidermal neoplasms that are often elevated above the skin and often appear papillary. Histologically, there is

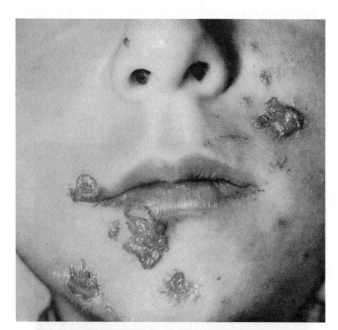

FIGURE 45-5 Impetigo of the face. (Abner Kurten, *Folia Dermatologica*. No. 2. Geigy Pharmaceuticals.) (From Sauer G. C., Hall J. C. [1996]. *Manual of skin diseases* [7th ed.]. Philadelphia: Lippincott-Raven.)

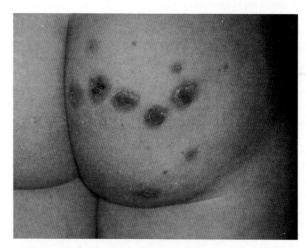

FIGURE 45-6 Ecthyma on the buttocks of a 13-year-old boy. (Glaxo-Wellcome Co.) (From Sauer G. C., Hall J. C. [1996]. *Manual of skin diseases* [7th ed.]. Philadelphia: Lippincott-Raven.)

an irregular thickening of the stratum spinosum and greatly increased thickening of the stratum corneum.

More than 50 types of HPV have been identified, a number of them capable of producing warts in humans.[6] Some HPVs, such as HPV type 16, have been associated with increased risk of genital (cervix, vulva, and penis) cancers (see Chapter 40). The skin warts caused by HPV types 1, 2, 3, 4, and 10 are not associated with malignant potential.[5] HPV transmission usually occurs through breaks in skin integrity. There are three main types of skin warts: verruca vulgaris, verruca plana, and plantar warts. *Verruca vulgaris,* also known as the *common wart,* is a papillary growth with a slightly raised surface (Fig. 45-7). They may be single or multiple and are most frequent on the surfaces of the hands or on the face. Common hand warts can be transmitted by biting the cuticles surrounding the nail. *Verruca plana,* or a flat wart, is a small flat papule that is often barely visible but can occur in clusters of 10 or more. They are commonly seen on the forehead and the dorsum of the hand. *Plantar warts* are flat to slightly raised, painful growths that extend deep into the skin on the plantar surfaces (*i.e.,* soles) of the feet. They are frequently transmitted to the abraded, softened heels of children in gym showers or swimming areas. Occasionally, similar lesions are found on palms of the hand (palmar warts).

Treatment of verrucae usually is directed at inducing a "wart-free" period without producing scarring. Warts resolve spontaneously when immunity to the virus develops. The immune response may be delayed for years. Removal is usually done by applying a keratolytic agent, such as salicylic acid, that breaks down the wart tissue, or by freezing with liquid nitrogen (cryotherapy). Various types of laser surgery, electrosurgery, and the use of cytotoxic or antiviral therapy also have been successful in wart eradication.[7] Occluding warts with duct tape has also been reported as an effective treatment that is painless and inexpensive.[8] Although the mechanism of action for duct tape is unknown, it has been hypothesized that the local irritation caused by the duct tape may stimulate the immune response.

Herpes Simplex. Herpes simplex virus (HSV) infections of the skin and mucous membrane (*i.e.,* cold sore or fever blister) are common. Two types of herpesviruses infect humans: type 1 and type 2. HSV-1 usually is confined to the oropharynx, and the organism is spread by respiratory droplets or by direct contact with infected saliva.[9,10] Genital herpes usually is caused by HSV-2 (see Chapter 40), although HSV-1 also can cause genital herpes.

Infection with HSV-1 may present as a primary or recurrent infection. Primary infections are usually asymptomatic, except for the vesicular lesions. Symptomatic primary infections are uncommon and are usually seen in children and young adults. Symptoms include fever, sore throat, painful vesicles, and ulcers of the tongue, palate, gingiva, buccal mucosa, and lips. Primary infection results in the production of antibodies to the virus so that recurrent infections are more localized and less severe. After an initial infection, the herpesvirus persists in the trigeminal and other dorsal root ganglia in the latent state. It is likely that many adults were exposed to HSV-1 during childhood and therefore have antibodies to the virus.

The recurrent lesions of HSV-1 infection usually begin with a burning or tingling sensation. Vesicles and erythema follow and progress to pustules, ulcers, and crusts before healing (Fig. 45-8). The lesions are most common on the lips, face, and mouth. Pain is common, and healing takes place within 10 to 14 days. Precipitating factors include stress, sunlight exposure, menses, or injury. Individuals who are immunocompromised may have severe attacks.

There is no cure for oropharyngeal herpes simplex; most treatment measures are largely palliative. Penciclovir cream, a topical antiviral agent, applied at the first symptom may be used to reduce the duration of an attack.[10] Application of over-the-counter topical preparations containing antihistamines, antipruritics, and anesthetic agents along with aspirin or acetaminophen may be used to relieve pain. Oral antiviral drugs that inhibit HSV replication may be used prophylactically to prevent recurrences. Sunscreen preparations applied to the lips can prevent sun-induced herpes simplex.

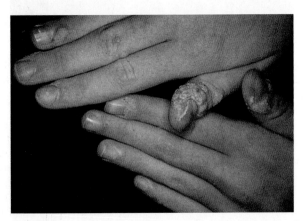

FIGURE 45-7 Common and periungual warts. (Reed & Carnrick Pharmaceuticals.) (From Sauer G. C., Hall J. C. [1996]. *Manual of skin diseases* [7th ed.]. Philadelphia: Lippincott-Raven.)

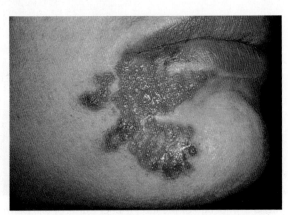

FIGURE 45-8 Recurrent herpes simplex of the face. (Dermik Laboratories, Inc.) (From Sauer G. C., Hall J. C. [1996]. *Manual of skin diseases* [7th ed.]. Philadelphia: Lippincott-Raven.)

Herpes Zoster. Herpes zoster (shingles) is an acute, localized vesicular eruption distributed over a dermatomal segment of the skin. It is caused by the varicella-zoster virus, the same herpesvirus that causes chickenpox. It is believed to result from reactivation of a latent form of the virus that remained dormant in a sensory dorsal root ganglia since a childhood infection.[9,11] During an episode of herpes zoster, the reactivated virus travels from the ganglia to the skin of the corresponding dermatome. Although herpes zoster is not as contagious as chickenpox, the reactivated virus can be transmitted to nonimmune contacts.

The incidence of herpes zoster increases with age; it occurs most frequently in persons older than 60 years.[12] The normal age-related decrease in cell-mediated immunity is thought to account for the increased viral activation in this age group. Other persons at increased risk because of impaired cell-mediated immunity are persons with conditions such as HIV infection and certain malignancies, and those receiving long-term corticosteroid treatment, cancer chemotherapy, and radiation therapy.

The lesions of herpes zoster typically are preceded by a prodrome consisting of a burning pain, tingling sensation, extreme sensitivity of the skin to touch, and pruritus along the affected dermatome. This may be present for 1 to 3 days or longer before the appearance of the rash. During this time, the pain may be mistaken for a number of other conditions, such as heart disease, pleurisy, various musculoskeletal disorders, or gastrointestinal disorders.

The lesions appear as an eruption of vesicles with erythematous bases that are restricted to skin areas supplied by sensory neurons of a single or associated group of dorsal root ganglia (Fig. 45-9). In immunosuppressed persons, the lesions may extend beyond the dermatome. Eruptions usually are unilateral in the thoracic region, trunk, or face. New crops of vesicles erupt for 3 to 5 days along the nerve pathway. The vesicles dry, form crusts, and eventually fall off. The lesions usually clear in 2 to 3 weeks, although they may persist up to 6 weeks in some elderly persons.

Serious complications can accompany herpes zoster. Eye involvement can result in permanent blindness and occurs in a large percentage of cases involving the ophthalmic division of the trigeminal nerve. Pain can persist for several months after the rash disappears. Postherpetic neuralgia, which is pain that persists longer than 1 to 3 months after the resolution of the rash, is an important complication of herpes zoster[12] (see Chapter 34). It is seen most commonly in persons who are 50 years of age or older. Affected persons complain of sharp, burning pain that often occurs in response to non-noxious stimuli. Even the slightest pressure of clothing and bed sheets may elicit pain. It usually is a self-limited condition that persists for months, with symptoms abating over time.

The treatment of choice for herpes zoster is the administration of an antiviral agent. The treatment is most effective when started within 72 hours of rash development. There are three antiviral agents available for treatment of herpes zoster: acyclovir, famciclovir, and valacyclovir.[12] Acyclovir, which is the least expensive, is usually given five times a day, whereas famciclovir and valacyclovir

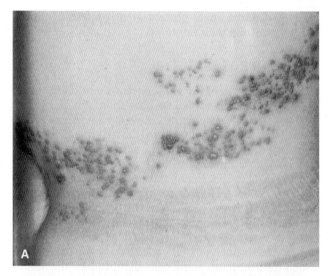

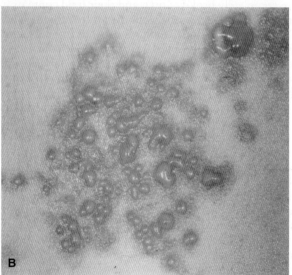

FIGURE 45-9 (**A**) Herpes zoster in a common presentation, with involvement of a single dermatome. (**B**) Herpes zoster is characterized by various sizes of vesicles. Vesicles of herpes simplex are uniform in size. (From Habif T. P. [1996]. *Clinical dermatology* [3rd ed., pp. 351 and 353]. St. Louis: C. V. Mosby, with permission from Elsevier Science.)

are given three times a day. Narcotic analgesics, tricyclic antidepressants or anticonvulsant drugs, and nerve blocks may be used for the management of postherpetic neuralgia. Oral corticosteroids sometimes are used to reduce the inflammation that may contribute to the pain.

There is current interest in developing a vaccine for preventing or modifying the course of herpes zoster in the elderly. The intent of the vaccine would be to prevent the establishment and reactivation of latent zoster.

A major concern regarding childhood vaccination against chickenpox is that it could result in an increase in herpes zoster in later life because of decreased exposure to the virus in vaccinated populations.[13] The rationale for this is that reexposure to the zoster virus from infected children might protect latently infected individuals by boosting their immunity.

ACNE AND ROSACEA

Acne is a disorder of the pilosebaceous unit (hair follicle and sebaceous gland).[5] The hair follicle is a tubular invagination of the epidermis in which hair is produced. The sebaceous glands empty into the hair follicle, and the pilosebaceous unit opens to the skin surface through a widely dilated opening called a *pore* (see Chapter 44, Fig. 44-5). The sebaceous glands produce a complex lipid mixture called *sebum,* from the Latin word meaning "tallow" or "grease." Sebum consists of a mixture of free fatty acids, triglycerides, diglycerides, monoglycerides, sterol esters, wax esters, and squalene. Sebum production occurs through what is called a *holocrine process,* in which the sebaceous gland cells that produce the sebum are completely broken down and their lipid contents are emptied through the sebaceous duct into the hair follicle. The amount of sebum produced depends on two factors: the size of the sebaceous gland and the rate of sebaceous cell proliferation. The sebaceous glands are largest on the face, scalp, and scrotum, but are present in all areas of the skin except for the soles of the feet and palms of the hands. Sebaceous cell proliferation and sebum production are uniquely responsive to direct hormonal stimulation by androgens. In men, testicular androgens are the main stimulus for sebaceous activity; in women, adrenal and ovarian androgens maintain sebaceous activity.

Acne lesions consist of *comedones* (whiteheads and blackheads), papules, pustules, nodules, and, in severe cases, cysts.[5] *Whiteheads* are pale, slightly elevated papules with no visible orifice. *Blackheads* are plugs of material that accumulate in sebaceous glands that open to the skin surface. The color of blackheads results from melanin that has moved into the sebaceous glands from adjoining epidermal cells. *Papules* are raised areas less than 5 mm in diameter. *Pustules* have a central core of purulent material. *Nodules* are larger than 5 mm in diameter and may become suppurative or hemorrhagic. Suppurative nodules often are referred to as *cysts* because of their resemblance to inflamed epidermal cysts. Acne lesions are divided into noninflammatory and inflammatory lesions. Noninflammatory acne consists primarily of comedones. Inflammatory acne consists of papules, pustules, nodules, and cysts.

Two types of acne occur during different stages of the life cycle: acne vulgaris, which is the most common form among adolescents and young adults, and acne conglobata, which develops later in life.[1] Other types of acne occur in association with various etiologic agents and influences.

Acne Vulgaris

Acne vulgaris is a common skin condition of adolescents and young adults. The condition is so common during adolescence that it is often regarded as a normal part of the maturing process. Acne vulgaris lesions, which consist of comedones (whiteheads and blackheads) or inflam-

matory lesions (pustules, nodules, or cysts), are found primarily on the face and neck and, to a lesser extent, on the back, chest, and shoulders (Fig. 45-10).

The cause of acne vulgaris remains unknown. Several factors are believed to contribute to acne, including (1) the influence of androgens on sebaceous cell activity; (2) increased proliferation of the keratinizing epidermal cells that form the sebaceous cells; (3) increased sebum production in relation to the severity of the disease; and (4) the presence of the *Propionibacterium acnes,* the microorganism responsible for the inflammatory stage of the disorder.[5,6] These factors probably are interrelated. Increased androgen production results in increased sebaceous cell activity, with a resultant plugging of the pilosebaceous ducts. The excessive sebum provides a medium for the growth of *P. acnes.* The *P. acnes* organism contains lipases that break down the free fatty acids that produce the acne inflammation.

The diagnosis of acne is based on history and physical examination. The severity of the acne is generally assessed by the number, type, and distribution of lesions.[14,15] Mild acne is usually characterized by the presence of a small number (generally <10) of open and closed comedones, with a few inflammatory papules; moderate acne by the

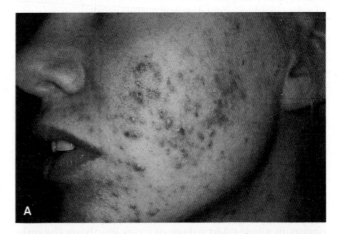

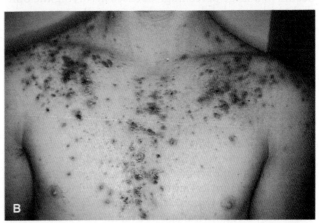

FIGURE 45-10 **(A)** Acne of the face and **(B)** acne of the chest. (From Hall J. C. [1999]. *Sauer's manual of skin diseases* [8th ed., p. 118]. Philadelphia: Lippincott Williams & Wilkins.)

presence of a moderate number (10 to 40) of erythematous papules and pustules, usually limited to the face; and moderately severe acne by the presence of numerous papules and pustules (40 to 100) and occasionally larger and deeper nodular inflamed lesions involving the face, chest, and back. Acne conglobata (to be discussed) is a severe chronic form of acne.

Treatment of acne focuses on clearing up existing lesions, preventing new lesions from forming, and limiting scar formation.[14–17] Treatment methods include the use of topical antimicrobials, oral antibiotics, topical retinoids, and isotretinoin. Soaps are usually not effective in treating acne, and unless the skin is exceptionally oily, a mild soap should be used to avoid additional irritation that will limit the effectiveness of other topicals. Mild acne is usually treated with a topical preparation containing a combination of erythromycin or clindamycin and benzoyl peroxide. Topical antibiotics do not affect existing lesions but decrease the amount of *P. acnes* on the skin, thereby reducing subsequent inflammation resulting from free fatty acid release and breakdown. Benzoyl peroxide, which is a bactericide, does not induce resistance, and when used with topical and oral antibiotics it protects against the development of this problem. Azelaic acid, products containing sodium sulfacetamide and sulfur, and salicylic acid preparations are also available. These agents are usually not considered as first-line therapies, but may be used in persons who cannot tolerate other topical agents.

Moderate to severe cases of acne may be managed with systemic antibiotics (*e.g.,* tetracycline), topical vitamin A derivatives (retinoids), or oral retinoids (isotretinoin). Systemic antibiotics decrease *P. acnes* colonization and have intrinsic anti-inflammatory effects. The action of topical vitamin A (*e.g.,* tretinoin) has been attributed to decreased cohesiveness of epidermal cells and increased epidermal cell turnover. This is thought to result in increased extrusion of open comedones and transformation of closed comedones into open ones. Isotretinoin is approved for treatment of recalcitrant cases of acne and cystic acnes. Although the exact mode of action is unknown, isotretinoin decreases sebaceous gland activity, prevents new comedones from forming, reduces the *P. acnes* count through sebum reduction, and has an anti-inflammatory effect. Because of its many side effects, it is used only in persons with severe acne. The oral retinoids are known teratogens and must not be used in women who are pregnant or may become pregnant.

Acne Conglobata

Acne conglobata occurs later in life and is a chronic form of acne. Comedones, papules, pustules, nodules, abscesses, cysts, and scars occur on the back, buttocks, and chest. Lesions occur to a lesser extent on the abdomen, shoulders, neck, face, upper arms, and thighs.[18] The comedones have multiple openings. Their discharge is odoriferous, serous, and purulent or mucoid. Healing leaves deep keloidal lesions. Affected persons have anemia with increased white blood cell counts, erythrocyte sedimentation rates, and

neutrophil counts. The treatment is difficult and stringent. It often includes debridement, systemic corticosteroid therapy, oral retinoids, and systemic antibiotics.

Rosacea

Rosacea is a chronic skin disorder of middle-aged and older persons. The disease has a variety of clinical manifestations (blushing, presence of telangiectatic vessels, eruption of inflammatory papules and pustules) that primarily affect the central areas of the face. In the early stage of rosacea development, there are repeated episodes of blushing.[18–20] The blush eventually becomes a permanent dark red erythema on the nose and cheeks that sometimes extends to the forehead and chin. This stage often occurs before 20 years of age. Ocular problems occur in at least 50% of persons with rosacea. Prominent symptoms include eyes that are itchy, burning, or dry; a gritty or foreign body sensation; and erythema and swelling of the eyelid. As the person ages, the erythema persists, and telangiectasia with or without acne components (*e.g.,* comedones, papules, pustules, nodules, erythema, edema) develops. After years of affliction, acne rosacea may develop into an irregular bullous hyperplasia (thickening of the skin) of the nose, known as *rhinophyma* (Fig. 45-11). Although rosacea is more common in women, rhinophyma is more common in men.

The cause of rosacea remains unknown. It is seen more commonly in fair-skinned persons and has been called "the curse of the Celts." Some persons identify exacerbating factors, particularly in regard to flushing, such as heat, alcohol, sunlight, hot beverages, stress, menstruation, and certain medications and foods. The common misconception that both the facial redness and rhinophyma associated with rosacea are due to excessive alcohol consumption makes rosacea a socially stigmatizing condition for many persons.[18]

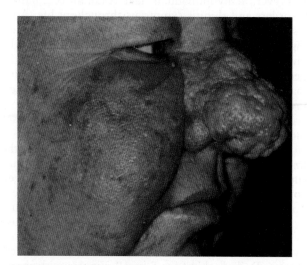

FIGURE 45-11 Chronic rosacea with rhinophyma. (Hoechst Marion Roussel Pharmaceuticals, Inc.) (From Sauer G. C., Hall J. C. [1996]. *Manual of skin diseases* [7th ed.]. Philadelphia: Lippincott-Raven.)

Persons with rosacea are usually heat sensitive. They are instructed to avoid vascular-stimulating agents such as heat, sunlight, hot liquids, foods, and alcohol. Treatment measures are similar to those used for acne vulgaris. Topical metronidazole and azelaic acid have been effective. Rhinophyma can be treated in a number of surgical ways, including electrosurgery, laser ablation, dermabrasion, cryosurgery, and scalpel excision.

ALLERGIC AND HYPERSENSITIVITY DERMATOSES

Allergic and hypersensitivity dermatoses involve an immunologic response to exogenous and endogenous agents. They include atopic and nummular eczema, urticaria, and drug-induced skin eruptions. Allergic contact dermatitis is discussed in Chapter 15.

Atopic Eczema

Atopic eczema (atopic dermatitis) is an itchy, inflammatory skin disorder that occurs in two clinical forms, infantile and adult.[1] It is usually associated with a type I hypersensitivity reaction (see Chapter 15), although some cases do not have demonstrable hypersensitivity to allergens.[21,22] There usually is a family history of asthma, hay fever, or atopic dermatitis, with asthma being a frequent comorbidity.

The infantile form of atopic dermatitis is characterized by poorly defined erythema, with edema, vesicles, and weeping in the acute stage and skin thickening (lichenification) in the chronic stage. It usually begins in the cheeks and may progress to involve the scalp, arms, trunk, and legs (Fig. 45-12). The skin of the cheeks may be paler, with extra creases under the eyes called *Dennie-Morgan folds.* The infantile form may become milder as the child grows older, often disappearing by the age of 15 years. However, many individuals have resultant eczematous disorders and rhinitis symptoms throughout life. Adolescents and adults usually have dry, leathery and hyperpigmented or hypopigmented lesions located in the antecubital and popliteal areas. These may spread to the neck, hands, feet, eyelids, and behind the ears. Itching may be severe with both forms. There is marked follicle involvement in darker-skinned persons with lesions that are hypopigmented, hyperpigmented, or both. Secondary infections are common.

Treatment of atopic eczema is designed to target the underlying abnormalities, such as skin dryness, pruritus, superinfection, and inflammation. It involves allergen control, basic skin care, and medications. Avoiding exposure to environmental irritants and foods that cause exacerbation of the symptoms is recommended. Because dry skin and pruritus often exacerbate the condition, hydration of the skin is essential to treating atopic dermatitis. Daily bathing for 5 to 10 minutes with warm (not hot) water is recommended. Although bathing dries the skin, it is important to maintain a low level of microorganisms to prevent infection. The use of soap should

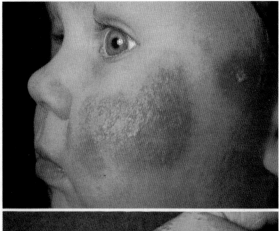
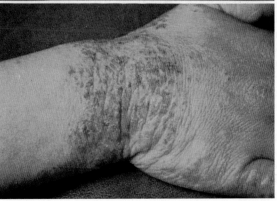

FIGURE 45-12 Atopic eczema on an infant's face and on a wrist. (Dome Chemicals.) (From Sauer G. C., Hall J. C. [1996]. *Manual of skin diseases* [7th ed.]. Philadelphia: Lippincott-Raven.)

be avoided as much as possible. An emollient should be applied immediately after bathing and before the skin is completely dry. Ointments are superior to creams and lotions, but they are greasy and often poorly tolerated.[21] Mild or healing lesions may be treated with lotions containing a mild antipruritic agent. Acute weeping lesions are treated with soothing lotions, soaks, or wet dressings. Soaks in sodium bicarbonate or emollient bath preparations such as those containing colloidal oatmeal can be used to treat pruritus. Persons with atopic dermatitis are advised to avoid temperature changes and stress to minimize vascular and sweat responses. Wool and scratchy clothing may be irritating and should be avoided.

Topical corticosteroids have been the standard of treatment, but can cause local and systemic side effects. The potency of topical corticosteroids is classified by the potential for vasoconstriction—a marker for clinical efficacy and skin thinning. In general, only weak or low-potency preparations are used on the face and genitals, whereas those that have moderate to high potency are used on other areas of the body.[21] Because of their side effects, systemic corticosteroids usually are reserved for severe cases. Persistent pruritus can be treated with antihistamines or tricyclic antidepressants.

Topical immune modulators (tacrolimus and pimecrolimus) are demonstrating positive outcomes in atopic dermatitis without the primary side effect of corticosteroid therapy (dermal atrophy).[22–24] Immune modulators are immunosuppressive agents that have been used systemically for the prevention of organ rejection. Tacrolimus is believed to control atopic dermatitis by inhibiting activation of immune cells involved in atopic dermatitis: T lymphocytes, dendritic cells, mast cells, and keratinocytes.[22,24] In March 2005, the U.S. Food and Drug Administration (FDA) issued an alert to health care professionals concerning a potential link between topical tacrolimus and pimecrolimus and cancer (mainly lymphoma and skin cancer) based on animal studies, case reports, and knowledge of how these drugs work. The alert emphasizes the importance of using these drugs only as labeled and when first-line therapy has failed or cannot be tolerated.[22]

Nummular Eczema

Nummular eczema is a rather common and distinctive eczematous condition, characterized by coin-shaped (nummular) papulovesicular patches mainly involving the arms and legs (Fig. 45-13). Lichenification and secondary bacterial infections are common. It is not unusual for the initial lesions seemingly to heal, followed by a secondary outbreak of mirror-image lesions on the opposite side of the body. Most nummular eczema is chronic, with weeks to years between exacerbations. Exacerbations occur more frequently in the cold winter months. The exact cause of nummular eczema is unknown. There usually is a history of asthma, hay fever, or atopic dermatitis. Treatment is largely palliative. Frequent bathing should be avoided. Topical corticosteroids, coal tar preparations, and oral antihistamines are prescribed as necessary.

Urticaria

Urticaria, or hives, is a common skin disorder characterized the development of edematous wheals accompanied by intense itching.[25] The lesions typically appear as raised pink or red areas surrounded by a paler halo. They blanch

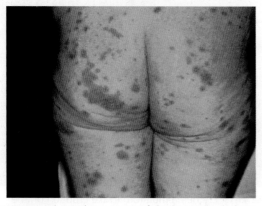

FIGURE 45-13 Nummular eczema of the buttocks. (Johnson & Johnson.) (From Sauer G. C., Hall J. C. [1996]. *Manual of skin diseases* [7th ed.]. Philadelphia: Lippincott-Raven.)

with pressure and vary in size from a few millimeters to centimeters. Angioedema, which can occur alone or along with urticaria, is characterized by nonpitting, nonpruritic, well-defined edematous swelling that involves subcutaneous tissues of the face, hands, feet, or genitals.[26] Occasionally there may be swelling of the tongue and upper airways. Angioedema tends to occur in the face and can cause significant disfigurement.

Urticaria can be acute or chronic and due to known or unknown causes. Numerous factors, both immunologic and nonimmunologic, can be involved in its pathogenesis. The urticarial wheal results from liberation of histamine from mast cells and basophils. Histamine causes hyperpermeability of the microvessels of the skin and surrounding tissue, allowing fluid to leak into the tissues, causing edema and wheal formation.

Acute immunologic urticaria is commonly the result of an immunoglobulin E (IgE)–mediated immune reaction that usually occurs within 1 hour of exposure to an antigen.[25] The most common causes of acute urticaria are foods or drinks, medications (most notably penicillin and cephalosporin), insect stings, viral infections, dust mites, and exposure to pollens or chemicals. Food is the most common cause of acute urticaria in children. Although nonsteroidal anti-inflammatory drugs, including aspirin, do not normally cause urticaria, they may exacerbate the condition.

Chronic urticaria primarily affects adults and is twice as common in women as in men. Usually its cause cannot be determined despite extensive laboratory tests. It appears to be an autoimmune disorder in a substantial number of persons. Approximately 40% to 50% of persons with chronic urticaria have circulating IgG antibodies to a subunit of the IgE receptor or to the IgE molecule. These antibodies activate basophils and mast cells to release histamine.[26] In rare cases, urticaria is a manifestation of underlying disease, such as certain cancers, collagen diseases, and hepatitis. There is an association between chronic urticaria and autoimmune thyroid disease (*e.g.,* Hashimoto thyroiditis, Graves disease, toxic multinodular thyroiditis).[27] A hereditary deficiency of a C1 (complement 1) inhibitor also can cause urticaria and angioedema.

The physical urticarias constitute another form of chronic urticaria.[27] Physical urticarias are intermittent, usually last less than 2 hours, are produced by appropriate stimuli, have distinctive appearances and locations, and are seen most frequently in young adults. Dermographism, or skin writing, is one form of physical urticaria in which wheals appear in response to simple rubbing of the skin (Fig. 45-14). The wheals follow the pattern of the scratch or rubbing, appearing within 10 minutes, and dissolving completely within 20 minutes. Other types of physical urticaria are induced by exercise (cholinergic), cold, delayed pressure, sunlight (solar), water (aquagenic), vibration, and heat (external localized). Appropriate challenge tests (*e.g.,* application of an ice cube to the skin to initiate development of cold urticaria) are used to differentiate physical urticaria from chronic urticaria due to other causes.

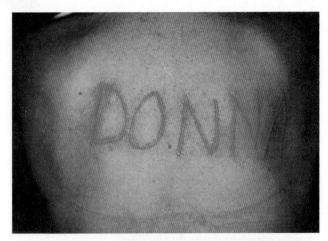

FIGURE 45-14 Dermographism on a patient's back. (Dermik Laboratories, Inc.) (From Sauer G. C., Hall J. C. [1996]. *Manual of skin diseases* [7th ed.]. Philadelphia: Lippincott-Raven.)

Most types of urticaria are treated with antihistamines, drugs that block histamine type 1 (H_1) receptors and, less frequently, H_1 in combination with histamine type 2 (H_2) receptors.[27,28] They control urticaria by inhibiting vasodilatation and the escape of fluid into the surrounding tissues. Usually nonsedating antihistamines that alleviate pruritus and decrease the incidence of hives without producing drowsiness are used. Leukotriene antagonists (zafirlukast and montelukast) may also be used.[27,28] Starch or colloid-type (*e.g.,* Aveeno) baths may be used as comfort measures. Persons who experience angioedema of the larynx and pharynx can be counseled to carry a prescription of epinephrine in an autoinjectable form (*e.g.,* EpiPen).[28] Oral corticosteroids may be used in the treatment of refractory urticaria. Tricyclic antidepressant drugs, particularly those with antihistamine actions, also may be used.

Drug-Induced Skin Eruptions

Almost any drug can cause a localized or generalized skin eruption. Topical drugs usually are responsible for a localized contact dermatitis type of rash, whereas systemic drugs cause generalized skin lesions. Although many drug-induced skin eruptions are morbilliform (*i.e.,* measles-like) or exanthematous, they may mimic almost any of the skin disorders described in this chapter. Because the lesions from drug sensitization vary greatly, diagnosis depends almost entirely on accurate patient report as well as a full drug history. Early recognition and discontinuation of the drug is essential. Management of mild cases is aimed at eliminating the offending drug while treating the symptoms. More severe cases, such as Steven-Johnson syndrome and toxic epidermal necrolysis, which are variants of erythema multiforme, require prompt medical treatment.

Erythema multiforme is an acute inflammatory skin disease that is divided clinically into minor and major types based on clinical findings. Erythema multiforme minor may be drug induced, but it more frequently occurs after infections, especially with HSV.[5,6] Erythema multiforme major (Steven-Johnson syndrome) is marked by toxicity and involvement of two or more mucosal surfaces (often oral and conjunctival) and most often is caused by drugs, especially sulfonamides, nonsteroidal anti-inflammatory drugs, and anticonvulsants, such as phenytoin.[29] A variant of erythema multiforme major, toxic epidermal necrolysis, results in diffuse necrosis and sloughing of epidermal surfaces, producing a clinical situation similar to that of extensive burns.[6]

The lesions of erythema multiforme minor and Stevens-Johnson syndrome are similar. The primary lesion of both is a round, erythematous papule, resembling an insect bite. Within hours to days, these lesions change into several different patterns. The individual lesions may enlarge and coalesce, producing small plaques, or they may change to concentric zones of color appearing as "target" or "iris" lesions (Fig. 45-15). The outermost rings of the target lesions usually are erythematous; the central portion usually is opaque white, yellow, or gray (dusky). In the center, small blisters on the dusky purpuric macules may form, giving them their characteristic target-like appearance. Although there is wide distribution of lesions over the body surface area, there is a propensity for them to occur on the face and trunk. With Stevens-Johnson syndrome, there is more skin detachment. Toxic epidermal necrolysis is the most serious drug reaction, with mortality rates of 30% to 35%.[30] There is a prodromal period of malaise, low-grade fever, and sore throat. Within a few days, widespread erythema and large, flaccid bullae appear, followed by loss of the epidermis, leaving a denuded and painful dermis. The skin surrounding the large denuded areas may have the typical target-like lesions seen with Stevens-Johnson syndrome. The application of lateral pressure often causes the surrounding skin to separate easily from the dermis (*Nikolsky's sign*).

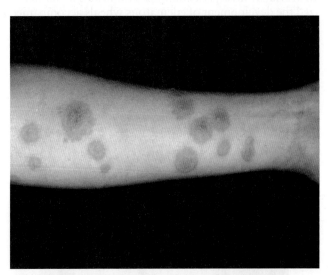

FIGURE 45-15 Erythema multiforme–like eruption on the patient's arm. Notice the dusky, target-like appearance. (Dermik Laboratories, Inc.) (From Sauer G. C., Hall J. C. [1996]. *Manual of skin diseases* [7th ed.]. Philadelphia: Lippincott-Raven.)

Usually the epithelium of mucosal surfaces, especially that of the mouth and eyes, is also involved.

Initially, these three types of bullous skin eruptions are quite similar. The diagnostic boundary for erythema multiforme minor is that it usually occurs after a HSV infection and is self-limiting. Precise diagnostic boundaries between Stevens-Johnson syndrome and toxic epidermal necrolysis have not been established. However, there is some general agreement that cases involving less than 10% of the body surface area are called Stevens-Johnson syndrome, and detachment of more than 30% of the epidermis is labeled toxic epidermal necrolysis, with a 10% to 30% overlap of diagnoses.[31]

Treatment of erythema multiforme minor and less severe cases of Stevens-Johnson syndrome includes relief of symptoms using compresses, antipruritic drugs, and topical anesthetics. Corticosteroid therapy may be indicated in moderate cases, although its use is controversial. For severe cases of Stevens-Johnson syndrome and toxic epidermal necrolysis, hospitalization is required for fluid replacement, administration of antibiotics, respiratory care, analgesics, and moist dressings. When large areas of skin are detached, the care is similar to that of thermal burn patients. Intravenous immunoglobulin may hasten the healing response of the skin. Generally, healing is a slow process, taking 6 weeks or more to regenerate skin. The mucous membranes heal more slowly, and follow-up treatment is often needed for ophthalmologic and mucous membrane sequelae. Avoidance of the responsible drug and chemically related compounds is essential.

PAPULOSQUAMOUS DERMATOSES

Papulosquamous dermatoses are a group of skin disorders characterized by scaling papules and plaques. Among the major papulosquamous diseases are psoriasis, pityriasis rosea, and lichen planus.

Psoriasis

Psoriasis is a common inflammatory skin disease characterized by circumscribed, red, thickened plaques with an overlying silvery-white scale.[6] Psoriasis occurs worldwide, although the incidence is lower in warmer, sunnier climates. It affects 1% to 2% of people in the United States.[6] The average age of onset is in the third decade; its prevalence increases with age. Approximately one third of patients have a genetic history, indicating a hereditary factor. Childhood onset of the disease is more strongly associated with a family history than psoriasis occurring in adults older than 30 years of age. There also appears to be an association between psoriasis and arthritis. Psoriatic arthritis occurs in 5% to as much as 20% of people with psoriasis and can account for a considerable amount of joint damage[32] (see Chapter 43).

The cause of psoriasis remains poorly understood and is probably multifactorial. There is evidence of a genetic component.[32] The more severe the disease, the greater is the likelihood of a familial background.[5] Environmental factors may also play a role. A variety of stimuli, such as physical injury, infections, use of certain drugs, and photosensitivity, may precipitate the development or exacerbation of lesions in people who are predisposed to the disease. The reaction of the skin to an original trauma of any type is called the *Köbner reaction*.[5] There is also evidence to suggest that deregulation of epidermal proliferation and an abnormality in the microcirculation of the dermis are responsible for the development of psoriatic lesions.

Although the factors that contribute to the generation of psoriatic lesions remain obscure, there is increasing evidence of a T-lymphocyte–based immunopathogenesis.[5,6,33] It is thought that a T-lymphocyte–mediated reaction results in the production of chemical messengers that stimulate abnormal growth of keratinocytes and dermal blood vessels. Accompanying inflammatory changes are caused by infiltration of neutrophils and monocytes.

Histologically, psoriasis is characterized by increased epidermal cell turnover with marked epidermal thickening, a process called *hyperkeratosis*. The granular layer (stratum granulosum) of the epidermis is thinned or absent, and neutrophils are found in the stratum corneum. There also is an accompanying thinning of the epidermal cell layer that overlies the tips of the dermal papillae (suprapapillary plate), and the blood vessels within dermal papillae become tortuous and dilated. These capillary beds show permanent damage even when the disease is in remission or has resolved. The close proximity of the abnormal vessels in the dermal papillae to the hyperkeratotic scale accounts for multiple, minute bleeding points that are seen when the scale is lifted.

There are several variants or types of psoriasis, including plaque-type psoriasis, guttate psoriasis, and pustular psoriasis.[34,35] *Plaque-type psoriasis (psoriasis vulgaris)*, the most common type, is a chronic stationary form of psoriasis. The lesions may occur anywhere on the skin, but most often involve the elbows, knees, and scalp (Fig. 45-16). The primary lesions are sharply demarcated, thick, red plaques with a silvery scale that vary in size and shape. In darker-skinned persons, the plaques may appear purple. There may be excoriation, thickening, or oozing from the lesions. A differential diagnostic finding is that the plaques bleed from minute points when scale is removed, which is known as the *Auspitz sign*. *Guttate psoriasis* is characterized by teardrop-shaped, pink to salmon, scaly lesions, and occurs in children and young adults. Its lesions are usually limited to the upper trunk and extremities. This form of psoriasis usually is brought on by a streptococcal infection. It generally responds to treatments such as ultraviolet B (UVB) phototherapy, only to return with recurrent streptococcal infections.[35] *Pustular psoriasis* is characterized by papules or plaques studded with pustules. Localized pustular psoriasis usually is limited to the palms of the hands and soles of the feet. Generalized pustular psoriasis is characterized by more general involvement and may be associated with systemic symptoms such as fever, malaise, and diarrhea. The person may or may not have had preexisting psoriasis.

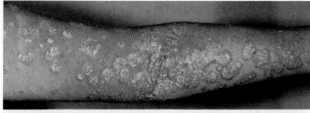
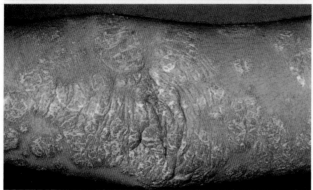

FIGURE 45-16 Psoriasis on the elbows of a 17-year-old girl. (Roche Laboratories.) (From Sauer G. C., Hall J. C. [1996]. *Manual of skin diseases* [7th ed.]. Philadelphia: Lippincott-Raven.)

Treatment. There is no cure for psoriasis. The goal of treatment is to suppress the signs and symptoms of the disease: hyperkeratosis, epidermal inflammation, and abnormal keratinocyte differentiation. Treatment depends on the severity of the disease, as well as the person's age, gender, treatment history, and level of treatment compliance. Treatment measures are divided into topical and systemic approaches. Usually, topical agents are used first in any treatment regimen and when less than 20% of the body surface is involved.[34] Combination therapies that are tailored to the needs of the client are most effective. Also, rotating various therapies may decrease the side effects of any one therapy.

Topical agents include emollients, keratolytic agents, coal tar products, anthralin, corticosteroids, and calcipotriene. Emollients hydrate and soften the psoriatic plaques. Petroleum-based products are more effective than water-based ones, but they are often less acceptable cosmetically to persons with psoriasis. Keratolytic agents are peeling agents, of which salicylic acid is the most widely used. It softens and removes plaques, and has been used alone or in conjunction with other topical agents. Coal tar, the byproduct of the processing of coke and gas from coal, is one of the oldest yet more effective forms of treatment. The skin is covered with a film of coal tar for up to several weeks. The exact mechanism of action of the tar products is unknown, but side effects of the treatment are few. Newer preparations of coal tar lotions and shampoos are more aesthetically pleasing, but the odor remains a problem. Anthralin, a synthesized product of Goa powder from Brazilian araroba tree bark, has remained a topical treatment of choice. It acts by reducing epidermal mitosis and has been effective in resolving lesions in approximately 2 weeks. A disadvan-

tage to anthralin is that it stains the uninvolved skin and clothes brown or purple.

Topical corticosteroids are widely used and relatively effective. Although the corticosteroids are rapidly effective in the treatment of psoriasis, they are associated with flare-ups after discontinuation, and they have many potential side effects. Their effectiveness is increased when used under occlusive dressings, but there is an increase in side effects.

Calcipotriene, a topical vitamin D derivative, has been effective for the treatment of psoriasis. It inhibits epidermal cell proliferation and enhances cell differentiation. *Tazarotene,* a synthetic retinoid, also has been effective. It is classified as a pregnancy category X drug and should be avoided in women of childbearing age.

Systemic treatments include phototherapy, photochemotherapy, methotrexate, retinoids, corticosteroids, and cyclosporine. Phototherapy with ultraviolet B (UVB) radiation is a widely used treatment. Newly developed narrow-band UVB is reportedly more effective than broadband UVB.[35] Photochemotherapy involves using a light-activated form of the drug methoxsalen. Methoxsalen, a psoralen, exerts its actions when exposed to ultraviolet A (UVA) radiation in 320- to 400-nm wavelengths. The combination treatment regimen of psoralen and UVA is known by the acronym PUVA. Methoxsalen is given orally before UVA exposure. Activated by the UVA energy, methoxsalen inhibits DNA synthesis, thereby preventing cell mitosis and decreasing the hyperkeratosis that occurs with psoriasis. Although viewed as one of the safest therapies since its introduction in the 1970s, PUVA increases the risk for squamous cell carcinoma, and it may increase the risk for development of melanoma.

Systemic corticosteroids have been effective in treating severe or pustular psoriasis. However, they cause severe side effects, including Cushing syndrome. Intralesional injection of triamcinolone has proven effective in resistant lesions.

The retinoids are another class of systemic psoriasis therapy. These drugs, which are derivatives of vitamin A, are only moderately effective as monotherapy and are associated with numerous mucocutaneous side effects such as hair loss, cheilitis, and thinning of the nails. However, when used as a short-term adjunct in combination with UVB phototherapy or PUVA, low-dose acitretin has been shown to be effective, allowing substantial clearing of lesions with fewer mucocutaneous side effects.[35] Teratogenicity limits use of retinoids in women of childbearing potential.

Methotrexate, which is used for cancer treatment, is an antimetabolite that inhibits DNA synthesis and prevents cell mitosis. Oral methotrexate has been effective in treating psoriasis when other approaches have failed. The drug has many side effects, including nausea, malaise, leukopenia, thrombocytopenia, and liver function abnormalities. Cyclosporine is a potent immunosuppressive drug used to prevent rejection of organ transplants. It suppresses inflammation and the proliferation of T cells in persons with psoriasis. Its use is limited to severe psoriasis because of serious side effects, including nephrotoxicity, hypertension, and increased risk of cancers. Intralesional cyclosporine also has been effective. New biologic agents (infliximab, etanercept, and alefacept) that target the activity of T lymphocytes and cytokines responsible for the inflammatory nature of psoriasis have proven effective not only for the skin lesions, but in halting the effects of the arthritis associated with psoriasis.[36,37]

Pityriasis Rosea

Pityriasis rosea is a rash that primarily affects young adults.[38] The origin of the rash is unknown, but it is believed to be caused by an infective agent. Numerous viruses have been investigated, but no conclusive evidence has been found linking them with the condition. The incidence is highest in winter. Cases occur in clusters and among persons who are in close contact with each other, indicating an infectious spread. However, there are no data to support communicability. It may be an immune response to any number of agents.

The characteristic lesion is an oval macule or papule with surrounding erythema (Fig. 45-17). The lesion spreads with a central clearing, much like tinea corporis. The initial lesion is a solitary lesion called the *herald patch* and is usually on the trunk or neck. As the lesion enlarges and begins to fade (2 to 10 days), successive crops of lesions appear on the trunk and neck. The lesions on the back have a characteristic "Christmas tree" pattern. The lesions may also involve the extremities, face, and scalp. Mild to severe pruritus may occur.

The disease is self-limited and usually disappears within 6 to 8 weeks. Treatment measures are palliative and include topical steroids, antihistamines, and colloid baths. Systemic corticosteroids may be indicated in severe cases.

Lichen Planus

The term *lichen* is of Greek origin and means "tree moss." The term is applied to skin disorders characterized by small (2 to 10 mm), flat-topped papules with irregular,

angulated borders (Fig. 45-18). Lichen planus is a relatively common chronic, pruritic disease. It involves inflammation and papular eruption of the skin and mucous membranes. There are variations in the pattern of lesions (*e.g.*, annular, linear) and differences in the sites (*e.g.*, mucous membranes, genitalia, nails, scalp). The characteristic lesion is a purple, polygonal papule covered with a shiny, white, lacelike pattern. The lesions appear on the wrist, ankles, and trunk of the body. Most persons who have skin lesions also have oral lesions, appearing as a milky white lacework on the buccal mucosa or tongue. Other mucosal surfaces, such as the genital, nasal, laryngeal, otic, gastric, and anal areas, may also be affected.

Lichen planus is believed to be caused by an abnormal immune response in which epithelial cells are recognized as foreign. The disorder involves the epidermal-dermal junction with damage to the basal cell layer. Lichen planus has been linked in many cases to hepatitis C virus infection or medication use. The most common medications implicated include gold, antimalarial agents, thiazide diuretics, beta blockers, nonsteroidal anti-inflammatory drugs, quinidine, and angiotensin-converting enzyme inhibitors.[39]

Diagnosis is based on the clinical appearance of the lesions and the histopathologic findings from a punch biopsy. For most persons, lichen planus is a self-limited disease. Treatment measures include discontinuation of all medications, followed by treatment with topical corticosteroids. An occlusive dressing may be used to enhance the effect of topical medications. Antipruritic agents are

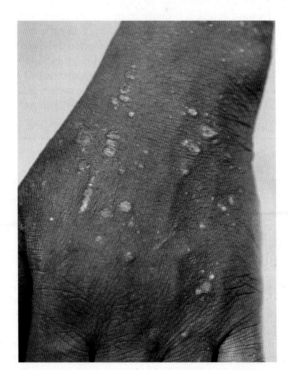

FIGURE 45-18 Lichen planus of the dorsum of the hand and wrist. Notice the violaceous color of the papules and the linear Köbner reaction. (From Sauer G. C., Hall J. C. [1996]. *Manual of skin diseases* [7th ed.]. Philadelphia: Lippincott-Raven.)

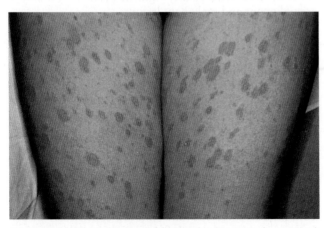

FIGURE 45-17 Pityriasis rosea of the thighs. (Syntex Laboratories.) (From Sauer G. C., Hall J. C. [1996]. *Manual of skin diseases* [7th ed.]. Philadelphia: Lippincott-Raven.)

helpful in reducing itch. Systemic corticosteroids may be indicated in severe cases. Intralesional corticosteroid injections also may be used. Acitretin, an orally administered retinoid agent, also may be effective. Because retinoids are teratogenic, they should be avoided in women of childbearing age.

In summary, primary skin disorders are those originating in the skin. They include infectious processes, acne and rosacea, allergic and hypersensitivity disorders, and papulosquamous dermatoses. The skin is subject to invasion by a number of microorganisms, including fungi, bacteria, and viruses. The superficial fungal infections, more commonly known as *tinea* or *ringworm*, invade only the superficial keratinized tissue. Tinea can affect the whole body (tinea corporis), scalp (tinea capitis), hands (tinea manus), feet (tinea pedis), or nails (tinea unguium). The deep fungal infections invade the skin more deeply and go into living tissue, and are also capable of involving other organs. Impetigo, which is caused by staphylococci aureus or group A β-hemolytic streptococci, is the most common superficial bacterial infection. Viruses are responsible for verrucae (warts), herpes simplex type 1 lesions (cold sores or fever blisters), and herpes zoster (shingles).

Noninfectious inflammatory skin conditions include acne and rosacea and the papulosquamous dermatoses. Acne is a disorder of the pilosebaceous unit. Acne vulgaris, which is a common skin disorder of adolescents and young adults, is thought to reflect increased sebum production and the presence of *P. acnes*. The papulosquamous dermatoses, which are characterized by scaling papules and plaques, include psoriasis, pityriasis rosea, and lichen planus. Allergic and hypersensitivity skin responses involve the body's immune system and are caused by hypersensitivity reactions to allergens, environmental agents, drugs, and other substances.

Ultraviolet Radiation, Thermal, and Pressure Injury

SKIN DAMAGE CAUSED BY ULTRAVIOLET RADIATION

The skin is the protective shield against harmful ultraviolet rays from the sun. Skin cancers and other skin disorders such as early wrinkling and aging have been attributed to the damaging effects of sunlight.

Sunlight is measured in wavelengths ranging from approximately 290 nm in the ultraviolet region up to approximately 2500 nm in the infrared region. Ultraviolet radiation (UVR) is divided into three types: ultraviolet C (UVC), UVB, and UVA. UVC rays are short (100 to 290 nm) and do not pass through the earth's atmosphere. However, they can be produced artificially and are damaging to the eyes. UVB rays are 290 to 320 nm. These are the rays that are primarily responsible for nearly all the skin effects of sunlight. They are more commonly referred to as *sunburn rays*. UVA rays are 320 to 400 nm. A comparable dose of UVA is less likely to produce a similar degree of erythema compared with UVB. Unlike UVB, however, UVA penetrates the dermal layer and may cause harmful effects not caused by UVB.[40] Artificial sources of UVA and UVB, such as tanning salons, may produce the same effects as UVR from natural sunlight. The average tanning bulb emits 95% UVA radiation and 5% UVB radiation.[41]

With UVR exposure, skin cells release vasoactive and injurious chemical mediators. Within the first 24 hours of exposure, UVR produces erythema and, depending on dosage, sunburn.[41,42] Melanin in the stratum corneum absorbs UVR as a means of preventing destruction of the lower skin layers; the skin responds to UVR exposure with an increase in melanin content and development of a suntan. Immediate pigment darkening begins during actual exposure to UVR and the oxidation of existing melanin in the epidermis. The degree of immediate pigment darkening depends on the duration and intensity of UVR exposure, extent of previous tanning (amount of preexisting melanin), and the skin type of the individual. Delayed tanning occurs 48 to 72 hours after UVR exposure and is the result of increased melanin production.[40]

Repetitive exposure to UVR can have multiple deleterious effects on the skin, including premature aging and increased risk for development of cutaneous malignancies. Photoaging, or premature aging of the skin, involves skin changes that are different from those associated with normal chronologic aging. Normal aging of the skin involves fine wrinkling, atrophy of the dermis, and a decrease in the amount of subcutaneous adipose tissue.[40] Photodamaged skin is wrinkled, yellowed, and sagging. Mildly affected skin becomes irregularly pigmented, rough, and dry, with mild wrinkles. Moderately affected skin becomes deeply wrinkled, sagging, thickened, and leathery, with vascular lesions. Severely affected skin becomes deeply furrowed, permanently and irregularly pigmented, and may manifest premalignant and malignant lesions.

The carcinogenic effects of UVR are thought to be at least twofold: (1) UVR causes direct DNA damage, and (2) it suppresses the cutaneous immune response. The number of immune cells is decreased, and their activity is lessened by UVR exposure. It is believed these effects prevent the immune system from detecting and removing sun-damaged cells with malignant potential.[42]

Sunburn

Sunburn is caused by excessive exposure of the epidermal and dermal layers of the skin to UVR, resulting in an erythematous inflammatory reaction.[40,41] Sunburn can range from mild to severe. A mild sunburn consists of various degrees of skin redness. Inflammation, vesicle eruption, weakness, chills, fever, malaise, and pain accompany more severe forms of sunburn. Scaling and peeling follow any overexposure to sunlight. Black skin also burns and may appear grayish or gray-black.

Severe sunburns are treated with wet Burow's solution soaks and topical creams and lotions to limit inflammation and pain. Extensive second- and third-degree burns may require hospitalization and specialized burn care techniques.

Drug-Induced Photosensitivity

Some drugs are classified as photosensitive drugs because they produce an exaggerated response to ultraviolet light. Examples include some of the anti-infective agents (fluoroquinolones, doxycycline, demeclocycline, nalidixic acid), tricyclic antidepressants, thiazide diuretics, nonsteroidal anti-inflammatory drugs, and quinidine.[43] Severe sunburn can result when persons taking these drugs are exposed to sunlight.

Drug-induced photosensitivity, such as UVA photosensitivity induced by the psoralens, may be used in treating skin conditions, such as psoriasis, that respond well to UVR exposure. Because an increased incidence of cancerous lesions has been reported in people who have been treated with these agents, their use requires caution and careful surveillance.

Sunscreens and Other Protective Measures

The ultraviolet rays of sunlight or other sources can be completely or partially blocked from the skin surface by sunscreens. The FDA requires a *sun protection factor* (SPF) rating on all commercial preparations based on their ability to obstruct UVR absorption. The ratings usually are on a scale of 1 to 30+, with the higher ratings indicating greater blocking of UVR.[40] Products with a higher SPF screen out more UVB rays, which are primarily responsible for acute sun damage.

There are two primary types of sunscreens available on the market—chemical (soluble) agents and physical (insoluble) agents.[40] Chemical agents (*e.g.*, para-aminobenzoic acid [PABA]) protect the skin from absorbing sunlight, and physical agents (*e.g.*, micronized titanium dioxide and microfine zinc) work by reflecting sunlight.

Other protective measures include knowledge about sunlight and how to protect the skin. Shielding the skin with protective clothing and hats or head coverings helps decrease UVR exposure.

THERMAL INJURY

About 1.2 million people in the United States require medical care for burns each year, with 51,000 requiring hospitalization. Between 30% and 40% of these are children younger than 15 years of age, with an average age of 32 months.[44]

The effects and complications of burns serve as a prime example of the essential function the skin performs as it protects the body from the many damaging elements in the environment while maintaining the constancy of the body's internal environment. Extensive loss of skin tissue

not only predisposes to attack by microorganisms in the environment, it allows for the massive loss of body fluids and their contents, interferes with temperature regulation, challenges the immune system, and imposes excessive demands on the metabolic and reparative processes that are needed to restore the body's interface with the environment.

Burns are caused by a number of sources. Flame burns occur because of exposure to direct fire. Scald burns result from hot liquids spilled or poured on the skin surface. In a child, a scald burn may indicate child abuse. Chemical burns occur from industrial agents used in occupational sites. Electrical burns occur from contact with live electrical wires outdoors or in the home. Electrical burns are usually more extensive because of internal tissue injury as well as entrance and exit wounds (see Chapter 2, Fig. 2-5). Lightning, electromagnetic radiation, and ionizing radiation also can cause skin burns.

Classification of Burns

Burns are typically classified according to the depth of involvement as first-degree, second-degree, and third-degree burns.[44–46] The depth of a burn is largely influenced by the duration of exposure to the heat source and the temperature of the heating agent.

First-degree burns (superficial partial-thickness burns) involve only the outer layers of the epidermis. They are red or pink, dry, and painful. There usually is no blister formation. A mild sunburn is an example. The skin maintains its ability to function as a water vapor and bacterial barrier and heals in 3 to 10 days. First-degree burns usually require only palliative treatment, such as pain relief measures and adequate fluid intake. Extensive first-degree burns on infants, the elderly, and persons who receive radiation therapy for cancer may require more extensive treatment measures.

Second-degree burns involve both the epidermis and dermis. *Second-degree partial-thickness burns* involve

KEY CONCEPTS

Burns

➤ Burns represent heat-induced injuries of the skin and subcutaneous tissues.

➤ The extent and depth of injury, the effect on physiologic functioning, and the degree and mechanism of healing are determined by the length of time exposed to the heat source, the temperature of the healing agent, and the amount of surface area that is involved.

➤ Burns affecting the epidermis heal by regeneration, whereas burns involving the deeper dermal and subcutaneous tissues heal by scar tissue replacement.

the epidermis and various degrees of the dermis. They are painful, moist, red, and blistered. Underneath the blisters is weeping, bright pink or red skin that is sensitive to temperature changes, air exposure, and touch. The blisters prevent the loss of body water and superficial dermal cells. It is usually important to maintain intact blisters after injury because they serve as a bandage and may help promote wound healing. These burns heal in approximately 1 to 2 weeks.

Second-degree full-thickness burns involve the entire epidermis and dermis. Structures that originate in the subcutaneous layer, such as hair follicles and sweat glands, remain intact. These burns can be very painful because the pain sensors remain intact. Tactile sensors may be absent or greatly diminished in the areas of deepest destruction. These burns appear as mottled pink, red, or waxy white areas with blisters and edema. The blisters resemble flat, dry tissue paper, rather than the bullous blisters seen with superficial partial-thickness injury. After healing, in approximately 1 month, these burns maintain their softness and elasticity, but there may be a loss of some sensation. Scar formation is usual. These burns require supportive medical care aimed at preventing further tissue damage, providing adequate hydration, and ensuring that the granular bed is adequate to support reepithelialization.

Third-degree full-thickness burns extend into the subcutaneous tissue and may involve muscle and bone. Thrombosed vessels can be seen under the burned skin, indicating that the underlying vasculature is involved. Third-degree burns vary in color from waxy white or yellow to tan, brown, deep red, or black. These burns are hard, dry, and leathery. Edema is extensive in the burn area and surrounding tissues. There is no pain because the nerve sensors have been destroyed. However, there is no such thing as a "pure" third-degree burn. Third-degree burns are almost always surrounded by second-degree burns, which are surrounded by an area of first-degree burns. The injury sometimes has an almost target-like appearance because of the various degrees of burn. Full-thickness burns wider than 1.5 inches usually require skin grafts because all the regenerative (*i.e.,* dermal) elements have been destroyed. Smaller injuries usually heal from the margins inward toward the center, the dermal elements regenerating from the healthier margins. However, regeneration may take many weeks and leave a permanent scar, even in smaller burns.

In addition to the depth of the wound, the extent of the burn also is important. Extent is measured by estimating the percentage of total body surface area (TBSA) involved. Several tools exist for estimating the TBSA. For example, the *Rule of Nines* counts anatomic body parts as multiples of 9% (the head is 9%, each arm 9%, each leg 18%, anterior trunk 18%, posterior trunk 18%), with the perineum 1%. The Lund and Browder chart includes a body diagram table that estimates the TBSA by age and anatomic part.[44,47] Children are more accurately assessed using this method because it takes into account the difference in relative size of body parts. The estimates of TBSA are then converted to the American Burn Association Classification of Extent of Injury (Table 45-2).

Other factors, such as age, body location, other injuries, and preexisting conditions, are taken into consideration for a full assessment of burn injury.[44–47] These factors can increase the severity of the assessed burn injury and the length of treatment. For example, a first-degree burn is reclassified as a more severe burn if other factors exist, such as burns to the hands, face, and feet; inhalation injury; electrical burns; other trauma; or coexistence of psychosocial problems. Genital burns almost always require hospitalization because edema may cause difficulty voiding and the location complicates maintenance of a bacteria-free environment.

TABLE 45-2	**American Burn Association Grading System for Burn Severity and Disposition**		
	Type of Burn		
	Minor	**Moderate**	**Major**
Criteria	<10% TBSA in adult	10%–20% TBSA in adult	>20% TBSA in adult
	<5% TBSA in young (<10 years) or old (>50 years)	5%–10% TBSA in young or old	>10% TBSA in young or old
	<2% Full-thickness burn	2%–5% Full-thickness burn	>5% Full-thickness burn
		High-voltage injury	High-voltage burn
		Suspected inhalation injury	Known inhalation injury
		Circumferential burn	Any significant burn to face, eyes, ears, genitalia, hands, feet, or major joints
		Concomitant medical problem predisposing to infection (*e.g.*, diabetes, sickle cell disease)	Significant associated injuries (*e.g.*, major trauma)
Disposition	Outpatient management	Hospital admission	Referral to burn center

TBSA, total body surface area.
(From American Burn Association. [1990]. Hospital and prehospital resources for optimal care of patients with burn injury: Guidelines for development and operation of burn centers. *Journal of Burn Care and Rehabilitation* 11, 98–104.)

Systemic Complications

Burn victims often are confronted with hemodynamic instability, impaired respiratory function, a hypermetabolic response, major organ dysfunction, and sepsis.[48–50] The magnitude of the response is proportional to the extent of injury, usually reaching a plateau when approximately 60% of the body is burned. In addition to loss of skin, burn victims often have associated injuries or illnesses. The treatment challenge is provision of immediate resuscitation efforts coupled with long-term maintenance of physiologic function. Pain and emotional problems are additional challenges faced by persons with burns.

Hemodynamic Instability. Hemodynamic instability begins almost immediately with injury to capillaries in the burned area and surrounding tissue. Fluid is lost from the vascular, interstitial, and cellular compartments. Because of a loss of vascular volume, major burn victims often present in the emergency department in a form of hypovolemic shock (see Chapter 19) known as *burn shock*. The patient has a decrease in cardiac output, increased peripheral vascular resistance, and impaired perfusion of vital organs. Electrical injuries that cause burns can produce cardiac arrhythmias that require immediate attention.

Respiratory System Dysfunction. Another injury commonly associated with burns is smoke inhalation and post-burn lung injury. Victims often are trapped in a burning structure and inhale significant amounts of smoke, carbon monoxide, and other toxic fumes. Water-soluble gases, such as ammonia, sulfur dioxide, and chlorine, that are found in smoke from burning plastics and rubber react with mucous membranes to form strong acids and alkalis that induce damage to the mucosal lining of the respiratory tract, bronchospasm, and edema. Lipid-soluble gases, such as nitrous oxide and hydrogen chloride, are transported to the lower airways, where they damage lung tissue. There also may be thermal injury to the respiratory passages. Manifestations of inhalation injury include hoarseness, drooling, an inability to handle secretions, hacking cough, and labored and shallow breathing. Serial blood gases show a fall in PO_2. Signs of mucosal injury and airway obstruction often are delayed for 24 to 48 hours after a burn. It is necessary continually to monitor the patient for early signs of respiratory distress. Other pulmonary conditions, such as pneumonia, pulmonary embolism, or pneumothorax, may occur secondarily to the burn.

Hypermetabolic Response. The stress of burn injury increases metabolic and nutritional requirements. Secretion of stress hormones such as catecholamines and cortisol is increased in an effort to maintain homeostasis. Heat production is increased in an effort to balance heat losses from the burned area. Hypermetabolism, characterized by increased oxygen consumption, increased glucose use, and protein and fat wasting, is a characteristic response to burn trauma. The hypermetabolic state peaks at approximately 7 to 17 days after the burn, and tissue breakdown diminishes as the wounds heal. Nutritional support is essential to recovery from burn injury. Enteral and parenteral hyperalimentation may be used to deliver sufficient nutrients to prevent tissue breakdown and post-burn weight loss.

Dysfunction of Other Organ Systems. Burn shock results in impaired perfusion of vital organs. The patient may have impaired function of the kidneys, gastrointestinal tract, and nervous system. Although the initial insult often is one of hypovolemic shock and impaired organ perfusion, sepsis may contribute to impaired organ function after the initial resuscitation period.

Renal insufficiency can occur in burn patients as a result of the hypovolemic state, damage to the kidneys at the time of the burn, or from drugs that are administered. Immediately after the burn, there is often a short period of relative anuria, followed by a phase of hypermetabolism characterized by increased urine output and nitrogen loss.

The effects of burn injury on the gastrointestinal tract include gastric dilatation and decreased peristalsis. These effects are compounded by immobility and narcotic analgesics. Burn victims are observed carefully for vomiting and fecal impaction. Acute ulceration of the stomach and duodenum (called *Curling's ulcer*) is a potential complication in burn victims and is thought to be the result of stress and gastric ischemia. It is largely controlled by the prophylactic administration of H_2 antagonists or proton pump inhibitors. Enteral feeding tubes are usually inserted early in the course of treatment for severe burns. Tube feeding is intended to mitigate ulcer formation, maintain the integrity of the intestinal mucosa, and provide sufficient calories and protein for the hypermetabolic state.

Neurologic changes can occur from periods of hypoxia. Neurologic damage may result from head injuries, drug or alcohol abuse, carbon monoxide poisoning, fluid volume deficits, and hypovolemia. With an electrical burn, the brain or spine can be directly injured. The responses to physiologic damage may include confusion, memory loss, insomnia, lethargy, and combativeness.

Musculoskeletal effects include fractures that occur at the time of the accident, deep burns extending to the muscles and bone, hypertrophic scarring, and contractures. The hypermetabolic state increases tissue catabolism and leads to severe protein and fat wasting without proper nutritional support.

Sepsis. A significant complication of the acute phase of burn injury is sepsis. It may arise from the burn wound, pneumonia, urinary tract infection, infection elsewhere in the body, or the use of invasive procedures or monitoring devices. Immunologically, the skin is the body's first line of defense. When the skin is no longer intact, the body is open to bacterial infection. Destruction of the skin also prevents the delivery of cellular components of the immune system to the site of injury. There also is a loss of normal protective skin flora and a shift to colonization by more pathogenic flora.

Emergency and Long-Term Treatment

Regardless of the type of burn, the first step in any burn situation is preventing the causal agent from producing further tissue damage.[47-50] Copious amounts of water over the burned area can be extremely helpful. Immediate submersion is more important than removal of clothing, which may delay cooling the involved areas. The application of ice is not recommended because it can further limit blood flow to an area, turning a partial-thickness into a full-thickness burn.

Depending on the depth and extent of the burn, medical treatment is necessary. Emergency care consists of resuscitation and stabilization with intravenous fluids while maintaining cardiac and respiratory function. Once hospitalized, the immediate treatment regimen focuses on continued maintenance of cardiorespiratory function, pain alleviation, wound care, and emotional support. Intermediate and long-term treatments depend on the extent of injury.

After hemodynamic and pulmonary stability have been established, treatment is directed toward initial care of the wound. Treatment of the burn wound focuses on protection from desiccation and further injury of those burn areas that reepithelialize in 7 to 10 days (superficial second-degree burns). "Nature's own blister" is the best protection for these burns. Topical antimicrobial preparations (*e.g.*, silver sulfadiazine) and dressings are used to cover the wound when the blister has been broken. Wounds that will not heal spontaneously in 7 to 10 days (deep second-degree and third-degree burns) are usually treated by excision and skin grafts. The sloughed tissue, or *eschar*, produced by the burn is excised as soon as possible. This decreases the chance of infection and allows the skin to regenerate faster.

Burns that encircle the entire surface of the body or a body part (*e.g.*, arms, legs, torso) act as tourniquets and can cause major tissue damage to the muscles, tendons, and vasculature under the area of the leathery eschar skin. These burns are called *circumferential burns*. The eschar is incised longitudinally (escharotomy), and sometimes a fasciotomy (surgical incision through the fascia of the muscle) is performed. The timing of these incisions is important. Incision is done after the patient's circulatory condition stabilizes to some degree, thereby limiting some of the massive fluid loss. However, the incisions must occur before the eschar formation can cause hypoxia and necrosis of the tissues and organs under it. This is extremely important when torso burns occur because the pressure placed on a chest can compromise respiratory function and decrease blood return to the heart.

Systemic infection remains a leading cause of morbidity among persons with extensive burns. Continuous microbiologic surveillance is necessary; protective isolation measures are often instituted. There is an increasing trend toward use of prophylactic antibiotic treatment in persons with major burns.

Skin grafts are surgically implanted as soon as possible, often at the same time the burn tissue is excised, to promote new skin growth, limit fluid loss, and act as a dressing. Skin grafts can be permanent or temporary and split-thickness or full-thickness. Permanent skin grafts are used over newly excised tissue. Temporary skin grafts are used to cover a burned area until the tissue underneath it has healed.

Various sources of skin grafts exist: *autograft* (skin obtained from the person's own body), *homograft* (skin obtained from another human being, alive or recently dead), and *heterograft* (skin obtained from another species, such as the pig). The best choice is autografting when there is enough uninterrupted skin on the person's body. The thickness of these grafts depends on the donor site and the needs of the burn patient. A *split-thickness skin graft* is one that includes the epidermis and part of the dermis. A split-thickness skin graft can be sent through a skin mesher that cuts tiny slits into the skin, allowing it to expand up to nine times its original size. These grafts are used frequently because they can cover large surface areas and there is less autorejection. *Full-thickness skin grafts* include the entire thickness of the dermal layer. They are used primarily for reconstructive surgery or for deep, small areas. The donor site of a full-thickness skin graft requires a split-thickness skin graft to help it heal.

Two-layered synthetic skin grafts (*Apligraf*, *Integra*) are now available and approved by the FDA.[51] Synthetic skin grafts generally are composed of a layer of silicone, mimicking the properties of the epidermis, and a layer or matrix of fibers. Skin cells attach to the fibers, enabling dermal skin growth. Once the dermal skin has regenerated, the silicone layer is removed and a thin epidermal skin graft is applied, thus requiring less skin grafting overall.

Other treatment measures include positioning, splinting, and physical therapy to prevent contractures and maintain muscle tone. Because the normal body response to disuse is flexion, the contractures that occur with a burn are disfiguring and cause loss of limb or appendage use. Once the wounds have healed sufficiently, elastic pressure garments, sometimes for the full body, often are used to prevent excessive scarring.

PRESSURE ULCERS

Pressure ulcers are ischemic lesions of the skin and underlying structures caused by unrelieved pressure that impairs the flow of blood and lymph. Pressure ulcers often are referred to as *decubitus ulcers* or *bedsores*. The word *decubitus* comes from the Latin term meaning "lying down." However, a pressure ulcer may result from pressure exerted in the seated as well as the lying position. Pressure ulcers are most likely to develop over a bony prominence, but they may occur on any part of the body that is subjected to external pressure, friction, or shearing forces. Several subpopulations are at particular risk, including persons with quadriplegia, elderly persons with restricted activity and hip fractures, and persons in the critical care setting.

Pressure ulcers are costly in terms of human suffering, financial expense, and allocation of health care resources.[52,53] The prevention and treatment of pressure ulcers is a public health issue and is addressed in *Healthy People 2010,* a national public health policy statement, which has set a target of a 50% decrease in prevalence of pressure ulcers in nursing home residents.[54]

Mechanisms of Development

Four factors contribute to the development of pressure ulcers: (1) pressure, (2) shear forces, (3) friction, and (4) moisture.[52] External pressures that exceed capillary pressure interrupt blood flow in the capillary beds. When the pressure between a bony prominence and a support surface exceeds the normal capillary filling pressure, capillary flow essentially is obstructed. If this pressure is applied constantly for 2 hours, oxygen deprivation coupled with an accumulation of metabolic end products leads to irreversible tissue damage. Although 32 mm Hg of pressure has been traditionally accepted as the amount necessary to compress capillaries and interrupt blood flow, this is highly variable among individuals.[52] Persons with impaired circulation require less pressure to interrupt circulation. The same amount of pressure causes more damage when it is distributed over a small area than when it is distributed over a larger area.

Whether a person is sitting or lying down, the weight of the body is borne by tissues covering the bony prominences. More than 95% of pressure ulcers are located on the lower part of the body, most often over the sacrum, the coccygeal areas, the ischial tuberosities, and the greater trochanter.[53] Pressure over a bony area is transmitted from the surface to the underlying dense bone, compressing all of the intervening tissue. As a result, the greatest pressure occurs at the surface of the bone and dissipates outward in a conelike manner toward the surface of the skin (Fig. 45-19). Thus, extensive underlying tissue damage can be present when a small superficial skin lesion is first noticed.

Altering the distribution of pressure from one skin area to another prevents tissue injury. Pressure ulcers most commonly occur in persons with conditions such as spinal cord injury in which normal sensation and movement to effect redistribution of body weight are impaired. Normally, persons unconsciously shift their weight to redistribute pressure on the skin and underlying tissues. For example, during the night, people turn in their sleep, preventing ischemic injury of tissues that overlie the bony prominences that support the weight of the body; the same is true for sitting for any length of time. The movements needed to shift the body weight are made unconsciously, and only when movement is restricted do people become aware of discomfort.

Shearing forces are caused by the sliding of one tissue layer over another with stretching and angulation of blood vessels, causing injury and thrombosis. Shear occurs when the skeleton moves, but the skin remains fixed to an external surface such as occurs with transfer from a stretcher to a bed or pulling a person up in bed. The same thing happens when the head of the bed is elevated, causing the torso to move toward the foot of the bed while friction and moisture cause the skin to remain fixed to the bed linens. *Friction* contributes to pressure ulceration by damaging the skin at the epidermal-dermal interface. This occurs as persons who are bedridden use their elbows and heels to aid themselves in movement. *Moisture* contributes to pressure ulcer formation by weakening the cell wall of individual skin cells and by changing the protective pH of the skin. This makes the skin more susceptible to pressure, shear, and friction injury.

Prevention

The prevention of pressure ulcers is preferable to treatment. In 1992, a special panel of the Agency for Health Care Policy and Research (AHCPR; now the Agency for Healthcare Research and Quality), the Panel for the Prediction and Prevention of Pressure Ulcers in Adults, released their clinical practice guideline, *Pressure Ulcers in Adults: Prediction and Prevention.* The panel recommended four overall goals: (1) identifying at-risk persons who need preventative measures and the specific factors placing them at risk; (2) maintaining and improving tissue tolerance to prevent injury; (3) protecting against the adverse effects of external mechanical forces (*i.e.,* pressure, friction, and shear); and (4) reducing the incidence of pressure ulcers through educational programs.[55] A 1994 publication of the AHCPR made specific recommendations for assessment of the person with pressure ulcers, management of tissue load, ulcer care, managing

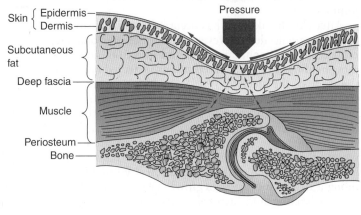

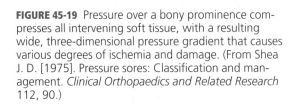

FIGURE 45-19 Pressure over a bony prominence compresses all intervening soft tissue, with a resulting wide, three-dimensional pressure gradient that causes various degrees of ischemia and damage. (From Shea J. D. [1975]. Pressure sores: Classification and management. *Clinical Orthopaedics and Related Research* 112, 90.)

bacterial colonization and infection, operative repair, and education and quality control.[56]

Risk factors identified as contributing to the development of pressure ulcers were those related to sensory perception (*i.e.*, ability to respond meaningfully to pressure-related discomfort), level of skin moisture, urine and fecal continence, nutrition and hydration status, mobility, circulatory status, and presence of shear and friction forces.

Methods for preventing pressure ulcers include frequent position change, meticulous skin care, and frequent and careful observation to detect early signs of skin breakdown. Moisture macerates and injures skin. Sources of moisture include sweat, wound drainage, and urine and feces. Both urinary and fecal incontinence increase the risk of pressure ulcers. Food crumbs, intravenous tubing, and other debris in the bed can greatly increase local skin pressure points. Adequate hydration of the stratum corneum appears to protect the skin against mechanical insult.[55] The prevention of dehydration improves the circulation. It also decreases the concentration of urine, thereby minimizing skin irritation in persons who are incontinent, and it reduces urinary problems that contribute to incontinence. Maintenance of adequate nutrition is important. Anemia and malnutrition contribute to tissue breakdown and delay healing after tissue injury has occurred.

Staging and Treatment

Pressure ulcers can be staged using four categories.[56,57] *Stage I ulcers* are characterized by a defined area of persistent redness in lightly pigmented skin or an area of persistent redness with blue or purple hues in darker-pigmented skin. *Stage II ulcers* represent a partial-thickness loss of skin involving epidermis or dermis, or both. The ulcer is superficial and presents clinically as an abrasion, a blister, or a shallow crater. *Stage III ulcers* represent a full-thickness skin loss involving damage and necrosis of subcutaneous tissue that may extend down to but not through underlying fascia. The ulcer manifests as a deep crater with or without undermining of adjacent tissue. *Stage IV ulcers* involve full-thickness skin loss and necrosis with extensive destruction or damage to the underlying subcutaneous tissues that may extend to involve muscle, bone, and supporting structures (*e.g.*, tendon or joint capsule).

After skin breakdown has occurred, special treatment measures are needed to prevent further ischemic damage, reduce bacterial contamination and infection, and promote healing. Treatment methods are selected based on the stage of the ulcer.[52,53,56–58] Stage I ulcers usually are treated with frequent turning and measures to remove pressure. Stage II or stage III ulcers with little exudate are treated with semipermeable or occlusive dressings. Occlusive dressings are credited with preventing the loss of wound fluid and maintaining a moist environment that is necessary for epithelial cell migration.[59] Wound fluid is thought to contain variety of growth factors that enhance wound healing. Occlusive dressings may also relieve wound pain and prevent bacterial contamination. There are several types of occlusive dressings available, including polymer films, hydrogels, hydrocolloids, biomembrane, and absorbing granules. The available products differ in their permeability to water vapor and wound protection and each has advantages and disadvantages.

Necrotic debris increases the possibility of bacterial infection and delays wound healing. Stage III ulcers with exudate and necrotic debris and stage IV ulcers usually require debridement (*i.e.*, removal of necrotic tissue and eschar). This can be done surgically, with wet-to-dry dressings, or through the use of proteolytic enzymes. Stage IV wounds often require packing to obliterate dead space and are covered with nonadherent dressings. Stage IV ulcers may require surgical interventions, such as skin grafts or myocutaneous flaps.

In summary, sunburn is caused by excessive exposure of the epidermal and dermal layers of the skin to UVR, resulting in an erythematous inflammatory reaction. Sunburn ranges from mild to severe. Sun exposure not only causes sunburn, but repeated exposure to the rays of the produces long-term damage to skin structures and predisposes to skin cancer. The ultraviolet rays of sunlight or other sources can be either completely or partially blocked from the skin surface by sunscreens.

Burns cause damage to skin structures, ranging from first-degree burns, which damage the epidermis, to third-degree full-thickness burns, which extend into the subcutaneous tissue and may involve muscle and bone. The extent of injury is determined by the thickness of the burn and the percentage of total body surface area involved. In addition to skin involvement, burn injury can cause hemodynamic instability with hypovolemic shock, inhalation injury with respiratory involvement, a hypermetabolic state, organ dysfunction, immune suppression and sepsis, pain, and emotional trauma. Treatment methods vary with the severity of injury and include immediate resuscitation and maintenance of physiologic function, wound cleaning and debridement, application of antimicrobial agents and dressings, and skin grafting. Efforts are directed toward preventing or limiting disfigurement and disability.

Pressure ulcers are caused by ischemia of the skin and underlying tissues. They result from external pressure, which disrupts blood flow, or shearing forces, which cause stretching and injury to blood vessels. Pressure ulcers are divided into four stages, according to the depth of tissue involvement. The prevention of pressure ulcers is preferable to treatment. The goals of prevention should include identifying at-risk persons who need prevention along with the specific factors placing them at risk; maintaining and improving tissue tolerance to pressure to prevent injury; and protecting against the adverse effects of external mechanical forces (*i.e.*, pressure, friction, and shear).

Nevi and Skin Cancers

NEVI

Nevi, or moles, are common congenital or acquired tumors of the skin that are benign. Almost all adults have nevi, some in greater numbers than others. Nevi can be pigmented or nonpigmented, flat or elevated, and hairy or nonhairy.

Nevocellular nevi are pigmented skin lesions resulting from proliferation of melanocytes in the epidermis or dermis. Nevocellular nevi are tan to deep brown, uniformly pigmented, small papules with well-defined and rounded borders. They are formed initially by melanocytes with their long dendritic extensions that are normally interspersed among the basal keratinocytes.[6] These melanocytes are transformed into round or oval melanin-containing cells that grow in nests or clusters along the dermal-epidermal junction. Because of their location, these lesions are called *junctional nevi* (Fig. 45-20). Eventually, most junctional nevi grow into the surrounding dermis as nests or cords of cells. *Compound nevi* contain epidermal and dermal components. In older lesions, the epidermal nests may disappear entirely, leaving a *dermal nevi*. Compound and dermal nevi usually are more elevated than junctional nevi.

Another form of nevi, the *dysplastic nevi*, are important because of their capacity to transform to malignant melanomas.[60] Although the association between dysplastic nevi and malignant melanoma was made more than 175 years ago, it was not until 1978 that the role of dysplastic nevi as a precursor of malignant melanoma was described in detail. Dysplastic nevi are larger than other nevi (often >5 mm in diameter). Their appearance is one of a flat, slightly raised plaque with a pebbly surface, or a target-like lesion with a darker, raised center and irregular border. They vary in shade from brown and red to flesh tones and have irregular borders. A person may have hundreds of these lesions. Unlike other moles or nevi, they occur on both sun-exposed and covered areas of the body. Dysplastic nevi have been documented in multiple members of families prone to the development of malignant melanoma.[6]

Because of the possibility of malignant transformation, any mole that undergoes a change warrants immediate medical attention. The changes to observe and report are changes in size, thickness, or color, and itching or bleeding.

SKIN CANCER

There has been an alarming increase in skin cancers during the past several decades. Since the 1970s, the incidence of malignant melanoma, the most serious form of skin cancer, has increased significantly. These increases are, on average, 4% per year, from 5.7 per 100,000 in 1973 to 13.8 per 100,000 in 1996, to approximately 59,580 new cases and 7700 deaths in 2005.[61] There also are approximately 1 million cases each year of highly curable basal cell and squamous cell cancers.[61]

The rising incidence of skin cancer has been attributed primarily to increased sun exposure associated with societal and lifestyle shifts in the United States. The thinning of the ozone layer in the earth's stratosphere is thought to be an important factor in this increased incidence. Society's emphasis on suntanning also is implicated. Many persons have more leisure time and spend increasing amounts of time in the sun with uncovered skin.

Although the factors linking sun exposure to skin cancer are incompletely understood, both total cumulative exposure and altered patterns of exposure (in the case of melanoma) are strongly implicated. Basal cell and squamous cell carcinomas tend to be associated with total cumulative UVR exposure, whereas melanomas are associated with intense intermittent exposure. Thus, basal cell and squamous cell carcinomas occur more commonly on maximally sun-exposed parts of the body, such as the face and back of the hands and forearms. In contrast, melanomas occur most commonly in areas of the body that are exposed to the sun intermittently, such as the back in men and the lower legs in women. They are also more common in persons with indoor occupations whose exposure to sun is limited to weekends and vacations.

Malignant Melanoma

Malignant melanoma is a malignant tumor of the melanocytes. It is a rapidly progressing, metastatic form of cancer. The increased incidence of melanoma that has occurred during the past several decades has been attributed to an increase in sun exposure. The risk is greatest in fair-skinned people, particularly those with blond or red hair who sunburn and freckle easily. Fortunately, the increased risk of melanoma has been associated with a concomitant increase in the 5-year survival rate, from approximately 40% in the 1940s to 90% at present.[62]

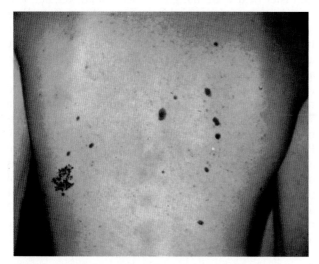

FIGURE 45-20 Junctional nevi of the back of a 16-year-old patient. (Owen Laboratories, Inc.) (From Sauer G. C., Hall J. C. [1996]. *Manual of skin diseases* [7th ed.]. Philadelphia: Lippincott-Raven.)

KEY CONCEPTS

Skin Cancers

➤ Increased and unprotected exposure to the ultra-violet rays of sunlight produces sunburn and increases the risk for development of skin cancer.

➤ The melanocytes, which protect against sunburn through increased production of melanin and suntanning, are particularly vulnerable to the adverse effects of unprotected exposure to ultraviolet light. Malignant melanoma, which is a malignant tumor of melanocytes, is a rapidly progressive and metastatic form of skin cancer.

➤ Basal cell carcinoma and squamous cell carcinoma, which also reflect the effects of increased sun exposure, are less aggressive forms of skin cancer and are more easily cured.

Public health screening measures, early diagnosis, increased knowledge of precursor lesions, and greater public knowledge of the disease may account for earlier intervention.

Severe, blistering sunburns in early childhood and intermittent intense sun exposures (trips to sunny climates) contribute to increased susceptibility to melanoma in young and middle-age adults. Roughly 90% of malignant melanomas in whites occur on sun-exposed skin. However, in African Americans and Asians, roughly 67% occur on non–sun-exposed areas, such as mucous membranes and subungual, palmar, and plantar surfaces.[63] Although sun exposure remains a significant risk factor for melanoma, other potential risk factors have been identified, including atypical mole/dysplastic nevus syndrome, immunosuppression, prior PUVA therapy, and exposure to UV light at tanning salons. Using statistical analysis, it has been determined that six factors independently influence the risk for development of malignant melanoma: family history of malignant melanoma, presence of blond or red hair, presence of marked freckling on the upper back, history of three or more blistering sunburns before 20 years of age, history of 3 or more years of an outdoor job as a teenager, and presence of actinic keratosis. Persons with two of these risk factors had a 3.5-fold increased risk of malignant melanoma, and those with three or more risk factors had a 20-fold increased risk.[63]

Malignant melanomas differ in size and shape. Usually, they are slightly raised and black or brown with irregular borders and uneven surfaces. Most seem to arise from pre-existing nevi or new molelike growths (Fig. 45-21). There may be surrounding erythema, inflammation, and tenderness. Periodically, melanomas ulcerate and bleed. Dark melanomas are often mottled with shades of red, blue, and white. These three colors represent three concurrent processes: melanoma growth (blue), inflammation and the body's attempt to localize and destroy the tumor (red), and scar tissue formation (white). Malignant melanomas can appear anywhere on the body. Although they frequently are found on sun-exposed areas, sun exposure alone does not account for their development. In men, they are found frequently on the trunk, head, neck, and arms; in women, they commonly are found on the legs.

Four types of melanomas have been identified: superficial spreading, nodular, lentigo maligna, and acral lentiginous.[64] *Superficial spreading melanoma* is characterized by a raised-edged nevus with lateral growth. It has a disorderly appearance in color and outline. This lesion tends to have biphasic growth, horizontally and vertically. It typically ulcerates and bleeds with growth. This type of lesion accounts for 70% of all melanomas and is most prevalent in persons who sunburn easily and have intermittent sun exposure. *Nodular melanomas,* which account for 15% to 30% of melanomas, are raised, dome-shaped lesions that can occur anywhere on the body. They are commonly a uniform blue-black color and tend to look like blood blisters. Nodular melanomas tend to invade the dermis rapidly from the start with no apparent horizontal growth phase. *Lentigo maligna* melanomas, which account for 4% to 10% of all melanomas, are slow-growing, flat nevi that occur primarily on sun-exposed areas of elderly persons. Untreated lentigo maligna tends to exhibit horizontal and radial growth for many years before it invades the dermis to become lentigo maligna melanoma. *Acral lentiginous melanoma,* which accounts for 2% to 8% of melanomas, occurs primarily on the palms of the hands, soles of the feet, nail beds, and mucous membranes. It has the appearance of lentigo maligna. Unlike other types of melanomas, it has a similar incidence in all ethnic groups.

Because virtually all the known risks of melanoma are related to susceptibility and magnitude of UV light exposure, protection from the sun's rays plays a critical role in the prevention of malignant melanoma. Early detection is critical with malignant melanoma. Regular self-examination of the total skin surface in front of a mirror under good lighting provides a method for early detection. It requires that a person undress completely and examine all areas of the body using a full mirror, handheld mirror, and handheld hair dryer (to examine the scalp). An *ABCD* rule was developed in 1985 to aid in early diagnosis and timely treatment of malignant melanoma.[65] The acronym stands for *asymmetry, border irregularity, color variegation,* and *diameter* greater than 0.6 cm (pencil eraser size). People should be taught to watch for these changes in existing nevi or the development of new nevi, as well as other alterations such as bleeding or itching. Because of the existence of small-diameter melanomas (*i.e.,* 6 mm or less in diameter), it has been suggested that the ABCD rule be expanded to include an "E" for an evolving change in the lesion over time.[65]

Diagnosis of melanoma is based on biopsy findings from a lesion. Consistent with other cancerous tumors, melanoma is commonly staged using the TNM (tumor, lymph node, and metastasis) staging system (see Chapter 5) or the Clark system, in which the tumor is rated I

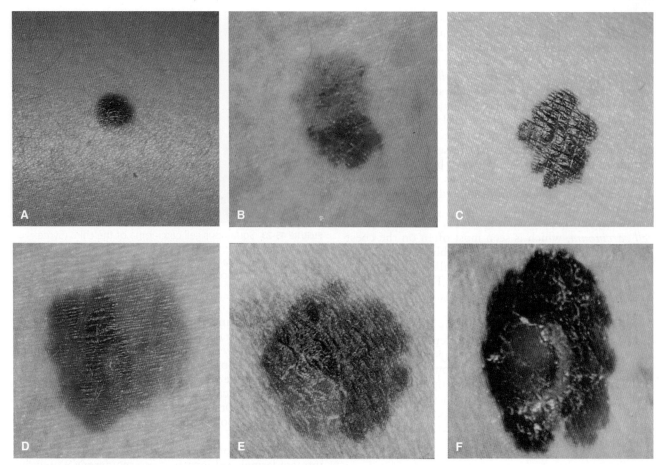

FIGURE 45-21 (**A**) Normal mole with even, round contour and sharply defined borders. (**B**) Changes in appearance of a mole: *asymmetry.* (**C**) Changes in appearance of a mole: *border irregularity.* (**D**) Changes in appearance of a mole: *color and uneven pigmentation.* (**E**) Changes in the appearance of a mole: *diameter greater than 6 mm.* (**F**) Changes in the surface of a mole: *scaliness, oozing, and bleeding.* (From American Cancer Society. [1995]. *What you should know about melanoma.* Dallas: Author.)

to V depending on the depth of tumor invasion.[64] Ulceration and invasion of the tumor into the deeper skin tissue result in poorer prognosis. Early diagnosis and treatment are of extreme importance.

Treatment is usually surgical excision, the extent of which is determined by the thickness of the lesion, invasion of the deeper skin layers, and spread to regional lymph nodes. Deep, wide excisions with elective removal of lymph tissue and use of skin grafts were once the hallmark of treatment.[66] A current capability allows for mapping lymph flow to a regional lymph node that receives lymphatic drainage from tumor sites on the skin. This lymph node, which is called the *sentinel lymph node*, is then sampled for biopsy. If tumor cells have spread from the primary tumor to the regional lymph nodes, the sentinel node will be the first node in which tumor cells appear. Therefore, sentinel biopsy can be used to test for the presence of melanoma cells and determine if radical lymph node dissection is necessary. When nodes are positive, consideration is given also to systemic adjuvant therapy.

Other cancer treatment, such as chemotherapy, is indicated when the disease becomes systemic. Interferon has been used for the treatment of melanoma.[67] An area of active research in melanoma therapy involves vaccine development or immunotherapy. Several types of vaccines have been developed and are under investigation.[67]

Basal Cell Carcinoma

Basal cell carcinoma is the most common skin cancer in humans, accounting for 75% of all nonmelanoma skin cancers.[68] Like other skin cancers, basal cell carcinoma has increased in incidence during the past several decades. Basal cell carcinoma usually occurs in persons who were exposed to great amounts of sunlight. The incidence is twice as high among men as women and greatest in the 55- to 75-year-old age group.

Basal cell carcinoma usually is a nonmetastasizing tumor that extends wide and deep if left untreated. These tumors are seen most frequently on sun-exposed areas of the body, such as the head and neck, but do occur on other skin surfaces that were not exposed to the sun (Fig. 45-22). Although there are several histologic types of basal cell carcinoma, nodular ulcerative and superficial basal cell carcinomas are the most frequently occurring types. *Nodular ulcerative basal cell carcinoma* is the most common type.[68] It is a nodulocystic structure that begins as a small, flesh-colored or pink, smooth, translucent nodule that enlarges with time. Telangiectatic vessels frequently are seen beneath the surface. Over the years, a central depression forms that progresses to an ulcer surrounded by the original shiny, waxy border. Basal cell carcinoma in darker-skinned persons usually is darkly pigmented and frequently misdiagnosed as other skin diseases, including melanoma.

The second most common form is *superficial basal cell carcinoma*, which is seen most often on the chest or back. It begins as a flat, nonpalpable, erythematous plaque. The red, scaly areas slowly enlarge, with nodular borders and telangiectatic bases. This type of skin cancer is difficult to diagnose because it mimics other dermatologic problems.

All suspected basal cell carcinomas should undergo biopsy for diagnosis. The treatment depends on the site and extent of the lesion. The most important treatment goal is complete elimination of the lesion. Also important is the maintenance of function and optimal cosmetic effect. Curettage with electrodesiccation, surgical excision, irradiation, and chemosurgery are effective in removing all cancerous cells. Patients should be checked at regular intervals for recurrences.

Squamous Cell Carcinoma

Squamous cell carcinomas are malignant tumors of the outer epidermis. They are commonly found on sun-exposed areas of the skin of people with fair complexions.[69,70] Metastasis is more common with squamous cell carcinoma than with basal cell carcinoma.

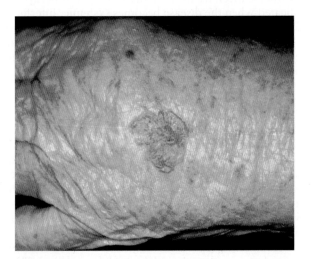

FIGURE 45-22 Basal cell carcinoma and wrinkling of the hand. (Syntex Laboratories.) (From Sauer G. C., Hall J. C. [1996]. *Manual of skin diseases* [7th ed.]. Philadelphia: Lippincott-Raven.)

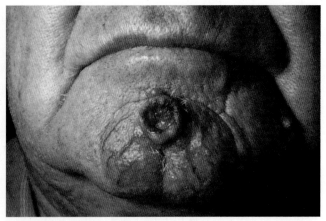

FIGURE 45-23 Squamous cell carcinoma of the chin. (Syntex Laboratories, Westwood Pharmaceuticals.) (From Sauer G. C., Hall J. C. [1996]. *Manual of skin diseases* [7th ed.]. Philadelphia: Lippincott-Raven.)

The mechanisms of squamous cell carcinoma development are unclear. Most squamous cell cancers occur in sun-exposed areas of the skin, and persons who spend much time outdoors, have lighter skin, and live in lower latitudes are more affected. The increase in the incidence of squamous cell carcinomas is consistent with increased UVR exposure. Other suspected causes include exposure to arsenic (*i.e.*, Bowen disease), gamma radiation, tars, and oils.

There are two types of squamous cell carcinoma: intraepidermal and invasive. *Intraepidermal squamous cell carcinoma* remains confined to the epidermis for a long time. However, at some unpredictable time, it may penetrate the basement membrane to the dermis and metastasize to the regional lymph nodes. It then converts to *invasive squamous cell carcinoma*. The invasive type can develop from intraepidermal carcinoma or from a premalignant lesion (*e.g.*, actinic keratoses). It may be slow growing or fast growing with metastasis.

Squamous cell carcinoma is a red-scaling, keratotic, slightly elevated lesion with an irregular border, usually with a shallow chronic ulcer (Fig. 45-23). Later lesions grow outward, show large ulcerations, and have persistent crusts and raised, erythematous borders. The lesions characteristically occur on the nose, forehead, helixes of the ears, lower lip, and back of the hands. In blacks, the lesions may appear as hyperpigmented nodules and occur more frequently on non–sun-exposed areas.

Treatment measures are aimed at the removal of all cancerous tissue using methods such as electrosurgery, excision surgery, chemosurgery, or radiation therapy. After treatment, the person is observed for the remainder of his or her life for signs of recurrence.

In summary, nevi are moles that usually are benign. Because they may undergo cancerous transformation, any mole that undergoes a change warrants immediate medical attention. There has been an alarming increase in skin cancers during the past few decades. Repeated exposure to the UV rays of the sun has been implicated as the principal cause of skin cancer.

Neoplasms of the skin include malignant melanoma, basal cell carcinoma, and squamous cell carcinoma. Malignant melanoma is a malignant tumor of the melanocytes. It is a rapidly progressing, metastatic form of cancer. The most important clinical sign is a change in size, shape, or color of a pigmented skin lesion, such as a mole. Early detection through skin self-examination is critical. Squamous cell carcinoma and basal cell carcinoma are of epidermal origin. Basal cell carcinomas are the most common form of skin cancer among whites. They are slow-growing tumors that rarely metastasize. Squamous cell carcinoma is common in pale-skinned elderly persons. The two types of squamous cell carcinoma are intraepidermal and invasive. Intraepidermal squamous cell carcinoma remains confined to the epidermis for a long time. Invasive squamous cell carcinoma can develop from intraepidermal carcinoma or from premalignant lesions such as actinic keratoses.

Age-Related Skin Manifestations

SKIN MANIFESTATIONS OF INFANCY AND CHILDHOOD

Skin Disorders of Infancy

Infancy connotes the image of perfect, unblemished skin. For the most part, this is true. However, several congenital skin lesions, such as mongolian spots, hemangiomas, and nevi, are associated with the early neonatal period. There are also several acquired skin conditions, including diaper dermatitis, prickly heat, and cradle cap, that are relatively common in infants.

Vascular and Pigmented Birthmarks. Pigmented and vascular lesions comprise most birthmarks.[71] Pigmented birthmarks represent abnormal migration or proliferation of melanocytes. Mongolian spots are caused by selective pigmentation. They usually occur on the buttocks or sacral area and are seen commonly in Asians and blacks. Nevi or moles are small, tan to brown, uniformly pigmented solid macules. *Nevocellular nevi* are formed initially from aggregates of melanocytes and keratinocytes along the dermal-epidermal border. *Congenital melanocytic nevi* are collections of melanocytes that are present at birth or develop within the first year of life. They present as macular, papular, or plaque-like pigmented lesions of various shades of brown, with a black or blue focus. The texture of the lesions varies and they may be with or without hair. They usually are found on the hands, shoulders, buttocks, entire arm, or trunk of the body. Some involve large areas of the body in garment-

like fashion. They usually grow proportionately with the child. Congenital melanocytic nevi are clinically significant because of their association with malignant melanoma.

Vascular birthmarks are cutaneous anomalies of angiogenesis and vascular development. Two types of vascular birthmarks commonly are seen in infants and small children: bright red, raised strawberry hemangiomas and flat, reddish-purple port-wine stains.

Strawberry hemangiomas begin as small, red lesions that are noticed shortly after birth. Hemangiomas are benign vascular tumors produced by proliferation of the endothelial cells. They are seen in approximately 5% to 10% of 1-year-old children.[72] Female infants are three times as likely as male infants to have hemangiomas, and there is an increased incidence in premature infants. Approximately 35% of these lesions are present at birth, and the remainder develop within a few weeks after birth. Hemangiomas typically undergo an early period of proliferation during which they enlarge, followed by a period of slow involution where the growth is reversed until complete resolution. Most strawberry hemangiomas disappear before 5 to 7 years of age without leaving an appreciable scar. Hemangiomas can occur anywhere in the body. Hemangiomas of the airway can be life threatening. Ulceration, the most frequent complication, can be painful and carries the risk of infection, hemorrhage, and scarring.[72]

Port-wine stains are pink or red patches that can occur anywhere on the body and are very noticeable (Fig. 45-24). They represent slow-growing capillary malformations that grow proportionately with the child and persist throughout life. Port-wine stains usually are confined to the skin, but may be associated with vascular malformations of the eye or leptomeninges over the cortex, leading to cognitive disorders, seizures, and other neurologic deficits.[72] Cover-up cosmetics are used in an attempt to conceal their disfiguring effects. Laser surgery has revolutionized the treatment of port-wine stains.

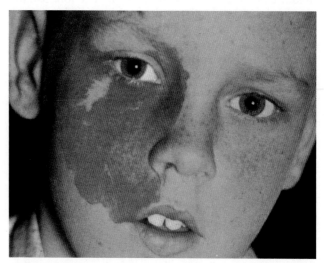

FIGURE 45-24 Port-wine stain on the face of a boy. (Ortho Dermatology Corp.) (From Sauer G. C., Hall J. C. [1996]. *Manual of skin diseases* [7th ed.]. Philadelphia: Lippincott-Raven.)

Diaper Dermatitis. Irritant diaper dermatitis or *diaper rash* is a form of contact dermatitis that is caused by the interaction of several factors, including prolonged contact of the skin with a mixture of urine and feces.[73,74] The wearing of diapers causes an increase in skin wetness and pH due to ammonia from urine. Prolonged wetness leads to softening and maceration of the skin, making it more susceptible to damage by friction from the surface of the diaper and local irritants. The contents of soiled diapers, if not changed frequently, can lead to contact dermatitis, bacterial infections, or other skin conditions. The proteases and lipases contained in feces are particularly irritating.

The appearance of *diaper rash* ranges from simple (*i.e.*, widely distributed macules on the buttocks and anogenital areas) to severe (*i.e.*, beefy, red, excoriated skin surfaces in the diaper area). Secondary infections with bacteria and yeasts are common; discomfort may be marked because of intense inflammation. Such conditions as contact dermatitis, seborrheic dermatitis, candidiasis, and atopic dermatitis should be considered when the eruption is persistent and recalcitrant to simple therapeutic measures.

Diaper dermatitis often responds to simple measures, including frequent diaper changes with careful cleansing of the irritated area to remove all waste products. Feces in particular should be removed from the skin as soon as possible after the diaper has been soiled. Since soap and lipid solvents will remove protective lipids from the stratum corneum, using water or an alcohol-free baby wipe is recommended. Exposing the irritated area to air is helpful. It has been shown that application of a barrier ointment after each diaper change is a valuable component of therapy. Topical corticosteroid therapy is generally effective, but should be used cautiously because infants absorb proportionally greater quantities through their skin than adults.[74] Antifungal therapy should not be used routinely, but only when *Candida* infection is established or suspected. Antibacterial agents should not be used because it is known that bacterial infections usually are not involved in diaper dermatitis, and the normal microflora should be preserved.

Selection of a barrier preparation is important. It is now clear that the barrier function of the skin is provided by the stratum corneum, whose main function is to minimize water loss and prevent inward penetration of toxic substances and microorganisms. Ideally, a barrier preparation should mimic the skin's natural function by forming a long-lasting barrier to increase protection against irritants and microorganisms and to maintain optimum moisture levels with the stratum corneum. Preparations should contain lipids that are similar to those naturally present in the stratum corneum. In general, water-in-oil formulations with a lipid content of 50% or greater provide a superior moisture barrier compared with lighter oil-in-water products.[74] For this reason, ointments are generally more effective than creams and lotions. Products containing nonessential ingredients such as perfumes can cause allergic contact dermatitis and should be avoided. Inclusion of an antiseptic is not necessary or desirable. Ideally, the safety and effectiveness of a barrier product should be clinically proven.

There is controversy regarding the effects of cloth versus disposable diapers in preventing diaper rash. In the early days of disposable diapers, infants who wore cloth diapers without plastic pants had fewer diaper rashes than those who wore disposable diapers. It has been suggested that this may not be true with the newer disposable diapers that have absorbent gelling material.[73,74] These superabsorbent diapers have the smallest increase in skin wetness compared with conventional disposable diapers and cloth diapers. When cloth diapers are used, they should be washed in gentle detergent and thoroughly rinsed to remove all traces of waste products. Plastic pants should be discouraged.

Intractable and severe cases of diaper dermatitis should be seen by a health care provider for treatment of any secondary infections. Secondary candidal (*i.e.*, yeast; Fig. 45-25) or other skin manifestations discussed in this chapter may occur in the diaper area. It is important to differentiate between normal diaper dermatitis and more serious skin problems.

Prickly Heat. *Prickly heat* (heat rash) results from constant maceration of the skin because of prolonged exposure to a warm, humid environment. Maceration leads to mid-epidermal obstruction and rupture of the sweat glands (Fig. 45-26). Although commonly seen during infancy, prickly heat may occur at any age. The treatment includes removing excessive clothing, cooling the skin with warm water baths, drying the skin with powders, and avoiding hot, humid environments.

Cradle Cap. *Cradle cap* is a greasy crust or scale formation on the scalp. It usually is attributed to infrequent and inadequate washing of the scalp. Cradle cap is treated using mild shampoo and gentle combing to remove the scales. Sometimes oil can be left on the head for minutes to several hours, softening the scales before scrubbing.

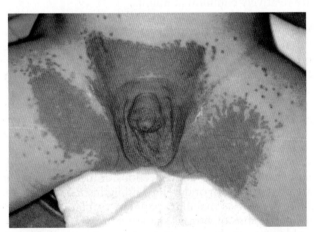

FIGURE 45-25 *Candida* intertrigo after a course of oral antibiotics in a 1-year-old child. (Owen Laboratories, Inc.) (From Sauer G. C., Hall J. C. [1996]. *Manual of skin diseases* [7th ed.]. Philadelphia: Lippincott-Raven.)

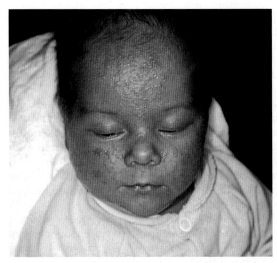

FIGURE 45-26 Prickly heat in 6-week-old infant. (From Hall J. C. [2000]. *Sauer's manual of skin diseases* [8th ed., p. 407]. Philadelphia: Lippincott Williams & Wilkins.)

Other emulsifying ointments or creams may be helpful in difficult cases. The scalp may need to be rubbed firmly to remove the buildup of keratinized cells. Recalcitrant cases should be seen by a health care practitioner because serious or chronic forms of seborrheic dermatitis may exist.

Skin Manifestations of Common Infectious Diseases

Infectious childhood diseases that produce rashes include roseola infantum (exanthem subitum), rubella, rubeola, and varicella. Although these diseases are seen less frequently because of successful immunization programs and the use of antibiotics, they still occur.

Roseola Infantum. *Roseola infantum* (exanthem subitum or sixth disease) is a contagious disease caused by human herpesviruses (HHV) 6 and 7.[44] HHV-6 is the etiologic agent in most cases and hence the condition is often referred as *sixth disease*. Primary HHV-6 infection occurs early in life, usually between 5 and 15 months. Roseola produces a characteristic maculopapular rash covering the trunk and spreading to the appendages. The rash is preceded by an abrupt onset of high fever ($\leq$105°F), inflamed tympanic membranes, and coldlike symptoms usually lasting 3 to 4 days. These symptoms improve at approximately the same time the rash appears. Unlike rubella, no cervical or postauricular lymph node adenopathy occurs. Roseola infantum frequently is mistaken for rubella. Rubella usually can be excluded by the age of the child and the absence of lymph node adenopathy. Less than half of HHV-6 infections in the United States are clinically recognizable as roseola.[44] In general, rubella does not develop in children younger than 6 months of age because they retain some maternal antibodies. Blood antibody titers may be taken to determine the actual diagnosis. In most cases, there are no long-term effects from this disease.

Rubella. *Rubella* (*i.e.*, 3-day measles or German measles) is a childhood disease caused by the rubella virus (a togavirus). It is characterized by a diffuse, punctate, macular rash that begins on the trunk and spreads to the arms and legs (Fig. 45-27). Mild febrile states occur; usually the fever is less than 100°F. Postauricular, suboccipital, and cervical lymph node adenopathy is common.[44] Coldlike symptoms usually accompany the disease in the form of cough, congestion, and coryza (*i.e.*, nasal discharge).

Rubella usually has no long-lasting sequelae; however, the transmission of the disease to pregnant women early in their gestation periods may result in congenital rubella syndrome. Among the clinical signs of congenital rubella syndrome are cataracts, microcephaly, mental retardation, deafness, patent ductus arteriosus, glaucoma, purpura, and bone defects. Most states have laws requiring immunization to prevent transmission of rubella. Immunization is accomplished by a live-virus vaccine. A single injection after 12 to 15 months of age has been shown to produce a 98% immunity response in immunized

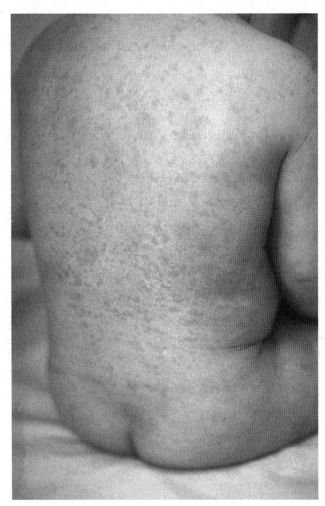

FIGURE 45-27 Rash of rubella on skin of a child's back. (From Centers for Disease Control and Prevention Public Health Image Library.)

children and is considered adequate in the prevention of rubella.[44] Many states require a second preschool or later dose of rubella vaccine to increase immunity. Cases and outbreaks of rubella occur in the United States, especially among foreign-born, unvaccinated adults.

Rubeola. *Rubeola* (measles, hard measles, 7-day measles) is an acute, highly communicable viral disease caused by a Morbillivirus. The characteristic rash is macular and blotchy; sometimes the macules become confluent (Fig. 45-28). The rubeola rash usually begins on the face and spreads to the appendages. There are several accompanying symptoms: a fever of 100°F or greater, *Koplik's spots* (*i.e.*, small, irregular red spots with a bluish-white speck in the center) on the buccal mucosa, and mild to severe photosensitivity.[44] The patient commonly has coldlike symptoms, general malaise, and myalgia. In severe cases, the macules may hemorrhage into the skin tissue or onto the outer body surface. This form is called *hemorrhagic measles*. The course of measles is more severe in infants, adults, and malnourished children. The World Health Organization recommends vitamin A treatment for measles in developing countries to reduce morbidity and mortality. There may be severe complications, including otitis media, pneumonia, and encephalitis. Antibody titers are determined for a conclusive diagnosis of rubeola.

Measles is a disease preventable by vaccine, and immunization is required by law in the United States. Immunization is accomplished by the injection of a live-virus vaccine. A single injection at 12 to 15 months of age is sufficient to produce initial immunity.[44] A second injection should be given on entry to primary school.

Varicella. *Varicella* (chickenpox) is a common communicable childhood disease. It is caused by the varicella-zoster virus, which also is the agent in herpes zoster (shingles). The characteristic skin lesion occurs in three stages: macule, vesicle, and granular scab. The macular stage is characterized by development within hours of macules over the trunk of the body, spreading to the limbs, buccal mucosa,

scalp, axillae, upper respiratory tract, and conjunctiva[44] (Fig. 45-29). During the second stage, the macules form vesicles with depressed centers. The vesicles break open and a scab forms during the third stage. Crops of lesions occur successively, so that all three forms of the lesion usually are visible by the third day of the illness.

Mild to extreme pruritus accompanies the lesions, which can lead to scratching and subsequent development of secondary bacterial infections. Chickenpox also is accompanied by coldlike symptoms, including cough, coryza, and sometimes photosensitivity. Mild febrile states usually occur, typically beginning 24 hours before lesion outbreak. Side effects, such as pneumonia, septic complications, and encephalitis, are rare.

Varicella in adults may be more severe, with a prolonged recovery rate and greater chances for development of varicella pneumonitis or encephalitis. Immunocompromised persons may experience a chronic, painful type.

Live attenuated varicella vaccine has been demonstrated to be 95% effective in the preventing of typical varicella and 70% to 90% effective in preventing all disease.[44] The vaccine is available in the United States and required by law in many states.

SKIN MANIFESTATIONS AND DISORDERS IN THE ELDERLY

Elderly persons experience a variety of age-related skin disorders and exacerbations of earlier skin problems. Skin aging is believed to involve a complex process of actinic (solar) damage, normal aging, and hormonal influences. Actinic changes primarily involve increased occurrence of lesions on sun-exposed surfaces of the body.

Normal Age-Related Changes

Normal aging consists of changes that occur on areas of the body that have not been exposed to the sun.[75] They include thinning of the dermis and the epidermis, diminu-

FIGURE 45-28 Child with rubeola displaying the characteristic red blotchy skin during the third day of the rash. (From Centers for Disease Control and Prevention Public Health Image Library.)

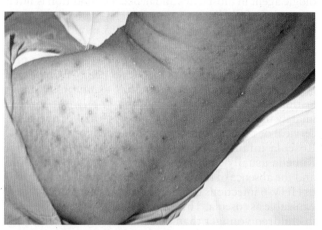

FIGURE 45-29 Blister-like rash on the back of a person with varicella-zoster (*i.e.*, chickenpox). (From Centers for Disease Control and Prevention Public Health Image Library.)

tion in subcutaneous tissue, a decrease in and thickening of blood vessels, and a decrease in the number of melanocytes, Langerhans cells, and Merkel cells. The keratinocytes shrink, but the number of dead keratinized cells at the surface increases. This results in less padding and thinner skin, with color and elasticity changes. The skin also loses its resistance to environmental and mechanical trauma. Tissue repair takes longer.

With aging, there is also less hair and nail growth, and there is permanent hair pigment loss. Hormonally, there is less sebaceous gland activity, although the glands in the facial skin may increase in size. Hair growth reduction also may be hormonally influenced. Although the reason is poorly understood, the skin in most persons older than 70 years of age becomes dry, rough, scaly, and itchy. When there is no underlying pathologic process, it is called *senile pruritus*. Itching and dryness become worse during the winter, when the need for home heating lowers the humidity.

The aging of skin, however, is not just a manifestation of age itself. Most skin changes associated with the elderly are the result of cumulative actinic or environmental damage. For example, the wrinkled, leathery look of aged skin, as well as odd scars and ecchymotic spots, are due to solar elastotic degenerative change.

Skin Lesions Common Among the Elderly

The most common skin lesions in the elderly are skin tags, keratoses, lentigines, and vascular lesions. Most are actinic manifestations; they occur as a result of exposure to sun and weather over the years.

Skin Tags. Skin tags are soft, brown or flesh-colored papules. They occur on any skin surface, but most frequently the neck, axilla, and intertriginous areas. They range in size from a pinhead to the size of a pea. Skin tags have the texture of normal skin. They are benign and can be removed with scissors or electrodesiccation for cosmetic purposes.

Keratoses. A *keratosis* is a horny growth or an abnormal growth of the keratinocytes. A *seborrheic keratosis* (*i.e.*, seborrheic wart) is a benign, sharply circumscribed, wartlike lesion that has a stuck-on appearance (Fig. 45-30). They vary in size up to several centimeters. They are usually round or oval, tan, brown, or black lesions. Less pigmented ones may appear yellow or pink. Keratoses can be found on the face or trunk, as a solitary lesion or sometimes by the hundreds. Seborrheic keratoses are benign, but they must be watched for changes in color, texture, or size, which may indicate malignant transformation to a melanoma.

Actinic keratoses are the most common premalignant skin lesions that develop on sun-exposed areas. The lesions usually are less than 1 cm in diameter and appear as dry, brown, scaly areas, often with a reddish tinge. Actinic keratoses often are multiple and more easily felt than seen (Fig. 45-31). They often are indistinguishable from squamous cell carcinoma without biopsy. A hyper-

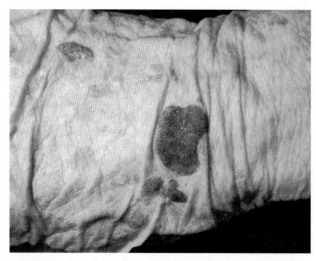

FIGURE 45-30 Large seborrheic keratoses on the hand of an 84-year-old woman. (From Sauer G. C., Hall J. C. [1996]. *Manual of skin diseases* [7th ed.]. Philadelphia: Lippincott-Raven.)

keratotic form also exists that is more prominent and palpable. Often, there is a weathered appearance of the surrounding skin. Slight changes, such as enlargement or ulceration, may indicate malignant transformation. Roughly 20% of actinic keratoses convert to squamous cell carcinomas. However, a current belief is that actinic keratoses do not convert or progress to cancerous cells, but that they are themselves the early malignancies.[76,77] Most actinic keratoses are treated with 5-fluorouracil cream, which erodes the lesions.

Lentigines. A *lentigo* is a well-bordered, brown to black macule, usually less than 1 cm in diameter. *Solar lentigines* are tan to brown, benign spots on sun-exposed areas. They are commonly referred to as *liver spots*. Creams and lotions containing hydroquinone (*e.g.*, Eldoquin,

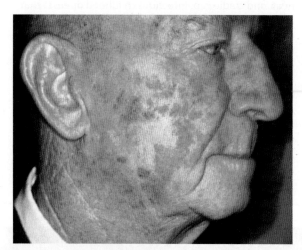

FIGURE 45-31 Multiple actinic keratoses of the face of an 80-year-old man. (Dermik Laboratories, Inc.) (From Sauer G. C., Hall J. C. [1996]. *Manual of skin diseases* [7th ed.]. Philadelphia: Lippincott-Raven.)

Solaquin) may be used temporarily to bleach the spots. These agents inhibit the synthesis of new pigment without destroying existing pigment. Higher concentrations are available by prescription. Successful treatment depends on avoiding sun exposure and consistent use of sunscreens. Liquid nitrogen applications have been successful in eradicating senile lentigines.

Lentigo maligna (*i.e.*, Hutchinson's freckle) is a slowly progressive (≤20 years) preneoplastic disorder of melanocytes. It occurs on sun-exposed areas, particularly the face. The lesion is a pigmented macule with a well-defined border and grows to 5 cm or sometimes larger. As it grows over the years, it may become slightly raised and wartlike. If untreated, a true malignant melanoma often develops. Surgery, curettage, and cryotherapy have been effective at removing the lentigines. Careful monitoring for conversion to melanoma is important.

Vascular Lesions. Vascular lesions are vascular tumors with chronically dilated blood vessels. The small blood vessels lie in the middle to upper dermis. *Senile angiomas* (cherry angiomas) are smooth, cherry-red or purple, dome-shaped papules. They usually are found on the trunk. *Telangiectases* are single dilated blood vessels, capillaries, or terminal arteries that appear on areas exposed to sun or harsh weather, such as the cheeks and the nose. The lesions can become large and disfiguring. Pulsed dye lasers have been effective in removing them. *Venous lakes* are small, dark blue, slightly raised papules that have a lakelike appearance. They occur on exposed body parts, particularly the backs of the hands, ears, and lips. They are smooth and compressible. Venous lakes can be removed by electrosurgery, laser therapy, or surgical excision if the person desires.

> **In summary,** some skin problems occur in specific age groups. Common in infants are diaper dermatitis, prickly heat, and cradle cap. Infectious childhood diseases that are characterized by rashes include roseola infantum, rubella, rubeola, varicella, and scarlet fever. Vaccines are available to protect against rubella, rubeola, and varicella. Changes in skin that occur with aging involve a complex process of actinic damage, normal aging, and hormonal influences. With aging, there is thinning of the dermis and the epidermis, diminution in subcutaneous tissue, lessening and thickening of blood vessels, and a slowing of hair and nail growth. Dry skin is common among the elderly, becoming worse during the winter months. Among the skin lesions seen in the elderly are skin tags, keratoses, lentigines, and vascular skin lesions.

Review Exercises

The mother of a 7-year-old-boy notices that he is scratching his head frequently. On close examination, she notices a grayish, round, and roughened area where the hair has broken off. Examination by the child's pediatrician produces a diagnosis of tinea capitis.

A. Explain the cause of the infection and propose possible mechanisms for its spread in school-age children, particularly during winter months.
B. Referring back to Chapter 12, explain the preference of the superficial mycoses (dermatophytes) for the skin-covered areas of the body.
C. What methods are commonly used in the diagnosis of superficial fungal infections?

A 75-year-old woman presents with severe, burning pain and a vesicular rash covering a strip over the rib cage on one side of the chest. She is diagnosed with herpes zoster or shingles.

A. What is the source of this woman's rash and pain?
B. Explain the dermatomal distribution of the lesions.

Psoriasis is a chronically recurring papulosquamous skin disorder, characterized by circumscribed, red, thickened plaques with an overlying silvery-white scale.

A. Explain the development of the plaques in terms of epidermal cell turnover.
B. Persons with psoriasis are instructed to refrain from rubbing or scratching the lesions. Explain the rationale for these instructions.
C. Among the methods used in treating psoriasis is the use of topical keratolytic agents and corticosteroid skin preparations. Explain how these two different types of agents exert their effect on the plaque lesions.

During the past several decades, there has been an alarming increase in the incidence of skin cancers, including malignant melanoma, which has been attributed to increased sun exposure.

A. Explain the possible mechanism(s) whereby UVR promotes the development of malignant skin lesions.
B. Cite two important clinical signs that aid in distinguishing a dysplastic nevus from a malignant melanoma.

REFERENCES

1. Hall J. C. (Ed.). (2000). *Sauer's manual of skin diseases* (8th ed., pp. 114–144, 198–222). Philadelphia: Lippincott Williams & Wilkins.
2. Murray P. R., Rosenthal K. S., Kobayashi G. S., et al. (2002). *Medical microbiology* (4th ed., pp. 639–650). St. Louis: Mosby.
3. Hainer B. L. (2003). Dermatophyte infections. *American Family Physician* 57, 101–108.
4. Weinstein A., Berman B. (2002). Topical treatment of common superficial tinea infections. *American Family Physician* 65, 2095–2102.
5. Storm C., Elder D. E. (2005). The skin. In Rubin E., Gorstein F., Rubin R., et al. (Eds.), *Rubin's pathology: Clinicopathologic foundations of medicine* (4th ed., pp. 1202–1267). Philadelphia: Lippincott Williams & Wilkins.
6. Murphy G. F., Sellheyer K., Mihm M. C. (2005). The skin. In Kumar V., Abbas A. K., Fausto N. (Eds.), *Robbins and Cotran pathologic basis of disease* (7th ed., pp. 1227–1271). Philadelphia: Elsevier Saunders.
7. Bacelieri R., Johnson S. M. (2005). Cutaneous warts: An evidence-based approach to therapy. *American Family Physician* 72, 647–652.
8. Focht D. R., Spicer C., Fairchok M. P. (2002). The efficacy of duct tape vs. cryotherapy in the treatment of verruca vulgaris (the common wart). *Archives of Pediatric and Adolescent Medicine* 156, 971–974.
9. Schwartz D., Genta R. M., Conner D. H. (2005). Infectious and parasitic diseases. In Rubin E., Gorstein F., Rubin R., et al. *Rubin's pathology: Clinicopathologic foundations of medicine* (4th ed., pp. 370–373). Philadelphia: Lippincott Williams & Wilkins.
10. Emmert D. H. (2000). Treatment of cutaneous herpes simplex virus infections. *American Family Physician* 61, 1697–1709.
11. Mounsey A. L., Mathew L. G., Slawson D. C. (2005). Herpes zoster and postherpetic neuralgia: Prevention and treatment. *American Family Physician* 72, 1075–1080.
12. Gilden D. H., Kleinschmidt-DeMasters B. K., LaGuardia J. J., et al. (2000). Neurologic complications of reactivation of varicella-zoster virus. *New England Journal of Medicine* 342, 635–645.
13. Edmunds W. J., Brisson M. (2002). The effect of vaccination on the epidemiology of varicella zoster virus. *Journal of Infection* 44, 211–219.
14. James E. D. (2005). Acne. *New England Journal of Medicine* 352, 1463–1472.
15. Feldman S., Careccia R. E., Barham K. L., et al. (2004). Diagnosis and treatment of acne. *American Family Physician* 69, 2123–2136.
16. Krowchuk D. P. (2000). Managing acne in adolescents. *Pediatric Clinics of North America* 47, 841–857.
17. Haiden A., Shaw J. C. (2004). Treatment of acne. *Journal of the American Medical Association* 292, 726–735.
18. Powell F. C. (2005). Rosacea. *New England Journal of Medicine* 352, 793–803.
19. Buechner S. A. (2005). Rosacea: An update. *Dermatology* 210, 100–108.
20. Blount B. W., Pelletter A. L. (2002). Rosacea: A common, yet commonly overlooked, condition. *American Family Physician* 66, 435–442.
21. Kristal L., Klein P. A. (2000). Atopic dermatitis in infants and children. *Pediatric Clinics of North America* 47, 877–894.
22. Williams H. C. (2005). Atopic dermatitis. *New England Journal of Medicine* 352, 2314–2324.
23. Leung D. Y., Boguniewicz M. (2003). Advances in allergic skin diseases. *Journal of Allergy and Clinical Immunology* 111, S805–S812.
24. Rico M. J., Lawrence I. (2002). Tacrolimus ointment for the treatment of atopic dermatitis: Clinical and pharmacologic effects. *Allergy and Asthma Proceedings*, 23, 191–197.
25. Yates C. (2002). Parameters for the treatment of urticaria and angioedema. *Journal of the American Academy of Nurse Practitioners* 14, 478–747.
26. Kaplan A. P. (2002). Chronic urticaria and angioedema. *New England Journal of Medicine* 346, 175–179.
27. Kozel M. M. A., Sabroe R. A. (2004). Chronic urticaria. *Drugs* 64, 2615–2636.
28. Muller B. A. (2004). Urticaria and angioedema: A practical approach. *American Family Physician* 69, 1123–1128.
29. Fritsch P. O., Sidoroff A. (2000). Drug-induced Stevens-Johnson syndrome/toxic epidermal necrolysis. *American Journal of Clinical Dermatology* 1, 349–360.
30. Roujeau J. C., Stern R. S. (1994). Severe adverse cutaneous reactions to drugs. *New England Journal of Medicine* 331, 1272–1284.
31. Odom R. B., James W. D., Berger T. G. (2000). *Andrew's diseases of the skin: Clinical dermatology* (pp. 186, 486, 488). Philadelphia: W. B. Saunders.
32. Schon M. P., Boehncke W. H. (2005). Psoriasis. *New England Journal of Medicine* 352, 1899–1912.
33. Galadari H., Fuchs B., Lebwohl M. (2003). Newly available treatments for psoriatic arthritis and their impact on skin psoriasis. *International Journal of Dermatology* 42, 231–237.
34. Pardasani A. G., Feldman S. R., Clark A. R. (2000). Treatment of psoriasis: An algorithm based approach for primary care physicians. *American Family Physician* 61, 725–733, 736.
35. Lebwohl M. (2003). Psoriasis. *Lancet* 363, 1197–1204.
36. Weinberg J. M., Saini R., Tutrone W. D. (2002). Biologic therapy for psoriasis—the first wave: Infliximab, etanercept, efalizumab, and alefacept. *Journal of Drugs in Dermatology* 1, 303–310.
37. Galadari H., Fuchs B., Lebwohl M. (2003). Newly available treatments for psoriatic arthritis and their impact on skin psoriasis. *International Journal of Dermatology* 42, 231–237.
38. Stulberg D. L., Wolfrey J. (2004). Pityriasis rosea. *American Family Physician* 69, 87–94.
39. Katta R. (2000). Lichen planus. *American Family Physician* 61, 3319–3324, 3327–3328.
40. Ives T. J. (2005). Photosensitivity and burns. In Koda-Kimble M. A., Young L. Y. (Eds.), *Applied therapeutics: The clinical use of drugs* (7th ed., pp. 1–14, 41). Philadelphia: Lippincott Williams & Wilkins.
41. Scarlett W. L. (2003). Ultraviolet radiation, sun exposure, tanning beds, and vitamin D levels: What you need to know and how to decrease the risk of skin cancer. *Journal of the American Osteopathic Association* 103, 371–375.
42. Granstein R. D. (2004). UV radiation–induced immunosuppression and skin cancer. *Cutis* 74(Suppl. 5), 10–13.
43. Monson W. L. (2004). Photosensitivity. *New England Journal of Medicine* 350, 1111–1117.
44. Behrman R. E., Kliegman R. M, Jenson H. B. (Eds). (2004). *Nelson textbook of pediatrics* (17th ed., pp. 330–337, 1026–1034, 1057–1059, 1069–1072). Philadelphia: Elsevier Saunders.

45. Morgan E. D., Bledsoe S. C., Barker J. (2000). Ambulatory management of burns. *American Family Physician* 62, 2015–2026, 2029–2030.

46. Mertens D. M., Jenkins M. E., Warden G. D. (1997). Outpatient burn management. *Nursing Clinics of North America* 32(2), 343–346.

47. Jordon B. S., Harrington D. T. (1997). Management of the burn wound. *Nursing Clinics of North America* 32, 251–273.

48. Monafo W. W. (1996). Initial management of burns. *New England Journal of Medicine* 335, 1581–1585.

49. Allison K., Porter K. (2004). Consensus on the prehospital approach to burns: Patient management. *Emergency Medicine Journal* 21, 112–114.

50. Gordon M., Goodwin C. W. (1997). Burn management: Initial assessment, management, and stabilization. *Nursing Clinics of North America* 32, 237–249.

51. Parenteau N. (1999). Skin: The first tissue-engineered products. *Scientific American* 280(4), 83–84.

52. Arnold M. C. (2003). Pressure ulcer prevention and management. *AACN Clinical Issues* 14, 411–428.

53. Maklebust J. (2005). Pressure ulcers: The great insult. *Nursing Clinics of North America* 40, 365–389.

54. National Institutes of Health. (2000). *Healthy people 2010.* [On-line]. Available: www.health.gov/healthypeople.

55. Panel for the Prediction and Prevention of Pressure Ulcers in Adults. (1992). *Pressure ulcers in adults: Prediction and prevention.* Clinical practice guideline no. 3. AHCPR publication no. 92-0047. Rockville, MD: Agency for Health Care Policy and Research, Public Health Service, U.S. Department of Health and Human Services.

56. Bergstrom N., Bennett M. A., Carlson C. E., et al. (1994). *Treatment of pressure ulcers.* Clinical practice guideline no. 15. AHCPR publication no. 95-0652. Rockville, MD: U.S. Department of Health and Human Services. Public Health Service, Agency for Health Care Policy and Research.

57. National Pressure Ulcer Advisory Panel. (2003). Staging report. [On-line]. Available: www.npuap.org/positn6.html. Accessed September 22, 2005.

58. Cannon B. C., Cannon J. P. (2004). Management of pressure ulcers. *American Journal of Health-System Pharmacists* 61, 1895–1905.

59. Thomas D. R. (2001). Prevention and treatment of pressure ulcers: What works? What doesn't? *Cleveland Clinic Journal of Medicine* 68, 704–722.

60. Naeyaert J. M., Brochez L. (2003). Dysplastic nevi. *New England Journal of Medicine* 349, 2233–2240.

61. Jemad A., Ward E., Tiwari R. C., et al. (2005). Cancer statistics, 2005. *CA: A Cancer Journal for Clinicians* 55, 10–30.

62. Rigel D. S., Carucci J. A. (2000). Malignant melanoma: Prevention, early detection, and treatment in the 21st century. *CA: A Cancer Journal for Clinicians* 50, 215–236.

63. Mikkilineni R., Weinstock M. A. (2001). Epidemiology. In Sober A. J., Haluska F. G. (Eds.), *American Cancer Society atlas of clinical oncology: Skin cancer* (pp. 1–15). Hamilton, Ontario: BC Decker.

64. Urist M. M., Heslin M. J., Miller D. M. (2001). Malignant melanoma. In Lenhard R. E., Osteen R. T., Gansler T. (Eds.), *The American Cancer Society's clinical oncology* (pp. 553–556). Atlanta: American Cancer Society.

65. Abbasi N. R., Shaw H. M., Rigel D. S., et al. (2004). Early diagnosis of cutaneous melanoma. *Journal of the American Medical Association* 292, 2771–2776.

66. Lens M. B., Dawes M., Goodacre T., et al. (2002). Excision margins in the treatment of primary cutaneous melanoma: A systematic review of randomized controlled trials comparing narrow vs wide excision. *Archives of Surgery* 137, 1101–1105.

67. Yang S., Haluska F. G. (2001). Immunotherapy for melanoma. In Sober A. J., Haluska F. G. (Eds.), *American Cancer Society atlas of clinical oncology: Skin cancer* (pp. 225–252). Hamilton, Ontario: BC Decker.

68. Menaker G. M., Chiu D. S. (2001). Basal cell carcinoma. In Sober A. J., Haluska F. G. (Eds.), *American Cancer Society atlas of clinical oncology: Skin cancer* (pp. 60–71). Hamilton, Ontario: BC Decker.

69. Carucci J. A., Rigel D. S., Friedman R. J. (2001). Basal cell and squamous cell skin cancer. In Lenhard R. E., Osteen R. T., Gansler T. (Eds.), *The American Cancer Society's clinical oncology* (pp. 553–556). Atlanta: American Cancer Society.

70. Robinson J. K. (2001). Squamous cell carcinoma. In Sober A. J., Haluska F. G. (Eds.), *American Cancer Society atlas of clinical oncology: Skin cancer* (pp. 72–84). Hamilton, Ontario: BC Decker.

71. Dohil M. A., Baugh W. P., Eichenfield L. F. (2000). Vascular and pigmented birthmarks. *Pediatric Clinics of North America* 47, 783–810.

72. Drolet B. A., Esterly N. B., Frieden I. J. (1999). Hemangiomas in children. *New England Journal of Medicine* 341, 173–181.

73. Kazaks E. L., Lane A. T. (2000). Diaper dermatitis. *Pediatric Clinics of North America* 47, 909–918.

74. Atherton D. J. (2004). A review of the pathophysiology, prevention and treatment of irritant diaper dermatitis. *Current Medical Research and Opinions* 20, 645–649.

75. Bolognia J. L. (1995). Aging skin. *American Journal of Medicine* 98, 99S–103S.

76. Lober B. A., Lober C. W. (2000). Actinic keratosis is squamous cell carcinoma. *Southern Medical Journal* 93, 650–655.

77. Cockerell C. J. (2000). Histopathology of incipient intraepidermal squamous cell carcinoma ("actinic keratosis") [comment]. *Journal of the American Academy of Dermatology* 42, 11–17.

Glossary

Abduction: The act of abducting (moving or spreading away from a position near the midline of the body or the axial line of a limb) or the state of being abducted.

Abrasion: The wearing or scraping away of a substance or structure, such as the skin, through an unusual or abnormal mechanical process.

Abscess: A collection of pus that is restricted to a specific area in tissues, organs, or confined spaces.

Accommodation: The adjustment of the lens (eye) to variations in distance.

Acromion: The lateral extension of the spine of the scapula, forming the highest point of the shoulder. (Noun: acromial)

Acuity: The clearness or sharpness of perception, especially of vision.

Adaptation: The adjustment of an organism to its environment, physical or psychological, through changes and responses to stress of any kind.

Adduction: The act of adducting (moving or drawing toward a position near the midline of the body or the axial line of a limb) or the state of being adducted.

Adhesin: The molecular components of the bacterial cell wall that are involved in adhesion processes.

Adrenergic: Activated by or characteristic of the sympathetic nervous system or its neurotransmitters (i.e., epinephrine and norepinephrine).

Aerobic: Growing, living, or occurring only in the presence of air or oxygen.

Afferent: Bearing or conducting inward or toward a center, as an afferent neuron.

Agglutination: The clumping together of particles, microorganisms, or blood cells in response to an antigen-antibody reaction.

Agonist: A muscle whose action is opposed by another muscle (antagonist) with which it is paired; or a drug or other chemical substance that has affinity for or stimulates a predictable physiologic function.

Akinesia: An abnormal state in which there is an absence or poverty of movement.

Allele: One of two or more different forms of a gene that can occupy a particular locus on a chromosome.

Alveolus: A small saclike structure, as in the alveolus of the lung.

Amine: An organic compound containing nitrogen.

Amblyopia: A condition of vision impairment without a detectable organic lesion of the eye.

Amorphous: Without a definite form; shapeless.

Amphoteric: Capable of reacting chemically as an acid or a base.

Ampulla: A saclike dilatation of a duct, canal, or any other tubular structure.

Anabolism: A constructive metabolic process characterized by the conversion of simple substances into larger, complex molecules.

Anaerobic: Growing, living, or occurring only in the absence of air or oxygen.

Analog: A part, organ, or chemical having the same function or appearance but differing in respect to a certain component, such as origin or development.

Anaplasia: A change in the structure of cells and in their orientation to each other that is characterized by a loss of cell differentiation, as in cancerous cell growth.

Anastomosis: The connection or joining between two vessels; or an opening created by surgical, traumatic, or pathologic means.

Androgen: Any substance, such as a male sex hormone, that increases male characteristics.

Anergy: A state of absent or diminished reaction to an antigen or group of antigens.

Aneuploidy: A variation in the number of chromosomes within a cell involving one or more missing chromosomes rather than entire sets.

Aneurysm: An outpouching or dilation in the wall of a blood vessel or the heart.

Ankylosis: Stiffness or fixation of separate bones of a joint, resulting from disease, injury, or surgical procedure. (Verb: ankylose)

Anorexia: Lack or loss of appetite for food. (Adjective: anorexic)

Anoxia: An abnormal condition characterized by the total lack of oxygen.

Antagonist: A muscle whose action directly opposes that of another muscle (agonist) with which it is paired; or a drug or other chemical substance that can diminish or nullify the action of a neuromediator or body function.

Anterior: Pertaining to a surface or part that is situated near or toward the front.

Antigen: A substance that generates an immune response by causing the formation of an antibody or reacting with antibodies or T cell receptors.

Apex: The uppermost point, the narrowed or pointed end, or the highest point of a structure, such as an organ.

Aphagia: A condition characterized by the refusal or the loss of ability to swallow.

Aplasia: The absence of an organ or tissue due to a developmental failure.

Apnea: The absence of spontaneous respiration.

Apoptosis: A mechanism of programmed cell death, marked by shrinkage of the cell, condensation of chromatin, formation of cytoplasmic blebs, and fragmentation of the cell into membrane-bound bodies eliminated by phagocytosis.

Apraxia: Loss of the ability to carry out familiar, purposeful acts or to manipulate objects in the absence of paralysis or other motor or sensory impairment.

Articulation: The place of connection or junction between two or more bones of a skeletal joint.

Ascites: An abnormal accumulation of serous fluid in the peritoneal cavity.

Asepsis: The condition of being free or freed from pathogenic microorganisms.

Astereognosis: A neurologic disorder characterized by an inability to identify objects by touch.

Asterixis: A motor disturbance characterized by a hand-flapping tremor, which results when the prolonged contraction of groups of muscles lapses intermittently.

Ataxia: An abnormal condition characterized by an inability to coordinate voluntary muscular movement.

Athetosis: A neuromuscular condition characterized by the continuous occurrence of slow, sinuous, writhing movements that are performed involuntarily. (Adjective: athetoid)

Atopy: Genetic predisposition toward the development of a hypersensitivity or an allergic reaction to common environmental allergens.

Atresia: The absence or closure of a normal body orifice or tubular organ, such as the esophagus.

Atrophy: A wasting or diminution of size, often accompanied by a decrease in function, of a cell, tissue, or organ.

Autocrine: A mode of hormone action in which a chemical messenger acts on the same cell that secretes it.

Autosome: Any chromosome other than a sex chromosome.

Axillary: Of or pertaining to the axilla, or armpit.

Bacteremia: The presence of bacteria in the blood.

Bactericide: An agent that destroys bacteria. (Adjective: bactericidal)

Bacteriostat: An agent that inhibits bacterial growth. (Adjective: bacteriostatic)

Ballismus: An abnormal condition characterized by violent flailing motions of the arms and, occasionally, the head, resulting from injury to or destruction of the subthalamic nucleus or its fiber connections.

Baroreceptor: A type of sensory nerve ending such as those found in the aorta and the carotid sinus that is stimulated by changes in pressure.

Basal: Pertaining to, situated at, or forming the base; or the fundamental or the basic.

Benign: Not malignant; or of the character that does not threaten health or life.

Bipolar neuron: A nerve cell that has a process at each end—an afferent process and an efferent process.

Bolus: A rounded mass of food ready to swallow or such a mass passing through the gastrointestinal tract; or a concentrated mass of medicinal material or other pharmaceutic preparation injected all at once intravenously for diagnostic purposes.

Borborygmus: The rumbling, gurgling, or tinkling noise produced by the propulsion of gas through the intestine.

Bruit: A sound or murmur heard while auscultating an organ or blood vessel, especially an abnormal one.

Buccal: Pertaining to or directed toward the inside of the cheek.

Buffer: A substance or group of substances that prevents change in the concentration of another chemical substance.

Bulla: A thin-walled blister of the skin or mucous membranes greater than 5 mm in diameter containing serous or seropurulent fluid.

Bursa: A fluid-filled sac or saclike cavity situated in places in the tissues at which friction would otherwise develop, such as between certain tendons and the bones beneath them.

Cachexia: A condition of general ill health and malnutrition, marked by weakness and emaciation.

Calculus: A stony mass formed within body tissues, usually composed of mineral salts.

Capsid: The protein shell that envelops and protects the nucleic acid of a virus.

Carcinogen: Any substance or agent that causes the development or increases the incidence of cancer.

Carpal: Of or pertaining to the carpus, or wrist.

Caseation: A form of tissue necrosis in which the tissue is changed into a dry, amorphous mass resembling crumbly cheese.

Catabolism: A metabolic process through which living organisms break down complex substances to simple compounds, liberating energy for use in work, energy storage, or heat production.

Catalyst: A substance that increases the velocity of a chemical reaction without being consumed by the process.

Catecholamines: Any one of a group of biogenic amines having a sympathomimetic action and composed of a catechol molecule and the aliphatic portion of an amine.

Caudal: Signifying an inferior position, toward the distal end of the spine.

Cellulitis: An acute, diffuse, spreading, edematous inflammation of the deep subcutaneous tissues and sometimes muscle, characterized most commonly by an area of heat, redness, pain, and swelling, and occasionally by fever, malaise, chills, and headache.

Cephalic: Of or pertaining to the head, or to the head end of the body.

Cerumen: The waxlike secretion produced by vestigial apocrine sweat glands in the external ear canal.

Cheilosis: A noninflammatory disorder of the lips and mouth characterized by chapping and fissuring.

Chelate: A chemical compound composed of a central metal ion and an organic molecule with multiple bonds, arranged in ring formation, used especially in treatment of metal poisoning.

Chemoreceptor: A sensory nerve cell activated by chemical stimuli, as a chemoreceptor in the carotid that is sensitive to changes in the oxygen content in the bloodstream and reflexly increases or decreases respiration and blood pressure.

Chemotaxis: A response involving cell orientation or cell movement that is either toward (positive chemotaxis) or away from (negative chemotaxis) a chemical stimulus.

Chimeric: Relating to, derived from, or being an individual possessing one's own immunologic characteristics and that of another individual; a phenomenon that can occur as the result of procedures such as a bone marrow graft.

Chondrocyte: Any one of the mature polymorphic cells that form the cartilage of the body.

Chromatid: One of the paired threadlike chromosome filaments, joined at the centromere, that make up a metaphase chromosome.

Chromosome: Any one of the structures in the nucleus of a cell containing a linear thread of DNA, which functions in the transmission of genetic information.

Chyme: The creamy, viscous, semifluid material produced during digestion of a meal that is expelled by the stomach into the duodenum.

Cilia: A minute, hairlike process projecting from a cell, composed of nine microtubules arrayed around a single pair. Cilia beat rhythmically to move the cell around in its environment or they move mucus or fluids over the surface.

Circadian: Being, having, pertaining to, or occurring in a period or cycle of approximately 24 hours.

Circumduction: The active or passive circular movement of a limb or of the eye.

Cisterna: An enclosed space, such as a cavity, that serves as a reservoir for lymph or other body fluids.

Clone: One or a group of genetically identical cells or organisms derived from a single parent.

Coagulation: The process of transforming a liquid into a semisolid mass, especially of blood clot formation.

Coarctation: A condition of stricture or contraction of the walls of a vessel.

Cofactor: A substance that must unite with another substance in order to function.

Colic: Sharp, intermittent abdominal pain localized in a hollow or tubular organ, resulting from torsion, obstruction, or smooth muscle spasm. (Adjective: colicky)

Collagen: The protein substance of the white, glistening, inelastic fibers of the skin, tendons, bone, cartilage, and all other connective tissue.

Collateral: Secondary or accessory rather than direct or immediate; or a small branch, as of a blood vessel or nerve.

Complement: Any one of the complex, enzymatic serum proteins that are involved in physiologic reactions, including antigen-antibody reaction and anaphylaxis.

Confluent: Flowing or coming together; not discrete.

Congenital: Present at, and usually before, birth.

Conjugate: To pair and fuse in conjugation; or a form of sexual reproduction seen in unicellular organisms in which genetic material is exchanged during the temporary fusion of two cells.

Contiguous: In contact or nearly so in an unbroken sequence along a boundary or at a point.

Contralateral: Affecting, pertaining to, or originating in the opposite side of a point or reference.

Contusion: An injury of a part without a break in the skin, characterized by swelling, discoloration, and pain.

Convolution: An elevation or tortuous winding, such as one of the irregular ridges on the surface of the brain, formed by a structure being infolded upon itself.

Corpuscle: Any small mass, cell, or body, such as a red or white blood cell.

Costal: Pertaining to a rib or ribs.

Crepitus: A sound or sensation that resembles a crackling or grating noise.

Cutaneous: Pertaining to the skin.

Cyanosis: A bluish discoloration, especially of the skin and mucous membranes, caused by an excess of deoxygenated hemoglobin in the blood.

Cytokine: Any of a class of polypeptide immunoregulatory substances that are secreted by cells, usually of the immune system, that affect other cells.

Cytology: The study of cells, including their origin, structure, function, and pathology.

Decibel: A unit for expressing the relative power intensity of electric or acoustic signal power that is equal to one tenth of a bel.

Defecation: The evacuation of feces from the digestive tract through the rectum.

Deformation: The process of adapting in form or shape; also the product of such alteration.

Degeneration: The deterioration of a normal cell, tissue, or organ to a less functionally active form. (Adjective: degenerative)

Deglutition: The act or process of swallowing.

Degradation: The reduction of a chemical compound to a compound less complex, usually by splitting off one or more groups.

Dehydration: The condition that results from excessive loss of water from the body tissues.

Delirium: An acute, reversible organic mental syndrome characterized by confusion, disorientation, restlessness, incoherence, fear, and often illusions.

Dendrite: One of the branching processes that extends and transmits impulses toward a cell body of a neuron. (Adjective: dendritic)

Depolarization: The reduction of a cell membrane potential to a less negative value than that of the potential outside the cell.

Dermatome: The area of the skin supplied with afferent nerve fibers of a single dorsal root of a spinal nerve.

Desmosome: A small, circular, dense area within the intercellular bridge that forms the site of adhesion between intermediate filaments and cell membranes.

Desquamation: A normal process in which the cornified layer of the epidermis is shed in fine scales or sheets.

Dialysis: The process of separating colloids and crystalline substances in solution, which involves the two distinct physical processes of diffusion and ultrafiltration; or a medical procedure for the removal of urea and other elements from the blood or lymph.

Diapedesis: The outward passage of red or white blood corpuscles through the intact walls of the vessels.

Diaphoresis: Perspiration, especially the profuse perspiration associated with an elevated body temperature, physical exertion, exposure to heat, and mental or emotional stress.

Diarthrosis: A specialized articulation that permits, to some extent, free joint movement. (Adjective: diarthrodial)

Diastole: The dilatation of the heart; or the period of dilatation, which is the interval between the second and the first heart sound and is the time during which blood enters the relaxed chambers of the heart from the systemic circulation and the lungs.

Differentiation: The act or process in development in which unspecialized cells or tissues acquire more specialized characteristics, including those of physical form, physiologic function, and chemical properties.

Diffusion: The process of becoming widely spread, as in the spontaneous movement of molecules or other particles in solution from an area of higher concentration to an area of lower concentration, resulting in an even distribution of the particles in the fluid.

Diopter: A unit of measurement of the refractive power of lenses equal to the reciprocal of the focal length in meters.

Diploid: Pertaining to an individual, organism, strain, or cell that has two full sets of homologous chromosomes.

Disseminate: To scatter or distribute over a considerable area.

Distal: Away from or being the farthest from a point of reference.

Diurnal: Of, relating to, or occurring in the daytime.

Diverticulum: A pouch or sac of variable size occurring naturally or through herniation of the muscular wall of a tubular organ.

Dorsum: The back or posterior. (Adjective: dorsal)

Dysgenesis: Defective or abnormal development of an organ or part, typically occurring during embryonic development. (Also called dysgenesia.)

Dyslexia: A disturbance in the ability to read, spell, and write words.

Dyspepsia: The impairment of the power or function of digestion, especially epigastric discomfort following eating.

Dysphagia: A difficulty in swallowing.

Dysphonia: Any impairment of the voice that is experienced as a difficulty in speaking.

Dysplasia: The alteration in size, shape, and organization of adult cell types.

Eburnation: The conversion of bone or cartilage, through thinning or loss, into a hard and dense mass with a worn, polished, ivorylike surface.

Ecchymosis: A small hemorrhagic spot, larger than a petechia, in the skin or mucous membrane caused by the extravasation of blood into the subcutaneous tissues.

Ectoderm: The outermost of the three primary germ layers of the embryo, and from which the epidermis and epidermal tissues, such as nails, hair, and glands of the skin, develop.

Ectopic: Relating to or characterized by an object or organ being situated in an unusual place, away from its normal location.

Edema: The presence of an abnormal accumulation of fluid in interstitial spaces of tissues. (Adjective: edematous)

Efferent: Conveyed or directed away from a center.

Effusion: The escape of fluid from blood vessels into a part or tissue, as an exudation or a transudation.

Embolus: A mass of clotted blood or other formed elements, such as bubbles of air, calcium fragments, or a bit of tissue or tumor, that circulates in the bloodstream until it becomes lodged in a vessel, obstructing the circulation. (Plural: emboli)

Empyema: An accumulation of pus in a cavity of the body, especially the pleural space.

Emulsify: To disperse one liquid throughout the body of another liquid, making a colloidal suspension, or emulsion.

Endocytosis: The uptake or incorporation of substances into a cell by invagination of its plasma membrane, as in the processes of phagocytosis and pinocytosis.

Endoderm: The innermost of the three primary germ layers of the embryo, and from which epithelium arises.

Endogenous: Growing within the body; or developing or originating from within the body or produced from internal causes.

Endoscopy: The visualization of any cavity of the body with an endoscope.

Enteropathic: Relating to any disease of the intestinal tract.

Enzyme: A protein molecule produced by living cells that catalyzes chemical reactions of other organic substances without itself being destroyed or altered.

Epiphysis: The expanded articular end of a long bone (head) that is separated from the shaft of the bone by the epiphyseal plate until the bone stops growing, the plate is obliterated, and the shaft and the head become united.

Epithelium: The covering of the internal and the external surfaces of the body, including the lining of vessels and other small cavities.

Erectile: Capable of being erected or raised to an erect position.

Erythema: The redness or inflammation of the skin or mucous membranes produced by the congestion of superficial capillaries. (Adjective: erythematous)

Etiology: The study or theory of all factors that may be involved in the development of a disease, including susceptibility of an individual, the nature of the disease agent, and the way in which an individual's body is invaded by the agent; or the cause of a disease.

Eukaryotic: Pertaining to an organism with cells having a true nucleus; that is, a highly complex, organized nucleus surrounded by a nuclear membrane containing organelles and exhibiting mitosis.

Euploid: Pertaining to an individual, organism, strain, or cell with a balanced set or sets of chromosomes, in any number, that is an exact multiple of the normal, basic haploid number characteristic of the species; or such an individual, organism, strain, or cell.

Evisceration: The removal of the viscera from the abdominal cavity, or disembowelment; or the extrusion of an internal organ through a wound or surgical incision.

Exacerbation: An increase in the severity of a disease as marked by greater intensity in any of its signs and symptoms.

Exfoliation: Peeling and sloughing off of tissue cells in scales or layers. (Adjective: exfoliative)

Exocytosis: The discharge of cell particles, which are packaged in membrane-bound vesicles, by fusion of the vesicular membrane with the plasma membrane and subsequent release of the particles to the exterior of the cell.

Exogenous: Developed or originating outside the body, as a disease caused by a bacterial or viral agent foreign to the body.

Exophthalmos: A marked or abnormal protusion of the eyeball.

Extension: A movement that allows the two elements of any jointed part to be drawn apart, increasing the angle between them, as extending the leg increases the angle between the femur and the tibia.

Extrapyramidal: Pertaining to motor systems supplied by fibers outside the corticospinal or pyramidal tracts.

Extravasation: A discharge or escape, usually of blood, serum, or lymph, from a vessel into the tissues.

Extubation: The process of withdrawing a previously inserted tube from an orifice or cavity of the body.

Exudate: Fluid, cells, or other substances that have been slowly exuded or have escaped from blood vessels and have been deposited in tissues or on tissue surfaces.

Fascia: A sheet or band of fibrous connective tissue that may be separated from other specifically organized structures, as the tendons, the aponeuroses, and the ligaments.

Febrile: Pertaining to or characterized by an elevated body temperature, or fever.

Fibrillation: A small, local, involuntary contraction of muscle, resulting from spontaneous activation of a single muscle fiber or of an isolated bundle of nerve fibers.

Fibrin: A stringy, insoluble protein formed by the action of thrombin on fibrinogen during the clotting process.

Fibrosis: The formation of fibrous connective tissue, as in the repair or replacement of parenchymatous elements.

Filtration: The process of passing a liquid through or as if through a filter, which is accomplished by gravity, pressure, or vacuum.

Fimbria: Any structure that forms a fringe, border, or edge or the processes that resemble such a structure.

Fissure: A cleft or a groove, normal or otherwise, on the surface of an organ or a bony structure.

Fistula: An abnormal passage or communication from an internal organ to the body surface or between two internal organs.

Flaccid: Weak, soft, and lax; lacking normal muscle tone.

Flatus: Air or gas in the intestinal tract that is expelled through the anus. (Adjective: flatulent)

Flexion: A movement that allows the two elements of any jointed part to be brought together, decreasing the angle between them, as bending the elbow.

Flora: The microorganisms, such as bacteria and fungi, both normally occurring and pathological, found in or on an organ.

Focal: Relating to, having, or occupying a focus.

Follicle: A sac or pouchlike depression or cavity.

Fontanel: A membrane-covered opening in bones or between bones, such as the soft spot covered by tough membranes between the bones of an infant's incompletely ossified skull.

Foramen: A natural opening or aperture in a membranous structure or bone.

Fossa: A hollow or depressed area, especially on the surface of the end of a bone.

Fovea: A small pit or depression in the surface of a structure or an organ.

Fundus: The base or bottom of an organ or the portion farthest from the mouth of an organ.

Ganglion: One of the nerve cell bodies, chiefly collected in groups outside the central nervous system. (Plural: ganglia)

Genotype: The entire genetic constitution of an individual, as determined by the particular combination and location of the genes on the chromosomes; or the alleles present at one or more sites on homologous chromosomes.

Glia: The neuroglia, or supporting structure of nervous tissue.

Globulin: One of a broad group of proteins classified by solubility, electrophoretic mobility, and size.

Gluconeogenesis: The formation of glucose from any of the substances of glycolysis other than carbohydrates.

Glycolysis: A series of enzymatically catalyzed reactions, occurring within cells, by which glucose is converted to adenosine triphosphate (ATP) and pyruvic acid during aerobic metabolism.

Gonad: A gamete-producing gland, as an ovary or a testis.

Gradient: The rate of increase or decrease of a measurable phenomenon expressed as a function of a second; or the visual representation of such a change.

Granuloma: A small mass of nodular granulation tissue resulting from chronic inflammation, injury, or infection. (Adjective: granulomatous)

Hapten: A small, nonproteinaceous substance that is not antigenic by itself but that can act as an antigen when combined with a larger molecule.

Haustrum: A structure resembling a recess or sacculation. (Plural: haustra)

Hematoma: A localized collection of extravasated blood trapped in an organ, space, or tissue, resulting from a break in the wall of a blood vessel.

Hematopoiesis: The normal formation and development of blood cells.

Hemianopia: Defective vision or blindness in half of the visual field of one or both eyes.

Heterozygous: Having two different alleles at corresponding loci on homologous chromosomes.

Heterogeneous: Consisting of or composed of dissimilar elements or parts; or not having a uniform quality throughout. (Noun: heterogeneity)

Histology: The branch of anatomy that deals with the minute (microscopic) structure, composition, and function of cells and tissue. (Adjective: histologic)

Homolog: Any organ or part corresponding in function, position, origin, and structure to another organ or part, as the flippers of a seal that correspond to human hands. (Adjective: homologous)

Homozygous: Having two identical alleles at corresponding loci on homologous chromosomes.

Humoral: Relating to elements dissolved in the blood or body fluids.

Hydrolysis: The chemical alteration or decomposition of a compound into fragments by the addition of water.

Hypercapnia: Excess amounts of carbon dioxide in the blood.

Hyperemia: An excess or engorgement of blood in a part of the body.

Hyperesthesia: An unusual or pathologic increase in sensitivity of a part, especially the skin, or of a particular sense.

Hyperplasia: An abnormal multiplication or increase in the number of normal cells of a body part.

Hypertonic: A solution having a greater concentration of solute than another solution with which it is compared, hence exerting more osmotic pressure than that solution.

Hypertrophy: The enlargement or overgrowth of an organ that is due to an increase in the size of its cells rather than the number of its cells.

Hypesthesia: An abnormal decrease of sensation in response to stimulation of the sensory nerves. (Also called hypoesthesia.)

Hypocapnia: A deficiency of carbon dioxide in the blood.

Hypotonic: A solution having a lesser concentration of solute than another solution with which it is compared, hence exerting less osmotic pressure than that solution.

Hypoxia: An inadequate supply of oxygen to tissue that is below physiologic levels despite adequate perfusion of the tissue by blood.

Iatrogenic: Induced inadvertently through the activity of a physician or by medical treatment or diagnostic procedures.

Idiopathic: Arising spontaneously or from an unknown cause.

Idiosyncrasy: A physical or behavioral characteristic or manner that is unique to an individual or to a group. (Adjective: idiosyncratic)

Incidence: The rate at which a certain event occurs (e.g., the number of new cases of a specific disease during a particular period of time in a population at risk).

Inclusion: The act of enclosing or the condition of being enclosed; or anything that is enclosed.

Infarction: Necrosis or death of tissues due to local ischemia resulting from obstruction of blood flow.

Inotropic: Influencing the force or energy of muscular contractions.

In situ: In the natural or normal place; or something, such as cancer, that is confined to its place of origin and has not invaded neighboring tissues.

Interferon: Any one of a group of small glycoproteins (cytokines) produced in response to viral infection and which inhibit viral replication.

Interleukin: Any of several multifunctional cytokines produced by a variety of lymphoid and nonlymphoid cells, including immune cells, that stimulate or otherwise affect the function of lymphopoietic and other cells and systems in the body.

Interstitial: Relating to or situated between parts or in the interspaces of a tissue.

Intramural: Situated or occurring within the wall of an organ.

Intrinsic: Pertaining exclusively to a part or situated entirely within an organ or tissue.

In vitro: A biologic reaction occurring in an artificial environment, such as a test tube.

In vivo: A biologic reaction occurring within the living body.

Involution: The act or instance of enfolding, entangling, or turning inward.

Ionize: To separate or change into ions.

Ipsilateral: Situated on, pertaining to, or affecting the same side of the body.

Ischemia: Decreased blood supply to a body organ or part, usually due to functional constriction or actual obstruction of a blood vessel.

Juxtaarticular: Situated near a joint or in the region of a joint.

Juxtaglomerular: Near to or adjoining a glomerulus of the kidney.

Karyotype: The total chromosomal characteristics of a cell; or the micrograph of chromosomes arranged in pairs in descending order of size.

Keratin: A fibrous, sulfur-containing protein that is the primary component of the epidermis, hair, and horny tissues. (Adjective: keratinous)

Keratosis: Any skin condition in which there is overgrowth and thickening of the cornified epithelium.

Ketosis: A condition characterized by the abnormal accumulation of ketones (organic compounds with a carboxyl group attached to two carbon atoms) in the body tissues and fluid.

Kinesthesia: The sense of movement, weight, tension, and position of body parts mediated by input from joint and muscle receptors and hair cells. (Adjective: kinesthetic)

Kyphosis: An abnormal condition of the vertebral column, characterized by increased convexity in the curvature of the thoracic spine as viewed from the side.

Lacuna: A small pit or cavity within a structure, especially bony tissue; or a defect or gap, as in the field of vision.

Lateral: A position farther from the median plane or midline of the body or a structure; or situated on, coming from, or directed towards the side.

Lesion: Any wound, injury, or pathologic change in body tissue.

Lethargy: The lowered level of consciousness characterized by listlessness, drowsiness, and apathy; or a state of indifference.

Ligament: One of many predominantly white, shiny, flexible bands of fibrous tissue that binds joints together and connects bones or cartilages.

Ligand: A group, ion, or molecule that binds to the central atom or molecule in a chemical complex.

Lipid: Any of the group of fats and fatlike substances characterized by being insoluble in water and soluble in nonpolar organic solvents, such as chloroform and ether.

Lipoprotein: Any one of the conjugated proteins that is a complex of protein and lipid.

Lobule: A small lobe.

Lordosis: The anterior concavity in the curvature of the lumbar and cervical spine as observed from the side.

Lumen: A cavity or the channel within a tube or tubular organ of the body.

Luteal: Of or pertaining to or having the properties of the corpus luteum.

Lysis: Destruction or dissolution of a cell or molecule through the action of a specific agent.

Maceration: Softening of tissue by soaking, especially in acidic solutions.

Macroscopic: Large enough to be visible with the unaided eye or without the microscope.

Macula: A small, flat blemish, thickening, or discoloration that is flush with the skin surface. (Adjective: macular)

Malaise: A vague feeling of bodily fatigue and discomfort.

Manometry: The measurement of tension or pressure of a liquid or gas using a device called a manometer.

Marasmus: A condition of extreme protein-calorie malnutrition that is characterized by growth retardation and progressive wasting of subcutaneous tissue and muscle and occurs chiefly during the first year of life.

Matrix: The intracellular substance of a tissue or the basic substance from which a specific organ or kind of tissue develops.

Meatus: An opening or passage through any body part.

Medial: Pertaining to the middle; or situated or oriented toward the midline of the body.

Mediastinum: The mass of tissues and organs in the middle of the thorax, separating the pleural sacs containing the two lungs.

Meiosis: The division of a sex cell as it matures, so that each daughter nucleus receives one half of the number of chromosomes characteristic of the somatic cells of the species.

Mesoderm: The middle layer of the three primary germ layers of the developing embryo, lying between the ectoderm and the endoderm.

Metabolism: The sum of all the physical and chemical processes by which living organisms are produced and maintained, and also the transformation by which energy is provided for vital processes and activities.

Metaplasia: Change in type of adult cells in a tissue to a form that is not normal for that tissue.

Metastasis: The transfer of disease (e.g., cancer) from one organ or part to another not directly connected with it. (Adjective: metastatic)

Miosis: Contraction of the pupil of the eye.

Mitosis: A type of indirect cell division that occurs in somatic cells and results in the formation of two daughter nuclei containing the identical complements of the number of chromosomes characteristic of the somatic cells of the species.

Molecule: The smallest mass of matter that exhibits the properties of an element or compound.

Morbidity: A diseased condition or state; the relative incidence of a disease or of all diseases in a population.

Morphology: The study of the physical form and structure of an organism; or the form and structure of a particular organism. (Adjective: morphologic)

Mosaicism: In genetics, the presence in an individual or in an organism of cell cultures having two or more cell lines that differ in genetic constitution but are derived from a single zygote.

Mutagen: Any chemical or physical agent that induces a genetic mutation (an unusual change in form, quality, or some other characteristic) or increases the mutation rate by causing changes in DNA.

Mydriasis: Physiologic dilatation of the pupil of the eye.

Myoclonus: A spasm of a portion of a muscle, an entire muscle, or a group of muscles.

Myoglobin: The oxygen-transporting pigment of muscle consisting of one heme molecule containing one iron molecule attached to a single globin chain.

Myopathy: Any disease or abnormal condition of skeletal muscle, usually characterized by muscle weakness, wasting, and histologic changes within muscle tissue.

Myotome: The muscle plate or portion of an embryonic somite that develops into a voluntary muscle; or a group of muscles innervated by a single spinal segment.

Necrosis: Localized tissue death that occurs in groups of cells or part of a structure or an organ in response to disease or injury.

Neutropenia: An abnormal decrease in the number of neutrophilic leukocytes in the blood.

Nidus: The point where a morbid process originates, develops, or is located.

Nociception: The reception of painful stimuli from the physical or mechanical injury to body tissues by nociceptors (receptors usually found in either the skin or the walls of the viscera).

Nosocomial: Pertaining to or originating in a hospital, such as a nosocomial infection; an infection acquired during hospitalization.

Nystagmus: Involuntary, rapid, rhythmic movements of the eyeball.

Oncogene: A gene that is capable of causing the initial and continuing conversion of normal cells into cancer cells.

Oocyte: A primordial or incompletely developed ovum.

Oogenesis: The process of the growth and maturation of the female gametes, or ova.

Opsonization: The process of making cells, such as bacteria, more susceptible to the action of phagocytes.

Organelle: Any one of the various membrane-bound particles of distinctive morphology and function present within most cells, as the mitochondria, the Golgi complex, and the lysosomes.

Orthopnea: An abnormal condition in which a person must be in an upright position in order to breathe deeply or comfortably.

Osmolality: The concentration of osmotically active particles in solution expressed in osmols or milliosmols per kilogram of solvent.

Osmolarity: The concentration of osmotically active particles in solution expressed in osmols or milliosmols per liter of solution.

Osmosis: The movement or passage of a pure solvent, such as water, through a semipermeable membrane from a solution that has a lower solute concentration to one that has a higher solute concentration.

Osteophyte: A bony project or outgrowth.

Palpable: Perceptible by touch.

Papilla: A small nipple-shaped projection, elevation, or structure, as the conoid papillae of the tongue.

Papule: A small, circumscribed, solid elevation of the skin less than one centimeter in diameter. (Adjective: papular)

Paracrine: A mode of hormone action in which a chemical messenger that is synthesized and released from a cell acts on nearby cells of a different type and affects their function.

Paralysis: An abnormal condition characterized by the impairment or loss of motor function due to a lesion of the neural or muscular mechanism.

Paraneoplastic: Relating to alterations produced in tissue remote from a tumor or its metastases.

Parenchyma: The basic tissue or elements of an organ as distinguished from supporting or connective tissue or elements. (Adjective: parenchymal)

Paresis: Slight or partial paralysis.

Paresthesia: Any abnormal touch sensation, which can be experienced as numbness, tingling, or a "pins and needles" feeling, often in the absence of external stimuli.

Parietal: Pertaining to the outer wall of a cavity or organ; or pertaining to the parietal bone of the skull or the parietal lobe of the brain.

Parous: Having borne one or more viable offspring.

Pathogen: Any microorganism capable of producing disease.

Pedigree: A systematic presentation, such as in a table, chart, or list, of an individual's ancestors that is used in human genetics in the analysis of inheritance.

Peptide: Any of a class of molecular chain compounds composed of two or more amino acids joined by peptide bonds.

Perfusion: The process or act of pouring over or through, especially the passage of a fluid through a specific organ or an area of the body.

Peripheral: Pertaining to the outside, surface, or surrounding area of an organ or other structure; or located away from a center or central structure.

Permeable: A condition of being pervious, or permitting passage, so that fluids and certain other substances can pass through, as a permeable membrane.

Pervasive: Pertaining to something that becomes diffused throughout every part.

Petechia: A tiny, perfectly round, purplish red spot that appears on the skin as a result of minute intradermal or submucous hemorrhage. (Plural: petechiae)

Phagocytosis: The process by which certain cells engulf and consume foreign material and cell debris.

Phalanx: Any one of the bones composing the fingers of each hand and the toes of each foot.

Phenotype: The complete physical, biochemical, and physiologic makeup of an individual, as determined by the interaction of both genetic makeup and environmental factors.

Pheresis: A procedure in which blood is withdrawn from a donor, a portion (plasma, leukocytes, etc.) is separated and retained, and the remainder is reperfused into the donor. It includes plasmapheresis and leukopheresis.

Pili: Hair; or in microbiology, the minute filamentous appendages of certain bacteria. (Singular: pilus)

Plexus: A network of intersecting nerves, blood vessels, or lymphatic vessels.

Polygene: Any of a group of nonallelic genes that interact to influence the same character in the same way so that the effect is cumulative, usually of a quantitative nature, as size, weight, or skin pigmentation. (Adjective: polygenic)

Polymorph: One of several, or many, forms of an organism or cell. (Adjective: polymorphic)

Polyp: A small, tumor-like growth that protrudes from a mucous membrane surface.

Polypeptide: A molecular chain of more than two amino acids joined by peptide bonds.

Presbyopia: A visual condition (farsightedness) that commonly develops with advancing years or old age in which the lens loses elasticity causing defective accommodation and inability to focus sharply for near vision.

Prevalence: The number of new and old cases of a disease that are present in a population at a given time or occurrences of an event during a particular period of time.

Prodrome: An early symptom indicating the onset of a condition or disease. (Adjective: prodromal)

Prokaryotic: Pertaining to an organism, such as bacterium, with cells lacking a true nucleus and nuclear membrane that reproduces through simple fission.

Prolapse: The falling down, sinking, or sliding of an organ from its normal position or location in the body.

Proliferation: The reproduction or multiplication of similar forms, especially cells.

Pronation: Assumption of a position in which the ventral, or front, surface of the body or part of the body faces downward. (Adjective: prone)

Propagation: The act or action of reproduction.

Proprioception: The reception of stimuli originating from within the body regarding body position and muscular activity by proprioceptors (sensory nerve endings found in muscles, tendons, joints).

Prosthesis: An artificial replacement for a missing body part; or a device designed and applied to improve function, such as a hearing aid.

Proteoglycans: Any one of a group of polysaccharide-protein conjugates occurring primarily in the matrix of connective tissue and cartilage.

Protooncogene: A normal cellular gene that with alteration, such as by mutation, becomes an active oncogene.

Proximal: Closer to a point of reference, usually the trunk of the body, than other parts of the body.

Pruritus: The symptom of itching, an uncomfortable sensation leading to the urge to rub or scratch the skin to obtain relief. (Adjective: pruritic)

Purpura: A small hemorrhage, up to about 1 cm in diameter, in the skin, mucous membrane, or serosal surface; or any of several bleeding disorders characterized by the presence of purpuric lesions.

Purulent: Producing or containing pus.

Quiescent: Quiet, causing no disturbance, activity, or symptoms.

Reflux: An abnormal backward or return flow of a fluid, such as stomach contents, blood, or urine.

Regurgitation: A flow of material that is in the opposite direction from normal, as in the return of swallowed food into the mouth or the backward flow of blood through a defective heart valve.

Remission: The partial or complete disappearance of the symptoms of a chronic or malignant disease; or the period of time during which the abatement of symptoms occurs.

Resorption: The loss of substance or bone by physiologic or pathologic means, for example, the loss of dentin and cementum of a tooth.

Retrograde: Moving backward or against the usual direction of flow; reverting to an earlier state or worse condition (degenerating); catabolic.

Retroversion: A condition in which an entire organ is tipped backward or in a posterior direction, usually without flexion or other distortion.

Rhabdomyolysis: Destruction or degeneration of muscle, associated with myoglobinuria (excretion of myoglobin in the urine).

Rostral: Pertaining to or resembling a beak.

Sacroiliitis: Inflammation in the sacroiliac joint.

Sclerosis: A condition characterized by induration or hardening of tissue resulting from any of several causes, including inflammation, diseases of the interstitial substance, and increased formation of connective tissues.

Semipermeable: Partially but not wholly permeable, especially a membrane that permits the passage of some (usually small) molecules but not of other (usually larger) particles.

Senescence: The process or condition of aging or growing old.

Sepsis: The presence in the blood or other tissues of pathogenic microorganisms or their toxins; or the condition resulting from the spread of microorganisms or their products. (Adjective: septic)

Serous: Relating to or resembling serum; or containing or producing serum, such as a serous gland.

Shunt: To divert or bypass bodily fluid from one channel, path, or part to another; a passage or anastomosis between two natural channels, especially between blood vessels, established by surgery or occurring as an abnormality.

Soma: The body of an organism as distinguished from the mind; all of an organism, excluding germ cells; the body of a cell.

Spasticity: The condition characterized by spasms or other uncontrolled contractions of the skeletal muscles. (Adjective: spastic)

Spatial: Relating to, having the character of, or occupying space.

Sphincter: A ringlike band of muscle fibers that constricts a passage or closes a natural orifice of the body.

Stenosis: An abnormal condition characterized by the narrowing or stricture of a duct or canal.

Stria: A streak or a linear scarlike lesion that often results from rapidly developing tension in the skin; or a narrow bandlike structure, especially the longitudinal collections of nerve fibers in the brain.

Stricture: An abnormal temporary or permanent narrowing of the lumen of a duct, canal, or other passage, as the esophagus, because of inflammation, external pressure, or scarring.

Stroma: The supporting tissue or the matrix of an organ as distinguished from its functional element, or parenchyma.

Stupor: A lowered level of consciousness characterized by lethargy and unresponsiveness in which a person seems unaware of his or her surroundings.

Subchondral: Beneath a cartilage.

Subcutaneous: Beneath the skin.

Sulcus: A shallow groove, depression, or furrow on the surface of an organ, as a sulcus on the surface of the brain, separating the gyri.

Supination: Assuming the position of lying horizontally on the back, or with the face upward. (Adjective: supine)

Suppuration: The formation of pus, or purulent matter.

Symbiosis: Mode of living characterized by close association between organisms of different species, usually in a mutually beneficial relationship.

Sympathomimetic: An agent or substance that produces stimulating effects on organs and structures similar to those produced by the sympathetic nervous system.

Syncope: A brief lapse of consciousness due to generalized cerebral ischemia.

Syncytium: A multinucleate mass of protoplasm produced by the merging of a group of cells.

Syndrome: A complex of signs and symptoms that occur together to present a clinical picture of a disease or inherited abnormality.

Synergist: An organ, agent, or substance that aids or cooperates with another organ, agent, or substance.

Synthesis: An integration or combination of various parts or elements to create a unified whole.

Systemic: Pertaining to the whole body rather than to a localized area or regional portion of the body.

Systole: The contraction, or period of contraction, of the heart that drives the blood onward into the aorta and pulmonary arteries.

Tamponade: Stoppage of the flow of blood to an organ or a part of the body by pathologic compression, such as the compression of the heart by an accumulation of pericardial fluid.

Teratogen: Any agent or factor that induces or increases the incidence of developmental abnormalities in the fetus.

Thrombus: A stationary mass of clotted blood or other formed elements that remains attached to its place of origin along the wall of a blood vessel, frequently obstructing the circulation. (Plural: thrombi)

Tinnitus: A tinkling, buzzing, or ringing noise heard in one or both ears.

Tophus: A chalky deposit containing sodium urate that most often develops in periarticular fibrous tissue, typically in individuals with gout. (Plural: tophi)

Torsion: The act or process of twisting in either a positive (clockwise) or negative (counterclockwise) direction.

Trabecula: A supporting or anchoring stand of connective tissue, such as the delicate fibrous threads connecting the inner surface of the arachnoid to the pia mater.

Transmural: Situated or occurring through the wall of an organ.

Transudate: A fluid substance passed through a membrane or extruded from the blood.

Tremor: Involuntary quivering or trembling movements caused by the alternating contraction and relaxation of opposing groups of skeletal muscles.

Trigone: A triangular-shaped area.

Ubiquitous: The condition or state of existing or being everywhere at the same time.

Ulcer: A circumscribed excavation of the surface of an organ or tissue, which results from necrosis that accompanies some inflammatory, infectious, or malignant processes. (Adjective: ulcerative)

Urticaria: A pruritic skin eruption of the upper dermis, usually transient, characterized by wheals (hives) of various shapes and sizes.

Uveitis: An inflammation of all or part of the uveal tract of the eye.

Ventral: Pertaining to a position toward the belly of the body; or situated or oriented toward the front or anterior of the body.

Vertigo: An illusory sensation that the environment or one's own body is revolving.

Vesicle: A small bladder or sac, as a small, thin-walled, raised skin lesion, containing liquid.

Visceral: Pertaining to the viscera, or internal organs of the body.

Viscosity: Pertaining to the physical property of fluids, caused by the adhesion of adjacent molecules, that determines the internal resistance to shear forces.

Zoonosis: A disease of animals that may be transmitted to humans from its primary animal host under natural conditions.

Appendix *A*
Laboratory Values

Prefixes Denoting Decimal Factors

Prefix	Symbol	Factor
mega	M	10^6
kilo	k	10^3
hecto	h	10^2
deci	d	10^{-1}
centi	c	10^{-2}
milli	m	10^{-3}
micro	μ	10^{-6}
nano	n	10^{-9}
pico	p	10^{-12}
femto	f	10^{-15}

Hematology

Test	Conventional Units	SI Units
Erythrocyte count (RBC count)	M. 4.2–$5.4 \times 10^6/\mu L$	M. 4.2–$5.4 \times 10^{12}/L$
	F. 3.6–$5.0 \times 10^6/\mu L$	F. 3.6–$5.0 \times 10^{12}/L$
Hematocrit (Hct)	M. 40–50%	M. 0.40–0.50
	F. 37–47%	F. 0.37–0.47
Hemoglobin (Hb)	M. 14.0–16.5 g/dL	M. 140–165 g/L
	F. 12.0–15.0 g/dL	F. 120–150 g/L
Mean corpuscular hemoglobin (MHC)	27–34 pg/cell	0.40–0.53 fmol/cell
Mean corpuscular hemoglobin concentration (MCHC)	31–35 g/dL	310–350 g/L
Mean corpuscular volume (MCV)	80–100 fL	
Reticulocyte count	1.0–1.5% total RBC	
Leukocyte count (WBC count)	4.8–$10.8 \times 10^3/\mu L$	4.8–$10.8 \times 10^9/L$
Basophils	0–2%	
Eosinophils	0–3%	
Lymphocytes	24–40%	
Monocytes	4–9%	
Neutrophils (segmented [Segs])	47–63%	
Neutrophils (bands)	0–4%	

Blood Chemistry*

Test	Conventional Units	SI Units
Alanine aminotransferase (ALT, SGPT, GPT)[†]	7–56 U/L	0.14–1.12 μkat/L
Alkaline phosphatase	41–133 U/L	0.7–2.2 μkat/L
Ammonia	18–60 μg/dL	11–35 μmol/L
Amylase[†]	20–110 U/L[†]	0.33–1.83 μkat/L
Aspartase aminotransferase (AST, SGOT, GOT)[†]	0–35 U/L[†]	0–0.58 μkat/L
Bicarbonate	24–31 mEq/L	24–31 mmol/L
Bilirubin (total)	0.1–1.2 mg/dL	2–21 μmol/L
Direct	0.1–0.5 mg/dL	<8 μmol/L
Indirect	0.1–0.7 mg/dL	<12 μmol/L
Blood urea nitrogen (BUN)	8–20 mg/dL	2.9–7.1 mmol/L
Calcium (Ca^{2+})	8.5–10.5 mg/dL	2.1–2.6 mmol/L
Carbon dioxide	24–29 mEq/L	24–29 mmol/L
Chloride	98–106 mEq/L	98–106 mmol/L
Creatine kinase (CK)[†]	32–267 U/L[†]	0.53–4.45 μkat/L
Creatine kinase (MB)[†]	<16 IU/L[†] or 4% of total CK	<0.27 μkat/L
Creatinine (serum)[‡]	0.6–1.2 mg/dL[‡]	50–100 μmol/L
Gamma-glutamyl-transpeptidase (GGT)[†]	9–85 U/L[†]	0.15–1.42 μkat/L
Glucose (blood)	60–110 mg/dL	3.3–6.3 mmol/L
Glycosylated hemoglobin (HbA$_{1c}$)[†]	3.9–6.9%	
Lactate dehydrogenase (LDH)[†]	88–230 U/L[†]	1.46–3.82 μkat/L[†]
Lipids		
Cholesterol	<200 mg/dL (desirable)	<5.2 mmol/L
Triglycerides	<165 mg/dL	<1.65 g/L
Lipase	0–160 U/L[†]	0.266 μkat/L
Magnesium	1.80–3.0 mg/dL	0.75–1.25 mmol/L
Osmolality	280–295 mOsm/kg H_2O	280–295 mmol/kg H_2O
Phosphorus (inorganic)	2.5–4.5 mg/dL	0.80–1.45 mmol/L
Potassium	3.5–5.0 mEq/L	3.5–5.0 mmol/L
Prostate specific antigen (PSA)	0–4 ng/mL	0–4 μg/L
Protein total	6.0–8.0 g/dL	60–80 g/L
Albumin	3.4–4.7 g/dL	34–47 g/L
Globulin	2.3–3.5 g/dL	23–35 g/L
A/G ratio	1.0–2.2	1.0–2.2
Thyroid Tests		
Thyroxine (T_4) total[†]	5.0–11.0 μg/dL	64–142 nmol/L
Thyroxine, free (FT$_4$)	9–24 pmol/L[†]	
Triiodothyronine (T_3) total	95–190 ng/dL	1.5–2.9 nmol/L
Thyroid stimulating hormone (TSH)	0.4–6.0 μU/mL	0.4–6.0 mU/mL
Thyroglobin	3–42 ng/mL	3–42 μg/L
Sodium	135–145 mEq/L	135–145 mmol/L
Uric acid	M. 2.4–7.4 mg/dL	M. 140–440 μmol/L
	F. 1.4–5.8 mg/dL	F. 80–350 μmol/L

U, units.

*Values may vary with laboratory. The values supplied by the laboratory performing the test should always be used since the ranges may be method specific.

[†]Laboratory and/or method specific

[‡]Varies with age and muscle mass

(Values obtained from Tierney LM., McPhee S.J., Papadakis M.A. [2006]. *Current medical diagnosis and treatment* [45th ed.]. New York: Lange Medical Books/McGraw-Hill, pp. 1736–1743; Fischbach F. [2004]. *A manual of laboratory and diagnostic tests* [7th ed.]. Philadelphia: Lippincott Williams & Wilkins, and other sources.)

Index

Note: Page numbers followed by the letter f refer to figures; those followed by the letter t refer to tables, and those followed by the letter c refer to charts.

Prefixes

a-, an- without, lack of
apnea (without breath)
anemia (lack of blood)

ab- separation, away from
abductor (leading away from)
aberrant (away from the usual course)

ad- to, toward, near to
adductor (leading toward)
adrenal (near the kidney)

ana- up, again, excessive
anapnea (to breathe again)
anasarca (severe edema)

ante- before, in front of
antecubital (in front of the elbow)
antenatal (occurring before birth)

anti- against, counter
anticoagulant (opposing coagulation)
antisepsis (against infection)

ap-, apo- separation, derivation from
apocrine (type of glandular secretion
that contains cast-off parts of the
secretory cell)

aut-, auto- self
autoimmune (immunity to self)
autologous (pertaining to self graft or
blood transfusion)

bi- two, twice, double
biarticulate (pertaining to two joints)
bifurcation (two branches)

brady- slow
bradyesthesia (slowness or dullness of
perception)

cata- down, under, lower, negative,
against
catabolism (breaking down)
catalepsy (diminished movement)

circum- around, about
circumflex (winding around)
circumference (surrounding)

contra- against, counter
contraindicated (not indicated)
contralateral (opposite side)

de- away from, down from, remove
dehydrate (remove water)
deaminate (remove an amino group)

dia- through, apart, across, completely
diapedesis (ooze through)
diagnosis (complete knowledge)

dis- apart, reversal, separation
discrete (made up of separated parts)
disruptive (bursting apart)

dys- difficulty, faulty, painful
dysmenorrhea (painful menstruation)
dyspnea (difficulty breathing)

e-, ex- out from, out of
enucleate (remove from)
exostosis (outgrowth of bone)

ec- out from
eccentric (away from center)
ectopic (out of place)

ecto- outside, situated on
ectoderm (outer skin)
ectoretina (outer layer of retina)

em-, en- in, on
empyema (pus in)
encephalon (in the brain)

endo- within, inside
endocardium (within heart)
endometrium (within uterus)

epi- upon, after, in addition
epidermis (on skin)
epidural (upon dura)

eu- well, easily, good
eupnea (easy or normal respiration)
euthyroid (normal thyroid function)

exo- outside
exocolitis (inflammation of outer coat
of colon)
exogenous (originating outside)

extra- outside of, beyond
extracellular (outside cell)
extrapleural (outside pleura)

hemi- half
hemialgia (pain affecting only one side
of the body)
hemilingual (affecting one side of the
tongue)

hyper- extreme, above, beyond
hyperemia (excessive blood)
hypertrophy (overgrowth)

hypo- under, below
hypotension (low blood pressure)
hypothyroidism (underfunction of
thyroid)

im-, in- in, into, on
immersion (act of dipping in)
injection (act of forcing fluid into)

im-, in- not
immature (not mature)
inability (not able)

infra- beneath
infraclavicular (below the clavicle)
infraorbital (below the eye)

inter- among, between
intercostal (between the ribs)
intervene (come between)

intra- within, inside
intraocular (within the eye)
intraventricular (within the ventricles)

intro- into, within
introversion (turning inward)
introduce (lead into)

iso- equal, same
isotonia (equal tone, tension, or activity)
isotypical (of the same type)

juxta- near, close by
juxtaglomerular (near an adjoining
glomerulus in the kidney)
juxtaspinal (near the spinal column)

macro- large, long, excess
macrocephaly (excessive head size)
macrodystrophia (overgrowth of a part)

mal- bad, abnormal
maldevelopment (abnormal growth or
development)
malfunction (to function imperfectly or
badly)

mega- large, enlarged, abnormally large
size
megaprosopous (having a large face)
megasoma (great size and stature)

meso- middle, intermediate, moderate
mesoderm (middle germ layer of
embryo)
mesocephalic (pertaining to a skull with
an average breadth–length index)

meta- beyond, after, accompanying
metacarpal (beyond the wrist)
metamorphosis (change of form)

micro- small size or amount
microbe (a minute living organism)
microtiter (a titer of minute quantity)

neo- new, young, recent
neoformation (a new growth)
neonate (newborn)

oligo- few, scanty, less than normal
oligogenic (produced by a few genes)
oligospermia (abnormally low number
of spermatozoa in the semen)

para- beside, beyond
paracardiac (beside the heart)
paraurethral (near the urethra)

per- through
perforate (bore through)
permeate (pass through)

peri- around
peribronchia (around the bronchus)
periosteum (around bone)

poly- many, much
polyphagia (excessive eating)
polytrauma (occurrence of multiple
injuries)

post- after, behind in time or place
postoperative (after operation)
postpartum (after childbirth)

pre-, pro- in front of, before in time or
place
premaxillary (in front of the maxilla)
prognosis (foreknowledge)

pseud-, pseudo- false, spurious
pseudocartilaginous (made up of a
substance resembling cartilage)
pseudopregnancy (false pregnancy)